CLINICAL VETERINARY ADVISOR

The Horse

Editor-in-Chief

David A. Wilson

DVM, MS, DACVS

Professor, Equine Surgery
Section Head, Equine Medicine & Surgery
Hospital Director
Veterinary Medical Teaching Hospital
Department of Veterinary Medicine & Surgery
College of Veterinary Medicine
University of Missouri
Columbia, Missouri

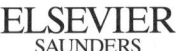
ELSEVIER
SAUNDERS

3251 Riverport Lane
St. Louis, Missouri 63043

CLINICAL VETERINARY ADVISOR: THE HORSE   ISBN: 978-1-4160-9979-6

International Standard Book Number: 978-1-4160-9979-6

Vice President and Publishing Director: Linda Duncan
Publisher, Veterinary Medicine: Penny Rudolph
Developmental Editor: Lauren Harms
Publishing Services Manager: Patricia Tannian
Project Manager: Carrie Stetz
Design Direction: Paula Catalano

Printed in the United States of America
Last digit is the print number: 9 8 7 6 5 4 3 2 1

Erratum: July 2011

P406 – Nutritional myopathy: Chronic treatment
The dosage is misstated at 3 mg/kg body weight IM or SC. The correct
dosage is 0.06 mg/kg body weight IM or SC.

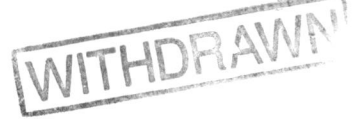

Editor-in-Chief

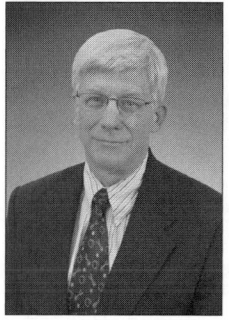

David A. Wilson, DVM, MS, DACVS
Skin
Professor, Equine Surgery
Section Head, Equine Medicine & Surgery
Hospital Director
Veterinary Medicine Teaching Hospital
Department of Veterinary Medicine & Surgery
College of Veterinary Medicine
University of Missouri
Columbia, Missouri

Editors

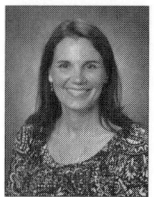

Michelle Henry Barton, DVM, PhD, DACVIM
Liver
Fuller E. Callaway Endowed Chair
Professor, Large Animal Internal Medicine
Department of Large Animal Medicine
College of Veterinary Medicine
The University of Georgia
Athens, Georgia

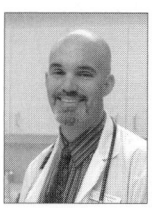

Jeffrey N. Bryan, DVM, MS, PhD, DACVIM
Oncology
Assistant Professor
Department of Veterinary Clinical Sciences
College of Veterinary Medicine
Washington State University
Pullman, Washington

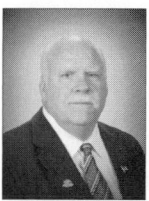

Daniel J. Burke, PhD
Nutrition
Director of Equine Nutrition
Tribute Equine Nutrition/Kalmbach Feeds, Inc.
Upper Sandusky, Ohio

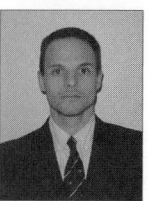

James L. Carmalt, MA, VetMB, MVetSc, FRCVS, DABVP(Eq), DACVS
Dentistry
Associate Professor
Department of Large Animal Clinical Sciences
Western College of Veterinary Medicine
University of Saskatchewan
Saskatoon, Saskatchewan, Canada

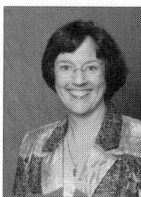

Patricia M. Dowling, DVM, MSc, DACVIM, DACVCP
Pharmacologic Principles
Professor, Veterinary Clinical Pharmacology;
Director, Canadian gFARAD
Western College of Veterinary Medicine
University of Sasketchewan
Saskatoon, Sasketchewan, Canada

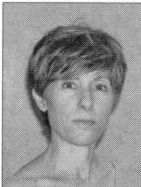

Mary M. Durando, DVM, PhD, DACVIM (Large Animal)
Cardiovascular System
Equine Sports Medicine Consultants, LLC
Landenberg, Pennsylvania

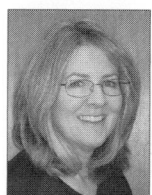

Cynthia L. Gaskill, DVM, PhD
Toxicology
Associate Professor
Veterinary Clinical Toxicology
Veterinary Diagnostic Laboratory
University of Kentucky
Lexington, Kentucky

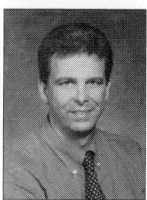

Brian C. Gilger, DVM, MS, DACVO
Ophthalmology
Professor of Ophthalmology
Department of Clinical Sciences
College of Veterinary Medicine
North Carolina State University
Raleigh, North Carolina

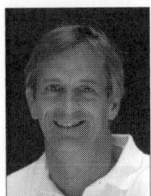

R. Reid Hanson, DVM, DACVS, DACVECC
Emergency and Critical Care
Professor of Surgery
J.T. Vaughan Teaching Hospital
Department of Clinical Sciences
College of Veterinary Medicine
Auburn University
Auburn, Alabama

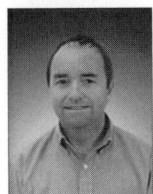

Philip J. Johnson, BVSc(Hons), MS, DACVIM, DECEIM, MRCVS
Laminitis
Professor and Instructional Leader
Equine Medicine and Surgery
Department of Veterinary Medicine and
 Surgery
College of Veterinary Medicine
University of Missouri
Columbia, Missouri

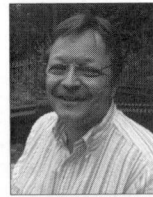

Andris J. Kaneps, DVM, PhD, DACVS, DACVSMR
Musculoskeletal
Staff Surgeon
New England Equine Medical and Surgical
 Center
Dover, New Hampshire

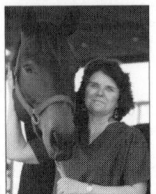

Maureen T. Long, DVM, PhD, DACVM
Infectious Diseases
Associate Professor, Large Animal Medicine
Department of Infectious Diseases and
 Pathology
College of Veterinary Medicine
University of Florida
Gainesville, Florida

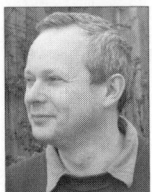

Tim Mair, BVSc, PhD, DEIM, DESTS, DECEIM, MRCVS
Gastrointestinal
Partner
Bell Equine Veterinary Clinic
Mereworth, Maidstone
Kent, United Kingdom

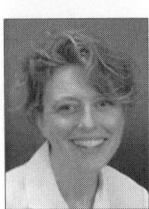

Melissa R. Mazan, DVM, DACVIM
Lower Respiratory Disorders
Associate Professor
Director, Issaam Fares Equine Sports Medicine
 Program
Department of Clinical Sciences
Sports Medicine
Cummings School of Veterinary Medicine
Tufts University
North Grafton, Massachusetts

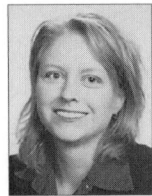

Amelia Munsterman, DVM, MS, DACVS, DACVECC
Emergency & Critical Care
Clinical Instructor
Equine Critical Care Medicine and Surgery
Department of Clinical Sciences
College of Veterinary Medicine
Auburn University
Auburn, Alabama

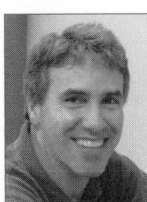

Eric J. Parente, DVM, DACVS
Upper Respiratory Disorders
Associate Professor
Department of Clinical Studies
New Bolton Center
University of Pennsylvania
School of Veterinary Medicine
Kennett Square, Pennsylvania

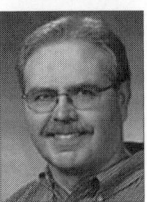

Stephen M. Reed, DVM, DACVIM
Neurology
Associate Veterinarian
Internal Medicine
Rood & Riddle Equine Hospital
Lexington, Kentucky

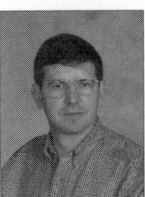

Juan C. Samper, DVM, MSc, PhD, DACT
Reproduction
Veterinary Reproductive Services
Langley, British Columbia, Canada

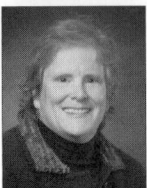

Elizabeth M. Santschi, DVM, DACVS
Foals
Associate Professor
Equine Surgery
Department of Veterinary Clinical Sciences
College of Veterinary Medicine
The Ohio State University
Columbus, Ohio

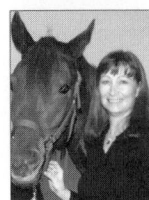

Debra C. Sellon, DVM, PhD, DACVM
Infectious Diseases
Professor, Equine Medicine
Department of Veterinary Clinical Sciences
College of Veterinary Medicine
Associate Dean, Graduate School
Washington State University
Pullman, Washington

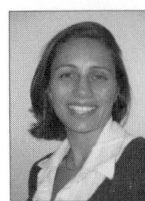

Ceri Sherlock, B Vet Med, MRCVS, DACVS
Gastrointestinal
Large Animal Surgery Clinical Instructor
Department of Large Animal Medicine
College of Veterinary Medicine
The University of Georgia
Athens, Georgia

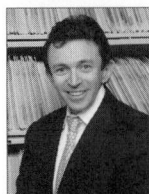

Nathan Slovis, DVM, DACVIM, CHT (Certified Hyperbaric Technologist)
Section VI: Drug Formulary
Director
Hagyard Equine Medical Insititute
McGee Critical Care and Medical Center
Lexington, Kentucky

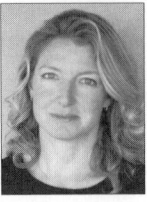

Phoebe A. Smith, DVM, DACVIM
Foals
Riviera Equine
Internal Medicine & Consulting
Santa Ynez, California

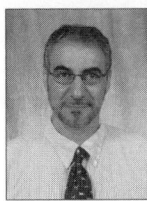

Ahmed Tibary, DMV, MS, DSc, PhD, DACT
Reproduction
Professor
Department of Veterinary Clinical Sciences
College of Veterinary Medicine
Washington State University
Pullman, Washington

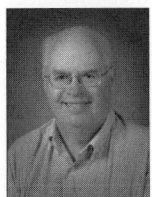

Ian Tizard, BVMS, BSc, PhD, DACVIM
Immunology
Professor of Immunology
Department of Veterinary Pathobiology
College of Veterinary Medicine
Texas A&M University
College Station, Texas

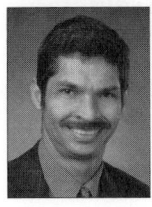

Ramiro E. Toribio, DVM, MS, PhD, DACVIM
Endocrinology
Associate Professor
Department of Veterinary Clinical Sciences
College of Veterinary Medicine
The Ohio State University
Columbus, Ohio

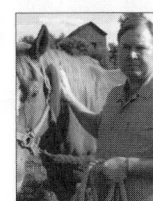

**Bryan M. Waldridge, DVM, MS, DABVP
(Equine Practice), DACVIM**
Urinary
Kentucky Equine Research
Versailles, Kentucky

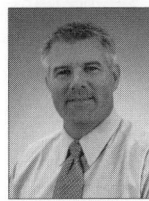

Charles Wiedmeyer, DVM, PhD, DACVP
Laboratory Tests
Assistant Professor, Veterinary Clinical
  Pathology
Department of Veterinary Pathobiology
College of Veterinary Medicine
University of Missouri
Columbia, Missouri

CONTRIBUTORS

Katie S. Amend, DVM
Resident
Department of Clinical
 Sciences
College of Veterinary
 Medicine and Biomedical
 Sciences
Colorado State University
Fort Collins, Colorado

**C. Scott Bailey, DVM, MS,
 DACT**
Assistant Professor,
 Theriogenology
Department of Clinical
 Sciences
College of Veterinary
 Medicine
North Carolina State
 University
Raleigh, North Carolina

Heidi Banse, DVM
Resident
Equine Internal Medicine
Department of Veterinary
 Clinical Sciences
College of Veterinary
 Medicine
Oklahoma State University
Stillwater, Oklahoma

**Robert M. Baratt, DVM, MS,
 FAVD**
Salem Valley Veterinary Clinic
Salem, Connecticut

**Anne Barger, DVM, MS,
 DACVP**
Clinical Associate Professor
Department of Pathobiology
College of Veterinary
 Medicine
University of Illinois
Urbana, Illinois

**Michelle Henry Barton
 DVM, PhD, DACVIM**
Fuller E. Callaway Endowed
 Chair
Professor, Large Animal
 Internal Medicine
Department of Large Animal
 Medicine
College of Veterinary
 Medicine
The University of Georgia
Athens, Georgia

**Lance H. Bassage, II, VMD,
 DACVS**
Staff Surgeon
Rhinebeck Equine, LLP
Rhinebeck, New York

Brenda T. Beerntsen, PhD
Associate Professor
Department of Veterinary
 Pathobiology
College of Veterinary
 Medicine
University of Missouri
Columbia, Missouri

**Alicia L. Bertone, DVM,
 PhD, DACVS**
Trueman Family Endowed
 Chair and Professor
Department of Veterinary
 Clinical Sciences
College of Veterinary
 Medicine
The Ohio State University
Columbus, Ohio

Eric K. Birks, DVM, PhD
Equine Sports Medicine
 Consultants, LLC
Newark, Delaware

**Karyn Bischoff, DVM, MS,
 DABVT**
Diagnostic Toxicologist
Associate Professor
New York State Animal
 Health Diagnostic Center
College of Veterinary
 Medicine
Cornell University
Ithaca, New York

**Karen Blissitt, BVSc,
 MRCVS, PhD, DVA,
 DECVAA**
Senior Lecturer
Department of Veterinary
 Clinical Studies
Royal (Dick) School of
 Veterinary Studies
Easter Bush Veterinary Centre
University of Edinburgh
Edinburgh, United Kingdom

**John D. Bonagura, DVM,
 MS, DACVIM (Cardiology,
 Internal Medicine)**
Professor
Department of Veterinary
 Clinical Sciences
College of Veterinary
 Medicine;
Cardiology Service Head
Veterinary Hospital;
Member
Davis Heart & Lung Research
 Institute
The Ohio State University
Columbus, Ohio

**Melissa Bourgeois, DVM,
 PhD**
Emerging Infectious Disease
 Fellow
Centers for Disease Control
 and Prevention
Atlanta, Georgia

**Jennifer A. Brown, DVM,
 DACVS**
Veterinary Sports Medicine
 and Surgery
Tampa, Florida

Jason W. Brumitt, DVM, MS
Veterinary Imaging Specialists
St. Louis, Missouri

**Jeffrey N. Bryan, DVM, MS,
 PhD, DACVIM**
Assistant Professor
Department of Veterinary
 Clinical Sciences
College of Veterinary
 Medicine
Washington State University
Pullman, Washington

Rikke Buhl, DVM, PhD
Associate Professor
Department of Large Animal
 Sciences
Faculty of Life Sciences
Large Animal Medicine
University of Copenhagen
Copenhagen, Denmark

Daniel J. Burke, PhD
Director of Equine Nutrition
Tribute Equine Nutrition/
 Kalmbach Feeds, Inc.
Upper Sandusky, Ohio

Melinda S. Camus, DVM
Clinical Pathology Resident
Department of Pathology
College of Veterinary Medicine
The University of Georgia
Athens, Georgia

**Igor Frederico Canisso,
 DVM, MSc**
Theriogenology Resident
Department of Clinical
 Sciences
College of Veterinary Medicine
Cornell University
Ithaca, New York

Kelly L. Carlson, DVM
Veterinary Resident Instructor
Large Animal Clinical Sciences
College of Veterinary
 Medicine & Biomedical
 Sciences
Texas A&M University
College Station, Texas

**James L. Carmalt, MA,
 VetMB, MVetSc, FRCVS,
 DABVP(Eq), DACVS**
Associate Professor
Department of Large Animal
 Clinical Sciences
Western College of Veterinary
 Medicine
University of Saskatchewan
Saskatoon, Saskatchewan,
 Canada

Leeah R. Chew, DVM
Theriogenology Resident
Department of Large Animal
 Clinical Sciences
Virginia-Maryland Regional
 College of Veterinary
 Medicine
Blacksburg, Virginia

Cameon M. Childers, DVM
Equine Internal Medicine
 Resident
Department of Clinical
 Sciences
College of Veterinary Medicine
Kansas State University
Manhattan, Kansas;
Equine Internal Medicine
 Resident
Rood and Riddle Equine
 Hospital
Lexington, Kentucky

Michelle Cora, DVM
Postdoctoral Fellow in
 Toxicological Pathology
National Institutes of
 Environmental Health
 Sciences
Research Triangle Park, North
 Carolina

**Lais R. R. Costa, MV, MS,
 PhD, DACVIM-Large
 Animal, DABVP-Equine**
Assistant Professor
Large Animal Medicine
Department of Clinical
 Sciences
Cummings School of
 Veterinary Medicine
Tufts University
North Grafton, Massachusetts

Marco A. Coutinho da Silva, DVM, MS, PhD, DACT
Assistant Professor
Department of Veterinary Clinical Sciences
College of Veterinary Medicine
The Ohio State University
Columbus, Ohio

Gabriel Borges Couto, DMV, DES, MSc
Department of Clinical Sciences
Faculté de Médicine Vétérinaire
Université de Montréal
Québec, Canada

Laura C. Cregar, DVM
Resident
Veterinary Clinical Pathology
Veterinary Pathobiology
College of Veterinary Medicine
University of Missouri
Columbia, Missouri

Antonio M. Cruz, DVM, MVM, MSc, Dr Vet Med, DACVS, DECVS
Associate Professor
Department of Clinical Studies
Ontario Veterinary College
University of Guelph
Guelph, Ontario, Canada

John J. Dascanio, VMD, DACT, DABVP
Professor, Theriogenology
Ross University School of Veterinary Medicine
Basseterre, St. Kitts
West Indies

Elizabeth J. Davidson, DVM, DACVS
Assistant Professor in Sports Medicine
Department of Clinical Studies
New Bolton Center
University of Pennsylvania
Kennett Square, Pennsylvania

Heather Davis, DVM
Equine Surgery Resident
College of Veterinary Medicine
Auburn University
Auburn, Alabama

Mary S. DeLorey, DVM
Northwest Equine Dentistry, Inc.
Washington and Idaho

Catherine A. DeLuca, DVM, MS, DACT
Lecturer
Department of Large Animal Clinical Sciences
College of Veterinary Medicine
University of Florida
Gainesville, Florida

Shane F. DeWitt, DVM, DACVIM (LAIM)
Associate
Internal Medicine
Woodside Equine Clinic, Inc.
Ashland, Virginia

Monica Dias Figueiredo, DVM, PhD, DACVIM
Senior Veterinary Scientist
Merial Ltd.
Athens, Georgia

Mouhamadou K. Diaw, DVM
Resident
Theriogenology
Veterinary Medical Center
Large Animal Hospital
University of Florida
Gainesville, Florida

Roberta Di Terlizzi, DVM, MRCVS, DACVP
Assistant Professor of Clinical Pathology
Department of Pathobiology
School of Veterinary Medicine
University of Pennsylvania
Philadelphia, Pennsylvania

Patricia M. Dowling, DVM, MSc, DACVIM, DACVCP
Professor, Veterinary Clinical Pharmacology;
Director, Canadian gFARAD
Western College of Veterinary Medicine
University of Sasketchewan
Saskatoon, Sasketchewan, Canada

Norm G. Ducharme, DMV, MSc, DACVS
James Law Professor of Surgery
Medical Director
Equine and Farm Animal Hospital
Department of Clinical Sciences
College of Veterinary Medicine
Cornell University
Ithaca, New York

Ghislaine Dujovne, DVM
Equine Theriogenology Resident
Department of Clinical Sciences
College of Veterinary Medicine
Auburn University
Auburn, Alabama

Mary M. Durando, DVM, PhD, DACVIM (Large Animal)
Equine Sports Medicine Consultants, LLC
Landenberg, Pennsylvania

Steven Duren, DVM
Performance Horse Nutrition, LLC
Weiser, Idaho

Edward T. Earley, DVM, FAVD/Eq
Laurel Highland Farm & Equine Service, LLC
Williamsport, Pennsylvania

Sarah E. Eaton, DVM, DACT
Associate Veterinarian
Animal Care Hospital
Williams Lake, British Columbia, Canada

Randy Eggleston, DVM, DACVS
Associate Clinical Professor
Large Animal Surgery
Department of Large Animal Medicine
College of Veterinary Medicine
The University of Georgia
Athens, Georgia

Johanna Elfenbein, DVM
Resident
Large Animal Internal Medicine
Department of Large Animal Clinical Sciences
College of Veterinary Medicine
University of Florida
Gainesville, Florida

Steve Ensley, DVM, PhD
Clinical Veterinary Toxicologist
Veterinary Diagnostic and Production Animal Medicine
College of Veterinary Medicine
Iowa State University
Ames, Iowa

Kira L. Epstein, DVM, DACVS
Clinical Assistant Professor
Department of Large Animal Medicine
College of Veterinary Medicine
The University of Georgia
Athens, Georgia

Tim J. Evans, DVM, PhD, DACT, DABVT
Assistant Professor
Department of Veterinary Pathobiology;
Toxicology Section Leader
Veterinary Medical Diagnostic Laboratory
College of Veterinary Medicine
University of Missouri
Columbia, Missouri

Kelly Farnsworth, MS, DVM, DACVS
Assistant Professor
Department of Veterinary Clinical Sciences
College of Veterinary Medicine
Washington State University
Pullman, Washington

Maria S. Ferrer, Vet., MS, DACT
Assistant Professor
Department of Clinical Sciences
School of Veterinary Medicine
Kansas State University
Manhattan, Kansas

Ryan A. Ferris, DVM, MS
Clinical Instructor
Department of Clinical Sciences
College of Veterinary Medicine & Biomedical Sciences
Colorado State University
Fort Collins, Colorado

Janean L. Fidel, DVM, DACVRO, DACVIM (Oncology)
Associate Professor
Department of Veterinary Clinical Sciences
College of Veterinary Medicine
Washington State University
Pullman, Washington

José M. García-López, VMD, DACVS
Associate Professor of Large Animal Surgery
Department of Clinical Sciences
Cummings School of Veterinary Medicine
Tufts University
North Grafton, Massachusetts

Bridget C. Garner, DVM, PhD, DACVP
Assistant Professor
Department of Pathology
College of Veterinary Medicine
The University of Georgia
Athens, Georgia

Cynthia L. Gaskill, DVM, PhD
Associate Professor
Veterinary Clinical Toxicology
Veterinary Diagnostic Laboratory
University of Kentucky
Lexington, Kentucky

Mathew P. Gerard, BVSc, PhD, DACVS
Clinical Associate Professor
Large Animal Surgery
Department of Clinical Sciences
College of Veterinary Medicine
North Carolina State University
Raleigh, North Carolina

Liberty M. Getman, DVM, DACVS
Lecturer in Large Animal Surgery
Department of Clinical Studies
New Bolton Center
University of Pennsylvania
Kennett Square, Pennsylvania

Brian C. Gilger, DVM, MS, DACVO
Professor of Ophthalmology
Department of Clinical Sciences
College of Veterinary Medicine
North Carolina State University
Raleigh, North Carolina

Lyndi L. Gilliam, DVM, DACVIM
Assistant Professor
Department of Veterinary Clinical Sciences
College of Veterinary Medicine
Oklahoma State University
Stillwater, Oklahoma

Shir Gilor, DVM, MSc
Clinical Pathology Resident
Department of Pathobiology
College of Veterinary Medicine
University of Illinois
Urbana, Illinois

Elizabeth A. Giuliano, DVM, MS, DACVO
Associate Professor
Department of Veterinary Medicine and Surgery
College of Veterinary Medicine
University of Missouri
Columbia, Missouri

Sara Gomez-Ibanez, DVM
Intern
Large Animal Medicine and Surgery
Department of Large Animal Medicine
College of Veterinary Medicine
The University of Georgia
Athens, Georgia

Patty Graham-Thiers, PhD
Professor
Equine Studies Department
Virginia Intermont College
Bristol, Virginia

François-Xavier Grand, DVM, IPSAV
Large Animal Theriogenology Resident
Department of Clinical Sciences
Faculté de médicine vétérinaire
Université de Montréal
Montréal, Québec
Canada

Britton Grasperge, DVM, DACVP
PhD Candidate
Department of Pathobiological Sciences
School of Veterinary Medicine
Louisiana State University
Baton Rouge, Louisiana

Tanya M. Grondin, DVM, DACVP
Clinical Pathologist
HPA Laboratories, Inc.
Ashland, Virginia

Erin S. Groover, DVM, DACVIM-LAIM
Visiting Clinical Assistant Professor
Department of Clinical Sciences
College of Veterinary Medicine
Auburn University
Auburn, Alabama

Alisha M. Gruntman, DVM
Resident in Large Animal Medicine
Department of Clinical Sciences
Cummings School of Veterinary Medicine
Tufts University
North Grafton, Massachusetts

Sharon Gwaltney-Brant, DVM, PhD, DABVT, DABT
Vice President & Medical Director
ASPCA Animal Poison Control Center
Adjunct Instructor
Department of Biosciences
College of Veterinary Medicine
University of Illinois
Urbana, Illinois

R. Reid Hanson, DVM, DACVS, DACVECC
Professor of Surgery
J.T. Vaughan Teaching Hospital
Department of Clinical Sciences
College of Veterinary Medicine
Auburn University
Auburn, Alabama

Kelsey A. Hart, DVM, PhD, DACVIM
Large Animal Internal Medicine Clinician
Department of Large Animal Medicine
College of Veterinary Medicine
The University of Georgia
Athens, Georgia

Kevin K. Haussler, DVM, DC, PhD
Assistant Professor
Orthopedic Research Center
Department of Clinical Sciences
College of Veterinary Medicine & Biomedical Sciences
Colorado State University
Fort Collins, Colorado

Jan F. Hawkins, DVM, DACVS
Associate Professor of Large Animal Surgery
Department of Veterinary Clinical Sciences
School of Veterinary Medicine
Purdue University
West Lafayette, Indiana

Shelby Hayden, DVM
Department of Large Animal Clinical Sciences
College of Veterinary Medicine and Biomedical Sciences
Texas A&M University
College Station, Texas

Jonathan Hayles, DVM, MVS, DACVR
Radiology Resident
Department of Veterinary Clinical Sciences, Radiology
College of Veterinary Medicine
Washington State University
Pullman, Washington

Don Henneke, PhD
Director of Equine Science
Tarleton State University
Stephenville, Texas

Christina Hewes, DVM, MS, DACVS
Clinical Instructor
Equine Surgery
Department of Clinical Sciences
Large Animal Teaching Hospital
College of Veterinary Medicine
Auburn University
Auburn, Alabama

Sara A. Hill, DVM
Resident in Veterinary Clinical Pathology
Department of Veterinary Clinical Sciences
College of Veterinary Medicine
University of Minnesota
St. Paul, Minnesota

Melissa T. Hines, DVM, PhD, DACVIM
Associate Professor
Equine Medicine
Department of Veterinary Clinical Sciences
College of Veterinary Medicine
Washington State University
Pullman, Washington

Siddra Hines, DVM
Resident, Equine Internal Medicine
Department of Veterinary Clinical Sciences
College of Veterinary Medicine
Washington State University
Pullman, Washington

Brent Hoff, DVM, DVSc, Dip. Tox.
Clinical Pathologist/Clinical Toxicologist
Animal Health Laboratory
Laboratory Services Division
University of Guelph
Guelph, Ontario, Canada

Andrew M. Hoffmann, DVM, DVSc
Associate Professor
Cummings School of
   Veterinary Medicine
Tufts University
North Grafton, Massachusetts

Rhonda M. Hoffman, PhD, PAS, DACAN
Associate Professor
School of Agribusiness and
   Agriscience
Middle Tennessee State
   University
Murfreesboro, Tennessee

Gilbert Reed Holyoak, DVM, PhD, DACT
Professor
Bullock Professorship of
   Equine Theriogenology
Department of Veterinary
   Clinical Sciences
Center for Veterinary Health
   Sciences
Oklahoma State University
Stillwater, Oklahoma

Amanda Martabano House, DVM, DACVIM
Assistant Professor
Large Animal Clinical Sciences
College of Veterinary
   Medicine
University of Florida
Gainesville, Florida

Samuel D. A. Hurcombe, BSc, BVMS (Hons), MS, DACVIM
Clinical Assistant Professor
Equine Emergency & Critical
   Care/Internal Medicine
Galbreath Equine Center
Veterinary Clinical Sciences
The Ohio State University
Columbus, Ohio

Paula M. Imerman, PhD, MS
Clinician/Analytical
   Toxicologist
Veterinary Diagnostic and
   Production Animal Medicine
College of Veterinary
   Medicine
Iowa State University
Ames, Iowa

Florien Jenner, Dr Med Vet, DACVS
Lecturer
Large Animal Surgery
Department of Veterinary
   Surgery
University College Dublin
Belfield, Dublin, Ireland

Sophy A. Jesty, DVM, DACVIM (Cardiology and Large Animal Internal Medicine)
Clinical Fellow
Department of Clinical
   Sciences
Cornell University Hospital
   for Animals
Cornell University
Ithaca, New York

Aime K. Johnson, DVM, DACT
Assistant Professor
Department of Clinical
   Sciences
J.T. Vaughan Large Animal
   Teaching Hospital
College of Veterinary
   Medicine
Auburn University
Auburn, Alabama

Philip J. Johnson, BVSc(Hons), MS, DACVIM, DECEIM, MRCVS
Professor and Instructional
   Leader
Equine Medicine and Surgery
Department of Veterinary
   Medicine and Surgery
College of Veterinary
   Medicine
University of Missouri
Columbia, Missouri

Kelly L. Kalf, DVM, DACVIM
Lecturer in Large Animal
   Internal Medicine
George D. Widener Hospital
   for Large Animals
New Bolton Center
University of Pennsylvania
Kennett Square, Pennsylvania

Andris J. Kaneps, DVM, PhD, DACVS, DACVSMR
Staff Surgeon
New England Equine Medical
   and Surgical Center
Dover, New Hampshire

Chris Kawcak, DVM, MS, PhD, DACVS
Associate Professor
Department of Clinical
   Sciences
College of Veterinary
   Medicine and Biomedical
   Sciences
Colorado State University
Fort Collins, Colorado

Kevin Keegan, DVM, MS, DACVS
Professor
Department of Veterinary
   Medicine and Surgery
College of Veterinary
   Medicine
University of Missouri
Columbia, Missouri

Alana King, DVM, DACT
Hagyard Equine Medical
   Institute
Lexington, Kentucky

Anthony P. Knight, BVSc, MS, DACVIM
Professor
Large Animal Medicine
Department of Clinical
   Sciences
College of Veterinary
   Medicine and Biomedical
   Sciences
Colorado State University
Fort Collins, Colorado

Joanne Kramer, DVM, DACVS
Assistant Teaching Professor
Department of Veterinary
   Medicine
University of Missouri
Columbia, Missouri

Paula M. Krimer, DVM, DVSc, DACVP
Assistant Professor
Athens Veterinary Diagnostic
   Laboratory
College of Veterinary
   Medicine
The University of Georgia
Athens, Georgia

Laura V. Lane, DVM
Resident
Veterinary Clinical Pathology
Department of Veterinary
   Pathobiology
Oklahoma State University
Stillwater, Oklahoma

Kara M. Lascola, DVM, MS, DACVIM
Assistant Professor
Department of Veterinary
   Clinical Medicine
College of Veterinary
   Medicine
University of Illinois
Urbana, Illinois

Laurie M. Lawrence, PhD
Professor
Department of Animal
   Sciences
College of Agriculture
University of Kentucky
Lexington, Kentucky

Rejean Cléophas Lefebvre, DVM, IPSAV, PhD, DACT
Associate Professor
Department of Clinical
   Sciences
Faculté de Médecine
   Vétérinaire
Université de Montréal
Montréal, Québec
Canada

Alfredo Sanchez Londoño, MV, MS, DACVIM (LAIM)
Ambulatory Clinician
Assistant Professor
Cummings School of
   Veterinary Medicine
Tufts University
Woodstock, Connecticut

Maureen T. Long, DVM, PhD, DACVM
Associate Professor, Large
   Animal Medicine
Department of Infectious
   Diseases and Pathology
College of Veterinary
   Medicine
University of Florida
Gainesville, Florida

Charles C. Love, DVM, PHD, DACT
Associate Professor
Clinical Theriogenologist
Department of Large Animal
   Clinical Sciences
College of Veterinary
   Medicine
Texas A&M University
College Station, Texas

Tim Mair, BVSc, PhD, DEIM, DESTS, DECEIM, MRCVS
Partner
Bell Equine Veterinary Clinic
Mereworth, Maidstone
Kent, United Kingdom

Chelsea Makloski, DVM, MS, DACT
Assistant Professor
Clinical Theriogenologist
Department of Veterinary
   Clinical Sciences
Center for Veterinary Health
   Sciences
Oklahoma State University
Stillwater, Oklahoma

John S. Mattoon, DVM, DACVR
Professor
Chief of Radiology
Department of Veterinary Clinical Sciences
College of Veterinary Medicine
Washington State University
Pullman, Washington

Melissa R. Mazan, DVM, DACVIM
Associate Professor
Director, Issaam Fares Equine Sports Medicine Program
Department of Clinical Sciences
Sports Medicine
Cummings School of Veterinary Medicine
Tufts University
North Grafton, Massachusetts

Hernán J. Montilla, DVM
Theriogenology Resident
Department of Clinical Sciences
College of Veterinary Medicine
Oregon State University
Corvallis, Oregon

Sandra E. Morgan, DVM, MS, DABVT
Associate Professor
Veterinary Toxicologist
Physiological Sciences
Oklahoma Animal Disease Diagnostic Laboratory
Oklahoma State University
Center for Veterinary Health Sciences
Oklahoma State University
Stillwater, Oklahoma

Peter R. Morresey, BVSc, MACVSc, DACT, DACVIM (Large animal)
Associate
Internal Medicine
Rood and Riddle Equine Hospital
Lexington, Kentucky

Michelle S. Mostrom, DVM, MS, PhD, DABVT, ABT
Veterinary Toxicologist
Veterinary Diagnostic Laboratory
North Dakota State University
Fargo, North Dakota

Amelia Munsterman, DVM, MS, DACVS, DACVECC
Clinical Instructor
Equine Critical Care Medicine and Surgery
Department of Clinical Sciences
College of Veterinary Medicine
Auburn University
Auburn, Alabama

Lisa A. Murphy, VMD, DABT
Assistant Professor of Toxicology
Department of Pathobiology
School of Veterinary Medicine
New Bolton Center
University of Pennsylvania
Kennett Square, Pennsylvania

Mike Murphy, DVM, PhD, JD
Professor Emeritus
College of Veterinary Medicine
University of Minnesota
St. Paul, Minnesota

Dana A. Neelis, DVM
Radiology Resident
Department of Veterinary Clinical Sciences
College of Veterinary Medicine
Washington State University
Pullman, Washington

Rose Nolen-Walston, DVM, DACVIM (LAIM)
Assistant Professor of Medicine
Department of Clinical Studies
New Bolton Center
University of Pennsylvania
Kennett Square, Pennsylvania

Joan Norton, VMD
Section of Medicine
Department of Clinical Studies
New Bolton Center
University of Pennsylvania
Kennett Square, Pennsylvania

Yvette S. Nout, DVM, MS, PhD, DACVIM, DACVECC
Assistant Researcher
Department of Neurological Surgery
University of California
San Francisco, California

Nicole H. Passler, DVM, MS
Instructor
Department of Clinical Sciences
College of Veterinary Medicine
Auburn University
Auburn, Alabama

Julia A. Paxson, DVM, PhD, DACVIM (LA)
Post-Doctoral Fellow
Department of Clinical Sciences
Cummings School of Veterinary Medicine
Tufts University
North Grafton, Massachusetts

Erwin G. Pearson, DVM, MS, DACVIM
Professor Emeritus
Large Animal Medicine
College of Veterinary Medicine
Oregon State University
Corvallis, Oregon

Lisa K. Pearson, DVM
Resident
Large Animal Theriogenology
Department of Veterinary Clinical Sciences
College of Veterinary Medicine
Washington State University
Pullman, Washington

Alessandra Pellegrini-Masini, DVM, PhD, DACVIM
Clinical Assistant Professor
Department of Large Animal Medicine
College of Veterinary Medicine
The University of Georgia
Athens, Georgia

Annette Petersen, Dr Med Vet, DACVD (Dermatology)
Assistant Professor of Dermatology
Department of Small Animal Clinical Sciences
College of Veterinary Medicine
Michigan State University
East Lansing, Michigan

Nelson I. Pinto, DVM, MS
Intern, Specialty Ophthalmology
Department of Small Animal Medicine and Surgery
College of Veterinary Medicine
The University of Georgia
Athens, Georgia

Ida Piperisova, DVM
Clinical Pathology Resident
Department of Population Health and Pathobiology
College of Veterinary Medicine
North Carolina State University
Raleigh, North Carolina

Tracy Plough, DVM, JCS
Veterinary Reproductive Services
St. Langley British Columbia, Canada

Sarah M. Puchalski, DVM, DACVR
Assistant Professor
Department of Surgical and Radiological Sciences
School of Veterinary Medicine
University of California–Davis
Davis, California

Birgit Puschner, DVM, PhD, DABVT
Professor of Veterinary Toxicology
Department of Molecular Biosciences
California Animal Health and Food Safety Laboratory System
School of Veterinary Medicine
University of California–Davis
Davis, California

Ignacio Raggio, DMV, DES, MSc
Department of Clinical Sciences
Faculté de Médicine Vétérinaire
Université de Montréal
Montréal, Québec, Canada

Merl F. Raisbeck, DVM, MS, PhD
Professor of Veterinary Toxicology
Wyoming State Veterinary Laboratory
College of Veterinary Medicine
University of Wyoming
Laramie, Wyoming

Stephen M. Reed, DVM, DACVIM
Associate Veterinarian
Internal Medicine
Rood and Riddle Equine Hospital
Lexington, Kentucky

Thomas J. Reilly, PhD
Clinical Assistant Professor
Department of Veterinary
  Pathobiology
College of Veterinary
  Medicine
University of Missouri
Columbia, Missouri

**Janelle S. Renschler, DVM,
PhD**
Lecturer in Clinical Pathology
Department of Population
  Health and Pathobiology
College of Veterinary
  Medicine
North Carolina State
  University
Raleigh, North Carolina

**Theresa E. Rizzi, DVM,
DACVP**
Clinical Assistant Professor
Department of Veterinary
  Pathogiology
Center for Veterinary Health
  Sciences
College of Veterinary
  Medicine
Oklahoma State University
Stillwater, Oklahoma

**Gregory D. Roberts, DVM,
MS, DACVR**
Clinical Associate Professor
Department of Veterinary
  Clinical Sciences
College of Veterinary
  Medicine
Washington State University
Pullman, Washington

**Jacobo S. Rodriguez, MV,
MS, DACT**
Resident
Department of Veterinary
  Clinical Sciences
College of Veterinary
  Medicine
Washington State University
Pullman, Washington

**Angela B. Royal, DVM, MS,
DACVP (Clinical
Pathology)**
Clinical Instructor
Department of Veterinary
  Pathobiology
College of Veterinary
  Medicine
University of Missouri
Columbia, Missouri

**Juan C. Samper, DVM, MSc,
PhD, DACT**
Veterinary Reproductive
  Services
Langley, British Columbia,
  Canada

**Francesca Sampieri, Dr
Med Vet, MS, MRCVS**
Resident
Veterinary Clinical
  Pharmacology
Veterinary Biomedical
  Sciences
Western College of Veterinary
  Medicine
Saskatoon, Saskatchewan,
  Canada

**Elizabeth M. Santschi,
DVM, DACVS**
Associate Professor
Clinical Equine Surgery
Department of Veterinary
  Clinical Sciences
College of Veterinary
  Medicine
The Ohio State University
Columbus, Ohio

Maria Clara Sardoy, Vet.
Equine Medicine and Surgery
  Intern
Veterinary Medical Teaching
  Hospital
College of Veterinary
  Medicine
Kansas State University
Manhattan, Kansas

**Swanand R. Sathe, BVSc &
AH, MVSc**
Resident
Theriogenology/Equine
  Reproduction
Department of Veterinary
  Clinical Medicine
Veterinary Teaching Hospital
College of Veterinary
  Medicine
University of Illinois
Urbana, Illinois

Susan Schommer, PhD
Assistant Professor
Department of Veterinary
  Pathobiology
Veterinary Medical Diagnostic
  Laboratory
College of Veterinary
  Medicine
University of Missouri
Columbia, Missouri

**John Schumacher, DVM,
MS, DACVIM**
Professor
Department of Clinical Sciences
College of Veterinary
  Medicine
Auburn University
Auburn, Alabama

**Colin C. Schwarzwald,
Dr Med Vet, PhD, DACVIM**
Senior Lecturer
Equine Department
Vetsuisse Faculty
University of Zurich
Zurich, Switzerland

**Olga Seco Diaz, Licenciada
en Veterinaria, MRCVS**
Adjunct Assistant Professor
Department of Clinical
  Studies
New Bolton Center
University of Pennsylvania
Kennett Square, Pennsylvania

**Kathy K. Seino, DVM, MS,
PhD**
Assistant Professor
Equine Internal Medicine
Department of Veterinary
  Clinical Sciences
College of Veterinary Medicine
Washington State University
Pullman, Washington

**Debra C. Sellon, DVM, PhD,
DACVIM**
Professor, Equine Medicine
Department of Veterinary
  Clinical Sciences
College of Veterinary Medicine;
Associate Dean, Graduate
  School
Washington State University
Pullman, Washington

**Kim A. Selting, DVM, MS,
DACVIM (Oncology)**
Assistant Teaching Professor
Department of Veterinary
  Medicine and Surgery
College of Veterinary
  Medicine
University of Missouri
Columbia, Missouri

David Senter, DVM, DACVD
Dermatologist
Veterinary Allergy and
  Dermatology Clinic, LLC
Overland Park, Kansas;
Adjunct Assistant Clinical
  Professor
College of Veterinary Medicine
University of Missouri
Columbia, Missouri

**Ceri Sherlock, B Vet Med,
MRCVS, DACVS**
Large Animal Surgery Clinical
  Instructor
Department of Large Animal
  Medicine
College of Veterinary
  Medicine
The University of Georgia
Athens, Georgia

Paul D. Siciliano, PhD
Associate Professor
Department of Animal
  Science
College of Agriculture and
  Life Sciences
North Carolina State University
Raleigh, North Carolina

**Phoebe A. Smith, DVM,
DACVIM**
Riviera Equine
Internal Medicine &
  Consulting
Santa Ynez, California

**Laura Ann Snyder, DVM,
DACVP (Clinical
Pathology)**
Assistant Clinical Professor
Clinical Pathology
Department of Veterinary
  Clinical Sciences
College of Veterinary
  Medicine
University of Minnesota
St. Paul, Minnesota

**Ted S. Stashak, DVM, MS,
DACVS**
Emeritus Professor of Equine
  Surgery
Department of Clinical
  Sciences
College of Veterinary
  Medicine and Biomedical
  Sciences
Colorado State University
Fort Collins, Colorado

**Allison J. Stewart,
BVSc(hons), MS, DACVIM-
LAIM, DACVECC**
Associate Professor
Department of Clinical
  Sciences
College of Veterinary
  Medicine
Auburn University
Auburn, Alabama

Carolyn L. Stull, MS, PhD
Animal Welfare Extension
  Specialist
School of Veterinary Medicine
University of California–Davis
Davis, California

**Kenneth E Sullins, DVM,
MS, DACVS**
Professor of Surgery
Marion duPont Scott Equine
  Medical Center
Virginia-Maryland Regional
  College of Veterinary
  Medicine
Virginia Tech
Leesburg, Virginia

W. Wesley Sutter, DVM, MS, DACVS
Surgeon
Department of Surgery
Ocala Equine Hospital
Ocala, Florida

Jennifer Taintor, DVM, MS, DACVIM
Assistant Professor
Department of Clinical Sciences
College of Veterinary Medicine
Auburn University
Auburn, Alabama

Patricia A. Talcott, DVM, PhD, MS, DABVT
Associate Professor
Diagnostic Toxicologist
Veterinary Comparative Anatomy
Pharmacology and Physiology
Washington Animal Disease Diagnostic Lab
College of Veterinary Medicine
Washington State University
Pullman, Washington

Brett Tennent-Brown, BVSc, MS, DACVIM, DACVECC
Assistant Professor
Department of Large Animal Medicine
College of Veterinary Medicine
The University of Georgia
Athens, Georgia

Christine Théorêt, DVM, PhD, DACVS
Professor, Equine Surgical Anatomy
Faculté de Médecine Vétérinaire
Université de Montréal
Montréal, Québec, Canada

Ahmed Tibary, DMV, MS, DSc, PhD, DACT
Professor
Department of Veterinary Clinical Sciences
College of Veterinary Medicine
Washington State University
Pullman, Washington

Peter J. Timoney, MVB, MS, PhD, FRCVS
Professor
Gluck Equine Research Center
Department of Veterinary Science
University of Kentucky
Lexington, Kentucky

Ian Tizard, BVMS, BSc, PhD, DACVIM
Professor of Immunology
Department of Veterinary Pathobiology
College of Veterinary Medicine
Texas A&M University
College Station, Texas

Ramiro E. Toribio, DVM, MS, PhD, DACVIM
Associate Professor
Department of Veterinary Clinical Sciences
College of Veterinary Medicine
The Ohio State University
Columbus, Ohio

Chelsea D. Tripp, DVM
Resident, Oncology
Department of Veterinary Clinical Sciences
College of Veterinary Medicine
Washington State University
Pullman, Washington

Mats H. T. Troedsson, DVM, PhD, DACT, DECAR
Chairman and Director
Gluck Equine Research Center
Department of Veterinary Science
University of Kentucky
Lexington, Kentucky

Beth A. Valentine, DVM, PhD, DACVP
Professor
Department of Biomedical Sciences
College of Veterinary Medicine
Oregon State University
Corvallis, Oregon

Gunther van Loon, DVM, PhD, DECEIM
Professor
Large Animal Internal Medicine
Faculty of Veterinary Medicine
Ghent University
Merelbeke, Ghent, Belgium

Karsten Velde, DVM, DACVS, DECVS
Surgeon
Clinic for Large Animal Surgery and Orthopaedics
Veterinary University of Vienna
Vienna, Austria

Dawna L. Voelkl, DVM, DACT
Assistant Teaching Professor
Department of Veterinary Medicine and Surgery
College of Veterinary Medicine
University of Missouri
Columbia, Missouri

Bryan M. Waldridge, DVM, MS, DABVP (Equine Practice), DACVIM
Kentucky Equine Research
Versailles, Kentucky

Lori K. Warren, PhD, MS
Assistant Professor
Department of Animal Sciences
College of Veterinary Medicine
University of Florida
Gainesville, Florida

Kimberly Weber, DVM
Teaching Associate
Department of Pathobiology
College of Veterinary Medicine
University of Illinois
Urbana, Illinois

Marlyn S. Whitney, DVM, PhD, DACVP (Clinical Pathology)
Clinical Associate Professor
Veterinary Medical Diagnostic Laboratory
Department of Veterinary Pathobiology
College of Veterinary Medicine
University of Missouri
Columbia, Missouri

Charles Wiedmeyer, DVM, PhD, DACVP
Assistant Professor
Veterinary Clinical Pathology
Department of Veterinary Pathobiology
College of Veterinary Medicine
University of Missouri
Columbia, Missouri

Robyn R. Wilborn, DVM, MS, DACT
Assistant Professor
Department of Clinical Sciences
College of Veterinary Medicine
Auburn University
Auburn, Alabama

Pamela Wilkins, DVM, PhD, ACIVM-LA, ACVEC
Professor
Veterinary Clinical Medicine
Section Head
Equine Medicine and Surgery
College of Veterinary Medicine
University of Illinois
Urbana, Illinois

Tom Wilkinson, DVM
Moore Equine Veterinary Centre
Calgary, Alberta, Canada

Carey A. Williams, PhD
Department of Animal Sciences
School of Environmental and Biological Sciences
Rutgers, The State University of New Jersey
New Brunswick, New Jersey

Jarred Williams, DVM, MS
Equine Surgery Resident
Department of Veterinary Clinical Sciences
College of Veterinary Medicine
The Ohio State University
Columbus, Ohio

Christine L. Wimer, MS, DVM
Postdoctoral Associate
Department of Population Medicine and Diagnostic Sciences
College of Veterinary Medicine
Cornell University
Ithaca, New York

L. Nicki Wise, DVM
Graduate Research Assistant, Equine Medicine
Department of Veterinary Clinical Sciences
College of Veterinary Medicine
Washington State University
Pullman, Washington

Lesley E. Young, BVSc, DVA, DVC, DECEIM, PhD, MRCVS
RCVS Recognized Specialist in Veterinary Cardiology
Specialist Cardiology Services
Newmarket, Suffolk
United Kingdom

This textbook is dedicated to my wife, Christina; my daughters, Erin, Emily, and Megan; and my two grandchildren, Ava and Anthony, who have given me support and inspiration throughout its production.

PREFACE

Keeping pace with the growing body of knowledge in any one part of veterinary medicine, let alone staying current in all of them, is an enormous challenge. As veterinarians, we see the extremes of the spectrum for published veterinary resources. On one end of the spectrum are definitive, peer-reviewed manuscripts in specialty publications that are the gold standard for accuracy. For a busy practitioner, however, these sources may contain too much detail to be immediately useful in a daily clinical setting. On the other end of the spectrum, simplified information may be more accessible, but the appeal can be hollow if the information is not peer reviewed or, in some cases, not even scientifically defensible. The purpose of the *Clinical Veterinary Advisor* is to provide an entry point between these two extremes by using a template-based format, photographs, and a multisection approach. It aims to present a concise review of the most useful information while covering six of the major facets of equine practice: diseases and disorders, procedures and techniques, differential diagnoses, algorithm-based decision making, laboratory tests, and medications. As a bridge between the comprehensive coverage of a specialty text and a quick reference guide, the *Clinical Veterinary Advisor* has been created to present the information that practitioners seek when we turn to a reference for help.

Section I, Diseases and Disorders, describes the most important elements of commonly encountered illnesses and presenting complaints of horses. The material is presented in a way that follows the natural progression of a typical case: background information is presented first, including the definition of the topic, synonyms, and epidemiologic facts. Next, the chief complaint at the time the appointment was made and typical history are presented. The remainder of the material in a Diseases and Disorders topic is likewise presented according to the process followed during the veterinary visit or in the veterinary hospital. For example, diagnostic testing is presented in two parts. Initial database tests come first; these are diagnostic tests that are routinely performed in an initial workup. Immediately afterward comes advanced or confirmatory testing, which encompasses the more-specific tests that may be indicated based on initial results or tests that may require more expensive equipment or advanced techniques. These are sometimes done in a general practice and in other cases require referral to a university hospital or specialty center. Similarly, treatment is described as acute treatment first, followed by chronic treatment. Drug dosages and routes of administration are included so the reader does not have to leaf through the Drug Formulary for every medication. The end of each topic includes a section for clinical tips, which are the most useful nuggets of information according to the experience of the author and editor—points we want to bring to the reader's attention, easily made mistakes to avoid, or other useful insights.

Section II is Procedures and Techniques. This section describes more than 80 diagnostic and therapeutic procedures specific to equine practice. The procedures range in complexity from the relatively simple, such as urinary catheterization or skin biopsy, to the advanced, such as intracytoplasmic sperm injection or metered-dose inhalation therapy. Here, too, the material is presented in a streamlined and formatted way by specialists who either have pioneered these procedures or are proficient in their use. The intent is to allow a reader to feel prepared to perform the procedures if his or her training and skills are otherwise adequate, or else to understand what is involved in a procedure when preparing to refer a patient to another practice or institution.

Section III, Differential Diagnosis, provides tables of differential diagnoses for many of the most common abnormalities encountered in equine practice. This section is perhaps most useful for students and young veterinarians, or for any veterinarian reviewing the breadth of potential explanations for a particular disorder. It represents a compilation of lists that cover a broad range of topics in equine practice.

Section IV, Laboratory Tests, presents a concise summary of clinical pathology tests and relevant information for the clinician. As in other parts of the book, the information is arranged alphabetically and the essential aspects of each test are described. This approach presents laboratory-based information in a clinically applicable format.

Section V, Clinical Algorithms, approaches the management of some of the most common or challenging disorders in equine practice in a "decision tree" format. This format can be enormously useful to some and of limited value to others. Younger veterinarians or those looking for information in an unfamiliar area of equine veterinary medicine may find this section most helpful because it represents a starting point of information in a direct, succinct manner. This basic, streamlined approach provides an initial framework for addressing a particular disorder.

Finally, the Drug Formulary in Section VI is presented from a practitioner's perspective. Medications in common use or that are emerging in practice are described in a tabular format. Space constraints preclude a very detailed description, so the most important elements of each have been selected and included.

Our goal was to provide readers with a solid summary of the information needed to properly handle most of what is encountered in practice—from the old to the new, from the routine to the exceptional. The governing principles have been to make the material accurate, practical, and rapidly accessible. I hope it will provide you with a convenient, reliable reference that will help support you in your practice every day.

ACKNOWLEDGMENTS

It is with great pleasure that I thank the editors for their excellent job in selecting the authors and in providing or refining the content for the book. Their efforts and cooperation allowed us to put together a superb list of authors, and their editorial efforts made each of their sections concise and relevant.

I would also like to thank each author for his or her contribution to the book. I am pleased that we were able to get support from many world-renowned specialists to produce the focused content of this book in its rather unique format.

I would also like to thank Dr. Joanne Kramer for her assistance in editing the final manuscript, and Emily Wilson, my daughter, for her assistance in helping organize the chapter submissions.

There are many people at Elsevier who helped during the preparation of the book. A few should be thanked individually. Jolynn Gower, Managing Editor, initially approached me about the project and convinced me it would be a great idea. Penny Rudolph, Publisher, and Lauren Harms, Developmental Editor, helped with the organization and provided motivation and technical support throughout the book's development. Carrie Stetz, Project Manager, provided the support and guidance to organize the final stages of the manuscript and shepherded the project through to publication. To everyone at Elsevier I owe my extreme gratitude. Thank you for your assistance and guidance throughout the entire production.

CONTENTS

xx Contents

SECTION II PROCEDURES AND TECHNIQUES

SECTION V CLINICAL ALGORITHMS

SECTION VI DRUG FORMULARY

SECTION I

Diseases and Disorders

Abortion, Equine Infectious

BASIC INFORMATION

DEFINITION

Pregnancy loss after placental development around 40 to 45 days (may be more correctly termed "stillbirth" in term pregnancies after 320 days). Causes include bacterial, fungal, and viral organisms.

EPIDEMIOLOGY

RISK FACTORS

Risk factors vary by inciting cause:

- Viral abortions, including equine herpes virus (EHV) and equine arteritis virus (EAV), may occur sporadically or as "abortion storms." Contact with aborting animals and negative vaccine status are important risk factors for viral abortions.
- Environmental conditions, such as standing water in pastures, and contact with wildlife are known risk factors for leptospiral abortions.
- Poor perineal conformation and trauma to the reproductive tract may be risk factors for bacterial or fungal placentitis. Other sources of vaginal or cervical contamination, including iatrogenic contamination during reproductive examination, may also represent risk factors.

CONTAGION AND ZOONOSIS

- Direct contact with infected, viremic animals or with aborted tissue is the primary mechanism of transmission for viral diseases. Additionally, EAV may be transmitted by aerosol across short distances. Leptospiral organisms may be transmitted in urine or via the abortus; however, most leptospiral abortions are sporadic. Bacterial abortions are not known to be contagious.
- The zoonotic potential for equine viral or bacterial abortificants (or abortifacients) is low; however, appropriate personal protection should be used when handling fetal or placental tissue of aborted animals.
- *Leptospira* spp. are known to be zoonotic and cause human disease. Transmission from horses to humans has not been documented to the author's knowledge.

GEOGRAPHY AND SEASONALITY

- Viral abortions occur worldwide.
- Abortions caused by nocardioform organisms are most commonly seen in Kentucky but have also been reported in Florida, Europe, and South Africa.
- Abortions are more common in mid to late gestation (20–44 weeks), generally coinciding with the winter months; however, no direct seasonal influences have been identified.
- Leptospiral abortions are more prevalent in locations or seasons with heavy rainfall and standing water.

ASSOCIATED CONDITIONS AND DISORDERS

- Placentitis (ascending bacterial placentitis or nocardioform placentitis)
- Respiratory disease (EHV)
- Dystocia
- Retained fetal membranes

CLINICAL PRESENTATION

DISEASE FORMS/SUBTYPES

- Bacterial
- Viral
- Fungal

HISTORY, CHIEF COMPLAINT

- Acute abortion or stillbirth
- Precocious mammary development
- Vulvar discharge
- Premature separation of fetal membranes at birth

PHYSICAL EXAM FINDINGS

- Blood-tinged perineal area; protruding membranes from vulvar area or in vagina.
- Physical parameters of mares are generally within normal limits.
- The fetus may be fresh or autolyzed.

ETIOLOGY AND PATHOPHYSIOLOGY

- The pathophysiology of the disease is poorly understood for most causative organisms.
- Abortion may be associated with clinical disease in the mare (EAV, EIA) or in the absence of clinical disease.
- Ascending placentitis is generally induced by opportunistic organisms ascending from the vagina though the cervix. The bacteria colonize the fetal membranes and penetrate to the allantoic and amniotic fluids, gaining access to the foal either by fetal swallowing and respiratory movements or by umbilical penetration. Bacterial invasion initiates a cascade of hormonal and physical changes that precipitate premature parturition. At the time of parturition, the fetus may be premature, precociously mature, or septic.
- It has not been established how nocardioform organisms reach the uterus, but they are characteristically found at the most ventral aspect of the uterus. Nocardioform placentitis results in disruption of placental function and fetal hypoxia but is not known to cause fetal sepsis.

DIAGNOSIS

DIFFERENTIAL DIAGNOSIS

- Ascending bacterial placentitis: *Streptococcus equi* subsp. *zooepidemicus*, *Escherichia coli*, *Pseudomonas aeruginosa*, *Klebsiella pneumoniae* associated with placentitis, funisitis, and fetal sepsis; the fetus may be fresh or autolyzed.
- Nocardioform placentitis: *Crosiella equi*, *Lentzea kentuckyensis*, *Amycolatopsis* spp., and *Cellulosimicrobium cellulans* cause chronic placentitis and placental insufficiency without fetal sepsis; foals may be born alive but underdeveloped and emaciated.
- Leptospiral abortion: *Leptospira kennewick* (formerly *Leptospira pomona*), *Leptospira grippotyphosa*, *Leptospira bratislava* (host adapted to equines); associated with abortion of autolyzed fetal tissue, mild diffuse placentitis, and funisitis; the fetus may be icteric.
- Viral abortion: EHV, EAV, rarely EIA; fetuses may be fresh (EHV) or autolytic (EAV).
- Fungal abortion: *Aspergillus* spp., *Mucor* spp., *Candida* spp. associated with placental insufficiency or fetal infection; *Histoplasma* spp. are a rare cause of abortion.
- Mare reproductive loss syndrome results in fetal death and abortion or mummification early in pregnancy (day 45–60) and rarely in late-term abortion. The syndrome is associated with ingestion of Eastern tent caterpillars. The cetae (hairs) of tent caterpillars are capable of penetrating the intestinal tract and serving as vectors for opportunistic intestinal organisms.
- Other infectious causes of abortion: *Taylorella equigenitalis* (contagious equine metritis), *Neorickettsia risticii* (Potomac horse fever), *Salmonella abortus equi*.
- Noninfectious causes of abortion: Twin pregnancy, umbilical torsion, fetal malformation.

INITIAL DATABASE

- Complete blood count and chemistry panel are usually normal but may be indicated to determine other organ involvement.
- Electrolyte content of milk may be useful to predict timing to parturition in mares with precocious mammary development and milk production.

- A progesterone (estimating total progestagens) or estrogen assay may be useful to predict timing to parturition or severity of disease in some cases.
- Transrectal palpation and ultrasonography should be performed to confirm the presence of a fetus if premonitory signs are noted or to confirm the complete evacuation of the uterus in a mare that presents after abortion.
- A thorough genital examination, including a culture swab of the uterus and a speculum examination of the caudal genital tract, may guide post-abortion treatment.

ADVANCED OR CONFIRMATORY TESTING

- Serologic tests for EHV, EAV, *Leptospira* spp., and *Neorickettsia* on maternal serum are available and may aid in the diagnosis of etiology after abortion.
- Necropsy of the fetus and fetal membranes represents the highest chance of achieving a diagnosis.

TREATMENT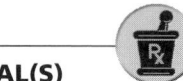

THERAPEUTIC GOAL(S)

- Maintaining pregnancy to term (if premonitory signs are noted)
- Maximizing fertility of subsequent breeding attempts
- Preventing transmission of contagious organism to susceptible animals

ACUTE GENERAL TREATMENT

- See "Parturition, Premature Signs of" in this section for treatment of pregnant mares with suspected placentitis.
- Isolation of mares after abortion and removal of fetal tissues and fluids from the presence of other pregnant mares may reduce the risk of multiple abortions.
- Large-volume uterine lavage (30–40 L of nonsterile saline) may be warranted

to evacuate retained fetal membranes or fetal tissues or to enhance bacterial clearance from the uterus.
- Antibiotic or antiinflammatory therapy may be warranted based on examination findings.

POSSIBLE COMPLICATIONS

- Dystocia
- Retained fetal membranes
- Retention of a dead fetus is a rare complication but warrants examination. A retained fetus that is undetected may result in mummification or maceration, which is associated with metritis and severe maternal disease or chronic infertility.

RECOMMENDED MONITORING

- Mares and abortuses, including the fetal membranes, should be examined carefully at the time of abortion to achieve an accurate diagnosis.
- Mares should receive regular nursing care, including monitoring of the rectal temperature to enhance diagnosis of secondary complications, such as retained fetal membranes and metritis.
- If clinically normal, mares should be examined by transrectal ultrasonography 5 to 8 days after abortion to monitor uterine involution.
- A complete breeding soundness examination may be warranted before subsequent breeding attempts.

PROGNOSIS AND OUTCOME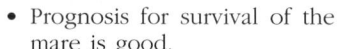

- Prognosis for survival of the mare is good.
- Prognosis for future fertility is good in the absence of predisposing anatomic conditions or secondary complications (eg, dystocia with ensuing damage to the reproductive tract, retained fetal membranes).

- Infection does not result in protective antibody formation for future pregnancies in most cases (except EAV).

PEARLS & CONSIDERATIONS

PREVENTION

- Vaccination of pregnant mares at 5, 7, and 9 months of gestation prevents abortion storms caused by EHV.
- Vaccination of at-risk horses reduces the transmission of EAV.
- Pregnant animals should be separated from young animals and competition animals to avoid transmission of disease.

CLIENT EDUCATION

Although there are no known strategies to prevent bacterial placentitis, client education regarding the importance of premonitory signs, including vaginal discharge and precocious mammary development, as well as routine diagnostic ultrasonography of late-pregnant mares may lead to a reduction in the incidence of abortion.

SUGGESTED READING

Donahue JM, Williams NM: Emergent causes of placentitis and abortion. *Vet Clin North Am Equine* 16(3):443, 2000.
Holyoak GR: Equine viral arteritis: current status and prevention. *Theriogenology* 70:403–414, 2008.
Macpherson ML, Bailey CS; A clinical approach to managing the mare with placentitis. *Theriogenology* 70:435–440, 2008.
Sebastian MM, Bernard WV, Riddle TW, et al: Mare reproductive loss syndrome. *Vet Pathol* 45(5):710–722, 2008.

AUTHOR: **C. SCOTT BAILEY**

EDITOR: **JUAN C. SAMPER**

Abscess, Perirectal

BASIC INFORMATION

DEFINITION

Abscessation around the aboral rectum and the anus

EPIDEMIOLOGY

RISK FACTORS Anorectal lymphadenopathy can progress to abscessation. Anorectal lymphadenopathy is more common in horses 3 to 15 months of age.

CLINICAL PRESENTATION

DISEASE FORMS/SUBTYPES The abscesses can be located anywhere circumferentially around the rectum and anus.

HISTORY, CHIEF COMPLAINT
- Mild colic signs
- Depression
- Inappetence
- Decreased fecal output
- Tenesmus
- Dyschezia
- Dysuria

PHYSICAL EXAM FINDINGS

- Temperature is variable depending on the severity of the lesion; it is often elevated.
- Heart rate may be normal or may be elevated.
- Mucous membranes are variable depending on severity of compromise; they are often pale pink and moist.
- Colic signs are variable.

ETIOLOGY AND PATHOPHYSIOLOGY
- Progression of anorectal lymphadenopathy

- Rectal puncture
- Rectal tears, especially those in the aboral nonperitoneal rectum
- Rectal inflammation
- Migration of an abscess after an intramuscular gluteal injection

DIAGNOSIS

DIFFERENTIAL DIAGNOSIS

- Anorectal lymphadenopathy
- Small colon impaction
- Rectal tear
- Nonstrangulating small colon or rectal obstruction
- Rectal neoplasia
- Rectal hematoma
- Urinary tract infection

INITIAL DATABASE

- Complete blood count: Leukopenia and leukocytosis are common; occasionally normal.
- Rectal evaluation: The firm abscess may be palpated in the perianal area or under the submucosa of the rectum.
- Ultrasonography: May see a well-circumscribed subcutaneous or submucosal mass.

ADVANCED OR CONFIRMATORY TESTING

- Perirectal abscess aspiration: This can be performed percutaneously or transrectally.
- Submit any aspirated fluid for cytology, culture, and sensitivity.
- *Escherichia coli* and *Streptococcus equi* subsp. *zooepidemicus* are commonly isolated.

TREATMENT

THERAPEUTIC GOAL(S)

- Systemic and local analgesia and antiinflammatories

- Abscess drainage
- Laxative diet
- Antibiotics based on culture and sensitivity

ACUTE GENERAL TREATMENT

- Occasionally abscessed anorectal lymph nodes in young horses can be treated with antibiotics, antiinflammatories, and laxative diets alone.
- Anorectal abscesses refractory to medical management or those in older horses frequently require surgical drainage.
  ○ Perform caudal epidural anesthesia with lidocaine (0.22 mg/kg)
  ○ Drain abscess
    ▪ Lateral abscesses can be drained lateral to the anus.
    ▪ Dorsal abscesses can be drained into the rectum.
    ▪ Ventral abscesses can be drained into the vagina in mares or ventral to the anus in males.
  ○ Administer nonsteroidal antiinflammatory drugs (flunixin meglumine, 1.1 mg/kg).
  ○ Depending on the invasiveness of surgery, consider administering broad-spectrum antibiotics while awaiting the results of culture and sensitivity.
  ○ Feed a laxative diet and administer mineral oil via nasogastric tube.
  ○ Occasionally, abscesses extend into the abdominal cavity; these may require exploratory celiotomy and marsupialization or drainage into the vagina or rectum.

CHRONIC TREATMENT

- Analgesia and antiinflammatories
- Antibiotics
- Laxative diet and mineral oil
- Lavage daily with dilute antiseptic solution to open abscesses

POSSIBLE COMPLICATIONS

- Peritonitis
- Endotoxemia
- Laminitis
- Adhesions
- Colic
- Stricture formation
- Jugular thrombophlebitis
- Recurrence of abscess
- Perianal fistula
- Rectovaginal fistula

RECOMMENDED MONITORING

- Pain
- Fecal output and consistency and any blood on feces
- Signs of endotoxemia
- Colic

PROGNOSIS AND OUTCOME

- Prognosis for abscesses without abdominal involvement is favorable.
- Abdominal involvement reduces the prognosis as there is a higher risk of complications.

SUGGESTED READING

Freeman D: Rectum and anus. In Auer JA, Stick JA, editors: *Equine surgery*, ed 3. St Louis, 2006, Saunders Elsevier, pp 479–491.

Magee AA, Ragle CA, Hines MT, et al: Anorectal lymphadenopathy causing colic, peritoneal abscesses or both in five young horses. *J Am Vet Med Assoc* 210:804–807, 1997.

Schumacher J: Disease of the small colon and rectum. In Mair TS, Divers T, Ducharme N, editors: *Manual of equine gastroenterology*. St Louis, 2002, WB Saunders, pp 299–315.

AUTHOR: **CERI SHERLOCK**

EDITORS: **TIM MAIR** and **CERI SHERLOCK**

Actinobacillosis

BASIC INFORMATION

DEFINITION

- *Actinobacillus* spp. is a gram-negative group of bacteria that causes a variety of clinical syndromes in horses.
- *Actinobacillus equuli* subsp. *equuli*
- *Actinobacillus equuli* subsp. *haemolyticus*

EPIDEMIOLOGY

SPECIES, AGE, SEX All species of horses are susceptible. *A. equuli* is associated with sepsis of foals and is a common bacteria isolated from abortions caused by the eastern tent caterpillar (ETC).

RISK FACTORS

- ETC (*Malacosoma americanum*) ingestion and intoxication

- Failure of passive transfer of immunoglobulin in foals

GEOGRAPHY AND SEASONALITY ETC infestation of the environment may fluctuate from year to year and is associated with fruiting trees, hatching in the spring.

ASSOCIATED CONDITIONS AND DISORDERS Mare reproductive loss syndrome (MRLS)

CLINICAL PRESENTATION

DISEASE FORMS/SUBTYPES
- Opportunistic infections of many organs and body systems of adults
- Septicemia of foals

HISTORY, CHIEF COMPLAINT
- Adults: History and chief complaint referable to the affected system: MRLS—abortion, pericarditis
- Neonates: Neonatal sepsis within the first 2 weeks of life

PHYSICAL EXAM FINDINGS
- Adults: Examination referable to the organ system affected consisting of abortion, metritis, mastitis, septicemia, arthritis, endocarditis, meningitis, pneumonia, and pleuritis
- Foals: Weakness, failure to suckle, hypothermia, and congested mucous membranes. If overwhelming liver infection is present, the foal may be icteric. Often fatal in foals.

ETIOLOGY AND PATHOPHYSIOLOGY
- *A. equuli* subsp. *equuli*: Causative agent of highly fatal septicemia in foals.
- *A. equuli* subsp. *haemolyticus*: Associated with opportunistic infections causing various diseases.
- Both subspecies are associated with abortion and pericarditis of mares with MRLS.
- Common commensal of the equine oral, pharyngeal, and intestine mucous membranes.
- Invasion of body cavities.
- With MRLS, it is hypothesized that ingestion of the ETC results in mucosal absorption of the exoskeleton and setae of the caterpillar. This allows concomitant bacterial infection of the pericardium and placenta.
- Neonatal sepsis likely occurs through ascending vaginal infections before and after foaling through the umbilical structures and respiratory and alimentary tracts.

DIAGNOSIS

DIFFERENTIAL DIAGNOSIS
Other bacterial and viral infections that cause primary syndromes

INITIAL DATABASE
- Complete blood count: Leukopenia, hyperfibrinogenemia
- Serum biochemical analysis: Changes are a reflection of the organ system affected

ADVANCED OR CONFIRMATORY TESTING
- Aerobic culture and identification of body fluids or tissues from the affected site
- Blood culture of both adults and foals

TREATMENT

THERAPEUTIC GOAL(S)
- Antimicrobial treatment
- Supportive care depending on the body system affected

ACUTE GENERAL TREATMENT
- Broad-spectrum parenteral antibiotics pending culture and sensitivity
- Potassium penicillin G (22,000 IU/kg IV q6h) or procaine penicillin (22,000 IU/kg IM q12h) combined with appropriate aminoglycoside depending on the age of the horse. Many *A. equuli* isolates are susceptible to these antibiotics.
- Nonsteroidal antiinflammatory therapy: Flunixin meglumine (0.25–0.50 mg/kg IV q6–8h)
- Fluid and nutritional support as needed

CHRONIC TREATMENT
- As indicated by type of infection
- See "Pericarditis" in this section for treatment of pericardial effusion.

POSSIBLE COMPLICATIONS
A. equuli has several toxins in addition to the lipopolysaccharide components of the gram-negative cell wall that mediate signs of cardiovascular collapse, organ necrosis, and sudden death.

RECOMMENDED MONITORING
- Impending abortion of pasture mates, early foalings with weak foals

- Cardiovascular status
- Joints for bacterial infection in foals with sepsis

PROGNOSIS AND OUTCOME

- Prognosis and outcome in adults depend on the clinical syndrome.
  - Peritonitis is highly responsive if treated in the acute stage.
  - The prognosis for recovery from pericarditis and pleuritis is highly guarded.
- Prognosis for recovery of foals with *A. equuli* infection is guarded; the condition often is rapidly fatal.
- Prognosis for recovery of foals with localized infection such as joint sepsis is good to guarded.

PEARLS & CONSIDERATIONS

COMMENTS
Early recognition and treatment with penicillin combined with gram-negative antimicrobial therapy are essential.

PREVENTION
Preventative measures for MRLS are associated with control of ETC.

CLIENT EDUCATION
- Mare and foal care
- Farm hygiene
- Preventive measures for MRLS

SUGGESTED READING
Christensen H, Bisgaard M: Revised definition of *Actinobacillus sensu stricto* isolated from animals. A review with special emphasis on diagnosis. *Vet Microbiol* 99:13, 2004.

Donahue JM, Sells SF, Bolin DC: Classification of *Actinobacillus* spp isolates from horses involved in mare reproductive loss syndrome. *Am J Vet Res* 67:1426–1432, 2006.

AUTHOR: **MAUREEN T. LONG**

EDITORS: **DEBRA C. SELLON** and **MAUREEN T. LONG**

Adenovirus

BASIC INFORMATION

DEFINITION
A virus causing respiratory disease and occasionally diarrhea primarily in Arabian foals with severe combined immunodeficiency syndrome (SCID)

EPIDEMIOLOGY
SPECIES, AGE, SEX
- Primarily affects Arabian foals with SCID, infecting the respiratory tract, gastrointestinal (GI) tract, liver, pancreas, and bladder.
- SCID foals are generally clinically affected by adenovirus at 1 to 3 months of age.
- Immunosuppression may predispose other foals to susceptibility to adenovirus, and adenovirus may contribute to development of bacterial pneumonia.
- There is a possible role in respiratory disease in adult horses.
- Coinfection with equine herpesvirus-1 or -4 or equine rhinitis virus may result in clinical respiratory disease in normal foals.
- Concurrent infection with rotavirus is often observed in foals affected with diarrhea.
- About 70% of yearlings and 2-year-old horses are seropositive.
- This is not a zoonotic disease.

CLINICAL PRESENTATION
PHYSICAL EXAM FINDINGS
- Infection is usually subclinical in normal foals and adult horses.
- Affected foals demonstrate signs of acute respiratory infection, including nasal discharge, conjunctivitis, and eventually bronchopneumonia (Figure 1).
- Thoracic auscultation is likely abnormal.
- The horse may be febrile and depressed.
- Infection of the GI tract results in low-grade diarrhea unless concurrent rotavirus infection is present, which then leads to severe diarrhea.

ETIOLOGY AND PATHOPHYSIOLOGY
- Two isolates have been identified: EAdV1 (associated with respiratory disease) and EAdV2 (associated with diarrhea).
- Transmitted by close-contact aerosolization or physical interaction.
- The virus replicates in respiratory epithelial cells, resulting in sloughing of cells and a hyperplastic response.

DIAGNOSIS

DIFFERENTIAL DIAGNOSIS
- *Streptococcus equi* subsp. *zooepidemicus*
- *Pasteurella* spp.
- *Bordetella bronchiseptica*
- *Rhodococcus equi*
- *Actinobacillus equuli*
- *Klebsiella pneumoniae*
- Aberrant parasite migration
- Equine influenza
- Equine herpesvirus
- Equine viral arteritis

INITIAL DATABASE
- Diagnosis primarily focuses on diagnosing SCID (characteristic signalment coupled with diagnostic test results).
- Foals with SCID have severe lymphopenia.
- Thoracic radiographs are consistent with pneumonia.

ADVANCED OR CONFIRMATORY TESTING
Diagnosis of SCID:
- Definitive diagnosis by genetic testing
- Persistent lymphopenia (<1000/μL)
- After 4 weeks of age, serial radial immunodiffusion may be performed to evaluate for the presence of immunoglobulin M (IgM) in the bloodstream.
- Hypoplasia of lymphoid tissue at necropsy
- If diagnosed with adenovirus, a lack of antibody response, as indicated by convalescent adenoviral titers to adenovirus, indicates SCID.

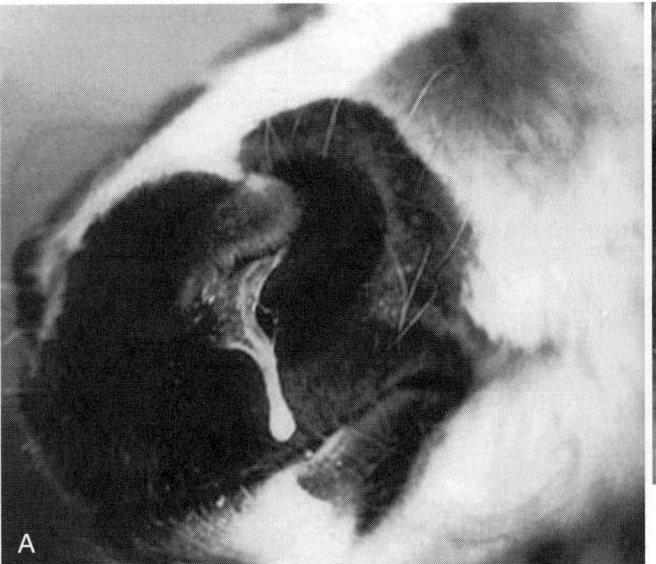
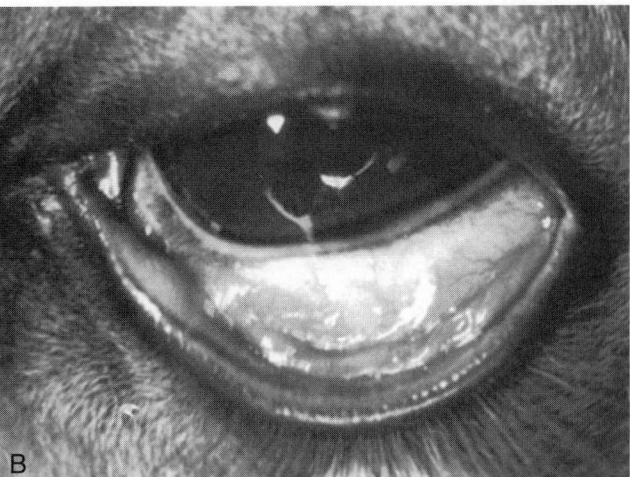

FIGURE 1 **A,** Nasal discharge in a 9-week-old specific-pathogen-free (SPF) foal 6 days after experimental intranasal/intraocular infection with EAdVI. **B,** Conjunctivitis in the same foal 6 days after infection. (From Sellon DC, Long MT: *Equine infectious diseases.* St Louis, Saunders Elsevier, 2007.)

Diagnosis of adenovirus:
- Detect adenovirus in feces by electron microscopy with negative staining.
- Viral isolation may be performed with variable results from nasopharyngeal, conjunctival, or rectal swabs.
- A possible polymerase chain reaction test is in development.
- Antibody response can be evaluated with hemagglutination inhibition assays, and the virus can be typed based on serum neutralization assays.
- Immune precipitation and complement fixation tests have also been used for diagnosis.
- Histopathology: may be evaluated antemortem in nasal or conjunctival tissue; intranuclear inclusions observed.

TREATMENT

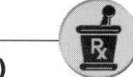

THERAPEUTIC GOAL(S)
Supportive treatment for non-SCID foals

ACUTE GENERAL TREATMENT
- No specific treatment is directed at the adenovirus itself.

- Foals with SCID will die despite any treatment.
- Foals without SCID should be placed on broad-spectrum antimicrobials because of the association with bacterial pneumonia.
- Foals without SCID with diarrhea may require supportive treatment consisting of IV fluids, plasma therapy, and possibly parenteral nutritional support.

POSSIBLE COMPLICATIONS
Foals without SCID may be predisposed by adenovirus infection to developing bacterial pneumonia.

PROGNOSIS AND OUTCOME

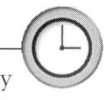

- Foals with SCID invariably die from their inability to respond to pathogens.
- Foals without SCID generally recover with appropriate treatment.

PEARLS & CONSIDERATIONS

PREVENTION
- Avoid breeding SCID foals. A genetic test is available to identify carriers of the SCID gene. One in four foals born to two carriers of the gene will be affected by SCID, and two of four will be genetic carriers.
- Ensure adequate passive transfer in foals without SCID.
- No vaccine is available.

SUGGESTED READING
Studdert MJ: Miscellaneous viral respiratory diseases. In Sellon DC, Long MT, editors: *Equine infectious diseases.* St Louis, 2006, Saunders Elsevier, pp 313–316.
Wilkins PA: Adenovirus. In Brown CM, Bertone JJ, editors: *The 5-minute veterinary consult equine.* Baltimore, 2009, Lippincott Williams & Wilkins, pp 56–57.

AUTHOR: **SIDDRA HINES**

EDITORS: **MAUREEN LONG** and **DEBRA SELLON**

Adhesions, Abdominal

BASIC INFORMATION

DEFINITION
Fibrous connection between intraabdominal organs or intraabdominal organs and the body wall

EPIDEMIOLOGY
SPECIES, AGE, SEX Foals are predisposed; however, adhesions are also seen in adult horses.
GENETICS AND BREED PREDISPOSITION Anecdotally, miniature horses are predisposed.
RISK FACTORS
- Foals
- Peritoneal inflammation
- Ischemic bowel
- Distended bowel
- Surgical manipulation
- Drying of the bowel during surgery
- Abrasion of the bowel during surgery
- Hemorrhage
- Peritonitis
- Presence of foreign material
- Bowel puncture

CLINICAL PRESENTATION
HISTORY, CHIEF COMPLAINT
- Horses with adhesions may be asymptomatic.

- Horses with adhesions may also present with inappetence, lethargy, and signs of colic.
- A high index of suspicion is necessary if the horse has a history of exploratory celiotomy.

PHYSICAL EXAM FINDINGS
- The heart rate is variable depending on the severity of the colic signs.
- The temperature is generally normal.
- Borborygmi are often reduced.
- The mucous membranes are generally pink and moist, but they may become tacky.
- Hydration is variable depending on the severity of colic.

ETIOLOGY AND PATHOPHYSIOLOGY
- Damage to the parietal or visceral peritoneum increases adhesion formation in two ways:
  - Increase in fibrin formation and deposition
  - Decrease in fibrinolytic activity
- Mechanism: disruption of the mesothelial cells leads to exposure of underlying connective tissue, blood vessels, collagen, lymphocytes, fibroblasts, mast cells, macrophages, and plasma cells.
  - Release of vasoactive substances (prostaglandin E2, serotonin, bradykinin, and histamine) from the

exposed submesothelial tissue leads to increased vascular permeability and extravasation of a fibrinogen-rich inflammatory exudate.
  - Release of thromboplastin (tissue factor) and exposure of subendothelial collagen activate the intrinsic and extrinsic clotting cascade, leading to thrombin-mediated conversion of fibrinogen to fibrin.
    - Normally, fibrin tags are lysed by plasmin in 2 to 5 days and the mesothelial layer repairs, but inadequate fibrinolysis allows fibroblasts to produce collagen by day 4, leading to fibrous adhesions.
    - Increased production of plasminogen activator inhibitor reduces the conversion of plasminogen to plasmin.

DIAGNOSIS

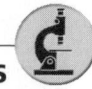

DIFFERENTIAL DIAGNOSIS
- Nonstrangulating small intestinal lesions:
  - Impaction at an anastomosis site
  - Postoperative ileus
  - Stricture formation
  - Ileal impaction

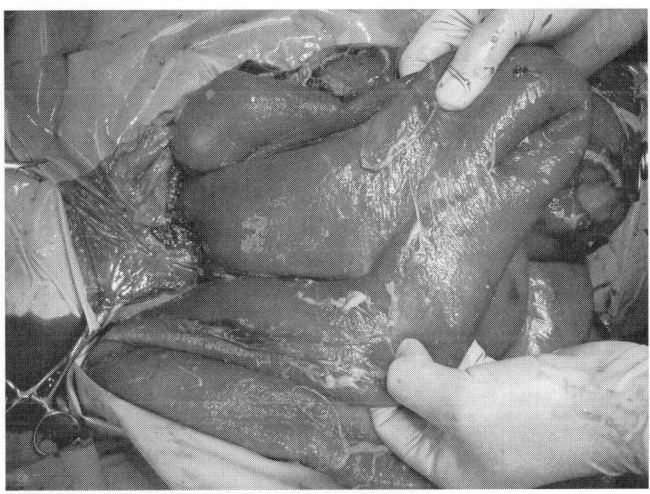

FIGURE 1 Fibrinous adhesions associated with septic peritonitis (appearance at exploratory laparotomy).

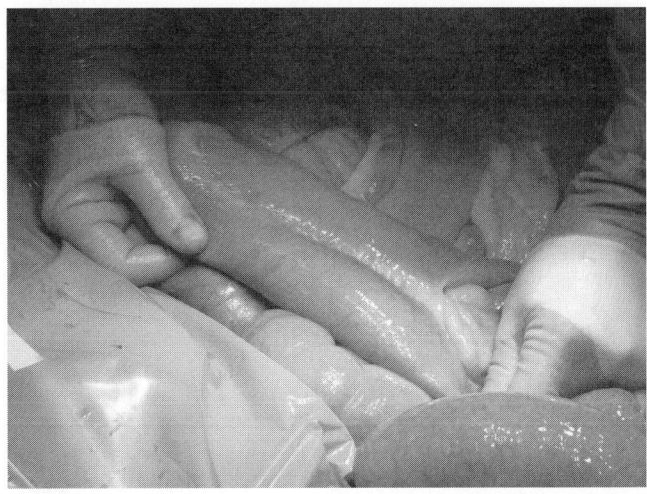

FIGURE 2 Mature fibrous adhesions, secondary to previous colic surgery, causing adherence and kinking of adjacent segments of jejunum (appearance at exploratory laparotomy; horse presented with recurrent colic).

- Very occasionally, adhesions cause strangulating lesions (ie, of the small intestine).

INITIAL DATABASE

- Complete blood count: Frequently normal
- Peritoneal fluid: frequently normal; occasionally, mild increases in total protein and nucleated cell counts; very rarely, serosanguineous
- Rectal palpation: adhesions are rarely palpable but their consequences are often felt (ie, distended small intestine)
- Reflux production: variable
- Transabdominal ultrasonography: occasionally reveals a fixed segment of intestine with adjacent hyperechoic material; however, most frequently just reveals the consequences of the adhesions (ie, small intestinal distension)

TREATMENT

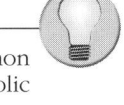

THERAPEUTIC GOAL(S)

- Stabilize the patient.
- Facilitate passage of food past the area obstructed by the adhesion.
  - Frequently attempted medically with a low-residue diet.
  - Repeat exploratory laparotomy or laparoscopy if the patient is nonresponsive to medical management.

ACUTE GENERAL TREATMENT

- Medical management
  - Withhold feed and administer IV balanced polyionic fluid therapy.
  - Administer flunixin meglumine (1.1 mg/kg).
  - Decompress the stomach every 3 hours.

- If unresponsive, surgical intervention may be necessary.
  - Repeat exploratory celiotomy to break down adhesions and aggressive prevention of recurrence.
    - Atraumatic tissue handling
    - 1% carboxymethylcellulose gel application during bowel manipulations
    - Use of a bioresorbable hyaluronic acid–carboxymethylcellose membrane
    - Heparin (40 IU/kg) intraperitoneally, IV, or SC
    - Perioperative antibiotics and anti-inflammatory drugs
    - Dimethyl sulfoxide (200 mg/kg) in a 10% solution IV
    - Peritoneal lavage
  - Laparoscopic adhesiolysis and aggressive prevention of recurrence

CHRONIC TREATMENT

- Medical management
  - Low-residue diet (ie, no hay)
    - Grass diet only
    - Pelleted complete food diet only

POSSIBLE COMPLICATIONS

- Repeat adhesion formation
- Incisional infection
- Ileus
- Peritonitis
- Endotoxemia
- Reobstruction
- Jugular thrombophlebitis
- Diarrhea
- Pyrexia
- Recurrent colic

RECOMMENDED MONITORING

- Abdominal pain
- Incisional swelling, pain, or discharge

- Mentation
- Fecal output

PROGNOSIS AND OUTCOME

- Adhesions have been implicated as a cause of postoperative pain or colic in 22% of horses undergoing small-intestine surgery.
- The long-term survival rate after repeat celiotomy is poor.

PEARLS & CONSIDERATIONS

- One of the most common complications after colic surgery
- Second most common reason for repeat exploratory celiotomy in horses with colic
- More common after small intestinal surgery

SUGGESTED READING

Fubini SL: Abdominal adhesions. In Mair TS, Divers T, Ducharme N, editors: *Manual of equine gastroenterology.* St Louis, 2002, Saunders, pp 209–211.

Haupt JL, McAndrews AG, Chaney KP, et al: Surgical treatment of colic in the miniature horse: a retrospective study of 57 cases (1993–2006). *Equine Vet J* 40:363–367, 2008.

Stick JA: Abdominal surgery. In Auer JA, Stick JA, editors: *Equine surgery.* St Louis, 2006, Saunders Elsevier, pp 506–507.

AUTHOR: CERI SHERLOCK

EDITORS: TIM MAIR and **CERI SHERLOCK**

Adrenal Insufficiency, Relative

BASIC INFORMATION

DEFINITION

Relative adrenal insufficiency (RAI) is a condition in which the adrenal gland, notably the adrenal cortex, is unable to respond (ie, secrete cortisol) to an appropriate level given the stimulus. RAI is often observed in patients with critical illness such as sepsis, in which adrenal hypofunction is considered part of the multiple organ dysfunction complex.

SYNONYM(S)

- Adrenal exhaustion
- Adrenal hypofunction

SPECIES, AGE, SEX

Premature foals have been shown to have hypofunctional hypothalamic-pituitary-adrenal axis (HPAA) responses, possibly due to underdevelopment; however, foals with sepsis or severe stress may have RAI, with a reported incidence of up to 52%.

RISK FACTORS

- Critical illness such as systemic inflammatory response syndrome (SIRS), sepsis, septic shock, endotoxemia, and trauma
- Long-term administration of anabolic steroids
- Prematurity

ASSOCIATED CONDITIONS AND DISORDERS

- SIRS
- Sepsis
- Septic shock
- Chronic stress responses
- Prematurity

CLINICAL PRESENTATION

HISTORY, CHIEF COMPLAINT Variable, based on the primary disease or disorder that causes RAI

PHYSICAL EXAM FINDINGS

- Referable to the primary illness: SIRS, sepsis, endotoxemia, or prematurity.
- Neurologic impairment, seizures, collapse, or other findings may be related to specific electrolyte abnormalities.

ETIOLOGY AND PATHOPHYSIOLOGY

- Prolonged or severe systemic illness leads to HPAA stimulation to yield increased cortisol concentrations.
- Diseases causing systemic inflammation and hypotension significantly increase HPAA responses.
- Excessive stimulation of the adrenal cortex (notably the zona fasciculata) results in an inability to secrete cortisol at an appropriate concentration for the stimulus (eg, adrenocorticotropin [ACTH])

- HPAA underdevelopment associated with neonatal prematurity may result in similar findings.
- In humans, subnormal cortisol responses have been associated with refractory hypotension and correlated with nonsurvival in certain patient populations (eg, septic shock).

DIAGNOSIS

DIFFERENTIAL DIAGNOSIS

Absolute adrenal insufficiency (true hypoadrenocorticism; Addison's disease), in which signs of mineralocorticoid deficiency exist, such as clinically relevant hyponatremia

INITIAL DATABASE

- Accurate diagnosis of the primary illness
  - Blood culture
  - Complete blood count
  - Serum chemistry
  - Fibrinogen concentration
  - Immunoglobulin G concentration in neonates
- Endogenous ACTH and cortisol concentrations
  - Highly variable values
  - An increased ACTH concentration with a concomitantly decreased or normal cortisol concentration may be suggestive of RAI
- Endogenous aldosterone concentration
  - Low concentrations are suggestive of mineralocorticoid deficiency, especially if concurrent with expected electrolyte derangements
- Hyponatremia, hyperkalemia, hypochloremia, and a sodium/potassium ratio <27 may be suggestive of mineralocorticoid deficiency
  - This is very unspecific because conditions such as uroperitoneum often have similar changes in electrolyte profiles

ADVANCED OR CONFIRMATORY TESTING

- ACTH stimulation test: Test of adrenocortical function
  - Administer exogenous ACTH (cosyntropin) and measure serial cortisol concentrations
  - In foals: 10 to 100 µg/51 kg body weight IV at time 0.
    - Serum cortisol measurements should be obtained at baseline and 30 minutes after injection.

- A minimum twofold increase in cortisol concentration is expected.
- Subnormal responses are diagnostic for RAI.
- Reportedly, there is no difference in the 30-minute cortisol concentration response in normal foals with a 10 or 100 µg/51 kg dosing regimen.
  - Cosyntropin may also be dosed based on weight: 0.2 to 2 µg/kg IV.

TREATMENT

THERAPEUTIC GOAL(S)

- Limited information exists regarding the treatment of RAI in sick horses.
- Treating the primary disease is integral to a successful outcome (eg, in neonatal sepsis).
- Corticosteroid replacement is controversial due to lack of controlled studies.

ACUTE GENERAL TREATMENT

- Glucocorticoid treatment:
  - Prednisolone 0.5 to 1.0 mg/kg, q12–24h IV/PO, then lowered to every other day based on follow-up laboratory data (electrolyte concentrations).
  - If the RAI is reversible, gradual reduction in steroid administration is recommended over a period of weeks.
  - Follow-up ACTH stimulation testing should be performed at the end of therapy to assess adrenocortical function.
- Mineralocorticoid treatment:
  - Fludrocortisone administration may be beneficial.
  - Fludrocortisone effects have not been assessed extensively in horses.
  - Suggested dose rate based on case reports in horses and for the treatment of canine hypoadrenocortical crisis is 15 to 25 µg/kg/day as needed.
- Treatment indicated in life-threatening hyperkalemia
  - Calcium gluconate IV
  - IV sodium chloride (0.9% solution)
  - IV dextrose (2.5% to 5% solution)
  - Insulin
  - IV sodium bicarbonate
- Treatment of hyponatremia:
  - Hypertonic saline solutions (0.9%, 3%, 7.2%)
    - Aim to increase the serum sodium concentration by up to 15 mEq/L/day (0.5 mEq/L/h maximum)

- Excessively fast sodium replacement has been reported to cause demyelinating central nervous system disorders in hyponatremic humans (central pontine myelinolysis)

CHRONIC TREATMENT

Ensure adequate sodium in the diet

RECOMMENDED MONITORING

- Serum electrolyte concentrations (sodium, potassium, chloride) should be monitored frequently (q6–12h), especially if the patient has received corticosteroids.
- ACTH stimulation testing should be reassessed at the end of corticosteroid therapy to confirm adequate adrenocortical function.
  - At least 12 to 24 hours after the last administration of prednisolone because it may interfere with test accuracy

PROGNOSIS AND OUTCOME

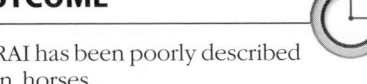

- RAI has been poorly described in horses.
- Based on preliminary work, foals with severe septicemia are more likely to have HPAA dysregulation, including RAI.
  - These foals are also more likely to die.
- RAI has been correlated to nonsurvival in critically ill humans, notably patients who do not respond to exogenous corticosteroid therapy.
- The prognosis in horses must be in part based on the primary illness (eg, sepsis or prematurity).

PEARLS & CONSIDERATIONS

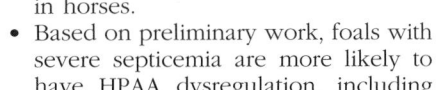

- RAI is not well described in the equine literature.
- For the moment, treatment is largely empirical until further studies provide

treatment guidelines for this condition in horses.
- RAI should be considered in critically ill horses with persistent catecholamine-resistant hypotension or unexplainable electrolyte derangements.

SUGGESTED READING

Couetil LL, Hoffman AM: Adrenal insufficiency in a neonatal foal. *J Am Vet Med Assoc* 212:1594, 1998.

Hart KA, Ferguson DC, Heusner GL, et al: Synthetic adrenocorticotropic hormone stimulation test in healthy neonatal foals. *J Vet Intern Med* 21:314–321, 2007.

Hurcombe SDA, Toribio RE, Slovis N, et al: Blood arginine vasopressin, adrenocorticotropin hormone, and cortisol concentrations at admission in septic and critically ill foals and their association with survival. *J Vet Intern Med* 22:639–647, 2008.

Hart KA, Slovis NM, Barton MH, et al: Hypothalamic-pituitary-adrenal axis dysfunction in hospitalized neonatal foals. *J Vet Intern Med* 23:901–912, 2009.

AUTHOR: **SAMUEL D.A. HURCOMBE**

EDITORS: **R. REID HANSON** and **AMELIA MUNSTERMAN**

Aflatoxin Toxicosis

BASIC INFORMATION

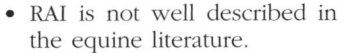

DEFINITION

Aflatoxins are hepatotoxic mycotoxins (mold toxins) produced by various *Aspergillus* spp. and other fungi, most commonly *A. flavus* and *A. parasiticus*. Aflatoxin can contaminate a wide variety of nutritious feedstuffs, including but not limited to corn, peanuts, sorghum, wheat, rice, cottonseed, sweet potatoes, and potatoes. The four major forms of aflatoxin in feedstuffs are aflatoxin B1, B2, G1, and G2. Aflatoxicosis has been reported in numerous species, including humans, dogs, cattle, swine, poultry, and fish, but there have been relatively few cases reported in horses.

SYNONYM(S)

Synonyms for aflatoxin poisoning are aflatoxicosis, hepatitis X (dogs), and X disease (turkeys).

EPIDEMIOLOGY

SPECIES, AGE, SEX Neonates may be more sensitive.
RISK FACTORS A protein-deficient diet may enhance the hepatotoxic effects of aflatoxins. Dietary vitamin A, carotene, selenium, and antioxidants decrease the effects.

GEOGRAPHY AND SEASONALITY Preharvest contamination occurs in tropical and temperate climates. Contamination of stored grain occurs worldwide.

CLINICAL PRESENTATION

DISEASE FORMS/SUBTYPES
- Chronic aflatoxin poisoning is the most common form in large animals.
- Acute aflatoxicosis may occur if high concentrations of aflatoxins are present in the feed.

HISTORY, CHIEF COMPLAINT
- Affected horses usually have a history of grain in the diet, most commonly corn.
- Clinical signs of chronic aflatoxicosis may be subtle at first, including decreased weight gain or weight loss and poor haircoat. Signs may progress to anorexia, depression, icterus, and hepatic encephalopathy.
- Acute clinical aflatoxicosis is associated with anorexia, depression, diarrhea, gastrointestinal hemorrhage, and icterus.

PHYSICAL EXAM FINDINGS
- Chronic
  - General unthriftiness
  - Icterus
- Acute
  - Coagulopathy
  - Icterus

ETIOLOGY AND PATHOPHYSIOLOGY
Aflatoxin is metabolized in the liver to an active compound that binds with cellular components such as nucleic acids, proteins, and subcellular organelles, disrupting cellular function.

DIAGNOSIS

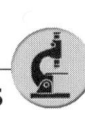

DIFFERENTIAL DIAGNOSIS

- Other hepatotoxins cause similar clinical signs and lesions
  - Pyrrolizidine alkaloids
  - Carboxyatractyloside from *Xanthium* spp. (cockleburs)
  - *Lantana* spp.
  - Cyanobacterial toxins (microcystin)
  - Mushroom toxins (amanitin)
  - Phenolics and coal tar derivatives
  - Iron overdose
- Other causes
  - Theiler's disease
  - Inflammatory hepatitis

INITIAL DATABASE

Serum chemistry:
- Elevated gamma-glutamyl transpeptidase early with low doses
- Elevated alanine transaminase with higher doses
- Increased serum bilirubin

- Activated prothrombin time may be increased

ADVANCED OR CONFIRMATORY TESTING

- Analysis for aflatoxin
  - Feed analysis
- Black-light analysis is used to check for the presence of *Aspergillus* spp. The absence of fluorescence does not guarantee that aflatoxin is absent nor does the presence of fluorescence guarantee the presence of aflatoxin.
- Commercially available bench-top enzyme-linked immunosorbent assays (ELISAs) for aflatoxin.
- Gas chromatography/mass spectrometry (GC/MS) and liquid chromatography/mass spectrometry (LC/MS) are the definitive quantitative analysis for aflatoxin in tissues.
- GC/MS or LC/MS is used to detect aflatoxin in blood, liver, or milk.
- False-negative results are common.
- Pathology:
  - Hepatocellular degeneration and necrosis, megalocytosis, and hepatic fibrosis and bile duct proliferation have been reported on histology.
  - Hemorrhagic enteritis has been reported.
  - Cerebral edema has been reported.

TREATMENT

THERAPEUTIC GOAL(S)

- Early detoxification
- Symptomatic and supportive care
- Hepatoprotectants and supplement glutathione scavenging

ACUTE TREATMENT

- Early detoxification for large ingestions of feed highly contaminated by aflatoxin
  - Activated charcoal
- Symptomatic and supportive
  - Maintain blood volume and electrolyte balance

- Vitamin K1 for coagulopathy
- Gastroprotection
- Hepatoprotectants and supplement glutathione scavenging
  - *N*-acetylcysteine
  - *S*-adenosyl-L-methionine
  - Milk thistle

CHRONIC TREATMENT

Maintain the patient on a high-quality diet.

POSSIBLE COMPLICATIONS

Long-term liver damage may occur.

RECOMMENDED MONITORING

- Liver enzymes
- Bilirubin
- Activated prothrombin time

PROGNOSIS AND OUTCOME

The prognosis depends on the concentration of aflatoxin in the feed and the duration of exposure. Severe liver damage and death are possible outcomes.

PEARLS & CONSIDERATIONS

COMMENTS

- Toxic dose of aflatoxin:
  - Aflatoxin was lethal to ponies dosed with 2 mg/kg once.
  - Approximately 3.8 ppm in the diet was lethal to some ponies after 37 to 39 days.
  - Clinical signs have been reported with dietary aflatoxin concentrations of 500 ppb (0.50 ppm).
- Although the United States Food and Drug Administration (FDA), which regulates mycotoxins in foods and feeds, does not give a specific limit for the concentration of aflatoxin that may be present in horse feed, the limit is 20 ppb (0.02 ppm) for human and

animal feeds that are not covered by other FDA recommendations.

PREVENTION

- Keep horses on a high-quality nutritionally balanced diet.
- Avoid feeding poor-quality or visibly moldy feeds.
- Screen feeds for aflatoxins.

CLIENT EDUCATION

- Horses with clinical aflatoxicosis typically have a guarded to poor prognosis depending on the concentration of aflatoxin in the feed and the amount ingested over time.
- It is often difficult to diagnose aflatoxicosis based on aflatoxin concentrations in the feed because:
  - Aflatoxin is not evenly distributed within the feed, and sampling error may occur.
  - The contaminated feed may be completely consumed before the clinical signs are apparent.
- It is difficult to diagnose aflatoxicosis from biologic (non-feed) samples because of the extremely low concentrations that remain in tissues. False-negative test results are common.
- It is best to prevent aflatoxicosis.

SUGGESTED READING

Committee on Nutrient Requirements of Horses, National Research Council: *Nutrient requirements of the horse*, 6th rev ed. Washington, DC, National Academies Press, 2007, p 62.

Food and Drug Administration: *Action levels for poisonous or deleterious substances in human food and animal feed*. Available at http://www.cfsan.fda.gov/~lrd/fdaact.html#afla.

Meerdink GL: Aflatoxins. In Plumlee KH, editor: *Clinical veterinary toxicology*. St Louis, 2003, Mosby Elsevier, pp 231–365.

Osweiler GD: Mycotoxins, *Vet Clin North Am Eq Pract* 17:547–566, 2001.

AUTHOR: KARYN BISCHOFF

EDITOR: CYNTHIA L. GASKILL

African Horse Sickness

BASIC INFORMATION

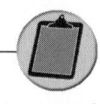

DEFINITION

- African horse sickness (AHS) is caused by a double-stranded, nonenveloped RNA virus that affects members of the family Equidae and is transmitted by midges (*Culicoides* spp.). Horses and mules are the most severely affected.

- There are nine distinct serotypes, with types 5 and 9 most commonly occurring outside of the endemic sub-Saharan Africa. Four major forms of the disease exist: peracute or pulmonary (95% mortality rate), subacute or cardiac (50% mortality rate), mixed (70% mortality rate), and horse sickness fever (recovery). The onset of disease in the severe forms is characterized by a high fever followed by respiratory failure with a frothy to serosanguineous nasal discharge or nondependent edema of the head and neck with petechiations of the conjunctiva. There is no effective treatment.

- A polyvalent vaccine exists that provides protection for all serotypes. Quarantine, constant monitoring, and vector control are necessary. This disease has not been documented in North America and is a World Organisation for Animal Health (OIE)–reportable disease.

EPIDEMIOLOGY

SPECIES, AGE, SEX

- Horses are most susceptible to infection, with a mortality rate of 70% to 95% depending on the form of the disease.
- Mules are slightly less susceptible, with a mortality rate of 50% to 70%.
- Donkeys and zebras develop subclinical disease.
- There does not appear to be an age predilection. Foals born to immune mares may receive passive immunity that disappears at age 4 to 6 months.
- There is no sex predilection.

GENETICS AND BREED PREDISPOSITION Horses indigenous to certain areas of North and West Africa appear to have acquired resistance to infection with AHS. There is no breed disposition.

CONTAGION AND ZOONOSIS The only known incident of humans contracting AHS occurred in a laboratory setting. AHS is not considered a zoonotic disease in the natural setting; however, veterinarians dealing with suspected cases of AHS should still follow universal precautions.

GEOGRAPHY AND SEASONALITY

- AHS is considered to be enzoonotic in eastern and central Africa, with yearly incursions of the disease into southern Africa. Documented and confirmed epidemics have occurred in North Africa, the Middle East, Turkey, Afghanistan, Pakistan, India, Spain, and Portugal. To date, the virus has never been documented in North America.
- Transmission
  - AHS is biologically transmitted by midges of the *Culicoides* genera. *Culicoides imicola* and *Culicoides bolitinos* appear to be the most important vectors in Africa. Other vectors, including ticks and mosquitoes, have been shown to transmit AHS under experimental conditions; however, they have never been shown to transmit the virus under natural conditions. Mechanical transmission of the virus may occur through biting flies and iatrogenic incidents. In the United States, *Culicoides sonorensis* and *Culicoides variipennis* (which are responsible for blue-tongue virus transmission) have been shown to transmit AHS under experimental conditions.
  - Transmission of AHS corresponds with peak vector activity. In Africa, this depends on climatic conditions, in which heavy rains followed by warm, dry periods favor the survival

of *Culicoides* individuals. Cold weather and frosts kill *Culicoides* spp. and thus decrease or stop AHS transmission. This effect of climate on AHS transmission is especially evident in AHS epidemics, when the virus makes incursions into South Africa. The wet, warm months of February, March, and April have the highest case rates of AHS, with cases of AHS disappearing after the first frosts in April or May. Epidemics also occur when individuals having a high viral load are transported to countries with *Culicoides* vectors capable of transmitting the virus. Epidemics have also been reported with the windborne spread of infected vectors.

- Maintenance of AHS in the environment.
  - The exact mechanism of the maintenance of AHS in the environment is uncertain. The short incubation period accompanied by the high mortality rate in horses and mules make it unlikely that these animals can serve as effective reservoirs for maintaining the virus.
  - Continuous transmission between zebras and *Culicoides* midges was demonstrated in South Africa in Kruger National Park. Thus large populations of zebras and donkeys are likely to be one of the major reservoirs of AHS.
  - Dogs have been shown to be susceptible to AHS when fed raw horse meat infected with AHS. Other populations of animals have yet to be investigated for their possible role in the maintenance of AHS.

CLINICAL PRESENTATION

DISEASE FORMS/SUBTYPES

- Pulmonary ("dunkop"): Peracute form
- Cardiac ("dikkop"): Subacute form
- Mixed: Most common form
- Horse sickness fever: Mildest form

HISTORY, CHIEF COMPLAINT Horses may present with a variety of clinical signs depending on the form of disease. These include a fever of 102° to 106° F, depression, supraorbital edema, and respiratory distress.

PHYSICAL EXAM FINDINGS

- Pulmonary/dunkop form: The peracute form of AHS appears in naive animals and is the most severe form of AHS, with a 95% mortality rate. The incubation period is 3 to 4 days. There is a sudden onset of a high fever (104°–106° F) with tachypnea (>50 beats/min) and dyspnea marked by expiratory distress and a heave line. Profuse sweating, coughing, and recumbency usually follow with a frothy to serosanguineous nasal discharge. The onset of dyspnea is

usually followed by death within a few hours. The clinical course of this form of the disease lasts only a few days.

- Cardiac/dikkop form: The subacute form of AHS has a 50% mortality rate with an incubation period of 5 to 7 days. A fever (102°–106° F) that persists for 3 to 4 days first appears. After the fever begins to subside, supraorbital edema appears and is quickly followed by nondependent edema of the head and neck. Dyspnea and cyanosis may occur as a result of the edema. Signs of colic may be present. Petechiations (conjunctiva and ventral tongue) are a poor sign, and death usually follows. The clinical course of this form of the disease lasts 3 to 8 days.
- Mixed form: This is the most common form of AHS and has a 70% average mortality rate. A fever (102°–106° F) develops that persists for 1 to 4 days. Two courses of the disease may then develop. In the first, mild pulmonary signs are followed by edema and cardiac failure. In the second, edema and subclinical cardiac disease are followed by the sudden onset of dyspnea, nasal discharge, and death. The clinical course of this form of the disease lasts 3 to 6 days.
- Horse sickness fever: This is the mildest form of AHS and the form that usually appears in zebras and donkeys, with an incubation period of 5 to 9 days. There is a gradual increase in temperature to 104° F over 4 days and then a return to normal. Mild clinical signs of the cardiac and pulmonary forms may occur.

ETIOLOGY AND PATHOPHYSIOLOGY

- AHS is a double-stranded, nonenveloped RNA virus in the genus *Orbivirus*, family Reoviridae.
- Closely related to blue-tongue virus and equine encephalosis virus.
- Has seven structural (VP1-7) and three nonstructural (NS1-3) proteins.
  - VP2 is responsible for antigenic variation.
  - VP7 and NS3 are important in vaccination.
- Nine serotypes have been identified.
  - Most types are restricted to sub-Saharan Africa.
  - Types 4 and 9 are responsible for most outbreaks outside sub-Saharan Africa.
  - Types 5 and 9 are neurotropic.
  - Cross-protection occurs between serotypes.
- Initial infection occurs through the bite of an infected *Culicoides*.
  - Replication occurs in the local lymph nodes.
  - A primary viremia occurs, leading to the dissemination of the virus to

target organs (lungs, spleen, lymphoid tissue, cecum, pharynx, choroid plexus).
- Replication of AHS then occurs in the endothelial cells of the target organs, leading to edema and effusions.
- A secondary viremia then occurs with fever and clinical signs.
- Horses have an average viremia of 4 to 8 days (≤21 days) with a $TCID_{50}$ of 10^5 PFU/mL.
- Zebras have an average viremia of 21 days (≤40 days) with a $TCID_{50}$ of 10^3 PFU/mL.
- Gross pathologic changes include:
  - Heavy, noncollapsible lungs
  - Yellow, gelatinous edema of the subcutaneous and intramuscular tissue
- Especially the nuchal ligament: Edema
- Lungs, supraorbital fossae, head, neck, thorax
  - Hydrothorax
  - Hydropericardium
  - Diffuse hemorrhage and petechiation
  - Lymphadenomegaly

DIAGNOSIS

DIFFERENTIAL DIAGNOSIS

- Equine encephalosis: Foreign animal disease not yet documented in North America
- Equine infectious anemia (EIA)
- *Streptococcus equi* subsp. *equi*: Strangles, bastard strangles, purpura hemorrhagica
- Piroplasmosis
- Equine viral arteritis
- Influenza
- Equine herpesviruses (EHV-1 and EHV-4)
- Bacterial pneumonia
- Pleuropneumonia
- Interstitial pneumonia
- Infectious heart disease: endocarditis, myocarditis, pericarditis
- Congestive heart failure

INITIAL DATABASE

- Complete blood count
  - Leukopenia
  - Thrombocytopenia
  - Increased packed cell volume
- Clotting tests
  - Increased fibrin degradation products
  - Prolonged prothrombin
  - Prolonged activated partial thromboplastin
  - Prolonged thrombin

ADVANCED OR CONFIRMATORY TESTING

- Viral isolation:
  - Cell culture
  - Intracerebral inoculation of suckling mice
- Serotyping of virus:
  - Virus neutralization
  - Complement fixation
  - Agar gel immunodiffusion
  - Indirect fluorescence antibody
  - Enzyme-linked immunosorbent assay (ELISA)
  - Polymerase chain reaction (RT-PCR)
- Antibody testing: ELISA
- Antigen testing:
  - ELISA
  - RT-PCR

TREATMENT

THERAPEUTIC GOAL(S)

Supportive care

ACUTE GENERAL TREATMENT

- Treatment should be aimed at making the horse comfortable with appropriate supportive care.
- It is extremely important that all affected equids are rested because exertion can lead to death. This rest should continue for at least 1 month after the cessation of clinical signs.

PROGNOSIS AND OUTCOME

- The prognosis for recovery from infection from AHS depends on the form that the equine contracts. In general, donkeys, horses, and mules from endemic areas have a much better prognosis for survival. Naive horses and mules have a moderate to poor prognosis depending on the form of AHS contracted.
- For the pulmonary or peracute form, there is a 5% chance of survival; for the cardiac or subacute form, there is a 50% chance of survival; and for the mixed form, there is a 30% chance of survival.

PEARLS & CONSIDERATIONS

COMMENTS

AHS is an OIE-reportable disease. Any suspect case in North America should be immediately reported to the United States Department of Agriculture (USDA).

PREVENTION

- Vaccination
  - Annually in endemic areas
  - Onderstepoort Laboratories (attenuated) in two components that should be administered 3 weeks apart
    - Trivalent: Serotypes 1, 3, and 4
    - Quadrivalent: Serotypes 2, 6, 7, and 8 (cross-protection for serotypes 5 and 9)
- Vector control
  - Stable 1 hour before dusk to 1 hour after dawn
  - Move only during daylight
  - Cover with day sheets
  - Apply insect repellant daily
  - Take rectal temperatures twice a day
  - Stable in insect-free stalls
- Decontamination:
  - Effective disinfectants: Virkon, acetic acid, bleach, formalin, β-propiolactone, acetyl-ethyleneimine derivatives
  - Susceptible to radiation
- Quarantine and import regulations by the USDA: All equids from AHSV endemic countries must have:
  - Resided in the country of interest for 60+ days
  - During this time found to be free of disease
  - Not been vaccinated in the 14 days before export
  - Not been on premises where AHSV has occurred in the 60 days preceding export
- Upon shipment to the United States, equines from countries with endemic AHSV must be quarantined for 60 days and watched for signs of illness.

SUGGESTED READING

Guthrie A: African horse sickness. In Sellon D, Long M, editors: *Equine infectious diseases*. St Louis, 2007, Saunders Elsevier, pp 164–171.

Mellor P, Hamblin C: African horse sickness. *Vet Res* 35(4):445–466, 2004.

World Organisation for Animal Health: *African horse sickness*. Available at http://www.oie.int/eng/maladies/fiches/a_A110.htm.

AUTHOR: MELISSA BOURGEOIS

EDITORS: DEBRA C. SELLON and **MAUREEN T. LONG**

Aggressive Stallion Behavior

BASIC INFORMATION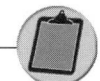

DEFINITION

- Aggressive behavior is defined as the overt display of dangerous reactions that may endanger people or other animals.
- Aggressive behavior by the stallion toward itself is possible and is discussed under self-mutilation.

SYNONYM(S)

Unruly stallions, rowdy stallions

EPIDEMIOLOGY

RISK FACTORS

- Poor training or handling
- Housing conditions (proximity to other breeding stallions)
- Lack of exercise
- Conditions associated with high testosterone
- Proximity to other stallions or estrous mares

GEOGRAPHY AND SEASONALITY Aggressive behavior may be exacerbated during the breeding season.

ASSOCIATED CONDITIONS AND DISORDERS Cryptorchidism, interstitial cell tumors (increased testosterone secretion)

CLINICAL PRESENTATION

HISTORY, CHIEF COMPLAINT

- History of recent introduction to the breeding shed
- History of abusive treatment
- Most common complaints:
  - Biting, kicking, or striking at the handler or mare
  - Rushing or charging the mare or dummy

ETIOLOGY AND PATHOPHYSIOLOGY

- The cause is often multifactorial.
- The pathophysiology is often considered to involve either a high level of testosterone or a complex chain of behavioral responses to specific conditions.
- Most of these cases are exacerbated by inadequate training.

DIAGNOSIS

DIFFERENTIAL DIAGNOSIS

- Progressively worsening or sudden development of aggressive behavior in stallions may reflect a painful condition associated with the genital tract such as abdominal or inguinal testicles, painful erection, or pelvic or back pain during breeding.

INITIAL DATABASE

- Detailed examination of the genital system.
- Measurement of serum testosterone levels may be helpful.

TREATMENT

THERAPEUTIC GOAL(S)

- Reduce the behavior through stallion and handler training.
- Reduce the urge to rush.
- Reduce the testosterone level.

ACUTE GENERAL TREATMENT

- Adequate training of the handler and stallion
  - Avoid explosive punishment if the stallion displays overt reactions, kicks, or rears.
  - Use calm estrous mares during training.
  - Work in several short sessions with the stallion.
  - Use appropriate negative reinforcement (verbal reprimands, shank chain pressure, occasional slaps on the shoulders).
  - Use positive reinforcement.
  - Keep terms, cues, and the environment consistent.
- Reduce the desire to rush.
  - Provide exercise.
  - Allow several breedings in rapid succession.
- Medical treatment is aimed at reducing testosterone or the libido and may be useful in nonbreeding stallions.
  - Immunization against gonadotropin-releasing hormone: Equity (Pfizer Animal Health; not available in the United States)
  - Progestogen: Altrenogest (0.088 mg/kg PO q24h)

POSSIBLE COMPLICATIONS

Stallions may become extremely dangerous if the situation is not handled properly.

RECOMMENDED MONITORING

Avoid changes in handlers and breeding routine.

PROGNOSIS AND OUTCOME

Very good in the majority of stallions

PEARLS & CONSIDERATIONS

COMMENTS

- Most of these problems are created by handlers.
- Knowledge of normal behavior of stallions in free mating as well as in-hand mating situations is paramount in understanding sexual behavioral alterations.
- Judicious use of disciplinary action is very important, particularly in stallions that are used for breeding and are still performing.

PREVENTION

Proper handling and socialization at a young age

CLIENT EDUCATION

- Stallion handling is a skill that requires a thorough understanding of stallion behavior and proper use of discipline.
- Avoid rough or excessive discipline of stallions during performance.
- Use judicious behavioral modification techniques to train stallions.

SUGGESTED READING

McDonnell SM: Stallion sexual behavior. In Samper JC, editor: *Equine breeding management and artificial insemination.* St Louis, 2009, Saunders Elsevier, pp 41–46.

McDonnell SM, Diehl NK, Oristaglio Turner RM, et al: Modification of unruly breeding behavior in stallions. *Compend Contin Ed Pract Vet* 17:411, 1994.

Stout TAE: Modulating reproductive activity in stallions: a review. *Anim Reprod Sci* 89:93, 2005.

Tibary A: Stallion reproductive behavior. In Samper JC, Pycock, JF, McKinnon AO, editors: *Current therapy in equine reproduction.* St Louis, 2007, Saunders Elsevier, pp 174–184.

AUTHORS: **LISA K. PEARSON, JACOBO S. RODRIGUEZ,** and **AHMED TIBARY**

EDITOR: **JUAN C. SAMPER**

Airway Obstruction, Recurrent

BASIC INFORMATION

DEFINITION

- A respiratory disease more frequently seen in middle-aged to older adult horses that is characterized clinically by recurrent episodes of airway obstruction when horses are exposed to organic dust or other particulate matter.
- Horses exhibit severe coughing and exaggerated respiratory effort that is more evident on expiration than inspiration. These attacks are initiated by an influx of neutrophils into the airways and by bronchoconstriction associated with excessive mucus and airway smooth muscle. At least in the initial stages, attacks of airway obstruction can be reversed by environmental remediation.

SYNONYMS

Chronic obstructive pulmonary disease (COPD), heaves, chronic bronchiolitis, bronchitis

EPIDEMIOLOGY

Middle-aged to older Equids
GENETICS AND BREED PREDISPOSITION There is evidence for a familial basis in Lipizaners and Warmbloods for recurrent airway obstruction (RAO), although the precise mode of inheritance is unknown.
RISK FACTORS Living in barns, exposure to organic dusts or moldy hay
GEOGRAPHY AND SEASONALITY
- Typically affects animals that have spent most of their lives in barns eating hay and housed in dusty environments.
- It is also seen in summer months when pastures are very dry or when there is excessive mold bloom in the pastures.

ASSOCIATED CONDITIONS AND DISORDERS Horses with RAO are predisposed to pulmonary hypertension.

CLINICAL PRESENTATION

HISTORY, CHIEF COMPLAINT
- Typically presents initially with a seasonal cough that worsens over a period of years.
- As the disease progresses, the cough is accompanied by tachypnea and evident respiratory distress.
- During an exacerbation of more severe disease, the horse will have flared nostrils and evident abdominal press seen more in expiration but also evident on inspiration.

- Hypertrophy of the expiratory muscles may result in a "heaves line."
- A marked nasal discharge is usually seen, ranging from serous to mucopurulent.
- Horses in advance stages of disease may be cachectic because their work of breathing exceeds their ability to eat.
- There is no history of fever.

PHYSICAL EXAM FINDINGS
- Physical examination findings usually are concordant with the above history. A moderate tachycardia may also be auscultated.
- Thoracic auscultation may reveal either loud bronchovesicular sounds or widely dispersed crackles and wheezes.
- In very severe cases, the lungs may be strangely silent because of the very small amount of airflow that the animal is able to achieve. In these cases, auscultation of the trachea is compatible with the presence of mucus.
- Lung fields are often enlarged because of air trapping, so percussion will reveal larger than normal lung fields.

ETIOLOGY AND PATHOPHYSIOLOGY

- RAO is akin to environmentally induced asthma in humans in that it is caused by chronic exposure to organic and inorganic dusts.
- Organic dusts are replete with endotoxin, β-glucans from mold, and various allergens. This exposure results in an outpouring of neutrophils into the horse's airways.
  - With acute exposure, there is endoscopically visible edema in the airways.
  - With chronic exposure, there is increased mucus production and poorer mucus clearance as well as airway wall remodeling, with smooth muscle hyperplasia and hypertrophy, peribronchial inflammation, and fibrosis. The combination of airway wall remodeling and increased responsiveness of the airway smooth muscle to various stimuli results in bronchoconstriction. It is unclear to what extent an allergic response is involved.
- Cytokine profiles in horses with RAO are not consistent, with some associated with a Th1 and others with a Th2 (allergic) response. The most likely explanation is that this is a very complex disease that develops differently in horses with differing genetic backgrounds and levels of exposure to particulates.

DIAGNOSIS

DIFFERENTIAL DIAGNOSIS

- Septic bronchitis
- Pneumonia
- Chronic interstitial diseases
- Toxicoses, including inhaled toxins (silicosis, various gases) as well as systemically ingested substances such as perilla mint
- Neoplastic disease, including primary tumors of the respiratory tract or, more commonly, distant metastases

INITIAL DATABASE

- Complete blood count and serum chemistry profile usually demonstrate no abnormalities.
- Arterial blood gas analysis reveals hypoxemia during exacerbation. Depending on the severity of the disease, $PaCO_2$ may be normal or elevated. The abnormalities in blood gas will be commensurate with the severity of the disease.
- Airway sampling is best done by bronchoalveolar lavage. Normal horses have no more than 10% neutrophils in the bronchoalveolar (BAL) fluid, and the ratio of alveolar macrophages to lymphocytes is approximately 60:40.
  - Neutrophils commonly comprise 50% to 100% of the BAL fluid cytology. The neutrophils are generally nondegenerate, and there is no evidence of bacterial infection.
  - Mucus is often prominent and fibrillar. Large amounts of neutrophils are commonly trapped within the mucus.
  - Although a transtracheal aspirate may also be performed to evaluate the airways, it does not reliably reflect the lower airways.
- Lung function testing reveals increased pleural pressures, reflecting the elevated work of breathing, as well as increased pulmonary and respiratory resistance and dynamic compliance. Lung function testing is not necessary for making a diagnosis in an exacerbation of RAO.
  - Noninvasive methods of lung function testing, such as open plethysmography or forced oscillatory maneuvers, can be very useful in determining whether the horse has a normal response to bronchodilators.
  - In horses in remission, lung function testing is used in conjunction with histamine bronchoprovocation to probe the status of the small

airways. In this procedure, small amounts of histamine are given while lung function is measured. Horses in remission are difficult to distinguish from normal horses on the basis of resting tests; however, horses in remission respond to much lower doses of histamine with a rapid increase in respiratory resistance.

ADVANCED OR CONFIRMATORY TESTING

- Radiography can be very helpful in determining whether disease is complicated (eg, whether there is coexisting bronchiolitis or pneumothorax caused by a ruptured bulla).
- Lung biopsy or bronchial biopsy reveals typical changes such as goblet cell and airway smooth muscle hyperplasia, as well as peribronchial fibrosis. Although a diagnostic sample is not always obtained with bronchial biopsy, it is associated with less risk than lung biopsy (eg, hemorrhage, pneumothorax).

TREATMENT

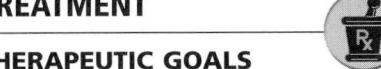

THERAPEUTIC GOALS

Treatment of RAO is three-pronged: effect bronchodilation, reduce inflammation, and remediate the environment.

ACUTE GENERAL TREATMENT

- The immediate goal of treatment in the face of RAO exacerbation is bronchodilation. This is best achieved by using a quickly acting β-adrenergic drug such as albuterol (5 puffs) via inhaler using a device such as the Aero-Hippus. If albuterol is not available, atropine may also be given IV (0.01–0.02 mg/kg); however, this treatment may induce ileus.
- Bronchodilation alone does not address the underlying problem, which is the reduction of inflammation. Therefore treatment with a corticosteroid should be initiated. Most horses in exacerbation require paren-

teral use of corticosteroids initially followed by inhaled corticosteroid therapy.
  ○ Multiple different glucocorticoids have been used for treatment of horses with RAO. The most commonly used are dexamethasone PO, IV, or IM (0.1 mg/kg) once daily for 5 to 7 days with a gradual reduction over 2 to 4 weeks and prednisolone (0.8 mg/kg) PO twice daily for 1 week, tapering gradually over 4 weeks.
  ○ The most commonly used inhaled glucocorticoids include fluticasone (Flovent 220) beginning with 9 to 12 puffs twice daily or QVAR (8 to 10 puffs twice daily) using the Aero-Hippus, with a gradual reduction over 2 to 3 weeks. A reasonable aim is to have the horse on an every other day treatment within 4 weeks. Inhaled glucocorticoids are expensive and not within the financial realm of all owners.

CHRONIC TREATMENT

Longer term goals involve reduction of inflammation through environmental remediation.
- This involves turnout in a nondusty paddock or if the horse cannot be turned out, reducing the dust in bedding and feed.
- Useful approaches include using a pelleted diet, ensiled hay (haylage), dengie (baked hay), or if this is not possible, soaking the hay for at least 1 hour.
- Although clean, bright straw has been shown to be low in organic dusts, it is very difficult to find.
- Pelleted bedding and shredded cardboard or paper are the lowest in dusts.
- Dust in the air is highest when there is a lot of human activity, especially during cleaning and feeding times, so ideally, horses are removed from the stable at that time.
- The first approach to dust is to dampen or sprinkle the aisleways with water before watering, and make sure that

indoor and outdoor arenas are kept moist to reduce dust.

RECOMMENDED MONITORING

BAL and lung function testing 1 month after initiating treatment with corticosteroid is valuable in monitoring progress and response to drugs and environmental remediation.

PROGNOSIS AND OUTCOME

- Prognosis for uncomplicated RAO is good provided that vigorous efforts at environmental remediation are made and there is good compliance with the treatment plan.
- In long-standing disease, it is unlikely that chronic remodeling of the airways will ever be reversed; these horses may have respiratory compromise even in the face of appropriate management.

PEARLS & CONSIDERATIONS

Interstitial pneumonia of donkeys has recently been linked to asinine herpesvirus-2 and -5. The exact role of γ-herpesviridae in Equids is still unclear.

SUGGESTED READING

DeLuca L, Erb HN, Young JC, et al: The effect of adding oral dexamethasone to feed alterations on the airway cell inflammatory gene expression in stabled horses affected with recurrent airway obstruction. *J Vet Intern Med* 22(2):427–435, 2008.
Miskovic M, Couetil LL, Thompson CA: Lung function and airway cytologic profiles in horses with recurrent airway obstruction maintained in low-dust environments. *J Vet Intern Med* 21(5):1060–1066, 2007.

AUTHORS: **MELISSA R. MAZAN** and **IAN TIZARD**

EDITOR: **MELISSA R. MAZAN**

Algal Toxicosis

BASIC INFORMATION

DEFINITION

Acute intoxication of the liver (microcystin) or central nervous system (anatoxins) subsequent to algal toxin exposure

SYNONYM(S)
- Microcystin toxicosis
- Anatoxin-a toxicosis
- Blue-green algae intoxication
- Cyanobacteria toxicosis

EPIDEMIOLOGY

RISK FACTORS
- Algal bloom prevalence is increased with elevated water temperature and nutrient concentrations in the water.
- Steady winds that propel toxic blooms to shore allow ingestion by drinking animals.

GEOGRAPHY AND SEASONALITY

More common in the summer and fall when water temperature is increased

CLINICAL PRESENTATION

DISEASE FORMS/SUBTYPES

- Acute hepatotoxicosis subsequent to microcystin exposure
- Acute onset of neurologic signs subsequent to anatoxin-a exposure
- Rapid onset of excessive salivation and neurologic signs subsequent to anatoxin-a(s) exposure

HISTORY, CHIEF COMPLAINT

- Microcystins: diarrhea and weakness within hours of exposure to water
- Anatoxin-a: rapid onset of muscle rigidity, muscle tremors, and convulsions within minutes to a few hours of exposure to water
- Anatoxin-a(s): rapid onset of excessive salivation, diarrhea, tremors, and convulsions within minutes of exposure to water

PHYSICAL EXAM FINDINGS

- Microcystins: microcystin intoxication should be suspected in cases of acute hepatotoxicosis with clinical signs of diarrhea, nasogastric reflux, weakness, pale mucous membranes, and shock. Although most animals die within a few hours of exposure, some animals may live for several hours and develop hyperkalemia, hypoglycemia, nervousness, recumbency, and convulsions. Animals that survive the acute intoxication may develop hepatogenous photosensitization.
- Anatoxin-a: clinical signs of anatoxin-a poisoning include a rapid onset of rigidity and muscle tremors followed by paralysis, cyanosis, and death. Death usually occurs within minutes to a few hours. In most cases, the animal is found dead.
- Anatoxin-a(s): animals poisoned with anatoxin-a(s) show a rapid onset of excessive salivation ("s" stands for salivation), lacrimation, diarrhea, and urination. Nicotinic overstimulation results in tremors, incoordination, convulsions, recumbency, and respiratory arrest. Animals often die within 30 minutes of exposure and thus are often found dead.

ETIOLOGY AND PATHOPHYSIOLOGY

- Microcystins are cyclic heptapeptides that inhibit protein phosphatases, which leads to hepatocyte necrosis. There are more than 80 different microcystins worldwide produced by various genera of cyanobacteria, such as *Microcystis, Anabaena, Planktothrix, Nostoc, Oscillatoria,* and *Anabaenopsis.*
- Anatoxin-a is a potent cholinergic agonist at nicotinic acetylcholine receptors in neurons and at the neuro-muscular junctions. Anatoxin-a is produced worldwide by cyanobacteria genera such as *Anabaena, Plantkothrix, Oscillatoria, Microcystis, Aphanizomenon, Cylindorspermum,* and *Phormidium.*
- Anatoxin-a(s) is a naturally occurring irreversible acetylcholinesterase inhibitor produced by cyanobacteria species such as *Anabena flosaquae, Anabena lemmermannii,* and *Anabena spiroides.*

DIAGNOSIS

DIFFERENTIAL DIAGNOSIS

- Microcystins: other causes of acute liver failure such as iron, amanitins, aflatoxins, cocklebur, alsike clover, Theiler's disease, and Tyzzer's disease
- Anatoxin-a: cyanide, yew, oleander, poison hemlock, insecticides, ionophore antibiotics, intestinal compromise (eg, torsion)
- Anatoxin-a(s): organophosphorus and carbamate insecticides, slaframine

INITIAL DATABASE

- Microcystins: elevated serum gamma-glutamyl transpeptidase, aspartate aminotransferase, bile acids, alkaline phosphatase; hypoglycemia; hyperkalemia
- Anatoxin-a and a(s): no abnormalities

ADVANCED OR CONFIRMATORY TESTING

Confirmatory testing is needed to reach an accurate diagnosis of algal intoxication.

- Identification of the algae in the suspect water source or stomach contents. However, positive identification does not confirm intoxication because the toxicity of the cyanobacteria is strain specific, and morphologic observations alone cannot predict the hazard level.
- Detection of microcystins and anatoxin-a in water and gastric contents is provided by select veterinary toxicology laboratories.
- Detection of anatoxin-a(s) in water and gastric contents can also be provided by select laboratories. In addition, determination of blood acetylcholinesterase activity can aid in the diagnostic workup.

TREATMENT

THERAPEUTIC GOAL(S)

There is no specific antidote for algal toxins. Despite the evaluation of numerous treatment options, no specific therapy has been proven to be effective.

ACUTE GENERAL TREATMENT

- Provide symptomatic and supportive care to treat hypovolemia and electrolyte imbalances.
- Although no studies have evaluated the efficacy of specific decontamination procedures, administration of activated charcoal has been recommended.
- Microcystins: because microcystins can enhance oxidative stress, antioxidants such as vitamin E and selenium appear to be beneficial.
- Anatoxin-a: seizure control with benzodiazepine, phenobarbital, or pentobarbital.
- Anatoxin-a(s): atropine should be given. Determine its efficacy in animals with life-threatening clinical signs with an initial test dose. After the test dose, atropine can be given repeatedly until cessation of salivation.

CHRONIC TREATMENT

Protect from sun exposure if hepatogenous photosensitization develops subsequent to microcystin intoxication.

POSSIBLE COMPLICATIONS

In many cases, the rapid onset of acute intoxication does not allow timely therapeutic intervention, and mortality rates are high.

RECOMMENDED MONITORING

Close monitoring of serum electrolytes, liver function, body temperature, and central nervous system signs

PROGNOSIS AND OUTCOME

- Prognosis is poor. Animals with algal toxin intoxication are often found dead.
- Animals that survive acute microcystin intoxication may develop photosensitization.

PEARLS & CONSIDERATIONS

COMMENTS

- Algal toxin exposure in horses is rarely reported but may result in acute liver disease or neurologic signs. Mortality rates are high.
- Proper diagnostic workup of suspect blue-green algae poisoning cases is necessary to prevent additional exposures.
- Therapeutic measures are limited, so it is prudent to take measures for avoiding exposure to algal toxins.
- Worldwide, the frequency and intensity of harmful cyanobacterial blooms appear to be increasing, and it is likely

that blue-green algae poisonings will become more common in animals as a result of accidental exposure.

PREVENTION
- Deny horses access to water with visible algal bloom.
- Reduce fertilizer run-off and applications in fields surrounding ponds used for drinking water.

CLIENT EDUCATION
- The increased incidence of blue-green algal blooms is partly a consequence of nutrient pollution.
- Inform clients that prognosis is poor for animals exposed to algal toxins.

SUGGESTED READING
Puschner B, Galey FD, Johnson B, et al: Blue-green algae toxicosis in cattle. *J Am Vet Med Assoc* 13:1605–1607, 1998.

Puschner B, Hoff B, Tor ER, et al: Diagnosis of anatoxin-a poisoning in dogs from North America. *J Vet Diagn Invest* 20:89–92, 2008.

Puschner B, Humbert J-F: Cyanobacterial (blue-green algae) toxins. In Gupta RC, editor: *Veterinary toxicology—basic and clinical principles.* San Diego, 2007, Academic Press, pp 714–724.

AUTHOR: **BIRGIT PUSCHNER**

EDITOR: **CYNTHIA L. GASKILL**

Alopecia Areata

BASIC INFORMATION

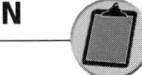

DEFINITION
A cell-mediated autoimmune disorder resulting in round patches of hair loss

EPIDEMIOLOGY
GENETICS AND BREED PREDISPOSITION A hereditary factor has been suggested.

CLINICAL PRESENTATION
HISTORY, CHIEF COMPLAINT Acute or insidious onset of patches of hair loss
PHYSICAL EXAM FINDINGS
- Focal or multifocal, noninflammatory, well-circumscribed, annular areas of hair loss. Areas of hair regrowth may be lighter than normal.

- Thinning of the mane and tail.
- The animal is otherwise healthy.

ETIOLOGY AND PATHOPHYSIOLOGY
T-lymphocyte disruption of the hair matrix, root sheath, and epithelium of the hair follicles

DIAGNOSIS

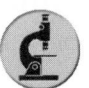

DIFFERENTIAL DIAGNOSIS
- Dermatophytosis
- Dermatophilosis
- Anagen defluxion
- Occult sarcoid

ADVANCED OR CONFIRMATORY TESTING
Histopathologic examination of skin biopsy shows accumulation of lymphocytes around the hair bulbs, the presence of "miniature" hair follicles, and possibly defective keratinization (chronic lesions).

PROGNOSIS AND OUTCOME

Spontaneous recovery has been recorded.

SUGGESTED READING
Pascoe RRR, Knottenbelt DC: Immune-mediated/allergic diseases. In Pascoe RRR, Knottenbelt DC, editors: *Manual of equine dermatology.* London, 1999, WB Saunders, pp 168–169.

AUTHOR: **JENNIFER TAINTOR**

EDITOR: **DAVID A. WILSON**

Alphaviruses

BASIC INFORMATION

DEFINITION
The Togaviridae include the major causes of infectious arthropod-borne equine encephalitides and are divided into two main groups: the Alphaviridae—including Eastern equine encephalitis (EEE), Western equine encephalitis (WEE), and Venezuelan equine encephalitis (VEE)—and the Flaviviridae, including West Nile virus (WNV).

SYNONYM(S)
EEE, WEE, and VEE viruses are members of the *Alphavirus* genus of the family Togaviridae and were formerly referred to as Arbovirus group A of the Togaviridae.

EPIDEMIOLOGY
SPECIES, AGE, SEX Generally any age or breed and either sex. Disease is uncommon in suckling foals younger than 3 months.
RISK FACTORS
- Lack of protective vaccination. Widespread vaccination programs in North America have markedly reduced incidence of EEE and WEE.
- Disease is limited to the summer in temperate regions but is year-round in subtropical to tropical areas.
CONTAGION AND ZOONOSIS
- Although these viruses cause similar clinical syndromes in horses, the consequences of the infections they cause in humans differ.
- EEE is the most severe of the arboviral encephalitides, with case fatality rates

of 50% to 70% and neurologic sequelae common in survivors.
- WEE virus appears to be less neuroinvasive but has pathology similar to EEE in patients with encephalitis.
- In adults, the VEE virus usually causes an acute, febrile, incapacitating disease with prolonged convalescence. In children, severe encephalitis may result from VEE.
GEOGRAPHY AND SEASONALITY
- As with most of the alphaviruses, EEE, WEE, and VEE are transmitted by mosquitoes and maintained in cycles with various vertebrate hosts. Environmental factors that affect the interactions of the relevant mosquito and reservoir host populations control the natural epidemiology of these viruses. Some overlap of geographic extent exists.

- Outbreaks of EEE virus have occurred in most eastern states and in south-eastern Canada but have been concentrated along the eastern and Gulf coasts.
- Outbreaks of WEE have been reported in the western and north-central United States, as well as Saskatchewan and Manitoba in Canada. Predominates west of the Mississippi River.
- VEE was originally reported in Venezuela, Colombia, Peru, and Ecuador before spreading to all of Central America and subsequently continuing north to Mexico and into Texas. Between active epizootics, it is not possible to isolate the equine virulent viruses with several attenuated, antigenically different VEE strains isolated instead. These enzootic strains can be differentiated among themselves and from the epizootic strains.

CLINICAL PRESENTATION

HISTORY, CHIEF COMPLAINT

- EEE, WEE, and VEE present with similar clinical signs, including an inapparent, generalized febrile response.
- Encephalomyelitis may occur singly or in combination.
- Horses may present with colic or vague signs of diffuse brain involvement.

PHYSICAL EXAM FINDINGS

- Clinical signs not pathognomonic
- Fever associated with viremia in majority of infected horses
- Initial hyperexcitability, progressing to depression and recumbency
- Blindness
- Head pressing
- Ataxia
- Compulsive walking, circling
- Seizure activity
- Permanent neurologic deficits may occur in survivors
- Early neurologic signs reflect diffuse, multifocal cortical disease
- Mortality ranges from 75% to 90% for EEE, 19% to 50% for WEE, and 40% to 90% for VEE

ETIOLOGY AND PATHOPHYSIOLOGY

- Birds are the primary reservoir for EEE, WEE, and VEE. Transfer of infection depends on an interplay between migratory bird patterns and vector seasonal population fluctuations. EEE may be found year-round in the southeastern United States. Small rodents can harbor VEE.
- Virus replication occurs within arthropod vector (mosquitoes *Culex*, *Aedes*, *Anopheles*, and *Culiseta*).
- After inoculation into the equine host, local replication occurs in the subcutaneous tissue at the site of inoculation.
- Lymphatic spread to the spleen and liver.

- Short-lived viremia ensues in the majority of infected animals. Viremia of EEE and WEE is too low to infect vectors, so the horse is a dead-end host. However, VEE titers are sufficient to infect vectors.
- In a small number of infected horses, the blood-brain barrier is crossed and encephalomyelitis results.
- Infected EEE and WEE horses do not cause direct or indirect lateral spread.
- Widespread neuronal necrosis throughout the central nervous system, especially the cerebrum.

DIAGNOSIS

DIFFERENTIAL DIAGNOSIS

- Bacterial encephalomyelitis
- Hepatic encephalopathy
- Equine protozoal myeloencephalitis
- Rabies
- WNV
- Verminous encephalomyelitis
- Diffuse brain trauma

INITIAL DATABASE

- Cerebrospinal fluid: Neutrophilic pleocytosis, increased protein; may be xanthochromic
- Antibodies: Detection of IgM or IgG in serum. May already have high levels in acute sera, complicating diagnosis by a fourfold increase between acute and convalescent sera.

ADVANCED OR CONFIRMATORY TESTING

- Histology
  - EEE: Neutrophilic-endothelial cuffing
  - WEE: lymphocytic-plasmocytic
  - VEE: Lymphocytic-neutrophilic
- Gross pathology: Cerebral malacia, patchy hemorrhage, swelling
- Brain: Viral culture, antigen and antibody detection

TREATMENT

THERAPEUTIC GOAL(S)

Treatment for the alphavirus encephalitides is centered on the control of central nervous system inflammation and supportive therapies.

ACUTE GENERAL TREATMENT

- Antiinflammatories: Nonsteroidal antiinflammatory drugs are preferred over corticosteroids by some veterinarians.
- Dimethyl sulfoxide: 1 g/kg IV as 10% solution
- Seizure control: Benzodiazepines
- Intensive supportive therapies: IV fluids, nutrition, general nursing
- Antimicrobial therapy for secondary bacterial infections (if present)

CHRONIC TREATMENT

- Management of secondary complications: Recumbency, aspiration pneumonia, decubital ulcers
- Avoidance of self-trauma during encephalitic phase or as a result of residual deficits

POSSIBLE COMPLICATIONS

- Decubital ulceration
- Self-mutilation
- Aspiration pneumonia
- Residual neurologic deficits: Ataxia, depression

PROGNOSIS AND OUTCOME

- Unvaccinated horses are likely to succumb to infection.
- Prognosis is poor with the onset of encephalitic signs.
- Grave prognosis for EEE and VEE. Survival in EEE is reported with previous but insufficient vaccine exposure, resulting in a modified disease with slow progression and spinal cord or brainstem lesions.
- WEE survival is occasionally reported with permanent neurologic deficits (depressed mentation, spinal ataxia).

PEARLS & CONSIDERATIONS

COMMENTS

- Vaccinate horses in the face of outbreak: Antibody increase noted 3 days after vaccination
- If VEE vaccination is required, use trivalent vaccine because the response is poorer in horses previously vaccinated against EEE and WEE.

PREVENTION

- Inactivated vaccines are available and highly efficacious. The duration of immunity is short (4–6 months), which may be less than vector season; repeated vaccinations are therefore necessary. Four monthly vaccinations may be necessary in areas where disease is common.
- Vaccinate in early spring and summer. Time the program to precede the encephalitis season by several months.
- Vaccinate pregnant mares 1 month before foaling to boost colostral protection of the foal; antibody persists up to 6 months.
- Vaccination can begin at any age; must repeat after 6 months of age.
- Vector control: Removal of mosquito breeding areas (stagnant water).

SUGGESTED READING

Bertone JJ: Togaviral encephalitis. In Reed S, Bayly W, Sellon D, editors: *Equine internal medicine*, ed 2. St Louis, 2004, Saunders, pp 631–635.

Goehring L: Viral diseases of the nervous system. In Furr M, Reed S, editors: *Equine neurology*. Ames, IA, 2008, Blackwell Publishing, pp 169–186.

Mayhew IG: Infectious, inflammatory and immune diseases. In Mayhew IG, editor: *Large animal neurology*, ed 2. Ames, IA, 2009, Wiley Blackwell, pp 225–293.

AUTHOR: **PETER R. MORRESEY**

EDITOR: **STEPHEN M. REED**

Amanitin Toxicosis

BASIC INFORMATION

DEFINITION

Acute hepatotoxicity subsequent to amanitin-containing mushroom exposure

SYNONYM(S)

- Amanita toxicosis
- Death cap intoxication
- Amatoxin poisoning
- Hepatotoxic mushroom poisoning
- Amanitin poisoning

EPIDEMIOLOGY

GEOGRAPHY AND SEASONALITY
Amanita phalloides mushrooms are found throughout North America, commonly in association with oaks and birch. The large fruiting bodies appear in the summer and fall. Local mycologic societies can provide detailed information on the occurrence of toxic mushrooms in certain regions.

CLINICAL PRESENTATION

DISEASE FORMS/SUBTYPES
- Severe gastrointestinal (GI) signs such as colic and diarrhea
- Acute hepatotoxicosis
- Fulminant multiorgan failure

HISTORY, CHIEF COMPLAINT
- Colic and diarrhea within 24 hours of amanitin-containing mushroom exposure
- Lethargy, icterus, ataxia, seizures, and coma approximately 36 to 48 hours after exposure to amanitins

PHYSICAL EXAM FINDINGS
- The clinical course of amanitin exposure can be divided into four phases. Physical examination findings are different for each phase.
  - The initial phase is a latency period of approximately 8 to 12 hours without any clinical signs after ingestion of amanitin-containing mushrooms.
  - During the second phase (6 to 24 hours after mushroom ingestion), the animal develops severe GI signs such as colic and diarrhea.
  - The third phase is a period of several hours to a few days during which the animal appears to have recovered. During this phase, close

monitoring of liver and kidney function is essential to prevent misdiagnosis.
  - The final stage begins approximately 36 to 84 hours after exposure to amanitins. In this stage, fulminant liver, renal, and multiorgan failure may occur, and affected animals may be icteric, lethargic, and ataxic and have seizures or coma. If large amounts of amanitin-containing mushrooms were ingested, it is feasible that the animal will die acutely within 24 hours and may simply be found dead.

ETIOLOGY AND PATHOPHYSIOLOGY

- Amanitins (α-, β-, γ-, and ϵ-amanitins) are bicyclic octapeptides and are found in three different mushroom genera: *Amanita*, *Galerina*, and *Lepiota* spp.
- The most toxic cylopeptide-containing mushrooms are *A. phalloides*, the ubiquitous "death cap" or "death angel," and *Galerina sulpices*. *A. phalloides* is found throughout North America, commonly in association with oaks and birch. *G. sulpices* is most commonly found in Europe.
- Amanitins inhibit nuclear RNA polymerase II, ultimately leading to decreased protein synthesis and cell death.
- Cells with a high metabolic rate, such as hepatocytes, crypt cells, and proximal convoluted tubules of the kidneys, are most commonly affected.

DIAGNOSIS

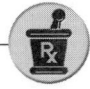

DIFFERENTIAL DIAGNOSIS

- Other causes of acute liver failure: iron, microcystins, aflatoxins, cocklebur, alsike clover, Theiler's disease, and Tyzzer's disease
- Other causes of gastroenteritis

INITIAL DATABASE

Approximately 24 hours after exposure: Elevated serum gamma-glutamyl transpeptidase, aspartate aminotransferase, bile acids, alkaline phosphatase, total bilirubin; hypoglycemia; prolonged prothrombin time, and partial thromboplastin time.

ADVANCED OR CONFIRMATORY TESTING

Confirmatory testing is needed to reach an accurate diagnosis of amanitin intoxication:

- Identification of mushroom pieces in gastric contents. Accurate mushroom identification requires consultation with an experienced mycologist and may include DNA sequencing.
- Detection of amanitins in the serum, urine, gastric contents, liver, or kidney: This testing is provided by select veterinary toxicology laboratories. In live symptomatic animals, urine is likely to be of superior diagnostic use to serum. Postmortem, the kidney contains higher concentrations than the liver and is considered the sample of choice.

TREATMENT

THERAPEUTIC GOAL(S)

- Close monitoring, fluid replacement, and supportive care are essential treatment components in amanitin poisoning.
- Even with supportive measures, the reported mortality rate from *Amanita* poisoning in humans is 20% to 40%. No data on horses are available, but amanitin intoxication requires prompt and aggressive treatment measures to improve prognosis.

ACUTE GENERAL TREATMENT

- Close monitoring and fluid replacement. There is no specific antidote for amanitins. Despite the evaluation of numerous treatment options, no specific therapy has proven to be effective.
- As part of vigorous supportive care, IV fluids, correction of hypoglycemia and electrolyte imbalances, vitamin K1, and plasma transfusions should be considered, depending on the severity of the clinical presentation.
- There is controversy about the efficacy of activated charcoal.
- Silibinin (the main component of milk thistle) may be beneficial, but controlled studies are lacking.

- *N*-acetylcysteine, cimetidine, and ascorbic acid may be given as antioxidants.

CHRONIC TREATMENT

If the animal survives all four phases of amanitin intoxication, close monitoring of liver and kidney function is necessary.

POSSIBLE COMPLICATIONS

- In many cases, the rapid onset of severe hepatotoxicosis does not allow for timely therapeutic intervention.
- Amanitin-containing mushrooms may initially cause GI signs followed by an apparent recovery. Therefore any animal presenting with GI signs after a suspected or known history of mushroom ingestion must be evaluated carefully and treated promptly.

RECOMMENDED MONITORING

Close monitoring of serum electrolytes, liver and kidney function, body temperature, and central nervous system signs

PROGNOSIS AND OUTCOME

Prognosis is poor. Animals with amanitin intoxication are often presented when severe liver damage has already occurred.

PEARLS & CONSIDERATIONS

COMMENTS

- Hepatotoxic mushroom ingestion in horses is rarely reported but may result in severe liver disease.
- Proper diagnostic workup of suspect amanitin poisonings is necessary to prevent additional exposures and to rule out other causes of acute liver disease.
- Therapeutic measures are limited, so it is essential to take measures to avoid exposing horses to toxic mushrooms.

PREVENTION

Deny horses access to areas where toxic mushrooms grow.

CLIENT EDUCATION

Inform clients that the prognosis is poor for animals exposed to toxic mushrooms. Inform clients that an accurate diagnostic workup is needed to confirm suspected amanitin exposure. Advise clients to contact local mycologic societies for occurrence of toxic mushrooms to prevent exposures.

SUGGESTED READING

Enjalbert F, Rapior S, Nouguier-Soulé J, et al: Treatment of amatoxin poisoning: 20-year retrospective analysis. *J Toxicol Clin Toxicol* 40:715–757, 2002.

Filigenzi MS, Poppenga RH, Tiwary AK, et al: The determination of alpha-amanitin in serum and liver by multistage linear ion trap mass spectrometry. *J Agric Food Chem* 55:2784–2790, 2007.

Puschner B: Mushroom toxins. In Gupta RC, editor: *Veterinary toxicology–basic and clinical principles.* San Diego, 2007, Academic Press, pp 915–925.

AUTHOR: **BIRGIT PUSCHNER**

EDITOR: **CYNTHIA L. GASKILL**

Aminoglycoside Toxicosis

BASIC INFORMATION

DEFINITION

The aminoglycosides are large molecules with numerous amino acid groups, making them basic polycations that are highly ionized at physiologic pHs. These physical properties are important in their known toxicities: nephrotoxicity, ototoxicity, and neuromuscular blockade.

EPIDEMIOLOGY

SPECIES, AGE, SEX All ages and sexes are affected, but neonates and geriatrics are more at risk because of their reduced renal function.

RISK FACTORS

- Prolonged aminoglycoside therapy (>7–10 days)
- Acidosis and electrolyte disturbances (hypokalemia, hyponatremia)
- Volume depletion (shock, endotoxemia)
- Concurrent therapy with nephrotoxic drug (eg, nonsteroidal antiinflammatory drugs [NSAIDs]) or diuretics
- Preexisting renal disease
- Elevated plasma trough concentrations

CLINICAL PRESENTATION

HISTORY, CHIEF COMPLAINT

- Nonoliguric renal failure
- Hearing loss
- Neuromuscular blockade

PHYSICAL EXAM FINDINGS Usually related to the original disease for which the aminoglycoside was being administered

ETIOLOGY AND PATHOPHYSIOLOGY Nephrotoxicity is caused by accumulation of the drug in the renal tubular epithelial cells.

- Aminoglycosides enter the renal tubule after filtration through the glomerulus.
- Cationic aminoglycoside molecules bind to anionic phospholipids on the proximal tubular cells.
- The aminoglycoside is taken into the cell by carrier-mediated pinocytosis and translocated into cytoplasmic vacuoles, which fuse with lysosomes.
- With additional pinocytosis, drug continues to accumulate within the lysosomes.
- The accumulated aminoglycoside interferes with normal lysosomal function, and the overloaded lysosomes eventually swell and rupture.
- Lysosomal enzymes, phospholipids, and the aminoglycoside are released

into the cytosol of the proximal tubular cell, disrupting other organelles and causing cell death.

- Neomycin is the most nephrotoxic, and streptomycin and dihydrostreptomycin are the least nephrotoxic.
- Amikacin is often recommended in critical patients over gentamicin because it is considered less nephrotoxic.

Ototoxicity:

- Occurs by the same mechanisms as nephrotoxicity
  - Not typically diagnosed in horses because of failure to identify partial hearing losses
- Toxicity varies with the drug
  - Vestibular damage (balance): Streptomycin, gentamicin
  - Cochlear damage (hearing): Amikacin, kanamycin, neomycin
  - Both: Tobramycin

Neuromuscular blockade:

- Rapid IV administration causes bradycardia, reduced cardiac output, and hypotension through an effect on calcium metabolism. These effects are of minor significance.
- Paralysis of skeletal muscles
  - A rare effect
  - From blockade of acetylcholine at the nicotinic cholinergic receptor

○ Most often seen when anesthetic agents are administered concurrently

DIAGNOSIS

DIFFERENTIAL DIAGNOSIS

NSAID-induced and other drug-induced renal failure

INITIAL DATABASE

- Serum chemistries
  - ○ Increased serum urea nitrogen and creatinine (Cr) confirm nephrotoxicity but are not seen for 7 days after significant renal damage has occurred.
- Urine gamma glutamyl transferase (GGT) and Cr
  - ○ The urine GGT and urine GGT/urine Cr ratio increase.
  - ○ The urine GGT/urine Cr ratio may increase to two to three times baseline within 3 days of a nephrotoxic dose.
- Urinalysis
  - ○ Proteinuria is the next best indicator of nephrotoxicity after the urine GGT/urine Cr ratio and is easily determined in a practice setting with urine dipstick tests.
  - ○ Hyposthenuria, polyuria, hematuria, and cylindruria (presence of casts in the urine) may also be seen.

ADVANCED OR CONFIRMATORY TESTING

Histopathology of renal biopsy or post-mortem samples: lesions of acute tubular necrosis

TREATMENT

THERAPEUTIC GOAL(S)

Aminoglycoside nephrotoxicity is best prevented by appropriate dosing and a high-protein, high-calcium diet.

ACUTE GENERAL TREATMENT

- Discontinuation of aminoglycoside therapy
- Nephrotoxicity
  - ○ Diuresis with balanced IV fluids and correction of metabolic acidosis and electrolyte abnormalities.
  - ○ Although peritoneal dialysis is useful in lowering Cr and serum urea nitrogen, it may not be effective in significantly increasing the elimination of the accumulating aminoglycoside.
- Neuromuscular blockade
  - ○ Prompt treatment with parenteral calcium chloride at 10 to 20 mg/kg IV or calcium gluconate at 30 to 60 mg/kg IV or neostigmine given slowly IV at 100 to 200 µg/kg

to reverse dyspnea from muscle response depression.
  - ○ Edrophonium at 0.5 mg/kg IV will also reverse neuromuscular blocking effects.

DRUG INTERACTIONS

- Aminoglycosides are inactivated if combined in vitro with other drugs because of pH incompatibilities.
- The aminoglycosides are synergistic against streptococci, *Pseudomonas* spp., and other gram-negative bacteria if combined with β-lactam antibiotics because of disruption of the bacterial cell wall by the β-lactam antibiotic.
- Halothane anesthesia causes significant changes in the pharmacokinetics of gentamicin in horses: total body clearance and volume of distribution decrease, and half-life of elimination increases. A longer gentamicin dosing interval after anesthesia may help correct the changes, but serious consideration should be given to choice of another antimicrobial.
- Neuromuscular blocking agents or drugs with neuromuscular blocking activity should not be used concurrently with aminoglycosides because they may increase the risk of neuromuscular blockade, particularly during anesthesia.
- Other nephrotoxic drugs and diuretics should be avoided when possible during aminoglycoside therapy.
- Concurrent administration of phenylbutazone with gentamicin decreases the elimination half-life of gentamicin by 23% and decreases the volume of distribution by 26%; the pharmacokinetics of phenylbutazone is not altered.

POSSIBLE COMPLICATIONS

- Chronic renal failure
- Death

RECOMMENDED MONITORING

- Individual horses differ widely in the serum concentrations produced from the same aminoglycoside dosage regimen.
  - ○ There is a tendency to underdose neonatal patients, especially those that are receiving aggressive fluid therapy.
- Therapeutic drug monitoring may reduce toxicity and confirm therapeutic concentrations.
  - ○ To allow for the distribution phase, blood sampling for the peak concentration is done at 0.5 to 1 hour after administration, and the trough sample is usually taken before the next dose.
  - ○ The peak and trough concentrations can then be used to estimate

the elimination half-life for the individual patient.
  - ○ If using a once-daily regimen, a blood sample just before the next dose will be well below the recommended trough concentrations and may even be below the limit of detection of the assay. For these patients, an 8-hour postdose sample will provide a more accurate estimate of the elimination half-life.
  - ○ Serum concentrations of drug should be 0.5 to 2.0 µg/mL before the next dose (gentamicin, tobramycin) or less than 6 µg/mL for amikacin.
  - ○ An increase in the elimination half-life during therapy with increasing trough concentrations is a very sensitive indicator of early tubular insult.

PROGNOSIS AND OUTCOME

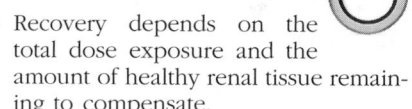

- Recovery depends on the total dose exposure and the amount of healthy renal tissue remaining to compensate.
- Progression to oliguric or anuric renal failure is infrequent, and most horses recover.

PEARLS & CONSIDERATIONS

COMMENTS

- Uptake and accumulation of aminoglycosides into renal tubular epithelium demonstrate saturable kinetics.
- Because nephrotoxicity is related to aminoglycoside accumulation in the renal proximal tubular cells, it is logical that peak concentrations are not related to toxicity and that longer dose intervals result in less total drug exposure to the renal brush border membrane.
- High-dose, once-daily dosing of aminoglycosides has now become common in human and veterinary medicine. This dosing regimen takes advantage of the concentration-dependent killing and long postantibiotic effect of these drugs, and avoids first exposure adaptive resistance and toxicity.

PREVENTION

- Calcium supplementation reduces the risk of nephrotoxicity.
- The risk of nephrotoxicity can also be decreased by feeding a high-protein, high-calcium diet such as alfalfa because protein and calcium cations compete with aminoglycoside cations

for binding to renal tubular epithelial cells. High dietary protein also increases the glomerular filtration rate and renal blood flow, reducing aminoglycoside accumulation.

SUGGESTED READING

Bucki EP, Giguère S, Macpherson M, et al: Pharmacokinetics of once-daily amikacin in healthy foals and therapeutic drug monitoring in hospitalized equine neonates. *J Vet Intern Med* 18:728–733, 2004.

Riviere JE, Coppoc GL, Hinsman EJ, et al: Species dependent gentamicin pharmacokinetics and nephrotoxicity in the young horse. *Fundam Appl Toxicol* 3:448–457, 1983.

Schumacher J, Wilson RC, Spano JS, et al: Effect of diet on gentamicin-induced nephrotoxicosis in horses. *Am J Vet Res* 52:1274–1278, 1991.

van der Harst MR, Bull S, Laffont CM, et al: Gentamicin nephrotoxicity—a comparison of in vitro findings with in vivo experiments in equines. *Vet Res Commun* 29:247–261, 2005.

AUTHOR: **PATRICIA M. DOWLING**

EDITOR: **CYNTHIA M. GASKILL**

Amyloidosis

BASIC INFORMATION

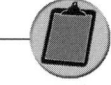

DEFINITION

Progressive systemic or cutaneous disease resulting from excessive deposition of insoluble protein polymers known as amyloid in various organs, especially the kidneys. This leads to progressive organ failure.

EPIDEMIOLOGY

SPECIES, AGE, SEX
- An uncommon disease that develops in older horses
- No sex or breed predilections

RISK FACTORS
- Visceral amyloidosis develops secondary to chronic infections, severe strongylid parasitism, or excessive immune stimulation. It is a significant problem in horses used in the commercial production of hyperimmune serum.
- Cutaneous amyloidosis is not associated with chronic inflammation but possibly with the presence of malignant histiocytic lymphoma.

ASSOCIATED CONDITIONS AND DISORDERS
- Renal failure
- Protein-losing nephropathy
- Specific organ failure depends on the location of amyloid deposits

CLINICAL PRESENTATION

DISEASE FORMS/SUBTYPES
- Most visceral cases are detected incidentally at necropsy.
- Protein-losing nephropathy and renal failure secondary to deposition of amyloid within glomeruli present as nephritic syndrome with massive proteinuria.
- Rarely involves the upper respiratory tract, including the nasal cavity, pharynx, larynx, guttural pouch, and associated lymph nodes.
- Cutaneous disease is associated with development of tumorlike amyloid nodules; papules and plaques; and subcutaneous amyloid deposits present on the head, neck, and chest.

HISTORY, CHIEF COMPLAINT
- Disease of gradual insidious onset
- Secondary amyloidosis develops gradually in response to chronic inflammation in osteomyelitis, abscesses, traumatic pericarditis, or tuberculosis.
- Insidious signs of progressive liver and kidney failure
- Chronic weight loss leading to emaciation
- In renal failure, the animal is uremic and becomes comatose
- Amyloidosis of the gut wall may result in diarrhea
- Cutaneous amyloidosis is a nodular disease of the skin

PHYSICAL EXAM FINDINGS
- Visceral: Depends on the organs affected; may include mild splenomegaly or hepatomegaly, ascites or edema secondary to renal failure (see "Renal Failure, Chronic" in this section), or severe weight loss
- Cutaneous: Firm, nonpainful, nonpruritic swellings with normal overlying skin

ETIOLOGY AND PATHOPHYSIOLOGY
- Serum amyloid A is an acute-phase protein produced in large amounts in chronic inflammation.
- Misfolded serum amyloid A forms β-pleated sheets. β-pleated sheets are highly insoluble and are deposited in organs as AA amyloid.
- Deposition of AA amyloid in glomeruli leads to loss of glomerular function and progressive renal failure.
- Deposition of AA amyloid in the liver and spleen leads to organ enlargement.
- Very rarely, excessive immunoglobulin light chain production in myelomas or other monoclonal gammopathies may lead to deposition of AL amyloid. AL amyloid is a degradation product of immunoglobulin light chains.

DIAGNOSIS

DIFFERENTIAL DIAGNOSIS

Systemic
- Protein-losing nephropathy
- Nephritic syndrome
- Renal failure
- Pyelonephritis

Cutaneous
- Nodular necrobiosis
- Cutaneous lymphosarcoma

INITIAL DATABASE
- Hematology: Unremarkable
- Chemistry profile: Evidence of renal failure
- Urinalysis: Massive proteinuria if amyloid is deposited in glomeruli
- Imaging: Often unremarkable

TREATMENT

THERAPEUTIC GOAL(S)
- Visceral: Identification and removal of the underlying inflammatory cause
- Treatment of renal failure

ACUTE GENERAL TREATMENT
- Stabilization and treatment of any urinary crisis
- Treatment of protein-losing nephropathy
- Stop hyperimmunization

CHRONIC TREATMENT
- Management of concurrent inflammatory disease or neoplasm
- Maintenance of renal function
- Cutaneous: No effective treatment

RECOMMENDED MONITORING

Urine protein/creatinine ratio, urinalysis, serum albumin, and creatinine levels should be measured every 3 months after the patient is stabilized.

PROGNOSIS AND OUTCOME

- Poor to bad
- Largely determined by the degree of renal damage
- Elimination of the source of inflammation will reduce the rate of disease progression and improve prognosis.

PEARLS & CONSIDERATIONS

COMMENTS

Some amyloidosis is present in all elderly horses. This may have no detectable effect on renal function.

PREVENTION

Prevent the development of persistent inflammatory foci such as abscesses and chronic osteomyelitis.

SUGGESTED READING

Buxbaum J: The genetics of the amyloidoses: interactions with immunity and inflammation. *Genes Immun* 7:439–449, 2006.

Gliatto JM, Alroy J: Cutaneous amyloidosis in a horse with lymphoma. *Vet Rec* 137:68–69, 1995.

Hawthorne TB, Bolon B, Meyer DJ: Systemic amyloidosis in a mare. *J Am Vet Med Assoc* 196:323–325, 1990.

Kim DY, Taylor HW, Eades SC, et al: Systemic AL amyloidosis associated with multiple myeloma in a horse. *Vet Pathol* 42:81–84, 2005.

van Andel AC, Gruys E, et al: Amyloid in the horse: a report of nine cases. *Equine Vet J* 20:277–285, 1988.

AUTHOR & EDITOR: **IAN TIZARD**

Anagen/Telogen Defluxion

BASIC INFORMATION

DEFINITION

- Telogen defluxion is hair loss associated with the telogen phase (resting phase) of hair growth.
- Anagen defluxion is the loss of hair during the anagen phase (active phase) of hair growth.

EPIDEMIOLOGY

RISK FACTORS

- Telogen defluxion: Stressors such as pregnancy, illness, and shock
- Anagen defluxion: Stressors such as antimitotic drugs, malnutrition, and metabolic and endocrine disorders

CLINICAL PRESENTATION

HISTORY, CHIEF COMPLAINT

- Telogen defluxion: History of stressor
- Anagen defluxion: History of stressor, administration or antimitotic drug, malnutrition, or metabolic or endocrine disorder

PHYSICAL EXAM FINDINGS Acute hair loss

ETIOLOGY AND PATHOPHYSIOLOGY

- In telogen defluxion, there is a premature cessation of hair growth as a result of a stress, such as pregnancy, high fever, severe illness, or shock, that leads to synchronous shedding of telogen hairs 2 to 3 months later.
- Anagen defluxion is a result of similar stresses as telogen defluxion plus the use of antimitotic drugs, malnutrition, and endocrine and metabolic disorders that interfere with the anagen phase of hair growth. This interference leads to hair loss and breaking of anagen phase hairs at the epidermal surface.

DIAGNOSIS

DIFFERENTIAL DIAGNOSIS

- Seasonal molting
- Dermatophilosis
- Dermatophytosis
- Sarcoidosis
- Pemphigus foliaceus
- Alopecia areata
- Mercurial poisoning
- Anhidrosis
- Selenium poisoning

ADVANCED OR CONFIRMATORY TESTING

- Microscopic examination of hairs is needed to confirm the diagnosis.
- Telogen hairs are characterized by a uniform shaft diameter; clubbed, non-pigmented root ends; and a lack of root sheaths.
- Anagen hairs are characterized by an irregular shaft diameter, deformity of the shaft, and ragged points or ends that easily break.

TREATMENT

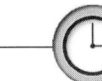

ACUTE GENERAL TREATMENT

Resolves after removal or treatment of underlying cause

PROGNOSIS AND OUTCOME

Good

SUGGESTED READING

Milne E, Rowland AC: Anagen defluxion in two horses. *Vet Dermatol* 3:139–143, 1992.

Pascoe RRR, Knottenbelt DC: Iatrogenic and idiopathic disorders. In Pascoe RRR, Knottenbelt DC, editors: *Manual of equine dermatology*. London, 1999, WB Saunders, pp 199–200.

AUTHOR: **JENNIFER TAINTOR**

EDITOR: **DAVID A. WILSON**

Anaphylaxis

BASIC INFORMATION

DEFINITION

A life-threatening acute immediate hypersensitivity reaction occurring as a result of the rapid release of inflammatory mediators from mast cells. Affected horses may develop acute respiratory distress, cardiovascular collapse, and death.

SYNONYM(S)

- Anaphylactic shock
- Acute anaphylaxis
- Type I hypersensitivity

EPIDEMIOLOGY

RISK FACTORS

- Previous exposure and sensitization to antigens suspected to cause allergies increases the risk, but this is not always recognized.
- May be triggered by antigens in vaccines, hormones, antibiotics, or antiparasitic agents.
- IV penicillin may trigger acute anaphylaxis in horses.
- Geography and seasonality: Insect-related anaphylaxis may be a summer disease.

CLINICAL PRESENTATION

DISEASE FORMS/SUBTYPES

- Anaphylactoid reactions: Under some circumstances, mast cell degranulation may occur in the absence of immunoglobulin E (IgE) antibodies and without prior sensitization. Thus these reactions do not require previous exposure to antigens.
- Anaphylactic reactions: Occur when an antigen (allergen) binds to IgE molecules located on the mast cell surface. These IgE molecules are induced by prior exposure to allergens.

HISTORY, CHIEF COMPLAINT

- Recent exposure to an inciting allergen
- Severe pruritus with urticaria
- Severe respiratory distress
- Excitement and ataxia
- Collapse
- Angioneurotic edema and laminitis may also develop

PHYSICAL EXAM FINDINGS

- Generalized wheals
- Weakness
- Poor pulse quality
- Tachycardia
- Severe dyspnea
- Collapse and coma

ETIOLOGY AND PATHOPHYSIOLOGY

Anaphylactic reactions
- Initial exposure to an allergen results in a Th2 response and the production of IgE antibodies. These antibodies bind to Fc receptors on the surface of mast cells and basophils.
- Subsequent exposure of the primed animal to the antigen results in antigen binding to the bound IgE and signaling to the mast cells and basophils, resulting in their rapid degranulation.
- Granules release the primary mediators, notably histamine and heparin.
- Degranulated cells synthesize secondary mediators, namely prostaglandins and leukotrienes, through the arachidonic acid cascade.
- Within a few hours, degranulated cells synthesize multiple cytokines, notably interleukin (IL)-4 and IL-13.
- The initial stages include acute hypotension combined with pulmonary arterial hypertension coinciding with histamine release. In a second phase, beginning about 3 minutes after exposure, venous blood pressure increases, coinciding with serotonin release. About 8 to 12 minutes after exposure, a third phase begins characterized by a reflex increase in blood pressure and alternating apnea and dyspnea. Subsequently, prostaglandin and leukotriene release lead to a phase of prolonged hypotension.
- The changes in vascular tone, increased vascular permeability, and bronchospasm lead to pulmonary congestion, edema, emphysema, and eventual death from hypoxia.

Anaphylactoid reactions
- Exposure to antigen leads to activation of the complement system, leading to the production of the peptides C3a and C5a.
- These peptides trigger mast cell and basophil degranulation and the release of mediator molecules.
- Mediator molecules, especially histamine, cause rapid smooth muscle contraction, especially in the respiratory and digestive tracts.
- Bronchoconstriction causes dyspnea, suffocation, collapse, and death.
- Severe rapid constriction of gastrointestinal smooth muscle leads to acute abdominal discomfort and colic.
- Heparin may prevent blood coagulation and lead to subsequent hemorrhage.
- Mast cell release of mediators within the skin may lead to localized swelling, urticaria, and pruritus.

DIAGNOSIS

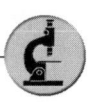

- Diagnosis is based on history and physical examination findings.
- Anaphylaxis may cause severe dyspnea, distress, recumbency, and convulsions.
- Death may occur in less than 10 minutes but more commonly takes about 1 hour. Time is of the essence.

DIFFERENTIAL DIAGNOSIS

- Shock
- Pulmonary edema
- Heart disease
- Acute colic

INITIAL DATABASE

The complete blood count may show an increase in packed cell volume and neutropenia. Serum electrolytes may show high potassium.

TREATMENT

THERAPEUTIC GOAL(S)

- Remove the offending allergen.
- Provide respiratory and cardiovascular support.
- Antagonize allergic mediators.

ACUTE GENERAL TREATMENT

- Initiate treatment immediately. Delay may be fatal.
- Epinephrine (0.1 mg/kg) to treat hypotension and bronchoconstriction. Give IM or one-fifth of the dose IV. This often works very rapidly, and the effect persists for 1 to 3 hours.
- Corticosteroids may potentiate the effects of epinephrine.
- Establish an airway in horses with upper airway obstruction or laryngeal edema.
- Give oxygen therapy.
- Bronchodilation if dyspnea persists after epinephrine administration: Aminophylline (15 mg/kg PO twice daily).

CHRONIC TREATMENT

- If the patient shows only mild signs of dyspnea or skin lesions, treatment may include:
  - Glucocorticoid therapy: Dexamethasone sodium phosphate
  - Antihistamine therapy (of questionable utility)

POSSIBLE COMPLICATION

Cardiac arrhythmias

RECOMMENDED MONITORING

- Monitor frequently for 24 hours after reaction.
- Monitor heart rate, respiratory rate and effort, pulse rate and quality, and mucous membrane color.

PROGNOSIS AND OUTCOME

Immediate recognition and prompt epinephrine therapy are critical to success. Death may occur within minutes in severe cases.

PEARLS & CONSIDERATIONS

PREVENTION

- Administer all IV medications slowly.
- Be aware that many therapeutic agents, especially those containing proteins such as vaccines, may cause anaphylaxis.
- It is best not to administer potential allergens to patients with a history of allergic reactions to an agent.

CLIENT EDUCATION

After an animal is sensitized, allergen avoidance is the only sure method of prevention.

SUGGESTED READING

Eyre P: Preliminary studies of pharmacological antagonism of anaphylaxis in the horse. *Can J Comp Med* 40:149–152, 1976.

Hanna CJ, Eyre P, Wells PW, et al: Equine immunology 2: immunopharmacology—biochemical basis of hypersensitivity. *Equine Vet J* 14:16–24, 1982.

Nielsen IL, Jacobs KA, Huntington PJ, et al: Adverse reaction to procaine penicillin G in horses. *Aust Vet J* 65:181–185, 1988.

AUTHOR & EDITOR: **IAN TIZARD**

Anemia, Equine Infectious

BASIC INFORMATION

DEFINITION

Equine infectious anemia (EIA) A viral infection of Equids caused by a lentivirus and characterized by inapparent infections and occasional clinical disease with recurrent episodes of fever, lethargy, inappetence, thrombocytopenia, and anemia

SYNONYM(S)

- Swamp fever
- Coggins disease
- EIA

EPIDEMIOLOGY

SPECIES, AGE, SEX

- No known age, gender, or breed predisposition
- Affects horses, ponies, donkeys, mules, and zebras

CONTAGION AND ZOONOSIS

- Spread by transfer of blood or body fluids
  - Most commonly transmitted by large biting horseflies and deerflies.
  - Stable flies may also be involved in transmission.
  - Insects are mechanical vectors, and the virus lives only a limited amount of time on vector mouthparts.
  - Iatrogenic infections are common through use of common needles or contaminated equipment.
  - A recent outbreak in Ireland suggests the possibility of direct or indirect horse-to-horse transmission without vectors or iatrogenic infection.
- Not zoonotic

GEOGRAPHY AND SEASONALITY

- Present worldwide
- Prevalence highest in regions with warm climates and large numbers of potential vector insects
- In the United States, most common in Gulf Coast states

CLINICAL PRESENTATION

DISEASE FORMS/SUBTYPES

- Acute disease causes fever, lethargy, and inappetence with mild thrombocytopenia.
- Inapparent infection with no recognizable clinical signs is most common.
- Chronic disease is associated with recurrent episodes of fever with weight loss, ventral edema, and petechial hemorrhages.

HISTORY, CHIEF COMPLAINT

- Fever, weight loss, petechial hemorrhages
- Inapparent carriers often identified at time of routine surveillance testing

PHYSICAL EXAM FINDINGS

- Acute disease: Fever, lethargy
- Inapparent carrier: Minimal recognizable clinical signs
- Chronic disease: Fever, ventral nonpainful pitting edema, petechial hemorrhages, poor body condition

ETIOLOGY AND PATHOPHYSIOLOGY

- EIA virus is a member of the lentivirus genus of the Retroviridae family.
- Establishes persistent, lifelong infection in Equids.
- The virus undergoes antigenic variation with resultant recurring episodes of fever and viremia.
- The immune system ultimately controls viral replication in most horses, resulting in inapparent carriers with minimal signs of disease.
- Uncontrolled viral replication results in signs of chronic disease.
- Anemia and thrombocytopenia probably result from immune- and non–immune-mediated peripheral destruction of erythrocytes and platelets as well as impaired bone marrow production of new cells.

DIAGNOSIS

DIFFERENTIAL DIAGNOSIS

- Any chronic infectious or inflammatory disease
- Purpura hemorrhagica
- Equine viral arteritis
- African horse sickness

INITIAL DATABASE

- Acute disease: Thrombocytopenia most common; possibly mild anemia
- Inapparent carriers: Minimal abnormalities on routine bloodwork; possible mild hyperglobulinemia
- Chronic disease: Evidence of chronic infection, inflammation
  - Anemia
  - Leukocytosis caused by mature neutrophilia
  - Hyperfibrinogenemia
  - Hyperglobulinemia
  - Monocytosis
  - Thrombocytosis

ADVANCED OR CONFIRMATORY TESTING

- In the United States, all testing must be done at diagnostic laboratories approved by the U.S. Department of Agriculture (USDA).
- A positive serologic infection confirms infection in adult horses. Foals from

seropositive mares may be seropositive from passive antibody transfer for up to 12 months.

- Serologic assays must be approved by the USDA for diagnosis.
  - Agar gel immunodiffusion (AGID or Coggins' test): Rare false-negative results
  - Enzyme-linked immunosorbent assay (ELISA): Occasional false-positive results
  - Western immunoblot: May be used as a confirmatory test for horses with equivocal AGID or ELISA results

TREATMENT

THERAPEUTIC GOAL(S)

- Supportive and symptomatic care may be considered during febrile, viremic episodes.
- Most seropositive, infected horses are euthanized.

ACUTE GENERAL TREATMENT

- No effective antiviral therapy is available.
- General, supportive care depending on the severity of clinical signs should be provided.

PROGNOSIS AND OUTCOME

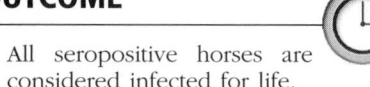

- All seropositive horses are considered infected for life.
- Most seropositive horses show minimal clinical signs and may live a normal life span with the infection.
- In the United States, federal and state laws dictate the response to a positive serologic test.
  - Seropositive horses must be placed under quarantine within 24 hours after the positive test results are known.
  - The quarantine area must provide at least 200 yards of separation from all other Equids.
  - A confirmatory test is performed.
  - Seropositive reactor horses must be permanently identified using the

National Uniform Tag code number assigned by the USDA to the state in which the reactor was tested followed by the letter A. This identification may take the form of a hot brand, chemical brand, freeze marking, or lip tattoo and must be applied by a USDA representative.
  - Reactor horses must be separated and removed from the herd by euthanasia, slaughter, or quarantine at the premises of origin.
  - Reactor horses may only move interstate under official permit to a federally inspected slaughter facility, to a federally approved diagnostic or research facility, or to return to the premises of origin.
  - After a reactor is detected in a herd and removed, testing for the disease must be performed on all horses on the premises and repeated until all remaining Equids on the premises test negative. These horses must be retested at 30- to 60-day intervals until no new cases are found.
  - Quarantine on the premises is released when test results for the entire herd have been negative at least 60 days after the reactor Equids have been removed.

PEARLS & CONSIDERATIONS

PREVENTION

- There is no effective vaccine to prevent EIA.
- The United States has an established federal and state prevention plan based on serosurveillance:
  - All Equids being moved interstate must have been tested for EIA with a negative result within 12 months before movement.
  - All Equids sold, traded, or donated within a state must have been tested negative for EIA no more than 12 months before a change in ownership and, preferably, no more than 60 to 90 days.
  - All Equids entering horse auctions or sales markets are required to

have a negative test result before sale or the horse must be held in quarantine within the state until the test results are known.
- It is recommended that horse owners implement the following EIA control measures.
  - Test all horses at least every 12 months as part of a routine health program. More frequent testing may be indicated in some areas with a high incidence.
  - Owners of Equids entering exhibitions or competitive events should present proof to event officials of a negative EIA test result.
  - All new Equids introduced into a herd should have a negative EIA test result before entry or be isolated on the farm while test results are pending.
  - Vector control practices, including application of insecticides and repellants and environmental insect control, should be implemented.
  - Good hygiene and disinfection principles should be maintained to prevent iatrogenic infection of horses with contaminated needles, syringes, or equipment.

CLIENT EDUCATION

All horse owners should be advised of the importance of maintaining an EIA prevention program as described above and encouraged to test all horses at least annually.

SUGGESTED READING

Mealey RH: Equine infectious anemia. In Sellon DC, Long MT, editors: *Equine infectious diseases*, St Louis, 2007, Elsevier, pp 396–404.

United States Department of Agriculture, Animal and Plant Health Inspection Service: *Equine infectious anemia: uniform methods and rules*. Available at http://www.aphis.usda.gov/vs/nahss/equine/eia/eia_umr_jan_10_2007.pdf.

AUTHOR: DEBRA C. SELLON

EDITORS: DEBRA C. SELLON and **MAUREEN T. LONG**

Anemia, Immune-Mediated

BASIC INFORMATION

DEFINITION

Anemia resulting from a loss of erythrocytes caused by increased destruction by autoantibodies and complement.

SYNONYM(S)

- Autoimmune hemolytic anemia
- Immune-mediated hemolytic anemia (IMHA)

EPIDEMIOLOGY

- Acute anemia resulting from autoimmune attack by antibodies directed against erythrocyte membrane antigens.

- May be triggered by infection with *Streptococcus fecalis*. In these cases, immunoglobulin M (IgM) cold agglutinins clump red blood cells (RBCs) from normal horses when chilled.
  - May occur in horses with lymphosarcoma and melanoma

ASSOCIATED CONDITIONS AND DISORDERS Thrombocytopenia (see "Thrombocytopenia, Immune-Mediated" in this section)

CLINICAL PRESENTATION

HISTORY, CHIEF COMPLAINT
- Pallor, weakness, depression, anorexia
- Anemia, lethargy, weakness
- Inappetence and anorexia
- Icterus
- Discolored urine (hemoglobinuria)

PHYSICAL EXAM FINDINGS
- Weakness and depression
- Pale mucous membranes
- Icterus
- Tachycardia
- Tachypnea or dyspnea
- Chronic anemia may result in cardiac dilation and development of a hemic murmur
- Pyrexia
- Splenomegaly
- Hemoglobinuria

ETIOLOGY AND PATHOPHYSIOLOGY
- Most cases are the result of apparently spontaneous production of anti-erythrocyte autoantibodies. These autoantibodies bind to erythrocytes and trigger their destruction.
- Some cases may be associated with infections or the presence of lymphoid neoplasia.
- Antibodies may target erythrocyte antigens directly (primary IMHA).
- Alternatively, antibodies may target modified erythrocyte membranes. These membranes may be modified by drugs or other infectious agents (secondary IMHA).
- Extravascular hemolysis may result in splenomegaly.
- Intravascular hemolysis may also occur.
- Liver and other organ damage may result from ischemia.

DIAGNOSIS

DIFFERENTIAL DIAGNOSIS
- Blood loss for other reasons
- Bleeding disorder
- Bone marrow failure
- Anemia of chronic disease
- Hepatitis
- Biliary obstruction
- Hemolytic toxins

INITIAL DATABASE
- Complete blood count with packed cell volume (PCV), erythrocyte number, hemoglobin content, and RBC morphology. Reticulocyte counts are not usually informative.
- Check for autoagglutination, spherocytosis, polychromasia, anisocytosis, reticulocytosis, and increased erythrocyte fragility.
- Serum may be discolored because of hemoglobinemia.
- Serum chemistry profile with total protein, baseline bilirubin, serum electrolytes, and serum liver and kidney enzymes.
- Urinalysis as a measure of renal function.
- Coagulation panel.

ADVANCED OR CONFIRMATORY TESTING

Direct antibody test (Coomb's test) or flow cytometry

TREATMENT

THERAPEUTIC GOAL(S)
- Maintenance of oxygen-carrying capacity
- Prevention of additional RBC loss
- Replacement of lost RBCs
- Immunosuppression

ACUTE GENERAL TREATMENT
- Packed RBC transfusion if anemia is severe (tachycardia, tachypnea, weakness)
- Dexamethasone sodium phosphate solution (0.08 mg/kg) PO once daily. After a response is obtained, progressively decrease to 0.02 mg/kg/day.
- Alternatively, 1 mg/kg/day PO prednisolone
- IV crystalloids

CHRONIC TREATMENT

Continued immunosuppression with dexamethasone and tapering doses if hematocrit remains stable

POSSIBLE COMPLICATIONS
- Adverse drug side-effects.
- Steroid-induced laminitis.
- In extreme cases of anemia, irreversible renal damage may prevent complete recovery.

RECOMMENDED MONITORING
- During acute crisis, PCV should be assessed two to three times daily.
- After the patient is stabilized, PCV should be monitored weekly for at least 1 month.

PROGNOSIS AND OUTCOME

Animals generally respond well, so the prognosis is good; however, relapses are common.

PEARLS & CONSIDERATIONS

Clients should be counseled to watch for signs of relapse.

SUGGESTED READING

Davis EG, Wilkerson MJ, Rush BR: Flow cytometry: clinical applications in equine medicine. *J Vet Intern Med* 16:404–410, 2002.

McConnico RS, Roberts MC, Tompkins M: Penicillin-induced immune-mediated hemolytic anemia in a horse. *J Am Vet Med Assoc* 201:1402–1403, 1992.

Robbins RL, Wallace SS, Brunner CJ, et al: Immune-mediated hemolytic disease after penicillin therapy in a horse. *Equine Vet J* 25:462–465, 1993.

Thomas HL, Livesey MA: Immune-mediated hemolytic anemia associated with trimethoprim-sulphamethoxazole administration in a horse. *Can Vet J* 39:171–173, 1998.

Weiss DJ, Moritz A: Equine immune-mediated hemolytic anemia associated with *Clostridium perfringens* infection. *Vet Clin Pathol* 32:22–26, 2003.

Wilkerson MJ, Davis E, Shuman W, et al: Isotype-specific antibodies in horses and dogs with immune-mediated hemolytic anemia. *J Vet Intern Med* 14:190–196, 2000.

AUTHOR & EDITOR: IAN TIZARD

Angular Limb Deformity

BASIC INFORMATION

DEFINITION

Angular limb deformities (ALDs) result in a limb deviation in the frontal plane either toward (varus) or away (valgus) from the body. They are often bilateral and are usually associated with growth centers, especially the epiphysis, but they can be diaphyseal. Not all ALDs are abnormal.

SYNONYM(S)

- Knock knees
- Cow hocks
- Toeing in or toeing out

EPIDEMIOLOGY

GENETICS AND BREED PREDISPOSITION

- Anecdotal evidence suggests ALD is genetic, but this is unproven.
- ALDs are most common in light-breed horses with fast growth rates such as Thoroughbreds and Quarter Horses, but they may occur in any breed.

RISK FACTORS

- Prematurity or dysmaturity, ligamentous laxity.
- For "windswept" foals, small uterine size in the mother and a lack of fetal activity are considered possible causes.

ASSOCIATED CONDITIONS AND DISORDERS
Some degree of limb rotation is often associated with ALD. Inward rotation is usually associated with varus and outward rotation with valgus. Although most ALDs are bilaterally symmetrical, an uncommon manifestation of congenital ALD is windswept foals, in which paired limbs are deviated in one direction. Rarely, ALDs are the result of severe congenital developmental bone disorders.

CLINICAL PRESENTATION

DISEASE FORMS/SUBTYPES

- The most common congenital ALD is carpal valgus followed by fetlock valgus and varus.
- Much rarer is tibial valgus followed by varus.

HISTORY, CHIEF COMPLAINT

- Congenital ALD may worsen during the first week of life because of the effects of gravity and asymmetric weight bearing.
- Severely affected foals may have difficulty nursing and ambulating.

PHYSICAL EXAM FINDINGS
Uncomplicated ALD in a neonate should not result in lameness or periarticular swelling. If caused by epiphyseal or physeal dysplasia, the limb examination results are normal but the deviation cannot be corrected manually. If caused by epiphyseal ligamentous laxity, the deviation can be corrected manually.

ETIOLOGY AND PATHOPHYSIOLOGY

- Most congenital ALDs are caused by some degree of immaturity of soft and hard tissues of limbs and possibly in utero positioning.
- The impact of genetics is more likely the result of breed influence for slender limbs and fast growth rather than an individual parent's impact.

DIAGNOSIS

DIFFERENTIAL DIAGNOSIS

- Uncomplicated limb deviations
- ALD caused by severe laxity
- ALD caused by prematurity or dysmaturity
- Congenital limb malformation

INITIAL DATABASE

The limbs should be checked for ligamentous laxity and foot balance. Radiographs should be obtained of severe deviations or in foals in which cuboidal bone hypoplasia is suspected.

ADVANCED OR CONFIRMATORY TESTING

Computed tomography or magnetic resonance imaging can be used to characterize deviations in cross-sectional anatomy but is rarely necessary.

TREATMENT

THERAPEUTIC GOAL(S)

- Most ALDs improve as the foal matures, as long as there is no persistent uneven limb loading. Allowing appropriate exercise is the most important management strategy in the treatment of ALDs (Figure 1).
- Foals with severe ligamentous laxity should have splints or casts applied to properly align the limb and protect the lax ligaments from additional stretching. Coaptation will also protect bones from asymmetric loading that may result in added stretching and bone crushing (Figure 2).

ACUTE GENERAL TREATMENT

- Balance the foot.
- Provide enough exercise to promote musculoskeletal development but not enough to result in excessive asymmetric weight bearing and further

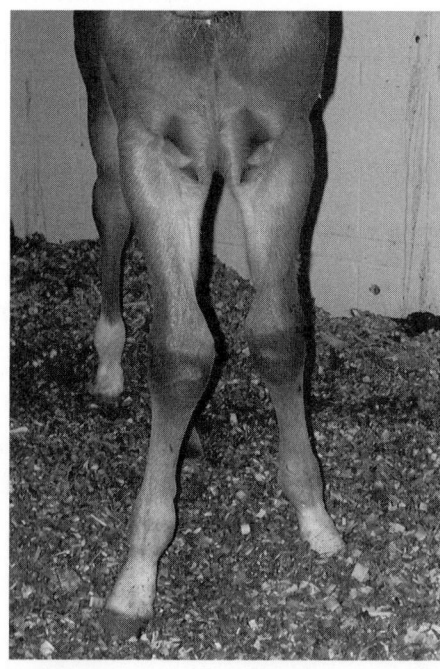

FIGURE 1 Six-week-old foal with significant bilateral carpal valgus deformity; right worse than left with outward rotation deviations. Full evaluation of these deviations requires radiography. (Courtesy Dr. Joanne Kramer.)

DISEASES AND
DISORDERS

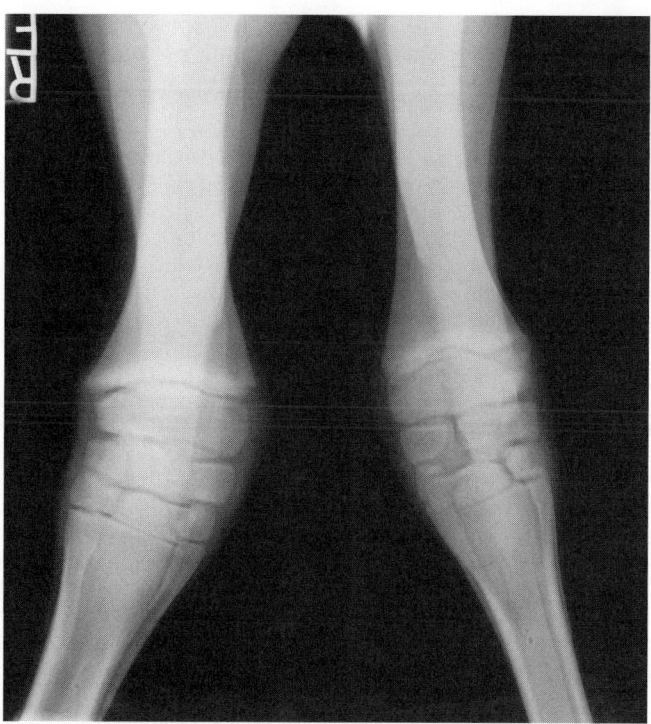

FIGURE 2 Dorsopalmar radiograph of both forelimbs of the foal in Figure 1. Abnormalities apparent include greater than 20 degrees of carpal valgus and mild crushing of the lateral aspect of the epiphysis and the lateral styloid process of the right forelimb and approximately 10 degrees of carpal valgus in the left forelimb. (Courtesy Dr. Joanne Kramer.)

bone damage. Foals with hypoplastic carpal bones should have exercise limited to a large stall and may require external coaptation if immaturity is severe to protect the delicate cartilage model for the mature bone.
- For fetlock inward deviations, the addition of lateral hoof augmentation to promote central foot breakover and to limit lateral hoof wall wear can be curative if applied early enough.
- Foals with ligamentous laxity require splints or casts to protect the limb and require stall confinement.

CHRONIC TREATMENT
- Surgical therapy may be helpful later in life for some congenital ALDs.
- If maturation and exercise restriction are not sufficient to correct the limb

deviation, either periosteal elevation (PE) or transphyseal bridging (TB) may be used to correct limb deviations. PE can be done at any age and may have some mild corrective effect. TB is done usually no sooner than 14 days of age because the bone must mature enough to hold the implants. The efficacy of both procedures relies on remaining growth potential in the growth plate, which is greater in younger foals. For distal metacarpal or metatarsal deformities, procedures should be done at less than 60 days. For distal radial deformities, correction can be obtained as late as 12 months, although moderate to severe deformities require earlier intervention.

POSSIBLE COMPLICATIONS
The most severe complication of ALD is permanent deformation of the bones of the limb, which will result in lifelong lameness and abnormal locomotion.

RECOMMENDED MONITORING
No specific monitoring besides visual examination is necessary for most foals with ALD. However, if limb deviations do not improve, radiographic examination is warranted.

PROGNOSIS AND OUTCOME
- The vast majority of carpal valgus in foals will correct as the foals mature. Fetlock and carpal varus deviations are more problematic and may require more aggressive intervention.
- Foals with hypoplastic bones or ligamentous laxity must be treated early and carefully to avoid permanent limb deformity.

PEARLS & CONSIDERATIONS

COMMENTS
ALDs are very common in young foals, and most self-correct. Intervention is only necessary in a small number of cases.

CLIENT EDUCATION
All foals should have a veterinary examination within 24 hours of birth to asses their overall health and determine appropriate passive transfer. Also important is a musculoskeletal examination to determine the foals' suitability for exercise.

SUGGESTED READING
Santschi EM, Leibsle SR, Morehead JP, et al: Carpal and fetlock conformation of the juvenile Thoroughbred from birth to yearling auction. *Eq Vet J* 38:604–609, 2006.

AUTHOR: **ELIZABETH M. SANTSCHI**

EDITORS: **PHOEBE A. SMITH** and **ELIZABETH M. SANTSCHI**

Anthrax

BASIC INFORMATION

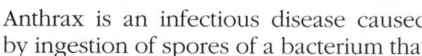

DEFINITION
Anthrax is an infectious disease caused by ingestion of spores of a bacterium that

multiplies upon inoculation or ingestion and secretes lethal toxins. A spore is a refractile or stainable structure of a microorganism formed as a hypobiotic stage in the organism's life cycle that

allows survival in environmental extremes. The vegetative form is a structure of a microorganism that develops when environmental conditions allow asexual reproduction or multiplication.

SYNONYM(S)

Wool sorter's disease, carbon fever, splenic fever

EPIDEMIOLOGY

SPECIES, AGE, SEX No predilection. Susceptibility to disease is greatest for cattle followed by sheep and then horses and goats. Pigs frequently develop clinical anthrax after exposure to *Bacillus anthracis* but are the only species that may spontaneously recover (many still die).

RISK FACTORS Geography, soil, water conditions

CONTAGION AND ZOONOSIS

- The zoonotic risk of *B. anthracis* cannot be minimized, and the occupational risk of infection of veterinarians is very high compared with the risk of intentional human-to-human transmission. Personal protection when handling anthrax-suspected animals should be complete, including gloves, boots, protective suits, and respiratory and eye protection. This protection must be maintained throughout all environmental and equipment decontamination processes. Complete bathing is recommended after handling any tissues or animals.
- In some situations, prophylactic antibiotic therapy is recommended if exposure is thought to be high or inadvertent through improper attention to personal protection. Animal hide, hair, and wool can contain spores, and people at occupational risk should seek immediate medical attention if skin or respiratory signs occur.

GEOGRAPHY AND SEASONALITY

- Climatic stressors allow reliable prediction of anthrax outbreaks. With climatic change, outbreaks of anthrax occur in infection cycles. A harbinger of infection or primary infection cycle occurs with the sudden death of one or two animals that have been recently introduced into an area. These infected carcasses contaminate the soil with *B. anthracis*. The secondary infection cycle involves multiple animals that develop anthrax after exposure to contaminated soil or carcasses from the primary infection cycle.
- Anthrax in local cattle is usually observed within the same time period.

CLINICAL PRESENTATION

DISEASE FORMS/SUBTYPES

- Cutaneous
- Respiratory
- Septicemic
- Sudden death

HISTORY, CHIEF COMPLAINT Sudden death in an appropriate geographic location

PHYSICAL EXAM FINDINGS

- Although not as frequently diagnosed with *B. anthracis* infection as cattle, horses do develop disease and die from anthrax. After an incubation period of about 3 to 7 days (can be as short as 1 day or as long as 7 days), horses usually develop the acute form of anthrax, although sudden death may occur. Initial clinical signs frequently include colic with presenting signs that may resemble those of acute enteritis. These horses rapidly progress to high fever with dyspnea. Subcutaneous edema of the ventral neck, thorax, and abdomen may be seen, especially with mediastinal involvement. Ventral edema involving the prepuce and mammary gland is postulated to be secondary to local transmission from insects.
- If an animal dies of disease consistent with anthrax in an endemic area, it is best not to open the carcass. Not only is this important for human safety, but it is also exceptionally important for long-term control by minimizing environmental contamination. Collection of blood in a closed system or a splenic aspirate obtained percutaneously is recommended to facilitate confirmation of the diagnosis. Blood clots poorly in affected animals, so a sample may be obtained for an extended time after death.
- Postmortem analysis is not recommended. The pathologic hallmark of anthrax is the absence of rigor mortis, with passage of blood from body orifices. Petechiae and ecchymoses are widespread, with large quantities of blood-stained serous fluid within body cavities. Severe mediastinal edema, enteritis, and splenomegaly are common. In particular, the spleen has a "blackberry jam" appearance.

ETIOLOGY AND PATHOPHYSIOLOGY

- *B. anthracis* infection
- Evasion of the immune system, rapid vegetative proliferation, and elaboration of toxin are critical steps in the pathogenesis of anthrax.
- The mammalian incubation period is 1 to 7 days for respiratory and gastrointestinal anthrax.
- Ingestion is likely the primary route of inoculation, with a break in the mucous membranes important.
- There is an initial round of primary replication in the regional lymph nodes.
- The organism enters the bloodstream through lymphatic drainage, with resultant bacteremia, septicemia, toxemia, and dissemination to all major organs.
- Anthrax toxin has three components: Protective antigen (PA), lethal factor (LF), and edema factor (EF).
  - PA molecule binds to the cell surface and is the target of antiserum.
  - LF mediates the fatal effect of *B. anthracis*.
  - EF causes extravasation of intercellular fluids into subcutaneous and peritoneal compartments and interstitial spaces.
  - A combination of PA and LF must be present for lethality.
  - Complexing of EF and PA produces edema.
  - When all three toxin components are present, the organism causes necrosis of cells with edema and is lethal.

DIAGNOSIS

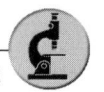

DIFFERENTIAL DIAGNOSIS

- Sudden death
- Sepsis
- Systemic inflammatory response syndrome (SIRS) or endotoxemia

INITIAL DATABASE

- With sudden death or a short course of fatal disease in suspect cases, a blood smear is safest.
- New methylene blue stain shows chains of large, square, gram-positive rods.

ADVANCED OR CONFIRMATORY TESTING

- If a sample for culture is obtained, initial identification of *B. anthracis* is through the basic microbiologic features discussed.
- Much safer for laboratory personnel is the inoculation of guinea pigs for lethality or fluorescent antibody testing of smears of froth, blood, or splenic aspirate.
- Serologic and molecular-based techniques are important for identification of the specific strain of *B. anthracis*.
- Strain typing to determine the origin of exposure in humans is a priority when bioterrorism is suspected.
- Molecular-based techniques have been developed for environmental monitoring and likely pose an alternative to inadvertent culture of body fluids.

TREATMENT

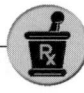

THERAPEUTIC GOAL(S)

Prevent death

ACUTE GENERAL TREATMENT

- Anthrax is rapidly fatal in horses, and it is unlikely that there would be an opportunity for therapy of an animal showing clinical signs at diagnosis.

- Careful examination of other exposed animals for disease should be performed. Close monitoring of any exposed horses may result in timely administration of antimicrobial agents.
- Antimicrobials recommended for prevention and treatment of anthrax include penicillin, tetracyclines, and fluoroquinolones.
- Recent outbreaks in humans support the use of fluoroquinolones as a first-line antimicrobial in suspected *B. anthracis* infection.
- IV administration is highly recommended. Single or short-duration administration of prophylactic antibiotics is recommended for exposed humans and is an option for horses.
- Supportive care is essential and consists of cardiovascular support in the form of fluid and oncotic therapy. Intranasal oxygen may alleviate signs of dyspnea.

RECOMMENDED MONITORING
- Limit access to body fluids.
- Limit access to hemolymphatic system.
- Do not perform a necropsy.

PROGNOSIS AND OUTCOME

Extremely poor

PEARLS & CONSIDERATIONS

PREVENTION
- Vaccines are available for the prevention of anthrax in cattle in some countries outside the United States.
- Cattle vaccines in horses are not recommended in the guidelines of the American Association of Equine Practitioners. Injection site reactions and severe edema after vaccination have been described.
- If *B. anthracis* is identified or suspected in horses, implement methods to prevent additional disease in horses and to minimize risk of human disease.
- Animals should have all external debris removed by thorough bathing with soap and water.
  - May use a 0.5% hypochlorite solution.

- Move animals away from sites that have been exposed to anthrax-laden carcasses.
- The World Health Organization recommends incineration of closed carcasses as the best method of disposal.
- Ensure complete incineration, including the ventral parts of the carcass.
- The soil from the site can be burned separately from the carcass or actually torched.

CLIENT EDUCATION
- Education regarding veterinarian evaluation of animals that die inexplicably and suddenly
- Education on zoonoses for persons living in endemic areas

SUGGESTED READING
American Veterinary Medical Association: *Anthrax Facts.* Available at http://www.avma.org/public_health/biosecurity/anthrax_facts.asp.

AUTHOR: MAUREEN T. LONG

EDITORS: **DEBRA C. SELLON** and **MAUREEN T. LONG**

Aortic Aneurysm

BASIC INFORMATION

DEFINITION
Localized abnormal dilation of the aorta that can be congenital or acquired. May occur at the aortic sinus or in the thoracic or abdominal aorta.

EPIDEMIOLOGY
SPECIES, AGE, SEX More common in males than females

CLINICAL PRESENTATION
DISEASE FORMS/SUBTYPES
- Intact aneurysm: May not cause clinical signs.
- Ruptured aneurysms: Clinical signs vary depending on the location (intracardiac, thoracic, or abdominal).

HISTORY, CHIEF COMPLAINT
- Depends on the location and etiopathology:
  - Sinus of Valsalva: Condition is asymptomatic until the aneurysm ruptures (see "Aortocardiac Fistula" in this section)
  - Intrathoracic: Signs of right-sided congestive heart failure, recumbency, shortness of breath, distress,

collapse, cardiovascular collapse, or sudden death
  - Intraabdominal: Colic, lameness, or sudden death

PHYSICAL EXAM FINDINGS
- Intact aneurysm: may be found incidentally; may or may not have a murmur
- Clinical signs depend on the site of rupture:
  - Intracardiac
    - Acute onset of right-sided heart failure: Ventral edema, jugular vein distension, jugular pulses, congested mucous membranes, decreased capillary refill time, weak arterial pulses
    - Ventricular arrhythmias: Result of disruption of the conduction system
    - Sudden death
  - Intrathoracic
    - Signs of right-sided heart failure: Ventral edema, jugular vein distension, jugular pulses, congested mucous membranes, decreased capillary refill time, weak arterial pulses
    - Sudden death

  - Intraabdominal
    - Hindlimb lameness and colic
    - Sudden death

ETIOLOGY AND PATHOPHYSIOLOGY
- Sinus of Valsalva aneurysms are congenital defects in the media of the wall of the aorta at the right sinus of Valsalva.
- The pathogenesis of equine aortic aneurysms is unknown.
  - Damage to the aortic wall (degeneration of the media followed by degeneration of the elastic tissue) secondary to septic thrombosis, parasitic migration, trauma, arteriosclerosis, bacterial or mycotic infections, cystic or laminar medial necrosis, or a dissecting aneurysm have all been suggested.
- Tears in the aorta may occur at any level.
  - Intracardiac rupture produces an aortocardiac fistula.
  - Rupture within the pericardium produces acute cardiac tamponade and sudden death.
  - Rupture of the extrapericardial aorta leads to fatal hemorrhage or a systemic-to-pulmonary shunt.

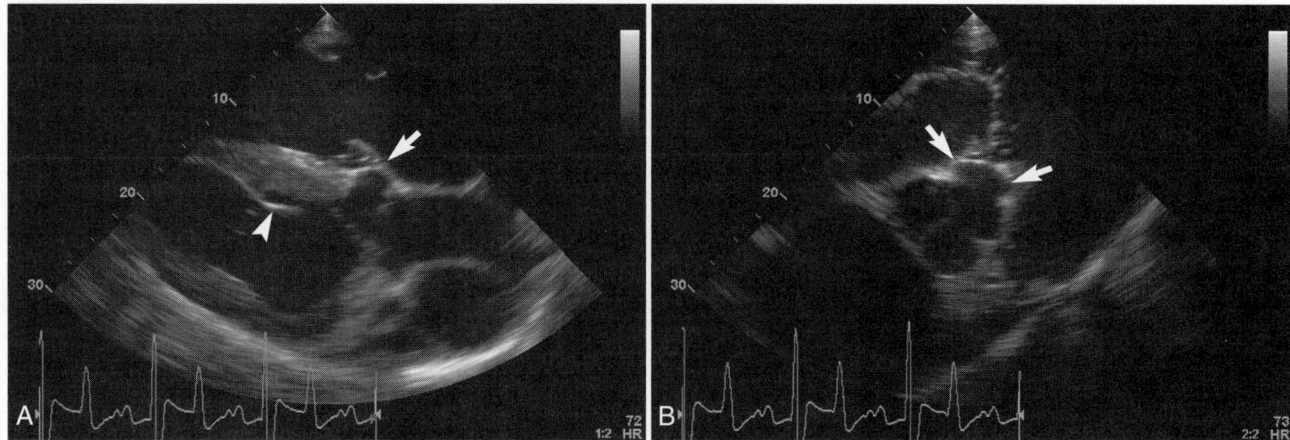

FIGURE 1 Right parasternal echocardiograms of the left ventricular outflow tract. **A,** Long-axis view. Note the thin membranous sac protruding from the sinus of Valsalva into the right atrium (*arrow*) and the dissection of blood along the left ventricular side of the interventricular septum (*arrowhead*). **B,** Short-axis view. Note the thin membranous sac protruding from the sinus of Valsalva into the right atrium (*arrows*).

DIAGNOSIS

DIFFERENTIAL DIAGNOSIS

- Heart failure from other causes
- Abdominal pain

INITIAL DATABASE

Radiology: May detect enlargement of a dilated aortic aneurysm in the aortic arch

ADVANCED OR CONFIRMATORY TESTING

- Echocardiography: Used to detect sinus of Valsalva aneurysm, which is visualized as a thin membranous sac protruding from the sinus of Valsalva at the junction of the membranous septum and the aortic root (Figure 1). Aneurysms of the ascending aorta may be detected with echocardiography.
- Transesophageal echocardiography: May detect aneurysms in the aortic arch and descending aorta.
- Aneurysms in the thoracic or abdominal aorta are usually a postmortem diagnosis.

TREATMENT

THERAPEUTIC GOAL(S)

- There is no treatment for intact aneurysms; horses are not safe to ride.

ACUTE GENERAL TREATMENT

Only symptomatic treatment for intracardiac rupture of a sinus of Valsalva aneurysm (see "Aortocardiac Fistula" in this section)

RECOMMENDED MONITORING

Horses with documented aortic aneurysms should have their attitude, appetite, and vital signs (heart rate and rhythm, respiratory rate and rhythm, and pulse quality) regularly monitored by their owners. In addition, these horses should be periodically auscultated for the presence of new murmurs or a change in character of existing murmurs. Any changes should prompt a complete cardiac workup, including echocardiography and electrocardiography, by a veterinarian.

PROGNOSIS AND OUTCOME

- Extremely grave
- Grave prognosis after identification of an aneurysm because of the high risk of sudden death
- Grave prognosis after rupture of the aneurysm
  - If the aorta ruptures into the thoracic or abdominal cavities, death occurs from rapid hypovolemic shock.
  - If the aorta ruptures into the pericardial sac, hemopericardium, cardiac tamponade, and death occur.
- Horses with intact aneurysms may live for years; however, they are not safe to use as performance horses because of risk of rupture and sudden death.

PEARLS & CONSIDERATIONS

A horse with an aortic aneurysm, regardless of the location, should not be used for riding because of the high risk of sudden death.

SUGGESTED READING

Okamoto M, Kamitani M, Tunoda N, et al: Mycotic aneurysm in the aortic arch of a horse associated with invasive aspergillosis. *Vet Rec* 160:268–270, 2007.

Reef VB: Cardiovascular ultrasonography. In Reef VB, editor: *Equine diagnostic ultrasound*, Philadelphia, 1998, WB Saunders, pp 215–272.

Shirai W, Momotani E, Sato T, et al: Dissecting aortic aneurysm in a horse. *J Comp Path* 120:307–311, 1999.

AUTHOR: **OLGA SECO DIAZ**

EDITOR: **MARY M. DURANDO**

Aortic/Pulmonic Regurgitation, Acquired

BASIC INFORMATION

DEFINITION

- Aortic regurgitation is common in older horses, and the aortic valve is the most common valve diagnosed with pathologic changes (usually nodular or general fibrous thickening of the valve leaflets).
- Pulmonic regurgitation is extremely rarely diagnosed by auscultation; it seldom results in an audible murmur because the pressure difference between the pulmonary circulation and the right ventricle in diastole is too low to produce significant turbulence that will cause a murmur. In addition, only rarely are clinical signs associated with pulmonic regurgitation in horses. Therefore most pulmonic regurgitation is of no relevance for clinicians unless it is severe or associated with bacterial endocarditis. This entry focuses primarily on aortic regurgitation.
- For both the pulmonic and the aortic valve, mild regurgitation detected by Doppler echocardiography occurs in a high proportion of Standardbred and Thoroughbred racehorses (Figure 1). Training-induced myocardial hypertrophy is the most likely reason for this minor regurgitation.

SYNONYM(S)

- Aortic or pulmonic insufficiency
- Aortic or pulmonic valve disease
- Semilunar valve insufficiency or regurgitation

EPIDEMIOLOGY

SPECIES, AGE, SEX Aortic regurgitation occurs commonly in older horses.
GENETICS AND BREED PREDISPOSITION There is no genetic predisposition, but the prevalence of very mild regurgitation is higher in Standardbreds and Thoroughbreds compared with the general horse population.
RISK FACTORS Aortic regurgitation: fenestrations of the aortic valves, membranous ventricular septal defect (VSD), and endocarditis

CLINICAL PRESENTATION

DISEASE FORMS/SUBTYPES

- Aortic regurgitation incidentally diagnosed in clinically normal horses (eg, during a pre-purchase examination)
- Aortic regurgitation causing clinical signs of heart failure, ataxia, or collapse during strenuous exercise in severe cases

HISTORY, CHIEF COMPLAINT

- Aortic regurgitation seldom causes reduced performance or other clinical changes that the owner will notice.
- However, if more severe, exercise intolerance may be reported.

PHYSICAL EXAM FINDINGS

- Diastolic cardiac murmur with the point of maximal intensity (PMI) over the aortic valve at the basal area of the left hemithorax: Because the aortic valve is located centrally in the heart, the murmur is often also heard over the right hemithorax and may radiate over the entire thorax. The murmur is often holosystolic or pansystolic with a decrescendo musical quality and is relatively easy to diagnose in these cases. A fenestration or vibrating portion of the leaflet is usually responsible for the musical quality, which is easily heard. However, the murmur may be harsh or blowing, and if the heart sounds are engulfed by the murmur, it may be difficult to differentiate from a systolic murmur. In these cases, simultaneous palpation of the peripheral pulse is helpful. The intensity of the murmur does not always correlate with the severity of the disease.
- Depending on the severity, one or more of the following signs may also be observed:
  - Systolic murmur on the left hemithorax over the mitral valve area is indicative of mitral regurgitation.
  - Palpation of the facial artery may reveal a bounding ("water hammer") pulse caused by a large difference between the systolic and the low diastolic pressure. This indicates more hemodynamically significant disease with an enlarged left ventricle.
  - Cardiac arrhythmias
  - Rarely, signs of heart failure may be observed, including one or more of the following: resting tachycardia and tachypnea, distension of the jugular veins, dependent edema, increased respiratory sounds caused by pulmonary edema, prolonged capillary refill time, or weight loss.

ETIOLOGY AND PATHOPHYSIOLOGY

- Most commonly, valvular changes arise because of normal progressive degeneration from aging. The condition is likely to deteriorate with time, but the rate of progression in individual horses is impossible to predict. For older horses, however, this seldom results in clinical signs of poor performance, and the eventual cause of death or euthanasia is seldom because of cardiac disease.
- When aortic regurgitation is diagnosed in younger horses (<10 years), it indicates premature aortic valve disease that may be caused by either complicating factors predisposing to development of aortic regurgitation or valvular malformations. In these situations, a VSD is often present and the right coronary cusp of the aortic valve prolapses into the septal defect, leading to aortic regurgitation. Because the aortic valve seals the septal defect, the

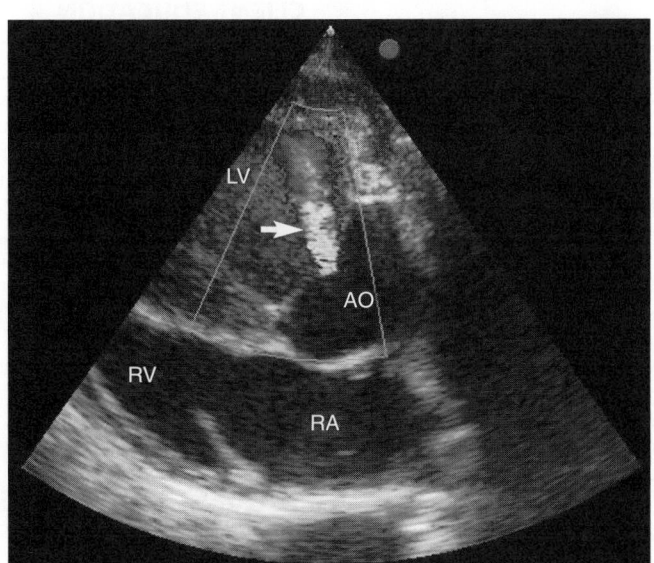

FIGURE 1 Long-axis color-flow Doppler echocardiogram of the aorta obtained from the left cardiac window showing mild aortic regurgitation (*arrow*). *AO*, Aorta; *LV*, left ventricle; *RA*, right atrium; *RV*, right ventricle.

typical murmur associated with a VSD may not be heard.
- Progression of aortic regurgitation leads to volume overload of the left ventricle and dilation and eccentric ventricular hypertrophy with a subsequent increasing myocardial oxygen demand. Blood supply for the myocardium is delivered during diastole via the coronary arteries just above the aortic valve, and as a result of the rapid decrease of diastolic blood pressure, coronary perfusion is reduced. Ischemia of the ventricles may lead to potentially fatal ventricular arrhythmias.
- Secondary to volume overload of the left ventricle, dilation of the mitral valve annulus may occur, leading to mitral valve regurgitation. If this becomes severe, pulmonary hypertension and right heart failure may develop.
- The aortic valve, along with the mitral valve, is the most common location of endocarditis (see "Endocarditis, Infective" in this section); however, the disease is not commonly encountered.
- Murmurs of aortic, mitral, and tricuspid regurgitation are often detected in Standardbred and Thoroughbred racehorses. These murmurs may develop in response to training, and their prevalence increases with age and training. However, the regurgitations are generally mild, the severity remains unchanged over time, and no negative effect on racing performance has been documented.

DIAGNOSIS

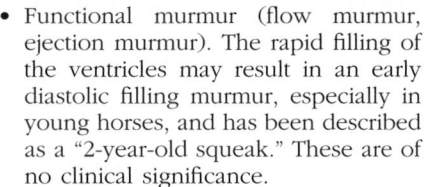

DIFFERENTIAL DIAGNOSIS
- Functional murmur (flow murmur, ejection murmur). The rapid filling of the ventricles may result in an early diastolic filling murmur, especially in young horses, and has been described as a "2-year-old squeak." These are of no clinical significance.
- Endocarditis

INITIAL DATABASE
- Definitive diagnosis of aortic or pulmonic regurgitation requires echocardiographic examination with the regurgitant jet visualized with Doppler echocardiography (see Figure 1).
- The severity of the disease must be assessed by echocardiography. Nodular thickening of the valve is not necessarily related to severity. The most important echocardiographic variables to measure are degree of left ventricular dilation, contractility of the left ventricle, and severity of mitral regurgitation. If mitral regurgitation is

severe, left atrial enlargement is important to note. The size and severity of the regurgitant jet can be estimated by Doppler echocardiography.
- Electrocardiography (ECG) at rest and during exercise is recommended if the horse is used for riding purposes.
- Complete blood count and serum biochemistry are usually unremarkable.

ADVANCED OR CONFIRMATORY TESTING
- Direct or indirect blood pressure measurements should be performed.
- Cardiac output monitoring provides information on the effect of regurgitation and cardiac function on hemodynamic status.

TREATMENT

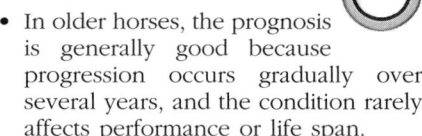

THERAPEUTIC GOAL(S)
- In most equine patients with aortic or pulmonic valve disease, specific therapy is not indicated, and management is aimed at periodic monitoring of the disease progression and cardiac function and providing client information. Because there is a potential risk of developing arrhythmias in association with significant aortic regurgitation, serial echocardiography and exercising ECG are indicated.
- Heart failure rarely develops because of aortic regurgitation, but if it does, supportive therapy may be considered. In general, because of the poor prognosis, treatment of horses in heart failure is often not considered. But for some valuable breeding horses or horses in which the owner has sentimental attachment, treatment can be tried.

ACUTE GENERAL TREATMENT
Supportive treatment of patients in heart failure includes diuretics to reduce congestion (furosemide 1–2 mg/kg IV q12h) in combination with a vasodilator such as an angiotensin-converting enzyme (ACE) inhibitor (enalapril 0.5 mg/kg IV q24h or quinapril 0.25 mg/kg PO q24h). ACE inhibitors have not been extensively studied in horses, although quinapril has been shown to be effective in horses with mitral regurgitation. If severe tachycardia is present, rate control with digoxin can be used at a dose of 0.0022 mg/kg IV q12h or 0.011 mg/kg PO q24h. For more detail on treatment regimens, see "Cardiac Failure" in this section.

CHRONIC TREATMENT
Similar to acute treatment, with drugs and dosages tailored to the individual.

Oral treatment regimens are preferred, if possible (see "Cardiac Failure" in this section).

POSSIBLE COMPLICATIONS
- Reoccurrence of heart failure or no effect of treatment
- Ventricular arrhythmia
- Atrial fibrillation
- Sudden cardiac death

RECOMMENDED MONITORING
- Clinical examination findings such as attitude, appetite, weight, respiratory rate and effort, heart rate, and exercise tolerance should be monitored by the owner regularly. Any changes should prompt a veterinary reexamination.
- Periodic echocardiography to assess progression of regurgitation or heart failure.
- Periodic exercising ECG to determine safety for use as a riding horse.

PROGNOSIS AND OUTCOME

- In older horses, the prognosis is generally good because progression occurs gradually over several years, and the condition rarely affects performance or life span.
- For young and middle-aged horses, the prognosis is more difficult to determine, but if no volume overload or mitral regurgitation is present and the progression during subsequent examinations is slow, the prognosis is considered good.

PEARLS & CONSIDERATIONS

CLIENT EDUCATION
- Regular echocardiographic monitoring and exercising ECG are recommended for horses with aortic regurgitation that are used for riding purposes; the horse should be retired from work when severe left ventricular dilation develops or ventricular arrhythmias occur during exercise.
- Most insurance companies insert a proviso in case of aortic valve regurgitation in young horses. In addition, resale may be considered more risky than for horses without regurgitation. Therefore the sale prices are often reduced in horses with valvular regurgitation greater than mild.

SUGGESTED READING
Buhl R, Ersbøll AK, Eriksen L, et al: Use of color Doppler echocardiography to assess the development of valvular regurgitation in Standardbred Trotters. *J Am Vet Med Assoc* 227:1630–1635, 2005.

Else RW, Holmes JR: Cardiac pathology in the horse. Microscopic pathology. *Equine Vet J* 4:57–62, 1972.

Marr CM: Cardiac murmurs: acquired valvular disease. In Marr CM, editor: *Cardiology of the horse.* Philadelphia, WB Saunders, 1999, pp 232–255.

AUTHOR: **RIKKE BUHL**

EDITOR: **MARY M. DURANDO**

Aortocardiac Fistula

BASIC INFORMATION

DEFINITION

An aortocardiac fistula is a defect in the wall of the aorta at the right aortic sinus. The defect can take the form of a tract dissecting through the aortic ring to the right ventricle (RV), right atrium (RA), or interventricular septum (IVS), or it may occur from aneurysmal dilation of the right aortic sinus (or more rarely in the noncoronary portion of the sinus) rupturing in the RA or RV or creating tracts dissecting through the myocardial septum.

SYNONYM(S)

- Aortic root rupture
- Ruptured aortic sinus aneurysm
- Tear of the aortic root

EPIDEMIOLOGY

SPECIES, AGE, SEX More common in middle-aged and older stallions, although it may affect geldings and mares as well
DISEASE FORMS/SUBTYPES
- Acute rupture
  - Sudden death
  - Distress, ventricular tachycardia, and right-sided murmur
- Subacute or chronic: Right-sided continuous murmur
  - Fistula opening in the RV or RA: Severe RA and RV volume overload leading to right-sided heart failure
  - Fistula dissecting down into the IVS: Form subendocardial tract along the septum that may rupture into RV, LV, or both, causing RV or LV volume overload

HISTORY, CHIEF COMPLAINT

- Acute distress sometimes mistaken for abdominal pain: Restlessness, sweating, and recumbency
- Exercise intolerance
- A murmur detected during routine examination
- Sudden death

PHYSICAL EXAM FINDINGS

- Extreme distress
- Right-sided, loud, continuous murmur
- Tachycardia
- Rapid, weak arterial pulses with pulse deficits
- Bounding arterial pulses
- Jugular venous pulses
- Tachypnea

ETIOLOGY AND PATHOPHYSIOLOGY

- May be congenital or acquired
  - A congenital sinus of Valsalva aneurysm is the underlying defect that precedes aortic rupture in some cases. The defect is believed to be an absence of the tunica media of the aorta in the area of the right sinus of Valsalva (see "Aortic Aneurysm" in this section).
  - May be an acquired lesion caused by increased intraaortic pressure that occurs during strenuous exercise such as racing or breeding in stallions that could be coupled with preexisting degeneration of the aortic media.
  - Degenerative aortic medionecrosis may predispose to aortic ring rupture.
- Aortic rupture into the right side of the heart usually causes severe right heart overload, leading to right heart failure.
- Aortic rupture dissecting through the ventricular septum causes widespread damage to the cardiac conduction system, resulting in rhythm disturbances (usually monomorphic ventricular tachycardia).

DIAGNOSIS

DIFFERENTIAL DIAGNOSIS

- Abdominal pain
- Other congenital or acquired cardiac anomalies

INITIAL DATABASE

- Auscultation: Tachycardia and loud right-sided continuous murmur
- Electrocardiography: Sustained monomorphic ventricular tachycardia with heart rate (HR) of 120 to 240 beats/min in horses presented soon after rupture

ADVANCED OR CONFIRMATORY TESTING

- Echocardiography: Defect in the aortic wall usually affecting the right aortic sinus or ruptured aneurysmal dilation of the aortic wall at this site. The ruptured aneurysm is visualized as a thin membrane fluttering into the RA or RV as blood shunts through the defect (Figure 1). Fistulas may extend to the RV, RA, or LV or dissect along the septal myocardium, appearing as anechoic blood between the septal endocardium and myocardium (Figure 2). The ventricles may appear enlarged from biventricular volume overload.
- Color-flow, pulsed, and continuous-wave Doppler echocardiography: High-velocity continuous blood flow through the aortocardiac fistula into the RA or RV
- Contrast echocardiography: Negative contrast jet from the left side into the right cardiac chambers that otherwise appears echogenic after the injection of the contrast solution into the jugular vein

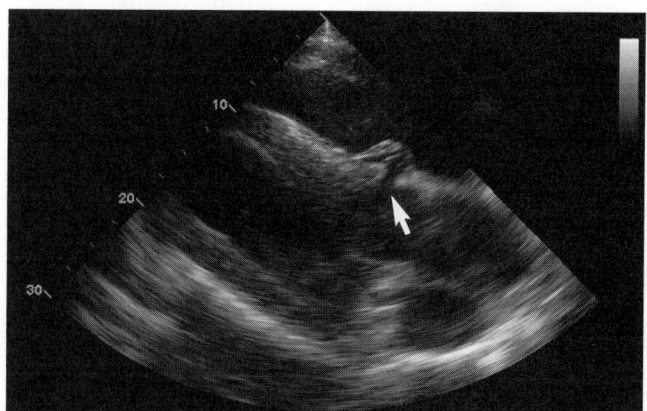

FIGURE 1 Right parasternal long-axis echocardiogram of the left ventricular outflow tract. Note the defect in the wall of the aorta at the right aortic sinus (*arrow*) that appears as a tract dissecting through the aortic ring to the right ventricle.

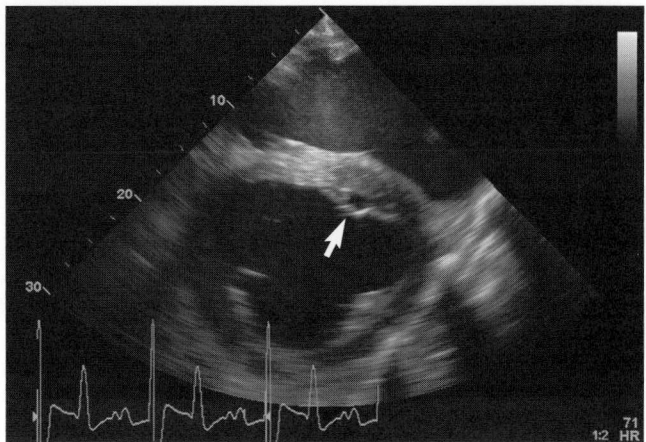

FIGURE 2 Right parasternal short-axis echocardiogram of the left ventricle. Note the dissection of blood between the endocardium (*arrow*) and myocardium along the left ventricular side of the interventricular septum.

TREATMENT

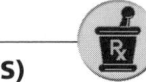

THERAPEUTIC GOAL(S)

- Stabilize the patient in the acute phase.
- Treatment is only symptomatic.

ACUTE GENERAL TREATMENT

Antiarrhythmic drugs to treat ventricular tachycardia when present (sometimes it resolves spontaneously): Treat if the HR is greater than 100 to 120 beats/min, clinical signs of cardiovascular collapse are present, or multiform or R on T phenomenon is present (see "Antiarrhythmic Drugs" in Section VI).

CHRONIC TREATMENT

- No specific treatment
- If heart failure develops (for detailed therapy recommendations, see "Cardiac Failure" in this section):
  - Diuretic therapy, such as furosemide: 1–2 mg/kg as needed IM or IV
  - Digoxin: 0.011–0.0175 mg/kg PO q12h
  - Angiotensin-converting enzyme inhibitor therapy such as enalapril: 0.5 mg/kg PO q12h
  - Hydralazine: 0.5–1.5 mg/kg PO q12h

POSSIBLE COMPLICATIONS

- RV and LV overload and myocardial dysfunction or failure leading to development of congestive heart failure
- Sudden death from cardiac arrhythmias
- Aortic regurgitation from loss of aortic root support from the aneurysm or after the aneurismal rupture, leading to further LV volume overload

RECOMMENDED MONITORING

- Acute event
  - Clinical signs pertaining to the cardiovascular system (HR, respiratory rate, arterial pulse quality, jugular pulses, or distension)
  - Telemetric electrocardiography to monitor heart rhythm
- Chronic monitoring
  - HR and rhythm, respiratory rate and effort, change in existing murmurs, attitude, and appetite should be monitored by owner. Any changes could signify a deterioration of status and should prompt a veterinary reexamination.
  - Periodic echocardiography (every 6–12 months) to monitor for progression of disease or sooner if any of the above clinical signs any noted.

- Guarded to grave prognosis
  - Death usually occurs acutely or soon after vessel rupture.
  - Some horses survive the acute event. The majority of these survive weeks to months (depending on the site and size of the rupture), although some horses survive for years after the acute rupture without developing congestive heart failure.
- The prognosis for performance is poor because these horses are not safe to ride or use.

PEARLS & CONSIDERATIONS

COMMENTS

- Aortic root rupture should be suspected in any horse presenting with acute distress; tachycardia with a HR greater than 80 beats/min; and a loud, continuous heart murmur.
- Horses with aortocardiac fistulas are not safe to ride for any kind of performance because they have a high risk of sudden death.

CLIENT EDUCATION

- Regular cardiac auscultation should be performed in middle-aged stallions, and if a continuous heart murmur is detected, a cardiac examination should be performed.
- Horses with aortocardiac fistulas are unsafe to use because of a high risk of sudden death.

SUGGESTED READING

Marr CM, Reef VB, Brazil TJ, et al: Aortocardiac fistulas in seven horses. *Vet Radiol Ultrasound* 39:22–31, 1998.

Piercy RJ, Marr CM: Collapse. In Marr CM, editor: *Cardiology of the horse.* Philadelphia, 1999, WB Saunders, pp 268–288.

Reef VB: Cardiovascular ultrasonography. In Reef VB, editor: *Equine diagnostic ultrasound.* Philadelphia, 1998, Saunders, pp 215–272.

Sleeper MM, Durando MM, Miller M, et al: Aortic root disease in four horses. *J Am Vet Med Assoc* 219(4):491–496, 2001.

AUTHOR: **OLGA SECO DIAZ**

EDITOR: **MARY M. DURANDO**

Aortoiliac Thrombosis

BASIC INFORMATION

DEFINITION

Total or partial occlusion of the terminal portion of the aorta or the internal or external iliac arteries by masses of well-organized and vascularized fibrous tissue containing hemorrhagic, necrotic, and sometimes calcified areas with large thrombi around them. Often these masses also affect the popliteal and femoral arteries or other branches of the iliac arteries.

SYNONYM(S)

- Vascular obstruction of the hindlimbs
- Aortoiliac obstruction
- Aortoiliac-femoral thrombosis

EPIDEMIOLOGY

SPECIES, AGE, SEX
- All ages reported
- Both sexes (although there is greater incidence of clinical disease in males because collateral circulation is thought to be more efficient in females)

GENETICS AND BREED PREDISPOSITION
- A hereditary predisposition has been suggested in one report, but there is little evidence to support it.
- Light breeds appear to be more commonly affected than heavy breeds.

CLINICAL PRESENTATION

DISEASE FORMS/SUBTYPES Clinical signs vary depending on the size, location of the thrombus, and amount of occlusion of the blood vessel.

HISTORY, CHIEF COMPLAINT
- Poor performance
- Chronic progressive hindlimb lameness that worsens with exercise
- Sexual dysfunction in stallions
- May be subclinical in nonathletic horses

PHYSICAL EXAM FINDINGS
- Lameness that becomes evident during exercise, is aggravated by work, and resolves after a brief rest
- May show weakness in the pelvic limbs, ataxia, collapse after strenuous work in advanced cases, reluctance to put a hind leg down, or tendency to cow-kick after exercise
- Absence of sweating in the affected limb with profuse sweating of the remainder of the body and respiratory distress after exercise
- May have reduced skin temperature of the affected distal hind limb after exercise
- May have reduced pulse in the femoral or plantar digital arteries after exercise
- May have prolonged medial saphenous vein filling time in the affected limb shortly after work; the veins in the affected leg are indistinct
- May have gluteal atrophy on the affected side
- Failure to ejaculate in stallions

ETIOLOGY AND PATHOPHYSIOLOGY
- Unknown
- Possible causes:
  - Organization of thromboembolisms caused by migrating forms of *Strongylus vulgaris* with incorporation of the thrombi into the arterial wall and centripetal development of progressive thrombosis
  - Damage to the arterial endothelium at points of turbulence or branching leading to plaque formation and overlying thrombosis
  - Spontaneous degenerative vascular disease at the aortic quadrification that may result in thrombosis and thromboembolism
  - Secondary to coagulopathies
  - Secondary to bacterial infection
  - Direct trauma attributable to falling or parturition

DIAGNOSIS

DIFFERENTIAL DIAGNOSIS
- Postexercise myopathy
- Cervical vertebral malformation
- Spinal or pelvic trauma (back disorders)
- Musculoskeletal lameness

INITIAL DATABASE
- Plasma and serum muscle enzymes are usually normal before and after exercise, although creatine kinase may be increased in severe cases with marked muscle damage.

- Rectal palpation: May feel a firm area of the aorta or iliac arteries with reduced pulsations and enlargement of the iliac arteries. The rectal examination may also be unremarkable.

ADVANCED OR CONFIRMATORY TESTING
- Transrectal ultrasound examination: Heterogeneous mass in the terminal aorta or iliac arteries (or both) (Figure 1)
- Arteriography: Invasive and technically difficult; unnecessary since the advent of rectal ultrasonography
- Nuclear angiography: Marked reduction or absence of blood flow through the affected iliac arteries

TREATMENT

THERAPEUTIC GOAL(S)
- Improve collateral circulation
- Prevent additional thrombus formation
- Encourage thrombolysis
- Provide analgesia

ACUTE GENERAL TREATMENT
- No drugs are effective to eliminate a formed thrombus; treatment is based on pain relief and antiinflammatory drugs, platelet inhibitors, antihelmintics, fibrinolytic agents, and anticoagulant drugs. Some of the medical treatments reported include phenylbutazone, aspirin, isoxsuprine, IV sodium gluconate, and ivermectin.
- Intraluminal arterial thrombectomy for total or partial removal of the thrombus may improve clinical signs if a portion of the thrombus is removed; however, recurrence is high.

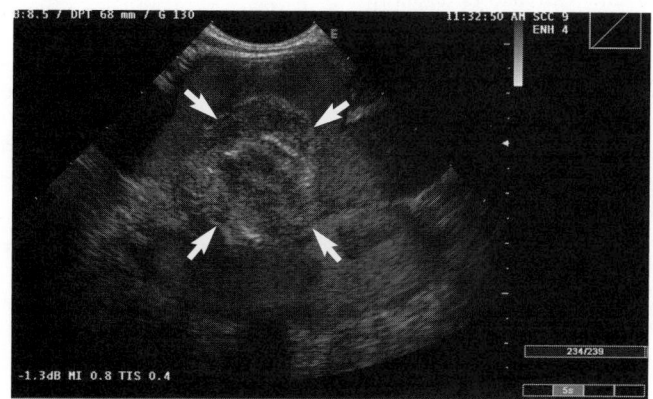

FIGURE 1 Transverse ultrasound of the terminal aorta using a rectal approach. A large heterogeneous mass is seen within the lumen of the aorta (*arrows*).

CHRONIC TREATMENT

Continued exercise to encourage and maintain collateral circulation

POSSIBLE COMPLICATIONS

- Progressive lameness unresponsive to analgesia.
- Acute thrombosis of one of the external iliac arteries may result in necrosis of the muscles in the affected limb.
- Progressive occlusion of the major arterial branches and embolism of the peripheral hind limb vessels that may cause initial mild lameness or large areas of muscle ischemia.
- Death from spontaneous rupture of an ischemic rectum has been reported.
- Reduced fertility in stallions.
- Death.

PROGNOSIS AND OUTCOME

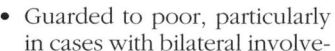

- Guarded to poor, particularly in cases with bilateral involve-

ment. No treatment consistently improves outcome. Successful treatment is based on development of collateral circulation.
- Poor prognosis for return to previous levels of athletic performance.

PEARLS & CONSIDERATIONS

- Rectal ultrasonography is the best diagnostic technique for a definitive diagnosis of this disorder.
- The severity of clinical signs depends on the degree of vascular occlusion. Complete vascular occlusion of the arteries may result in death caused by ischemic necrosis.
- Serum muscle enzymes, neurologic examination, and diagnostic regional anesthesia may rule out other disorders.
- Any improvement in clinical signs is most likely attributable to development of effective collateral circulation.

SUGGESTED READING

Dyson SJ: Pelvic injuries in the non-racehorse. In Ross MW, Dyson SJ, editors: *Diagnosis and management of lameness in the horse.* St Louis, 2003, Saunders Elsevier, pp 497–498.

Hilton H, Aleman M, et al: Ultrasound-guided balloon thrombectomy for treatment of aorto-iliac-femoral thrombosis in a horse. *J Vet Intern Med* 22:679–683, 2008.

MacLeay JM: Diseases of the musculoskeletal system. In Reed SM, Bayly WM, Sellon DC, editors: *Equine internal medicine.* St Louis, 2004, Saunders Elsevier, pp 505–507.

Maxie MG, Physick-Sheard PW: Aorto-iliac thrombosis in horses. *Vet Pathol* 22:238–249, 1985.

Ross MW, Maxson AD, Stacy VS, et al: First-pass radionuclide angiography in the diagnosis of aortoiliac thrombosis in a horse. *Vet Radiol Ultrasound* 38(3):226–230, 1997.

AUTHOR: OLGA SECO DIAZ

EDITOR: MARY M. DURANDO

Arsenic Toxicosis

BASIC INFORMATION

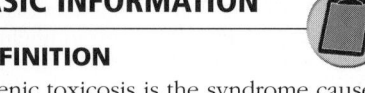

DEFINITION

Arsenic toxicosis is the syndrome caused by exposure to injurious amounts of inorganic arsenic (trivalent arsenic, pentavalent arsenate) or organic arsenic (aliphatic, aromatic, and phenylarsenic compounds). Exposure can be by ingestion or by dermal contact. Possible sources of arsenic include older formulation of some insecticides, rodenticides, herbicides, fungicides, and defoliants or desiccants; ashes from arsenic-treated lumber; contaminated water and soil sources; and feed additives for poultry and swine. Arsenic can also be found in mine tailings and ores, old paints and other industrial chemicals, and some drugs. Arsenic is naturally found in soil, rocks, and some water sources.

EPIDEMIOLOGY

SPECIES, AGE, SEX

- Debilitated animals and young animals are more sensitive.
- The phenylarsonic feed additives are less likely to be a problem in horses and cause problems mainly in swine and pigs.

RISK FACTORS

- Access to old barns or sheds that may contain older pesticides or chemicals

- Access to dump or burn piles containing burned lumber
- Proximity to mining and manufacturing operations that may contribute to ground and water contamination

CLINICAL PRESENTATION

DISEASE FORMS/SUBTYPES

- Peracute or acute toxicosis: Single toxic dose
- Subacute toxicosis: Lower repeated doses over a longer period
- Phenylarsonic toxicosis: Mainly seen in swine and poultry, not horses

HISTORY, CHIEF COMPLAINT

- Exposure to arsenic-containing product
- Peracute death (no premonitory clinical signs)
- Acute: Severe gastrointestinal (GI) signs, colic, ataxia, recumbency, shock, and death
- Subacute: Persistent watery diarrhea and signs of renal dysfunction
- Phenylarsonics: Peripheral neuropathy with low mortality rate

PHYSICAL EXAM FINDINGS Acute toxicosis:

- High morbidity and mortality rates
- Drooling
- Trembling
- GI pain or stasis
- Colic (sudden onset)

- Diarrhea (green to black and severe)
- Dehydration
- Weak pulse
- Recumbency

Subacute toxicosis:

- Persistent GI signs (watery diarrhea)
- Depression
- Anorexia

Signs associated with severe shock:

- Dehydration
- Oliguria, polyuria, anuria
- Weakness
- Ataxia
- Metabolic acidosis
- Hyperemic mucous membranes
- Tachycardia

ETIOLOGY AND PATHOPHYSIOLOGY

- Arsenic reacts with sulfhydryl groups in cells. As a result, sulfhydryl enzyme systems essential to cellular metabolism are impaired. The net effect is the blocking of fat and carbohydrate metabolism and cellular respiration.
- Tissues most affected are those rich in oxidative enzymes (GI tract, endothelium, lung, kidney, liver, and epidermis).
- Disruption of capillary integrity is the effect on the GI tract, resulting in necrosis and hemorrhagic enteritis.
- Endothelial damage with fluid loss into interstitium, hypovolemia, hypotension, and pulmonary edema.

- Hepatic and renal damage from direct effect of arsenic or secondary to hypovolemia and organ hypoperfusion.
- Toxicity varies with physical form, solubility, and valence.
- Inorganic arsenic (eg, arsenic trioxide) is more toxic than organic forms (eg, arsanilic acid).
- Trivalent arsenic (arsenite) is more toxic than pentavalent forms (arsenate).
- Highly soluble forms (arsenic acid) are more toxic than insoluble forms.
- Single lethal dose of sodium arsenite = 1 to 25 mg/kg of body weight
- Arsenic trioxide is three to 10 times less toxic than sodium arsenite.

DIAGNOSIS

DIFFERENTIAL DIAGNOSIS

- Other heavy metal toxicosis (eg, lead, mercury)
- Poisonous plants
- Salmonellosis
- Caustic agents
- Zinc phosphide toxicosis

INITIAL DATABASE

If the horse survives the acute phase:
- Azotemia
- Hypokalemia
- Hyponatremia
- Hypochloremia
- Hyperglycemia
- Hyperbilirubinemia
- Increased glutamate dehydrogenase and lactate dehydrogenase

ADVANCED OR CONFIRMATORY TESTING

- Normal renal and hepatic arsenic concentrations are less than 1 ppm; definitive diagnosis of arsenic toxicosis is based on liver and kidney arsenic concentrations greater than 10 ppm (wet weight).

- Antemortem urine arsenic concentrations greater than 10 mg/L indicate excessive exposure.
- Postmortem lesions include generalized or localized redness, edema, and necrosis of gastric and intestinal mucosa with massive accumulation of fluid in dilated and atonic intestine.
- Organic arsenicals target the nervous system with edema and necrosis.

TREATMENT

THERAPEUTIC GOAL(S)

- Control life-threatening signs.
- Prevent systemic absorption.
- Provide chelation therapy.
- Manage GI effects.

ACUTE GENERAL TREATMENT

- Provide decontamination with activated charcoal if no clinical signs are present.
- Provide aggressive fluid therapy.
- Administer sodium thiosulfate orally to bind unabsorbed arsenic.
- Administer arsenic chelators such as dimercaprol or D-penicillamine (marginally useful).
- Provide other sources of sulfhydryl groups (cysteine, acetylcysteine).
- Give antibiotics for secondary bacterial infection.
- Monitor renal and hepatic function.

CHRONIC TREATMENT

- Provide general supportive care
- Manage renal insufficiency as needed
- Provide supportive care for possible hepatic dysfunction

POSSIBLE COMPLICATIONS

Renal failure

RECOMMENDED MONITORING

- Hydration and electrolyte status
- Hematocrit, total solids
- Acid-base status

- Biochemical profile, especially renal values

PROGNOSIS AND OUTCOME

Most horses die within 12 to 24 hours of ingestion of lethal doses.

PEARLS & CONSIDERATIONS

COMMENTS

- Toxicosis is less common now because of decreased use of arsenic-containing products, but occasional cases are still seen.
- Horses with extensive damage to the GI mucosa are unlikely to recover fully.
- The destruction of crypt cells may prevent regeneration of the mucosa needed for proper absorption of nutrients.

PREVENTION

- Avoid arsenic-containing products where horses are kept.
- Ensure ashes from arsenic-treated wood are not disposed of where horses are kept.

SUGGESTED READING

Gwaltney-Brant SM: Arsenic toxicosis. In Coté E, editor: *Clinical veterinary advisor: dogs and cats.* St. Louis, 2007, Mosby Elsevier, pp 81–82.

Pace LW, Turnquist SE, Casteel SW, et al: Acute arsenic toxicosis in five horses. *Vet Pathol* 34:160–164, 1997.

Plumlee KH: Pesticide toxicosis in the horse. *Vet Clin North Am Equine Pract* 17(3): 491–500, vii, 2001.

AUTHOR: BRENT HOFF

EDITOR: CYNTHIA L. GASKILL

Arteritis, Equine Viral

BASIC INFORMATION

DEFINITION

Equine viral arteritis (EVA) is a contagious arterivirus disease of horses named for the characteristic vascular lesions that develop.

EPIDEMIOLOGY

SPECIES, AGE, SEX
- Disease of horses, but antibodies have been found in donkeys

- Disease depends on age and sex
- Inapparent infection, especially in mares
- Persistent infection only in stallions (testosterone dependent)

GENETICS AND BREED PREDISPOSITION
- Seroprevalence varies by country, breed, and age. EVA is endemic in Standardbreds (75%–80% seropositive) but has a low prevalence in Thorough-

breds, with a 1% to 5% seropositive rate. Many European Warmblood stallions are seropositive.
- Genetic differences conferring resistance to infection may be a factor but have not been proven.

RISK FACTORS
- Stallions may be inapparent carriers and can shed virus in the semen for years. Cooled or frozen serum can still retain infective virus.

- Infected mares and/or vaccinated mares bred to infected stallions can become infected and shed the virus.

CONTAGION AND ZOONOSIS

- EVA is an arterivirus in the family of Arteriviridae. The first Bucyrus strain was isolated in 1953. Virulence is variable in terms of clinical disease and abortion of viral isolates, but all strains are neutralized by polyclonal antiserum from the highly virulent Bucyrus strain.
- There is no known zoonotic potential.

GEOGRAPHY AND SEASONALITY

Worldwide except for Iceland and Japan

CLINICAL PRESENTATION

HISTORY, CHIEF COMPLAINT

- Anorexia, depression, edema (ventral limbs, preputial [male], mammary [mare]), abortion storms, urticaria.
- Most infections are subclinical or inapparent.

PHYSICAL EXAM FINDINGS

- Variable clinical signs (depend on age, condition of horse, viral strain, environmental conditions)
- Usually inapparent infection, particularly in mares
- Systemic disease: Fever (105°–106° F), anorexia, depression, edema (ventrum, periorbital, distal limbs, prepuce, mammary), urticaria, conjunctivitis, rhinitis, cough/dyspnea
- Less common: Icterus, photophobia, corneal opacity, abdominal pain, diarrhea, ataxia, petechiation, lymphadenopathy
- Abortion (3–10 months' gestation) with no premonitory signs
- Neonates: Fulminant severe interstitial pneumonia or fibrinonecrotic enteritis
- Stallions: Temporary subfertility, decreased libido, decreased sperm motility, concentration, and morphology up to 7 weeks
- Stallions with persistent infection: No change in semen quality after acute recovery

ETIOLOGY AND PATHOPHYSIOLOGY

- Transmission is primarily by inhalation of aerosolized virus from respiratory secretions and contact with venereal secretions, urine, or exposure to aborted fetus or placenta. Indirect transmission of the virus with fomites is possible.
- Incubation is 3 to 14 days; the virus then spreads to the lungs and bronchial lymph nodes.
- The circulatory system spreads it through rest of body, with infection and replication of virus occurring in the endothelial cells.
- Increased vascular permeability, hemorrhage, and edema with degeneration

and necrosis of the tunica media of small arteries (>1 mm).

- Mares remain infective for up to 2 weeks after infection, with shedding of the virus in nasal secretions.
- Transplacental infection of the fetus is possible if the mare is infected in late pregnancy.
- Virus is not isolated from horses after 28 days except for stallions.
- Persistent infection in stallions
  - Unknown mechanism, testosterone dependent
  - Virus lives in the accessory sex glands of stallions, with the highest titers found in the ampulla of the vas deferens
  - Variable duration
    - Short term: A few weeks after acute infection
    - Intermediate: 3 to 7 months
    - Long term (30%–35% of stallions): Lifelong, continual shedders or may spontaneously stop shedding

DIAGNOSIS

DIFFERENTIAL DIAGNOSIS

- Equine herpesvirus-1 and -4
- Influenza
- Equine rhinitis A and B viruses
- Equine adenovirus
- Equine infectious anemia
- Purpura hemorrhagica
- Urticaria
- Leptospirosis
- African horse sickness
- Hoary alyssum toxicosis

INITIAL DATABASE

- Leukopenia
- Thrombocytopenia

ADVANCED OR CONFIRMATORY TESTING

- Virus isolation using whole blood (ethylenediamine tetraacetic acid or citrate only; heparin will inhibit the virus), nasopharyngeal or conjunctival swabs, placental or fetal tissues/fluid, vaginal secretions, semen.
  - Virus cannot be isolated after 28 days of infection except in semen or carrier stallions.
  - Virus is detected in the nasopharynx (2–14 days), buffy coat (2–19 days), or serum or plasma (7–9 days).
- Paired (acute and convalescent) serology using serum taken 3 to 4 weeks apart with four-fold increase; this is the gold standard set by the World Organisation for Animal Health.
- Antigen detection: Immunohistochemistry.
- Polymerase chain reaction (PCR) (realtime PCR, nested) is still being vali-

dated and standardized.

- Diagnosis of carrier stallions: (1) Test breed to two seronegative mares and monitor for seroconversion; (2) isolate virus from sperm-rich fraction of semen.

TREATMENT

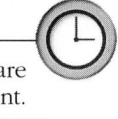

THERAPEUTIC GOAL(S)

- Symptomatic and supportive care to maintain general health and well-being.
- Decrease distal edema.
- Prevent or treat secondary bacterial infections.

ACUTE GENERAL TREATMENT

- Symptomatic treatment (rest, antipyretics) as for other viral respiratory infections
- Symptomatic treatment for distal edema (diuretics, support wraps)
- No effective treatment for foals with EVA-induced interstitial pneumonia or enteritis; antibiotics for secondary bacterial infection
- Only way to eliminate persistent infection in stallions is by castration

PROGNOSIS AND OUTCOME

- Majority of EVA infections are subclinical or inapparent. Mortality is rare in adult horses.
- Fatal interstitial pneumonia may occur in neonates.

PEARLS & CONSIDERATIONS

COMMENTS

EVA is an important disease in terms of its economic impact on the equine industry from abortion losses, export restrictions of seropositive horses, and performance-related losses.

PREVENTION

- No domestic program for EVA prevention or control exists, but the U.S. Department of Agriculture and Animal and Plant Health Inspection Services have guidelines and standards outlining preventative vaccination and control measures.
- Modified live virus vaccine is available in the United States.
- Vaccinate foals before puberty (at 6 months of age), then annually.
- Vaccinate seronegative stallions 28 days before breeding season and isolate after vaccination. Stallions should be screened before primary

immunization. Neutralization titer of 1:4 or greater is positive for EVA.
- Nonvaccinated seropositive stallions should be tested for virus shedding by virus isolation every 12 months or by test breeding with two seronegative mares monitored for seroconversion at 14 and 28 days after breeding.
- Pony/outrider horses or any horses with potential contact with multiple horses should be vaccinated annually for EVA.
- Carrier stallions and confirmed semen shedders should be isolated, collected separately, and bred to mares that are seropositive or vaccinated at least 3 weeks before breeding.
- Mares bred to shedding stallions or inseminated with infective semen should be isolated for 3 weeks from seronegative or nonvaccinated horses.

Mares should be vaccinated 3 weeks before breeding to shedding stallions.

CLIENT EDUCATION
- The increasing number of outbreaks and apparent global dissemination of EVA likely reflect the rapid national and international movement of horses for competition and breeding as well as increased recognition of the importance of EVA infection.
- Prevention of outbreaks of EVA relies on raising the awareness of the disease in owners, identification of persistently infected stallions, and institution of management practices (eg, vaccines, biosecurity).
- If an outbreak of EVA is suspected:
  ○ Notify the state veterinarian.
  ○ Institute quarantine of premises by isolating affected and in-contact horses, stopping traffic movement

on and off the farm, vaccinating at-risk horses, and stopping breeding activity.
  ○ Confirm diagnosis of EVA with laboratory testing.
  ○ Properly disinfect affected premises.
  ○ End the quarantine when no more clinical cases of EVA or serologic evidence of infection is observed for 3 consecutive weeks.

SUGGESTED READING
Holyoak GR, et al: Equine viral arteritis: current status and prevention. *Theriogenology* 70:403-414, 2008.
USDA Animal and Plant Health Inspection Services (APHIS): *Equine viral arteritis.* Available at http://www-mirror.aphis.usda.gov/animal_health/animal_diseases/eva/.

AUTHOR: **KATHY K. SEINO**

EDITORS: **MAUREEN T. LONG** and **DEBRA C. SELLON**

Arytenoid Chondritis and Chondropathy

BASIC INFORMATION

DEFINITION
A progressive, acute or chronic, predominately infectious process resulting in exercise intolerance or upper airway noise caused by thickening of the arytenoid cartilage, the surrounding soft tissue, or both

SYNONYM(S)
- Arytenoid granuloma is a granulating mass and may be a component of the lesion.
- *Arytenoid chondroma* is a term used previously for granuloma.
- Neoplasia is uncommon and not part of this disease.

EPIDEMIOLOGY
SPECIES, AGE, SEX
- Racing breeds during active training
- Former race horses, including broodmares
- A milder, predominately self-limiting form observed in yearlings
- Less frequently affects horses of any breed or occupation
RISK FACTORS
- Mucosal surface trauma caused by contact of arytenoid cartilages during exercise
  ○ Laryngeal hemiplegia
  ○ Enlargement of the opposite arytenoid cartilage

- Mucosal disruption has been experimentally demonstrated to cause the disease
CONTAGION AND ZOONOSIS Not considered contagious
GEOGRAPHY AND SEASONALITY
- The incidence can be variably higher from particular regions or racetracks within a region.
  ○ Racing surface, air quality, and training methods must be considered.
  ○ Arytenoid chondritis is very uncommon where racing is predominately on turf.
ASSOCIATED CONDITIONS AND DISORDERS
- May be observed concurrently with laryngeal hemiplegia, presumably because of mucosal surface trauma from collapse of the paretic cartilage.
- Either or both cartilages may be affected.

CLINICAL PRESENTATION
DISEASE FORMS/SUBTYPES
- Acute or chronic progression of:
  ○ Arytenoid mucosal ulceration
  ○ Arytenoid axial surface granulation
  ○ Arytenoid full- or partial-thickness intracartilaginous septic tracts
  ○ Intracartilaginous or pericartilaginous abscessation: The arytenoid cartilage may be axially displaced by abaxial extracartilaginous abscessation, producing airway obstruction without actual invasion of the arytenoid cartilage.

  ○ Arytenoid cartilage enlargement or distortion
HISTORY, CHIEF COMPLAINT
- Variable exercise intolerance
- Variable upper respiratory noise
- Occasionally presents as a respiratory emergency caused by airway obstruction at rest because of abscessation or granulation tissue masses
- Often becomes more severe in nonathletes because it remains undetected until the obstruction is complete
PHYSICAL EXAM FINDINGS
- Generally outwardly normal horse
- Physical examination usually normal; possible exceptions:
  ○ Upper airway inspiratory stertor at rest in severe cases; however, with persistent stenosis, the stertor is audible on expiration as well.
  ○ Dysphagia is uncommon but may be associated with severe perilaryngeal or pharyngeal inflammation.
ETIOLOGY AND PATHOPHYSIOLOGY
- Most often presumed to be mucosal disruption leading to deeper infection or inflammation, causing thickening of the arytenoid cartilage or swelling of the surrounding tissue.
- Arytenoid abduction is mechanically prevented by cartilage distortion or adjacent soft tissue swelling.
- Arytenoid distortion or axial compression of the arytenoid may be observed without a visible mucosal disruption.
- Hematogenous seeding of infection must be considered a possibility,

although a previously undetected mucosal lesion could have healed.

DIAGNOSIS

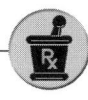

DIFFERENTIAL DIAGNOSIS

- Laryngeal hemiplegia
  - There should be no thickening or mucosal lesion with left laryngeal hemiplegia
  - May occur concurrently
- Retropharyngeal abscess
- Ventricular mucocele
- Has been observed after ventricular ablation without resection
- Neoplasia

INITIAL DATABASE

- External laryngeal palpation is most commonly normal.
- Arytenoid chondritis may occur concurrently with laryngeal hemiplegia, so cricoarytenoideus dorsalis muscle atrophy may be palpable.

ADVANCED OR CONFIRMATORY TESTING

- Nasopharyngeal endoscopy provides the diagnosis for almost all cases.
  - Affected arytenoid cartilage(s) will be thickened with or without mucosal swelling. Both may be subtle.
  - There is often a contact (kissing) lesion on the contralateral cartilage from contact with the enlarged cartilage or a granulation tissue mass from the affected cartilage (Figure 1). Arytenoid chondritis may be bilateral.
  - Retroflexion of the scope within the trachea allows detection of thicken-

ing of the caudal arytenoid body or changes in mobility, particularly during swallowing.
- Ultrasonography may demonstrate:
  - Cartilage thickening or abscessation
  - Extracartilaginous abscess or mucocele
- Magnetic resonance imaging: Demonstrative but not likely to be necessary

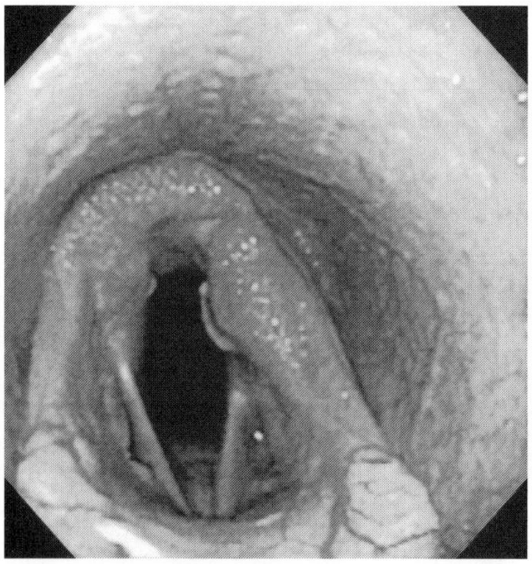

TREATMENT

THERAPEUTIC GOAL(S)

- Restoration of normal upper airway function
- Restoration of an airway to save the life of the horse

ACUTE GENERAL TREATMENT

- Provide an airway for emergency situations.
  - Tracheotomy
  - More likely during warm weather or when the horse is stressed
- Medical therapy may be successful in horses without arytenoid deformity or airway compromise.
  - Broad-spectrum or specific antibacterial therapy: Duration, 10 to 30 days depending on severity and chronicity
  - Local and systemic antiinflammatory therapy
    - Topical antiinflammatory throat spray
    - Systemic nonsteroidal antiinflammatory drug therapy
    - Systemic steroid therapy unless acute infection is too active
- Horses with permanent arytenoid deformity or adjacent thickening that compromises the airway must undergo a partial arytenoidectomy (removing all but the muscular process of the arytenoid cartilage).
  - Acute inflammation should be relieved with medical therapy as much as possible before surgery. The applicable procedure or the need for any surgery at all may change after medical therapy.
  - Successful partial arytenoidectomy can be performed with or without mucosal closure.
- Horses with less-affected arytenoid cartilages or resolvable adjacent soft tissue lesions may undergo successful (standing) debridement of the affected areas accompanied by medical therapy.
  - The lesion is accessed through a trocar placed in the cricothyroid membrane and performed with a laser and conventional instruments. Culture of the lesion is recommended.
  - Debridement may lead to drainage of arytenoid or adjacent abscesses,

thereby rapidly reducing the deformity.
  - Case selection is critical for success because the potential for arytenoid abduction must be present after the inflammation has resolved.
    - Evaluation of cartilage morphology and mobility can be improved by digital palpation through a standing laryngotomy.
    - The caudal margin, mid-body through the lateral ventricle and rostral body abaxial and caudal to the corniculate process should be palpated.
- Horses with only surface granulomas may respond favorably to standing removal of the mass followed by local and systemic antiinflammatory and antibacterial therapy.
- The author's opinion is that all but the most obviously superficial lesions should be probed for deeper tracts that may be debrided or drained before permanent arytenoid deformity occurs.

POSSIBLE COMPLICATIONS

- Partial arytenoidectomy may be followed by a variable degree of aspiration of food into the trachea, causing mild or serious aspiration pneumonia, although this seems to be less common.
- Horses undergoing bilateral partial arytenoidectomy do not commonly remain functional athletes.
- The most serious complication of arytenoid debridement is failure to restore function and a subsequent need for partial arytenoidectomy.

PROGNOSIS AND OUTCOME

- Partial arytenoidectomy has been reported in the older literature to fail to return horses to their previous athletic ability.
- More recent experience and reports have been more favorable.
- Success of arytenoid debridement in appropriate cases has been quite favorable.

PEARLS & CONSIDERATIONS

COMMENTS

- When the arytenoid cartilage is affected in an area containing a medullary cavity, the axial and abaxial laminae of the cartilage may be split apart. The axial lamina may separate during partial arytenoidectomy, leaving an incomplete removal. The surgeon should watch for this situation.

FIGURE 1 Left arytenoid chondropathy. The right arytenoid is fully abducted, but the left is not. The left corniculate is abnormally shaped and has a mucosal lesion on its medial surface. All are consistent with a left arytenoid chondropathy.

- Subtotal arytenoidectomy (leaving the corniculate and muscular process) has been reported in older literature but has been shown to be insufficient for return to substantial athletic performance.

SUGGESTED READING

Barnes AJ, Slone DE, Lynch TM: Performance after partial arytenoidectomy without mucosal closure in 27 Thoroughbred racehorses. *Vet Surg* 33:398, 2004.

Goodall CLM, Birks EK, Sullins KE: Prosthetic laryngoplasty or partial arytenoidectomy for the treatment of laryngeal hemiplegia in horses. *Vet Surg* 37:E14, 2008.

Parente EJ: Arytenoid chondropathy. In McGorum B, Dixon P, Robinson NE, et al, editors: *Equine respiratory medicine and surgery.* Philadelphia, 2007, Elsevier, p 515.

Radcliffe CH, Woodie JB, Hackett RP, et al: A comparison of laryngoplasty and modified partial arytenoidectomy as treatments for laryngeal hemiplegia in exercising horses. *Vet Surg* 35:643, 2006.

Wereszka M, Sullins K: Evaluation of standing minimally invasive laser-assisted and/or simple debridement technique for treatment of equine arytenoid chondritis in 27 horses. *Vet Surg* 36:E28, 2007.

AUTHOR: **KENNETH E. SULLINS**

EDITOR: **ERIC J. PARENTE**

Ascariasis

BASIC INFORMATION

DEFINITION

Mange caused by a variety of mites, including the chorioptic (leg mange) and psoroptic families

SYNONYM(S)

Mange

EPIDEMIOLOGY

GENETICS AND BREED PREDISPOSITION Chorioptic mange typically affects draft breeds with heavy feathering in their legs but may occasionally affect light breeds with thin hair coats. Psoroptic mange typically affects young horses of any breed.

RISK FACTORS

Young, stabled horses are at increased risk of being affected by psoroptic mange. When introduced into a new barn, they can transmit the disease to older horses. Horses affected by chorioptic mange can be asymptomatic carriers.
CONTAGION AND ZOONOSIS Neither psoroptic nor chorioptic mange is considered a zoonotic disease. Both psoroptic and chorioptic mange are reportable diseases in the United States.
GEOGRAPHY AND SEASONALITY Both chorioptic and psoroptic mange are more frequently seen in the cooler months of the year. Psoroptic mange has been eradicated from horses in the United States but is still present in other areas.
ASSOCIATED CONDITIONS AND DISORDERS Psoroptic mange has been associated with tail rubbing and otic irritation, which may lead to head shaking. Chorioptic mange may cause weight loss, irritability, and decreased exercise tolerance.

CLINICAL PRESENTATION

DISEASE FORMS/SUBTYPES Psoroptic and chorioptic mange

HISTORY, CHIEF COMPLAINT

- Psoroptic mange is characterized by severe pruritus, head shaking, and tail rubbing. Papules, crusts, and alopecia are frequently seen at the base of the mane, tail, ears, and submandibular area, and it may then spread to the rest of the body.
- Chorioptic mange lesions are typically seen in the pastern area, but in severe cases, the infection may spread to the ventral abdomen or even become generalized. Pruritus in chorioptic mange is variable, and severe thickening of the skin with secondary bacterial infection may result from self-trauma.

PHYSICAL EXAM FINDINGS Moderate to severe pruritic dermatitis in the ears, mane, body, and tail head ("rat tail" appearance), head shaking, and irritability are characteristic of psoroptic mange. Irritation, moderate pruritus with significant discomfort of the legs characterized by foot stamping and biting at the lower legs, patchy alopecia, and scaling are also common in chorioptic mange.

ETIOLOGY AND PATHOPHYSIOLOGY

- Mites *Psoroptes equi* and *Chorioptes equi*, both of which are relatively host specific, live on the surface of the epidermis.
- Both *P. equi* and *C. equi* normally have a 2-week lifespan.
- If there are favorable conditions of temperature, moisture, and humidity in the environment, *P. equi* can live away from its host for up to 3 weeks, but *C. equi* can live away from its host for just a few days.

DIAGNOSIS

DIFFERENTIAL DIAGNOSIS

- Dermatophilosis
- Dermatophytosis
- Trombiculidiasis
- Lice infestation
- *Culicoides* hypersensitivity
- Parasitic dermatitis
- Pastern dermatitis

INITIAL DATABASE

- *P. equi:* Demonstration of mites in skin scrapings and ear swabs from affected animals; round, elongated bodies with segmented pedicles
- *C. equi:* Demonstration of mites in skin scrapings from the pastern area and plantar or palmar area of the cannon bone

TREATMENT

THERAPEUTIC GOAL(S)

- Eliminate both eggs and adults of the parasites
- Decrease the risk of contamination of other animals in the barn

ACUTE GENERAL TREATMENT

- Psoroptic mange: Topical insecticides, including deltamethrin, coumaphos, diazinon, malathion, toxaphene, and lime sulphur, should be used. Ivermectin has also been used, but it does not always eliminate live mites from all animals. The contaminated environment also needs to be treated to prevent infection of other animals. It is important to continue treatment for at least 1 month.
- *C. equi:* Lime sulfur or fipronil applied once a week for at least 1 month is recommended. Lesions should be clipped and scabs removed before the affected areas are scrubbed with insecticidal shampoo or powder. Oral ivermectin given twice at 2-week intervals may be effective.

CHRONIC TREATMENT

Ascariasis may be difficult to eradicate after it becomes established in a stable.

PROGNOSIS AND OUTCOME

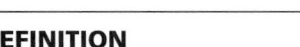

- If diagnosed and appropriately treated early in the course of the disease, the prognosis is favorable.

- After it has been established in the barn, the disease may be difficult to eradicate.

PEARLS & CONSIDERATIONS

Not zoonotic diseases, but reportable

SUGGESTED READING

White SD: Parasitic skin diseases. In Smith BP, editor: *Large animal internal medicine.* St Louis, 2009, Mosby Elsevier, pp 1321–1322.

AUTHOR: **ALFREDO SANCHEZ LONDOÑO**

EDITOR: **DAVID A. WILSON**

Ascites

BASIC INFORMATION

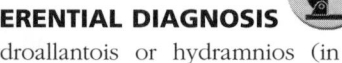

DEFINITION

Accumulation of peritoneal fluid (transudative effusion) in the peritoneal cavity

CLINICAL PRESENTATION

HISTORY, CHIEF COMPLAINT
- Abdominal distension
- Inappetence, mild colic, and lethargy are frequently reported.

PHYSICAL EXAM FINDINGS
- Ventral abdominal or distal limb edema is often present.
- Other clinical signs are variable and depend on the cause of ascites.
  - Poor body condition and signs of abdominal pain are often present if ascites occurs with abdominal neoplasia.
  - Jugular vein distension and pulsation, exercise intolerance, tachycardia, and a heart murmur may be present if right heart failure is the inciting cause.
- Rectal examination may be abnormal, with organ enlargement, intestinal distension, or palpable masses if intraabdominal neoplasia is the cause.

ETIOLOGY AND PATHOPHYSIOLOGY
- Abdominal neoplasia may result in obstruction of abdominal lymphatics or production of excess peritoneal fluid (especially with mesothelioma) and may result in ascites.
- Right-sided heart failure causes congestion of the venous circulation and increases capillary hydrostatic pressure, resulting in a transudative abdominal effusion.
- Hypoproteinemia may result from protein-losing enteropathy or protein-losing nephropathy, causing a decrease in colloid oncotic pressure that results in loss of fluid from the vascular space.
- However, clinically apparent ascites is uncommonly seen with right heart failure or hypoproteinemia in horses because of the large capacity of the equine peritoneal cavity.

- Also, in contrast to other species, ascites rarely accompanies hepatic disease in horses.

DIAGNOSIS

DIFFERENTIAL DIAGNOSIS
- Hydroallantois or hydramnios (in a broodmare)
- Chronic peritonitis
- Uroperitoneum
- Hemoperitoneum

INITIAL DATABASE
- Complete blood count: Variable; may be normal or may show evidence of chronic inflammation (mild anemia, leukocytosis, hyperfibrinogenemia) or abnormal leukocyte distribution or morphology if neoplasia is the inciting cause.
- Serum biochemistry profile: Variable; may be normal or hypoproteinemia or hypoalbuminemia may be present.
- Urinalysis: Should be performed in hypoproteinemic patients to rule out protein-losing nephropathy. Significant proteinuria should warrant further evaluation for glomerular disease.
- Transabdominal ultrasonography.
  - A large amount of hypoechoic free peritoneal fluid is visible in the ventral abdomen.
  - Evidence of intestinal disease (eg, inflammatory bowel disease causing protein-losing enteropathy) or intraabdominal neoplasia with intestinal thickening or intraabdominal masses may be apparent.
- Peritoneal fluid analysis.
  - Fluid is typically clear and watery but is occasionally cloudy or red-tinged if abdominal neoplasia is the cause.
  - The nucleated cell count and total protein concentration are usually within reference intervals (<10,000 cells/µL and 1.5 mg/dL, respectively). Occasionally, the fluid is

more consistent with a modified transudate (ie, mildly increased cell count and total protein concentration) in neoplastic disease.
  - Cytologic evaluation of the peritoneal fluid may be within normal limits or neoplastic cells may be seen.
  - Measurement of peritoneal fluid creatinine concentration may be performed to help rule out uroperitoneum. In ascites, peritoneal fluid creatinine is comparable to or lower than plasma creatinine.
- Cardiac ultrasonography should be performed if clinical evidence of right heart failure is present or if an alternative cause of ascites cannot be identified.

TREATMENT

THERAPEUTIC GOAL(S)
- Manage or treat primary disease if possible.
- Remove accumulated fluid.

ACUTE GENERAL TREATMENT
- Management of primary disease
  - Right heart failure may be managed with diuretics and positive inotropes (see "Cardiac Failure" in this section).
  - Plasma transfusion or administration of synthetic colloids may be indicated in hypoproteinemic patients.
  - Specific therapy for disseminated abdominal neoplasia resulting in ascites is usually palliative in horses. Dexamethasone (0.05–0.10 mg/kg IV or IM q24h) may result in transient clinical improvement in some neoplasias, especially lymphosarcoma.
- Drainage of accumulated peritoneal fluid
  - Not indicated unless large volume accumulation and associated clinical signs (abdominal pain, colic) are present.

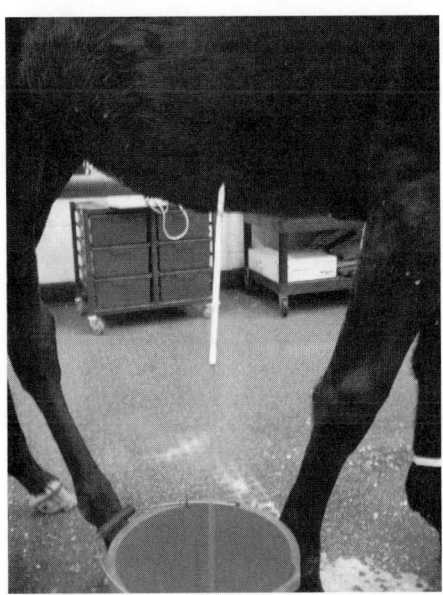

FIGURE 1 Drainage of peritoneal fluid with a chest drain from the abdomen of a yearling with ascites secondary to neoplasia.

◦ May be performed with a teat cannula as for an abdominocentesis or chest drain, but fluid removal should be done slowly and an equivalent volume of IV fluids administered simultaneously to avoid hypovolemic shock.

PROGNOSIS AND OUTCOME

Guarded to poor because the inciting causes of ascites in horses are usually difficult to impossible to treat

PEARLS & CONSIDERATIONS

Because ascites is uncommon in horses, it is vital to rule out uro-

peritoneum in horses with abdominal distension and a large volume of free hypoechoic peritoneal fluid. The concurrent presence of azotemia or electrolyte derangements, such as hyponatremia or hyperkalemia, should warrant a comprehensive evaluation of the urogenital tract.

SUGGESTED READING

Mair T: Abdominal distension in the adult horse. In Mair T, Divers T, Ducharme N, editors: *Manual of equine gastroenterology.* London, 2002, WB Saunders, pp 317–322.

AUTHOR: **KELSEY A. HART**

EDITOR: **TIM MAIR**

Atonic/Hypotonic Bladder

BASIC INFORMATION

DEFINITION

Dysuria or incontinence caused by sensory and motor deficits of the nervous system

SYNONYM(S)

Atonic or paralytic bladder, lower motor neuron bladder, spastic bladder, upper motor neuron bladder

EPIDEMIOLOGY

RISK FACTORS

- Feeding or exposure to sorghum or sudan grass
- Illicit tail blocking

CONTAGION AND ZOONOSIS Infectious agents incriminated include equine herpesvirus-1 (EHV-1), *Sarcocystis neurona*, and *Neospora hughesi*.

ASSOCIATED CONDITIONS AND DISORDERS

- Affected animals have a history or suspicion of a congenital disorder, spinal cord trauma, sacral trauma, or evidence of a concurrent inflammatory or degenerative neurologic disorder.
- Sabulous urolithiasis.

CLINICAL PRESENTATION
DISEASE FORMS/SUBTYPES

- Upper motor neuron or spastic bladder: Lack of descending inhibition, turgid bladder, increased urethral sphincter tone, periodic uncontrolled high-pressure urine production, and incomplete bladder emptying. The bladder is difficult to express by transrectal compression. The urethra is difficult to catheterize because of increased tone.
- Lower motor neuron or paralytic bladder: Loss of sensory fibers signaling bladder wall stretching that normally initiates urination. Detrusor muscle innervation and contractility are lost. The bladder fills to capacity and then passively overflows. The bladder is easily compressed per rectum, allowing urine voiding.
- Automatic bladder: Spinal cord damage cranial to the sacrum. Bladder filling and uncontrolled reflex emptying caused by loss of upper motor neuron influence. Higher sensation of bladder fill is lost, and emptying is incomplete.

HISTORY, CHIEF COMPLAINT

- Urinary incontinence
- May have concurrent neurologic disease

PHYSICAL EXAM FINDINGS

- Urine scalding over the perineum and between the hind legs.
- Frequent attempts to urinate or uncontrolled voiding.
- Perineal analgesia, loss of tail tone, loss of anal tone, fecal incontinence.
- Abnormalities of pelvic limb gait and regional muscle wasting may occur.
- Signs referable to more widespread neurologic dysfunction may be present.

ETIOLOGY AND PATHOPHYSIOLOGY

- Sympathetic, parasympathetic, and somatic branches of the central nervous system are required to coordinate bladder function.
  ◦ Sympathetic innervation: Hypogastric nerve (L1–L4) via the caudal mesenteric ganglion. Postganglionic fibers innervate the bladder wall (β_2 receptors) and proximal urethra (α_1 with some α_2 receptors).
  ◦ Parasympathetic innervation: The pelvic nerve (sacral segments) innervates the detrusor smooth muscle.
  ◦ Somatic innervation: The pudendal nerve (S1–S2) supplies the striated musculature of the urethra.

- Normal bladder function consists of bladder filling, urine storage, and evacuation. Extrapolation from other species is used to model bladder function in horses.
  - During bladder filling, tone increases in the external (pudendal nerve) and internal (sympathetic) urethral sphincters to hold urine. The detrusor muscle relaxes because of α-receptor–mediated inhibition of pelvic nerve afferent input and smooth muscle β_2-receptor stimulation caused by stretch receptors in the bladder wall acting on pelvic nerve afferents stimulating the hypogastric nerve. This allows an increased volume of urine storage in the bladder without a corresponding increase in pressure.
  - Evacuation of the bladder results from pelvic nerve afferent impulses transmitted to higher (intracranial) control centers in response to detrusor muscle stretch. Detrusor contraction is initiated by pelvic nerve impulses, spreading throughout the smooth muscle of the bladder and allowing coordinated contraction. Inhibition of pudendal and hypogastric nerve input also occurs, allowing more complete detrusor muscle contraction and urethral sphincter relaxation. Bladder emptying ceases when stretch receptors sense the bladder is no longer full. Pudendal and hypogastric nerve activity is then no longer inhibited, allowing detrusor muscle relaxation and increased urethral sphincter tone.

DIAGNOSIS

DIFFERENTIAL DIAGNOSIS

- Congenital anomaly: Ectopic ureter
- Cystolithiasis
- Cystitis
- Sabulous urolithiasis
- Nonneurogenic or myogenic bladder: Degenerative detrusor muscle changes
- Idiopathic incontinence of geldings
- Parturient urethral trauma of mares: Physical trauma to the pelvic urethra and pelvic nerves
- Musculoskeletal disorders: Pain preventing posturing to urinate

INITIAL DATABASE

- Complete blood count with fibrinogen concentration
- Serum chemistries
- Rectal palpation: Bladder size and tone, ease of manual expression
- Transrectal ultrasonography: Bladder size and content
- Urethral catheterization: May be difficult with increased urethral tone (upper motor neuron bladder)
- Cystoscopy, urethroscopy: To rule out nonneurogenic problems

ADVANCED OR CONFIRMATORY TESTING

- Suspected meningitis: Cerebrospinal fluid analysis ± culture
- Suspected viral infection: EHV-1 polymerase chain reaction, serology
- Suspected pelvic or sacral fracture (pain, compressive myelopathy): Radiography, scintigraphy, ultrasonography
- Suspected degenerative conditions (equine degenerative myelopathy, equine motor neuron disease): Vitamin E levels, muscle or peripheral nerve biopsy

TREATMENT

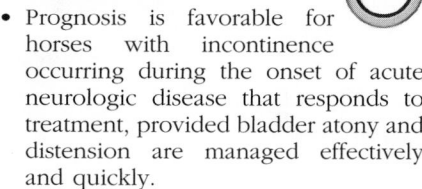

THERAPEUTIC GOAL(S)

- Management of primary neurologic disorder
- Management of bladder distension and urolithiasis
- Management of urine scalding from chronic overflow
- Management of cystitis and ascending infection of kidneys, if present

ACUTE GENERAL TREATMENT

- Drainage of urine by catheterization
- Appropriate antimicrobial therapy if cystitis is present
- Management of secondary complications: Urine scald
- Management of concurrent neurologic or musculoskeletal disorders

CHRONIC TREATMENT

- Long-term bladder catheterization
- Long-term antimicrobial or antiinflammatory therapy for appropriate cases
- Management of underlying neurologic or musculoskeletal disorder may be necessary

- Prevention and treatment of dermatitis secondary to urine scald

PROGNOSIS AND OUTCOME

- Prognosis is favorable for horses with incontinence occurring during the onset of acute neurologic disease that responds to treatment, provided bladder atony and distension are managed effectively and quickly.
- Prognosis is poor for horses with urinary incontinence resulting from chronic bladder dysfunction caused by a persistence of underlying neurologic factors or onset of sabulous urolithiasis.
- Chronically overdistended bladders are unlikely to respond to treatment.

PEARLS & CONSIDERATIONS

COMMENTS

- Prognosis depends on the anatomic location of any neurogenic cause of dysfunction.
- Treatment options are limited and similar, regardless of the origin of the problem.
- Secondary changes (cystitis, detrusor muscle degeneration) may be irreversible in advanced cases.

CLIENT EDUCATION

Neurologic bladder dysfunction may not resolve and requires long-term management.

SUGGESTED READING

Bayly WM: Urinary incontinence and bladder dysfunction. In Reed S, Bayly WM, Sellon DC, editors: *Equine internal medicine*, ed 2. St Louis, 2004, Saunders Elsevier, pp 1290–1294.

Furr M, Sampieri F: Differential diagnosis of urinary incontinence and cauda equine syndrome. In Furr M, Reed S, editors: *Equine neurology*. Ames, IA, 2008, Blackwell Publishing, pp 119–126.

Mayhew IG: Urinary bladder distension, dilated rectum and anus, and atonic tail: cauda equine syndrome. In Mayhew IG, editor: *Large animal neurology*, ed 2. Ames, IA, 2009, Wiley Blackwell, pp 163–166.

AUTHOR: **PETER R. MORRESEY**

EDITOR: **BRYAN M. WALDRIDGE**

Atrial Fibrillation

BASIC INFORMATION

DEFINITION

Supraventricular arrhythmia characterized by very rapid and chaotic, self-sustaining atrial electrical activity with an irregularly irregular ventricular response.

SYNONYM(S)

Auricular fibrillation

EPIDEMIOLOGY

SPECIES, AGE, SEX

- Large breeds are more susceptible than small breeds.
- Rarely occurs in ponies unless severe cardiac pathology is present.

RISK FACTORS

- Underlying cardiovascular pathology leading to:
  - Atrial dilation: Chronic valvular regurgitation (eg, mitral regurgitation), congenital heart disease (eg, ventricular septal defect)
  - Structural lesions of the atrial myocardium (eg, fibrosis caused by heart failure or pressure overload)
- Frequent occurrence of atrial premature beats (eg, caused by electrolyte disturbances, structural lesions, viral disease, myocardial stretch [exercise])
- Electrolyte disturbances
- High vagal tone (leads to dispersion in refractoriness of the atrial myocardium)

ASSOCIATED CONDITIONS AND DISORDERS

- Epistaxis during vigorous exercise
- Occasionally associated with ventricular ectopy

CLINICAL PRESENTATION

DISEASE FORMS/SUBTYPES

- Regarding etiology:
  - Primary or "lone" atrial fibrillation (AF): No underlying cardiac pathology. This form is much more common in horses than in other species.
  - Secondary AF: Underlying cardiac or noncardiac disease.
- Regarding duration:
  - Persistent (sustained) AF: Can only convert to sinus rhythm with treatment (most frequently in horses).
  - Paroxysmal AF (terminates spontaneously). Occasionally seen in racehorses (Thoroughbreds, Standardbreds) during (sub)maximal exercise. Within minutes, hours, or days, spontaneous conversion to sinus rhythm occurs.

HISTORY, CHIEF COMPLAINT

- Obvious signs of performance loss in horses working at maximal speed: Pulling up during race with signs of respiratory distress, ataxia, or even collapse
- Less pronounced signs of decreased performance in jumping and dressage horses or horses working at lower levels
- May be an incidental finding in pleasure horses, breeding horses, or horses at rest
- Epistaxis during exercise
- Signs of heart failure in horses with severe underlying cardiac disease and secondary AF

PHYSICAL EXAM FINDINGS

- Irregular pulse with pulse deficits
- Auscultation
  - Irregularly irregular rhythm
  - No atrial sound; loud first heart sound
  - Normal heart rate at rest or tachycardia in case of cardiac failure
- Signs of underlying cardiac disease
  - Cardiac murmur
  - Signs of heart failure (edema, jugular pulsation, tachypnea, weight loss)

ETIOLOGY AND PATHOPHYSIOLOGY

- Mechanism
  - During AF, depolarization waves spread continuously and in a rapid and chaotic manner over the atrial myocardium (usually 350–450/min). These depolarization waves originate from reentry or from rapidly firing foci and result in a continuous source of electrical activity independent of the sinoatrial node.
  - During AF, a (reversible) loss of atrial contractile function occurs.
  - At rest and when no severe underlying cardiac disease is present, high vagal tone causes the atrioventricular (AV) node to block most of the electrical pulses, thereby maintaining a normal heart rate. Conduction toward the ventricle occurs randomly resulting in an irregularly irregular cardiac rhythm.
  - Decreases in vagal tone (stress, exercise, heart failure, colic) results in an exacerbated increase in heart rate.
- Etiology
  - To be sustained, AF depends on a trigger to start the arrhythmia (atrial premature beat or rapidly firing focus) and a substrate to maintain it (atrial myocardium). Factors in favor of AF are:

  - A high trigger burden, that is, a high number of atrial premature beats: induced by stretch (eg, high atrial pressure during exercise), myocardial lesions, or electrolyte disturbances.
  - A suitable substrate, that is, the atrial myocardium: large atrial size, high vagal tone, short refractoriness of the myocardium and structural lesions.
  - In general, once initiated, AF rapidly (hours to days) becomes permanent, that is, it will never convert to sinus rhythm without therapy. In particular, during the first weeks to months the arrhythmia becomes increasingly stable.
  - Occasionally paroxysmal AF occurs during exercise, most commonly in racehorses. A potential cause is a high trigger burden during (sub)maximal exercise, while the myocardium is not suited to maintain the arrhythmia for a prolonged period (due to its size, electrophysiologic properties). Spontaneous conversion generally occurs within the first 72 hours.
- Impact:
  - In horses with lone AF:
    - At rest: no impairment of cardiac function (long diastolic time renders ventricular filling sufficient).
    - During exercise: impaired cardiac function occurs because of impaired ventricular filling as a result of (1) an absent atrial contractile function and (2) a disproportionate increase in heart rate. Some horses may present with epistaxis because of effects on pulmonary vascular pressures.
  - In horses with severe underlying cardiac disease: exacerbation of clinical signs because of a further decrease in cardiac function.

DIAGNOSIS

DIFFERENTIAL DIAGNOSIS

- Second-degree AV block: regularly irregular on auscultation with presence of the atrial sound (S4).
- Frequently and irregularly occurring atrial and/or ventricular premature beats.

INITIAL DATABASE

- AF may be strongly suspected on auscultation: an irregularly irregular

rhythm, a loud first heart sound, and absence of the atrial sound.
- Final diagnosis is made with an electrocardiogram (ECG) by the typical characteristics (Figures 1 and 2):
  - No P waves
  - Presence of f (fibrillation) waves. Changes between coarse (clearly undulating baseline) and fine (minor deflections of the baseline) fibrillation waves frequently occur on the same ECG.
  - Irregular RR interval (less obvious at high heart rates)
  - QRS morphology is normal but often shows minor alterations because of superposition with the f waves. The T wave may change after short RR intervals.
- Assess for signs of underlying cardiac disease such as a cardiac murmur, ventral edema, jugular pulsations, and tachycardia.

ADVANCED OR CONFIRMATORY TESTING

- Cardiac ultrasonography is essential to distinguish between lone and secondary AF (eg, atrial dilation, valvular regurgitation, congenital heart disease, congestive heart failure).
- Electrolyte imbalance (serum and fractional excretions) especially for recent-onset AF.
- Myocardial markers (cardiac troponin I) when myocardial damage is suspected.
- ECG (long-term telemetric or 24-hour Holter monitoring) to monitor for concurrent ventricular premature beats (Figure 3).

TREATMENT

- Do not treat for the first 72 hours after onset of AF because spontaneous conversion may occur (especially in racehorses).

- Check electrolyte status before treatment.

THERAPEUTIC GOAL(S)

- Lone AF: Medical or electrical conversion to sinus rhythm; no treatment in horses at rest.
- Secondary AF: Medical therapy to improve cardiac function, reduce ventricular response rate (furosemide, digoxin, angiotensin-converting enzyme inhibitors). Cardioversion should not be attempted in horses with heart failure.

ACUTE GENERAL TREATMENT

- Medical treatment: Perform in a quiet environment and have IV access available. Continuous ECG monitoring is necessary.
  - Quinidine sulphate via nasogastric tube: 22 mg/kg q2h until:
    - Conversion to sinus rhythm: Terminate treatment.

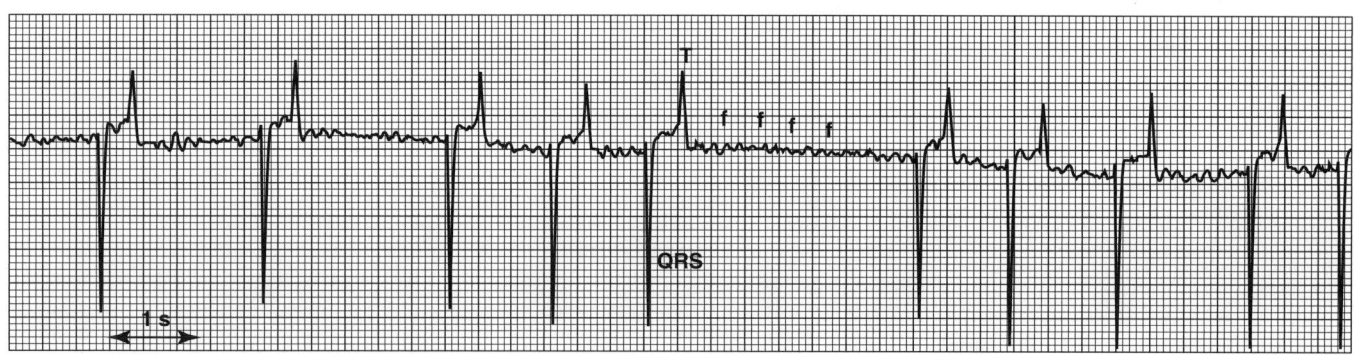

FIGURE 1 Atrial fibrillation (AF). During AF, P waves are absent and replaced by (coarse and fine) fibrillation waves (f waves). QRS complexes have a normal morphology, but RR intervals are irregularly irregular.

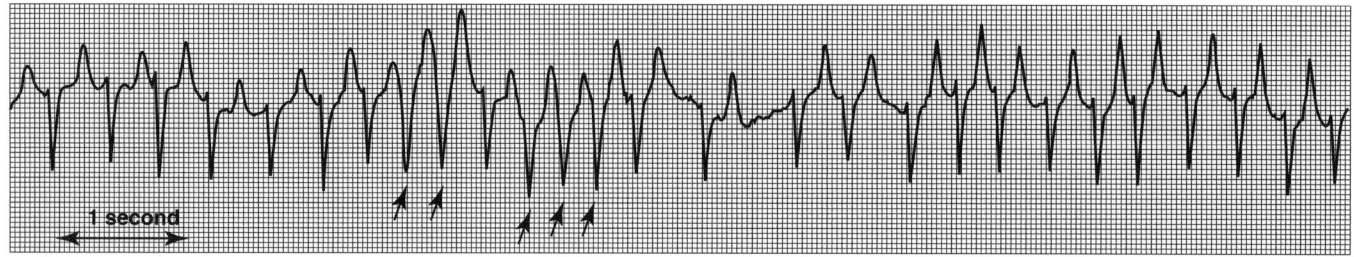

FIGURE 2 Transvenous electrical cardioversion (TVEC). Surface electrocardiogram during TVEC of a horse with atrial fibrillation (AF) of 10 weeks' duration. A 150-J biphasic shock (*arrow*), synchronized with the R wave (*arrowheads*), converts AF (f waves) instantaneously to sinus rhythm (P waves).

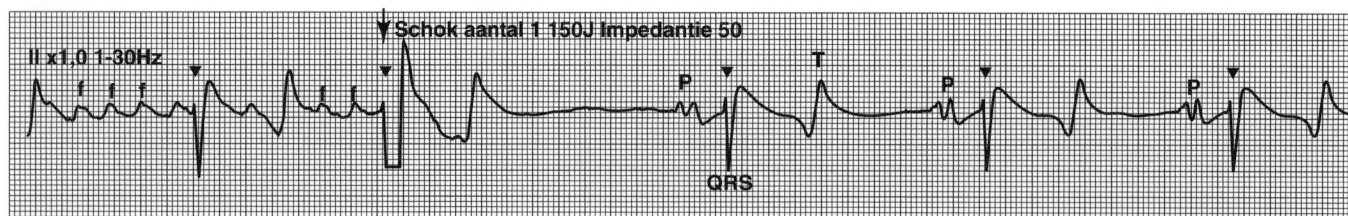

FIGURE 3 Atrial fibrillation with ventricular tachycardia. During exercise, rhythm remains irregular, although differences in RR intervals are smaller and less obvious because of the high heart rate. The horse presents with a run of wide QRS complexes (*arrows*) and shows the R-on-T phenomenon. The abnormal QRS complexes are caused by ventricular ectopy or aberrant conduction.

- Maximal daily dose of 132 mg/kg: Continue the same treatment for the second (or third) day.
- Mild toxic signs occur such as tachycardia below 100 beats/min, depression, anorexia, nasal edema, mild discomfort: Increase the interval between treatments (q3–4h) or administer q6h (half-life of quinidine).
- Severe toxic signs such as a ventricular rate in excess of 100 beats/min, QRS duration increased by 25%, colic, diarrhea, laminitis, hypotension, collapse: Terminate quinidine treatment.
  - Administer isotonic sodium bicarbonate (1 mEq/kg IV) to increase protein binding.
  - If tachycardia is supraventricular: Digoxin (2.2 μg/kg IV) (because of protein binding, the risk for adverse effects might be increased) or propranolol (0.03 mg/kg IV) or if no severe signs of hypotension are present, an IV α_2-agonist (eg, detomidine 5.0–7.5 μg/kg). Diltiazem may prove useful for ventricular rate control but has not been proven in horses with AF.
  - If tachycardia is ventricular: Magnesium sulphate IV (4 mg/kg q2min up to a total of 50 mg/kg). Treat life-threatening ventricular tachycardia with lidocaine IV (0.25–0.5 mg/kg q5min to a total dose of 2–4 mg/kg) or procainamide (1 mg/kg/min IV; maximal dose, 20 mg/kg).
  - In case of hypotension: Crystalloids and phenylephrine IV (0.1–0.2 g/kg/min up to 0.01 mg/kg)
- If quinidine plasma levels can be monitored: Therapeutic plasma concentration is 2 to 5 μg/mL.
- If cardioversion is not achieved, a second treatment might be attempted after 1 week. Combine treatment with digoxin if treatment failure occurred because of tachycardia.
  - Quinidine gluconate IV: 1.0 to 1.5 mg/kg q10min until conversion, toxic side effects occur, or a total dose of 12 mg/kg
    - Particularly useful for recent-onset AF
    - Increased risk of side effects
  - Amiodarone IV: 5 mg/kg administered over 1 hour followed by continuous infusion of 0.83 to 1.90 mg/kg/min over 1 to 3 days
    - Side effects include diarrhea and hindlimb weakness.

- Lower efficacy than oral quinidine sulphate.
- Especially useful in horses when therapeutic quinidine levels cannot be achieved because of toxic side effects.
  - Flecainide IV at 0.2 mg/kg/min over 10 minutes. Should not be used because of low efficacy and high risk for life-threatening ventricular arrhythmias.
- Transvenous electrical cardioversion
  - Requires general anesthesia, specialized equipment, and expertise
  - A biphasic synchronized direct-current shock is delivered via two transvenously inserted cardioversion catheters (with a large surface area electrode)
    - Preparation in the standing horse
      - Check and correct electrolyte disorders.
      - Insert and position catheters under ultrasonographic guidance.
        - Position one cardioversion catheter in the left branch of the pulmonary artery.
        - Position one cardioversion catheter in the right atrium.
      - An additional pacing catheter may be inserted into the right ventricular apex.
      - Administration of an antiarrhythmic drug may decrease the risk for immediate recurrence of AF after cardioversion.
    - After induction of general anesthesia
      - Take precautions to avoid injury because of the horse's limb movement during shock delivery.
      - Avoid any direct or indirect (urine, table) contact between individuals and the horse during shock delivery.
      - Check catheter position by ultrasongraphy or radiography and correct if necessary.
      - Connect both catheters and a surface ECG (avoid alcohol as a coupling agent!) to the defibrillator.
      - Carefully check R-wave detection by the defibrillator. In case of T-wave detection, always reposition surface electrodes to avoid T-wave detection. There is no unique electrode position that avoids T-wave detection.
      - Deliver biphasic synchronized shocks (simultaneous with the R wave of the surface ECG) at incremental energy levels (125–360 J with 50-J steps). Cardioversion usually occurs

between 150 and 250 J (see Figure 3).
  - In case of temporary asystole, ventricular pacing is performed via the right ventricular pacing electrode.
  - In case of conversion failure, cardioversion catheters should be repositioned to repeat the cardioversion procedure. Simultaneous administration of antiarrhythmic drugs (eg, IV amiodarone) may increase the success rate.
  - After successful cardioversion, wait for 10 minutes before gentle retraction of the catheters. Atrial premature beats might easily reinduce AF.

DRUG INTERACTIONS

Quinidine and digoxin are both highly protein bound with narrow therapeutic windows. Their concurrent use increases effective plasma levels of both drugs, increasing the risk of adverse effects.

POSSIBLE COMPLICATIONS

- Quinidine sulphate complications
  - Laminitis, diarrhea, hypotension, collapse, sudden death (ventricular proarrhythmia).
  - Permanent venous access and permanent ECG monitoring should be available during treatment.
- Amiodarone complications
  - Hindlimb weakness, weight shifting, and diarrhea.
  - Terminate amiodarone treatment; treat with 6000 IU of vitamin E PO.
  - Symptoms of weight shifting resolve within a few hours.
  - Diarrhea may last for about 1 to 10 days. Treat with supportive therapy.
- Transvenous electrical cardioversion complications
  - Related to anesthesia
  - Related to catheterization (premature beats, embolism, and thrombosis)
  - Related to shock delivery
    - T wave on the surface ECG is detected as an R wave. Shock delivery on a T wave holds a very high risk for induction of ventricular fibrillation (fatal). Reposition surface electrodes (no standard location) so that the T wave is no longer detected by the defibrillator.
    - Atrial or ventricular ectopy: Minimize risk by shock synchronization with R wave and by using lowest energy levels.
    - Temporary asystole: Perform temporary right ventricular pacing via the temporary pacing catheter (inserted before induction of anesthesia)

- Myocardial damage: Keep applied energy to a minimum.
  - Related to catheter withdrawal: Atrial or ventricular premature beats, which might result in immediate recurrence of AF.
    - Wait for 10 minutes after cardioversion before withdrawing catheters.
    - Simultaneous use of antiarrhythmic drugs during electrical cardioversion reduces the risk for immediate recurrence or may lower the cardioversion threshold.

RECOMMENDED MONITORING

- In case of successful cardioversion
  - Wait at least 5 days after cardioversion to perform 24-hour ECG monitoring.
    - Presence of frequently occurring atrial premature beats might increase the risk for AF recurrence.
    - Presence of ventricular premature beats
  - Rest period:
    - (Sub)acute AF (days to weeks): May rest similar to the duration of AF
    - If AF duration is more than 2 months: May rest for 1 to 2 months
  - Check heart rhythm before returning to work.
  - Teach the owner to palpate apex beat or auscultate with a stethoscope. Check every 3 to 6 months or when recurrence is suspected.
- In case of cardioversion failure
  - Horse at rest: No further monitoring unless underlying cardiac disease is present.
  - Horses intended for exercise: An exercise ECG during a thorough exercise test, compatible with the level of work the horse will be used for, is strongly recommended. Horses presenting with extremely high ventricular rates with abnormal QRS morphology (R-on-T) should

not be used for intense work because of an increased risk for collapse or sudden death and an inability to perform that work level.
  - Horses with AF cannot perform strenuous exercise such as racing.

PROGNOSIS AND OUTCOME

- Lone AF: Good prognosis if sinus rhythm can be restored, particularly if present for a short duration before conversion attempts. Horses return to previous level of performance when sinus rhythm is restored. The recurrence rate of AF is approximately 15% to 20%.
- Lone AF with concurrent ventricular ectopy: Guarded as long as ventricular premature beats persist.
- Secondary AF: Poor prognosis; depends on the underlying cardiac disease.

PEARLS & CONSIDERATIONS

COMMENTS

- Inform owners about the possible risk of the treatment, especially medical treatment (all antiarrhythmic drugs have the potential to be proarrhythmic).
- AF is very well tolerated when horses are not put into work and may be well tolerated if the work is not strenuous.
- Paroxysmal AF may be difficult to discover when it only occurs during maximal exercise. ECG monitoring during exercise is necessary and may show extremely high rates (commonly >250 beats/min). At such high rates, the irregularity in RR interval becomes difficult to detect.

PREVENTION

There is no prevention for AF. However, there may be some benefit to being extremely cautious if using diuretics in

racehorses that have had a prior episode of AF because electrolyte disturbances arising from diuretic use may potentiate AF.

CLIENT EDUCATION

For successfully converted horses, the owner should be trained how to palpate the apex beat or auscultate with a stethoscope. A change in exercise tolerance should also prompt a recheck evaluation by a veterinarian.

SUGGESTED READING

De Clercq D, van Loon G, Baert K, et al: Effects of an adapted intravenous amiodarone treatment protocol in horses with atrial fibrillation. *Equine Vet J* 39:344–349, 2007.

De Clercq D, van Loon G, Baert K, et al: Intravenous amiodarone treatment in horses with chronic atrial fibrillation. *Vet J* 172:129–134, 2006.

De Clercq D, van Loon G, Schauvliege S, et al: Transvenous electrical cardioversion of atrial fibrillation in six horses using custom made cardioversion catheters. *Vet J* 177:198–204, 2008.

McGurrin MKJ, Physick-Sheard PW, Kenney DG, et al: Transvenous electrical cardioversion of equine atrial fibrillation: technical considerations. *J Vet Intern Med* 19:695–702, 2005.

McGurrin MKJ, Physick-Sheard PW, Kenney DG: Transvenous electrical cardioversion of equine atrial fibrillation: patient factors and clinical results in 72 treatment episodes. *J Vet Intern Med* 22:609–615, 2008.

Reef VB, Reimer JM, Spencer PA: Treatment of atrial fibrillation in horses: new perspectives. *J Vet Intern Med* 9:57, 1995.

Schwarzwald CC, Bonagura JD, Luis-Fuentes V: Effects of diltiazem on hemodynamic variables and ventricular function in healthy horses. *J Vet Intern Med* 19:703–711, 2005.

van Loon G: *Atrial pacing and experimental atrial fibrillation in equines* [doctoral thesis]. Belgium, Ghent University, 2001, pp 1–258.

van Loon G, De Clercq D, Tavernier R, Amory H, Deprez P: Transient complete atrioventricular block following transvenous electrical cardioversion of atrial fibrillation in a horse. *Vet J* 170:124–127, 2005.

AUTHOR: GUNTHER VAN LOON

EDITOR: MARY M. DURANDO

Atrial Flutter

BASIC INFORMATION

DEFINITION

Supraventricular arrhythmia characterized by rapid, regular atrial depolarizations that are caused by a self-sustaining,

single-circuit reentry mechanism. The atrial rate is approximately 180 to 250 contractions per minute with an irregular ventricular response.

SYNONYM(S)

Auricular flutter

EPIDEMIOLOGY

SPECIES, AGE, SEX

- Large breeds are more susceptible than small breeds.
- Rarely occurs in ponies.

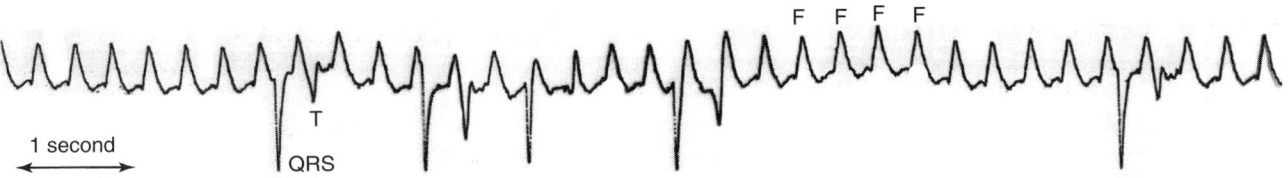

FIGURE 1 Atrial flutter is characterized by continuous, rapid, regular, sawtooth flutter waves (F waves). The ventricular rate at rest is normal, but the ventricular rhythm is irregular. Slight changes in QRS and T-wave morphology occur because of superposition of the flutter waves.

RISK FACTORS
- Similar to atrial fibrillation (AF)
- Underlying cardiovascular pathology leading to atrial dilation or atrial myocardial structural lesions
- Atrial premature contractions
- Electrolyte disturbances
- High vagal tone

CLINICAL PRESENTATION
DISEASE FORMS/SUBTYPES
- Spontaneous, sustained atrial flutter occurs on rare occasions in horses. In most animals, the arrhythmia quickly turns into AF.
- Atrial flutter is frequently encountered during quinidine treatment in horses, as an intermediate rhythm between AF and sinus rhythm.

HISTORY, CHIEF COMPLAINT
- Performance loss
- Occurs during quinidine treatment

PHYSICAL EXAM FINDINGS
- Irregular pulse
- Auscultation
  - Irregular rhythm (normal rate at rest)
  - Rapid atrial sounds rarely detected

ETIOLOGY AND PATHOPHYSIOLOGY
- A single-circuit reentry is induced by atrial premature beats and results in a regular, rapid atrial rate independent of the sinus node.
- Irregular conduction of the atrial impulses through the atrioventricular (AV) node results in an irregular ventricular response.
- Chronic atrial flutter leads to a loss of atrial contractile function caused by tachycardiomyopathy.
- Generally, no or only mild underlying cardiac pathology is present. Horses with severe cardiac disease generally do not develop atrial flutter but rather AF.

DIAGNOSIS

DIFFERENTIAL DIAGNOSIS
- Atrial tachycardia: Generally produces a slower or irregular atrial rate (or both). However, regular atrial tachycardia at a high rate may be impossible to differentiate from atrial flutter.
- AF: Fibrillation waves are found on the surface electrocardiogram (ECG).
- Advanced second-degree AV block: At rest, P waves occur at a rate of 24 to 120/min; isoelectric segments are present; normal QRS morphology with (ir)regular RR intervals.
- Third-degree AV block: At rest, the surface ECG presents P waves (24–120/min); isoelectric segments are present; normal or abnormal QRS morphology with (ir)regular RR intervals.

INITIAL DATABASE
- Auscultation: Irregularly irregular rhythm
- ECG:
  - Typical sawtooth flutter waves replace the P waves and isoelectric segments
  - Irregular RR intervals
  - QRS morphology is supraventricular but shows small alterations because of superposition with the flutter waves
- Evaluate for signs of underlying cardiac disease

ADVANCED OR CONFIRMATORY TESTING
- Cardiac ultrasonography
- Electrolyte status
- Myocardial markers

TREATMENT

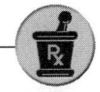

THERAPEUTIC GOAL(S)
Conversion of sustained atrial flutter to sinus rhythm

ACUTE GENERAL TREATMENT
- Similar treatment as for AF.
- Atrial burst pacing in standing horses has been described.
  - A temporary pacing catheter is placed in the right atrium and connected to a pacing device.
  - Burst pacing (pulses of 5.0–7.5 V and 0.5–1.0 ms) at a rate slightly faster than the flutter rate is performed to entrain and terminate the reentry mechanism.

RECOMMENDED MONITORING
Similar to AF

PROGNOSIS AND OUTCOME
Good prognosis if sinus rhythm is restored

SUGGESTED READING
Bonagura JD, Reef VB, Schwarzwald CC: Cardiovascular diseases. In Reed SM, Bayly WM, Sellon DC, editors: *Equine internal medicine*, ed 3. St Louis, 2010, Saunders, pp 378–487.

Buchanan JW: Spontaneous arrhythmias and conduction disturbances in domestic animals. *Ann N Y Acad Sci* 127:224–238, 1965.

van Loon G, Jordaens L, Muylle E, et al: Intracardiac overdrive pacing as a treatment of atrial flutter in a horse. *Vet Rec* 142:301–303, 1998.

van Loon G, Jordaens L, Muylle E: Temporary transvenous atrial pacing in horses: threshold determination. *Equine Vet J* 33:290–295, 2001.

AUTHOR: GUNTHER VAN LOON

EDITOR: MARY M. DURANDO

Atrial Premature Complexes and Atrial Tachycardia

BASIC INFORMATION

DEFINITION

- Atrial premature complex (APC): A premature depolarization that originates from the atrial myocardium, resulting in a P′ wave on the surface electrocardiogram (ECG) (Figure 1).
- Atrial tachycardia (AT): Three or more consecutive atrial premature beats, usually with regular P′P′ intervals.
- Depending on their prematurity, the premature beats may or may not be conducted to the ventricles.

SYNONYM(S)

- Atrial premature contractions
- Atrial premature beats
- Atrial premature depolarizations
- Atrial extrasystoles
- Atrial ectopy

EPIDEMIOLOGY

RISK FACTORS

- Atrial dilation
- Atrial myocardial disease
- Electrolyte and metabolic disturbances
- Hypoxia, anemia
- Fever
- High sympathetic tone or administration of sympathomimetics

CLINICAL PRESENTATION

DISEASE FORMS/SUBTYPES

- Isolated atrial premature contractions versus AT
- Paroxysmal (short, self-terminating bout) versus sustained (continuous) AT

HISTORY, CHIEF COMPLAINT

- Usually no complaints; incidental finding during auscultation or ECG
- Occasionally, poor performance
- Complaints related to underlying disease (eg, respiratory or gastrointestinal disease, atrial dilation caused by mitral regurgitation)
- Drug administration

- Previous episodes of atrial fibrillation (paroxysmal AF or successfully converted AF)

PHYSICAL EXAM FINDINGS

- APCs
  - Generally result in an irregular cardiac rhythm on auscultation; the intensity of the first heart sound is usually normal or decreased.
  - Nonconducted, interlaced APCs may produce a soft atrial sound or may not be heard on auscultation at all.
- AT
  - May result in a fast but regular ventricular response when 1:1 or 2:1 atrioventricular conduction occurs
  - May result in an irregular ventricular response because of irregular atrioventricular conduction
- Pulse deficits or weak pulses may be palpated.
- Signs of underlying disease that produces hypoxia, electrolyte imbalance, atrial dilation (eg, heart murmur, heart failure)

ETIOLOGY AND PATHOPHYSIOLOGY

- Atrial dilation
- Atrial myocardial lesions
- Electrolyte and metabolic disturbances
- Hypoxia, anemia
- Fever
- Drug administration (halothane, dobutamine)
- Endocarditis, pericarditis
- Iatrogenic during cardiac catheterization
- An electrical impulse is generated in the atrial myocardium and depolarizes both atria.
- Hemodynamic effects of isolated APCs, especially nonconducted APCs, are minimal. Frequent occurrence of conducted APCs, bouts of AT, or sustained AT reduce cardiac output and affect performance.
- APCs may increase, decrease, or disappear altogether during exercise.

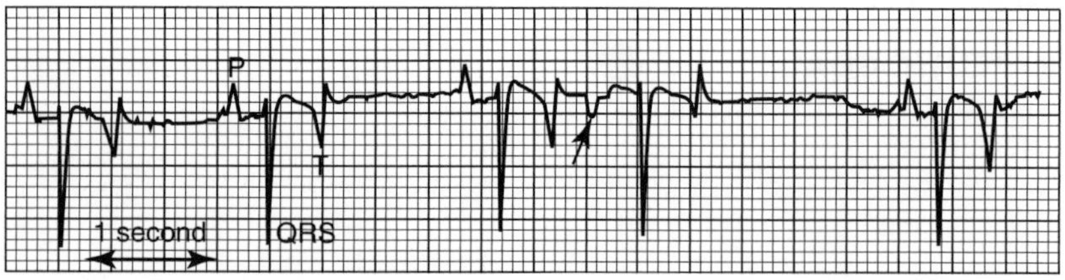

DIAGNOSIS

DIFFERENTIAL DIAGNOSIS

- Sinus tachycardia: Regularly occurring P waves (>50–60/min) because of stress, exercise, pain, drugs, or underlying disease.
- Atrial flutter: Regularly occurring sawtooth flutter waves at about 180 to 250/min.
- Atrial fibrillation: Fibrillation waves replace P waves.
- Ventricular premature contractions (VPCs): Depending on the prematurity of a VPC, the intensity of the first heart sound may be normal or reduced (indistinguishable from APC) or increased (in contrast to an APC). ECG is needed for the final diagnosis.
- Ventricular tachycardia: (Ir)regular RR intervals, QRS complexes with abnormal duration and morphology, and not associated with a preceding P wave

INITIAL DATABASE

- Ambulatory ECG
  - APC:
    - P′ occurs earlier than expected (premature) but may be buried in the preceding QRS or T.
    - P′ morphology may be normal or abnormal.
    - If conducted to the ventricles, QRS morphology is normal; T-wave morphology might change with a shortened RR interval (for a short RR interval, the T wave becomes opposite to the QRS complex).
    - The P′Q interval may be slightly different.
    - P′ is:
      - Usually followed by a noncompensatory pause (the RR interval of three consecutive sinus complexes [normal–normal–normal] is longer than that of the normal–premature–normal complexes because of resetting of the sinus node by the APC).
      - Occasionally followed by a compensatory pause (the RR interval of three consecutive sinus complexes is equal to that of the normal–premature–normal complexes because resetting of the sinus node did not occur)
      - Occasionally interlaced (P′ is not conducted to the ventri-

FIGURE 1 An atrial premature contraction presents as a P′ wave that occurs too early. In this case, the P′ wave has a different morphology. The QRS complex that follows has a normal morphology and duration.

cles, does not reset the sinus node, and therefore does not disturb the underlying rhythm)
○ AT:
- Three or more consecutive APCs, usually with a fairly regular $P'P'$ interval, and a rate of ±50 to 160/ min.
- P' waves that conduct to the ventricles result in a normal QRS morphology (abnormal QRS morphology caused by bundle branch block is probably rare in horses).
- Paroxysmal (self-terminating) or sustained.
- Intermittent conduction (2:1 or 3:1) or irregular conduction results in a normal or moderately elevated ventricular rate or an irregular ventricular rate.
- When every P' is conducted (1:1 conduction), the ventricular rate is high and regular. Because of their high vagal tone, horses rarely present with a high (>120 beats/min) ventricular response rate and 1:1 conduction at rest except when sympathetic tone is increased (stress, exercise, hypotension, heart failure, hypoxia).
- Exercise ECG is needed (unless the condition of the horse precludes an exercise test) to look at the response of APC or AT during exercise and to find out if paroxysmal atrial fibrillation develops during (sub)maximal exercise.
- Echocardiography to identify atrial structural lesions or predisposing cardiac disease.
- Electrolyte status (serum, fractional excretion).
- Complete blood cell count and biochemistry to look for underlying disease.

ADVANCED OR CONFIRMATORY TESTING
- Arterial blood gas analysis.
- Vitamin E and selenium levels.
- Myocardial markers (cardiac troponin I, CK-MB).
- Long-term ambulatory ECG recordings (24-hour Holter monitor) should be made to monitor the frequency of APC or AT.
- Repeated monitoring of electrolyte status to look for a correlation with the arrhythmia.
- Right atrial myocardial biopsies may be taken, especially when generalized myocardial disease is suspected (not commonly performed in horses).

TREATMENT

THERAPEUTIC GOAL(S)
- No treatment in case of occasional and asymptomatic APCs
- Rest
- Treatment of underlying, predisposing disorders
- Antiinflammatory drugs in case of suspected myocardial disease

ACUTE GENERAL TREATMENT
- No treatment is required if APCs are infrequent and asymptomatic and disappear during exercise.
- Treat electrolyte imbalances.
- Terminate drug administration (eg, dobutamine).
- If APCs occur only during exercise or if APCs are frequent at rest and exercise and there is exercise intolerance, rest for 4 to 8 weeks. If no response, the rest period can be combined with prednisolone therapy when there is no indication of infection (1 mg/kg PO SID for 1 week; 0.5 mg/kg PO SID for 1 week; 0.5 mg/kg SID every other day for 1 week).
- If AT with normal ventricular rate: Rest for 4 to 8 weeks (may be combined with steroids)
- If AT with persistent high ventricular response rate at rest (rare): Treat with propranolol, diltiazem, or digoxin.
- Repeated resting ECGs, 24-hour Holter monitoring, and exercise ECG need to be performed before the horse returns to full exercise.

RECOMMENDED MONITORING
Telemetric ECG monitoring during treatment with propranolol, diltiazem, or digoxin (rarely indicated)

PROGNOSIS AND OUTCOME
- APCs and AT are a possible trigger for induction of atrial fibrillation, although the exact prevalence is unknown.
- Horses with occasional and asymptomatic APCs have a fairly good prognosis.
- Occasional APCs at rest that disappear during exercise are not likely to be associated with poor performance and carry a fairly good prognosis.
- If APCs occur frequently during exercise, APCs are frequent at rest and exercise, or the APCs are related to paroxysmal AF during exercise:
  ○ Prognosis is guarded until repeated ECG monitoring shows improvement of the condition.
  ○ Prognosis is guarded in case of myocardial disease (fibrosis, calcification, neoplasia), endocarditis, and pericarditis.
- Prognosis depends on the underlying cause (hypoxia, anemia, renal disorders).

PEARLS & CONSIDERATIONS
APCs or AT represent a risk factor for development of sustained or paroxysmal atrial fibrillation (generally during [sub]maximal exercise).

SUGGESTED READING
Martin BB Jr, Reef VB, Parente EJ, Sage AD: Causes of poor performance of horses during training, racing, or showing: 348 cases (1992–1996). *J Am Vet Med Assoc* 216:554–558, 2000.

Reef VB: Arrhythmias. In Marr CM, editor: *Cardiology of the horse*. London, 1999, WB Saunders, pp 179–209.

Schwarzwald CC, Hamlin RL, Bonagura JD, et al: Atrial, SA nodal, and AV nodal electrophysiology in standing horses: normal findings and electrophysiologic effects of quinidine and diltiazem. *J Vet Intern Med* 21:166–175, 2007.

AUTHOR: **GUNTHER VAN LOON**

EDITOR: **MARY M. DURANDO**

Atrioventricular Block, First Degree

BASIC INFORMATION

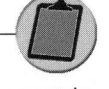

DEFINITION
Delayed conduction of the supraventricular impulse at the level of the atrioventricular (AV) node, resulting in a prolonged PQ interval.

SYNONYM(S)
First-degree AV block, first-degree heart block

EPIDEMIOLOGY
GENETICS AND BREED PREDISPOSITION More common in horses than in ponies

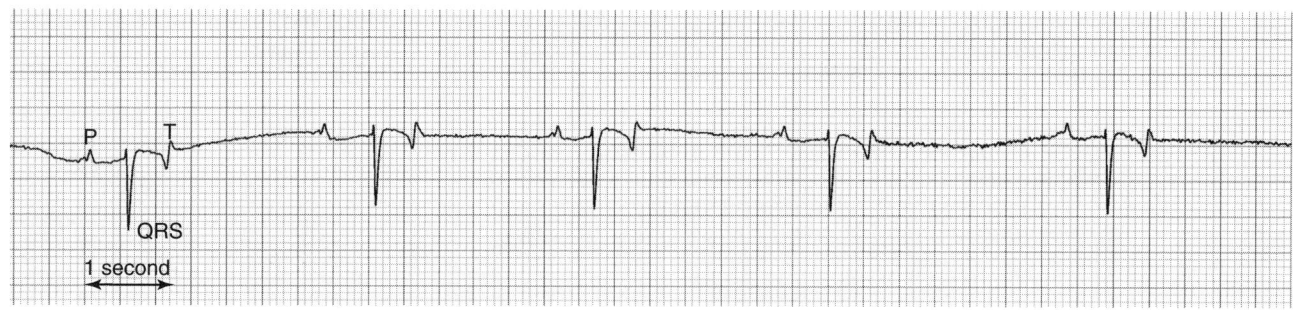

FIGURE 1 First-degree atrioventricular (AV) block. During first-degree AV block, conduction of the atrial impulse (P wave) through the AV node is delayed, resulting in an increased PQ interval (>500 ms).

RISK FACTORS
- High vagal tone
- Drug administration (eg, α_2 agonists, digoxin)

ASSOCIATED CONDITIONS AND DISORDERS Other vagally induced arrhythmias such as sinus arrhythmia, sinus block, second-degree AV block

CLINICAL PRESENTATION
HISTORY, CHIEF COMPLAINT
- Usually no complaints
- Drug administration

PHYSICAL EXAM FINDINGS Auscultation: Normal or slow heart rate. The atrial sound is clearly separated from the first heart sound.

ETIOLOGY AND PATHOPHYSIOLOGY
- High vagal tone
- Drug administration (eg, α_2 agonists such as detomidine or xylazine or calcium channel blockers such as verapamil or digoxin)
- Electrolyte disorders

DIAGNOSIS

INITIAL DATABASE
- Electrocardiography (Figure 1):
  - Prolonged PQ interval (>500 ms). The duration of the PQ interval often increases and decreases.
  - Normal P wave and QRS morphology.
  - P wave is followed by QRS complex.
  - Disappears upon decreased vagal tone (eg, stress, physical activity, atropine administration).

ADVANCED OR CONFIRMATORY TESTING
Ultrasound: The M-mode of the mitral valve often shows a presystolic opening.

SUGGESTED READING
Holmes JR: Cardiac rhythm irregularities in the horse. *Equine Pract* 2:15–25, 1980.

Kojouri GA, Rezakhani A, Torki E: The effects of verapamil hydrochloride on electrocardiographic (ECG) parameters of domestic donkey (*Equus asinus*). *J Equine Vet Sci* 27:499–503, 2007.

Wagner AE, Muir WW, Hinchcliff KW: Cardiovascular effects of xylazine and detomidine in horses. *Am J Vet Res* 52:651–657, 1991.

AUTHOR: GUNTHER VAN LOON

EDITOR: MARY M. DURANDO

Atrioventricular Block, Second Degree

BASIC INFORMATION

DEFINITION
The supraventricular impulse is intermittently blocked at the level of the atrioventricular (AV) node, resulting in a "missed" ventricular beat. At rest, this arrhythmia occurs in about 45% of healthy horses.

SYNONYM(S)
- Second-degree AV block
- Second-degree heart block
- The term *high-grade* or *high-degree AV block* is used for both advanced second- and third-degree AV block.

EPIDEMIOLOGY
RISK FACTORS
- High vagal tone
- Drug administration (eg, α_2 agonists)

ASSOCIATED CONDITIONS AND DISORDERS Other vagally induced arrhythmias such as sinus arrhythmia, sinus block, first-degree AV block

CLINICAL PRESENTATION
DISEASE FORMS/SUBTYPES
- Physiologic second-degree AV block (most common arrhythmia in healthy horses)
  - Mobitz type I (Wenckebach): The PQ interval progressively prolongs until a P wave is blocked. Variations in pp intervals are often present.
  - Mobitz type II: Constant PQ interval with an intermittently blocked P wave.
- Advanced (high-grade or high-degree) second-degree AV block (pathologic): Three or more consecutive P waves are blocked, resulting in a large difference between atrial and ventricular rate. AV conduction is still present.

HISTORY, CHIEF COMPLAINT
- Usually no complaints
- Drug administration
- For advanced second-degree AV block: Exercise intolerance, weakness, and occasionally syncope

PHYSICAL EXAM FINDINGS
- Heart rate normal or decreased
- Pulse deficit (missing pulse)
- Auscultation
  - A dropped beat: Beat-to-beat interval is double the preceding intervals.
  - An atrial sound (S4) is often heard during the pause.
  - The irregularity often appears at regular intervals (eg, every 4 or 5 beats).
  - The irregularity abolishes with stress, exercise, or vagolytic agents.
- In case of advanced second-degree AV block: Slow or normal heart rate. Weakness or exercise intolerance may be present. Multiple dropped beats in a row that may not disappear with exercise or vagolytic agents may occur.

ETIOLOGY AND PATHOPHYSIOLOGY

- Caused by high vagal tone: This is a regulatory mechanism at rest whereby a beat-to-beat increase in blood pressure leads to a blocked beat to maintain a stable blood pressure.
- Drug administration: α_2 agonists (detomidine, xylazine) or calcium channel blockers (verapamil).
- Electrolyte imbalance.
- Toxicity (digitalis, injection of iron preparations).
- Structural lesions of the AV node (degeneration, inflammation, fibrosis). In these cases, advanced second-degree AV block may progress to third-degree AV block.
- Immediately after delivery of an intracardiac direct current electrical shock (eg, treatment of atrial fibrillation [AF]), advanced second-degree AV block may occur temporarily.
- Idiopathic.
- Second-degree AV block does not produce any clinical signs unless it results in a very slow heart rate (ie, advanced second-degree AV block).

DIAGNOSIS

DIFFERENTIAL DIAGNOSIS

- Sinus block: Missing beat without a P wave
- Sinus arrest: Longer pause without the presence of a P wave
- AF: Irregularly irregular RR intervals, absence of P waves, presence of fibrillation waves
- Third-degree AV block: No relationship between P waves and QRS complexes; QRS morphology often abnormal; RR intervals often irregular

INITIAL DATABASE

- Auscultation: A dropped beat with the presence of an atrial sound (this cannot always be heard)
- Electrocardiography (ECG)
  - Intermittently, the P wave is blocked at the AV node and therefore not followed by a QRS complex (Figure 1).
  - In between the blocked beats, the underlying rhythm is regular.
  - The PQ interval can progressively prolong until it is blocked (Mobitz I) or can be fixed (Mobitz II).
  - QRS complexes are preceded by a P wave, have a normal (or slightly prolonged) PQ interval, and have a normal morphology.
  - Advanced second-degree AV block: Three or more consecutively blocked P waves (Figure 2).
- ECG during stress or exercise or after administration of vagolytic drugs (eg, atropine or glycopyrrolate):
  - The arrhythmia is usually physiologic and disappears.
  - Persistence of the arrhythmia is pathologic.
- Electrolyte status

ADVANCED OR CONFIRMATORY TESTING

- Echocardiography to look for structural lesions:
  - It is normal to detect a brief regurgitant flow at the AV valves after a blocked P wave.
  - It is normal to detect a small amount of regurgitation at the semilunar valves at the end of diastole after a blocked P wave.
- Myocardial markers (eg, cardiac troponins)

TREATMENT

THERAPEUTIC GOAL(S)

- No treatment is required for physiologic second-degree AV block
- Advanced second-degree AV block
  - Reduce inflammation
  - Increase heart rate

ACUTE GENERAL TREATMENT

- Physiologic second-degree AV block: No treatment is required.
- Advanced second-degree AV block:
  - Complete rest
  - Correction of electrolyte status
  - Antiinflammatory treatment. Corticosteroids are generally used (if no infection is present): Dexamethasone (0.05–0.2 mg/kg IV followed by longer term oral prednisolone)
  - Signs of weakness or syncope
    - Vagolytic drugs such as atropine or glycopyrrolate at 0.001 to 0.01 mg/kg to determine if an increase in AV node conduction can occur (treatment may induce colic)
    - Isoproterenol at 0.05 to 0.2 μg/kg/min: Should be used with care because it may induce ventricular tachyarrhythmias
    - Temporary pacing or permanent pacemaker implantation

CHRONIC TREATMENT

- Advanced second-degree AV block
  - Prolonged oral prednisolone treatment
  - Response to medical treatment to increase heart rate often unrewarding

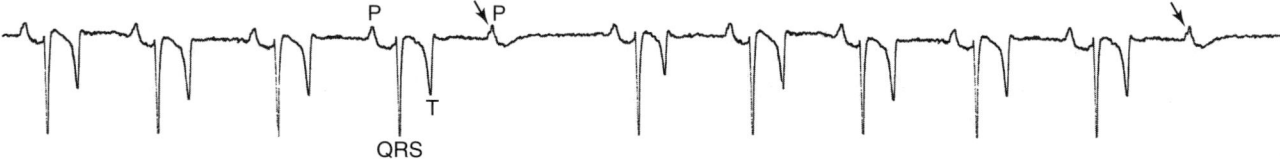

FIGURE 1 Second-degree atrioventricular (AV) block. During second-degree AV block, the atrial impulse is intermittently blocked at the AV node; the P wave (*arrow*) is not followed by a QRS complex.

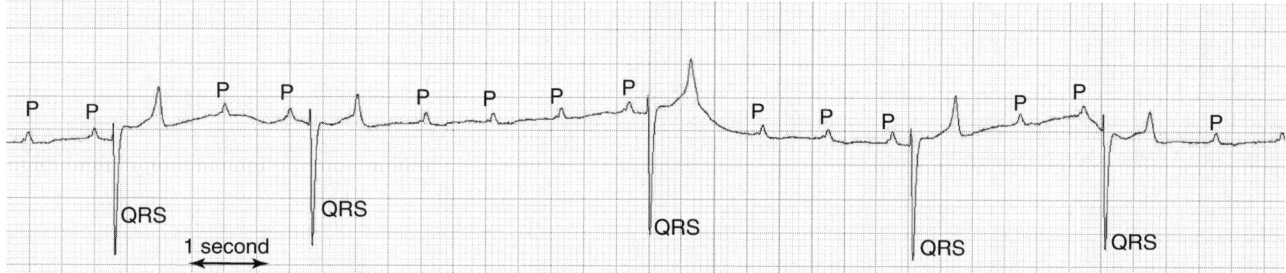

FIGURE 2 Advanced second-degree atrioventricular (AV) block. The term *advanced second-degree AV block* is used when three or more consecutive P waves are blocked at the AV node while AV conduction is still present. The latter implies that QRS complexes are preceded by conducted P waves and that the PQ interval is fixed.

- Pacemaker implantation (see "Atrioventricular Block, Third Degree" in this section)

POSSIBLE COMPLICATIONS

Advanced second-degree AV block, even with no clinical signs at rest, may suddenly deteriorate to third-degree AV block with severe signs of syncope.

RECOMMENDED MONITORING

- Advanced second-degree AV block
  - Monitor heart rate
  - Monitor exercise tolerance
  - Monitor ECG to assess response to medical treatment

PROGNOSIS AND OUTCOME

- Excellent for physiologic second-degree AV block

- Guarded to severe for advanced second-degree AV block that does not respond to steroid therapy

PEARLS & CONSIDERATIONS

For advanced second-degree AV block, the client should be aware of the risk of syncope or collapse. These animals should not be ridden because the risk to the rider is significant. The horse's environment should be adjusted to minimize trauma in case syncope occurs.

SUGGESTED READING

Holmes JR: Cardiac rhythm irregularities in the horse. *Equine Pract* 2:15–25, 1980.
Kiryu K, Kaneko M, Satoh H: Cardiopathological observations on histopathogenesis of incomplete atrioventricular block in horses. *Nippon Juigaku Zasshi* 39:425–436, 1977.
Kojouri GA, Rezakhani A, Torki E: The effects of verapamil hydrochloride on electrocardiographic (ECG) parameters of domestic donkey (*Equus asinus*). *J Equine Vet Sci* 27:499–503, 2007.
Schwarzwald CC, Hamlin RL, Bonagura JD, et al: Atrial, SA nodal, and AV nodal electrophysiology in standing horses: Normal findings and electrophysiologic effects of quinidine and diltiazem. *J Vet Intern Med* 21:166–175, 2007.
Wagner AE, Muir WW, Hinchcliff KW: Cardiovascular effects of xylazine and detomidine in horses. *Am J Vet Res* 52:651–657, 1991.
Yamaya Y, Kubo K, Amada A, Sato K: Intrinsic atrioventricular conductive function in horses with a second degree atrioventricular block. *J Vet Med Sci* 59:149–151, 1997.

AUTHOR: GUNTHER VAN LOON

EDITOR: MARY M. DURANDO

Atrioventricular Block, Third Degree

BASIC INFORMATION

DEFINITION

Total dissociation between the atrial (P waves) and ventricular (QRS complexes) rhythm because there is no conduction through the atrioventricular (AV) node. The ventricles depend on their own (slow) escape rhythm.

SYNONYM(S)

- Third-degree AV block
- Third-degree heart block
- Complete heart block
- The term *high-grade* or *high-degree AV block* is used for both advanced second- and third-degree AV block.

EPIDEMIOLOGY

RISK FACTORS Anesthetized foals with uroperitoneum

CLINICAL PRESENTATION

HISTORY, CHIEF COMPLAINT

- Marked exercise intolerance
- Weakness
- Syncope or collapse

PHYSICAL EXAM FINDINGS

- Progressive filling of the jugular vein during long diastolic pauses with visible pulsation secondary to right atrial contractions.
- Auscultation
  - Bradycardia
  - Regular or irregular rhythm
  - Loud first heart sound
  - Soft atrial sounds can often be heard, usually at an increased rate (>60/min)

- Signs of congestive heart failure may be found.
- Intermittent syncope or presyncope caused by long diastolic pauses. Immediately before syncope, the horse briefly shows an increased respiratory effort. Horses usually fall backward, sideways, or both.
- Lifting the head of a bradycardic horse may induce syncope.
- Syncopal episodes are usually short (seconds) and, after a few moments, the horse is able to stand again and looks relatively normal.

ETIOLOGY AND PATHOPHYSIOLOGY

- Etiology
  - Structural lesions of the AV node (fibrosis, inflammation, degeneration) that may be associated with endocarditis, myocarditis, or infiltrative processes
  - Severe hyperkalemia
  - Intoxication (rattlesnake envenomation)
  - Immediately after delivery of an intracardiac direct current electrical shock (eg, treatment of atrial fibrillation), a temporary high-degree AV block may occur
  - Idiopathic
- Pathophysiology
  - Clinical signs of weakness and intermittent syncope are related to the ability of the ventricles to generate their own (slow) escape rhythm.
  - The escape rhythm may emanate from pacemaker cells from the distal AV node, His bundle, or ventricle.

  - Bradycardia results in low blood pressure and a reflex increase in the atrial rate (commonly 60–120/min).
  - Lifting the horse's head seems to further decrease blood flow to the brain and may elicit syncope.

DIAGNOSIS

DIFFERENTIAL DIAGNOSIS

- Causes of fainting or collapse
  - Other cardiovascular causes such as tachyarrhythmias, structural cardiovascular disease (congenital defects, aortocardiac fistula, cardiomyopathy), severe pulmonary hypertension, systemic hypertension, embolism, intracardiac neoplasia.
  - Intracranial disease.
  - Narcolepsy (cataplexy): A narcoleptic episode usually starts with lowering the head and buckling at the knees and may progress to collapse.
  - Vasovagal syncope.
  - Metabolic (eg, hypoglycemia).
- Causes of bradycardia
  - Sinus bradycardia: Slow rate of P waves, normal AV conduction.
  - Sinus arrest: Pause without P wave or QRS complex; AV conduction is normal.
  - Advanced second-degree AV block: Three or more consecutive P waves are blocked at the AV node; AV conduction is still present.
- Electrocardiographic (ECG) features: Atrial flutter (or high-rate atrial tachy-

cardia). The PQ interval may vary; there are more P waves than QRS complexes and a clear relation between atrial and ventricular complexes is not present. However, the atrial rate (≈180–250/min) is much higher than in horses with third-degree AV block (≈60–120/min).

INITIAL DATABASE

- A good history: Knowing the manner in which the horse collapses and other associated events and timing of collapse helps to differentiate between the different causes of collapse.
- ECG to confirm the diagnosis (Figure 1)
  - P waves generally occur at an increased rate (>60/min) and have no relationship to the QRS complexes. PQ intervals have a variable duration.
  - Ventricular rate is slow (bradycardia).
  - QRS complexes have a normal (AV nodal or His bundle origin) or abnormal (ventricular origin) morphology and duration and occur at a slow rate.
  - RR intervals are regular (usually monomorphic QRS, idionodal rhythm) or irregular (monomorphic or polymorphic QRS, idioventricular rhythm).
- Echocardiography: To look for structural cardiovascular disease.

ADVANCED OR CONFIRMATORY TESTING

- Myocardial markers (eg, cardiac troponin I).
- Complete blood count, serum biochemistry. These are usually normal. Congestive heart failure may result in increased γ-glutamyltransferase, creatinine, or lactate concentrations.

TREATMENT

THERAPEUTIC GOAL(S)

- Increase heart rate
- Increase blood pressure
- Reduce inflammation

ACUTE GENERAL TREATMENT

- Medical treatment: Unrewarding in most cases
  - Vagolytic drugs such as atropine or glycopyrrolate IV (0.01 mg/kg): Usually no effect (risk for colic).
  - Corticosteroids (if no infectious underlying process): Dexamethasone IV (0.05–0.2 mg/kg) followed by oral prednisolone.
  - Isoproterenol at 0.05 to 0.2 μg/kg/min to stimulate ectopy should be used with care because it may induce ventricular tachyarrhythmias.

- Some horses regain AV conduction but still have advanced second-degree AV block. These animals are at risk for recurrence of third-degree AV block because part of their conductive tissue might remain nonfunctional.
- Temporary pacing until a permanent pacemaker can be implanted
  - Insert the temporary pacing catheter in the lower jugular vein and position the catheter tip in right ventricular apex under ultrasound guidance.
  - Connect electrodes to a temporary pacing device fixed to the horse's back.
  - Start ventricular pacing at two or three times the threshold at a rate of about 40 beats/min.
  - Prepare for permanent pacemaker implantation.
- Permanent pacemaker implantation.

CHRONIC TREATMENT

- Permanent pacemaker implantation can be performed in the standing horse. Temporary pacing is performed during the procedure to prevent bradycardia and syncope.
  - Depending on the pacemaker type, one or two pacemaker leads are inserted via the cephalic vein or the jugular vein.
  - The lead tip is positioned in the right atrium, right ventricle, or both under ultrasound guidance.
  - A fixation mechanism at the lead tip preserves endomyocardial contact. Fixation of the atrial lead is the most difficult part of the procedure because it more easily dislodges and is more difficult to visualize on ultrasonography.
  - The leads are connected to a pacemaker that is implanted in a subcutaneous pocket at the chest.
  - Via the electrode(s), the pacemaker is able to sense intrinsic activity of the myocardium and to stimulate the myocardium by delivering an electrical pulse.
- Pacemaker types (in order of complexity)
  - Ventricular (single-chamber) pacemaker: One lead is implanted in the right ventricle. The pacemaker prevents bradycardia by maintaining a minimal ventricular rate.
  - Ventricular rate-adaptive pacemaker: Ventricular pacemaker with an activity sensor. When physical activity is detected, the paced heart rate progressively increases and decreases.
  - Dual-chamber pacemaker (Figure 2): One lead is implanted in the right ventricle, and one lead is implanted in the right atrium. Both

chambers can be sensed and paced. The pacemaker is programmed to stimulate the ventricle each time an atrial depolarization is sensed, which results in a physiologic adaptation of heart rate. This type of pacemaker provides the best result with third-degree AV block.
  - Dual-chamber rate-adaptive pacemaker: Dual-chamber pacemaker is able to adapt heart rate when it senses physical activity of the horse. This type is indicated more for sinus bradycardia and sick sinus syndrome.

POSSIBLE COMPLICATIONS

- Complications associated with syncope, such as trauma
- Complications associated with temporary pacing: Embolism, lead dislodgement, loss of capture, infection
- Complications associated with pacemaker implantation: Lead dislodgement, loss of capture (fibrosis around lead tip), infection

RECOMMENDED MONITORING

- Periodic monitoring of heart rate, exercise tolerance, and ECG for horses with third-degree AV block that reverts to second-degree AV block

PROGNOSIS AND OUTCOME

- Fair to good with permanent pacemaker implantation.
- Fair to good for horses in which third-degree AV block reverts to normal conduction. In some horses, recurrence of third-degree AV block may occur.
- Grave when third-degree AV block persists and when a pacemaker cannot be implanted. The condition leads to congestive heart failure and death.

PEARLS & CONSIDERATIONS

Inform the client of the risk of a collapsing horse. These horses should never be ridden because of the danger to the rider.

SUGGESTED READING

Reef VB, Clark ES, Oliver JA, Donawick WJ: Implantation of a permanent transvenous pacing catheter in a horse with complete heart block and syncope. *J Am Vet Med Assoc* 189:449–452, 1986.

Hamir AN, Reef VB: Complications of a permanent transvenous pacing catheter in a horse. *J Comp Pathol* 101:317–326, 1989.

Lawler JB, Frye MA, Bera MM, et al: Third-degree atrioventricular block in a horse

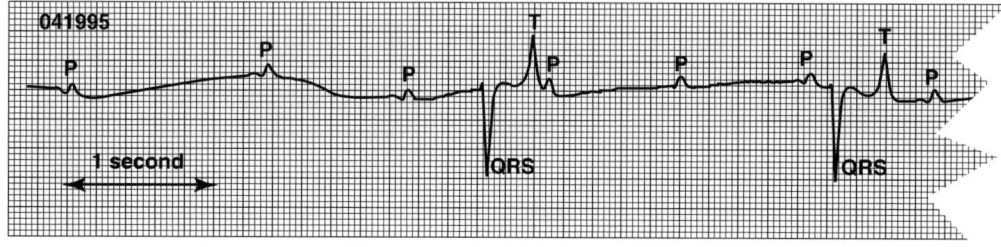

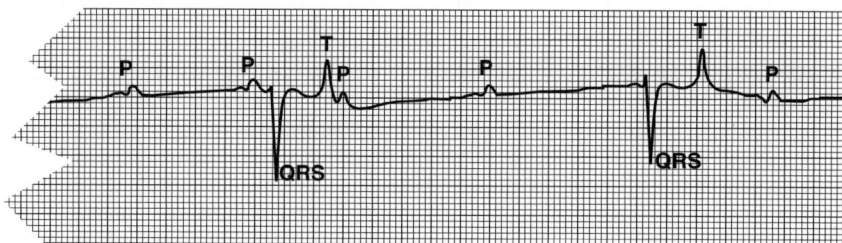

FIGURE 1 Third-degree atrioventricular (AV) block. AV conduction is completely absent during third-degree AV block, resulting in dissociation between atrial and ventricular rhythm. The atrial and ventricular rates were 65 and 23 beats/min, respectively.

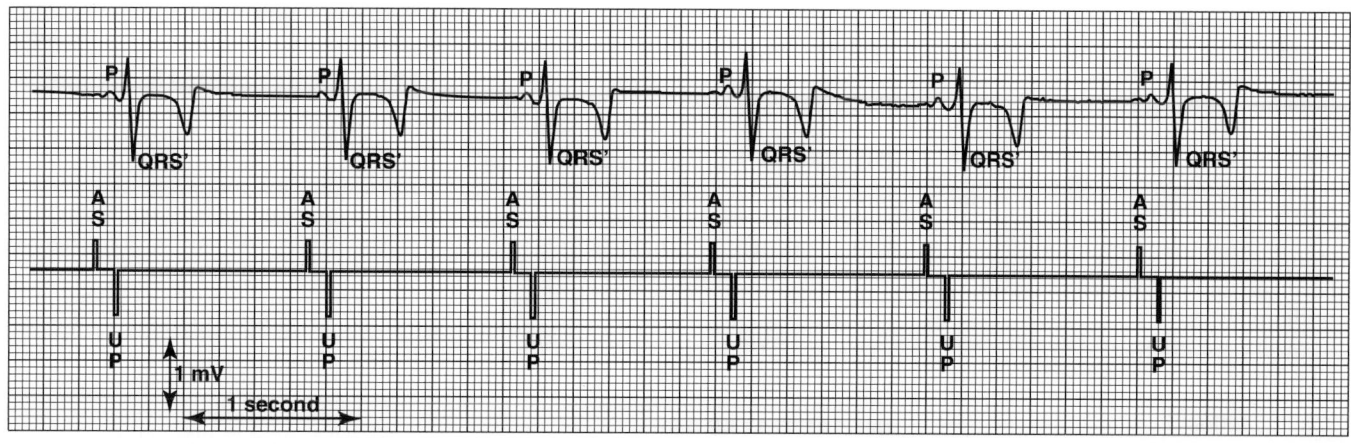

FIGURE 2 Pacemaker. Surface electrocardiogram (*upper trace*) and marker channel (*lower trace*) of a horse with a dual-chamber pacemaker. The pacemaker is programmed to pace the ventricle after each sensed atrial depolarization; each spontaneous P wave is sensed and triggers a ventricular pace (VP), which results in a QRS' complex. Because ventricular pacing is performed in the right ventricular apex, the QRS' complex has an abnormal morphology and duration. *AS,* Atrial sense.

secondary to rattlesnake envenomation. *J Vet Intern Med* 22:486–490, 2008.

Sugiyama A, Takeuchi T, Morita T, et al: Mediastinal lymphoma with complete atrioventricular block in a horse. *J Vet Med Sci* 70:1101–1105, 2008.

van Loon G, De Clercq D, Tavernier R, et al: Transient complete atrioventricular block following transvenous electrical cardioversion of atrial fibrillation in a horse. *Vet J* 170:124–127, 2005.

van Loon G, Fonteyne W, Rottiers H, et al: Dual chamber pacemaker implantation via the cephalic vein in healthy equids. *J Vet Intern Med* 15:564–571, 2001.

van Loon G, Fonteyne W, Rottiers H, et al: Implantation of a dual-chamber, rate-adaptive pacemaker in a horse with suspected sick sinus syndrome. *Vet Rec* 151:541–545, 2002.

van Loon G, Laevens H, Deprez P: Temporary transvenous atrial pacing in horses: threshold determination. *Equine Vet J* 33: 290–295, 2001.

AUTHOR: GUNTHER VAN LOON

EDITOR: MARY M. DURANDO

Back Pain (Thoracolumbar Dysfunction)

BASIC INFORMATION

DEFINITION
Abnormal function of the thoracolumbar region caused by pain, muscle hypertonicity, or stiffness. Severe cases include neurologic deficits.

SYNONYM(S)
• Thoracolumbar hyperesthesia
• Thoracolumbar hyperpathia
• Cold back syndrome

EPIDEMIOLOGY
SPECIES, AGE, SEX Congenital vertebral malformations are more likely to be observed in young horses.
GENETICS AND BREED PREDISPOSITION
• Hyperkalemic periodic paralysis (HyPP) in Quarter Horses
• Hereditary equine regional dermal asthenia (HERDA) or hyperelastosis cutis in Quarter Horses
• Polysaccharide storage myopathy (PSSM) in Quarter Horse–related breeds, Warmbloods, and draft horses
• Breed predisposition for dorsal spinous process impingement or overriding in Thoroughbreds and lordosis in Saddlebreds

RISK FACTORS
• Vertebral column malformations
• Trauma or flipping over backward
• Exercise-induced myopathies
• Poor musculoskeletal conditioning or overuse
• Pelvic limb lameness
• Improper or poorly fitting saddle, saddle pads, or harness
• Unskilled or overweight riders

CONTAGION AND ZOONOSIS Supraspinous bursitis (fistulous withers) has a zoonotic potential caused by *Brucella abortus* infection.

ASSOCIATED CONDITIONS AND DISORDERS
• Poor performance
• Lameness or altered gait

CLINICAL PRESENTATION

DISEASE FORMS/SUBTYPES
• Congenital: Vertebral malformations, ankylosis
• Degenerative: Osteoarthritis, spondylosis
• Acquired: Dorsal spinous process impingement
• Traumatic: Pressure sores from ill-fitting tack, spinous process or vertebral body fractures
• Infectious: Equine protozoal myeloencephalitis (EPM), equine herpesvirus type 1 (EHV-1) myeloencephalitis
• Metabolic: PSSM
• Iatrogenic: Improper or ill-fitting saddle, saddle pads, or harness

HISTORY, CHIEF COMPLAINT
• Skin lesions or bumps in the saddle region
• Asymmetric sweat marks on the back or dirt patterns on the saddle pad
• Painful or stiff back
• Change in spinal posture or soft tissue swelling
• Resentment to grooming, saddle placement, or tightening of the girth or cinch
• History of flipping over backward
• Bucking and rearing when mounted or ridden
• Pins ears or swishes tail when mounted or ridden
• Poor performance and vague gait abnormalities
• Difficulty with collection
• Reluctance to jump

PHYSICAL EXAM FINDINGS

- Dermatitis or skin lesions
- Alopecia or white hairs in the region of saddle or harness
- Increased heat or palpable swelling
- Pain elicited on palpation of the thoracolumbar soft tissues or dorsal spinous processes
- Thoracic lordosis, lumbar kyphosis, or scoliosis
- Flattened and widened dorsal contour of the withers
- Dorsally prominent or laterally deviated dorsal spinous process
- Reduced active and passive range of spinal motion in lateral bending or extension
- Generalized lack of muscle development or local muscle atrophy
- Epaxial muscle hypertonicity or fasciculations
- Exaggerated cutaneous trunci reflex or spinal reflexes
- Ataxia, spasticity, or weakness (in pelvic limbs only)
- Reduced dorsoventral spinal mobility at the walk, trot, or canter
- Poor pelvic limb engagement and propulsion during the canter
- Precipitated or aggravated back problem only when ridden

ETIOLOGY AND PATHOPHYSIOLOGY

Numerous tissues may be the source of back pain or stiffness:

- Soft tissue
  - Trauma: Poorly fitting saddle, muscle strain, postanesthetic myopathy
  - Inflammation: Supraspinous ligament desmitis, thoracolumbar fasciitis
  - Infection: Dermatitis (bacterial or fungal)
  - Metabolic: PSSM
  - Endocrine: Hyperadrenocorticism
  - Genetic: HERDA or hyperelastosis cutis, PSSM, HyPP
  - Nutritional: Vitamin E and selenium deficiency (nutritional myodegeneration or white muscle disease, equine rhabdomyolysis)
- Vertebral column
  - Congenital: Hemivertebrae or block vertebrae
  - Degeneration: Osteoarthritis, spondylosis
  - Trauma: Dorsal spinous process or vertebral body fractures
  - Infection: Vertebral osteomyelitis, discospondylitis
- Neurologic
  - Trauma: Thoracolumbar spinal cord compression
  - Infection: EPM, EHV-1 myeloencephalitis
  - Neoplasia (space-occupying mass): Malignant melanoma
  - Nutritional: Vitamin E deficiency (equine degenerative myeloencephalopathy (EDM), equine motor neuron disease (EMND)

DIAGNOSIS

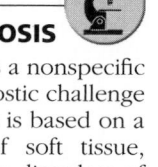

DIFFERENTIAL DIAGNOSIS

Back pain or dysfunction is a nonspecific clinical sign and is a diagnostic challenge for practitioners. Diagnosis is based on a diagnosis of exclusion of soft tissue, orthopedic, and neurologic disorders of the thoracolumbar region. For specific differential diagnoses, see "Etiology and Pathophysiology" above.

INITIAL DATABASE

- Inspection of trunk conformation, posture, muscle symmetry, and development
- Gait evaluation to assess limb lameness, propulsion, and dorsoventral spinal mobility
- Saddle fit assessment
- Evaluation of ridden exercise or athletic activity
- Neurologic examination
- Soft tissue and bony palpation
- Active and passive joint range of motion in flexion-extension and lateral bending
- Spinal and cutaneous trunci reflexes
- Rectal examination
- Thoracolumbar spinal radiography
- Microbial culture and sensitivity of any draining wounds
- Serum vitamin E and selenium levels
- Serum potassium levels
- Urinalysis to assess myoglobinuria

ADVANCED OR CONFIRMATORY TESTING

- Diagnostic local anesthesia of dorsal spinous processes, articular facets, or intertransverse joints
- Nuclear scintigraphy
- Ultrasonography of supraspinous ligament, dorsal spinous processes, or articular processes
- Transrectal ultrasonography to assess the lumbosacral joint and intervertebral disc space
- Serum creatine kinase and aspartate aminotransferase levels before and after exercise
- Muscle biopsies for histologic and histochemical analysis
- Pressure algometry to assess mechanical nociceptive thresholds
- Therapeutic trial with high dosage of nonsteroidal antiinflammatory drugs (NSAIDs) for 7 to 10 days
- Cerebrospinal fluid analysis
- Electromyography
- Thermography
- Serology and virus isolation
- Genetic testing: HyPP, PSSM, and HERDA

TREATMENT

THERAPEUTIC GOALS

- Eliminate or reduce pain so that affected horses can resume regular training programs
- Reduce muscle hypertonicity
- Promote full joint range of thoracolumbar motion in flexion-extension and lateral bending
- Eliminate any sources of infection
- Establish proper saddle fit and ridden exercise
- Develop effective therapeutic exercise and training programs
- Increase muscle mass and symmetry
- Restore athletic and performance capabilities

ACUTE GENERAL TREATMENT

- Stall confinement or exercise restriction, only as needed
- Controlled hand walking
- Slow and prolonged warmup period
- Temporary reduction in intensity, duration, or frequency of exercise or training program
- Passive thoracolumbar mobilization
- Cryotherapy to reduce heat, swelling, or pain
- Antiinflammatory drugs: NSAIDs, corticosteroids, dimethyl sulfoxide
- Muscle relaxants
- Periarticular or interspinous space corticosteroid injections
- Low-level light or laser therapy
- Electroacupuncture and mesotherapy
- Electric muscle stimulation
- Surgical exploration or debridement of puncture wounds or draining tracts
- Tiludronate

CHRONIC TREATMENT

- Active and passive thoracolumbar range of motion and stretching exercises
- Core stabilization and strengthening exercises
- Moist heat therapy
- Acupuncture
- Chiropractic treatment to reduce pain and muscle hypertonicity, increase spinal mobility, and restore symmetric spinal motion
- Daily physical therapy and rehabilitation
- Massage therapy
- Electromagnetic stimulation
- Extracorporeal shock-wave therapy
- Antioxidant supplementation with vitamin E
- Surgical resection of refractory impinged dorsal spinous processes
- Warmup or flexibility exercises: "long and low," circles, figure-8, serpentine
- Ground poles, cavalletti, and incline work
- Maintain proper body conditioning

DRUG INTERACTIONS

- Complications associated with excessive dosages or long-term phenylbutazone use in horses include gastrointestinal ulceration, renal medullary crest necrosis leading to acute or chronic renal failure, and ulceration of the right dorsal colon.
- NSAIDs should not be used in conjunction with corticosteroids.

POSSIBLE COMPLICATIONS

- Worsening or recurrence of clinical signs
- Adverse reaction to antiinflammatory medications
- Development of behavioral issues related to chronic pain

RECOMMENDED MONITORING

- Monitor signs of pain, muscle tone, and flexibility daily.
- Repeat physical and chiropractic examination to assess response to therapy or rehabilitation.
- Periodically modify and increase therapeutic exercise and training programs.
- Repeat saddle fit assessment during changes in body condition and muscle development.

PROGNOSIS AND OUTCOME

- Highly variable depending on the specific cause and the severity of the underlying disease process
- Dependent on the type, severity, and number of concurrent spinal lesions present
- Dependent on the rider's ability to correctly use the horse and to engage its back

PEARLS & CONSIDERATIONS

COMMENTS

- Long-term rest or pasture turnout without active rehabilitation is often contraindicated.
- Localization of pain to affected structures requires detailed physical and chiropractic examinations.
- Active and passive trunk range of motion is useful for identifying affected vertebral levels and laterality of the thoracolumbar dysfunction.

PREVENTION

- Turnout as much as possible
- Establish proper saddle fit and saddle pad use
- Importance of maintaining trunk flexibility and range of motion exercises
- Nutritional management with a high-fat, low-carbohydrate diet
- DNA testing and selective breeding to noncarriers of genetic-based diseases

CLIENT EDUCATION

- Owner should monitor recurrence of signs that warrant repeat examination.
- Avoid riding exercise in any horse with neurologic deficits.
- Proper saddle fit is difficult in horses with fractured withers and displaced dorsal spinous processes.
- If an appropriate therapeutic response is not noted with conservative care, then additional diagnostics and advanced imaging techniques are warranted.

SUGGESTED READING

Denoix JM, Dyson SJ: Thoracolumbar spine. In Ross MW, Dyson SJ, editor: *Diagnosis and management of lameness in the horse.* St Louis, 2003, Elsevier, pp 509–521.

Haussler KK, Stover SM, Willits NH, et al: Pathologic changes in the lumbosacral vertebrae and pelvis in Thoroughbred racehorses. *Am J Vet Res* 1999;60:143–153, 1999.

Jeffcott LB: Disorders of the thoracolumbar spine of the horse—a survey of 443 cases. *Equine Vet J* 1980;12:197–210, 1980.

Landman MAAM, de Blaauw JA, van Weeren PR, et al: Field study of the prevalence of lameness in horses with back problems. *Vet Rec* 2004;155:165–168, 2004.

Sullivan KA, Hill AE, Haussler KK, et al: The effects of chiropractic, massage and phenylbutazone on spinal mechanical nociceptive thresholds in horses without clinical signs of back pain. *Equine Vet J* 2008;40:14–20, 2008.

AUTHOR: **KEVIN K. HAUSSLER**

EDITOR: **ANDRIS J. KANEPS**

Biliary Atresia

BASIC INFORMATION

DEFINITION

In horses, biliary atresia is a rare congenital absence of the common bile duct.

EPIDEMIOLOGY

SPECIES, AGE, SEX Considered a congenital disease; the signalment is a newborn to 1-month-old foal.

ASSOCIATED CONDITIONS AND DISORDERS

- Clinical signs of biliary atresia are associated with hepatic insufficiency and are generally nonspecific.
- Differential diagnoses for hepatic disease, gastrointestinal disease, or septicemia should be excluded.

CLINICAL PRESENTATION

HISTORY, CHIEF COMPLAINT Nonspecific clinical signs include lethargy, decreased appetite, failure to thrive, colic, icterus, fever, polydipsia, and polyuria.

PHYSICAL EXAM FINDINGS Physical examination findings are nonspecific and include fever, icterus, poor body condition, abdominal pain, and lethargy.

ETIOLOGY AND PATHOPHYSIOLOGY Extrahepatic biliary atresia is a congenital absence of the entrance to common bile duct or absence of the duct itself in neonatal foals, resulting in intrahepatic biliary hypertrophy that displaces hepatocytes and causes periportal or perilobular hepatocellular damage, fibrosis, and ultimately liver failure.

DIAGNOSIS

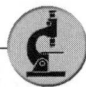

DIFFERENTIAL DIAGNOSIS

- Portosystemic shunt
- Biliary obstruction secondary to duodenal stricture

INITIAL DATABASE

- Complete Blood count with fibrinogen: Normal or consistent with acute or chronic inflammation
- Sorbitol dehydrogenase (SDH) activity: Normal to mildly increased
- Gamma glutamyltransferase (GGT): Markedly increased
- Serum conjugated bilirubin concentration: Increased
- Serum bile acids concentration: Markedly increased

ADVANCED OR CONFIRMATORY TESTING

- Ultrasound examination of the liver and abdomen
- Liver biopsy reveals extensive biliary proliferation with absence of bile, degenerative hepatocytes, and fibrosis
- Nuclear hepatobiliary scintigraphy (see "Diagnostic Imaging of the Liver" in Section II)

TREATMENT

Therapeutic options are not currently available for congenital biliary atresia in horses.

PROGNOSIS AND OUTCOME

Biliary atresia is accompanied by a fatal prognosis.

SUGGESTED READING

van der Luer RJ: Biliary atresia in a foal. *Equine Vet J* 14:91, 1982.
Witzelben CL, Buck BE, Schnaufer L, Brzosko WJ: Studies on the pathogenesis of biliary atresia. *Lab Invest* 38:525, 1978.

AUTHOR: **ERIN S. GROOVER**

EDITOR: **MICHELLE HENRY BARTON**

Biliary Obstruction

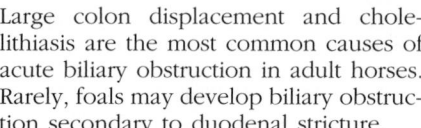

BASIC INFORMATION

DEFINITION

Large colon displacement and cholelithiasis are the most common causes of acute biliary obstruction in adult horses. Rarely, foals may develop biliary obstruction secondary to duodenal stricture.

EPIDEMIOLOGY

SPECIES, AGE, SEX
- Middle-aged to older horses
- Neonatal foals secondary to duodenal stricture

CLINICAL PRESENTATION

HISTORY, CHIEF COMPLAINT
- Depression, anorexia, and colic.
- Bruxism and salivation may be present in foals.

PHYSICAL EXAM FINDINGS
- Fever, variable icterus, and colic.
- Clinical signs of hepatoencephalopathy and photosensitization may also be present.
- Clinical signs may be intermittent if a partial obstruction is present.
- Foals with duodenal stricture may have excessive gastric reflux.

ETIOLOGY AND PATHOPHYSIOLOGY
- Obstruction of the biliary tract in a mature horse may be attributable to cholelithiasis, right dorsal colon displacement, neoplasia, hepatic torsion, or portal vein thrombosis. Duodenal stricture in foals may be secondary to duodenal ulceration.
- Acute biliary obstruction causes cholestasis, biliary distension, and variable pain.
- Chronic biliary obstruction results in hepatic fibrosis, originating around the obstructed biliary branch(es).

DIAGNOSIS

DIFFERENTIAL DIAGNOSIS
- Cholelithiasis
- Pyrrolizidine alkaloid toxicity
- Chronic active hepatitis
- Biliary atresia in foals

INITIAL DATABASE
- The diagnosis of obstruction of the common bile duct in horses is difficult. Exploratory celiotomy may be necessary to identify the possible location or cause of the obstruction.
- The presence of concentric fibrosis around intrahepatic bile ducts on histopathology supports obstruction of the common bile duct.

ADVANCED OR CONFIRMATORY TESTING
- Hepatic ultrasonography may reveal hepatomegaly, increased echogenicity of the liver parenchyma, and bile duct dilation.
- The visualization of well-defined hyperechoic foci with acoustic shadows within dilated bile ducts confirms the diagnosis of biliary obstruction caused by the presence of choleliths.
- Rectal examination may be helpful in the diagnosis of a right dorsal colon displacement.
- Evidence of delayed gastric emptying in foals is supportive evidence for duodenal stricture.

TREATMENT

THERAPEUTIC GOAL(S)
Treatment should be directed to the underlying cause.

ACUTE GENERAL TREATMENT
General and supportive care with IV balanced fluids.

PROGNOSIS AND OUTCOME

The prognosis depends on the extent of liver involvement, severity of clinical signs, degree of secondary hepatic fibrosis, and number and location of the biliary obstruction.

SUGGESTED READING

Gardner RB, Nydam DV, Mohammed HO, et al: Serum gamma glutamyl transferase activity in horses with right or left dorsal displacements of the large colon. *J Vet Intern Med* 19:761–764, 2005.
Peek SF, Divers TJ: Medical treatment of cholangiohepatitis and cholelithiasis in mature horses: 9 cases (1991–1998). *Equine Vet J* 32:301, 2000.

AUTHOR: **MONICA DIAS FIGUEIREDO**

EDITOR: **MICHELLE HENRY BARTON**

Black Walnut Toxicosis

BASIC INFORMATION

DEFINITION

- Black walnut trees are large (50–100 feet) deciduous forest trees often planted as ornamentals.
- The demand for black walnut lumber has increased, and the wood shavings are sold for animal bedding. Shavings that contain even a small percentage of black walnut can cause laminitis when used as bedding for horses. Colic and respiratory distress have been reported in horses after they have chewed on black walnut bark.

SYNONYM(S)

Walnut family, including English walnut, butternuts, hickories, and pecans

EPIDEMIOLOGY

SPECIES, AGE, SEX Foals and yearling horses are often unaffected or recover quickly.

RISK FACTORS

- Horses that are bedded on more than 5% to 20% walnut shavings may develop laminitis (Figures 1 and 2).
- Not all black walnut trees have naturally occurring toxicity.

GEOGRAPHY AND SEASONALITY Black walnut (*Juglans nigra*) is a common hardwood species that ranges from the Great Plains to the east coast of North America. The species has been widely planted outside of its natural range and can be found all over North America. Laminitis may occur any time of the year, whenever walnut bedding is used.

ASSOCIATED CONDITIONS AND DISORDERS Consumption of the shavings or bark may cause laminitis as well as mild colic. Horses on pasture may show mild respiratory signs from chewing on bark, pollen, or fallen leaves.

CLINICAL PRESENTATION

DISEASE FORMS/SUBTYPES

- Laminitis
- Limb edema
- Respiratory distress
- Colic

HISTORY, CHIEF COMPLAINT

- History of new bedding material introduced with dark-colored shavings.
- Horses (often several animals in a stable) with clinical signs of laminitis.
- Signs usually develop within 8 to 18 hours of contact.
- Affected horses become unwilling to move or have their feet picked up, are often depressed, and may have limb edema.

PHYSICAL EXAM FINDINGS

- Laminitis
- Edema of the legs ("stocking up")
- Anorexia and depression
- Increased heart rate, respiratory rate, body temperature, and coronary band and hoof temperature
- Pounding digital pulse

ETIOLOGY AND PATHOPHYSIOLOGY

- The toxic principle is not known. Juglone was once believed to be involved because it was found in high concentrations in the hull of the nut. However, aqueous extracts of black walnut heartwood, which contain no juglone, consistently induce laminitis.
- The toxin appears to be absorbed through the coronary band and skin.
- The pathogenesis is not completely understood but is believed to be similar to other causes of acute laminitis.

- Black walnut shavings or aqueous extract induce alterations in the hemodynamics of blood flow to the hoof.
- Overall, blood flow to the foot is increased, and perfusion to the hoof is decreased.
- The toxin appears to act by causing a sensitization of vessels of the foot to the effects of adrenergic agonists, leading to an acute reduction in the functional blood flow to the foot that reaches the dorsal laminae.

DIAGNOSIS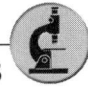

DIFFERENTIAL DIAGNOSIS

- Other causes of acute laminitis.
- If the hind legs are involved, affected horses have a gait that resembles "tying up," or myositis.

INITIAL DATABASE

- The complete blood count reveals a transient neutropenia in horses given an aqueous extract of black walnut orally at approximately 4 hours before the onset of the initial stages of laminitis.
- A sustained increase in plasma cortisol levels.

ADVANCED OR CONFIRMATORY TESTING

- Severity of the laminitis can be determined by radiography of the feet.
- Identification of shavings should be performed by a specialist in wood science.
- Histopathology is typical of acute laminitis, with necrosis of the dorsal laminae followed by mitotic activity in an effort to repair the damage.

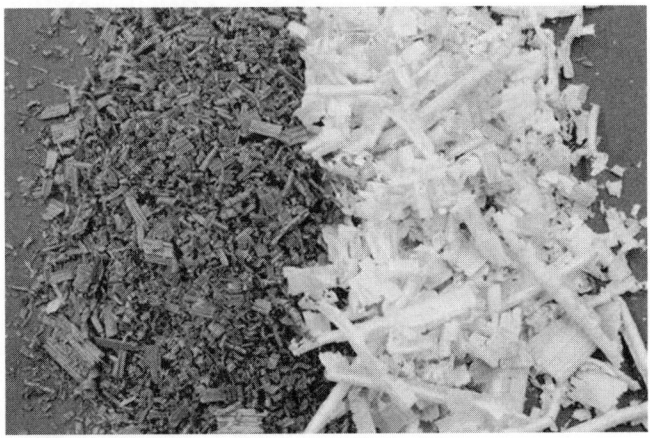

FIGURE 1 Pine and spruce wood shavings (*right*) and walnut wood shavings (*left*).

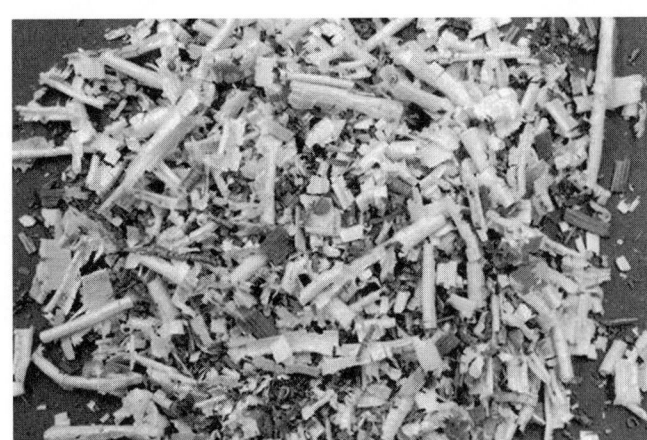

FIGURE 2 Pine shavings contaminated with walnut wood shavings.

TREATMENT

THERAPEUTIC GOAL(S)

- Begin treatment immediately.
- Remove all horses from the bedding and remove the bedding.
- Treatment is symptomatic and supportive; no specific antidote exists.

ACUTE GENERAL TREATMENT

- Wash the legs with mild detergent to remove any remaining residues.
- Conduct gastrointestinal decontamination with mineral oil or activated charcoal.
- Provide symptomatic therapy to control pain (eg, phenylbutazone administration).
- Give acepromazine or a more specific α-blocker to restore circulation to the dorsal laminae.
- Heparin may be used to prevent microthrombi formation.
- Refer to "Laminitis, Acute" and "Laminitis, Chronic" in this section for more information on therapy.

CHRONIC TREATMENT

- Place affected animals in sand stalls for relief of pain.
- Consider removing the shoes.

POSSIBLE COMPLICATIONS

Rotation of the third phalanx through the sole with permanent damage and sloughing of the hoof.

RECOMMENDED MONITORING

Radiography of the hoof

PROGNOSIS AND OUTCOME

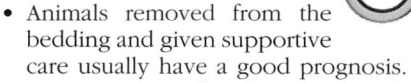

- Animals removed from the bedding and given supportive care usually have a good prognosis.
- Symptoms usually disappear within a few days after the shavings are removed.
- Horses with severe laminitis and rotation of P3 have a very guarded prognosis.

PEARLS & CONSIDERATIONS

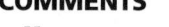

COMMENTS

- Horses on pasture may show mild respiratory signs from chewing on bark, pollen, or fallen leaves.
- Remember that the other members of the walnut family may also be a problem for horses.

PREVENTION

Do not use fresh shavings from black walnut trees or any of the walnut family for bedding.

CLIENT EDUCATION

Bedding from a hardwood mill or a furniture factory may contain black walnut shavings that can be very harmful to horses. If you are not sure, contact an expert with a sample of the shavings.

SUGGESTED READING

Black walnut (*Juglans nigra*). In Knight AP, Walter RG, editors: *A guide to plant poisoning of animals in North America*. Jackson, WY, 2001, Teton NewMedia, pp 301–302.

Galey FD: Black walnut. In Plumlee KH, editor: *Clinical veterinary toxicology*. St Louis, 2003, Mosby Elsevier, pp 425–427.

MacDaniels LH: Perspective on the black walnut toxicity problem—apparent allergies to man and horse. *Cornell Vet* 73:204–207, 1983.

Uhlinger C: Black walnut toxicosis in ten horses. *J Am Vet Med Assoc* 195:343–344, 1989.

AUTHOR: **BRENT HOFF**

EDITOR: **CYNTHIA GASKILL**

Black Widow Spider Toxicosis

BASIC INFORMATION

DEFINITION

The female black widow spider, *Latrodectus* spp., is recognized by its characteristic red hourglass marking on the adult ventral abdomen. Only the bite of the female spider is of toxicologic importance.

SYNONYM(S)

- Brown widow, red-legged spider, hourglass spider

EPIDEMIOLOGY

SPECIES, AGE, SEX Although cases are not well documented in horses, all are potentially susceptible.

RISK FACTORS

GEOGRAPHY AND SEASONALITY Distributed throughout North America, found in barns and other structures and outdoor wood and brush piles.

CLINICAL PRESENTATION

HISTORY, CHIEF COMPLAINT Black widow spider envenomation generally results in neuromuscular signs.

PHYSICAL EXAM FINDINGS Muscle fasciculations and rigidity, ataxia, and flaccid paralysis can progress to an ascending paralysis. The muscles of respiration may eventually become involved, leading to dyspnea and other breathing abnormalities. Restlessness, pain, abdominal rigidity, and cramping of the large muscle masses may also be observed.

ETIOLOGY AND PATHOPHYSIOLOGY The most important toxin in black widow spider venom is α-latrotoxin, a biologically active protein neurotoxin. Both calcium-dependent and -independent mechanisms lead to the release of numerous neurotransmitters because of increased movement of synaptic vesicles to the presynaptic neuronal membranes.

DIAGNOSIS

DIFFERENTIAL DIAGNOSIS

Colic, tying up, botulism, tetanus

INITIAL DATABASE

Elevated creatine kinase and aspartate transaminase levels may be detected.

ADVANCED OR CONFIRMATORY TESTING

Identification of the spider (if found)

TREATMENT

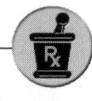

THERAPEUTIC GOAL(S)

- Respiratory and cardiac monitoring
- Pain management

ACUTE GENERAL TREATMENT

Administration of a 10% calcium gluconate solution is recommended in most veterinary references for the reversal of muscle fasciculations and weakness, although its efficacy appears to be inconsistent in humans. Initial symptomatic treatment for human patients instead typically consists of morphine and diazepam.

PROGNOSIS AND OUTCOME

Most animals completely recover within days to weeks with symptomatic and supportive care.

PEARLS & CONSIDERATIONS

Several antivenin products have been developed and may be extremely useful for patients that do not adequately respond to symptomatic care alone and are commonly administered to severely affected humans either IV or IM. The newer antivenins have fewer human allergic reactions because of a lack of protein impurities. The efficacy and adverse effects of these products in horses have not been documented.

SUGGESTED READING

Peterson ME: Toxic exotics. *Vet Clin North Am Exot Anim Pract* 11:375–287, 2008.
Roder JD: Spiders. In Plumlee KH, editor: *Clinical veterinary toxicology.* St Louis, 2004, Mosby Elsevier, pp 112–113.

AUTHOR: **LISA A. MURPHY**

EDITOR: **CYNTHIA L. GASKILL**

Blister Beetle Toxicosis

BASIC INFORMATION

DEFINITION

Blister beetles (*Epicauta* spp.) are insects that contain the toxin cantharidin, a potent vesicating agent that is readily absorbed from the gastrointestinal (GI) tract and skin. Cantharidin is a direct irritant that can cause shock and death within 4 hours after a massive dose or affect various organ systems, depending on the dose.

SYNONYM(S)

- Cantharidin toxicosis
- Cantharidiasis

EPIDEMIOLOGY

RISK FACTORS Feeding hay, pellets, or cubes that contain alfalfa, particularly after it has been crimped

GEOGRAPHY AND SEASONALITY
- Beetles can be a variety of colors, depending on their location (eg, black, gray with black spots, orange with black spots). Striped blister beetles, *Epicauta lemniscata,* are often found in alfalfa hay in the southwestern United States (Figure 1).
- Most blister beetles live in the South.
- Most cases occur in the winter when more hay is fed.
- Cases can occur year round if contaminated alfalfa products are fed.
- Cases can occur anywhere contaminated alfalfa is shipped.

CLINICAL PRESENTATION

DISEASE FORMS/SUBTYPES
- Acute: Massive dose
- Subacute: Lower dose

HISTORY, CHIEF COMPLAINT
- Sudden death: The horse is found dead in the morning after appearing normal when fed the previous night
- Depressed
- Anorectic

- Any clinical signs associated with colic
- Playing in water with muzzle
- Client's observation that animal is "not acting right"

PHYSICAL EXAM FINDINGS
Not all horses exhibit all the following clinical signs:
- Increased pulse
- Increased respiratory rate
- Diaphragmatic flutter
- Muscle fasciculations
- Tachycardia
- Sweating
- Frequent painful urination
- Depression
- Colic
- Diarrhea
- Oral lesions
- Salivation
- Restlessness
- Congested mucous membranes
- Increased capillary refill time
- Stiff gait
- Hematuria
- Fever

ETIOLOGY AND PATHOPHYSIOLOGY
- Cantharidin is a powerful vesicant.
- Concentration depends on the species, sex, and whether the insects have mated.
- Found in the hemolymph of male blister beetles.
- Transferred to females during mating.
- Affects mitochondrial membrane permeability.
- Has a direct irritant effect on entire GI tract.
- Rapidly absorbed from the GI tract.
- Excreted unchanged in the kidney and may cause irritation of the urinary system.
- May cause myocardial necrosis.
- Four grams of dried beetles may be lethal to a horse, with approximately 0.5 to 0.1 mg of cantharidin per kilogram of body weight being the estimated lethal dose.

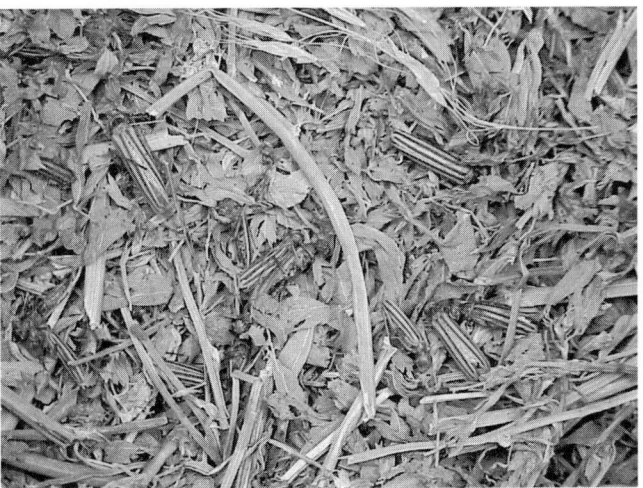

FIGURE 1 Blister beetles in alfalfa hay.

DIAGNOSIS

DIFFERENTIAL DIAGNOSIS

- Other types of colic
- Ionophore toxicosis

INITIAL DATABASE

- Decreased serum calcium
- Decreased serum magnesium

ADVANCED OR CONFIRMATORY TESTING

- Examination of alfalfa hay for the presence of beetles.
- Detection of cantharidin in urine by gas chromatography/mass spectrometry (GC/MS) or high-performance liquid chromatography (HPLC).
- Possible detection of cantharidin in serum, GI content, liver, or kidney, but these are not the specimens of choice.
- Cantharidin has been detected in pelleted feed and hay cubes.
- Postmortem lesions range from none to severe irritation and ulceration from the mouth throughout the entire GI tract and urinary bladder. White streaks have been observed on the heart. Gastroenteritis, nephrosis, cystitis, urethritis, and myocarditis have been seen microscopically.

TREATMENT

THERAPEUTIC GOAL(S)

- Reduce the absorption and enhance elimination of the toxin.
- Control pain.
- Control diarrhea.
- Reinoculate the gut.

ACUTE GENERAL TREATMENT

Aggressive therapy (day 1):
- Fluids
- Calcium in the form of calcium gluconate 23% solution 0.1 mL/kg/h IV

(large amounts in fluids until levels become normal)
- Magnesium in the form of magnesium sulfate 50 mg/kg IV diluted in 1 L of fluids for the first hour followed by continuous-rate infusion of 25 mg/kg/h
- Activated charcoal
- Nonsteroidal antiinflammatory drugs (NSAIDs)

CHRONIC TREATMENT

Days 2 to 5:
- NSAIDs
- Fluids
- Calcium, magnesium
- Diatomaceous earth
- Omeprazole
- Probiotics

POSSIBLE COMPLICATIONS

- Nephrosis
- Cardiac dysfunction

RECOMMENDED MONITORING

Serum calcium and magnesium

PROGNOSIS AND OUTCOME

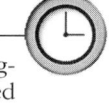

- Prognosis is good if recognized early and treated aggressively.
- Prognosis is guarded to poor if high dose, the animal is not diagnosed early, or therapy is not aggressive.

PEARLS & CONSIDERATIONS

COMMENTS

- The owner's observation that horse that has been eating alfalfa is "just not right," low serum calcium, diaphragmatic flutter, and playing in the water should initiate aggressive therapy.

- Diagnostic confirmation can be done in 4 to 24 hours.
- Cantharidin is very stable in hay and hay products.
- Contamination can occur even if blister beetles have not been observed. It is not practical to check every inch of hay.

PREVENTION

- Do not feed alfalfa hay, pellets, or cubes.
- Purchase hay that has not been crimped before baling and that has been baled before bloom stage or after a frost to decrease the incidence of beetle contamination.

CLIENT EDUCATION

- Clients can learn to identify blister beetles.
- Beetles tend to swarm, so multiple beetles generally can be observed in individual flakes of hay.

SUGGESTED READING

Helman RG, Edwards WC: Clinical features of blister beetle poisoning in equids: 70 cases (1983–1996). *J Am Vet Med Assoc* 211(8):1018–1021, 1997.

Gwaltney-Brandt S, Dunayer EK, Youssef HY: Terrestrial zootoxins. In Gupta RC, editor: *Veterinary toxicology.* New York, 2007, Elsevier, pp 791–793.

Stair EL, Plumlee KH: Blister beetles. In Plumlee KH, editor: *Clinical veterinary toxicology.* St Louis, 2004, Mosby Elsevier, pp 101–103.

Toribio RE: Disorders of calcium and phosphorus. In Reed SM, Bayly WM, Sellon DC, editors: *Equine internal medicine,* ed 3. St Louis, 2010, Saunders Elsevier, pp 1277-1291.

Toribio RE: Magnesium and disease. In Reed SM, Bayly WM, Sellon DC, editors: *Equine internal medicine,* ed 3. St Louis, 2010, Saunders Elsevier, pp 1291-1295.

AUTHOR: **SANDRA E. MORGAN**

EDITOR: **CYNTHIA GASKILL**

Borna Disease

BASIC INFORMATION

DEFINITION

- Borna disease virus (BDV) is an enveloped, single-stranded RNA virus that causes polioencephalomyelitis in horses.
- Transmission most likely occurs through contact with infected nasal, lacrimal, or salivary secretions with viral ascent through the olfactory (and

possibly trigeminal) nerve. The incubation period is extended, and infection appears to be restricted to the central nervous system (CNS).
- Affected horses present with alterations in behavior, sensorium, and consciousness that may progress to cranial nerve abnormalities, spinal cord abnormalities, and death. There is no effective treatment or vaccine. The prevalence and incidence of the disease worldwide are unknown.

SYNONYM(S)

Hot-headed disease, brain fever, subacute meningoencephalitis, hypersomnia of horses

EPIDEMIOLOGY

SPECIES, AGE, SEX

- There is no species or sex predilection.
- Age may be a factor in clinical disease because there is a high rate of sero-

prevalence but a low rate of disease in endemic areas.

GENETICS AND BREED PREDISPOSITION Genetics may be a factor in clinical disease because there is a high rate of seroprevalence but a low rate of disease in endemic areas.

RISK FACTORS Exposure to affected horses

CONTAGION AND ZOONOSIS

- The route of transmission of BDV is unknown. The virus has been detected in nasal, lacrimal, and salivary secretions of affected animals, so it is postulated that direct and indirect contact with infected horses can spread the virus.
- Whether BDV is a zoonotic agent that causes overt illness in humans is unknown. It does appear that humans can be affected by either the Borna virus or a Borna-like virus. Seroprevalence studies have revealed BDV antibodies in humans with psychiatric disorders and in humans without disease (similar to horses). However, the exact pathology of the virus in humans, whether it is transmitted to humans from horses, and whether it is a causative agent of disease in people, is unknown at this time.
- Veterinarians should take universal precautions when handling and performing necropsies on horses with any neurologic disease.

GEOGRAPHY AND SEASONALITY

- Clinical BDV has been recognized in horses in Germany, Switzerland, Liechtenstein, and Austria. Seroprevalence studies in Germany reveal that there is a large discrepancy between the incidence of disease (low) and the prevalence of BDV-specific antibodies (11%–20% normally; 55% during outbreaks). New occurrences of disease may occur anywhere from 2 months to several years after the initial outbreak. There is no seasonal trend to the virus.
- BDV is not likely restricted to Europe. Seroprevalence studies have revealed BDV antibodies in horses worldwide, including Europe, Turkey, the Middle East (Israel and Iran), Asia (Japan and China), Australia, and the United States. However, the incidence of disease caused by BDV infection in these countries is unknown.

CLINICAL PRESENTATION

DISEASE FORMS/SUBTYPES Peracute, acute, subacute, chronic polioencephalomyelitis

HISTORY, CHIEF COMPLAINT Horses present initially with alterations in behavior and consciousness.

PHYSICAL EXAM FINDINGS

- Initial clinical signs involve changes in personality and sensorium. Move-

ments are deliberate and slow and include general hypokinesia, postural unawareness, and slow eating or chewing with no food in the mouth. Many horses demonstrate rhythmic or repetitive movements and often yawn frequently and head press. Changes in personality and mental status, including hyperexcitability, fear, aggression, lethargy, somnolence, and stupor, may also occur. Loss of the cutaneous trunci reflex may also be noted early in the disease. A fever refractive to nonsteroidal antiinflammatory drugs may also occur.

- As the disease progresses, neurologic deficits increase. Cranial nerve abnormalities are often seen, including alterations in cranial nerve (CN) III (strabismus and miosis), CN V/VII (bruxism, trismus), CN VII/XI (nystagmus), CN VIII (head tilt), CN IX/X (dysphagia, pharyngeal paralysis), and CN XII (tongue paralysis). Spinal cord abnormalities are also present, including ataxia, imbalance, abnormal postures, hyporeflexia of spinal reflexes, and proprioceptive deficits. Changes in personality may progress.

- In the latter, end stages of BDV, the horse appears extremely unbalanced and often stops eating or drinking. Neurogenic torticollis accompanied by dystonia of the neck muscles with or without circular walking is often present. Head tremors, convulsions, head pressing, loss of the pupillary light reflex, and comatose states occur.

ETIOLOGY AND PATHOPHYSIOLOGY

- BDV mainly affects horses and sheep, although it has also been found to affect other equids, cattle, goats, and rabbits.
- The incubation period is extended and ranges from 2 weeks to several months (average, 2–3 months) after exposure.
- Enveloped negative-sense, single-stranded RNA virus.
- Released by budding from the cell.
- Initial infection most likely occurs through direct contact with viral particles from an infected animal or fomite.
- The virus appears to remain restricted to the CNS.
- The virus may invade the CNS through the following:
  - Intranasal infection through the olfactory nerve
  - Oral infection through the trigeminal nerve
- The virus migrates along the olfactory or trigeminal axons and replicates in the neuron cell bodies and glial cells of the limbic system.
- Over time, the virus disseminates throughout the CNS and then spreads

to the peripheral nervous system and retina.

- This coincides with the progression of clinical signs.
- Pathologic changes are indicative of polioencephalomyelitis.
  - Mainly involves the gray matter of the CNS and spinal cord
  - Retinal changes may also be seen.
  - Histopathologically, perivascular cuffing, parenchymal inflammation, astrocytosis, and loss of pyramidal cells may be seen.

DIAGNOSIS

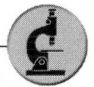

DIFFERENTIAL DIAGNOSIS

- Viral
  - Alphavirus encephalitis (Eastern equine encephalitis, Western equine encephalitis, Venezuelan equine encephalitis)
  - Flavivirus encephalitis (West Nile virus, Kunjin virus,* Japanese encephalitis,* Murray Valley fever*)
  - Rabies
  - Equine herpesvirus type 1
  - Equine encephalosis virus*
  - Nipah virus*
- Bacterial: Botulism
- Parasitic
  - *Halicephalobus gingivalis*
  - Setaria
  - *Strongylus vulgaris*
  - Equine protozoal myeloencephalitis
- Noninfectious
  - Hypocalcemia
  - Tremorgenic toxicities
  - Hepatoencephalopathy
  - Leukoencephalomalacia

INITIAL DATABASE

- Cerebrospinal fluid (CSF)
  - Increased proteins (>70 mg/dL)
  - Increased cell count (lymphomonocytic pleocytosis)
  - Chronic cases: CSF is usually normal except with elevated lactate levels
- Complete blood count and serum chemistries
  - Normal
  - Hyperbilirubinemia from decreased food intake

ADVANCED OR CONFIRMATORY TESTING

- BDV antibody detection: Titer ranges between 1:2 and 1:1280
- There is no correlation between disease severity and antibody titers.
- May or may not be present early in the course of disease or in corticosteroid-treated horses

---

*Foreign animal diseases not yet documented in North America.

- Tests
  - Enzyme-linked immunosorbent assay
  - Western immunoblot
  - Indirect immunofluorescence assay
- Postmortem testing
  - Histopathology
  - Immunohistochemistry
  - Western immunoblot
  - Reverse transcription polymerase chain reaction

TREATMENT

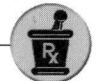

THERAPEUTIC GOAL(S)

Supportive care

ACUTE GENERAL TREATMENT

- There is no known effective treatment for BDV.
- Treatment strategies should focus on supportive care and the relief of anxiety.
  - Corticosteroids
  - Mannitol (0.25–2.0 g/kg q24h IV) may relieve brain edema.

PROGNOSIS AND OUTCOME

- Infection with BDV leads to death approximately 1 to 4 weeks after the onset of clinical signs in approximately 80% of animals.
- Approximately 10% of infected horses demonstrate a chronic, recurrent course of disease.
- With less severe cases, recovery can occur. There may be a persistent CNS infection.

PEARLS & CONSIDERATIONS

COMMENTS

- The prevalence and incidence of the disease outside of Europe is not known.
- Thus quarantine and having BDV on the differential list for horses with any neurologic disease is important.

PREVENTION

- There is no licensed vaccine for the prevention of BDV.
- The environment should be decontaminated with standard decontaminating agents.
- Affected horses and new arrivals should be quarantined.
- Proper universal precautions should be taken by all humans in contact with affected or suspect horses.

SUGGESTED READING

Richt J, Grabner A, Herzog S, et al: Borna disease. In Sellon D, Long M, editors: *Equine infectious diseases.* St Louis, 2007, Saunders Elsevier, pp 207–213.

AUTHOR: **MELISSA BOURGEOIS**

EDITORS: **MAUREEN T. LONG** and **DEBRA C. SELLON**

Bots

BASIC INFORMATION

DEFINITION

Infection with larvae of one or more species of botfly. Second- and third-stage larvae of *Gasterophilus intestinalis* and *Gasterophilus nasalis* cause focal mucosal irritation in the equine stomach or intestine, where they attach.

EPIDEMIOLOGY

RISK FACTORS Exposure to adult botflies and ingestion of eggs laid on the horse's hair.

CONTAGION AND ZOONOSIS

- Bots are not directly contagious from horses to people.
- There are occasional reports of human infection with horse botfly larvae, several of which involved patients with known exposure to horses.
- Migration of first-stage larvae is associated with cutaneous and ocular myiasis in humans.
- The burrowing of larvae beneath the skin may produce a tortuous path with severe pruritus.

GEOGRAPHY AND SEASONALITY

- Infection with botfly larvae occurs in horses worldwide.
- *G. intestinalis* and *G. nasalis* are the most common species in North America.
- *G. pecorum* is found in Asia.

- Adult fly activity is most common in the summer and fall.
- Larvae persist in the stomach and intestine through the winter and spring.

CLINICAL PRESENTATION

DISEASE FORMS/SUBTYPES Bot larvae cause minimal pathology in most horses.

HISTORY, CHIEF COMPLAINT

- Most horses show no recognizable clinical signs.
- Abnormal behavior may be caused by attempts at fly evasion.
- Signs associated with minor gingival irritation and necrosis, including increased salivation, abnormal mastication, and swallowing.
- Signs of colic and endotoxemia in the rare horse with gastric ulceration and rupture, gastritis, peritonitis secondary to gastroduodenal perforation, or gastroesophageal reflux.
- Aberrant larval migration may cause more unusual clinical signs.

PHYSICAL EXAM FINDINGS

- Most horses show no abnormalities on physical examination that can be directly related to botflies except for the presence of botfly eggs attached to the hairs.
- Physical examination findings consistent with abdominal pain and endo-

toxemia in rare horses with gastric ulceration and rupture, gastritis, peritonitis secondary to gastroduodenal perforation, and gastroesophageal reflux.
- Gingival hyperemia and necrosis on oral examination.
- *G. pecorum* infection may cause esophageal constriction and hypertrophy of muscles of the oropharynx and esophagus with resultant dysphagia and death. It may also cause epidemic deaths of horses resulting from attachment of large numbers of bots to the soft palate.

ETIOLOGY AND PATHOPHYSIOLOGY

- Adult botflies are similar in size and appearance to honeybees.
  - The common horse botfly (*G. intestinalis*) lays yellow to gray eggs on the hairs of the forelegs, mane, and flanks.
  - Throat botfly eggs (*G. nasalis*) are attached to the long hairs beneath the mandible and chin.
  - Nose botfly eggs (*G. haemorrhoidalis*) are deposited on hairs around the muzzle.
- Hatching of eggs is stimulated by warmth and moisture associated with licking the eggs during normal grooming behavior.
- Larvae spend about 3 weeks migrating in soft tissue of the oral cavity and

then migrate to the stomach or small intestine, where they attach to the mucosa.

- Larvae remain in the stomach until spring or early summer, when they detach, are passed in feces, enter the soil below the manure pile, and pupate.
- In weeks to months, adult flies emerge.
- Adult *G. pecorum* bots lay eggs in batches on grass, and eggs are ingested when horses graze.

DIAGNOSIS

DIFFERENTIAL DIAGNOSIS

- Definitive diagnosis is by visual identification of parasites, usually by gastroscopy.
- Bot larvae are occasionally identified in gastroesophageal reflux fluid.
- Internal larval presence should be highly suspect in horses that have not recently received avermectin anthelminthics and that have obvious botfly eggs attached to the hairs of their legs or face.

TREATMENT

THERAPEUTIC GOAL(S)

Eliminate all botfly larvae.

ACUTE GENERAL TREATMENT

- Avermectin anthelminthic treatment
- Physical removal of botfly eggs from hairs

PROGNOSIS AND OUTCOME

Prognosis is excellent for most horses.

PEARLS & CONSIDERATIONS

COMMENTS

The most effective time to administer boticides is in the late fall after the first

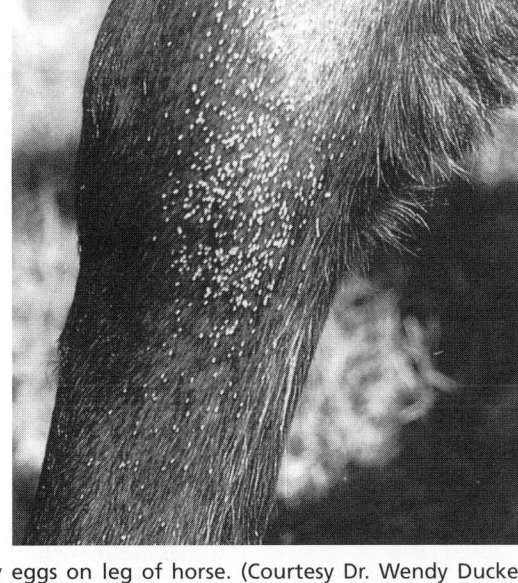

FIGURE 1 Botfly eggs on leg of horse. (Courtesy Dr. Wendy Duckett. From Sellon DC, Long MT: *Equine infectious diseases.* St Louis, 2007, Mosby Elsevier.)

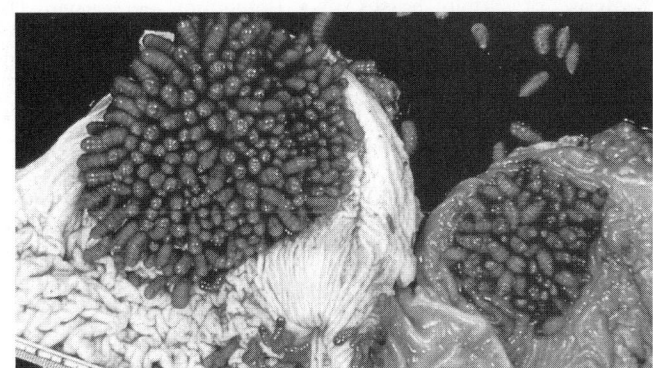

FIGURE 2 Botfly larvae attached to a gastric mucosa of a horse. (Courtesy Dr. Wendy Duckett. From Sellon DC, Long MT: *Equine infectious diseases.* St Louis, 2007, Mosby Elsevier.)

hard frost, when adult fly activity has ceased.

CLIENT EDUCATION

Instruct clients that regular grooming to remove bot eggs from the horse's hair is helpful.

SUGGESTED READING

Sellon DC: Miscellaneous parasitic diseases. In Sellon DC, Long MT, editors: *Equine infectious diseases.* St Louis, 2007, Elsevier, pp 473–480.

AUTHOR: **DEBRA C. SELLON**

EDITORS: **MAUREEN T. LONG** and **DEBRA C. SELLON**

Botulism

BASIC INFORMATION

DEFINITION

A neuromuscular disorder of horses and other mammals caused by neurotoxins of *Clostridium botulinum.* Toxicoinfectious

botulism occurs through oral ingestion of botulism and elaboration in the intestine of affected animals.

SYNONYM(S)

Shaker foal syndrome, forage poisoning, grass sickness

EPIDEMIOLOGY

SPECIES, AGE, SEX Botulism neurotoxins type B and C are most commonly reported in foals. Shaker foal syndrome (toxicoinfectious) is associated with 1- to 3-month-old foals but may occur as early as age 7 days. In adult horses, a form of adult toxicoinfectious botulism (grass sickness) occurs in Europe.

RISK FACTORS

- Decaying vegetable matter in food and water
- Feeding practices including silage, haylage, round baled hay, animal tissue contamination of feeds, bird and animal contamination of standing water sources

GEOGRAPHY AND SEASONALITY

Equine botulism is most frequently observed in Kentucky and the mid-Atlantic region of the eastern United States, although the disease has been reported worldwide. Botulism type B can be found throughout United States but is more predominant in the north and central east. Type A botulinum is isolated from soil primarily in western and northwestern states. Botulism type C occurs in Florida.

CLINICAL PRESENTATION

DISEASE FORMS/SUBTYPES

- Flaccid paralysis of adult horses (wound and forage poisoning)
- Shaker foal syndrome (toxicoinfectious)
- Grass sickness (Europe)

HISTORY, CHIEF COMPLAINT

- Sudden, unexplained death
- Clinically affected horse with intermittent paralysis

PHYSICAL EXAM FINDINGS

- The time to onset of clinical signs after exposure to toxin varies from 12 hours to several days. Sudden, unexplained death of one or more horses may be the initial signal of the onset of an outbreak.
- Decreased eyelid, tongue, and tail tone may be observed early in disease. Horses that walk may have a stilted, short-strided gait without ataxia. Muscle trembling and weakness may be apparent, particularly in foals.
- Pupillary dilation with sluggish pupillary light reflexes is common.
- There is normal cutaneous sensation with depressed spinal reflexes.
- Pharyngeal paralysis is frequently observed in adult horses with botulism and may be confirmed by endoscopic examination of the upper airway.
- Clinical signs may rapidly progress to recumbency.
- Tachycardia may occur, particularly in foals. Foals may appear or become constipated and dysuric.
- Signs of colic may be associated with diminished gastrointestinal (GI) motility.
- Dyspnea and cyanosis may be present initially or terminally.
- Death is generally attributed to respiratory failure secondary to respiratory muscle paralysis.

ETIOLOGY AND PATHOPHYSIOLOGY

- *Clostridium botulinum*
- Neurotoxins A, B, C, and D
- Three methods of toxin exposure in horses:
  - Forage poisoning: Ingestion of preformed toxin elaborated in feedstuffs by vegetative form of *C. botulinum*
  - Toxicoinfectious: Ingestion of spores, formation of vegetative state, multiplication, and elaboration of toxins within the GI tract after in vivo toxin production
  - Wound botulism: Contamination of a wound with spores, formation of vegetative state, multiplication, and elaboration of toxins within the tissues after in vivo toxin production
- Botulism intoxication occurs by a multistep process: binding to the target cell and internalization, translocation, and inhibition of neurotransmitter release.
- Botulinum neurotoxin (BoNT) prevents exocytosis of acetylcholine at the neuromuscular synapse by the cleavage of soluble N-ethylmaleimide sensitive factor attachment receptor proteins involved in the fusion of synaptic vesicles with the plasma membrane.
- The clinical effect is flaccid paralysis of large motor neuron units with lower motor neuron disease of the limbs, respiratory intercostal muscles, and pharyngeal muscles.
- Without intervention and supportive care, respiratory paralysis and death occur.
- Overwhelming exposure may result in death.

DIAGNOSIS

DIFFERENTIAL DIAGNOSIS

- Foals
  - Hypocalcemia
  - Severe electrolyte imbalances
  - Cranial trauma if recumbent
- Adults
  - West Nile virus: May have intermittent weakness and paralysis
  - Equine protozoal myeloencephalitis: Should have muscle wasting
  - Early onset of rabies
  - Pharyngeal disorders, including choke and trauma
  - Tick paralysis

INITIAL DATABASE

- Complete blood count: Normal
- Serum biochemical analysis: Normal
- Urinalysis: Normal

ADVANCED OR CONFIRMATORY TESTING

- Electromyography: May demonstrate lower motor neuron abnormalities. Negative findings should not rule out the disease.
- Definitive diagnosis: Detection of toxin in serum, feces, GI contents, or feed)
  - Format detection: Enzyme-linked immunosorbent assay, radioimmunoassay, polymerase chain reaction
  - Specific toxin activity: Mouse inoculation test
- Isolation of *C. botulinum* from serum, feces, GI contents, or feed

TREATMENT

THERAPEUTIC GOAL(S)

- Blockade of remaining circulating toxin
- Supportive care

ACUTE GENERAL TREATMENT

- Botulism antitoxin: Equine-origin polyvalent (anti-B and anti-C) botulism antitoxin (Botulism Laboratory, New Bolton Center, Kennett Square, PA) or monovalent (anti-B) botulinum antitoxin (Veterinary Dynamics, Templeton, CA)
- Adults and foals with mild respiratory failure (normal pH and mild to moderate increase in arterial carbon dioxide tension [$PaCO_2$]) may frequently be treated with intranasal oxygen insufflation, positioning in sternal recumbency, and repeated arterial blood gas (ABG) monitoring to detect worsening respiratory failure.
- Mechanical ventilation may ameliorate ABG abnormalities and allow time for the patient to recover cholinergic neuromuscular control.
- Antimicrobial administration, although not required for treatment unless wound botulism is suspected, is frequently used in an effort to prevent or reduce some of the complications of the disease, such as aspiration pneumonia caused by dysphagia.

CHRONIC TREATMENT

- Nutritional management must be considered in horses with botulism and can generally be achieved in foals by feeding milk or milk replacer via indwelling nasogastric or nasoesophageal tubes (Kangaroo, 12-Fr, 43-inch enteral feeding tube, Sherwood Medical, St. Louis, MO) as small, frequent meals (every 2 hours).
- In adult horses, periodic nasogastric intubation of slurry meals can be provided. In prolonged cases, it may be beneficial to consider commercially

available liquid diets. Parenteral nutrition is generally not necessary.
- Nursing care is an important part of treatment, and equine patients should be protected as much as possible from development of decubital ulcers, corneal ulcers, and inadvertent aspiration.
- Ocular examination should be performed at least daily and ocular lubricant ointments used to prevent exposure keratitis.

DRUG INTERACTIONS

Antimicrobial drugs that might potentiate neuromuscular blockage (eg, procaine penicillin, aminoglycosides, and tetracyclines) should be avoided.

POSSIBLE COMPLICATIONS

Close ABG monitoring is required for the first 24 to 48 hours of treatment.

RECOMMENDED MONITORING

- Close ABG monitoring is required for the first 24 to 48 hours of treatment because administration of botulinum antitoxin does not remove toxin already bound to receptors within the terminal neuromuscular junction of the axon, and the equine patient may deteriorate further during this period.
- ABG analysis should also be performed if the patient's condition appears to change; these horses may suddenly alter their respiratory rate and pattern as respiratory failure worsens.
- Increased nostril flare, decreased chest excursion, and restlessness may be physical indicators of worsening respiratory failure.
- Adult horses with botulism that remain standing have a good prognosis for recovery; however, it may require several weeks to months before affected horses regain sufficient strength to return to work.
- Horses that become recumbent have a poorer prognosis even with antitoxin administration and excellent nursing care. This is related in part to their size and the secondary effects of prolonged recumbency.

- The degree of respiratory compromise can be severe, and long-term (days) mechanical ventilation of adult horses is a difficult undertaking.

PROGNOSIS AND OUTCOME

- The survival rate for botulinum neurointoxication in appropriately treated foals younger than 6 months of age is greater than 90%.
- Approximately 50% of affected foals require some form of ventilatory support, ranging from intranasal oxygen insufflation to mechanical ventilation, and all affected foals should have repeated ABG analysis performed during the first 48 hours of treatment.

PEARLS & CONSIDERATIONS

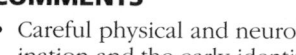

COMMENTS

- Careful physical and neurologic examination and the early identification and treatment with antitoxin is essential for successful outcome of clinical botulism in horses.
- In standing but weak horses, endoscopic examination and assessment of pharyngeal function should be performed.
- Abnormal pharyngeal function in the presence of neuromuscular weakness should lead to botulism as a top differential diagnosis.

PREVENTION

- Vaccination (*C. botulinum* type B toxoid, Neogen, Tampa, FL) is thought to be almost 100% protective in adult horses.
- Vaccination of pregnant mares is the most efficient way to protect foals in endemic areas; however, foals from vaccinated mares have developed disease.

- Passively transferred antibody levels may be variable and have variable decay rates in individuals.
- Adults
  - Broodmares: Initial three-dose series at 30-day intervals with the last dose 4 to 6 weeks before anticipated parturition date, and annually thereafter, 4 to 6 weeks prepartum.
  - Other adult horses: Should consider vaccination, particularly if in endemic regions. Initial three-dose series and then annual booster.
- Foals
  - From vaccinated mares: Three-dose series of toxoid at 1-month intervals starting at 2 to 3 months of age
  - From unvaccinated mares: Foals may benefit from (1) toxoid at 2, 4, and 8 weeks of age; (2) transfusion of plasma from a vaccinated horse; or (3) antitoxin (efficacy needs further study).

CLIENT EDUCATION

- Vaccination procedures should be reviewed in endemic areas.
- Proper feeding and storage of hay and grain are essential.
- Avoidance of silage and haylage in equines is recommended.
- If bulked baled hay is an important source of feed, education of clients of recognition of poor hay quality and hay management from supplies is important.

SUGGESTED READING

Wilkins PA, Palmer JE: Botulism in foals less than 6 months of ages: 30 cases (1989–2002). *J Vet Intern Med* 17:702–707, 2003.

Wilkins PA, Palmer JE: Mechanical ventilation in foals with botulism: 9 cases (1989–2002). *J Vet Intern Med* 17:708–712, 2003.

Wylie CE, Proudman CJ: Equine grass sickness: epidemiology, diagnosis, and global distribution. *Vet Clin North Am Equine Pract* 25:381–389, 2009.

AUTHOR: **PAMELA WILKINS**

EDITOR: **MAUREEN T. LONG** and **DEBRA C. SELLON**

Bracken Fern and Horsetail Toxicosis

BASIC INFORMATION

DEFINITION

Bracken fern and horsetails cause neurotoxicity in horses as a result of thiamine depletion.

SYNONYM(S)

- Bracken or bracken fern (*Pteridium aquilinum*)
- Horsetail, field or western horsetail, scouring rush (*Equisetum arvense*)
- Scouring rush horsetail (*Equisetum hyemale* or *Hippochaete hyemalis*)

EPIDEMIOLOGY

RISK FACTORS Poor-quality hay containing these plants is a risk to hungry horses.

GEOGRAPHY AND SEASONALITY
- Bracken fern is distributed throughout the world except in very low-precipitation areas.

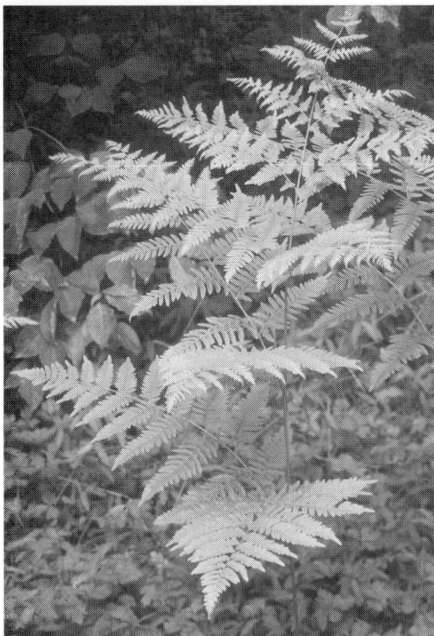

FIGURE 1 Bracken fern (*Pteridium aquilinum*).

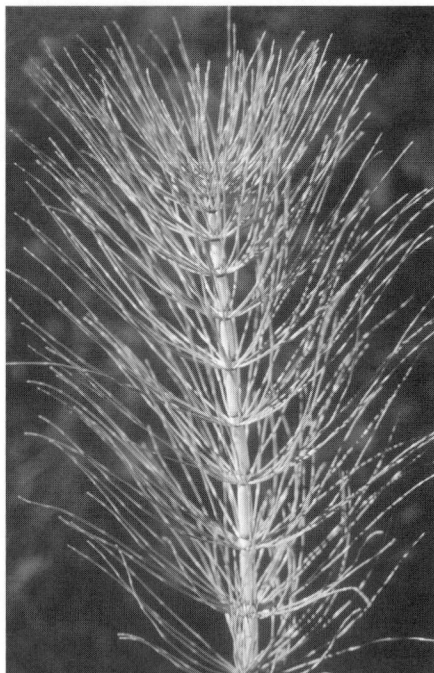

FIGURE 2 Horsetail (*Equisetum arvense*).

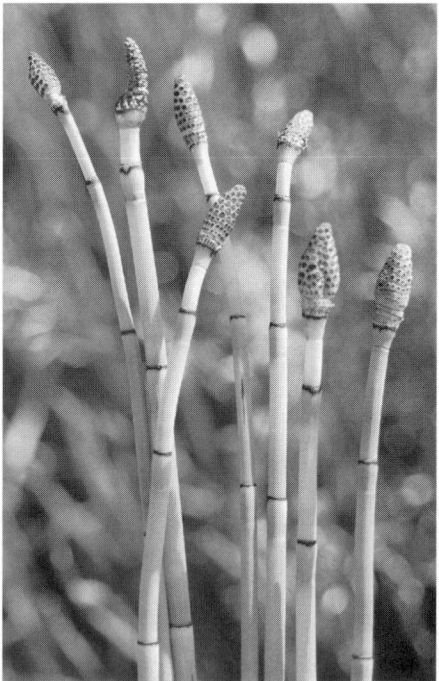

FIGURE 3 Scouring rush horsetail (*Equisetum hyemale* or *Hippochaete hyemalis*).

- Bracken fern is a deciduous perennial that develops from a black extensive root system with erect, triangular-shaped fronds 3 to 5 feet in height. The stems are smooth and green except at the base. Reproduction occurs via spores formed on the underside of fronds following the edge of the leaflets (Figure 1).
- Horsetail is widely distributed in North America, preferring moist areas. It is an invasive, deciduous perennial plant that forms large colonies from branching rhizomatous roots. The stems are erect, hollow, ribbed, and jointed. The leaves are vestigial (scale-like) in whorls at the nodes. Some species have branches in whorls at the nodes. Horsetails are flowerless and reproduce from spore-forming cones at the ends of fertile stems (Figures 2 and 3).

CLINICAL PRESENTATION

HISTORY, CHIEF COMPLAINT Gradual onset over several days of weakness, depression, and incoordination leading to difficulty standing and recumbency. Seizures can occur terminally.

PHYSICAL EXAM FINDINGS
- Weight loss, incoordination, muscle tremors, and crouching stance when the head is raised.
- Recumbency followed by seizures and eventually death.
- Appetite may initially be good.

ETIOLOGY AND PATHOPHYSIOLOGY
- The primary toxin in bracken fern responsible for the neurologic syndrome in horses is thiaminase. Thiaminase creates a thiamin deficiency by breaking down thiamin and competitively inhibiting thiamin activity.
- Consumption of a diet of 20% to 25% bracken fern for 3 weeks or more is necessary to produce signs.
- Dried plant material retains its toxicity.
- Ruminants are not affected by the thiaminase because their rumen microflora degrades it.
- Bracken fern also contains ptaquiloside, which is carcinogenic and causes thrombocytopenia and hemangiomas of the bladder in cattle. This is not reported in horses.
- The rhizomes and rapidly growing young fronds are the most toxic.
- The toxin in *Equisetum* spp. is also a thiaminase.
- Most poisoning occurs in horses fed hay contaminated with horsetail.
- Consumption of hay with 20% or more horsetail for 2 to 3 weeks is necessary to cause poisoning.

DIAGNOSIS

DIFFERENTIAL DIAGNOSIS
- Equine leukoencephalomalacia
- Encephalitis: Rabies, West Nile virus, Eastern and Western equine encephalitis virus
- Equine herpesvirus
- Sage poisoning
- Pyrrolizidine alkaloid toxicity

INITIAL DATABASE
Serum pyruvate and lactate increase due to inhibition of pyruvate dehydrogenase.

ADVANCED OR CONFIRMATORY TESTING
- Blood thiamine levels in horses decrease to 25 to 30 µg/L.
- Postmortem findings are generally nonspecific, with congestion of the brain and other organs.
- Histologically, necrosis of neurons may be seen.
- Response to thiamine treatment may be the only practical confirmatory test.

TREATMENT

THERAPEUTIC GOAL(S)
Replenish thiamine.

ACUTE GENERAL TREATMENT
- Thiamine (vitamin B_1): 0.5 to 1.0 g/d parenterally, decreasing the dose over several days
- Provide a palatable and nutritious diet.

RECOMMENDED MONITORING
Monitor serum pyruvate, lactate, and thiamine levels.

PROGNOSIS AND OUTCOME

If the condition is recognized and treatment initiated before the horse becomes recumbent, recovery in a few days is likely.

PEARLS & CONSIDERATIONS

COMMENTS

Bracken fern and horsetail poisoning in horses is unusual and is often the result of feeding poor-quality hay.

PREVENTION

Feed weed-free hay

CLIENT EDUCATION

Recognition of green and dried bracken fern and horsetail is essential.

SUGGESTED READING

Burrows GE, Tyrl RJ: Pteridium. In *Toxic plants of North America.* Ames, IA, 2001, Iowa State Press, pp 415–422.

Knight AP, Walter RG. *A guide to plant poisoning of animals in North America.* Jackson, WY, 2001, Teton NewMedia, pp 194–197, 222–224.

Meyer P: Thiaminase activities and thiamine content of Pteridium aquilinum, Equisetum ramosissimum, Malva parviflora, Pennisetum clandestinum and Medicago sativa. *Onderstepoort J Vet Res* 56(2):145–146, 1989.

Radostits OM, Gay CC, Blood DC, Hinchcliff KW: *Veterinary medicine,* ed 9. Edinburgh, 2000, Elsevier, pp 1556–1558, 1659.

AUTHOR: **ANTHONY P. KNIGHT**

EDITOR: **CYNTHIA L. GASKILL**

Branchial Cysts

BASIC INFORMATION

DEFINITION

Branchial cysts are congenital epithelial cysts that arise as malformations of the branchial arches during embryogenesis. They are uncommon, but when they are present, they are described most often in and around the head and neck from a failure of obliteration of the second branchial cleft.

SYNONYM(S)

Lateral cervical cyst

EPIDEMIOLOGY

SPECIES, AGE, SEX
- Clinical signs may not be immediately apparent, but when the cysts are large or surround critical structures such as the larynx or esophagus, they may be apparent very soon after birth.
- Branchial cysts are rare, and no gender predisposition has been noted.

GENETICS AND BREED PREDISPOSITION This is a congenital abnormality, but no genetic or breed predisposition has been established.

ASSOCIATED CONDITIONS AND DISORDERS
- Surrounding vascular, neural, and anatomic structures may be affected and should be examined as part of the preoperative planning.
- Cysts may become infected and develop abscesses.
- Aspiration pneumonia may be present.

CLINICAL PRESENTATION

HISTORY, CHIEF COMPLAINT Unilateral or bilateral retropharyngeal, laryngeal, or cervical swelling, which may rapidly increase in size over a short period

PHYSICAL EXAM FINDINGS
- Firm, nonpainful mass in the area of the caudal mandible to mid-cervical region.
- Unilateral or bilateral mucopurulent discharge may be present.
- Respiratory crackles may be present upon thoracic auscultation.
- Dyspnea.
- Inspiratory stridor.

ETIOLOGY AND PATHOPHYSIOLOGY
- During the fourth week of embryonic life, the development of branchial (or pharyngeal) clefts results in five ridges known as the branchial (or pharyngeal) arches, which contribute to the formation of various structures of the head, neck, and thorax.
- The second arch grows caudally and, ultimately, covers the third and fourth arches. The buried clefts become ectoderm-lined cavities, which normally involute around week 7 of development.
- If a portion of the cleft fails to involute completely, the entrapped remnant forms an epithelium-lined cyst with or without a sinus tract to the overlying skin.

DIAGNOSIS

DIFFERENTIAL DIAGNOSIS
- Salivary mucocele
- Cervical abscess
- Lymphadenopathy

INITIAL DATABASE
- Complete blood count to evaluate concurrent disease.
- Survey radiographs of the laryngeal and cranial cervical regions.
- Endoscopy of the pharynx, larynx, guttural pouches, and trachea may aid in the detection of affected structures and further preoperative planning.

ADVANCED OR CONFIRMATORY TESTING
- A sinogram may be obtained. If a sinus tract exists, radiopaque dye can be injected to delineate the course and to examine the size of the cyst.
- Ultrasonography helps delineate the cystic nature of these lesions.
- A contrast-enhanced computed tomography scan shows a cystic and enhancing mass in the neck. It may aid preoperative planning and identify compromise of local structures.
- Magnetic resonance imaging allows finer resolution during preoperative planning. The wall of the cyst may be enhanced on gadolinium scans.

HISTOPATHOLOGY
- Most branchial cleft cysts are lined with stratified squamous epithelium with keratinous debris within the cyst.
- The cyst may be lined with respiratory (ciliated columnar) epithelium.
- Lymphoid tissue is often present outside the epithelial lining.
- In infected or ruptured lesions, inflammatory cells are seen within the cyst cavity or the surrounding stroma.

TREATMENT

THERAPEUTIC GOAL(S)

Complete removal of cyst and cystic epithelial lining

ACUTE GENERAL TREATMENT
- Surgical incision and drainage of abscesses are indicated, if present, usually along with concurrent antimicrobial therapy.
- Percutaneous aspiration and surgical drainage of cysts are considered inappropriate because most cysts will reappear if any epithelium remains.
- Injection of cysts with a sclerosing agent may be considered if surgery is not possible.

POSSIBLE COMPLICATIONS
- Untreated lesions may cause difficulty swallowing and breathing and are prone to recurrent infection and

- abscess formation with resultant scar formation and possible compromise of local structures.
- Complications of surgical excision result from damage to nearby vascular or neural structures.

RECOMMENDED MONITORING

Postoperatively, patients should be monitored for recurrence.

PROGNOSIS AND OUTCOME

- Prognosis is good after complete removal of the cystic epithelial lining.

- In humans, recurrence is uncommon after surgical excision, with a risk estimated at 3% unless previous surgery or recurrent infection has occurred, in which case it may be as high as 20%. The data are unknown in horses.

PEARLS & CONSIDERATIONS

The owner should be reminded that this is a benign, congenital problem. No genetic or breed disposition has been established.

SUGGESTED READING

Hance SR, Robertson JT, Wicks JR: Branchial cyst in a filly. *Equine Vet J* 24(4):329–331, 1992.

Slovis NM, Watson JL, Couto SS: Marsupialization and iodine sclerotherapy of a branchial cyst in a horse. *J Am Vet Med Assoc* 219(3):338–340, 2001.

AUTHOR: **JARRED WILLIAMS**

EDITORS: **ELIZABETH M. SANTSCHI** and **PHOEBE A. SMITH**

Bronchopneumonia, Bacterial

BASIC INFORMATION

DEFINITION

Bacterial infection and inflammation of the airways, lung parenchyma, or both

EPIDEMIOLOGY

GENETICS AND BREED PREDISPOSITION

- There is no genetic or breed predisposition, except in cases in which horses are immune compromised (eg, Arabian foals with combined immunodeficiency disorder).
- Performance horses (Thoroughbred racehorses and show jumpers) have an increased risk of developing pneumonia, most likely reflecting an increase in several risk factors (eg, long-distance transport, strenuous exercise, and increased exposure to respiratory viruses).

RISK FACTORS Any disease or situation that compromises the respiratory defenses or increases the risk of aspiration:
- Compromised respiratory defenses (more common)
  - Strenuous exercise
  - Long-distance transport with the head elevated
  - Concurrent respiratory viral infection (equine influenza; equine herpesvirus [EHV] -1, -2, and -4; equine arteritis virus; equine rhinovirus A and B)
  - Mechanical ventilation (general anesthesia)
  - Exercise-induced pulmonary hemorrhage
- Increased risk of aspiration: Laryngeal or pharyngeal dysfunction (less common)

  - Primary neuropathy of cranial nerve IX or X (equine protozoal myeloencephalitis, botulism, *Streptococcus equi*, subsp. *equi* infection, guttural pouch mycoses)
  - Primary myopathy of pharyngeal, laryngeal or esophageal musculature (vitamin E and selenium deficiencies, megaesophagus)
  - Physical limitation of laryngeal function after tie-back surgery
  - Esophageal obstruction (choke)

ASSOCIATED CONDITIONS AND DISORDERS Lung abscesses, pleuropneumonia

CLINICAL PRESENTATION

HISTORY, CHIEF COMPLAINT

- The chief complaint may be related to pneumonia or to a predisposing condition. The history may include recent long-distance transportation, exposure to horses with respiratory viruses, or recent esophageal obstruction.
- Pneumonia
  - In acute stages, some animals will not have obvious clinical signs related to respiratory tract disease.
  - Exercise intolerance is sometimes the earliest and only complaint at presentation.
  - May include vague history of fever, depression, and inappetence.
  - Cough
  - Weight loss
  - Mucopurulent nasal discharge.
- Laryngeal or pharyngeal dysfunction
  - Dysphagia
  - Inspiratory stridor
  - Cough

PHYSICAL EXAM FINDINGS

- Physical examination findings are variable and depend on the stage, severity, and cause of the disease. A lack of physical examination findings referable to the respiratory system cannot definitively rule out bronchopneumonia.
- Crackles and wheezes (focal or diffuse): Lung sounds should be assessed both before and after application of a rebreathing bag (if no respiratory distress is present) because the deep breaths achieved after rebreathing can be invaluable in more accurately ausculting the presence and degree of abnormal lung sounds.
- Mucopurulent nasal discharge
- Fever
- Tachypnea or respiratory distress
- Tachycardia
- Cough
- Depression

ETIOLOGY AND PATHOPHYSIOLOGY

- In adult horses, bacterial pneumonia occurs most frequently as a sequela to a predisposing condition or disease that reduces the respiratory immune defenses, limits ciliary clearance of bacteria from the lower respiratory tract, or increases the aspiration or inhalation of bacteria.
- These conditions result most commonly in polymicrobic infections of bacteria that normally inhabit the upper respiratory tract or gastrointestinal tract.
  - The most common gram-positive bacterial isolates include *Streptococcus equi* subsp. *zooepidemicus*,

Staphylococcus aureus, and *Streptococcus pneumoniae.*

- ○ The most common gram-negative bacterial isolates include *Pasteurella* and *Actinobacillus* spp., *Escherichia coli, Klebsiella pneumoniae,* and *Bordetella bronchiseptica.*
- ○ The most common anaerobic bacterial isolates include *Bacteroides fragilis, Peptostreptococcus anaerobius,* and *Fusobacterium* spp.
- Compromised respiratory defenses: Strenuous exercise
- Increased bacterial contamination of the lower airway (10- to 100-fold increase in bacterial counts from tracheal washes after a single bout of high-intensity exercise)
- Reduced mucociliary clearance
- Alterations of systemic immune defenses, predisposing animals to both viral and bacterial pulmonary infections: Long-distance transport
- Reduced mucociliary clearance when the head is tied
- As little as 6 hours of elevated head position during transport increases pulmonary neutrophilic inflammation and accumulation of *Actinobacillus, Pasteurella,* and *Streptococcus* bacterial species
- Reduced efficacy of systemic antimicrobial defenses (such as reduced phagocytosis by peripheral blood mononuclear cells): Concurrent respiratory viral infection
- Damage to respiratory epithelial cells enhances bacterial attachment
- Reduced mucociliary clearance and alveolar macrophage dysfunction for up to 30 days after infection: Mechanical ventilation (general anesthesia)
- Increased risk of aspiration: Laryngeal or pharyngeal dysfunction
  - ○ Increased aspiration of bacteria secondary to dysphagia is a less common cause of bacterial pneumonia in adult horses.
  - ○ Most often associated with esophageal obstruction in horses with poor dental health.
  - ○ Other causes of dysphagia should also be considered and include neuropathy of cranial nerve IX or X (equine protozoal myeloencephalitis, botulism, *S. equi* infection, guttural pouch mycoses) and primary myopathy of pharyngeal, laryngeal, or esophageal musculature (vitamin E and selenium deficiencies, megaesophagus).

DIAGNOSIS

DIFFERENTIAL DIAGNOSIS

- Noninfectious lower airway diseases such as inflammatory airway disease,

recurrent airway obstruction, and idiopathic pulmonary fibrosis
- Fungal pneumonia (especially if unresponsive to antimicrobial therapy)
- Pulmonary neoplasia
- Respiratory parasites

INITIAL DATABASE

- Complete blood count (CBC): Leukocytosis and neutrophilia (with or without left shift) may be present, although neutropenia may be present in cases of severe gram-negative bacterial pneumonia (associated with the effects of endotoxin). Hyperfibrinogenemia, hyperglobulinemia, and anemia of chronic disease are compatible with chronic bacterial pneumonia.
- Serum biochemistry profile: Usually normal
- Thoracic radiography: Alveolar and interstitial patterns in dependent areas of the lung

ADVANCED OR CONFIRMATORY TESTING

- Tracheal wash: Degenerative neutrophils, intracellular bacteria
- Tracheal wash culture: Isolation of pathogenic bacteria
- Arterial blood gas analysis: Hypoxemia may be present and is generally indicative of more severe lower airway disease
- Upper airway endoscopic examination: Possible laryngeal or pharyngeal dysfunction
- Other tests for underlying laryngeal dysfunction (eg, EHV1 polymerase chain reaction or enzyme-linked immunosorbent assay, or serum vitamin E or selenium level

TREATMENT

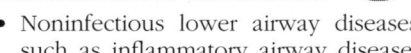

THERAPEUTIC GOAL(S)

- Eliminate pathogenic bacteria.
- Correct any underlying laryngeal or pharyngeal dysfunction.

ACUTE GENERAL TREATMENT

- Broad-spectrum antimicrobial therapy until culture results are available and antimicrobial therapy can be tailored. Any combination should at least initially cover both aerobic and anaerobic bacteria.
  - ○ For more severely affected animals, use IV antibiotic combinations such as potassium penicillin (22,000 IU/kg IV q6h) or ceftiofur (4.4 mg/kg IV q12h) and an aminoglycoside (gentamicin is most cost effective in adults; 6.6 mg/kg IV q24h) or fluoroquinolone (enrofloxacin, 5–10 mg/kg IV q24h). Metronidazole can also be added to increase

anaerobic coverage (15 mg/kg PO q6h), especially against the penicillin-resistant *B. fragilis.*
  - ○ Because the most commonly isolated bacteria in cases of mild bacterial pneumonia is *S. equi* subsp. *zooepidemicus,* treatment of mild cases before return of sensitivity panels might be limited to ceftiofur because this antibiotic has good efficacy against *S. equi* subsp. *zooepidemicus* as well as several common gram-negative species.
  - ○ In less severe cases, oral antibiotics may be sufficient, such as potentiated sulfonamides (trimethoprim-sulfadiazine 30 mg/kg PO q12h, although the efficacy of this antibiotic against *S. equi* subsp. *zooepidemicus* in vivo for the treatment of pulmonary infections has been recently challenged despite good in vitro sensitivity), chloramphenicol (50 mg/kg PO q12h), or doxycycline (10 mg/kg PO q12h).
- Nonsteroidal antiinflammatory drugs (NSAIDs) such as flunixin meglumine can be given for pain (0.5–1.1 mg/kg IV or PO q12h) and for antiendotoxic effects (0.25 mg/kg IV or PO q6h).
- Maintain adequate hydration, especially important if aminoglycosides or NSAIDs are used in treatment. IV fluids may be necessary if the animal is depressed and not drinking sufficiently.
- Intranasal oxygen, bronchodilators (eg, inhaled albuterol 600–720 μg puffs q4–6h) and laminitis prophylaxis measures may be necessary depending on the type and severity of disease.
- Provide palatable food choices to maintain appetite.

CHRONIC TREATMENT

- Identification and resolution of any underlying disease with increased risk of aspiration pneumonia.
- Continuation of antibiotic therapy at least 1 week past the resolution of clinical signs and significant improvement of thoracic radiographic abnormalities.
- Some horses with laryngeal or pharyngeal dysfunction may require placement of an esophagostomy tube for feeding to avoid continued aspiration until the dysfunction resolves.

POSSIBLE COMPLICATIONS

- Lung abscessation
- Pleuropneumonia
- Laminitis from severe gram-negative infection

RECOMMENDED MONITORING

- Clinical signs: Animals should be reevaluated in 48 to 72 hours for signs

of improvement. Lack of improvement in this period may indicate the necessity for an antibiotic change.
- Thoracic radiographs should be reevaluated 7 to 10 days after the initiation of treatment and may lag behind clinical signs by 2 to 3 days.
- Repeat arterial blood gas analysis: For severe pneumonia, repeated analysis of gas exchange may provide information about the response to treatment.
- CBC: Resolution of neutrophilia or neutropenia should occur within 7 to 10 days.

PROGNOSIS AND OUTCOME

- The prognosis is variable and depends on the severity of the disease and the predisposing factors; however, the prognosis is generally good if early aggressive treatment is initiated.
- The risk of recurrence is high for animals with unresolved underlying disease.
- The prognosis is guarded if complications such as lung abscesses or pleuropneumonia are present.

PEARLS & CONSIDERATIONS

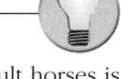

COMMENTS

- Bacterial pneumonia in adult horses is usually the result of an underlying disease or stressor.
- Therefore any adult equid that presents with bacterial pneumonia should be carefully evaluated for underlying risk factors.

PREVENTION

- Preventive measures involve reducing the occurrence of risk factors.
  - Avoid long-distance transport, especially with head restraint. Studies have shown that simple measures such as increased rest stops and trailer cleaning can minimize or eliminate respiratory insult during long-distance transport.
  - Adequate immunization against respiratory viral diseases (EHV, equine influenza) that can predispose animals to the development of secondary bacterial pneumonia.
  - Adequate dental care in older horses to avoid esophageal obstruction.

CLIENT EDUCATION

Clients should be informed of possible risk factors and advised on appropriate measures to avoid recurrence.

SUGGESTED READING

Ainsworth D, Cheetham J: Disorders of the respiratory system. In Reed S, Bayly W, Sellon D, editors: *Equine internal medicine*, ed 3. St Louis, 2010, Saunders Elsevier, pp 290–371.

Giguere S: Bacterial pneumonia and pleuropneumonia in adult horses. In Smith B, editor: *Large animal internal medicine*, ed 4. St Louis, 2008, Mosby Elsevier, pp 500–510.

Oikawa M, Hobo S, Oyamada T, Yoshikawa H: Effects of orientation, intermittent rest and vehicle cleaning during transport on development of transport-related respiratory disease in horses. *J Comp Pathol* 132 (2–3):153–168, 2005.

Racklyeft D, Love D: Bacterial infection of the lower respiratory tract in 34 horses. *Aust Vet J* 78:549, 2000.

Wilkins P: Lower airway diseases of the adult horse. *Vet Clin North Am Equine Pract* 19:101, 2003.

AUTHOR: JULIA A. PAXSON

EDITOR: MELISSA R. MAZAN

Brucellosis

BASIC INFORMATION

DEFINITION

- An infectious disease caused by infection with species of the genus *Brucella*, especially *Brucella abortus* and *Brucella suis*. *B. abortus* has a predilection for the tendons, muscles, bones, and joints of horses.
- It is most often associated with septic bursitis of the supraspinous bursa over the second and third dorsal vertebral spinous processes (fistulous withers) or supraatlantal bursa over the first and second cervical vertebra (poll evil).

SYNONYM(S)

- Fistulous withers
- Poll evil

EPIDEMIOLOGY

SPECIES, AGE, SEX Most infected horses are older than 3 years.
RISK FACTORS Most affected horses have a history of contact with cattle.
CONTAGION AND ZOONOSIS
- Brucellosis is considered a zoonotic disease, but reports of disease in

humans in contact with infected horses are rare.
- Numerous reports of accidental infection of veterinarians with *B. abortus* from strain 19 vaccine.
- Infection in humans may result in subclinical, acute, localized, or chronic disease or relapsing infection.
- Acute disease is characterized by malaise, chills, sweats, fatigue, weakness, fever, myalgia, weight loss, and arthralgia.
- Localized infection may occur at almost any site.
- Chronic infection is characterized by persistent fatigue, malaise, and depression.
- Relapse may occur after apparent successful antimicrobial treatment. Relapse may occur as long as 2 years after initial treatment.

GEOGRAPHY AND SEASONALITY
- It has been reported in horses worldwide, but *B. abortus* has been effectively eradicated from several European countries, Japan, and Israel.

CLINICAL PRESENTATION
DISEASE FORMS/SUBTYPES
- *B. abortus* infections are more common than *B. suis* infections.
- *B. abortus* is associated with:
  - Septic supraspinous bursitis
  - Atlantal bursitis
  - Other bursal infections
  - Septic arthritis
  - Vertebral osteomyelitis
  - Rarely, abortion
- *B. suis* has been isolated from:
  - Septic bursitis
  - Aborted equine fetuses
  - The internal organs of one mare with no clinical signs of disease

HISTORY, CHIEF COMPLAINT
- Most affected horses have a history of exposure to cattle.
- Many seropositive horses show no recognizable clinical signs.
- The onset of clinical signs may be sudden or insidious.
- Lethargy and general stiffness in movement are seen.
- Pain, heat, and swelling of the withers or poll that may progress to obvious external fistulation or exudate.
- Rarely, the chief complaint may be abortion.

- Lameness may be the primary complaint with some infections.

PHYSICAL EXAM FINDINGS

- Pain, heat, and swelling of the withers or poll
- May progress to obvious external fistulation or exudate
- May be apparent healing, fibrosis, and refistulation as disease progresses
- Clinical signs of bursitis, tenosynovitis, arthritis, or osteomyelitis, depending on the site of infection
- Evidence of recent abortion (rare)

ETIOLOGY AND PATHOPHYSIOLOGY

- *Brucella* spp. are nonmotile, aerobic, intracellular gram-negative cocci or short rods that require complex media for growth in culture.
- Transmission may occur by ingestion, inhalation, or direct contact through skin abrasions or mucous membranes.
- The organism may be shed in equine feces and urine and in tissues from aborted equine fetuses.

DIAGNOSIS

DIFFERENTIAL DIAGNOSIS

Bacterial infections and abscesses caused by other organisms

INITIAL DATABASE

- Complete blood count and serum biochemical profile to assess systemic health
- Culture of exudate sampled aseptically from deep within the initial site of infection

TREATMENT

THERAPEUTIC GOAL(S)

- Eliminate the causative bacteria.
- Facilitate healing of affected tissues.

ACUTE GENERAL TREATMENT

- Many *Brucella* spp. are sensitive to tetracyclines, chloramphenicol, streptomycin, and selected sulfonamides.
- Long-term treatment solely with antimicrobials is rarely effective.
- Lavage of draining tracts with antiseptic or antimicrobial solutions may be beneficial.
- Aggressive surgery to remove diseased tissue is recommended if possible.
- Postsurgical healing is often slow and may not be complete.
- Administration of *Brucella* vaccine may be an effective extralabel treatment for horses with *B. abortus* infection; however, SC administration of the vaccine is associated with severe local and systemic reactions, and IV vaccine administration resulted in death in three of four treated horses.

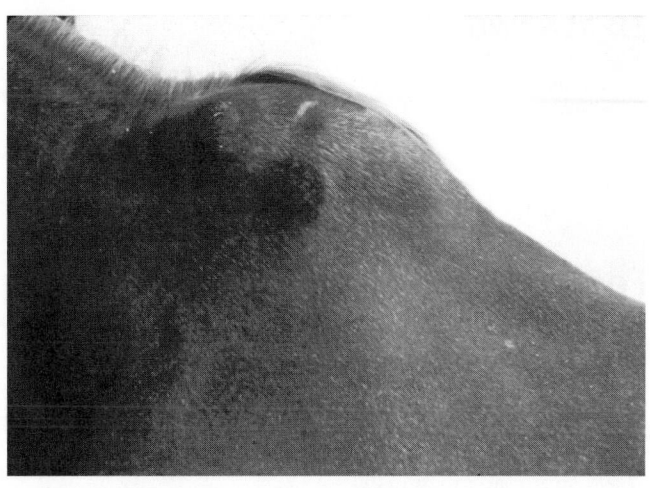

FIGURE 1 Chronic fistulous withers with multiple tracts in horse infected with *Brucella abortus*. (From Sellon DC, Long MT: *Equine infectious diseases*. St Louis, 2007, Saunders.)

CHRONIC TREATMENT

All horses with brucellosis require chronic treatment as outlined above.

POSSIBLE COMPLICATIONS

Even with aggressive surgical and antimicrobial treatment, recovery may not be complete.

PROGNOSIS AND OUTCOME

Prognosis is guarded even with aggressive therapy, with the potential for poor and incomplete healing.

PEARLS & CONSIDERATIONS

COMMENTS

- In geographic areas with a low prevalence of *B. abortus* infection in cattle, *B. abortus* is rarely isolated from horses with fistulous withers.
- Although horses are a potential source of *B. abortus* infection for cattle, experimental infections indicate that horses do not excrete the organism in sufficient numbers to efficiently infect cattle in close contact.
- Horses with fistulous withers that are seropositive to *B. abortus* are significantly more likely than seronegative horses with fistulous withers to have radiographic evidence of osteomyelitis of underlying dorsal spinous processes.
- Confirmation of diagnosis by bacterial culture may be difficult because other bacteria are frequently found in exudates and may overgrow *B. abortus*. Culture of aspirates from deep inside lesions or from affected tissues col-

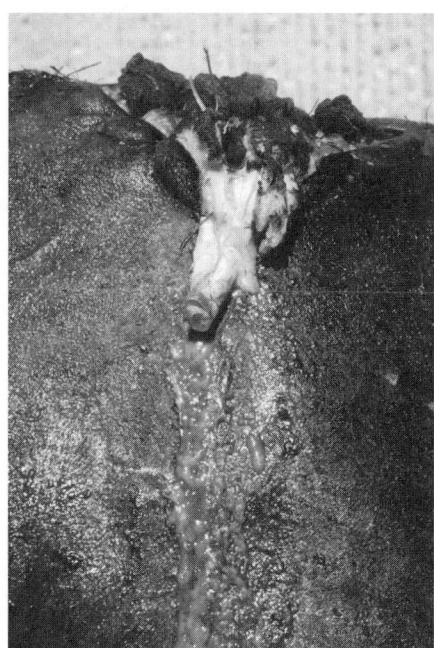

FIGURE 2 Severe postsurgical lesions and exudation in horse with fistulous withers. (From Sellon DC, Long MT: *Equine infectious diseases*. St Louis, 2007, Saunders.)

lected at surgery or necropsy is indicated to attempt confirmation of the diagnosis.

PREVENTION

- Avoid comingling of horses with seropositive cattle.
- Use properly fitted saddles and harnesses to minimize trauma to the withers and poll.
- Effective parasite control programs to eliminate *Onchocerca* spp. and control fly populations may also be beneficial.

SUGGESTED READING

Cohen ND, Carter GK, McMullan WC: Fistulous withers in horses: 24 cases (1984–1990). *J Am Vet Med Assoc* 201(1):121–124, 1992.

Nicoletti PL: Brucellosis. In Sellon DC, Long MT, editors: *Equine infectious diseases.* St Louis, 2007, Elsevier, pp 348–350.

AUTHOR: **DEBRA C. SELLON**

EDITORS: **MAUREEN T. LONG** and **DEBRA C. SELLON**

Bufo Toad Toxicosis

BASIC INFORMATION

DEFINITION

Exposure to *Bufo* spp. toads may result in the acute onset of severe cardiovascular and neurologic signs.

SYNONYM(S)

Cane, giant, or marine toad (*Bufo marinus*), Colorado River toad (*Bufo alvarius*)

EPIDEMIOLOGY

RISK FACTORS Most cases in the literature describing *Bufo* toad intoxications involve dogs and cats rather than horses and other large domestic animals. Although young or curious horses might mouth *Bufo* toads, a more likely route of exposure for most horses is the contamination of food or water sources by live or dead toads.

GEOGRAPHY AND SEASONALITY
- *Bufo* toads are primarily found in Florida, Texas, Colorado, Arizona, and Hawaii.
- These toads breed during warmer, wetter months and tend to hibernate during the colder, dryer months, making wintertime exposures less likely. Toads appear to be most active around dusk and at night and after rainstorms.

CLINICAL PRESENTATION

HISTORY, CHIEF COMPLAINT Oral contact with a *Bufo* toad is rapidly followed by hypersalivation, tachypnea, and disorientation. Severe exposures may progress to seizures, collapse, and cardiac arrhythmias.

PHYSICAL EXAM FINDINGS
- In addition to hypersalivation, hyperemic oral mucous membranes may also be observed.
- Horses should be examined for cardiovascular and neurologic abnormalities. Neurologic abnormalities reported in dogs include seizures, stupor, ataxia, nystagmus, opisthotonos, and extensor rigidity.

ETIOLOGY AND PATHOPHYSIOLOGY
- Many biologically active compounds, including dopamine, epinephrine, norepinephrine, serotonin, bufotenine, bufagenins, bufotoxins, and indolealkylamines, are secreted from the toad's large parotid glands. These compounds are readily absorbed across mucous membranes or through open wounds.
- Bufotenine is a pressor substance that may have hallucinogenic properties.
- Bufagenins and bufotoxins are cardiac glycosides that cross-react with digoxin, binding to and inhibiting Na/K-ATPase. These changes inhibit normal myocardial conduction and function.

DIAGNOSIS

DIFFERENTIAL DIAGNOSIS
- Other cardiac glycosides, including digoxin and digitoxin
- Seizure disorders
- Head trauma
- Other toxicoses: Metaldehyde, methylxanthines, oleander, anticholinesterase insecticides, hallucinogenic plants or mushrooms

INITIAL DATABASE

The initial examination should include determination of heart rate, thoracic auscultation, and evaluation of perfusion. Diagnosis of *Bufo* toad toxicity typically relies on the presence of compatible clinical signs and a history of exposure to toads.

ADVANCED OR CONFIRMATORY TESTING
- Horses with significant cardiac or neurologic abnormalities should have at least an initial electrocardiographic evaluation.
- When available, polyclonal (but not monoclonal) digoxin immunoassays may assist in confirming exposure, although results do not appear to correlate well with clinical effects.
- Some diagnostic laboratories may also be able to identify toad toxins from gastrointestinal contents and other samples using gas or liquid chromatography/mass spectrometry.

TREATMENT

THERAPEUTIC GOAL(S)
- Decontaminate the oral cavity.
- Control seizure activity.
- Evaluate and correct cardiac arrhythmias.
- Provide general supportive care.

ACUTE GENERAL TREATMENT
- Initially, the oral cavity should be flushed with copious amounts of water.
- If present, seizures should be controlled with diazepam.
- Crystalloid electrolyte solutions can be given intravenously.
- The cardiac status should be evaluated and treated symptomatically.
- Severely affected animals may benefit from digoxin-specific Fab fragments. Although used successfully in humans, this treatment has not been thoroughly evaluated in animals.

POSSIBLE COMPLICATIONS

Hyperkalemia may develop and require treatment. Administration of calcium should be avoided.

RECOMMENDED MONITORING

Careful cardiac monitoring is indicated, and hyperthermia may occur as a sequela of seizure activity.

PROGNOSIS AND OUTCOME

Many animals can fully recover with early intervention and treatment.

PEARLS & CONSIDERATIONS

There is also good evidence that *Bufo* toads' eggs are toxic and could be another potential source of exposure for horses.

SUGGESTED READING

Licht LE: Death following possible ingestion of toad eggs. *Toxicon* 5:141–142, 1967.

Peterson ME: Toxic exotics. *Vet Clin North Am Exot Anim Pract* 11:375–387, 2008.
Roberts BK, Aronsohn MG, Moses BL: Bufo marinus intoxication in dogs: 94 cases (1997–1998). *J Am Vet Med Assoc* 216(12):1941–1944, 2000.
Roder JD: Toads. In Plumlee KH, editor: *Clinical veterinary toxicology.* St Louis, 2004, Mosby Elsevier, p 113.

AUTHOR: **LISA A. MURPHY**

EDITOR: **CYNTHIA L. GASKILL**

Burns

BASIC INFORMATION

DEFINITION

A lesion caused by contact with heat or fire

EPIDEMIOLOGY

SPECIES, AGE, SEX

- Barn fires are one of the most common causes of burn in horses of any age.
- Horses housed in at-risk barns (no fire detection or protection systems) are more predisposed to burn injury.

CLINICAL PRESENTATION

DISEASE FORMS/SUBTYPES

- Burns are classified by the depth of the injury:
  - First-degree burns involve only the most superficial layers of the epidermis. These burns are painful and are characterized by erythema, edema, and desquamation of the superficial layers of the skin. The germinal layer of the epidermis is spared, and these burns heal without complication.
  - Second-degree burns involve the epidermis and may be superficial or deep.
    - Superficial second-degree burns involve the stratum corneum, stratum granulosum, and a few cells of the basal layer. Tactile and pain receptors remain intact. Because the basal layers remain relatively uninjured, superficial second-degree burns heal rapidly with minimal scarring, within 14 to 17 days.
    - Deep second-degree burns involve all layers of the epidermis, including the basal layers. These burns are characterized by erythema and edema at the epidermal-dermal junction, necrosis of the epidermis, accumulation of white blood cells at the basal layer of the burn, eschar (slough produced by a thermal burn) formation, and minimal pain. The only germinal cells spared are those within the ducts of sweat glands and hair follicles. Deep second-degree wounds may heal spontaneously in 3 to 4 weeks if care is taken to prevent further dermal ischemia that may lead to full-thickness necrosis. In general, deep second-degree wounds, unless grafted, heal with extensive scarring.
  - Third-degree burns are characterized by loss of the epidermal and dermal components, including the adnexa (Figure 1). The wounds range in color from white to black. There is fluid loss and a marked cellular response at the margins and deeper tissue, eschar formation, lack of pain, shock, wound infection, and possible bacteremia and septicemia. Healing is by contraction and epithelialization from the wound margins or acceptance of an autograft. These burns are frequently complicated by infection.
  - Fourth-degree burns involve all of the skin and underlying muscle, bone, ligaments, fat, and fascia.

HISTORY, CHIEF COMPLAINT Burn injury to the horse of various depths, usually the result of barn fire and falling asphalt shingles on the dorsum

PHYSICAL EXAM FINDINGS

- Because heat is slow to dissipate from burn wounds, it is often difficult to accurately evaluate the amount of tissue damage in the early phase of injury. Whereas the extent of the burn depends on the size of the area exposed, the severity relates to the maximum temperature the tissue attains and the duration of overheating. This explains why skin injury often extends beyond the original burn.
- Burns are most commonly seen on the back and face.
  - Erythema, pain, vesicles, and singed hair are present depending on the extent of the injury.
  - Increases in heart and respiratory rates are present in association with abnormal discoloration of mucous membranes.
  - The burned horse may have blepharospasm, epiphora, or both, signifying corneal damage.
  - Coughing may indicate smoke inhalation, and a fever signals or confirms a systemic response.
  - Whereas the percentage of total body surface area involved usually correlates with death, the depth of the burn determines morbidity.

ETIOLOGY AND PATHOPHYSIOLOGY

- After severe burns, a dramatic cardiovascular effect termed *burn shock* occurs, which resembles hypovolemic shock. A dramatic increase in local and systemic capillary permeability occurs as a result of heat and the release of cytokines, prostaglandins, nitric oxide, vasoactive leukotrienes, serotonin,

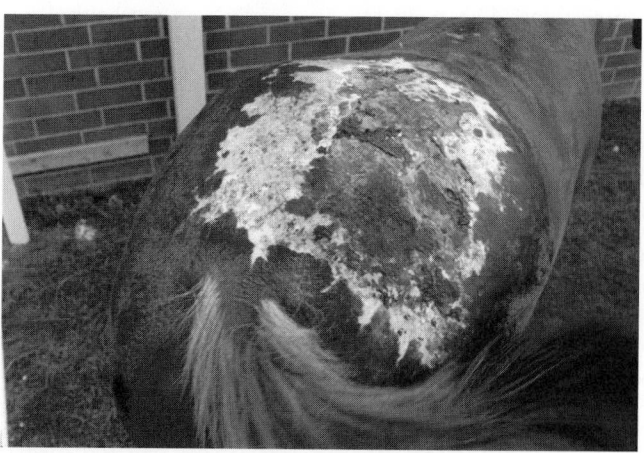

FIGURE 1 Third-degree burn of the dorsal gluteal region incurred during a barn fire caused by hot asphalt roof shingles falling on the horse. The central burn area is surrounded by deep and superficial second-degree burns.

histamine, and oxygen radicals. Local tissue damage results from massive protein coagulation and cellular death.

- Inhalation injury is a common sequela of closed-space fires and develops through three mechanisms: direct thermal injury, carbon monoxide poisoning, and chemical insult. Direct thermal injury causes edema and obstruction of the upper airway, but because of the efficient heat exchange capacity of the nasopharynx and oropharynx, superheated air is cooled before entering the lower respiratory tract.

DIAGNOSIS

DIFFERENTIAL DIAGNOSIS

Chemical burn injury

INITIAL DATABASE

- Complete blood count
- Serum chemistry panel
- Serial arterial blood gas analyses
- Upper airway endoscopy

ADVANCED OR CONFIRMATORY TESTING

- Thoracic radiographs
- Transtracheal washes for cytology and culture

TREATMENT

THERAPEUTIC GOAL(S)

Cardiovascular support to avoid circulatory collapse from burn shock in patients with greater than 15% of the total body surface area affected

ACUTE GENERAL TREATMENT

- Isotonic fluids should be given at a rate of 2 to 4 mL/kg body weight for each percentage of body surface area burned. Give a half dose in the first 24 hours and the other half the next day.
  - Fluid resuscitation is best titrated to maintain a stable and adequate blood pressure.
  - If there has been smoke or heat inhalation injury, crystalloids should be limited to the amount that normalizes circulatory volume and blood pressure.
- Two to 10 L of plasma is an effective albumin source as well as an exogenous source of antithrombin III for coagulopathies.

- Flunixin meglumine (0.25–1.0 mg/kg q12–24h IV) and pentoxifylline (8.0 mg/kg q12h IV) are effective analgesics and improve blood flow in the small capillary networks.
- Dimethyl sulfoxide (DMSO) (1 g/kg, diluted to <20% IV) for the first 24 hours may decrease inflammation and pulmonary edema.
- Dexamethasone may be administered once at 0.5 mg/kg IV if pulmonary edema is present and is unresponsive to DMSO.

CHRONIC TREATMENT

- First-degree burns:
  - Are generally not life threatening and are simply managed.
  - Topical therapy in the form of cool compresses, cold-water baths, and wound coverings may provide relief.
  - Pain control may be accomplished with nonsteroidal antiinflammatory drugs or narcotics.
- Second degree burns:
  - Are associated with vesicles and blisters.
  - These vesicles should be left intact for the first 24 to 36 hours after formation because blister fluid provides protection from infection, and the presence of a blister is less painful than the denuded exposed surface.
  - After this interval, the blister is partially excised, and an antibacterial dressing is applied to the wound or an eschar is allowed to form.
- Third-degree burns:
  - May be difficult to manage.
  - Destruction of the dermis leaves a primary collagenous structure called an eschar.
  - Dry exposure is a treatment method that operates under the principle that bacteria do not thrive on a dry surface.
    - The goals of therapy are to keep the wound dry and protected from mechanical trauma.
    - Heat and water loss from the uncovered wound, however, are a disadvantage.
    - The eschar is covered with silver sulfadiazine in a 1% water miscible cream twice daily.
  - The exposed bed can then be grafted or allowed to contract.

DRUG INTERACTIONS

- Povidone-iodine causes some patient discomfort.

- Its hyperosmolality causes severe hypernatremia and acidosis because of water loss such that it should not be used on extensive burns where systematic absorption is likely.
  - Immune system depression has also been reported in humans.
- Gentamicin is excellent for serious gram-negative infections but should be used only in selected cases because resistance can develop, and it may be nephrotoxic in patients with renal problems.
- Neomycin, bacitracin, and polymixin B
  - Generally associated with the rapid development of bacterial resistance and systemic toxicity
  - Not recommended for routine use in long-term wound care

POSSIBLE COMPLICATIONS

- Systemic antibiotics do not favorably influence wound healing, fever, or mortality, and they may encourage the emergence of resistant microorganisms.
- Many burned equine patients are pruritic, and measures must be taken to prevent self-mutilation of the wound.
- Reserpine may be effective in decreasing the urge to scratch by successfully breaking the itch-scratch cycle.

PROGNOSIS AND OUTCOME

Delayed healing and poor epithelialization and complications of second intention healing may limit return of the animal to previous uses.

PEARLS & CONSIDERATIONS

COMMENTS

- Extensive thermal injuries in horses may be difficult to manage.
- The large surface of the burn dramatically increases the potential for loss of fluids, electrolytes, and calories.

SUGGESTED READING

Hanson RR. Burn injuries. In Stashak TS, Theoret C, editors: *Equine wound management*, ed 2. Ames, IA, 2008, Blackwell, pp 569–584.

AUTHOR & EDITOR: R. REID HANSON

CO-EDITOR: AMELIA MUNSTERMAN

Candidiasis

BASIC INFORMATION

DEFINITION

Candida spp. are opportunistic fungal pathogens that can cause a variety of localized and systemic infections in neonatal and adult horses that have been immunocompromised for any reason.

SYNONYM(S)

Thrush

EPIDEMIOLOGY

GENETICS AND BREED PREDISPOSITION Horses with genetic conditions leading to immune compromise (eg, severe combined immunodeficiency of Arabians) are at increased risk.

RISK FACTORS

- Prolonged broad-spectrum antibiotic therapy
- Disruption of cutaneous or mucosal barriers by burns, surgery, cytotoxic agents, or trauma
- Any immune deficiency or immunosuppression produced by genetic defects, disease states such as sepsis, or administration of drugs such as glucocorticoids
- Low birth weight, premature foals
- Long-term placement of indwelling IV or urinary catheters or endotracheal tubes
- Prolonged parenteral nutrition

CONTAGION AND ZOONOSIS Although humans may develop a variety of infections from *Candida* spp., infection acquired from handling affected horses is probably unlikely unless the person is immunocompromised.

ASSOCIATED CONDITIONS AND DISORDERS Any other condition associated with immune deficiency

CLINICAL PRESENTATION

DISEASE FORMS/SUBTYPES
- Oral candidiasis or thrush
- Systemic candidiasis with variable organ localization
- Endometritis

HISTORY, CHIEF COMPLAINT History and chief complaint vary depending on the risk factors present, the reason for immunocompromise, and the site of infection.

PHYSICAL EXAM FINDINGS
- Physical examination findings vary depending on the risk factors present, the reason for immunocompromise, and the site of infection.

- Oral candidiasis (thrush) manifests as white plaques on the oral mucosa and tongue.
- Systemic candidiasis may present with nonspecific signs of fever or with signs related to the site of infection of the infection (eg, arthritis, meningitis, omphalophlebitis, pneumonia).
- Mares with uterine candidiasis may present with vaginal discharge or failure to conceive.

ETIOLOGY AND PATHOPHYSIOLOGY
- *Candida* is acquired as part of the normal flora as neonates pass through the birth canal.
- It colonizes the mucosal and mucocutaneous surfaces of the gastrointestinal, respiratory, and genitourinary tracts.
- Under most circumstances, overgrowth of *Candida* spp. is inhibited by normal microflora.
- Opportunistic infections occur when immune defenses are altered by disease or various interventional strategies.
- Mucocutaneous forms such as thrush are often related to defects in cell-mediated immunity; systemic spread is more likely to be associated with neutropenia.

DIAGNOSIS

DIFFERENTIAL DIAGNOSIS

Other bacterial or fungal infection

INITIAL DATABASE
- Complete blood count and serum biochemical profile to assess systemic health and identify possible sites of infection or reasons for immunocompromise
- Cytologic evaluation or culture of appropriate clinical samples (eg, blood, synovial fluid, cerebrospinal fluid, scrapings from mucosal surfaces)

TREATMENT

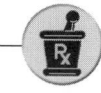

THERAPEUTIC GOAL(S)
- Eliminate infection.
- Resolve underlying reasons for immunodeficiency.

ACUTE GENERAL TREATMENT
- Treat any underlying diseases and discontinue administration of immune suppressive medications.

- Antifungal therapy with fluconazole as a loading dose of 8 mg/kg PO followed by 4 mg/kg q12–24h
- Resistant strains may be treated with itraconazole at 3–6 mg/kg PO.
- Intrauterine infections (endometritis) may be treated with large-volume uterine flush followed by intrauterine infusion of nystatin (0.5–2.5 million units), clotrimazole (500–700 mg), fluconazole (100 mg), or miconazole (200 mg) in a small volume of solution.
- Supportive care should be provided as appropriate depending on the site of infection and underlying disease processes.

PROGNOSIS AND OUTCOME

Prognosis is guarded because many cases are complicated by serious underlying immunosuppressive conditions.

PEARLS & CONSIDERATIONS

- Treatment of septic arthritis caused by *Candida* spp. must be aggressive and include successive joint lavage and arthroscopic flush procedures to facilitate physical removal of accumulated fibrin.
- Patients with systemic candidiasis may have embolic colonization and microabscess formation in lung, kidneys, joints, eyes, liver, brain, or myocardium.

SUGGESTED READING

Carrillo NA: Candidiasis. In Sellon DC, Long MT, editors: *Equine Infectious Diseases.* St Louis, 2007, Elsevier, pp 406–408.
McClure JJ, Addison JD, Miller RI: Immunodeficiency manifested by oral candidiasis and bacterial septicemia in foals. *J Am Vet Med Assoc* 186:1195–1197, 1985.
Reilly LK, Palmer JE: Systemic candidiasis in four foals. *J Am Vet Med Assoc* 205:464, 1994.

AUTHOR: **DEBRA C. SELLON**

EDITORS: **MAUREEN T. LONG** and **DEBRA C. SELLON**

Cardiac Failure

BASIC INFORMATION

DEFINITION

Clinical syndrome resulting from an acute or chronic impairment of cardiac function characterized by a reduction in cardiac output, inadequate perfusion of vital organs, heightened neurohumoral activity, renal sodium and fluid retention, and accumulation of fluid in tissues and body cavities

SYNONYM(S)

- Acute heart failure
- Chronic heart failure
- Congestive heart failure (CHF)

EPIDEMIOLOGY

SPECIES, AGE, SEX

- May occur at any age.
  - The majority of affected patients are older horses with severe valvular heart disease.
  - Foals and younger horses may develop heart failure secondary to congenital malformations.

ASSOCIATED CONDITIONS AND DISORDERS

- Heart failure develops in foals and adult horses as a sequela to severe cardiac disease.
- Underlying conditions include congenital malformations, valvular heart disease, pericardial disease, myocardial disease, rupture of large vessels, severe pulmonary disease, or chronic cardiac arrhythmias.

CLINICAL PRESENTATION

DISEASE FORMS/SUBTYPES

- May be acute (eg, chordal rupture, bacterial endocarditis) or chronic (eg, degenerative valve disease)
- Early heart failure: May be subclinical at rest. Signs may include poor performance and delayed recovery after exercise.
- Acute or advanced chronic heart failure: Clinical signs are evident at rest. Even in chronic disease, sudden onset of clinical signs is common.
- CHF is characterized by volume overload, elevation of venous pressures, and fluid accumulation in tissues and in body cavities.
- CHF is uncommon in horses.
- Left ventricular failure is characterized by pulmonary venous congestion and pulmonary edema. Slowly progressive left heart disease often goes unnoticed until the right heart fails in response to chronic pulmonary hypertension (PH), leading to biventricular failure.
- Right ventricular and biventricular failure are characterized by systemic venous congestion, ventral edema, and effusion in body cavities.

HISTORY, CHIEF COMPLAINT

- Clinical signs may be subtle and depend on the stage of disease and the underlying cause.
- Early complaints: Poor performance, exercise intolerance, and delayed recovery after exercise.
- Advanced disease may lead to anxiety, weight loss, lethargy, tachypnea, cough, foamy nasal discharge, ventral edema, distension of the jugular veins, weakness, ataxia, syncope, or collapse.

PHYSICAL EXAM FINDINGS

- Early heart failure: May be unremarkable
- Advanced heart failure: Tachycardia, weak arterial pulses, pale mucous membranes, prolonged capillary refill time, and cool extremities. Cardiac cachexia (weight loss or loss of muscle mass) may also be seen.
- Cardiac auscultation may reveal:
  - Cardiac murmurs
  - Irregular cardiac rhythm
  - Muffled heart sounds or friction rubs, indicating pericardial disease
  - A loud third heart sound, indicating a severe increase in filling pressures
  - A prominent or split second heart sound, indicating PH
- Left ventricular failure: Tachypnea, increased respiratory effort, dyspnea, cough, nasal discharge, and abnormal lung sounds (crackles, wheezes) on auscultation. The pulmonary edema of pure left-sided congestive heart failure is frequently misdiagnosed as pneumonia, especially in foals with congenital heart disease.
- Right ventricular or biventricular heart failure: Distension of superficial veins; jugular venous pulsation; and generalized ventral, preputial, and pectoral edema. Isolated limb edema and ventral edema in the absence of generalized venous distension are not consistent with CHF.
- Fever may indicate an inflammatory or infectious process such as endocarditis, valvulitis, pericarditis, or myocarditis.

ETIOLOGY AND PATHOPHYSIOLOGY

- May result from any structural or functional heart disease.
- The pathophysiology is complex and affects many body systems.
- Exact mechanisms have not been extensively studied in horses but are likely similar to those reported in other species.
- The failing heart is characterized by:
  - Poor myocardial contractility
  - Decreased preload reserve (diminished response to volume loading)
  - Increased sensitivity to ventricular afterload (wall tension, primarily determined by ventricular geometry and systemic blood pressures)
- Systolic failure occurs because of reduced cardiac pump function.
- Diastolic failure occurs because of impaired cardiac relaxation and ventricular filling.
- Impairment of ventricular filling and reduction of cardiac pump function results in inadequate perfusion of vital organs.
- Inadequate organ perfusion leads to an activation of multiple neurohumoral pathways, including:
  - Sympathetic nervous system
  - Renin-angiotensin-aldosterone system
  - Other hormones, including vasopressin (antidiuretic hormone), endothelin, and natriuretic peptides
- Initially, neurohumoral activation is compensatory and beneficial. An increase in heart rate, contractility, and circulating blood volume allow support of cardiac pump function, and arteriolar vasoconstriction results in redistribution of blood flow to vital organs.
- With disease progression, the compensatory capacity of the cardiovascular system is exceeded, leading to development of overt congestive heart failure. Chronic neurohumoral activation results in exacerbation of clinical signs and heart failure.
  - Sodium and water retention contribute to volume overload, resulting in organ congestion.
  - Catecholamines exert proarrhythmic effects, promote myocardial remodeling, and are toxic to myocytes.
  - Aldosterone causes endothelial dysfunction and myocardial fibrosis.
  - Proinflammatory cytokines contribute to weight loss and apoptotic cell loss in myocardial tissues.
- Strenuous work, anemia, fever, or pregnancy increase the demands for cardiac output and may precipitate heart failure in a compensated patient.
- Development of atrial fibrillation in a horse with underlying structural disease may also cause sudden deterioration in a compensated patient.
- Left-sided heart failure: The left ventricle undergoes remodeling, leading

to dilation and hypertrophy, with decreased myocardial perfusion and potential myocardial ischemia. Ventricular dilation may result in worsening of mitral regurgitation, exacerbating pulmonary congestion.

- Chronic left-sided CHF in horses causes interstitial lung edema, remodeling of the pulmonary vasculature, and PH.
- PH leads to dilation of the pulmonary artery and development of pulmonic and tricuspid regurgitation (see "Pulmonary Hypertension" in this section).
- Biventricular failure may result from chronic right ventricular overload.
- In severe (but rare) cases, rupture of the dilated pulmonary artery is possible.

DIAGNOSIS

DIFFERENTIAL DIAGNOSIS

- Other systemic diseases resulting in fever, weight loss, and tachycardia.
- For left-sided failure: Other causes of respiratory distress such as acute respiratory distress syndrome, recurrent airway obstruction, or severe pneumonia or pleuropneumonia.
- For right-sided heart failure: Other causes of venous distension and edema such as a mediastinal or thoracic mass or other space-occupying masses.
- Causes of left-sided or biventricular failure include:
  - Mitral regurgitation: Severe degenerative valve disease, valvulitis, bacterial endocarditis, chordal rupture (see "Mitral/Tricuspid Regurgitation" and "Endocarditis, Infective" in this section)
  - Aortic regurgitation: Severe degenerative valve disease, valvulitis, bacterial endocarditis, rupture or fenestration of aortic valve leaflet (see "Aortic/Pulmonic Regurgitation, Acquired" in this section)
  - Myocardial disease: Dilated cardiomyopathy, ionophore toxicity, white muscle disease, myocarditis, myocardial ischemia, myocardial necrosis (see "Myocarditis" and "Cardiomyopathy" in this section)
  - Vascular rupture (see "Aortocardiac Fistula" in this section)
  - Chronic tachyarrhythmia
  - Congenital heart disease: Ventricular septal defect, patent ductus arteriosus, and other malformations (see "Congenital Heart Disease" in this section and "Comments" below)
- Causes of right-sided failure include:
  - Tricuspid or pulmonary valve lesions: severe degenerative valve disease, valvulitis, bacterial endo-

carditis, chordal rupture (see "Mitral/Tricuspid Regurgitation" and "Endocarditis, Infective" in this section)
  - Pericardial disease: Pericardial effusion, constrictive pericarditis (see "Pericardial Disease" in this section)
  - Severe primary lung disease or pulmonary vascular disease, leading to PH (cor pulmonale)
  - Congenital heart disease: Tricuspid valve atresia, atrial septal defect, and other malformations (see "Congenital Heart Disease" in this section)
- The most common cause of CHF in horses is valvular heart disease, often complicated by atrial fibrillation.
- Biventricular failure often occurs because of progression of left-sided heart disease to CHF.

INITIAL DATABASE

- Thorough medical history, including current use, athletic condition, and exercise capacity
- Complete physical examination, including careful assessment of mucous membranes, palpation of peripheral pulses, and inspection of venous filling; cardiac auscultation; thoracic auscultation; thoracic percussion; and observation of edema and body condition

ADVANCED OR CONFIRMATORY TESTING

- Echocardiography:
  - Detection of underlying structural heart disease
  - Identification of abnormal blood flow patterns (eg, valvular insufficiencies, shunts)
  - Detection of cardiomegaly and volume overload
  - Evaluation of myocardial function
  - Diagnosis of PH
- Electrocardiography:
  - Assessment of cardiac rhythm disturbances
  - Atrial fibrillation is commonly seen in association with CHF
  - Other arrhythmias such as supraventricular or ventricular premature depolarizations or supraventricular or ventricular tachycardia may also occur
- Thoracic radiography:
  - To identify pulmonary edema and evaluate response to treatment.
  - Limited in its ability to demonstrate mild forms of congestion.
  - Clinical signs do not always correlate with radiographic findings.
  - Mild congestion may be characterized by an interstitial pattern and pulmonary venous congestion.
  - Acute heart failure and severe congestion are characterized by an

alveolar pattern and air bronchograms; the cardiac silhouette may be rounded or enlarged, and pleural effusion may be identified.
- Thoracic and abdominal ultrasonography: to identify pleural effusion, ascites, and hepatic congestion
- Complete blood count and plasma fibrinogen concentration: Diagnosis of underlying inflammatory conditions such as endocarditis, valvulitis, pericarditis, or myocarditis
- Serum biochemistry profile:
  - To assess the severity of renal compromise (prerenal or renal azotemia)
  - To identify serum electrolyte disturbances
  - To assess the degree of hepatic damage secondary to congestion
- Blood or plasma lactate concentration to assess peripheral perfusion deficiencies
- Cardiac troponin I (cTnI) or cardiac troponin T (cTnT): Sensitive and specific markers of myocardial cell damage (see "Troponins, Cardiac" in Section IV)
- Blood culture and susceptibility testing: mandatory with suspected bacterial endocarditis (see "Endocarditis, Infective" in this section)
- Ultrasound-guided pericardiocentesis, cytologic evaluation and culture and sensitivity testing: In cases with pericardial effusion (see "Pericardiocentesis" in Section II)
- Exercise testing
  - In horses with early heart failure that are subclinical at rest
  - To document exercise intolerance and poor performance
- Blood pressure monitoring (direct or indirect): To assess the degree of hypotension or response to treatment
- Intracardiac and pulmonary vascular pressure measurements:
  - Cardiac chamber pressure, pulmonary artery pressure, capillary wedge pressure
  - To document PH and increased filling pressures
  - Invasive procedure that is rarely performed in clinical practice

TREATMENT

THERAPEUTIC GOAL(S)

- General goals:
  - Reduction of congestion and edema
  - Improvement of cardiac output and tissue perfusion
  - Inhibition of deleterious neurohumoral activation
- If possible, treat the underlying condition
  - Pericardiocentesis and drainage of pericardial effusion

○ Antimicrobial therapy in bacterial endocarditis

○ Antiarrhythmics to control chronic tachyarrhythmias

○ Addressing treatable causes of myocarditis or cardiomyopathy

ACUTE GENERAL TREATMENT

- Acute heart failure or acute worsening of chronic heart failure:
  ○ Diuretics (eg, furosemide): 0.5 to 3.0 mg/kg SC, IM, or IV q8–12h or as a bolus of 0.12 mg/kg IV followed by a constant rate infusion (CRI) at a rate of 0.12 mg/kg/hr; doses should be adjusted as needed to produce a diuretic effect.
  ○ Positive inotropes (eg, dobutamine): CRI at doses of 1 to 5 µg/kg/min, uptitrated to effect or until development of adverse reactions (eg, arrhythmias, tachycardia, extreme anxiety). Administer 2 to 4 µg/kg/min.
  ○ Intranasal oxygen
- Vasodilators:
  ○ Used to reduce pulmonary congestion, lower ventricular afterload, and improve tissue perfusion
  ○ Hydralazine (arterial dilator; 0.5–1.5 mg/kg PO q12h), nitroglycerin (venodilator), milrinone (inotropic vasodilator)
  ○ Data on efficacy and safety of these drugs in horses with heart failure are lacking
- Cardiac tamponade:
  ○ Requires a different approach.
  ○ Initial management includes pericardiocentesis and drainage of the effusion (see "Pericardiocentesis" in Section II).
  ○ IV fluid administration (as opposed to diuresis) may be necessary to ensure adequate volume loading of the ventricles.
- Life-threatening tachyarrhythmias:
  ○ May require immediate antiarrhythmic treatment after careful consideration of potential adverse effects (see "Antiarrhythmic Drugs" in Section VI)
  ○ Criteria for immediate antiarrhythmic treatment include:
    ▪ Severe hemodynamic compromise
    ▪ Sustained heart rates greater than 100 to 120 beats/min
    ▪ Presence of multiforme ventricular complexes or R-on-T phenomenon (when the succeeding QRS complex is essentially continuous with the preceding T wave, increasing the likelihood of inducing ventricular fibrillation)

CHRONIC TREATMENT

- In clinical practice, therapy is often limited to furosemide and digoxin.
  ○ Furosemide (0.5–2.0 mg/kg SC, IM, or IV q8–12h, titrated to effect), to alleviate volume overload, congestion, and edema.
  ○ Digoxin (0.011 mg/kg q12h PO, titrated to effect) to increase myocardial contractility and to slow ventricular response rate in patients with rapid atrial fibrillation.
  ○ Oral potassium supplementation to prevent the occurrence of furosemide-induced hypokalemia that could potentiate the toxic effects of digoxin.
- Angiotensin-converting enzyme (ACE) inhibitors:
  ○ Decrease renal sodium and water reabsorption, reduce volume overload, counteract the development of diuretic resistance, cause vasodilation with a decrease in myocardial oxygen demand, and are considered to be cardioprotective by decreasing myocardial remodeling and fibrosis.
  ○ Enalapril (0.5 mg/kg PO q12h), ramipril (0.05 mg/kg PO q24h), and quinapril (0.25 mg/kg PO q24h) have been used in horses.
  ○ The pharmacology of ACE inhibitors in horses has not been fully investigated, and the efficacy for prophylaxis and treatment of heart failure is unknown.
- β-adrenergic inhibitors, aldosterone antagonists, or inodilators such as pimobendan are commonly used in humans and in dogs with CHF. The use of these agents in the treatment of heart failure has not been investigated in horses to date.
- Pericardectomy: Potential treatment option in horses with severe constrictive pericarditis
- Long-term IV, broad-spectrum antibiotic treatment:
  ○ Indicated for bacterial endocarditis or infective pericarditis.
  ○ The antibiotic choice should be adapted based on the results of bacterial culture and susceptibility testing.
- Antiarrhythmics:
  ○ Lidocaine, magnesium sulphate, procainamide, quinidine, propafenone, phenytoin, and diltiazem
  ○ Used for treatment of severe arrhythmias after careful consideration of the benefits and potential risks of treatment

DRUG INTERACTIONS

- Simultaneous administration of quinidine and digoxin increases the steady-state serum concentration of digoxin and may promote toxic concentrations

because of the narrow therapeutic window.

- Furosemide is potassium wasting, which can potentiate the toxic effects of digoxin.

POSSIBLE COMPLICATIONS

- Furosemide (long-term administration): Hyponatremia, hypokalemia, hypomagnesemia, and metabolic alkalosis
- Positive inotropes: Dose-dependent tachycardia, ventricular arrhythmias, and vasoconstriction leading to hypertension and increases in ventricular afterload
- Digoxin: Depression, anorexia, colic, diarrhea, sinus bradycardia, atrioventricular block, as well as supraventricular and ventricular arrhythmias (eg, bigeminy)
- ACE inhibitors: Cough, impairment of renal function, hyperkalemia, and hypotension
- Vasodilators: Severe hypotension, reflex tachycardia, and weakness
- Antiarrhythmics: Proarrhythmic, cardiodepressant, and hypotensive effects

RECOMMENDED MONITORING

- Clinical monitoring: Periodic reevaluation of mentation and behavior, heart rate, respiratory rate and effort, mucous membranes, peripheral arterial pulses, jugular veins, lung sounds, ventral edema, and exercise capacity.
- Monitoring for signs of adverse drug effects.
- Furosemide, dobutamine, and digoxin should be titrated to effect; improved perfusion, decreased edema, reduced respiratory effort and respiratory rate, decreased heart rate and increased exercise capacity indicate clinical efficacy.
- Serum digoxin concentrations:
  ○ Periodic monitoring required because of the marked interindividual pharmacokinetic variation
  ○ Recommended digoxin peak (1–2 hours) and trough (12 hours) concentrations at steady state: 0.8 to 2.0 ng/mL (1.0–2.6 nmol/L)
- Electrocardiographic changes: monitored to detect potential proarrhythmic effects of dobutamine and digoxin
- Serum electrolyte concentrations and serum creatinine concentration:
  ○ Periodic monitoring is advisable during diuretic therapy to avoid electrolyte disturbances and prerenal azotemia.
  ○ Important because renal dysfunction may affect digoxin excretion and abnormalities in serum sodium, potassium, magnesium, and calcium concentrations may alter the sensitivity to digoxin.

PROGNOSIS AND OUTCOME

- Usually, management of CHF is only effective in the short and medium term (2 to 6 months).
- The prognosis is usually guarded to poor when irreversible structural heart disease is the cause of CHF. Euthanasia is often elected because of the poor prognosis at the time of diagnosis.
- The prognosis may be fair for horses with potentially reversible diseases such as pericarditis, myocarditis, acute myocardial ischemia, or sustained ventricular tachycardia.

PEARLS & CONSIDERATIONS

COMMENTS

- Clinical detection of CHF should prompt the veterinarian to perform a complete cardiovascular workup to identify the cause of heart failure.
- At the time of detection of CHF, the underlying cardiac disease is usually advanced and severe.

- Treatment options are limited in horses. The appropriate treatment may vary depending on the underlying cause.
- The prognosis is guarded to poor in most cases. Selected horses with a potentially reversible cause may have a fair prognosis.

CLIENT EDUCATION

- Congestive heart failure is a serious, life-threatening condition resulting from severe heart disease.
- Immediate treatment or euthanasia is required at the time of diagnosis.
- Treatment is usually only effective in the short and medium term (maximum, 2–6 months), and the prognosis is usually guarded to poor.
- Horses with CHF should not be worked or ridden. There may be a risk of syncope (collapse) or sudden death because of severe ventricular arrhythmia or pulmonary artery rupture.
- Breeding of animals with controlled CHF may be possible under close supervision through the veterinarian. However, pregnancy may trigger sudden deterioration of a compensated condition, and breeding could trigger pulmonary artery rupture in a stallion.

SUGGESTED READING

Bonagura JD, Reef VB, Schwarzwald CC: Cardiovascular diseases. In Reed SM, Bayly WM, Sellon DC, editors: *Equine internal medicine,* ed 3. St Louis, 2010, Saunders Elsevier, pp 372–487.

Davis JL, Gardner SY, Schwabenton B, et al: Congestive heart failure in horses: 14 cases (1984–2001). *J Am Vet Med Assoc* 220:1512–1515, 2002.

Marr CM: Heart failure. In Marr CM, editor: *Cardiology of the horse.* London, 1999, WB Saunders, pp 289–311.

Reef VB: Cardiovascular system. In Orsini JA, Divers TJ, editors: *Manual of equine emergencies: treatment and procedures,* ed 2. Philadelphia, 2003, Saunders Elsevier, pp 130–188.

Reef VB: Severe mitral regurgitation in horses: clinical, echocardiographic and pathological findings. *Equine Vet J Suppl* 30:18, 1998.

Schwarzwald CC, Bonagura JD, Muir WW: The cardiovascular system. In Muir WW, Hubbell JAE, editors: *Equine anesthesia,* ed 2. St Louis, 2009, Saunders Elsevier, pp 37–100.

Schwarzwald CC: Cardiovascular pharmacology. In Robinson NE, editor: *Current therapy in equine medicine,* ed 6. St Louis, 2009, Saunders Elsevier, pp 182–191.

AUTHOR: **COLIN C. SCHWARZWALD**

EDITOR: **MARY M. DURANDO**

Cardiomyopathy

BASIC INFORMATION

DEFINITION

A myocardial disease process resulting in decreased myocardial function. In horses, this often results in dilation and decreased contractility, which can lead to congestive heart failure, arrhythmias, or both. Myocarditis is often a precursor to cardiomyopathy.

SYNONYM(S)

Dilated cardiomyopathy

EPIDEMIOLOGY

RISK FACTORS Any cause of myocarditis that does not completely resolve has the potential to progress to cardiomyopathy (see "Myocarditis" in this section).

GEOGRAPHY AND SEASONALITY Cardiomyopathy associated with selenium deficiency is most common in young horses (see "Myocarditis" in this section).

CLINICAL PRESENTATION

DISEASE FORMS/SUBTYPES Acute, subacute, and chronic: These subtypes

have not been well characterized in horses.

HISTORY, CHIEF COMPLAINT
- Exercise intolerance
- Signs of left-sided heart failure: Tachypnea, dyspnea, cough, nostril flare, weakness
- Signs of right-sided heart failure: Jugular pulses, jugular distension, edema, abdominal distension
- Syncope, sudden death

PHYSICAL EXAM FINDINGS
- Tachycardia, arrhythmias, gallop rhythm
- Cardiac murmurs
- Tachypnea, dyspnea, nostril flare, cough
- Exercise intolerance
- Weak pulses, jugular pulses, jugular distention, ventral (pectoral) edema
- Abdominal distension
- Syncope
- Nonspecific signs include weight loss (cardiac cachexia), depression, anorexia, weakness

ETIOLOGY AND PATHOPHYSIOLOGY
- Causes of myocarditis that become chronic may progress to cardiomyopathy.

- Most often leads to decreased systolic function and chamber dilation, with subsequent arrhythmias.
- Arrhythmogenic right ventricular cardiomyopathy is also seen in horses, rarely.

DIAGNOSIS

DIFFERENTIAL DIAGNOSIS

- For exercise intolerance, lethargy, weakness, weight loss: Abnormalities in respiratory, neuromuscular, gastrointestinal systems
- For arrhythmias: Arrhythmias secondary to severe valvular or congenital heart disease with cardiac enlargement; systemic disease; electrolyte abnormalities
- For heart failure: Primary valvular, pericardial, or congenital heart disease
- For respiratory signs: Primary pulmonary or pleural disease

INITIAL DATABASE

- The complete blood count may be normal or may show characteristics of concurrent disease.
- Chemistry panel: Changes consistent with passive congestion from right-sided heart failure (increased liver enzymes) or changes consistent with organ dysfunction caused by decreased cardiac output (azotemia). Elevations in creatine kinase in horses with selenium deficiency may be seen. Elevations in lactate associated with poor tissue perfusion may be seen.
- Thoracic radiography: Evidence of pulmonary edema (interstitial or alveolar pattern may be seen), cardiomegaly, pleural effusion.
- Electrocardiogram (ECG): Sinus tachycardia with any additional arrhythmias.
- Echocardiogram: Will show evidence of dilated cardiomyopathy, including dilated atria and ventricles possibly with thin walls, decreased systolic function (low fractional shortening), spontaneous contrast indicating a low flow state, and distended pulmonary artery suggesting pulmonary hypertension. The left ventricle will appear hypokinetic, with an increased septal–E point separation. Doppler evaluation may show valvular regurgitation. There may be evidence of infiltrative cardiomyopathy (thick walls, heteroechogenicity of myocardium) (Figure 1).
- Cardiac troponin I: Likely elevated in cases of cardiomyopathy associated with active myocardial necrosis.

ADVANCED OR CONFIRMATORY TESTING

- Evaluation of pasture for toxic plants and feed for ionophore antimicrobials

- Blood selenium concentrations
- Pursuit of heavy metal exposure
- Pursuit of potential infectious cause, as for myocarditis (see "Myocarditis" in this section)

TREATMENT

THERAPEUTIC GOAL(S)

- Resolve congestive heart failure (address fluid retention, provide inotropic support, and control arrhythmias)
- Improve quality of life
- Treat underlying disease

ACUTE GENERAL TREATMENT

- Arrhythmias: Treat life-threatening arrhythmias with antiarrhythmics drugs (AAD).
- Congestive heart failure: Furosemide (1–2 mg/kg IV q12h or as needed), positive inotropes (eg, dobutamine), and vasodilators (eg, hydralazine) (see "Cardiac Failure" in this section).
- Intranasal oxygen supplementation.
- Minimize stress.
- Suspect recent intoxication: remove all suspected contaminated feed, and remove the horse from the pasture. Administer activated charcoal or mineral oil via nasogastric intubation.
- Suspect monensin intoxication: administer high levels of vitamin E and selenium to stabilize cell membranes.
- Address mineral deficiencies, such as selenium and vitamin E supplementation.

CHRONIC TREATMENT

- Arrhythmias: AAD can be given orally if necessary to treat persistent ventricular arrhythmias. It is contraindicated to convert atrial fibrillation (AF) to sinus rhythm when it is associated with dilated cardiomyopathy and congestive heart failure, but rate control to slow the ventricular response, if excessive, is critical. Drugs such as quinidine are negative inotropes, hypotensive agents, and vagolytic (increase ventricular rate), all of which are detrimental in heart failure. AF alone is unlikely to result in the horse's death and will not cause significant progression of heart failure.
- Diuretics: Furosemide as needed to control edema. It is not well absorbed in horses orally, so it is best if given SC, IM, or IV (see "Cardiac Failure" in this section).
- Digoxin as a positive inotrope: The initial dose is 0.011 mg/kg PO q12h; this may need to be adjusted based on therapeutic drug monitoring of peak and trough serum concentrations (therapeutic range, 0.5–2.0 ng/mL) and clinical signs. Renal function and electrolytes should also be monitored closely. Decreased renal function will increase digoxin levels, potentially into the toxic range, and hypokalemia may precipitate digoxin toxicity. Horses receiving furosemide are more likely to become hypokalemic, particularly if anorectic, and may require potassium supplementation (see "Cardiac Failure" in this section).
- Angiotensin-converting enzyme (ACE) inhibitors such as enalapril (0.5–1.0 mg/kg q12h PO), although this is not well absorbed orally in horses and does not result in significant decrease in ACE activity (see "Cardiac Failure" in this section).
- Strict stall rest for as long as clinical signs remain (a minimum of 2 months).
- Supplement with selenium and vitamin E, if indicated.
- Treat the primary disease process.
- Provide supportive care to improve quality of life.

DRUG INTERACTIONS

- Digoxin should not be used in cases of monensin intoxication because both increase intracellular calcium; this may enhance myocardial cell death, leading to arrhythmias.
- Furosemide treatment may lead to hypokalemia, which may lead to arrhythmias and potentiate digoxin toxicity. Serum potassium concentrations should be monitored and supplemented orally as needed.
- Corticosteroids should only be used after active infections have been ruled out.

POSSIBLE COMPLICATIONS

- Any AAD can be proarrhythmic and have other cardiovascular side effects such as hypotension.

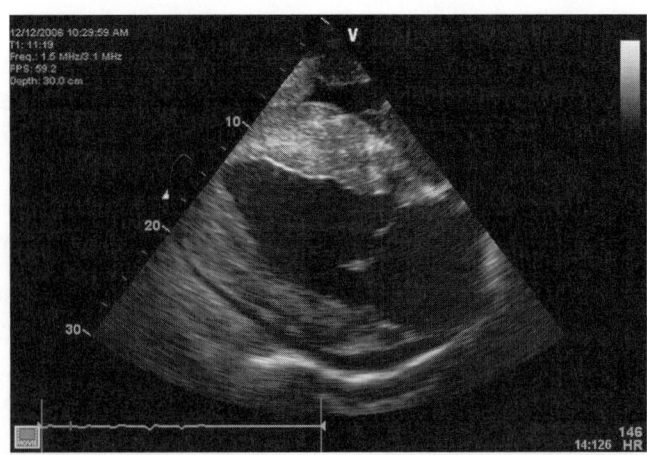

FIGURE 1 Right-sided parasternal longitudinal four-chamber echocardiographic view of a horse with cardiomyopathy secondary to monensin intoxication. Note the thick heteroechoic myocardial walls from active inflammation and the mild pericardial effusion. Systolic function was significantly decreased. This scan was acquired at 1.5 MHz and a depth of 30 cm.

- Sudden death (fatal arrhythmia).
- Dilated cardiomyopathy will likely progress to congestive heart failure unless it is mild or discovered early.

RECOMMENDED MONITORING

- Initial monitoring:
  - Arrhythmias: Continuous ECG monitoring using radiotelemetry (particularly if arrhythmia is being treated).
  - Serum lactate concentrations may be used as an indicator of tissue perfusion.
  - Central venous pressure monitoring may be used to assess preload and cardiac function.
  - Cardiac catheterization will show severe increases in right ventricular and pulmonary artery systolic, mean, and diastolic pressures in cases nearing heart failure.
  - Cardiac output monitoring will show decreased cardiac output.
- Chronic monitoring:
  - Horse should have activity level, appetite, attitude, heart rate, respiratory rate and effort, and edema monitored by the owner after discharge. Any changes in these may indicate a progression of disease.
  - Repeat echocardiograms should be performed every 3 to 6 months after discharge or sooner if any of the above clinical signs are noted by the owner. These should continue until normal echocardiograms are seen.
  - 24-hour continuous ECG (Holter) monitoring should be performed intermittently after discharge or if the above clinical signs are noted.
  - If clinical and echocardiographic abnormalities resolve, the horse must have an exercising electrocardiogram performed before it is determined if the horse is safe to

ride. Significant arrhythmias occurring during exercise may lead to syncope or collapse and injury or death to the rider or horse.
  - Cardiac troponin I may reflect changes in the degree of myocardial cell injury or necrosis and may be monitored intermittently.
  - Renal parameters and electrolyte status should be monitored at home, particularly if the horse is on chronic furosemide and digoxin therapy.
  - Therapeutic drug monitoring of digoxin levels should be done until the horse is stable. This should be repeated if any change in status such as anorexia, diarrhea, depression, or colic or changes in heart rate occur.

PROGNOSIS AND OUTCOME

- Prognosis is guarded to poor in most situations because it is often not recognized until disease is fairly advanced. Treatment is usually palliative and aimed at increasing the comfort level and lifespan of the horse.
- If the cause is recognized early and can be removed (eg, early removal of monensin, early recognition of selenium deficiency), the prognosis may be fair.

PEARLS & CONSIDERATIONS

COMMENTS

- In cases of monensin intoxication, the initial echocardiogram has prognostic value.

- Horses with normal left ventricular function have an excellent prognosis for life and performance.
- Horses with mild systolic dysfunction have a good prognosis for life and a fair prognosis for performance.
- Horses with significant systolic dysfunction have a poor prognosis for life and performance.

PREVENTION

- Monensin intoxication: use a reputable feed supplier, preferably one that does not mix equine feed in the same location as poultry or steer feed.
- Plant intoxications: know the content of pastures on which horses are kept.
- Selenium deficiency: know the status of soil and pastures.

CLIENT EDUCATION

- Horses with dilated cardiomyopathy leading to chamber enlargement and pulmonary hypertension are at risk for collapse or sudden death secondary to fatal arrhythmias or pulmonary artery rupture (rare).
- These horses should never be ridden because of this risk.

SUGGESTED READING

Martin BB, Reef VB, Parente EJ, et al: Causes or poor performance of horses during training, racing, or showing: 348 cases (1992–1996). *J Am Vet Med Assoc* 216:554–558, 2000.

Reef VB: A monensin outbreak in horses in the eastern United States: pathogenesis, clinical signs, and epidemiology. *Proceedings of the Eighth Annual Veterinary Medicine Forum*, 1990:126–128.

AUTHOR: **SOPHY A. JESTY**

EDITOR: **MARY M. DURANDO**

Cardiotoxic Plants

BASIC INFORMATION

DEFINITION

Cardiac disease subsequent to exposure to toxic plants

SYNONYM(S)

- Oleander poisoning (*Nerium oleander*)
- Summer pheasant's eye poisoning (*Adonis aestivalis*)

- Grayanotoxin intoxication (*Azalea* spp., *Rhododendron* spp; see "Rhododendron Toxicosis" in this section.)
- Yew poisoning (*Taxus* spp; see "*Taxus* Toxicosis" in this section.)
- Avocado poisoning (*Persea* spp.)
- Cardiac glycoside intoxication (*N. oleander*, *Digitalis* spp., *Asclepias* spp.)

EPIDEMIOLOGY
RISK FACTORS

- Fresh cardiotoxic plants have low palatability. Animals are more likely

to ingest dried cardiotoxic plant material.
- Plant trimmings present the most common source for oleander and yew poisoning.
- Contamination of hay or hay cubes with cardiotoxic plants is a great risk.
- The Guatemalan race of avocados and the Fuerte hybrid are reportedly toxic. The Mexican race has low toxicity.

GEOGRAPHY AND SEASONALITY

- Oleander exposure is a year-round risk. Oleander poisoning is common

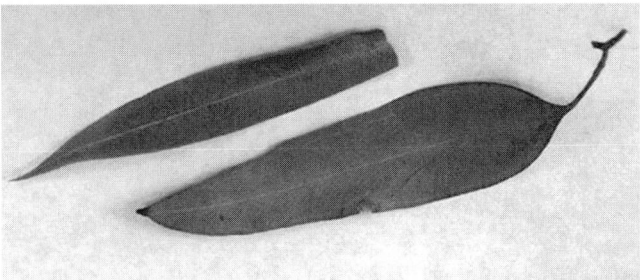

FIGURE 1 Oleander leaf (*top*) and eucalyptus leaf (*bottom*).

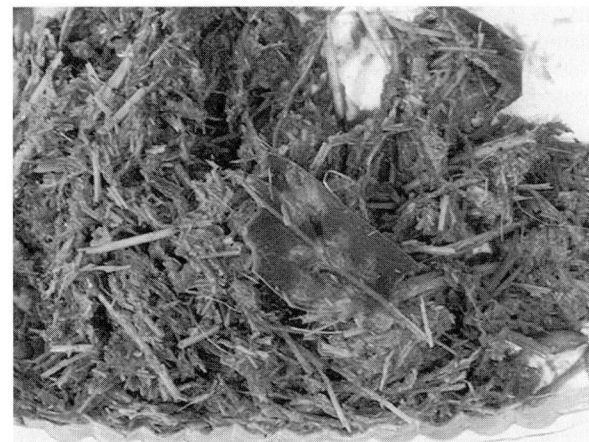

FIGURE 2 Oleander leaf in stomach contents.

in horses, especially in California, Arizona, and Texas. Ingestion of dried oleander clippings often causes poisoning.
• Summer pheasant's eye has been limited to some northern California counties.
• Grayanotoxin-containing plants have the highest toxin concentrations in the leaves.
• Ingestion of yew clippings is the most common cause for poisonings with *Taxus* spp. All species of *Taxus*, including *T. baccata* (English yew), *T. cuspidata* (Japanese yew), and *T. brevifolia* (Pacific or Western yew), are considered toxic.
• Avocado is extensively cultivated in California and Florida but can also be found as an ornamental in the Gulf Coast areas. Avocado leaves are especially toxic.
• Some cardiotoxic plants are most abundant in the spring and summer, depending on the location

CLINICAL PRESENTATION
DISEASE FORMS/SUBTYPES
• Acute cardiotoxicity subsequent to exposure to cardiotoxic plants.
• Acute death from ingestion of oleander, yew, summer pheasant's eye, avocado, or azaleas. Animals are often found dead.
• Cardiac changes include bradyarrhythmias, tachyarrhythmias, atrioventricular (AV) blocks, ectopic beats, and gallop rhythms.
HISTORY, CHIEF COMPLAINT
• Clinical signs of colic are often seen within hours of exposure.
• Other clinical signs include weakness, tremors, excessive salivation, incoordination, dyspnea, and sometimes convulsions. Progression of signs may be rapid.
• Animals exposed to oleander may be anorectic for several days.

PHYSICAL EXAM FINDINGS
• Oleander: Irregular fast pulse with tachycardia, ventricular arrhythmias, or gallop rhythms; anorexia and colic; occasionally diarrhea
• Summer pheasant's eye: Gastrointestinal (GI) stasis, feed refusal, dyspnea, and cardiac arrhythmias
• Grayanotoxins: Depression, salivation, abdominal pain, possibly diarrhea; in severe cases: recumbency, seizures, tachycardia, tachypnea, and pyrexia
• Yew: Incoordination, nervousness, difficulty in breathing, bradycardia, diarrhea, and convulsions. Sudden death is often all that is seen.
• Avocado: Subcutaneous edema of the head and chest, submandibular edema, respiratory dyspnea, and cardiac arrhythmias

ETIOLOGY AND PATHOPHYSIOLOGY
• Oleander contains cardiotoxic glycosides, such as oleandrin. Cardiac glycosides inhibit Na$^+$/K$^+$ ATPase, which leads to increased intracellular Ca^{2+} concentrations and a subsequent positive inotropic effect. In addition, direct effects on the sympathetic nervous system are seen.
• Summer pheasant's eye contains cardiotoxic glycosides.
• Grayanotoxins, found in azaleas and rhododendrons, are diterpenes that bind to sodium channels in excitable cell membranes (skeletal and myocardial muscle, nerves, and central nervous system). Excitable cells are maintained in a state of depolarization. Additionally, increased intracellular sodium results in an exchange with extracellular calcium, which affects the control of transmitter release.
• Yews contain taxine alkaloids (such as taxine A and B) that are inotropic and change AV conduction. Yews also contain ephedrine, nitriles, and irritant oils that are likely to be responsible for colic and diarrhea.

• Avocado contains persin, but the exact mechanism of toxic action is not known.

DIAGNOSIS

DIFFERENTIAL DIAGNOSIS
• Toxic plants that can cause sudden death, such as poison hemlock, water hemlock, tree tobacco, lupine
• Monensin and other ionophore antibiotics
• Cyanide poisoning
• Organophosphorus or carbamate intoxication
• Acute intestinal disease
• Myocarditis
• Endocarditis

INITIAL DATABASE
• Serum chemistry changes are often limited.
• In horses with oleander poisoning, azotemia may be present.
• Myocardial damage may lead to hyperkalemia and elevated lactate dehydrogenase, creatinine kinase, aspartate aminotransferase, and cardiac troponin I.

ADVANCED OR CONFIRMATORY TESTING
• Visual and microscopic examination of stomach or intestinal contents for plant fragments often aids in the diagnosis.
• Postmortem lesions, such as reddening of the mucosa of the GI tract and congestion of organs, are generally nonspecific.
  ○ Horses with oleander poisoning may have fluid in the pericardium and body cavities, endocardial hemorrhages, and multifocal myocardial degeneration and necrosis.
  ○ *Taxus* poisoning may result in mild to moderate endocardial hemorrhages.

○ Avocado-poisoned horses may have fluid accumulation in the pericardial sac and in the thoracic and abdominal cavities, edema of the gallbladder and perirenal tissues, and a flabby, pale heart.

- Confirmatory testing is often needed to reach an accurate diagnosis of cardiotoxic plant intoxication.
  ○ Oleander: Detection of oleandrin and other cardiac glycosides in serum, urine, stomach, cecal or colon contents, liver, and myocardium; detection of oleandrin in hay or other source material
  ○ Summer pheasant's eye: Detection of the aglycone strophanthidin in source material or stomach, cecal, or colon contents
  ○ Grayanotoxins: Grayanotoxin detection in source material or stomach, cecal, or colon contents
  ○ Yew: Taxine alkaloid detection in source material or stomach, cecal, or colon contents
  ○ Avocado: Confirmatory testing not available

TREATMENT

THERAPEUTIC GOAL(S)

- There is no specific antidote for plant cardiotoxins. The recommended treatment of exposed animals is symptomatic and supportive and should include administration of IV fluids and antiarrhythmics.
- Adsorption of toxins with activated charcoal is recommended; multidose activated charcoal is beneficial in oleander intoxications.
- Atropine may be given in cases of severe bradycardia.

ACUTE GENERAL TREATMENT

- Oleander: Activated charcoal is the adsorbent of choice in horses with oleander toxicosis.
- Cardiac effects are best treated after careful cardiac evaluation. Atropine and propranolol have been used successfully.

- Digoxin-specific Fab antibody fragments have been effective in cross-reacting with cardiac glycosides in oleander, but Fab antibodies have not been studied in horses and dosages are empirical.
- Avocado: If edema is present in avocado poisoning, administration of diuretics is recommended.

POSSIBLE COMPLICATIONS

- In many cases, the rapid onset of acute intoxication does not allow timely therapeutic intervention, so mortality rates are high.
- Potassium should not be administered in fluids if hyperkalemia is present.

RECOMMENDED MONITORING

Close monitoring of serum electrolytes and electrocardiogram

PROGNOSIS AND OUTCOME

- Horses are often found dead after exposure to cardiotoxic plants.
- Progression of animals with cardiotoxic plant poisoning is rapid, and treatment is often too late.
- In horses with oleander and yew intoxications, the prognosis is poor.
- If treatment is initiated promptly after the onset of clinical signs, the prognosis is fair.
- Animals that survive the acute poisoning may have myocardial damage and may be more prone to stress.

PEARLS & CONSIDERATIONS

COMMENTS

- Cardiotoxic plants can be deadly if they are grazed upon or unintentionally incorporated into hay or baleage. The ability to recognize the presence of poisonous plants in hay or forage

may help prevent additional animal poisonings.
- Oleander is cultivated widely in the southern United States and is most commonly associated with plant poisonings in horses.
- The treatment of most cardiotoxic plants intoxications is nonspecific. Awareness of poisonous plants growing in a certain geographic region and their associated clinical signs are instrumental in making a diagnosis and initiating treatment.
- Proper and rapid diagnostic workup of suspect cardiotoxic plant poisonings is necessary to prevent additional exposures.

PREVENTION

- Recognize cardiotoxic plants of concern in the geographic location and prevent access by horses.
- Provide adequate forage to limit ingestion of toxic plants.

CLIENT EDUCATION

- If poisonous weed contamination is suspected, hay should be tested before feeding.
- Oleander poisoning in horses is common and often lethal. Oleander plants should be removed from the environment of horses.

SUGGESTED READING

Galey FG: Cardiac glycosides. In Plumlee KH, editor: *Clinical veterinary toxicology.* St Louis, 2004, Mosby Elsevier, pp 386–388.

Oelrichs PB, Ng JC, Seawright AA, et al: Isolation and identification of a compound from avocado (*Persea americana*) leaves which causes necrosis of the acinar epithelium of the lactating mammary gland and the myocardium. *Nat Toxins* 3:344–349, 1995.

Puschner B: Grayanotoxins. In Plumlee KH, editor: *Clinical veterinary toxicology,* St Louis, 2004, Mosby Elsevier, pp 412–415.

Woods LW, Filigenzi MS, Booth MC, et al: Summer pheasant's eye (*Adonis aestivalis*) poisoning in three horses. *Vet Pathol* 41:215–220, 2004.

AUTHOR: **BIRGIT PUSCHNER**

EDITOR: **CYNTHIA L. GASKILL**

Cataracts

BASIC INFORMATION

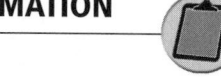

DEFINITION

Cataracts are opacities of the eye's crystalline lens or lens capsule.

EPIDEMIOLOGY

GENETICS AND BREED PREDISPOSITION Horses prone to developing recurrent uveitis are at risk for developing cataracts.

RISK FACTORS

- Any type of ocular trauma
- Chronic or recurrent uveitis

ASSOCIATED CONDITIONS AND DISORDERS

- Chronic or recurrent uveitis
- Ocular trauma

CLINICAL PRESENTATION

DISEASE FORMS/SUBTYPES Diseases of the equine lens may be congenital

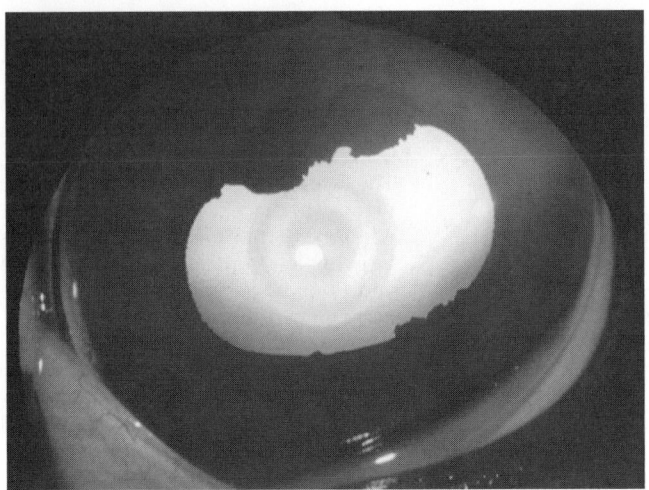

FIGURE 1 Equine congenital nuclear cataract.

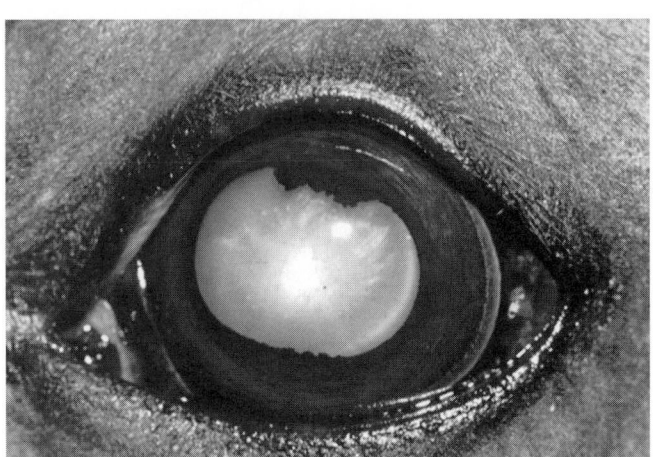

FIGURE 2 Diffuse mature cataract in an adult horse.

or acquired and generally involve malformation, malposition, or lens opacity (cataract). The most common and significant lens disorder is cataract formation.

HISTORY, CHIEF COMPLAINT Cataracts are the most common congenital ocular anomaly in horses, and development of cataracts in adult horses is a common cause of vision loss, with or without associated uveitis.

PHYSICAL EXAM FINDINGS

- Cataracts are classified according to age at onset (congenital, juvenile, senile), cause (e.g., hereditary; secondary to uveitis, trauma, metabolic disease), or location within the lens (anterior polar, anterior subcapsular, anterior cortical, equatorial, peripheral cortical, nuclear, posterior cortical, posterior subcapsular, and posterior polar).
- Congenital cataracts may be unilateral or bilateral, and they may be focal or diffuse (Figures 1 and 2). Focal opacities involving the anterior or posterior suture lines are often nonprogressive, but progression does occur in some cases. A nuclear cataract may appear as a ringlike opacity, a hollow sphere, or a solid opacity in the center (nucleus) of the affected lens. These cataracts rarely progress and often decrease in size relative to total lens size as new layers of normal cortical fiber are produced throughout life. The location, density, and size of a focal cataract determine its effect on vision.

ETIOLOGY AND PATHOPHYSIOLOGY Aqueous humor, which acts to supply metabolic needs of intraocular structures, is produced constantly by the ciliary body of the equine eye. In uveitis, the aqueous humor is altered, which affects the lens metabolism. Abnormal lens metabolism results in cataract formation.

DIAGNOSIS

DIFFERENTIAL DIAGNOSIS

- Chronic uveitis
- Lens rupture caused by penetrating ocular trauma
- Nuclear sclerosis
- Lens luxation

INITIAL DATABASE

A thorough and complete ophthalmic examination with mydriasis should be done to help differentiate the cause of the cataracts and to rule out other causes of ocular opacity such as keratitis.

ADVANCED OR CONFIRMATORY TESTING

If cataract surgery is being considered, an ocular ultrasound and electroretinogram should be considered to determine if the remainder of the eye is healthy.

TREATMENT

THERAPEUTIC GOAL(S)

- Prevent progression of cataracts
- Improve visual function

ACUTE GENERAL TREATMENT

- Control ocular inflammation with use of topical and systemic antiinflammatory medications.
- Cataract dissolving medications have not been demonstrated to be effective in any animal, including horses.

CHRONIC TREATMENT

Equine cataract surgery: Phacoemulsification and aspiration of cataracts in horses through a small corneal incision with intraocular lens implantation are becoming routine procedures.

POSSIBLE COMPLICATIONS

Vision loss is common because the disease is progressive. Both eyes are at risk and should be monitored.

RECOMMENDED MONITORING

Examine monthly to determine lens progression.

PROGNOSIS AND OUTCOME

- Prognosis is guarded for saving vision.
- Cataract surgery has a success rate of more than 80%.

PEARLS & CONSIDERATIONS

COMMENTS

- Both eyes are at risk and should be monitored.
- Photographing the eye with the pupil dilated will help monitor cataract progression.

PREVENTION

- Minimizing ocular and corneal trauma may help prevent the development of ocular inflammation.
- Use of a quality fly mask is recommended.
- Feeding hay on the ground is recommended to minimize ocular trauma.

SUGGESTED READING

Matthews AG: Lens opacities in the horse: a clinical classification. *Vet Ophthalmol* 3: 65–71, 2000.

Whitely RD: Diseases and surgery of the lens. In Gilger BC, editor: *Equine ophthalmology.* St Louis, 2005, Elsevier, pp 269–284.

AUTHOR & EDITOR: **BRIAN C. GILGER**

Cecal Impaction

BASIC INFORMATION

DEFINITION

Distension of the cecum with feed material or fluid (or both) associated with mechanical or functional obstruction to flow of ingesta

EPIDEMIOLOGY

SPECIES, AGE, SEX It appears that older horses (>15 years in one study) are predisposed to cecal impaction. Cecal impaction in hospitalized patients may not have the same age predisposition.

GENETICS AND BREED PREDISPOSITION One report indicated predisposition in Arabians, Appaloosas, and Morgans. Other studies have not reported any breed predisposition.

RISK FACTORS Proposed risk factors have included:

- Dietary factors: Poor-quality or coarse roughage, Bermuda grass hay
- Poor dentition
- Decreased water consumption
- Parasitism: Parasite-induced thromboembolism, tapeworm (*Anoplocephala perfoliata*) infestation
- Change in exercise: Lack of exercise with use of nonsteroidal antiinflammatory drugs (NSAIDs)
- Hospitalization with or without surgery and anesthesia, frequently for nongastrointestinal (GI) disease (especially musculoskeletal problems)

GEOGRAPHY AND SEASONALITY There has been some suggestion that horses in regions with Bermuda grass hay are predisposed. No seasonality has been established.

CLINICAL PRESENTATION

DISEASE FORMS/SUBTYPES Cecal impactions are frequently divided into two types: impaction with firm ingesta causing a mechanical obstruction and distension with fluid ingesta without any apparent mechanical obstruction. Motility dysfunction has been proposed in horses with distension with fluid ingesta.

HISTORY, CHIEF COMPLAINT

- Horses with cecal impactions often show signs of mild colic (lying down, flank watching) for several days to weeks. Horses with fluid cecal impaction or dysfunction may have acute and increased signs of pain.
- Decreased appetite is one of the first clinical signs in many horses with cecal impactions. Horses frequently have decreased fecal output or changes in fecal consistency (soft or firm small fecal balls). Historical findings may indicate any of the risk factors identified in the epidemiology section.
- It is important to note that cecal perforation may occur in horses with cecal impaction with little to no signs of colic (see "Cecal Perforation" in this section).

PHYSICAL EXAM FINDINGS

- Physical examination in horses with cecal impaction often reveals vital signs within normal limits with the exception of tachycardia during episodes of colic. Horses with fluid cecal impaction or dysfunction may have more pronounced tachycardia.
- Affected horses frequently have decreased borborygmi. Horses with fluid cecal impaction or dysfunction may show signs of endotoxemia.
- If perforation occurs, clinical signs will worsen rapidly (see "Cecal Perforation" in this section).

ETIOLOGY AND PATHOPHYSIOLOGY

- Impaction with dry, firm feed material may have a similar pathogenesis to large colon impactions (see "Large Colon Impaction" in this section). Risk factors described above may affect motility, particle size of feed material, and water content of ingesta, resulting in accumulation of dry, firm feed material in the cecum.
- Motility dysfunction has been proposed in horses with distension with fluid ingesta. Anesthesia, NSAID administration, diet changes, and parasites (especially tapeworms) have been proposed to alter GI motility. Administration of NSAIDs may mask the mild clinical signs associated with cecal impactions and contribute to ulceration and predispose to cecal perforation.

DIAGNOSIS

DIFFERENTIAL DIAGNOSIS

- Other causes of mild abdominal pain are simple or nonstrangulating obstructions of the GI tract such as feed or sand impaction of the large colon, enterolithiasis, large colon displacements, large intestinal intraluminal obstructions, tympany, small colon impactions, and ileal impactions.
- Other causes of a firm, digesta-filled viscus in the right dorsal abdomen include feed or sand impaction of the large colon, right dorsal colon impaction with a right dorsal displacement, nonstrangulating infarction of the cecum, and cecocecal or cecocolic intussusception.

INITIAL DATABASE

- Examination per rectum is the most useful diagnostic test for cecal impactions. Early in the course of the disease or if impaction is restricted to the cupula, the most significant finding on examination per rectum will be a tight, sometimes thickened ventral band of the cecum (coursing from the right caudodorsal abdomen cranioventrally). As impaction of the body and base of the cecum progresses, the round cecal base is palpable in the right caudodorsal abdomen. Differentiation of the cecum from the colon can be difficult. If the distended structure is the cecum, the examiner should not be able to pass his or her hand over the impaction dorsally because the cecum is attached to the dorsal body wall. As the disease progresses, the colon empties, and the cecum becomes heavier. This may result in inability to diagnose the cecal impaction during examination per rectum. Careful evaluation of the thickness of the cecal wall and the texture of the contents may help differentiate between the two types of impaction (firm ingesta causing mechanical obstruction versus fluid ingesta associated with dysfunction).
- Nasogastric reflux is uncommon.
- Bloodwork is generally normal or consistent with mild to moderate dehydration (prerenal azotemia, elevated packed cell volume, elevated total protein).
- Abdominal fluid analysis is generally within normal limits. Horses with fluid cecal impaction or dysfunction may have elevation in total protein. It is important to remember that intestinal compromise may occur with little to no change in peritoneal fluid with cecal disease.

TREATMENT

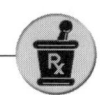

THERAPEUTIC GOAL(S)

Passage or removal of impacted ingesta

ACUTE GENERAL TREATMENT

- Treatment of cecal impactions remains controversial. The controversy is associated with the risk of rupture without warning of worsening clinical signs and the difficulty in appropriately identifying which type of impaction is present to better judge the likelihood of resolution with medical treatment and the risk of recurrence. Horses with fluid cecal impaction or dysfunction are believed to be less likely to respond to medical management and are at risk for continued dysfunction after resolution, resulting in some surgeons electing to perform bypass procedures during surgery.

- Medical management of cecal impactions is similar to medical treatment of large colon impactions. Horses should be held off feed. IV and oral fluid administration is combined with laxatives or cathartics such as mineral oil; $MgSO_4$, dioctyl sodium sulfosuccinate, and psyllium have been recommended. Judicious administration of analgesics (flunixin meglumine most commonly) may be helpful. Careful monitoring with repeated physical and rectal examinations is important to ensure that analgesics are not masking progression of the disease and the need for surgery. The administration of prokinetics has been suggested by some clinicians, but the safety and efficacy are unknown.
- Surgical treatment is recommended in cases with marked signs of colic at presentation, very firm ingesta or fluid ingesta, signs of systemic compromise, increasing signs of colic during treatment, or lack of improvement or progression of impaction during medical treatment. Typhlotomy with evacuation of the contents is the mainstay of surgical treatment. A surgeon may elect to perform a bypass procedure (complete or incomplete jejunocolic or ileocolic anastomosis) in cases of recurrent cecal impaction or fluid cecal impaction or dysfunction.
- Refeeding after resolution of cecal impaction should be done slowly and monitored closely with repeat examination per rectum to identify any recurrence of impaction.

POSSIBLE COMPLICATIONS

The two most important complications associated with cecal impaction are cecal perforation (see "Cecal Perforation" in this section) and recurrence of impac-

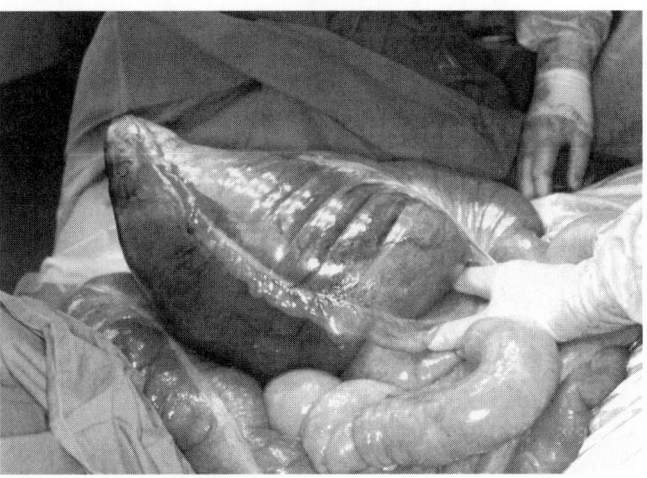

FIGURE 1 Cecal impaction as identified at exploratory laparotomy; distension by fluid and gas secondary to cecal dysfunction.

tion. Cecal perforation has been reported in 25% to 57% of cases with cecal impaction. Reported recurrence rates range from 13% to 29%.

PROGNOSIS AND OUTCOME

Reported success rates for cecal impactions are quite variable. Most recent reports indicate that both medical and surgical treatment may result in successful outcomes with up to 90% survival. However, when discussing prognosis with owners, it is important to address the significant risks of perforation and recurrence.

PEARLS & CONSIDERATIONS

COMMENTS

- Cecal impaction should be considered as a differential diagnosis in horses with mild signs of colic, decreased appetite, and changes in fecal production.
- Horses hospitalized for non-GI diseases may be predisposed to cecal impaction.

- Early identification and close monitoring are required for successful treatment of cecal impaction.

PREVENTION

Hospitalized horses should be monitored closely for any change in attitude, appetite, or fecal production. Handwalking may stimulate GI motility in horses on stall rest.

SUGGESTED READING

Dabareiner RM: Impaction of the ascending colon and cecum. In White NA, Moore JN, editors: *Current techniques in equine surgery and lameness.* Philadelphia, 1998, WB Saunders, pp 270–273.

Plummer AE, Rakestraw PC, Hardy J, et al: Outcome of medical and surgical treatment of cecal impaction in horses: 114 cases (1994–2004). *J Am Vet Med Assoc* 231:1378–1385, 2007.

Rakestraw PC, Hardy J: Large intestine. In Auer JA, Stick JA, editors: *Equine surgery.* St Louis, 2006, Saunders Elsevier, pp 436–478.

Ross MW: Diseases of the cecum. In Colahan PT, Merritt AM, Moore JN, et al, editors: *Equine medicine and surgery.* St Louis, 1999, Mosby, pp 735–740.

AUTHOR: KIRA L. EPSTEIN

EDITORS: TIM MAIR and CERI SHERLOCK

Cecal Intussusception

BASIC INFORMATION

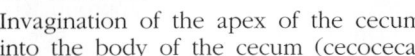

DEFINITION

Invagination of the apex of the cecum into the body of the cecum (cecocecal

intussusception) or through the cecocolic orifice into the right ventral colon (cecocolic intussusception)

EPIDEMIOLOGY

SPECIES, AGE, SEX Increased incidence has been reported in young (<3 years old) horses, although it can occur in all ages.

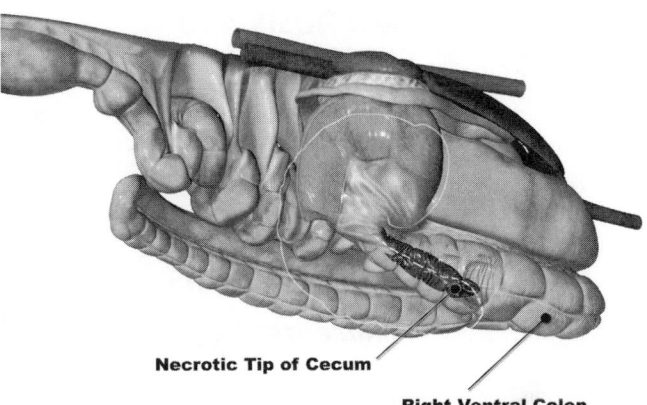

FIGURE 1 Diagram demonstrating cecocolic intussusception. (Courtesy The Glass Horse Equine Colic CD.)

Necrotic Tip of Cecum

Right Ventral Colon

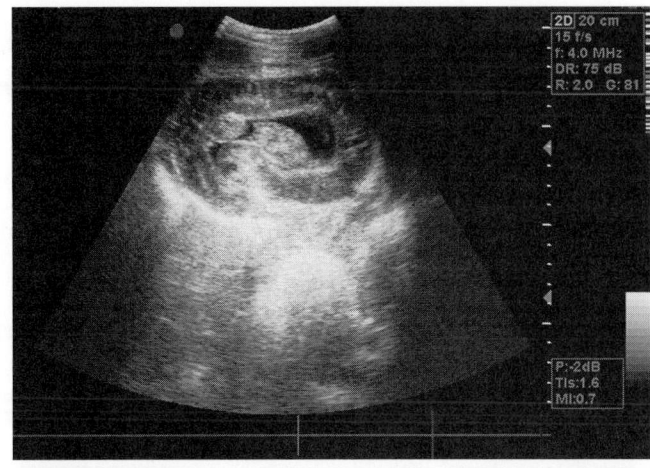

FIGURE 2 Transcutaneous ultrasonogram (4 MHz) of the right ventral abdomen showing the typical bull's eye appearance of a cecal intussusception.

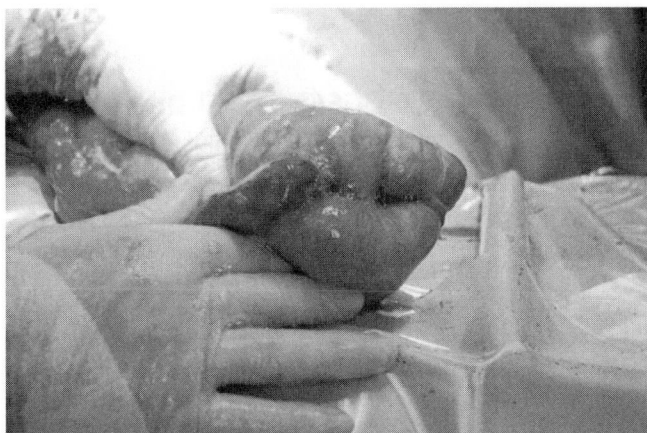

FIGURE 3 Cecocecal intussusception at exploratory laparotomy.

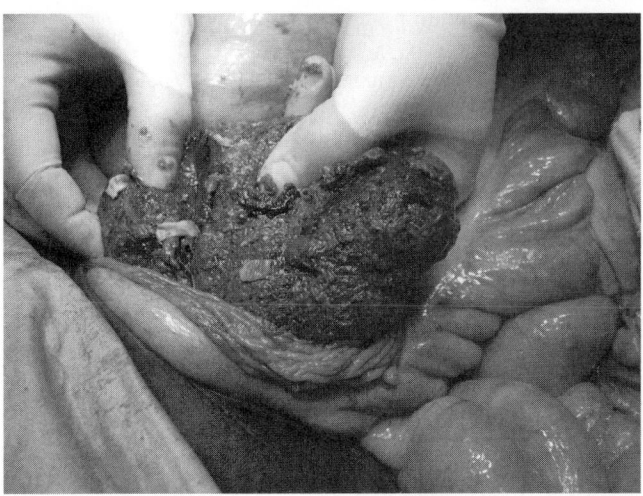

FIGURE 4 Cecocolic intussusception at exploratory laparotomy. The mucosal surface of the necrotic tip of the intussuscepted cecal apex is visible through a colotomy of the right ventral colon. Several tapeworms are present on the mucosa.

GENETICS AND BREED PREDISPOSITION Increased incidence has been reported in Standardbreds.

RISK FACTORS A number of risk factors have been proposed. Proposed infectious risk factors include abscessation of the cecal wall and infection with *Salmonella* spp., *Emeria leuckarti*, *Strongylus vulgaris*, cyathostomins, or *Anoplocephala perfoliata*. Other possible risk factors include dietary changes and use of organophosphates or parasympathomimetic drugs.

CLINICAL PRESENTATION

DISEASE FORMS/SUBTYPES

- Cecal intussusceptions can be separated into cecocecal and cecocolic intussusception.
- There appear to be three forms of cecal intussusception: acute (requiring immediate surgical intervention), subacute (clinical signs persisting 3–8

days), and chronic (clinical signs persisting 6–120 days). Acute is the most common form followed by subacute and then chronic. Whereas cecocolic intussusception is more likely to result in ischemia of the apex of the cecum and an acute presentation, cecocecal intussusception is more likely to result in partial obstruction without ischemia and result in a more chronic presentation.

HISTORY, CHIEF COMPLAINT Clinical signs are variable depending on the degree of obstruction and intestinal compromise. Horses with the acute form have rapid onset of moderate to severe abdominal pain. Horses with the subacute form have intermittent mild to moderate signs of colic and soft feces or diarrhea. Horses with the chronic form have a history of intermittent mild abdominal pain, scant feces, and weight loss.

PHYSICAL EXAM FINDINGS Physical examination findings also depend on the degree of obstruction and intestinal viability. As ischemia and obstruction worsens, signs of progressive tachycardia and cardiovascular compromise (eg, prolonged capillary refill time, decreased jugular refill, cold extremities) occur. Fever is common in horses with the chronic form of cecal intussusception.

ETIOLOGY AND PATHOPHYSIOLOGY The most likely cause of cecal intussusception is abnormal motility associated with the proposed risk factors discussed in the etiology section.

DIAGNOSIS

DIFFERENTIAL DIAGNOSIS

- Other causes of abdominal pain include feed or sand impaction of the large colon, enterolithiasis, large colon displacements, large intestinal intraluminal obstructions, tympany, small colon impactions, and ileal impactions.

- Other causes of a firm viscus in the right dorsal abdomen include feed or sand impaction of the large colon, right dorsal colon impaction with a right dorsal displacement, nonstrangulating infarction of the cecum, and cecal impaction.
- Other causes of change in fecal production and character include infectious and sand colitis and cecal impactions.
- Other causes of abdominal pain associated with fever include infectious and sand colitis and small colon impactions.

INITIAL DATABASE

- Examination per rectum may be within normal limits or reveal an abnormality in palpation of the cecum. The abnormal findings vary and include a firm, edematous viscus in the right dorsal abdomen, malpositioning of the cecum, and inability to palpate the cecum.
- Nasogastric reflux is uncommon because the small intestine is generally not obstructed.
- Bloodwork varies with the degree of intestinal compromise. Progressive dehydration (prerenal azotemia, elevated packed cell volume, elevated total protein) and metabolic acidosis may occur with worsening ischemia.

- Because the damaged intestine is sequestered from the abdomen, abdominocentesis is insensitive for cecal intussusception and may be normal even with ischemic bowel. Elevations in nucleated cell count, total protein, and color (serosanguinous) may occur over time with increased severity.
- Abdominal ultrasonography of the cecum and right dorsal colon may reveal a bull's-eye pattern of bowel within bowel typical of an intussusception.

TREATMENT

THERAPEUTIC GOAL(S)

- Reduction of the intussusception with resection of ischemic bowel as necessary
- Supportive care

ACUTE GENERAL TREATMENT

Exploratory celiotomy is required to treat cecal intussusception. Cecocecal intussusceptions are easier to reduce than cecocolic intussusceptions. Reduction of cecocolic intussusceptions may require an enterotomy into the right dorsal colon with or without resection of damaged cecum within the colon before reduction.

CHRONIC TREATMENT

If *A. perfoliata* or *A. cyathostomin* larvae are identified at the time of surgery, appropriate deworming is recommended.

PROGNOSIS AND OUTCOME

The prognosis appears good if resection of the damaged portion of the cecum is possible.

PEARLS & CONSIDERATIONS

COMMENTS

- Cecal intussusception is an uncommon cause of abdominal pain in horses.
- Acute, subacute, and chronic forms of the disease occur. Clinical signs and diagnostic findings are variable depending on the form of the disease and the severity of obstruction and intestinal compromise.
- Prognosis is good with surgical treatment.

SUGGESTED READING

Martin BB, Jr, Freeman DE, Ross MW, et al: Cecocecal and cecocolic intussusception in horses: 30 cases (1976–1996). *J Am Vet Med Assoc* 214:80–84, 1999.

Rakestraw PC, Hardy J: Large intestine. In Auer JA, Stick JA, editors: *Equine surgery*. St Louis, 2006, Saunders Elsevier, pp 436–478.

Ross MW: Diseases of the cecum. In Colahan PT, Merritt AM, Moore JN, et al, editors: *Equine medicine and surgery*. St Louis, 1999, Mosby, pp 735–740.

AUTHOR: **KIRA L. EPSTEIN**

EDITORS: **TIM MAIR** and **CERI SHERLOCK**

Cecal Perforation

BASIC INFORMATION

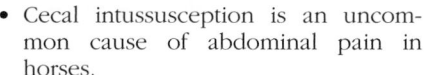

DEFINITION

Loss of integrity of the cecal wall associated with leakage of intestinal contents into the abdomen

SYNONYM(S)

Cecal rupture

EPIDEMIOLOGY

SPECIES, AGE, SEX

- In one form of cecal perforation, the disease occurs solely in broodmares at the time of parturition.
- In other forms of cecal perforation, there is no known age or sex predisposition.

RISK FACTORS In broodmares with cecal perforation at the time of parturi-

tion, dystocia appears to be a risk factor. In other forms of cecal perforation, risk factors including hospitalization, nonsteroidal antiinflammatory drug (NSAID) administration, and anesthesia have been identified.

ASSOCIATED CONDITIONS AND DISORDERS Cecal perforation has been reported in association with infestation with *Anoplocephala perfoliata*.

CLINICAL PRESENTATION

DISEASE FORMS/SUBTYPES Cecal perforation occurs in several forms:

- Cecal perforation has been identified in broodmares at the time of parturition with no evidence of cecal outflow obstruction or dysfunction.
- Cecal perforation occurs in 25% to 57% of horses with cecal impaction.

- Cecal perforation has been reported in horses hospitalized for non-gastrointestinal (GI) disease without evidence of cecal impaction with feed. However, it is important to note that horses with fluid cecal impactions or dysfunction may not show signs of colic before perforation and would not have evidence of impaction with feed at the time of necropsy.
- Cecal perforation has been reported with infestation with *A. perfoliata*.

HISTORY, CHIEF COMPLAINT Broodmares with cecal perforation may show signs of abdominal pain shortly after parturition. In general, horses with cecal perforation show signs referable to endotoxemia. Owners may note pain, muscle fasciculations, and sweating. Sudden collapse and death are also possible.

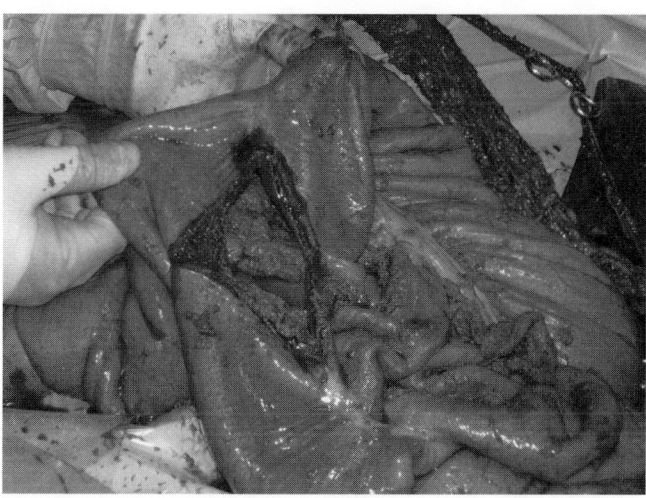

FIGURE 1 Cecal perforation identified at exploratory laparotomy.

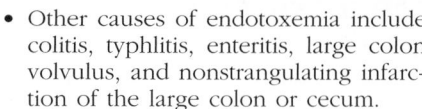

PHYSICAL EXAM FINDINGS Horses with cecal perforation are in endotoxemic shock. Typical findings on physical examination include tachycardia, tachypnea, toxic mucous membranes, prolonged capillary refill time, cold extremities, and poor pulse quality.

ETIOLOGY AND PATHOPHYSIOLOGY
- The proposed pathophysiology for broodmares with periparturient cecal perforation is cecal distension caused by altered motility that ruptures because of increased abdominal pressure during parturition.
- The pathophysiology of cecal perforation in hospitalized horses administered NSAIDs may be related to ulceration or masking clinical signs of fluid cecal impaction or dysfunction.
- The pathophysiology of cecal perforation associated with *A. perfoliata* is unknown.
- The pathophysiology of cecal perforation secondary to cecal impaction is discussed in "Cecal Impaction" in this section.

DIAGNOSIS

DIFFERENTIAL DIAGNOSIS
- Other causes of endotoxemia include colitis, typhlitis, enteritis, large colon volvulus, and nonstrangulating infarction of the large colon or cecum.
- Other causes of septic peritonitis include gastric rupture and idiopathic peritonitis.

INITIAL DATABASE
- Examination per rectum is consistent with pneumoperitoneum. In cases of pneumoperitoneum, the rectum will tightly surround the arm during palpation, and as the person performing palpation moves his or her arm, there is a floating sensation. Additional findings on examination per rectum may include roughening of the surface of the intestines caused by ingesta and fibrin formation and crepitus over the cecum associated with perforation.
- Nasogastric reflux may occur because of ileus secondary to endotoxemia and peritonitis.
- Bloodwork is consistent with endotoxemic shock, including hemoconcentration, leukopenia caused by a neutropenia with a left shift, azotemia, and hyperlactatemia.
- Abdominal fluid reveals a mixed population of intracellular bacteria and plant material. Intracellular bacteria ensure that the fluid is not the result of enterocentesis. Ultrasound guidance during collection of abdominal fluid may help prevent enterocentesis.
- Abdominal ultrasonography reveals increased abdominal fluid. The fluid has a mixed echogenicity and may have hyperechoic, shadowing gas bubbles.

TREATMENT

THERAPEUTIC GOAL(S)
Relieve suffering

ACUTE GENERAL TREATMENT
There is no viable treatment for gross fecal contamination of the abdomen secondary to cecal perforation. Horses should be humanely euthanized.

PROGNOSIS AND OUTCOME

For humane reasons, horses should be euthanized.

PEARLS & CONSIDERATIONS

COMMENTS
- Cecal perforation should be considered as a differential diagnosis in horses with signs of severe endotoxemic shock and septic peritonitis.
- Broodmares at the time of parturition and hospitalized horses may be at increased risk.

PREVENTION
- Hospitalized horses should be monitored closely for any change in attitude, appetite, and fecal production. Handwalking may stimulate GI motility in horses on stall rest.

SUGGESTED READING
Rakestraw PC, Hardy J: Large intestine. In Auer JA, Stick JA, editors: *Equine surgery*. St Louis, 2006, Saunders Elsevier, pp 436–478.

Ross MW: Diseases of the cecum. In Colahan PT, Merritt AM, Moore JN, et al, editors: *Equine medicine and surgery*. St Louis, 1999, Mosby, pp 735–740.

AUTHOR: **KIRA L. EPSTEIN**

EDITORS: **TIM MAIR** and **CERI SHERLOCK**

Cecal Tympany

BASIC INFORMATION

DEFINITION
Accumulation of gas in the cecum

SYNONYM(S)
Cecal dilation

CLINICAL PRESENTATION
DISEASE FORMS/SUBTYPES Cecal tympany can be separated into primary and secondary subtypes. Cecal tympany occurs most commonly secondary to obstructions of the large colon such as feed or sand impactions, large colon displacements, large colon tympany, and large colon intraluminal obstructions. The history, clinical signs, diagnostic findings, treatment, and prognosis for cecal tympany secondary to nonstrangulating obstructions of the large colon are related to the primary disease (see entries on respective conditions). This entry focuses on the less common primary cecal tympany.

HISTORY, CHIEF COMPLAINT Abdominal pain and distension (primarily right sided)

PHYSICAL EXAM FINDINGS
- Cardiovascular parameters are generally stable. Elevations of heart rate may be associated with pain, abdominal distension, decreased or absent borborygmi, and signs of mild dehydration.
- Uncommonly, severe distension may result in compromise to the cardiovascular and respiratory systems.

ETIOLOGY AND PATHOPHYSIOLOGY
Overproduction of gas because of diet changes, changes in bacterial flora, or alterations in motility resulting in decreased passage of gas through the cecum may result in increased gas accumulation in the cecum.

DIAGNOSIS

DIFFERENTIAL DIAGNOSIS
- Other causes of mild to moderate abdominal pain are simple or nonstrangulating obstructions of the gastrointestinal tract such as feed or sand impaction of the large colon, enterolithiasis, large colon displacements, large intestinal intraluminal obstructions, cecal impaction, small colon impactions, and ileal impactions.
- Other causes of cecal distension on examination per rectum include typhlitis; nonstrangulating infarction of the cecum; and nonstrangulating obstructions of the large colon, such as feed or sand impaction, enterolithiasis, large colon tympany, other large colon displacements, large colon volvulus, and other intraluminal obstructions resulting in secondary distension of the cecum.

INITIAL DATABASE
- Examination per rectum reveals a variable degree, possibly severe, of gas distension of the cecum.
- Nasogastric reflux is uncommon.
- Bloodwork may be normal or consistent with mild dehydration (prerenal azotemia, elevated packed cell volume, elevated total protein).
- Abdominal fluid analysis is within normal limits.

TREATMENT

THERAPEUTIC GOAL(S)
- Pain management
- Supportive care

ACUTE GENERAL TREATMENT
- Withhold feed.
- Most horses with cecal tympany have a good response to analgesics (flunixin meglumine, α_2 agonists, butorphanol). Analgesics minimize sympathetic inhibition of motility.
- Some horses may benefit from IV fluids to support cardiovascular status and treat any dehydration.
- Trocarization of the cecum (right flank) can relieve pain from cecal tympany. Because of the potential for complications (peritonitis, abscess formation), clinicians should choose the patient carefully. Before performing trocarization, the clinician should take into account the cardiovascular status of the horse and the potential for referral and surgery.

RECOMMENDED MONITORING
- During treatment, horses should be monitored for signs of unrelenting pain, nasogastric reflux, progressive abdominal distension, and systemic deterioration (increasing heart rate, cardiovascular compromise).
- Progression of signs may indicate an inability to resolve the gas distension medically or that the cecal tympany is secondary to a primary large intestinal disease. Surgical exploration may be required.

PROGNOSIS AND OUTCOME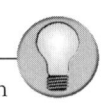

Prognosis is excellent.

PEARLS & CONSIDERATIONS

- Primary cecal tympany is an uncommon cause of colic.
- Cecal tympany occurs more frequently secondary to disease of the large colon.

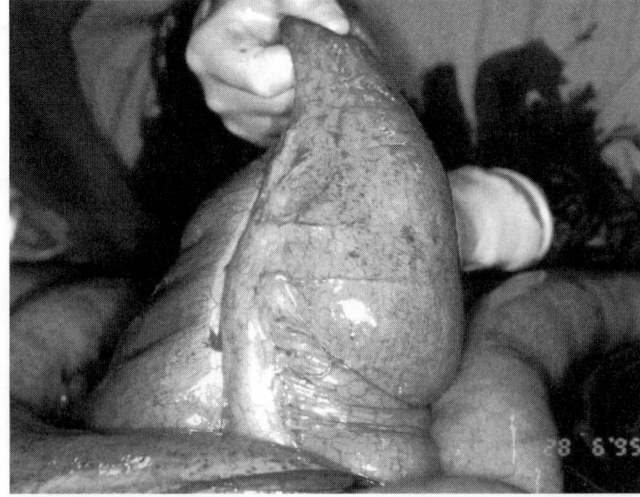

FIGURE 1 Cecal tympany (secondary to colon displacement) identified at exploratory laparotomy.

SUGGESTED READING

Ross MW: Diseases of the cecum. In Colahan PT, Merritt AM, Moore JN, et al, editors: *Equine medicine and surgery.* St Louis, 1999, Mosby, pp 735–740.

AUTHOR: **KIRA L. EPSTEIN**

EDITORS: **TIM MAIR** and **CERI SHERLOCK**

Cecal Volvulus

BASIC INFORMATION

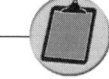

DEFINITION

Rotation of the cecum around the mesenteric axis (which is also the long axis of the cecum)

SYNONYM(S)

Cecal torsion

EPIDEMIOLOGY

ASSOCIATED CONDITIONS AND DISORDERS Cecal volvulus has been associated with congenital abnormalities of the cecocolic fold and dorsal body wall attachments of the cecum.

CLINICAL PRESENTATION

DISEASE FORMS/SUBTYPES Cecal volvulus can be separated into primary and secondary subtypes. Cecal volvulus occurs most commonly secondary to large colon volvulus. The history, clinical signs, diagnostic findings, treatment, and prognosis for cecal volvulus secondary to large colon volvulus are consistent with a large colon volvulus (see "Large Colon Volvulus"). This entry focuses on the less common primary cecal volvulus.

HISTORY, CHIEF COMPLAINT Horses with cecal volvulus present with acute, severe signs of colic.

PHYSICAL EXAM FINDINGS Physical examination findings depend on the duration and degree of cecal compromise and distension. Early in the disease, physical examination may reveal tachycardia and decreased or absent borborygmi. As ischemia and distension progress, cardiovascular compromise and endotoxemia will occur. Signs of endotoxemia or hypovolemia on physical examination may include hyperemic or toxic mucous membranes, prolonged or increased capillary refill time, poor pulse quality, cold extremities, and decreased jugular refill.

ETIOLOGY AND PATHOPHYSIOLOGY

- As noted above, cecal volvulus may be associated with abnormalities of the cecocolic ligament or dorsal body wall attachments of the cecum. These abnormalities allow an increased range of motion of the cecum, resulting in a greater potential for rotation.
- In cases in which no congenital abnormality is identified, the etiology of cecal volvulus is unknown. As with large colon volvulus, it is possible that changes in motility or distension are the cause of the volvulus.

DIAGNOSIS

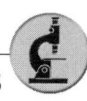

DIFFERENTIAL DIAGNOSIS

- Other causes of severe colic include large colon volvulus; severe colitis; and strangulating lesions of the small intestine such as small intestinal volvulus, epiploic foramen entrapment, and strangulating lipoma.
- Other causes of cecal distension on examination per rectum include cecal tympany, typhlitis; nonstrangulating infarction of the cecum; and nonstrangulating obstructions of the large colon resulting in secondary distension of the cecum such as feed or sand impaction, enterolithiasis, large colon tympany, other large colon displacements, large colon volvulus, and other intraluminal obstructions.
- Other causes of endotoxemia include colitis, typhlitis, enteritis, and nonstrangulating infarction of the large colon or cecum.

INITIAL DATABASE

- Findings on examination per rectum are nonspecific. A variable degree of cecal distension may be palpable.
- Nasogastric reflux is unlikely.
- Bloodwork will vary depending on the degree of cardiovascular compromise and endotoxemia. Progressive increase in packed cell volume, decrease in total protein, and leukopenia caused by neutropenia with a left shift indicate increased severity of systemic compromise. Hyperlactatemia is associated with poor perfusion and ischemia of the strangulated region.
- Increases in abdominal fluid total protein or nucleated cell count are possible.
- Thickening of the wall of the cecum may be evident on ultrasonography of the right paralumbar fossa. However, the severity of pain may make ultrasound evaluation difficult, and it is unnecessary to make the decision that surgery is required.
- Surgical exploration is often required for diagnosis.

TREATMENT

THERAPEUTIC GOAL(S)

- Correction of volvulus and resection of compromised cecum as necessary
- Supportive care

ACUTE GENERAL TREATMENT

- If cardiovascular compromise is present, rapid fluid resuscitation should be performed before anesthesia.
- At surgery, the volvulus is corrected, and the viability of the cecum is assessed. All nonviable tissue should be resected. Complete typhlectomy is possible but requires a rib resection.

POSSIBLE COMPLICATIONS

If cecal volvulus is associated with a congenital abnormality of the cecocolic ligament or the dorsal body wall attachments of the cecum, recurrence is possible.

PROGNOSIS AND OUTCOME

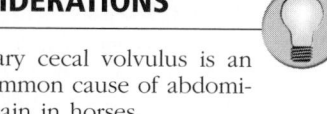

- Prognosis is likely related to the severity of compromise and the amount of cecum involved.
- One report indicated a 60% survival after partial typhlectomy.

PEARLS & CONSIDERATIONS

- Primary cecal volvulus is an uncommon cause of abdominal pain in horses.
- Affected horses show signs of acute, severe pain with progressive cardiovascular collapse and endotoxemia.

SUGGESTED READING

Dart A, Hodgson DR, Snyder JR: Caecal disease in equids. *Aust Vet J* 75:552–557, 1997.

Rakestraw PC, Hardy J: Large intestine. In Auer JA, Stick JA, editors: *Equine surgery.* St Louis, 2006, Saunders Elsevier, pp 436–478.

Ross MW: Diseases of the cecum. In Colahan PT, Merritt AM, Moore JN, et al, editors: *Equine medicine and surgery,* ed 3. St Louis, 1999, Mosby, pp 735–740.

AUTHOR: **KIRA L. EPSTEIN**

EDITORS: **TIM MAIR** and **CERI SHERLOCK**

Cecum: Nonstrangulating Infarction

BASIC INFORMATION

DEFINITION

Loss of blood supply to the cecum not associated with strangulation

EPIDEMIOLOGY

RISK FACTORS High parasite load and inappropriate deworming programs may predispose to infestation with *Strongylus vulgaris* or larval cyathostomins.

CLINICAL PRESENTATION

HISTORY, CHIEF COMPLAINT Affected horses may have mild signs of colic that progress over approximately 24 hours (most commonly reported) or acute, severe abdominal pain. Horses may also have a history of diarrhea.

PHYSICAL EXAM FINDINGS Physical examination findings vary depending on the amount of cecum affected and the severity of vascular compromise. Variable tachycardia, tachypnea, and fever are associated with pain and endotoxemia. Cardiovascular collapse and endotoxemic shock may occur with hyperemic or toxic mucous membranes, prolonged or decreased capillary refill time, poor pulse quality, cold extremities, and decreased jugular refill.

ETIOLOGY AND PATHOPHYSIOLOGY

- One proposed cause is verminous arteritis associated with *S. vulgaris* infestation (see "Large Colon: Nonstrangulating Infarction" in this section).
- Multifocal infarction secondary to infestation with larval cyathostomins has also been proposed as a cause.

DIAGNOSIS

DIFFERENTIAL DIAGNOSIS

- Other causes of colic include feed or sand impaction, enterolithiasis, large colon tympany, other large colon displacements, large intestinal intraluminal obstructions, small colon impactions, ileal impactions, strangulating small intestinal obstructions, large colon volvulus, and colitis.
- Other causes of a firm viscus in the right dorsal abdomen include feed or sand impaction of the large colon, right dorsal colon impaction with a right dorsal displacement, cecal intussusception, and cecal impaction.
- Other causes of endotoxemia include colitis and large colon volvulus.
- Other causes of peritonitis include idiopathic gastrointestinal (GI) rupture and other strangulating GI lesions such as small intestinal or large colon volvulus.
- Other causes of change in fecal production and character include infectious and sand colitis and cecal impactions.

INITIAL DATABASE

- Examination per rectum may be within normal limits or may reveal a firm viscus in the right dorsal abdomen.
- Nasogastric reflux is not expected.
- Findings on routine blood work are variable. Chronic parasitism may be associated with anemia, hypoalbuminemia (if associated with protein-losing enteropathy), or hyperglobulinemia (if associated with chronic inflammation). Endotoxemia is frequently accompanied by leukopenia, specifically neutropenia with left shift.
- Abdominal fluid is frequently consistent with peritonitis with changes in color (serosanguinous), increased total nucleated cell count, and increased total protein.
- If the ischemic region is edematous, abdominal ultrasonography may reveal a thickened, hypoechoic bowel wall.

TREATMENT

THERAPEUTIC GOAL(S)

- Remove ischemic bowel.
- Provide supportive care.

ACUTE GENERAL TREATMENT

Depending on the amount of the cecum that is affected, surgical resection may be curative. Although total typhlectomy has been described, it does not appear necessary in most cases.

CHRONIC TREATMENT

Affected horses should be placed on a good deworming program.

POSSIBLE COMPLICATIONS

If the condition is progressive, additional portions of the cecum may become necrotic after surgical resection is performed.

PROGNOSIS AND OUTCOME

- Prognosis appears good with partial typhlectomy in the limited number of cases reported in the literature.
- It is likely that prognosis would decrease when total typhlectomy is required.

PEARLS & CONSIDERATIONS

COMMENTS

- Nonstrangulating infarction of the cecum is an uncommon cause of colic in horses.
- Nonstrangulating infarction may be associated with verminous arteritis or multifocal infarction caused by larval cyathostomins.

PREVENTION

- Appropriate deworming may decrease the potential for nonstrangulating infarction of the cecum associated with *S. vulgaris* and larval cyathostomins.

SUGGESTED READING

Dart A, Hodgson D, Snyder J: Caecal disease in equids. *Aust Vet J* 75:552, 1997.

Rakestraw PC, Hardy J: Large intestine. In Auer JA, Stick JA, editors: *Equine surgery,* ed 3. St Louis, 2006, Saunders Elsevier, pp 436–478.

Ross MW: Diseases of the cecum. In Colahan PT, Merritt AM, Moore JN, Mayhew IG, editors: *Equine medicine and surgery.* St Louis, 1999, Mosby, pp 735–740.

AUTHOR: **KIRA L. EPSTEIN**

EDITORS: **TIM MAIR** and **CERI SHERLOCK**

Cerebellar Diseases

BASIC INFORMATION

DEFINITION

- The cerebellum provides regulation of range, rate, and strength of skeletal movement, as well as coordination of balance and posture. Diseases of the cerebellum often have profound effects on posture and gait but fortunately are rare in horses.
- Diseases of the equine cerebellum include cerebellar abiotrophy and degeneration; congenital brain malformation (Dandy-Walker–like syndrome); developmental diseases (eg, cerebellar hypoplasia, cerebellar dysplasia, cerebellar hypoplasia with internal hydrocephalus); infection caused by *Sarcocystis neurona, Streptococcus equi* subsp. *equi*, equine herpesvirus type 1, or *Halicephalobus gingivalis*; and miscellaneous conditions (eg, Gomen disease, cerebellar herniation, methyl mercurial poisoning, hematoma of the fourth ventricle reported in two Thoroughbred foals). Most of the diseases are very rare, and interested readers are referred to literature describing the specific diseases.

EPIDEMIOLOGY

SPECIES, AGE, SEX

- Cerebellar abiotrophy and degeneration
  - Abiotrophy: Arabian, Gotland pony, and Oldenburg horse breeds; degeneration: Thoroughbred and Paso Fino horses
  - Clinical signs develop between the time of birth and 6 months of age. Foals are often born without abnormalities and develop the disease later.
- Dandy-Walker syndrome
  - Thoroughbred and Arabian horses
  - Foals are born with signs of the defect

GENETICS AND BREED PREDISPOSITION

- Cerebellar abiotrophy and degeneration: This is a genetic neurologic disease with a recessive mode of inheritance, meaning that a horse can carry the disease gene but not be affected by the disease. Arabian and part-Arabian horses are affected most frequently. Cerebellar abiotrophy in Oldenburg horses is progressively fatal with histologic lesions similar to those of Arabian foals. The disease is not usually fatal in Arabian foals.

RISK FACTORS A high degree of inbreeding of affected Arabian foals has been shown on pedigree analysis.

CLINICAL PRESENTATION
HISTORY, CHIEF COMPLAINT

- Cerebellar abiotrophy and degeneration: Affected foals appear normal at birth but develop intentional head tremor (vertical or horizontal) and a lack of balance equilibrium (ataxia) at around 6 weeks of age.
- Dandy-Walker syndrome: Difficulty rising, seizures shortly after birth in Arabian or Thoroughbred foals

PHYSICAL EXAM FINDINGS

- Cerebellar abiotrophy and degeneration: Clinical signs include ataxia, wide-based stance and gait, dysmetria, spasticity, and intentional head tremor. Nystagmus is almost never reported. Mentation is not affected. A menace reflex is often diminished or absent. Gait abnormalities are generally symmetric and can be exacerbated with blindfolding or by having the foal travel over obstacles. The signs vary in severity.
- Dandy-Walker syndrome
  - Foals are often abnormal from birth, with seizures, difficulty rising, ataxia, nystagmus, and absent suckle reflex.
  - Excessively domed forehead.
  - Aggression and difficulties in training can be seen as the foal ages.

ETIOLOGY AND PATHOPHYSIOLOGY Cerebellar abiotrophy and degeneration is a genetic condition with a recessive mode of inheritance.

DIAGNOSIS

DIFFERENTIAL DIAGNOSIS

- Cranial malformations
- Congenital spinal malformations (atlantoaxial malformation and stenotic myelopathy)
- Inflammation or infection of the cerebellum
- Trauma

INITIAL DATABASE

- Cerebellar abiotrophy and degeneration
  - Antemortem diagnosis is based on history and clinical signs in appropriate breeds.
  - Completed blood count and serum biochemistries are normal.
  - Cerebrospinal fluid analysis: Elevated creatine kinase activity

(6.6–62 IU/μL; normal, 0–8 IU/μL); associated with neural necrosis or degeneration. Total protein is elevated (226 mg/dL; normal, 0–180 mg/dL), but this elevation is not specific for cerebellar abiotrophy.
  - Electroencephalographic (EEG) abnormalities may be observed; this is primarily useful to exclude seizure disorders as the cause of tremors (ie, EEG would likely be normal in the case of seizure disorders).
  - Skull and cervical radiographs are unremarkable.
- Dandy-Walker syndrome: Diagnosis is made using computed tomography or on postmortem examination.

ADVANCED OR CONFIRMATORY TESTING

- Ancillary testing is of limited value.
- Although the clinical signs are distinctive, the only definitive confirmation for a diagnosis of cerebellar abiotrophy is to examine the brain histologically after euthanasia.

TREATMENT

THERAPEUTIC GOAL(S)

Cerebellar diseases are untreatable.

PROGNOSIS AND OUTCOME

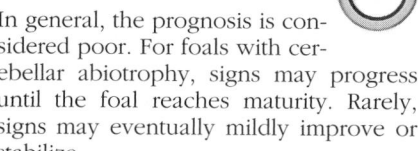

In general, the prognosis is considered poor. For foals with cerebellar abiotrophy, signs may progress until the foal reaches maturity. Rarely, signs may eventually mildly improve or stabilize.

PEARLS & CONSIDERATIONS

CLIENT EDUCATION

- Cerebellar abiotrophy and degeneration
  - Breeding between two carrier horses will produce an affected foal 25% of the time.
  - At the time of this writing, research to identify the defective gene and create a DNA-based test is ongoing at University of California, Davis Veterinary Genetics Laboratory. Interested readers are advised to go to the following websites to learn if the test is available at the current time:

- To order tests: http://www.vgl.ucdavis.edu/services/horse.php
- For more information: http://www.vgl.ucdavis.edu/genomic/cerebellar/

SUGGESTED READING

Byrne BA: Diseases of the cerebellum. In Reed SM, Bayly WM, Sellon DC, editors: *Equine Internal Medicine*, ed 3. St Louis, 2010, Saunders Elsevier, pp 598–603.

DeBowes RM, Leipold HW, Turner-Beatty M: Cerebellar abiotrophy. *Vet Clin North Am Equine Pract* 345–352, 1987.

Scarratt WK: Cerebellar disease and disease characterized by dysmetria and tremors. *Vet Clin Food Anim* 20:275–286, 2004.

AUTHOR: **NICOLE H. PASSLER**

EDITOR: **STEPHEN M. REED**

Cervix, Defects of

BASIC INFORMATION

DEFINITION

Cervical defects in mares may be caused by congenital, traumatic, or aging processes and may include malformations, muscle defects (healed cervical lacerations), adhesions, or failure to dilate due to fibrosis.

EPIDEMIOLOGY

SPECIES, AGE, SEX Mares of any age may present with a cervical problem, but the average age that most mares are diagnosed with cervical defects is approximately 13 years of age; these mares are most often pluriparous.

GENETICS AND BREED PREDISPOSITION These defects may be seen in any breed, but Thoroughbreds appear to be overrepresented in the literature.

RISK FACTORS

- Middle-aged (older than 12 years of age), pluriparous mares are predisposed to muscle defects and cervical adhesions.
- Middle-aged (older than 12 years of age), maiden mares, and donor mares that have not carried a foal in 3 or more years are predisposed to a cervix that fails to dilate.
- History of previous foaling (eutocia or dystocia), abortion, stillbirth, or the birthing of foals with congenital musculoskeletal abnormalities
- Rarely, congenital or breeding injuries

ASSOCIATED CONDITIONS AND DISORDERS Persistent or chronic endometrial infections, inability to conceive, early embryonic death, ascending placentitis, abortion, failure for the cervix to dilate at time of parturition, septic foals, maladjustment syndrome in neonates

CLINICAL PRESENTATION

DISEASE FORMS/SUBTYPES

- Cervical muscle defect or healed cervical lacerations
- Cervical adhesion

- Cervical fibrosis
- Cervical malformation

HISTORY, CHIEF COMPLAINT Mares with cervical defects are generally middle-aged, pluriparous mares that have been diagnosed with chronic, persistent endometrial infections and the inability to conceive and carry a foal to term.

PHYSICAL EXAM FINDINGS

- The physical examination results are often normal. Transrectal palpation and ultrasound examination of the reproductive tract may reveal evidence of uterine fluid and edema associated with an inflammatory response but may be normal.
- Digital examination of the cervix is necessary to assess for muscle defects in the external os, cervical body, or internal os of the cervix as well as intraluminal or extraluminal adhesions or cervical fibrosis.

ETIOLOGY AND PATHOPHYSIOLOGY

- Cervical muscle defects and adhesions are generally associated with trauma to the cervix during foaling and occasionally may be seen after natural mating or iatrogenically induced with aggressive cervical manipulation.
- Cervical fibrosis may be caused by trauma or aging changes.
- Cervical malformation is generally a congenital condition but may be secondary to cervical trauma.

DIAGNOSIS

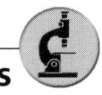

DIFFERENTIAL DIAGNOSIS

- Persistent or chronic endometrial infection
- Endometrial or periglandular fibrosis
- Ascending placentitis (pregnancy)

INITIAL DATABASE

- Good reproductive history
- Transrectal palpation and ultrasonography
- Vaginal speculum examination
- Digital examination of the cervix

ADVANCED OR CONFIRMATORY TESTING

- Although digital examination of the cervix is generally the gold standard test to diagnose a cervical defect, the following tests should be considered to determine if the mare is a good candidate for surgery or if she should be treated for an endometrial infection before surgical intervention.
  - Endometrial culture
  - Endometrial cytology
  - Endometrial biopsy

TREATMENT

THERAPEUTIC GOAL(S)

Improve integrity of the cervix, thus improving the fertility of the mare.

ACUTE GENERAL TREATMENT

Acute treatment of cervical lacerations is based on decreasing inflammation with nonsteroidal antiinflammatory drugs and the incidence of infection with systemic antibiotics. Surgical intervention is not attempted until the tissue has healed.

CHRONIC TREATMENT

- Surgical intervention for the correction of the incompetent cervix is the gold standard treatment for cervical muscle defects and adhesions.
- Cervical fibrosis may be treated with prostaglandin E_2 topical creams 1 to 2 hours before breeding to allow for optimal cervical dilatation and then a postbreeding uterine lavage 4 to 6 hours after mating to promote uterine clearance and decrease intraluminal uterine debris. Ecbolics such as oxytocin and prostaglandin $F_{2\alpha}$ may assist in uterine clearance as well.
- Surgical treatment for cervical fibrosis and malformation is rarely beneficial.

POSSIBLE COMPLICATIONS

Minimal

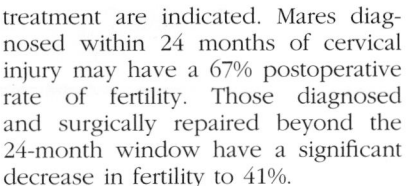

RECOMMENDED MONITORING

- Postsurgical correction of the cervix should not be manipulated for 2 to 4 weeks to allow the incision(s) to heal.
- Incisional adhesions may occur and should be bluntly dissected. The use of glucocorticoid creams or hyaluronic suppositories may be useful in decreasing adhesion formation after surgery.

PROGNOSIS AND OUTCOME

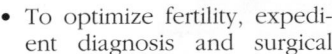

- To optimize fertility, expedient diagnosis and surgical

treatment are indicated. Mares diagnosed within 24 months of cervical injury may have a 67% postoperative rate of fertility. Those diagnosed and surgically repaired beyond the 24-month window have a significant decrease in fertility to 41%.
- Recurrence rate of cervical defects after surgical intervention is approximately 20%.

SUGGESTED READING

Blanchard T, Evans L, Kenney R, et al: Congenitally incompetent cervix in a mare. *J Am Vet Med Assoc* 181:266, 1982.

Blanchard T, Varner D, Schumacher J, et al: *Manual of Equine Reproduction.* St Louis, 2003, Mosby, pp 190–191.

Brown J, Varner D, Hinrichs K, Kenney R: Surgical repair of the lacerated cervix in the mare. *Theriogenology* 22:351–359, 1984.

Makloski-Cohorn C: *Post-Operative Fertility in Mares with Cervical Defects*, Unpublished thesis. Oklahoma State University, 2009.

Miller C, Embertson R, Smith S: Surgical repair of cervical lacerations in thoroughbred mares: 53 cases (1985–1995). *Proc Am Assoc Equine Pract* 42:154–155, 1996.

AUTHOR: **CHELSEA MAKLOSKI**

EDITOR: **JUAN C. SAMPER**

Cervical Vertebral Stenotic Myelopathy

BASIC INFORMATION

DEFINITION

Cervical vertebral stenotic myelopathy (CVM, CVSM, CSM, CVCM) is characterized by compression of the spinal cord in the cervical region at the site of two adjacent vertebrae. Compression of the spinal cord results in chronic or repetitive trauma with blockage of normal conduction pathways, axon damage, and eventual loss with resulting signs of weakness and ataxia.

SYNONYM(S)

Wobbler, CVM, CSM, CVSM, CVCM

EPIDEMIOLOGY

- Horses affected with CVSM often present at a young age (younger than age 2 years), although some horses may not be identified until 5 years or older.
- Some investigators suggest bony malformation may be a result of developmental abnormalities such as osteochondrosis affecting the articular process joints of the cervical vertebral column with subsequent instability and hypertrophy of the soft tissues such as the ligamentum flavum and other support structures associated with the vertebral column.
- Osteochondrosis is a disturbance in endochondral ossification in rapidly growing animal species and humans. Diet appears to be a factor in this condition as well as in other developmental orthopedic problems affecting the appendicular skeleton of horses.
- The higher incidence in Thoroughbreds and a few other breeds suggests an inherited basis, although character-

ization of the mode of inheritance has not been completed to date. In addition to diet and a role of genetic predisposition, gender, rate of growth, endocrine dysfunction, and biomechanical stress have also been incriminated.

SPECIES, AGE, SEX The condition appears more often in males than in females, although it affects both genders. The age of affected horses is generally younger than 2 years of age, although it may present at a later time.

GENETICS AND BREED PREDISPOSITION Because the problem has a higher incidence in Thoroughbred horses, a genetic predisposition is suspected, although an exact mode of inheritance has not been identified.

RISK FACTORS

- Important risk factors are described above; however, a very important factor appears to be diet. In some studies, the incidence of osteochondrosis affecting the vertebral articular process joints of the cervical vertebrae was nearly six times as frequent in foals born to mares fed and foals raised on diets lower in copper than in a similar group fed a diet much higher in copper.
- Other important factors are the glycemic index of the diet, the gender of the foals, trauma, and the rate of growth.

GEOGRAPHY AND SEASONALITY This condition is recognized worldwide, and horses may present at any time during their lives, although many animals are recognized during periods of growth. The condition often consists of episodes of ataxia, which often appear most obvious after a period of rapid growth after a period of quiescence.

ASSOCIATED CONDITIONS AND DISORDERS Horses affected with CVSM often have concurrent signs of developmental orthopedic conditions affecting the appendicular skeleton such as osteochondritis dissecans of some long bones of the horse along with evidence of epiphysitis and physitis of some long bones.

CLINICAL PRESENTATION

DISEASE FORMS/SUBTYPES

- This condition is observed as a developmental disease in which malformation and malarticulation of cervical vertebrae result in compression of the spinal cord. The condition appears to be multifactorial, and the higher incidence in Thoroughbred horses suggests a genetic predisposition.
- The observation of the problem most often in young growing horses, male more often than female, that are fed high-carbohydrate diets that may be deficient in copper or contain excess zinc supports the idea of a multifactorial cause for this condition.
- The second group of affected horses are generally older and have osteoarthritic enlargements of the articular processes.

HISTORY, CHIEF COMPLAINT

- Ataxia (often symmetrical)
- Paresis
- Hypometria
- Dysmetria of all limbs with signs usually most severe in the pelvic limbs
- In a few cases, signs may progress to recumbency.
- Cases may be either acute or insidious, but in many horses, the signs often appear episodic with intermittent

worsening of signs followed by periods of improvement.

PHYSICAL EXAM FINDINGS

• Ataxia, paresis (often symmetrical), or both, which are a result of upper motor neuron and general proprioceptive tract damage as a result of spinal cord compression. Damage to these tracts results in ataxia, incoordination, and weakness along with inappropriate limb rigidity.

• The horse should be evaluated by careful observation of the gait while walking on a nonslippery surface as well as while walking in circles and walking on a slope or other maneuvers to help demonstrate the presence of signs in all limbs.

ETIOLOGY AND PATHOPHYSIOLOGY

• Clinical signs result from compression of the spinal cord as a result of vertebral canal stenosis.

• Canal stenosis may result from elongation of the dorsal laminae (vertebral arch) with a relative shortening of the vertebral body.

• This may contribute to vertebral instability with either lordotic or kyphotic deviations of the vertebrae along with flare of the caudal epiphysis of the vertebral body.

• Degenerative osteoarthritis of the articular process joints

• Vertebrae will be narrowed from dorsal to ventral at the cranial and caudal orifice of the vertebral foramen.

• Soft tissue changes such as hypertrophy of the ligamentum flavum, thickening of the joint capsules, or synovial cyst formation may also result in or contribute to spinal cord compression.

DIAGNOSIS

DIFFERENTIAL DIAGNOSIS

• Equine degenerative myelopathy
• Equine herpesvirus-1 myelopathy
• Equine protozoal myeloencephalitis
• Spinal cord trauma
• Cervical vertebral osteoarthropathy

INITIAL DATABASE

• Neurologic examination
• Cervical vertebral radiographs
• Cervical vertebral myelography (Figure 1)
• Cerebrospinal fluid (CSF) analysis for cytologic evaluation
• Serum and CSF testing for equine protozoal encephalomyelitis

ADVANCED OR CONFIRMATORY TESTING

• Radiography of the cervical vertebrae
• Myelographic examination of the cervical vertebrae (see Figure 1)
• CSF analysis and cytology

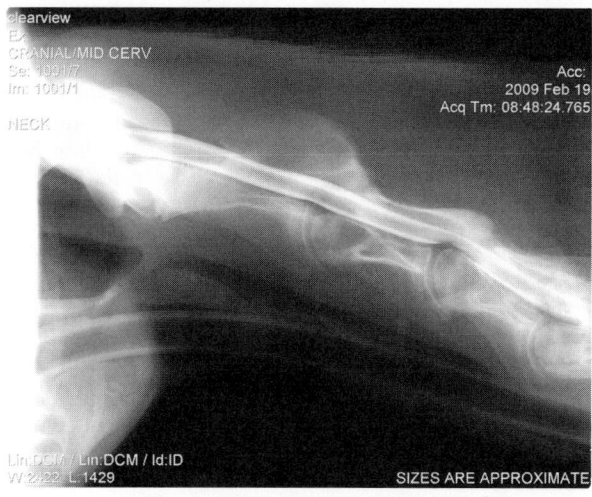

FIGURE 1 Lateral view myelogram of the cranial half of the cervical vertebrae illustrating a compressive lesion at C3–C4.

• Postmortem examination with histopathologic evaluation.

TREATMENT

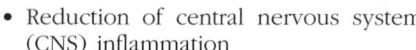

THERAPEUTIC GOAL(S)

• Reduction of central nervous system (CNS) inflammation
• Ventral stabilization to stop spinal cord compression
• Supportive care until the horse can improve neurologic function

ACUTE GENERAL TREATMENT

• Corticosteroids: Dexamethasone (0.05–0.2 mg/kg IV q12–24h) or methylprednisolone sodium succinate (1.0–2.5 mg/kg IV q6h). The dose and interval depend on the severity of the clinical signs.
• Flunixin meglumine: 1.1 mg/kg IV q12–24h
• Dimethyl sulfoxide (0.5–1.0 g/kg IV q12–24h) must be diluted to a 10% solution or less in an isotonic balanced electrolyte solution.
• Surgical correction using ventral stabilization at the affected site(s)

CHRONIC TREATMENT

• In young horses (younger than 1 year of age and preferably younger than 6 months of age) may try dietary management to affect the rate of growth and vertebral canal development.
• Antiinflammatory medications such as flunixin meglumine (0.5–1.1 mg/kg PO q12–24h), phenylbutazone (1–2 mg/kg PO q12–24h), prednisolone (0.5–1.0 mg/kg PO q12–24h), or dexamethasone (0.05–0.2 mg/kg PO q12–24h) as needed for CNS inflammation.
• Horses that are unable to stand or get up on their own need to be placed into a sling periodically.

RECOMMENDED MONITORING

Periodic repeat neurologic examinations to assess response to therapy

PROGNOSIS AND OUTCOME

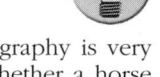

• The overall prognosis for complete recovery is guarded.
• Horses that survive may have permanent neurologic deficits.

PEARLS & CONSIDERATIONS

COMMENTS

• Cervical vertebral radiography is very helpful to determine whether a horse has a narrow vertebral canal.
• Myelography is recommended before attempting surgical correction.
• CSF testing is strongly indicated to eliminate other causes of spinal ataxia.

PREVENTION

• Careful observation of young, growing horses for signs of ataxia
• Use of cervical vertebral radiography at an early age to evaluate the canal diameter
• Careful attention to diet in young, growing foals

CLIENT EDUCATION

• Make clients aware of important risk factors as well as the important diagnostic tests essential for diagnosis of canal stenosis.

SUGGESTED READING

Knight DA, Weisbrode SA, Schmall LM, et al: The effects of copper supplementation on the prevalence of cartilage lesions in foals. *Equine Vet J* 22(6):426–432, 1990.

Mayhew IG: Cervical vertebral malformation and malarticulation of horses. In *Large Animal Neurology*, ed 2. West Sussex, UK, 2009, Blackwell, pp 394–404.

Moore BR, Reed SM, Biller DS, et al: Assessment of vertebral canal diameter and bony malformations of the cervical part of the spine in horses with cervical stenotic myelopathy. *Am J Vet Res* 55:5–13, 1994.

Nout YS, Reed SM: Cervical vertebral stenotic myelopathy. *Equine Vet Ed* 15:212–223, 2003.

Stewart RH, Reed SM, Weisbrode SE: Frequency and severity of osteochondrosis in horses with cervical vertebral stenotic myelopathy. *Am J Vet Res* 52:873–879, 1991.

AUTHOR & EDITOR: **STEPHEN M. REED**

Choanal Atresia

BASIC INFORMATION

DEFINITION

Choanal atresia is a congenital abnormality resulting in unilateral or bilateral obstruction of the choanae. Choanal atresia is caused by failure of the bucconasal membrane to rupture. The obstruction can be membranous or fibrocartilaginous.

EPIDEMIOLOGY

SPECIES, AGE, SEX There is no known breed or sex predilection, although most of the reported cases have been in Standardbreds. Foals with choanal atresia are diagnosed at birth if the case is bilateral. Horses with unilateral choanal atresia may not be diagnosed until they are placed into training.

CLINICAL PRESENTATION

HISTORY, CHIEF COMPLAINT

- Foals affected with bilateral choanal atresia are unable to breathe at birth and present with acute respiratory distress. Foals with bilateral choanal atresia usually die unless an emergency tracheotomy or orotracheal intubation is performed. Placement of the hands over the nares reveals no air movement from the nares.
- Unilateral choanal atresia may not be clinically evident until the horse is placed into athletic training. Affected horses make a respiratory noise and develop exercise intolerance. An additional abnormality is failure to pass a nasogastric tube on the affected side(s).

PHYSICAL EXAM FINDINGS

- The diagnosis of choanal atresia is suspected based on clinical signs of nasal obstruction or severe dyspnea in foals at birth. Evaluation of airflow from the nares reveals no air movement from the affected side(s).
- Endoscopy is the best method to confirm choanal atresia. Endoscopic findings compatible with choanal atresia include failure to pass the endoscope into the nasopharynx and the presence of a sheet of tissue at the caudal aspect of the junction between the ethmoid turbinates, nasal septum, and caudal nasal conchae. Because of the obstructing membrane, the nasopharynx cannot be visualized.

ETIOLOGY AND PATHOPHYSIOLOGY

- Choanal atresia results from failure of the bucconasal membrane to separate from the primitive buccal or oral cavity from the nasal pits during embryologic development.
- This membrane can be complete, consisting of bone or fibrocartilage, or membranous. In horses, the majority of affected cases are membranous.
- Bilateral choanal atresia results in dyspnea at birth and may result in death if an emergency tracheotomy is not performed.
- Unilateral choanal atresia is typically not diagnosed until the horse is placed into training and is not life threatening.

DIAGNOSIS

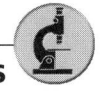

DIFFERENTIAL DIAGNOSIS

- Epiglottic entrapment
- Epiglottitis
- Dorsal displacement of the soft palate
- Epiglottic retroversion
- Rostral displacement of the palatopharyngeal arch
- Laryngeal hemiplegia
- Arytenoid chondritis
- Tracheal collapse
- Nasal passage obstruction

INITIAL DATABASE

- Physical examination: Subjective evaluation of airflow from each nasal passage. Unilaterally affected horses have no airflow from the affected side. Foals with bilateral choanal atresia are dyspneic.
- Endoscopy: Endoscopic examination reveals an obstructing membrane between the caudal aspect of the nasal septum, ventral aspect of the ethmoid turbinates, and nasal conchae. No nasopharyngeal structures can be visualized through the membrane.

- Radiography: Contrast radiography with contrast media being instilled into the affected nasal passage can highlight the obstructing membrane with no communication between the nasal passage and nasopharynx.

TREATMENT

THERAPEUTIC GOAL(S)

- Foals with bilateral choanal atresia must have an emergency tracheotomy as soon as possible after birth. Alternatively, if moribund, the foal can be intubated orally.
- After the tracheotomy, treatment options can be discussed with the owner.
- Horses with unilateral choanal atresia require surgical creation of a new opening via the obstructing membrane from the nasal passage into the nasopharynx.
- The problem with either of the surgical techniques is after resection or ablation of the obstructing membrane, stricture of the new opening is common and should be expected to occur to some degree. To help minimize the chances for stricture, the choanae should be stented for 2 to 3 weeks. The authors currently recommend ablation of the obstructing membrane with a noncontact, diode laser (50 W). After the choanae has been opened with the noncontact laser, the new opening is stented with a shortened nasotracheal tube for at least 2 to 3 weeks.

ACUTE GENERAL TREATMENT

- Few cases of choanal atresia have been reported in the veterinary literature. This makes treatment recommendations difficult because of the lack of experience with the condition.
- There are basically two methods of surgical management: Resection of the membrane through unilateral or bilateral nasal osteoplastic flaps and ablation of the membrane with a diode or Nd:YAG surgical laser.

○ When using osteoplastic nasal bone flaps, the margins of the membrane are resected to establish an opening between the nasal passage and nasopharynx. In horses with a small nasal passage, resection of turbinates and the caudal aspect of the nasal septum may be considered to ensure an adequate airway.

○ Standing laser ablation of the obstructing membrane can be performed with a noncontact, diode laser. Personal experience has shown that the noncontact laser ablation has several advantages over contact laser techniques. These advantages include less hemorrhage and a larger opening secondary to latent thermal necrosis at the margins of the laser ablation. The minimum power setting for this application is 50 W, with the laser fiber being discharged for 3 seconds and off for 1 second.

- Regardless of the surgical technique used, the newly created opening should be stented with a shortened nasotracheal tube for a minimum of 2 to 3 weeks. Postoperative stricture is not unusual after surgical ablation, and owners should be apprised of this potential complication.
- Some horses may require follow-up surgical procedures to ensure an adequate airway diameter. These procedures may include repeat laser ablation or incision of strictured opening or

partial resection of the nasal septum with an osteoplastic flap. Radial incisions at the stricture in conjunction with bougienage have also been successful.

POSSIBLE COMPLICATIONS

The most significant complication after surgical correction of choanal atresia is stricture of the new opening.

RECOMMENDED MONITORING

Surgically treated horses should be monitored with endoscopy at 1- to 2-month intervals after surgical correction. This is done in an effort to address stricture if it occurs.

PROGNOSIS AND OUTCOME

- The prognosis for choanal atresia is poor unless the new choanal opening remains patent.
- Horses with unilateral choanal atresia may be successfully treated and return to athletic activity.
- However, the majority of horses with choanal atresia have a guarded prognosis for athletic activity, especially racing.
- Horses with small nasal passages and problems with stricture of the choana after surgery have a guarded prognosis.

PEARLS & CONSIDERATIONS

- Standing noncontact laser surgical ablation of the obstructing membrane is preferred over contact techniques.
- Stenting of the newly created opening is very important to maintain the patency of the new opening.
- The stricture can be resolved with follow-up surgical procedures if necessary.

SUGGESTED READING

Aylor MK, Campbell ML, Goring RL, et al: Congenital bilateral choanal atresia in a Standardbred foal. *Equine Vet J* 16:396–398, 1984.

Crouch GM, Morgan SJ: Bilateral choanal atresia in a foal. *Compend Contin Educ Pract Vet* 5(suppl):S206–S211, 1983.

Goring RL, et al: Surgical correction of congenital bilateral choanal atresia in a foal. *Vet Surg* 13:211–216, 1984.

Hogan PM, Embertson RM, Hunt RJ: Unilateral choanal atresia in a foal. *J Am Vet Med Assoc* 207:471–473, 1995.

James FM, Parente EJ, Palmer JE: Management of bilateral choanal atresia in a foal. *J Am Vet Med Assoc* 229:1784–1789, 2006.

Richardson JL, Lane JG, Day MJ: Congenital choanal restriction in 3 horses. *Equine Vet J* 26:162–165, 1994.

Sprinkle FP, Crowe MW, Swerczek TW: Choanal atresia in foals. *Mod Vet Pract* 65:306, 1984.

AUTHOR: **JAN F. HAWKINS**

EDITOR: **ERIC J. PARENTE**

Cholangiohepatitis, Chronic, and Biliary Fibrosis

BASIC INFORMATION

DEFINITION

Cholangiohepatitis is an inflammatory process of the walls of the bile ducts and the adjacent liver parenchyma. A bacterial infection (primary or secondary) is a common component of cholangiohepatitis, which frequently presents with biliary stasis and sometimes cholelithiasis. With chronicity, ongoing inflammation triggers the onset and progression of liver fibrosis.

EPIDEMIOLOGY

RISK FACTORS

- Gastroduodenal ulcers and duodenal strictures in foals.
- Anterior enteritis in adult horses.
- Enterocolitis.
- Cholelithiasis.

- In a case series of cholangiohepatitis in horses, broodmares were overrepresented, but the low number of subjects in the study did not allow making an association. In human medicine, pregnancy (and particularly the cholestatic effect of estrogens) is suspected to predispose to biliary tract diseases.
- Sepsis in neonatal foals.

ASSOCIATED CONDITIONS AND DISORDERS

- The form of chronic active hepatitis characterized by neutrophilic infiltration, cholangitis, and cholestasis is consistent with chronic cholangiohepatitis.
- Cholelithiasis, defined by the presence of calculi within the biliary ducts, is commonly accompanied by cholangiohepatitis and biliary fibrosis.
- Bacterial hepatitis.

CLINICAL PRESENTATION

DISEASE FORMS/SUBTYPES

- Most commonly subtle and gradual in onset
- Manifestation of clinical signs can be acute

HISTORY, CHIEF COMPLAINT Depressed mentation, inappetence, weight loss, signs of abdominal discomfort, loose stools

PHYSICAL EXAM FINDINGS

- Fever.
- Icterus.
- Dehydration.
- Colic or diarrhea may be directly related to cholangiohepatitis or may be secondary to an underlying gastrointestinal disease.
- Signs of hepatic failure (photosensitization, mucosal petechiation, hepatic encephalopathy) are less commonly present.

ETIOLOGY AND PATHOPHYSIOLOGY

- The most common isolates are enteric bacteria:
  - Gram negative: *Salmonella* spp., *Escherichia coli, Enterobacter* spp., *Citrobacter* spp., *Actinobacillus* spp.
  - Anaerobes: *Bacteroides* spp.
- Hypotheses of pathogenesis:
  - Bacterial infection ascends the bile ducts from the lumen of the small intestine and is secondary to any condition that is associated with cholestasis (eg, right dorsal colon displacement, anterior enteritis, enterocolitis, duodenal stricture in foals).
  - Bacterial translocation of intestinal microorganisms into the blood stream drained by the portal vein with secondary bacterial infection of the portal triad and cholangitis.
  - Cholelithiasis: Bilirubin precipitates with calcium, forming calcium bilirubinate, with secondary bile stasis, cholangitis, and bacterial infection. However, it is more likely that choleliths may be a consequence, rather than a cause, of chronic cholangiohepatitis.
  - Hematogenous spread secondary to septicemia in neonatal foals.
  - With any form of chronic cholangiohepatitis, hepatic fibrosis may ensue and progress.

DIAGNOSIS

DIFFERENTIAL DIAGNOSIS

- Biliary obstruction secondary to acute or chronic colon displacement
- Cholelithiasis
- Bacterial hepatitis
- Chronic active hepatitis
- Chronic megalocytic hepatopathy
- Biliary atresia in neonates
- Hepatic neoplasia
- Amyloidosis
- Liver parasites

INITIAL DATABASE

- Packed cell volume: Normal or increased because of hemoconcentration or erythrocytosis induced by liver disease
- Total protein concentration: Normal or increased (hyperglobulinemia)
- White blood cell count: Normal or increased
- Fibrinogen concentration: Normal or increased
- Sorbitol dehydrogenase (SDH) and aspartate aminotransferase (AST) activity: Normal or increased
- Gamma glutamyltransferase (GGT) and alkaline phosphatase (ALP) activity: Moderately to markedly increased

- Total bilirubin: Increased
- Direct (conjugated) fraction: >25% of total bilirubin
- Serum bile acids concentration: Increased; may be normal

ADVANCED OR CONFIRMATORY TESTING

- Plasma ammonia may be increased.
- Clotting profile: prothrombin time and activated partial thromboplastin time may be increased.
- Transabdominal ultrasonographic examination of the liver (see "Diagnostic Imaging of the Liver" in Section II):
  - Liver size may be increased.
  - Increased liver parenchyma echogenicity, localized or generalized.
  - Lack of homogenicity in the ultrasonographic appearance of the liver parenchyma.
  - Biliary distension.
  - Hyperechoic "sludge-like" material within the biliary tract.
  - Hyperechoic shadow-casting foci within the bile ducts are consistent with choleliths.
- Transabdominal ultrasonographic examination of the abdomen may reveal increased peritoneal fluid volume.
- Abdominocentesis may be consistent with a transudate or nonseptic inflammation.
- Ultrasound-guided liver biopsy:
  - Histopathology
    - Suppurative inflammation characterized by neutrophils infiltrating the lumen of the bile ducts, the biliary walls, and the liver parenchyma (most pronounced in the portal area)
    - Hepatocellular degeneration, necrosis, or both
    - Biliary hyperplasia
    - Fibrosis may be incipient in early stages and more pronounced in chronic cases, up to the point of connecting one portal triad to another (bridging fibrosis)
  - Bacterial culture of liver tissue: gram-negative enteric bacteria most commonly cultured

TREATMENT

THERAPEUTIC GOAL(S)

The goal of medical therapy is treatment of the underlying bacterial infection. Supportive care and dietary manipulation may be required to maintain hydration and provide nutrition while minimizing liver workload.

ACUTE GENERAL TREATMENT

- IV fluids if the horse is febrile and dehydrated.

- Flunixin meglumine (1.1 mg/kg IV) to control signs of abdominal pain or pyrexia.
- Long-term antimicrobial therapy.
  - Potentiated sulfonamides, ceftiofur, penicillin and gentamicin, enrofloxacin, ampicillin, or chloramphenicol.
  - Metronidazole may be added for improved anaerobic coverage.
- Antimicrobial therapy should be administered until GGT and ALP activity has normalized for 2 to 4 weeks.

CHRONIC TREATMENT

- Dimethylsulfoxide 1 g/kg IV (diluted in a 5% solution in fluids) q24h for 5 to 7 days may act as a solvent for calcium bilirubinate calculi.
- Surgical procedures (manual lithotripsy or choledocholithomy) have been reported to successfully treat complete biliary obstruction in horses with persistent signs.

ADDITIONAL TREATMENTS

- Also see treatment for "Hepatic Encephalopathy."
- S-adenosylmethionine (SAMe): 5 g PO q24h; the bioavailability of crushed pills is questionable in horses.

PREVENTION OF LIVER FIBROSIS

- Pentoxifylline: 8–16 mg/kg PO q8–12h
- Colchicine: 0.03 mg/kg PO q24h; there have been anecdotal reports of presumed toxicity

POSSIBLE COMPLICATIONS

- Diarrhea
- Peritonitis

RECOMMENDED MONITORING

- GGT or ALP activity
- Serum bile acids concentration
- Repeat liver biopsy

PROGNOSIS AND OUTCOME

- Good prognosis with early diagnosis and treatment of bacterial infection and suppurative hepatitis
- Guarded to poor prognosis with biliary fibrosis
- Typically a grave prognosis when bridging fibrosis is present

PEARLS & CONSIDERATIONS

A transient increase in serum GGT may be observed in the initial phase of medical treatment, possibly consistent with response to therapy and biliary epithelium regeneration and hyperplasia.

SUGGESTED READING

Davis JL, Jones SL: Suppurative cholangiohepatitis and enteritis in adult horses. *J Vet Intern Med* 17:583, 2003.

Peek SF: Cholangiohepatitis. In Mair T, Divers N, Ducharme N, editors: *Manual of equine gastroenterology.* St Louis, 2002, Saunders, pp 386–388.

Peek SF, Divers TJ: Medical treatment of cholangiohepatitis and cholelithiasis in mature horses: 9 cases (1991–1998). *Equine Vet J* 32(4):301, 2000.

AUTHOR: **ALESSANDRA PELLEGRINI-MASINI**

EDITOR: **MICHELLE HENRY BARTON**

Cholelithiasis

BASIC INFORMATION

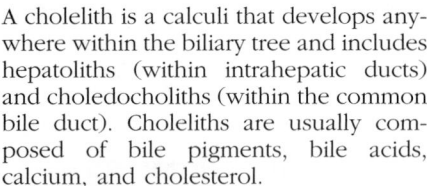

DEFINITION

A cholelith is a calculi that develops anywhere within the biliary tree and includes hepatoliths (within intrahepatic ducts) and choledocholiths (within the common bile duct). Choleliths are usually composed of bile pigments, bile acids, calcium, and cholesterol.

SYNONYM(S)

Bile stones

EPIDEMIOLOGY

SPECIES, AGE, SEX
- Broodmares may be at greater risk
- Middle age (6–15 years)

RISK FACTORS
- Cholangiohepatitis
- Any condition resulting in cholestasis.
- Pregnancy may be a risk factor.

ASSOCIATED CONDITIONS AND DISORDERS Clinical signs of cholelithiasis may be indistinguishable from other liver disorders, including cholangiohepatitis, chronic megalocytic hepatopathy, clover toxicity, chronic active hepatitis, hepatic abscessation, and hepatic neoplasia.

CLINICAL PRESENTATION

DISEASE FORMS/SUBTYPES
- Chronic: Intermittent weight loss, anorexia, colic, fever, icterus
- Acute: Hepatoencephalopathy, fever, colic

HISTORY, CHIEF COMPLAINT Owners may observe intermittent colic, weight loss, anorexia, depression, icterus, or fever.

PHYSICAL EXAM FINDINGS Icterus, fever, low-grade colic, photosensitization, hepatoencephalopathy, petechiae (rarely).

ETIOLOGY AND PATHOPHYSIOLOGY
- The exact mechanism is unknown.
- Excreted conjugated bilirubin becomes unconjugated bilirubin and combines with calcium to form calcium bilirubinate, which precipitates, resulting in cholelith formation.
- Often associated with ascending cholangitis or cholangiohepatitis, especially with gram-negative enteric bacteria.

DIAGNOSIS

DIFFERENTIAL DIAGNOSIS
- Cholangiohepatitis
- Chronic megalocytic hepatopathy
- Chronic active hepatitis
- Clover toxicity
- Hepatic abscess
- Hepatic neoplasia

INITIAL DATABASE
- Leukocytosis characterized by neutrophilia
- Hyperfibrinogenemia
- Gamma glutamyltransferase (GGT) activity: Increased
- Alkaline phosphatase (ALP) activity: Increased
- Serum bile acids concentration: Increased
- Total bilirubin concentration: Increased
- Direct bilirubin concentration: Increased, usually >25% of total
- Sorbitol dehydrogenase (SDH) activity: Variable degree of increase
- Hyperglobulinemia
- Bilirubinuria

ADVANCED OR CONFIRMATORY TESTING
- Coagulation times, particularly prothrombin time, may be prolonged.
- Blood ammonia concentration may be increased.
- Ultrasonography: Increased echogenicity of hepatic parenchyma, hepatomegaly, distended bile ducts. Choleliths typically appear as hyperechoic foci and may cast anacoustic shadows (see "Diagnostic Imaging of the Liver" in Section II).
- Liver biopsy: Periportal fibrosis, biliary hyperplasia, bile stasis, concentric fibrosis around intrahepatic bile ducts, cholangitis
- Liver culture: Gram-negative enteric bacteria are often isolated.

TREATMENT

THERAPEUTIC GOAL(S)
- With medical treatment, the clinical signs may resolve. Choledocholiths may be amenable to surgical removal.

ACUTE GENERAL TREATMENT
- IV fluids may be required in animals that are febrile and dehydrated.
- Antiinflammatory drugs: Flunixin meglumine (1.1 mg/kg PO q12h).
- Nutritional support: Low-protein diet with high content of branched-chain amino acids.
- See treatment for "Hepatic Encephalopathy" in this section.

CHRONIC TREATMENT
- Nutritional support
- Antiinflammatory drugs
- Antifibrotic agents: pentoxifylline (8–16 mg/kg PO q8–12h)
- Dimethyl sulfoxide has been shown to dissolve calcium bilirubinate stones in humans.
- Long-term antimicrobial therapy as guided by liver culture (enrofloxacin, 5.0–7.5 mg/kg PO q24h; trimethoprim-sulfa, 20–30 mg/kg PO q12h; procaine penicillin G, 22,000 U/kg IM q12h) and gentamicin (6.6 mg/kg IM q24h); ceftiofur (2.2–4.4 mg/kg IM q12h); ampicillin (20 mg/kg IV q6–8h); chloramphenicol (50 mg/kg PO q6h)
- Surgical exploration is the only way to confirm obstruction of the common bile duct. Choledocholiths may be removed by external manual pressure to crush the stones, with subsequent dislodgement into the duodenum. Choledocholithotripsy and choledochotomy have been performed in horses.

POSSIBLE COMPLICATIONS

Hepatic encephalopathy, photosensitivity dermatitis, rupture of the common bile duct and fatal bile peritonitis, hepatic fibrosis

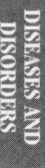

RECOMMENDED MONITORING

- Monitor liver enzymes every 2 to 3 weeks until GGT returns to within normal limits.
- Serial liver biopsies (q2–3mo).

PROGNOSIS AND OUTCOME

Guarded to good prognosis, depending on the degree of hepatic fibrosis and success of cholelith removal

PEARLS & CONSIDERATIONS

- It has been recommended to continue antimicrobial therapy until GGT activity returns to normal and there is complete resolution of clinical and laboratory evidence of inflammation.
- Horses with recurrent colic or signs of hepatic disease should be considered as candidates for exploratory celiotomy to rule out obstruction of the common bile duct.

SUGGESTED READING

Johnson JK, Divers TJ, Reef VB, et al: Cholelithiasis in horses: ten cases (1982–1986). *J Am Vet Med Assoc* 194:405, 1989.
Peek SF, Divers TJ: Medical treatment of cholangiohepatitis and cholelithiasis in mature horses: 9 cases (1991–1998). *Equine Vet J* 32:301, 2000.

AUTHOR: **HEIDI BANSE**

EDITOR: **MICHELLE HENRY BARTON**

Cleft Palate

BASIC INFORMATION

DEFINITION
A congenital defect resulting in the partial or complete failure of closure of the palatal folds in early embryologic development

SYNONYM(S)
Palatoschisis

EPIDEMIOLOGY
RISK FACTORS Influence of teratogens, genetic factors, and malnutrition around the forty-seventh day of gestation
ASSOCIATED CONDITIONS AND DISORDERS
- As with other congenital diseases, concurrent congenital malformations or defects may be present.
- Most often, coughing or aspiration of milk develops soon after birth and may lead to life-threatening aspiration pneumonia.

CLINICAL PRESENTATION
DISEASE FORMS/SUBTYPES
- The extent of clinical signs depends on the size of the defect and ranges from mild to severe.
- Both the soft and the hard palates may be involved. If the defect is small and only involves the caudal aspect of the soft palate, clinical signs may be mild and aspiration pneumonia may not be obvious for several weeks (if left untreated). These foals may eventually grow more slowly than healthy foals and appear unthrifty.
- Foals with a larger defect in the soft palate or with a cleft hard palate develop much more severe signs within days, prompting the owners to consult a veterinarian immediately.

HISTORY, CHIEF COMPLAINT Owners may observe milk running out of both nostrils immediately after nursing. Affected foals show signs of aspiration of milk (coughing, dyspnea) and may be weak and lethargic.
PHYSICAL EXAM FINDINGS
- Milk draining from both nostrils after nursing, coughing, dyspnea
- Later, signs of aspiration pneumonia and possibly fever
ETIOLOGY AND PATHOPHYSIOLOGY
- Not yet completely understood.
- Closure of the palatal folds occurs around the forty-seventh day of gestation.
- Genetic, nutritional, and teratogenic factors that are present around this time may be responsible for the development of a cleft palate.

DIAGNOSIS

DIFFERENTIAL DIAGNOSIS
- Other causes of aspiration in newborn foals, such as:
  - Fourth branchial arch anomaly
  - Epiglottic entrapment
  - Esophageal inclusion cyst
  - Pharyngeal dysfunction

INITIAL DATABASE
- Drainage of milk from both nostrils after nursing in a newborn foal.
- Coughing
- Dyspnea
- Observation of the cleft palate by oral examination (most often only possible with a hard palate defect).
- Digital palpation (hard or possibly soft palate defect).
- Diagnosis is confirmed, and the extent of the defect may be described by endoscopy. The epiglottis is positioned between the two edges of the soft palate and appears to be "dropped down" in the oropharynx.

ADVANCED OR CONFIRMATORY TESTING
If the defect involves only the caudal part of the soft palate, the epiglottis may still cover the cleft. Swallowing should be initiated during the endoscopic examination to be able to visualize the caudal aspect of the soft palate.

TREATMENT

THERAPEUTIC GOAL(S)
- Prevention of further aspiration.
- Surgical reconstruction (palatoplasty) of the palate as a salvage procedure.
- Treatment attempts should not be done if more than 20% of palatal tissue is missing.

ACUTE GENERAL TREATMENT
- Because no medical treatment option exists, the foal should be stabilized with supportive therapy and the signs of aspiration should be treated to decrease the risk for general anesthesia.
  - Broad-spectrum antimicrobial agents
  - Nonsteroidal antiinflammatory drugs (NSAIDs)
  - IV fluids if needed
  - Parenteral nutrition
- The ultimate treatment is the surgical reconstruction of the palate by mandibular symphysiotomy, laryngotomy, or pharyngotomy, or transoral reconstruction (endoscopic assisted). Broad-spectrum antimicrobial agents, NSAIDs, and enteral nutrition via a nasogastric tube or parenteral nutrition should be continued postoperatively as needed.

POSSIBLE COMPLICATIONS

- Dehiscence of the repair (partial or complete) is common.
- The severity of already established aspiration pneumonia can be life ending.

RECOMMENDED MONITORING

- If the repaired defect was small, an alternative way of feeding (nasogastric tube, parenteral nutrition) may not be necessary. In these rare cases, recurrence of clinical signs (milk drainage from the nose after nursing, coughing) must be monitored.
- If the foal is not allowed to nurse after surgery, the integrity of the repair should be monitored endoscopically.
- Signs of aspiration pneumonia should be monitored in both cases (endoscopy, lung auscultation, chest radiography, leukocyte counts, and fibrinogen).

PROGNOSIS AND OUTCOME

- The prognosis depends on the size and symmetry of the defect.
- If the defect involves both the hard and the soft palate, the prognosis decreases significantly (<20%).

- Even in the best-case scenario (ie, minimal tissue loss and a defect on the midline), successful repair may not exceed 50%.
- Because cleft palate repair is considered a salvage procedure, a successful outcome is reached when the animal can eat, swallow, and breathe normally.

PEARLS & CONSIDERATIONS

COMMENTS

- Repair of a cleft palate is a surgical procedure with a high failure rate. This may be because of the congenital nature of the defect. The surgeon must adapt tissue that has never been joined together before. Unlike tissue that was separated by trauma, a cleft palate represents a defect that may not only be repaired with considerable tension along the suture line, but the direction of the muscle fibers is changed. The muscle fibers of the levator veli palatini muscle in foals with a cleft palate do not insert at midline but rather at the caudal aspect of the hard palate. If possible, this false insertion should be severed and attempts should be undertaken to reconstruct the so-called *levator sling*.

- Horses with even small defects should be treated because chronic aspiration of milk and later other food material will decrease the quality of life of the affected animal to an extent that may not be tolerable.
- The only alternative to surgical treatment of a cleft palate is euthanasia.

CLIENT EDUCATION

- Clients must understand that cleft palate is a severe, potentially life-threatening disease that should not be left untreated.
- Palatoplasty is a salvage procedure, and the animal may never become an athlete.
- Horses that are successfully treated should be excluded from the gene pool because the disease is congenital in nature.

SUGGESTED READING

Kirkham LE, Vasey JR: Surgical cleft soft palate repair in a foal. *Aust Vet J* 80:143–146, 2002.
Krause HR, Koene M, Rustemeyer J: Transoral endoscopically assisted closure of cleft palate in foals. *Plast Reconstr Surg* 122:166e–167e, 2008.
Sullivan EK, Parente EJ: Disorders of the pharynx. *Vet Clin North Am Equine Pract* 19:159–167, 2003.

AUTHOR: KARSTEN VELDE

EDITOR: ERIC J. PARENTE

Clostridiosis, Enteric

BASIC INFORMATION

DEFINITION

Enteric disease caused by infection with clostridial species, primarily *Clostridium perfringens* and *Clostridium difficile*

SYNONYM(S)

- Necrotizing enterocolitis (typically associated with *C. perfringens*)
- Pseudomembranous colitis (typically associated with *C. difficile*)

EPIDEMIOLOGY

RISK FACTORS Antimicrobial use
CONTAGION AND ZOONOSIS

- Occurrence is often sporadic, but outbreaks have been described on farms and in veterinary hospitals. Therefore isolation of affected horses and use of barrier precautions, such as dedicated clothes and gloves, are recommended.
- Both *C. perfringens* and *C. difficile* are recognized enteropathogens in humans. Although direct transmission

between horses and humans has not been documented, horses should be treated as if infectious and control measures implemented (barrier precautions, hand hygiene, disinfectants).

CLINICAL PRESENTATION

DISEASE FORMS/SUBTYPES

- Variable signs depending on several factors, including the region of the gastrointestinal (GI) tract that is affected
- Acute colitis most common
- Proximal enteritis

HISTORY, CHIEF COMPLAINT

- Diarrhea is the most common complaint
- Colic
- Occasionally, sudden death

PHYSICAL EXAM FINDINGS

- Colitis
  - Diarrhea
  - Anorexia, pyrexia
  - Variable degrees of dehydration, toxemia, colic

- Cases that involve only the small intestine or cecum may exhibit similar signs without diarrhea.
- Cases that involve the proximal small intestine may present with significant reflux.

ETIOLOGY AND PATHOPHYSIOLOGY

- Gram-positive, anaerobic bacteria in the genus *Clostridium*, primarily *C. difficile* and *C. perfringens*.
- Transmission is by ingestion; disease is caused by the proliferation of toxigenic strains in the intestinal tract.
- Toxin production results in enterocolitis.
- *C. difficile*: primarily toxin A (enterotoxin) and toxin B (cytotoxin).
  - Approximately 13% of equine isolates do not produce any toxin and are nonpathogenic; most pathogenic isolates produce both toxin A and B.
  - Age influences colonization rates: subclinical carriage of *C. difficile* has been reported in 29% of foals younger than 14 days of age but in

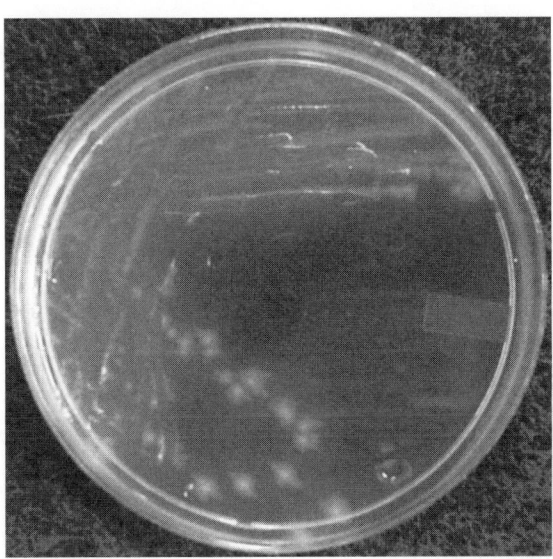

FIGURE 1 Colony morphology of *Clostridium difficile* on a cycloserine-cefoxitin fructose agar, a selective and differential culture medium used for isolation of *C. difficile*. (From Sellon DC, Long MT: *Equine infectious diseases*. St. Louis, Saunders, 2007.)

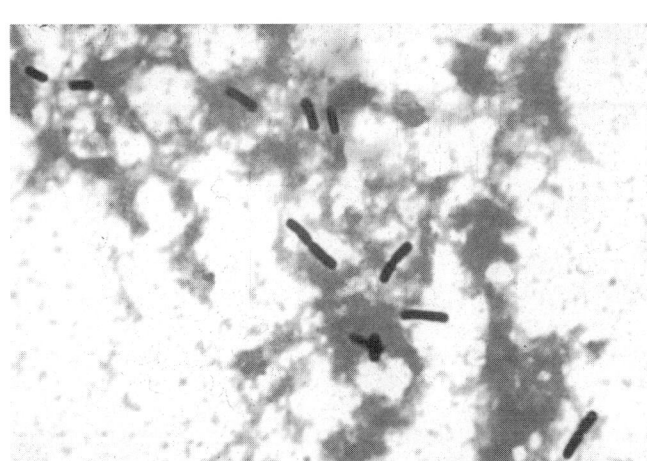

FIGURE 3 Gram stain appearance of *Clostridium perfringens*, demonstrating the characteristic appearance of short, thick, gram-positive rods. (From Sellon DC, Long MT: *Equine infectious diseases*. St. Louis, Saunders, 2007.)

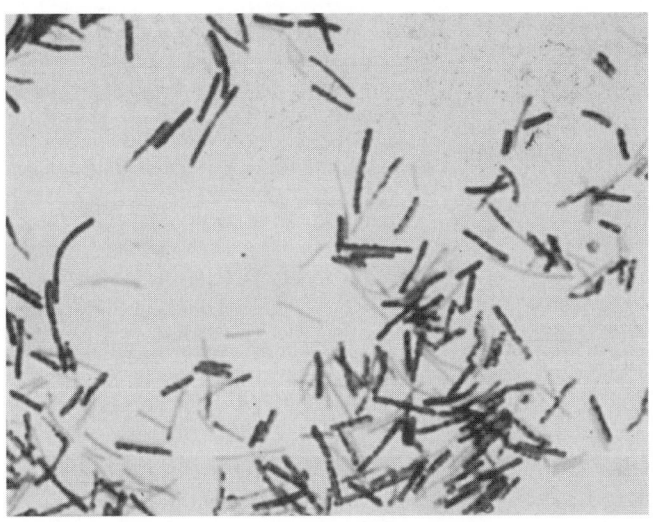

FIGURE 2 Gram stain morphology of *Clostridium difficile*. Note the long, thin rods. The variable staining appearance may be encountered in cultures over 48 hours or longer. (From Sellon DC, Long MT: *Equine infectious diseases*. St. Louis, Saunders, 2007.)

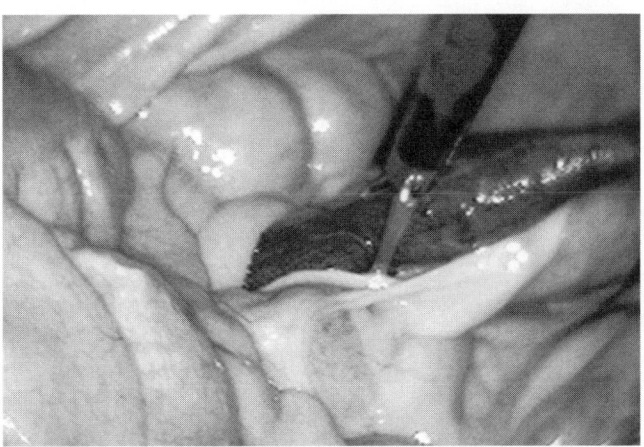

FIGURE 4 *Clostridium difficile* colitis. Note the widespread petechial and ecchymotic hemorrhages consistent with disseminated intravascular coagulation. (From Sellon DC, Long MT: *Equine infectious diseases*. St. Louis, Saunders, 2007.)

less than 1% of older foals and normal adults.
- *C. perfringens*: classified into different types based on the pattern of toxin production; β-2 toxin and enterotoxin may be the most important clinically.
  - A normal inhabitant of the equine GI tract found in 19% to 35% of broodmares and more than 90% of 3-day-old foals
  - Type A: predominant type in normal horses and horses with diarrhea
  - Type C: has been associated with severe enterocolitis, especially in foals
  - Limited reports of disease associated with types B and D

DIAGNOSIS

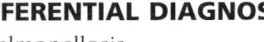

DIFFERENTIAL DIAGNOSIS
- Salmonellosis
- *Neorickettsia risticii* (Potomac horse fever)
- Cantharidin toxicity
- Parasitism
- *Aeromonas*, *Campylobacter*, and *Lawsonia* spp.
- Other antibiotic-associated diarrhea
- Sand
- Thromboembolic disease
- Anaphylaxis
- Undiagnosed colitis
- Additional differentials in foals
  - Rotavirus, coronavirus
  - Foal heat diarrhea
  - Cryptosporidiosis
  - Associated with septicemia
  - Secondary lactose intolerance

INITIAL DATABASE
- Clinicopathologic abnormalities: non-specific; consistent with dehydration and endotoxemia from diarrhea and mucosal damage
  - Leukopenia, neutropenia
  - Elevated packed cell volume (PCV), variable total protein (TP); hypoproteinemia often develops
  - Acid-base and electrolyte abnormalities consistent with diarrhea
- Although clostridial diarrhea in neonatal foals is not generally associated with failure of passive transfer, it is

recommended to evaluate affected foals for antibody concentration and the presence of septicemia.
- Abdominal ultrasonography may reveal ileus or a thickened intestinal wall; occasionally, intramural gas is seen (may also be seen radiographically in foals).

ADVANCED OR CONFIRMATORY TESTING

- Culture: not diagnostic by itself because of the presence of nonpathogenic isolates and the presence in some normal horses, especially with *C. perfringens*; culture samples should be handled anaerobically.
- *C. difficile* toxin detection in feces (toxins stable in refrigerated or frozen samples)
  - Cell cytotoxicity assay (toxin B): Considered the gold standard but not available in some laboratories
  - Enzyme immunoassays (EIA) to detect toxin A or B: Rapid and frequently used, but sensitivity and specificity in horses are not well established
  - Polymerase chain reaction for toxin genes after culture
- *C. perfringens*
  - Genotyping of isolates to determine the strain and, identify specific toxin genes
  - Detection of toxin in feces: Commercial EIA for enterotoxin; sensitivity and specificity in horses are not known

TREATMENT

THERAPEUTIC GOAL(S)

- Resolution of enterocolitis
- Maintenance of physiologic homeostasis of water and electrolyte balance
- Amelioration of clinical effects of systemic inflammatory response syndrome

ACUTE GENERAL TREATMENT

- Specific antimicrobial therapy: Drug choice is most often based on historical information because antimicrobial sensitivity testing for *Clostridium* spp. is not routine in many laboratories. However, antimicrobial resistance has been documented in *Clostridium* spp., and sensitivity testing is recommended in refractory cases.
  - Metronidazole (15 mg/kg PO q8h): Generally considered the drug of

choice; resistance has been identified infrequently
  - Vancomycin has been used in cases with metronidazole resistance; consider use carefully because of the importance of vancomycin in the treatment of resistant bacteria in human medicine
  - Zinc bacitracin is effective against *C. perfringens* but resistance is common in *C. difficile*
- Di-tri-octahedral smectite (BioSponge, Platinum Performance, Belton, CA.) adsorbs clostridial toxins and endotoxin in vitro.
- *Saccharomyces boulardii* (25 g PO q12h) may be useful in the management of horses with acute enterocolitis.
- Supportive care for diarrhea
  - Treatment for dehydration and electrolyte and acid-base abnormalities
  - Treatment for associated systemic inflammatory response syndrome (endotoxemia).
  - Broad-spectrum systemic antibiotic therapy in horses with colitis is controversial.
    - Sometimes used to prophylactically control potential bacteremia from translocation of bacteria across the damaged intestinal mucosa.
    - If diarrhea developed while the horse is on antibiotics, discontinuing or changing those antibiotics is suggested.

POSSIBLE COMPLICATIONS

- Laminitis
- Thrombophlebitis
- Peritonitis

RECOMMENDED MONITORING

- Attitude, vital parameters, diarrhea
- PCV, TP
- Hydration status, renal function
- Acid-base and electrolyte abnormalities

PROGNOSIS AND OUTCOME

- Prognosis is variable depending on the strain and host factors.
- A mortality rate of up to 42% has been reported with *C. difficile*; prognosis may be worse in adults than foals.

- Prognosis is guarded in foals with *C. perfringens*, especially type C; the mortality rate is approximately 50%.

PEARLS & CONSIDERATIONS

COMMENTS

Enteric clostridiosis is an important cause of enterocolitis in horses, accounting for approximately 40% of cases in some studies.

PREVENTION

- Careful use of antimicrobials.
- Clostridial spores are often present in the environment; good management practices, including regular cleaning and disinfection of stalls and equipment, will limit the environmental burden.
- There is no approved vaccine for horses. Anecdotally, vaccines approved in other species for the prevention of *C. perfringens*–associated disease have been used in horses; no data currently support their use.

CLIENT EDUCATION

Clients should be made aware of the risk of antibiotic-associated diarrhea and should be counseled to call their veterinarian if diarrhea occurs.

SUGGESTED READING

Baverud V: Clostridium difficile diarrhea: infection control in horses. *Vet Clin North Am Equine Pract* 20:615, 2004.

Lawler JB, Hassel DM, Magnuson RJ, et al: Adsorptive effects of di-tri-octahedral smectite on *Clostridium perfringens* alpha, beta, and beta-2 exotoxins and equine colostral antibodies. *Am J Vet Res* 69:233–239, 2008.

Magdesian KG, Dujowich M, Madigan JE, et al: Molecular characterization of *Clostridium difficile* isolates from horses in an intensive care unit and association of disease severity with strain type. *J Am Vet Med Assoc* 228:751–755, 2006.

Weese JS, Staempfli HR, Prescott JF: A prospective study of the roles of *Clostridium difficile* and enterotoxigenic *Clostridium perfringens* in equine diarrhea. *Equine Vet J* 33:403–409, 2001.

Weese JS, Toxopeus L, Arroyo L: *Clostridium difficile* associated diarrhoea in horses within the community: predictors, clinical presentation and outcome. *Equine Vet J* 38:185–188, 2006.

AUTHOR: MELISSA T. HINES

EDITORS: MAUREEN T. LONG and **DEBRA C. SELLON**

Clover Toxicosis

BASIC INFORMATION

DEFINITION

Clover toxicity is caused by ingestion of alsike clover (*Trifolium hybridum*) or red clover (*Trifolium pratense*), resulting in signs of photosensitivity and liver failure.

SYNONYM(S)

- Dew poisoning
- Trifoliosis
- Big liver disease

EPIDEMIOLOGY

RISK FACTORS Consumption of pasture or hay containing alsike or red clover

GEOGRAPHY AND SEASONALITY

- Found mainly in Canada and the northwestern United States
- Most cases occur from April to November
- Associated with a wet spring

CLINICAL PRESENTATION

DISEASE FORMS/SUBTYPES

- Photosensitization
- Chronic hepatic disease
- Chronic wasting and failure to thrive

HISTORY, CHIEF COMPLAINT

- Owners may observe a necrotizing dermatitis primarily affecting white skin, weakness, weight loss, anorexia, ataxia, and behavior changes.
- History of consumption of alsike or red clover hay or pasture.

PHYSICAL EXAM FINDINGS Icterus, photosensitivity dermatitis, ulceration of mucous membranes, hepatic encephalopathy, weight loss

ETIOLOGY AND PATHOPHYSIOLOGY

- Alsike or red clover ingestion resulting in bile duct proliferation and perilobular (periportal) fibrosis.
- Photosensitization is the result of systemic accumulation of the chlorophyll metabolite phylloerythrin that is not removed by the diseased liver. Phylloerythrin is a photodynamic agent that absorbs ultraviolent radiation, particularly in unpigmented skin, leading to skin necrosis.
- Signs develop 2 to 4 weeks after ingestion.

- The exact toxin(s) are not known, although fungal infection of the clover with *Cymodothea trifolii* increases the risk of liver disease.

DIAGNOSIS

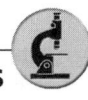

DIFFERENTIAL DIAGNOSIS

- Chronic megalocytic hepatopathy
- Aflatoxicosis
- Cholelithiasis
- Chronic active hepatitis
- Cholangiohepatitis
- Any cause of primary or secondary photosensitization

INITIAL DATABASE

- Complete blood count: Typically normal
- Gamma glutamyltransferase (GGT), alkaline phosphatase (ALP, aspartate aminotransferase (AST), and sorbitol dehydrogenase (SDH) activity: Increased
- Hyperglobulinemia: May be present if chronic
- Serum bile acids concentration: Increased
- Total bilirubin concentration: Increased
- Direct bilirubin concentration: Increased; often more than 25% of total
- Coagulation times: May be prolonged
- Plasma ammonia concentration: May be increased
- Urinalysis: Bilirubinuria

ADVANCED OR CONFIRMATORY TESTING

- Ultrasonography: Hepatomegaly or a small, difficult-to-find liver; distended bile ducts
- Liver biopsy: Periportal, centrolobular to perilobular fibrosis that typically spares the sinusoids; biliary hyperplasia, bile stasis, mild megalocytosis, and inflammatory cells may be present

TREATMENT

THERAPEUTIC GOAL(S)

Palliative

ACUTE GENERAL TREATMENT

- See treatment for "Hepatic Encephalopathy" in this section.
- For photosensitization, avoid sunlight. Topical or systemic antiinflammatory or antimicrobial agents (or both) may be necessary if skin lesions are severe.

CHRONIC TREATMENT

See treatment for "Hepatic Encephalopathy" in this section.

POSSIBLE COMPLICATIONS

Hepatic encephalopathy, photosensitivity dermatitis

RECOMMENDED MONITORING

- Monitor GGT activity and serum bile acid concentrations.
- Perform serial liver biopsies.

PROGNOSIS AND OUTCOME

Fair to grave, depending on the degree of hepatic fibrosis

PEARLS & CONSIDERATIONS

COMMENTS

A diet with 20% alsike clover hay has been associated with disease.

PREVENTION

Ensure clover hay is less than 20% of the diet (avoid completely if possible).

CLIENT EDUCATION

Remove the source of alsike clover (herbicidal treatment and reseed pasture; provide new source of hay)

SUGGESTED READING

Nation NP: Alsike clover poisoning: a review. *Can Vet J* 30:410, 1989.
Talcott P: Alsike clover (*Trifolium hybridum*) and red clover (*Trifolium pratense*) poisonings in horses. *18th ACVIM Forum Proceedings* 161–162, 2000.

AUTHOR: HEIDI BANSE

EDITOR: MICHELLE HENRY BARTON

Coccidioidomycosis

BASIC INFORMATION

DEFINITION

A systemic fungal infection of equids and other mammals that may result in pneumonia, osteomyelitis, mastitis, abortion, or superficial or internal abscessation.

EPIDEMIOLOGY

CONTAGION AND ZOONOSIS

- Horses and humans acquire disease by inhalation of arthroconidia or rarely through the skin.
- Horse-to-horse and horse-to-human transmission is very rare. However, there is one report of a veterinarian developing fatal disease after attending the necropsy of a horse with disseminated coccidioidomycosis.

GEOGRAPHY AND SEASONALITY

- Indigenous to the southwestern and western United States and areas of Mexico, Central America, and South America between 40 degrees south latitude and 40 degrees north latitude
- Areas with significant problems often have hot, dry summers with relatively mild winters and moderate rainfall.
- Cases are most common in late summer and fall.

CLINICAL PRESENTATION

DISEASE FORMS/SUBTYPES

- Respiratory disease is common because infection is usually acquired by inhalation.
- Systemic dissemination may occur, leading to disease in a variety of locations.
- Cutaneous inoculation may cause localized subcutaneous infection.

HISTORY, CHIEF COMPLAINT

- Fever, weight loss
- Signs reflecting an internal site of infection
  - Respiratory tract infection: Increased respiratory rate, cough, dyspnea
  - Osteomyelitis: Pain, lameness, neurologic signs
  - Abdominal infection: Colic
  - Subcutaneous infection: Abscess, chronic draining tracts
  - Respiratory tract: Abortion, placentitis

PHYSICAL EXAM FINDINGS Vary to reflect the site of infection

ETIOLOGY AND PATHOPHYSIOLOGY

- *Coccidioides immitis* is a diphasic, pleomorphic mold and fungus.
- The saprobic phase is found in nature and in culture.
  - Hyphae differentiate into chains of arthroconidia (spores).
  - Mammalian infection occurs by inhalation of arthroconidia.
- Inside the host, arthroconidia transform to spherules, which release endospores to form more spherules.
- Spherules and endospores induce a neutrophil and macrophage response with development of suppurative-granulomatous lesions.
- Growth elicits host antibody response to chitinase enzyme that is released as spherules mature and release endospores.

DIAGNOSIS

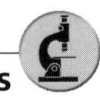

DIFFERENTIAL DIAGNOSIS

- Respiratory infection
  - Bacterial pneumonia, pleuropneumonia
  - Other fungal pneumonias
  - Pulmonary abscess
  - Interstitial pneumonia
  - Pulmonary nodular fibrosis (equine herpesvirus-5)
- Systemic infection
  - Abdominal abscess
  - Strangles (*Streptococcus equi* subsp. *equi*)
  - Pigeon fever (*Corynebacterium pseudotuberculosis*)
  - Other bacterial or fungal forms of osteomyelitis
  - Abortion secondary to bacterial or fungal endometritis, nocardioform infection, leptospirosis
- Cutaneous infection
  - Subcutaneous bacterial or fungal abscesses
  - Sporotrichosis
  - *Corynebacterium pseudotuberculosis*

INITIAL DATABASE

- Mild to moderate anemia
- Leukocytosis caused by mature neutrophilia
- Hyperfibrinogenemia
- Hyperglobulinemia
- Monocytosis
- Thrombocytosis

ADVANCED OR CONFIRMATORY TESTING

- Imaging such as radiography or ultrasonography depending on the site of suspected infection
- Direct demonstration of organism in tracheobronchial aspirates, exudates, or tissues
- Culture of appropriate tissues, exudates, or tracheobronchial aspirates

- Serum antibody testing by immuno-diffusion or enzyme immunoassay. Higher titers are seen in horses with disseminated disease or pneumonia with thoracic effusion compared with horses with abortion, bone involvement only, or cutaneous infection.

TREATMENT

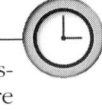

THERAPEUTIC GOAL(S)

Eliminate infection through a combination of surgical and medical therapy.

ACUTE GENERAL TREATMENT

- Surgical removal of lesions if possible
- Preferred antifungal therapy may be fluconazole (10 mg/kg PO loading dose followed by 5 mg/kg PO q24h).
- Alternative antifungal medications include amphotericin B, ketoconazole, itraconazole, and voriconazole.

CHRONIC TREATMENT

Antifungal therapy may be required for months or years.

POSSIBLE COMPLICATIONS

Amphotericin B is nephrotoxic and irritating when administered IV and should be used with caution.

RECOMMENDED MONITORING

Increasing serum antibody titer generally indicates worsening disease.

PROGNOSIS AND OUTCOME

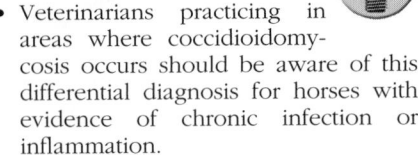

- Guarded prognosis; successful treatment may require considerable time and expense.
- Horses with higher titers may have a poorer prognosis.

PEARLS & CONSIDERATIONS

- Veterinarians practicing in areas where coccidioidomycosis occurs should be aware of this differential diagnosis for horses with evidence of chronic infection or inflammation.
- Rising titers in a horse with evidence of chronic infection or inflammation should be considered diagnostic of

coccidioidomycosis even if the actual site of infection cannot be identified.

SUGGESTED READING

Higgins JC, Leith GS, Pappagianis D, Pusterla N: Treatment of *Coccidioides immitis* pneu-monia in two horses with fluconazole. *Vet Rec* 159:349, 2006.

Higgins JC, Pusterla N, Pappagianis D: Comparison of *Coccidioides immitis* serological antibody titers between forms of clinical coccidioidomycosis in horses. *Vet J* 173:118, 2007.

Pappagianis D, Higgins J: Coccidioidomycosis. In Sellon DC, Long MT, editors: *Equine Infectious Diseases.* St Louis, 2007, Elsevier, pp 396–404.

AUTHOR & EDITOR: DEBRA C. SELLON

Cocklebur Toxicosis

BASIC INFORMATION

DEFINITION

Cockleburs (*Xanthium* spp.) are common weeds throughout North America with the capability of causing acute liver failure in pigs, cattle, sheep, poultry, and occasionally horses. Pigs are most frequently affected.

SYNONYM(S)

There are three species of cocklebur: *Xanthium strumarium*, *Xanthium spinosum*, and *Xanthium ambrosioides*. Common names include ditch bur, sheep bur, bur thistle, and abrojo.

EPIDEMIOLOGY

RISK FACTORS
- Young animals
- Cocklebur seedlings in the spring

GEOGRAPHY AND SEASONALITY
- The most common cocklebur, *X. strumarium*, is found throughout North America.
- Poisoning in animals occurs most often in the spring and summer when growing conditions favor germination of the seedlings.
- The mature plants are prolific bur producers; consequently, massive numbers of seedlings may germinate at once, increasing the potential for poisoning to occur.
- Cockleburs are annual erect, branching plants up to 6 feet in height with a taproot. The leaves are large and simple and alternate with serrated edges. Flowers are produced in leaf axils or terminally on branches. Characteristic burs turn brown when mature (Figure 1).

ASSOCIATED CONDITIONS AND DISORDERS
- Cocklebur poisoning can mimic other hepatotoxins, including alsike clover and cyanobacteria toxin poisoning.
- Animals that survive acute cocklebur poisoning may develop chronic liver disease that may mimic pyrrolizidine alkaloid poisoning.

CLINICAL PRESENTATION

HISTORY, CHIEF COMPLAINT
- Owners may observe acute onset of anorexia, depression, weakness, and colic.
- Death may be the only presenting sign.

PHYSICAL EXAM FINDINGS
- Anorexia, depression, weakness, ataxia, spasms of the cervical muscles, dyspnea, and convulsions may be observed.
- Death may occur within hours of the onset of signs.
- Animals that survive acute poisoning often develop signs of chronic liver disease.

ETIOLOGY AND PATHOPHYSIOLOGY
- Cocklebur poisoning generally causes acute liver failure.
- Carboxyatractyloside, a sulfated diterpene glycoside, is the primary hepatotoxin. It primarily acts by inhibiting oxidative phosphorylation at the mitochondria.
- The two-leafed (cotyledonary) stage of the seedling poses the highest risk, with the highest toxin concentrations in the two cotyledons within the bur (0.46%).
- Ingestion of 0.75 to 3.0% of body weight of cotyledonary seedlings causes acute toxicity.

- As seedlings develop past the two-leafed stage, their toxicity rapidly decreases.
- Mature plants with multiple burs are toxic but are rarely palatable.

DIAGNOSIS

DIFFERENTIAL DIAGNOSIS
- Ingestion of Alsike clover, *Nolina texana, Agave lechuguilla, Phyllanthus abnormis,* and *Lantana camara*
- Ingestion of Klein grass
- Ingestion of plants containing pyrrolizidine alkaloids
- Ingestion of cyanobacteria (blue-green algae)
- Ingestion of gossypol

INITIAL DATABASE
- Blood glucose: Severe hypoglycemia
- Serum hepatic enzymes: Markedly elevated

ADVANCED OR CONFIRMATORY TESTING
- Assay for carboxyatractyloside in stomach contents, blood, urine, and aqueous humor
- Gross necropsy: Swollen liver, pulmonary edema, hydrothorax, hydropericardium

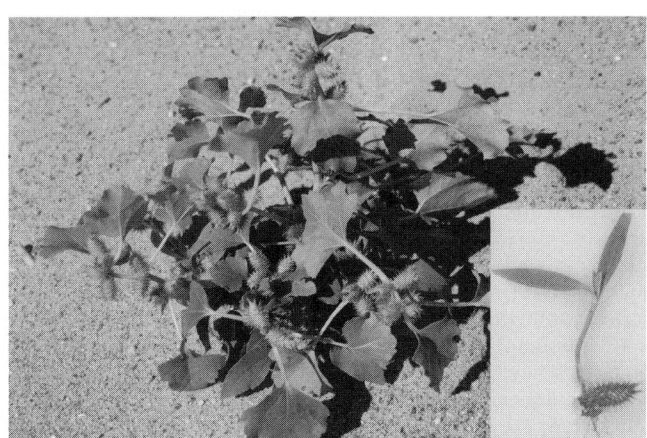

FIGURE 1 Cocklebur and two-leafed seedling (inset).

- Histology: Severe diffuse centrilobular hepatocellular necrosis

TREATMENT

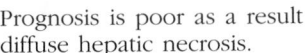

THERAPEUTIC GOAL(S)

Acute cocklebur poisoning is seldom treatable because of the acute nature of the toxicity.

ACUTE GENERAL TREATMENT

Early treatment with activated charcoal via a nasogastric tube may decrease absorption of the toxin.

CHRONIC TREATMENT

Supportive therapy

PROGNOSIS AND OUTCOME

Prognosis is poor as a result of diffuse hepatic necrosis.

PEARLS & CONSIDERATIONS

COMMENTS

Cocklebur poisoning in horses is rarely reported, but because of the invasiveness of the plants the potential for poisoning can be high. Germination of massive numbers of cocklebur seedlings in late summer in the muddy shores of ponds or flooded areas poses a high risk.

CLIENT EDUCATION

- Learn to recognize cocklebur plants and burs.
- Remove the plants before they produce seeds.
- Mechanically cultivate, mow, or use appropriate herbicides on the seedlings.

SUGGESTED READING

Burrows GE, Tyrl RJ: Xanthium. In Burrows GE, Tyrl RJ, editors: *Toxic plants of North America.* Ames, IA, 2001, Iowa State University Press, pp 214–218.

Knight AP, Walter RG: *A guide to poisoning of animals in North America.* Jackson, WY, 2001, Teton New Media, pp 167–168.

Stuart BP, Cole RJ, Gosser HS: Cocklebur (*Xanthium strumarium* L. var. *strumarium*) intoxication in swine: review and redefinition of the toxic principle. *Vet Pathol* 18:368–383, 1981.

Witte ST, Osweiler GD, Stahr HM, et al: Cocklebur toxicosis in cattle associated with the consumption of mature *Xanthium strumarium. J Vet Diag Invest* 2:263–267, 1990.

AUTHOR: **ANTHONY P. KNIGHT**

EDITOR: **CYNTHIA L. GASKILL**

Colitis, Antimicrobial Associated

BASIC INFORMATION

DEFINITION

Colitis or diarrhea that occurs during or shortly after administration of antimicrobial drugs

EPIDEMIOLOGY

RISK FACTORS

Antimicrobial administration:
- May occur with any antimicrobial drug but most often associated with:
  - Macrolides and lincosamides (erythromycin, clarithromycin, azithromycin, lincomycin, and clindamycin) in adult horses and foals older than 6 months of age
    - Diarrhea has also been reported in mares whose young foals were receiving erythromycin for treatment of *Rhodococcus equi* infection, presumably because of exposure to erythromycin in the foals' feces.
  - Trimethoprim-sulfamethoxazole
  - Ceftiofur
  - Metronidazole
  - Doxycycline or enrofloxacin, although development of diarrhea with these antimicrobials seems to have some regional specificity
- Changing from one class of antimicrobial to another or concurrent hospitalization, surgery, or gastrointestinal

disease may increase the likelihood of development of antimicrobial-associated diarrhea.

CLINICAL PRESENTATION

HISTORY, CHIEF COMPLAINT
- Recent or ongoing antimicrobial administration
- Inappetence, colic, fever and diarrhea are most common, as for other causes of colitis (see "Colitis/Diarrhea, Acute" in this section).

PHYSICAL EXAM FINDINGS As for other causes of colitis (see "Colitis/Diarrhea, Acute" in this section)

ETIOLOGY AND PATHOPHYSIOLOGY
- Antimicrobial-associated diarrhea presumably results from alteration in the normal colonic bacterial flora, allowing overgrowth of or colonization with a pathogenic bacterial species.
- Overgrowth of toxin-producing *Clostridium difficile* strains has been documented in some horses with antimicrobial-associated colitis, although salmonellosis or diarrhea caused by an overgrowth of an unidentified pathogen may also occur.
- Infection with a pathogenic bacterial species results in damage to and disruption of the colonic mucosal barrier as for other causes of diarrhea (see "Colitis/Diarrhea, Acute" and "Diarrhea, Clostridial" in this section), resulting in fluid, electrolyte, and

protein losses and diarrhea as well as signs of endotoxemia and colic.
- Clinical signs are typically, but not always, seen within 1 to 7 days of initiating antimicrobial therapy.

DIAGNOSIS

DIFFERENTIAL DIAGNOSIS

Other causes of colitis (see "Colitis/Diarrhea, Acute" in this section)

INITIAL DATABASE

As for other causes of colitis (see "Colitis/Diarrhea, Acute" in this section)

ADVANCED OR CONFIRMATORY TESTING

A presumptive diagnosis of antimicrobial-associated diarrhea is made when a horse develops signs of acute colitis during antimicrobial therapy. However, testing for clostridial toxin production and *Salmonella* infection should be performed (see "Diarrhea, Clostridial" and "Salmonellosis" in this section).

TREATMENT

THERAPEUTIC GOAL(S)

- Provide supportive care.
- Promote reestablishment of normal colonic flora.

ACUTE GENERAL TREATMENT

- Provide fluid and colloidal support, antiinflammatory and antiendotoxic therapy, and other supportive care as for other causes of colitis (see "Colitis/Diarrhea, Acute" in this section).
- Current antimicrobial therapy should be discontinued and antimicrobials avoided even in severely leukopenic patients if at all possible, with the potential exception of:
  - Metronidazole (15–25 mg/kg PO or PR q8h), which is indicated if the horse was not on metronidazole when the signs developed or if clostridial toxins are detected in the feces.
- Dietary support is critical because provision of adequate roughage in the form of pasture, hay, or easily digestible fiber will aid in facilitating reestablishment of normal colonic flora. All efforts should be made to encourage the horse to eat and to stimulate its appetite.
- Other therapy, including probiotics (eg, *Saccharomyces boulardii*), or di-tri-octahedral smectite (Bio-Sponge), may be beneficial in antimicrobial-associated colitis as for other causes of colitis (see "Colitis/Diarrhea, Acute" and "Diarrhea, Clostridial" in this section).

POSSIBLE COMPLICATIONS

As for other causes of colitis (see "Colitis/Diarrhea, Acute" in this section)

PROGNOSIS AND OUTCOME

- Fair to good with good clinical response to discontinuing antimicrobials and supportive care
- Guarded to poor with colitis associated with macrolide or lincosamide administration in adult horses (which is often rapidly fatal)

PEARLS & CONSIDERATIONS

- Even though *C. difficile* is considered to play a role in many cases of antimicrobial-associated colitis, some horses do develop diarrhea while taking metronidazole. In these cases, another pathogen (or potentially a metronidazole-resistant strain of *Clostridium* spp.) may be the cause of the diarrhea, so metronidazole should be discontinued and fecal testing for clostridial toxins performed.
- Vancomycin has been effective in treating metronidazole-resistant clostridial organisms in horses, although its use in veterinary medicine is controversial.

SUGGESTED READING

Jones SJ: Medical disorders of the large intestine: acute diarrhea. In Smith BP, editor: *Large Animal Internal Medicine.* St Louis, 2009, Mosby, pp 745–774.

AUTHOR: **KELSEY A. HART**

EDITOR: **TIM MAIR**

Colitis/Diarrhea, Acute

BASIC INFORMATION

DEFINITION

Inflammation of the colon

EPIDEMIOLOGY

RISK FACTORS

- Stress: shipping, routine changes, illness, hospitalization
- Recent diet changes
- Recent antimicrobial administration
- Nonsteroidal antiinflammatory drug (NSAID) therapy

CLINICAL PRESENTATION

HISTORY, CHIEF COMPLAINT

- Usually, the horse has a history of depression, fever, inappetence, and mild colic signs, with or without diarrhea, lasting hours to days.
- Occasionally, the horse has an acute onset of severe colic signs and rapid systemic deterioration in the absence of diarrhea. Rarely, in peracute cases, horses are simply found dead.

PHYSICAL EXAM FINDINGS

- Depression
- Variable signs of abdominal pain ranging from none to mild colic or inappetence to severe intractable colic
- Pyrexia
- Variable tachycardia (normal to 80–100 beats/min)
- Variable tachypnea
- Mucous membranes are often injected and may vary in color from bright pink to purple-gray.
- Capillary refill time may range from brisk (<1 second) in the early stages to dramatically prolonged (4–5 seconds) as severe dehydration and endotoxic or septic shock progress.
- There may be evidence of hypovolemia and poor peripheral perfusion (cold extremities, poor jugular refill) in severe cases.
- Hypermotile, "fluidy" gastrointestinal borborygmi
- Gross abdominal distension is occasionally present, especially in severe or peracute cases.
- Diarrhea may be absent or range from soft, formed feces to profuse, watery, or hemorrhagic diarrhea.
- Rectal examination
  - Should be performed in all horses with signs of colic or abdominal distension because concurrent colonic displacements or large or small colon impactions may occur in horses with colitis.
  - Edematous rectal mucosa and fluid colonic contents are often appreciated even when rectal findings are otherwise normal.

ETIOLOGY AND PATHOPHYSIOLOGY

- Initially, the colonic mucosal barrier is damaged focally or diffusely by one of the following:
  - Bacteria in the intestinal lumen, including:
    - Invasion of a primary pathogen (eg, *Salmonella*, *Neorickettsia risticii*)
    - Overgrowth of or toxin production from a potentially pathogenic organism normally present in low numbers (*Clostridium difficile* and *Clostridium perfringens*) caused by alterations in normal enteric flora associated with stress, dietary changes, or antimicrobial administration
  - Intestinal parasitic infection
  - Toxin ingestion (cantharidin)
  - Altered colonic mural perfusion and mucus production with NSAID therapy
  - Colonic sand accumulation
- Loss of the colonic mucosal barrier allows intraluminal bacteria and bacterial toxins (eg, endotoxin) to invade the colonic wall, stimulating mural inflammation and edema.

- Bacteria and bacterial toxins are also then able to enter the intestinal lymphatic system and systemic circulation, resulting in clinical signs of endotoxemia and the systemic inflammatory response syndrome (fever, tachycardia, tachypnea, congested mucous membranes, and altered hemodynamic status and peripheral perfusion).
- In addition, the damaged mucosal barrier compromises colonic absorptive capacity, resulting in loss of water and electrolytes in the feces, and may permit loss of plasma proteins if the damage is severe.
- See sections "Cyathostominosis," "Salmonellosis," "Diarrhea, Clostridial," "Potomac Horse Fever," "Nonsteroidal Antiinflammatory Drug Toxicity," "Colitis, Antimicrobial Associated," "Colitis X," "Blister Beetles," and "Sand Enteropathy" in this section for more details.

DIAGNOSIS

DIFFERENTIAL DIAGNOSIS

- Salmonellosis
- Clostridial diarrhea
- Potomac horse fever
- Cyathostominosis
- NSAID toxicity
- Antimicrobial-associated colitis
- Colitis X
- Cantharidin toxicity
- Sand enteropathy

INITIAL DATABASE

- Complete blood count
  - Leukopenia characterized by neutropenia with increased band neutrophils and toxic changes in neutrophils is typically seen.
  - The hematocrit varies with hydration status but may be markedly increased (>60%) in severe cases.
  - Thrombocytopenia is occasionally present in severe cases with concurrent disseminated intravascular coagulation.
- Serum biochemistry profile
  - Variable electrolyte derangements are common, with hypokalemia, hyponatremia, hypochloremia, and hypocalcemia most common.
  - Serum total protein concentration may be increased with dehydration or normal or low with enteric loss.
  - Variable azotemia is common and may be caused by prerenal or renal causes (or both).
  - Hyperlactatemia (>2 mmol/L) suggests impaired peripheral perfusion and tissue oxygenation caused by hypovolemia.
  - Metabolic acidosis is often present and may be associated with hyper-

lactatemia, bicarbonate loss in the feces, or both.
- Transabdominal ultrasonography
  - Fluid contents in the colon or cecum are often appreciated.
  - Colonic mural thickness may be increased (>5 mm) focally or diffusely.
- Peritoneal fluid analysis
  - Should be performed in horses that have persistent signs of colic, fever, or leukopenia because peritonitis resulting from translocation of intestinal bacteria or, less often, infarction of the colonic vasculature may occur in severe colitis.
  - In most horses with colitis, grossly normal-appearing peritoneal fluid with a normal nucleated cell count and mildly increased protein concentration (>2 g/dL) is observed.

ADVANCED OR CONFIRMATORY TESTING

- Diagnostic testing for specific causes of colitis in adult horses should include the following:
  - Fecal flotation for intestinal parasites
  - Fecal polymerase chain reaction (PCR) or culture for *Salmonella* spp.
  - Fecal Gram stain and fecal toxin assays for *C. perfringens* and *C. difficile* toxins
  - Serology or whole-blood PCR for Potomac horse fever
  - Fecal sedimentation and abdominal radiography for sand accumulation
  - Positive or negative urinanalysis for cantharidin
- See sections "Cyathostominosis," "Salmonellosis," "Diarrhea, Clostridial," "Potomac Horse Fever," "Sand Enteropathy," and "Blister Beetles" in this section for more details.

TREATMENT

THERAPEUTIC GOAL(S)

- Supportive care: fluid support, antiinflammatory therapy
- Specific therapy for certain causes

ACUTE GENERAL TREATMENT

- IV fluid therapy
  - Fluid resuscitation with hypertonic saline (2–4 mL/kg IV bolus) or hydroxyethyl starch (Hetastarch) (5–10 mL/kg IV bolus) is indicated in severely dehydrated patients.
  - This should be followed by isotonic balanced polyionic crystalloid fluids (eg, Normosol-R or Plasmalyte) at 50 to 150 mL/kg/day, depending on the degree of dehydration and ongoing losses in diarrhea.
  - Supplementation with potassium chloride (10–40 mEq/L with the rate not to exceed 0.05 mEq/kg/h),

23% calcium gluconate (1–2 mL/kg/day), or magnesium sulfate (20–25 g/450 kg/day) is often necessary to correct electrolyte derangements.
  - Administration of sodium bicarbonate may be necessary with severe metabolic acidosis (pH ≤7.1; serum bicarbonate concentration <15 mmol/L), but correction of dehydration often sufficiently corrects metabolic acidosis without the need for additional bicarbonate supplementation.
  - Colloidal support with equine plasma (20–40 mL/kg IV) or hydroxyethyl starch (5–10 mL/kg IV bolus q24–48h or 1 mL/kg/h IV continuous rate infusion [CRI]) is indicated in patients with hypoproteinemia. (Note: Patients with initially normal total protein concentrations may have hypoproteinemia after rehydration.)
  - Horses with colitis are particularly prone to thrombophlebitis. Long-term polyethylene IV catheters should be used and removed at the first sign of a problem with the catheter or vein.
- Antiinflammatory and analgesic therapy
  - Flunixin meglumine: 0.5 to 1.1 mg/kg IV q12h for colic; then decrease to 0.25 mg/kg IV q6–8h for antiinflammatory effects when signs of colic resolve. **Do not use in NSAID toxicity.**
  - Lidocaine: 1.3 mg/kg IV as a slow bolus; then 0.05 mg/kg/min IV CRI for persistent colic or as a primary analgesic in NSAID toxicity
  - Pentoxifylline: 8 mg/kg PO q8–12h (may decrease inflammatory cytokine production and may promote microvascular blood flow by rheologic and antiplatelet effects)
  - Dimethylsulfoxide (90% solution): 20 to 100 mg/kg diluted to less than 10% solution in IV fluids q12h for 1 to 3 days (may scavenge free radicals and limit oxidative injury)
- Antiendotoxic therapy
  - Equine plasma (2–4 L IV or more if hypoproteinemic, regular equine plasma, or hyperimmune plasma with antiendotoxin antibodies may be used) or hyperimmune antiendotoxin serum (Endoserum, 1–2 mL/kg diluted in 3–5 L isotonic fluids IV)
  - Polymyxin-B: 2000 to 6000 IU/kg (diluted in 500–1000 mL 0.9% saline) IV q12h for 1 to 3 days after the patient is hydrated and if renal function is adequate
- Laminitis prophylaxis
  - Placement of frog supports and maintenance in deep bedding should be initiated immediately.

- Periodic or continuous maintenance in ice boots during initial therapy may be helpful in preventing laminitis, although this is not universally accepted.
- If signs of laminitis occur, treatment should be rapid and aggressive (see "Laminitis, Acute" in this section).
- Intestinal absorbents
  - Bio-Sponge (di-tri-octahedral smectite) has been shown to absorb clostridial toxins and may absorb other bacterial toxins as well.
  - Activated charcoal or bismuth subsalicylate (4.5 mL/kg by nasogastric tube q6–12h) may provide similar benefits, although there is less evidence to support their use.
- Diet and nutritional support
  - It is important to encourage appetite and provide adequate nutritional support to horses with colitis. In general, horses with colitis that maintain a good appetite generally have a better prognosis than persistently inappetent or anorectic horses.
  - Early on, minimize concentrates and provide adequate roughage with good-quality grass hay and access to fresh pasture or grass if at all possible.
  - If NSAID toxicity or protracted diarrhea is present, provide a low-residue, easily digestible fiber source such as a complete pelleted equine senior feed.
  - Evaluation for or treatment of gastric ulceration should be considered in horses that are persistently inappetent.
- Antimicrobial therapy
  - Controversial because it can prevent reestablishment of normal enteric flora and does not appear to improve prognosis in most adult horses with colitis.
  - Specific antimicrobial therapy for clostridial diarrhea and Potomac horse fever and occasionally for salmonellosis is indicated (see "Potomac Horse Fever," "Diarrhea, Clostridial," and "Salmonellosis" in this section).
  - Broad-spectrum antimicrobial therapy is indicated in patients with peritonitis or in profoundly neutropenic patients (which are at greater risk of developing secondary infections such as pneumonia or septic thrombophlebitis). This therapy may include:
    - Potassium penicillin: 22,000 IU/kg IV q6h and gentamicin (6.6 mg/kg IV q24h) or enrofloxacin (5 mg/kg IV q24h)
    - Metronidazole: 15 to 25 mg/kg PO or PR may be used to provide

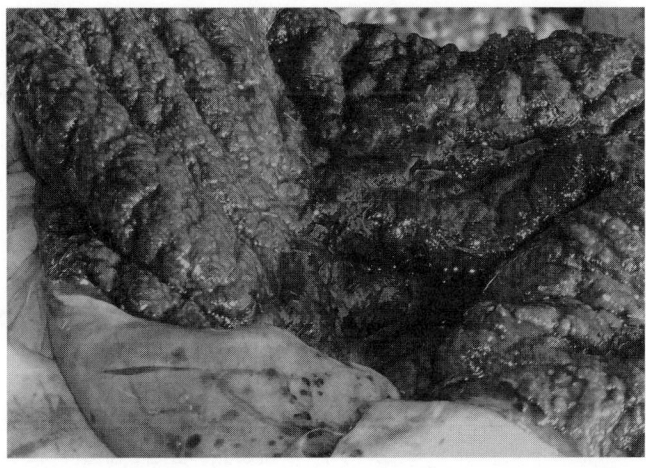

FIGURE 1 Acute colitis. Postmortem appearance of large colon showing severe inflammation and edema of the mucosa.

additional anaerobic coverage and may be beneficial in patients with suspected clostridial or antimicrobial-induced colitis.

- Other
  - Isolate the patient if at all possible. Minimize exposure of other horses to feces from the patient, clean the patient's stall last, and disinfect tools and equipment used on the affected horse.
  - Loosely wrapping or bagging the tail and daily cleaning of the hind limbs is necessary to prevent scald with severe diarrhea.
  - Probiotic therapy is controversial and not proven to be effective in equine diarrhea, although there is some evidence to support the use of products containing *Saccharomyces boulardii* in horses with colitis (see "Diarrhea, Clostridial" in this section).
  - Some evidence suggests that some horses with severe colitis may be hypercoagulable because of subclinical disseminated intravascular coagulation and thus are at greater risk of thrombotic complications. Heparin (20–40 IU/kg IV or SC q8h) may be beneficial in these cases.

POSSIBLE COMPLICATIONS
- Laminitis
- Thrombophlebitis
- Peritonitis
- Colonic infarction
- Colonic fibrosis and chronic diarrhea

RECOMMENDED MONITORING
Monitor the packed cell volume, total protein concentration, serum creatinine, and serum electrolyte concentrations closely during initial therapy and tailor fluid therapy accordingly.

PROGNOSIS AND OUTCOME
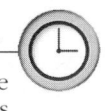

- Fair to good with adequate supportive care in patients that maintain a good appetite
- Guarded with concurrent laminitis or peritonitis
- Guarded to poor with severe abdominal distension, persistent colic, or serosanguineous peritoneal fluid

PEARLS & CONSIDERATIONS
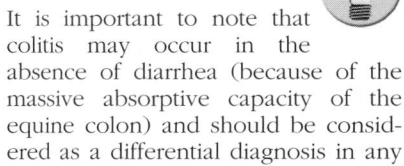

- It is important to note that colitis may occur in the absence of diarrhea (because of the massive absorptive capacity of the equine colon) and should be considered as a differential diagnosis in any horse with colic or fever of unknown origin.
- Even though colitis is successfully managed medically in the majority of cases, exploratory celiotomy should be considered in horses with suspected colitis that have persistent and severe colic signs to rule out an obstructive lesion and evaluate the integrity of the colon.

SUGGESTED READING
David JB: Diarrheal diseases. In Orsini JA, Divers TJ, editors: *Equine Emergencies: Treatment and Procedures.* St Louis, 2008, Saunders Elsevier, pp 159–165.

AUTHOR: **KELSEY A. HART**

EDITOR: **TIM MAIR**

Colitis X

BASIC INFORMATION

DEFINITION

Peracute colitis, endotoxic shock, and anaphylaxis of unknown etiology

EPIDEMIOLOGY

CONTAGION AND ZOONOSIS Although an infectious or toxic cause is suspected, disease typically occurs in an individual horse on a farm rather than as an outbreak.

HISTORY, CHIEF COMPLAINT
- Severe colic, fever, and acute collapse with or without diarrhea are most often observed.
- Some horses are simply found dead without observation of prior illness.

PHYSICAL EXAM FINDINGS
- Severe depression to obtundation or severe, intractable colic.
- Pyrexia is common, but hypothermia may be present in terminal cardiovascular collapse.
- Tachycardia
- Tachypnea
- Red to purple mucous membranes and dramatically prolonged capillary refill time.
- Mild to severe abdominal distension.
- Decreased to absent gastrointestinal borborygmi.
- Severe (± hemorrhagic) diarrhea, soft feces, or scant manure may be noted.
- Rectal examination usually reveals edema in the rectum and colon wall. Occasionally, large colonic gas distension may be present.

ETIOLOGY AND PATHOPHYSIOLOGY
- The cause of colitis X is unknown, although an infectious or toxic cause is suspected.
- The severe colonic edema and mucosal damage observed in horses with colitis X is believed to be a specific organ

manifestation of anaphylaxis in response to an unknown antigen.

DIAGNOSIS

DIFFERENTIAL DIAGNOSIS
- Peracute salmonellosis
- Clostridial diarrhea
- Cantharidin toxicity
- See "Salmonellosis," "Diarrhea, Clostridial," and "Blister Beetles" in this section

INITIAL DATABASE
- Other causes of colitis (see "Colitis/Diarrhea, Acute" in this section)
- Leukopenia and typical electrolyte derangements are usually seen, but the presentation occasionally may be so acute that clinicopathologic abnormalities are not observed.
- Transabdominal ultrasonography typically reveals moderate to severe focal or diffuse edema in the colon wall (>5–10 mm thick).

ADVANCED OR CONFIRMATORY TESTING
- Testing for other causes of colitis (see "Colitis/Diarrhea, Acute" in this section) should be performed.
- A diagnosis of colitis X is made based on the peracute presentation and typical clinical signs in conjunction with characteristic pathologic findings and the absence of detection of a specific pathogen.
- Gross and histopathologic findings at necropsy include severe, segmental, or diffuse colonic edema with or without focal regions of mural hemorrhage. Evidence of endotoxic shock and cardiovascular collapse is also noted.

TREATMENT

THERAPEUTIC GOAL(S)
Supportive care

ACUTE GENERAL TREATMENT
- Fluid and colloidal support, antiinflammatory and antiendotoxic therapy, and other supportive care should be initiated as for other causes of colitis (see "Colitis/Diarrhea, Acute" in this section).
- However, affected horses usually do not respond or respond only transiently to treatment and die despite aggressive therapy.

PROGNOSIS AND OUTCOME

Grave

PEARLS & CONSIDERATIONS

Horses with peracute salmonellosis or clostridial colitis may present very similarly. Thus isolation of affected horses and comprehensive testing for these pathogens should be performed because of the potential risk of disease in herdmates and other exposed horses.

SUGGESTED READING
Divers TJ: Acute diarrhea. In Orsini JA, Divers TJ, editors: *Manual of equine emergencies: treatment and procedures.* Philadelphia, 2003, Saunders Elsevier, pp 251–260.

AUTHOR: KELSEY A. HART

EDITOR: TIM MAIR

Compartment Syndrome

BASIC INFORMATION

DEFINITION

An increase in pressure in a confined anatomic space that leads to ischemic damage to the tissue

EPIDEMIOLOGY
RISK FACTORS
- Anesthesia
- Fracture
- Puncture wound
- Infection (ie, *Clostridium* spp.)
- Soft tissue trauma
- Circumferential burns
- External bandage, cast, or splint

- Reperfusion injury
- Arterial or venous obstruction
- Intense exercise
- Envenomation

ASSOCIATED CONDITIONS AND DISORDERS
- Most commonly occurs in soft tissue structures that are bounded by fascia and bony structures

- May occur with any condition in which perfusion pressure decreases below tissue pressure in a closed anatomic space

CLINICAL PRESENTATION

HISTORY, CHIEF COMPLAINT History of anesthesia, trauma, infection, burns, perfusion abnormalities, intense exercise, or snakebite

PHYSICAL EXAM FINDINGS

- The most common clinical sign is tense muscle swelling with a decreased range of motion of the affected area.
- Paraesthesia with pain that is more than expected with the diagnosed injury may be noted.
- Pulselessness is recognized in humans and may be present in horses as well.

ETIOLOGY AND PATHOPHYSIOLOGY

- Soft tissue injury results in swelling in the confined space.
- Tissue pressures increase because of edema and hemorrhage.
- When the tissue pressure increases above the diastolic blood pressure, circulation is impaired, leading to decreased tissue oxygenation and alterations in cell metabolism.
- Cells may be irreversibly damaged with severe oxygen depletion because of release of inflammatory mediators and histamine.
- Muscle and nervous tissue are the most sensitive to the negative effects of compartment syndrome.

DIAGNOSIS

DIFFERENTIAL DIAGNOSIS

- Avascular necrosis
- Venous thrombosis

INITIAL DATABASE

- Intracompartmental pressure measurements are useful for diagnosis in humans.
  - No methods have been developed to measure compartmental pressures consistently in horses.
  - Diagnosis is made from clinical signs and history.

TREATMENT

THERAPEUTIC GOAL(S)

Restore perfusion to the soft tissues.

ACUTE GENERAL TREATMENT

- Remove any constricting bandages or casts.
- Place the limb at the level of the heart if the patient is recumbent.
- Change the recumbency of the patient (ie, from left lateral to right lateral) every 3 to 4 hours.
- Corticosteroids and anticoagulants may be beneficial. Vascular structures must be patent for medications to have effect.
- Surgical decompression via a fasciotomy is the gold standard (Figure 1). Perform a large longitudinal incision with scissors or a scalpel blade.

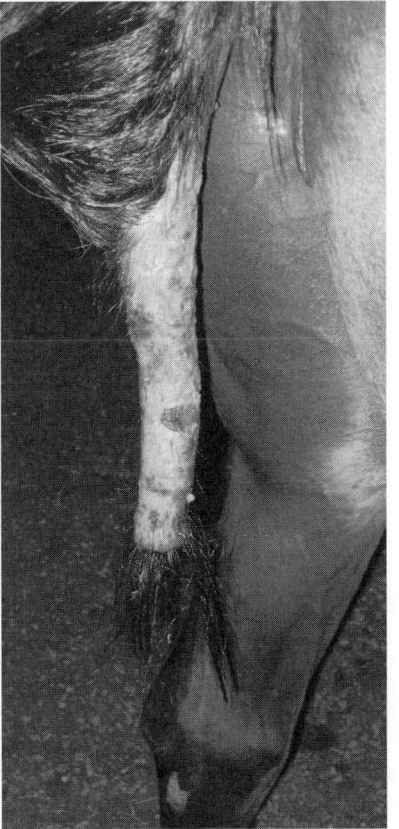

FIGURE 1 Compartment syndrome occurring after a constricting tail wrap. Approximately 75% of the tail was affected. Fasciotomy was performed twice with daily debridement, and the wounds covered with silver sulfadiazine to allow for moist healing. The tail fully healed without amputation. Sensation and hair follicles were preserved.

- Avoid vessels or nerves.
- Ensure release of all constricting fascia.
- Remove necrotic tissue.
- Direct muscle visualization is recommended in humans. Cover the fasciotomy with a moist, sterile dressing.
- Three to 5 days after fasciotomy, the incision can be closed if the patient is doing well.

POSSIBLE COMPLICATIONS

- Complications associated with fasciotomy include scarring, infection, hematoma, deep vein thrombosis, and neurovascular injury.
- An incomplete fasciotomy may cause chronic stiffness and muscle contracture.

PROGNOSIS AND OUTCOME

Long-term prognosis for the horse is good for life as long as the inciting cause for the compartment syndrome has been addressed and corrected.

PEARLS & CONSIDERATIONS

COMMENTS

If left untreated, postischemic scarring and contracture may occur.

SUGGESTED READING

Clanton TL, Klawitter PF: Adaptive responses of skeletal muscle to intermittent hypoxia: the known and the unknown [review]. *J Appl Physiol* 90:2476–2487, 2001.

Konstantakos EK, Dalstrom DJ, Nelles ME, et al: Diagnosis and management of extremity compartment syndromes: an orthopaedic perspective. *Am Surg* 73(12):1199–1209, 2007.

Ouellette EA: Compartment syndromes in obtunded patients. *Hand Clin* 14:431–450, 1998.

Taxter AJ, Konstantakos EK, Ames DW: Lateral compartment syndrome of the lower extremity in a recreational athlete: a case report. *Am J Emerg Med* 26(8):973, 2008.

AUTHOR: **CHRISTINA HEWES**

EDITORS: **R. REID HANSON** and **AMELIA MUNSTERMAN**

Congenital Heart Disease

BASIC INFORMATION

DEFINITION

Congenital heart disease (CHD) is caused by malformations of the heart or great vessels related to abnormal formation of the embryonic heart that are present at birth. Anatomic defects range from simple to complex and from trivial to life threatening. CHD is potentially heritable.

SYNONYM(S)

- Congenital heart defects
- Cardiac malformations

EPIDEMIOLOGY

SPECIES, AGE, SEX

- Most commonly recognized in foals and yearlings but may also be identified in older horses.
- Severe, complex, or multiple malformations often cause clinical signs in foals.

GENETICS AND BREED PREDISPOSITION The prevalence of CHD is unknown, but cardiac defects were identified in 3.5% of foals examined at necropsy. It is possible that some defects carry a genetic liability. Arabian horses may be predisposed to ventricular septal defect (VSD) and tetralogy of Fallot.

RISK FACTORS There are no proven associations for CHD in horses. Potential but unproven causes include drugs, viral infection, environmental toxins, and nutritional disorders.

ASSOCIATED CONDITIONS AND DISORDERS CHD generally occurs in isolation but may be associated with persistent fetal circulation or respiratory infection.

CLINICAL PRESENTATION

DISEASE FORMS/SUBTYPES

- Various classification schemes can be used to categorize CHD, including systems assessing segmental concordance of veins, atria, ventricles, and great vessels along with morphologic lesions of the valves and cardiac septae. A clinical classification includes:
  - Shunts: Communications between systemic and pulmonary circulations at the level of the atria (atrial septal defect [ASD]), ventricle (VSD), or ductus arteriosus (patent ductus arteriosus [PDA]).
    - VSDs are considered the most common heart malformation and can be single, multiple, small, or large. The aorta may be malaligned and override the septum.
    - In most cases, a VSD is paramembranous (perimembranous), meaning the hole is dorsal and involves the fibrous component of the septum. Echocardiographically, these defects are below the right and noncoronary cusps of the aortic valve, adjacent to the tricuspid valve, and ventral to the supraventricular crest ("subcristal").
    - Other locations include muscular ("apical," "trabecular"); right ventricular inlet septum (ventral to the septal tricuspid leaflet); and subarterial, below each semilunar valve ("supracristal").
    - Cardiac auscultation and echocardiographic examination findings are influenced by the location of the defect.
    - Aortic regurgitation may develop from aortic root prolapse.
  - Valvular malformations are rare.
    - Stenosis or atresia of the pulmonic and tricuspid valves leads to right-to-left intracardiac shunting across an ASD or VSD, causing cyanosis.
    - Aortic valve, mitral valve, and associated left ventricular malformations may lead to shock or congestive heart failure (CHF).
  - Complex CHD in horses includes endocardial cushion defects, common atria, single ventricle, tetralogy of Fallot, and malformation or malposition of the great vessels. The latter include double-outlet right ventricle, persistent truncus arteriosus, and transposition of the great vessels generally associated with one or more defects in the cardiac septae.

HISTORY, CHIEF COMPLAINT

- Many affected animals demonstrate no overt clinical signs other than a heart murmur.
- Complex CHD or severe defects may cause exercise intolerance or signs of CHF, including tachypnea and ventral edema.
- Failure to grow or unthriftiness may be evident.
- Atrial fibrillation (AF) may develop from cardiac enlargement.

PHYSICAL EXAM FINDINGS

- CHD should be considered in any horse with a prominent heart murmur and should be suspected in foals and yearlings with loud murmurs or a palpable precordial thrill.
- Cardiac murmurs are characterized by timing, point of maximal intensity, loudness or grade, radiation, and character (see "Cardiac Auscultation" in Section II).
- The typical holosystolic murmur of a paramembranous VSD is loudest over the right, ventral-cranial thorax. An ejection murmur may be heard over the craniodorsal heart base on the left.
- Subarterial VSD is often loudest over the pulmonic valve area and left craniodorsal heart base.
- Diastolic murmurs typically indicate the presence of aortic regurgitation.
- Continuous murmurs may be caused by persistent PDA.
  - Tachypnea, exercise intolerance, or cyanosis in foals is most often caused by respiratory disease or infection; however, CHD should also be considered.
  - Tricuspid or pulmonary atresia often produces profound cyanosis.
  - Potential signs of CHF include tiring, tachypnea, and respiratory distress.
  - Jugular venous distension, ventral edema, pleural effusion, and resting tachycardia are typical signs of right-sided or biventricular CHF.

ETIOLOGY AND PATHOPHYSIOLOGY

- The pathophysiology of VSD is caused by left-to-right shunting with volume overload of the left ventricle. Right-sided enlargement depends on the size of the defect and the presence of obstruction to right ventricular outflow.
  - A large VSD creates a functional "common ventricle," and shunting occurs along the path of lowest resistance.
  - When pulmonary vascular resistance is normal, signs relate to high pulmonary blood flow with risk of left-sided or biventricular CHF.
  - When complicated by pulmonic stenosis, pulmonary atresia, or high pulmonary vascular resistance, a right-to-left shunt may occur, and clinical signs stem from limited cardiac output and arterial hypoxemia.
- Complex abnormalities of segmental discordance also follow these general rules, and signs relate largely to the amount of pulmonary over- or undercirculation.
- Clinical signs in primary valvular malformation are similar to those observed in other species.
- Superimposition of AF in moderate to severe CHD may impair exercise capacity or precipitate CHF.

DIAGNOSIS

DIFFERENTIAL DIAGNOSIS

- Functional ejection murmurs are ubiquitous and may pose a diagnostic dilemma. An ejection murmur loudest over the great vessels is found with some cardiac defects, but in most cases, a left basilar ejection murmur simply represents a functional (flow) disturbance unrelated to heart disease (see "Cardiac Auscultation" in Section II).
- The differential diagnosis of a loud heart murmur (with or without CHF) includes CHD, infective endocarditis, degenerative valvular disease, valvulitis, ruptured chordae tendineae, myocarditis, cardiomyopathy, tachyarrhythmia-induced cardiomyopathy, and aorto-cardiac fistula (ruptured aortic sinus into the heart). Pericarditis may create a friction rub.

INITIAL DATABASE

- Complete physical examination
- Auscultation of the heart and lungs
- Examination of the precordium for thrills, cardiac displacement, or increased area of cardiac dullness
- Inspection of mucous membranes
- Palpation of the arterial pulse
- Visual assessment of jugular venous pulse and pressure
- Two-dimensional imaging of the heart for enlargement and overt lesions

ADVANCED OR CONFIRMATORY TESTING

- Echocardiography complemented by Doppler studies is the gold standard for diagnosis of CHD.
  - Quantitation of defect or heart size is useful for identifying moderate to severe defects. VSD measuring less than 2.5 cm across the greatest diameter (in mature horses) is often well tolerated. Right ventricular wall hypertrophy suggests pulmonary stenosis, vascular disease, or a functionally common ventricle. Moderate to severe left atrial dilatation suggests a hemodynamically important shunt, mitral valve disease, or left ventricular failure.
  - Contrast echocardiography with agitated saline may identify a right-to-left shunt.
  - Color Doppler studies can identify abnormal flow patterns from shunting or valvular disease.
  - Spectral continuous wave Doppler can quantify pressure differences. A VSD flow of greater than 4.5 m/s indicates a small (restrictive) defect. High-velocity tricuspid regurgitation (>4 m/s) indicates right ventricular

outflow obstruction or pulmonary hypertension.
- An electrocardiogram should be recorded if an arrhythmia is evident.
- Arterial blood gas and packed cell volume are indicated in cases of cyanosis.
- Thoracic radiography, thoracic ultrasonography, airway endoscopy, or cytologic evaluation of tracheal wash fluid should be considered when there are signs of primary lung or pleural disease.

TREATMENT

THERAPEUTIC GOAL(S)

- Definitive therapy for VSD involves cardiopulmonary bypass surgery; however, new "hybrid" procedures involving catheter devices delivered by a transventricular approach and guided by epicardial echocardiography are possible, although perhaps not practical.
- Medical management of CHF or of arrhythmias associated with CHD may be considered.
- Breeding of affected animals should be discouraged, especially in Arabian horses.

ACUTE GENERAL TREATMENT

If CHF develops, initial treatment includes IV digoxin and furosemide.

CHRONIC TREATMENT

- Exercise capacity should be assessed and exercise limited if indicated. In many cases, the lesion does not create an obvious problem.
- Chronic therapy of CHF if deemed appropriate (see "Cardiac Failure" in this section)
- Horses with AF can be treated with quinidine or electrocardioversion if indicated. Significant cardiomegaly reduces success and predisposes to reversion to AF.
- Horses with severe malformations should not be used or bred. When clinical signs are severe, persistent, or associated with poor quality of life, euthanasia may be suggested.

DRUG INTERACTIONS

- Drugs increasing pulmonary vascular resistance worsen right-to-left shunting.
- Drugs increasing systemic vascular resistance increase left-to-right shunting.

POSSIBLE COMPLICATIONS

Sudden death, progressive cardiomegaly, CHF, arrhythmias, and arterial hypoxemia

RECOMMENDED MONITORING

- Horses with mild to moderate CHD should be reevaluated at least yearly by history, auscultation, and echocardiography. Cases of moderate to severe CHD should be examined more often.
- Exercise intolerance, tachypnea, tachycardia, or ventral edema should prompt immediate reassessment.

PROGNOSIS AND OUTCOME

- Prognosis is highly variable, depending on the lesion and severity.
- Potential outcomes for VSD include tolerance, partial or complete closure by adherence of the tricuspid valve or fibrous tissue, or from aortic valve prolapse; progressive aortic regurgitation; AF; CHF; pulmonary hypertension; or reversal of the shunt with arterial hypoxemia and cyanosis.

PEARLS & CONSIDERATIONS

COMMENTS

- The rare occurrence of aortic and pulmonic stenosis reduces the indication for echocardiography in horses with soft to moderate ejection murmurs over the left craniodorsal heart base. In most of these cases, the murmur is functional.
- Many murmurs of VSD are loudest at the right ventral thorax.
- One cannot prognosticate from the loudness of a murmur.
- When a cardiac malformation is found in a foal, the mare should also be auscultated for possible CHD.
- Consultation with a specialist experienced in CHD is helpful.

PREVENTION

Do not breed horses with known CHD.

CLIENT EDUCATION

CHD can negatively impact the life, use, and value of a foal and cast doubt on the genetic reliability of the mare or stallion.

SUGGESTED READING

Bonagura JD: Congenital heart disease. In Robinson NE, editor: *Current therapy in equine medicine*, ed 5. Philadelphia, 2003, Saunders Elsevier, pp 591–601.

Schwarzwald CC: Sequential segmental analysis: a systemic approach to the diagnosis of congenital cardiac defects. *Equine Vet Educ* 20:305–309, 2008.

AUTHOR: **JOHN D. BONAGURA**

EDITOR: **MARY M. DURANDO**

Contagious Equine Metritis

BASIC INFORMATION

DEFINITION

Contagious equine metritis (CEM) is a nonsystemic, highly contagious venereal infection of members of the family Equidae caused by *Taylorella equigenitalis*, a bacterium unrecognized before 1977.

EPIDEMIOLOGY

GENETICS AND BREED PREDISPOSITION To date, there is no evidence of variation among horse breeds with respect to susceptibility to *T. equigenitalis* infection. This also applies to different breeds of ponies that have been investigated. Based on experimental findings, donkey jennies can be successfully infected with *T. equigenitalis*, although the associated clinical signs tended to be less pronounced and of shorter duration than observed in pony mares.

RISK FACTORS

- Direct or indirect venereal contact with *T. equigenitalis*
- Occurrence of the carrier state in the stallion and the mare
- International or national movement of stallions and mares and shipment of semen
- Certain management practices (eg, "vanning in" or "walking-in" of mares to be bred naturally or by artificial insemination [AI])
- Failure to observe appropriate sanitary measures when breeding stallions naturally or when collecting semen for AI

CONTAGION AND ZOONOSIS

- Transmission of CEM occurs primarily by the venereal route through:
  - Direct genital contact between an infected mare and a stallion or vice versa
  - AI with semen from a carrier stallion. The risk of transmission by AI is significantly reduced by the use of extenders containing appropriate antibiotics. Spread of CEM through cryopreserved semen remains to be determined.
  - Indirect genital contact with fomites contaminated with *T. equigenitalis*, such as vaginal specula, forceps, obstetrical sleeves, and tail bandages used in examination of the reproductive tract of the mare. Failure to observe appropriate sanitary measures when handling the external genitalia of stallions has also been implicated in the indirect

transmission of CEM. Among the items believed of major importance as potential sources of contagion in stallion collection centers is the external covering of the phantom, artificial vaginas, and wash buckets.

- Transplacental infection of the fetus
- Contact of the external genitalia of the foal with a *T. equigenitalis*–positive placenta or clitoral area of an infected mare at the time of foaling
- Exposure of the external genitalia of postpartum foal to bedding or pasture contaminated with *T. equigenitalis* infective placental fluids or vaginal discharge
- Transmission between stallions and colts through the use of common sponges or cloths contaminated with *T. equigenitalis* to wash the external genitalia
- CEM is not a zoonotic disease.

GEOGRAPHY AND SEASONALITY

- CEM has been reported to have occurred in some 29 countries worldwide since the disease was initially recognized in 1977. In countries where it is currently known or believed to occur, the infection is endemic largely in non-Thoroughbred breeds.
- Outbreaks of CEM and infection with *T. equigenitalis* invariably occur during the breeding season, whether in the Northern or Southern Hemispheres. On the other hand, carrier stallions or mares can be detected at any time either when undergoing pre- or post-entry testing required by an importing country or as part of a pre-breeding season screening program to identify carrier animals.

ASSOCIATED CONDITIONS AND DISORDERS Clinical signs of CEM in mares can closely mimic those caused by several serotypes of *Klebsiella pneumoniae* (1, 2, and 5 and possibly types 7 and 39), *Pseudomonas aeruginosa*, *Streptococcus equi* subsp. *zooepidemicus*, *Escherichia coli*, and (uncommonly) sporadic infections caused by other miscellaneous bacteria.

CLINICAL PRESENTATION

DISEASE FORMS/SUBTYPES

- CEM is an acute venereally transmissible disease that is restricted to the reproductive tract in mares. It is a non–life-threatening infection that is characterized by short-term infertility and very rarely, abortion around 7 months' gestation.
- The clinical outcome after primary exposure in a mare can vary consider-

ably from overt disease to asymptomatic infection. *T. equigenitalis* exists as a commensal on the external genitalia of the stallion, causing neither a local nor systemic inflammatory reaction.

HISTORY, CHIEF COMPLAINT

- After an incubation period of 2 to 13 days, typically affected mares may present with an odorless, greyish-white, mucopurulent vulvar discharge of uterine origin. This can vary in amount and may persist for 2 weeks or longer. The discharge is accompanied by an endometritis, cervicitis, and vaginitis of varying severity.
- Irrespective of the presence or absence of clinical signs of infection, most mares fail to conceive after primary exposure to *T. equigenitalis* and return to estrus after a shortened diestrus period. The resultant infertility is short term with no long-term adverse effects on a mare's fertility. Persistence of *T. equigenitalis* in the reproductive tract of the mare need not compromise the maintenance of a normal pregnancy and birth of a healthy foal.

PHYSICAL EXAM FINDINGS

- Clinical signs of the disease are only found in mares, with stallions being asymptomatic carriers of the organism. In clinical cases of infection, affected mares develop a severe, diffuse acute endometritis along with inflammation of the cervix and vagina.
- Acutely or chronically infected mares are afebrile without displaying any clinical signs of systemic illness. Typical cases of CEM have a mucopurulent vulvar discharge, which may be so profuse as to run down the hindquarters, wetting the entire perineal area and inside the thighs and matting the tail hairs. In contrast, other mares may merely have a bead of discharge at the lower commissure of the vulva. Intrauterine fluid accumulation can often be detected on ultrasonographic examination of affected mares. On vaginoscopic examination, discharge can be observed seeping between the folds of the external os of the cervix and accumulating on the floor of the vagina. Affected mares have a concomitant cervicitis and vaginitis, which may be more severe than seen in other bacterial infections of the reproductive tract in the mare.

ETIOLOGY AND PATHOPHYSIOLOGY

- *T. equigenitalis* is a gram-negative, non–acid-fast coccobacillus.
- The bacterium has fastidious growth requirements, growing best on choco-

latized blood agar under microaerophilic conditions of incubation.

- Two biotypes of *T. equigenitalis* exist, those that are sensitive and those that are resistant to streptomycin.
- *T. equigenitalis* is nonfermentative and nonproteolytic but is cytochrome oxidase, catalase, and alkaline phosphatase positive.
- In late 1997 and early 1998, a second species of *Taylorella* spp., *Taylorella asinigenitalis*, was identified in several donkeys, horse mares, and a stallion in the United States. This bacterium has yet to be confirmed as a cause of venereal disease in donkey jennies or mares.
- Mares acutely affected with CEM develop a severe diffuse endometritis and cervicitis, with accumulation of exudate between the endometrial folds that are edematous and congested.
- Mild multifocal salpingitis was a frequently observed feature in one experimental study on CEM.
- Cellular infiltration of the endometrium, which initially is primarily neutrophilic, becomes predominantly plasmacytic by 14 days.
- Subsequently, a mild diffuse or multifocal lymphocytic infiltration supervenes that can persist for up to 3 to 4 months after infection.

DIAGNOSIS

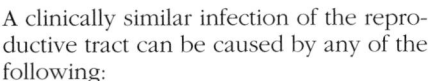

DIFFERENTIAL DIAGNOSIS

A clinically similar infection of the reproductive tract can be caused by any of the following:

- *K. pneumoniae* (types 1, 2, 5 and possibly types 7 and 39)
- *P. aeruginosa*
- *S. equi*, subsp. *zooepidemicus*
- *E. coli*
- Miscellaneous other bacteria

INITIAL DATABASE

- Vaginoscopic and ultrasound examination of the reproductive tract of the mare
- Smears of endometrial and cervical swabs, and any vaginal discharge for cytologic examination using a rapid differential staining technique. The presence of numerous neutrophils, desquamated epithelial cells, and bacteria morphologically similar to *T. equigenitalis*, either free or phagocytosed within neutrophils, is strongly suggestive, although not confirmatory of CEM.
- Collection of individual endometrial or cervical swabs together with swabs from the clitoral fossa and clitoral

sinuses and a specimen of vaginal discharge (if present) for bacteriologic culture and polymerase chain reaction (PCR) examination
- Screening stallions for *T. equigenitalis* is based on collecting individual swabs from the urethral fossa, urethral diverticulum, terminal urethra, and external surface of the penis and sheath for bacteriologic culture and PCR examination.
- Mares and stallions should be swabbed three times with at least 3 days between each sampling.
- It is very important that the culture sites in the mare and the stallion are appropriately sampled, the swabs immediately transferred to individual tubes of Amie's transport medium with charcoal, and the specimens kept refrigerated and plated out in the laboratory within 48 hours of collection.

ADVANCED OR CONFIRMATORY TESTING

- Bacteriologic culture is still the most widely accepted means of confirming the presence of *T. equigenitalis* in mares and stallions. It provides the opportunity to determine the cultural, antimicrobial sensitivity, and pathogenic and antigenic characteristics of isolates of the organism. It is a sensitive although somewhat lengthy means of diagnosing CEM.
- The PCR assay may provide a more rapid and sensitive method of demonstrating *T. equigenitalis* on swabs collected from mares or stallions. Preliminary data on the reliability of this assay in detecting the bacterium in extended or cryopreserved semen, although promising, requires additional verification.
- Test breeding is highly reliable for confirming the carrier state in stallions. It is based on demonstration of *T. equigenitalis* in the reproductive tract in one or both test mares or the development of CF antibodies to the organism within 15 to 40 days after breeding.
- Serology or the development of CF antibodies to *T. equigenitalis* is only of value in confirming recent infection in mares. Stallions do not mount a detectable humoral antibody response to the bacterium.

TREATMENT

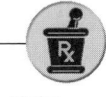

THERAPEUTIC GOAL(S)

The goals of treatment of CEM are twofold:

- Promote more rapid resolution of clinical signs of the disease in the mare.

- Eliminate *T. equigenitalis* from the sites of persistence in the carrier stallion and the mare.

ACUTE GENERAL TREATMENT

- Although *T. equigenitalis* is sensitive to a wide range of antimicrobial drugs in vitro, currently, no one treatment necessarily guarantees both rapid resolution of clinical signs and clearance of the carrier state in mares.
- Mares with acute endometritis can be effectively treated by the intrauterine infusion of ampicillin (2 g in 60-mL saline or gentamicin [buffered] for each of 3 to 5 days); this may be combined with systemic treatment with sulfamethoxazole-trimethoprim (30 mg/kg PO for 5 days).

CHRONIC TREATMENT

- Treatment of clitoral carrier mares requires prior removal of any smegma-type material from the clitoral sinuses by flushing them with a cerumenolytic agent followed by irrigation with 4% chlorhexidine gluconate before packing them with 0.2% nitrofurazone or 1% silver sulphadiazine ointment.
- The clitoral fossa and sinuses are scrubbed for 4 more days with 4% chlorhexidine and packed with 0.2% nitrofurazone or 1% silver sulphadiazine ointment.
- Topical treatment of the distal reproductive tract of the mare may be combined with systemic treatment with sulfamethoxazole-trimethoprim (30 mg/kg PO for 5 days), and if dealing with a uterine carrier, with intrauterine infusion of ampicillin (2 g in 60-mL saline or gentamicin [buffered] for 3 to 5 days).
- In the case of carrier stallions, the external genitalia are scrubbed once a day for 5 days with 4% chlorhexidine scrub and the penis and sheath liberally covered with 0.2% nitrofurazone or 1% silver sulphadiazine ointment, with care being taken to pack the ointment into the urethral fossa and urethral sinus.
- Treatment of the external genitalia of the stallion may be combined with systemic administration of sulfamethoxazole-trimethoprim (30 mg/kg PO for 7 days).

POSSIBLE COMPLICATIONS

- Treatment of some carrier mares and stallions may have to be repeated one or more times before *T. equigenitalis* is finally eliminated from the reproductive tract.
- Carrier mares refractive to repeated treatments may have to undergo surgical ablation of the clitoral sinuses.

RECOMMENDED MONITORING

- After treatment, mares and stallions need to be retested by bacteriologic culture of the sampling sites prescribed for each, beginning no less than 21 days after the last day of topical treatment and no less than 7 days after completion of systemic treatment.
- In the case of mares, three sets of swabs must be collected at a sampling interval of not less than 3 days within a 7- to 12-day period to confirm the absence of infection.
- Treated stallions must be swabbed at least once before being test bred to two mares and confirmed culture negative for *T. equigenitalis*. Both test mares must remain culturally and serologically negative for infection up to 21 days after being test bred.
- Swabs from mares and stallions may also be subjected to PCR testing, with similar negative results for evidence of *T. equigenitalis*.

PROGNOSIS AND OUTCOME

- Clinical signs of CEM in the mare will resolve in time even without recourse to treatment.
- Although most mares acutely infected with *T. equigenitalis* clear the organism from their reproductive tract after resolution of signs of the disease, a percentage remain asymptomatically infected for months or years, the great majority as clitoral carriers and a much smaller number as uterine carriers.
- A clinically inapparent carrier state can be established in a significant percentage of stallions exposed to *T. equigenitalis*. Preferred sites of persistence of the organism are the urethral fossa and associated sinus. The carrier state can persist in the untreated stallion for years.
- Elimination of *T. equigenitalis* from the reproductive tract of the carrier mare and stallion can be successfully achieved after one or more courses of treatment.

PEARLS & CONSIDERATIONS

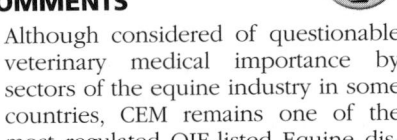

COMMENTS

- Although considered of questionable veterinary medical importance by sectors of the equine industry in some countries, CEM remains one of the most regulated OIE-listed Equine diseases in terms of international trade.
- *T. equigenitalis* has the potential to cause significant economic loss in previously unexposed breeding populations.
- The ease with which CEM can be spread internationally through the movement of carrier stallions and mares represents a continuing risk for countries with established freedom from the disease.
- Although evidence suggests that transmission of CEM can occur through the use of extended semen, the risks associated with the use of cryopreserved semen from a carrier stallion remain to be determined.
- Additional research may reveal that certain strains of the closely related bacterium *T. asinigenitalis* also have the potential to cause venereal disease in mares and donkey jennies.

PREVENTION

- CEM should be made a notifiable or if nonnotifiable, a reportable disease.
- Availability of laboratories with proven ability to provide a fully reliable diagnostic service for CEM
- More stringent standards of management and hygiene on breeding farms and at stallion collection centers
- Use of disposable or sterile equipment and materials in breeding sheds and at collection centers
- Comprehensive screening of stallions and mare populations to detect carrier animals
- Stallions and mares cultured positive for *T. equigenitalis* should not be used for breeding until proven free from the bacterium.
- Comprehensive postentry testing all stallions and mares imported from

countries in which CEM is known or suspected to occur
- Currently, there is no vaccine against CEM.

CLIENT EDUCATION

- Availability of educational materials on CEM to increase awareness of the salient features of the disease among stallion and mare owners and breeders
- Seminars on how to improve breeding practices and management of stallions and mares to minimize the risk of spread of CEM and other venereal infections on farms and at stallion collection centers
- Through meetings and educational releases, emphasize:
  - The potential economic importance of CEM and not just in terms of international trade
  - The insidious nature of the disease in that many first-time infected mares will not develop overt clinical signs other than a period of temporary infertility lasting one or two estrous cycles.

SUGGESTED READING

Heath P, Timoney PJ: Contagious equine metritis. In *OIE manual of diagnostic tests and vaccines for terrestrial animals*, vol 2. Paris, 2008, Office International des Epizooties, pp 838–844.

Jang SS, Donahue JM, Arata AB, et al: *Taylorella asinigenitalis* sp. *nov.*, A bacterium isolated from the genital tract of male donkeys (*Equus asinus*). *Int J Syst Evol Microbiol* 51:971, 2001.

Kristula M: Contagious equine metritis. In Sellon DC, Long MT, editors: *Equine infectious diseases*. St Louis, 2007, Saunders Elsevier, pp 351–353.

Platt H, Atherton JG, Dawson FL, Durrant DS: Developments in contagious equine metritis. *Vet Rec* 102:19, 1978.

Wakely PR, Errington J, Hannon S, et al: Development of a real time PCR for the detection of *Taylorella equigenitalis* directly from genital swabs and discrimination from *T. asinigenitalis*. *Vet Microbiol* 118:247, 2006.

AUTHORS: **MATS H.T. TROEDSSON** and **PETER J. TIMONEY**

EDITOR: **JUAN C. SAMPER**

Corneal Ulcers, Superficial Nonhealing

BASIC INFORMATION

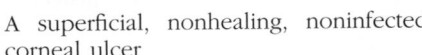

DEFINITION

A superficial, nonhealing, noninfected corneal ulcer

SYNONYM(S)

Indolent ulcer

EPIDEMIOLOGY

RISK FACTORS

- Any type of ocular trauma
- Feeding hay from hay bags, nets, or balls

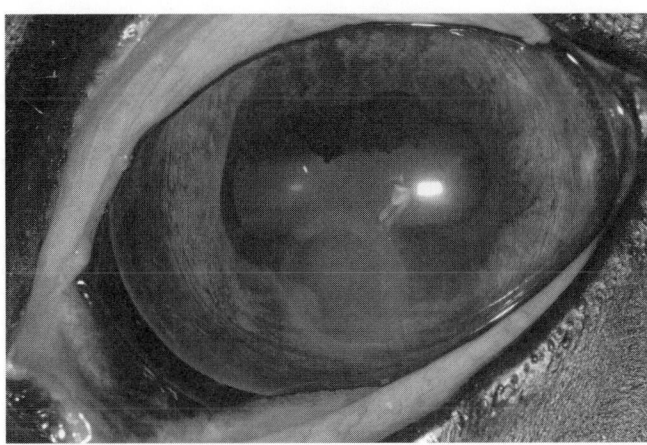

FIGURE 1 Superficial nonhealing corneal ulcer in a horse.

CLINICAL PRESENTATION

DISEASE FORMS/SUBTYPES Superficial nonhealing corneal ulcer

HISTORY, CHIEF COMPLAINT Chronic, nonhealing corneal ulcer that is nonresponsive to topical medications

PHYSICAL EXAM FINDINGS Indolent corneal ulcers in horses are similar to small animal indolent ulcers. The characteristic appearance is a superficial ulcer with a redundant epithelial border. Other signs include minimal corneal neovascularization, focal edema, and moderate discomfort (Figure 1).

ETIOLOGY AND PATHOPHYSIOLOGY

- Superficial nonhealing cornea ulcers are chronic ulcers in which the corneal epithelium will not adhere to the underlying corneal stroma.
- A defect of the superficial corneal stroma is suspected.

DIAGNOSIS

DIFFERENTIAL DIAGNOSIS

Other causes of corneal ulceration should be ruled out before a diagnosis is made.
- Foreign body (eg, burdock bristles)
- Ectopic cilia, distichiasis
- Infectious keratitis
- Viral keratitis
- Lagophthalmos (eg, facial nerve paralysis)
- Neurotrophic keratitis (lack of cranial nerve V innervation)
- Chronic trauma

INITIAL DATABASE

A bacterial and fungal culture should be submitted from all corneal ulcers in the horse. Cultures should be obtained from the margin of the ulcer itself before any therapeutic or diagnostic agents are distilled in the eye. After a culture has been obtained and the cornea has been fluorescein stained, topical anesthetic is applied, and a scraping is obtained from the ulcer for cytologic examination. The cells are placed on a glass slide and stained to examine for bacteria, fungal hyphae, and cell types. Gram, Giemsa, and Diff-Quik stains work well for examination. Only epithelial cells and a few neutrophils are typical of chronic superficial nonhealing corneal ulcers.

ADVANCED OR CONFIRMATORY TESTING

Corneal biopsy after superficial keratectomy

TREATMENT

THERAPEUTIC GOAL(S)

Treatment of indolent ulcers includes searching for the cause (foreign bodies, ectopic cilia, eyelid abnormality, repeated trauma) and promoting adherence of the epithelium to the corneal stroma.

ACUTE GENERAL TREATMENT

Treatment options reported in horses include
- Medical therapy
  - Topical broad-spectrum antimicrobials (eg, oxytetracycline)
  - Topical atropine if secondary uveitis
  - Systemic nonsteroidal antiinflammatory drugs to assist in pain control
- Surgical therapy (if nonresponsive to medical therapy)
  - Superficial keratectomy
  - Grid keratotomy has *not* been shown to be beneficial for healing in horses.

CHRONIC TREATMENT

Superficial keratectomy: Results in healing within 10 to 14 days

POSSIBLE COMPLICATIONS

The most common complication is bacterial or fungal keratitis caused by a chronic corneal ulcer.

RECOMMENDED MONITORING

Examine daily until the cornea has healed.

PROGNOSIS AND OUTCOME

Generally good with time

PEARLS & CONSIDERATIONS

COMMENTS

These ulcers are frustrating to treat and generally take up to 4 to 6 weeks to heal.

PREVENTION

- Minimizing ocular and corneal trauma may help prevent the development of infected corneal ulcers.
- Use of a quality fly mask is recommended.
- Feeding hay on the ground is recommended to minimize ocular trauma.

CLIENT EDUCATION

Client communication is essential so that expectations are not too high for quick healing of the corneal ulcer.

SUGGESTED READING

Andrew S, Willis M: Diseases of the cornea and sclera. In Gilger BC, editor: *Equine ophthalmology.* St Louis, 2005, Elsevier.

Michau TM, Schwabenton B, Davidson MG, Gilger B: Superficial, nonhealing corneal ulcers in horses: 23 cases (1989–2003). *Vet ophthalmol* 6(4):291–297, 2003.

AUTHOR & EDITOR: BRIAN C. GILGER

Corynebacterium Pseudotuberculosis Infection

BASIC INFORMATION

DEFINITION

Corynebacterium pseudotuberculosis causes suppurative processes and abscesses in several species. The biotype *equi* affects horses and occasionally cattle.

SYNONYM(S)

- For external abscesses: Pigeon fever, dryland distemper, false strangles
- For corynebacterial folliculitis: Contagious acne

EPIDEMIOLOGY

SPECIES, AGE, SEX

- May affect horses of any age (ranging from 3 months to 28 years), but young horses (ages 1 to 5 years) appear more susceptible.
- No sex predilection, although mares might be overrepresented

RISK FACTORS Other cases on the premises

CONTAGION AND ZOONOSIS

- Not contagious between horses; however, abscesses serve as source of environmental contamination
- Zoonotic potential exists; humans can develop lymphadenitis and pneumonia.

GEOGRAPHY AND SEASONALITY

- Endemic areas include the Southwestern United States, Australia, and Brazil.
- Soil-borne organism found worldwide; infection can occur any time of the year.
- Cases of external and internal abscesses occur mostly in endemic areas, and more frequently during fall and early winter, especially after heavy rainfall.
- Seasonal incidence appears to associate with presence of biting insects (eg, *Haematobia irritans, Musca domestica, Stomoxys calcitrans,* and *Culicoides* spp).

ASSOCIATED CONDITIONS AND DISORDERS

- *C. pseudotuberculosis* infection is characterized by a suppurative process and abscessation in several animal species but is recognized as the cause of specific disease syndromes only in horses and small ruminants.
- *C. pseudotuberculosis* infection in sheep and goats is known as caseous lymphadenitis.
- Organisms survive in soil for long periods (endemic farms), leading to insidious, often recurring disease that causes significant economic losses.

CLINICAL PRESENTATION

DISEASE FORMS/SUBTYPES

There are four syndromes:

- External abscesses: Deep subcutaneous infection often located in pectoral, ventral abdomen, axillary, and inguinal or mammary areas
- Internal abscess
- Ulcerative lymphangitis: An excoriating, suppurating inflammation of the lymphatics usually confined to the distal limbs
- Corynebacterial folliculitis

HISTORY, CHIEF COMPLAINT

- Previous case on the premises
- Insidious onset

PHYSICAL EXAM FINDINGS

- External abscesses: Painful and warm swelling in the pectoral, ventral abdomen, axillary, and inguinal or mammary areas; systemic signs such as fever, lethargy, and decreased appetite are common.
- Internal abscesses: Prominent signs of systemic illness (persistent or recurring fever, lethargy, and poor appetite) are associated with weight loss, tachycardia, tachypnea, abdominal discomfort, and signs of organ dysfunction associated with the location of the internal abscess. It may occur in association with external abscesses.
- Ulcerative lymphangitis: Swelling of the distal limb associated with non–weight-bearing lameness generally affects one limb, most commonly a hindlimb. The affected limb is usually very edematous, with subcutaneous nodules that ulcerate, releasing green-tinged pus. The ulcers are slow to heal and are generally below the fetlock.
- Corynebacterial folliculitis: Pustules form in areas of the skin in contact with tack and harness; thought to originate from contamination of traumatized skin with the organism.

ETIOLOGY AND PATHOPHYSIOLOGY

- The portal of entry of the organism is thought to be abrasions of the skin. Many insects have been incriminated as vectors for the transmission of *C. pseudotuberculosis,* including *H. irritans, M. domestica, S. calcitrans,* and *Culicoides* species.
- The incidence of the disease varies from year to year presumably because of environmental factors and vectors.
- *C. pseudotuberculosis* is a gram-positive, pleomorphic rod-shaped, facultative intracellular, facultative anaerobic bacterium.
- The organism contains corynomycolic acid in the cell wall (confers the ability to resist lysosomal digestion and survive within macrophages) and produces several exotoxins, including phospholipase D and sphingomyelinase (degrade endothelial cell wall leading to increased vascular permeability), that facilitate carriage of the bacteria by lymphatic drainage from the site of infection to regional lymph nodes. The abscess formation in regional lymph nodes is an important feature of the infection.
- Incubation period is 3 to 4 weeks.

DIAGNOSIS

DIFFERENTIAL DIAGNOSIS

- For lymphangitis or cellulitis
  - Sporadic bacterial lymphangitis or cellulitis caused by:
    - *Streptococcus* spp.
    - *Staphylococcus* spp.
    - *Pseudomonas aeruginosa*
    - *Rhodococcus equi*
  - Sporotrichosis by *Sporothrix schenckii*
  - Phycomycosis by *Pythium insidiosum, Basidiobolus* spp.
  - Insect or arthropod bite
  - Other causes
  - Cutaneous glanders by *Burkholderia* (*Pseudomonas*) *mallei* (exotic in the United States and reportable)
  - Epizootic lymphangitis by *Histoplasma farciminosum* (outside the United States)
- For external abscesses
  - Strangles (*Streptococcus equi* subsp. *equi*)
  - Abscess by other bacteria (eg, *Streptococcus* spp., *R. equi*)
  - Hematoma
  - Seroma
  - Foreign body
  - Neoplasia
- For internal abscesses
  - Bastard strangles (*S. equi* subsp. *equi*)
  - Internal abscess by other bacteria (eg, *Streptococcus* spp., *R. equi*)
  - Neoplasia
- For corynebacterial folliculitis
  - Staphylococcal folliculitis
  - Dermatophilosis
  - Dermatophytosis

INITIAL DATABASE

- Complete blood cell count (CBC), serum biochemistry profile, and fluid analysis of abdominal fluid
- CBC often reveals normocytic normochromic anemia (chronic disease), leu-

kocytosis, and neutrophilia, particularly in cases of internal abscesses.
- Hyperproteinemia, hyperglobulinemia, and hyperfibrinogenemia are common, especially in cases of internal abscesses.
- Biochemistry profile: Abnormalities indicating dysfunction corresponding to the organ involved (eg, liver dysfunction associated with hepatic abscessation).
- Peritoneal fluid analysis: Increased protein and nucleated cell count often associated with suppurative inflammation; present in cases of abdominal abscesses.

ADVANCED OR CONFIRMATORY TESTING

- Abscesses deep in the musculature or internal organs or body cavities might require ultrasonography for detection or localization.
- Evaluation of the specimen from the abscess, peritoneal fluid, or transtracheal wash by:
  - Gram stain: Gram-positive, rod-shaped pleomorphic bacteria
  - Aerobic bacterial culture (biochemistry and Gram stain)
- Serologic titer by synergistic hemolysis inhibition (SHI) test: Measures IgG to the exotoxin phospholipase D and indicates chronicity and severity of the infection and antibody response
  - SHI titer up to 1:128 indicates exposure; SHI titer of 1:512 or higher strongly suggests infection.
  - Low SHI titer does not rule out the disease.
  - Many horses with external abscess have low SHI titers before drainage of the abscess.
  - Almost all horses with internal abscesses have SHI titers of 1:512 or higher.

TREATMENT

THERAPEUTIC GOAL(S)

- Main goals are to eliminate suppurative exudates and provide pain management as needed. The infective exudates should be disposed of properly to minimize environmental contamination.
- Treatment depends on the form and the location of lesions.

ACUTE GENERAL TREATMENT

Variable according to the form and location of lesions
- Eliminate suppurative exudates.
  - Establish drainage of external and internal abscesses.
  - For best drainage, the abscess must be allowed to mature.
  - External abscesses
    - Hot compresses, warm soaks, and poultices expedite abscess maturation.
    - When the abscess is mature, lance at the most ventral portion.
  - Internal abscesses: Marsupialization if possible
  - Clean lesions in ulcerative lymphangitis and folliculitis.
  - If possible, lavage with antiseptic solution should be performed.
- Provide analgesia and antiinflammatory treatment as needed, especially if lameness is present in cases of ulcerative lymphangitis.
- Antibiotic therapy
  - Recommended in cases of internal abscesses and ulcerative lymphangitis
  - Controversial in cases of external abscesses
  - Warranted if signs of severe systemic illness
  - Organism has broad antibiotic susceptibility in vitro (penicillins, cephalosporins, trimethoprim-sulfonamide, tetracyclines):
    - Potassium penicillin G: 22,000 IU/kg IV q6h
    - Procaine penicillin: 22,000 IU/kg IM q12h
    - Ceftiofur: 2.2 to 4.4 mg/kg IV or IM q12h
    - Trimethoprim-sulfamethoxazole: 30 mg/kg PO q12h
  - Drug penetration can limit the effectiveness of antimicrobial therapy.
  - Rifampin in addition to one of the above drugs or chloramphenicol are good alternatives to improve penetration.
    - Rifampin: 5 mg/kg PO q12h
    - Chloramphenicol: 50 mg/kg PO q12h
    - Length of treatment is variable.

CHRONIC TREATMENT

- Prolonged antimicrobial treatment is required for:
  - Ulcerative lymphangitis: 30 days
  - Internal abscesses: At least 6 weeks; up to 14 weeks
- Antimicrobial choice must take into consideration the lengthy course of treatment.

POSSIBLE COMPLICATIONS

- Antibiotic therapy might be problematic because:
  - Abscesses have thick capsule.
  - Drugs must be able to penetrate well and able to kill intracellular bacteria.
  - The organism might show antibiotic susceptibility in vitro but not in vivo.

- In cases of external abscesses, systemic antimicrobial therapy is thought to prolong the course of disease (ie, delay resolution).

RECOMMENDED MONITORING

Internal abscesses require repeated evaluation (eg, imaging of abscess, CBC and fibrinogen, abdominocentesis and fluid analysis, bacterial culture).

PROGNOSIS AND OUTCOME

- Prognosis depends on the form and the location of lesions.
  - For external abscesses: Good
  - For internal abscesses: Guarded (mortality rate of 30%–40% despite treatment; 100% if untreated)
  - For ulcerative lymphangitis: Guarded (because of disfigurement and debilitation)
  - If diagnosed and appropriately treated early in the course of the disease, the prognosis improves.
- Resolution of external abscesses
  - If drainage and no systemic antimicrobials: Average of 3 weeks after drainage, up to 60 to 90 days
  - If systemic antimicrobial and drainage: Average of 30 days
- Resolution of internal abscesses: Variable, averaging 2 months; can take as long as 4 to 6 months

PEARLS & CONSIDERATIONS

COMMENTS

When infection is established in the premises, the disease is likely to occur again.

PREVENTION

- Isolation of infected animal, particularly after drainage has been established
- Good sanitation and disposal of contaminated materials
- Insect control
- Vaccination with autogenous bacterin toxoid is limited to endemic areas.

CLIENT EDUCATION

Ulcerative lymphangitis is thought to be associated with poor hygiene and an abundance of biting insect vectors.

SUGGESTED READING

Aleman, M, Spier SJ: *Corynebacterium pseudotuberculosis* infection. In Smith BP, editor: *Large Animal Internal Medicine*, ed 4. St Louis, 2009, Mosby Elsevier, pp 1184–1188.

Scott DW, Miller WH Jr: Corynebacterial infections. In *Equine dermatology.* St Louis, 2003, Elsevier, pp 228–232.

White SD: Bacterial diseases: equine *Corynebacterium pseudotuberculosis* cellulitis. In Smith BP, editor: *Large animal internal medicine,* ed 4. St. Louis, 2009, Mosby Elsevier, p 1314.

AUTHOR: **LAIS R. R. COSTA**

Cryptorchidism

BASIC INFORMATION

DEFINITION
A state in which a stallion has one or both testes in a location other than the scrotum

SYNONYM(S)
Retained testicles, rigs, ridgelings, or originals

EPIDEMIOLOGY
SPECIES, AGE, SEX Horses are one of domestic animal species with the highest prevalence rate of cryptorchidism. The overall prevalence is about 3% to 4%, with a much higher percentage in certain breeds.

GENETICS AND BREED PREDISPOSITION
- Percherons, American Saddlebreds, and American Quarter Horses have a higher risk than Thoroughbreds, Standardbred, Morgans, Tennessee Walking Horses, and Arabians.
- Unilateral testis retention occurs more often than bilateral. The right testis is more often retained in the inguinal canal and the left testis is more commonly retained in the abdomen cavity.

RISK FACTORS
- Familial: Cryptorchidism recurs in families and displays variability in the degree of manifestation (inguinal, abdominal, ectopic testes) and in the pattern of occurrence (breed differences).
- Drugs: The vulnerability of testicular descent to estrogenic and antiandrogenic influence in certain species (eg, pigs) should raise questions when potential hormones or drugs with hormone-like effects (eg, estradiol, diethylstilbestrol, progestagens, cimetidine, flutamide, finasteride) are considered during pregnancy.

ASSOCIATED CONDITIONS AND DISORDERS Increased risk of testicular neoplasia is associated with the retained testicle. Teratomas are the most common testicular tumor associated with a retained testicle in young horses.

CLINICAL PRESENTATION
DISEASE FORMS/SUBTYPES Depending on the precise location of the retained testicle, different nomenclature may be used.
- Inguinal cryptorchid (high flanker) is defined as a stallion with one testis that did not pass the superficial inguinal ring.
- Complete abdominal cryptorchid has both the testis and the epididymis in the abdominal cavity.
- In partial abdominal cryptorchid, a portion of the epididymis lies in the inguinal canal.
- Ectopic retained testicles are located subcutaneously and cannot move toward the scrotum.

HISTORY, CHIEF COMPLAINT
- A good case history is very important to reduce the risk of errors.
- On visual examination of a stallion, one or two testicles are missing from the scrotum.
- Castrated stallion with a nebulous history and suspicious male-like behavior.

PHYSICAL EXAM FINDINGS The conformation of the scrotum is meticulously assessed for the presence of testicles and for signs of castration scars. If no evidence of a testicle is noticed, the animal should be sedated (xylazine) to ensure good relaxation of the cremaster muscle revealing the testicle. In addition to the visual examination, palpation of the scrotum and the inguinal area is essential.

ETIOLOGY AND PATHOPHYSIOLOGY
- Sex differential events are generally influenced by multigenetic and multi-environmental factors.
- Failure of the testis to regress in size, overstretching of the gubernaculum, or insufficient abdominal pressure could mechanically prevent the engagement of the testis in the vaginal ring and further stop the testis' advance through the inguinal canal.
- Defective hypothalamic-pituitary axis and deficiency of gonadotrophin hormone have been proposed.
- Factors such as Müllerian inhibiting substance (MIS), genitofemoral nerve and calcitonin gene-related peptides, and insulin-like factor-3 could play a role in cryptorchidism.
- Definitive experimental evidence has yet to be obtained.

DIAGNOSIS

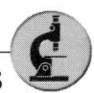

DIFFERENTIAL DIAGNOSIS
- Unilateral cryptorchid (ectopic, inguinal, and abdominal)
- Bilateral cryptorchid (ectopic, inguinal, and abdominal)
- Behavioral problem
- Gonadal agenesis (extremely rare)
- Intersex: XY sex reversal (rare)

INITIAL DATABASE
- History
- Palpation (scrotum and inguinal area)
- Transrectal palpation
- Deep palpation of the inguinal canal often allows the location of the testis in an inguinal cryptorchid. Differentiation between subcutaneous fat and testicular tissue is important.
- Palpation of the inguinal region is completed by transrectal palpation. The vaginal ring or internal inguinal ring is relatively easy to find, and one or two fingers may be inserted. Transrectal palpation of the ductus deferens in the inguinal ring suggests a testis located in the inguinal canal or in the scrotum. Contrarily, the absence of the ductus deferens suggests an abdominal location of the retained testis.
- In the absence of one or both testicles in the scrotum, the persistence of stallion-like behavior (erection, mounting, and sexually aggressive behavior) of an otherwise assumed castrated male could be the main complaint.

ADVANCED OR CONFIRMATORY TESTING
- Ultrasonographic examination (inguinal, transabdominal, and transrectal)
- Hormone essay
- Systematic transabdominal ultrasonography (3.5-MHz transducer) in both caudal abdominal and inguinal regions can locate the retained testis. Transabdominal ultrasonography is a diagnostic technique with high sensitivity (93.2%) and specificity (100%). A systematic and meticulous transabdominal craniocaudal scanning method of the area of the caudal aspect of the abdomen from midline to the flank and of the inguinal area is performed. The hyperechoic albuginea and the

central vein of the testis or the epididymis are readily identified. When the testis is not found, transrectal ultrasonography is a method to precisely locate the testis.

- Endocrinologic profiling is a useful diagnostic tool when ultrasonography (transabdominal, inguinal or transrectal) is not available or did not enable a confident diagnosis of cryptorchidism. The endocrinologic profile includes baseline testosterone or estrone sulphate concentrations and human chorionic gonadotropin (hCG) stimulation test for testosterone. The baseline testosterone level in geldings (<40 pg/mL) is significantly lower than in stallions (>100 pg/mL). With uncertain results, testosterone levels after hCG stimulation could be used to confirm the diagnosis of cryptorchidism. A blood sample is obtained at 0, 60, and 120 minutes after hCG administration (10000 IU), and the testosterone concentration is compared with the baseline level at time 0 (94.6% accurate test). Some cryptorchids show a late response (48 to 72 hours after hCG stimulation). Practically, blood should be sampled at 0, 1, 2, 48, and 72 hours after hCG injection and the samples taken at 0, 1, and 2 hours sent to the laboratory. When suspicious cryptorchidism is not confirmed, the 48- and 72-hour samples could be sent later. Test result interpretation is based on specific reference range from individual laboratories.
- In geldings, the estrogen sulfate baseline concentrations is expected to be low (<50 pg/mL), but cryptorchids show high concentrations (>400 pg/mL). Excluding horses younger than 3 years old and donkeys, 96% accuracy has been reported.

TREATMENT

THERAPEUTIC GOAL(S)

- Removal of the retained and descended testes

ACUTE GENERAL TREATMENT

- The appropriate surgical approach can be selected depending on different factors:
  - Location of the retained testis
  - Temperament of the horse
  - Health of the horse
  - Function of the horse
  - Experience or preference of the surgeon
  - Cost of the surgical approach
- The different surgical approaches are:
  - Inguinal approach for inguinal and abdominal retained testicles
  - Parainguinal approach when the vaginal process cannot be located or when the testis is too big to be removed by the inguinal canal
  - Paramedian approach for bilateral cryptorchids or animals with stallion-like behavior that are unreliable and dangerous to work with or with an unknown castration history. Flank and laparoscopic approaches for abdominal retained testicles.

CHRONIC TREATMENT

Medical treatment as described for humans is not recommended because of the heritable nature of the condition.

POSSIBLE COMPLICATIONS

- Hemorrhage
- Evisceration
- Edema
- Septic funiculitis
- Clostridial infection
- Septic and nonseptic peritonitis
- Hydrocele
- Continued masculine behavior (false rigs)

RECOMMENDED MONITORING

Activity should be restricted to hand-walking for the first 3 weeks.

PROGNOSIS AND OUTCOME

Return to normal behavior within 3 to 4 weeks after surgery and prognosis for life are excellent.

PEARLS & CONSIDERATIONS

CLIENT EDUCATION

Keep good records.

PREVENTION

Remove affected animals from the breeding program.

SUGGESTED READING

Brinsko SP: Neoplasia of the male reproductive tract. *Vet Clin North Am Equine Pract* 14:517–533, 1998.

Brinsko SP: Surgery of the stallion reproductive tract. In Blanchard TL, Varner DD, Schumacher J, Love CC, Brinsko SP, Rigby SL, editors: *Manual of equine reproduction*, ed 2. St Louis, 2003, Mosby Elsevier, pp 199–203.

Cox JE, Redhead PH, Dawson FE: Comparison of the measurement of plasma testosterone and plasma oestrogens for the diagnosis of cryptorchidism in the horse. *Equine Vet J* 18:179–182, 1986.

Hayes HM: Epidemiological features of 5009 cases of equine cryptorchism. *Equine Vet J* 18:467–471, 1986.

Schambourg MA, Farley JA, Marcoux M, Laverty S: Use of transabdominal ultrasonography to determine the location of cryptorchid testes in the horse. *Equine Vet J* 38:242–245, 2006.

AUTHORS: **RÉJEAN CLÉOPHAS LEFEBVRE, FRANÇOIS-XAVIER GRAND, GABRIEL BORGES COUTO,** and **IGNACIO RAGGIO**

EDITOR: **JUAN C. SAMPER**

Cryptosporidiosis

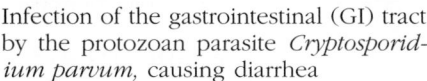

BASIC INFORMATION

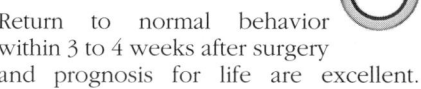

DEFINITION

Infection of the gastrointestinal (GI) tract by the protozoan parasite *Cryptosporidium parvum,* causing diarrhea

SPECIES, AGE, SEX

Horses of any age may potentially be affected, but clinical disease is most common in foals.

RISK FACTORS

- Immunodeficiency: Clinical disease is most often identified in association with the stress of hospitalization and concurrent infection or in foals with severe combined immunodeficiency.
- Risk factors for fecal shedding include:
  - Age younger than 6 months
  - History of diarrhea in the past 30 days
  - Residence on specific breeding farms

CONTAGION AND ZOONOSIS

- Transmission is by the fecal-oral route.
- Strains are transmissible between species.
- Zoonotic; may cause severe diarrhea in humans.

CLINICAL PRESENTATION

DISEASE FORMS/SUBTYPES
- Many infections are subclinical.
- May result in severe disease.

HISTORY, CHIEF COMPLAINT Diarrhea

PHYSICAL EXAM FINDINGS
- Diarrhea of variable severity
- Dehydration
- Fever

ETIOLOGY AND PATHOPHYSIOLOGY
- Oocysts are sporulated and infectious at the time they are excreted in the feces and may persist in the environment.
- Infection occurs by ingestion of oocysts.
- Cryptosporidia develop in the GI epithelial cells and cause damage to microvilli, which may result in malabsorption, maldigestion, and diarrhea.
- Short prepatent period (72–96 hours)

DIAGNOSIS

DIFFERENTIAL DIAGNOSIS
- Enteric clostridiosis
- Salmonellosis
- Rotavirus, coronavirus
- Foal heat diarrhea
- Parasitic diarrhea
- Septicemia

INITIAL DATABASE
- Laboratory findings are nonspecific; evidence is often found of dehydration along with acid-base and electrolyte abnormalities consistent with diarrhea.

- Evaluate neonatal foals for passive transfer of antibody and septicemia.

ADVANCED OR CONFIRMATORY TESTING
- Identification of *C. parvum* in feces (oocysts are smaller than those of most coccidia—4–5 μm)
  - Microscopic examination with special staining (acid-fast, acridine orange, modified Ziehl-Neelsen)
  - Immunofluorescence assay
  - Flow cytometry
- Histopathology: Villous atrophy; organisms may be visualized

TREATMENT

THERAPEUTIC GOAL(S)
Resolution of diarrhea

ACUTE GENERAL TREATMENT
- Supportive care for diarrhea should be provided.
- No data are available regarding specific therapy for *C. parvum* infection in horses.
- Pharmacologic control has been difficult in other species.
- Drugs that may be effective include nitazoxanide, paromomycin, and azithromycin.

PROGNOSIS AND OUTCOME

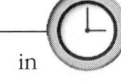

- Generally self-limiting in immunocompetent hosts.

- Severe cases may result in marked dehydration, weakness, and death.

PEARLS & CONSIDERATIONS

COMMENTS
- This is an uncommon cause of diarrhea in horses but should be considered, especially in hospitalized, stressed, and immunocompromised foals.
- Highly transmissible to humans.

PREVENTION
- Oocysts resistant to most common disinfectants. Exposure to 5% ammonia solution or 10% formalin for 18 hours will kill oocysts; freezing, thorough drying, and moist heat may also be effective.
- Removal of manure may limit oocysts in the environment.

CLIENT EDUCATION
Good hygiene is essential when handling foals with diarrhea.

SUGGESTED READING
Cole DJ, Cohen ND, Snowden K, et al: Prevalence of and risk factors for fecal shedding of *Cryptosporidium parvum* oocysts in horses. *J Am Vet Med Assoc* 213:1296, 1998.
Coleman SU, Klei TR, French DD, et al: Prevalence of *Cryptosporidium* sp in equids in Louisiana. *Am J Vet Res* 50:575, 1989.

AUTHOR: **MELISSA T. HINES**

EDITORS: **MAUREEN LONG** and **DEBRA C. SELLON**

Cushing's Disease (Pituitary Pars Intermedia Dysfunction)

BASIC INFORMATION

DEFINITION
A clinical condition of old horses associated with hirsutism, laminitis, depression, polyuria (PU) and polydipsia (PD), muscle wasting, weight loss, docility, polyphagia, and recurrent infections

SYNONYM(S)
- Pituitary pars intermedia dysfunction (PPID) is the appropriate term.
- Pituitary adenoma
- Pars intermedia adenoma
- Pituitary-dependent hyperadrenocorticism

EPIDEMIOLOGY

SPECIES, AGE, SEX
- Horses older than 7 years of age (range, 7–40 years)
- More prevalent in ponies

GEOGRAPHY AND SEASONALITY
More evident in the spring and summer when horses with PPID fail to shed their hair coat

CLINICAL PRESENTATION

HISTORY, CHIEF COMPLAINT Hirsutism (60%–80%) is the most frequent clinical sign in affected horses.

PHYSICAL EXAM FINDINGS
- Chronic laminitis is a consistent finding in these horses.
- PU and PD have been reported in up to 75% of horses.

- Failure to shed hair coat in spring or summer is a consistent finding.
- Weight loss, lethargy, increased docility
- Secondary infections (dermatitis, sinusitis, pneumonia), dental disease
- Excessive sweating (hyperhidrosis) and lack of sweating (anhidrosis)
- Redistribution of fat deposits
- Pendulous abdomen, sway back, and loss of muscle mass
- Other clinical signs include abnormal estrus cycles and neurologic signs (seizures, narcolepsy).

ETIOLOGY AND PATHOPHYSIOLOGY
- The hypothalamus, via dopamine, inhibits cells (melanotropes) of the pars intermedia of the pituitary gland.
- Hypothalamic neuronal oxidative damage results in loss of dopaminer-

gic inhibition of melanotropes, which leads to hyperplasia, adenoma formation, and excessive production of adrenocorticotropic hormone (ACTH), α-melanocyte-stimulation hormone (α-MSH), and β-endorphin
- Excessive ACTH leads to increased cortisol concentrations (hyperadrenocorticism) and clinical signs of the disease.
- Increased α-MSH concentrations may be responsible for abnormal hair shedding.
- Increased β-endorphin concentrations appear to be responsible for the calm behavior of these horses.
- High cortisol concentrations lead to hyperglycemia, insulin resistance, laminitis, immunosuppression, and secondary infections.
- Adenoma enlargement may result in additional hypothalamic damage.
- Neuronal degeneration may be responsible for seizures.
- PPID is a better term for this disease because unlike humans and dogs with Cushing's disease in which the adenoma is in the pars distalis (anterior lobe), the adenoma is in the pars intermedia in horses.

DIAGNOSIS

DIFFERENTIAL DIAGNOSIS
- Equine metabolic syndrome
- Obesity and laminitis
- Hyperadrenocorticism
- Hypothyroidism

INITIAL DATABASE
- Dexamethasone suppression test (DST)*

---

*The resting ACTH, DST, TRH stimulation test, and combined DST/TRH stimulation test are well accepted among practitioners.

- Thyrotropin-releasing hormone (TRH) stimulation test*
- Resting plasma ACTH concentrations*
- Resting cortisol concentrations
- Urinary corticoid:creatinine ratio
- Combined DST-TRH test*
- Hyperglycemia and increased insulin concentrations are a common finding in these horses.
- Domperidone response test
- Plasma α-MSH concentrations (human assays can be used; use a control horse)
- It is important to know seasonal variations when collecting samples for diagnosis.
- ACTH and α-MSH concentrations in healthy horses are increased at the end of summer and early fall (may lead to misdiagnosis).
- Cortisol concentrations after the DST in healthy horses are higher in late summer and early fall.

TREATMENT

ACUTE GENERAL TREATMENT
- Pergolide (0.2–5.0 mg PO SID), a dopamine D2 receptor agonist, is the drug of choice. Most horses show improvement with doses of 0.75 to 1.5 mg/d of pergolide.
- In Europe, bromocriptine (0.03–0.09 mg/kg BID PO or SC) is an alternative dopamine agonist.
- Improvement is evident by 6 weeks of treatment and includes shedding of the hair coat, a decrease in plasma ACTH concentration, and a decrease in glucose concentration.
- Cyproheptadine (0.25 mg/kg PO SID), a serotonin antagonist, has been used with some success.
- Combinations of pergolide and cyproheptadine have been used.

CHRONIC TREATMENT
- These drugs do not cure PPID, and horses with clinical improvement should be treated for life.
- Clipping the hair coat may be necessary in hot weather.
- Avoid stressful conditions.
- Decrease intake of soluble carbohydrates (concentrates, sweet feed, corn).
- Provide specific treatment of chronic laminitis or solar abscesses.

PROGNOSIS AND OUTCOME
- Depends on clinical signs. Treatment is palliative.
- PPID is an incurable disease.
- Horses with mild laminitis and specific treatment can live for many years.
- Horses with severe laminitis or secondary infections have a guarded prognosis.

PEARLS & CONSIDERATIONS

CLIENT EDUCATION
- The disease is incurable.
- Secondary infections are common.
- Avoid heat exposure.
- Treatment can be expensive.

SUGGESTED READING
McFarlane D: Pituitary and hypothalamus. In Smith BP, editor: *Large animal internal medicine*, ed 4. St Louis, 2009, Mosby Elsevier, pp 1339–1344.
McFarlane D, Toribio RE: Pituitary pars intermedia dysfunction (equine Cushing's disease). In Reed SM, Bayly WM, Sellon DC, editors: *Equine internal medicine*, ed 3. St Louis, 2010, Saunders Elsevier, pp 1262–1270.

AUTHOR & EDITOR: **RAMIRO E. TORIBIO**

Cyanide Toxicosis

BASIC INFORMATION

DEFINITION
Cyanide poisoning in animals usually results from ingestion of plants containing cyanogenic glycosides. Poisoning may also occur when cyanide is inhaled as gaseous hydrogen cyanide or is ingested in the chemical forms of sodium and potassium cyanide, but these causes are very uncommon in animals. Cyanide poisoning is rare in horses.

SYNONYM(S)
- Prussic acid poisoning
- Hydrogen cyanide (HCN) poisoning

EPIDEMIOLOGY
SPECIES, AGE, SEX All ages and species of mammals are susceptible to cyanide poisoning.
GEOGRAPHY AND SEASONALITY There are at least 2500 plant species in many plant families, including the Asteraceae, Chenopodiaceae, Euphorbiaceae, Fabaceae, Juncaginaceae, Linaceae, Poaceae, and Rosaceae, that are known to contain cyanogenic glycosides. A few of the more common plants with cyanogenic potential include service berry, elderberry, Johnson grass, Sudan grass, arrow grass, corn, cherry laurel, wild cherry, and chokecherry.

CLINICAL PRESENTATION
DISEASE FORMS/SUBTYPES
- Acute cyanide poisoning
- Chronic cyanide poisoning is discussed in "Sorghum and Sudan Grass Toxicosis" in this section

HISTORY, CHIEF COMPLAINT Sudden death is usually the presenting feature of cyanide poisoning.

PHYSICAL EXAM FINDINGS
- Severe dyspnea, open-mouthed breathing, staggering gait, prostration
- Mucous membranes initially are congested and bright red, becoming cyanotic near death.
- A lethal dose of cyanide results in death within a few minutes to 1 hour.

ETIOLOGY AND PATHOPHYSIOLOGY
- Cyanide reversibly inhibits mitochondrial cytochrome oxidase and blocks electron transport, resulting in decreased oxidative metabolism and oxygen utilization.
- Plant-associated cyanide toxicity depends on enzymatic hydrolysis of cyanogenic glycosides that liberates the toxic cyanide ion responsible for toxicity. Plants do not contain free HCN because the cyanogenic glycosides and the hydrolyzing enzymes are compartmentalized in the plant.
- Damage to the plant cell compartments is necessary to start the hydrolytic process. Optimally, this occurs at a pH greater than 4 or when the plants are damaged as a result of drought, wilting, freezing, or crushing.
- Plant-induced acute cyanide poisoning in horses is poorly documented in the literature, but cyanide poisoning in ruminants is well documented. This species difference is related to the ability of rumenal digestive microflora to rapidly hydrolyze cyanogenic glycosides and the low pH of the horse's stomach in contrast to the more alkaline pH of the rumen.
- Plant cyanide-producing potential is highest in new growth and declines significantly as leaves mature.

DIAGNOSIS

DIFFERENTIAL DIAGNOSIS
- Other causes of sudden death
- Ionophore toxicity
- Carbon monoxide poisoning
- Yew (*Taxus* spp.) poisoning
- Milkweed (*Asclepias* spp.) poisoning
- Oleander (*Nerium oleander*) poisoning
- Perilla mint (*Perilla frutescens*) poisoning
- Electrocution
- Malicious poisoning with chemicals such as fluoroacetate or zinc phosphide

INITIAL DATABASE
Venous blood and mucous membranes may be bright red

ADVANCED OR CONFIRMATORY TESTING
- Lactic acidosis occurs as a consequence of anaerobic metabolism.
- No gross abnormalities are evident on postmortem examination.
- Stomach contents should be collected immediately after death, frozen in an air-tight container, and submitted for cyanide detection. Tissues such as spleen, liver, and muscle can also be analyzed for cyanide. Autolyzed tissues can give false-positive cyanide results.
- Refrigerated blood from live animals can be tested for cyanide. Blood cyanide levels above 1 ppm are highly suggestive of acute toxicity.
- Suspect plant material that the animal has been consuming should be collected for cyanide analysis. Plant cyanide levels above 200 ppm are potentially toxic.
- Rapid testing for cyanide in plant or stomach contents can be done with Cyantesmo paper (Macherey-Nagel, Dueren, Germany).

TREATMENT

THERAPEUTIC GOAL(S)
- Avoid stressing the animal as much as possible.
- Provide antidotal treatment and supportive care
- Remove the source of cyanide.

ACUTE GENERAL TREATMENT
- Sodium thiosulfate administered IV is an antidotal therapy for cyanide poisoning.
- A combination of sodium thiosulfate and sodium nitrite can also be used but may not be as safe. Sodium nitrite causes the formation of methemoglobin that binds with cyanide to form cyanmethemoglobin, and the formation of methemoglobin further compromises oxygen carrying capacity of the red blood cells.
- Hydroxocobalamin (Cyanokit) is the preferred treatment for cyanide poisoning in humans and has been used in dogs, but its use is not yet documented in horses.

PROGNOSIS AND OUTCOME

Animals surviving more than 1 hour after the onset of signs often recover.

PEARLS & CONSIDERATIONS

COMMENTS
Cyanide poisoning was initially thought to be involved in the Mare reproductive loss syndrome (MRLS) reported from central Kentucky in 2001. Eastern tent caterpillars feeding on cherry tree leaves and subsequently eaten by horses grazing the pastures where the caterpillars were prevalent in massive numbers were thought to have poisoned the mares. Extensive experiments in which caterpillars were fed to horses showed that cyanide was apparently not the cause of MRLS. However, the eastern tent caterpillar appears to be involved in MRLS, possibly through an as yet unidentified toxin or by causing damage to the intestinal mucosa, allowing bacteria to enter the blood and affect the fetus (see "Actinobacillosis" in this section).

PREVENTION
- Reduce exposure to known cyanogenic glycoside-containing plants.
- Feed a balanced ration to ensure that horses do not exclusively eat potentially toxic plants.
- Do not plant cherry trees in or around horse pastures.

SUGGESTED READING
Burrows GE, Tyrl RJ: Xanthium. In Burrows GE, Tyrl RJ, editors: *Toxic plants of North America.* Ames, IA, 2001, Iowa State University Press, pp 1043–1074.

Dalefield RR: Rapid method for the detection of cyanide gas release from plant material using CYANTESMO paper. *Vet Human Toxicol* 42:356–357, 2000.

Jackson T: Cyanide poisoning in two donkeys. *Vet Hum Toxicol* 37:567–568, 1995.

Salkowski AA, Penney DG: Cyanide poisoning in animals and humans: a review. *Vet Hum Toxicol* 36:455–465, 1994.

Smeathers DM, Gray E, James JH: Hydrocyanic acid potential of black cherry leaves as influenced by aging and drying. *Agron J* 65:775–777, 1973.

Vetter J: Plant cyanogenic glycosides. *Toxicon* 38:11–36, 2000.

AUTHOR: ANTHONY P. KNIGHT

EDITOR: CYNTHIA L. GASKILL

Cyathostominosis

BASIC INFORMATION

DEFINITION

Parasitic infection in the large colon or cecum with cyathostomes (small strongyles)

SYNONYM(S)

- Larval cyathostomiasis
- Cyathostomiasis

EPIDEMIOLOGY

SPECIES, AGE, SEX Most common in horses between ages 1 and 6 years, which have less resistance to parasitic infection

GEOGRAPHY AND SEASONALITY Commonly occurs in winter and spring

CLINICAL PRESENTATION

DISEASE FORMS/SUBTYPES

- Subclinical infestation
- Clinical disease (see below)

HISTORY, CHIEF COMPLAINT

- Weight loss
- Inappetence
- Diarrhea
- Colic (of variable severity)
- Fever may or may not be present
- Ventral edema

PHYSICAL EXAM FINDINGS

- Poor body condition and rough hair coat
- Variable pyrexia
- Ventral edema frequently present
- Other findings as for other causes of colitis (See "Colitis/Diarrhea, Acute" in this section)
- Rectal examination
  - Usually as for other causes of colitis, with rectal mucosal edema and fluid colonic contents.
  - Occasionally, live larvae (small red or white worms) may be seen grossly in the feces or on the rectal sleeve.
  - Rarely, mesenteric lymphadenopathy or irregularities in the colonic surface are palpable per rectum in severe cases.
  - Intestinal intussusceptions are occasionally associated with cyathostominosis and may be palpable per rectum as a firm mass, usually in the right caudal abdomen. Alternatively, distension of the large or small intestine may be noted with such intestinal obstruction.

ETIOLOGY AND PATHOPHYSIOLOGY

- The life cycle of cyathostomes is directly regulated by environmental temperature.
  - Eggs are passed in the feces and develop into L1, L2, and then infective L3 larvae in the environment in temperate weather (45° to 85° F). Development is impaired by hot, dry weather or freezing temperatures.
  - L3 larvae are ingested by horses on pasture and enter a period of dormancy (weeks to years) by encysting in the cecal and colonic wall.
  - When environmental conditions are favorable for further development, these hypobiotic larvae emerge from their cysts and develop in the colonic lumen into mature (L4 and L5) larvae, which lay eggs that are then passed in the feces.
- In most climates, emergence of encysted larvae and clinical cyathostominosis occurs in the late winter and early spring, but in hotter climates, clinical disease may be seen in the late fall.
- Associated clinical signs (weight loss, diarrhea, colic, fever, and hypoproteinemia) are attributable to disruption of the colonic mucosal barrier caused by penetration or reemergence of large numbers of encysted larvae.
- Intestinal intussusception (most often cecocolic, cecocecal, or colocolic) associated with cyathostominosis may result from abnormal peristaltic contractions because of severe mural inflammation associated with encysted larvae.

DIAGNOSIS

DIFFERENTIAL DIAGNOSIS

Other causes of colitis (see "Colitis/Diarrhea, Acute" in this section)

INITIAL DATABASE

- In general, as for other causes of colitis (see "Colitis/Diarrhea, Acute" in this section).
- Leucocytosis and neutrophilia are common findings.
- Hypoproteinemia and hypoalbuminemia are fairly consistent findings.
- Transabdominal ultrasonography may reveal multifocal or diffuse increased mural thickness (>5 mm) in the cecum or colon in patients with large numbers of encysted larvae. An intussusception may be visualized ultrasonographically, appearing as a "bull's eye," with an intestinal wall or walls visible within the lumen of another segment of intestine.
- The presence of serosanguineous peritoneal fluid or persistent signs of abdominal pain in a horse with sus-

pected or confirmed cyathostominosis should prompt consideration of an intussusception and may warrant exploratory celiotomy.

ADVANCED OR CONFIRMATORY TESTING

- Fecal flotation
  - Large numbers of strongyle larvae or eggs are consistent with cyathostominosis.
  - However, strongyle eggs may not be seen even in severe cases because clinical disease typically occurs during the prepatent period.
- Testing for other causes of colitis is also warranted, as detailed in "Colitis/Diarrhea, Acute" in this section.

TREATMENT

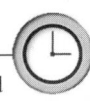

THERAPEUTIC GOAL(S)

- Eliminate encysted and intraluminal larvae.
- Provide supportive care.

ACUTE GENERAL TREATMENT

- Fluid and colloidal support, antiinflammatory and antiendotoxic therapy, and other supportive care as for other causes of colitis (see "Colitis/Diarrhea, Acute" in this section)
- Anthelmintic therapy
  - Fenbendazole: 10 mg/kg PO q24h for 5 days (widespread resistance to benzimidazoles may limit the efficacy of this treatment).
  - Moxidectin: 0.4 to 0.5 mg/kg PO once (not for use in foals <4 to 6 months old).
  - Ivermectin and pyrantel pamoate are not effective against encysted cyathostomes but are effective against the intraluminal stages.

POSSIBLE COMPLICATIONS

Intestinal intussusception

PROGNOSIS AND OUTCOME

Fair to good with aggressive and appropriate therapy

PEARLS & CONSIDERATIONS

COMMENTS

- It is important to note that a negative fecal flotation result does not rule

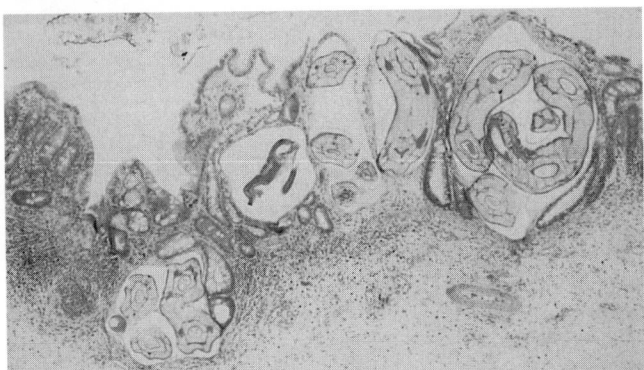

FIGURE 1 Histologic appearance of the colon showing multiple encysted cyathostomin larvae.

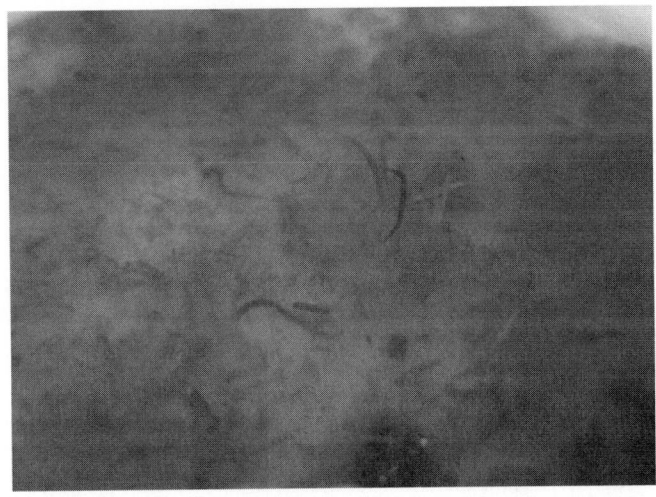

FIGURE 2 Cyathostomin larvae in fecal sample of horse affected by larval cyathostominosis.

out cyathostominosis as a cause of colitis.
- Empiric larvicidal deworming should be considered in equine colitis cases in which weight loss is an accompanying clinical sign or in which another specific cause is not determined.

PREVENTION
- Seasonal larvicidal deworming with fenbendazole or moxidectin during the early winter (or late summer in hot climates) may decrease the incidence of clinical cyathostominosis. However, fecal egg counts should be monitored and deworming strategies determined for individual farms to minimize the development of anthelmintic resistance.
- Appropriate manure and pasture management (with limited horse density) is also helpful in reducing transmission and parasite loads.

SUGGESTED READING
Fleming SA: Parasite control programs. In Smith BP, editor: *Large animal internal medicine*, St Louis, 2009, Mosby Elsevier, pp 1624–1625.

AUTHOR: **KELSEY A. HART**

EDITOR: **TIM MAIR**

Cystitis, Bacterial

BASIC INFORMATION

DEFINITION
Bacterial infection of the urinary bladder

EPIDEMIOLOGY
RISK FACTORS
- Urolithiasis
- Neoplasia
- Incontinence
- Iatrogenic contamination (eg, passage of endoscopes, catheters)

ASSOCIATED CONDITIONS AND DISORDERS
- Sabulous urolithiasis
- Urolithiasis
- Urethral damage
- Incontinence

CLINICAL PRESENTATION
HISTORY, CHIEF COMPLAINT
- Pollakiuria
- Hematuria
- Incontinence
- Mild chronic colic
- Frequently posturing to urinate

PHYSICAL EXAM FINDINGS
- Dysuria
- Urine scalding or crystals on the perineum or hind limbs
- Hematuria
- Incontinence

ETIOLOGY AND PATHOPHYSIOLOGY
- Usually secondary to urine retention
- Decreased urine flow allows for bacterial colonization.
- Hematuria occurs when the bladder or urethral mucosa is eroded or severely irritated.
- Common infectious agents of cystitis include:
  - *Escherichia coli*
  - *Proteus mirabilis*
  - *Pseudomonas aeruginosa*
  - *Corynebacterium renale*
  - *Klebsiella* spp.
  - *Enterobacter* spp.
  - *Streptococcus* spp.
  - *Staphylococcus* spp.
  - *Candida* spp. (fungal pathogen more common in neonates on antimicrobial therapy)

DIAGNOSIS

DIFFERENTIAL DIAGNOSIS
- Estral behavior in mares
- Urolithiasis
- Pyelonephritis

INITIAL DATABASE
- Complete blood count (CBC) and serum chemistries
  - CBC is usually within normal limits.
  - Serum chemistries may reveal azotemia.
- Urinalysis: High number of white blood cells, epithelial cells, erythrocytes, and intracellular and extracellular bacteria
- Urine culture
- Palpation per rectum: Thickened bladder

ADVANCED OR CONFIRMATORY TESTING
- Quantitative urine culture (>10,000 CFU/mL is significant)
- Cystoscopy

- Transrectal or transabdominal ultrasound examination

TREATMENT

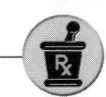

THERAPEUTIC GOAL(S)

- Correct any predisposing problems.
- Resolve bacterial infection.

ACUTE GENERAL TREATMENT

- Antimicrobials based on culture and sensitivity results, especially those that are eliminated into the urine
  - Antibiotics should be administered for at least 1 week.
  - Trimethoprim-sulfonamides: 15 to 30 mg/kg PO q12h
  - Penicillin and an aminoglycoside (provided creatinine is normal)
- Procaine penicillin G: 22,000 to 44,000 IU/kg IM q12h
- Potassium penicillin: 22,000 IU/kg IV q6h
- Gentamicin: 6.6 mg/kg IV q24h
  - Ceftiofur: 2.2 to 4.4 mg/kg IM q24h or IV q12h
  - Enrofloxacin: 7.5 mg/kg PO or 5.5 mg/kg IV q24h
- Catheterization of the bladder if urinary retention is a predisposing factor

CHRONIC TREATMENT

- A 4- to 6-week course of antimicrobials may be necessary in some cases.
- Lavage the bladder with sterile saline ± antiseptics.
- Oral salt administration (50–75 g/d) to increase water intake
- Urinary acidification (efficacy is questionable)
  - Ammonium chloride: 20 mg/kg/d
  - Vitamin C: 10 to 20 g/d
  - $CaSO_4$ (gypsum): 100 g/d
  - Potassium magnesium aspartate: 2.5 g PO q12h

RECOMMENDED MONITORING

- Repeated urinalysis and urine culture
- Cystoscopy may be necessary to assess healing of the mucosa.

PROGNOSIS AND OUTCOME

- Experimental models of bacterial cystitis showed spontaneous recovery in 2 to 4 weeks, but complete resolution was seen in 3 to 6 days with treatment.
- Chronic infections may result in sabulous cystitis or pyelonephritis.

PEARLS & CONSIDERATIONS

COMMENTS

- Primary bacterial cystitis is uncommon.
- Predisposing conditions that lead to urinary retention or cystitis (urolithiasis) must be ruled out and treated as necessary.

PREVENTION

- Aseptic technique should be used whenever urinary catheters or other instruments are used within the urinary tract.
- Prophylactic antibiotic therapy may be effective whenever any surgery is performed or any instrument is introduced into the urinary tract.

SUGGESTED READING

Divers TJ: Urinary tract infections. In Smith BP, editor: *Large Animal Internal Medicine*. St Louis, 2009, Saunders Elsevier, pp 934–935.
Schott HC: Urinary tract infections. In Reed S, Bayly W, Sellon D, editors: *Equine Internal Medicine*, ed 3. St Louis, 2010, Saunders Elsevier, pp 1199–1200.

AUTHOR: **JOAN NORTON**

EDITOR: **BRYAN M. WALDRIDGE**

Death Camas Toxicosis

BASIC INFORMATION

DEFINITION

Death camas (*Zigadenus* spp.) is native to North America and is poisonous to humans and other animals.

SYNONYM(S)

Star lily

EPIDEMIOLOGY

GENETICS AND BREED PREDISPOSITION Horses and livestock eating the new growth or bulbs are at risk for poisoning.
RISK FACTORS Early spring grazing when the death camas shoots emerge before grasses
GEOGRAPHY AND SEASONALITY Perennial plants growing from an onion-like bulb with long, narrow, V-shaped basal leaves appearing in early spring. Flowers are radially symmetrical, bisexual, and six-tepalled (three petals and three sepals identical) and are generally white or yellowish-green. There are at least 14 recognized species in North America (Figure 1).
ASSOCIATED CONDITIONS AND DISORDERS A plant of the southeastern states, *Amianthium muscaetoxicum* (crow poison, fly poison, or stagger grass, as it is variously known) contains similar hypotensive and neurotoxic alkaloids to those found in *Zigadenus* spp. (Figure 2).

CLINICAL PRESENTATION

HISTORY, CHIEF COMPLAINT Excessive salivation, colic, and depression are the primary signs.
PHYSICAL EXAM FINDINGS Depending on the amount of death camas consumed, signs can be mild to severe with depression, colic, and excessive salivation being the most common findings in horses. Intestinal peristalsis may be increased in severe cases, resulting in diarrhea.
ETIOLOGY AND PATHOPHYSIOLOGY
- Both *Zigadenus* and *Amianthium* spp. contain varying quantities of cevanine alkaloids similar to those found in *Veratrum* spp. These alkaloids have

hypotensive and neurotoxic effects and increase reflex activity.
- In sheep, death results from central respiratory depression.

DIAGNOSIS

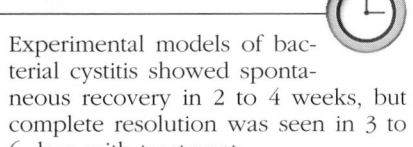

DIFFERENTIAL DIAGNOSIS

Ionophore toxicity

INITIAL DATABASE

Hematology and serum biochemistry values are often normal.

ADVANCED OR CONFIRMATORY TESTING

Cevanine alkaloid detection in stomach contents

TREATMENT

ACUTE GENERAL TREATMENT

- If horses are seen grazing the plants or soon after signs are recognized,

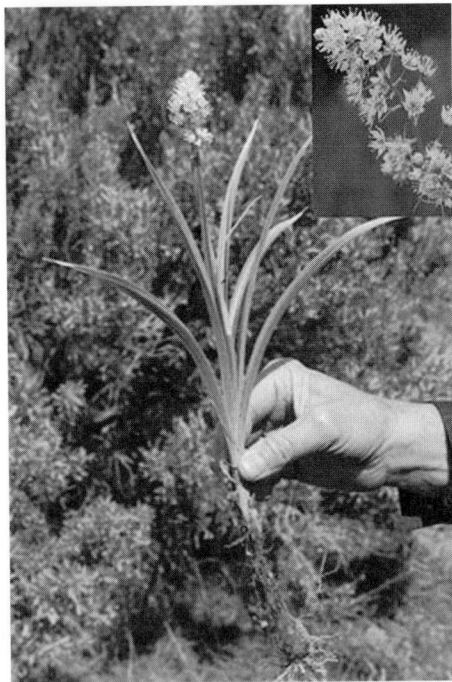

FIGURE 1 Meadow death camas (*Zigadenus venenosus*).

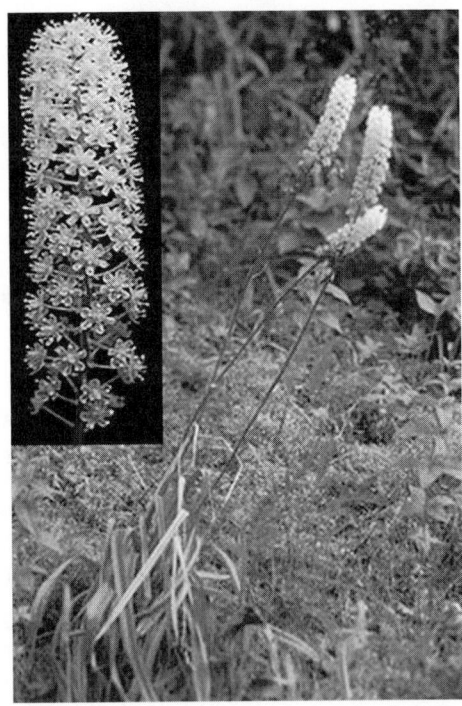

FIGURE 2 Crow or fly poison (*Amianthium muscaetoxicum*).

activated charcoal via nasogastric tube is beneficial.
• Supportive treatment should be provided as necessary.

PROGNOSIS AND OUTCOME

Horses rarely eat sufficient quantities of the plant to induce serious toxicity and generally recover within 2 to 3 days after ingesting death camas.

PEARLS & CONSIDERATIONS

COMMENTS
• Death camas and fly poison are native plants that may be concentrated in some pastures, making toxicity more likely.
• Death camas and fly poison are both toxic to humans, especially when the bulbs are mistakenly eaten for wild onion bulbs.

PREVENTION
Where the density of plants is high, selective herbicides may be useful in removing the plants.

CLIENT EDUCATION
Recognition of the plants aids in preventing toxicity.

SUGGESTED READING
Collet S, et al: Deaths of 23 adult cows attributed to intoxication of the alkaloids of *Zigadenus venenosus* (meadow death camas). *Agri Pract* 17:5–9, 1996.
Majak W, et al: Content of zygacine in *Zigadenus venenosus* at different stages of growth. *Phytochem* 31:3417–3418, 1992.
Panter KE, et al: Death camas: early grazing can be hazardous. *Rangelands* 11:147–149, 1989.

AUTHOR: ANTHONY P. KNIGHT

EDITOR: CYNTHIA GASKILL

Dehydration

BASIC INFORMATION

DEFINITION
A state in which fluid losses (apparent losses as well as insensible losses combined) outpace fluid intake

SYNONYM(S)
• Hypovolemia
• Negative fluid balance

EPIDEMIOLOGY
SPECIES, AGE, SEX Foals are particularly at risk because of their high body water content and surface-to-volume ratio.
CONTAGION AND ZOONOSIS Dehydration is not contagious itself; however, some of the diseases that cause it may be communicable to others (eg, colitis caused by *Salmonella* spp. or rabid encephalitis).

GEOGRAPHY AND SEASONALITY
• Cold weather may limit access to water because of freezing of water sources or reduced intake because of the decreased palatability of cold water.
• Hot weather may increase fluid and electrolyte losses through sweat.
ASSOCIATED CONDITIONS AND DISORDERS Diseases that increase fluid losses in excess of the horse's ability to take in fluids, toxins that increase vascular leakage, disruption of the protective

dermis by burn injury, as well as disorders that inhibit the horse's ability to drink and swallow may cause dehydration.

CLINICAL PRESENTATION

DISEASE FORMS/SUBTYPES
- Hypertonic dehydration
- Isotonic dehydration
- Hypotonic dehydration

HISTORY, CHIEF COMPLAINT Variable because of the diverse etiology

PHYSICAL EXAM FINDINGS
- Depression; lethargy; tachycardia; reduced pulse quality; increased duration of skin tent test; dry mucous membranes; increased capillary refill time (CRT); cool extremities; mucus-covered fecal balls; or dry, scant feces (Figures 1 and 2)
- Weight loss is the gold standard for determining the percent of body weight lost to dehydration.
- The approximate percent dehydration can be estimated from physical examination findings as follows:
  - Heart rate 40 to 60 beats/min, CRT <2: approximately 6% dehydration
  - Heart rate 61 to 80 beats/min, CRT <3: approximately 8% dehydration
  - Heart rate 81 to 100 beats/min, CRT <4: approximately 10% dehydration
  - Heart rate 101+ beats/min, CRT >4, packed cell volume (PCV) >50%: approximately >10% dehydration; the horse is in hypovolemic shock

ETIOLOGY AND PATHOPHYSIOLOGY
- Pathophysiology: Dehydration results in a reduction of relative circulating volume. Decreased tissue perfusion reduces oxygen delivery to the tissues, increasing anaerobic metabolism and reducing tissue pH through acid accumulation and lactate production.
- Reduced intake
  - Environmental: Weather, lack of available water
  - Mechanical obstruction: Jaw fracture, pharyngeal injury, choking
  - Neurologic disorders causing dysphagia
  - Gastrointestinal disease: Gastric outflow obstruction, small intestinal obstruction, or ileus
- Increased losses
  - Enterocolitis
  - Primary renal disease
  - Significant nasogastric reflux caused by enteritis
  - Severe burns
  - Endotoxemia
- Relative dehydration: Salt toxicity

DIAGNOSIS

DIFFERENTIAL DIAGNOSIS
Dehydration is a secondary condition to a number of primary diseases and disorders.

INITIAL DATABASE
- Complete blood count
- PCV and total protein (TP)
- Blood lactate
- Serum chemistry
- Urinalysis

ADVANCED OR CONFIRMATORY TESTING
Based on physical examination findings and the initial database, system specific tests may be applicable:
- Oral or pharyngeal disorders: Oral examination, endoscopy, radiography
- Neurologic disease: Neurologic examination, cerebrospinal fluid analysis, serum titers, computed tomography, radiography, liver biopsy
- Gastrointestinal disease: Abdominocentesis, abdominal ultrasonography, rectal examination, nasogastric intubation, fecal culture (aerobic, anaerobic), fecal clostridial toxin screening
- Renal disease: Fractional electrolyte excretion tests, renal biopsy

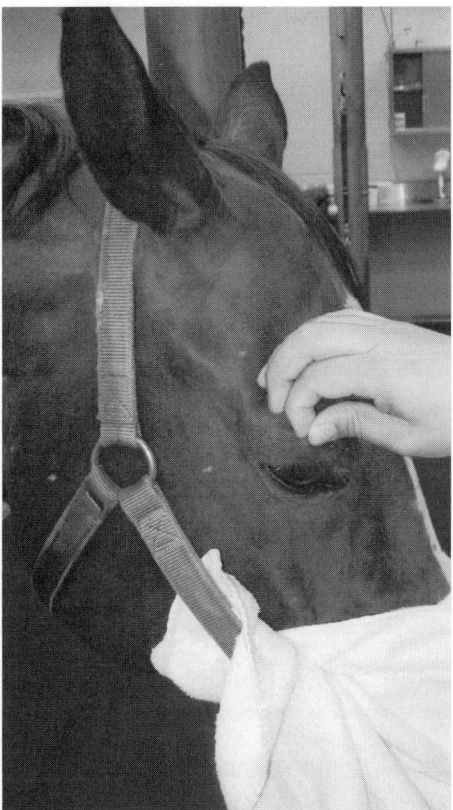

FIGURE 1 Skin tent test for dehydration using the upper eyelid of the horse. This test may also be performed on the neck dorsal to the cervical vertebrae and cranial to the shoulder.

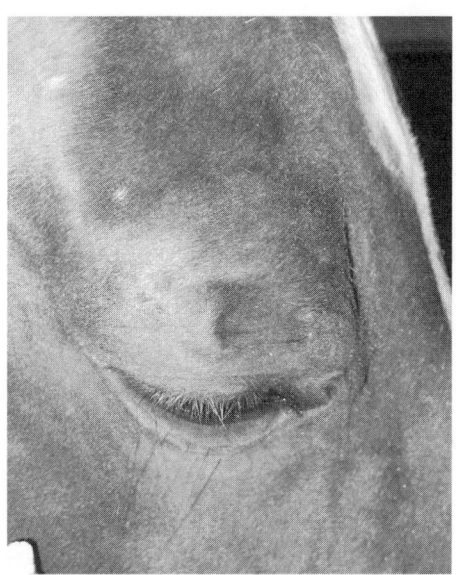

FIGURE 2 Prolonged skin tent test of >4 seconds. Based on the complete physical examination, this horse was more than 10% dehydrated.

TREATMENT

THERAPEUTIC GOAL(S)

- Replacement of the circulating volume
- Normalization of electrolyte abnormalities
- Resolution of acid-base disorders
- Treatment of the underlying disease

ACUTE GENERAL TREATMENT

Fluid therapy:
- Generally administered IV or by nasogastric intubation in boluses or by constant-rate infusion. Oral fluids are not absorbed if the horse is more than 8% dehydrated.
- Dehydration is corrected in the first 24 hours, and then maintenance fluids are administered.
- Isotonic fluid requirements for dehydration are determined by the following calculation:

  Volume (L) = Estimated dehydration
  + Estimated acute loss
  + Maintenance rate

in which:
- ○ Estimated dehydration = % Dehydration × Body weight (kg)
- ○ Dehydration is in decimal form (eg, 8% = 0.08)
- ○ Adult maintenance fluid rate = 60 mL/kg/day divided by 1000 mL for liters of fluid required
- Isotonic crystalloids (Normosol R, Plasmalyte, lactated Ringer's solution) are typically used.
  - ○ Hypertonic saline or colloids may complement the crystalloid plan in hypovolemic shock in adults.
  - ○ Hypertonic saline should never be administered to foals because of a risk of demyelination.
- Fluid therapy should be reassessed q12h to update losses and reassess response.
- Electrolyte supplementation may be required for electrolyte derangements or to provide maintenance electrolytes in fluids administered for longer than 48 hours.
  - ○ Potassium
    - Maximum administration rate: 0.5 mEq/kg/h
    - Maintenance rate: 20 mEq/L in potassium-poor crystalloids
  - ○ Magnesium: 50 to 100 mg/kg IV q24h
  - ○ Sodium
    - Serum concentration should not change more than 0.5 mEq/h.
    - Serum sodium should not be corrected faster than 10 mmol/L over 24 hours.
  - ○ Calcium
    - 10 to 25 mL 23% calcium gluconate/L
    - Maintenance rate: 10 mL calcium gluconate/L in calcium-poor crystalloids
  - ○ Bicarbonate therapy is typically unnecessary. Acidosis usually corrects with fluid therapy alone.

CHRONIC TREATMENT

Depends on the underlying disease

DRUG INTERACTIONS

Bicarbonate may precipitate in calcium-containing fluids

POSSIBLE COMPLICATIONS

- Tissue edema: May result from overhydration, increased vascular permeability with endotoxemia, or cardiac dysfunction resulting in pulmonary hypertension. Colloids may be required to maintain colloid oncotic pressures and intravascular fluid.
- Hemodilution: May occur with overhydration; complicates monitoring.
- Cerebral edema and demyelination: May occur with extreme changes in sodium concentration.

RECOMMENDED MONITORING

- First 24 hours:
  - ○ PCV and TP q6h
  - ○ Urine output
  - ○ Blood urea nitrogen and creatinine q24h
  - ○ Electrolyte values q4–6h (if there is a severe derangement initially)
  - ○ Physical examination q4h (heart rate, respiratory rate and character, mucous membranes, skin tent test, peripheral temperature)
  - ○ Central venous pressure: May identify overhydration; low sensitivity in monitoring dehydration
- If therapy is sufficient and the patient is stable, monitoring may become less frequent.

PROGNOSIS AND OUTCOME

Good prognosis if primary disease can be resolved

PEARLS & CONSIDERATIONS

COMMENTS

- Horses should be monitored closely the first 24 hours of therapy to allow adjustments in administration rates and to ensure that the rehydration plan is adequate.
- The skin tent test may be a poor predictor of dehydration in old horses and neonates because of decreased organized dermal collagen.

PREVENTION

- Ensure adequate access to fresh, clean water in normal horses.
- Refer to specific disease processes for prevention.

CLIENT EDUCATION

- Fresh, clean water should be available at all times.
- Foals may dehydrate quickly and should be assessed by a veterinarian immediately if not nursing.

SUGGESTED READING

Palmer JE: Fluid therapy in the neonate: not your mother's fluid space. *Vet Clin North Am Equine Pract* 20:63–75, 2004.

Schott HC: Fluid therapy: a primer for students, technicians, and veterinarians in equine practice. *Vet Clin North Am Equine Pract* 22:1–14, 2006.

AUTHOR: **AMELIA MUNSTERMAN**

EDITORS: **R. REID HANSON** and **AMELIA MUNSTERMAN**

Dental Avulsions

BASIC INFORMATION

DEFINITION

Teeth that have been traumatically removed from their alveoli (section of the parent bone) may be salvageable for reimplantation.

SYNONYM(S)

Dental fracture

EPIDEMIOLOGY

SPECIES, AGE, SEX Young horses (median age, 6 years) in one published study

ASSOCIATED CONDITIONS AND DISORDERS Mandibular fractures

CLINICAL PRESENTATION

HISTORY, CHIEF COMPLAINT
- Acute presentation with missing teeth or clear malocclusions
- Hemorrhage

PHYSICAL EXAM FINDINGS
- Incisor avulsion portion of the incisive plate.
- Feed may be packed around the avulsed tooth roots and alveolar bone.
- Some teeth may be retained solely by a portion of the gingiva.

ETIOLOGY AND PATHOPHYSIOLOGY These fractures are usually the result of the inquisitive nature of horses such as entrapment of the teeth under a wire or fence and ensuing panic. The horse pulls back, and the teeth are avulsed.

DIAGNOSIS

DIFFERENTIAL DIAGNOSIS
- Dental fracture
- Mandibular fracture

INITIAL DATABASE
Oral and radiographic examination to include intraoral ventrodorsal projections

TREATMENT

THERAPEUTIC GOAL(S)
Incisor reattachment (incisive plate)

ACUTE GENERAL TREATMENT
- Sedation or general anesthesia, depending on the degree of soft tissue discomfort
- Removal of putrefying feed
- Wiring of teeth (bone) back to the mandible or maxilla; this may require an intraoral splint, depending on the fracture configuration

CHRONIC TREATMENT
Incisor removal if reattachment fails

POSSIBLE COMPLICATIONS
- Fixation failure
- Infection

RECOMMENDED MONITORING
Recheck in 6 weeks. Possible wire removal at this stage.

PROGNOSIS AND OUTCOME

Good

PEARLS & CONSIDERATIONS

If there is a possibility that the tooth may be saved, however tenuous, it is better to try to save it and possibly succeed rather than remove every tooth at the first examination.

SUGGESTED READING
Auer JA: Craniomaxillofacial disorders. In Auer JA, Stick JA, editors: *Equine surgery*, ed 3. New York, 2006, Saunders Elsevier, pp 1341–1362.
Baker GJ: Dental trauma. In Baker GJ, Easley J, editors: *Equine dentistry*, ed 2. New York, 2005, Saunders Elsevier, pp 87–90.

AUTHOR & EDITOR: JAMES L. CARMALT

Dentigerous Cysts

BASIC INFORMATION

DEFINITION
A cystic structure, typically present at the base of the ear, containing either dental remnants or complete teeth

SYNONYM(S)
Temporal teratoma

EPIDEMIOLOGY
SPECIES, AGE, SEX Young horses, but the cyst may enlarge with age as dental elements mature

CLINICAL PRESENTATION
HISTORY, CHIEF COMPLAINT A non-healing draining tract producing milky white or cream-colored fluid situated at the base of the ear
ETIOLOGY AND PATHOPHYSIOLOGY A congenital defect arising as an embryonic failure to close the first branchial cleft containing, by definition, dental elements

DIAGNOSIS

DIFFERENTIAL DIAGNOSIS
Pathognomonic lesion and presentation

INITIAL DATABASE
Palpation and radiographic evaluation

TREATMENT

THERAPEUTIC GOAL(S)
No treatment is necessary unless the intermittent drainage is cosmetically undesirable. If so, complete extirpation of the cyst is necessary

ACUTE GENERAL TREATMENT
General anesthesia and surgical removal

POSSIBLE COMPLICATIONS
- Damage to the auriculopalpebral nerve and associated musculature
- Damage to the calvarium during removal

PROGNOSIS AND OUTCOME

Excellent

PEARLS & CONSIDERATIONS

COMMENTS
Attempt to avoid opening the cyst.

PREVENTION
Congenital lesion; prevention is impossible

SUGGESTED READING
Carr EA: Skin conditions amenable to surgery. In Auer JA, Stick JA, editors: *Equine surgery*, ed 3. New York, 2006, Saunders Elsevier, pp 309–320.
Knottenbelt DC, Kelly DF: Oral and dental tumors. In Baker GJ, Easley J, editors: *Equine dentistry*, ed 2. New York, 2005, Saunders Elsevier, pp 127–148.

AUTHOR & EDITOR: JAMES L. CARMALT

Depigmentation Disorders (Vitiligo)

BASIC INFORMATION

DEFINITION

- Leukoderma: Depigmentation of the skin
- Leukotrichia: Depigmentation of the hair
- Reticulated leukotrichia: Cross-hatched or netlike pattern of leukotrichia
- Spotted leukotrichia: Individual small areas of leukotrichia

SYNONYM(S)

- Vitiligo: Idiopathic depigmentation; this is an overall term that includes both leukoderma and leukotrichia
- "Snowflakes"

EPIDEMIOLOGY

SPECIES, AGE, SEX

- Most common in horses but may be seen in other Equidae as well.
- Mostly in young horses but may be seen in any age
- Genetics and breed predisposition
  - Most commonly seen in (gray) Arabian horses and Shires, but any breed can be affected
  - The condition may be hereditary.

ASSOCIATED CONDITIONS AND DISORDERS A subform of equine vitiligo: Arabian fading syndrome or "pinky syndrome"

CLINICAL PRESENTATION

DISEASE FORMS/SUBTYPES

- Idiopathic vitiligo
- Leukoderma
- Leukotrichia
- Asymptomatic reticulated leukotrichia
- Hyperesthetic leukotrichia: A painful subform of reticulated leukotrichia. This may be an unusual form of erythema multiforme (associated with herpes virus infection or vaccinations).

HISTORY, CHIEF COMPLAINT Various degrees of depigmentation affecting the hair, skin, or both

PHYSICAL EXAM FINDING

- Gradually expanding depigmented macules
- Distribution of lesions may be symmetrical or segmental.
- Lesions typically affect the lips, muzzle, and eyelids; less commonly, the anus, vulva, sheath, and hooves may be affected or lesions may be generalized.
- Leukotrichia without leukoderma is common.
- No preexisting lesions in affected areas

- Pruritus is absent.
- Depigmentation may wax and wane but is usually permanent.
- Occasionally, lesions become repigmented.
- Usually nonpainful except in the early stages of hyperesthetic leukotrichia during which crusts may be present that get replaced by white hair
- Arabian fading syndrome: A form of equine vitiligo that develops in young (1–2 years of age) Arabians, more commonly in grey animals. It is characterized by round, depigmented macules at mucocutaneous junctions and is commonly permanent. If a mare develops the condition during pregnancy or shortly after parturition, the foal may be at higher risk for future development of vitiligo.

ETIOLOGY AND PATHOPHYSIOLOGY

- Vitiligo is assumed to be genetically programmed depigmentation, but to the author's knowledge, the pathophysiology of vitiligo, leukoderma, and leukotrichia in horses remains unknown.
- Three hypotheses for pigment loss in human vitiligo have been advanced:
  - Autotoxicity hypothesis: Reactive melanin precursor molecules are thought to predispose melanocytes to destruction, possibly because of inhibition of thioredoxin reductase, a free radical scavenger associated with the melanocyte cell membrane.
  - Neural hypothesis: Melanocytes originate from the neural crest and have characteristics of nerve cells; thus, neural injury has been advanced to explain dermatomally distributed vitiligo.
  - Autoimmune hypothesis: Melanocytes can be destroyed by humoral or cellular immune mechanisms; in humans and horses with vitiligo, autoantibodies against melanocytes have been found, but it is unclear whether these antibodies are the cause or a result of the disease.
- Multiple mechanisms may contribute to development of vitiligo in individual horses.

DIAGNOSIS

DIFFERENTIAL DIAGNOSIS

- Acquired depigmentation through external factors, often at sites of previous inflammation leading to the

destruction or nonfunctioning of the melanocytes
- Examples include pressure wounds, freeze branding, chemical burns, local anesthetic with epinephrine for nerve blocks, radiation, discoid or systemic lupus erythematosus, infectious bites (eg, onchocerciasis, dourine [*Trypanosoma equiperdum*], *Culicoides* spp.), aural plaques, coital exanthema (equine herpesvirus-3), and excessive amounts of exogenous thyroid hormone supplementation leading to presumed vitamin A deficiency.

INITIAL DATABASE

- Detailed history to rule out external causes (especially previous injuries)
- Physical examination: Normal appearance of hair and skin (except the lack of pigment)

ADVANCED OR CONFIRMATORY TESTING

Biopsies for histopathologic examination show normal skin (with absence of melanin).

TREATMENT

THERAPEUTIC GOAL(S)

- Repigmentation of hair and skin (can rarely be achieved)
- Prevention of sunburn of depigmented skin

ACUTE GENERAL TREATMENT

- Observation only (benign neglect) is the preferred treatment.
- Daily application of sunscreen (zinc oxide) before turning the horse out, stabling during daylight hours, or covering of affected areas (fly mask)

CHRONIC TREATMENT

- Reports of treatment for equine vitiligo are anecdotal.
  - Vitamin A (large quantities of carrots) in cases of excessive thyroid hormone supplementation
  - Copper supplementation (copper is important for the rate-limiting enzyme in melanogenesis)
  - Other treatments adapted from humans (unproven to be either safe or effective in horses)
  - Topical corticosteroids: High-potency fluorinated corticosteroids (eg, fluocinolone with dimethyl sulfoxide, Synotic) applied to lesions for 1 to 2 months and then

changed to a less potent corticosteroid; if there is no response after 3 months, treatment is discontinued; repigmentation 4 months or longer in humans; may recur after treatment is discontinued; side effects may include skin atrophy (treatment is reported to be 64% effective in childhood vitiligo).

- Topical tacrolimus (Protopic, 0.03% ointment): Use has not been described in horses; safe and effective for treatment of vitiligo in children (86% showed some repigmentation after 12 weeks of treatment).

PROGNOSIS AND OUTCOME

Usually a cosmetic disease only. Some horses repigment within 1 year; others may wax and wane, but most often the depigmentation is permanent.

PEARLS & CONSIDERATIONS

CLIENT EDUCATION

For affected show horses, it is possible to dye the depigmented hair.

PREVENTION

Because of potential heritability of equine vitiligo, breeding of affected horses is not recommended

SUGGESTED READING

Pigmentary abnormalities. In Scott DW, Miller WH, editors: *Equine dermatology.* St Louis, 2003, Saunders Elsevier Science, pp 587–599.

AUTHOR: **ANNETTE PETERSEN**

EDITOR: **DAVID A. WILSON**

Dermatitis, Atopic

BASIC INFORMATION

DEFINITION

A hypersensitivity disorder in which the patient becomes sensitized to inhaled or percutaneously absorbed allergens such as dust, pollens, and molds, causing pruritus or urticaria.

SYNONYM(S)

Allergic inhalant dermatitis, allergies, atopy

EPIDEMIOLOGY

SPECIES, AGE, SEX Age of onset is 1 to 6 years, although it can occur in older horses that have moved to different botanical zones.
GENETICS AND BREED PREDISPOSITION Familial, Thoroughbreds, and Arabians may be predisposed.
RISK FACTORS Genetic predisposition and sensitization to allergens at a young age
GEOGRAPHY AND SEASONALITY May be seasonal or nonseasonal and may be more common or severe in warmer areas with longer pollen seasons
ASSOCIATED CONDITIONS AND DISORDERS Insect hypersensitivity, eosinophilic granulomas, allergic airway disease, chronic obstructive pulmonary disease, or head shaking

CLINICAL PRESENTATION

DISEASE FORMS/SUBTYPES Pruritus, urticaria, or pruritic urticaria
HISTORY, CHIEF COMPLAINT Seasonal or nonseasonal pruritus or urticaria
PHYSICAL EXAM FINDINGS Alopecia and excoriations of the face, ears, neck, legs, or ventrum secondary bacterial folliculitis

ETIOLOGY AND PATHOPHYSIOLOGY A type 1 hypersensitivity reaction in which an allergen is inhaled, ingested, or percutaneously absorbed, resulting in the production of allergen-specific IgE. When the IgE fixed on the surface of mast cells reacts with the offending allergen, mast cell degranulation occurs, causing release and production of various pruritogenic compounds such as histamine, leukotrienes, and prostaglandins.

DIAGNOSIS

DIFFERENTIAL DIAGNOSIS

Insect hypersensitivity, food hypersensitivity, contact dermatitis, mange mites, storage mites, pediculosis, trombiculosis, oxyuriasis

INITIAL DATABASE

Diagnosis is made by history, clinical findings, response to therapies, and ruling out other differentials.

ADVANCED OR CONFIRMATORY TESTING

- Histopathology is supportive but not confirmative: Superficial and deep perivascular dermatitis with eosinophils.
- Intradermal allergy testing: Preferred
- Serological allergy testing: Unreliable

TREATMENT

THERAPEUTIC GOAL(S)

Ameliorate the clinical signs. Atopy cannot be cured, only managed.

ACUTE GENERAL TREATMENT

- Corticosteroids
  - Prednisone or prednisolone: 1 to 2 mg/kg/d PO; then tapered to the lowest possible alternate day dose
  - Dexamethasone: 0.1 to 0.2 mg/kg/d PO; then tapered to the lowest possible q72h dose.
- Antihistamines
  - Hydroxyzine: 1 to 2 mg/kg PO BID to TID
  - Doxepin: 1 mg/kg PO BID
  - Amitriptyline: 1 mg/kg PO BID
  - Chlorpheniramine: 0.25 to 0.5 mg/kg PO BID
  - Diphenhydramine: 1 to 2 mg/kg PO BID to TID
- Shampoos and rinses (eg, oatmeal soaks, pramoxine, glucocorticoids)
- Fatty acid supplements

CHRONIC TREATMENT

- Allergen-specific immunotherapy (preferably based on intradermal testing) is the most specific treatment.
- Symptomatic therapy with antihistamines, low alternate-day dose prednisolone, or topical antipruritics

POSSIBLE COMPLICATIONS

Secondary bacterial infection must be identified and eliminated with antibacterial shampoos and systemic antibiotics.

RECOMMENDED MONITORING

- Monitor and control infections.
- Decrease exposure to insects if the patient has concurrent insect hypersensitivity.

PROGNOSIS AND OUTCOME

Prognosis is good for control of the disease, although cure is not possible.

PEARLS & CONSIDERATIONS

COMMENTS

If symptoms exist longer than 2 months out of the year, then immunotherapy is the safest, most specific, and often the least expensive treatment option. There are no drug residues to be concerned about for show animals.

PREVENTION

- Affected animals should not be considered for breeding

- Avoidance of the offending allergens is beneficial but often impractical.

SUGGESTED READING

Rees CA: Response to immunotherapy in six related horses with urticaria secondary to atopy. *J Am Vet Med Assoc* 218:753, 2001.

Scott D, Miller WH: Skin immune system and allergic skin disease. *Equine dermatology.* St Louis, 2003, WB Saunders, pp 395–449.

AUTHOR: **DAVID SENTER**

EDITOR: **DAVID A. WILSON**

Dermatitis, Contact

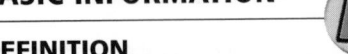

BASIC INFORMATION

DEFINITION

Rare form of hypersensitivity associated to contact with potential allergens. Substances that have been identified as potential sources are soaps, shampoos, plants, bedding material, topical medications, insect and fly repellents, leather, disinfectants, dyes, blankets, and pads.

SYNONYM(S)

Contact hypersensitivity

EPIDEMIOLOGY

GEOGRAPHY AND SEASONALITY
Contact dermatitis may be either seasonal or nonseasonal, depending on the inciting agent.

CLINICAL PRESENTATION

HISTORY, CHIEF COMPLAINT Frequently, the complaint is the presence of vesicles or papules over the specific contact area. After the vesicles rupture, an erythematous area with serous discharge is found. Pruritus and pain are rare and minimal if present.

PHYSICAL EXAM FINDINGS
- Localized inflammatory reactions occur where the foreign material has been in contact. Generally, the lesions are very well localized, but multiple areas are occasionally affected.
- Areas of self-mutilation or secondary bacterial contamination may be present in the lesions.

ETIOLOGY AND PATHOPHYSIOLOGY
- In general, the particles that create the hypersensitivity are nonallergenic on their own, but when in contact with the skin, they penetrate through the epidermis and bind to carrier pro-

teins, resulting in allergic contact dermatitis.
- The resulting type of sensitivity is a type IV hypersensitivity reaction.
- Some horses have more sensitivity reactions to fly sprays, and it can be exacerbated by applying these products before saddling and tacking because the pressure of the saddle and tack compress the offending chemical between equipment and hot sweaty skin.

DIAGNOSIS

DIFFERENTIAL DIAGNOSIS

- Parasitic hypersensitivity
- Culicoides hypersensitivity
- Pastern dermatitis
- Food hypersensitivity
- Drug eruptions
- Sarcoptic or psoroptic mange
- Ectoparasites

INITIAL DATABASE

The history, clinical signs, and physical examination can lead to a preliminary diagnosis.

ADVANCED OR CONFIRMATORY TESTING

Patch testing is confirmatory of contact dermatitis. It involves applying the suspected affecting substance on a cloth that is then applied to the skin with adhesive tape for 48 hours. If a marked reaction is present, it is suggestive of contact dermatitis. It is important to consider the possibility of reaction to the tape or the cloth material. A blank negative should be used to identify a positive reaction.

TREATMENT

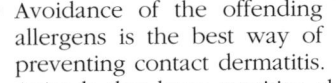

THERAPEUTIC GOAL(S)

Eliminate the source of reaction and decrease skin reaction as quickly as possible.

ACUTE GENERAL TREATMENT

- Remove the horse from the environment or source of the allergen.
- Administering oral or topical corticosteroids will decrease the clinical signs but will not cure the problem.

PROGNOSIS AND OUTCOME

- Excellent prognosis after the allergen is identified and removed from the environment of the horse
- Minimal scarring is expected after small localized lesions, but if larger areas are affected, some scarring is to be expected.

PEARLS & CONSIDERATIONS

- Avoidance of the offending allergens is the best way of preventing contact dermatitis.
- Animals that have sensitive skin may react to different types of substances, so it is important to consider the different active ingredients in products when selecting shampoos, insect repellents, and soaps.

SUGGESTED READING

Pascoe RR, Knottenbelt DC: *Manual of equine dermatology.* London, 1999, WB Saunders, pp 173–174.

Scott DW: *Equine dermatology.* St Louis, 2003, Saunders Elsevier, pp 449–453.

AUTHOR: **ALFREDO SANCHEZ LONDOÑO**

EDITOR: **DAVID A. WILSON**

Dermatophilosis

BASIC INFORMATION

DEFINITION

Common acute and chronic exudative dermatitis caused by an actinomycete. Commonly seen during rainy and humid periods.

SYNONYM(S)

Rain rot, rain scald, mud rash, mud fever

EPIDEMIOLOGY

Horses, cattle, sheep, goats and occasionally humans can be affected.

RISK FACTORS

- Horses that live outdoors and have minimal to no shelter are at a higher risk of developing the disease. Very wet and humid summers can also predispose horses to be affected because of the moisture that is maintained in the hair coat, which provides the appropriate conditions for the organism to proliferate.
- Debilitated, immunocompromised, or malnourished horses are more susceptible to developing the disease, but in general, any horse can develop the disease.

CONTAGION AND ZOONOSIS Mechanical transmission by both biting and nonbiting flies and ticks is possible, and fomites (blankets, brushes) can also cause the disease. Humans, especially those who are immunocompromised, can occasionally be affected by the disease.

GEOGRAPHY AND SEASONALITY The disease is seen worldwide and generally during very rainy seasons, mostly in the fall and winter or very rainy summers.

CLINICAL PRESENTATION

HISTORY, CHIEF COMPLAINT Presence of lesions over the dorsum of the horse that look like large drops have scalded the horse. These lesions typically exude, causing hair mats that can form a plaque. These lesions can be very painful but are rarely pruritic.

PHYSICAL EXAM FINDINGS Multiple lesions, usually less than 2 cm in diameter, over the rump, loin, and saddle area of the horse, occasionally on the face and in some cases on the legs. In severe cases, horses may show signs of systemic disease and require parenteral antibiotic treatment.

ETIOLOGY AND PATHOPHYSIOLOGY

- The etiologic agent is *Dermatophilus congolensis*, a gram-positive actinomycete bacterium. It is a non–acid-fast, branching, filamentous aerobic bacterium that is seen as parallel rows of coccoid zoospores.
- A carrier animal, moisture, and skin abrasions are necessary conditions for development of the disease.
- The primary source of infection is chronically affected animals. When the lesions in these animals are moistened, the infective stage zoospores are released. The moisture causes epidermal maceration and the organism to be infective.
- The organism can be isolated from the environment of the affected horse.

DIAGNOSIS

DIFFERENTIAL DIAGNOSIS

- Dermatophytosis
- Folliculitis caused by *Staphylococcus aureus* or *Corynebacterium pseudotuberculosis* infection
- Pemphigus foliaceus
- Viral infections
- Severe urticaria
- Generalized granulomatous disease

INITIAL DATABASE

- Complete history, physical examination, and distribution of lesions
- Removal of "paintbrush" lesions made of a scab with the undersurface covered with exudates is typically diagnostic.
- Bacterial or fungal culture of the exudates under the scab
- Gram stain identification of the filamentous organism with its classic alignment in parallel rows of 2×8 coccoid zoospores, giving it the appearance of railroad tracks
- Culture can be helpful if fresh lesions are submitted but not for old ones.
- Biopsies help differentiate it from other diseases. Findings include neutrophilic folliculitis and intraepidermal pustules.

TREATMENT

THERAPEUTIC GOAL(S)

- Remove horse from wet environment; keep the horse dry and protected from biting insects.
- Control worsening of the disease by transmission to other horses.
- Remove infective crusts and appropriately dispose of them because the organism can persist for up to 4 years.
- Prevent systemic disease.
- Provide appropriate skin hygiene.

ACUTE GENERAL TREATMENT

- Removal of crusts: This can be extremely painful, and depending on the severity of lesions, the horse may require sedation to successfully remove them.
- In severe and chronic cases in which systemic involvement is suspected, use of procaine penicillin at 22,000 IU/kg IM BID or trimethoprim sulfa at 30 mg/kg PO BID for a minimum of 7 days may be required.
- Use of shampoos containing chlorhexidine or iodine may be beneficial to soften the scabs and allow for easier removal and to prevent secondary bacterial infection.

CHRONIC TREATMENT

- Use of antibacterial shampoos is beneficial in decreasing the bacterial load.
- In hot and humid climates where rainfall amounts are large, use of insect repellent on a daily basis is recommended.

DRUG INTERACTIONS

Use of long-term antibiotics may cause digestive disturbances, so daily monitoring of fecal consistency is recommended.

PROGNOSIS AND OUTCOME

- The prognosis is good, but animals can be chronically infected and either develop the disease or be sources of infection for other animals.

- No permanent scarring will be left from removal of the scabs, but the horse can be painful shortly after removal of all the scabs and during the recovery period until normal, healthy skin is present.
- No immunity will be developed by affected horses, so relapses are possible if the appropriate conditions are present.

PEARLS & CONSIDERATIONS

COMMENTS
- Removal and appropriate disposal of the scabs is important in prevention of the disease. The scabs should not be removed and disposed of on the ground because the organism has been shown to live for up to 4 years if adequate conditions are present.
- Use of gloves when removing scabs and when treating affected horses is important to decrease the possibility of human contagion.

PREVENTION
Provide adequate shelter so that the animal is protected from severe weather. If the animal still gets extremely wet, try to dry the horse as best as possible to minimize the risk of developing the disease because of appropriate moisture and humidity in the skin.

SUGGESTED READING
Pilsworth RC, Knottenbelt D: Dermatophilosis (rain scald). *Equine Vet Ed* 19(4):212–214, 2007.
White SD: Bacterial diseases. In Smith BP, editor: *Large animal internal medicine*. St Louis, 2009, Elsevier, pp 1312–1313.

AUTHOR: **ALFREDO SANCHEZ LONDOÑO**

EDITOR: **DAVID A. WILSON**

Dermatophytosis

BASIC INFORMATION

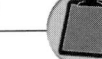

DEFINITION
Highly contagious superficial fungal infection of skin, hair, or hooves of horses and cattle and occasionally sheep and goats

SYNONYM(S)
Ringworm

EPIDEMIOLOGY
SPECIES, AGE, SEX
- Commonly seen in horses and cattle, less frequently in goats, and rarely in sheep
- Young animals are more susceptible to the infection. This increased susceptibility is because of their lack of immunity and potentially poor nutrition.

RISK FACTORS Overcrowding of animals, poor nutrition, and warmth and humidity are important risk factors in development of the disease.

CONTAGION AND ZOONOSIS Horses can get infected through direct contact with infected hair, animals, or fomites. Zoonoses are possible if direct contact with affected animals occurs.

GEOGRAPHY AND SEASONALITY The disease is seen worldwide and is commonly seen during the winter months because of overcrowding, which provides adequate conditions for the organism to grow.

CLINICAL PRESENTATION
HISTORY, CHIEF COMPLAINT Presence of multiple circular alopecic lesions, mostly on the face, legs, girth, shoulder, and chest

PHYSICAL EXAM FINDINGS
- The classic appearance in horses is a ring lesion with the central area often showing signs of healing. Scaling and crusting of these lesions can be variable, and pruritus is minimal or absent and may become exudative. The lesions may expand and start coalescing, creating large patches of alopecia. Some of these lesions may show a silver tinge to them, hyperpigmentation, and lichenification.
- Multiple lesions are typically present, but solitary lesions may rarely be present.
- Immunocompromised foals or horses may be severely affected and may develop generalized dermatophytosis.

ETIOLOGY AND PATHOPHYSIOLOGY
- *Trichophyton equinum, Microsporum equinum, Trichophyton mentagrophytes*, and *Trichophyton verrucosum* infection
- Direct or indirect transmission may occur. Contaminated grooming equipment, blankets, and tack may be a source of transmission, as can insects.
- Stress or concurrent disease may predispose horses to development of dermatophytosis.
- The incubation period is between 2 and 3 weeks. During this period, other horses very likely are already infected and starting to show signs of disease.
- Dermatophytes only invade fully keratinized and nonliving tissues, which leads to weak hair shafts and alopecia.

- Superficial infections are the most common and develop thick crusts and a classic moth-eaten appearance and a ring pattern.
- Erythema is not usually seen and can be difficult to identify in pigmented skin.
- Most infections are self-limiting over a 5- to 10-week period, but treatment is recommended to limit the spread of infection.

DIAGNOSIS

DIFFERENTIAL DIAGNOSIS
- *Staphylococcus folliculitis*
- Dermatophilosis
- *Pemphigus foliaceus*
- *Culicoides* or insect hypersensitivity
- Mange
- Generalized granulomatous disease
- Alopecia areata
- Anhidrosis
- Occult or flat sarcoid
- Chronic skin rubs
- Abrasions
- Mercury poisoning
- Wound or exudative scalding

INITIAL DATABASE
- Direct microscopic examination of infected hairs with follicles attached from the periphery of lesions
- Skin scrapings from alopecic areas
- The most reliable diagnostic tool is fungal culture, but this can take up to 4 weeks. Use of Sabouraud's medium with phenol red dye can help in the diagnosis because the agar will change to a bright red color within a few days

if the dermatophyte is present in the sample.
- Biopsy is rarely used but can be done to rule out other diseases and identify fungal spores.

TREATMENT

THERAPEUTIC GOAL(S)
- Limit the spread of the disease to other horses by isolating affected horses from the herd.
- Eliminate infective spores in the environment.
- Use fungicidal treatment on the horse and sporicidal treatment of the environment.
- Treat all at-risk or in-contact horses.
- Prevent zoonotic transmission.
- Clean and disinfect all tack, blankets, and grooming equipment.

ACUTE GENERAL TREATMENT
- Clip affected areas but be sure to disinfect clippers after use to prevent infection of other areas.
- Chlorhexidine- or miconazole-based shampoos are very effective and should be used as needed depending on the severity of the disease. Povidone-iodine–based shampoos can also be effective in eliminating infective spores.
- Lime sulphur (1 cup to 1 gallon of water) and bleach 1:10 with water are very effective but need to be measured appropriately; otherwise, they can be either extremely irritating to the

skin or completely ineffective against the fungus.
- The environment should be cleaned with a 6% bleach solution or alternatively sporicidal disinfectants such as halogenated peroxygen agents (Virkon) or quaternary ammonium compounds (Trigene).

CHRONIC TREATMENT
- Refractory cases may require use of systemic griseofulvin (5–10 mg/kg/d for 30–60 days). Griseofulvin therapy can be extremely expensive.
- Use of 20% sodium iodide given IV (250 mL/500 kg once or twice every 7 days) has been attempted.

DRUG INTERACTIONS
- Griseofulvin should not be used in pregnant mares because of its teratogenic effects.
- Sodium iodide treatment is contraindicated in pregnant mares because it can cause abortion.

PROGNOSIS AND OUTCOME

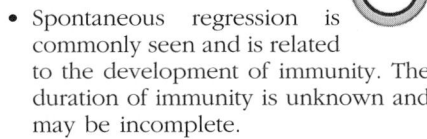

- Spontaneous regression is commonly seen and is related to the development of immunity. The duration of immunity is unknown and may be incomplete.
- Horses have a good prognosis if appropriate treatment is instituted early in the course of the disease and

appropriate environmental management is instituted.

PEARLS & CONSIDERATIONS

COMMENTS
- Younger horses take a longer time to recover from the disease than older ones because of their lack of resistance.
- Outbreaks may occur on premises that have previously been infected.

CLIENT EDUCATION
- Always use gloves when applying treatment to the affected areas to decrease the risk of human transmission.
- Do not share equipment with any other horses until the equipment has been disinfected. All tack, blankets, and grooming equipment should be disinfected before use on other horses.
- Infections in humans are typically self-limiting and respond effectively to antifungal treatments.

SUGGESTED READING
Pilsworth RC, Knottenbelt D: Dermatophytosis (ringworm). *Equine Vet Ed* 19(3):151–154, 2007.
White SD: Fungal diseases. In Smith BP, editor: *Large animal internal medicine*. St Louis, 2009, Elsevier, pp 1318–1319.

AUTHOR: **ALFREDO SANCHEZ LONDOÑO**

EDITOR: **DAVID A. WILSON**

Diarrhea, Chronic

BASIC INFORMATION

DEFINITION
Persistent or intermittent diarrhea of at least 1-month duration

CLINICAL PRESENTATION
HISTORY, CHIEF COMPLAINT
- Persistent or intermittent diarrhea for longer than 1 month
- Variable appetite
- Variable signs of abdominal pain; diarrhea often occurs in the absence of colic or inappetence
- ± Weight loss

PHYSICAL EXAM FINDINGS
- Poor body condition is often noted.
- Other findings are quite variable. No abnormalities other than diarrhea may be present, or clinical signs of dehydration and toxemia, as for acute

colitis (see "Colitis/Diarrhea, Acute" in this section), may be noted.
- Rectal examination:
  - Often within normal limits.
  - Thickened rectal or colonic mucosa may be noted.
  - Rarely, mural or intraluminal intestinal masses are palpated.

ETIOLOGY AND PATHOPHYSIOLOGY
A variety of distinct etiologies can manifest with chronic diarrhea via a variety of mechanisms, including:
- Partial large colonic obstruction, such as an enterolith or mural intestinal neoplasia. This may irritate the colonic mucosa or intermittently partially obstruct the colonic lumen, only allowing passage of softer fecal material around the obstruction.
- Sand enteropathy: sand irritates and inflames the colonic mucosa.

- Infectious causes, such as parasitism or salmonellosis, or rotavirus in foals. These also result in damage to and chronic inflammation of the colonic mucosa.
- Primary infiltrative or inflammatory intestinal disease impairs the normal absorptive capacity of the colonic mucosa.
- Colonic fibrosis secondary to previous severe acute colitis. This also impairs the normal absorptive capacity of the colonic mucosa.
- Gastroduodenal ulcer disease in foals is presumed to alter the absorptive function of the small intestine, which may overwhelm the colonic absorptive capacity in the less mature colon of a foal.
- Maldigestion or abnormal fermentative function of colonic flora may be

caused by slight alterations in the non-pathogenic colonic flora population, resulting in altered volatile fatty acid synthesis or absorption, which may impair colonic water and electrolyte absorption.

- Other systemic disease, such as hepatic disease and congestive heart failure may cause portal hypertension, altering fluid dynamics in the colonic vasculature and impairing water absorption.

DIAGNOSIS

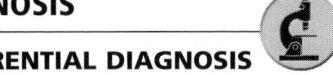

DIFFERENTIAL DIAGNOSIS

- Partial large colonic obstruction (enterolith or mural intestinal neoplasia)
- Sand enteropathy
- Infectious causes: parasitism, salmonellosis
- Colonic fibrosis secondary to previous severe acute colitis
- Primary infiltrative or inflammatory intestinal disease
- Abnormal fermentative function of colonic flora (altered volatile fatty acid synthesis or absorption)
- Gastroduodenal ulcer disease in foals
- Rotavirus in foals
- Hepatic disease
- Congestive heart failure

INITIAL DATABASE

- Complete blood count: may be within normal limits or may show evidence of chronic inflammation with leukocytosis, mild anemia, and hyperfibrinogenemia
- Serum biochemistry profile:
  - Metabolic acidosis caused by bicarbonate loss and variable electrolyte derangements may be present (hypokalemia, hyponatremia, hypochloremia, and hypocalcemia, as for acute colitis) but are not consistent findings.
  - Serum total protein concentration may be increased because of hyperglobulinemia with chronic inflammation or may be decreased because of enteric protein loss (hypoalbuminemia).
  - Liver function should be evaluated by assessment of serum sorbitol dehydrogenase and gamma glutamyltransferase activity and serum bile acid concentration. Inflammatory intestinal disease may result in mild hepatic inflammation and mild increase in hepatocellular enzymes, but marked increases and increased serum bile acids are suggestive of primary hepatic dysfunction.
- Transabdominal ultrasound examination:

- Fluid contents in the colon or cecum are often appreciated.
- Colonic mural thickness may be increased (>5 mm) focally or diffusely.
- Concurrent small intestinal mural thickening (>5 mm) is suggestive of diffuse inflammatory or infiltrative intestinal disease.
- Peritoneal fluid analysis: may be grossly and cytologically normal or may reveal a mildly increased nucleated cell count and protein concentration consistent with intestinal inflammation.

ADVANCED OR CONFIRMATORY TESTING

Determining a definitive diagnosis in cases of chronic diarrhea is difficult. Diagnostic testing for specific etiologies may include the following:

- Fecal flotation for parasites.
- Serial fecal polymerase chain reaction or cultures for salmonellosis (five to 15 samples may be needed).
- Abdominal radiography for sand enteropathy.
- Gastroduodenoscopy in foals.
- D-Glucose or D-xylose absorption test, if weight loss, hypoalbuminemia, or small intestinal mural thickening is present. Although this test assesses small intestinal rather than colonic absorptive function, it can provide information as to whether malabsorptive disease is diffuse or confined to the large colon.
- Rectal mucosal biopsy: In some cases of inflammatory or infiltrative intestinal disease, a diagnosis can be obtained via rectal mucosal biopsy. However, a normal rectal biopsy result does not rule out inflammatory intestinal disease confined to the more proximal intestinal tract. In addition, many causes of intestinal inflammation may result in nonspecific inflammation on rectal mucosal biopsy.
- Exploratory celiotomy and intestinal biopsy:
  - Intestinal biopsies may be obtained via laparotomy or laparoscopically from some locations. Several sites should be biopsied, and samples should be evaluated histopathologically and cultured for *Salmonella* spp.
  - May be indicated if above test results are negative or inconclusive.
  - Laparotomy allows possible resolution of some causes, such as sand enteropathy, enterolith, or resection of focal intestinal neoplasia.
  - However, if diarrhea is caused by altered colonic fermentative function, no gross or histopathologic

abnormalities will be noted on exploratory or intestinal biopsy.

TREATMENT

THERAPEUTIC GOAL(S)

- Eliminate the primary cause.
- Alter the colonic flora to support resolution of diarrhea.

ACUTE GENERAL TREATMENT

- If a specific etiology is determined, treatment may include:
  - Larvicidal deworming for parasites with fenbendazole (10 mg/kg PO q24h for 5 days) or moxidectin (0.4–0.5 mg/kg PO once). Concurrent administration of flunixin meglumine (0.5 to 1.1 mg/kg PO or IV q12–24h) may decrease concurrent colonic inflammation associated with deworming in heavily parasitized horses.
  - Administration of laxative therapy or laparotomy and pelvic flexure enterotomy for sand enteropathy (see "Sand Enteropathy" in this section).
  - Enrofloxacin (5 mg/kg IV or 7.5 mg/kg PO q24h) for chronic salmonellosis.
  - Immunosuppressive therapy with corticosteroids for inflammatory bowel disease (see "Inflammatory Bowel Disease" in this section).
  - Surgical removal of an enterolith or resection of focal intestinal neoplasia.
  - Gastroprotectants for gastroduodenal ulcer disease in foals (see "Gastric Ulceration in Foals" in this section).
- If a specific cause is not determined, therapy may include:
  - Presumptive larvicidal deworming (because encysted cyathastomes may not produce a patent infection)
  - Administration of bismuth subsalicylate (4–5 mL/kg PO or via nasogastric tube q6–12h) for 5 to 7 days may be helpful in some horses.
  - Empiric diet change to alter the colonic flora and volatile fatty acid production. Often, changing to a complete pelleted ration results in slow but successful resolution of the diarrhea, although improvement may take 6 to 8 weeks.
  - Administration of iodochlorhydroxyquin (10–20 mg/kg PO q24h) is reportedly successful in some horses, although the beneficial effects may be transient. The mechanism is unknown, but it is presumed to alter the colonic flora. If effective, the horse should be

maintained on it because diarrhea tends to recur when the drug is discontinued.

PROGNOSIS AND OUTCOME

Variable, depending on the primary cause

PEARLS & CONSIDERATIONS

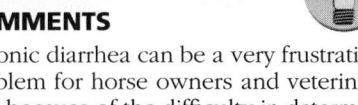

COMMENTS

Chronic diarrhea can be a very frustrating problem for horse owners and veterinarians because of the difficulty in determining a definitive diagnosis. If a diagnosis is not determined with noninvasive diagnostic testing, empiric diet change as above may be warranted before exploratory celiotomy or intestinal biopsy.

SUGGESTED READING

Jones SJ: Medical disorders of the large intestine: Chronic diarrhea. In Smith BP, editor: *Large animal internal medicine.* St Louis, 2009, Mosby Elsevier, pp 749–750.

AUTHOR: KELSEY A. HART

EDITOR: TIM MAIR

Diarrhea, Clostridial

BASIC INFORMATION

DEFINITION
Colitis or diarrhea caused by *Clostridium perfringens* or *Clostridium difficile*

RISK FACTORS
Treatment with antimicrobial agents (*C. difficile*)

CLINICAL PRESENTATION
DISEASE FORMS/SUBTYPES
- *C. perfringens:*
  - Common fecal isolate from normal horses and foals
  - Clinical disease more common in foals
- *C. difficile:*
  - Rarely isolated from adult horses but appears to cause subclinical infection in many healthy foals (<1 month old)
  - May play a role in antimicrobial-associated colitis in adult horses and may be associated with some cases of proximal enteritis (see "Enteritis, Proximal" in this section)

HISTORY, CHIEF COMPLAINT
- Inappetence, colic, fever, and diarrhea are most common, as for other causes of colitis (see "Colitis/Diarrhea, Acute" in this section).

PHYSICAL EXAM FINDINGS
- As for other causes of colitis (see "Colitis/Diarrhea, Acute").
- Hemorrhagic diarrhea is seen frequently (but not always) in horses with colitis caused by *C. perfringens.*
- In some cases, the initial findings are more consistent with proximal enteritis than colitis (see "Enteritis, Proximal" in this section), with moderate- to large-volume gastric reflux and small intestinal distension on rectal examination.

ETIOLOGY AND PATHOPHYSIOLOGY
- Clostridial organisms are anaerobic, spore-forming, gram-positive rods.
- Many clostridial species, including some strains of *C. difficile* and *C. perfringens*, may be normal enteric flora in horses.
- Clinical disease occurs as a result of overgrowth of, or infection with, toxin-producing strains.
  - *C. difficile* can produce at least five toxins, of which type A (enterotoxin) and type B (cytotoxin) are best understood.
  - *C. perfringens* can also produce several toxins. The two most common isolates identified in clinical disease in horses include type A, which produces the α toxin, and type C, which produces the α and β toxins. Some strains may also produce enterotoxin, which has also been associated with clinical disease.
- Overgrowth of toxin-producing strains of *C. difficile* has been associated with antimicrobial-associated colitis in adult horses.
- Infection may also occur with ingestion of clostridial organisms or spores from the environment or from the feces of clinically or subclinically infected animals.
- Clostridial toxins directly damage enterocytes by a variety of mechanisms, resulting in inflammation and necrosis of colonic epithelial cells, damaging the mucosal barrier, resulting in systemic exposure to bacterial toxins and loss of fluid, electrolytes, and plasma proteins into the intestinal lumen, as for other causes of colitis (see "Colitis/Diarrhea, Acute" in this section).

DIAGNOSIS

DIFFERENTIAL DIAGNOSIS
Other causes of colitis (see "Colitis/Diarrhea, Acute" in this section)

INITIAL DATABASE
- As for other causes of colitis (see "Colitis/Diarrhea, Acute" in this section).
- With *C. perfringens* infection in foals, intramural gas (hyperechoic regions casting acoustic shadows) in the wall of the colon or small intestine may be seen on transabdominal ultrasonography.

ADVANCED OR CONFIRMATORY TESTING
- Confirmation of clostridial colitis requires detection of the toxin(s) in the feces.
  - Enzyme-linked immunosorbent assays (ELISAs) for *C. difficile* A and B toxin and *C. perfringens* enterotoxin are commercially available.
  - Toxin production can also be determined by polymerase chain reaction or bioassay, although these tests are not available in all laboratories.
  - The duration and frequency of toxin production are unknown in equine clostridial diarrhea, so testing of serial samples may be warranted if clostridial infection is strongly suspected.
- Fecal Gram stain findings can be supportive of a diagnosis of clostridial diarrhea if large numbers of gram-positive rods are seen.
- Similarly, fecal culture yielding a pure culture of *C. difficile* or *C. perfringens* may be supportive, although toxin production should still be documented as above.
- Testing to rule out other causes of colitis is also warranted as detailed in "Colitis/Diarrhea, Acute" in this section.

TREATMENT

THERAPEUTIC GOAL(S)

- Supportive care
- Antimicrobial therapy

ACUTE GENERAL TREATMENT

- Fluid and colloidal support, antiin-flammatory and antiendotoxic therapy, and other supportive care as for other causes of colitis (see "Colitis/Diarrhea, Acute" in this section)
- Antimicrobial therapy: metronidazole (15–25 mg/kg PO or PR q8h)
- This is effective in most cases, although sporadic metronidazole resistance has been reported. Vancomycin has been effective in treating metronidazole-resistant clostridial strains, although use of this agent in veterinary medicine is controversial.
- Other therapy:
  - *Saccharomyces boulardii*, a non-pathogenic yeast organism, is effective in the treatment of clostridial diarrhea in humans and may decrease the severity of diarrhea in horses with colitis from many causes. Products containing *S. boulardii* are available commercially for use in horses.
  - Di-tri-octahedral smectite (Bio-Sponge) has been documented to bind clostridial toxins in vitro and may also be helpful in clostridial diarrhea in horses.

POSSIBLE COMPLICATIONS

As for other causes of colitis (see "Colitis/Diarrhea, Acute" in this section)

PROGNOSIS AND OUTCOME

- Fair with early therapy and supportive care
- Guarded with *C. difficile* infection secondary to antimicrobial administration in adult horses

PEARLS & CONSIDERATIONS

Because of the lack of availability of assays for all clostridial toxins and thus the difficulty in reaching a rapid and definitive diagnosis, presumptive treatment with 3 to 7 days of metronidazole therapy may be appropriate in many cases of equine diarrhea in which another specific cause is not determined. However, the potential for development of metronidazole resistance should also be considered with such empiric therapy.

SUGGESTED READING

Jones SJ: Medical disorders of the large intestine: acute diarrhea. In Smith BP, editor: *Large animal internal medicine*. St Louis, 2009, Mosby Elsevier, pp 745–747.

AUTHOR: **KELSEY A. HART**

EDITOR: **TIM MAIR**

Diarrhea of the Neonatal Foal

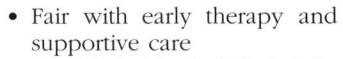

BASIC INFORMATION

DEFINITION

Loose or watery fecal consistency

EPIDEMIOLOGY

RISK FACTORS
- Sepsis
- Failure of passive transfer
- Peripartum asphyxia syndrome
- Pica

CONTAGION AND ZOONOSIS Salmonellosis

CLINICAL PRESENTATION

DISEASE FORMS/SUBTYPES
- Noninfectious
  - Foal heat diarrhea
  - Asphyxia-associated gastroenteropathies: peripartum asphyxia syndrome
  - Necrotizing enterocolitis
  - Mechanical enterocolitis
  - Dietary intolerances
- Infectious
  - Clostridial enteritis
  - Salmonellosis
  - Enterotoxigenic *Escherichia coli*
  - Rotavirus
  - *Cryptosporidium parvum*

HISTORY, CHIEF COMPLAINT
- Loose manure
- Decreased appetite, lethargy
- Normal attitude and appetite in foal heat diarrhea

- Ingestion of foreign material may be observed or suspected

PHYSICAL EXAM FINDINGS
- Temperature: Hyperthermic or hypothermic
- Heart rate: Often tachycardic
- Mentation: Depressed, lethargic, decreased affinity for the dam
- Mucous membranes: Injected, tacky, bright, muddy; prolonged capillary refill time
  - Perineum: Wet with diarrhea unless very projectile; inspect walls of the horse's stall for evidence of diarrhea.
  - Hydration: Severely dehydrated foals have sunken eyes, sluggish jugular refill, and cool extremities.
  - Foal heat diarrhea: Foals are hydrated; afebrile; and have normal mentation, attitude, and appetite.

ETIOLOGY AND PATHOPHYSIOLOGY
- Noninfectious
  - Foal heat diarrhea: Unknown; believed to be related to maturational changes of the gastrointestinal (GI) tract; occurs between approximately 5 and 15 days of age.
  - Asphyxia-associated gastroenteropathies: Hypoxic insult to the GI tract and hypoperfusion; possibly reperfusion injury sustained during hypoxic event (umbilical cord compression, dystocia, red bag delivery).

  - Necrotizing enterocolitis: Unknown; necrotizing insult to the GI tract; suspected to be associated with prematurity or hypoxia.
  - Mechanical enterocolitis: Ingestion of sand, dirt, bedding, or the dam's tail hair may result in mechanical irritation of the GI mucosa.
  - Dietary intolerances: Feeding a milk replacer often results in diarrhea; lactase deficiency occurs with the loss of the mucosal brush border of the small intestine. (*Clostridium difficile* and rotavirus infections are especially associated with lactase deficiency.)
- Infectious
  - Clostridial enteritis: *C. difficile* and *Clostridium perfringens* are most commonly involved; both can be primary pathogens to foals without preceding risk factors.
  - Salmonellosis: bacteremia and sepsis are common with GI tract salmonellosis.
  - *E. coli*: enterotoxigenic strains may result in bacteremia and diarrhea.
  - Rotavirus: affects the small intestine by causing blunting of the microvilli and secondary maldigestion and malabsorption; decreased absorption and increased secretion result in diarrhea. Loss of lactase production adds an osmotic component to

diarrhea by allowing lactose to enter the colon.
- ○ *C. parvum*: occurs more frequently in immunocompromised (severe combined immunodeficiency) foals but occurs rarely in immunocompetent foals.

DIAGNOSIS

DIFFERENTIAL DIAGNOSIS
Infectious versus noninfectious diarrhea

INITIAL DATABASE
- Complete blood count (CBC)
  - ○ Leukopenia or leukocytosis is common in horses with infectious diarrhea.
  - ○ CBC is normal in foal heat diarrhea.
  - ○ Normal CBC results alone do not rule out an infectious cause of diarrhea.
- Lactate
  - ○ A handheld measurement device has been validated for use in horses.
  - ○ Lactate level above 2.0 mmol/L in horses with hypovolemia, dehydration, and sepsis.
- Serum biochemical profile
  - ○ Normal in foal heat diarrhea
  - ○ Electrolyte derangements, metabolic acidosis: GI losses
  - ○ Azotemia: prerenal in dehydration
  - ○ Hypoglycemia: caused by decreased milk ingestion and increased glucose consumption in horses with sepsis

ADVANCED OR CONFIRMATORY TESTING
- Fecal culture (aerobic and anaerobic)
- Fecal smear with Gram stain
- Radiography of the abdomen to rule in or out sand ingestion
- Lactose tolerance test or response to lactase supplementation
- Polymerase chain reaction for toxins of *C. perfringens*
- Immunoassay for toxins of *C. difficile*
- Immunoassay or electron microscopy for rotavirus
- Acid-fast staining oocytes on fecal smear, immunofluorescence assay, or electron microscopy for *C. parvum*

TREATMENT

THERAPEUTIC GOAL(S)
- Maintain hydration.
- Maintain adequate organ system perfusion.
- Normalize acid-base balance.
- Normalize electrolytes.
- Provide nutrition as dictated by GI tract disease.

- Prevent sepsis from translocated bacteria across compromised bowel wall.
- Direct treatment of the causative agent when appropriate.

ACUTE GENERAL TREATMENT
- IV crystalloids and colloids for volume resuscitation
  - ○ Boluses of 10 to 20 mL/kg crystalloids given over 20 to 30 minutes until hypovolemia is resolved and urine is produced.
  - ○ Maintenance rate of crystalloids depends on rate of ongoing losses (2–6 mL/kg/h).
  - ○ Colloids (hetastarch, plasma) should be used if protein is decreased. Doses of 3 to 5 mL/kg can be used effectively in foals to maintain adequate colloidal oncotic pressure.
- Metabolic acidosis may be caused by hypoperfusion (hyperlactatemia) or relative hyperchloremia.
  - ○ Restore adequate circulating volume with crystalloids, colloids, and pressors if needed.
  - ○ Treat relative hyperchloremia with sodium bicarbonate; calculate the amount needed as $0.3 \times$ Body weight (kg) $\times$ Base deficit; administer 50% of the calculated deficit over 2 to 4 hours and the remainder over the next 12 to 18 hours.
- Direct treatment
  - ○ Metronidazole for clostridial enteritis
  - ○ Removal of foreign material in the environment if ingestion is suspected

CHRONIC TREATMENT
- Systemic antimicrobial agents
  - ○ Aminoglycoside (gentamicin, 8.8 mg/kg IV q24h, or amikacin, 22 mg/kg IV q24h) plus a β-lactam such as potassium penicillin (22,000 IU/kg IV q6h) or procaine penicillin (20,000 IU/kg IM q12h) or a cephalosporin, such as ceftiofur (2.2–1.00 mg/kg IV or IM q6–12h)
- GI protectants
  - ○ Kaolin or pectin compounds and bismuth subsalicylate: 0.5–4.0 mL/kg PO q6–24h
  - ○ Stagger these medications from other oral medications
- Gastric ulcer prophylaxis
  - ○ Controversial but recommended by the author
  - ○ Omeprazole (4 mg/kg PO q24h), ranitidine (6.6 mg/kg PO q8h or 1.5 mg/kg IV q8–12h), or famotidine (2.8 mg/kg PO q12h or 0.3 mg/kg IV q12h)
- Nutrition
  - ○ Foals with abdominal distension, ileus, reflux, colic, profuse, or watery diarrhea and foals with

likely lactose deficiency or osmotic diarrhea should be withheld from milk temporarily.
- ○ Dextrose in IV crystalloids (4–8 mg/kg/min or 240 mL/h of a 5% dextrose solution for a 50-kg foal) with frequent measurement of blood glucose) may be used for 12 to 24 hours.
- ○ Prolonged intolerance of milk may necessitate parenteral nutrition.

POSSIBLE COMPLICATIONS
- Septicemia from translocation of bacteria across compromised bowel
- Localization of bacteria in sepsis cases to bone, joint, eye, lung, and so on

RECOMMENDED MONITORING
- Packed cell volume and total solids
- Blood glucose, lactate, electrolytes, and gases
- Urine specific gravity
- Therapeutic drug monitoring in foals on aminoglycosides

PROGNOSIS AND OUTCOME

Prognosis is directly affected by the severity of disease. It is the author's opinion that most foals survive with few to no complications when treated rapidly and aggressively.

PEARLS & CONSIDERATIONS

COMMENTS
- Quarantine and adherence to isolation protocols in suspected infectious diarrhea cases is imperative to limit transmission of disease.
- Disinfection of the foal's environment after disease is resolved is also imperative. (Phenol disinfectants are useful against rotavirus and many bacteria.)

PREVENTION
- Disinfection of foaling stalls between mares
- Quarantine of affected foals
- Disinfection of environment

SUGGESTED READING
Lester GD: Foal diarrhea. In Robinson NE, editor: *Current therapy in equine medicine*, ed 5. Philadelphia, 2003, Saunders, pp 677–680.

Magdesian G: Neonatal foal diarrhea. Neonatal Medicine and Surgery. *Vet Clin North Am Equine Pract* 21(2):295–312, 2005.

AUTHOR: **PHOEBE A. SMITH**

EDITORS: **ELIZABETH M. SANTSCHI** and **PHOEBE A. SMITH**

Diastema Formation

BASIC INFORMATION

DEFINITION

Diastema (Greek: an interval; *pl.* diastemata): a space between two adjacent teeth in the same dental arch. As pertaining to the equine cheek teeth, this is, by definition, pathologic.

EPIDEMIOLOGY

ASSOCIATED CONDITIONS AND DISORDERS Periodontal disease

CLINICAL PRESENTATION

DISEASE FORMS/SUBTYPES
- Congenital or acquired
- Two subtypes: Open and closed (valved)

HISTORY, CHIEF COMPLAINT
- Acute or chronic weight loss
- Quidding
- Reluctance to drink cold water
- Halitosis
- Nasal discharge

PHYSICAL EXAM FINDINGS
- Feed packed between the cheek teeth despite oral lavage
- Gingivitis: Reddened gums, pain on palpation, and possible gingival recession
- Increased gingival sulcus depth adjacent to the teeth

ETIOLOGY AND PATHOPHYSIOLOGY
- Etiology:
  - Congenital: Abnormal spacing or absence of adjacent dental buds; polyodontia or oligodontia; rotation or incorrect angulation of emerging teeth may also be a factor
  - Acquired: Dental displacements, fractured crowns, and tooth loss; iatrogenic by premature removal of deciduous teeth
  - Irrespective of the cause, there are two forms of disease:
    - Open diastemata: Bounding teeth are vertical such that the resulting space resembles a rectangle with the long sides formed by the

rostral and caudal teeth and the short sides formed by the gingival margin and the buccal cavity.
- Closed (valved) diastemata: Bounding teeth are sloped such that the space resembles an inverted triangle. The apex of the triangle is at the buccal cavity, and the base is the gingival margin. A narrow ingress into this space acts as a valve, allowing partially masticated feed into the space; however, no egress occurs. Putrefaction occurs with subsequent associated gingivitis and periodontal disease.

DIAGNOSIS

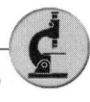

DIFFERENTIAL DIAGNOSIS

Dental fracture

INITIAL DATABASE

- Complete oral examination: sedation, full-mouth speculum, light source and mirror
- Radiographic examination: lateral, bilateral oblique, and dorsoventral projections

ADVANCED OR CONFIRMATORY TESTING

Oral endoscopy

TREATMENT

THERAPEUTIC GOAL(S)

- Diastema widening to allow feed ingress and egress
- Treatment of associated periodontal disease

ACUTE GENERAL TREATMENT

- Sedation (or general anesthesia, depending on the degree of soft tissue discomfort)
- Removal of putrefying feed

- Mechanical widening of diastema using a conical burr
- Lowering of the excessive transverse ridge that commonly develops on the opposing tooth (because of a failure of occlusion)

POSSIBLE COMPLICATIONS

- Inadequate widening of the diastema
- Failure to remove the excessive transverse ridge on the opposing tooth
- Inadvertent entry into the caudal pulp chambers of the rostral tooth and the rostral pulp chambers of the caudal tooth
- Oromaxillary fistulation in chronic cases

RECOMMENDED MONITORING

Recheck in 3 to 6 months. Ensure resolution of associated periodontal disease, feed egress, and repeat lowering of the developing excessive transverse ridge on the opposing tooth.

PEARLS & CONSIDERATIONS

PREVENTION

Complete, competent oral examination every 6 to 12 months

CLIENT EDUCATION

Complete, competent oral examination every 6 to 12 months

SUGGESTED READING

Carmalt JL: Understanding the equine diastema. *Equine Vet Educ* 15:34, 2003.
Carmalt JL, Wilson DG: Treatment of a valve diastema in two horses. *Equine Vet Educ* 16:188, 2004.
Dixon PM, Barakzai S, Collins N, et al: Treatment of equine cheek teeth by mechanical widening of diastemata in 60 horses (2000–2006). *Equine Vet J* 40:22–28, 2008.

AUTHOR & EDITOR: **JAMES L. CARMALT**

Disseminated Intravascular Coagulation

BASIC INFORMATION

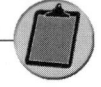

DEFINITION

Disseminated intravascular coagulation (DIC) is a thrombohemorrhagic syn-

drome resulting from the inappropriate systemic activation of the coagulation system caused by systemic inflammation. Disproportionate endothelial cell activation causes intravascular fibrin formation and microangiopathic thrombosis, result-

ing in organ ischemia, necrosis, reperfusion injury, and multiorgan dysfunction. Concurrent widespread hemorrhage may occur because of consumption of coagulation factors, fibrinogen, and platelets.

SYNONYMS

- DIC
- Consumptive coagulopathy
- Dysfibrinogen syndrome

EPIDEMIOLOGY

RISK FACTORS Any primary disorder that causes systemic inflammation, including endotoxemia, sepsis, shock, trauma, hemorrhage, neonatal hypoxic-ischemic encephalopathy syndrome, local infections (endometritis), envenomation, neoplasia, immune-mediated disease (purpura hemorrhagica), gastrointestinal disease (large colon volvulus, colitis), and heatstroke

ASSOCIATED CONDITIONS AND DISORDERS

- A component of the massive and inappropriate inflammatory response resulting from traumatic or septic conditions
- Has been linked to endotoxemia

CLINICAL PRESENTATION

DISEASE FORMS/SUBTYPES

- DIC progresses through three continuous, overlapping stages:
  - Hypercoagulation: Not noted clinically
  - Compensated or subclinical stage: May see alterations in coagulation profiles or end-organ dysfunction
  - Fulminant or uncompensated stage: Fulminant coagulopathy and signs of hemorrhage

HISTORY, CHIEF COMPLAINT

- Typically indistinct
- Varies based on the primary disease process
- Hemorrhage noted in end-stage DIC

PHYSICAL EXAM FINDINGS

- Depend on primary disease process, the location and severity of fibrin deposition, and the extent of clotting factor depletion
- May not see overt clinical signs in patients with subclinical DIC
  - Pale mucous membranes
  - Tachycardia
  - Tachypnea
  - Petechia, progressing to diffuse bruising (ecchymosis)
  - Hematuria
  - Melena
  - Epistaxis
  - Icterus
  - Venous thrombosis
  - Colic

ETIOLOGY AND PATHOPHYSIOLOGY

- DIC may be initiated by one of three methods.
  - Procoagulants (tissue factor or a specific neoplastic procoagulant) expressed by adenocarcinoma or lymphoma directly stimulate coagulation pathways.
  - Bacterial endotoxins (gram-negative bacteria) or exotoxins (gram-positive bacteria) present in severe sepsis, stimulating the release of inflammatory cytokines that initiate an imbalance of coagulation.
  - Trauma, releasing inflammatory mediators and tissue factor, and causing direct damage to endothelial cells that initiates a systemic inflammatory response.
- In systemic inflammation, the disrupted endothelium and activated mononuclear cells produce proinflammatory cytokines that initiate an imbalance of coagulation.
  - Tissue factor is expressed by mononuclear cells and endothelium, initiating the extrinsic coagulation pathway.
  - Intravascular fibrin formation is promoted because of disruption of anticoagulant mechanisms.
- Anticoagulation pathways are inhibited by downregulation of antithrombin III (ATIII), thrombomodulin, and protein C.
- Abnormal coagulation is promoted by consumption of anticlotting factors, including thrombomodulin and antithrombin III.
  - Fibrinolysis is inhibited by plasminogen activator inhibitor type 1 released by the endothelium.
  - Thrombocytopenia and consumption of coagulation factors may occur as DIC progresses, initiating the hemorrhagic phase.
- Thrombosis causes local ischemia, acidosis, necrosis, and reperfusion injury, which perpetuates DIC and may lead to multiorgan failure.

DIAGNOSIS

DIFFERENTIAL DIAGNOSIS

- Anticoagulant or rodenticide exposure
- Severe thrombocytopenia
- Inherited or acquired platelet dysfunction
- Hydroxyethyl starch administration (prolonged clotting times)
- Liver failure

INITIAL DATABASE

- Initial testing is focused on identification of the disease process or a risk factor linked to DIC. A complete blood count, platelet count, and blood smear evaluation should be performed.
  - Platelet counts are usually decreased in patients with acute coagulopathy because of consumption or immune-mediated destruction.
  - Platelet function tests may indicate subclinical DIC caused by reduced function by fibrinogen degradation products (FDPs) or fibrin binding to platelets.
- Serum chemistry profile
- Urinalysis
- Chest and abdominal ultrasonography
- Abdominocentesis

ADVANCED OR CONFIRMATORY TESTING

- The presence of DIC is supported by an identified risk factor through the initial database plus abnormal coagulation test results, positive fibrinolysis results, clot inhibitor consumption results, or end-organ failure.
- No single test is confirmatory for DIC; however, three abnormal coagulation test results and clinical signs of hemorrhage or thrombosis are indicative of this condition.
  - Procoagulant and coagulation tests: require age-matched control subjects because activated partial thromboplastin time (APTT) and prothrombin time (PT) are commonly increased in normal neonates.
- PT
  - Tests the extrinsic and common coagulation pathways
  - Increase of 20% compared with age-matched control subjects is significant
  - Highly indicative of survival in horses with colic
- APTT
  - Tests the intrinsic and common pathways
  - Sensitive for identification of subclinical DIC but not specific
  - Both PT and APTT may be increased in normal neonates
- Fibrinogen
  - Large production capacity by the liver in horses
  - Not commonly decreased in horses with fulminant DIC; reductions are suspicious
- Thromboelastography
  - Viscoelastic method of assessing clot formation in vitro using a vibrating sensor
  - Significantly increased in foals with coagulation abnormalities; associated with increased mortality
- Fibrinolysis activation tests
  - D-Dimer or fibrin/FDP concentrations
  - Produced by plasmin degradation of fibrinogen or cross-linked fibrin
  - Typically increased in DIC indicative of fibrinolysis
  - Poor prognostic indicator in horses
- Clot inhibitor consumption tests
  - ATIII activity
    - May increase in the peritoneal cavity with strangulating lesions
    - Typically decreased in DIC
    - Associated with a negative outcome

- End-organ damage or failure tests
  - Lactate: May be increased with hypercoagulation, indicating decreased tissue perfusion
  - Creatinine: Azotemia may occur because of decreased renal perfusion and end-organ failure
- Necropsy may provide a definitive diagnosis
  - Microthrombi noted in one or more organs is indicative of DIC
  - Tissues must be fixed rapidly after death to identify microthrombi or the clots dissolve

TREATMENT

THERAPEUTIC GOAL(S)

Diagnose and correct the primary condition, reverse coagulopathies, restore normal hemostasis, and prevent end-organ failure caused by thrombosis.

ACUTE GENERAL TREATMENT

- Treat the primary condition
  - Ensure adequate tissue perfusion with IV fluid therapy.
  - If the patient is anemic, administer whole blood transfusion or polymerized hemoglobin solution.
  - Supplemental nasal oxygen may be indicated.
- Address endotoxemia
  - Low-dose flunixin meglumine to reduce prostaglandin release: 0.25 mg/kg q8h IV
  - Polymixin B to bind to endotoxin and prevent cell activation: 6000 IU/kg q8–12h IV
  - Risk of nephrotoxicity in dehydrated horses
- Address consumptive coagulation disorders
  - Fresh-frozen plasma for supplemental ATIII and coagulation factors; repeated doses may be required
  - Platelet-rich plasma
- Address thrombosis
  - Heparin
  - Unfractionated sodium heparin
    - Increases activity of ATIII, inactivates Xa, inhibits conversion of prothrombin to thrombin.

- Higher doses inactivate thrombin and act as a cofactor to ATIII-mediated inhibition of factors IX, X, XI, and XII.
- 5 to 80 U/kg bolus; then 5 to 25 U/kg/h continuous-rate infusion or 40 to 80 IU/kg q8h SC or IV.
- May cause thrombocytopenia and erythrocyte agglutination.
- Administer plasma concurrently if ATIII activity is less than 60% of normal.
  - Low-molecular-weight heparin
    - More reliable effects and a longer half-life without the side effects of unfractionated heparin
    - Dalteparin (Fragmin): 5 to 100 U/kg q24h SC
    - Enoxaparin (Lovenox): 40 to 80 U/kg q24h SC
    - Cost may limit use
  - Aspirin
    - Inhibits cyclooxygenase enzymes, reducing thromboxane A2 production and platelet aggregation
    - 15 to 100 mg/kg q8h PO or 30 mg/kg q24–48h PO

DRUG INTERACTIONS

- Avoid aspirin, heparin, and hydroxyethyl starches in patients in fulminant hemorrhagic DIC or with prolonged clotting times or thrombocytopenia.
- Ensure adequate hydration and renal function before administering nonsteroidal medications or polymixin B.

RECOMMENDED MONITORING

- Serial platelet counts and in vitro clotting times.
- Repeated serum chemistries to monitor organ function.
- Serial lactate monitoring for signs of decreased tissue perfusion.
- With unfractionated heparin therapy, monitor for hemorrhage, decreasing platelet count or packed cell volume, and excessive prolongation of in vitro clotting times.
- Low-dose sodium heparin is antithrombotic without affecting APTT and is recommended over calcium heparin, which prolongs the APTT and reduces hematocrit.

PROGNOSIS AND OUTCOME

Guarded to poor

PEARLS & CONSIDERATIONS

COMMENTS

- Recognition of the risk factors that may lead to the development of DIC is required to provide early and adequate monitoring for patients with DIC.
- Therapy for patients with DIC in the fulminant stage is difficult and will not be successful without resolution of the primary disease.

PREVENTION

Timely therapy and resolution of the disease processes that can lead to DIC is the key to prevention.

CLIENT EDUCATION

The development of DIC represents a severe, and often fatal, complication of systemic disease.

SUGGESTED READING

Cotovio M, Monreal L, Navarro M, et al: Detection of fibrin deposits in tissues from horses with severe gastrointestinal disorders. *J Vet Intern Med* 21(2):308–313, 2007.

Dallap BL: Coagulopathy in the equine critical care patient. *Vet Clin North Am Equine Pract* 20(1):231–251, 2004.

Dolente BA, Wilkins PA, Boston RC: Clinicopathologic evidence of disseminated intravascular coagulation in horses with acute colitis. *J Am Vet Med Assoc* 220(7):1034–1038, 2002.

Levi M: Current understanding of disseminated intravascular coagulation. *Br J Haematol* 124:567–576, 2003.

AUTHOR: AMELIA MUNSTERMAN

EDITORS: R. REID HANSON and AMELIA MUNSTERMAN

Dorsal Displacement of the Soft Palate

BASIC INFORMATION

DEFINITION

Intermittent dorsal displacement of the soft palate (DDSP) is a purely dynamic upper airway obstruction occurring during exercise. In this clinical presentation, the caudal edge of the soft palate is located dorsal to the epiglottic cartilage, resulting in an obstruction during exhalation as air is being diverted through the oropharynx. Permanent dorsal displacement of the soft palate is seen at rest and may be accompanied by dysphagia. This clinical presentation thus leads to early interference with ventilation during exercise and may be accompanied by lower airway infection in its more severe form.

SYNONYM(S)

Palate displacement

EPIDEMIOLOGY

SPECIES, AGE, SEX Higher prevalence in younger horses (ages 2 to 3 years)
GENETICS AND BREED PREDISPOSITION It is unknown if there is a genetic predisposition to this disease, although racehorses (Standardbred and Thoroughbreds) are more commonly affected; it cannot be determined if the high prevalence in those breeds is really breed related or related to their being subjected to the most strenuous exercise conditions.
RISK FACTORS Racing conditions and upper airway inflammation
ASSOCIATED CONDITIONS AND DISORDERS Aside from the aforementioned upper airway inflammation, associated conditions include various epiglottic abnormalities such as shortened or deformed epiglottic cartilage, appearance of epiglottic flaccidity, and subepiglottic masses (cysts or granulomas). Similarly, palatal abnormalities such as cysts or granulomas are occasionally seen with dorsal displacement of the soft palate.

CLINICAL PRESENTATION
DISEASE FORMS/SUBTYPES
- Intermittent displacement of the soft palate
- Permanent displacement of the soft palate

HISTORY, CHIEF COMPLAINT
- Typically, racehorses with intermittent DDSP experience a sudden decrease in performance in the last half of the race. The trainer, driver, or jockey generally reports a "gurgling" sound during exercise or as the horse slows down. Sport horse riders report a respiratory noise more marked with collection, which may or may not be accompanied by a decrease in performance.
- Horses with permanent DDSP have the same abnormal upper respiratory noise starting with initiation of exercise. In addition, signs of dysphagia can be seen with this presentation.

PHYSICAL EXAM FINDINGS
- The most common sign of this condition is auditory (ie, hearing an abnormal fluttering noise). However, some horses with dorsal displacement of the soft palate do not make an abnormal upper respiratory sound; the percentage of "silent" displacers has been estimated to be as high as 38%.

- Few other signs of DDSP are seen on external physical examination except for evidence of upper airway inflammation (enlarged submandibular lymph node, bilateral nasal discharge) or billowing of the cheeks during exercise as airflow is diverted through the mouth.

ETIOLOGY AND PATHOPHYSIOLOGY
- Decreased neuromuscular control of the intrinsic nasopharyngeal muscles, specifically the palatinus and palatopharyngeus
- Caudal position of the larynx
- Results in resistive breathing during exhalation with no measurable airway obstruction during inhalation

DIAGNOSIS

DIFFERENTIAL DIAGNOSIS
- Epiglottic entrapment
- Nasopharyngeal collapse
- Alar fold paralysis
- Recurrent laryngeal neuropathy

INITIAL DATABASE
- Videoendoscopic examination at rest allows identification of predisposing factors such as changes in epiglottic shape, nasopharyngeal masses, or inflammation. The value of resting examination in predicting intermittent DDSP at exercise is low because approximately 80% of horses with confirmed DDSP at exercise do not show abnormalities at rest. In addition, almost all horses can be made to displace their soft palates at rest, so this observation solely at rest is not sufficient for the diagnosis of intermittent DDSP at exercise.
- Permanent DDSP can be diagnosed at rest and may be associated with evidence of tracheal aspiration of feed material.
- Laryngeal ultrasonography indicates that the position of the basihyoid of a horse with DDSP is more ventral. However, the actual mean difference in the depth of the basihyoid varies approximately 3 mm (probably too sensitive to measurement error). At the time of this writing, this diagnostic modality is promising but still premature.
- Sound analysis during exercise reveals a concentration of spectral energy in the range of 20 to 90 Hz.

ADVANCED OR CONFIRMATORY TESTING
Videoendoscopy at exercise (either during treadmill exam or with wireless videoendoscopy) allowing the observation of the soft palate dorsal to the epiglottis for more than 8 continuous seconds is the gold standard of diagnosis.

TREATMENT

THERAPEUTIC GOAL(S)
- Reduce upper airway inflammation so that intrinsic neuromuscular tone is restored.
- Remove structural abnormalities interfering with subepiglottic position of the soft palate.
- Prevent caudal and ventral movement of the larynx during exercise. This can be achieved with a change in tack or by surgical intervention.

ACUTE GENERAL TREATMENT
No treatment is needed at the termination of exercise; postexercise hypernea will restore arterial blood gases hemostasis.

CHRONIC TREATMENT
- Reduce abnormal upper airway inflammation with a course of systemic steroids (dexamethasone or prednisolone).
- Rest if upper airway inflammation is present.
- Use of tongue-tie or external device that displaces the laryngohyoid structures forward, dorsally, or both.
- Remove or reduce palatal or epiglottic masses.
- Surgical alteration of laryngohyoid position (sternothyroid muscle–tendon transection and laryngeal tie-forward).

POSSIBLE COMPLICATIONS
Dysphagia if staphylectomy is used as a modality of treatment

RECOMMENDED MONITORING
- Abnormal upper respiratory noise during exhalation
- Monitor abrupt decreases in performance during exercise with endoscopic examination

PROGNOSIS AND OUTCOME

The prognosis is fair, with 60% to 75% of horses responding to treatment.

PEARLS & CONSIDERATIONS

COMMENTS
Dorsal displacement of the soft palate is the most common cause of upper airway obstruction during exercise.

PREVENTION

Decrease upper airway inflammation with proper vaccination and reduce exposure to infective agents.

CLIENT EDUCATION

This is a common cause of airway obstruction during exhalation and is akin to snoring in humans in terms of noise. The cause is decreased neuromuscular control of the pharynx and position of the laryngohyoid apparatus.

SUGGESTED READING

Cheetham J, Pigott JH, Thorson LM, et al: Racing performance following the laryngeal tie-forward procedure: a case-controlled study. *Equine Vet J* 40:501–507, 2008.

Franklin SH, Price C, Burn J: The displaced equine soft palate as a source of abnormal respiratory noise during expiration. *Equine Vet J* 36:590–594, 2004.

Holcombe SJ, Derksen FJ, Stick JA, et al: Effect of bilateral blockade of the pharyngeal branch of the vagus nerve on soft palate function in horses. *Am J Vet Res* 59:504–508, 1998.

Parente EJ, Martin BB, Tulleners EP, et al: Dorsal displacement of the soft palate in 92 horses during high-speed treadmill examination (1993–1998). *Vet Surg* 31:507–512, 2002.

Woodie JB, Ducharme NG, Hackett RP, et al: Can an external device prevent dorsal displacement of the soft palate during strenuous exercise? *Equine Vet J* 37:425–429, 2005.

AUTHOR: **NORM G. DUCHARME**

EDITOR: **ERIC J. PARENTE**

Early Embryonic Loss

BASIC INFORMATION

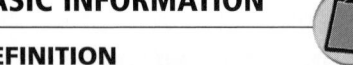

DEFINITION

The failure to maintain pregnancy between fertilization and day 40 of gestation. This stage corresponds to the time of transition from the embryonic to the fetal stage of conceptus development.

SYNONYM(S)

Early embryonic death (EED), early pregnancy loss (EPL)

EPIDEMIOLOGY

SPECIES, AGE, SEX

- EEL is usually seen in very young yearling mares or older mares in a range of 2.5% to 24%, with the highest incidence seen in mares older than 18 years of age.
- Younger mares usually experience EEL between days 15 and 35 of gestation.
- Older mares experience much higher embryonic losses during both oviductal (days 0–6) and the early uterine period (days 6–16).
- The effect of age on fertility usually originates in the oocyte, and embryos from the oviducts of especially older mares have shown to have significantly fewer cells and poor morphology.

GENETICS AND BREED PREDISPOSITION

- Chromosomal abnormalities such as chromosomal translocations and trisomy
- Thoroughbred mares in particular are proven to have low reproductive efficiency with EEL cited as the main reason for low production.

RISK FACTORS

- Endometrial disease
- Progesterone insufficiency

- Maternal age
- Maternal chromosomal abnormalities
- Anatomic defects such as poor perineal conformation, urine pooling, and so on predisposing to infectious endometritis.
- Venereal infections
- Foal heat breeding
- Poor nutrition

ASSOCIATED CONDITIONS AND DISORDERS

- Abortion
- Failure to conceive
- Endometritis
- Metritis

CLINICAL PRESENTATION

HISTORY, CHIEF COMPLAINT

- Failure to maintain pregnancy
- Return to estrus after a previous positive diagnosis for pregnancy

PHYSICAL EXAM FINDINGS

- Transrectal palpation results in failure to detect a chorionic vesicle at the base of either horn at or after 28 days of gestation. There may be a loss or decrease in uterine tone.
- Transrectal ultrasonography may reveal a sudden disappearance of the embryonic vesicle between examinations without evidence of premonitory signs. Other findings include signs of impending embryo loss such as an irregularly shaped embryonic vesicle, prolonged embryonic mobility (beyond day 16), signs of estrus such as excessive endometrial edema despite presence of the embryo, underdeveloped or small for their age embryos, absence of embryonic heartbeat, dislodgement of the vesicle with loss of fluid, increased echogenicity of fluid within the conceptus, or abnormal development of embryonic membranes.

- None, mucoid, or mucopurulent vulvar discharge

ETIOLOGY AND PATHOPHYSIOLOGY

- Infectious causes
  - Contagious equine metritis caused by *Taylorella equigenitalis* may cause embryonic loss after initial infection (see "Contagious Equine Metritis" in this section).
  - Bacterial endometritis may be caused by several species of bacteria, the most important being *Streptococcus equi* subsp. *zooepidemicus*. Others include *Escherichia coli*, *Klebsiella pneumoniae* (capsule 1, 2, and 5), *Pseudomonas aeruginosa*, and *Bacteroides fragilis* (especially in postpartum and foal heat mares).
  - These organisms cause abnormal fluid retention and endometritis resulting in the release of complement, leukotriene B4, prostaglandin E, and prostaglandin $F_{2\alpha}$ (PG $F_{2\alpha}$) and premature lysis of the corpus luteum. This causes subsequent progesterone deficiency and embryonic mortality.
- Hormonal causes
  - Progesterone deficiency caused by the failure of the primary CL to develop adequately or because of luteolysis caused by PG $F_{2\alpha}$ release triggered because of endotoxemia of the gastrointestinal tract or other systemic illness
  - Anecdotal evidence of endocrine disorders such as hypothyroidism
- Genetic causes: Chromosomal abnormalities such as autosomal translocations and trisomy may produce unbalanced gametes, resulting in early embryonic loss.

DIAGNOSIS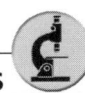

DIFFERENTIAL DIAGNOSIS

- Conception failure: Failure to detect a 14-day pregnancy by transrectal ultrasound examination.
- Differentiate from structures such as endometrial cysts and intrauterine fluid. Paraovarian structures can be confused with follicles but not with pregnancy because they are not in the uterus.

INITIAL DATABASE

- Complete blood count, serum biochemistry, and urinalysis are generally not indicated unless concurrent systemic illness is suspected.
- Maternal progesterone assays by enzyme-linked immunosorbent assay or radioimmunoassay. It is generally desirable to have levels above 4 ng/mL to maintain pregnancy. However, levels may vary depending on the reference laboratory.
- Serial ultrasound examination of mares with a history of EEL to monitor conceptus development as well as detect premonitory signs of impending embryo loss
- Maternal triiodothyronine (T3) and thyroxine (T4) levels in cases of suspected hypothyroidism

ADVANCED OR CONFIRMATORY TESTING

- Breeding soundness examination of old, barren mares or mares with a history of EEL
- Endometrial cytology or culture and endometrial biopsy in mares suspected of having endometritis
- Color Doppler ultrasonography to detect alterations in blood flow to the pregnant uterus and determine the uterine index. Low uterine index values are indicative of reduced blood supply to the pregnant horn and impending or ongoing embryonic mortality.
- Cytogenetic studies such as karyotyping may be indicated in mares suspected of having chromosomal abnormalities

TREATMENT

THERAPEUTIC GOAL(S)

- Minimize contamination during breeding to prevent infectious endometritis.
- Careful monitoring of embryonic development
- Treatment of concurrent illnesses
- Progestin supplementation in case of impending embryo loss

ACUTE GENERAL TREATMENT

- Prevention and treatment of postbreeding endometritis
  - Optimizing breeding management by breeding close to ovulation or inducing ovulation by administration of human chorionic gonadotropin or gonadotropin-releasing hormone analogues, thus reducing the need for more than one mating or insemination during estrus
  - Judicious use of uterine lavage, ecbolics such as oxytocin, and antibiotics after breeding to evacuate uterine fluid and stimulate uterine contractions
- Progesterone supplementation may be indicated in mares displaying signs of impending embryonic loss or in mares with a history of repeated EEL.
  - Altrenogest (Regumate; Hoechst-Roussel Agri-Vet) a synthetic progestin (0.044–0.088 mg/kg PO q24h starting 4–6 days after ovulation and continuing until day 120 of gestation). The dose may decline gradually over a 14-day period at the end of its administration.
  - Administration of 100 to 150 mg progesterone in oil q24h (available from compounding pharmacies) is also adequate to maintain pregnancy. The drawback is the need for daily injections.
- Surgical correction of anatomic defects to prevent urine pooling and fecal contamination of the genital tract

POSSIBLE COMPLICATIONS

- Abortion and high-risk pregnancy in later stages of gestation.
- Progesterone should not be used if infectious endometritis is suspected concurrently because this may prevent physical clearance of the infection from the uterus.

RECOMMENDED MONITORING

- Periodic monitoring of embryonic development by transrectal ultrasonography
- Monitoring maternal serum progesterone levels

PROGNOSIS AND OUTCOME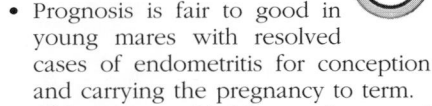

- Prognosis is fair to good in young mares with resolved cases of endometritis for conception and carrying the pregnancy to term.
- Older mares with history of repeated EEL and severe endometritis have a guarded to poor prognosis.

- Mares with chromosomal abnormalities do not respond to treatment and carry a poor prognosis to maintain pregnancy.

PEARLS & CONSIDERATIONS

COMMENTS

- EEL remains a cause of significant economic loss to the breeding industry. There is no cure for genetic causes of EEL such as chromosomal abnormalities; however, fertility and pregnancy rates can be considerably improved by using minimal-contamination breeding techniques and promptly and aggressively treating postbreeding endometritis.
- Although exogenous progesterone helps maintain high-risk pregnancies, serial monitoring is essential to confirm embryo viability because retention of the conceptus after death may result from continued treatment.

PREVENTION

- Optimal breeding management and treatment of endometritis
- Judicious use of hormonal medication in bred mares
- Karyotyping and early identification of mares suspected of having chromosomal abnormalities

CLIENT EDUCATION

- Educate clients regarding proper use of altrenogest, such as wearing gloves and washing the hands after use because this product can be absorbed through the skin.
- Help clients understand the genetic and age-related aspects and their refractoriness to treatment.

SUGGESTED READING

Allen WR: Luteal deficiency and embryo mortality in the mare. *Reprod Domest Anim* 36:121–131, 2001.

Causey RC: Making sense of uterine infections: the many faces of physical clearance. *Vet J* 172:405–421, 2006.

Chen YH, Stolla R: Using "Uterine Index" to diagnose embryonic death in mares. *J Equine Vet Sci* 26(5):219–224, 2006.

Lear TL, Lundquist J, Zent WW, et al: Three autosomal chromosome translocations associated with repeated early embryonic loss (REEL) in the domestic horse (*Equus caballus*). *Cytogenet Genome Res* 120:117–122, 2008.

Vanderwall DK: Early embryonic loss in the mare. *J Equine Vet Sci* 28(11):691–702, 2008.

AUTHOR: SWANAND R. SATHE

EDITOR: JUAN C. SAMPER

Ehrlichiosis

BASIC INFORMATION

DEFINITION

Ehrlichiosis is caused by a variety of gram-negative bacteria of the *Anaplasmataceae* in which the primary infection is composed of intracellular infection of the hemolymphatic system. Hemolymphatic disease indicates disorders that affect the red and white blood cells, platelets, endothelial cells, or lymphoid cells and tissues.

SYNONYM(S)

Equine granulocytic ehrlichiosis (formerly *Ehrlichia equine*), human granulocytic ehrlichiosis

EPIDEMIOLOGY

SPECIES, AGE, SEX Younger animals (<4 years) are less severely affected

CONTAGION AND ZOONOSIS *Anaplasma equi* may be transmitted by ticks to a variety of animals and humans. Horses do not directly transmit this pathogen to humans, but there is a potential that horses may be infectious to ticks during their short ehrlichemic phase. Horses, similar to humans, are considered a dead-end host, and infection is considered acute without chronic carrier status after an acute episode.

GEOGRAPHY AND SEASONALITY

*   Associated geographically with *Ixodes* spp., *Ixodes Pacificus*, and *Ixodes scapularis*
*   Equine disease has been reported in Washington, Oregon, New Jersey, New York, Colorado, Illinois, Minnesota, Connecticut, Florida, and Wisconsin and outside the United States in Canada and Brazil.
*   In northern Europe, *Ixodes ricinus* likely transmits the organism.

CLINICAL PRESENTATION

DISEASE FORMS/SUBTYPES

*   Subclinical
*   Clinical
*   Febrile vasculopathy
*   Febrile acute ataxia

HISTORY, CHIEF COMPLAINT Development of febrile syndrome of depression, partial anorexia, limb edema, petechiation, icterus, ataxia, and reluctance to move

PHYSICAL EXAM FINDINGS

*   The total clinical course of the disease ranges from 3 to 16 days. The horse has an initial high fever, fluctuating from 39.4° to 41.3° C (102.9°–106.3° F).

*   The first clinical signs may be reluctance to move, distal limb and ventral edema, ataxia, depression, anorexia, icterus (Figure 1), and petechiation of the nasal septum mucosa. Severe weakness, staggering, or ataxia may occur with falling, recumbency, and injury; this may be severe to the point that horses sustain fractures after falling.
*   More severe signs of disease develop by days 3 to 5, with fever and illness lasting 10 to 14 days if untreated. With the onset of more severe disease, there is an increase in the rectal temperature, an increase in the heart rate (50–60 beats/min), and often an increase in the respiratory rate. Rarely, cardiac arrhythmias consisting of ventricular tachycardia and premature ventricular contractions occur. The disease is normally self-limiting in untreated horses.
*   Mortality is usually caused by sequelae consisting of secondary infection and injury. Abortion has not been observed in pregnant mares nor has laminitis been a reported feature of the clinical syndrome.
*   Milder signs, including moderate fever, depression, moderate limb edema, and ataxia, develop in horses <4 years.
*   Fever is usually the only clinical feature in horses <1 year.

ETIOLOGY AND PATHOPHYSIOLOGY

*   *A. phagocytophilum* infection
*   Poorly understood pathogenesis
*   Tick infestation, bite, inoculation, and spread
*   Infection of granulocytes, including platelets and neutrophils
*   Inflammation of the spleen, liver, and lungs and damage caused by proinflammatory events

*   Loss of granulocytic cell lines
*   Development of clinical signs associated with widespread vasculitis, anemia, and thrombocytopenia
*   Vascular inflammation leading to edema, cardiac impairment, and neurologic signs

DIAGNOSIS

DIFFERENTIAL DIAGNOSIS

*   Acute viral infection, especially equine viral arteritis and equine infectious anemia virus
*   Viral encephalitides
*   Purpura hemorrhagica
*   Disseminated intravascular coagulation
*   Pancytopenia secondary to myelophthisic disease or drug toxicity

INITIAL DATABASE

*   Complete blood count demonstrating anemia, thrombocytopenia, and leukopenia
*   Cytologic evaluation of peripheral blood smear or buffy coat for detection of morulae in cytoplasm of neutrophils and eosinophils
*   Electrolytes, blood urea nitrogen, and creatinine to assess cardiovascular status
*   Bleeding profile is usually normal
*   Liver function tests
*   Blood ammonia

ADVANCED OR CONFIRMATORY TESTING

*   The presence of three inclusion bodies in one blood smear or buffy coat preparation is definitive.

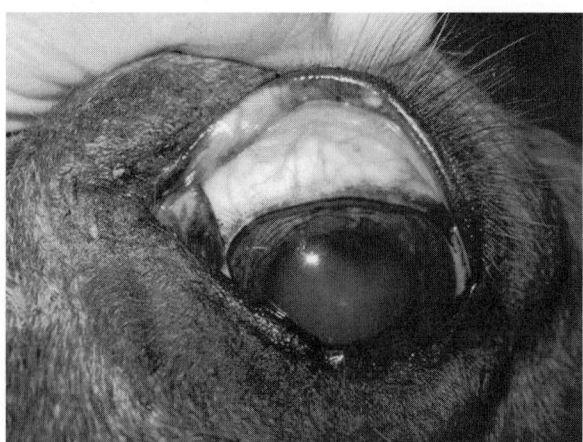

FIGURE 1 Horse infected with *Anaplasma phagocytophila*. (From Sellon DC, Long MT (eds): *Equine infectious diseases*. St Louis, 2007, Saunders Elsevier.)

- Polymerase chain reaction (PCR) for detection of *A. phagocytophilum* DNA in smear
- Fourfold increase in endpoint serum titer measured by the indirect fluorescent antibody test

TREATMENT

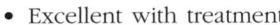

THERAPEUTIC GOAL(S)

- Antimicrobial agent to treat organism
- Antiinflammatory agents to address vasculitis and fever
- Fluid therapy to address hypovolemia
- Prevention of self-trauma

ACUTE GENERAL TREATMENT

- Oxytetracycline: 7 mg/kg q24h for 5 to 7 days
- IV fluid and electrolyte therapy if indicated
- Flunixin meglumine: 0.5 to 1.1 mg/kg IV q12–24h
- Support wraps for distal limb edema
- Stall confinement
- Protective head gear

CHRONIC TREATMENT

Does not cause chronic disease

DRUG INTERACTIONS

The combination of tetracycline and non-steroidal antiinflammatory drugs may

result in injury to the renal system, with a higher risk in hypovolemic patients.

POSSIBLE COMPLICATIONS

- Fractures
- Exacerbation of preexisting conditions such as lymphedema and chronic cellulitis

RECOMMENDED MONITORING

- A dramatic response to therapy in terms of the animal's appetite and activity should occur within 12 hours.
- If no response is seen with two doses of tetracycline, then consideration of other causes of the clinical signs is highly warranted.

PROGNOSIS AND OUTCOME

- Excellent with treatment
- Many horses recover spontaneously, and no long-term sequelae are expected, even in untreated horses.

PEARLS & CONSIDERATIONS

COMMENTS

- Direct blood film visualization and analysis should be a cornerstone of veterinary practice.

- After tetracycline therapy has been instituted, PCR is of limited value.
- Always obtain extra purple top and red top tubes upon the horse's first visit and before treatment.
- Titers increase very quickly, and a fourfold increase in titer can be observed within the first 5 days of clinical signs.

PREVENTION

No vaccine is available, so tick control is the only prevention.

CLIENT EDUCATION

- Tick control on farms is important.
- Avoid heavily infested locations during the summer, fall, and winter months.

SUGGESTED READING

Pusterla N, Chae JS, Kimsey RB, et al: Transmission of *Anaplasma phagocytophila* (human granulocytic ehrlichiosis agent) in horses using experimentally infected ticks (*Ixodes scapularis*). *J Vet Med B* 49:484, 2002.

Pusterla N, Madigan JE: *Anaplasma phagocytophila*, In Sellon DC, Long MT, editors: *Equine infectious diseases*. St Louis, 2007, Saunders Elsevier, pp 354–357.

AUTHOR: **MAUREEN T. LONG**

EDITORS: **DEBRA C. SELLON** and **MAUREEN T. LONG**

Ejaculatory Dysfunction

BASIC INFORMATION

DEFINITION

- Ejaculation is the process of sperm transport from the epididymis to the urethral meatus, resulting in expulsion of semen. Ejaculation is divided in two phases: seminal emission, which occurs at high arousal, and propulsatile ejaculation.

SYNONYMS

- Aspermia, anejaculation, retrograde ejaculation, urospermia, premature ejaculation

EPIDEMIOLOGY

SPECIES, AGE, SEX Males of any age
ASSOCIATED CONDITIONS AND DISORDERS
- Musculoskeletal disorders (sore back, lameness, degenerative joint, lameness after breeding, myositis, laminitis)

- Neurologic diseases (EPM)
- Vascular lesions (aortoiliac thrombosis)
- Cystic remnant of Müllerian ducts (uterus masculinus)

CLINICAL PRESENTATION

DISEASE FORMS/SUBTYPES

- Ejaculation failure (aspermia, anejaculation): The most common cause of ejaculatory dysfunction. It is an intermittent or continuous failure of emission of semen and ejaculation in spite of normal sexual arousal and persistent mounting and thrusting.
- Sperm accumulation syndrome (spermiostasis/spermastasis): Abnormal accumulation of sperm within the ductal system.
- Urospermia: Emission of variable quantities of urine during ejaculation.
- Premature ejaculation: Very rare affliction in which ejaculation occurs before adequate insertion.

- Retrograde ejaculation: Process by which semen passes backward through the bladder neck into the bladder. It can be partial or total.

HISTORY, CHIEF COMPLAINT

- Poor breeding performance
- Difficulty in collecting semen
- Poor semen quality (intermittent or permanent)

PHYSICAL EXAM FINDINGS

- Possibly none; findings are variable depending on cause.
- Musculoskeletal or neurologic dysfunctions during mating or semen collection, such as failure to couple squarely and thrust; asymmetric hind limb weight bearing and thrusting; lateral instability; falling during thrusting or dismount; reluctance to mount or dismount; early dismount.
- Acute or chronic sources of pain affecting the urogenital tract (eg, epididymitis, scrotal inflammation).

- Acute or chronic lesions of the penis.
- Ultrasonographic examination of:
  - The accessory sex glands could show dilated (fluid filled) and/or hyperechoic areas of the ampullae.
  - Arteries: For aortoiliac thrombosis.

ETIOLOGY AND PATHOPHYSIOLOGY

- Ejaculation failure:
  - Acute or chronic pain of musculoskeletal origin (back pain, painful hind limb, lameness)
  - Urogenital tract problem (pain of the bladder, the penis, testis, or accessory sex gland)
  - Neurologic dysfunction (penile nerve damage, "tail nerving," incomplete spinal injury)
  - Vascular problems (aortoiliac thrombosis)
  - Psychogenic causes, such as poor handling (excessive punishment such as overuse of the chain shank or bit, overuse of the stallion, poor or inappropriate breeding environment (unstable phantom, slippery breeding shed floor), which induces pain, fear, or unpleasant experience.
- Sperm accumulation syndrome: Stallions with large testicles and high daily sperm production that are sexually rested for long periods. The sperm has a lower motility, reduced longevity, and poorer morphology.
- Urospermia: Unknown cause. Associated conditions include:
  - Neurologic dysfunction (cauda equina syndrome or equine herpesvirus-1 infection)
  - Poor or inadequate closure of the bladder neck
  - Neoplastic changes
  - Sorghum toxicosis
  - Sequelae of fractures and osteomyelitis
- Premature ejaculation: Unknown cause
- Retrograde ejaculation: Extremely rare
  - Impairment of the muscles or nerves of the bladder neck prohibit closure during ejaculation
  - Trauma or surgery of the bladder, prostate, or pelvic urethra
  - Congenital defect in the urethra or bladder
- Disease affecting the nervous system

DIAGNOSIS

DIFFERENTIAL DIAGNOSIS

- Must ensure that the stallion is having a complete ejaculation
- Aspermia from blockage or testicular dysfunction

INITIAL DATABASE

- Low number of sperm in the ejaculate

- Azoospermia
- Ultrasonographic examination of:
  - Accessory sex glands: Could show dilated (fluid filled) and/or hyperechoic areas of the ampullae
  - Arteries: For aortoiliac thrombosis

ADVANCED OR CONFIRMATORY TESTING

Measurement of seminal plasma alkaline phosphatase (SPAP) levels: SPAP >1000 IU/L (typically >3000 IU/L): fluid from the epididymis and testicles are present (complete ejaculate). SPAP <100 IU/L: the sample does not contain fluid from the epididymis and testicles (either failure to ejaculate or mechanical blockage preventing the semen from exiting the urethra, such as ampullary blockage). SPAP between 100 and 1000 IU/L, partial ejaculate, or partial blockage of the excurrent duct may suggest severe testicular or epididymal pathology.

TREATMENT

THERAPEUTIC GOAL

- Regaining fertility for natural breeding or managing condition through artificial reproductive techniques

ACUTE GENERAL TREATMENT

- Ejaculation failure:
  - Proper management: Expose the stallion to a mare in natural heat in a quiet environment and for a long period before collection.
  - To reduce pain:
    - Correctly adjust the phantom and ensure good footing in the shed
    - Nonsteroidal antiinflammatory drugs combined with acupuncture can also help if pain is the origin of the dysfunction (eg, phenylbutazone 2.2 mg/kg PO q12h for 3–5 days prior)
  - Maximize the conditions to the preferences of the stallion: Temperature and pressure of the artificial vagina, application of hot towels to the base of the penis.
  - In stallions that have difficulty mounting, collection can be made on the ground either by use of an artificial vagina or manual stimulation. Treatment with gonadotropin-releasing hormone to enhance arousal (50 μg Cystorelin SC 1 and 2 hours before breeding) or Diazepam to reduce anxiety (0.05 mg/kg slow IV, up to a maximum of 20 mg, regardless of weight) are used. Xylazine and imipramine are recommended to induce ejaculation without sexual excitement or stimulation (2.2 mg/kg imipramine PO

followed 2 hours later by 0.66 mg/kg xylazine IV).
- Retrograde ejaculation:
  - Increase the tone of the bladder neck (sympathetic activity) or decrease parasympathetic activity
  - Imipramine 1.76 mg/kg PO q12h starting 4 days before collection
- Sperm accumulation syndrome:
  - Vigorous massage per rectum of the ampullae
  - Oxytocin (10-20 IU IV) just before collection
  - Prostaglandin $F_{2\alpha}$ is helpful to achieve ejaculation (0.01 to 0.15 mg/kg IM)
  - Collect often and frequently until sperm numbers are in line with predicted daily sperm production; then collect regularly to prevent reoccurrence.
- Urospermia:
  - Collect semen using an open artificial vagina immediately after urination, which can be obtained naturally in a fresh clean stall by a diuretic such as furosemide. Catheterization of the bladder may cause bacterial cystitis if used too often.
  - Imipramine, combined with draining of the bladder, can reduce the signs of urospermia in an affected stallion for a limited period.
- Premature ejaculation
  - Use cold water to wash the penis
  - Deflect the penis ventrally (or laterally) until insertion

POSSIBLE COMPLICATIONS

- May lose the stallion for breeding depending on cause and severity of problem

PROGNOSIS AND OUTCOME

- Depending on the condition, spermiostasis has a good prognosis; however, the prognosis could be guarded for psychogenic problems.

PEARLS & CONSIDERATIONS

- Spermiostasis must stress the importance of frequent breeding or collection

SUGGESTED READING

McDonnell SM: Techniques for extending the breeding career of aging and disabled stallions. *Clin Tech Equine Pract* 269:276, 2005.
Martin BB, McDonnell SM, Love CC: Effects of musculoskeletal and neurologic diseases on breeding performance in stallions. *Compendium* 1159:1168, 1998.

Samper JC: Techniques for artificial insemination. In Youngquist RS, Threlfall WR, editors: *Large animal theriogenology*. St Louis, 2007, Elsevier, pp 37–42.

Turner RM, et al: Use of imipramine hydrochloride for treatment of urospermia in a stallion with a dysfunctional bladder. *J Am Vet Med Assoc* 1602:1607, 1995.

Turner RM: Current techniques for evaluation of stallion fertility. *Clin Tech Equine Pract* 257:268, 2005.

AUTHOR: **MOUHAMADOU K. DIAW**

EDITOR: **JUAN C. SAMPER**

Encephalopathy, Hypoxic-Ischemic

BASIC INFORMATION

DEFINITION

Syndrome of central nervous system (CNS) disease in foals with onset in the first 3 days of life, excluding infectious and traumatic causes and congenital and genetic defects

SYNONYMS

Perinatal asphyxia syndrome; neonatal maladjustment syndrome; "dummy," "wanderer," or "barker" foals

EPIDEMIOLOGY

SPECIES, AGE, SEX Onset is within the first 3 days of life.
RISK FACTORS Presumably, any cause of neonatal asphyxia (maternal illness, placental disease, dystocia, cesarean section, "red bag" delivery)

CLINICAL PRESENTATION

DISEASE FORMS/SUBTYPES
- Delayed onset of CNS signs
- Abnormal at birth

HISTORY, CHIEF COMPLAINT
- Delayed onset of CNS signs: Foal born normally, stands and nurses normally, appears normal for first 12 to 48 hours before the onset of behavioral abnormalities
- Abnormal at birth: Foals born with risk factors for hypoxic-ischemic encephalopathy (HIE), do not stand and nurse normally, and do not show normal CNS function.

PHYSICAL EXAM FINDINGS
- Abnormal behavior: Decreased affinity for the dam, restlessness or somnolence, hyperresponsive to handling, abnormal posture, tongue protrusion, star gazing, head pressing, recumbency, abnormal breathing patterns, seizures
- Temperature, pulse, respiration, and mucous membranes are typically normal in most foals.

ETIOLOGY AND PATHOPHYSIOLOGY Unknown, but believed to be the result of hypoxic injury of the CNS neurons. The syndrome may occur without any risk factors. Damage to organ systems other than the CNS (renal, hepatic, gastrointestinal) suggests that global hypoxia-ischemia may play a role, but this has not been proven.

DIAGNOSIS

DIFFERENTIAL DIAGNOSIS

- Sepsis
- CNS trauma
- Bacterial meningitis
- Hypoglycemia, severe electrolyte derangements
- Kernicterus
- Hepatoencephalopathy
- Congenital CNS defects

INITIAL DATABASE

- Complete blood count, serum chemistry panel, serum electrolytes, glucose
- Blood work results are normal unless HIE is complicated by a comorbid disease (eg, sepsis and HIE)

ADVANCED OR CONFIRMATORY TESTING

Cerebrospinal fluid assessment: May be normal or xanthochromic

TREATMENT

THERAPEUTIC GOAL(S)

- General support
- Control of seizures
- Prevention of infection

ACUTE GENERAL TREATMENT

- Treatment recommendations vary widely, even among seasoned clinicians with respect to direct treatment of the CNS disease. Empirical treatments include flunixin meglumine (1.1 mg/kg IV q12–24h), Magnesium sulphate (MgSO$_4$; 0.05 mg/kg/h loading dose, then 0.025 mg/kg/h), thiamine (5 mg/kg IV slowly or SC q24h), vitamin E (20 IU/kg SC or PO q24h), mannitol (0.5–2.0 mg/kg IV over 45 minutes q6h)
- General treatment is dictated by the severity of CNS disease.
  - Recumbent foals require padding and maintenance in sternal recumbency.
  - Foals with seizures require anticonvulsant therapy plus padded walls or head protection.
  - Some foals may require bladder catheterization
  - Many foals with HIE require feeding through a nasogastric tube.
- Seizure control: Diazepam for short-term control (0.1–0.2 mg/kg IV once or twice); if seizures persist, phenobarbital (10–20 mg/kg IV over 30 minutes loading dose followed by 5–7 mg/kg IV or PO q24h) or midazolam CRI (0.1–0.2 mg/kg/h)
- Prevention of infection: Broad-spectrum antimicrobial agents

PROGNOSIS AND OUTCOME

- Uncomplicated cases are generally those that experience a delayed onset of clinical signs. With appropriate treatment, these foals respond very well and do not have residual CNS deficits.
- Complicated cases, especially foals that show CNS signs at birth and HIE foals that have multiple organ system dysfunction generally have a poor prognosis.

PEARLS & CONSIDERATIONS

Diagnosis of HIE is one of exclusion. There is no definitive diagnostic test, so one must rely on history and physical findings coupled with exclusion of other differentials.

SUGGESTED READING

Wilkins PA: Disorders of foals. In Reed SM, Bayly WM, Sellon DC, editors: *Equine internal medicine*, ed 3. St Louis, 2010, Saunders Elsevier, pp 1311–1363.

AUTHOR: **PHOEBE A. SMITH**

EDITORS: **ELIZABETH M. SANTSCHI** and **PHOEBE A. SMITH**

Endocarditis, Infective

BASIC INFORMATION

DEFINITION

Endocarditis is usually the result of infections of the endocardial surface of the heart, either involving the valves (valvular endocarditis) or the walls (mural endocarditis) of the heart.

SYNONYM

Bacterial endocarditis

EPIDEMIOLOGY

SPECIES, AGE, SEX
- Endocarditis is rare in horses.
- It is seen in both young and adult horses; males are predisposed.

RISK FACTORS There are no reported risk factors, although right-sided endocarditis has been associated with jugular vein thrombophlebitis after transvenous catheterization.

CLINICAL PRESENTATION

DISEASE FORMS/SUBTYPES
- Endocarditis can be categorized as acute, subacute, or chronic; bacterial or nonbacterial in origin; and valvular or mural (involving the endocardial walls), but most equine cases appear to be subacute or chronic and bacterial in origin and involve valvular structures (Figure 1).
- Rarely, parasitic infections may also result in endocarditis in horses.
- The left-sided valves (ie, mitral and aortic valve) are most frequently affected followed by the tricuspid and finally the pulmonic valve.

HISTORY, CHIEF COMPLAINT
- Most frequent presenting complaints: fever and associated clinical signs (eg, anorexia, depression), although fever may be intermittent or even absent in some patients
- Weight loss
- Signs of congestive heart failure, including tachypnea, coughing, edema, and complaints of severe exercise intolerance are possible
- Lameness (embolization into muscles or joint)

PHYSICAL EXAM FINDINGS
- Cardiac murmurs are heard in most patients, but endocarditis is not always accompanied by a detectable murmur, especially if nonvalvular structures are involved.
- Often, the endocardial lesions result in valvular regurgitation, but valvular stenosis may also occur.
- The classification of the murmur depends on the valves affected and whether a valvular regurgitation or stenosis is present. If the mitral or tricuspid valves are involved leading to regurgitation, a systolic murmur will be heard on either the left or right hemithorax. If the aortic valve is affected, often a diastolic murmur is heard because of valvular regurgitation. Valvular stenosis may also be a consequence of space-occupying lesions on the affected valves. In this case, a diastolic murmur may be ausculted over the tricuspid or mitral valves and a systolic murmur over the heart base if the aortic or pulmonic valve is stenotic.

- With heart failure, clinical signs such as tachycardia, tachypnea, coughing, harsh lung sounds caused by pulmonary edema, distension of the jugular veins, ventral pectoral or preputial edema, and weight loss may be encountered.

ETIOLOGY AND PATHOPHYSIOLOGY
- Occurs primarily in a subacute or chronic form and requires a complex interaction between endothelium, immune response, and circulating bacteria. After initial trauma to the endothelial cells and depositions of platelets and fibrin, a nonbacterial thrombotic lesion develops. During bacteremia, colonization with microorganisms occurs, creating a bacterial endocarditis visualized as a vegetative mass, leading to valvular regurgitations or stenosis and a cardiac murmur.
- Although a bacteremia is required, endocarditis may develop with no current or recent history of septic foci.
- The most frequently isolated bacteria are *Staphylococcus* spp., *Streptococcus* spp., *Actinobacillus* spp., *Pasteurella* spp., and *Escherichia coli*.
- Parasitic lesions caused by the nematode *Strongylus vulgaris* have also been reported (although rarely), primarily involving the aortic valves as well as the endothelium within the aorta and coronary arteries.

DIAGNOSIS

DIFFERENTIAL DIAGNOSIS
- Diagnosis is based on clinical findings of pyrexia, depression, weight loss, and possibly signs of heart failure and is supported by the presence of a cardiac murmur on auscultation. However, these signs are nonspecific and may reflect inflammation in any organ. An exact diagnosis is obtained by a positive blood culture result and echocardiographic examination showing vegetative lesions on the affected valves.
- Any disease resulting in systemic illness with fever, depression, and weight loss.
- Fibrotic and nodular thickening of the valves are incidentally visualized on echocardiography in horses. These structures generally have no inflammatory component but often result in a cardiac murmur. These findings can be difficult to differentiate echocardiographically from endocarditis lesions. However, these horses do not nor-

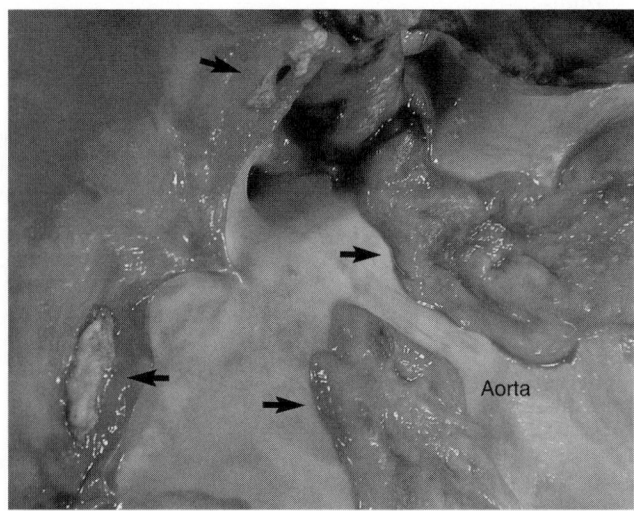

FIGURE 1 Heart with an opened left ventricle showing endocardial lesions of the aorta and aortic valves (*arrows*). (Courtesy Dr. H.E. Jensen, University of Copenhagen, Denmark.)

mally have clinical or hematologic signs of infection unless they have an infection in another organ system. When in doubt, diagnostic testing and treatment for endocarditis should be initiated.

INITIAL DATABASE

- Hematology shows nonspecific signs of a chronic infection (eg, leukocytosis with neutrophilia, hyperfibrinogenemia, hyperproteinemia, and anemia).
- Blood cultures may be positive for bacteria. Ideally, three separate blood samples taken at least 1 hour apart should be submitted for culture before initiating antibiotic treatment. If the patient is severely ill, the samples can be taken in intervals of 5 to 10 minutes before initiating treatment. Often, patients have been treated initially with antibiotics because of fever and depression, so bacterial culture results may be negative. However, for optimal treatment, it is essential to attempt to isolate the bacterial organism.
- Two-dimensional echocardiography provides an accurate diagnosis by visualizing masses of different size, often with an irregular surface on the endocardium (Figure 2). Doppler echocardiography is used to quantify the severity of valvular regurgitation or stenosis.
- If infection with *S. vulgaris* is suspected, the lesions will be caused by aberrant migration of parasitic larvae. At this stage of infection, the parasites have not yet returned to the intestine, so fecal egg counts and larval cultures will have no diagnostic value.

ADVANCED OR CONFIRMATORY TESTING

Some horses develop severe cardiac arrhythmias along with endocarditis (eg, ventricular tachycardia, supraventricular or ventricular premature complexes, and atrial fibrillation). Therefore horses with endocarditis should have electrocardiograms (ECGs) recorded regularly. If indicated, these horses should be monitored with continuous telemetric ECG.

TREATMENT

THERAPEUTIC GOAL(S)

- Provide effective antimicrobial treatment to eliminate infection.
- Provide supportive therapy if heart failure is present.
- Provide antiarrhythmic drugs if clinically significant dysrhythmias are present.

ACUTE GENERAL TREATMENT

- Initially, parenteral broad-spectrum antimicrobial agents should be instituted, pending results of blood culture and antimicrobial sensitivity testing. A common first choice is potassium penicillin (50,000 IU/kg IV q8h or 22,000 IU/kg IV q6h) in combination with gentamicin (6.6 mg/kg IV q24h). If possible, antibiotics with good penetration into fibrinous tissue should be chosen.
- Supportive treatment should be provided for patients in heart failure, including diuretics to reduce congestion (eg, furosemide 1–2 mg/kg IV q12h) in combination with a vasodilator such as an angiotensin-converting

enzyme (ACE) inhibitor (eg, enalapril 0.5 mg/kg IV q12–24h or quinapril 0.25 mg/kg PO q24h). These drugs have not been completely investigated in horses in heart failure, although the latter has shown efficacy in horses with mitral regurgitation. If severe tachycardia is present, digoxin can be given at a dosage of 0.0022 mg/kg IV q12h or 0.011 mg/kg PO q24h. (For more details on treatment of patients with heart failure, see "Cardic Failure" in this section.)

- Significant persistent dysrhythmias that contribute to clinical signs or are likely to progress to fatal dysrhythmias (eg, rapid ventricular tachycardia) should be addressed.
- If infection with *S. vulgaris* is suspected, anthelmintic treatment with ivermectin (200 µg/kg PO), moxidectin (400 µg/kg PO), or a 5-day course of fenbendazole (10 mg/kg PO) may be used to kill the migrating larvae.
- Nonsteroidal antiinflammatory drugs should be given to decrease fever and improve the patient's comfort level.
- Aspirin therapy has been recommended to decrease potential thrombus formation; however, neither that sequela nor the efficacy of aspirin in its prevention has been well documented in horses.
- Provide general supportive care to encourage the patient's appetite.

CHRONIC TREATMENT

- Continuation of antibiotic treatment is essential. The initial treatment may need to be altered according to the sensitivity pattern of the bacteria isolated.
- The horse should be treated with antibiotics for at least 5 to 6 weeks even if blood culture results are negative.
- Results of the complete blood count (CBC), serum chemistry panel, and echocardiography can be used to monitor the treatment duration.

POSSIBLE COMPLICATIONS

- Emboli originating from the vegetations may affect the lungs, brain, kidneys, joints, myocardium, and spleen, resulting in clinical signs associated with these organs.
- Cardiac arrhythmias may be seen secondary to extension of the inflammatory response in the area or because of embolic spreading to the myocardium.

RECOMMENDED MONITORING

- Clinical signs: fever, attitude, and appetite.
- Heart rate and rhythm.
- Character of murmur.
- CBC, fibrinogen, and globulin concentrations.

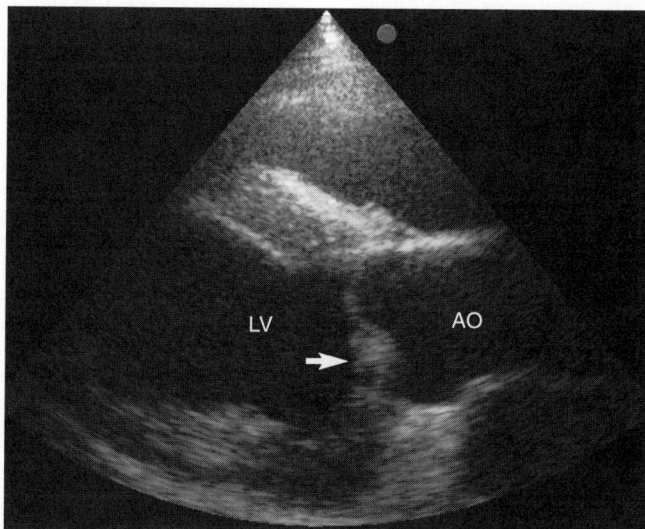

FIGURE 2 Long-axis echocardiogram of the aorta obtained from the right cardiac window showing a vegetative process on the left coronary cusp of the aortic valve (*arrow*). *AO*, Aorta; *LV*, left ventricle.

- Periodic echocardiographic assessment of valvular lesions and severity of valvular regurgitation or stenosis to determine response to therapy.
- Monitoring should be continued after antimicrobial treatment has been discontinued to determine if relapses have occurred. If significant valvular abnormalities exist after therapy has been completed, the horse should be monitored for the possibility of development of congestive heart failure (clinical signs and echocardiography).

PROGNOSIS AND OUTCOME

- The prognosis is guarded because of the risk of embolic spreading and the risk of developing congestive heart failure. Although a bacteriologic cure may be achieved, the valves may remain incompetent or stenotic from scarring, leading to a worsening of valvular function over time and progression to heart failure.

- For horses with mitral and aortic valve endocarditis, the prognosis is generally regarded as worse than for tricuspid and pulmonic valve endocarditis because of the consequences of left-sided volume overload, heart failure, and pulmonary edema.
- The effect of treatment should be monitored by echocardiography. The lesions should diminish in size, and the surface of the vegetations should become smoother in response to treatment.

PEARLS & CONSIDERATIONS

COMMENTS
In horses with signs of infection and a cardiac murmur, it is essential to identify whether the murmur is recent in onset or has been longstanding and was present on earlier examinations of the horse before signs of infection occurred. A longstanding murmur is likely caused by noninfectious endocardial thickening

and should therefore not be suspected as endocarditis.

CLIENT EDUCATION
Owners should be informed that the prognosis may be poor (especially for horses with aortic and mitral valve lesions), the treatment is prolonged and may be expensive, and the horse may not return to full athletic performance.

SUGGESTED READING
Aalbaek B, Ostergaard S, Buhl R, et al: *Actinobacillus equuli* subsp *equuli* associated with equine valvular endocarditis. *APMIS* 12:1437–1442, 2007.
Buergelt CD, Cooley AJ, Hines SA, et al: Endocarditis in six horses. *Vet Pathol* 22:333–337, 1985.
Maxson AD, Reef VB: Bacterial endocarditis in horses: ten cases (1984–1985). *Equine Vet J* 29(5):394–399, 1997.
Sage AM, Worth L: Fever: endocarditis and pericarditis. In Marr CM, editor: *Cardiology of the horse*. Philadelphia, 1999, WB Saunders, pp 256–259.

AUTHOR: RIKKE BUHLE

EDITOR: MARY M. DURANDO

Endometritis

BASIC INFORMATION

DEFINITION
Endometritis is inflammation of the endometrium and has many causes such as semen, bacteria, air, or foreign objects.

EPIDEMIOLOGY
SPECIES, AGE, SEX Physiologic postbreeding endometritis is seen in all mares. Pathologic endometritis is seen more commonly in older mares (especially postbreeding endometritis) but can occur in any age mare if uterine contamination with a sexually transmitted disease occurs or after insemination with frozen semen.
RISK FACTORS
- Older mares have an increased incidence of prolonged postbreeding endometritis from multiple factors.
- Mares with poor perineal conformation or a history of wind sucking are anatomically predisposed to uterine contamination with fecal and vaginal bacteria.
- Older (>12 years) maiden mares may be predisposed to excessive postbreeding endometritis because of a fibrotic, nonrelaxing cervix.
- In addition, urine pooling may lead to a sterile endometritis because of cranial urine flow into the uterus.

- Mares with compromised immune systems (caused by diseases such as Cushing disease) have a higher incidence of endometritis.
CONTAGIOUS AND ZOONOSIS Endometritis is not usually a contagious disease with the exception of certain sexually transmitted organisms, including *Taylorella equigenitalis*, some subtypes of *Pseudomonas aeruginosa*, and *Klebsiella pneumoniae*.

CLINICAL PRESENTATION
DISEASE FORMS/SUBTYPE
- Physiologic endometritis: The normal inflammatory response that occurs after breeding or parturition to allow for the expulsion of contaminants such as dead sperm or lochia.
- Mating-induced endometritis: The inflammatory response triggered by insemination. Normal inflammation allows for the phagocytosis and expulsion of unnecessary sperm, debris, and any bacteria that were introduced and should resolve within 24 hours of breeding.
- Persistent mating-induced: A continuation of mating-induced endometritis that persists for >72 hours after breeding. It is clinically relevant if the inflammation persists for >24 hours after breeding.

- Chronic endometritis: Endometritis that has persisted for more than one estrous cycle without resolution.
- Endometrosis: Chronic, degenerative changes to the endometrium that are irreversible and untreatable.
HISTORY, CHIEF COMPLAINT The chief complaint of mares with endometritis or endometrosis is often a failure to conceive ("repeat breeder"). Mares with endometritis may present 0 to 72 hours after breeding with vaginal discharge or tail rubbing or showing persistent estrus. Mares may also be found to have intrauterine fluid >24 hours after ovulation or at the pregnancy examination. In addition, endometritis may be an incidental finding on transrectal palpation or ultrasonography because of the lack of external signs.
PHYSICAL EXAM FINDINGS
- Mating-induced: Inflammation is seen after breeding. Vaginal discharge may be present but should be only a small amount. On ultrasonography, fluid may be present in the uterine lumen, and uterine edema may be increased compared with previous examinations. Physiologic inflammation should resolve within 24 hours of breeding.
- Persistent mating-induced: A continuation of mating-induced endometritis that persists >72 hours after breeding

but is clinically relevant if it persists for >24 hours after breeding. Physical examination and ultrasound findings are similar to those of mating-induced endometritis but are often more severe.

- Chronic endometritis: Many mares with clinical endometritis are asymptomatic but fail to conceive after repeat breedings. Ultrasound findings may show intrauterine fluid or edema but may also be within normal limits. Further diagnostic testing (see below) may be necessary to identify mares with chronic endometritis.
- Endometrosis: Mares with endometrosis are asymptomatic or are repeat breeders.

ETIOLOGY AND PATHOPHYSIOLOGY

- Insults to the endometrium (sperm, bacteria, debris) lead to an inflammatory cell influx into the tissue and lumen.
- Physiologic inflammation to insemination should resolve within 24 hours.
- Resolution of endometritis involves physiologic inflammation, increased mucous secretion, and mechanical clearance.
- Mares susceptible to endometritis have delayed uterine clearance.
- The most common organism isolated from mares with endometritis is *Streptococcus equi* subsp. *zooepidemicus*. The most common gram-negative bacteria is *Escherichia coli*.
- Fungal endometritis is rare but is more common in mares that have been treated extensively for bacterial endometritis. *Candida* is the most common fungal agent.

DIAGNOSIS

DIFFERENTIAL DIAGNOSIS

- Clinical signs: Tail rubbing caused by discharge or insect hypersensitivity
- Ultrasound findings: Early pregnancy (<22 days) or endometrial cysts

INITIAL DATABASE

- Ultrasound findings suggestive of endometritis include endometrial fluid, endometrial edema that is asynchronous with the stage of the estrous cycle, and poor uterine tone after ovulation or during diestrus.
- Endometritis is diagnosed by finding a significant number of neutrophils in the uterine lumen either via a double-guarded swab (positive result is >5% neutrophils), low-volume lavage (positive result is >15% neutrophils), or endometrial biopsy (positive result is >2 neutrophils per high power field). In addition, a uterine culture should be performed to identify the causative agent.

- The gold standard for diagnosis of endometritis is the culture of uterine biopsy tissue taken through a vaginal speculum to minimize secondary bacterial contamination. Culture results should be correlated with histopathology findings.
- The diagnosis of endometrosis is made by the evaluation of a uterine biopsy. Mares with endometrosis have chronic degenerative endometrial changes such as glandular nesting and fibrosis, lymphatic lacunae, and diffuse or perivascular fibrosis. Inflammation may or may not be present.

ADVANCED OR CONFIRMATORY TESTING

The culture of certain organisms such as *T. equigenitalis*, anaerobic bacteria, or fungi may require special media, storage, and transportation.

TREATMENT

THERAPEUTIC GOAL(S)

The goal of treatment is to resolve the inflammation by removing the inciting cause. In a breeding situation, resolution of endometritis is time sensitive. Treatment for endometritis must be aggressive because it needs to be resolved by day 3 after ovulation to minimize negative effects on the embryo.

ACUTE GENERAL TREATMENT

- Treatment generally varies depending on the severity of the inflammation, the mare's history, and the clinician's experience. Some mares may only require a single treatment; others may need to be managed intensively before and after breeding.
- Treatment options
  - Uterine lavage until efflux fluid is clear to help remove intrauterine debris, decrease the bacterial load, and gently dilate the uterus to allow removal of debris from endometrial glands and folds. Warmed (39°–45° C) sterile saline or lactated Ringer's solution is infused into the uterus 1 to 2 L at a time and then collected via gravity flow. The resulting fluid is evaluated for color and turbidity and can be spun down for cytology or culture. Uterine lavage should be performed within 4 to 6 hours but no later than 12 hours of insemination to avoid affecting subsequent pregnancy rates.
  - Ecbolics as needed to help with uterine evacuation. The most commonly used drug is oxytocin (20–40 IU IV or IM) given every 1 to 4 hours. If oxytocin is administered at very high doses (80–100 IU) or very

frequently, it can lead to spastic uterine contractions that do not help evacuate fluid through the cervix. Carbetocin, a long-acting analogue of oxytocin, has been used in doses of 100 to 200 µg slowly IV for a longer duration of uterine contractility (1–2 hours).

  - Cloprostenol (250 µg/mL, 1 mL IM), a prostaglandin analogue, may be used before breeding to induce longer acting uterine contractions, but should not be given more than 12 hours after ovulation because it can have negative effects on the developing corpus luteum.
  - Mares with a fibrotic cervix require uterine lavage to help remove excess sperm and bacteria. In addition, prostaglandin E (100–200 µg in a small amount of sterile lubricant) can be applied topically to the cervix to aid in cervical dilatation.
  - Antibiotics or antifungals if necessary to help decrease the organism load within the uterus. Table 1 shows commonly used antibiotics and antifungals. The choice of antibiotic and route of administration depend on the organism cultured and its sensitivity, the mare's temperament, client cooperation, and cost. References for less commonly used antibiotics and antifungals are listed in the suggested reading.
  - Ancillary therapies in research include glucocorticoids (to suppress the immune inflammatory response) and mycobacterial cell wall extracts IU or IV (to modulate the inflammatory response). Recent studies describe different treatment and dosing regimens for glucocorticoid use, and further research is ongoing. Caslick's surgery should be performed on mares with poor perineal conformation or a history of fecal-

---

TABLE 1 Antibiotics and Antifungal Agents Commonly Used to Treat Endometritis*

Amikacin[†]

Potassium penicillin

Procaine penicillin

Trimethoprim sulfa

Gentamicin[†]

Ticarcillin with clavulanate

Enrofloxacin

Fluconazole (antifungal)[†]

Amphotericin B (antifungal)[†]

*Further dosing information can be found in "Endometritis, Bacterial and Fungal" in this section.
[†]Care should be taken when using antibiotics or antifungals known to be nephrotoxic or hepatotoxic. Owners should be advised of risks, and blood work should be monitored as necessary.

vaginal contamination. This can be done after therapy is complete or during the pregnancy examination.

POSSIBLE COMPLICATIONS

Caution should be used when introducing drugs and solutions into the uterus because high or low pH levels can damage the endometrium and lead to permanent fibrosis and adhesions.

RECOMMENDED MONITORING

Mares with a history of repeat breeding, pooling fluid after breeding, or other clinical signs of endometritis should be closely monitored on subsequent breeding cycles and treated if needed.

PROGNOSIS AND OUTCOME

- The treatment of mares with infectious endometritis caused by a sexually transmitted

disease is generally rewarding and does not affect long-term fertility.
- Mares with chronic or repeated endometritis will have decreased fertility. The Kenney-Doig biopsy score can be used as a prognosticator for clients.
- Endometrosis is a chronic, degenerative disease. Therapy is aimed at minimizing the amount of inflammation, but the permanent fibrosis will decrease the mare's fertility.

PEARLS & CONSIDERATIONS

COMMENTS

- The treatment for endometritis is very variable by animal. Clinicians should use their personal knowledge, the client's financial investment in the case, and the history of the patient to plan a treatment regimen.
- Ideally, a stallion with high fertility should be chosen for "problem" mares

to minimize extrinsic causes for the mare's subfertility.

CLIENT EDUCATION

Clients should be informed about the increased cost of breeding a mare with endometritis as well as the decrease in pregnancy rate compared with noninflamed mares.

SUGGESTED READING

Dascanio JJ: Antibiotics in mare reproduction. *Clin Therio* 1:169, 2009.

LeBlanc MM, Causey RC: Clinical and subclinical endometritis in the mare: both threats to fertility. *Reprod Domest Anim* 44:10, 2009.

Wolfsdorf K, Caudle AB: Inflammation of the tubular reproductive tract of the mare. In Youngquist RS, Threlfall WR, editors: *Current therapy in large animal theriogenology 2.* St Louis, 2007, Saunders Elsevier, pp 158–167.

AUTHOR: SARAH E. EATON

EDITOR: JUAN C. SAMPER

Endometritis, Bacterial and Fungal

BASIC INFORMATION

DEFINITION

Inflammation of the uterine lining (endometrium) caused by the presence of bacterial or fungal organisms, creating an environment unsuitable for an embryo

SYNONYMS

Acute endometritis, chronic endometritis, uterine infection, uterine inflammation

EPIDEMIOLOGY

SPECIES, AGE, SEX Older (>15 years) mares are predisposed to bacterial infections

GENETICS AND BREED PREDISPOSITION Saddlebreds are predisposed to development of fungal infections.

RISK FACTORS

- Less than two thirds of the vulva below the brim of the pelvis
- Poor or decreased muscular tone to the vulva
- Poor conformation to the perineum
- Cervical abnormalities (trauma, adhesions, fibrosis)
- Abnormalities of the vulva (trauma)
- Decreased uterine contractility
- Exposure to pathogens during breeding
- Chronic intrauterine antibiotic administration
- Pendulous uterus

- Wind sucking: Aspiration of air into the reproductive tract
- Equine pituitary pars intermedia dysfunction
- Poor body condition (body condition score <4 of 9)

CONTAGION AND ZOONOSIS Exposure of a mare to venereal pathogens (*Taylorella equigenitalis, Pseudomonas aeruginosa, Klebsiella pneumonia*)

GEOGRAPHY AND SEASONALITY Uterine infections can occur at any time during the year and are not restricted geographically.

ASSOCIATED CONDITIONS AND DISORDERS

- Infertility
  - Low pregnancy rate
  - Increased pregnancy loss rate
- Systemic illness is rare

CLINICAL PRESENTATION

DISEASE FORMS/SUBTYPES

- Acute infectious endometritis
- Chronic infectious endometritis

HISTORY, CHIEF COMPLAINT

- Subfertility
- Shortened interovulatory period
- Vulvar discharge

PHYSICAL EXAM FINDINGS

- Mares appear systemically healthy.
- Intrauterine fluid present on transrectal ultrasound examination
- Vaginal discharge or fluid in the vaginal vault

- Speculum examination: Reddened cervix and cervical discharge

ETIOLOGY AND PATHOPHYSIOLOGY

- Normally, the mare's uterus can rapidly clear infections if exposed to bacteria or fungi.
- Any breakdown in the defense mechanisms of the reproductive tract predisposes a mare to a uterine infection.
  - Conformation: Abnormalities of the perineum, vestibulovaginal seal, or cervix may allow increased numbers of pathogens to reach the uterus.
  - Uterine clearance: Decreased ability of the mare's uterus to contract, reducing clearance of fluid and contaminants from the uterus.
  - Innate immune system: Breakdown in the response toward pathogens in the uterus
- Exposure during breeding to a venereal pathogen

DIAGNOSIS

DIFFERENTIAL DIAGNOSIS

For intrauterine fluid:

- Urine pooling in the vaginal vault and uterus
- Mating- or postmating-induced endometritis
- Pyometra
- Pneumouterus (wind sucking) may allow bacteria to be carried into the

uterus. In addition, air is a local irritant to the endometrium.
- Mucus associated with estrus
- Heavy edema, inducing an exudate

INITIAL DATABASE
- Uterine culture via double-guarded uterine culture swab
  - Identifies microbiologic agent(s).
  - A negative culture result may not always indicate an absence of intrauterine bacteria.
- Uterine cytology
  - Sample of endometrial cells and intraluminal contents.

BOX 1 Etiologic Agents Detected in the Equine Uterus

Bacteria Known to Be Pathogenic
Streptococcus spp.
  β-hemolytic
  equi subsp. *zooepidemicus*
Escherichia coli
Pseudomonas spp.
  aeruginosa
  fluorescens
Klebsiella spp.
  pneumoniae

Bacteria with Questionable Pathogenicity
Methicillin-resistant *Staphylococcus aureus*
Streptococcus spp.
  α-hemolytic
  nonhemolytic
  faecalis
  equisimilis
Bordetella bronchiseptica
Proteus spp.
  mirabilis
  vulgaris
Staphylococcus spp.
  aureus
  albus
  intermedius
Serratia spp.
Corynebacterium spp.
Citrobacter spp.
Enterobacter spp.
Bacillus spp.
Acinetobacter spp.
Micrococcus spp.
Pasteurella spp.
Anaerobic
Bacteroides fragilis
Fusobacterium spp.
Clostridium spp.
  perfringens
  difficile
Mycoplasma spp.
Chlamydia spp.
Fungal
Candida spp.
  albicans
  other
Aspergillus spp.
Actinomyces spp.
  fumigatus
Cryptococcus spp.
Fusarium spp.
Mucor spp.

- Commonly collected using a culture swab or brush and rolled onto a glass microscope slide and stained with Diff-Quik
  - Polymorphic neutrophils (PMNs) indicate active inflammation in the endometrium.
- Interpretation
  - Positive culture result with a positive cytology result is diagnostic of a uterine infections.
  - Negative culture with a positive cytology result suggests inflammation not caused by an infectious agent (postmating-induced endometritis, pneumovagina, urine pooling). However, intrauterine bacteria are not always cultured using standard techniques.
- In some cases, bacterial and fungal organisms may be seen on a cytology slide, and the uterine culture results are negative.
  - Positive culture result with a negative cytology result may be observed with some uterine bacterial infections (eg, *Escherichia coli*); may not always be associated with an inflammatory response.
  - Combination of bacterial culture of a single organism with the presence of more than 5 PMNs per 40× field confirms bacterial infection.

ADVANCED OR CONFIRMATORY TESTING
- Small-volume lavage with culture or cytology of centrifuge pellet: Provides a more representative sample of the entire uterus
- Uterine biopsy for histopathology: Determines the presence or absence of endometritis when clinical and bacteriologic findings are inconclusive
- Uterine biopsy for culture: Has been suggested to be more diagnostic than a traditional culture
- Uterine biopsy for cytology: An alternative to traditional cytology sampling technique

TREATMENT

THERAPEUTIC GOAL(S)
- To aid the uterus in clearing infectious agents and inflammatory debris
- Administration of appropriate antibiotic or antifungal agent based on antimicrobial sensitivity determined from uterine culture

ACUTE GENERAL TREATMENT
- Aid in uterine clearance
- Uterine lavage
  - 0.9% saline or lactated Ringer's solution to reduce the numbers

---

TABLE 1 Common Intrauterine Antibiotics Used in the Treatment of Bacterial Endometritis

Antibiotic	Daily Recommended Intrauterine Dose	Spectrum
Amikacin should be buffered	1–2 g	Gram negative
Ampicillin	1–3 g	Gram positive
Gentamicin should be buffered	1–3 g	Gram negative
Potassium penicillin	5 million IU	Primarily *Streptococcus* spp.
Ticarcillin	3–6 g	Broad spectrum
Ticarcillin/clavulanic acid	3–6 g	Broad spectrum
Ceftiofur sodium	1 g	Broad spectrum

TABLE 2 Common Intrauterine Antibiotics Used in the Treatment of Fungal Endometritis

Antifungal	Daily Recommended Intrauterine Dose	Purpose
Amphotericin B	100–200 mg	Polyene antibiotic altering the permeability of the fungal cytoplasmic membrane; dilute in 100 mL
Nystatin	0.5–2.5 million U	Polyene antibiotic altering the permeability of the fungal cytoplasmic membrane; *do not* mix with saline, which may cause precipitation
Clotrimazole	500–700 mg	Disruption of nutrient exchange across the fungal cell wall and membrane
Fluconazole	100 mg	Disruption of nutrient exchange across the fungal cell wall and membrane
Miconazole	500–700 mg	Disruption of nutrient exchange across the fungal cell wall and membrane

of infectious agents and remove inflammatory debris from the uterus
- Enhances luminal defense mechanisms by inducing local irritation and influx of PMNs into the uterine lumen
- Mycotic infections: Anecdotal evidence suggests the addition of dimethyl sulfoxide (10%–20%), dilute iodine (0.5%), or white vinegar (1%–2%) to the lavage solution may be beneficial.
- Ecbolics
  - Oxytocin: 5 to 20 IU administered IM or IV
  - Cloprostenol: 250 µg IM
- Appropriate intrauterine antibiotic or antifungal agent
- Bacterial infections are typically treated once daily for 3 to 5 days during estrus when the cervix is open.
- Fungal infections are also typically treated during estrus once daily for 7 to 10 days.
- Appropriate systemic antibiotics
- Often more expensive to reach minimum inhibitory concentrations within uterine tissues than with intrauterine administration
- May be used when antibiotic sensitivity warrants treatment with antibiotics not appropriate for intrauterine use (eg, enrofloxacin)

CHRONIC TREATMENT

- Repair of abnormal conformation or damaged reproductive anatomy. Common surgeries are a Caslick's procedure, perineal body reconstruction, or cervical laceration repair.
- Surgical repair should be performed before treatment with antibiotics.
- Good hygiene should be practiced by personnel and stallions when breeding mares.

POSSIBLE COMPLICATIONS

- Mares with repeated uterine infections may have an increase in development of uterine fibrosis (scar tissue). This has been shown to lead to decreased fertility rates.
- Enrofloxacin should not be used for intrauterine treatment.
- Avoid administration of prostaglandins after ovulation or during formation of the corpus luteum because it could adversely affect corpus luteum development and decrease pregnancy rates.

RECOMMENDED MONITORING

- Ultrasound examination as the mare comes back into estrus for the presence of intrauterine fluid
- Recheck uterine culture and cytology during posttreatment estrus.

PROGNOSIS AND OUTCOME

- Bacterial
  - If the initial inciting cause of the infection can be prevented, appropriate treatment will allow the mare to return to her previous level of fertility.
- Fungal
  - Treatment of fungal and more specifically yeast infections are often unrewarding. Reoccurrence of yeast infections is common. Also, the amount of intrauterine damage sustained during the infection leads to decreased fertility.
  - Mares with a fungal infection commonly have a secondary bacterial infection concurrently or after treatment for fungal organisms.

SUGGESTED READING

Dascanio JJ: Antibiotics in mare reproduction. *Proc Soc Their* 169–176, 2009.

Dascanio JJ: Treatment of fungal endometritis. In Samper JC, Pycock JF, McKinnon AO, editors: *Current therapy in equine reproduction.* St Louis, 2007, Saunders Elsevier, pp 116–120.

Lu KG, Morresey PR: Reproductive tract infections in horses. *Vet Clin Equine* 22:519–552, 2006.

AUTHOR: **RYAN A. FERRIS**

EDITOR: **JUAN C. SAMPER**

Enteritis, Focal Eosinophilic

BASIC INFORMATION

DEFINITION

Recently described syndrome characterized by focal or circumferential regions of eosinophilic inflammatory infiltration in the small intestinal wall

SYNONYM

Idiopathic focal eosinophilic enteritis

CLINICAL PRESENTATION

HISTORY, CHIEF COMPLAINT Acute colic
PHYSICAL EXAM FINDINGS The initial evaluation of horses with focal eosinophilic enteritis is identical to that of horses presenting for other causes of nonstrangulating small intestinal obstruction, with moderate to severe abdominal pain, tachycardia, small intestinal disten-sion on rectal examination, and gastric reflux.

ETIOLOGY AND PATHOPHYSIOLOGY

- The specific cause and the reason for the focal or circumferential nature of the inflammatory infiltrate are unknown.
- The inciting cause is likely similar to other causes of inflammatory bowel disease (see "Inflammatory Bowel Disease" in this section).
- Because of the predominance of eosinophils in the inflammatory infiltrate, a parasitic or allergic cause has been proposed, although evidence to support this is currently lacking.
- The inflammatory infiltrate and associated fibrosis creates an intramural mass or a circumferential mural band that obstructs the small intestinal lumen, resulting in acute colic.

DIAGNOSIS

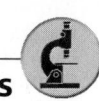

DIFFERENTIAL DIAGNOSIS

Other causes of nonstrangulating or strangulating small intestinal obstruction

INITIAL DATABASE

- No significant abnormalities other than mild dehydration are typically found on complete blood count.
- Serum biochemistry profile
  - Hypoproteinemia and hypoalbuminemia are frequently seen.
  - Globulin concentrations may be low, normal, or increased.
- Transabdominal ultrasonography: Moderate to severe small intestinal distension consistent with an obstructive pattern is frequently seen. A thickened small intestine is not usually appreciated.
- Peritoneal fluid analysis: Variable. In most cases, peritoneal fluid is either normal or has a mildly elevated nucle-

ated cell count and total protein concentration.

ADVANCED OR CONFIRMATORY TESTING

- Exploratory celiotomy and histopathology
  - Reveal characteristic focal region or regions of intramural masses or mural bands in the small intestine with small intestinal distension oral to the lesion(s).
  - Resection of the affected regions is necessary. Histopathologic analysis reveals characteristic eosinophilic inflammatory infiltrates with variable fibrosis.

TREATMENT

THERAPEUTIC GOAL(S)

Surgical resection of affected intestine

ACUTE GENERAL TREATMENT

- Exploratory celiotomy is indicated because of colic signs associated with small intestinal obstruction that are refractory to medical management. Surgical resection of affected segments and anastomosis of unaffected jejunum is associated with a good prognosis.
- Medical management with immunosuppressive therapy as for other types of inflammatory bowel disease may have the potential to be effective but is usually not possible because of severe colic signs.
- Immunosuppressive therapy after surgery does not appear to be necessary because the lesions do not tend to recur.

POSSIBLE COMPLICATIONS

Small intestinal or gastric rupture if surgery is not performed

PROGNOSIS AND OUTCOME

Fair to good with surgical resection of affected intestine

PEARLS & CONSIDERATIONS

It is not clear whether this syndrome is an emerging phenomenon or is simply being recognized more frequently.

SUGGESTED READING

Davis JL: Medical disorders of the small intestine: inflammatory bowel disease. In Smith BP, editor: *Large animal internal medicine.* St Louis, 2009, Mosby Elsevier, pp 730–731.

Southwood, Kawcak CE, Trotter GW, et al: Idiopathic focal eosinophilic enteritis associated with small intestinal obstruction in 6 horses. *Vet Surg* 29(5):415–419, 2000.

AUTHOR: **KELSEY A. HART**

EDITORS: **TIM MAIR** and **CERI SHERLOCK**

Enteritis, Proximal

BASIC INFORMATION

DEFINITION

Inflammatory disease of the duodenum and proximal jejunum resulting in excessive enteric fluid and electrolyte secretion and large-volume enterogastric reflux

SYNONYMS

- Anterior enteritis
- Duodenitis-proximal jejunitis (DPJ)

EPIDEMIOLOGY

CONTAGION AND ZOONOSIS Although infectious or toxic agents may contribute to proximal enteritis, the disease typically occurs in an individual horse on a farm rather than as an outbreak.

CLINICAL PRESENTATION

HISTORY, CHIEF COMPLAINT Depression, inappetence, fever, and variable signs of colic (mild to severe)

PHYSICAL EXAM FINDINGS

- Depression
- Pyrexia is commonly observed.
- Variable tachycardia and tachypnea
- Variable signs of colic, which are almost always relieved by passage of a nasogastric tube and gastric decompression
  - A significant volume of gastric reflux (5–25 L) is usually obtained initially. Reflux volume may increase with therapy when the patient is rehydrated.
  - The reflux may be orange to dark brown in color and often has a fetid odor. Hemorrhagic gastric reflux is occasionally encountered.
- Injected, hyperemic mucous membranes with a "toxic line" are usually encountered.
- Moderate to severe dehydration, with prolonged capillary refill time, prolonged skin tent, and poor jugular refill.
- Decreased to absent gastrointestinal borborygmi.
- Mild abdominal distension may be present.
- Rectal examination:
  - Mild to moderately distended or thickened small intestine is usually appreciated.
  - Concurrent large colonic gas distension is occasionally noted with severe, diffuse intestinal ileus.

ETIOLOGY AND PATHOPHYSIOLOGY

- The specific cause of proximal enteritis is unknown, although several infectious or toxic agents have been proposed. It is likely that a variety of causes result in a similar clinical syndrome.
  - Toxigenic *Clostridium difficile* is the pathogen most often isolated from horses with proximal enteritis, although *C. difficile* infection is not documented in all cases.
  - *Clostridium perfringens* and *Salmonella* spp. infection also occasionally manifest with signs consistent with proximal enteritis.
  - Cantharidin toxicity may result in small intestinal as well as colonic damage, and affected horses may present with clinical signs of proximal enteritis.
  - Lesions consistent with proximal enteritis have been produced experimentally in horses exposed to toxins produced by *Fusarium moniliforme.* However, neurologic signs and central nervous system lesions typical of leukoencephalomalacia were also observed in those horses and are not described in most cases of proximal enteritis.
- Regardless of the specific inciting cause, the gross pathologic findings in horses with proximal enteritis include duodenal and proximal jejunal serositis with mucosal and submucosal hyperemia and edema. Histopathologic findings include loss of intestinal villi and necrosis of epithelial cells with neutrophilic infiltration and sub-

mucosal and serosal hemorrhages and fibrinopurulent exudates.

- Several factors may contribute to the large-volume enterogastric reflux in proximal enteritis.
  - With severe intestinal mural inflammation and epithelial cell necrosis, fluid, electrolytes, and plasma protein are lost passively through the damaged mucosa.
  - In addition, an active secretory component may be induced by bacterial toxins and likely plays a role in most cases, resulting in further enteric fluid and electrolyte loss.
  - Intestinal mural edema and inflammation and villus loss also decrease the small intestinal absorptive capacity and inhibit normal peristalsis, resulting in enterogastric reflux.
  - Finally, in some cases of proximal enteritis, pancreatic secretions are increased because of concurrent pancreatitis.
- Bacterial toxins enter the systemic circulation through the compromised enteric mucosal barrier or via the portal circulation, resulting in the clinical signs of endotoxemia and the systemic inflammatory response syndrome.

DIAGNOSIS

DIFFERENTIAL DIAGNOSIS

- Strangulating or nonstrangulating small intestinal obstruction
- Ulcerative duodenitis or gastric outflow obstruction (see "Ulcerative Duodenitis" and "Pyloric Stenosis" in this section)

INITIAL DATABASE

- Complete blood count
  - Leukopenia characterized by a neutropenia with increased band neutrophils and toxic changes in neutrophils is typically seen.
  - The hematocrit varies with hydration status but can be markedly increased in severe cases (>60%).
  - Thrombocytopenia is occasionally present in severe cases with concurrent disseminated intravascular coagulation (DIC).
- Serum biochemistry profile
  - Variable electrolyte derangements are common, with hypokalemia, hyponatremia, hypochloremia, and hypocalcemia most common
  - Serum total protein (TP) concentration may be increased with dehydration or normal or low with enteric loss
  - Some degree of azotemia is common and may be caused by prerenal or renal causes (or both).

- Metabolic acidosis and hyperlactatemia (>2 mmol/L) suggests impaired peripheral perfusion and tissue oxygenation caused by hypovolemia.
- Transabdominal ultrasonography
  - Mild to severe small intestinal distension with increased small intestinal mural thickness (>5 mm) is usually appreciated.
  - The duodenum is typically dilated and hypomotile with increased mural thickness (>5 mm).
- Peritoneal fluid analysis
  - Variable. In most cases, peritoneal fluid is grossly normal with a mildly increased nucleated cell count and TP concentration.
  - However, exudative fluid with a more substantially increased nucleated cell count may be seen if concurrent peritonitis has occurred because of bacterial translocation.
  - In severe cases, peritoneal fluid can be grossly serosanguineous, which may make it difficult to differentiate proximal enteritis from a strangulating intestinal obstruction.

ADVANCED OR CONFIRMATORY TESTING

- Diagnostic testing for specific causes of proximal enteritis should include the following.
  - Polymerase chain reaction or culture for *Salmonella* spp. on gastric reflux and feces
  - Gram stain and toxin assays for *C. perfringens* and *C. difficile* toxins on gastric reflux and feces.
  - ±Urine analysis for cantharidin if historical exposure
- Gastroduodenoscopy may be indicated to rule out ulcerative duodenitis and pyloric outflow obstruction, but visualization of the pylorus and duodenum may be difficult with large-volume gastric reflux.

TREATMENT

THERAPEUTIC GOAL(S)
Supportive care

ACUTE GENERAL TREATMENT

- An indwelling nasogastric tube should be maintained and the patient monitored for gastric reflux q2–3h to maintain gastric decompression and prevent gastric rupture. A careful record of gastric reflux volume can direct fluid therapy to meet ongoing fluid losses.
- IV fluid therapy
  - Fluid resuscitation with hypertonic saline (2–4 mL/kg IV bolus) or hydroxyethyl starch (5–10 mL/kg

IV bolus) or both is indicated in severely dehydrated patients.
  - This should be followed by isotonic balanced polyionic crystalloid fluids (eg, Normosol-R or Plasmalyte) at 50 to 150 mL/kg/day, depending on the degree of dehydration and ongoing losses in gastric reflux.
  - Supplementation with potassium chloride (10–40 mEq/L with the rate not to exceed 0.5 mEq/kg/h), 23% calcium gluconate (1–2 mL/kg/day) or magnesium sulfate (20–25 g/450 kg horse/day) is often necessary to correct electrolyte derangements.
  - Colloidal support with equine plasma (20–40 mL/kg IV) or hydroxyethyl starch (5–10 mL/kg IV bolus q24–48h or 1 mL/kg/h IV continuous rate infusion [CRI]) is indicated in hypoproteinemic patients. (Note: Patients with initially normal TP concentrations may have hypoproteinemia after rehydration.)
  - Horses with inflammatory intestinal diseases such as proximal enteritis are particularly prone to thrombophlebitis. Long-term polyethylene IV catheters should be used and removed at the first sign of a problem with the catheter or vein.
- Antiinflammatory and analgesic therapy
  - Flunixin meglumine: 0.5 to 1.1 mg/kg IV q12h for analgesic and antiinflammatory effects; may be decreased to 0.25 mg/kg IV q6–8h
  - Lidocaine: 1.3 mg/kg IV as a slow bolus; then 0.05 mg/kg/min IV CRI for analgesic and prokinetic effects
  - ± Dimethylsulfoxide (90% solution): 20 to 100 mg/kg diluted to less than 10% solution in IV fluids q12h for 1 to 3 days (may scavenge free radicals and limit oxidative injury)
- Antiendotoxic therapy
  - Equine plasma (2–4 L IV or more if hypoproteinemic; regular equine plasma or hyperimmune plasma with antiendotoxin antibodies) or hyperimmune antiendotoxin serum (Endoserum, 1–2 mL/kg diluted in 3–5 L isotonic fluids IV)
  - Polymixin-B: 2000 to 6000 IU/kg (diluted in 500–1000 mL 0.9% saline) IV q12h for 1 to 3 days after the patient is hydrated and if renal function is adequate
- Laminitis prophylaxis
  - Placement of frog supports and maintenance in deep bedding should be initiated immediately.
  - Periodic or continuous maintenance in ice boots during initial therapy may be helpful in preventing laminitis, although this is not universally accepted.

○ If signs of laminitis occur, treatment should be rapid and aggressive (see "Laminitis, Acute" in this section).

- Oral medications and intestinal absorbants should be avoided because of likely poor absorption and the risk of gastric rupture.
- Nutritional support
  ○ Addition of 1% to 2.5% dextrose to IV fluids during early therapy may help meet some of the patient's initial energy requirements.
  ○ Parenteral nutrition should be considered in protracted cases with persistent gastric reflux for several days or more.
- Antimicrobial therapy
  ○ Controversial because a specific infectious cause is often difficult to determine, and most horses recover without specific antimicrobial therapy.
  ○ Metronidazole (15–25 mg/kg by rectum) is indicated if clostridial toxin assay results are positive.
  ○ Broad-spectrum antimicrobial therapy is indicated in patients with peritonitis or in profoundly neutropenic patients (which are at greater risk of development of secondary infections such as pneumonia or septic thrombophlebitis). May include potassium penicillin 22,000 to 44,000 IU/kg IV q6h *and* genta-

micin (6.6 mg/kg IV q24h) or enrofloxacin (5 mg/kg IV q24h)
- Other
  ○ Some evidence suggests that some horses with proximal enteritis may be hypercoagulable because of subclinical DIC and thus are at greater risk for thrombotic complications. Heparin (20–40 IU/kg IV or SC q8h) may be beneficial in these cases.
  ○ Some horses show signs of persistent abdominal pain despite gastric decompression and analgesic therapy. Exploratory celiotomy is warranted in these cases to rule out a small intestinal obstructive lesion.

POSSIBLE COMPLICATIONS

- Thrombophlebitis
- Laminitis
- Intestinal infarction
- Gastroduodenal ulcers with prolonged anorexia
- Increased risk of intraabdominal adhesions if laparotomy is necessary

PROGNOSIS AND OUTCOME

- Fair with normal peritoneal fluid, good response to sup-

portive care, and avoidance of laminitis
- Guarded with concurrent peritonitis or serosanguineous peritoneal fluid, concurrent laminitis, or if laparotomy is necessary

PEARLS & CONSIDERATIONS

It can be difficult to differentiate between proximal enteritis and a strangulating small intestinal obstruction in some cases. Peritoneal fluid analysis should be performed in these cases and exploratory celiotomy considered if signs of colic persist after gastric decompression.

SUGGESTED READING

Davis JL: Medical disorders of the small intestine: duodenitis-proximal jejunitis. In Smith BP, editor: *Large animal internal medicine.* St Louis, 2009, Mosby Elsevier, pp 725–728.

AUTHOR: **KELSEY A. HART**

EDITORS: **TIM MAIR** and **CERI SHERLOCK**

Enterolithiasis

BASIC INFORMATION

DEFINITION

Obstruction of the flow of ingesta or gas associated with the presence of an enterolith(s)

SYNONYMS

Stone, rock

EPIDEMIOLOGY

SPECIES, AGE, SEX Almost all reported cases of enterolithiasis are in horses >4 years, with most between 5 and 10 years of age. However, isolated reports of younger horses exist (eg, a 2-year-old Quarter Horse filly and an 11-month-old Miniature Horse).
GENETICS AND BREED PREDISPOSITION Arabians are overrepresented. Other breeds with reported predisposition include Arabian crosses, Morgans, American Saddlebreds, donkeys, and Miniature Horses.
RISK FACTORS Risk factors include diets high in alfalfa hay, wheat bran, and

magnesium and phosphorus content and horses that are kept indoors more than 50% of the time.
GEOGRAPHY AND SEASONALITY States with high prevalence of enterolithiasis include California, Florida, and the Southern states.

CLINICAL PRESENTATION

HISTORY, CHIEF COMPLAINT

- Clinical signs of enterolithiasis are variable depending on the location and size of the enterolith(s). In general, horses present with mild to moderate abdominal pain (colic) and decreased or absent fecal production.
- Horses may have a history of repeated episodes of mild colic associated with intermittent partial obstruction.
- Diet, geographic location, and signalment consistent with enterolithiasis should be recognized.

PHYSICAL EXAM FINDINGS

- Horses with enterolithiasis have physical examination findings similar to horses with other simple obstructions of the large or small colon.

- If transmural pressure necrosis occurs, clinical signs will be consistent with intestinal perforation or rupture, including progression toward cardiovascular collapse, peracute peritonitis, and severe endotoxemia.

ETIOLOGY AND PATHOPHYSIOLOGY

- Enteroliths form around small niduses (eg, pieces of wire, nails, sand, pebbles, rope).
- The dominant mineral within enteroliths is struvite (ammonium magnesium phosphate).
- Diets high in magnesium (water or feed; wheat bran, alfalfa) and protein (eg, alfalfa with high concentrations of ammonium and nitrogen in the large colon) have been implicated in the pathogenesis of enterolithiasis. However, other factors must play a role because horses fed similar diets in parts of the country where enteroliths are not prevalent do not develop them.
- The most common site of obstruction with enteroliths is the junction of the right dorsal colon and the transverse

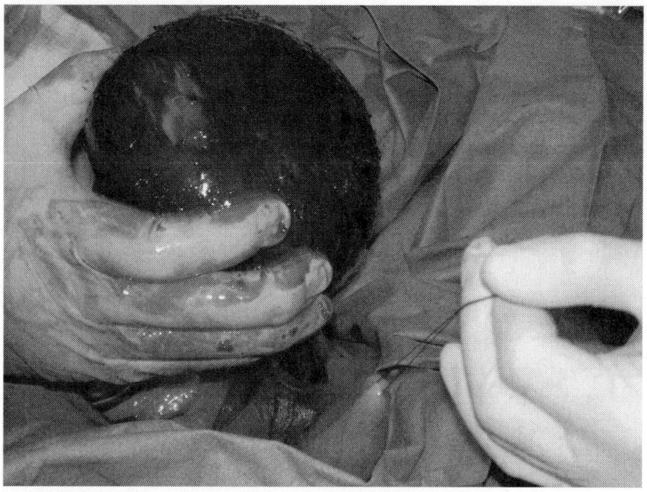

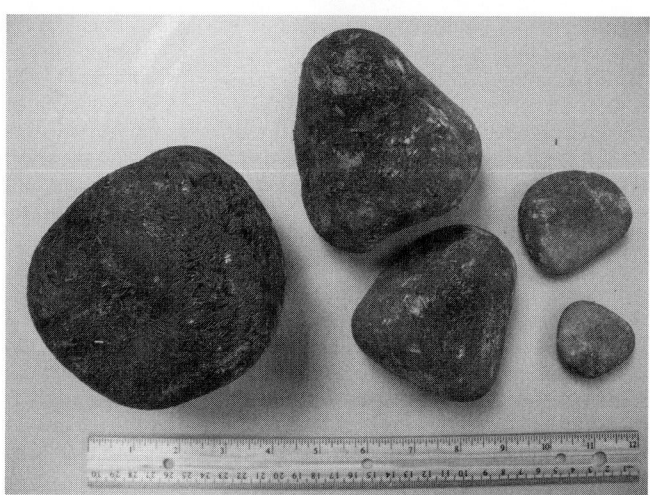

FIGURE 1 Enterolith being removed by colotomy in the right dorsal colon at exploratory laparotomy.

FIGURE 2 Typical appearance of enteroliths.

colon. Less frequently, obstruction occurs in the transverse colon or the small colon. Enteroliths have also been found in the right ventral colon and diaphragmatic flexure.

DIAGNOSIS

DIFFERENTIAL DIAGNOSIS

- Other causes of mild to moderate abdominal pain are simple or non-strangulating obstructions of the gastrointestinal tract such as large colon impactions (feed and sand), large colon displacements, large intestinal intraluminal obstructions, tympany, small colon impactions, and ileal impactions.
- Other causes of large intestinal distension on examination per rectum include tympany, large colon impactions (feed and sand), large colon displacements, and other intraluminal obstructions.

INITIAL DATABASE

- Horses may pass small enteroliths in their feces, but this is not necessarily correlated with the presence of obstructive enteroliths.
- Findings on examination per rectum depend on the location of the impaction. Distension of the large colon and cecum is common with the addition of distension of the small colon if the enterolith is within the small colon. It is uncommon to palpate an enterolith per rectum.
- Nasogastric reflux is uncommon but can occur.
- Bloodwork may be normal or consistent with mild to moderate dehydration (prerenal azotemia, elevated packed cell volume, elevated total protein [TP]). If transmural necrosis

has occurred, the leukogram may reveal a leukopenia with or without a left shift.
- Abdominal fluid analysis is generally within normal limits. Elevations in TP and total nucleated cell counts indicate compromise to the intestinal wall.
- Abdominal radiography may be useful for identifying enteroliths. Radiographs are more likely to identify enteroliths in the large colon than the small colon and have a better positive predictive value than negative predictive value. Radiographs are likely more useful in areas with a high prevalence of enterolithiasis.

TREATMENT

THERAPEUTIC GOAL(S)

Remove the enterolith(s)

ACUTE GENERAL TREATMENT

- Surgical exploration and removal may be performed. If pressure necrosis is present, resection of the affected bowel may be required.
- Provide perioperative supportive care as required.

CHRONIC TREATMENT

- The recurrence rate of enteroliths is unknown.
- Prevention of recurrence focuses on dietary modifications. Recommendations include avoiding high-risk feeds such as alfalfa and wheat bran; preventing ingestion of material that may serve as a nidus, including sand and gravel; offering alternative water sources in areas with high mineral content in the water; and providing diets with a dietary cation-anion balance between 200 and 300 mEq/kg, such as grass hays and cereal grains.

Acidification with cider vinegar (1 cup twice daily) and administration of psyllium has also been recommended.

PROGNOSIS AND OUTCOME

- Prognosis is considered excellent if surgical removal is pursued and no pressure necrosis has occurred.
- Prognosis with pressure necrosis depends on the location of the enterolith (ie, if resection and anastomosis are possible).

PEARLS & CONSIDERATIONS

COMMENTS

- Enterolithiasis should be considered as a differential diagnosis in horses with signs of simple obstruction of the large or small colon in regions with a high prevalence of the disease.
- Surgical removal is the recommended treatment for obstruction associated with an enterolith.

PREVENTION

Changes in management as described in chronic treatment may also serve as methods of prevention.

CLIENT EDUCATION

Client education may be useful in prevention.

SUGGESTED READING

Cohen ND, Vontur C, Rakestraw PC: Risk factors for enterolithiasis among horses in Texas. *J Am Vet Med Assoc* 216:1787, 2000.

Hassel DM, Langer DL, Snyder JR, et al: Evaluation of enterolithiasis in equids: 900 cases (1973–1996). *J Am Vet Med Assoc* 214:233, 1999.

Johnston JK, Freeman DE: Diseases and surgery of the large colon. *Vet Clin North Am Equine Pract* 13(2):317, 1997.
Rakestraw PC, Hardy J: Large intestine. In Auer JA, Stick JA, editors: *Equine surgery*. St Louis, 2006, Saunders Elsevier, pp 436–478.

AUTHOR: **KIRA L. EPSTEIN**

EDITORS: **TIM MAIR** and **CERI SHERLOCK**

Epiglottic Entrapment

BASIC INFORMATION

DEFINITION

Epiglottic entrapment occurs when aryepiglottic tissue envelops the epiglottis.

EPIDEMIOLOGY

SPECIES, AGE, SEX Most common in young racehorses
GENETICS AND BREED PREDISPOSITION The disorder is most commonly identified in Thoroughbred and Standardbred racehorses. Between 0.7% and 2% of racehorses have epiglottic entrapment, and as many as 8% of horses with upper airway obstruction have the disorder.
RISK FACTORS
- Racing or in race training
- Hypoplastic epiglottis
- Upper airway inflammation
ASSOCIATED CONDITIONS AND DISORDERS Affected horses are more likely to have concurrent epiglottic hypoplasia. Epiglottic flaccidity and dorsal displacement of the soft palate may also be noted.

CLINICAL PRESENTATION

HISTORY, CHIEF COMPLAINT Most affected horses are exercise intolerant and make an abnormal upper respiratory noise during exercise. Occasionally, epiglottic entrapment is an incidental finding. Rarely dysphagia, cough, or nasal discharge are noted.
PHYSICAL EXAM FINDINGS Normal
ETIOLOGY AND PATHOPHYSIOLOGY
- The cause is unknown. Entrapment may be precipitated by inflammation of the redundant aryepiglottic tissue. Epiglottic hypoplasia may be a predisposing factor because as many as 30% of affected horses have some degree of epiglottic hypoplasia.
- Onset of hard work in racehorses has been incriminated.

DIAGNOSIS

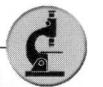

DIFFERENTIAL DIAGNOSIS

Dorsal displacement of the soft palate

INITIAL DATABASE

- The clinical pathology is normal.
- Examination of affected horse during exercise may elicit abnormal upper respiratory noise.

ADVANCED OR CONFIRMATORY TESTING

- Endoscopic evaluation of the upper airway confirms the diagnosis. The general shape of the epiglottis is visible; however, the normal serrated edge of the epiglottis and dorsal epiglottic vasculature are obscured by entrapping aryepiglottic tissue.
- Exercising endoscopic evaluation of the upper airway may be necessary for identification of intermittent or speed-induced disorder.
- Radiographic abnormalities of the larynx include excessive soft tissue density surrounding the epiglottis. Smaller thyroepiglottic length is common.

TREATMENT

THERAPEUTIC GOAL(S)

Relieve the entrapment by transecting or resecting the enveloping aryepiglottic tissue.

ACUTE GENERAL TREATMENT

- Surgical techniques for treatment include transendoscopic laser axial division, transnasal or transoral axial division using a curved bistoury, transendoscopic electrosurgical axial division, or excision through a laryngotomy or pharyngotomy.
- Phenylbutazone (4.4 mg/kg) and dexamethasone (0.04 mg/kg) should be given once before surgery.
- Topical antiinflammatory solution can be sprayed twice a day using a nasopharyngeal catheter after surgery.
- Stall confinement and handwalking are recommended for 7 days after surgical correction.

CHRONIC TREATMENT

Horses with excessively thickened, ulcerated, or fibrotic appearing entrapping aryepiglottic tissues may not be good candidates for axial division. Surgical excision of the affected tissue through a laryngotomy may be required.

POSSIBLE COMPLICATIONS

- The recurrence rate after surgical correction is 5% to 10%.
- Intermittent or permanent dorsal displacement of the soft palate occurs postoperatively in 5% to 15% of cases.
- Lacerations of the nasopharynx, soft palate, and epiglottis have occurred during transnasal axial transection of the entrapping membrane with a bistoury if the horse swallows or moves during the procedure.

RECOMMENDED MONITORING

- Endoscopic evaluation of the upper airway should be performed immediately after surgical correction and before resuming training.
- Endoscopic evaluation of the upper airway is recommended if clinical signs of exercise intolerance or abnormal upper respiratory noise recur.

PROGNOSIS AND OUTCOME

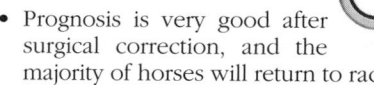

- Prognosis is very good after surgical correction, and the majority of horses will return to racing.
- Horses with concurrent epiglottic hypoplasia or dorsal displacement of the soft palate are less likely to race after surgery.
- Horses with severely ulcerated aryepiglottic tissue requiring resection through a laryngotomy have the worst prognosis.

PEARLS & CONSIDERATIONS

COMMENTS

Epiglottic entrapment is a common cause of poor performance and abnormal respiratory noise in horses. It is readily diagnosed during endoscopic evaluation of the upper airway. Most affected horses require surgical correction.

CLIENT EDUCATION

After identification during upper airway endoscopy, surgical correction is recommended, and the majority of horses will maintain or improve performance after surgery.

SUGGESTED READING

Holcombe SJ, Ducharme NG: Epiglottic entrapment. In Hinchcliff KW, Kaneps AJ, Geor RJ, editors: *Abnormalities of the upper airway.* Philadelphia, 2004, Saunders Elsevier, pp 573–575.

Ross MW, Gentile DG, Evans LE: Transoral axial division, under endoscopic guidance, for correction of epiglottic entrapment in horses. *J Am Vet Med Assoc* 203:416–420, 1993.

Tulleners EP: Transendoscopic contact neodymium:yttrium aluminium garnet laser correction of epiglottic entrapment in standing horses. *J Am Vet Med Assoc* 196: 1971–1980, 1990.

AUTHOR: **ELIZABETH J. DAVIDSON**

EDITOR: **ERIC J. PARENTE**

Equine Protozoal Myeloencephalitis

BASIC INFORMATION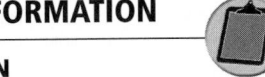

DEFINITION

A central nervous system (CNS) disorder resulting from infection with a protozoan parasite, either *Sarcocystis neurona* or *Neospora hughesi*

SYNONYMS

EPM, protozoal myelitis, protozoal encephalomyelitis

EPIDEMIOLOGY

SPECIES, AGE, SEX Foals <6 months old and adults >12 years appear to be more often affected.

RISK FACTORS

- Many horses are exposed to the causative organism for EPM, but very few become infected, and most horses exposed to *S. neurona* ultimately control or eliminate the parasite.
- Exposure to the definitive host, the opossum (*Didelphis virginiana*) is important, although the exact mechanism for how the organism enters the CNS as well as what factors related to the role of the equine immune system are not fully understood.
- The high levels of serum antibody in many horses showing signs of clinical disease suggest that antibody is not sufficient to prevent disease. Other risk factors include season of the year (fall more than spring, and summer more than winter), and the presence of opossums on the premises along with previous diagnosis of EPM on the premises.
- Stress from sales, transportation, and concurrent disease are other risk factors.

CONTAGION AND ZOONOSIS

- Infections take place in incidental hosts as a result of exposure to the causative organism from the definitive host. The definitive host becomes infected by ingestion of sarcocysts contained within the muscle tissues of intermediate hosts, including rac-coons, armadillos, cats, skunks, and sea otters. The intermediate host may exhibit clinical neurologic symptoms from infection with *S. neurona*.
- The disease is not contagious from horse to horse, and horses are considered an aberrant host because sarcocysts are not formed in this species, failing to complete the life cycle.

GEOGRAPHY AND SEASONALITY The disease is observed most often during the warmer months of the year, likely as a result of travel and exposure to the organism. States that do not have opossums have many fewer horses infected with this organism. For example, in a study conducted on serum collected from wild horses in a state outside the range of wild opossums, there was a seroprevalence rate of only 6.5% using immunoblot assay.

ASSOCIATED CONDITIONS AND DISORDERS Horses that develop EPM are often under some sort of stress, either as a result of concurrent disease or immunosuppression secondary to transportation.

CLINICAL PRESENTATION

DISEASE FORMS/SUBTYPES

- Most EPM cases are sporadic cases with an insidious onset and often progressive signs of disease, although subclinical EPM is often suspected in horses that are not performing well or up to the expected level of training.
- Clinical signs in many horses may vary from mild to severe ataxia with muscle atrophy. Cranial nerve deficits may occur.

HISTORY, CHIEF COMPLAINT

- Ataxia (often asymmetrical)
- Cranial nerve deficits (dysphagia, head tilt, circling)
- Depression
- Paresis
- Recumbency
- Seizures (occasional)
- Muscle atrophy
- Nonspecific hindlimb lameness

- Most cases are insidious, although the disease may sometimes be rapidly progressive.

PHYSICAL EXAM FINDINGS

- Ataxia or paresis (often asymmetrical)
- Behavioral changes
- Cranial nerve deficits: Blindness, circling, dysphagia, head tilt
- Possible muscle atrophy

ETIOLOGY AND PATHOPHYSIOLOGY

- Clinical signs may result from direct damage to neural tissue or from resultant inflammatory response as a result of infection with either *S. neurona* or less commonly *N. hughesi.*
- The organism is sometimes found in the CNS of the horse in the asexual forms of schizonts or merozoites. Sarcocysts have never been identified in horse tissues after either natural or experimental infection.
- Infection of horses is via the oral route, and organisms can sometimes be found in the nervous tissues. In most cases, no organisms are identified, although histopathologic lesions may be detected.

DIAGNOSIS

DIFFERENTIAL DIAGNOSIS

- Cervical vertebral malformation
- Equine degenerative myelopathy
- Equine herpesvirus-1 myelopathy
- Cerebrospinal nematodiasis
- Leukoencephalomalacia
- Meningitis
- Neoplasia
- Temporohyoid osteoarthropathy
- Trauma
- Viral encephalidities (Eastern equine myeloencephalitis, Western equine myeloencephalitis, Venezuelan equine myeloencephalitis, rabies, West Nile virus)

INITIAL DATABASE

- Complete blood count
- Serum chemistries
- Neurologic examination

- Cerebrospinal fluid (CSF) analysis
- Testing for IgG antibodies in serum, CSF, or both
  - Western blot
  - Modified Western blot
  - Indirect fluorescent antibody test
  - Enzyme-linked immunosorbent assay (ELISA) based on SAG-2 or a blend of SAG-4/3 antigens
  - ELISA based on SAG-1 antigen

ADVANCED OR CONFIRMATORY TESTING

- Radiography of the skull, cervical spine, or both to rule out other disorders
- CSF analysis and cytology to rule out other disorders and to test for EPM
- Magnetic resonance imaging: Lesions detected in a few cases of suspected EPM have been confirmed post-mortem.
- Postmortem examination, histopathology, and microscopic identification of protozoal organisms are most useful for a definitive diagnosis.

TREATMENT

THERAPEUTIC GOAL(S)

- Kill protozoal parasites.
- Control and reduce CNS inflammation.
- Provide supportive care until the horse's neurologic function improves.

ACUTE GENERAL TREATMENT

- Ponazuril: 5 mg/kg PO q24h for 28 to 60 days
- Diclazuril: 1 mg/kg PO q24h for 28 days (pending Food and Drug Administration approval)
- Pyrimethamine (1 mg/kg) and sulfadiazine (20 mg/kg) PO q24h for 60 to 90 days

- Flunixin meglumine: 1.1 mg/kg IV q12–24h
- Dimethyl sulfoxide (0.5–1.0 g/kg IV q12–24h) must be diluted to a 10% solution or less in an isotonic balanced electrolyte solution
- IV fluids in recumbent, dehydrated, or dysphagic horses

CHRONIC TREATMENT

- Ponazuril, diclazuril, or pyrimethamine and sulfadiazine PO for longer periods.
- Horses that are unable to stand or get up on their own need to be placed into a sling periodically.

RECOMMENDED MONITORING

Periodic repeat neurologic examinations to assess response to therapy

PROGNOSIS AND OUTCOME

- The overall prognosis for complete recovery is guarded to good.
- Horses that are recumbent or unable to stand or support themselves in a sling for longer than 2 to 3 days are unlikely to recover.
- Horses that survive may have permanent neurologic deficits.

PEARLS & CONSIDERATIONS

COMMENTS

EPM remains an important cause of neurologic disease in horses, and diagnosis depends on careful and often repeated neurologic examinations along with evaluation of antibodies in the blood and CSF as well as response to treatment.

PREVENTION

- To date, no effective course of medication for prevention has been established.
- However, good and proper hygiene with regard feed storage along with elimination of dead carrion from the environment as well as avoidance of opossum exposure to feed and water areas used for horses are helpful.

SUGGESTED READING

Dubey JP, Davis SW, Speer CA, et al: *Sarcocystis neurona* n. sp (Protozoa: Apicomplexa), the etiologic agent of equine protozoal myeloencephalitis. *J Parasitol* 77(2):212–218, 1991.

Marsh AE, Barr BC, Lakritz J, et al: Experimental infection of nude mice as a model for *Sarcocystis neurona*-associated encephalitis. *Parasitol Res* 83:706–711, 1997.

Marsh AE, Barr BC, Madigan J, et al: Neosporosis as a cause of equine protozoal myeloencephalitis. *J Am Vet Med Assoc* 209(11):1907–1913, 1996.

Saville WJA, Reed SM, Morley PS, et al: Analysis of risk factors for the development of EPM in horses. *J Am Vet Med Assoc* 217(8):1174–1178, 2000.

Sofaly CD, Reed SM, Gordon JC, et al: Experimental induction of equine protozoal myeloencephalitis (EPM) in the horse: effect of *Sarcocystis neurona* dose on the development of clinical neurologic disease. *J Parasitol* 88:1164–1170, 2002.

AUTHOR & EDITOR: **STEPHEN M. REED**

Ergot-Related Toxicosis

BASIC INFORMATION

DEFINITION

Claviceps fungi ("ergot") produce a variety of toxins that can adversely affect the reproductive, circulatory, nervous, and musculoskeletal systems of horses. *Claviceps* fungi are visible as sclerotia or ergot bodies on susceptible grasses (Table 1) and small cereal grains such as wheat, barley, and oats (but not corn).

SYNONYMS

- Ergot, ergot poisoning, or ergotism
- Indole alkaloid mycotoxins

  - Ergot alkaloids (eg, ergocornine, ergocristine, ergocryptine, ergosine, ergotamine, ergovaline) and compounds related to lysergic acid (LSD) produced by *C. purpurea*
  - Indole-diterpene tremorgenic mycotoxins (ie, paspalinine; paspalitrems A, B, C) produced by *Claviceps paspali* and other species producing tremorgens

EPIDEMIOLOGY

SPECIES, AGE, SEX

- Except for agalactia and pregnancy abnormalities, horses are much less susceptible to ergotism than are cattle.

- The species and age of exposed horses may influence the amount of toxin ingested.
- Aged animals, especially mares, may have concurrent disease that is exacerbated by toxin exposure.
- Age influences the likelihood of mares cycling or becoming pregnant.
- Mares are particularly susceptible to the reproductive effects of ergopeptine alkaloids.

GENETICS AND BREED PREDISPOSITION

- Anecdotal reports suggest that individual animal differences in susceptibility exist.

TABLE 1 Common Grasses Susceptible to *Claviceps* Infection

Common Name of Susceptible Grasses	Latin Name of Susceptible Grasses	Claviceps spp.	Claviceps Toxins
Bahiagrass	*Paspalum notatum*	*Claviceps paspali*	Indole-diterpene alkaloids[a]
Bluegrasses	*Poa* spp.	*Claviceps purpurea*	Ergot alkaloids[b,c]
Bromegrasses	*Bromus* spp.	*C. purpurea*	Ergot alkaloids[b,c]
Canarygrasses	*Phalaris* spp.	*C. purpurea*	Ergot alkaloids[b,c]
Curlygrass[d]	*Hilaria jamesii*	*Claviceps cinerea*	Indole-diterpene alkaloids[a]
Dallisgrass	*Paspalum dilatatum*	*C. paspali*	Indole-diterpene alkaloids[a]
Fescue grasses	*Festuca* spp.	*C. purpurea*	Ergot alkaloids[b,c]
Junegrasses	*Koeleria* spp.	*C. purpurea*	Ergot alkaloids[b,c]
Lovegrasses	*Eragrostis* spp	*C. purpurea*	Ergot alkaloids[b,c]
Orchard grasses	*Dactylis* spp.	*C. purpurea*	Ergot alkaloids[b,c]
Pearl millet	*Pennisetum glaucum*	*C. fusiformis*	Ergot alkaloids[e]
Quack grasses	*Agropyron* spp.	*C. purpurea*	Ergot alkaloids[b,c]
Redtops	*Agrostis* spp.	*C. purpurea*	Ergot alkaloids[b,c]
Ryegrasses	*Lolium* spp.	*C. purpurea*	Ergot alkaloids[b,c]
Timothy grasses	*Phleum* spp.	*C. purpurea*	Ergot alkaloids[b,c]
Wild barleys	*Hordeum* spp.	*C. purpurea*	Ergot alkaloids[b,c]
Wild oats	*Avena* spp.	*C. purpurea*	Ergot alkaloids[b,c]
Wild ryes	*Elymus* spp.	*C. purpurea*	Ergot alkaloids[b,c]

[a]Especially the tremorgenic mycotoxins; paspalinine; and penitrems A, B, and C.
[b]Especially the ergopeptides, ergocornine, ergocristine, ergocryptine, ergosine, ergotamine, and ergovaline.
[c]LSD-related ergot alkaloids are also produced by *C. purpurea* and related species.
[d]Other *Hilaria* spp. can also be infected by *C. cinerea*.
[e]Somewhat different clinical signs in human outbreak; uncertain of specific ergot alkaloids.

- Possible differences in breed disposition might reflect influences of risk factors and geography.

RISK FACTORS

- Claviceps ergopeptine alkaloids:
  - Subacute to chronic consumption of the seed head stage of susceptible grasses or ergotized small grains or grass seed
  - Concurrent exposure to endophyte-infected tall fescue (see "Fescue-Related Toxicosis" in this section)
  - Early and particularly late gestation in mares
  - Mares in the spring transitional phase before the onset of normal cyclicity
  - "No till" farming practices
  - Cool, damp spring weather
  - Rye and triticale in horse rations
  - Pelletized rations, especially those incorporating screenings
  - History of laminitis
  - Hot or cold environmental temperatures
  - Forced exercise under hot and humid conditions
- *Claviceps* indole-diterpene tremorgenic mycotoxins
  - Several days' consumption of ergotized Dallisgrass (*Paspalum dilatatum*) or Bahiagrass (*Paspalum notatum*) in pasture or hay
  - Damp or wet disturbed soils favoring growth of *C. paspali* and related species
  - Concurrent exposure to endophyte (*Neotyphodium lolii*)-infected perennial ryegrass (*Lolium perenne*) hay or pasture or other tremorgenic mycotoxins
  - Forced exercise

CONTAGION AND ZOONOSIS Between grasses but not between animals and/or humans

GEOGRAPHY AND SEASONALITY

- *Claviceps* ergopeptine alkaloids
  - Seen worldwide, but predisposing weather conditions are common in the northern Great Plains and Pacific Northwest regions of North America (more sporadically in Midwestern and Atlantic coastal regions of the United States)
  - Cool, wet weather in the spring favors the *C. purpurea* life cycle
  - Reproductive ergotism is most common in spring when mares are being bred and are foaling.
  - Hyperthermic ergotism is most common during hot and humid summers.
  - Gangrenous ergotism is most common during extremely cold winters.
- *Claviceps* indole-diterpene tremorgenic mycotoxins
  - Southeastern United States, Central and South America, parts of Europe, Africa, Australia, and New Zealand
  - Clinical signs of nervous ergotism or "grass staggers" are most common when rainy or humid summers and autumns favor the *C. paspali* life cycle

ASSOCIATED CONDITIONS AND DISORDERS

- *Claviceps* ergopeptine alkaloids: Fescue toxicosis
- *Claviceps* indole–diterpene tremorgenic mycotoxins
  - Other "grass staggers" syndromes
  - Other tremorgenic mycotoxins

CLINICAL PRESENTATION

DISEASE FORMS/SUBTYPES

- *C. purpurea* ergopeptine alkaloids
  - Reproductive ergotism: Most common form in horses; observed at low dosages of toxins
  - Hyperthermic ergotism: Less common in horses; observed at higher toxin doses than reproductive ergotism
  - Gangrenous or cutaneous ergotism: Less common in horses; observed at higher toxin doses than reproductive ergotism
- *C. purpurea* LSD-like ergot alkaloids, especially *C. paspali* indole-diterpene tremorgenic mycotoxins: Nervous or convulsive ergotism

HISTORY, CHIEF COMPLAINT

- Generally, multiple animals are affected in instances of ergotism.
- Reproductive ergotism (indistinguishable from most common form of equine fescue toxicosis)
  - Agalactia or dysgalactia (may be observed in absence of any other clinical signs)
  - Prolonged gestation
  - Retained fetal membranes
  - Dystocia, premature placental separation (ie, "red bag")
  - Fetal dysmaturity/overmaturity
  - Abortion/stillbirth
  - Prolonged transitional phase before the first ovulation or abnormal cyclicity in the spring
  - Conception failure or early embryonic loss
- Hyperthermic ergotism
  - Heat intolerance
  - Increased sweating
  - Decreased feed intake and growth
  - Impaired athletic performance
  - Mortality
- Gangrenous or cutaneous ergotism
  - Lameness or possible laminitis characterized by ischemic necrosis of the hooves, as well as associated bones, joints, and soft tissues
  - Dry gangrene of the tips of the ears and tail
  - Mortality
- Nervous or convulsive ergotism
  - Confusion and ataxia with LSD-like ergot alkaloids
  - Exercise-exacerbated ataxia, tremors, convulsions, and occasional

deaths caused by misadventure associated with indole-diterpene tremorgens

PHYSICAL EXAM FINDINGS

- Reproductive ergotism
  - Little or no udder development within 14 days of the due date; this may be the only clinical sign seen
  - Aborted fetus or stillbirth
  - Dystocia with an abnormally large or malpositioned foal
  - Premature separation of the chorio-allantois ("red bag" presentation)
  - Thickened, edematous fetal membranes, possibly retained
  - Dysmature or overmature foal unable to suckle
  - Failure of passive transfer
  - Multiple, anovulatory follicles; failure to ovulate in a timely fashion
- Hyperthermic ergotism
  - Elevated body temperature and respiratory rate
  - Increased sweating
  - Mortality
- Gangrenous or cutaneous ergotism
  - Multiple limb lameness and possible laminitis, often beginning with swelling or reddening at the coronary band
  - Shifting leg lameness
  - Inflammation and ischemic necrosis in distal limbs, with possible secondary bacterial infections
  - Dry gangrene of the tips of the ears and tail
  - Mortality, generally because of complications
- Nervous or convulsive ergotism
  - Altered mentation and ataxic gait with *Claviceps* LSD-related ergot alkaloids
  - Nervousness or a belligerent attitude, as well as exercise-exacerbated tremors, ataxia, or convulsions associated with *Claviceps* indole-diterpene tremorgens
  - Mortality, generally through misadventure or trauma secondary to central nervous system effects

ETIOLOGY AND PATHOPHYSIOLOGY

- Reproductive ergotism caused by *C. purpurea* ergopeptine alkaloids: D2 dopamine receptor agonism-induced hypoprolactinemia (decreased prolactin secretion by the anterior pituitary) and altered uterofetoplacental progestagen metabolism
- Hyperthermic and gangrenous ergotism: Vasoconstriction caused by D1 dopaminergic receptor inhibition and partial adrenergic and serotoninergic receptor agonism
- *C. purpurea* LSD-related ergot alkaloids: Neurotransmitter imbalance in the pituitary and pineal glands
- *C. paspali* indole-diterpene tremorgenic mycotoxins: Impairment of

γ-aminobutyric acid and glycine-mediated inhibitory pathways

DIAGNOSIS

DIFFERENTIAL DIAGNOSIS

- Reproductive ergotism: Fescue toxicosis (horses are very sensitive to agalactia and pregnancy abnormalities)
- Hyperthermic ergotism
  - Fescue toxicosis (horses require higher dosages of toxins than cattle)
  - Noninfectious respiratory disease
  - Viral or bacterial respiratory diseases
  - Other potential causes of impaired athletic performance
- Gangrenous or cutaneous ergotism
  - Fescue toxicosis (potential association with laminitis)
  - Other causes of laminitis, cellulitis, or vasculitis
  - Thromboembolic events
  - Strangulating trauma to the distal limbs
  - Frostbite
- Nervous or convulsive ergotism
  - Other "staggers" or "grass staggers" syndromes (eg, Bermuda grass staggers, perennial rye grass staggers, stagger syndromes associated with the consumption of Tares [*Lolium temulentum*]
  - Other tremorgenic mycotoxins (eg, penitrem A, verruculogen) in contaminated feedstuffs
  - Plants associated with gait abnormalities and ataxia (sorghum ataxia, locoism, lathyrism)
  - Plants associated with tremorgenic or convulsive syndromes: Water hemlock, blue-green algae, poison hemlock, tobacco
  - Equine protozoal myelopathy
  - Equine herpes viral infections
  - Viral encephalitides
  - Pesticide exposures
  - Cervical vertebral instability ("wobblers" syndrome)
  - Trauma

INITIAL DATABASE

- *Claviceps* ergopeptine alkaloids
  - Agalactia or dysgalactia; failure to "wax"; no increase in calcium in mammary secretions before foaling; little or no milk production
  - Failure of passive transfer
  - Hemograms and biochemical profiles: Vary depending on the complicating secondary conditions
  - Sensitivity to hoof testers over tip of the coffin bone, frequently in more than one foot, indicative of laminitis
  - Radiographic evidence of rotation of the coffin bone, osteomyelitis, or other bony changes

- *Claviceps* LSD-related ergot alkaloids and *Claviceps* indole-diterpene tremorgenic mycotoxins: Changes in hemograms and routine biochemical profiles reflect secondary physiological abnormalities.

ADVANCED OR CONFIRMATORY TESTING

- Endocrine analyses
  - Hypoprolactinemia, especially in late-gestational mares
  - Decreased maternal progestagen concentrations in late-gestational mares (use cross-reactive progesterone radioimmunoassay to detect 5α-pregnanes)
  - Decreased maternal relaxin; variable alterations in circulating maternal estrogens in late-gestational mares
- Detection of *Claviceps* indole alkaloid mycotoxins in feedstuffs
- Pathologic findings for reproductive ergotism
  - Gross findings in foals are consistent with prolonged gestation (over-sized foal, eruption of the foal's incisors, increased eponychium on the foal's hooves, angular limb deformities), dystocia (limb trauma, meconium staining, possible ruptured bladder), agalactia, or failure of passive transfer (absence of colostrum or milk in the gastrointestinal tract, joint or umbilical cord infections).
  - Histopathologic findings in foals that are characteristic of ergopeptine alkaloid exposure, such as distended thyroid follicles lined by flat cuboidal epithelial cells, may be observed.
  - Nonspecific histopathologic findings in foals consistent with prolonged gestation
  - Fetal membranes grossly thickened, edematous, and possibly retained or prematurely separated
  - Gross findings in mares consistent with agalactia, dystocia (trauma to the reproductive and urinary tracts, retained fetal membranes, possible laminitis)
  - Histopathologic findings in mares consistent with sepsis and laminitis

TREATMENT

THERAPEUTIC GOAL(S)

- *Claviceps* ergopeptine alkaloids
  - Prevent further exposure to contaminated feedstuffs.
  - Counteract the mechanisms of action of ergopeptine alkaloids.
  - Provide supportive care and prevent complications.

- *Claviceps* LSD-related ergot alkaloids and *C. paspali* diterpene tremorgenic mycotoxins
  - Prevent further exposure to contaminated feedstuffs.
  - Decrease absorption of tremorgenic mycotoxins.
  - Control tremors and convulsions.
  - Provide supportive care and prevent complications.
  - Prevent death from misadventure.

ACUTE GENERAL TREATMENT

- Removal from source of toxins
- For agalactia, prolonged gestation, and cycling abnormalities: Antidotal treatment with domperidone, a D2 dopamine receptor antagonist (Equidone; Equi-tox, Inc., Central, SC), at 1.1 mg/kg PO q24h
- Need to adjust dosage or frequency of administration of domperidone if dripping of milk or leaking of colostrum occurs
- Potential extrapyramidal neurologic side effects with other D2 dopamine antagonists, such as fluphenazine and perphenazine
- Administration of activated charcoal in cases of LSD-related ergot alkaloids and tremorgens
- Supportive care for inflammation, infections, wounds, or pain caused by ergopeptine alkaloids
- Supportive care for tremors and convulsions caused by LSD-related ergot alkaloids or indole-diterpene tremorgenic mycotoxins

CHRONIC TREATMENT

Varies depending on the possible complications described below

POSSIBLE COMPLICATIONS

- Reproductive ergotism
  - In mares, trauma or rupture of the reproductive tract or its vasculature; bladder or bowel displacement; subsequent laminitis
  - Sepsis in mares or foals
  - Ruptured urinary bladder in foals secondary to dystocia
- Gangrenous ergotism: Chronic laminitis, lameness, and infections of bones and soft tissues
- Hyperthermic ergotism: Heat stroke; chronically impaired athletic performance
- Nervous ergotism: Trauma

RECOMMENDED MONITORING

- Depends on the observed clinical signs and complications
- Monitor udder development in pregnant mares; attend and assist with foaling.

PROGNOSIS AND OUTCOME

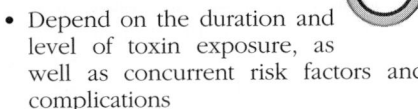

- Depend on the duration and level of toxin exposure, as well as concurrent risk factors and complications
- Possible mortality

PEARLS & CONSIDERATIONS

COMMENTS

Agalactia is the most sensitive indicator of ergopeptine alkaloid exposure in horses. Signs of hyperthermic or gangrenous ergotism are rarely seen in horses.

PREVENTION

- Mow pastures to prevent seed head stage of ergotized grasses.
- Ensure there are no grain or grass seed screenings in rations.
- Maintain careful breeding records and confirm pregnancy in regions where ergopeptine alkaloid exposure is common.
- Carefully inspect animals, especially udder development in late-gestational mares.
- Provide daily oral treatment with domperidone 10 to 14 days before the foaling due date.
- Attend and assist with foaling

CLIENT EDUCATION

Increased awareness of risk to horses from exposure to ergot-related toxins

SUGGESTED READING

Evans TJ, Gupta, RC: Tremorgenic mycotoxins. In Gupta RC, editor: *Veterinary toxicology: basic and applied principles.* New York, 2007, Academic Press Elsevier, pp 1004–1010.

Evans TJ, Rottinghaus GE, Casteel SW: Ergot. In Plumlee K, editor: *Clinical veterinary toxicology.* St Louis, 2004, Mosby Elsevier, pp 239–243.

Nicholson SS: Ergot. In Gupta RC, editor: *Veterinary toxicology: basic and applied principles.* New York, 2007, Academic Press Elsevier, pp 1015–1018.

AUTHOR: **TIM J. EVANS**

EDITOR: **CYNTHIA GASKILL**

Esophageal Cysts, Intramural

BASIC INFORMATION

DEFINITION

Inclusion cysts of the esophageal wall. Inclusion cysts are defined as a cyst formed by the implantation of epithelial tissue into another structure.

SYNONYM(S)

Intramural inclusion cysts

EPIDEMIOLOGY

SPECIES, AGE, SEX Foals and young adult horses

CLINICAL PRESENTATION

HISTORY, CHIEF COMPLAINT
- Clinical signs of esophageal obstruction, including hypersalivation and esophageal dysphagia
- Regurgitation
- Progressive swelling of the cervical esophagus as the cysts enlarge

PHYSICAL EXAM FINDINGS
- The findings of physical examination confirm the presenting signs, including dysphagia, hypersalivation, and retching.
- A visible or palpable soft tissue swelling of the cervical esophagus may be present.

ETIOLOGY AND PATHOPHYSIOLOGY Congenital inclusion cyst

DIAGNOSIS

DIFFERENTIAL DIAGNOSIS

- Other causes of dysphagia (especially abnormalities of the pharyngeal and esophageal phases of deglutition): Pharyngeal paralysis, pharyngeal cysts, pharyngeal compression by strangles abscesses and guttural pouch empyema, subepiglottic cyst, fourth branchial arch defect, esophageal obstruction, megaesophagus, esophageal stricture, esophageal rupture, equine grass sickness
- Other cysts involving the esophagus: Esophageal duplication cysts

INITIAL DATABASE

- The leukogram and hematology are likely to be normal.
- Confirmation of the intramural inclusion cyst is achieved by endoscopic examination (esophagoscopy reveals focal compression of the esophageal lumen) and radiography (positive or double-contrast esophagraphy). A filling defect is present on radiography.
- Ultrasonography demonstrates a soft tissue cystic structure in the esophageal wall.

TREATMENT

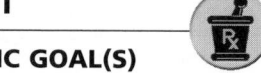

THERAPEUTIC GOAL(S)

Surgical excision of the cysts

ACUTE GENERAL TREATMENT

- Surgical removal of the cyst in its entirety is required. The cyst can be dissected from the esophageal wall after esophagomyotomy.

- Alternatively, the cyst can be marsupialized to the skin. (This procedure reduces the risk of inadvertently entering the esophageal lumen.)

CHRONIC TREATMENT

Frequent small meals of moistened pellets or fresh grass should be fed.

POSSIBLE COMPLICATIONS

- Complications of surgery include inadvertent esophagotomy and esophageal fistula formation.
- Other complications of surgical excision have included surgical trauma to the recurrent laryngeal nerve (resulting in laryngeal hemiplegia).

PROGNOSIS AND OUTCOME

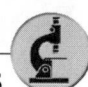

The prognosis appears to be fair to good with surgery.

PEARLS & CONSIDERATIONS

Persistent or recurrent signs of esophageal obstruction in a young horse should alert the clinician to the possibility of an intramural esophageal cyst.

SUGGESTED READING

Fubini SL: Esophageal diseases. In Mair T, Divers T, Ducharme N, editors: *Manual of equine gastroenterology.* London, 2002, Saunders Elsevier, pp 89–98.

Greet TR: Observations on the potential role of oesophageal radiography in the horse. *Equine Vet J* 14:73, 1982.

Sams AE, Weldon AD, Rakestraw P: Surgical treatment of intramural esophageal inclusion cysts in three horses. *Vet Surg* 22:135, 1993.

Sanchez LC: Esophageal diseases. In Reed SM, Bayly WM, Sellon DC, editors: *Equine internal medicine,* ed 3. St Louis, 2010, Saunders Elsevier, pp 830–838.

Scott ER, Snoy P, Prasse KW, et al: Intramural esophageal cyst in a horse. *J Am Vet Med Assoc* 171:652, 1977.

AUTHOR & EDITOR: TIM MAIR

Esophageal Diverticulum

BASIC INFORMATION

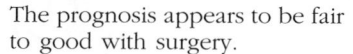

DEFINITION

Outpouching of the lumen of the esophagus

EPIDEMIOLOGY

RISK FACTORS

- Esophageal obstruction
- Trauma

ASSOCIATED CONDITIONS AND DISORDERS Esophageal diverticula may occur after esophageal obstruction, especially chronic obstruction, or trauma to the neck.

CLINICAL PRESENTATION

HISTORY, CHIEF COMPLAINT Some esophageal diverticula may be asymptomatic. Others can become impacted with food material and cause esophageal obstruction.

PHYSICAL EXAM FINDINGS The findings of physical examination are identical to those of esophageal obstruction. A moveable mass in the mid to distal cervical region may be noticeable before the onset of complete obstruction. The mass

may enlarge and reduce repeatedly over a long period of time.

ETIOLOGY AND PATHOPHYSIOLOGY

- There are two types of esophageal diverticula:
  - Traction or true diverticulum resulting from periesophageal fibrous scar tissue often secondary to a wound or previous surgery. This results in tenting of the wall of the esophagus. This condition is usually asymptomatic and appears as a wide neck on barium swallow esophagraphy.
  - Pulsion or false diverticulum, resulting from protrusion of mucosa and submucosa through a defect in the esophageal musculature. These diverticuli may be caused by external trauma or by some fluctuation in esophageal intraluminal pressure and overstretch damage to the esophageal muscle fibers by impacted feed stuff. A pulsion diverticulum appears spherical and flasklike on an esophagram. They may enlarge over time and may become impacted with food material.

DIAGNOSIS

DIFFERENTIAL DIAGNOSIS

- Other causes of dysphagia (especially abnormalities of the pharyngeal and esophageal phases of deglutition), including pharyngeal paralysis, pharyngeal cysts, pharyngeal compression by strangles abscesses and guttural pouch empyema, subepiglottic cyst, fourth branchial arch defect, esophageal obstruction, megaesophagus, esophagitis, intramural esophageal cysts, esophageal rupture, and equine grass sickness.
- Repeated bouts of esophageal obstruction should increase the suspicion of an underlying esophageal stricture or esophageal diverticulum.

INITIAL DATABASE

- The leukogram and hematology results are likely to be normal unless there is dehydration from chronic esophageal obstruction.
- The presence of a focal, firm, and moveable swelling over the esophagus is suspicious of a pulsion diverticulum.
- Confirmation of esophageal diverticulum can be made in some cases by

endoscopic examination (esophagoscopy).

ADVANCED OR CONFIRMATORY TESTING

Radiography, including contrast radiography or double-contrast radiography, may be necessary to identify an esophageal diverticulum. A traction diverticulum appears as a wide neck on a barium swallow esophagram. A pulsion diverticulum appears spherical and flasklike on an esophagram.

TREATMENT

THERAPEUTIC GOAL(S)

- Horses with traction diverticula rarely require any specific treatment.
- Horses with pulsion diverticula may require surgical closure.

ACUTE GENERAL TREATMENT

Acute treatment is required only in horses that develop complete esophageal obstruction (see treatment under "Esophageal Obstruction" in this section).

CHRONIC TREATMENT

- Pulsion diverticula may be corrected surgically by inverting or resecting

the prolapsed mucosa and closing the underlying defect in the esophageal wall.
- Diverticulectomy is the treatment of choice for a large pulsion diverticulum that has a narrow communication with the esophageal lumen or for a diverticulum that is inflamed and necrotic.

POSSIBLE COMPLICATIONS

Complications of esophageal surgery include esophageal impaction, stricture, and postsurgical dehiscence.

RECOMMENDED MONITORING

After surgical treatment, horses should be monitored for signs of infection or surgical dehiscence.

PROGNOSIS AND OUTCOME

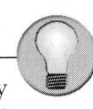

- The prognosis for horses with traction diverticuli is generally good, and they rarely require specific treatment.
- The prognosis for a pulsion diverticulum depends on its size.
- After surgical treatment, the prognosis is generally fair to good.

PEARLS & CONSIDERATIONS

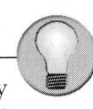

- Traction diverticuli are usually asymptomatic and do not require treatment.
- Pulsion diverticuli are usually amenable to surgical treatment.

SUGGESTED READING

Craig DR, Shivy DR, Pankowski RL, et al: Esophageal disorders in 61 horses: results of nonsurgical and surgical management. *Vet Surg* 18:432, 1989.

Frauenfelder HC, Adams SB: Esophageal diverticulectomy in a horse. *J Am Vet Med Assoc* 180:771, 1982.

Freeman DE: Esophageal surgery. In Robinson NE, Sprayberry KA, editors: *Current therapy in equine medicine*, ed 6. St Louis, 2009, Saunders Elsevier, pp 358–360.

Sanchez LC: Esophageal diseases. In Reed SM, Bayly WM, Sellon DC, editors: *Equine internal medicine*, ed 3. St Louis, 2010, Saunders Elsevier, pp 830–838.

Stick JH: Surgery of the equine esophagus. *Vet Clin North Am Large Anim Pract* 4:33, 1982.

AUTHOR: TIM MAIR

EDITORS: TIM MAIR and CERI SHERLOCK

Esophageal Duplication Cyst

BASIC INFORMATION

DEFINITION

A congenital cystic formation attached to or originating from the esophagus that has the same structure as the esophagus

EPIDEMIOLOGY

SPECIES, AGE, SEX Foals and young adult horses

CLINICAL PRESENTATION

HISTORY, CHIEF COMPLAINT

- Clinical signs of esophageal obstruction, including hypersalivation, esophageal dysphagia, and regurgitation.
- There is progressive swelling of the cervical esophagus as the cysts enlarge.

PHYSICAL EXAM FINDINGS

- The findings of physical examination confirm the presenting signs, including dysphagia, hypersalivation, and retching. A visible or palpable soft tissue swelling of the cervical esophagus may be present.

ETIOLOGY AND PATHOPHYSIOLOGY Congenital malformation

DIAGNOSIS

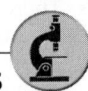

DIFFERENTIAL DIAGNOSIS

- Other causes of dysphagia (especially abnormalities of the pharyngeal and esophageal phases of deglutition), including pharyngeal paralysis, pharyngeal cysts, pharyngeal compression by strangles abscesses and guttural pouch empyema, subepiglottic cyst, fourth branchial arch defect, esophageal obstruction, megaesophagus, esophageal stricture, esophageal rupture, and equine grass sickness
- Other cysts involving the esophagus, including intramural esophageal cysts

INITIAL DATABASE

- The leukogram and hematology results are likely to be normal.
- Confirmation of the esophageal duplication cyst is achieved by endoscopic examination (esophagoscopy) and radiography (positive or double-contrast esophagraphy). On endoscopic examination, compression of the esophageal lumen may be identi-

fied; in some cases, a communication to the cyst may be demonstrated. A filling defect is present on radiography.
- Ultrasonography shows the presence of a soft tissue cystic lesion adjacent to the esophageal wall.

TREATMENT

THERAPEUTIC GOAL(S)

Surgical excision of the cyst

ACUTE GENERAL TREATMENT

- Surgical removal of the cyst in its entirety is required. The cyst can be dissected from the esophageal wall after esophagomyotomy.
- Alternatively, the cyst can be marsupialized to the skin. This procedure reduces the risk of inadvertently entering the esophageal lumen.

CHRONIC TREATMENT

Frequent small meals of moistened pellets or fresh grass should be fed.

POSSIBLE COMPLICATIONS

- Complications of surgery include inadvertent esophagotomy and esophageal fistula formation.
- Surgical damage to the recurrent laryngeal nerve or sympathetic trunk may result in laryngeal hemiplegia and Horner's syndrome, respectively.

PROGNOSIS AND OUTCOME

Prognosis appears to be fair to good with surgery.

PEARLS & CONSIDERATIONS

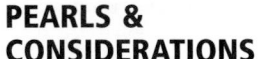

Persistent or recurrent signs of esophageal obstruction in a young horse should alert the clinician to the possibility of an esophageal duplication cyst.

SUGGESTED READING

Gaughan EM, Gift LJ, Frank RK: Tubular duplication of the cervical portion of the esophagus in a foal. *J Am Vet Med Assoc* 201:748, 1992.

Greet TR: Observations on the potential role of oesophageal radiography in the horse. *Equine Vet J* 14:73, 1982.

Orsini JA, Sepsey L, Donawick WJ, et al: Esophageal duplication cyst as a cause of choke in the horse. *J Am Vet Med Assoc* 193:474, 1988.

Peek SF, De Lahunta S, Hackett RP: Combined oesophageal and tracheal duplication cyst in an Arabian filly. *Equine Vet J* 27:475, 1995.

Sanchez LC: Esophageal diseases. In Reed SM, Bayly WM, Sellon DC, editors: *Equine internal medicine*, ed 3. St Louis, 2010, Saunders Elsevier, pp 830–838.

AUTHOR: **TIM MAIR**

EDITORS: **TIM MAIR** and **CERI SHERLOCK**

Esophageal Fistula

BASIC INFORMATION

DEFINITION

Permanent opening of esophagus draining to the skin surface

EPIDEMIOLOGY

RISK FACTORS
- Esophageal rupture
- Esophageal surgery

ASSOCIATED CONDITIONS AND DISORDERS Esophageal fistula may occur after esophageal surgery (failure of an esophagostomy incision to heal appropriately) or after esophageal rupture.

CLINICAL PRESENTATION

HISTORY, CHIEF COMPLAINT A chronic draining tract at the skin surface overlying the esophagus from which saliva and food drains

PHYSICAL EXAM FINDINGS Affected horses are usually normal apart from the presence of the draining tract. In the case of large fistulae, signs of dehydration and weight loss may occur. There may be localized cellulitis or swelling of the neck and excoriation of the skin around the fistula.

ETIOLOGY AND PATHOPHYSIOLOGY
- Inappropriate healing after esophageal perforation
- Inappropriate healing after esophageal surgery (esophagotomy)

DIAGNOSIS

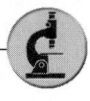

DIFFERENTIAL DIAGNOSIS

- Abscess or chronic draining tract caused by a foreign body
- Other causes of cellulitis of the neck

INITIAL DATABASE

- Bloodwork is usually normal, but for large fistulae, hemoconcentration, electrolyte abnormalities (hyponatremia, hypochloremia), and metabolic acidosis may be present.
- Physical examination confirms drainage of saliva from the tract. Saliva (with or without food material) will spontaneously drain if the horse is offered food. Water will drain when the horse drinks.

ADVANCED OR CONFIRMATORY TESTING

The presence of an esophageal fistula may be confirmed by esophagoscopy and contrast radiography (administration of barium suspension under pressure).

TREATMENT

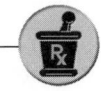

THERAPEUTIC GOAL(S)

Facilitate healing of the damaged esophageal wall and surrounding tissues.

ACUTE GENERAL TREATMENT

Surgical treatment: Resection of the sinus tract and closure of the stoma

POSSIBLE COMPLICATIONS

Complications include esophageal stricture, breakdown of the surgical repair, and reformation of esophageal fistula.

RECOMMENDED MONITORING

During treatment, horses should be monitored for signs of dehydration, weight loss, and electrolyte abnormalities.

PROGNOSIS AND OUTCOME

Prognosis appears to be fair to good after surgical resection.

PEARLS & CONSIDERATIONS

Failure to repair the fistula is likely to result in weight loss and fluid and electrolyte abnormalities.

SUGGESTED READING

Fubini SL: Esophageal diseases. In Mair T, Divers T, Ducharme N, editors: *Manual of equine gastroenterology*. London, 2002, Saunders Elsevier, pp 89–98.

AUTHOR: **TIM MAIR**

EDITORS: **TIM MAIR** and **CERI SHERLOCK**

Esophageal Obstruction

BASIC INFORMATION

DEFINITION
Obstruction of the esophageal lumen

SYNONYM
Choke

EPIDEMIOLOGY
RISK FACTORS
- Horses and ponies that have ravenous appetites or "bolt" their feed may be at increased risk.
- Older horses and ponies with poor dentition and young horses with erupting teeth may be at an increased risk because of poor mastication of food.
- A previous episode of esophageal obstruction may predispose to further episodes; some horses are affected by repeated episodes of esophageal obstruction as a result of stricture or diverticulum formation.

ASSOCIATED CONDITIONS AND DISORDERS Dental diseases, esophageal neoplasia, thyroid tumors, external compressive masses (eg, mediastinal lymphoma), and congenital abnormalities (eg, duplication cysts, megaesophagus, neuromuscular disorders) may predispose horses to esophageal obstruction.

CLINICAL PRESENTATION
DISEASE FORMS/SUBTYPES Esophageal obstructions may be caused by a primary intraluminal obstruction, or they may arise secondary to an extraluminal compressive mass or functional problem.

HISTORY, CHIEF COMPLAINT The most common presenting signs are acute onset of excessive salivation, retching (repeated flexion and extension of the neck), coughing, and copious discharge of saliva from the nostrils.

PHYSICAL EXAM FINDINGS
- Affected horses often sweat excessively and appear distressed, but the body temperature is usually normal.
- The heart rate may be mildly elevated.
- Mucous membranes may be mildly congested.
- There may be a palpable swelling in neck in the jugular groove or over the trachea (if the obstruction is in the cervical region). If the obstruction is in the cervical part of the esophagus, most affected horses will retch immediately after attempting to swallow. (There is often a 10- to 12-second delay between the swallow and the onset of retching if the obstruction is in the distal esophagus.)

ETIOLOGY AND PATHOPHYSIOLOGY
- The obstructing mass is usually food, especially dry pelleted food or dry sugar beet pulp. The dry, fibrous material swells with the absorption of saliva, and an expanding bolus occludes the esophageal lumen. Subsequent boluses compound the obstruction.
- Primary feed impactions may also be composed of roughage, especially leafy alfalfa hay, coarse grass hay, bedding, and even grass.
- Occasionally, foals and young horses may eat foreign bodies that lodge in the esophagus and initiate an obstruction.
- Eating too soon after sedation or general anesthesia (when coordinated muscular activity of the esophagus has not yet returned) may predispose horses to obstruction.
- The most common sites of esophageal obstruction are the proximal esophagus and just cranial to the thoracic inlet.

DIAGNOSIS

DIFFERENTIAL DIAGNOSIS
Other causes of dysphagia, especially abnormalities affecting the pharyngeal and esophageal phases of deglutition, including pharyngeal paralysis, pharyngeal cysts, pharyngeal compression by strangles abscesses and guttural pouch empyema, subepiglottic cyst, fourth branchial arch defect, megaesophagus, esophageal stricture, intramural esophageal cysts, esophageal rupture, and equine grass sickness

INITIAL DATABASE
- Bloodwork may be normal or consistent with mild to moderate dehydration (prerenal azotemia, elevated packed cell volume, elevated total protein).
- Mucous membranes may be mildly congested.
- Passage of a nasogastric tube is impeded by an obstruction in the esophagus. The horse may become distressed when attempting to swallow the nasogastric tube.

ADVANCED OR CONFIRMATORY TESTING
- Esophageal endoscopy allows identification of the type of material that is causing the obstruction. (Remember that any food that the horse has swallowed subsequent to the occurrence of the obstruction will be visualized by endoscopy, so the initial obstructing mass may not be visible.)
- Ultrasound examination can be used to confirm an obstruction and to identify any extraluminal masses (in the cervical region).
- Radiography (including contrast radiography) can be used to confirm the presence of an obstruction but is more useful in investigating possible strictures or diverticuli.

TREATMENT

THERAPEUTIC GOAL(S)
Treatments are aimed at relieving the obstruction and preventing secondary complications such as inhalation pneumonia.

ACUTE GENERAL TREATMENT
- If choke is suspected, the owners should be advised to remove all food and water immediately.
- Many "chokes" can be relieved by heavy sedation and the repeated administration of spasmolytic agents. This treatment can be continued for several hours or even days, but the distressed state of the patient and the likelihood of serious respiratory complications demand that conservative management should not be prolonged.
- The horse should be tranquillized with acepromazine, and further sedation should be provided with xylazine, detomidine, or romifidine to lower the animal's head (to allow drainage of feed and saliva from the nostrils and prevent aspiration).
- N-butylscopolammonium bromide (Buscopan; 0.3 mg/kg IV) may be used to relax the esophagus.
- Oxytocin (0.11–0.22 IU/kg IV q6h) may reduce esophageal smooth muscle tone (do not administer to pregnant mares).
- Lidocaine (30–100 mL of 2% solution) may be administered via nasogastric tube to aid relaxing the esophageal musculature.

CHRONIC TREATMENT
- Conservative treatments are frequently sufficient to relax the esophagus and allow the obstruction to pass within 4 to 6 hours. If conservative therapy fails

to relieve the obstruction after 24 hours, most clinicians advocate lavage under sedation (with the patient's head kept low) or general anaesthesia. Gentle lavage is performed via a nasogastric tube. Warm water is gently pumped or administered by gravity flow. The nasogastric tube must be maneuvered carefully to avoid iatrogenic damage to the esophagus.

- Intravenously administered crystalloids may be required in long-standing cases to prevent dehydration.
- Prophylactic antibiotics should be administered to prevent the development of inhalation pneumonia.
- After the obstruction has been resolved, the horse should be allowed access to water only for 24 to 48 hours before being fed a soft diet.
- If all attempts to resolve the obstruction fail, surgical intervention (esophagotomy) may be necessary.

POSSIBLE COMPLICATIONS

Inhalation pneumonia, esophageal rupture, esophageal stricture, esophageal diverticulum, reobstruction

RECOMMENDED MONITORING

During treatment, horses should be monitored for nasal discharge of saliva and retching. Resolution of these signs suggests that the obstruction has cleared. Passage of a nasogastric tube confirms clearance of the obstruction. Endoscopic examination may be helpful in identifying mucosal damage after resolution of the impaction.

PROGNOSIS AND OUTCOME

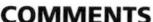

The prognosis for horses with simple esophageal obstruction is good, but the prognosis is poor if an esophageal stricture occurs.

PEARLS & CONSIDERATIONS

COMMENTS

- Do not leave food or water in the stall after esophageal obstruction occurs.

- Do not use mineral oil as a lubricant to lavage esophageal obstructions because of the risk of aspiration.
- Do not attempt to lavage the esophagus unless the horse's head is lowered.

CLIENT EDUCATION

Never feed dried beet pulp. Ensure that horses cannot gain access to dried beet pulp.

SUGGESTED READING

Divers TJ: Disorders of the esophagus. In Orsini JA, Divers TJ, editors: *Equine emergencies: treatments and procedures*, ed 3. St Louis, 2008, Saunders Elsevier, pp 117–121.

Elce YA: Esophageal obstruction. In Robinson NE, Sprayberry KA, editors: *Current therapy in equine medicine*, ed 6. St Louis, 2009, Saunders Elsevier, pp 351–353.

Fubini SL: Esophageal diseases. In Mair T, Divers T, Ducharme N, editors: *Manual of equine gastroenterology*. London, 2002, Saunders Elsevier, pp 89–98.

AUTHOR: **TIM MAIR**

EDITORS: **TIM MAIR** and **CERI SHERLOCK**

Esophageal Rupture

BASIC INFORMATION

DEFINITION

Rupture of the wall of the esophagus

SYNONYM

Esophageal perforation

EPIDEMIOLOGY

RISK FACTORS
- Chronic esophageal obstruction
- Kick wounds to the neck region

ASSOCIATED CONDITIONS AND DISORDERS Esophageal rupture may occur after esophageal obstruction, especially chronic obstruction, or as an extension of infection or injury from surrounding tissues.

CLINICAL PRESENTATION

HISTORY, CHIEF COMPLAINT Clinical signs of esophageal rupture include cervical swelling, cellulitis, abscess formation, and subcutaneous emphysema. With open perforations, there is a wound from which saliva and food may drain.

PHYSICAL EXAM FINDINGS In addition to the presenting signs listed above, affected horses may be febrile and have congested mucous membranes. Dyspnea may develop because of tracheal compression or obstruction or pleuritis.

ETIOLOGY AND PATHOPHYSIOLOGY

- Chronic obstruction of the esophagus may cause pressure-induced necrosis of the esophageal wall.
- Swallowed perforating foreign body
- Penetrating external wounds, especially kick wounds
- Repeated traumatic nasogastric intubation

DIAGNOSIS

DIFFERENTIAL DIAGNOSIS

- Other causes of cellulitis of the neck
- Other causes of subcutaneous emphysema (eg, thoracic wounds)
- Other causes of dyspnea

INITIAL DATABASE

- The leukogram may reveal a leukopenia with or without a left shift and hypoproteinemia.
- Confirmation of esophageal rupture may be aided by endoscopic examination (esophagoscopy). Ruptures of the cranial esophageal sphincter may be very difficult to visualize with esophagoscopy. The more distal esophageal ruptures are easier to see using esophagoscopy.

ADVANCED OR CONFIRMATORY TESTING

- Diagnosis can be aided by radiography and ultrasound examination. Survey radiographs may reveal emphysema and gas tracking along the fascial planes around the esophagus.
- Contrast radiography may show leakage of liquid contrast agents into the tissues surrounding the esophagus.
- Thoracic radiography may show pneumomediastinum or pneumothorax.

TREATMENT

THERAPEUTIC GOAL(S)

- Maintain a patent airway and treat dyspnea.
- Control infection.
- Facilitate healing of the damaged esophageal wall and surrounding tissues.

ACUTE GENERAL TREATMENT

- Acute (6–12 hours) perforations may be amenable to debridement and primary surgical closure if sufficient healthy esophageal tissue is present.
- Horses should receive nothing by mouth for 48 to 72 hours after surgery.

- Administer balanced polyionic fluids intravenously until the horse is eating and drinking again.
- Nonsteroidal antiinflammatory drugs should be administered.
- Tetanus prophylaxis should be administered if required.
- The horse may be so dyspneic (because of compression of the trachea by cellulitis or emphysema) that a tracheotomy is required.
- If pneumothorax is present, drainage of pleural air by a chest drain may be required.
- Broad-spectrum antibiotic treatment is indicated. A suitable antibiotic combination is sodium or potassium penicillin (22,000–44,000 IU/kg IV q6h) and gentamicin (6.6 mg/kg IV q24h). Metronidazole (15–25 mg/kg PO q6h) may be useful in treating anaerobic infections.

CHRONIC TREATMENT

- Most esophageal perforations have to heal by secondary intention. Adequate ventral drainage is essential to prevent migration of the infection to the thoracic inlet, and the wound is allowed to heal by contraction and epithelialization.

- The horse can be fed by placing an esophagotomy tube through the rupture site, allowing tissues to contract down around the tube.
- Alternatively, the patient can be fed through a tube placed distally to the esophageal perforation in a normal area of the esophagus.
- Some horses take a long time to granulate the wound and allow migration of esophageal mucosa over the granulating bed.
- Intermittent fluid therapy may be necessary.

POSSIBLE COMPLICATIONS

Complications include esophageal stricture, failure to heal with formation of esophageal fistula, esophageal impaction, septic mediastinitis, and pleuritis.

RECOMMENDED MONITORING

During treatment, horses should be monitored for signs of dehydration, weight loss, and septic pleuritis.

PROGNOSIS AND OUTCOME

- Prognosis appears to be fair for horses with acute esopha-

geal perforation if aggressive therapy is instituted early and the perforation is amenable to surgical closure.
- In chronic cases, the prognosis is more guarded because of the risk of complications.

PEARLS & CONSIDERATIONS

Prompt, aggressive treatment offers the best chance of complete healing without complications.

SUGGESTED READING

Craig DR, Shivy DR, Pankowski RL, et al: Esophageal disorders in 61 horses: results of nonsurgical and surgical management. *Vet Surg* 18:432, 1989.

Divers TJ: Disorders of the esophagus. In Orsini JA, Divers TJ, editors: *Equine emergencies: treatments and procedures*, ed 3. St Louis, 2008, Saunders Elsevier, pp 117–121.

Fubini SL: Esophageal diseases. In Mair T, Divers T, Ducharme N, editors: *Manual of equine gastroenterology*. London, 2002, Saunders Elsevier, pp 89–98.

Stick JH: Surgery of the equine esophagus. *Vet Clin North Am Large Anim Pract* 4:33, 1982.

AUTHOR: TIM MAIR

EDITORS: TIM MAIR and CERI SHERLOCK

Esophageal Stricture

BASIC INFORMATION

DEFINITION

Stricture (narrowing of the lumen) of the esophagus

SYNONYMS

Esophageal webs or rings

EPIDEMIOLOGY

RISK FACTORS
- Esophageal obstruction
- Esophagitis

ASSOCIATED CONDITIONS AND DISORDERS Esophageal stricture may occur after esophageal obstruction, especially chronic obstruction, or circumferential esophageal erosion or ulceration. Stricture may also occur after trauma to the neck. Congenital strictures have been reported rarely.

CLINICAL PRESENTATION

HISTORY, CHIEF COMPLAINT Clinical signs of esophageal stricture are similar to those of esophageal obstruction, including acute onset of excessive salivation, retching (repeated flexion and

extension of the neck), coughing, and copious discharge of saliva from the nostrils. Repeated bouts of esophageal obstruction may occur.

PHYSICAL EXAM FINDINGS The findings of physical examination are identical to those of esophageal obstruction.

ETIOLOGY AND PATHOPHYSIOLOGY
- Esophageal strictures may develop in three forms:
  - Mural lesions that involve only the adventitia and muscularis
  - Esophageal rings or webs that involve only the mucosa or submucosa
  - Annular stenosis that involves all layers of the esophageal wall

DIAGNOSIS

DIFFERENTIAL DIAGNOSIS

- Other causes of dysphagia (especially abnormalities of the pharyngeal and esophageal phases of deglutition), including pharyngeal paralysis, pharyngeal cysts, pharyngeal compression by strangles abscesses and guttural pouch empyema, subepiglottic cyst, fourth

branchial arch defect, esophageal obstruction, megaesophagus, esophagitis, intramural esophageal cysts, esophageal rupture, and equine grass sickness
- Repeated bouts of esophageal obstruction should increase the suspicion of an underlying esophageal stricture.

INITIAL DATABASE

- The leukogram and hematology results are likely to be normal unless there is dehydration from chronic esophageal obstruction.
- Confirmation of esophageal stricture can be made in some cases by endoscopic examination (esophagoscopy). Esophageal webs and rings can often be detected by endoscopy, but mural strictures or annular stenosis may not be visible.

ADVANCED OR CONFIRMATORY TESTING

Radiography, including contrast radiography or double-contrast radiography, may be necessary to identify an esophageal stricture.

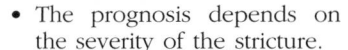

TREATMENT

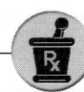

THERAPEUTIC GOAL(S)

Resolution of the stricture

ACUTE GENERAL TREATMENT

- Clinical and experimental studies indicate that stricture formation may occur as soon as 15 days after circumferential mucosal loss. There is little change in lumen diameter for the next 15 days.
- Between 30 and 60 days postinjury, the lumen diameter increases, with the largest change occurring between 30 and 45 days. Surgical treatment of a stricture should, therefore, be delayed until at least 60 days after the traumatic incident.
- Medical management (feeding a slurry diet and administration of nonsteroidal antiinflammatory drugs) may allow some strictures to resolve without the need for surgery. Pelleted mash has been found to be the most palatable feed. Alternatives include IV total parenteral or partial parenteral nutrition or extraoral alimentation using an esophagostomy tube.

CHRONIC TREATMENT

- Surgical therapy is indicated in cases in which the stricture fails to resolve and recurrent obstructions develop. The surgical management of an esophageal stricture depends on the layer of the esophagus that is involved, although this may not be known before surgery.
- Esophagomyotomy is indicated for an esophageal stricture confined to the muscularis and adventitia. A longitudinal incision is made through the adventitia and muscle, allowing mucosa and submucosa to bulge through the incision. A stomach tube is gently advanced to determine if the lumen will allow passage easily across the strictured site. In most instances, the myotomy is left open, and the rest of the surgical incision is drained and sutured in a routine manner.
- Partial esophageal resection is most appropriate for lesions confined to the mucosa and submucosa. The muscu-

laris and adventitia are incised in a longitudinal manner, and the strictured area of mucosa and submucosa is dissected free and resected. The mucosa is closed only if it is possible to do so without excessive tension. The muscularis is closed because it serves as a muscular tube upon which the mucosal defect can regenerate. It may be necessary to feed the horse through a separate esophagotomy site or via extraoral alimentation.
- Complete esophageal resection: Transection of the esophagus is performed in healthy tissue cranial and caudal to the lesion, and a two-layer anastomosis is performed. Extraoral alimentation or feeding by esophagostomy after surgery can be advantageous.
- Esophagoplasty: A longitudinal incision in the esophagus is closed in a transverse manner. This is only recommended for very small lesions (<2 cm in length).
- Patch grafting with local musculature has been described. A patch graft of the sternocephalicus tendon can be apposed to the mucosal defect left after resection of the stricture.
- Fenestration through a cicatrix: The esophagus is isolated, and an esophagotomy is performed through the strictured area followed by fenestration of the mucosal and submucosal cicatrix. An esophagostomy tube is passed through the defect and left in place until the site constricts down enough for the tube to be removed. The wound will heal with a small traction diverticulum.
- Bougienage is used in humans and small animals for treatment of esophageal stricture, but horses do not tolerate the technique well.

POSSIBLE COMPLICATIONS

Complications of esophageal surgery are common and include esophageal impaction, recurrence of stricture, and postsurgical dehiscence.

RECOMMENDED MONITORING

During treatment, horses should be monitored for signs of dehydration, weight loss, infection, and surgical dehiscence

PROGNOSIS AND OUTCOME

- The prognosis depends on the severity of the stricture.
- In strictures that fail to resolve with medical therapy, the prognosis is better if surgery is performed than if continued conservative management is attempted.

PEARLS & CONSIDERATIONS

Medical management of esophageal strictures early in the course of the disease (the first 60 days) is frequently successful.

SUGGESTED READING

Clabough DL, Roberts MC, Robertson I: Probable congenital esophageal stenosis in a thoroughbred foal. *J Am Vet Med Assoc* 199:483, 1991.

Craig DR, Shivy DR, Pankowski RL, et al: Esophageal disorders in 61 horses: results of nonsurgical and surgical management. *Vet Surg* 18:432, 1989.

Craig DR, Todhunter RJ: Surgical repair of an esophageal stricture in a horse. *Vet Surg* 16:251, 1987.

Freeman DE: Esophageal surgery. In Robinson NE, Sprayberry KA, editors: *Current therapy in equine medicine*, ed 6. St Louis, 2009, Saunders Elsevier, pp 358–360.

Hoffer RE, Barber SH, Kallfelz FA, et al: Esophageal patch grafting as a treatment for esophageal stricture in a horse. *J Am Vet Med Assoc* 171:350, 1977.

Knottenbelt DC, Harrison LJ, Peacock PJ: Conservative treatment of oesophageal stricture in five foals. *Vet Rec* 131:27, 1992.

Sanchez LC: Esophageal diseases. In Reed SM, Bayly WM, Sellon DC, editors: *Equine internal medicine*, ed 3. St Louis, 2010, Saunders Elsevier, pp 830–838.

Suann CJ: Oesophageal resection and anastomosis as a treatment for oesophageal stricture in the horse. *Equine Vet J* 14:163, 1982.

Todhunter RJ, Stick JA, Trotter GW, et al: Medical management of esophageal stricture in seven horses. *J Am Vet Med Assoc* 185:784, 1984.

AUTHOR: **TIM MAIR**

EDITORS: **TIM MAIR** and **CERI SHERLOCK**

Esophagitis

BASIC INFORMATION

DEFINITION
Inflammation of the wall of the esophagus; may be ulcerative or nonulcerative

SYNONYM
Reflux esophagitis

EPIDEMIOLOGY
RISK FACTORS
- Esophageal obstruction
- Gastric fluid regurgitation into the esophagus

ASSOCIATED CONDITIONS AND DISORDERS Esophagitis may occur after esophageal obstruction, especially chronic obstruction, or as a result of reflux of gastric fluid into the esophagus.

CLINICAL PRESENTATION
HISTORY, CHIEF COMPLAINT Clinical signs of esophagitis are nonspecific and are similar to those of esophageal obstruction and gastric ulcer disease. Affected horses present with signs of dysphagia or discomfort when swallowing, hypersalivation, bruxism, and inappetence.

PHYSICAL EXAM FINDINGS The findings of physical examination confirm the presenting signs, which include dysphagia, hypersalivation, and bruxism. Weight loss may occur in chronic cases.

ETIOLOGY AND PATHOPHYSIOLOGY
- Chronic obstruction of the esophagus may cause pressure-induced necrosis of the esophageal wall.
- Swallowed perforating foreign body
- Penetrating external wounds, especially kick wounds
- Repeated traumatic nasogastric intubation
- Repeated episodes of gastric fluid reflux into the distal esophagus (secondary to gastric ulcer disease, motility disorders, gastric outflow obstruction, intestinal ileus, proximal enteritis)
- Chemical injury from swallowed irritant substances

DIAGNOSIS

DIFFERENTIAL DIAGNOSIS
Other causes of dysphagia (especially abnormalities of the pharyngeal and esophageal phases of deglutition), including pharyngeal paralysis, pharyngeal cysts, pharyngeal compression by strangles abscesses and guttural pouch empyema, subepiglottic cyst, fourth branchial arch defect, esophageal obstruction, megaesophagus, esophageal stricture, intramural esophageal cysts, esophageal rupture, and equine grass sickness

INITIAL DATABASE
- The leukogram and hematology results are likely to be normal unless there is dehydration from chronic esophagitis or changes secondary to any underlying disease.
- Confirmation of esophagitis is achieved by endoscopic examination (esophagoscopy). Diffuse, patchy, linear, or coalescing areas of inflammation, erosion, or ulceration may be observed.

ADVANCED OR CONFIRMATORY TESTING
- Investigations should be undertaken to establish whether there is a primary underlying disease causing secondary esophagitis. The stomach should be examined endoscopically to establish the presence of gastritis, gastric ulceration, or gastric outflow abnormalities.
- Radiography, including contrast radiography, may be helpful in assessing esophageal motility and transit time.

TREATMENT

THERAPEUTIC GOAL(S)
- Control infection.
- Facilitate healing of the damaged esophageal wall and surrounding tissues.
- Treat any underlying primary disease.

ACUTE GENERAL TREATMENT
- Decrease or discontinue nonsteroidal antiinflammatory drug therapy if at all possible.
- Gastric acid suppression
  - Proton pump inhibitors
    - Omeprazole: 4 mg/kg PO q24h
    - Pantoprazole (1.5 mg/kg IV q24h) is available for patients in which oral omeprazole cannot be used but may be cost prohibitive
  - Histamine H2-receptor antagonists
    - Cimetidine: 16 to 25 mg/kg PO or 6.6 mg/kg IV q6–8h
    - Ranitidine: 6.6 mg/kg PO or 1.5 mg/kg IV q8h
    - Famotidine: 2.8 to 4.0 mg/kg PO or 0.23 to 0.5 mg/kg IV q8–12h
  - Antacids: Magnesium hydroxide, aluminum hydroxide

- Require frequent administration (q2–4h) to have any effect on increasing gastric pH; thus, they are not recommended
- Mucosal protectants: Sucralfate (20 mg/kg PO q6–8h). Efficacy has not been proven for esophageal ulcers.
- Broad-spectrum antibiotic treatment is indicated if there is infection of the esophageal wall or periesophageal tissues. A suitable antibiotic combination is sodium or potassium penicillin (22,000–44,000 IU/kg IV q6h) and gentamicin (6.6 mg/kg IV q24h). Metronidazole (15–25 mg/kg PO q6h) may be useful for treating anaerobic infections.
- Horses with reflux esophagitis caused by gastroduodenal ulcer disease, gastric paresis, or proximal enteritis may benefit from prokinetic drugs that act on the proximal gastrointestinal tract (eg, metoclopramide, 0.02–0.10 mg/kg SC q4–12h, or bethanechol, 0.025–0.035 mg/kg SC q4–24h)

CHRONIC TREATMENT
- Frequent small meals of moistened pellets or fresh grass should be fed.
- Severe esophagitis may require withholding food completely for several days.

POSSIBLE COMPLICATIONS
Complications include esophageal stricture and esophageal impaction.

RECOMMENDED MONITORING
During treatment, horses should be monitored for signs of dehydration and weight loss.

PROGNOSIS AND OUTCOME

- The prognosis depends on the presence and nature of any underlying primary disease.
- The prognosis appears to be fair to good for horses with acute esophagitis without any underlying primary disease.
- In chronic cases, the prognosis is more guarded because of the risk of complications.

PEARLS & CONSIDERATIONS

- Esophagitis is frequently secondary to an underlying

disease affecting the stomach or proximal intestinal tract.
- The nature and severity of any underlying primary disease is most important in determining the prognosis.

SUGGESTED READING

Greet TR: Observations on the potential role of oesophageal radiography in the horse. *Equine Vet J* 14:73, 1982.
Sanchez LC: Esophageal diseases. In Reed SM, Bayly WM, Sellon DC, editors: *Equine internal medicine*, ed 3. St Louis, 2010, Saunders Elsevier, pp 830–838.

AUTHOR: **TIM MAIR**

EDITORS: **TIM MAIR** and **CERI SHERLOCK**

Esophagus: Idiopathic Muscular Hypertrophy

BASIC INFORMATION

DEFINITION

Muscular hypertrophy of the small muscle layers of the distal esophagus

EPIDEMIOLOGY

ASSOCIATED CONDITIONS AND DISORDERS Idiopathic muscular hypertrophy of other regions of the gastrointestinal tract

CLINICAL PRESENTATION

HISTORY, CHIEF COMPLAINT In most cases, the disease is asymptomatic and is discovered as an incidental postmortem finding. In a small number of cases, the disease may be associated with esophageal dysphagia (hypersalivation, nasal discharge of saliva or food) or recurrent esophageal obstructions by feed. Affected horses may also present with weight loss.
PHYSICAL EXAM FINDINGS The findings of physical examination confirm the presenting signs, which include dysphagia, hypersalivation, and nasal discharge containing food material. Distension of the cervical esophagus may be visible or palpable.
ETIOLOGY AND PATHOPHYSIOLOGY Unknown cause. There is muscular hypertrophy of the tunica muscularis of the distal esophagus without fibrosis or inflammation.

DIAGNOSIS

DIFFERENTIAL DIAGNOSIS

- Other causes of dysphagia (especially abnormalities of the pharyngeal and esophageal phases of deglutition): Pharyngeal paralysis, pharyngeal cysts, pharyngeal compression by strangles abscesses and guttural pouch empyema, subepiglottic cyst, fourth branchial arch defect, esophageal obstruction, esophageal stricture, esophageal rupture, megaesophagus, and equine grass sickness
- Other obstructions of the esophagus: Intramural esophageal cysts, duplication cysts of the esophagus, esophageal neoplasia

INITIAL DATABASE

- The leukogram, hematology, and blood chemistry results are likely to be normal unless they reflect abnormalities associated with secondary aspiration pneumonia.
- Endoscopic examination (esophagoscopy) may reveal reduced esophageal peristaltic activity and dilatation of the lumen. There may be evidence of esophagitis.
- Fluoroscopy and contrast radiography can be used to demonstrate prolonged transit time of a bolus from the cervical esophagus to the stomach. Contrast radiography also demonstrates dilatation of the esophageal lumen and a thickened esophageal wall.

ADVANCED OR CONFIRMATORY TESTING

Confirmation is achieved by postmortem examination.

TREATMENT

THERAPEUTIC GOAL(S)

- Treat any secondary inhalation pneumonia
- Aid transit of food along the esophagus

ACUTE GENERAL TREATMENT

- Treat any secondary aspiration pneumonia with broad-spectrum antibiotics.
- Dietary modification may help esophageal transit of food boluses to the stomach. Feeding slurries of pellets and feeding from an elevated position may help.
- Metoclopramide or bethanechol may benefit patients with reflux esophagitis by increasing lower esophageal tone, increasing gastric emptying, and reducing gastroesophageal reflux.

CHRONIC TREATMENT

Frequent small meals of slurries or fresh grass should be fed.

POSSIBLE COMPLICATIONS

- Aspiration pneumonia
- Weight loss

PROGNOSIS AND OUTCOME

The prognosis is poor in most cases.

PEARLS & CONSIDERATIONS

Idiopathic muscular hypertrophy of the esophagus should be considered as a rare cause of chronic signs of esophageal dysphagia.

SUGGESTED READING

Benders NA, Veldhuis Kroeze EJ, van der Kolk JH: Idiopathic muscular hypertrophy of the oesophagus in the horse: a retrospective study of 31 cases. *Equine Vet J* 36:46, 2004.

AUTHOR: **TIM MAIR**

EDITORS: **TIM MAIR** and **CERI SHERLOCK**

Estrus, Prolonged

BASIC INFORMATION

DEFINITION
Estrous behavior lasting more than 12 days

SYNONYM(S)
Persistent estrus, nymphomania

EPIDEMIOLOGY
SPECIES, AGE, SEX Sexually mature mares
RISK FACTORS Endometritis
GEOGRAPHY AND SEASONALITY
- Prolonged estrus during spring transition between January and April (Northern Hemisphere)
- Hemorrhagic anovulatory follicles are more common during the fall

ASSOCIATED CONDITIONS AND DISORDERS
- Endometritis
- Ovarian disorders

CLINICAL PRESENTATION
HISTORY, CHIEF COMPLAINT Signs of estrus for >12 days (normal duration 5–7 days with a range of 2–12 days)
PHYSICAL EXAM FINDINGS Body condition generally good
ETIOLOGY AND PATHOPHYSIOLOGY
- Seasonality: Prolonged estrous behavior during spring transition or winter anestrus
- Granulosa theca cell tumor (GTCT): Increased production of estrogens or lack of progesterone
- Gonadal dysgenesis: 63,XO; 65,XXX; 64,XY mares
- Hormone imbalance: Older mares may fail to ovulate and exhibit prolonged estrus; possibly due to insufficient or ineffective leutinizing hormone release
- Previous ovariectomy
- Hemorrhagic anovulatory follicles (HAF): 14.3% remain as follicular structures with consequent signs of persistent estrus

DIAGNOSIS

DIFFERENTIAL DIAGNOSIS
- Frequent urination
  - Cystitis/urethritis
  - Bladder atony
- Frequent posturing and straining
  - Urovagina
  - Vaginitis
  - Pneumovagina
- Submissive behavior
- Missed shortened interestrus

- Psychogenic behavioral problem not associated with physiologic or pathologic causes of prolonged estrus

INITIAL DATABASE
- Teasing: Estrous behavior
- Transrectal palpation and ultrasound: Serial examinations may be needed to evaluate the estrous cycle and its association with behavior.
  - Anestrus: Small inactive ovaries, no uterine edema, relaxed cervix.
  - Spring transition: Active ovaries, 20 mm follicles, ±uterine edema, relaxed cervix.
  - GTCT: Asymmetric ovaries, no uterine edema, relaxed cervix; the affected ovary presents a multicystic or honeycombed appearance, with loss of ovulation fossa, but also could appear as a solid mass or a single large cyst. The contralateral ovary is generally inactive and small.
  - Gonadal dysgenesis: Small inactive ovaries, no uterine edema, relaxed cervix.
  - Hormone imbalance: Active ovaries with follicles, uterine edema, relaxed cervix.
  - HAF: Asymmetric ovaries, uterine edema, relaxed cervix. HAFs may be 5 to 15 cm in diameter and persist for up to 2 months. Fibrous (hyperechoic) bands or strands traversing the follicular lumen may be seen on ultrasound, but in some cases the only feature observed is a thickening of the follicular wall. The contralateral ovary is generally active.
- Speculum vaginal examination
  - Urovagina: Presence of urine in the lumen
  - Vaginitis: Irritation of the vaginal walls

ADVANCED OR CONFIRMATORY TESTING
- Inhibin, testosterone, and progesterone serum concentrations for GTCT
- Inhibin >0.7 ng/mL, testosterone >50 to 100 pg/mL, and progesterone <1 ng/mL
- Urinalysis to rule out cystitis
- Karyotyping for gonadal dysgenesis

TREATMENT

THERAPEUTIC GOAL(S)
Treat underlying cause

ACUTE GENERAL TREATMENT
- Winter anestrus: Progestogens will abolish estrous signs (Altrenogest

0.044 mg/kg PO q24h or progesterone in oil 150 mg IM q24h)
- Spring transition
  - Hastening the first ovulation of the year
    - Artificial lighting (14.5–16h of light daily, starting in December, extending the natural light in the evening, with an intensity of 10 lux or 1 foot-candle)
    - Progestogens will shorten and ease the transitional signs (Altrenogest 0.044 mg/kg PO q24h or progesterone in oil 150 mg IM q24h for 10–15 days during late transition; ovulation is expected 12–15 days after discontinuation of treatment)
- Estrus suppression
- GTCT: Unilateral ovariectomy.
- No known efficacious treatment for hormone imbalance. Induction of ovulation can be attempted by administration of human chorionic gonadotropin (hCG; 1500–3500 IU, IM, or IV) or Deslorelin (gonadotropin-releasing hormone analog; 1.5 mg IM) when a >35 mm follicle is present.
- HAF: Administration of hCG (1500–3500 IU, IM, or IV) or Deslorelin (1.5 mg IM) to induce ovulation or luteinization of the follicles (although they may not respond to such treatment) followed by administration of prostaglandin $F_{2\alpha}$ (Dinoprost 5–10 mg IM) 7 to 10 days later to induce luteolysis (repeated doses may be needed). Most HAFs regress spontaneously without treatment.
- Previous ovariectomy: Progestogens will abolish estrous signs (Altrenogest 0.044 mg/kg PO q24h or progesterone in oil 150 mg IM q24h).

POSSIBLE COMPLICATIONS
- Treatment with progestagens may decrease uterine defenses and lead to endometritis.
- Injections of progesterone may produce muscle soreness.

RECOMMENDED MONITORING
GTCT: Ultrasound examination to check for return to cyclicity of the remaining ovary starting 2 months after ovariectomy

PROGNOSIS AND OUTCOME
- GTCT: Good prognosis for life and fertility. Time to return to cyclicity of the contralat-

- eral ovary is 6 months on average (2–12 months)
- Guarded for fertility for hormonal imbalance
- Poor prognosis for fertility in mares with congenital disorders
- Once winter anestrus and spring transition are over, the mare is expected to cycle normally

PEARLS & CONSIDERATIONS

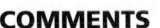

COMMENTS

- One complaint is that the mare constantly shows a behavior, interpreted as estrus, that interferes with the mare's performance. Often this complaint is not associated with an abnormality in cyclicity.

- Signs of discomfort, agitation, or submission can be confused with signs of estrus.
- Deslorelin is only available through compounding pharmacies in the United States.

CLIENT EDUCATION

Human safety must be considered when handling Altrenogest. Gloves must be worn while handling this product. Pregnant women or women who suspect they are pregnant should not handle this drug. Women of child-bearing age should exercise extreme caution when handling this product. Accidental absorption could lead to a disruption of the menstrual cycle or prolongation of pregnancy, uterine or abdominal cramping, increased or decreased uterine bleeding, and headaches.

SUGGESTED READING

Daels PF, Hughes JP: The abnormal estrous cycle. In Mc Kinnon AO, Voss JL, editors: *Equine reproduction.* Philadelphia, 1993, Lea & Febiger, pp 144–157.

Hinrichs K: Irregularities of the estrous cycle and ovulation in mares (including seasonal transition). In Younquist RD, Threlfall WR, editors: *Current therapy in large animal theriogenology.* St Louis, 2007, Saunders Elsevier, pp 144–152.

McCue P: Ovulation failure. In Samper JC, Pyckock JF, McKinnon AO, editors: *Current therapy in equine reproduction.* St Louis, 2007, Saunders Elsevier, pp 83-85.

AUTHOR: **MARIA CLARA SARDOY**

EDITOR: **JUAN C. SAMPER**

Ethmoid Hematoma, Progressive

BASIC INFORMATION

DEFINITION

- A well-encapsulated, non-neoplastic, and slowly growing mass that originates in the ethmoid turbinate region and less often within the paranasal sinuses
- The condition is most often unilateral, although 15% to 20% of reported cases have bilateral disease.

SYNONYM(S)

Ethmoid hematoma

EPIDEMIOLOGY

SPECIES, AGE AND SEX Although progressive ethmoid hematoma (PEH) is often considered a disease of middle-aged horses (10–12 years old), reported age ranges from <1 year to 20 years old.
GENETICS AND BREED PREDISPOSITION
- Any breed can be affected, although the condition is overrepresented in Thoroughbreds and Arabians.
- Standardbreds appear underrepresented.

CLINICAL PRESENTATION

DISEASE FORMS/SUBTYPES
Based on the origin of the PEH:
- Ethmoid turbinate
- Sphenopalatine sinus
- Maxillary sinus
- Other location within the paranasal sinus

HISTORY, CHIEF COMPLAINT

- Unilateral epistaxis, which is often mild and intermittent in nature.
- May occur spontaneously or after exercise.
- A respiratory noise may be heard at rest but more often during exercise.

PHYSICAL EXAM FINDINGS

- Epistaxis alone or mixed with mucopurulent nasal discharge.
- Respiratory noise may be present.
- Some uncommon findings during physical examination include coughing, halitosis, facial deformity, head shyness or shaking, dyspnea, and visualization of the mass at the level of the nostril.
- Small PEHs may not show any clinical signs.

ETIOLOGY AND PATHOPHYSIOLOGY

- The initiating cause is unknown.
- PEHs form because of an episode of hemorrhage in the submucosa of either an ethmoid turbinate or paranasal sinus, causing the mucosa to stretch and secondarily thicken creating a capsule.
- As the hematoma expands, the capsule becomes necrotic, which can leak or rupture, leading to episodes of mild and often intermittent epistaxis.

DIAGNOSIS

DIFFERENTIAL DIAGNOSIS

- Guttural pouch mycosis
- Paranasal sinus cysts

- Neoplasia of the ethmoids, paranasal sinuses, or guttural pouch
- Ulcerative or fungal rhinitis
- Skull fracture
- Foreign body
- Pulmonary abscess or pleuropneumonia

INITIAL DATABASE

- Physical examination
- Resting endoscopic examination will reveal a glistening yellow- to green-tinged mass either at the ethmoid turbinate or through the nasomaxillary opening. The absence of a mass in the nasal passages does not rule out PEH because PEHs can be found within the paranasal sinuses.
- Radiographs of the sinuses and nasal passage may reveal a smooth-walled and well-demarcated soft tissue density within the sinus cavity or in the nasal passage at times impinging on the nasal septum. Fluid lines within the sinuses may be present in some cases.
- Small lesions may fail to be identified radiographically.
- Bloodwork (complete blood count and chemistry profile) is usually normal, although it may reveal anemia in some cases.

ADVANCED OR CONFIRMATORY TESTING

- Computed tomography may provide an exact location, origin, and extent of the PEHs, as well as providing information regarding all other soft tissue structures within the skull. It can be very useful to accurately diagnose bilateral lesions as well.

- Nuclear scintigraphy may help differentiate a PEH from a cyst or a carcinoma. PEH typically appears scintigraphically as a poorly defined region of radioisotope uptake within the sinus or ethmoidal region. Cysts are usually well defined and within the maxillary or frontal sinus, and carcinomas invade bone, which will be shown scintigraphically as another region of radioisotope uptake.
- Biopsies taken transendoscopically in cases of PEH are typically of limited or no diagnostic benefit because of their thick capsule. Biopsies are usually more beneficial to rule in other conditions such as granulomas and carcinomas.

TREATMENT

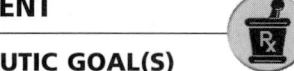

THERAPEUTIC GOAL(S)

To eliminate the PEHs and to minimize the chance of recurrence

ACUTE GENERAL TREATMENT

- Photoablation of the PEH with an Nd:YAG laser under endoscopic guidance
  - May be done with the horse standing or under general anesthesia.
  - Intranasal portion of the PEH.
  - The goal is to create thermal necrosis and obliteration of the mass.
  - Noncontact fiber.
  - May be necessary to perform several treatment sessions depending on the size of the lesion, usually 1 to 2 weeks apart to allow for the charred and necrotic material to slough.
- Chemical ablation of the PEH using 10% formalin (4% formaldehyde solution) under endoscopic guidance
  - Standing procedure.
  - Although used mostly for PEH with a nasal component, it may be used in PEHs within the sinus using a trephine opening.
  - Between 30 and 50 mL of formalin is injected using a commercially available catheter with guarded needle tip (Cook Veterinary Products, Spencer, IN) or homemade.
- PEH is injected until it begins to leak.
  - The method of action is desiccation and coagulation of the tissue by protein hydrolysis.
  - Several treatments are likely needed (range, 1–18) every 3 to 4 weeks.

- PEH removal via frontonasal bone flap
  - The goal is to remove the entire hematoma, including its origin.
  - May be done in combination with Nd:YAG laser.
  - Because of the need to access the ethmoid labyrinth or base of the sphenopalatine sinus, hemorrhage can be severe.
  - After removal of the PEH, the sinuses are packed with sterile gauze, exiting through a corner of the flap or through the nasal cavity and secured to the nostril. The packing is removed approximately 72 hours after surgery.

CHRONIC TREATMENT

Ablation of the PEH using either Nd:YAG laser or formalin injections usually requires several treatments spaced every week or 3 to 4 weeks, respectively, until the lesion is fully destroyed.

POSSIBLE COMPLICATIONS

- Although rare, there have been reports of significant complications after the use of intralesional formalin such as severe laminitis and erosion of the cribiform plate, allowing formalin to come in contact with the brain. In addition, formalin can induce significant nasal edema, which can lead to complete obstruction if bilateral lesions are simultaneously treated.
- Thermal damage to surrounding structures, including the brain, is possible when using the Nd:YAG laser. For this reason, it is very important to aim the laser beam at the center of the lesion and monitor the amount of energy used.
- Severe hemorrhage during surgical removal through a frontonasal bone flap is possible and should be discussed with the owner before surgery.

RECOMMENDED MONITORING

Repeat endoscopy or radiography of the skull is recommended every 6 months.

PROGNOSIS AND OUTCOME

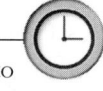

- Long-term prognosis is fair to guarded.
- The incidence of recurrence has been reported in up to 45% of cases.
- Bilateral lesions (43%) seem to have a significantly worse prognosis compared with unilateral lesions (8%) regarding long-term remission.

PEARLS & CONSIDERATIONS

COMMENTS

- It is important to examine both nasal passages to assess whether there is unilateral or bilateral involvement.
- Because of the chance of significant hemorrhage during surgical extirpation of the PEH, it is always recommended to have donor blood available. Alternatively, if a donor is not available, it is recommended to collect blood from the patient 2 to 4 weeks before surgery for an autotransfusion.
- In cases of mild to moderate hemorrhage, IV administration of aminocaproic acid (10–20 mg/kg) diluted in 100 mL of saline can be beneficial. The treatment can be given q6h for several days. It is important to monitor the hematocrit because it will artificially decrease (reason unknown, potentially rouleaux formation).
- Aminocaproic acid is an antifibrinolytic or antiproteolytic drug that works by blocking plasminogen activator factor. This keeps plasmin from being activated, which then cannot split fibrin.

CLIENT EDUCATION

Horse owners must be advised about the potential for several treatments and long-term regular follow-up to enhance the chances for a good long-term outcome.

SUGGESTED READING

Freeman DE: Sinus disease. In Parente EJ, editor: *The veterinary clinics of North America equine practice: respiratory disease.* Philadelphia, 2003, Saunders Elsevier, pp 218–222.

Frees KE, et al: Severe complications after administration of formalin for treatment of progressive ethmoid hematoma in a horse. *J Am Vet Med Assoc* 219:950–952, 2001.

Nickles FA: Nasal passages and paranasal sinuses. In Auer JA, Stick JA, editors: *Equine surgery.* St Louis, 2006, Saunders Elsevier, pp 537–540.

Tate LP: Noncontact free fiber ablation of equine progressive ethmoid hematoma. In Orsini JA, editor: *Clinical techniques in equine practice: the use of lasers in surgery.* Philadelphia, 2002, Saunders Elsevier, pp 22–27.

AUTHOR: JOSÉ M. GARCÍA-LÓPEZ

EDITOR: ERIC J. PARENTE

Ethylene Glycol Toxicosis

BASIC INFORMATION

DEFINITION
Condition caused by intoxication with ethylene glycol (EG) characterized by neurologic, acid-base, and renal disturbances

SYNONYM(S)
EG poisoning, antifreeze poisoning

EPIDEMIOLOGY
SPECIES, AGE, SEX The paucity of case reports suggests that EG toxicosis is uncommon in horses.

CLINICAL PRESENTATION
DISEASE FORMS/SUBTYPES Early acute onset of neurologic dysfunction and acidosis followed by renal insufficiency or failure.
HISTORY, CHIEF COMPLAINT Acute onset (10–30 minutes) of central nervous system (CNS) depression and ataxia, progression to profound CNS depression, subsequent polyuria, oliguria, or anuria may develop.
PHYSICAL EXAM FINDINGS Signs developing soon after ingestion include ataxia, CNS depression, tachypnea, sweating, tachycardia, hypothermia, decreased gut motility, colic, and seizure. Development of renal insufficiency occurs within 24 to 36 hours after exposure.
ETIOLOGY AND PATHOPHYSIOLOGY EG is metabolized via alcohol dehydrogenase to glycoaldehyde, glycolic acid, glyoxylic acid, and oxalic acid, resulting in severe systemic acidosis. Oxalic acid combines with serum calcium to form calcium oxalate crystals, which precipitate in the kidney and contribute to the renal injury caused directly from other EG metabolites.

DIAGNOSIS

DIFFERENTIAL DIAGNOSIS
- Other causes of acute onset of neurologic dysfunction: Viral and bacterial encephalidities, fumonisins, hepatic encephalopathy, and propylene glycol
- Other causes of renal injury: Soluble oxalate-containing plants, nonsteroidal antiinflammatory drug toxicosis, enterotoxemia, aminoglycoside toxicosis, myoglobinuria, and hemoglobinuria

INITIAL DATABASE
- Baseline serum chemistry and blood gases followed by repeat testing of renal function and serum calcium levels
  - Expect metabolic acidosis, increased anion gap, hypocalcemia, increased blood urea nitrogen, increased creatinine, and possibly hyperkalemia.
- EG levels can be measured in the blood with in-house test kits.

ADVANCED OR CONFIRMATORY TESTING
- Qualitative and quantitative testing for EG can be done at most diagnostic laboratories and at human hospitals.
- Gritty texture upon cutting the kidney at necropsy.
- Uremic ulcers in the oral cavity; gastric mucosal mineralization.
- Histopathologic examination of the kidney reveals proximal tubular necrosis associated with the presence of birefringent crystals in the lumens of tubules.

TREATMENT

THERAPEUTIC GOAL(S)
Manage acidosis, provide supportive care, enhance elimination, and prevent formation of toxic metabolites.

ACUTE GENERAL TREATMENT
- IV fluid diuresis at twice to three times maintenance rate (8.0–12.0 mL/kg/h IV) to enhance elimination of EG and metabolites.
- Ethanol: 4.4 mL/kg of 25% solution followed by 2.0 mL/kg IV q4h for 4 days.
- Administration of sodium bicarbonate IV as needed based on blood gas results.
- Provide a quiet, padded environment with minimal sensory stimuli.

CHRONIC TREATMENT
Long-term dietary alteration may be necessary if residual kidney dysfunction occurs.

POSSIBLE COMPLICATIONS
Pulmonary edema is possible.

RECOMMENDED MONITORING
Acid-base status, oxygen saturation, urine output (fluid ins/outs), renal values, serum calcium

PROGNOSIS AND OUTCOME

Prognosis is guarded to poor if there is evidence of renal dysfunction.

PEARLS & CONSIDERATIONS

COMMENTS
- Although some sources suggest the use of activated charcoal to adsorb glycols, the current consensus is that activated charcoal is a poor adsorbent for small molecules such as these and is of little benefit in EG exposures.
- There is no information on the efficacy (or lack thereof) of fomepizole causing inhibition of equine alcohol dehydrogenase; therefore, the usefulness of this modality in treating equine EG intoxication is not known.
- Some car antifreeze products contain fluorescein dye, which may cause fluorescence when a wood's lamp is used to visualize urine. Because not all EG products contain fluorescein, absence of urine fluorescence should not be construed as a negative test for EG.

PREVENTION
Keep horses away from areas where EG is being used.

SUGGESTED READING
Bailey EM, Garland T: Management of toxicoses. In Robinson NE, editor: *Current therapy in equine medicine*, ed 3. Philadelphia, 1992, WB Saunders, pp 346–352.
Swor TM, Aubrey P, Murphy ED, et al: Acute ethylene glyol toxicosis in a horse. *Equine Vet Educ* 14:234–239, 2002.

AUTHOR: SHARON GWALTNEY-BRANT

EDITOR: CYNTHIA L. GASKILL

Exercise-Induced Pulmonary Hemorrhage

BASIC INFORMATION

DEFINITION

Hemorrhage originating from small pulmonary vessels associated with strenuous exercise.

SYNONYM(S)

- EIPH
- Bleeders

EPIDEMIOLOGY

SPECIES, AGE, SEX

- Females are thought to have a slightly increased risk of epistaxis associated with EIPH.
- The incidence of EIPH is increased in older horses doing strenuous work.

RISK FACTORS

- Increased exercise intensity
- Previous EIPH episodes
- Extended time in training
- Existing airway inflammation
- Cardiac arrhythmias such as atrial fibrillation
- Significant upper airway obstruction

GEOGRAPHY AND SEASONALITY

Anecdotally, seasonal association with extreme environmental conditions (ie, cold, dry winter or hot, humid summer)

ASSOCIATED CONDITIONS AND DISORDERS

- Upper airway obstruction
- Lower airway inflammation: Infectious or noninfectious
- Cardiac dysrhythmia (especially atrial fibrillation)

CLINICAL PRESENTATION

DISEASE FORMS/SUBTYPES

- Blood visualized in trachea with endoscope. This is the most common method of diagnosing EIPH. The severity of EIPH is quantified by scores from 0 to 4.
  - Grade 0: No blood in the trachea
  - Grade 1: Small droplets of blood in the trachea
  - Grade 2: Narrow stream of blood (<5 mm wide) in the trachea
  - Grade 3: Confluent wider streams of blood in the trachea
  - Grade 4: Pooling of blood occupying the majority of the tracheal circumference
- Red blood cells (RBCs) seen microscopically in bronchoalveolar lavage (BAL) fluid in the absence of blood visible endoscopically in the trachea
- Epistaxis: Uncommonly observed (<1% of race starts); some association with higher bleeding scores

HISTORY, CHIEF COMPLAINT

- Reduced athletic performance
- Frank hemorrhage in trachea
- Epistaxis (rarely)

PHYSICAL EXAM FINDINGS

- None specific
- Epistaxis (rarely)

ETIOLOGY AND PATHOPHYSIOLOGY

- Horses undergoing strenuous exercise have very high pulmonary vascular and left atrial pressures. This predisposes the smaller vessels in the lungs to damage.
- Stress failure of pulmonary capillaries results when transmural forces exceed the strength of the capillary walls.
- Increased transmural forces can occur from both elevated pulmonary vascular pressures or increased swings in airway pressures during intense exercise.
- When this occurs, protein-rich fluid and then RBCs (hemorrhage) leak into the interstitium and alveoli.
- The blood in the alveoli eventually migrates to the trachea, where it may be seen with endoscopy. This blood can be engulfed and cleared by alveolar macrophages, which are seen on cytologic evaluation of BAL fluid as hemosiderophages. Very rarely, blood is seen at the nose (epistaxis). It may also be coughed up and swallowed.
- The RBCs remaining in the interstitium likely set up an inflammatory response in the lung parenchyma and may be responsible for ongoing damage and fibrosis in the lung.
- The capillaries in the dorsocaudal region of the lung are the most prominently affected, particularly in early episodes of EIPH.
- With time, the vessels in more cranial portions of the lung are affected, especially noted at the periphery of prior lesions. The ventral aspect of the lung is much less commonly involved.
- Other factors, including airway inflammation, limb loading and hoof impact, and cardiac disease, are thought to modify the extent or frequency of hemorrhage.

DIAGNOSIS

DIFFERENTIAL DIAGNOSIS

- Airway hemorrhage from other sources (eg, larynx, pharynx, nasal passages, ethmoids, guttural pouches, sinuses)
- Pulmonary hemorrhage not associated with exercise

INITIAL DATABASE

- Airway endoscopy for blood in the trachea or bronchi
- BAL for enumeration of erythrocytes in BAL fluid. RBCs may persist for at least 7 days after an episode in BAL fluid. Nucleated cell count and differential analysis or cytology to assess degree of airway inflammation are also important.
- The presence of hemosiderophages in BAL fluid indicates hemorrhage occurred sometime in the past (generally persist up to 3 weeks after an episode).
- The complete blood count is likely to be normal.
- Thoracic radiographs may show characteristic lesions (increased interstitial density) in the caudodorsal lung field. With chronicity, a bronchial pattern may be seen superimposed over the interstitial pattern; however, this is not a sensitive indicator of EIPH.
- Thoracic ultrasonography may show increased numbers of "comet tail" artifacts in the caudodorsal lung fields. This is neither sensitive nor specific for EIPH, but may be a way to monitor EIPH severity or pulmonary damage in horses with repeated episodes over time.

ADVANCED OR CONFIRMATORY TESTING

Scintigraphy with labeled RBCs may be used, but this is very technically demanding, not readily available, and may not accurately distinguish between hemorrhage and RBCs within vessels.

TREATMENT

THERAPEUTIC GOAL(S)

- Eliminate factors that may predispose the horse to increased severity of EIPH or increased number of episodes (eg, cardiac arrhythmias, airway inflammation, and upper airway obstruction)
- Rest to allow time for pulmonary lesions to heal

ACUTE GENERAL TREATMENT

- Many treatments have been used to limit EIPH or its severity; however, few have met with consistent success. Although some treatments do seem to work in individual horses under certain circumstances, none has been found to consistently decrease or prevent EIPH. Treatments fall under general categories of reduction of pulmonary artery (PA) pressures, decreasing airway resistance, proco-agulants, antiinflammatory agents, and other.

- Furosemide (Lasix, Salix): This is the only race day medication approved in all racing jurisdictions in the United States. Its primary mechanism is to reduce PA pressures (and body weight) through diuresis; however, it also has bronchodilatory as well as other effects. It is permitted a minimum of 4 hours before racing, using a dose range of 100 to 500 mg (variable between jurisdictions). There is no agreement that furosemide overall prevents EIPH, although anecdotally it may decrease severity in some situations. Studies report conflicting results as to its efficacy.
- Endothelin receptor antagonists: No effect on PA pressures or EIPH
- Nitric oxide (NO), NO donors, NO with type 5 phosphodiesterase (PDE) inhibitors: Conflicting results as to efficacy; most promising is a combination of NO and a selective type 5 PDE inhibitor; not commercially available or approved for race day use
- Nasal strip: Mechanism is to decrease nasal resistance. Studies show conflicting results regarding the ability to decrease EIPH.
- Bronchodilatory agents: Mechanism is to decrease airway resistance. However, airways of healthy horses are fully dilated during maximal exercise. These agents do not appear to directly influence EIPH. If a horse has inflammatory airway disease, these agents may affect EIPH; however, they are not approved as a race day medication.
- Various procoagulants (eg, herbal remedies, aminocaproic acid, conjugated estrogens, vitamin K) have not been shown to be efficacious.

- Antiinflammatory agents: The mechanism is to decrease airway inflammation; does not have a direct effect on EIPH; not approved as race day medication

CHRONIC TREATMENT

- Chronic treatment is aimed at reducing predisposing causes contributing to EIPH occurrence or severity.
- Management practices designed to decrease airway inflammation such as decreasing dust, irritants, and allergens in environment and use of corticosteroids may help to control EIPH if it is exacerbated by inflammation.
- Correction of upper airway obstructions that may contribute to increased inspiratory airway resistance
- Ensuring that cardiac function is normal
- Rest to allow time for pulmonary lesions to heal

POSSIBLE COMPLICATIONS

- Decreased pulmonary function over time if repeated episodes of severe bleeding with parenchymal damage and fibrosis occur.
- Bronchitis or pneumonia

PROGNOSIS AND OUTCOME

- Horses that are "severe" bleeders are likely to continue to have episodes. These horses are usually retired because of poor athletic performance related to EIPH.
- Horses that bleed more severely (grade 3 or 4) do not perform as well on the racetrack.
- All horses undergoing intense exercise on a regular basis bleed at some time during their athletic career. If the epi-

sodes are mild, this may not be a performance-limiting factor.

PEARLS & CONSIDERATIONS

COMMENTS

All athletic horses participating in intense exercise will bleed, although not all horses have detectable blood every time they exercise. Factors contributing to the variability seen in the diagnosis of EIPH are not known. This makes it difficult to assess treatment efficacy.

PREVENTION

- None
- As noted above, medications are used to attempt to limit EIPH, although their efficacy is mostly unproven.

SUGGESTED READING

Birks EK, Durando MM, McBride S, et al: Exercise-induced pulmonary hemorrhage. *Vet Clin Equine North Am* 19:87–100, 1997.
Birks EK, Durando MM, McBride S: Exercise-induced pulmonary hemorrhage. *Vet Clin Equine North Am* 19:87–100, 2003.
Hinchcliff KW, Jackson MA, Morley PS, et al: Association between exercise-induced pulmonary hemorrhage and performance in Thoroughbred racehorses. *J Am Vet Med Assoc* 227:768–774, 2005.
Newton JR: Epidemiology of EIPH. In Marlin DJ, Hinchcliff KW, Wade JF, editors: *Havemeyer proceedings of a workshop on exercise-induced pulmonary haemorrhage: state of current knowledge*. Newmarket, UK, 2008, R&W Communications, pp 3–7.
West JB, et al: Stress failure of pulmonary capillaries in racehorses with exercise-induced pulmonary hemorrhage. *J Appl Physiol* 75:1097–1109, 1993.

AUTHOR: MARY DURANDO

EDITOR: MELISSA R. MAZAN

Failure of Passive Transfer

BASIC INFORMATION

DEFINITION

- Failure of transfer of passive immunity (FPT) from the dam's colostrum to the foal. The most widely accepted definition of FPT is measurement of serum immunoglobulin G (IgG) concentrations less than 400 mg/dL at or after 24 hours of age.
- Partial failure of passive transfer (PFPT) is commonly defined as

IgG concentrations between 400 and 800 mg/dL.
- Adequate transfer of passive immunity is generally defined as IgG of 800 mg/dL or greater.

SYNONYM(S)

Failure of transfer of passive immunity

EPIDEMIOLOGY

SPECIES, AGE, SEX Foals younger than 1 month.

RISK FACTORS Prematurity, rejection by dam, peripartum asphyxia syndrome, geriatric dam, colostrum lost before parturition

ASSOCIATED CONDITIONS AND DISORDERS Sepsis

CLINICAL PRESENTATION

DISEASE FORMS/SUBTYPES

- FPT with secondary sepsis
- FPT without disease

HISTORY, CHIEF COMPLAINT

- Detection at routine new foal examination
- Foals that have not nursed adequately
- Foals rejected by dam
- Premature lactation of dam
- Weak, poor affinity for dam

PHYSICAL EXAM FINDINGS

- FPT without other illness: No abnormalities on physical examination
- FPT with illness: Signs of generalized disease (weakness, lethargy, poor affinity for dam) or localized disease (swollen joint, lameness) (see "Neonatal Sepsis" in this section)

ETIOLOGY AND PATHOPHYSIOLOGY

- Insufficient production
  - Premature birth of foal
  - Serious illness of dam
  - Ingestion of endophyte-infected fescue during third trimester of gestation
  - Premature lactation (as with placentitis, premature placental separation, twinning)
  - Variation of IgG concentration of colostrum among mares
- Insufficient ingestion
  - Weak foal
  - Congenital musculoskeletal abnormalities of foal
  - Rejection by dam
  - Separation of dam and foal (eg, foal rolls under a fence)
- Insufficient absorption
  - Concurrent disease
  - Hypoxic ischemic insult to enterocytes

DIAGNOSIS

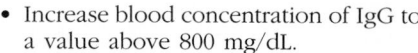

DIFFERENTIAL DIAGNOSIS

Sepsis with adequate transfer of passive immunity

INITIAL DATABASE

- Whole blood or serum for estimation of IgG concentration
  - Quantitative immunoassay (DVM stat) or semiquantitative (SNAP, IDEXX Laboratories, Westbrook, ME) immunoassays
  - Zinc sulphate turbidity (Equine FPT Test Kit, VmRD, Inc., Pullman, Wash.) or glutaraldehyde coagulation (Gamma-Check E, Plasvacc USA, Templeton, CA)

- Complete blood count (CBC): Aids in distinguishing FPT alone from FPT and sepsis

ADVANCED OR CONFIRMATORY TESTING

- Turbidimetric immunoassay (TIA)
- Single radial immunodiffusion: Most quantitatively accurate but requires 18 to 24 hours of incubation time

TREATMENT

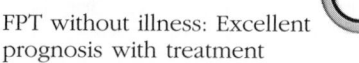

THERAPEUTIC GOAL(S)

- Increase blood concentration of IgG to a value above 800 mg/dL.
- Prevent infection in the lag time between the time of exposure to pathogens (at birth) and the development of a protective immune response.

ACUTE GENERAL TREATMENT

- Plasma is recommended for all foals older than 12 hours with IgG below 800 mg/dL.
- Foals with IgG between 400 and 800 mg/dL may not require treatment if a clean environment is maintained and the foal shows no physical or laboratory (CBC) abnormalities.
- Foals younger than 12 hours of age with inadequate nursing: Equine colostrum
  - Begin with 200 to 400 mL colostrum to ensure the gastrointestinal tract will tolerate feedings.
  - Feed via nasogastric tube to weak foals.
  - Total of 1 to 2 L of good-quality colostrum is recommended for the average 45-kg foal.
- Foals older than 12 hours of age: IV equine plasma
  - Administer United States Department of Agriculture–licensed products or plasma obtained from a local donor.
  - Administer slowly through a whole-blood filter set.

CHRONIC TREATMENT

- FPT with sepsis: See "Neonatal Sepsis" in this section for specific treatment recommendations.
- FPT without illness: Broad-spectrum oral or intramuscular antibiotics may be used prophylactically.

POSSIBLE COMPLICATIONS

- Transfusion reaction to plasma: Slow rate or stop transfusion; start at slower rate; or switch to another plasma donor if the patient is still reacting
- Focal infection
- Sepsis

RECOMMENDED MONITORING

- Recheck IgG after administering treatment to ensure sufficient concentration achieved. This can be done immediately after transfusion.
- Check septic foals IgG approximately weekly. Catabolism and distribution of immunoglobulins may differ from those of nonseptic foals.

PROGNOSIS AND OUTCOME

- FPT without illness: Excellent prognosis with treatment
- FPT with illness: Varied depending on the specific illness

PEARLS & CONSIDERATIONS

COMMENTS

- The appearance of colostrum is not reliably a good indicator of quality or IgG concentration.
- Colostrometers are available for measuring IgG (good-quality colostrum contains >3000 mg/dL IgG).
- Consumption of ingested IgG in sick foals may result in inadequate circulating concentrations.
- Immunoglobulins in plasma or serum are poorly absorbed when given orally.

CLIENT EDUCATION

The cost of testing for FPT is minimal compared with treating an infected foal with FPT.

SUGGESTED READING

Giguere S, Polkes AC: Immunologic disorders in neonatal foals. In Sanchez C, editor: *Neonatal medicine and surgery*, Philadelphia, 2005, Saunders Elsevier, pp 241–272.

AUTHOR: **PHOEBE A. SMITH**

EDITORS: **ELIZABETH M. SANTSCHI** and **PHOEBE A. SMITH**

Failure to Cycle

BASIC INFORMATION

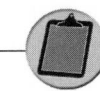

DEFINITION

Failure to show estrous behavior when expected during the breeding season

SYNONYMS

- Noncycling mare
- Anestrus

EPIDEMIOLOGY

SPECIES, AGE, SEX Sexually mature mares

RISK FACTORS

- Iatrogenic from the use of hormones
- Long-term chronic infections, such as pyometra

GEOGRAPHY AND SEASONALITY

- From October to February (Northern Hemisphere), most mares present physiologic anestrus.
- Mares that foal between January and early March under the natural photoperiod (Northern Hemisphere) are more predisposed to lactational anestrus, especially if they are in poor body condition.

ASSOCIATED CONDITIONS AND DISORDERS Poor body condition, negative energy balance, endometritis, photoperiod, pregnancy loss, pyometra

CLINICAL PRESENTATION

DISEASE FORMS/SUBTYPES

- Lack of ovarian activity
- Prolonged luteal activity
- Behavioral
- Iatrogenic

HISTORY, CHIEF COMPLAINT

- Absence of estrous behavior when expected during the breeding season
- Absence of follicular development during the breeding season

PHYSICAL EXAM FINDINGS Good/poor body condition, ± vulvar discharge

ETIOLOGY AND PATHOPHYSIOLOGY

- Lack of ovarian activity
  - Seasonality (winter anestrus): Decreased gonadotropin-releasing hormone (GnRH) secretion from increased melatonin secretion during darkness
  - Lactational anestrus: In mares that foal from January to March under the natural photoperiod and/or that are in poor body condition, the condition is likely related to the suppressive effect of the photoperiod on GnRH secretion and/or negative energy balance
  - Gonadal dysgenesis (63,XO; 65,XXX, 64,XY)
  - Ovarian tumors (eg, granulosa theca cell tumor [GTCT]): Produc-

tion of inhibin suppresses follicular activity through follicle-stimulating hormone suppression
  - Anabolic steroid treatment: Suppresses pituitary gonadotropin secretion
- Prolonged luteal activity
  - Persistent corpus luteum (CL): Can remain functional for up to 60 to 90 days if untreated
    - Pyometra: Failure to release prostaglandin $F_{2\alpha}$ ($PGF_{2\alpha}$) because of extensive damage to the endometrium
    - Insensitivity to released $PGF_{2\alpha}$: Diestrus ovulation after the tenth day postovulation
    - Pseudopregnancy: Embryonic death after the first luteal response to pregnancy (typically days 14 to 15 days postovulation)
  - Pregnancy: Persistent progesterone production by the CL after maternal recognition of pregnancy or progestogens from the fetoplacental unit
- Behavioral
  - Silent estrus: Absence of estrous behavior in spite of normal cyclicity
- Iatrogenic
  - Progestins: Suppress estrous behavior by inhibition at the level of the brain
  - Oxytocin treatment for estrus suppression: Prolongs luteal activity

DIAGNOSIS

DIFFERENTIAL DIAGNOSIS

See Etiology above

INITIAL DATABASE

- Teasing: No signs of estrous behavior
- Transrectal palpation and ultrasound:
  - Follicular activity, CL, no uterine edema, tight cervix: Prolonged luteal function
  - Small inactive ovaries, no uterine edema, no CL, relaxed cervix: Lack of ovarian activity
  - Asymmetric ovaries, no uterine edema, cervix relaxed: GTCT
  - Follicular activity, uterine edema, relaxed cervix: Silent estrus
  - Uterine contents
    - Conceptus: Pregnancy
    - Intrauterine fluid: Pyometra or endometritis

ADVANCED OR CONFIRMATORY TESTING

- Inhibin, testosterone, and progesterone serum concentrations for GTCT

  - Inhibin >0.7 ng/mL, testosterone >50 to 100 pg/mL, and progesterone <1 ng/mL in a nonpregnant mare are suggestive of GTCT
- Uterine culture and cytology for pyometra/endometritis
- Karyotyping for gonadal dysgenesis
- Progesterone test for detection of an active corpus luteum

TREATMENT

THERAPEUTIC GOALS

- Treat the underlying cause
- Induce ovarian activity
- Eliminate source of progesterone
- Induce estrous behavior

ACUTE GENERAL TREATMENT

- Induction of ovarian activity
  - Artificial lighting for advancing first ovulation of the year
    - 14.5 to 16 hours of light daily added after sunset, starting in December, with an intensity of 10 lux or 1 foot-candle.
    - Transition may last 40 to 60 days. Traditionally, it was advised to keep mares under lights until late spring, but it has been shown that mares resume cyclicity with only 35 days of light starting at winter solstice.
  - GnRH for induction of ovulation in anestrus mares
    - GnRH
      - Hourly infusion for 28 days (100 ng/kg SC via an osmotic minipump) induced ovulation and fertile estrus in 50% of mares. Mares in shallow seasonal anestrus were more likely to respond to GnRH infusion.
      - Administration of GnRH 167 µg q8h for 7 or 7.5 days induced normal follicular growth and luteinization in anestrous mares.
    - GnRH analogs (Cystorelin, Merial)
      - 10 to 40 µg, IM or SC, q12h for 3 to 4 weeks has been associated with ovulation rates of 26% in deep anestrus and 45% in transitional mares. The resulting pregnancies may be jeopardized because of the potential for dysfunctional primary CL.
      - The subcutaneous GnRH analogue implant (Ovuplant Peptech, Sydney, Australia)

designed to release 100 μg/day administered to transitional mares for 28 days resulted in 60% of mares ovulating 4 to 30 days after implant treatment.

- ○ Dopamine antagonists for lactational anestrus
  - Sulpiride (200 mg IM q12h) or domperidone (440 mg PO q24h) and 16 hours of daylight previous to starting the treatment. Treatment is unlikely to be effective if the mare has not presented estrous by 18 days.
- ○ No treatment for gonadal dysgenesis
- ○ Unilateral ovariectomy for GTCT
- ○ Discontinuation of treatment for exogenous anabolic steroids
- Elimination of source of progesterone
  - ○ Persistent CL
    - Dinoprost (5–10 mg IM), or cloprostenol (100–250 μg IM). Return to estrus is expected in 3 to 5 days (range, 2–12 days). Cloprostenol is not labeled for use in horses.
    - Pyometra: Several uterine lavages with saline or lactated Ringer's solution may be necessary to eliminate the uterine contents. Oxytocin and PGF$_{2\alpha}$ can be used to induce myometrial contractions.
  - ○ Termination of pregnancy: Method selected for termination of pregnancy depends on the stage of pregnancy
    - 5 to 33 days postovulation:
      - □ Dinoprost (5–10 mg IM) or cloprostenol (100–250 μg IM; not labeled for horses).
      - □ Before day 11 to 15, a single injection is generally effective. More injections may be needed later. Estrous behavior appears on average 3 to 5 days (range, 2–12 days) after treatment.
      - □ Intrauterine infusions of 100 mL saline or lavage with 1 to 3 L saline
      - □ Manual crushing of the vesicle (days 16–25)
      - □ Transvaginal ultrasound guided aspiration of fetal fluids (>20 days)
    - 34 to 120 days postovulation:
      - □ PGF$_{2\alpha}$ q6–24h for 3 to 5 days until pregnancy loss
      - □ Manual invasion of the cervix
      - □ Rupture of the chorioallantois
      - □ Manual extraction of the fetus and membranes
      - □ Transvaginal ultrasound guided aspiration of allantoic fluid (days 40–65)

- ≥120 days postovulation:
  - □ Multiple injections of PGF$_{2\alpha}$
  - □ Manual disruption of the fetal membranes and removal of the fetus after cervical dilatation with 17β-estradiol (6–10 mg IM 24 hours before induction of abortion) or PGE$_1$/misoprostol (200 μg, intracervical, once)
  - □ Oxytocin 10 to 20 IU IM or IV in 5-IU increments q15–20 min
  - □ Transabdominal ultrasound-guided fetal-cardiac puncture and injection of potassium chloride or potassium penicillin
  - □ Transcervical intra-allantoic injection of dexamethasone induced abortion within 3 days in treated mares
- Silent estrus
  - ○ Frequent transrectal palpation and ultrasound examination to monitor estrous cycles.
  - ○ Attempt change in estrus detection methods.
  - ○ The use of estradiol has been suggested for mares not allowing the stallion to mount, but studies on effect on fertility are not available. It is advised to use as last resource.
    - 0.5 to 10 mg 17β-estradiol IM 6 hours before breeding
    - 10 mg of estradiol cipionate IM 2 to 3 days before breeding
    - Cipionate is available through compounding pharmacies in the United States and needs to be administered 2 to 3 days in advance; estrous behavior starts in 2 to 3 days and persists for 3 to 4 days after injection
- Discontinuation of treatment for exogenous progestins

POSSIBLE COMPLICATIONS

- Endometritis from invasion of the uterus during pregnancy termination
- Dystocia, retained fetal membranes, trauma to the genital tract with termination of late pregnancy
- Treatment with PGF$_{2\alpha}$ or its analogues can produce undesirable side effects, including sweating, trembling, increased heart rate, and even signs of colic. These signs present within 15 minutes of administration and resolve within 1 hour.

RECOMMENDED MONITORING

- Anestrus and transitional mares should be monitored weekly until a CL is detected, indicative of the first ovulation of the year
- Return to estrus is expected in 3 to 5 days (range, 2–12 days) after PGF$_{2\alpha}$ administration

- Perform ultrasound examinations to check for return to cyclicity of the remaining ovary starting 2 months after ovariectomy for GTCT
- Estrus occurs 4 to 5 days after withdrawal of progestogens
- Return to cyclicity may be affected for up to 6 months after cessation of anabolic steroid administration

PROGNOSIS AND OUTCOME

- Pyometra has guarded prognosis for fertility from damage to the endometrium and good prognosis for life.
- Good prognosis for return to cyclicity for prolonged diestrus, winter anestrus, lactational anestrus.
- Poor prognosis for fertility in mares with congenital disorders.
- GTCT: Good prognosis for life and fertility. Time to return to cyclicity of the contralateral ovary averages 6 months (range, 2–12 months).

PEARLS & CONSIDERATIONS

COMMENTS

- Winter anestrus is a physiologic reproductive stage in mares, although 20% of mares do not undergo anestrus.
- Prolonged luteal phase may occur in 4% to 18% of cycles; in these cases the luteal phase may be prolonged for up to 60 days.

PREVENTION

Lactational anestrus: Mares with expected foaling dates before March 15 can be placed under artificial lights at the beginning of December; adequate feed intake should be available and monitored.

SUGGESTED READING

Hinrichs K: Irregularities of the estrous cycle and ovulation in mares (including seasonal transition). In Youngquist RD, Threlfall WR, editors: *Current therapy in large animal theriogenology*, St Louis, 2007, Saunders Elsevier, pp 144–152.

Pycock JF: Breeding management of the problem mare. In Samper JC, editor: *Equine breeding management and artificial insemination*, Philadelphia, 2000, Saunders, pp 203–208.

LeBlanc M: *An approach to the diagnosis of infertility in the mare.* Presented at the North American Veterinary Conference, Jan 8–12, 2005, Orlando, FL.

Minoia P, Mastronardi M: Use of GnRH to induce oestrus in seasonally anoestrous mares. *Equine Vet J* 19:241–242, 1987.

AUTHOR: MARIA CLARA SARDOY

EDITOR: JUAN C. SAMPER

False Dandelion/Flat Weed Toxicosis

BASIC INFORMATION

DEFINITION

- Stringhalt, a unique disease of horses characterized by spasmodic hyperflexion of one or both hind legs, has been associated with horses eating *Hypochaeris radicata* (cat's ear, flat weed).
- Other plants that have been associated with stringhalt include sweet peas (*Lathyrus* spp.), dandelion (*Taraxacum officinale*), and mallow (*Malva parviflora*).

SYNONYM(S)

- *H. radicata* is commonly known as cat's ear, hairy cat's ear, false dandelion, and flat weed.
- "Australian stringhalt" refers to a similar condition in horses in Australia associated with grazing the same plant.

EPIDEMIOLOGY

GENETICS AND BREED PREDISPOSITION All breeds may be affected, with Thoroughbreds being commonly affected and ponies rarely.

RISK FACTORS
- Overgrazed pastures with heavy infestation of false dandelion (flat weed)
- Poisoning is most common in late summer.

GEOGRAPHY AND SEASONALITY
- False dandelion is a perennial, native plant of most of North America, Australia, and New Zealand that has become a nuisance weed in some areas.

- Closely resembling the common dandelion, *H. radicata* has a rosette of basal leaves and multiple branching flower stems (Figure 1) in contrast to the single-flowered stems of the dandelion.

CLINICAL PRESENTATION

DISEASE FORMS/SUBTYPES Stringhalt may be intermittent and vary from mild to severe, resulting in an abnormal gait and lameness.

HISTORY, CHIEF COMPLAINT Unusual movement of one or both hindlimbs

PHYSICAL EXAM FINDINGS
- Hyperflexion of one or both hock joints
- In extreme cases, the foot is drawn up sharply to the abdomen and is then slapped to the ground.
- Turning, backing, and excitement exacerbate signs.
- The horse may have a hopping gait when both hind legs are affected.
- Atrophy of the lateral thigh muscles may occur in chronic cases.
- Laryngeal hemiplegia resulting in "roaring" may occur in some affected horses

ETIOLOGY AND PATHOPHYSIOLOGY
- The specific toxin in *H. radicata* responsible for stringhalt is not known.
- The condition can be reproduced experimentally by feeding horses a mean of 9.8 kg of green plant daily for 50 days.
- The toxin affects conduction in the long nerves in the body.
- Increased electromyographic activity is reported in the long digital extensor muscle.

DIAGNOSIS

DIFFERENTIAL DIAGNOSIS

- Upward fixation of the patella
- Injury to the lower pastern area or hind limb laminitis may mimic stringhalt.

INITIAL DATABASE

- Physical examination: Normal
- Hematology: Normal
- Serum biochemistry profile: Normal

ADVANCED OR CONFIRMATORY TESTING

- Electromyography of long digital extensor muscle
- Axonal degeneration of peripheral nerves histologically

TREATMENT

ACUTE GENERAL TREATMENT

- Phenytoin (15 mg/kg body weight PO for 2 weeks) may help shorten the recovery period.
- Thiamine has helped in recovery of Australian stringhalt.

CHRONIC TREATMENT

Horses with persisting signs may benefit from tenectomy of the lateral digital extensor(s).

PROGNOSIS AND OUTCOME

- There is a good prognosis with early diagnosis and removal of the plant from the horse's diet.
- Recovery may take a few weeks up to 18 months after horses are removed from the flat weed.
- Most horses recover after flat weed is removed from their diets.

PEARLS & CONSIDERATIONS

PREVENTION

Pasture management to prevent overgrazing in late summer when weeds such as *H. radicata* are abundant will prevent the occurrence of the stringhalt syndrome.

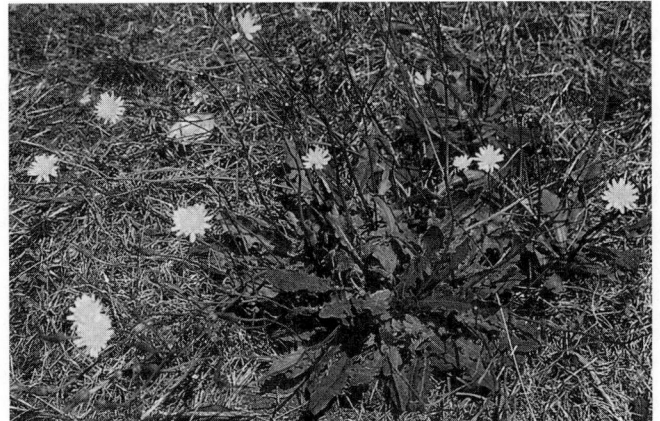

FIGURE 1 False dandelion, or flat weed (*Hypochaeris radicata*).

CLIENT EDUCATION

- Owner recognition of the plant and herbicides can be useful in controlling the plant.

SUGGESTED READING

Araujo JAS, et al: Stringhalt in Brazilian horses caused by *Hypochoeris radicata. Toxicon* 52:190–193, 2008.

Gardner SY, et al: Stringhalt associated with a pasture infested with *Hypochoeris radicata. Equine Vet Educ* June:154–158, 2005.

Gay CC, et al: *Hypochaeris*-associated stringhalt in North America. *Equine Vet J* 25:456–457, 1993.

Colorado State University: Guide to poisonous plants. Available at http://southcampus.colostate.edu/poisonous_plants.

AUTHOR: **ANTHONY P. KNIGHT**

EDITOR: **CYNTHIA L. GASKILL**

Fescue-Related Toxicosis

BASIC INFORMATION

DEFINITION

Toxins, such as ergovaline, produced by the tall fescue endophyte (*Neotyphodium coenophialum*; formerly *Acremonium coenophialum*), which is not externally visible on infected plants and grows symbiotically within the fescue grass (*Lolium arundinaceum*; formerly *Festuca arundinacea*)

SYNONYM(S)

- Fescue toxicosis
- Tall fescue toxicosis
- Ergopeptine alkaloid (ergovaline) toxicosis

EPIDEMIOLOGY

SPECIES, AGE, SEX

- Except for agalactia and pregnancy abnormalities, horses are less susceptible to fescue toxicosis than are cattle.
- There are possible differences between Equid species.

GENETICS AND BREED PREDISPOSITION
There have been anecdotal reports of individual differences in susceptibility, perhaps reflecting the influences of risk factors and geography

RISK FACTORS

- Generally subacute to chronic consumption of endophyte-infected fescue in pastures or hay
- Late-gestational mares (~270–300 days)
- Early-gestational mares
- Mares in the spring transitional phase before the onset of normal cyclicity
- Endophyte-infected fescue in the seed head stage
- Aberrant weather conditions (eg, flood, drought) that favor growth of endophyte-infected fescue
- High rate of application of nitrogen-containing fertilizers
- Concurrent exposure to *Claviceps purpurea* ergot in pastures, hay, grain, and especially pelletized rations incorporating "screenings" (see "Ergot-Related Toxicosis" in this section)

GEOGRAPHY AND SEASONALITY

- Upper Southeastern and lower Midwestern United States; the area of distribution is increasing in size
- Worldwide distribution in parts of South America, Europe, Africa, and Asia
- Spring when mares are cycling and being bred and when foals are being born
- Seasonal variation in toxin concentration occurs, with the riskiest time of year being late spring when the grass is in the seed head stage.

ASSOCIATED CONDITIONS AND DISORDERS
Ergot, ergot poisoning, or ergotism (see "Ergot-Related Toxicosis" in this section)

CLINICAL PRESENTATION

DISEASE FORMS/SUBTYPES

- Fescue toxicosis in mares
- "Summer slump": Much less common and less severe in horses than in cattle (see "Ergot-Related Toxins" in this section)
- "Fescue foot": Much less common and less severe in horses than in cattle (see "Ergot-Related Toxins" in this section)

HISTORY, CHIEF COMPLAINT

- Agalactia or dysgalactia may be observed in the absence of any other clinical signs.
- Prolonged gestation
- Retained fetal membranes
- Dystocia or premature placental separation (ie, "red bag")
- Fetal dysmaturity or overmaturity
- Abortion or stillbirth
- Prolonged transitional phase before the first ovulation or abnormal cyclicity in the spring
- Conception failure or early embryonic loss
- Impaired athletic performance in hot weather
- Laminitis
- See "Ergot-Related Toxicosis" in this section for other hyperthermic and gangrenous effects (uncommon in horses).

PHYSICAL EXAM FINDINGS

- Little or no udder development within 14 days of the due date; this may be the only clinical sign seen
- Aborted fetus or stillbirth
- Dystocia with an abnormally large or malpositioned foal
- Premature separation of the chorioallantois ("red bag" presentation)
- Thickened, edematous fetal membranes, possibly retained
- Dysmature or overmature foal unable to suckle
- Failure of passive transfer
- Multiple, anovulatory follicles; failure to ovulate in a timely fashion
- Increased sweating and heat intolerance during exercise in hot weather
- Multiple limb lameness or laminitis
- See "Ergot-Related Toxicosis" in this section for other hyperthermic and gangrenous effects (uncommon in horses).

ETIOLOGY AND PATHOPHYSIOLOGY

- Fescue toxins consist of a number of ergopeptine alkaloids, including ergovaline (the ergopeptine of highest concentration), and ergoline alkaloids, including lysergic acid.
- In mares, these toxins cause the following:
  - Decreased prolactin secretion by the anterior pituitary via D2 dopamine receptor agonism
  - Altered uterofetoplacental progestagen metabolism
  - Speculated direct or indirect inhibition of corticotropes in the fetal anterior pituitary
- See "Ergot-Related Toxicosis" in this section for hyperthermic and gangrenous effects.

DIAGNOSIS

DIFFERENTIAL DIAGNOSIS

- Reproductive signs
  - Reproductive ergotism
  - Idiopathic agalactia, prolonged gestation, or dystocia not associated with ergot alkaloid exposure

- Delayed fetal development for gestational age
- Infectious causes of abortion or stillbirth, placental abnormalities, or fetal septicemia
- Foal dysmaturity unrelated to ergot alkaloid exposure
- "Summer slump" (horses require higher dosages of ergovaline than cattle)
  - Hyperthermic ergotism
  - Other causes of altered athletic performance
- "Fescue foot" (horses require higher dosages of ergovaline than cattle; laminitis is most likely)
  - Gangrenous ergotism
  - Other causes of laminitis

INITIAL DATABASE

- Confirmation of prolonged gestation
- Agalactia or dysgalactia; failure to "wax"; no increase in calcium in mammary secretions before foaling; little or no milk production
- Failure of passive transfer
- Hemograms or biochemical profiles: Vary depending on the complicating secondary conditions

ADVANCED OR CONFIRMATORY TESTING

- Endocrine analyses
  - Hypoprolactinemia, especially in late-gestational mares
  - Decreased maternal progestagen concentrations in late-gestational mares (use cross-reactive progesterone radioimmunoassay to detect 5α-pregnanes)
  - Decreased maternal relaxin; variable alterations in circulating maternal estrogens in late-gestational mares
- Ultrasound imaging results
  - Placental thickening
  - Anovulatory ovarian follicles when mares should be cycling
  - Conception failure or embryonic loss
- Chemical analyses
  - Detection of ergopeptine alkaloids, especially ergovaline, in pasture or hay using a variety of analytical methods. Total dietary concentrations of ergopeptine alkaloids as low as 100 ppb have been associated with clinical cases of fescue toxicosis in late gestational mares, with some reports of concenratins as low as 50 ppb being associaed with agalactia.
  - ELISA analyses (Agrinostics, Inc., Watkinsville, GA) for ergot alkaloids (greater affinity for ergoline alkaloids than ergopeptine alkaloids) in forages or in urine samples from exposed animals. Ergot alkaloids are rapidly excreted after removal from the source.
- Pathology
  - Gross findings in foals consistent with prolonged gestation (oversized foal, eruption of the foal's incisors, increased eponychium on the foal's hooves, angular limb deformities), dystocia (limb trauma, meconium staining, possible ruptured bladder), agalactia or failure of passive transfer (absence of colostrum or milk in the gastrointestinal tract, joint or umbilical cord infections)
  - Histopathologic finding of distended thyroid follicles lined by flat, cuboidal epithelial cells
  - Grossly thickened or edematous, possibly retained or prematurely separated fetal membranes
  - Edematous fetal membranes
  - Gross findings in mares consistent with agalactia and dystocia (trauma to the reproductive and urinary tracts, retained fetal membranes, possible laminitis)
  - Histopathologic findings in mares consistent with sepsis and laminitis

TREATMENT

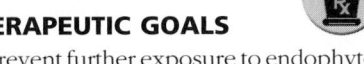

THERAPEUTIC GOALS

- Prevent further exposure to endophyte-infected fescue.
- Counteract the mechanisms of action of ergopeptine alkaloids.
- Provide supportive care.
- Prevent complications.

ACUTE GENERAL TREATMENT

- Removal of source of toxins
- For agalactia, prolonged gestation, and cycling abnormalities: Antidotal treatment with domperidone, a D2 dopamine receptor antagonist (Equidone; Equi-tox, Inc., Central, SC) at 1.1 mg/kg body weight q24h PO
- Need to adjust the dosage or frequency of administration of domperidone if dripping of milk or leaking of colostrum occurs
- Potential extrapyramidal neurologic side effects with other D2 dopamine antagonists, such as fluphenazine and perphenazine
- See "Ergot-Related Toxins" in this section for other hyperthermic and gangrenous effects.

CHRONIC TREATMENT

Depends on complications associated with fescue toxicosis

POSSIBLE COMPLICATIONS

- In mares, trauma or rupture of the reproductive tract or its vasculature; bladder or bowel displacement; subsequent laminitis
- Sepsis in mares or foals
- Ruptured urinary bladder in foals secondary to dystocia
- See "Ergot-Related Toxins" in this section for possible hyperthermic or gangrenous complications.

RECOMMENDED MONITORING

- Depends on the observed clinical signs and complications
- Monitor udder development in pregnant mares; attend and assist with foaling.

PROGNOSIS AND OUTCOME

Depend on the duration and level of toxin exposure, as well as concurrent risk factors and complications; possible death of the mare, foal, or both

PEARLS & CONSIDERATIONS

COMMENTS

- Agalactia is the most sensitive indicator of ergopeptine alkaloid exposure in horses; it may be observed in the absence of any other signs.
- With ergopeptine alkaloid toxicosis, parturition cannot be predicted by "waxing" or increased calcium concentrations in mammary secretions.
- Consider domperidone treatment in cases of prolonged pregnancies that are 345 days or longer with little or no udder development in regions where ergopeptine alkaloid exposure is common.
- Dystocia in late-gestational, agalactic mares is highly suggestive of exposure to ergopeptine alkaloids.

PREVENTION

- Maintain careful breeding records and confirmation of pregnancy in regions where ergopeptine alkaloid exposure is common.
- Withdraw pregnant mares from endophyte-infected fescue pasture or hay at least 30 days before the foaling due date (60–90 days before foaling is preferable, if possible).
- Carefully inspect animals, especially udder development in late-gestational mares.
- Provide oral treatment with domperidone 1.1 mg/kg q24h 10 to 14 days before the foaling due date, especially if the mare has agalactia or withdrawal from fescue is not possible.
- Attend and assist at the time of foaling.
- Keep pastures mowed to prevent seed head stage of tall fescue.

- Inspect pastures and hay for fescue and ergot.
- Overseed fescue pastures with legumes.
- Replace toxic endophyte-infected fescue with tall fescue infected with a genetically modified, "nontoxic" endophyte.

CLIENT EDUCATION

Increased awareness of risks to horses, especially late-gestational mares, associated with exposure to fescue-related endophytic toxins

SUGGESTED READING

Blodgett DJ: Fescue toxicosis. In Gupta RC, editor: *Veterinary toxicology: basic and applied principles*, New York, 2007, Academic Press Elsevier, pp 907–914.

Cross DL, et al: Equine fescue toxicosis; signs and solutions. *J Anim Sci* 73:899–908, 1995.
Evans TJ, Rottinghaus GE, Casteel SW: Ergot. In Plumlee K, editor: *Clinical veterinary toxicology*, St Louis, 2004, Mosby Elsevier, pp 239–243.
Evans TJ, Rottinghaus GE, Casteel SW: Fescue. In Plumlee K, editor: *Clinical veterinary toxicology*, St Louis, 2004, Mosby Elsevier, pp 243–250.

AUTHOR: **TIM J. EVANS**

EDITOR: **CYNTHIA L. GASKILL**

Fibrotic Myopathy

BASIC INFORMATION

DEFINITION

A mechanical lameness characterized by an abrupt shortening of the forward swing of one or both pelvic limbs with a characteristic "slapping" of the affected hoof onto the ground

SYNONYM(S)

Ossifying myopathy

EPIDEMIOLOGY

SPECIES, AGE, SEX
- Horses: Average age of 8.7 years in one study and 11.8 years in another study
- Mares are overrepresented in one study

GENETICS AND BREED PREDISPOSITION Quarter Horse–related breeds are predisposed because of Western performance activities.

RISK FACTORS
- Overstretching trauma to the thigh musculature associated with reining maneuvers such as sliding stops
- Abscesses, injection reactions, or wounds in the semitendinosus muscle

ASSOCIATED CONDITIONS AND DISORDERS An identical gait can be seen with hind limb denervating disease such as equine motor neuron disease and peripheral neuropathy and with myopathies such as polysaccharide storage myopathy.

CLINICAL PRESENTATION

DISEASE FORMS/SUBTYPES
- Most often affects the distal semitendinosus muscle with occasional involvement of the gracilis, biceps femoris, and semimembranosus muscles.
- Unilateral signs are most often caused by trauma, although early peripheral neuropathy is still possible.
- If bilateral, consider an underlying denervation or myopathy.

HISTORY, CHIEF COMPLAINT Prior trauma resulting in increased muscle tension (eg, sliding stops, slipping, catching a hind leg in a halter) or localized muscle damage caused by wounds or injections

PHYSICAL EXAM FINDINGS
- The abnormal gait is characteristic. The gait abnormality is most obvious at a walk, becomes less noticeable to absent at a trot, and is rarely seen at a canter.
- Palpable abnormalities such as fibrous to bony thickening may be present in the affected muscle, most often the distal semitendinosus muscle.

ETIOLOGY AND PATHOPHYSIOLOGY Reduced muscle elasticity from fibrosis secondary to physical trauma or chronic denervation or caused by myopathy, results in abnormal limb biomechanics.

DIAGNOSIS

INITIAL DATABASE

- Observation of gait
- Palpation of the hind limb musculature

TREATMENT

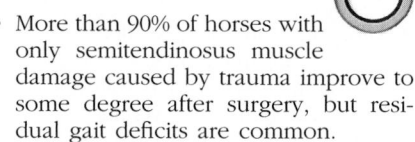

THERAPEUTIC GOAL(S)

Increase muscle elasticity to improve limb biomechanics

ACUTE GENERAL TREATMENT

Antiinflammatory (eg, nonsteroidal antiinflammatory drug) therapy if treated immediately after predisposing injury

CHRONIC TREATMENT

- Horses with traumatic injury resulting in fibrosis often respond to surgery (eg, semitendinosus myotenectomy, myotomy, or tenotomy).

- Cases caused by neuropathy or myopathy are less likely to respond to surgery.
- Horses with polysaccharide storage myopathy can be treated with diet and exercise (see "Polysaccharide Storage Myopathy" in this section).
- Horses with neuropathy caused by equine motor neuron disease can be treated with high doses (≥10,000 IU) of vitamin E.

POSSIBLE COMPLICATIONS

Wound dehiscence or infection after surgery

RECOMMENDED MONITORING

Regular examination

PROGNOSIS AND OUTCOME

- More than 90% of horses with only semitendinosus muscle damage caused by trauma improve to some degree after surgery, but residual gait deficits are common.
- Horses with traumatic damage to multiple muscles may not respond as well to surgery.
- Horses with polysaccharide storage myopathy improve with diet change.
- Horses with neuropathy are unlikely to respond to any therapy, and the disease process may progress.

PEARLS & CONSIDERATIONS

COMMENTS

Fibrotic myopathy is not a diagnosis; rather, it is a clinical sign of a mechanical lameness that may have a variety of causes.

PREVENTION

Minimize trauma to the caudal thigh muscles.

CLIENT EDUCATION

Fibrotic myopathy does not appear to be painful. Some degree of gait deficit may persist despite therapy, but horses can still be functional.

SUGGESTED READING

Gomez-Villamandos R, Santisteban J, Ruiz I, Avila I: Tenotomy of the tibial insertion of the semitendinosus muscle of two horses with fibrotic myopathy. *Vet Rec* 136:67–68, 1995.

Magee AA, Vatistas NJ: Standing semitendinosus myotomy for the treatment of fibrotic myopathy in 39 horses (1989–1997). *Proc Am Assoc Eq Pract* 44:263–264, 1998.

Turner AS, Trotter GW: Fibrotic myopathy in the horse. *J Am Vet Med Assoc* 184:335–338, 1984.

Valentine BA, Rousselle SD, Sams AE, et al: Denervation atrophy in three horses with fibrotic myopathy. *J Am Vet Med Assoc* 205:332–336, 1994.

AUTHOR: BETH A. VALENTINE

EDITOR: ANDRIS J. KANEPS

Flail Chest

BASIC INFORMATION

DEFINITION

Three or more consecutive fractured ribs, allowing a section of the rib cage to float freely

SYNONYM(S)

Multiple rib fractures

EPIDEMIOLOGY

SPECIES, AGE, SEX

- Rare in adult horses because of the magnitude of force required to fracture multiple ribs
- Foals may develop a flail segment secondary to rib fractures sustained in parturition.
- Flail chest is rare in foals; rib fractures are usually singular (one per rib).

ASSOCIATED CONDITIONS AND DISORDERS

- Pneumothorax
- Pneumomediastinum
- Hemothorax
- Pulmonary contusions
- Pleuritis
- Cardiac contusions

CLINICAL PRESENTATION

HISTORY, CHIEF COMPLAINT

- History
  - Trauma (eg, hit by car)
  - Dystocia
  - Thoracic wounds
- Chief complaint: Increased respiratory rate and effort

PHYSICAL EXAM FINDINGS

- Paradoxical movement of the flail segment
  - In with inspiration
  - Out with expiration
- Tachypnea, dyspnea
- Tachycardia, arrhythmias
- Circulatory compromise (pale mucous membranes, cool extremities, poor pulse quality)
- Crepitus or depression at the site of the fractures
- Wounds or other injuries related to the inciting cause

ETIOLOGY AND PATHOPHYSIOLOGY

- Fractured ribs are caused by trauma (external blunt force, penetrating injuries) or compression because of abnormal presentation during parturition.
- Respiratory dysfunction is likely caused by a pulmonary contusion, pneumothorax, or pleural effusion secondary to the initiating trauma rather than the flail segment itself.
- Pulmonary trauma results in atelectasis, edema, and hypoventilation, which results in hypoxemia through decreased diffusion of oxygen and ventilation-perfusion mismatching.
- Pain amplifies hypoxia through decreased tidal volume and hypoventilation.

DIAGNOSIS

DIFFERENTIAL DIAGNOSIS

Rib fractures without a flail chest

INITIAL DATABASE

- Physical examination, rebreathing exam, thoracic ultrasonography, arterial blood gas, serum lactate
- Complete blood count, serum chemistry indicated for evaluation of concurrent injury or infection

ADVANCED OR CONFIRMATORY TESTING

- Electrocardiography (ECG) for cardiac arrhythmias caused by cardiac contusion
- Thoracic radiographs are insensitive in identifying fractures in horses.

TREATMENT

THERAPEUTIC GOAL(S)

- Relieve pain
- Improve oxygenation
- Treat concurrent traumatic injuries

ACUTE GENERAL TREATMENT

- Analgesia
  - Nonsteroidal antiinflammatory drugs
    - Flunixin meglumine: 1.1 mg/kg IV q12h
    - Phenylbutazone: 2.2 mg/kg IV q12h
  - Opioids (may cause ileus)
    - Morphine: 0.05 to 0.1 mg/kg IV q12–24h up to q6h if IM
    - Combine with detomidine (5 µg/kg) or acepromazine (0.02–0.05 mg/kg) to reduce excitement
    - Butorphanol (13 µg/kg/h continuous rate infusion)
    - Variable pain relief
    - Fentanyl patch: Two to three 100-µg/h patches per 1000 lb
    - Absorption not consistent
  - Local anesthetic infusion: Caudal to rib; dorsal to fractures
    - Bupivacaine
    - Mepivacaine
- Respiratory and circulatory support
  - Nasal oxygen (5–15 L/min): Provides an FiO$_2$ of up to 40%
  - Mechanical ventilation: Indicated if PaO$_2$ remains below 60 mm Hg or SpO$_2$ remains below 90% despite oxygen therapy
  - Thoracocentesis for removal of pneumothorax or hemothorax
    - Required only if inhibiting oxygenation
    - Drainage of hemothorax may induce acute hemorrhage caused by clot disruption
  - Fluid therapy for cardiovascular shock (crystalloids, colloids, hypertonic saline)
- Wound management
  - Debridement, suturing, packing
  - Seal open chest wounds with stent bandages or plastic occlusive bandages or plastic wrap
  - Antibiotics
  - Tetanus prophylaxis

- Fracture stabilization in foals
  - Required only for fractures that risk cardiac perforation
  - Plate fixation ± cerclage wires

POSSIBLE COMPLICATIONS

- Concurrent head injury may necessitate ventilation because of central respiratory depression.

RECOMMENDED MONITORING

- Monitor for respiratory fatigue as an indication for mechanical ventilation.
  - Tachypnea or bradypnea
  - PaO_2 below 60 mm Hg on nasal oxygen
  - $PaCO_2$ above 60 mm Hg on nasal oxygen
  - PaO_2/FiO_2 ratio below 200
- Monitor arrhythmias with continuous ECG

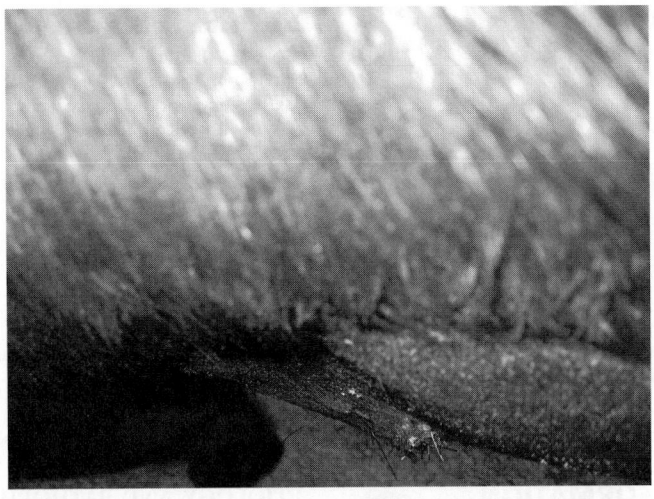

FIGURE 1 Flail chest. In this image of the left thorax, taken from above, note the depression where the flail segment lies.

PROGNOSIS AND OUTCOME

- Adult horses have a poor prognosis. The majority of adult horses succumb to the extensive trauma that caused the flail chest.
- Foals have a good prognosis with therapy. The extent of concurrent injuries may decrease the prognosis.

PEARLS & CONSIDERATIONS

Thoracic bandages may limit chest excursion and increase hypoxemia.

SUGGESTED READING

Bellezzo F, Hunt RJ, Provost R, et al: Surgical repair of rib fractures in 14 neonatal foals: case selection, surgical technique and results. *Equine Vet J* 36(7):557–562, 2004.
Hassel DH: Thoracic trauma in horses. *Vet Clin North Am Equine Pract* 23:67–80, 2007.

AUTHOR: **AMELIA MUNSTERMAN**

EDITORS: **REED HANSON** and **AMELIA MUNSTERMANN**

Fractures: Mandible and Maxilla

BASIC INFORMATION

DEFINITION

- Mandibular fractures are the most common type of fracture of the equine head. The incisive plate (rostral portion of the mandible), interdental space, horizontal ramus (caudal), and vertical ramus or the mandibular condyle (within the temporomandibular joint) can all be affected. Anatomical considerations when assessing these fractures should include the position of the parotid duct (emptying into the mouth adjacent to the fourth premolar (third cheek tooth, X08), the facial vein and artery, and the mental nerve foramen.
- Maxillary fractures are less common than mandibular fractures. Involvement of the premaxilla (incisive), frontal, nasal, and maxillary bones are most common. Paranasal sinus involvement may also complicate case management.

CLINICAL PRESENTATION

CLINICAL SIGNS

- Anorexia, difficulty prehending feed, quidding, ptyalism, halitosis, swelling, heat, pain
- In the case of maxillary fractures, there may only be a puncture wound or depression in the contour of the skull.

PHYSICAL EXAM FINDINGS

- Visual examination of incisor occlusion: In some fractures, disruption of the integrity of the mandible results in offset incisors (laterally), tipped lower incisors (relative to the maxilla), or missing teeth.
- Complete oral examination (sedation, full-mouth speculum, light source, and mirror): In some cases, because of the presence of significant pain, this can only be achieved using general anesthesia. Fractures are frequently open and significantly contaminated. It is important that injuries are not exacerbated during oral examination.

DIAGNOSIS

INITIAL DATABASE

Imaging Modalities

- Radiography: Adequately exposed radiographs should include at a minimum the lateromedial, dorsoventral, and two oblique projections. An offset dorsoventral projection is sometimes useful, especially in rostral fractures. This is achieved by moving the mandible across the midline immediately before exposure. This places the rostral portion of the horizontal ramus and incisor teeth in the middle of the radiograph to minimize the overlap by other bony anatomy. An intraoral ventrodorsal projection may also be of use.
- Computed tomography (CT): In complex fractures in which significant dental involvement is predicted by clinical and radiographic examination, CT examination before surgical intervention may augment surgical planning.

- Ultrasonography: Marginal and body fractures of the mandibular ramus as well as those of the maxilla can be imaged using ultrasonography. This is particularly useful where deep musculature may have splinted the fracture, leading to minimal swelling despite clinical and historical evidence of pain and anorexia. A 10-MHz linear probe is used by the author.

TREATMENT

ACUTE GENERAL TREATMENT

Fracture stabilization:
- Unilateral, nondisplaced fractures may be managed conservatively.
- Surgical intervention is required when the fracture fragments are displaced and there is instability. Techniques used include intraoral wiring, wiring combined with intramedullary pins or lag screws, and intraoral U-bar

or polymethylmethacrylate (PMMA) splints. Type I or II external fixator, lag screw, or orthopedic plate fixations may also be used.
- Involved teeth should not be automatically removed. They may provide essential stability to the resultant fracture fixation. Additionally (especially with incisor teeth), inclusion in a repair may result in dental retention. Every attempt should be made to *not* place an implant through the structure of a tooth (eg, a bone screw) during the fixation process. The hypsodont nature of the equine dentition is such that the process of continued eruption will be compromised, and future pathology is likely to occur.
- Maxillary fractures involving the paranasal sinuses: In some cases, minimally invasive elevation of fractured fragments may confer normality to the contour of the skull. In more extensive cases, repair can be achieved using cuttable bone plates.

POSSIBLE COMPLICATIONS

- Implant infection and loosening
- Sequestrum formation
- Dental loss and opposing tooth overgrowth

RECOMMENDED MONITORING

Recheck in 3 to 6 months. Ensure dental viability and eruption. Implant removal should be done if infected.

PROGNOSIS AND OUTCOME

Good, assuming stability has been conferred to the fractures

SUGGESTED READING

Auer JA: Craniomaxillofacial disorders. In Auer JA, Stick JA, editors: *Equine surgery*, ed 3, St Louis, 2006, Saunders Elsevier, pp 1341–1362.

AUTHOR & EDITOR: **JAMES L. CARMALT**

Fractures: Metacarpal/Metatarsal Condyles

BASIC INFORMATION

DEFINITION

Fractures of the distal condyles of the third metacarpus/metatarsus (MC/MT-III). Fractures originate at the distal articular surface and propagate proximally in the sagittal plane.

SYNONYMS

These fractures are simply referred to as *condylar fractures* or longitudinal fractures of the third metacarpal/metatarsal condyles.

EPIDEMIOLOGY

SPECIES, AGE, SEX Condylar fractures occur predominantly in young racehorses.
GENETICS AND BREED PREDISPOSITION Condylar fractures are most commonly seen in Thoroughbred racehorses. They also occur in Standardbred racehorses; racing Arabians; and occasionally polo ponies, steeplechasers, and eventers.
RISK FACTORS Racing plates with long toe grabs and harder dirt surfaces have been proposed as risk factors based on results of epidemiologic studies.

CLINICAL PRESENTATION

DISEASE FORMS/SUBTYPES
- Fractures may involve either the lateral or medial condyle.

  ○ Lateral condylar fractures are either incomplete or complete (exit the ipsilateral cortex). The majority of complete fractures are displaced.
  ○ Medial condylar fractures rarely exit the ipsilateral cortex and instead have a propensity to propagate proximally into the diaphysis or proximal metaphysis. They do so in either a spiral configuration or in a sagittal plane that changes abruptly in mid-diaphysis to take on a Y-shaped configuration. This type (Y configuration) is at risk of catastrophic failure.

HISTORY, CHIEF COMPLAINT
- Most horses present with an acute onset of moderate to severe lameness during or shortly after a race or a workout. In some cases, horses finish the race well with no "bad step" perceived by the rider. With some incomplete fractures, lameness is not noted until the following day.
- Some horses have a history of pain ("soreness") and inflammation (heat and effusion) in the associated fetlock joint at some point in the days or weeks leading up to fracture.

PHYSICAL EXAM FINDINGS
- Horses with condylar fractures generally bear full weight on the limb and exhibit mild to severe lameness at the walk. Lameness in many cases improves rapidly so that by 24 to 48

hours, there may be minimal lameness at the walk (most evident on turns).
- Fetlock effusion is invariably present and is typically marked. Horses with complete lateral condylar fractures often have noticeable soft tissue swelling along the lateral aspect of the distal metaphysis. Pain on lower limb (fetlock) flexion is typically moderate to severe in the acute stage.

ETIOLOGY AND PATHOPHYSIOLOGY
- Condylar fractures are fatigue fractures resulting from accumulated high-speed cyclic strains.
- Subchondral microdamage develops where stress is concentrated along the condylar groove (junction between the condyle and sagittal ridge).
- Overt fracture occurs acutely and begins in the distal palmar/plantar aspect of the articular surface and propagates proximally between or along the sagitally oriented "plates" of trabecular bone.

DIAGNOSIS

DIFFERENTIAL DIAGNOSIS

Other intraarticular fractures of the fetlock joint

INITIAL DATABASE

- Physical examination in the vast majority of cases reliably identifies the fetlock joint as the site of injury.

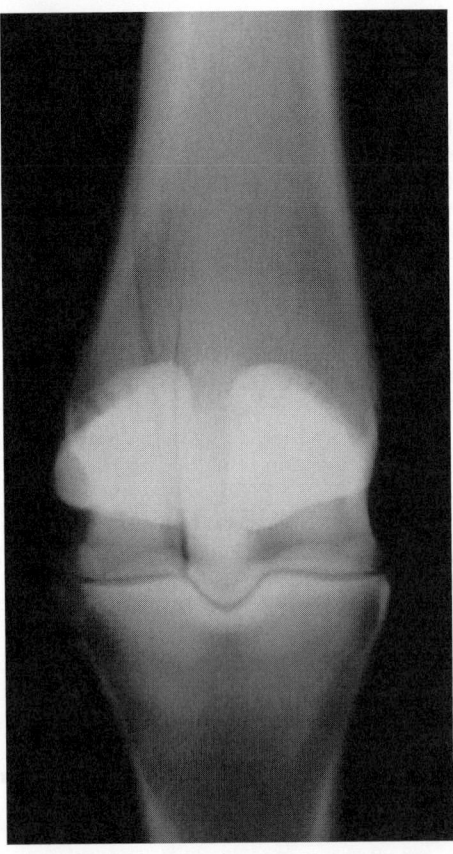

FIGURE 1 Dorsopalmar radiograph of the metacarpophalangeal joint of a horse with an incomplete lateral condylar fracture.

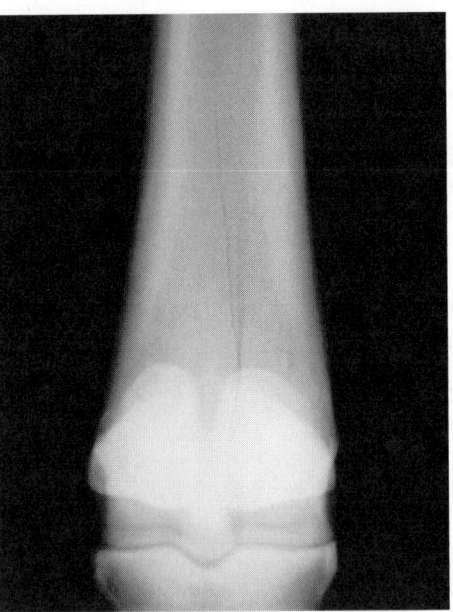

FIGURE 3 Dorsopalmar radiograph of the metacarpus of a horse with a medial condylar fracture.

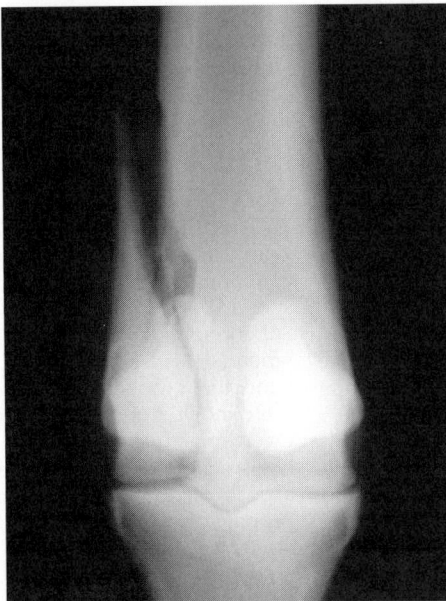

FIGURE 2 Dorsopalmar radiograph of the metacarpophalangeal joint of a horse with a complete, displaced, lateral condyle fracture.

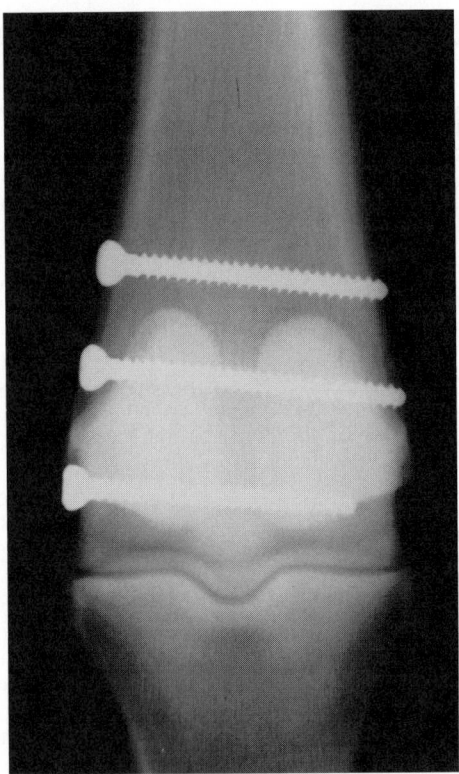

FIGURE 4 Postoperative dorsopalmar radiograph of the metacarpophalangeal joint of a horse following screw fixation of a lateral condylar fracture.

- Radiographs confirm the diagnosis.
- Radiographs should include the four standard views as well as a flexed dorsopalmar/plantar projection to aid in detection of articular comminution (Figures 1 to 3).

ADVANCED OR CONFIRMATORY TESTING

- In rare cases (typically short, chronic, incomplete fractures) diagnostic analgesia (low four-point block or IA anesthesia) is helpful to confirm the fetlock as the site of pain.
- Nuclear scintigraphy may prove useful in these same cases.

TREATMENT

THERAPEUTIC GOALS

- Promote fracture healing and minimize degenerative changes in the affected joint.
- With medial condylar fractures, avoiding catastrophic failure is also paramount.

ACUTE GENERAL TREATMENT

- Stall confinement, bandaging, and systemic antiinflammatory drugs.
- Rigid, full-limb external coaptation is indicated after diagnosis of any propagating medial condylar fracture.

CHRONIC TREATMENT

- Surgical repair using cortical screws in a lag fashion (Figure 4).
- Screws in lateral condylar fractures are inserted through individual stab incisions.
- Complete lateral condylar fractures are reduced under arthroscopic control.
- All medial condylar fractures with a mid-diaphyseal Y configuration or those with fracture lines that do not spiral and end abruptly in the mid-diaphysis should be repaired with a combination of lag screws and application of a dynamic compression plate or locking compression plate.
- Medial condylar fractures with a radiographically confirmed spiral configuration may be repaired with lag screws alone, but many surgeons opt for plate stabilization as added security.

- Nonsurgical management is an option for selected incomplete fractures.

POSSIBLE COMPLICATIONS

- The most devastating complication is a catastrophic failure in cases of medial condylar fracture.
- Insufficient fracture reduction and failure to accurately realign the articular surface in repairing displaced fractures invariably results in debilitating arthritis.

RECOMMENDED MONITORING

Follow-up radiographs are taken to monitor fracture healing.

PROGNOSIS AND OUTCOME

- The prognosis for nondisplaced condylar fractures is generally good to very good (70%–90% return to athletic soundness).
- The prognosis for displaced condylar fractures in the forelimbs of Thoroughbred racehorses is guarded to fair (<50% return to athletic soundness).
- The presence of degenerative joint disease, concurrent proximal sesamoid fracture, or other significant IA pathology imparts a lower prognosis.
- Concurrent axial fracture of a proximal sesamoid bone is almost always associated with a poor prognosis.

PEARLS & CONSIDERATIONS

COMMENTS

- Most horses can resume training 4 to 5 months after surgical repair.
- The author does not routinely remove screws before training commences, although some surgeons do.
- Plates must be removed from cases of medial condylar fracture if athletic use is anticipated.

PREVENTION

- Carefully monitor for early detection of pathology in and around the fetlock.
- Avoid shoes with long toe grabs.
- Have the horse race and train on grass or synthetic surfaces.

SUGGESTED READING

Bassage LH: Metacarpus/metatarsus. In Hinchcliff KW, Kaneps AJ, Geor RJ, editors: *Equine sports medicine and surgery*, London, 2004, Saunders Elsevier, pp 319–348.

Richardson DW: Metacarpal and metatarsal bones. In Auer JA, Stick JA, editors: *Equine surgery*, ed 3, St Louis, 2006, Saunders Elsevier, pp 1238–1253.

Schneider RK, Jackman BR: Fractures of the third metacarpus and metatarsus. In Nixon AJ, editor: *Equine fracture repair*, Philadelphia, 1996, Saunders Elsevier, pp 179–194.

AUTHOR: **LANCE H. BASSAGE II**

EDITOR: **ANDRIS J. KANE**

Fractures: Middle Phalanx

BASIC INFORMATION

DEFINITION

Fractures of the middle phalanx may be classified as osteochondral chip fractures, uniaxial or biaxial fracture of the medial or lateral eminence of the middle phalanx, axial fractures, or comminuted middle phalanx fractures

SYNONYM(S)

P2 fracture

EPIDEMIOLOGY

SPECIES, AGE, SEX Fractures of the middle phalanx occur in horses of all ages, including foals. However, fractures at this location happen most commonly in the hindlimbs of middle-aged (4–10 years) Western performance horses and polo horses.

GENETICS AND BREED PREDISPOSITION Quarter Horses are the most commonly represented breed, although all breeds may be affected.
RISK FACTORS Athletic activities that involve abrupt stops or turns such as those that occur during cutting, roping, barrel racing, pole bending, and polo

CLINICAL PRESENTATION

HISTORY, CHIEF COMPLAINT Acute moderate to severe lameness that may occur during athletic activity or in paddock turnout
PHYSICAL EXAM FINDINGS
- Osteochondral chip fractures
  - Mild to moderate lameness
  - May be an incidental finding
  - Respond to diagnostic anesthesia of the proximal interphalangeal joint
- Uniaxial palmar or plantar eminence fractures

  - Moderate to severe lameness
  - Pain on manipulation
  - Instability or crepitus (usually not present)
- Biaxial palmar or plantar eminence and comminuted fractures
  - Severe non–weight-bearing lameness
  - Pain on manipulation
  - Joint instability and crepitus

ETIOLOGY AND PATHOPHYSIOLOGY

- The hind limbs are more likely to sustain a fracture than the forelimbs.
- Comminuted fractures are the most common fracture type.
- Comminuted fractures result from the complex forces that occur when the horse pivots on the hind limb with the foot fixed relative to the digit.
- Eminence fractures may result from avulsion of the bony insertion of the superficial digital flexor tendon.

DIAGNOSIS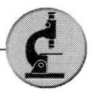

DIFFERENTIAL DIAGNOSIS

- Fracture of the proximal or distal phalanx
- Luxation of the proximal interphalangeal joint
- Sole abscess

INITIAL DATABASE

- Localization of the lameness with physical examination and manipulation of the distal limb
- Complete radiographic evaluation of the middle phalanx
- Complete blood count and serum biochemistry panel

ADVANCED OR CONFIRMATORY TESTING

Computed tomography or magnetic resonance imaging may help define fracture configuration and aid in fracture repair planning.

TREATMENT

THERAPEUTIC GOALS

- Restoration of limb function
- Restoration of the normal pastern joint angle
- Limit development of osteoarthritis in the distal interphalangeal joint

ACUTE GENERAL TREATMENT

First aid stabilization:
- With the limb held off the ground, a light padded bandage is applied from the proximal metacarpus/metatarsus to just distal to the coronary band. A rigid splint (polyvinyl chloride) is taped to the dorsum (forelimb) or plantar surface (hindlimb) of the bandage to maintain axial alignment of the dorsal cortices of the metacarpus/metatarsus and phalanges. The bandage and foot are then encased in fiberglass cast material to temporarily stabilize the fracture for transport.
- Osteochondral chip fractures are treated by removal of the osteochondral fragments with arthroscopy or an open technique.
- All other fracture types are best treated with internal fixation and arthrodesis of the proximal interphalangeal joint.
- Arthrodesis is generally recommended because of the high likelihood of developing performance limiting osteoarthritis.
- With comminuted fractures the aim of surgical repair is reconstruction of the proximal and distal articular surfaces of the middle phalanx to preserve the distal interphalangeal joint.
- Select cases of comminuted fractures may be treated with transfixation pin casting.

CHRONIC TREATMENT

- After internal fixation, the horse is maintained in a distal limb cast for 4 to 6 weeks.
- After cast removal, the horse is supported with either a heavy bandage or a bandage cast.
- The horse is stall confined for a total of 3 to 4 months until there is radiographic evidence of fracture healing and arthrodesis of the joint.
- Handwalking usually begins at 2 to 3 months after surgery depending on the degree of lameness.
- Complete healing generally requires 6 to 8 months.

POSSIBLE COMPLICATIONS

- Implant failure
- Osteoarthritis of the distal interphalangeal joint
- Infection
- Persistent lameness
- Contra-limb laminitis

RECOMMENDED MONITORING

Radiographic evaluation at intervals until healing is complete

PROGNOSIS AND OUTCOME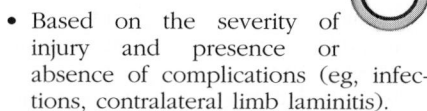

- Based on the severity of injury and presence or absence of complications (eg, infections, contralateral limb laminitis).
- Horses with osteochondral chip fractures have a good prognosis for return to soundness.
- Horses with uniaxial eminence fractures have a fair to favorable prognosis for return to athletic activity.
- Horses with biaxial eminence fractures have a fair prognosis for return to some level of athletic activity after arthrodesis.
- Horses with comminuted fractures have a guarded prognosis. Horses have returned to athletic activity, although some residual lameness is anticipated if there is inadequate reduction of the fracture fragments entering the distal interphalangeal joint.

PEARLS & CONSIDERATIONS

Comminuted unstable fractures are the most common fracture configuration and require early diagnosis and first aid and stabilization for transport to increase the likelihood of restoring some degree of athletic activity.

SUGGESTED READING

Nixon AJ: Phalanges and the metacarpophalangeal and metatarsophalangeal joints. In Auer JA, Stick JA, editors: *Equine surgery.* ed 3, Philadelphia, 2006, Saunders Elsevier, pp 1217–1222.

Watkins JP: Fractures of the middle phalanx. In Nixon AJ, editor: *Equine fracture repair*, Philadelphia, 1996, WB Saunders, pp 129–145.

AUTHOR: KELLY FARNSWORTH

EDITOR: ANDRIS J. KANEPS

Fractures: Physeal

BASIC INFORMATION

DEFINITION

Fractures of any bone involving the physis or growth plate

SYNONYM(S)

- Growth plate fracture
- Salter-Harris–type fracture

EPIDEMIOLOGY

ASSOCIATED CONDITIONS AND DISORDERS

- Angular limb deformity
- Juvenile arthritis
- Support limb breakdown
- Growth plate infection

CLINICAL PRESENTATION

DISEASE FORMS/SUBTYPES

The Salter-Harris fracture classification is a guide for determination of prognosis and treatment options:
- Type I: Fracture through the physis (involves only the zone of hypertrophied chondrocytes); most common

- Type II: Fracture across the physis and extends into a portion of the metaphysis
- Type III: Fracture involving the physis and epiphysis (this type extends into the joint)
- Type IV: Fracture involving the physis, epiphysis, and metaphysis (this type also extends into the joint)
- Type V: Compression injury of the physis
- Type VI: Periosteal bridging between the metaphysis and epiphysis

HISTORY, CHIEF COMPLAINT
- Lameness, swelling, limb deviation, recumbency, and reluctance to stand or bear weight on the affected limb

PHYSICAL EXAM FINDINGS
- Varying degree of lameness, but usually grade 3 to 5 of 5
- Pain upon palpation of the injured area
- Swelling
- Possible instability of the limb
- Possible angular deviation of the limb distal to the fracture

ETIOLOGY AND PATHOPHYSIOLOGY
The vast majority of physeal fractures are traumatic in origin. The physis is weaker than bone, ligament, tendons, and joint capsule. Therefore, the growth plate is the most vulnerable aspect of the immature musculoskeletal system. Bending, shearing, torsional, tensile, or compressive forces are sufficient to result in physeal fractures.

DIAGNOSIS

DIFFERENTIAL DIAGNOSIS
- Infectious physitis
- Infectious arthritis
- Joint luxation or subluxation
- Foot abscess

INITIAL DATABASE
- Physical examination and digital palpation
- Examination of locomotion

ADVANCED OR CONFIRMATORY TESTING
Radiographic evaluation

TREATMENT

THERAPEUTIC GOALS
- Stabilization of the fracture
- Immediate improvement of comfort level

- Even weight bearing across all limbs
- Minimal limb deformity

ACUTE GENERAL TREATMENT
- The neonate limb responds poorly to external coaptation; therefore, internal fixation is preferred.
- A major difficulty in surgical stabilization may be the small size of the epiphysis for implant purchase. This problem has been partially overcome with the use of cross pins, transfixation pins, tension-band wiring, or T-plates.
- Conservative management with external coaptation is often unsuccessful because it results in extreme limb laxity. Also, it is not possible in foals with femoral and proximal tibial physeal fractures.
- Returning a fractured limb to weight bearing as soon as possible is important to protect the other limbs (especially the contralateral limb) from overload. Young bones are very susceptible to maldevelopment if overloaded.

CHRONIC TREATMENT
- Monitor for signs of infection. Treat quickly and aggressively if suspected.
- Monitor for signs of inappropriate stabilization and remedy immediately if suspected.
- Assist in maintaining even weight bearing and appropriate levels of comfort (pain management drugs, including nonsteroidal antiinflammatory drugs and opioids).

POSSIBLE COMPLICATIONS
- Fracture fixation or implant failure
- Infection (septic physitis or osteomyelitis)
- Cast sores
- Residual lameness
- Muscle atrophy
- Tendon contracture or laxity
- Angular limb deformity of the contralateral limb
- Angular limb deformity of affected limb (rare)
- Limb length discrepancy (rare)

RECOMMENDED MONITORING
Monitor for signs of residual lameness, angular limb deformity, flexural limb deformity, and limb length discrepancy. Also monitor for signs of gastrointestinal discomfort caused by the stress and use of nonsteroidal drugs.

PROGNOSIS AND OUTCOME

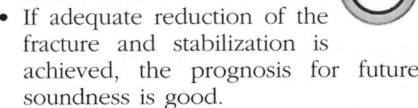

- If adequate reduction of the fracture and stabilization is achieved, the prognosis for future soundness is good.
- Types I and II Salter-Harris fractures are most common and involve the third metacarpal or metatarsal bones. The prognosis is good for healing without lameness.
- In general, prognosis decreases if the Salter-Harris classification number increases. However, other factors essential to prognosis include the severity of the trauma to the growth plate, the foal's age, the location of the injury, the time elapsed before treatment, the level of displacement, whether the injury is open or closed, and the integrity of the vasculature and accompanying soft tissue structures.

PEARLS & CONSIDERATIONS

COMMENTS
- Physeal fractures are the most common fracture in foals.
- Physeal fractures should be considered serious and addressed immediately because of the risk for abnormal or retarded growth patterns.

CLIENT EDUCATION
- Physeal fractures heal in approximately 50% of the time necessary for metaphyseal fractures.
- Younger foals appear to tolerate injury to the physis better than older foals.

SUGGESTED READING
Embertson RM, Bramlage LR, Herring DS, et al: Physeal fractures in the horse: II. Management and outcome. *Vet Surg* 15:230–236, 1986.

Hance SR, Bramlage LR: Fractures of the femur and patella. In Nixon AJ, editor *Equine fracture repair*, Philadelphia, 1996, WB Saunders, pp 284–293.

Watkins JP: Fractures of the tibia. In Nixon AJ, editor: *Equine fracture repair*, Philadelphia, 1996, WB Saunders, pp 273–283.

AUTHOR: JARRED WILLIAMS

EDITORS: ELIZABETH M. SANTSCHI and **PHOEBE A. SMITH**

Fractures: Proximal Phalanx

BASIC INFORMATION

DEFINITION

Fractures of the proximal phalanx may be broadly classified as proximal intraarticular osteochondral fractures and fractures involving the diaphyseal region of the proximal phalanx.

SYNONYM(S)

- P1 fractures
- Long pastern fractures

EPIDEMIOLOGY

SPECIES, AGE, SEX

- Osteochondral fractures involving the proximal dorsal rim of the proximal phalanx are common in racehorses.
- Osteochondral fractures involving the proximopalmar/plantar aspect of P1 are seen in young athletic horses and are classified as type 1 when they are avulsed from the axial portion of proximal P1 and are mostly articular. Type 2 lesions are abaxial, larger, and have limited articular cartilage and are most commonly seen in the hindlimbs.
- Diaphyseal fractures are seen in horses of all ages and are typically the result of trauma.

CLINICAL PRESENTATION

HISTORY, CHIEF COMPLAINT

- Osteochondral fractures involving the proximal dorsal rim of P1 typically present with a history of several days of moderate lameness that may improve with rest.
- Type 1 osteochondral fractures involving the proximopalmar/plantar aspect of P1 typically present for mild lameness that may only be evident at higher speeds.
- Type 2 lesions are often found only on radiographic evaluation, and most do not cause lameness.
- Horses with diaphyseal fractures most often have a history of trauma or acute injury.

PHYSICAL EXAM FINDINGS

- Small osteochondral fractures demonstrate significant joint effusion and moderate pain on flexion.
- Horses with diaphyseal fractures present for moderate to severe lameness depending on the severity of the fracture and the instability of the limb.

ETIOLOGY AND PATHOPHYSIOLOGY

- Osteochondral fractures involving the proximal dorsal rim of the P1 are seen most commonly in racehorses and result from hyperextension of the metacarpophalangeal joint with impact on the dorsal region of the metacarpus.
- Osteochondral fractures involving the proximopalmar/plantar aspect of P1 were thought to be the result of osteochondrosis; however, recent evidence supports a fracture etiology.
- Diaphyseal fractures result from compressive and torsional forces transmitted from the sagittal ridge of the cannon bone through the sagittal groove propagating distally.

DIAGNOSIS

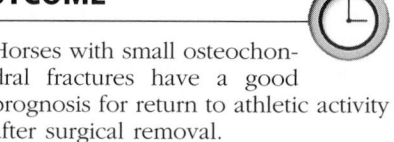

DIFFERENTIAL DIAGNOSIS

- Proximal sesamoid fractures
- Middle phalanx fractures
- Condylar fractures

INITIAL DATABASE

- Clinical examination localizing the lesion to the area.
- Complete radiographic evaluation.

ADVANCED OR CONFIRMATORY TESTING

Computed tomography may help with determining fracture configuration for surgical planning.

TREATMENT

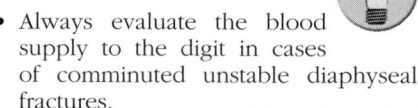

THERAPEUTIC GOAL(S)

- Restore limb function.
- Restore the normal metacarpophalangeal joint angle.
- Limit development of osteoarthritis.

ACUTE GENERAL TREATMENT

- Horses with osteochondral fractures involving the proximal dorsal rim of P1 are treated with arthroscopic removal of the fragments and cartilage debris.
- Horses with type 1 osteochondral fractures involving the proximopalmar/plantar aspect of P1 are treated with arthroscopic removal of the fragment when the lesions cause clinical lameness.
- Horses with type 2 lesions rarely require surgery; however, in select cases, surgical fixation of the fragment with a screw placed in lag fashion may be required.
- First aid stabilization of diaphyseal fractures
- With the limb held off the ground, a light padded bandage is applied from the proximal metacarpus or metatarsus to just distal to the coronary band. A rigid splint (polyvinyl chloride) is taped to the dorsum (forelimb) or plantar surface (hindlimb) of the bandage to maintain alignment of the dorsal cortices of the metacarpus or metatarsus and phalanges. The bandage and foot are then encased in fiberglass cast material to temporarily stabilize the fracture for transport.
- Diaphyseal fractures require treatment with internal fixation, external fixation, or a combination of both in many cases.
- Reconstruction of comminuted diaphyseal fractures requires at least one piece of intact bone spanning its length (also referred to as a *strut*) to which other fragments can be anchored.
- In severely comminuted fractures, external fixation alone may provide the best option.

PROGNOSIS AND OUTCOME

- Horses with small osteochondral fractures have a good prognosis for return to athletic activity after surgical removal.
- The prognosis for diaphyseal fractures depends on the fracture configuration and amount of displacement.
- Horses with minimally displaced fractures have a good prognosis for survival and return to work.
- Horses with displaced comminuted fractures have a guarded prognosis for survival and a poor prognosis for athletic activity.

PEARLS & CONSIDERATIONS

- Always evaluate the blood supply to the digit in cases of comminuted unstable diaphyseal fractures.
- Osteoarthritis is the likely sequela of any fracture where the joint surface cannot be perfectly reconstructed and may be the limiting factor in return to soundness.

SUGGESTED READING

Nixon AJ: Phalanges and the metacarpophalangeal and metatarsophalangeal joints. In Auer JA, Stick JA, editors: *Equine surgery.* ed 3, Philadelphia, 2006, Saunders Elsevier, pp 1223–1227.

Richardson DW: Fractures of the proximal phalanx. In Nixon AJ, editor: *Equine fracture repair*, Philadelphia, 1996, WB Saunders, pp 117–128.

AUTHOR: **KELLY FARNSWORTH**

EDITOR: **ANDRIS J. KANEPS**

Fractures: Proximal Sesamoid Bones

BASIC INFORMATION

DEFINITION

Fractures of the proximal sesamoid bones may be classified as apical, midbody, basilar, abaxial, axial, sagittal, or comminuted.

EPIDEMIOLOGY

SPECIES, AGE, SEX Common injuries in racing Thoroughbreds, Standardbreds, and Quarter Horses. The forelimbs are most commonly affected in Thoroughbreds (right front) and Quarter Horses. The hind limbs are most frequently affected in Standardbreds (left hind).

CLINICAL PRESENTATION

HISTORY, CHIEF COMPLAINT

- Moderate to severe lameness developing either during exercise or racing or within 24 hours
- Lameness may or may not improve with rest.

PHYSICAL EXAM FINDINGS

- All except abaxial nonarticular fractures result in metacarpophalangeal or metatarsophalangeal joint effusion and moderate to severe lameness.
- The horse may have soft tissue swelling around the sesamoid bones.
- Weight bearing on the toe is common.
- Mild to moderate pain on flexion of the fetlock joint is seen.

ETIOLOGY AND PATHOPHYSIOLOGY

- Occur as a result of excessive tension on the suspensory apparatus
- Hyperextension during maximal loading may produce tensile forces on the sesamoid bones, exceeding their internal strength.
- Sufficient exercise results in increased strength of the suspensory ligament, increasing the likelihood of sesamoid fractures versus injury to the suspensory ligament in unfit horses.

DIAGNOSIS

DIFFERENTIAL DIAGNOSIS

- Proximal phalanx fracture
- Third metacarpal or metatarsal condylar fracture
- Suspensory ligament injury

INITIAL DATABASE

- Complete radiographic evaluation, including standard dorsopalmar, lateral medial, and oblique projections
- Other views to consider include flexed lateral and a skyline view of the abaxial surface of the sesamoid bones.
- Evaluation of the blood supply to the digit if breakdown of the suspensory apparatus (identified as a dropped fetlock joint on weight bearing) is apparent

TREATMENT

THERAPEUTIC GOAL(S)

- Restoration of limb function
- Return to soundness

ACUTE GENERAL TREATMENT

- Most horses not intended for further athletic careers may be treated conservatively with support bandages, splinting, or casting with stall rest.
- Severe injuries in these horses may require use of a splint such as the Kimzey leg saver that places the horse on its toe and relieves suspensory tension.
- Apical fractures are almost always articular and treated with removal of the apical fragment up to one third of the proximodistal dimension via either arthroscopy or arthrotomy.
- Midbody fractures are repaired with internal fixation with either lag screw placement or circumferential wiring.
- Basilar fractures are repaired with internal fixation using circumferential wiring when they involve the entire base or by fragment removal when they are small.
- Abaxial fractures are usually nonarticular and do not require surgery. Articular abaxial fractures are treated with arthroscopic removal of the fragments.
- Sagittal fractures tend to occur in conjunction with other injuries to the fetlock joint; they are treated with lag screw fixation.
- Comminuted and biaxial fractures are best treated with fetlock arthrodesis.

CHRONIC TREATMENT

- Horses with apical fractures treated by removal of osteochondral fragments

are typically stall confined for 30 to 60 days, depending on the amount of suspensory ligament disruption, followed by a slow return to exercise.
- Internal fixation is usually supplemented with a lower limb cast for 1 to 4 weeks with a total convalescence of 10 to 12 months.

POSSIBLE COMPLICATIONS

- Implant failure
- Persistent lameness

RECOMMENDED MONITORING

- Periodic radiographic follow-up to determine the degree of repair if internal fixation was used
- Ultrasonographic evaluation of the suspensory ligament before initiating rehabilitative exercise

PROGNOSIS AND OUTCOME

- Horses with apical fractures have a good prognosis (~65%) for return to some degree of athletic activity with surgery.
- Horses with midbody fractures repaired with internal fixation also have a good chance of returning to athletic activity.
- Horses with basilar fractures that involve less than 25% of the base and can be removed surgically also have almost a 60% chance of returning to soundness.
- Horses with larger basilar fractures have a guarded prognosis for return to athletic activity.
- Horses with comminuted and biaxial fractures have a poor prognosis for return to soundness and typically require fetlock arthrodesis to salvage the animals as pets or for breeding.

PEARLS & CONSIDERATIONS

The suspensory ligament should be carefully evaluated with ultrasonography in all cases to determine the amount of damage to the ligament because suspensory desmitis may ultimately become the limiting factor in the horse's return to soundness.

SUGGESTED READING

Bertone AL: Fractures of the proximal sesamoid bones. In Nixon AJ, editor: *Equine fracture repair*, Philadelphia, 1996, WB Saunders, pp 163–171.

Nixon AJ: Phalanges and the metacarpophalangeal and metatarsophalangeal joints. In Auer JA, Stick JA, editors: *Equine surgery*, ed 3, Philadelphia, 2006, Saunders Elsevier, pp 1228–1230.

AUTHOR: **KELLY FARNSWORTH**

EDITOR: **ANDRIS J. KANEPS**

Fractures: Rib in the Neonate

BASIC INFORMATION

DEFINITION

Separation of a rib into two or more pieces under stress

SYNONYM(S)

- Broken rib
- Flail chest

EPIDEMIOLOGY

SPECIES, AGE, SEX Most occurrences are at the time of parturition.

RISK FACTORS
- Large birth weight of foal
- Dystocia

CLINICAL PRESENTATION

HISTORY, CHIEF COMPLAINT
- Rib fractures detected during routine well foal examination
- Tachypnea, flail chest
- Attitude and appetite are often normal.

PHYSICAL EXAM FINDINGS
- Groaning or grunting by the foal, subcutaneous edema over the ribs and axilla near the elbows, pain and crepitus on palpation of the affected rib(s)
- Flail chest: Paradoxical movement of a segment of the chest wall separated from the rest by multiple adjacent fractured ribs

ETIOLOGY AND PATHOPHYSIOLOGY
- Trauma to the ribcage during parturition is believed to be the most significant factor associated with rib fractures. Postnatal trauma could also result in rib fractures.
- Most fractures are located very near the costochondral junction. The distal piece of the fragmented rib typically displaces axially.
- Laceration of the myocardium and or great vessels is fatal.

DIAGNOSIS

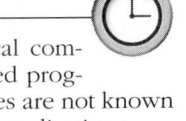

DIFFERENTIAL DIAGNOSIS

Displaced versus nondisplaced rib fractures

INITIAL DATABASE

- Careful palpation of the ribcage
- Thoracic ultrasonography: More sensitive than radiography in detecting rib fractures; hemothorax may be present if the rib fragment lacerates pulmonary tissue

TREATMENT

THERAPEUTIC GOALS

- Prevent fatal laceration by rib fragment.
- Prevent respiratory distress.
- Minimize pulmonary contusion.
- Prevent infection.

ACUTE GENERAL TREATMENT

- Confinement to a stall or small pen; minimize movement by use of sedation
- Use antiinflammatory drugs judiciously to maintain low activity level.
- Blood transfusion if laceration has resulted in signs of hypovolemia and hypoxia.
- Broad-spectrum antibiotics
- Surgical stabilization of rib fragments in cases of fragments near the heart

CHRONIC TREATMENT

Four to 6 weeks of confinement is recommended to allow for healing of the fracture

POSSIBLE COMPLICATIONS

- Myocardial, vascular, or pulmonary laceration
- Diaphragmatic hernia
- Hemothorax
- Pneumothorax
- Death

RECOMMENDED MONITORING

Serial ultrasound evaluations to determine healing of fracture

PROGNOSIS AND OUTCOME

Rib fractures with clinical complications have a guarded prognosis. Healed rib fractures are not known to result in long-term complications.

PEARLS & CONSIDERATIONS

Careful palpation of the ribcage during routine well foal examinations will allow for detection of rib fractures.

SUGGESTED READING

Sprayberry KA, et al: 56 Case of rib fractures in neonatal foals hospitalized in a referral center intensive care unit from 1997–2001. *Proc Am Assoc Equine Pract* 47:395, 2001.

AUTHOR: **PHOEBE A. SMITH**

EDITORS: **ELIZABETH M. SANTSCHI** and **PHOEBE A. SMITH**

Fractures: Small Splint Bones

BASIC INFORMATION

DEFINITION

Fractures and proliferative periostitis of the second and fourth metacarpal/metatarsal bones (MC/MT-II and MC/MT-IV).

SYNONYM(S)

- "Splint bone" fractures
- A proliferative periostitis lesion is commonly known as a *splint*.

EPIDEMIOLOGY

SPECIES, AGE, SEX Proliferative periostitis affecting MC-II (and less frequently MC-IV) is commonly seen in young horses in early training.

RISK FACTORS

- Poor conformation, particularly at the carpus and tarsus, is a risk factor for proliferative periostitis of MC/MT-II and MC/MT-IV.
- Carpus or tarsus valgus or varus, and "offset knees" or "bench knees" exacerbate strains on these bones. Base narrow, toe-out conformation of the forelimbs may exacerbate the tendency for interference, specifically trauma to the contralateral MC-II.

ASSOCIATED CONDITIONS AND DISORDERS Concurrent suspensory desmitis is often seen in horses with fractures of the distal aspect of the small metacarpal/metatarsal bones.

CLINICAL PRESENTATION

DISEASE FORMS/SUBTYPES Splint bone fractures are divided into three types based on location: Proximal, midshaft, and distal (Figures 1 to 3).

HISTORY, CHIEF COMPLAINT

- Horses with proliferative periostitis have a history of either gradual (insidious) or acute onset of lameness. Lameness may be unilateral or bilateral and is usually mild to moderate. Lameness improves with rest and anti-inflammatory treatment and recurs with resumption of exercise. Sometimes a cosmetic blemish (focal hard swelling) is the first sign noted by the owner or trainer.
- Horses with splint bone fractures often have a history of external trauma (eg, a kick). Lameness in these cases is invariably acute and typically moderate to severe. Horses with fractures of the distal aspect that are associated with internal trauma (repetitive strain) and possibly a concurrent suspensory branch desmitis have a more variable history with onset being either acute or gradual and ranging from mild-to-moderate (rarely severe). Some distal splint fractures are discovered as incidental findings.

PHYSICAL EXAM FINDINGS

- A "splint" is recognized as a focal swelling along the shaft of the affected bone that is smooth and firm to hard on palpation. In some cases, the swelling is located axially, and the lesion can only be detected by palpation (most effectively with the limb held in flexion). Single lesions are most common, but multiple lesions affecting the same bone are sometimes present. Multiple lesions are most common on MC-II in young horses associated with early training. In this group, splints are also commonly bilateral. Horses exhibit variable degrees of pain on palpation of the splint. Pain is most severe in the acute stages and does not always correlate well with the degree of swelling or exostosis. Chronic splints, or those that have healed clinically, are typically not sensitive to palpation.
- Horses with distal splint bone fractures generally have very mild to moderate local soft tissue inflammation. The degree varies with the chronicity of the injury. Fractures that are more than 1 or 2 weeks old may have minimal residual associated swelling. Suspensory enlargement, most commonly of the associated branch, may also be present. Focal pain is common on firm palpation of the fracture site. If the

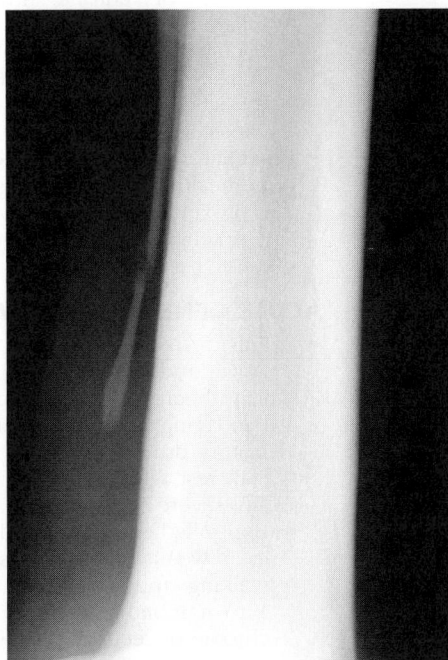

FIGURE 1 Dorsomedial-to-palmarolateral oblique radiograph of the left metacarpus of a horse with a typical fracture of the distal aspect of MC-II.

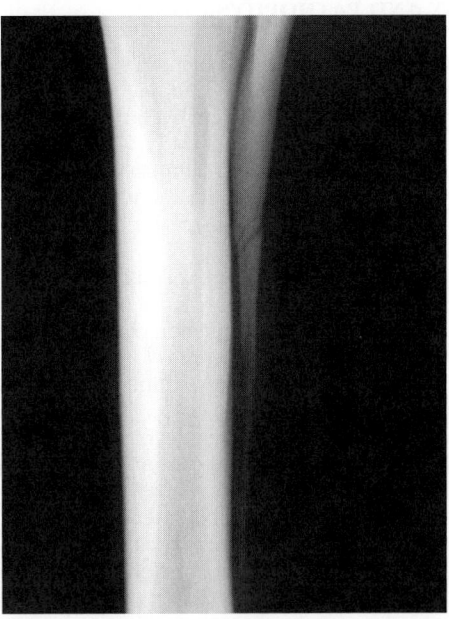

FIGURE 2 Dorsolateral-to-palmarolateral oblique radiograph of the left metatarsus of a horse with an acute fracture of the midshaft of MT-IV.

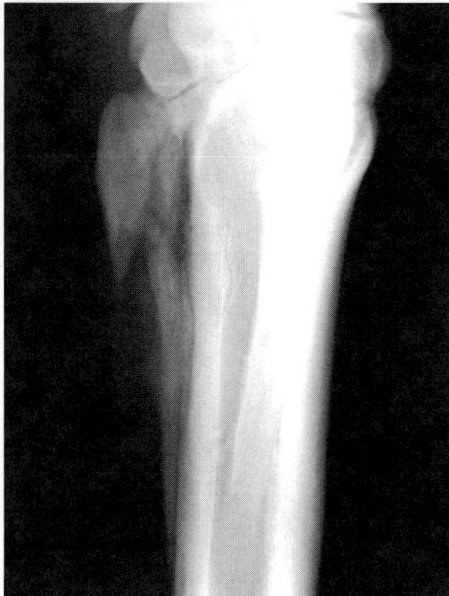

FIGURE 3 Dorsolateral-to-palmarolateral oblique radiograph of the right metacarpus of a horse with a displaced fracture of the proximal aspect of MC-II. This fracture is best treated with internal fixation using a small plate.

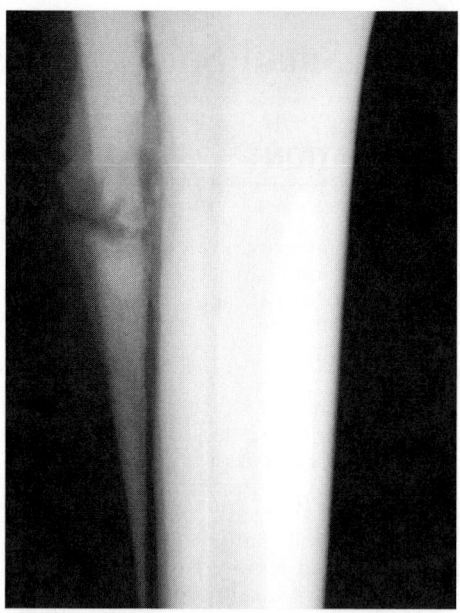

FIGURE 4 Dorsolateral-to-plantaromedial oblique radiograph of the right metatarsus of a horse with a chronic fracture of the mid-shaft of MT-IV. Note the extensive periosteal callus and persistent fracture gap typical of a delayed union or nonunion in this non-surgically managed fracture.

fracture is chronic, a callus can often be palpated along with instability if the distal tip or "button" is pressed axially.

- Variable degrees of soft tissue swelling and pain on palpation of the fracture site are the hallmarks of fractures of the more proximal portions of the splint bones. Open wounds or abrasions may be present if the fracture is the result of external trauma. Signs of soft tissue infection are common with chronic fractures associated with open wounds.

ETIOLOGY AND PATHOPHYSIOLOGY

- Splints
  - Caused by internal (most common) or external (less common) trauma
  - Internal trauma is the result of cyclic strains during exercise.
  - Initiated by tearing and inflammation of the interosseous ligament and underlying periosteum of the cannon and splint bones.
  - Focal desmitis and periostitis develop.
  - Swelling is initially a combination of soft tissue edema and fibrosis.
  - Progresses to periosteal new bone or exostosis.
  - Eventually, a synostosis often develops between the splint and cannon bone.
  - In contrast, splints caused by external trauma begin as a primary focal periostitis or osteitis of the affected bone.
  - In either case, if the exostosis becomes exuberant and projects

axially, a secondary, focal suspensory desmitis may develop.

- Splint bone fractures
  - Distal fractures: Cyclic axial compressive forces during loading and tensile strains imparted by the suspensory ligament
  - Middle and proximal fractures: Blunt external trauma
  - Some oblique fractures of the head of MC-II may be avulsion fractures or the result of internal torsional forces.

DIAGNOSIS

DIFFERENTIAL DIAGNOSIS

Splints and closed splint bone fractures are differentials for each other.

INITIAL DATABASE

- Physical examination
- Lameness examination, including diagnostic analgesia in selected cases
- Radiographs confirm the diagnosis.

ADVANCED OR CONFIRMATORY TESTING

- Nuclear scintigraphy may be helpful in selected cases.
- Ultrasound examination of the suspensory ligament in selected cases
- Synoviocentesis is indicated to rule in or rule out joint involvement in open fractures of the proximal aspect of the bone.

TREATMENT

THERAPEUTIC GOALS

- Splints: Reduce or eliminate the inciting cause, reduce inflammation, minimize the size of the exostosis, and allow the lesion to become quiescent or "set up."
- Fractures
  - Distal fractures: Eliminate the source of chronic irritation or inflammation.
  - Mid-shaft fractures: Minimize the convalescent time and prevent formation of exuberant callus or exostosis.
- Proximal fractures: Promote primary bone healing, preserve the stability of the proximal portion, and minimize the potential for degenerative joint disease.

ACUTE GENERAL TREATMENT

- Splints
  - Local and systemic antiinflammatory therapy (cold hosing or icing, bandaging, nonsteroidal antiinflammatory drugs)
  - Stall rest when lameness is unusually severe (ie, apparent at a walk)
  - Controlled exercise: Handwalking 2 to 6 weeks in most cases; handwalking and paddock turnout for 1 to 4 months in more severe or chronic or recurrent cases
  - Local corticosteroid injection

- Fractures
  - Stall rest and antiinflammatory therapy (as above) pending decisions on definitive treatment
  - Wound care and antimicrobial therapy in cases with open wounds or established infection

CHRONIC TREATMENT
- Splints
  - Corrective trimming and shoeing to reduce strains on the bone and minimize the tendency for interfering
  - Boots and protective bandages to offer protection from interference
  - Surgery (partial ostectomy) is reserved for refractory cases with chronic or recurrent lameness and those with exuberant exostoses.
- Fractures
  - Nonsurgical management may be effective in selected cases.
  - Surgery decreases the convalescent time and minimizes the potential for delayed or nonunion and exuberant callus formation (Figure 4).
  - Distal and mid-shaft fractures are generally best treated surgically by partial ostectomy.
  - Segmental ostectomy is an option for some mid-shaft fractures.
  - Simple debridement of comminuted fragments in open fractures is an option in some cases.

- Proximal fractures are treated with internal fixation when feasible to preserve joint integrity.
- Complete ostectomy of MT-IV is a viable option in selected cases.

POSSIBLE COMPLICATIONS
- Secondary suspensory desmitis is a concern in cases of splints or fractures with exuberant callus or exostosis formation.
- Septic arthritis is a potential complication with open fractures involving the carpometacarpal or tarsometatarsal joints.

RECOMMENDED MONITORING
Follow-up radiography to monitor fracture healing (non-ostectomy cases)

PROGNOSIS AND OUTCOME

- The prognosis for proliferative periostitis (splints) is very good to excellent in the majority of cases.
- The prognosis for splint bone fractures is also typically good to excellent if diagnosed early and properly treated.
- Exceptions: Cases with concurrent suspensory desmitis; cases of proximal

---

fractures with resultant osteoarthritis (chronic displacement or septic arthritis)

PEARLS & CONSIDERATIONS

Occasionally, a horse with a fractured splint bone resulting from blunt trauma will also have a hairline fracture of the cannon bone. Radiographs should be carefully scrutinized in these cases, particularly before general anesthesia.

SUGGESTED READING
Bassage LH: Metacarpus/metatarsus. In Hinchcliff KW, Kaneps AJ, Geor RJ, editors: *Equine sports medicine and surgery*, London, 2004, Saunders Elsevier, pp 319–348.

Doran R: Fractures of the small metacarpal and metatarsal (splint) bones. In Nixon AJ, editor: *Equine fracture repair*, Philadelphia, 1996, Saunders Elsevier, pp 200–207.

Dyson SJ: The metacarpal region. In Ross MW, Dyson SJ, editors: *Diagnosis and management of lameness in the horse*, St Louis, 2003, Saunders Elsevier, pp 362–376.

AUTHOR: **LANCE H. BASSAGE II**

EDITOR: **ANDRIS J. KANEPS**

Frostbite

BASIC INFORMATION

DEFINITION
Destruction of the skin, and often deeper tissues, by freezing temperatures

SYNONYM(S)
Cryopathy

EPIDEMIOLOGY
SPECIES, AGE, SEX Frostbite may affect any horse with prolonged exposure to below-freezing temperatures, particularly in conjunction with high humidity, low wind chill factors, and a wet haircoat or blanket. Debilitated animals and neonates are at particular risk.
RISK FACTORS Low ambient temperatures
ASSOCIATED CONDITIONS AND DISORDERS Hypothermia

CLINICAL PRESENTATION
HISTORY, CHIEF COMPLAINT
- History of exposure to cold climates
- Horses may not present with clinical signs until tissue sloughing is noted.

PHYSICAL EXAM FINDINGS
- Clinical signs include erythema and bulla formation superficially.
- Hemorrhagic blisters, ulceration, gangrene, anesthesia, or hyperesthesia may occur in the deeper subcutaneous tissues.
- There may be color change to the tissue beneath the hair from white to deep purple.

ETIOLOGY AND PATHOPHYSIOLOGY
- Cold temperatures induce vasoconstriction, infarction, and endothelial damage.
- Crystallization of water into ice in the tissue and capillaries leads to further tissue damage and ischemic necrosis.

- Further mechanical effects include free radical generation, production of prostaglandins and thromboxane A2, release of proteolytic enzymes, and generalized inflammation.

DIAGNOSIS

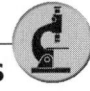

DIFFERENTIAL DIAGNOSIS
Any blistering disease

INITIAL DATABASE
- None required
- Specific tests may be dictated by the concurrent illness or injury that led to frostbite.

ADVANCED OR CONFIRMATORY TESTING
Doppler ultrasonography may provide a view of vascular flow to the affected region.

TREATMENT

THERAPEUTIC GOAL(S)

- Rewarm the affected region slowly.
- Treat the secondary effects of the cold-induced damage (tissue necrosis, infection).

ACUTE GENERAL TREATMENT

- Because rewarming followed by refreezing can be more harmful to the extremity than a delay in rewarming, protect the involved extremity and avoid rewarming until correct procedures can be performed.
  - In human patients, the affected tissue is warmed by placing it in water with 10% povidone-iodine at 40° C for about 20 minutes and elevating the region immediately afterward.
  - In horses, the tissue can be rewarmed with warm, damp towels (without rubbing, which can injure frozen cells), circulating warm water heating pads, warm water bottles, or forced warm air blankets and moving the animal to a warm environment out of the wind.
- Nonsteroidal antiinflammatory drugs (flunixin meglumine, 1.1 mg/kg q12h IV) should be used to control pain and decrease inflammation.

- Pentoxifylline (8.4 mg/kg q12h PO) can be used to improve microvascular circulation and prevent erythrocyte clumping.
- Aspirin (acetylsalicylic acid, 17 mg/kg, q12h PO) and low-molecular-weight heparin (50–80 U/kg, q24h SC) can be used to prevent microvascular thrombosis.
- Acepromazine can also be used for vasodilation.
- Antibiotics should be started if the patient is debilitated or young or if necrosis is anticipated.

CHRONIC TREATMENT

- Local tissue care is important to care for the skin.
  - Topical aloe vera gel should be applied to the skin three or four times daily.
  - Topical nitroglycerin may also help improve circulation to the affected tissue.

POSSIBLE COMPLICATIONS

- Skin and hoof sloughing may occur depending on the severity of the injury.
- Local infection may occur and may progress to sepsis if severe.

PROGNOSIS AND OUTCOME

Persistent edema and failure to rewarm are poor prognostic indicators for the affected tissues.

PEARLS & CONSIDERATIONS

Avoid exposure of debilitated animals to low ambient temperatures.

SUGGESTED READING

Bilgiç S, Ozkan H, Ozenç S, et al: Treating frostbite. *Can Fam Physician* 54(3): 361–363, 2008.

Divers TJ: Hypothermia and frostbite. In Orsini JA, Divers TJ, editors: *Equine emergencies treatment and procedures*, St Louis, 2008, Saunders Elsevier, pp 556–557.

Heggers JP, Robson MC, Manavalen K, et al: Experimental and clinical observations on frostbite. *Ann Emerg Med* 16(9):1056–1062, 1987.

McCauley RL, Heggers JP, Robson MC: Frostbite: methods to minimize tissue loss. *Postgrad Med* 88(8):67–68, 1990.

Patel NN, Patel DN: Frostbite. *Am J Med* 121(9):765–766, 2008.

AUTHOR: **CHRISTINA HEWES**

EDITORS: **R. REID HANSON** and **AMELIA MUNSTERMAN**

Fumonisin Toxicosis

BASIC INFORMATION

DEFINITION

Fumonisins are mycotoxins produced by field infections of primarily *Fusarium verticillioides* and *Fusarium proliferatum* in corn that cause leukoencephalomalacia, hepatotoxicity, and cardiovascular dysfunction in horses.

SYNONYM(S)

- Equine leukoencephalomalacia (ELEM)
- Moldy corn disease

EPIDEMIOLOGY

SPECIES, AGE, SEX Any horse of any gender or age is susceptible to the adverse effects of fumonisins.

RISK FACTORS

- Feeding corn screenings or broken corn kernels increases the risk of fumonisin toxicosis.
- Three main fumonisins in corn are responsible for toxicity:

  - Fumonisin B1 (FB1) and fumonisin B2 (FB2) are approximately equal in toxicity but naturally occur in a ratio of about 3:1 for FB1/FB2.
  - Fumonisin B3 (FB3) is much less toxic.
- The development of clinical signs depends on the dose. Horses fed high fumonisin concentrations can develop leukoencephalomalacia in 5 to 8 days, but it may require several months for clinical signs to appear at low fumonisin concentrations.
- The Food and Drug Administration's Center for Veterinary Medicine guidelines recommend maximum levels of total fumonisins (FB1 + FB2) in corn used for equine feed of 5 mg/kg (ppm) and in the final equine ration of 1 mg/kg (ppm).

GEOGRAPHY AND SEASONALITY Fumonisins occur worldwide, primarily in corn. Insect damage and adverse weather conditions, particularly drought during the corn-growing season followed by cool and moist conditions during pollination and kernel formation, favor fumonisin production.

CLINICAL PRESENTATION

DISEASE FORMS/SUBTYPES

- The clinical signs from fumonisin contamination of equine rations are probably related to the dose, duration of exposure, and tolerance of the individual horse. Although not truly distinct, two forms may appear in a herd outbreak or in an individual animal:
  - Equine leukoencephalomalacia or classic neurotoxic syndrome
  - Hepatic syndrome

HISTORY, CHIEF COMPLAINT

- The initial clinical signs may include a lack of appetite and neurologic signs, including aimless wandering, depression, hyperexcitability, or sudden death.
- The cardiovascular dysfunction includes decreases in heart rate and

- cardiac output, which may contribute to signs of dyspnea and edema.
- Horses with liver damage may show icterus, hemorrhage, and depression.
- The time from the onset of clinical signs to death may be 24 hours to 7 days. Typically, if only liver damage occurs and the fumonisin exposure stops, the liver lesions may be reversible.

PHYSICAL EXAM FINDINGS

- Horses with hepatic disease may display:
  - Icterus
  - Petechiae of mucous membranes
  - Hemorrhage
  - Depression
  - Swelling of the lips or muzzle
- Horses with ELEM may develop:
  - Aimless circling
  - Head pressing
  - Standing motionless for a period or displaying continuous repetitive movements until death
  - Paresis
  - Ataxia
  - Apparent blindness
  - Hyperexcitability
  - Facial paralysis
  - Coma
  - Tonic-clonic seizures
  - Death

ETIOLOGY AND PATHOPHYSIOLOGY

- Fumonisins inhibit key enzymes in the synthesis of sphingolipid and disrupt sphingolipid metabolism, increasing sphinganine and sphingosine and decreasing complex sphingolipids. Sphingolipids are involved in cell growth, cell-to-cell communication, differentiation, and neoplastic transformation. Elevated sphinganine-to-sphingosine ratios are associated with fumonisin toxicosis.
- Sphingosine inhibits L-type calcium channels in myocardial cells, decreasing cardiac contractility.
- Fumonisin toxicity in horses and resulting increases in sphingosine concentrations are associated with development of vasogenic cerebral edema as a direct result of increased blood-brain barrier permeability. It is hypothesized that increased sphingosine concentrations inhibit the calcium channels in cerebral arterioles, leading to altered cerebral blood pressure and vasogenic cerebral edema. Elevations

in protein, albumin, and immunoglobulin G (IgG) concentrations have been identified in the cerebrospinal fluid (CSF) of horses with ELEM.

DIAGNOSIS

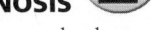

DIFFERENTIAL DIAGNOSIS

- Brain trauma, abscesses, and edema
- Cerebrospinal nematodiasis
- Hyperammonemia
- Acute lead toxicosis
- Poisonous plants causing pyrrolizidine alkaloid toxicosis
- Aflatoxicosis

INITIAL DATABASE

- Serum biochemical changes are related to the hepatotoxicity and include elevated liver enzymes, including aspartate aminotransferase, gamma-glutamyl transpeptidase, and alkaline phosphatase.
- CSF changes in horses with ELEM include increased concentrations in protein, albumin, and IgG.

ADVANCED OR CONFIRMATORY TESTING

- Hepatic lesions include a swollen, brownish liver with irregular nodules. Histologic changes include hepatocyte vacuolation, loss of hepatic architecture, periacinar necrosis, bile stasis, portal fibrosis, and bile ductule proliferation.
- ELEM lesions appear as softening and necrosis of subcortical cerebral white matter, with lesions ranging from very small to large cavitations and inward collapse of cortical gray matter. Hemorrhages may be evident. Lesions are generally not symmetrical or bilateral and can involve the thalamus, cerebellum, brainstem, and medulla oblongata.
- Suspect feed should be analyzed for fumonisins (FB1 and FB2). Typically, the analysis is by high-performance liquid chromatography or enzyme-linked immunosorbent assay.
- An increased sphingosine-to-sphinganine ratio in serum or urine is a sensitive early indicator of fumonisin toxicosis; however, this analysis is not common in diagnostic laboratories.

TREATMENT

THERAPEUTIC GOAL(S)

There is no antidote for fumonisins. Typically, the clinical onset is acute and progressive until death occurs.

ACUTE GENERAL TREATMENT

- The important action is to identify the source and stop exposure to fumonisins in the ration.
- Because of the delay in onset of clinical signs after the start of exposure, decontamination is generally of limited to no value.
- Horses with hepatic damage should be provided appropriate supportive care.

PROGNOSIS AND OUTCOME

The appearance of clinical signs from fumonisin exposure indicates a grave prognosis. The majority of horses with ELEM die. If an affected animal survives, significant neurologic damage may be a sequela.

PEARLS & CONSIDERATIONS

COMMENTS

- Corn and corn products in equine rations should be periodically analyzed for fumonisin concentrations.
- Distillers' grains are often contaminated with fumonisins at a concentration of concern for horses; therefore, feeding distillers' grains to horses is not recommended.

CLIENT EDUCATION

Emphasize to clients that corn screenings or broken corn kernels may contain toxic concentrations of fumonisins and produce fatal ELEM in horses.

SUGGESTED READING

Smith GW: Fumonisins. In Gupta RC, editor: *Veterinary toxicology*, New York, 2007, Elsevier, pp 983–996.

AUTHOR: MICHELLE S. MOSTROM

EDITOR: CYNTHIA L. GASKILL

Gasterophilus

BASIC INFORMATION

DEFINITION
The most common, although rarely clinically significant, gastric endoparasite in adult horses and foals

SYNONYM(S)
- "Bots," the bot fly larvae, are the stage found in the equine stomach.
- *Gasterophilus intestinalis* and *Gasterophilus nasalis* are most commonly found in horses; other less frequently identified species include *Gasterophilus haemorrhoidalis* and *Gasterophilus pecorum*.

EPIDEMIOLOGY
GEOGRAPHY AND SEASONALITY
- Found worldwide.
- Adult bot flies are present during the summer months and lay their eggs on the hairs of the horse's face and legs in the fall. The larvae overwinter in the equine stomach, are passed in the feces in the spring, and then pupate and mature into adult bot flies.

CLINICAL PRESENTATION
HISTORY, CHIEF COMPLAINT
Associated clinical signs are rare but may include signs similar to gastric ulceration (see "Gastric Ulceration" in this section) if large numbers are present in the stomach or signs consistent with gastric outflow obstruction (see "Gastric Impaction" in this section) if large numbers obstruct the duodenum.
PHYSICAL EXAM FINDINGS
- Usually within normal limits.
- In the fall, small, yellow bot fly eggs may be visible stuck to the hairs of the face and forelimbs.
ETIOLOGY AND PATHOPHYSIOLOGY
Direct life cycle:
- The adult bot fly lays eggs on the horse's hair coat (legs or head) during warm months. The eggs hatch on the hair coat, releasing first-stage larvae, which then enter the oral cavity by crawling there or are ingested by the horse during grooming behavior.
- First- and second-stage larvae develop in the oral cavity in the gingival tissue (*G. nasalis*) or tongue (*G. intestinalis*).
- Late second-stage larvae are swallowed and mature to third-stage larvae in the stomach. The third-stage larvae then attach to the gastric (*G. intestinalis*) or proximal duodenal (*G. nasalis*) mucosa, where they overwinter.
- Third-stage larvae detach from the gastric mucosa in the spring and are passed in the feces and pupate. Adult bot flies emerge during the summer and repeat the cycle.
- In general, *Gasterophilus* organisms are nonpathogenic, and related clinical disease is uncommon unless large numbers of larvae are present in the stomach, resulting in gastric mucosal pain or inflammation or in the duodenum, resulting in gastric outflow obstruction.

DIAGNOSIS

DIFFERENTIAL DIAGNOSIS
Gastric ulceration

INITIAL DATABASE
Complete blood count and serum biochemical profile: Usually within reference intervals

ADVANCED OR CONFIRMATORY TESTING
Gastroscopy:
- The larvae, which are usually yellow or tan, are seen attached to the gastric mucosa as solitary organisms or occasionally in clusters.
- The presence of bot fly larvae is often an incidental finding.

TREATMENT

THERAPEUTIC GOAL(S)
Eliminate the larval stage.

ACUTE GENERAL TREATMENT
- Ivermectin: 200 µg/kg PO once
  - *Gasterophilus* larvae are very susceptible to avermectins but are not eliminated by other classes of anthelmintics.
- Remove bot eggs from the hair coat in the fall using a bot knife.

PROGNOSIS AND OUTCOME

Good; rarely associated with clinical disease and easy to eliminate with ivermectin

PEARLS & CONSIDERATIONS

COMMENTS
Concurrent gastric ulceration is rarely present. If gastric ulceration is present in a horse with gastric *Gasterophilus* larvae, other inciting causes for ulcers should be suspected and investigated (see "Gastric Ulceration" in this section).

PREVENTION
Routine deworming should include administration of ivermectin in the winter months to eliminate *Gasterophilus* larval infestation.

SUGGESTED READING
Murray MJ: Stomach diseases of the foal. In Mair T, Divers T, Ducharme N, editors: *Manual of equine gastroenterology*, London, 2002, Saunders Elsevier, pp 469–476.

AUTHOR: KELSEY A. HART

EDITORS: TIM MAIR and CERI SHERLOCK

Gastric Dilation

BASIC INFORMATION

DEFINITION
Distension of the stomach with fluid or gas

CLINICAL PRESENTATION
HISTORY, CHIEF COMPLAINT
- Colic (often acute onset and severe)
- ± History of consumption of large volume of fermentable feed such as grain, grass clippings, or apples

PHYSICAL EXAM FINDINGS
- Tachycardia, tachypnea.
- Decreased to absent gastrointestinal borborygmi.
- Variable gross abdominal distension ranging from absent to dramatic.

- Depression, fever, dehydration, and hyperemic or injected mucous membranes are often seen if the underlying cause is inflammatory small intestinal disease (proximal duodenitis or jejunitis).

ETIOLOGY AND PATHOPHYSIOLOGY

- Primary gastric dilation: Occurs when large volumes of gas are rapidly produced after consumption of a large amount of highly fermentable material (grain, grass clippings, apples)
- Secondary gastric dilation: Caused by reflux of small intestinal fluid contents retrograde into the stomach because of small intestinal obstructive lesions or caused by excessive small intestinal fluid secretion and small intestinal dysmotility with proximal duodenitis or jejunitis, postoperative ileus, or equine grass sickness
- Emesis or spontaneous regurgitation of gastric contents into the esophagus is usually prevented in the horse with severe gastric dilation because of mechanical distortion of the cardia.

DIAGNOSIS

DIFFERENTIAL DIAGNOSIS

Gastric impaction

INITIAL DATABASE

Passage of a nasogastric tube yields a large volume of fluid (often 10–20 L) or gas and usually results in at least temporary resolution of the colic episode. This confirms the diagnosis of gastric dilation but does not help to differentiate primary from secondary gastric dilation.

ADVANCED OR CONFIRMATORY TESTING

- Should be undertaken to determine the underlying cause of gastric dilation and may include the following:
  - Complete blood count: Often within reference intervals, although leukopenia and significant hemoconcentration suggest small intestinal inflammatory disease as the underlying cause
  - Serum biochemistry profile: Hypochloremia, hyponatremia, and other electrolyte derangements are frequently observed.
  - Rectal examination: May be normal with primary gastric dilation, although caudal displacement of the spleen because of the marked

gastric distension is occasionally appreciated. Small intestinal distension or thickening is often noted in secondary gastric dilation.
  - Transabdominal ultrasonography: Caudal displacement of the gastric contour, beyond the 15th intercostal space, is often present. Small intestinal distension, hypomotility, and increased mural thickness (>5 mm) are often seen in secondary gastric dilation
  - Peritoneal fluid analysis: Usually within reference intervals in primary gastric dilation. Variable in secondary gastric dilation, depending on the inciting cause.
- Exploratory celiotomy is often indicated if colic persists or recurs after gastric decompression or if a primary small intestinal obstructive lesion is suspected.

TREATMENT

THERAPEUTIC GOAL(S)

- Remove excess gastric fluid or gas to prevent gastric rupture.
- Eliminate the underlying cause.

ACUTE GENERAL TREATMENT

- Gastric decompression via a nasogastric tube
  - If it is difficult to pass the tube through the cardia, instillation of 20 to 40 mL of 2% lidocaine down the nasogastric tube may promote sufficient cardiac relaxation to permit passage of the tube.
  - Maintenance of an indwelling nasogastric tube is often necessary to maintain gastric decompression. The tube may be capped and the horse monitored for reaccumulation of gastric fluid every 1 to 3 hours, or the tube may be left uncapped to allow gas and fluid to spontaneously escape.
  - A finger from a latex glove with a small opening cut in the end may be secured over the end of an uncapped nasogastric tube to allow gas or fluid efflux but prevent unwanted influx of air into the stomach.
- Gastric lavage (see "Gastric Impaction" and "Grain Overload" in this section) is indicated in primary gastric dilation to remove ingested fermentable feed if possible.

- The underlying cause of secondary gastric dilation should be investigated and treated appropriately.
- The horse should be kept NPO (nothing by mouth) until the inciting cause has resolved and continuous or intermittent gastric decompression is no longer necessary.

POSSIBLE COMPLICATIONS

Gastric rupture

PROGNOSIS AND OUTCOME

- Primary gastric dilation: The prognosis is good to excellent if gastric decompression is accomplished early and maintained.
- Secondary gastric dilation: The prognosis is variable and depends on the underlying inciting cause.

PEARLS & CONSIDERATIONS

- Passage of a nasogastric tube should be performed in any horse with signs of colic or unexplained tachycardia. If small intestinal distension is noted on rectal examination, enteral fluids or laxatives should not be administered (even if no significant reflux is obtained on initial examination), and the horse should be serially monitored for development of gastric reflux until the small intestinal distension is resolved.
- If transfer to a referral hospital is necessary in a horse with gastric dilation, it is imperative that the horse be shipped with a well-secured, uncapped indwelling nasogastric tube in place.

SUGGESTED READING

Mueller POE, Moore JN, Divers TJ: Disorders of the stomach. In Orsini JA, Divers TJ, editors: *Equine emergencies: treatments and procedures*, ed 3, St Louis, 2008, Saunders Elsevier, pp 121–122.

Murray MJ: Diseases of the stomach. In Mair T, Divers T, Ducharme N, editors: *Manual of equine gastroenterology*, London, 2002, Saunders Elsevier, pp 241–248.

AUTHOR: KELSEY A. HART

EDITORS: TIM MAIR and CERI SHERLOCK

Gastric Impaction

BASIC INFORMATION

DEFINITION
Distension of the stomach with feed or a phytobezoar or trichobezoar

EPIDEMIOLOGY
SPECIES, AGE, SEX Foals may be predisposed to indiscriminate hair ingestion, resulting in trichobezoar formation
RISK FACTORS
- Feeding poor-quality roughage or certain feed stuffs such as beet pulp and wheat bran, which may not be adequately hydrated by saliva and gastric fluid contents
- Poor dentition resulting in inadequate mastication
- Concurrent gastrointestinal (GI) disease, resulting in generalized decreased GI motility
- Pyloric outflow obstruction (see "Gastric Outflow Obstruction" in this section)

ASSOCIATED CONDITIONS AND DISORDERS Horses with acute or chronic hepatic disease have an increased incidence of gastric impaction, although the direct relationship between the two conditions is poorly understood.

CLINICAL PRESENTATION
HISTORY, CHIEF COMPLAINT
- Inappetence or anorexia
- Colic (variable severity)
PHYSICAL EXAM FINDINGS
- Variable; may be within normal limits.
- Mild to moderate tachycardia and tachypnea and evidence of mild to moderate dehydration (prolonged skin tent, tacky mucous membranes, and prolonged capillary refill time) are frequently observed.
- Gross abdominal distension is uncommon unless a concurrent distal intestinal obstruction is present.
- Rectal examination
  - Often within normal limits in primary gastric impaction, although caudal displacement of the spleen may be appreciated.
  - Small intestinal or large colonic distension may be noted if an accompanying distal intestinal obstruction has predisposed to the gastric impaction.
ETIOLOGY AND PATHOPHYSIOLOGY
- Feed material accumulates within the stomach with:
  - Consumption of large amounts of poor-quality roughage or dry feed stuffs
  - Dehydration or limited water intake

- Impaired gastric emptying caused by pyloric outflow obstruction or more distal intestinal obstruction
- Bezoar formation
  - Persimmon seed or hair ingestion may result in formation of a phytobezoar or trichobezoar, respectively.
  - A large bezoar may obstruct the pylorus, or a small bezoar may obstruct the duodenum, resulting in impaired gastric outflow.
- Idiopathic gastric impaction infrequently occurs as a primary cause of colic in the absence of a specific predisposing or concurrent cause.

DIAGNOSIS

DIFFERENTIAL DIAGNOSIS
Gastric dilation

INITIAL DATABASE
- Passage of a nasogastric tube
  - It is typically difficult to impossible to pass the tube through the cardia, and the horse may show signs of pain when this is attempted.
  - Significant gastric reflux is usually not present because the impacted material is usually dry and fibrous.
  - Gastric contents may have a stale, foul, fermentative odor.
- Complete blood count and serum biochemical profile
  - Usually within reference intervals or consistent with mild dehydration
  - Increased serum liver enzyme activity and bile acid concentration are present if the gastric impaction is secondary to hepatic disease.

ADVANCED OR CONFIRMATORY TESTING
Definitive diagnosis is difficult and is often made during exploratory laparotomy because of protracted and unrelenting abdominal pain.
- Transabdominal ultrasonography: Caudal displacement of the gastric contour beyond the left fifteenth intercostal space may be seen. However, the sonographic location of the gastric contour can vary dramatically and occasionally extends to this location in the absence of a gastric impaction.
- Gastroscopy
  - Useful for visualization of a phytobezoar or trichobezoar
  - Identification of feed material at the level of the cardia in a fasted horse is consistent with gastric impaction

- However, accurate determination of gastric size is not possible with gastroscopic examination.
- An apparently large amount of feed material is often visualized in the stomach of nonfasted horses and may appear endoscopically identical to a true gastric impaction.
- Thus, one-time gastroscopy may be misleading. The persistence of a large amount of feed material on serial examinations over 12 to 36 hours in a fasted horse is needed for a presumptive gastroscopic diagnosis of gastric impaction.

TREATMENT

THERAPEUTIC GOAL(S)
- Prevent further gastric distension or gastric rupture.
- Promote hydration of gastric contents to allow gastric emptying.
- Resolve inciting, concurrent intestinal obstruction, if present.

ACUTE GENERAL TREATMENT
- It is vital to withhold all feed, water, and oral medications because of the substantial risk of gastric rupture.
- Medical therapy: Promote hydration of gastric contents and breakdown of the impaction.
- Administer IV balanced polyionic fluids at 100 to 200 mL/kg/day.
- Intragastric administration of isotonic fluids and laxatives can be helpful but should be done in small volumes via gravity flow with great caution because gastric rupture is a potential consequence:
  - 8% dioctyl sodium sulfosuccinate (DSS): 100 to 200 mL once
  - ~1 L of isotonic fluids q4–8h
  - 1 L of mineral oil may be alternated with magnesium sulfate salts (8 oz/1 L water) q6–12h
- Administration should be ceased and administered fluids siphoned out if the horse shows any signs of discomfort during or after administration.
- Administration of 0.5 to 1 L of carbonated soda (eg, Coca-Cola) via nasogastric tube q12–24h can aid the breakdown of impacted material in both feed impactions and persimmon phytobezoars.
- Gastric lavage via a large-bore nasogastric tube
  - Perform gently q6–12h with instillation of small volumes of fluid (<1 L) via gravity flow at a time.

- If an equivalent or greater volume of fluid and gastric contents is not siphoned out on each attempt, gastric lavage should be discontinued to avoid further distension of the stomach.
- Analgesic therapy
  - Flunixin meglumine (0.5–1.1 mg/kg IV q12h) as needed to control pain
  - Sedation with α_2 adrenergic agonists or opioids should be minimized if possible to avoid potential decreased GI motility.
  - Prokinetic therapy is not recommended unless a pyloric or more distal intestinal obstruction has been ruled out.
- Surgical therapy
  - Exploratory celiotomy is indicated in horses with increasing or persistent abdominal pain or in those in which medical management over 2 to 4 days is ineffective.
  - If gastric impaction is diagnosed or confirmed at surgery, direct instillation of isotonic fluids and gastric massage can be performed to help soften the impaction.
  - Surgical resolution of a gastric impaction or removal of a gastric bezoar via gastrotomy is extremely challenging in adult horses because of limited surgical exposure and inability to exteriorize the stomach, resulting in the substantial risk for abdominal contamination at surgery.

CHRONIC TREATMENT

Horses with hepatic disease or pyloric outflow obstruction that are at risk for recurrent gastric impactions can be managed conservatively with low-bulk diets consisting of short clipped-pasture, complete pelleted feed, or both.

POSSIBLE COMPLICATIONS

Gastric rupture

RECOMMENDED MONITORING

Serial gastroscopy every 24 hours until resolution of the impaction: Before refeeding, endoscopic evaluation of the pylorus and proximal duodenum is recommended to ensure a mechanical obstruction is not present.

PROGNOSIS AND OUTCOME

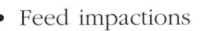

- Feed impactions
  - Guarded to fair with prompt medical therapy in primary gastric impactions
  - High likelihood of recurrence if occurs secondary to pyloric outflow obstruction
- Phytobezoars or trichobezoars: Guarded to poor because of difficulty resolving without surgery
- Poor if gastrotomy is required.

PEARLS & CONSIDERATIONS

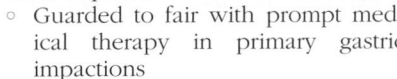

COMMENTS

- Gastric impaction should not be overlooked as a primary or secondary cause of colic, especially in horses in which difficulty passing a nasogastric tube through the cardia is noted.
- Definitive diagnosis can require exploratory laparotomy, but surgical resolution via gastrotomy carries substantial risk and should only be attempted if medical management is unsuccessful.

PREVENTION

- Ensure good-quality roughage, access to water, and appropriate dental care.
- Limit or prevent access to persimmon trees and persimmon fruit.

SUGGESTED READING

Murray MJ: Diseases of the stomach. In Mair T, Divers T, Ducharme N, editors: *Manual of equine gastroenterology*, London, 2002, Saunders Elsevier, pp 241–248.

AUTHOR: **KELSEY A. HART**

EDITORS: **TIM MAIR** and **CERI SHERLOCK**

Gastric Rupture

BASIC INFORMATION

DEFINITION

Full-thickness disruption of the gastric wall

EPIDEMIOLOGY

RISK FACTORS Gastric distension from any cause

CLINICAL PRESENTATION

HISTORY, CHIEF COMPLAINT

- Colic: Signs may improve or resolve temporarily immediately after gastric rupture occurs
- Inappetence
- Profuse sweating
- Tachypnea (often marked)

PHYSICAL EXAM FINDINGS

- Depressed mentation progressing to obtundation or recumbency
- Rectal temperature is variable, ranging from hypothermia caused by circulatory collapse and shock to pyrexia caused by endotoxemia.
- Marked tachycardia and tachypnea are usually noted.
- Mucous membranes are injected, muddy, purple to grey, and tacky or dry, with a prolonged capillary refill time.
- Decreased to absent gastrointestinal borborygmi
- ± Gross abdominal distension
- Rectal examination
  - Serosal surfaces often feel "gritty," and definition of the abdominal structures is often dramatically improved because of pneumoperitoneum.
  - Small intestinal distension may be present if gastric distension was secondary to a more distal intestinal obstruction.
  - May be normal

ETIOLOGY AND PATHOPHYSIOLOGY

- Any mechanical or functional lesion resulting in gastric outflow obstruction and gastric distension can ultimately culminate in gastric rupture (see "Gastric Dilation," "Gastric Impaction," "Gastric Outflow Obstruction," and "Grain Overload" in this section).
- Severe gastric ulceration causing perforation (uncommon; see "Gastric Ulceration in Adult Horses" and "Gastric Ulceration in Foals" in this section).

DIAGNOSIS

DIFFERENTIAL DIAGNOSIS

- Rupture of another gastrointestinal viscus
- Rarely, severe compromise to bowel with severe enterocolitis or protracted strangulating intestinal lesions can present similarly

INITIAL DATABASE

- Complete blood count
  - Significant polycythemia caused by hemoconcentration

- Variable leukogram; often leukopenic
- Lactate: Often marked hyperlactatemia (>5 mmol/L) caused by circulatory collapse
- Serum biochemical profile
  - Variable electrolyte derangements
  - Often marked hyperglycemia
  - Marked metabolic acidosis is common
  - Variable azotemia (prerenal)
- Abdominal ultrasonography
  - Evaluation of the dorsal abdomen may be obscured by pneumoperitoneum.
  - Increased free peritoneal fluid of variable echogenicity may be present.
  - Small intestinal distension or increased mural thickening may be noted if primary small intestinal disease is present.
  - Occasionally normal (in acute rupture).

ADVANCED OR CONFIRMATORY TESTING

- Abdominocentesis
  - Gross evaluation
    - Green/brown or hemorrhagic discolored fluid

- Feed material may be grossly visible.
- Often foul smelling
  - Cytological evaluation
    - Feed material present
    - Intra- and extracellular mixed bacterial population, usually in large numbers
    - The leukocyte count and total protein concentration may be markedly increased.
- Exploratory celiotomy: Necessary for antemortem confirmation of gastric rupture, although rapid systemic decompensation and welfare implications normally preclude this procedure

TREATMENT

THERAPEUTIC GOAL(S)

Treatment is not indicated because of the grave prognosis.

ACUTE GENERAL TREATMENT

Humane euthanasia

PROGNOSIS AND OUTCOME

Grave

PEARLS & CONSIDERATIONS

- The potential fatal consequences of marked gastric distension highlight the importance of passage of a nasogastric tube and maintenance of gastric decompression in horses with signs of colic or unexplained tachycardia.
- The administration of oral or intragastric fluids or laxatives to horses that are producing gastric reflux or have small intestinal distension should be avoided.

SUGGESTED READING

Mueller POE, Moore JN, Divers TJ: Disorders of the stomach. In Orsini JA, Divers TJ, editors: *Equine emergencies: treatments and procedures*, ed 3, St Louis, 2008, Saunders Elsevier, pp 121–122.

Murray MJ: Diseases of the stomach. In Mair T, Divers T, Ducharme N, editors: *Manual of equine gastroenterology*, London, 2002, Saunders Elsevier, pp 241–248.

AUTHOR: **KELSEY A. HART**

EDITORS: **TIM MAIR** and **CERI SHERLOCK**

Gastric Ulceration in Adult Horses

BASIC INFORMATION

DEFINITION

Disruption of the gastric mucosa, potentially extending into the lamina propria

EPIDEMIOLOGY

SPECIES, AGE, SEX Most common in race horses (estimated >90% prevalence) and performance horses in active training

RISK FACTORS

- High-concentrate diet
- Stress: Shipping, showing, racing, heavy training
- Gastrointestinal (GI) disease or other illness
- Anorexia or withholding of feed
- Nonsteroidal antiinflammatory drug (NSAID) and corticosteroid therapy

ASSOCIATED CONDITIONS AND DISORDERS

- Inflammatory bowel disease (IBD; idiopathic or autoimmune)
- Gastric outflow obstruction

CLINICAL PRESENTATION

HISTORY, CHIEF COMPLAINT

- Inappetence
- Colic: Usually mild and often associated with feeding
- Bruxism or hypersalivation
- Mild depression
- Weight loss may be noted if chronic or severe
- Behavior or performance issues are often presumptively or anecdotally associated but are not consistent findings. These may include:
  - Discomfort when girthing or mounting, reluctance to move forward, hypersensitivity to leg aids
  - Sudden or gradual decrease in performance
- Many adult horses have no clinical signs even with severe gastric ulceration.

PHYSICAL EXAM FINDINGS

- Usually within normal limits unless the patient has a concurrent predisposing disease.
- Moderately poor body condition and rough hair coat are sometimes present in severe cases. Marked weight loss in a horse that is diagnosed with gastric ulceration suggests concurrent predisposing disease such as IBD and warrants further diagnostic investigation for such a cause.
- Rectal examination: Usually normal unless ulceration is secondary to other GI disease such as IBD, a chronic or recurrent colonic displacement, or other partial intestinal obstruction.

ETIOLOGY AND PATHOPHYSIOLOGY

- Hydrochloric acid is continuously secreted by the parietal cells in the gastric glandular epithelium.
- The gastric mucosa is typically protected from the extremely acidic gastric contents by several mechanisms, including:
  - A mucus-bicarbonate barrier
  - Gastric mucosal blood flow, which is supported by prostaglandins such as prostaglandin E_2 (PGE_2)
  - Eating, which increases gastric pH by stimulating secretion of alkaline saliva and by absorption of gastric secretions by ingested roughage to prevent their contact with the gastric mucosa

- Anything that disrupts these innate protective mechanisms may result in gastric ulceration
  - High-concentrate diets, infrequent feeding and withholding of feed, and anorexia result in prolonged periods of low gastric pH, resulting in lesions in the poorly protected squamous mucosa.
  - NSAID and corticosteroid therapy (by decreased production of protective prostaglandins), intense exercise, and other systemic illness may result in alterations in mucosal blood flow, resulting in both squamous and glandular lesions.
- Bacterial causes of gastric ulceration (eg, *Helicobacter pylori*) have not been documented in horses.

DIAGNOSIS

DIFFERENTIAL DIAGNOSIS

- Gastric neoplasia
- Infectious (bacterial or fungal) gastritis (rare)

INITIAL DATABASE

- Complete blood count
  - Usually within reference intervals.
  - Mild anemia may be present with severe ulceration, but severe hemorrhage associated with gastric ulceration is uncommon in horses.
- Serum biochemical profile
  - Usually within reference intervals.
  - The presence of a hypochloremic metabolic alkalosis in conjunction with gastric ulceration should warrant investigation for a primary gastric outflow obstruction.
  - Severe hypoproteinemia or hypo-albuminemia may suggest more diffuse intestinal protein loss, as with malabsorptive diseases such as IBD or intestinal neoplasia, and warrants further investigation for these conditions.
- Fecal occult blood test: Neither sensitive nor specific for gastric ulceration and thus not recommended for diagnosis
- Transabdominal ultrasonography
  - A portion of the gastric wall is visualized in the left cranial flank, in the region of the ninth to fourteenth intercostal spaces, but it is not possible to image the entire gastric contour in horses, so gastric ulceration may be easily missed by transabdominal ultrasonography.
  - Focal or diffusely increased gastric mural thickness (>1 cm) or focal disruptions in the contour of the gastric wall may indicate gastric ulceration but can be difficult to differentiate from normal gastric rugal folds.

ADVANCED OR CONFIRMATORY TESTING

Gastroscopy:

- A 2- to 3-m flexible endoscope is necessary to fully evaluate the stomach in adult horses and most ponies.
- Twelve to 24 hours of fasting is required before gastroscopy to ensure sufficient visualization for complete evaluation.
- The most common location for gastric ulceration is in the squamous mucosa, just above the margo plicatus, although ulceration may occur anywhere in the squamous or glandular mucosa, including the pyloric region or cardia.
- Ulceration in the cardia and distal esophagus is often associated with gastroesophageal reflux and pyloric outflow obstructions.
- Gastric ulcers are graded on a scale of 0 to 3
  - 0 = Normal, no ulceration
  - 1 = Mild ulceration with single or multifocal hyperemic areas or small superficial ulcers
  - 2 = Moderate ulceration with moderately sized single or multifocal ulcers
  - 3 = Severe ulceration with large, multifocal, coalescing or diffuse, deep, often hemorrhagic ulcers
- Hyperkeratosis of the squamous mucosa in the absence of active ulceration is consistent with previous gastric ulceration.

TREATMENT

THERAPEUTIC GOALS

- Eliminate predisposing disease, stress, or dietary causes.
- Increase gastric pH to limit further mucosal damage.
- Promote mucosal blood flow and support healing.

ACUTE GENERAL TREATMENT

- Decrease or discontinue NSAID therapy if at all possible.
- Decrease or eliminate dietary concentrate and permit access to pasture if possible.
- Gastric acid suppression
  - Proton pump inhibitors
    - Omeprazole: 4 mg/kg PO q24h
      - Requires up to 72 hours to effectively increase gastric pH
      - A lower dose (2 mg/kg PO q24h) may be effective in treating gastric ulceration
      - Very effective, with a success rate greater than 95%
      - The parenteral form (Losec, 0.5 mg/kg IV q24h) may be useful in hospitalized patients in which gastric reflux pre-

vents oral administration (not available in the United States).
    - Pantoprazole (1.5 mg/kg IV q24h) is available for patients in which oral omeprazole cannot be used, but pantoprazole may be cost prohibitive.
  - Histamine H2-receptor antagonists
    - Cimetidine: 16 to 25 mg/kg PO or 6.6 mg/kg IV q6–8h
      - Inhibit hepatic cytochrome p450 oxidase, thus altering metabolism of other drugs; use with caution in patients on concurrent medications
    - Ranitidine: 6.6 mg/kg PO or 1.5 mg/kg IV q8h
    - Famotidine: 2.8 to 4.0 mg/kg PO or 0.23 to 0.5 mg/kg IV q8–12h
    - Because of the need for more frequent administration, these agents are most useful to rapidly increase gastric pH during the initial 72 hours of proton pump inhibitor therapy but may also be effective when used alone.
  - Antacids (magnesium hydroxide, aluminum hydroxide): Require frequent administration (q2–4h) to have any effect on increasing gastric pH; thus not recommended
- Mucosal protectants
  - Sucralfate: 20 mg/kg PO q6–8h
    - Adheres to ulcerated mucosa, providing protection from gastric acid, and stimulates local production of protective prostaglandins and cytokines to promote mucosal healing
    - Useful in improving comfort during initial therapy (3–7 days) in horses with severe gastric ulceration
  - Misoprostol: 2.5 to 5.0 µg/kg
    - A PGE_2 analogue that inhibits acid secretion, promotes mucosal blood flow, and enhances bicarbonate and mucus production
    - Useful in NSAID-induced gastric ulceration
    - Side effects may include abdominal pain and diarrhea.
    - Should not be used in pregnant mares or handled by women who are or may become pregnant

CHRONIC TREATMENT

Acid suppression therapy should be continued for 3 to 4 weeks to ensure complete mucosal healing.

DRUG INTERACTIONS

Sucralfate can prevent the absorption of other drugs and should not be given within 1 to 2 hours of other medications, particularly orally administered H2-receptor antagonists.

POSSIBLE COMPLICATIONS

Perforation of a gastric ulcer may occur but is very rare in adult horses.

RECOMMENDED MONITORING

- Improvement in clinical signs is often adequate for determining response to therapy.
- In asymptomatic horses or those with severe ulceration, gastroscopy should be repeated in 4 to 6 weeks to ensure complete resolution.
- Repeat gastroscopy is imperative in horses whose clinical signs do not improve with or recur after medical therapy. Biopsy of gastric lesions is warranted in these cases and can be performed transendoscopically.

PROGNOSIS AND OUTCOME

- Primary gastric ulceration carries a good prognosis with medical therapy of sufficient duration and appropriate diet and management changes.
- Recurrence is common in performance horses. Some horses may require intermittent or prolonged prophylactic therapy (see below).

PEARLS & CONSIDERATIONS

COMMENTS

Gastric ulceration in a pasture or pleasure horse or persistent or recurrent gastric ulceration despite appropriate medical therapy and dietary and management changes should prompt an extensive diagnostic search for an underlying and predisposing problem (eg, IBD, recurrent intestinal obstruction).

PREVENTION

- Dietary and routine management
  - Limit or eliminate concentrates or grain.
  - Feed small meals often and provide access to pasture or free-choice hay to prevent large fluctuations in or prolonged periods of low gastric pH.
  - Elimination of shipping and training stress is impossible in racehorses and performance horses, but provision of maximal turnout time and maintenance of a consistent routine are helpful and should be attempted.
  - Avoid long-term NSAID or corticosteroid therapy if possible.
- Medical ulcer prophylaxis
  - Omeprazole: 1 to 2 mg/kg PO q24h
  - Has been shown to effectively prevent gastric ulceration in race

horses in some studies but may not be necessary with above diet and routine changes
  - Efficacy at preventing NSAID-induced gastric ulceration is unknown
- Corn oil (45 mL PO qd on feed) has been shown to decrease gastric acid output and increase PGE2 synthesis in horses and thus may have some gastroprotective effects. However, it was ineffective in preventing experimentally induced gastric ulceration in one study.

SUGGESTED READING

Cargile JL, Burrow JA, Kim I, et al: Effect of dietary corn oil supplementation on equine gastric fluid acid, sodium, and prostaglandin E2 content before and during pentagastrin infusion. *J Vet Intern Med* 18:545–549, 2005.

Frank N, Andrews FM, Elliott SB, Lew J: Effects of dietary oils on the development of gastric ulcers in mares. *Am J Vet Res* 66:2006–2011, 2005.

McClure SR, White GW, Sifferman RL, et al: Efficacy of omeprazole paste for prevention of recurrence of gastric ulcers in horses in race training. *J Am Vet Med Assoc* 226:1685–1688, 2005.

Orsini JA, Mueller POE: Gastric ulcers. In Orsini HJ, Divers TJ, editors: *Equine emergencies: treatment and procedures.* St Louis, 2008, Saunders Elsevier, pp 155–157.

AUTHOR: KELSEY A. HART

EDITORS: TIM MAIR and **CERI SHERLOCK**

Gastric Ulceration in Foals

BASIC INFORMATION

DEFINITION

Disruption of the gastric mucosa, potentially extending into the lamina propria

SYNONYM(S)

Gastroduodenal ulcer disease (GDUD)

EPIDEMIOLOGY

SPECIES, AGE, SEX Most common in foals ages 1 to 6 months but is also occasionally seen in younger foals

RISK FACTORS

- Gastrointestinal (GI) disease, especially diarrhea
- Nonsteroidal antiinflammatory drug (NSAID) therapy
- Anorexia or withholding of enteral nutrition

ASSOCIATED CONDITIONS AND DISORDERS Neonatal encephalopathy (neonatal maladjustment syndrome) and sepsis in young foals

CLINICAL PRESENTATION

HISTORY, CHIEF COMPLAINT

- Colic
  - Variable severity but usually more severe than in adult horses with gastric ulceration.
  - May be manifest as increased periods of recumbency.
  - Young foals with gastric ulcers are often observed to roll onto their backs or lie in dorsal recumbency, but this may also be observed in foals with colic due to other causes.
- Bruxism
- Hypersalivation
- Inappetence
- Diarrhea is commonly associated with GDUD in foals in contrast to the case in adult horses.
- Poor condition if the case is chronic and severe.
- In contrast to adult horses, foals with GDUD almost always show related clinical signs.

PHYSICAL EXAM FINDINGS

- Tachycardia and tachypnea are common during colic episodes
- ± Fever
- ± Evidence of diarrhea
- Poor body condition and rough hair coat may be present in severe cases

ETIOLOGY AND PATHOPHYSIOLOGY

- Similar to adult horses, in which an imbalance between innate gastroprotective factors and injurious factors such as hydrochloric acid and proteolytic enzymes (pepsin) occurs
  - Innate gastroprotective factors include the mucus-bicarbonate barrier; adequate gastric mucosal blood flow; and nursing or eating, which rapidly increases gastric pH.
  - These protective mechanisms are easily disrupted in foals, with rapid decreases in gastric pH seen in healthy foals with more than 20 minutes of not nursing. This may result in lesions in the glandular mucosa.

- The gastric squamous mucosa undergoes rapid thickening and then desquamation in neonatal foals, which may also predispose them to squamous mucosal lesions.
  - Concurrent disease in foals, such as neonatal encephalopathy or sepsis, may significantly disrupt gastric mucosal blood flow and may result in or worsen both glandular and squamous gastric ulceration.
- Duodenal ulceration is uncommon in adult horses but occurs frequently in foals. This may be a direct result of impaired duodenal mucosal defenses and subsequent injury from exposure to gastric acid, or it may be related to more diffuse intestinal disease (bacterial enterocolitis).

DIAGNOSIS

DIFFERENTIAL DIAGNOSIS

- Infectious enterocolitis
- Pyloric stenosis (congenital)
- Small intestinal obstructive lesions

INITIAL DATABASE

- Complete blood count
  - Usually within reference intervals with primary GDUD.
  - Mild anemia may be present with severe ulceration, but severe hemorrhage is uncommon.
  - Abnormalities in the leukogram, such as leukopenia or leukocytosis, may be present in severe cases of GDUD or may reflect concurrent infectious enterocolitis, sepsis, or other illness.
- Serum biochemical profile
  - Usually within reference intervals.
  - The presence of a hypochloremic metabolic alkalosis should warrant investigation for a concurrent pyloric outflow obstruction.
- Fecal occult blood test: Neither sensitive nor specific for gastric ulceration and thus not useful for diagnosis.
- Transabdominal ultrasonography
  - A portion of the gastric wall is visualized in the left cranial flank in the region of the ninth to fourteenth intercostal spaces, but it is not possible to image the entire gastric contour, so gastric ulceration may be easily missed.
  - Focal or diffusely increased gastric mural thickness (>8–10 mm) or focal disruptions in the contour of the gastric wall may indicate gastric ulceration but can be difficult to differentiate from normal gastric rugal folds.

ADVANCED OR CONFIRMATORY TESTING

- Gastroduodenoscopy
  - A 2- to 3-m flexible endoscope is necessary to fully evaluate the stomach and duodenum in most foals.
  - Feed should be withheld and nursing prevented for approximately 1 hour before gastroduodenoscopy in very young foals and for 2 to 6 hours in older foals on solid feed.
  - Ulceration may occur anywhere in the squamous or glandular mucosa, pyloric region, or cardia. Glandular and pyloric mucosal lesions and duodenal ulcers are more common in foals than adults.
  - Ulceration in the cardia and distal esophagus is often associated with gastroesophageal reflux and pyloric outflow obstructions. Pyloric sphincter function should be evaluated carefully and further evaluation or treatment for gastric outflow obstructions pursued if indicated (see "Pyloric Stenosis" in this section).
  - A specific grading system has not been established for foals, but a similar grading system as for adult horses (see "Gastric Ulceration in Adult Horses" in this section) is often used.

TREATMENT

THERAPEUTIC GOAL(S)

- Eliminate predisposing causes and treat the underlying disease.
- Increase gastric pH to limit further mucosal damage.
- Promote mucosal blood flow and support healing.

ACUTE GENERAL TREATMENT

- Discontinue and avoid NSAID therapy.
- Promote frequent nursing or feed (roughage) intake in older foals to help increase gastric pH.
- Supportive care with IV fluids is indicated in dehydrated or anorectic foals.
- Acid suppression
  - Proton pump inhibitors
    - Omeprazole: 4 mg/kg PO q24h
      - Appears to increase gastric pH more rapidly (with one dose) in foals compared with adult horses (with approximately three doses).
      - The parenteral form (Losec, 0.5 mg/kg IV q24h) is useful in foals in which gastric reflux prevents PO administration (not available in the United States).
    - Pantoprazole: 1.5 mg/kg IV q24h
      - Has been shown to effectively increase gastric pH in foals
      - Available in the United States
  - Histamine H2-receptor antagonists
    - Cimetidine: 16 to 25 mg/kg PO or 6.6 mg/kg IV q6–8h
      - Inhibits hepatic cytochrome p450 oxidase and thus alters metabolism of other drugs; use with caution in patients on concurrent medications
    - Ranitidine: 6.6 mg/kg PO or 1.5 mg/kg IV q8h
    - Famotidine: 2.8 to 4.0 mg/kg PO or 0.23 to 0.5 mg/kg IV q8–12h
  - Antacids (magnesium hydroxide, aluminum hydroxide): Less effective than the above; not recommended
- Mucosal protectants
  - Sucralfate: 20 mg/kg PO q6–8h
    - Adheres to ulcerated mucosa, providing protection from gastric acid, and stimulates local production of protective prostaglandins and cytokines to promote mucosal healing
    - Appears to effectively improve comfort in foals with severe lesions
  - Misoprostol: 2.5 to 5.0 µg/kg PO q12–24h
    - A prostaglandin E2 (PGE2) analogue that inhibits acid secretion, promotes mucosal blood flow, and enhances bicarbonate and mucus production
    - Useful in NSAID-induced gastric ulceration
    - Side effects may include abdominal pain and diarrhea
    - Should not be handled by women who are or may become pregnant
- Analgesic therapy
  - Avoid NSAIDS!
  - Sedation with diazepam, α_2 adrenergic agonists, or opioids (butorphanol) may be beneficial in foals with severe colic.
  - Intragastric administration of 2% lidocaine may provide transient pain relief in severe cases (10–20 mL diluted to 60 mL with saline for an average foal; be careful not to exceed a total dose of ~7–8 mg/kg). IV lidocaine (1.5 mg/kg IV slow bolus; then 0.05 mg/kg/min IV continuous rate infusion) may also be beneficial for analgesic and prokinetic effects, but lidocaine safety and pharmacokinetics have not been determined in foals.
- Antimicrobial therapy
  - Not indicated in foals with uncomplicated primary GDUD
  - Broad-spectrum antimicrobial prophylaxis should be considered in

foals with severe GDUD with fever or concurrent diarrhea because a significant proportion of foals with diarrhea have bacteremia.

CHRONIC TREATMENT

Medical therapy should be continued for 3 to 4 weeks to ensure complete mucosal healing.

DRUG INTERACTIONS

Sucralfate can prevent the absorption of other drugs and should not be given within 1 to 2 hours of other oral medications, particularly orally administered H2-receptor antagonists.

POSSIBLE COMPLICATIONS

- Gastric or duodenal ulcer perforation
- Pyloric or duodenal stricture resulting in pyloric outflow obstruction

RECOMMENDED MONITORING

Gastroscopy should be repeated in approximately 4 weeks to ensure complete resolution and assess for development of pyloric or duodenal stricture formation.

PROGNOSIS AND OUTCOME

- Prognosis is good if foal shows a good clinical response within 3 to 5 days of initiating early and aggressive medical therapy.
- Prognosis is guarded to poor if pyloric outflow obstruction develops.

PEARLS & CONSIDERATIONS

COMMENTS

- Gastric acid provides an important protective mechanism in preventing GI bacterial invasion; thus increasing the gastric pH with acid suppression therapy is not innocuous.
  - Critically ill, recumbent neonatal foals do not appear to have extremely acidic gastric pH and may not need acid suppression therapy.
  - Sucralfate may provide adequate gastric ulcer prophylaxis in foals

that are at risk for but do not have active gastric ulceration.

- However, foals may be at greater risk for NSAID-induced gastric ulceration than adult horses.
  - Avoid NSAIDs in foals if possible.
  - If prolonged NSAID use is unavoidable, concurrent administration of sucralfate or omeprazole may be considered for ulcer prophylaxis, although the efficacy of omeprazole in preventing NSAID-induced ulceration has not been established experimentally.

SUGGESTED READING

Murray MJ: Stomach diseases of the foal. In Mair T, Divers T, Ducharme N, editors: *Manual of equine gastroenterology*, London, 2002, Saunders Elsevier, pp 469–476.

Orsini JA, Mueller POE: Gastric ulcers. In Orsini HJ, Divers TJ, editors: *Equine emergencies: treatment and procedures*, St Louis, 2008, Saunders Elsevier, pp 155–157.

AUTHOR: **KELSEY A. HART**

EDITORS: **TIM MAIR** and **CERI SHERLOCK**

Glanders

BASIC INFORMATION

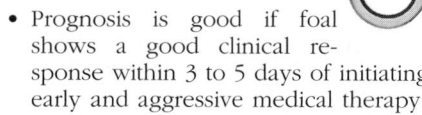

DEFINITION

A disease of horses caused by infection with the bacteria *Burkholderia mallei* that may affect the skin, nasal passages, or lungs

SYNONYM(S)

Farcy (cutaneous form)

EPIDEMIOLOGY

SPECIES, AGE, SEX

- Horses, donkeys, and mules are affected.
- Occasional cases are seen in cats, dogs, goats, sheep, and camels.
- Carnivores may be infected from ingestion of contaminated meat.

RISK FACTORS Poor sanitation, crowding, immunosuppression

CONTAGION AND ZOONOSIS

- Rare but serious zoonotic disease
- Enters via cutaneous exposure
- Cutaneous and systemic infections occur with mortality that may approach 95% in untreated humans

GEOGRAPHY AND SEASONALITY

- Restricted to Eastern Europe, Asia, Africa, the Middle East, Central America, and South America

- Endemic in some countries, including Iraq, Turkey, Pakistan, India, Mongolia, and China
- Eradicated from Europe, Australia, and North America

CLINICAL PRESENTATION

DISEASE FORMS/SUBTYPES

- Cutaneous form
- Nasal form
- Acute pulmonary form

HISTORY, CHIEF COMPLAINT

- Cutaneous swellings, erosions, ulcerations with exudate
- Lymphatic cording
- Depression, inappetence
- Dyspnea, nasal discharge, increased respiratory rate

PHYSICAL EXAM FINDINGS

- Cutaneous form ("farcy"): Nodules with subsequent development of ulcers and exudation. Swollen lymphatic vessels with cording and development of "farcy buds" that enlarge, ulcerate, and drain.
- Nasal form: Nodules on nasal septum develop into stellate scars with purulent nasal discharge. These may obstruct the nasopharynx with severe dyspnea.
- Acute pulmonary form: High fever, bronchopneumonia

ETIOLOGY AND PATHOPHYSIOLOGY

- Short, gram-negative, aerobic, facultative intracellular, nonmotile, non–spore-forming bacterial rods
- Host-adapted pathogen that does not persist long in the environment
- Probably enters horses through the mucous membranes with common feed and water the most likely sources of infection
- Subclinical infection in horses may contribute to spread in a group of horses
- Disease may be more severe in donkeys and mules

DIAGNOSIS

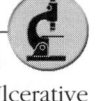

DIFFERENTIAL DIAGNOSIS

- Cutaneous form ("farcy"): Ulcerative lymphangitis (*Corynebacterium pseudotuberculosis*), sporotrichosis (*Sporothrix schenckii*), epizootic lymphangitis (*Histoplasma farciminosum*), melioidoses (*Burkholderia pseudomallei*)
- Nasal form: Strangles, neoplasia, upper respiratory tract infection
- Acute pulmonary form: Bacterial bronchopneumonia, African horse sickness, acute interstitial pneumonia

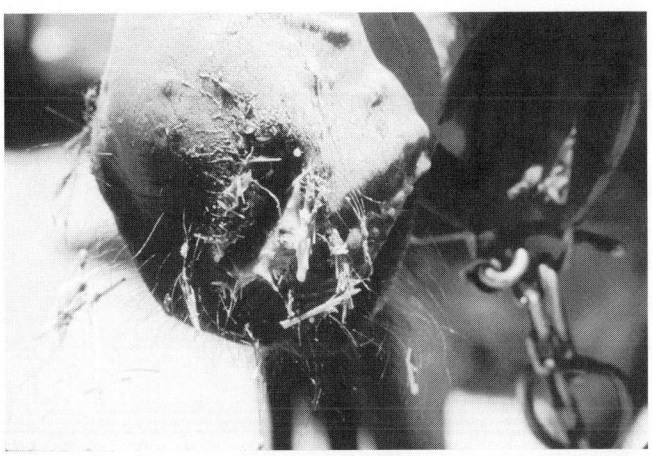

FIGURE 1 Nasal exudate in a horse with glanders. (From Sellon DC, Long MT: *Equine infectious diseases.* St Louis, 2007, Saunders Elsevier.)

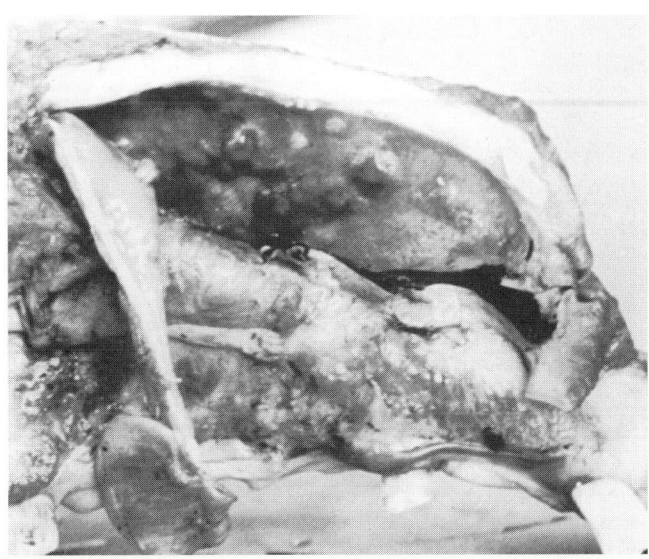

FIGURE 3 Pulmonary granulomas and marked congestion observed at necropsy of a horse with glanders. (From Sellon DC, Long MT: *Equine infectious diseases.* St Louis, 2007, Saunders Elsevier.)

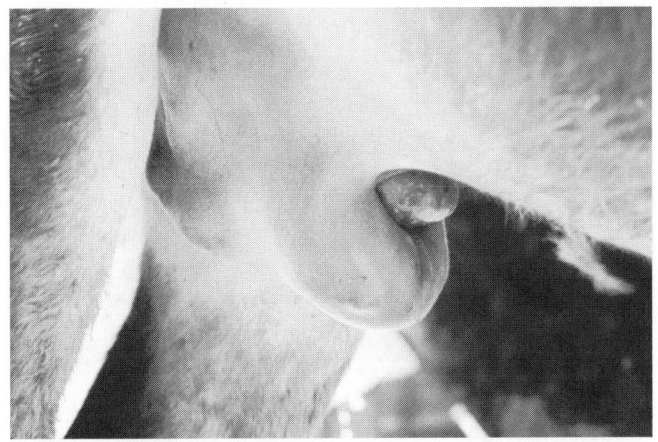

FIGURE 2 Swollen sheath in horse with orchitis caused by glanders. (From Sellon DC, Long MT: *Equine infectious diseases.* St Louis, 2007, Saunders Elsevier.)

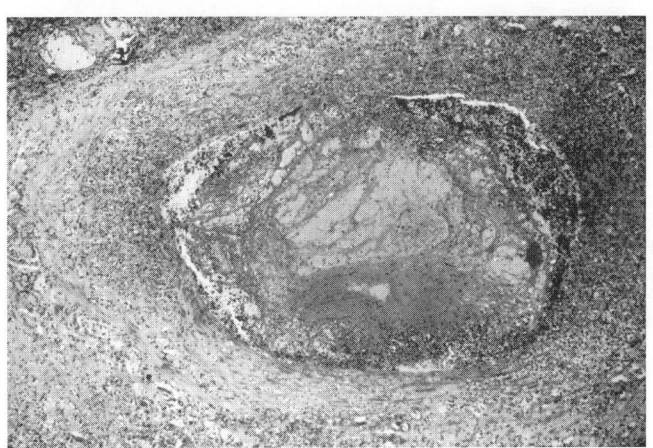

FIGURE 4 Photomicrograph of a typical nodule from a horse with glanders. (From Sellon DC, Long MT: *Equine infectious diseases.* St Louis, 2007, Saunders Elsevier.)

INITIAL DATABASE

Laboratory tests are consistent with acute or chronic infection.

ADVANCED OR CONFIRMATORY TESTING

- Mallein test: Intradermal injection of bacterial extract in the neck or eyelid with subsequent observation for hypersensitivity reaction. Reactions include fever higher than 104° F, local swelling of 35 mm in diameter after 48 to 72 hours, and lacrimation. False-negative and -positive reactions may occur.
- Serologic tests: Complement fixation, agglutination, enzyme-linked immunosorbent assay, and counter immunoelectrophoresis. Many false-positive and -negative results may occur.

- Culture or immunohistochemical staining to detect organism in tissues or exudates.

TREATMENT

THERAPEUTIC GOAL(S)

Eradication of the disease

ACUTE GENERAL TREATMENT

- The organism may be susceptible to enrofloxacin, ticarcillin-clavulanate, imipenem, chloramphenicol, doxycycline, rifampicin, and erythromycin.
- Treatment is rarely attempted.
- There has been a recent report of cure with 3-week treatment using combination treatment with IV enrofloxacin and trimethoprim-sulfadiazine.

PROGNOSIS AND OUTCOME

- Euthanasia or slaughter of infected Equids is strongly recommended and is mandatory in many countries, including the United States.
- No vaccine is available.

PEARLS & CONSIDERATIONS

There have been no naturally occurring cases of glanders in North America in more than 60 years.

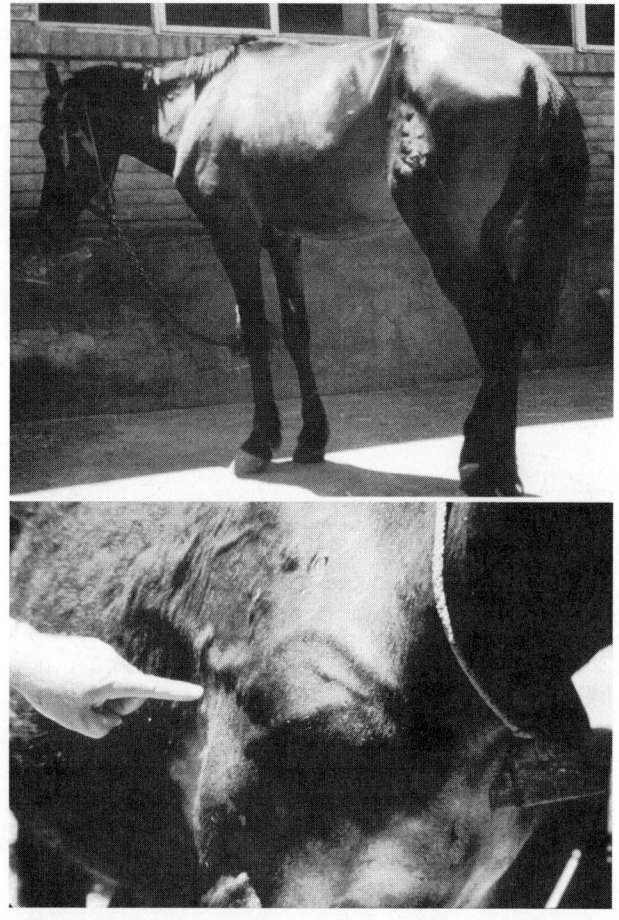

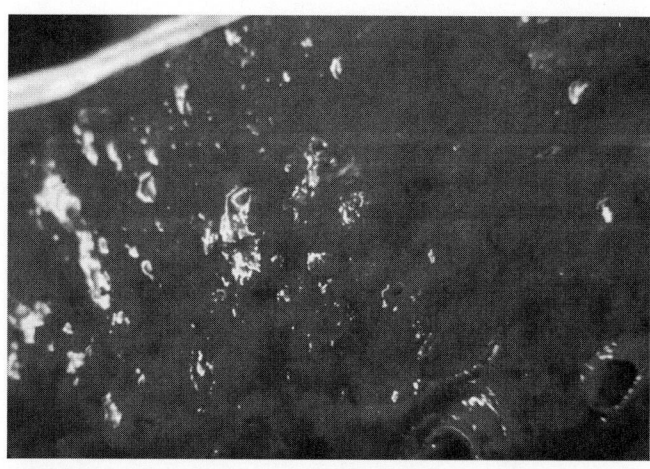

FIGURE 6 Granulomas and ulcers (stellate scar) in the nasal septum of a horse with glanders. (From Sellon DC, Long MT: *Equine infectious diseases.* St Louis, 2007, Saunders Elsevier.)

FIGURE 5 *Top* and *bottom,* Nodules, swollen cutaneous lymphatic vessels, and drainage typical of horses with glanders. (From Sellon DC, Long MT: *Equine infectious diseases.* St Louis, 2007, Saunders Elsevier.)

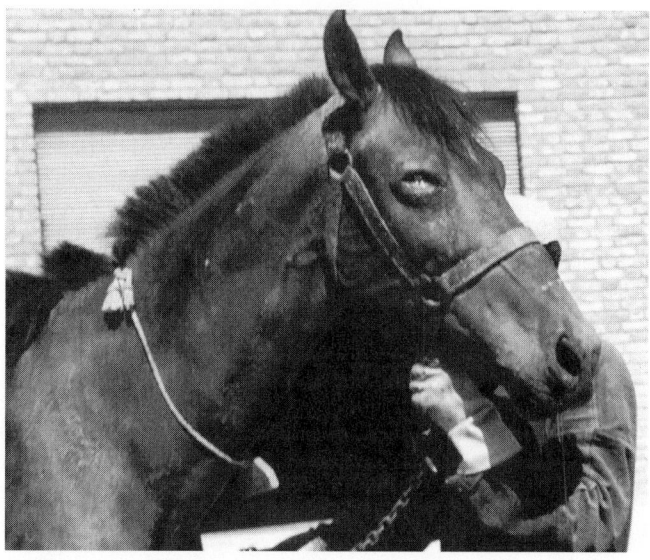

FIGURE 7 Positive ocular reaction to mullein. (From Sellon DC, Long MT: *Equine infectious diseases.* St Louis, 2007, Saunders Elsevier.)

SUGGESTED READING

Elschner MC, Klaus CU, Liebler-Tenorio E, et al: *Burkholderia mallei* infection in a horse imported from Brazil. *Equine Vet Educ* 21:147, 2009.

Nicoletti PL: Glanders. In Sellon DC, Long MT, editors: *Equine infectious diseases,* St Louis, 2007, Elsevier, pp 345–348.

AUTHOR: **DEBRA C. SELLON**

EDITORS: **MAUREEN T. LONG** and **DEBRA C. SELLON**

Glaucoma

BASIC INFORMATION

DEFINITION
Pathologic disease state associated with elevated intraocular pressure (IOP)

EPIDEMIOLOGY
GENETICS AND BREED PREDISPOSITION
Horses prone to developing recurrent uveitis are at risk for developing glaucoma.
RISK FACTORS
- Any type of ocular trauma
- Chronic or recurrent uveitis

ASSOCIATED CONDITIONS AND DISORDERS
Chronic or recurrent uveitis

CLINICAL PRESENTATION
DISEASE FORMS/SUBTYPES
- Primary glaucoma: No underlying or preceding ocular disease

- Secondary glaucoma: Any ocular abnormality, such as uveitis or neoplasia, that results in elevated IOP and glaucoma

HISTORY, CHIEF COMPLAINT

- The most common cause of glaucoma in horses is chronic or recurrent uveitis (a type of secondary glaucoma). Historically, these horses have multiple episodes of intraocular inflammation followed by a severe, unrelenting bout of ocular cloudiness and discomfort (as a result of the development of glaucoma) that does not respond to traditional uveitis therapy.
- Horses with primary glaucoma most commonly present with partial or diffuse corneal edema. These eyes may or may not be painful.

PHYSICAL EXAM FINDINGS

- Horses with secondary glaucoma associated with chronic uveitis have high IOP (40–80 mm Hg); diffusely edematous corneas; and signs of chronic intraocular inflammation, such as posterior synechia (adhesions), a miotic pupil, and cataract formation. These eyes may appear enlarged or normal sized (Figure 1).
- Horses with primary glaucoma most commonly present with partial or diffuse corneal edema. These eyes may or may not be painful. Early in the disease process, vision and pupil size may be normal. IOP may range from 35 to 80 mm Hg.
- With chronic primary glaucoma, vision decreases, the cornea becomes diffusely edematous, and other signs of chronic glaucoma may become evident (eg, diffuse corneal edema, corneal striae, retinal and optic nerve degeneration). In general, however, the horse tends to lose vision much later in the disease process compared with dogs and humans. An increased size of the eye (>40–45 mm anterior to posterior) and lens subluxation may also occur late in the disease.

ETIOLOGY AND PATHOPHYSIOLOGY

Aqueous humor, which acts to supply metabolic needs of intraocular structures, is produced constantly by the ciliary body of the equine eye. The fluid must also drain constantly from the eye through the iridocorneal and uveoscleral outflow pathways. Obstruction of this outflow of fluid may be the result of an abnormally developed drain (ie, primary glaucoma) or through damage to the drain from scarring, vascularization, or accumulation of debris (ie, secondary glaucoma). The result of this obstruction is retention of aqueous humor and a subsequent increase in the pressure within the eye. The pathologic disease state associated with elevated IOP is called glaucoma.

DIAGNOSIS

DIFFERENTIAL DIAGNOSIS

Other causes of corneal edema should be ruled out:

- Corneal ulcers
- Immune-mediated keratitis (IMMK), especially the endothelial form of IMMK
- Uveitis
- Primary endothelial disease
- Anterior lens luxation

INITIAL DATABASE

- A tonometer is essential for the diagnosis of equine glaucoma. Applanation tonometers must be used. The most practical and portable applanation tonometers are the Tonopen, Tonometer, and TonoVet Tonometer. For accurate tonometry, auriculopalpebral nerve blocks should be performed because tension on the eyelids may artificially elevate the IOP. In addition, tranquilization may artificially lower the IOP. The pressure measurement should be taken from the most normal, least edematous

location of the cornea if possible.

- A thorough and complete ophthalmic examination should also be done to help differentiate the cause of the glaucoma and to rule out other causes of corneal edema, such as keratitis. With glaucoma, the cornea is edematous, but rarely, yellow or creamy cellular infiltrate, epithelial loss (ie, corneal ulceration), or diffuse vascularization is present. These findings are more common with primary corneal disease. The complete ophthalmic examination will also determine if the glaucoma is primary or secondary. Glaucoma secondary to intraocular disease other than uveitis is rare but is possible with intraocular tumors and luxation of the lens.

ADVANCED OR CONFIRMATORY TESTING

Tonometry is needed for confirmation of glaucoma.

TREATMENT

THERAPEUTIC GOAL(S)

Lower the IOP

ACUTE GENERAL TREATMENT

Treatment options reported in the horse include:

- Topical timolol 0.5% (1 drop or 0.2 mL) BID
- If there is poor control with this therapy (after 7–10 days), the next choice is a combination of timolol 0.5% and dorzolamide HCl (1 drop or 0.2 mL q8h).
- Another option is brinzolamide HCl (1 drop or 0.2 mL q8h).
- Systemic nonsteroidal antiinflammatory drugs also seem to lower the IOP by an unknown mechanism.

CHRONIC TREATMENT

If there continues to be poor IOP control and there is potential for vision, then laser cycloablation (laser destruction of the ciliary body) is indicated.

POSSIBLE COMPLICATIONS

Vision loss is common because the disease is progressive. Both eyes are at risk and should be monitored.

RECOMMENDED MONITORING

Examine weekly until pressures are controlled and then every 3 months.

PROGNOSIS AND OUTCOME

Prognosis is guarded for saving the eye.

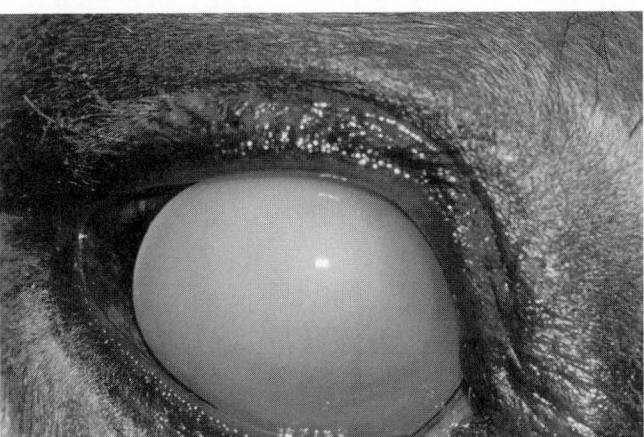

FIGURE 1 Equine glaucoma.

PEARLS & CONSIDERATIONS

COMMENTS

Both eyes are at risk and should be monitored.

PREVENTION

- Minimizing ocular and corneal trauma may help prevent the development of glaucoma.

- Use of a quality fly mask is recommended.
- Feeding hay on the ground is recommended to minimize ocular trauma.

CLIENT EDUCATION

Client communication is essential so it is understood that treatment is aimed at controlling, not curing, this condition. Persistent treatment is required to maintain vision.

SUGGESTED READING

Lassaline M, Brooks D: Equine glaucoma. In Gilger BC, editor: *Equine ophthalmology*, St Louis, 2005, Elsevier, pp 323–339.

AUTHOR & EDITOR: **BRIAN C. GILGER**

Glomerulonephritis

BASIC INFORMATION

DEFINITION

Glomerulonephritis is a renal disease in which immune-mediated glomerular damage is the initiating factor. The hallmark of glomerulonephritis is increased permeability of the glomerular barrier. Proliferative glomerulonephritis is characterized by proliferation of the mesangial cells with an influx of inflammatory cells. Membranous glomerulonephritis is characterized by accumulation of matrix and thickening of the glomerular basement membrane (GBM) and capillary wall.

SYNONYM(S)

Glomerulonephropathy, proliferative glomerulonephritis, membranous glomerulonephritis

EPIDEMIOLOGY

RISK FACTORS Glomerulonephritis has been reported with several underlying disease processes, including equine infectious anemia (75% of cases have histologic evidence of glomerulonephritis), *Streptococcus equi* subsp. *equi* and *Streptococcus equi* subsp. *zooepidemicus* infection, purpura hemorrhagica, and leptospirosis. Any chronic infection or neoplasia can be a predisposing cause of glomerulonephritis.
CONTAGION AND ZOONOSIS *S. equi* subsp. *equi* and *S. equi* subsp. *zooepidemicus* may cause poststreptococcal glomerulonephritis in humans.
ASSOCIATED CONDITIONS AND DISORDERS Hypercoagulability and thrombosis are common complications of glomerulonephritis.

CLINICAL PRESENTATION

DISEASE FORMS/SUBTYPES
- Proliferative or membranous glomerulonephritis
- Glomerulonephritis may cause subclinical or clinical disease.

HISTORY, CHIEF COMPLAINT
- Weight loss
- Polyuria
- Polydipsia
- ± Ventral edema
- ± Decreased appetite
- ± Lethargy

PHYSICAL EXAM FINDINGS
- Poor body condition
- ± Ventral edema

ETIOLOGY AND PATHOPHYSIOLOGY
- Circulating immune complexes are deposited along the glomerular capillaries or form in situ along the GBM.
- Rarely, glomerulonephritis results from true immune-mediated disease caused by antibodies against the GBM.
- Inflammatory cells infiltrate the glomerulus, releasing proteolytic enzymes and reactive oxygen species that further damage the glomerulus and increase glomerular permeability.
- Complement is activated by immune complexes (type III hypersensitivity), leading to platelet activation, thrombosis, and further glomerular damage.
- Mesangial cells proliferate, excess matrix is produced, and fibrosis occurs.
- The glomerular barrier may also be damaged as a result of ischemia, toxic insult, or infection.

DIAGNOSIS

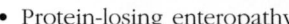

DIFFERENTIAL DIAGNOSIS

- Protein-losing enteropathy
- Protein-losing nephropathy (glomerulonephritis or acute tubular necrosis)
- Hepatic disease

INITIAL DATABASE

- Complete blood count and fibrinogen concentration
- Serum chemistries: Decreased total protein and albumin; may also have elevated blood urea nitrogen, creatinine, and triglyceride concentrations

- Urinalysis: Proteinuria; may also have hematuria and lipiduria
- Rectal examination: The left kidney may feel small if the patient has advanced renal disease.
- Renal ultrasonography: Loss of corticomedullary contrast with advanced renal disease

ADVANCED OR CONFIRMATORY TESTING

- Glucose or D-xylose absorption test: To rule out protein-losing enteropathy
- Urine protein:creatinine ratio: A value greater than 2:1 indicates glomerular protein loss
- Antithrombin III: Decreased in plasma and increased in urine
- Systemic complement concentration: Decreased
- Systemic blood pressure: May be increased
- Streptococcal M-protein titer: May be increased if *S. equi* infection is the underlying cause
- Coggins test: Positive result if equine infectious anemia is the underlying cause
- Renal biopsy: To confirm lesion and help determine prognosis
- Light microscopy, immunohistochemistry, or electron microscopy: To confirm lesion
- Immunofluorescence: To determine the underlying etiology. Granular, irregular staining indicates immune complex deposition, whereas linear staining indicates anti-GBM antibodies.

TREATMENT

THERAPEUTIC GOAL(S)

- Address underlying disease, if present
- Provide immune modulation
- Reduce hypercoagulability
- Reduce hypertension
- Decrease dietary protein intake

ACUTE/CHRONIC GENERAL TREATMENT

- Immunosuppressive therapy: Only if indicated for underlying disease. Corticosteroids are known to increase GFR, stimulate glomerular hypertrophy, and enhance matrix production in humans. They can also increase the risk of infection, thrombosis, and azotemia.
- Immune modulation: Supplement dietary omega-3 fatty acids, such as linseed oil (2–6 oz/d), canola oil, or commercial diets high in omega-3 fatty acids.
- Hypercoagulability: Low-dose aspirin therapy (4–12 mg/kg PO q24–48h).
- Hypertension: Angiotensin-converting enzyme (ACE) inhibitors, such as enalapril (0.5–1 mg/kg PO q12–24h), may be effective, if not cost prohibitive. Acepromazine (0.02 mg/kg PO q8–12h) is inferior to the ACE inhibitors but may be useful.
- Reduce dietary protein: 1.3 g of crude protein/kg/d is the lower end of protein requirement for horses. This can be accomplished by feeding 6.4 kg of grass hay and 2 kg of 12% protein senior-type feed per day.

POSSIBLE COMPLICATIONS

Long-term immunosuppressive treatment may increase the risk of concurrent disease and laminitis (if large doses of corticosteroids are administered).

RECOMMENDED MONITORING

Monitor the degree of proteinuria and azotemia as well as the horse's clinical condition.

PROGNOSIS AND OUTCOME

- The prognosis for long-term survival is poor, even with treatment.
- Horses with chronic low-grade azotemia may still be used for breeding and light riding.

PEARLS & CONSIDERATIONS

COMMENTS

- Renal changes caused by glomerulonephritis are common in horses, but clinical disease is rare.

- Glomerulonephritis is the most common cause of chronic renal failure in horses.
- Horses are the only domestic species in which anti-GBM complexes have been found in naturally occurring cases of disease.
- Horses are the only species to have focal glomerulosclerosis.

PREVENTION

Appropriate routine care and quarantine protocols may reduce the risk of infectious diseases that have been associated with glomerulonephritis.

SUGGESTED READING

Divers T: Proliferative glomerulonephritis. In Smith B, editor: *Large animal internal medicine*, St Louis, 2009, Mosby Elsevier, p 930.
Schott H: Chronic renal failure in horses. *Vet Clin Equine* 23:593–612, 2007.
Van Biervliet J, Divers TJ, Porter B, et al: Glomerulonephritis in horses. *Compend Contin Educ Pract Vet* 24:892, 2002.

AUTHOR: **KELLY L. CARLSON**

EDITOR: **BRYAN M. WALDRIDGE**

Grain Overload

BASIC INFORMATION

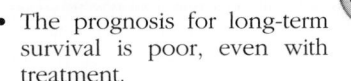

DEFINITION

Ingestion (almost always accidental) of a large quantity of grain

CLINICAL PRESENTATION

HISTORY, CHIEF COMPLAINT

- Recent consumption of a large amount of grain
- Well-educated horse owners may request evaluation and treatment immediately after discovering excessive grain ingestion before the development of clinical signs.
- Signs typically occur within 1 to 48 hours, depending on the amount and type of grain consumed, and usually include colic, profuse sweating, and trembling.
- Lameness caused by acute laminitis may also be observed.
- Diarrhea is sometimes reported but is less common.

PHYSICAL EXAM FINDINGS

- Early on, the physical examination results may be within normal limits.
- If clinical signs are present, they include some or all of the following:

  - Marked tachycardia and tachypnea
  - Variable rectal temperature, ranging from hypothermia because of poor perfusion or shock to pyrexia associated with endotoxemia
  - Hyperemic to purple mucous membranes, prolonged capillary refill time, cold extremities, poor jugular refill, prolonged skin tent
  - Severe gross abdominal distension, absent gastrointestinal borborygmi, or hypermotile or "fluidy" gastrointestinal sounds
  - Signs of laminitis: Bounding digital pulses, weight shifting, lameness, reluctance to move or pick up the feet, sensitivity to hoof testers over the toe
- Rectal examination
  - May be within normal limits early on.
  - Colonic gas distension with taut colonic bands is usually present by the time clinical signs have developed.

ETIOLOGY AND PATHOPHYSIOLOGY

Rapid consumption of an excessive amount of soluble carbohydrates has several consequences.

- Early on, especially if a very large volume of grain has been consumed, overdistension of the stomach and primary gastric dilatation caused by fermentation occurs (see "Gastric Dilation" in this section) and may result in gastric rupture in severe cases.
- As the ingested grain material enters the small intestine, the enteric carbohydrate digestive capacity is overwhelmed. Fermentation of this excess carbohydrate thus occurs in the cecum and large colon, resulting in rapid overgrowth of fermenting hindgut bacteria and death of normal fiber-digesting bacterial flora.
- This damages the colonic mucosal barrier, permitting bacterial byproducts, such as lactic acid, endotoxin, and exotoxins, to enter the systemic circulation and culminating in a massive systemic inflammatory response.
- The horse may succumb to the severe cardiovascular consequences of septic or endotoxic and hypovolemic shock or may develop laminar vascular disruption and inflammation culminating in laminitis.

DIAGNOSIS

INITIAL DATABASE

- Passage of a nasogastric tube: May yield significant volumes of fluid or gas if gastric dilatation is severe. An indwelling nasogastric tube should be left in place for at least 12 to 24 hours to maintain gastric decompression (see "Gastric Dilation" in this section).
- Complete blood count: Severe polycythemia and leukopenia characterized by neutropenia with a left shift and toxic changes in neutrophils is evident in symptomatic horses.
- Serum biochemistry profile and blood gas analysis
  - Moderate to severe lactic acidosis
  - Variable electrolyte derangements
  - Azotemia is frequently observed because of prerenal, renal, or combined factors.

ADVANCED OR CONFIRMATORY TESTING

- Transabdominal ultrasonography may reveal gastric, small intestinal, or large colonic distension or increased mural thickness.
- Peritoneal fluid analysis is usually within reference intervals, but if colonic damage is severe, evidence of intraperitoneal inflammation or ischemia (increased white blood cell count and total protein concentration, sanguinous appearance) may be apparent.

TREATMENT

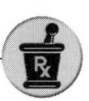

THERAPEUTIC GOAL(S)

- In acute ingestion, relieve gastric distension and remove grain from the stomach if possible.
- Prevent or limit colonic absorption of bacterial toxins.
- Provide supportive care for septic, endotoxic, and hypovolemic shock.
- Provide laminitis prophylaxis.

ACUTE GENERAL TREATMENT

- Asymptomatic horses
  - Gastric lavage (see "Gastric Impaction" in this section) is indicated if the horse is evaluated in the first 4 to 6 hours after grain ingestion or if a significant amount of feed remains in the stomach on initial evaluation.
  - If gastric reflux is absent, substances to bind bacterial toxins and promote colonic emptying should be administered via nasogastric tube and may include:
    - Activated charcoal: 0.5 lb in 1 L warm water once
    - Bio-Sponge powder: 1 to 2 lb in 1 L water q24h for 1 to 3 days

- Mineral oil: 2 to 3 L q24h for 1 to 3 days
  - Antiinflammatory and analgesic therapy: Flunixin meglumine (1.1 mg/kg IV once and then 0.25–0.3 mg/kg IV or PO q6-8h for 48–72 hours).
  - Remove all feed for 24 hours (permit free access to water) and then gradually reintroduce the horse to feed with small amounts of grass hay or short periods of pasture grazing over 24 to 48 hours.
- Symptomatic horses
  - Gastric lavage and bacterial toxin binders or laxative therapy as above
  - If cecal or colonic distension is severe, cecal trocharization may be necessary to relieve distension (see "Cecal Trocharization" in Section II).
  - Antiinflammatory and analgesic therapy
    - Flunixin meglumine: 1.1 mg/kg IV q12h initially for colic; then decreased to 0.25 mg/kg IV q6–8h for antiinflammatory effects when signs of colic resolve
    - Lidocaine: 1.3 mg/kg IV as a slow bolus and then 0.05 mg/kg/min IV continuous-rate infusion (promotes intestinal motility in addition to providing analgesic therapy)
    - ± Pentoxifylline: 8 mg/kg PO q8–12h (may decrease inflammatory cytokine production and promote laminar blood flow via rheologic and antiplatelet effects)
    - ± Dimethylsulfoxide (90% solution): 0.5 to 1.0 g/kg diluted to less than 10% solution in IV fluids q12h for 1 to 3 days (may scavenge free radicals and limit oxidative injury)
  - Antiendotoxic therapy
    - Equine plasma (2–4 L IV; may be regular equine plasma or hyperimmune plasma with antiendotoxin antibodies) or hyperimmune antiendotoxin serum (Endoserum, 1–2 mL/kg diluted in 3–5 L isotonic fluids IV)
    - Polymyxin-B: 2000 to 6000 IU/kg (diluted in 500–1000 mL 0.9% saline) IV q12h for 1 to 3 days after the patient is hydrated if renal function is adequate
  - Laminitis prophylaxis
    - Placement of frog supports, deep bedding, and maintenance in ice boots for 1 to 2 days should be initiated immediately even if no signs of laminitis are present.
    - If signs of laminitis occur, treatment should be rapid and aggressive (see "Laminitis, Acute" in this section).
  - IV fluid therapy

- Initial fluid resuscitation may include isotonic crystalloids (25–50 mL/kg IV bolus), hypertonic saline (2–4 mL/kg IV once), or Hetastarch (5–10 mL/kg IV bolus once).
  - Resuscitation fluids should be followed by balanced polyionic crystalloid IV fluids at 100 to 200 mL/kg/d until rehydration is established and then at 50 to 100 mL/kg/d for maintenance as needed.
  - Feed should be withheld until signs of colic, gastric distension, and gastric reflux have ceased and then should be reintroduced as for asymptomatic horses as above.
  - Antimicrobial therapy should be avoided because it may slow reestablishment of normal colonic bacterial flora.

POSSIBLE COMPLICATIONS

- Laminitis
- Gastric rupture
- Colonic rupture
- Death from cardiovascular collapse in endotoxic shock

PROGNOSIS AND OUTCOME

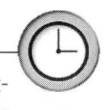

- Asymptomatic horses: Prognosis is good if early, aggressive treatment is initiated.
- Symptomatic horses: Prognosis is guarded to poor.
- Severe, persistent signs of colic and early development of laminitis are associated with a grave prognosis even with aggressive medical therapy.

PEARLS & CONSIDERATIONS

The absence of clinical signs on initial evaluation in a horse with grain overload does not imply that severe disease will not develop. Early and aggressive treatment is indicated in any horse that consumes a moderate to large amount of grain and can be very successful at preventing the potentially devastating sequelae associated with grain overload.

SUGGESTED READING

Mueller POE, Moore JN, Divers TJ: Disorders of the stomach. In Orsini JA, Divers TJ, editors: *Equine emergencies: treatments and procedures*, ed 3, St Louis, 2008, Saunders Elsevier, pp 121–122.

AUTHOR: **KELSEY A. HART**

EDITORS: **TIM MAIR** and **CERI SHERLOCK**

Granulosa Cell Tumor

BASIC INFORMATION

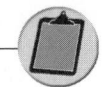

DEFINITION

A granulosa cell tumor (GCT) is a sex-cord stromal tumor of the ovary. It is by far the most common tumor of the equine ovary. When the tumor is composed primarily of granulosa cells, the term GCT is used; when both granulosa and theca cells are present, the term granulosa-theca cell tumor (GTCT) is used.

EPIDEMIOLOGY

SPECIES, AGE, SEX Intact equine females of any age. The mean age is 10.6 years with a range of 2 to 20 years. Juvenile cases have also been reported.
ASSOCIATED CONDITIONS AND DISORDERS Behavioral problems, infertility

CLINICAL PRESENTATION

DISEASE FORMS, SUBTYPES
- GCT
- GTCT

HISTORY, CHIEF COMPLAINT
- Behavioral abnormalities
  - Prolonged anestrus
  - Aggressive or stallion-like behavior
  - Persistent estrus
- Infertility

PHYSICAL EXAM FINDINGS The affected ovary is enlarged and firm, and the ovulation fossa is usually not palpable. The contralateral ovary is almost always small and inactive. Rarely, bilateral tumors have been reported.

ETIOLOGY AND PATHOPHYSIOLOGY
- GCT is a neoplasm of the sex cord stroma.
- It is the only ovarian abnormality in mares associated with inactivity of the contralateral ovary.
- Inactivity of the contralateral ovary is presumed to occur by suppression of pituitary follicle-stimulating hormone as a result of inhibin secretion from the neoplastic ovary.

DIAGNOSIS

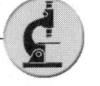

DIFFERENTIAL DIAGNOSIS

- Other causes of ovarian enlargement (hematoma; pregnancy; or other ovarian neoplasm, including cystadenoma, teratoma, or dysgerminoma). Some forms of ovarian enlargement (as during pregnancy or with an ovarian hematoma) resolve with time, but GCT does not. Most importantly, GCT/CTCT is the only cause of ovarian enlargement that is associated with inactivity of the contralateral ovary. In rare cases when the mare continues to cycle on the contralateral ovary, the tumors are thought to be in the early stages of development.
- Other causes of prolonged anestrus: Season, old or young age, chromosomal abnormality, persistent luteal tissue, pregnancy, progestin administration, anabolic steroid administration, gonadotropin-releasing hormone vaccination, or persistent endometrial cups
- Other causes of stallion-like behavior: Anabolic steroid administration, disorder of sexual differentiation (eg, male pseudohermaphroditism)

INITIAL DATABASE

- Ultrasonography of the affected ovary reveals a multicystic, honeycombed structure, but the tumor may also present as a solid mass or as a single large cyst. The contralateral ovary is small and inactive, but mares with GCT on one ovary and a functional contralateral ovary have been reported.
- Serum inhibin is elevated in 90% of cases. Serum testosterone is elevated in 50% to 60% of cases. Serum progesterone is baseline (<1.0 ng/mL) because normal follicular development, ovulation, and corpus luteum formation do not occur. Measurements of inhibin above 0.7 ng/mL, testosterone above 50 to 100 pg/mL, and progesterone below 1.0 ng/mL in a nonpregnant mare are suggestive of a GCT.

ADVANCED OR CONFIRMATORY TESTING

Definitive diagnosis is by histopathology, but a presumptive diagnosis can be made based on clinical examination and suggestive serum inhibin, testosterone, and progesterone concentrations.

TREATMENT

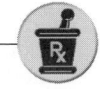

THERAPEUTIC GOALS

Surgical removal is recommended. The tumor will continue to grow and may eventually cause colic or other problems.

ACUTE GENERAL TREATMENT

Surgical removal of the affected ovary results in resolution of clinical signs. Surgical approaches include colpotomy, flank or ventral midline laparotomy, and laparoscopy. Follicular activity resumes in the unaffected ovary during the breeding season after surgery. Mares are suitable broodmares after normal cyclicity resumes.

POSSIBLE COMPLICATIONS

- Although uncommon, metastasis has been reported.
- Large GCT/GTCTs may cause colic or other gastrointestinal problems.
- Rupture of GCT/GTCTs has been reported, with intraabdominal hemorrhage.
- Adhesions of GCTs to abdominal viscera have been reported.
- Torsion of the ovary containing a GTCT has been described.

PROGNOSIS AND OUTCOME

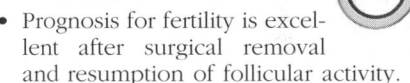

- Prognosis for fertility is excellent after surgical removal and resumption of follicular activity.
- Prognosis for survival is excellent after surgical removal.

PEARLS & CONSIDERATIONS

GCT/GTCT is the only ovarian abnormality in mares associated with inactivity of the contralateral ovary.

SUGGESTED READING

McCue PM: Equine granulosa cell tumors. *Proc 38th Ann Conv Am Assoc Equine Pract* 587–585, 1992.
McCue PM, Roser JF, Munro CJ, et al: Granulosa cell tumors of the equine ovary. *Vet Clin North Am Equine Pract* 22:799–817, 2006.
Stabenfelt GH, et al: Clinical findings, pathologic changes and endocrinological secretory patterns in mares with ovarian tumors. *J Reprod Fert* 27(suppl):277–285, 1979.

AUTHOR: **CATHERINE A. DeLUCA**

EDITOR: **JUAN C. SAMPER**

Grass Sickness

BASIC INFORMATION

DEFINITION

Neurologic disease primarily associated with the degeneration of neurons in the autonomic nervous system, particularly the enteric nervous system

SYNONYM(S)

Equine dysautonomia

EPIDEMIOLOGY

SPECIES, AGE, SEX Grass sickness most commonly affects horses between 2 and 7 years of age. Older horses rarely develop the disease, possibly because of the development of immunity or tolerance to the causative agent. The disease is very rare in foals and weanlings.

GENETICS AND BREED PREDISPOSITION All Equids appear to be susceptible to grass sickness, with the disease having been reported in horses, ponies, donkeys, and captive exotic Equidae. There is no breed predisposition.

RISK FACTORS

Numerous risk factors have been identified, including:

- Cool weather temperatures (7°–11° C) and dry weather with irregular ground frosts in the preceding 2 weeks
- Horses in good or fat body condition
- Higher numbers of horses and the presence of young horses on the premises
- Sandy soils and loam soils
- Increased levels of soil nitrogen
- Previous occurrence of grass sickness on the premises
- Grazing grass: The disease is extremely rare in horses with no access to grass. Co-grazing with ruminants gives some protection from the disease.
- Dietary change
- Movement or recent stress, especially movement to a new pasture in the preceding 2 to 4 weeks
- Pasture disturbance (eg, construction or mole activity)
- High-frequency use of anthelmintics and specific use of ivermectin for ultimate and penultimate treatments
- Mechanical removal of feces from the pasture
- Pasture cutting

GEOGRAPHY AND SEASONALITY

- The northeast region of Scotland has the highest incidence of grass sickness, but the disease is also recognized throughout the United Kingdom as well as in many other Northern European countries, including Norway, Sweden, Denmark, France, Switzerland, and Germany. The disease does not occur in Australasia, Asia, Africa, North America, or Ireland. A clinically and pathologically identical disease known as mel seco (dry sickness) occurs in South America.
- Cases of equine grass sickness may occur throughout the year, but there is a significant peak in incidence in the northern hemisphere in the spring and early summer.

CLINICAL PRESENTATION

DISEASE FORMS/SUBTYPES Grass sickness can be divided into three subdivisions—acute, subacute, and chronic—which are characterized clinically by varying degrees of gastrointestinal immotility and dysphagia, although it should be emphasized that there is a continuum. The acute and subacute forms of the disease are invariably fatal; however, a proportion of mildly affected horses with the chronic form may survive.

HISTORY, CHIEF COMPLAINT

- Acute form
  - The onset and progression of clinical signs is rapid, with death occurring in less than 48 hours.
  - Animals usually present with depression or somnolence, inappetence, and rapid progression to varying degrees of abdominal pain in many cases.
  - The degree of colic may, however, be relatively mild and inconsistent with the profound elevation in pulse rate.
- Subacute form
  - Clinical signs are generally similar to but less severe than those of acute cases. Their duration is longer, and the outline of the abdomen quickly develops a marked "tucked-up" appearance.
  - This finding does not appear to be entirely attributable to loss of body condition, although significant weight loss does become apparent.
- Chronic form
  - Clinical signs in the chronic form are more insidious in onset.
  - The most obvious signs include severe weight loss with the development of a distinct "tucked-up" abdomen. Affected horses often have a very base narrow stance, thus adopting the characteristic "elephant on a tub" posture.
  - Some horses show apparent weakness, and a reduced anterior phase to the stride results in occasional toe dragging.

PHYSICAL EXAM FINDINGS

- Acute form
  - Dehydration is usually present, which can be demonstrated by prolonged tenting of the skin. A generalized, marked reduction in intestinal motility is evident during abdominal auscultation.
  - Bilateral ptosis may or may not be present.
  - Muscle fasciculations of the triceps and quadriceps muscle groups may be observed, and sweating may be generalized or localized to the flanks, neck, and shoulder regions.
  - Dysphagia is almost invariably present but may be difficult to appreciate because of coexisting inappetence. It may be apparent, however, when observing the animal attempting to drink, when many affected horses flick their muzzles through the water or "paw" at the water bucket, presumably because of frustration.
  - Excessive dribbling of saliva is often present and probably results from a combination of excessive saliva production and a reduced ability to swallow.
  - Some horses show spontaneous gastric reflux with foul-smelling green or brown fluid exiting from both nostrils. As the disease progresses, abdominal distension becomes apparent in most cases.
- Subacute form
  - Affected animals are almost invariably dysphagic.
  - Persistent tachycardia is present with or without any evidence of abdominal pain.
  - Patchy sweating, usually around the flanks, neck, and shoulder, and muscle tremors of the triceps and quadriceps muscle groups are often present.
  - As the disease progresses, many subacute cases will exhibit worsening episodes of colic.
- Chronic form
  - Bilateral ptosis is often present resulting in a sleepy, depressed expression.
  - Persistent tachycardia is present; however, the heart rate is lower than in acute and subacute cases, rarely exceeding 60 beats/min.
  - Varying degrees of muscle tremor, patchy sweating, and abdominal pain are present.
  - Signs of colic are usually mild and transient.

- Varying degrees of dysphagia are common, but the associated reduction in appetite may make this difficult to appreciate.
- Frequently, affected horses accumulate chewed food between the cheeks and molar teeth, often resulting in a fetid odor to the breath.
- Many chronic cases will have severe rhinitis with the accumulation of dry hemorrhagic mucoid material on the nasal septum and nasal turbinates.
- Although this can be appreciated by close inspection of the rostral nasal septum using a pen torch (light), often the animal will make a distinctive "snuffling" sound during breathing that originates from the nasal cavity.

ETIOLOGY AND PATHOPHYSIOLOGY

- The cause of grass sickness is unknown. Numerous epidemiologic studies have found no evidence for a conventional infectious agent. Considerable evidence exists to suggest that a natural neurotoxin may be implicated, and the presence of a neurotoxic component in the plasma of acute cases has been demonstrated experimentally.
- Investigations into the possible role of toxic plants, viruses, fungal, chemical, and bacterial toxins have failed to identify the cause. The current leading hypothesis is that equine grass sickness results from a toxicoinfection with *Clostridium botulinum* types C and D, whereby toxin is produced locally within the horse's gastrointestinal tract by resident bacteria. Horses with equine grass sickness have lower serum concentrations of antibody against surface antigens of *C. botulinum* type C and one of its neurotoxins (BoNT/C) compared with co-grazing horses. Significantly higher levels of mucosal IgA antibodies against BoNT/C and BoNT/D (the neurotoxin produced by *C. botulinum* type D) have been identified in the small intestines of horses with acute grass sickness compared with control subject.

DIAGNOSIS

DIFFERENTIAL DIAGNOSIS

- Other causes of mild to moderate abdominal pain are simple or nonstrangulating obstructions of the gastrointestinal tract such as sand impaction, enterolithiasis, large colon displacements, large intestinal intraluminal obstructions, tympany, small colon impactions, and ileal impactions.

- Other causes of large intestinal distension on examination per rectum include sand impaction, enterolithiasis, tympany, large colon displacements, and other intraluminal obstructions.
- Dehydration of feed within the large intestine may occur secondary to small intestinal obstruction.

INITIAL DATABASE

- Acute form
  - The pulse is usually weak and may exceed 100 beats/min in many cases. Pyrexia (≤40° C) may be present.
  - Passage of a nasogastric tube invariably results in the retrieval of many liters of malodorous reflux.
  - Rectal examination reveals a dry rectal mucosa, and some horses strain excessively during the rectal examination.
  - Frequently, distension of the small intestine can be appreciated; consequently, the rectal findings in many acute cases may appear similar to those encountered in some surgical colic cases with associated small intestinal obstruction.
  - In some cases, a hard secondary impaction of the large colon can be palpated in the caudal abdomen. The distinct corrugated nature of this structure often distinguishes it from the relatively smooth outline of a primary colonic or cecal impaction.
- Subacute form
  - Nasogastric reflux and small intestinal distension are usually absent early on in the course of the disease; however, they may develop in a small number of horses as the disease progresses.
- Chronic form
  - Colonic and cecal impaction is common and readily appreciated during rectal examination. Abdominal auscultation usually reveals a reduction in intestinal motility.
  - Small intestinal distension and colonic impaction are rare, so rectal examination usually reveals a lack of contents within the palpable regions of the colon and cecum.
  - No alterations in blood clinical chemistry or hematologic parameters are pathognomonic for grass sickness. Because one of the major differential diagnoses of grass sickness is colic, most of the comparisons of clinical chemistry parameters have been made between horses with grass sickness, normal control subjects, and horses with colic.
  - Plasma cortisol, catecholamine, and histamine concentrations are significantly higher in horses with acute

and subacute grass sickness than in horses with colic and normal animals. The acute phase proteins haptoglobin and orosomucoid are increased in all three forms of grass sickness but not in the majority of colic cases. Also, the protein content of peritoneal fluid is higher in horses with grass sickness compared with horses with medical colic.

ADVANCED OR CONFIRMATORY TESTING

- There is no definitive noninvasive antemortem diagnostic test for equine grass sickness. In most cases, the diagnosis is based on the clinical signs and history. Repeated examinations may be necessary before a diagnosis can be made.
- Confirmation of a diagnosis of grass sickness can only be made by demonstrating the characteristic histopathologic lesions in the autonomic or enteric ganglia during postmortem examination or by ileal biopsy at laparotomy. This latter technique may be useful in the antemortem diagnosis of acute and subacute cases in which surgical colic is a major differential diagnosis. In chronic cases, however, where subsequent treatment is being considered, anesthesia and surgery are likely to adversely affect the outcome. Rectal biopsy is not yet a reliable technique in grass sickness because the enteric neurons in the rectum are only mildly affected, and only a small sample can be obtained.
- Esophageal endoscopy and barium swallow radiography may reveal defective esophageal motility. Reflux esophagitis may also be recognized by endoscopy.
- Topical application of phenylephrine eye drops (0.5%) to one eye with subsequent examination 30 minutes later often reveals reversal of ptosis in the ipsilateral eye, with an increase in angle between the corneal surface and the eyelash. It should be recognized that false-positive responses may occur with this test.

TREATMENT

THERAPEUTIC GOAL(S)

- Euthanasia may be required in many cases.
- Nursing treatment of selected horses with chronic grass sickness may be possible.

ACUTE GENERAL TREATMENT

- Acute form: The prognosis in acute cases is hopeless; therefore, euthanasia is required after this diagnosis has been made.

- Subacute form: Although a small number of cases that present initially as subacute cases will gradually progress to the chronic stage, the vast majority will die or require euthanasia within 7 days of the onset of signs.

CHRONIC TREATMENT

- Some horses affected by chronic grass sickness may survive. However, strict selection of treatment candidates and adherence to good management protocols are important. The suggested criteria for selection of cases for treatment include:
  - A willingness to attempt to drink and swallow food
  - Retention of some ability to drink and swallow food
  - Absence of continuous moderate to severe signs of colic
- Treatment involves intensive nursing care.
- High-energy, high-protein feeds are ideal and can be mixed with molasses, biscuits, and succulents (eg, apples and carrots) to improve palatability. The preference of the horse for a particular feed will often change from day to day. The frequent provision of feed is indicated with a recommendation of four to five feeds per day. Soaking the feeds may facilitate swallowing in some cases; however, whether to dampen the feed or not again depends the individual animal's preference.
- The energy content of the feed may be improved by the addition of up to 500 mL of corn oil, but this should be done gradually. The consumption of concentrate feed to minimize excess

weight loss is vital to the horse's survival.

- Nasogastric feeding has been attempted in some horses with extremely limited success, so the indication for such treatment remains questionable.
- The importance of nursing, frequent human contact, frequent grooming, and regular walking out and hand-grazing cannot be overemphasized. Occasionally, it may be necessary to handfeed some horses when their appetite is especially poor. In many cases, despite a moderate degree of food intake, the body weight will continue to decrease quite dramatically during the first 2 to 4 weeks. The prognosis, however, is considerably poorer if this decrease in body weight continues beyond 6 weeks' duration.
- Mild to moderate postprandial colic may occur, and this can be managed with phenylbutazone (2.2–4.4 mg/kg IV or PO q12h) or flunixin meglumine (0.5–1.1 mg/kg IV q12h) and omeprazole (4 mg/kg PO q24h).
- The use of gastrointestinal motility enhancers and appetite stimulants has been attempted in the past but with disappointing results.

RECOMMENDED MONITORING

During treatment, horses should be monitored for signs of pain and continued weight loss.

PROGNOSIS AND OUTCOME

Overall, the prognosis for equine grass sickness is extremely poor.

PEARLS & CONSIDERATIONS

COMMENTS

Only selected horses with chronic equine grass sickness can survive. Other horses should be euthanized on humane grounds.

PREVENTION

- Avoiding risk factors is a key to prevention.
- No vaccine is currently available, although work is currently being undertaken to evaluate the safety and immunogenicity of a recombinant protein-based vaccine against *C. botulinum* toxins.

CLIENT EDUCATION

Education of clients about risk factors may decrease the incidence of equine grass sickness.

SUGGESTED READING

Hunter LC, Miller JK, Poxton IR: The association of *Clostridium botulinum* type C with equine grass sickness: a toxicoinfection? *Equine Vet J* 31:492, 1999.

McGorum BC, Pirie RS: Grass sickness. In Robinson NE, Sprayberry KA, editors: *Current therapy in equine medicine*, ed 6. St Louis, 2009, Saunders Elsevier, pp 361–365.

Milne E, Wallis N: Nursing the chronic grass sickness patient. *Equine Vet Ed* 6:217–219, 1994.

Milne EM, Woodman MP, Doxey DL: Use of clinical measurements to predict the outcome in chronic cases of grass sickness (equine dysautonomia). *Vet Rec* 134:438, 1994.

Scholes SFE, Vaillant C, Peacock P, et al: Diagnosis of grass sickness by ileal biopsy. *Vet Rec* 133:7, 1993.

AUTHOR: **TIM MAIR**

EDITORS: **TIM MAIR** and **CERI SHERLOCK**

Guttural Pouch Empyema

BASIC INFORMATION

DEFINITION

Accumulation of purulent material within one or both of the guttural pouches. In some cases, chondroids, or concretions of inspissated purulent material, may also be present.

SYNONYMS

- Catarrh of the guttural pouch
- Strangles (if caused by infection with *Streptococcus equi* subsp. *equi*)

EPIDEMIOLOGY

SPECIES, AGE, SEX

- Seen most commonly in young horses and older horses with possible immune compromise (eg, Cushing's disease)
- Horses of any age or breed or both sexes can be affected.

RISK FACTORS

- Prior upper respiratory tract infection (especially with *S. equi* subsp. *equi* or *Streptococcus equi* subsp. *zooepidemicus*)

- Retropharyngeal lymph node abscessation and rupture
- Fracture of the stylohyoid bone
- Infusion of irritant substances into the guttural pouch
- Pharyngeal orifice stenosis or adhesions
- Pharyngeal perforation due to passage of a nasogastric tube
- Immune compromise secondary to pituitary disease

CONTAGION AND ZOONOSIS

- Approximately 30% of horses with guttural pouch empyema are culture positive for *S. equi* subsp. *equi.* This is the causative agent of strangles and is highly contagious.

- Horses with clinical signs of guttural pouch empyema should be handled with appropriate biosecurity precautions due to this risk until the results of bacterial culture and sensitivity or polymerase chain reaction (PCR) are obtained.

ASSOCIATED CONDITIONS AND DISORDERS
- Chondroids: Found in approximately 20% of horses with guttural pouch empyema
- Strangles
- Laryngeal hemiplegia
- Dysphagia
- Dyspnea

CLINICAL PRESENTATION
HISTORY, CHIEF COMPLAINT Persistent mucopurulent nasal discharge (unilateral or bilateral) is the most common presenting complaint.

PHYSICAL EXAM FINDINGS
- Mucopurulent nasal discharge
- Retropharyngeal swelling that is painful on palpation
- Other clinical signs: Cough, fever, anorexia, depression, dyspnea, dysphagia, respiratory noise, extended head and neck carriage, enlarged retropharyngeal ± submandibular lymph nodes

ETIOLOGY AND PATHOPHYSIOLOGY
- Guttural pouch empyema is most commonly caused by infection with β-hemolytic streptococci. *S. equi* subsp. *equi* or *S. equi* subsp. *zooepidemicus* species are the most common species
- Other isolates include *Escherichia coli*, *Klebsiella* spp., *Corynebacterium* spp., *Bordetella* spp., and *Salmonella* spp.
- Horses can be asymptomatic carriers of *S. equi* subsp. *equi* in their guttural pouches after an infection for an extended period of time.
- Chondroids form as a result of chronic inflammation within the guttural pouch and consist of epithelial cells, inflammatory products, and necrotic tissue. Their presence complicates treatment and may necessitate surgical intervention.

DIAGNOSIS

DIFFERENTIAL DIAGNOSIS
- Guttural pouch tympany
- Strangles
- Pharyngitis
- Upper or lower respiratory tract infection

INITIAL DATABASE
- Complete blood count: Normal or leukocytosis
- Fibrinogen: Increased
- Hematocrit: Normal
- Total protein: Normal or increased
- Upper airway endoscopy
  - Mucopurulent material ± chondroids in one or both guttural pouches
  - Retropharyngeal lymph node enlargement (seen on the floor of the guttural pouch; may cause dorsal pharyngeal collapse)
  - Mucosal hyperplasia, thickening, and discoloration of the pharyngeal ostium
  - Pharyngeal abnormalities: Lymphoid hyperplasia, narrowing, or edema
- Radiography (less sensitive than endoscopy)
  - Fluid line(s) within the affected pouch(es)
  - Chondroids
  - Retropharyngeal lymph node enlargement

ADVANCED OR CONFIRMATORY TESTING
- Bacterial culture and sensitivity testing of an aspirate from the guttural pouch or from a guttural pouch wash to determine the causative agent
- PCR testing for *S. equi* subsp. *equi* to rule out strangles

TREATMENT

THERAPEUTIC GOALS
- The hallmarks of treatment are guttural pouch drainage and lavage, systemic antimicrobial therapy, and systemic antiinflammatory treatment.
- Medical therapy alone is successful in the majority of cases; however, about 20% of cases require more extensive therapy, which may include surgical intervention.

ACUTE GENERAL TREATMENT
- Guttural pouch drainage and lavage
  - Transendoscopically or via devices placed into the guttural pouch (Chambers catheter, Foley catheter, male dog urinary catheter, polyethylene tubing, or commercially available guttural pouch catheters).
  - Horses should be heavily sedated to facilitate drainage and prevent aspiration pneumonia.
  - Lavage should be done daily for 5 to 10 days.
  - The lavage solution should be an isotonic electrolyte solution.
    - Noxious agents (iodine, hydrogen peroxide, antiseptics) are

contraindicated because they may cause severe inflammation and harmful side effects, such as dysphagia.
    - Antimicrobials may be added to the solution, but studies have not shown this to be any more effective than electrolyte solutions alone.
    - There are successful reports of the use of acetylcysteine in the lavage solution to break the disulfide bonds in the mucoproteins; however, some authors advise against this because it can also cause inflammation.
- Systemic antimicrobial therapy
  - Should be used as an adjunct to drainage and lavage and not as a sole treatment.
  - Also used to prevent the development of aspiration pneumonia.
  - Should be based on results obtained from bacterial culture and sensitivity testing.
  - Until those results are available, empirical therapy should be initiated.
    - The drug of choice for the most common isolates β-hemolytic streptococci) is a penicillin or cephalosporin.
      - Potassium penicillin (22,000 IU/kg, IV q6h) is the treatment of choice but may be cost prohibitive.
      - Procaine penicillin G (22,000 IU/kg IM q12h) is a cheaper alternative.
      - Ceftiofur (2 mg/kg IV or IM q12h) can also be used.
      - Potentiated sulfonamides should not be used empirically because about 75% of isolates in one study were resistant.
- Systemic antiinflammatory treatment: Phenylbutazone (2.2 mg/kg IV or PO q12h or 4.4 mg/kg IV or PO q24h) or flunixin meglumine (1.1 mg/kg IV or PO q12–24h).
- Horses in severe respiratory distress may require an emergency tracheotomy.

CHRONIC TREATMENT
- When chondroids are present, they must be removed.
- Nonsurgical removal (via endoscopic snares or baskets)
  - Successful in about 40% of cases
  - Can be extremely time consuming and necessitate increased hospitalization time and cost
- Surgical removal
  - Helps expedite the process of removing the chondroids, decreasing hospitalization time and cost.
  - Traditional techniques (Viborg's triangle, hyovertebrotomy, White-

house, and modified Whitehouse approaches) are performed under general anesthesia. Potential complications include iatrogenic nerve damage.
  ◦ A modified Whitehouse approach in standing horses was recently reported. It provides good drainage and avoids general anesthesia.
  ◦ Laser surgery: Creates a fistula in the pharyngeal opening to remove the chondroids. Avoids general anesthesia and decreases the risk of iatrogenic nerve damage.
• Horses with chronic dysphagia may require an esophagostomy to provide enteral nutrition until cranial nerve function returns.
• Horses with secondary aspiration pneumonia should be treated appropriately.

DRUG INTERACTIONS

For horses with chronic disease, creatinine values should be checked before treating the horse with nonsteroidal anti-inflammatory drugs or aminoglycoside antimicrobials.

POSSIBLE COMPLICATIONS

• Rupture of the guttural pouch has been reported as a complication of daily guttural pouch lavage.
• Nerve damage: Either from the inflammation caused by the empyema or from iatrogenic damage from lavage with noxious solutions or surgical intervention can be seen.
  ◦ Cranial nerves VII, IX, X, XI, and XII, as well as the pharyngeal branch of the vagus nerve, the cranial cervical ganglion, the cranial laryngeal nerve, and the cervical sympathetic stump, may be affected.

◦ Clinically, this may manifest as laryngeal hemiplegia, dysphagia, signs of facial nerve paralysis, persistent dorsal displacement of the soft palate, Horner's syndrome, and pharyngeal collapse.
  ◦ These deficits may improve over time but may be permanent.
• Aspiration pneumonia

RECOMMENDED MONITORING

• Repeat endoscopic evaluation should be performed to evaluate the success of daily lavage.
• Repeat PCR testing for *S. equi* subsp. *equi* should be performed in horses with positive test results to determine when biosecurity measures can be discontinued.

PROGNOSIS AND OUTCOME

• About 80% of horses with guttural pouch empyema respond favorably to medical treatment, with an average duration of hospitalization of 5 to 10 days and a good prognosis for return to previous use.
• About 20% of horses experience complications or have chondroids that necessitate more intensive treatment or surgical intervention.
  ◦ Horses with chondroids but without neurologic signs have a good prognosis, but treatment can be prolonged, and the associated costs are increased.
  ◦ Horses with neurologic deficits have a fair to poor prognosis, depending on the duration of clinical signs and the specific neurologic deficit. Treatment duration and cost

can be substantially increased in these horses.

PEARLS & CONSIDERATIONS

COMMENTS

• All horses with clinical signs of guttural pouch empyema should be cultured for strangles and treated with appropriate isolation and biosecurity protocols until the disease is ruled out.
• If medical management is not successful within 5 to 7 days or after chondroids are identified, surgical treatment is indicated and can decrease hospitalization time and cost if performed early on.

CLIENT EDUCATION

• Clients should be aware that any horse with persistent mucopurulent nasal discharge could be affected with guttural pouch empyema and possibly strangles.
• These horses should be kept isolated from other horses at the farm until they are examined by a veterinarian.

SUGGESTED READING

Perkins GA, et al: Diagnosing guttural pouch disorders and managing guttural pouch empyema in adult horses. *Compend Contin Educ Pract Vet* 25:966–973, 2003.
Perkins JD, Schumacher J, Kelly G, et al: Standing surgical removal of inspissated guttural pouch exudate (chondroids) in ten horses. *Vet Surg* 35:658–662, 2006.

AUTHOR: **LIBERTY M. GETMAN**

EDITOR: **ERIC J. PARENTE**

Guttural Pouch Mycosis

BASIC INFORMATION

DEFINITION

Fungal infection within the guttural pouch(es) that affects the neurovascular structures inside of the pouch, causing hemorrhage and neurologic deficits

EPIDEMIOLOGY

ASSOCIATED CONDITIONS AND DISORDERS Aspiration pneumonia, laryngeal hemiplegia, Horner syndrome

CLINICAL PRESENTATION

DISEASE FORMS/SUBTYPES

• Acute, severe epistaxis (unilateral or bilateral)
• Chronic neurologic deficits: Dysphagia, laryngeal or pharyngeal paralysis, esophageal obstruction, Horner's syndrome, facial nerve paralysis

HISTORY, CHIEF COMPLAINT

• The most common presenting complaint is moderate to severe epistaxis.
• Dysphagia is the second most common presenting complaint.

PHYSICAL EXAM FINDINGS

• Acute, moderate to severe epistaxis:
  ◦ Unilateral is most common, but it can also be bilateral
  ◦ Signs of hypovolemic or hemorrhagic shock
• Tachycardia, tachypnea, pale mucous membranes, weak peripheral pulses, anxious demeanor, weakness
• Neurologic deficits:
  ◦ Dysphagia: Horses may present with esophageal obstruction, aspiration pneumonia, or tongue protrusion or have feed material in the nares.

- Laryngeal or pharyngeal paralysis: A respiratory noise may be noted during exercise.
- Horner syndrome: Ptosis, meiosis, enophthalmos, patchy sweating, and nasal mucosa congestion on the affected side.
- Facial nerve paralysis: Ear droop, ptosis, lip droop, and inability to blink on the affected side.
- The inability to blink may lead to the development of corneal ulcers on the affected side.
- Other less common clinical signs: Nasal discharge, colic, blindness, unusual head carriage, parotid area pain, head shyness.

ETIOLOGY AND PATHOPHYSIOLOGY

- The most common etiologic agents recovered from horses with guttural pouch mycosis are *Emericella nidulans* and *Aspergillus fumigatus*.
- These fungi are ubiquitous and thrive in warm, moist areas such as bedding material containing urine and water.
- These fungi act as opportunistic pathogens, entering the guttural pouch through the pharyngeal orifice, where they incite an inflammatory response.
- This leads to the formation of a diphtheritic membrane, composed of necrotic tissue, cell debris, bacteria, and fungal mycelia.
- The fungi can penetrate deeper tissues, causing thromboarteritis, aneurysm, and hemorrhage.
  - This typically occurs in the internal carotid artery (two thirds of cases).
  - The external carotid artery, its branches, or the maxillary artery are affected in the other third of cases.
- Damage may occur to any of the nerves within the guttural pouch because of the acute inflammatory response or because of chronic fibrosis.
  - Cranial nerves VII, IX, X, XI, and XII; the pharyngeal branch of the vagus nerve; the cranial cervical ganglion; the cranial laryngeal nerve; and the cervical sympathetic stump may be affected.
  - Neurologic deficits are generally seen in the more chronic stages of the disease.

DIAGNOSIS

DIFFERENTIAL DIAGNOSIS

- Trauma to the nasal passages or sinuses
- Rupture of the ventral straight muscles of the head
- Masses of the nasal passages, sinuses, or guttural pouches
  - Progressive ethmoidal hematomas

- Neoplasia: Squamous cell carcinoma, fibrosarcoma, melanoma, hemangiosarcoma
  - Paranasal sinus cysts
- Exercise-induced pulmonary hemorrhage
- Bacterial or fungal sinusitis

INITIAL DATABASE

- Complete blood count: Normal
- Hematocrit: Normal in the acute stages (<24 hours after hemorrhage); decreased later
- Total protein: Normal in the subacute stages (<4–6 hours after hemorrhage); decreased later
- Fibrinogen: Normal, decreased (if substantial hemorrhage), or increased (chronic inflammation or infection)
- Platelet count: Normal or decreased after substantial hemorrhage
- Serum chemistry: Normal or azotemia (prerenal) if hypovolemic shock is present
- Upper airway endoscopy
  - Blood clot at the pharyngeal orifice of the affected pouch
  - Diphtheritic membrane along the roof or wall of the affected pouch
    - Internal carotid artery: The medial compartment of the affected pouch
    - External carotid artery, maxillary artery: The lateral compartment of the affected pouch
    - May not be able to identify the affected artery or arteries if there is active hemorrhage; the affected pouch will be filled with blood and clot material that inhibits visualization.
  - In chronic cases with neurologic deficits, there may be pharyngeal collapse, laryngeal hemiplegia, dorsal displacement of the soft palate, and feed material on the pharyngeal walls.

TREATMENT

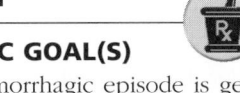

THERAPEUTIC GOAL(S)

- The first hemorrhagic episode is generally not fatal; however, after this occurs, prompt surgical intervention should be recommended because subsequent episodes of hemorrhage are often fatal and may occur within hours to days after the initial episode.
- Treatment should be aimed at stabilizing the horse hemodynamically to transport it to a referral center for surgery.
- Although medical therapy has been described, surgical occlusion of the affected artery or arteries is the treatment of choice and should be performed promptly after the first hemorrhagic episode.

ACUTE GENERAL TREATMENT

- Hemodynamic stabilization after an acute hemorrhagic episode
  - Crystalloid colloid fluid therapy until blood volume is restored
    - Fresh-frozen plasma (FFP) is the colloid of choice because it contains platelets and clotting factors and provides oncotic support.
    - Hetastarch should be avoided because of its potential for exacerbating coagulopathies and promoting hemorrhage.
    - Large-bore IV catheters can be placed in both jugular veins in cases of severe hemorrhage for large-volume resuscitation.
    - Normovolemia should be restored; fluid therapy should not be too aggressive because the resultant increase in blood pressure may dislodge a forming clot at the affected artery.
  - Blood transfusions
    - Do if packed cell volume is below 20% acutely or below 12% to 14% with chronic blood loss.
    - Perform cross-match if available.
      - In acute, severe bleeds, this may not be practical; a Quarter Horse or Standardbred gelding should be used as the donor.
      - 10 L can be collected safely from a 500-kg donor.
  - Treatments aimed at stopping hemorrhage
    - Aminocaproic acid (100 mg/kg IV) inhibits fibrinolysis
    - FFP (4–5 mL/kg IV): Monitor for transfusion reactions
- Broad-spectrum IV antimicrobial therapy to guard against secondary bacterial infections
- Antiinflammatory and analgesic therapy
- Phenylbutazone (2.2 mg/kg IV or PO q12h or 4.4 mg/kg IV or PO q24h) or flunixin meglumine (1.1 mg/kg IV or PO q12–24h)
- Medical therapy
  - Is not the treatment of choice; treatment is often prolonged, costly, and ineffective
  - If there is no surgical option, treatment consists of systemic and topical therapy.
    - Itraconazole: 3 mg/kg PO q12h for 4 to 5 months
    - Enilconazole: 60 mL of a 33.3-mg/mL solution flush q24h
- Surgical occlusion of the affected artery or arteries
  - Direct arterial ligation
    - Difficult to identify the proper artery or arteries to ligate if active hemorrhage obscures endoscopic visualization

- Increased morbidity and mortality versus newer surgical techniques
- No specialized equipment required
  ○ Balloon catheter occlusion
    - Decreased morbidity and mortality versus direct ligation
    - Difficult to identify the proper artery or arteries to ligate if active hemorrhage obscures endoscopic visualization
    - Does not stop hemorrhage from aberrant vasculature (if present)
  ○ Transarterial coil embolization
    - Lowest morbidity and mortality rates
    - Minimally invasive
    - Can detect affected vessels if active hemorrhage is present; does not rely on endoscopy
    - Can detect and occlude aberrant vessels
    - Need specialized equipment (fluoroscopy, coils, and a special surgery table)
    - Steep learning curve

CHRONIC TREATMENT

- After surgical occlusion of the affected artery or arteries, secondary complications may need to be addressed.
  ○ Dysphagia may necessitate placement of an esophagostomy tube for long-term enteral nutrition.
  ○ Aspiration pneumonia: IV antimicrobials as directed by the results of a bacterial culture and sensitivity taken from a transtracheal wash.

POSSIBLE COMPLICATIONS

- Dysphagia may be seen preoperatively or may develop postoperatively.

○ Poor prognostic indicator
○ May take 6 to 18 months to resolve or may be permanent
- Laryngeal hemiplegia is often permanent.
- Facial nerve paralysis and Horner's syndrome typically resolve within months.
- Surgical site infections: More common with direct ligation or balloon catheterization.

RECOMMENDED MONITORING

Repeat endoscopic evaluation of the affected guttural pouch.

PROGNOSIS AND OUTCOME

- Up to 50% of horses with hemorrhage caused by guttural pouch mycosis die because of hemorrhagic shock without treatment. This risk is greatly reduced with surgical intervention.
- Medical therapy is costly, prolonged, and often ineffective, with an approximate 35% fatality rate because of severe hemorrhage.
- Surgical therapy results in improved success rates:
  ○ About 20% of horses that undergo direct arterial ligation experience postoperative hemorrhage versus 10% of those that undergo balloon catheter occlusion and 6% of those that undergo transarterial coil embolization.
  ○ Transarterial coil embolization techniques result in improved survival rates (84%), decreased morbidity, and decreased hospitalization time.

- Neurologic deficits may persist for months to years and may contribute to postoperative morbidity and mortality.
- Dysphagia is a poor prognostic indicator.

PEARLS & CONSIDERATIONS

COMMENTS

Any horse with guttural pouch mycosis should be considered a surgical candidate, even if there is no active hemorrhage present at the time of endoscopic evaluation.

CLIENT EDUCATION

- Surgical therapy is ultimately more effective and often less costly than medical therapy.
- Clients should be made aware of the risk of development of neurologic deficits, especially if the horse is intended to be athletic after surgery.

SUGGESTED READING

Crotty E, et al: Managing guttural pouch disease in adult horses: surgical treatment of guttural pouch empyema and mycosis. *Compend Contin Educ Pract Vet* 708–717, 2005.

Freeman DE, Hardy J: Guttural pouch. In Auer JA, Stick JA, editors: *Equine surgery*, ed 3, St Louis, 2006, Saunders Elsevier, pp 591–608.

Lepage OM, et al: Transarterial coil embolization in 31 horses (1999–2002) with guttural pouch mycosis: a 2 year follow-up. *Equine Vet J* 37:430–434, 2005.

AUTHOR: **LIBERTY M. GETMAN**

EDITOR: **ERIC J. PARENTE**

Guttural Pouch Tympany

BASIC INFORMATION

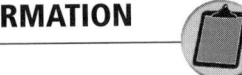

DEFINITION

A congenital abnormality causing air accumulation in the guttural pouch secondary to an abnormality involving the plica salpingopharyngea

EPIDEMIOLOGY

SPECIES, AGE, SEX The most commonly affected age is 1 year or younger, with fillies being more commonly affected.
GENETICS AND BREED PREDISPOSITION Arabians are the most commonly affected breed. In addition to Arabians,

other breeds, such as Thoroughbreds and Quarter Horses, can be affected.
ASSOCIATED CONDITIONS AND DISORDERS Air distension of the guttural pouch may result in respiratory noise, dyspnea, dysphagia, aspiration pneumonia, and secondary guttural pouch empyema.

CLINICAL PRESENTATION

HISTORY, CHIEF COMPLAINT The most common historical finding associated with guttural pouch tympanites is a soft, fluctuant, nonpainful, and elastic swelling in the parotid region. Affected horses may also exhibit unilateral or

bilateral mucopurulent nasal discharge secondary to guttural pouch empyema.
PHYSICAL EXAM FINDINGS Most horses with guttural pouch tympany without evidence of guttural pouch empyema have a normal rectal temperature and heart rate. Some horses with severe air distension of the guttural pouch may have tachypnea and dyspnea.
ETIOLOGY AND PATHOPHYSIOLOGY

- Tympany of the guttural pouch is the direct result of the entrapment of air within one or both guttural pouches.
- In normal horses, the guttural pouch openings open when the horse swallows, allowing passage of air in and out of the pouch.

- In horses affected with guttural pouch tympany, air is allowed into the guttural pouch via the plica salpingopharyngea but is not allowed to exit the guttural pouch.
- The cause of guttural pouch tympany is most likely secondary to redundancy or abnormal function of the plica salpingopharyngea. The plica salpingopharyngea is a soft tissue structure that lies just beneath the cartilaginous opening of the guttural pouch.
- A redundant plica salpingopharyngea can be congenital or secondary to chronic guttural pouch inflammation.

DIAGNOSIS

DIFFERENTIAL DIAGNOSIS

- Guttural pouch empyema
- Bronchopneumonia

INITIAL DATABASE

- Complete blood count: Typically normal unless the horse has aspiration pneumonia or severe guttural pouch empyema
- The diagnosis is readily made based on clinical signs alone. The characteristic nonpainful, pliable swelling in the parotid region is difficult to confuse with any other condition.
- The most challenging diagnostic dilemma is determining whether the condition is unilateral or bilateral, since a unilateral disorder will often result in a mild external swelling on the contralateral side.
- Methods of determining whether the condition is bilateral include passage of an endoscope into one or both guttural pouches, aspiration of air from the pouch with the most distension, and obtaining a dorsoventral radiographic view of the skull.
- In unilateral guttural pouch tympany, passage of the endoscope into the affected guttural pouch results in complete decompression of the guttural pouch. If the side with endoscope decompresses but the contralateral side does not, then the condition is bilateral. If there is no change in the external appearance of either guttural pouch, then the condition is most likely unilateral on the contralateral side.
- The second method of determination is to pass a Chambers catheter into the most distended guttural pouch under endoscopic guidance. The findings as described above hold true for this technique.
- Some authors have mentioned external needle decompression of the guttural pouch, but we do not recommend it because of the chance for iatrogenic damage to the neurovascular structures within the guttural pouch.
- The final method of determination of unilateral or bilateral disease is a dorsoventral radiographic view of the skull. Whereas unilateral guttural pouch tympany causes displacement of the affected medial septum of the guttural pouch toward the contralateral side, bilateral guttural pouch tympany results in bilateral air distension of each guttural pouch.
- Endoscopic findings compatible with guttural pouch tympanites include collapse of the dorsal pharyngeal wall, and if concurrent guttural pouch empyema is present, purulent exudate can be visualized exiting the guttural pouch opening.

TREATMENT

THERAPEUTIC GOAL(S)

Relief of air distension from the affected guttural pouch

ACUTE GENERAL TREATMENT

- The surgical management of horses with guttural pouch tympany is the only viable technique to resolve the clinical signs. The most important surgical consideration is the determination of unilateral versus bilateral disease. The surgical techniques for guttural pouch tympanites have been well described.
- Acceptable surgical techniques for unilateral guttural pouch tympany include fenestration of the median septum of the guttural pouch (allowing communication between the abnormal and normal pouch) with laser or traditional surgery, traditional surgical resection of the plica salpingopharyngea on the affected side, and laser plica salpingopharyngea fistula.
- Bilateral guttural pouch tympany can be managed with a combination of medial septum fenestration with resection of the plica salpingopharyngea on one side with laser fenestration of the median septum and unilateral laser plica salpingopharyngea fistula or with bilateral laser plica salpingopharyngea fistula.
- Fenestration of the median septum between the normal and abnormal pouch allows air to escape through the normal guttural pouch opening.
- The principle behind resection of the plica salpingopharyngea is to enlarge the normal opening into the guttural pouch. Laser fistulation through the plica salpingopharyngea allows for continuous decompression of the guttural pouch.

- The most significant complication of any of these techniques is stricture of the newly created openings. To lessen the risk for stricture formation, the newly created openings can be stented with indwelling Foley catheters exiting one or both nasal passages.
- Frequent monitoring after surgery is very important to determine whether stricture is occurring.

POSSIBLE COMPLICATIONS

Stricture of laser fenestration of the median septum and plica salpingopharyngea may occur and may require repeat fenestration. Dysphagia after laser fenestration of the median septum may occur and may be persistent. Concurrent guttural pouch empyema may require specific medical therapy.

RECOMMENDED MONITORING

The recurrence of air accumulation within the guttural pouch should be monitored. Recurrence may be secondary to stricture of surgically created fenestrations.

PROGNOSIS AND OUTCOME

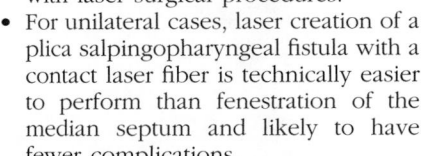

- The prognosis after surgical treatment of guttural pouch tympany is good, although in our experience, more than one surgical procedure may be required, especially if stricture develops.
- Foals affected by dysphagia or aspiration pneumonia in combination with guttural pouch tympany have a guarded to fair prognosis.

PEARLS & CONSIDERATIONS

- Guttural pouch tympany may be treated in a standing horse with laser surgical procedures.
- For unilateral cases, laser creation of a plica salpingopharyngeal fistula with a contact laser fiber is technically easier to perform than fenestration of the median septum and likely to have fewer complications.
- Horses with bilateral guttural pouch tympany are preferentially managed with laser fenestration of the median septum of the guttural pouch and creation of unilateral salpingopharyngea fistula.
- Horses treated with laser fenestration of the median septum or plica salpingopharyngea should be monitored at monthly intervals with endoscopy for postoperative stricture formation.

SUGGESTED READING

Bell C: Pharyngeal neuromuscular dysfunction associated with bilateral guttural pouch tympany in a foal. *Can Vet J* 48:192–194, 2007.

Blazyczek I, Hamann H, Deegen E, et al: Retrospective analysis of 50 cases of guttural pouch tympany in foals. *Vet Rec* 154:261-264, 2004.

Blazyczek I, Hamann H, Ohnesorge B, et al: Inheritance of guttural pouch tympany in the Arabian horse. *J Hered* 95:195–199, 2004.

Freeman DE: Guttural pouches. In Beech J, editor: *Equine respiratory disorders.* Philadelphia, 1991, Lea & Febiger, pp 305–330.

Tate LP Jr, Blikslager AT, Little ED, et al: Transendoscopic laser treatment of guttural pouch tympanites in eight foals. *Vet Surg* 24:367–372, 1995.

AUTHOR: **JAN F. HAWKINS**

EDITOR: **ERIC J. PARENTE**

Head Injury

BASIC INFORMATION

DEFINITION

Injury to the head caused by a sudden (mechanical and usually external) force. This entry focuses on the consequences to the central nervous system (CNS).

SYNONYM(S)

Traumatic brain injury (TBI)

EPIDEMIOLOGY

SPECIES, AGE, SEX

- Young animals are more prone to traumatic (training) accidents.
- Basilar bones fuse at around 5 years of age, so young animals may be more susceptible to basilar bone fractures.

GENETICS AND BREED PREDISPOSITION
Thoroughbred breeds may be more prone to traumatic accidents because of their temperament and the young age at which race training commences.

RISK FACTORS

- Temperament or disposition
- Management: Training and pasture group composition

ASSOCIATED CONDITIONS AND DISORDERS

- Sudden death
- Fractures of the basilar bones (Figure 1)
- Cranial nerve disorders
- Vestibular disease
- Cerebellar disease
- Temporohyoid osteoarthropathy: A pathologic process in which fusion between the temporal and stylohyoid bones occurs that may result in skull fractures with secondary traumatic damage to the vestibular apparatus, cranial nerve VII, or both

CLINICAL PRESENTATION

DISEASE FORMS/SUBTYPES

- Closed head injury: Skull remains intact
- Open head injury: Penetrating wound that causes skull fracture and brain damage

HISTORY, CHIEF COMPLAINT

- Down or recumbent
- External damage to the head: Wounds, fractures, hemorrhage
- Blood or cerebrospinal fluid (CSF) from the ear canals
- Signs of neurologic disease: Unresponsiveness, ataxia, blindness

PHYSICAL EXAM FINDINGS

- Varies depending on the severity of the insult
- Wounds or fractures of the skull
- Hemorrhage or CSF from the nostril, mouth, or ear canals
- Signs range from inapparent to recumbency with unconsciousness to death.
- Severe damage: Down, unresponsiveness, obtundation, respiratory abnormalities, cardiovascular instability, depression, inability to get up
- Milder damage: Ataxia, circling, blindness and pupillary abnormalities (signs are typically asymmetrical)
- Cranial nerve deficits (eg, cranial nerve VII)
- Signs of vestibular or cerebellar disease
- Altered behavior

ETIOLOGY AND PATHOPHYSIOLOGY

- Although head injury in horses is quite common, subsequent brain injury occurs only in 25% to 50% of cases.
- Primary damage: Initial mechanical disruption of vasculature and components of the CNS, such as cell bodies (neurons, astrocytes, oligodendrocytes) and axons
- Secondary damage: A complex cascade of molecular, cellular, and biochemical events that may occur for days to months after the initial insult, resulting in delayed tissue damage
- Systemic alterations further contribute to the tissue damage: Hypoxia, ischemia, brain swelling, alterations in intracranial pressure (ICP), hydrocephalus, infection, breakdown of blood-brain barrier, impaired energy metabolism, altered ionic homeostasis, changes in gene expression, inflam-

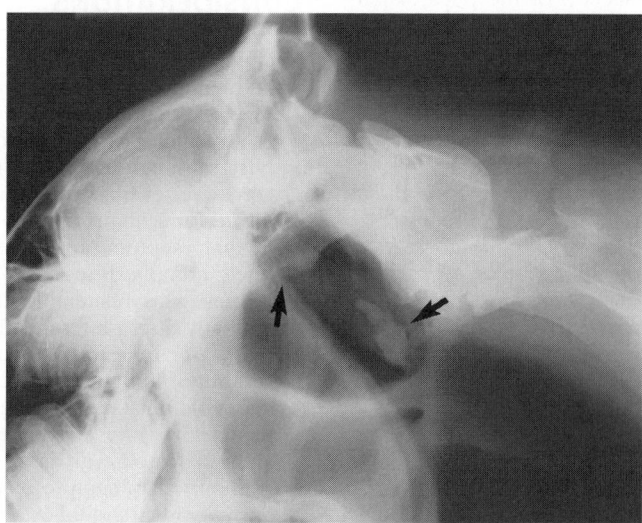

FIGURE 1 Lateral radiograph of the head showing an avulsion basilar skull fracture. *Arrows* point to the defect in the basisphenoid/basioccipital bone (*left*) and the avulsed fracture fragment (*right*).

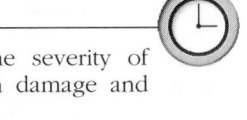

mation, and activation or release of autodestructive molecules occur and exacerbate the initial injury.

- Elevation of the ICP: Particularly a concern in closed head injury; an increase in ICP caused by, for example, a hematoma or edema will lead to a decreased cerebral perfusion pressure and subsequently decreased cerebral blood flow.

DIAGNOSIS

DIFFERENTIAL DIAGNOSIS

- Other causes of sudden death
  - Lightning strike
  - Cardiac disease
- Other causes of CNS disease with a neuroanatomic localization rostral to foramen magnum
  - Equine herpesvirus-1 myelopathy
  - Equine protozoal myeloencephalitis
  - Leukoencephalomalacia
  - Meningitis
  - Neoplasia
  - Temporohyoid osteoarthropathy
  - Trauma
  - Viral encephalitides (Eastern equine encephalomyelitis, Western equine encephalomyelitis, Venezuelan equine encephalomyelitis, rabies, West Nile virus)

INITIAL DATABASE

- History
- Complete physical and neurologic examination

ADVANCED OR CONFIRMATORY TESTING

- Imaging of the head: Radiography, computed tomography for bony lesions, magnetic resonance imaging for brain pathology
- CSF analysis: Hemorrhage
- Rule out other (infectious) disease through complete blood count, serum titers, and CSF analysis.

TREATMENT

THERAPEUTIC GOAL(S)

- Prevent further neurologic damage.
- Save or salvage undamaged or reversibly damaged components.
- Enhance recovery or regeneration.

ACUTE GENERAL TREATMENT

- Optimize oxygen delivery.
  - Optimize cerebral blood flow.
  - Optimize mean arterial blood pressure and hemoglobin concentration.
    - Fluid therapy
    - Vasopressor or inotropic support (or both)
  - Ensure that ICP is not elevated.
    - Mannitol: 20%; 0.25 to 2.0 mg/kg IV
    - Hypertonic saline: 3%, 5%, 7.5%: 4 to 6 mL/kg IV; 23.4%; monitor serum sodium
- Prevent or reduce elevated temperature.
  - Antiinflammatory drugs
    - Corticosteroids: Dexamethasone (0.1–0.25 mg/kg IV q6–24h) or methylprednisolone sodium succinate (0.5–2.5 mg/kg IV q6h); the dose and interval depend on the severity of clinical signs
    - Flunixin meglumine: 1.1 mg/kg IV q12–24h
    - Dimethyl sulfoxide: 0.5 to 1.0 g/kg IV q12–24h; must be diluted to a 10% solution or less in an isotonic balanced electrolyte solution
- Prevent or contain seizure activity.
  - Diazepam (0.05–0.2 mg/kg IV), midazolam (0.1–0.4 mg/kg IV; as a continuous rate infusion in 50-kg foals: 1–3 mg/hr)
  - Phenobarbital: 4 to 10 mg/kg PO q12h
- Antibiotic treatment with antimicrobials that penetrate into the CNS, particularly in open head injury

CHRONIC TREATMENT

- Provide adequate nutritional support.
- Provide sling support in horses that are unable to stand or get up on their own.
- Provide physiotherapy rehabilitation. Exercise has been shown to be beneficial for recovery of function after CNS damage in multiple animal models.

POSSIBLE COMPLICATIONS

Deterioration because of development of cerebral edema

RECOMMENDED MONITORING

- Periodic repeat neurologic examinations to assess response to therapy and recovery of function
- Monitor appetite and hydration status. Monitor urine and creatinine concentration if treating with possible nephrotoxic drugs.

PROGNOSIS AND OUTCOME

- Depend on the severity of sustained brain damage and early treatment
- Gauged by response to treatment; recovery can be remarkable
- In general, horses with basilar skull fractures and brainstem injuries have a grave prognosis.
- Horses with recumbency, tetraparesis, and severe dementia have a grave prognosis.

PEARLS & CONSIDERATIONS

COMMENTS

Particularly animals with suspect closed head injury may need thorough repeated evaluation because the damage may not be immediately obvious.

PREVENTION

Prevent injuries by increasing safety around horses and when handling horses.

CLIENT EDUCATION

Clients should be knowledgeable on topics such as (multiple) horse management and safe handling and training.

SUGGESTED READING

Feary DJ, Magdesian KG, Aleman MA, et al: Traumatic brain injury in horses: 34 cases (1994–2004). *J Am Vet Med Assoc* 231:259–266, 2007.

Feige K, Fürst A, Kaser-Hotz B, et al: Traumatic injury to the central nervous system in horses: occurrence, diagnosis and outcome. *Equine Vet Ed* 12:220–224, 2000.

Nout YS: Central nervous system trauma. In Reed SM, Furr MO, editors: *Equine neurology*, Ames, IA, 2007, Blackwell, pp 305–327.

AUTHOR: **YVETTE S. NOUT**

EDITOR: **STEPHEN M. REED**

Heart Murmur

BASIC INFORMATION

DEFINITION

- Murmurs are audible vibrations heard during a normally silent part of the cardiac cycle. Blood flow through the heart is generally laminar, but a number of circumstances may alter the normal laminar flow, causing turbulent flow to develop. This may cause vibration of cardiac structures, resulting in a murmur that can be heard with a stethoscope. Turbulence is most likely generated when blood viscosity is low, when the blood flow velocity is high, or when the diameter of the blood vessel is large. Three different types of murmurs exist, two of which are not associated with cardiac abnormalities.
  - Functional murmur (systolic flow murmur, systolic ejection murmur): These benign murmurs are common in horses, especially in racehorses, because the large stroke volume and large diameters of the great vessels induce turbulent blood flow in aortic and pulmonary artery roots in early systole.
  - Physiologic murmur: A number of conditions such as anemia and endotoxemia can lead to altered blood viscosity as well as increased cardiac output, which induces turbulent blood flow, leading to a benign systolic murmur. This is quite often heard in horses presented with substantial hemorrhage, high fever, or colic.
  - Pathologic murmur: Acquired or congenital cardiac malformations (eg, valvular regurgitations or ventricular septal defects [VSDs]) result in high-velocity blood flow, inducing a murmur.

SYNONYM(S)

- Cardiac murmur
- Murmur

EPIDEMIOLOGY

SPECIES, AGE, SEX Whereas degenerative valvular diseases are often seen in older horses, clinically significant congenital cardiac diseases are often discovered in young animals.

GENETICS AND BREED PREDISPOSITION

- A high proportion of both Thoroughbreds and Standardbreds have heart murmurs; these may be either functional murmurs or murmurs caused by acquired valvular regurgitation.

RISK FACTORS

- High stroke volume and large diameter of the vessel may lead to a benign functional murmur.
- Systemic conditions such as anemia and endotoxemia may result in a benign physiological heart murmur.
- Acquired or congenital cardiac diseases often result in heart murmurs.

ASSOCIATED CONDITIONS AND DISORDERS Variable, depending on the cause of the murmur and the severity of the situation inducing the murmur

CLINICAL PRESENTATION

DISEASE FORMS/SUBTYPES As defined above, heart murmurs can be divided into three different types with functional and physiologic murmurs considered to be benign. Pathologic murmurs may or may not have a clinical effect on the horse. Therefore two fundamental questions should be answered: What is the source of the murmur, and what is its clinical significance?

HISTORY, CHIEF COMPLAINT

- Heart murmur may be detected on routine examinations (eg, prepurchase examination, auscultation before sedation, vaccination or a general clinical examination) in otherwise healthy animals.
- Heart murmur may be detected in systemically ill patients (eg,. anemia, colic, endotoxemia). In this situation, it is important to rule out cardiac disease and to assess whether it is a physiologic murmur that will disappear after the primary disease has resolved.
- Heart murmurs detected in horses presented with signs of cardiac disease (eg, ventral edema, tachycardia, arrhythmia, tachypnea or dyspnea, exercise intolerance, or collapse).

PHYSICAL EXAM FINDINGS

- Before auscultation of the left hemithorax, palpation of the apex beat with the flat of the left hand should be performed because the point of maximal intensity (PMI) of the mitral valve is usually located in this area (apical area). The apical area lies above the point of the elbow at the caudal edge of the triceps musculature. In this region, the first (S1) and second (S2) heart sounds are of equal loudness. From this location, the stethoscope is advanced in a dorsocranial direction until S2 becomes more accentuated relative to S1 and the aortic and pulmonic valve area is identified (basal area).
- On the right hemithorax, the apex beat is rarely palpable unless the horse is thin and narrow chested or has enlargement of the right ventricle or atrium. The auscultation area is more cranially located compared with the apical area on the left side of the horse. Often the right forelimb should be placed cranial to the left forelimb to allow better access. The only valve auscultated on the right hemithorax is the tricuspid valve, and because of the anatomical location of the heart toward the left side of the thorax, the tricuspid valve may be difficult to hear in some horses.
- Murmurs are classified according to a number of different criteria.
  - Intensity: The intensity of a murmur is usually graded on a 6-point scale.
    - Grade I/VI is a very quiet murmur that can only be heard in a focal area after careful examination in a quiet area.
    - Grade II/VI is also a quiet murmur but is heard immediately at its PMI.
    - Grade III/VI is a moderately loud murmur that is easily appreciated.
    - Grade IV/VI is a loud murmur (particularly relative to S1 and S2) that is heard over a widespread area but has no obvious palpable prechordial thrill.
    - Grade V/VI is a loud murmur with a palpable thrill.
    - Grade VI/VI is loud enough that it can be heard with the stethoscope just off the chest wall and has an obvious palpable thrill.
  - Timing and duration: Murmurs should be classified as systolic, diastolic, or continuous when occurring in both systole and diastole. Simultaneous palpation of the peripheral pulse can help to differentiate timing if it is unclear with auscultation alone. They should also be classified as early, mid, or late systolic or diastolic. If the murmur is heard throughout systole or diastole but the heart sounds are still distinct, a holosystolic or a holodiastolic murmur is heard. *Pansystolic* or *pandiastolic* refers to a holosystolic or holodiastolic murmur that additionally engulfs the first, second, or both heart sounds.
  - PMI: The PMI of the murmur is where the murmur is most intense and indicates the likely source of the murmur. Identification of the

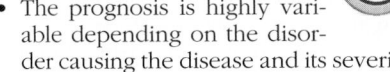
valve areas is therefore important, but in general, the heart is divided into the apical area (mitral and tricuspid valves) and the more dorsally located basal area (aortic and pulmonary valves).

○ Shape: The shape of the murmur describes its change in intensity over time. It is often described as crescendo (increasing in intensity); decrescendo (decreasing in intensity); or band shaped (plateau), which stays a constant intensity throughout the murmur. The shape can sometimes help to determine the cause of the murmur.

○ Quality: The quality of the murmur is related to the characteristic of the sound and can be described as soft, coarse or harsh, or musical. A musical murmur is harmonic and is often caused by a vibrating structure (fenestrated valve leaflet or ruptured chordae tendineae).

ETIOLOGY AND PATHOPHYSIOLOGY

- Functional and physiologic murmurs are generated by turbulence induced by noncardiac disease.
- Pathologic murmurs can be acquired or congenital. The most common congenital condition is a VSD. However, the majority of pathologic murmurs are caused by valvular regurgitation.
- It is important to note that valvular stenosis is extremely rare in horses and is therefore rarely considered as a differential diagnosis in adult horses.

DIAGNOSIS

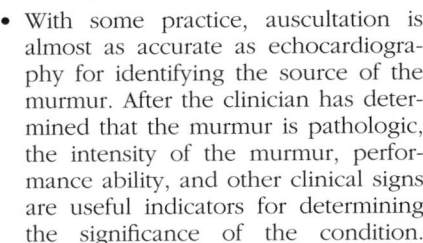

DIFFERENTIAL DIAGNOSIS

- With some practice, auscultation is almost as accurate as echocardiography for identifying the source of the murmur. After the clinician has determined that the murmur is pathologic, the intensity of the murmur, performance ability, and other clinical signs are useful indicators for determining the significance of the condition.

However, an exact diagnosis and quantification of the severity of the condition requires an echocardiographic examination.

- Situations in which physiologic murmurs may be present are typically those in which noncardiac explanations for the murmur exist (eg, anemia, colic, fever). In these situations, the horse should be reassessed after resolution of the primary condition.

INITIAL DATABASE

- Auscultation
- Complete blood count and serum chemistry, especially packed cell volume and inflammatory markers for systemic illness
- Echocardiography if indicated

TREATMENT

THERAPEUTIC GOAL(S)

There is no treatment for heart murmurs. The primary goals are to provide an accurate prognosis for both the life and performance to the owner and to monitor the horse regularly if indicated based on the cardiac diagnosis.

RECOMMENDED MONITORING

- Most murmurs associated with mild or moderate regurgitation that is not progressive do not require specific monitoring.
- However, the owner should always be aware of the horse's attitude, heart rate, and exercise tolerance. Any changes should prompt a veterinary examination.
- The characteristics of the murmur (eg, intensity, duration, quality), regardless of the cause, should be monitored on an annual basis by the regular veterinarian. Any changes, particularly if accompanied by changes in clinical parameters, should prompt an echocardiographic examination.
- Annual echocardiograms should be performed in horses that have murmurs

associated with pathology that has more potential to progress.

PROGNOSIS AND OUTCOME

- The prognosis is highly variable depending on the disorder causing the disease and its severity.
- Most valvular regurgitation has no clinical significance. Mild to moderate valvular regurgitation that does not progress is unlikely to impact either lifespan or most performance activity.
- In general, loud murmurs with palpable thrills are more likely to be clinically important than quiet ejection murmurs. However, the intensity of the murmur does not always correlate with the severity of the disease, and there are exceptions to this rule (eg, a loud murmur caused by a restrictive VSD may not be clinically significant, but a quiet murmur associated with a large VSD may indicate a large defect with low-velocity flow through the defect and a poor prognosis for life).

PEARLS & CONSIDERATIONS

Most horses with murmurs do not have clinically significant cardiac disease. However, if a murmur is associated with exercise intolerance, lethargy, respiratory signs, collapse, fever, or weight loss, veterinary attention should be sought immediately.

SUGGESTED READING

Blissitt KJ: Auscultation. In Marr CM, editor: *Cardiology of the horse*, Philadelphia, 1999, WB Saunders, pp 71–93.

Patteson M, Blissitt KJ: Evaluation of cardiac murmurs in horses. 1. Clinical examination. *In Practice* 367–373, 1996.

AUTHOR: **RIKKE BUHL**

EDITOR: **MARY M. DURANDO**

Hematuria

BASIC INFORMATION

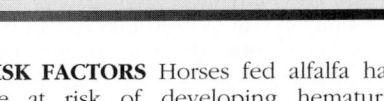

DEFINITION

Blood in the urine. Hematuria can be microscopic or macroscopic.

EPIDEMIOLOGY

SPECIES, AGE, SEX The age and sex of the affected horse may rule out some

possible causes of hematuria. Urethral rents as a cause of hematuria are reported only in geldings. Male horses are more commonly affected with cystic urolithiasis. Hematuria caused by a hematoma within the bladder and urachus has been reported in foals.

GENETICS AND BREED PREDISPOSITION Idiopathic hematuria is reported primarily in Arabian horses.

RISK FACTORS Horses fed alfalfa hay are at risk of developing hematuria caused by ingestion of blister beetles.

ASSOCIATED CONDITIONS AND DISORDERS

- Urolithiasis
- Blister beetle toxicosis (equine cantharidiasis)
- Urinary tract neoplasia

- Pyelonephritis
- Cystitis
- Urethral rents
- Vascular anomalies

CLINICAL PRESENTATION

HISTORY, CHIEF COMPLAINT

- The history and chief complaints vary with the cause of hematuria.
  - Urethral rents: Hemorrhage occurs immediately after urination.
  - Cystic calculi/urolith: Hematuria is likely to be more pronounced near the end of urination. Hematuria observed after exercise is the most common clinical sign displayed by horses affected with a cystic calculus and is virtually pathognomonic for the condition.
- Renal *Halicephalobus gingivalis* infections: Hematuria plus concomitant neurologic disease and osteomyelitis
- Cantharidin toxicosis: Hematuria plus signs of abdominal pain and a recent history of ingesting alfalfa.
- Miscellaneous: Dehydrated horses treated inappropriately with nonsteroidal antiinflammatory drugs (NSAIDs) may develop hematuria. Hematuria is observed occasionally in exercising horses, especially if the bladder has been emptied immediately before exercise.

PHYSICAL EXAM FINDINGS The
hindlimbs are often stained with urine or blood. The presence of a cystic calculus can usually be confirmed by palpation of the bladder per rectum.

ETIOLOGY AND PATHOPHYSIOLOGY

- Hemorrhage into the urethral lumen through a urethral rent occurs when pressure in the corpus spongiosum penis (CSP) increases with contraction of the bulbospongiosus muscle to expel urine remaining in the urethra after urination.
- Exfoliated epithelial cells may act as a nidus for formation of cystic calculi in horses because some horses with urinary calculi have infection of the upper urinary tract.
- A severe, often fatal, idiopathic hematuria is reported to occur in primarily Arabian horses. Some clinicians believe that this condition is caused by pyelonephritis, which is a suppurative bacterial infection of the renal pelvis and parenchyma.
- Hematuria in horses may be caused by renal infection with *H. gingivalis* (previously known as *Micronema deletrix*), a saprophytic nematode.
- Renal and vesicular neoplasia. Adenocarcinoma (renal cell carcinoma) and lymphosarcoma are the most common tumors affecting the kidney, but adenocarcinoma is more likely than lymphosarcoma to cause hematuria. Squamous cell and transitional cell

carcinomas of the bladder are also reported to cause hematuria in horses.
- Cantharidin, the toxic principle of blister beetles, is irritating to the digestive and urinary tracts. Irritation of the urinary tract may cause pollakiuria and hemorrhage of the urinary mucosa.
- Trauma to the umbilicus during the periparturient period with damage to the umbilical blood vessels may result in retrograde bleeding into the urachus and bladder and subsequent hematuria.
- Bacterial toxins or immune complexes may cause endothelial damage in glomerular capillary loops and small arterioles (glomerulonephritis), leading to renal failure, intravascular hemolysis, and renal hemorrhage.
- Chronic or excessive administration of NSAIDs causes decreased renal medullary blood flow that may result in medullary necrosis, leading to renal hemorrhage.
- Vascular anomalies, either congenital or acquired, are a rare cause of hematuria in horses.
- Repeated concussion of the bladder during exercise can be sufficient to cause mucosal damage and hemorrhage.

DIAGNOSIS

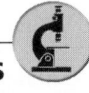

DIFFERENTIAL DIAGNOSIS

- Hematuria may be confused with hemoglobinuria, myoglobinuria, pigmenturia caused by ingestion of some plants (eg, red and white clover), drug-derived (rifampin, phenothiazine, nitazoxanide, and doxycycline) urinary pigments, and oxidizing agents (pyrocatechin) normally found in urine.
- Urolithiasis
- Blister beetle toxicosis (equine cantharidiasis)
- Urinary tract neoplasia
- Pyelonephritis
- Cystitis
- Urethral rents
- Vascular anomalies
- Glomerulonephritis
- NSAID toxicosis
- Exercise-induced hematuria
- Idiopathic hematuria

INITIAL DATABASE

- Complete blood cell count (CBC) and serum biochemistries, urinalysis, culture of urine collected by catheterization (failure to find bacteria or increased numbers of white blood cells during light microscopy does not rule out bacterial infection of the urinary tract), and palpation of the bladder and pelvic urethra per rectum

- The reproductive system of mares should be examined.
- Whereas an abundance of red blood cells (RBCs) found during microscopic examination of discolored urine suggests hematuria, an absence of RBCs suggests pigmenturia. RBCs may rupture if examination of urine, especially if it is dilute, is delayed (for as little as 1 to 2 hours), resulting in false hemoglobinuria. In this case, RBC ghosts may be seen during microscopic examination of sediment.
- Clinical signs of myopathy and markedly increased serum creatine kinase (CK) activity indicate myoglobinuria as a cause of urine discoloration. Activity of CK is increased to at least several thousand units per liter when significant muscle injury has occurred. Serum is clear if pigmenturia is caused by myoglobinuria.
- In contrast to hematuria and myoglobinuria, intravascular hemolysis causes discolored serum and urine.

ADVANCED OR CONFIRMATORY TESTING

- Endoscopy aids in the diagnosis of a cystic calculus, primary bacterial cystitis, and blood emanating from a ureteral opening (Figure 1).
- Endoscopic examination of a male urethra may identify a 5- to 10-mm linear defect on the convex surface of the urethra distal to the openings of the bulbourethral glands near the level of the ischial arch (Figure 2).
- Ultrasonography of the kidneys and bladder is indicated for cystic urolithiasis if blood is observed emanating from a ureteral orifice during cystoscopy or if no cause of hematuria is apparent.
- Endoscopic catheterization of the ureters for collection of urine if blood is thought to originate from a kidney

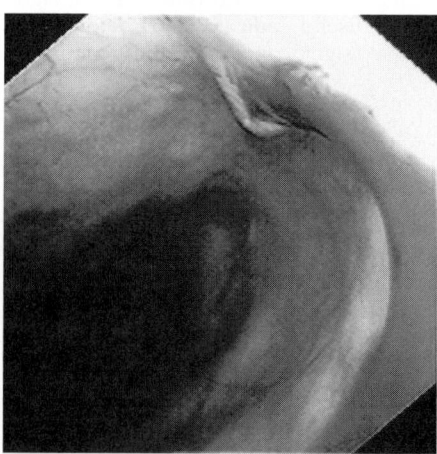

FIGURE 1 Cystoscopy showing blood from the right ureter in a horse with unilateral pyelonephritis.

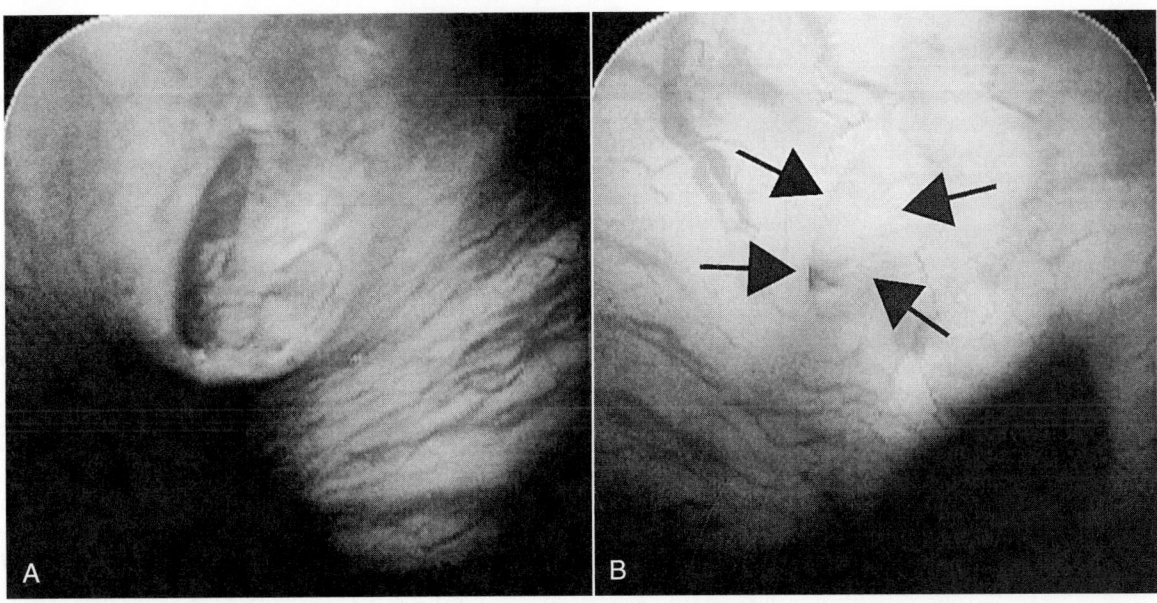

FIGURE 2 Endoscopic images of urethral defects or tears at the level of the ischial arch. **A,** A more acute lesion (hematuria of 2 weeks' duration) is surrounded by a raised rim of tissue. **B,** A chronic lesion (hematuria of 6 months' duration) is flat to recessed (between *arrows*). Evidence of inflammation around both lesions is minimal. (From Reed SM, Bayly WM, Sellon DC, editors: *Equine internal medicine*, ed 3. St Louis, 2010, Saunders Elsevier.)

- Kidney biopsy may be indicated if renal disease is the suspected cause of hematuria.
- If blister beetle toxicosis is suspected as the cause of hematuria, at least 500 mL of urine or 200 g of stomach contents should be submitted to a toxicology laboratory in a refrigerated container for identification of cantharidin. Samples should be collected early in the course of the condition. Suspect hay should also be inspected for possible blister beetles.

TREATMENT

THERAPEUTIC GOAL(S)

- The only treatment for cystic urolithiasis is surgical removal of the urolith.
- Nephrectomy is the treatment for horses with neoplasia of the kidney, but renal adenocarcinomas are usually inoperable because the neoplasm is often not diagnosed until the tumor has metastasized. Function of the contralateral kidney must be normal to perform a nephrectomy.
- Horses with hematuria associated with anuric or oliguric renal failure and intravascular hemolysis usually die, but treatment can be attempted with IV polyionic fluids, vasopressor agents, and diuretics to induce polyuria.

ACUTE GENERAL TREATMENT

- Urethral rents often heal without treatment, but surgical treatment may speed recovery. Affected geldings can be treated by temporary ischial urethrotomy or by an ischial incision that extends into the CSP but does not enter the lumen of the urethra.
- For horses with idiopathic hematuria, long-term antibiotic therapy may be appropriate. If renal hemorrhage is unilateral, then removal of the affected kidney may resolve the signs, but the remaining kidney may also begin to bleed.
- Horses suspected of having a renal infection of *H. gingivalis* should be treated with antiinflammatory drugs and a larvicidal anthelmintic agent.
- Treatment of horses with blister beetle toxicosis includes repeated administration of mineral oil by nasogastric tube because cantharidin is lipid soluble. Diuresis is indicated for affected horses with IV balanced polyionic fluids (with calcium added if the horse is hypocalcemic). Furosemide may be beneficial because cantharidin is excreted via the kidneys.
- Foals with cystic hematomas can be treated surgically by removing the cystic hematoma along with the umbilical remnants and bladder apex. Most affected foals respond to medical treatment with routine antimicrobial prophylaxis and IV fluids to promote diuresis.
- Some horses with severe renal hemorrhage and anemia may require blood transfusion.

CHRONIC TREATMENT

For horses with pyelonephritis, treatment for at least 3 weeks to several months with an appropriate antibiotic is indicated.

RECOMMENDED MONITORING

- Assessment of erythrocyte mass via periodic measurement of packed cell volume and urinalysis
- Horses with suspected pyelonephritis should have periodic CBCs and fibrinogen determinations, urinalyses, and a negative urine culture results before discontinuing antibiotics.
- Horses that have a kidney removed should have regular measurement of serum blood urea nitrogen and creatinine concentrations to monitor function of the remaining kidney.

PROGNOSIS AND OUTCOME

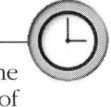

- The prognosis and outcome depend on the cause of hematuria.
- The generally favorable prognosis for horses with cystic urolithiasis has been questioned because of the high rate of recurrence in one large study and the finding that some of these horses may have concomitant pyelonephritis.
- Geldings with urethral rents respond favorably to an ischial incision that extends into the CSP.
- Horses with idiopathic hematuria or pyelonephritis often have recurrence of hematuria; affected horses may experience severe hematuria requiring blood transfusion for survival.
- Horses with hematuria caused by *H. gingivalis* usually die despite treatment.

- Horses with renal or vesicular neoplasia usually die or are euthanized, but removal of the affected portion of the bladder wall may result in survival of horses with vesicular neoplasia.

PEARLS & CONSIDERATIONS

The most common causes of hematuria in male horses are urolithiasis and urethral rents. Renal vascular anomalies, anuric or oliguric renal failure, and inappropriate administration of NSAIDs are rare causes of hematuria.

SUGGESTED READING

Schumacher J: Hematuria and pigmenturia of horses. *Vet Clin Equine* 23:655, 2007.

AUTHOR: **JOHN SCHUMACHER**

EDITOR: **BRYAN M. WALDRIDGE**

Hemoperitoneum

BASIC INFORMATION

DEFINITION
Hemorrhage into the peritoneal cavity

SYNONYM(S)
Hemoabdomen

EPIDEMIOLOGY
SPECIES, AGE, SEX Uterine or ovarian artery rupture occurs more often in aged multiparous broodmares than young or primiparous mares.
RISK FACTORS
- Late-term pregnancy or parturition
- Blunt abdominal trauma
- Recent abdominal surgery or percutaneous biopsy of abdominal organs (eg, liver, kidney, spleen)
- Coagulopathy

CLINICAL PRESENTATION
HISTORY, CHIEF COMPLAINT
- Colic (often severe)
- Sweating
- Trembling or muscle fasciculations
- ± Historical evidence of the above risk factors
PHYSICAL EXAM FINDINGS
- Clinical signs related to hypovolemia and hemorrhagic shock, including:
  - Tachycardia (often marked)
  - Tachypnea
  - Weak peripheral pulses, cool extremities, and poor jugular refill
  - Pale mucous membranes, prolonged capillary refill time
  - Weakness
  - ± Altered mentation (depression is typical, but violent behavior or severe colic may also be seen)
- Moderate to severe gross abdominal distension is often noted, especially in the later stages.
- A mesenteric or broad ligament hematoma may be palpated on rectal examination, although the rectal examination

is often within normal limits in horses with hemoperitoneum.

ETIOLOGY AND PATHOPHYSIOLOGY
- Rupture of an intraabdominal vessel or organ may occur with any of the following conditions:
  - Uterine or ovarian artery rupture with late-term pregnancy or parturition
  - Blunt external trauma, resulting in rupture of mesenteric vessels or the liver, spleen, or kidney. Rarely, displaced pelvic fractures may lacerate the iliac or pelvic arteries and result in hemoperitoneum.
  - Intraabdominal rupture of the umbilical vessels in neonatal foals
  - Iatrogenic hemorrhage after abdominal surgery (especially after enterotomy or intestinal resection and anastomosis) or biopsy of intraabdominal organs (liver, spleen, or kidney)
  - Intraabdominal neoplasia if invasion of intraabdominal blood vessels or spontaneous hemorrhage from highly vascular tumors occurs
  - Coagulopathy occasionally results in spontaneous hemoabdomen.
  - Rupture of an aortic or other vascular aneurysm is rare but has been described.
- Idiopathic hemoperitoneum also occurs with some frequency in adult horses with no historical risk factors or identifiable cause or source of hemorrhage.
- Rarely, hemorrhage may be confined to the mesentery; intestinal or uterine wall; or within the hepatic, splenic, or renal capsule. In these cases, horses may present with clinical and clinicopathologic findings consistent with acute intraabdominal hemorrhage, but the ultrasonographic findings and peritoneal fluid analysis may not demonstrate frank hemorrhage in the peritoneal cavity.

DIAGNOSIS

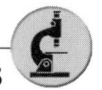

DIFFERENTIAL DIAGNOSIS
Strangulating intestinal obstruction (in horses with signs of severe abdominal pain)

INITIAL DATABASE
- Packed cell volume (PCV) and total solids (TS)
  - May be normal in acute stages. A disproportionate decrease in TS concentration is often noted before the PCV decreases significantly.
  - Within 6 to 24 hours of initial hemorrhage, decreased PCV and TS concentration are typically observed.
- Complete blood count
  - Variable hematocrit, as for PCV above.
  - Leukogram is usually normal or consistent with a stress response.
  - The platelet count is usually within reference intervals unless a concurrent coagulopathy (disseminated intravascular coagulation, immune-mediated thrombocytopenia) is present.
- Serum biochemistry profile and blood gas analysis
  - Hypocalcemia is frequently present because of loss of albumin-bound calcium. Ionized calcium may be normal or low.
  - Hypoproteinemia or hypoalbuminemia is usually present.
  - Variable azotemia (prerenal or renal) is often present and is reflective of poor renal perfusion because of hypovolemia.
  - Hyperlactatemia (>2 mmol/L) or low venous oxygen (PvO_2 <30 mm Hg or SvO_2 <50%) in an anaerobically collected sample indicates significantly decreased oxygen-carrying capacity.
- The coagulation profile should be performed to rule out an underlying coagulopathy.

- Transabdominal ultrasonography
  - A moderate to significant volume of homogeneously echogenic, swirling, free peritoneal fluid is usually visible in the ventral abdomen by the time clinical signs are present.
  - Ultrasonographic evidence of intra-abdominal neoplasia; mesenteric hematoma; or hepatic, splenic, or renal rupture may be apparent.
- Peritoneal fluid analysis: The peritoneal fluid is usually grossly hemorrhagic in appearance, with a PCV and TS concentration similar to the peripheral blood.
  - A very low PCV may indicate mild and resolving hemoperitoneum or intestinal compromise with a strangulating intestinal obstruction.
  - A PCV that is significantly higher than the peripheral blood is more consistent with splenocentesis than hemoperitoneum. Ultrasonographic visualization of the spleen at the site of the abdominocentesis is supportive of splenocentesis.
  - Cytologic evaluation of the peritoneal fluid may reveal platelets in acute or ongoing hemorrhage or hemosiderophages or erythrophagocytosis with previous or chronic hemorrhage (>6–12 hours' duration).

ADVANCED OR CONFIRMATORY TESTING

- Exploratory celiotomy
  - Because of the size and depth of the equine abdomen, surgical localization and ligation of the bleeding vessel or vessels is difficult to impossible in many cases. Thus medical management is usually preferable in most cases of hemoperitoneum.
  - Rarely, exploratory surgery may be indicated in horses exhibiting severe abdominal pain to confirm hemoperitoneum and rule out a concurrent intestinal lesion.

TREATMENT

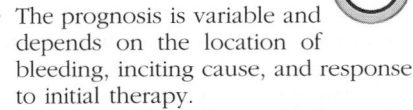

THERAPEUTIC GOAL(S)

- Support hemostasis
- Replace intravascular volume and oxygen-carrying capacity
- Provide pain relief
- Provide supportive care

ACUTE GENERAL TREATMENT

- Hemostatic support: Keep the patient quiet with strict stall confinement and a quiet atmosphere.
- Sedation should be avoided if possible unless the horse is violent because of alterations in blood pressure caused by commonly used sedatives.

- Aminocaproic acid (10–40 mg/kg IV slowly in 1 L of 0.9% saline q6h or 70 mg/kg in 1 L of 0.9% saline IV over 20–30 minutes; then IV continuous rate infusion [CRI] at 15 mg/kg/h) to inhibit fibrinolysis.
- Fresh or fresh-frozen plasma should be administered to provide clotting factors and platelets if a primary coagulopathy is present.
  - Drainage of the blood from the peritoneal cavity is rarely, if ever, indicated because the increasing abdominal pressure actually supports hemostasis. In addition, erythrocytes and plasma proteins may be reabsorbed from the peritoneal cavity as hemorrhage ceases.
- Fluid therapy and blood transfusion
  - Aggressive fluid resuscitation with hypertonic saline, hydroxyethyl starch, or bolus administration of isotonic crystalloids should be avoided because a rapid increase in blood pressure may perpetuate hemorrhage. However, reestablishment of normovolemia is vital, and conservative fluid therapy with isotonic crystalloids at 50 to 100 mL/kg/d is indicated in most cases. The decrease in PCV that will occur with crystalloid therapy is not concerning because peripheral perfusion and tissue oxygenation improve with the resultant volume expansion. Fluid therapy rates should be sufficient to maintain mean arterial pressure above 70 mm Hg and ensure normal urine production.
  - Whole-blood transfusion or administration of synthetic bovine hemoglobin (Oxyglobin) is indicated in horses exhibiting clinical signs of hypovolemia or hemorrhagic shock or clinicopathologic evidence of decreased oxygen-carrying capacity as above, regardless of the PCV.
- Analgesic therapy and supportive care
  - Flunixin meglumine: 0.5 to 1.1 mg/kg IV q12h
  - Lidocaine (1.3 mg/kg IV slow; then 0.05 mg/kg/min IV CRI) for refractory pain
  - Naloxone (0.01–0.03 mg/kg IV) is an opioid antagonist that may be beneficial in hemorrhagic shock. It should not be used in conjunction with butorphanol.
- Prophylactic broad-spectrum antimicrobial therapy with ceftiofur (2.2 mg/kg IV q12h) or with potassium penicillin (22,000 IU/kg IV q6h) and gentamicin (6.6 mg/kg IV q24h) or enrofloxacin (5 mg/kg IV q24h) should be initiated because intraperitoneal blood is an optimal medium for bacterial growth.

POSSIBLE COMPLICATIONS

- Acute renal failure may occur because of hypoxic injury to the kidneys.
- Laminitis is also a possible complication if hemorrhagic shock or hypoperfusion is severe.

RECOMMENDED MONITORING

- PCV and TS, venous lactate concentration, and venous oxygen saturation should be monitored to determine if transfusion(s) is necessary.
- Urine output and renal function should also be monitored carefully during initial therapy.

PROGNOSIS AND OUTCOME

- The prognosis is variable and depends on the location of bleeding, inciting cause, and response to initial therapy.
  - If hemorrhage is confined to the mesentery or broad ligament, the prognosis for recovery is generally good, although hemorrhage may recur in subsequent pregnancies in broodmares.
  - If hemostasis is established early on and good clinical response to aggressive medical therapy is noted, prognosis is generally good even if the source of bleeding is never identified (eg, in idiopathic hemoabdomen).
  - The prognosis with splenic or hepatic rupture or rupture of a large uterine or mesenteric artery or aortic aneurysm is usually guarded to poor because hemorrhage can occur at such a rapid rate that even early and aggressive medical therapy is futile.

PEARLS & CONSIDERATIONS

In horses with acute hemoperitoneum, the peripheral PCV and TS are often normal. Thus, transabdominal ultrasonography and serial monitoring of the PCV and TS are vital for making an early and accurate diagnosis of hemoperitoneum.

SUGGESTED READING

Bain FT: Hemoperitoneum. In Mair T, Diver T, Ducharme N, editors: *Manual of equine gastroenterology*, London, 2002, Saunders Elsevier, pp 332–334.

Divers TJ: Hemorrhage into body cavity. In Orsini JA, Divers TJ, editors: *Equine emergencies: treatments and procedures*, ed 3, St Louis, 2008, Saunders Elsevier, pp 253–255.

AUTHOR: **KELSEY A. HART**

EDITORS: **TIM MAIR** and **CERI SHERLOCK**

Hemorrhage

BASIC INFORMATION

DEFINITION
Loss of blood from the vascular space

SYNONYM(S)
- Extravascular blood loss
- Bleeding

EPIDEMIOLOGY
SPECIES, AGE, SEX Horses of any age are susceptible to blood loss because of a number of causes; however, vessel rupture and urolithiasis are more common in older horses, and idiopathic hematuria is limited to males.

GENETICS AND BREED PREDISPOSITION Genetic platelet disorders and coagulation factor dysfunction have been identified in horses, as well as a genetic predisposition to granulomatous gastrointestinal proliferation and urolithiasis.

RISK FACTORS
- Horses in race training are at risk for developing exercise-induced pulmonary hemorrhage.
- Horses taking nonsteroidal antiinflammatory drugs (NSAIDs; eg, phenylbutazone) are at risk for right dorsal colon ulceration and hemorrhage.

CONTAGION AND ZOONOSIS
- Certain infectious and parasitic causes of hematuria may be transferred between horses
  - Strongylus vulgaris
  - Streptococcus equi

CLINICAL PRESENTATION

DISEASE FORMS/SUBTYPES Hemorrhage can be classified by location (internal or external), duration (acute or chronic loss), vessel size (capillary and venuole or arteriole versus larger vessel), and cause (coagulation disorder versus traumatic vessel disruption)

HISTORY, CHIEF COMPLAINT
- Chief complaints are variable and depend on the amount of blood lost and how acute the loss is.
  - External signs of blood loss may be apparent (Figure 1).
  - Significant blood loss may cause pallor, colic, sweating, and depression.
  - Less significant blood loss or chronic loss of blood may be noted as lethargy and exercise intolerance.

PHYSICAL EXAM FINDINGS
- Hypothermia, cool extremities, sweating
- Tachypnea
- Tachycardia with extreme blood loss
- Pale mucous membranes

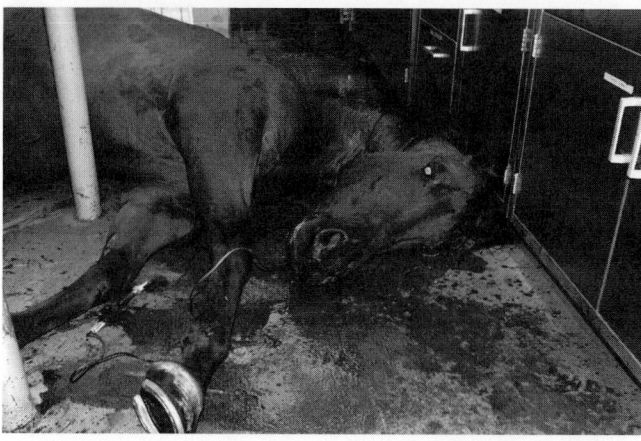

FIGURE 1 Fatal guttural pouch mycosis. Complete exsanguination occurred within 10 minutes after rupture of the internal carotid.

- Poor pulse quality
- Decreased gastrointestinal sounds, colic
- Petechia, ecchymosis

ETIOLOGY AND PATHOPHYSIOLOGY
- Traumatic vascular disruption occurs because of an injury that mechanically opens a vessel or vessels (caused by injury, disease, infection, or neoplasia) with a normal coagulation system that is unable or slow to repair the defect because of vessel size and blood pressure, repeated trauma, or systemic inflammation.
- Hemostatic bleeding disorders may occur by one of two pathways:
  - Primary hemostatic defects involve either a genetic failure of the platelets to functionally occlude a vascular leak or thrombocytopenia, which reduces effective platelet numbers. Both result in capillary and small vessel hemorrhage (petechia, ecchymosis).
  - Secondary hemostatic issues are related to coagulopathies caused by congenital defects, vitamin K deficiencies, hepatic disease, drug toxicity, envenomation, poisons, or consumption of coagulation factors (ie, disseminated intravascular coagulation). This results in overt hemorrhage into body cavities or externally.

DIAGNOSIS

DIFFERENTIAL DIAGNOSIS
- Degenerative disorders
  - Vessel rupture
    - Aorta
    - Middle uterine artery
- Anomalies
  - Idiopathic hematuria in geldings and stallions
  - Coagulation abnormalities
    - Genetic platelet function disorders
    - Coagulation factor disorders (von Willibrand disease)
- Neoplastic conditions
  - Paranasal sinus and skull neoplasia
  - Urogenital (renal, ureteral, bladder, uterine, perineal) neoplasia
  - Abdominal organ neoplasia
- Inflammatory
  - Infectious
    - Guttural pouch mycosis (Aspergillus spp.)
    - Pneumonia
    - Pleuritis
    - Paranasal sinus infection
    - Pyelonephritis
    - Cystitis
    - Urolithiasis
    - Abdominal abscess (Streptococcus equi)
  - Parasitic
    - Verminous arteritis
    - Gastrointestinal and ectoparasites
  - Noninfectious
    - Gastrointestinal ulceration
    - Hepatic failure (lack of coagulation factors)
    - Envenomation
    - Systemic inflammatory response syndrome
- Immune disorder: Granulomatous enteritis
- Trauma
  - Exercise-induced pulmonary hemorrhage
  - Head trauma, skull fracture
  - Ventral straight muscle (longus capitus and rectus capitis ventralis muscle) rupture: Poll trauma

- Thoracic trauma
- Rib fracture
- Abdominal trauma
  - Splenic rupture
  - Hepatic fracture
  - Mesenteric vessel rupture
- Iatrogenic trauma
  - Surgery
  - Nasogastric intubation
  - Percutaneous biopsy
- Wounds
- Foreign bodies
- Toxicity
  - NSAID (right dorsal colitis)
  - Rodenticides
  - Heparin overdose
  - High-dose colloid administration (hetastarch or dextran)

INITIAL DATABASE

- Physical examination: Determine the site or sites of hemorrhage.
- Packed cell volume (PCV) and total protein (may not reflect acute blood loss of <8 hours)
- Platelet count
- Arterial blood pressure (effective in identifying acute hemorrhage)
- Blood gas (pH, venous oxygen, base deficit)
- Central venous pressure

ADVANCED OR CONFIRMATORY TESTING

- Coagulation testing
  - Activated clotting time
  - Activated partial thromboplastin time
  - Prothrombin time
  - Thrombin clotting time
  - Protein C
  - D-dimers and fibrinogen
  - Thromboelastography

TREATMENT

THERAPEUTIC GOAL(S)

- Stop active bleeding
- Provide adequate tissue perfusion
- Increase the oxygen-carrying capacity of the blood

ACUTE GENERAL TREATMENT

- Hemostasis
  - Apply pressure to vessels (bandaging).
  - Seal vessels with cautery, ligation, or thrombin sealants.
  - Antifibrinolytic medications may assist inaccessible bleeding.
    - Aminocaproic acid: 3.5 mg/kg/min IV over 15 minutes; then continuous rate infusion of 0.25 mg/kg/min for up to 6 hours
    - Formalin (10%): 37 mL diluted to 1 L in 0.9% saline; bolus slowly
- Fluid resuscitation
  - Controlled hemorrhage: Shock dose fluid administration (see "Shock Dose Fluid Administration" in Section II)
    - Hypertonic saline, crystalloids, and colloids early
    - The goals of resuscitation is normalization of vital parameters to ensure microcirculation.
      - pH = 7.4
      - Lactate <2 mmol/L
      - Venous oxygen tension near 30 mm Hg
      - Urine production
      - Normal mentation
  - Uncontrolled hemorrhage: Hypotensive resuscitation
    - Administer fluid therapy (crystalloids only) to maintain a mean arterial pressure of 60 mm Hg.
      - Provides adequate tissue perfusion without disrupting the fibrin seal, promoting reactive vasoconstriction, or diluting clotting factors.
      - The goal of hypotensive resuscitation is to ensure minimal perfusion of the microcirculation.
        - pH >7.25
        - Lactate <4 mmol/L
        - Urine production
        - Normal mentation
- Normalization of hemostatic components
  - Indications for transfusion are lactate concentrations above 4 mmol/L, PCV below 12%, loss of 30% of the blood volume or uncontrolled hemorrhage, and persistent hypotension despite fluid resuscitation.
  - Goals of hemostatic transfusions are a PCV above 15% and platelets above 50,000/μL.
    - Plasma administration provides coagulation factors, albumin, and platelets.
    - Whole blood provides hemoglobin, coagulation factors, albumin, and platelets.
    - 2.2 mL/kg of whole blood increases PCV by approximately 1%.
    - Packed red blood cells provide hemoglobin only (for normotensive patients).

CHRONIC TREATMENT

Depends on the cause of hemorrhage

POSSIBLE COMPLICATIONS

Administration of colloids (hetastarch, dextrans) at high doses may inhibit coagulation through interference with von Willebrand factor and factor 8, as well as through further dilution of clotting factors.

RECOMMENDED MONITORING

- Depends on the cause of hemorrhage
- Monitor parameters of perfusion for severe hemorrhage (lactate, blood pressure, urination, mentation, pH).
- Monitor PCV.
- Monitor platelet count and coagulation profile.

PROGNOSIS AND OUTCOME

Related to the ability to stop acute hemorrhage, the horse's response to fluid resuscitation, and the ability to provide definitive therapy for the cause of bleeding

PEARLS & CONSIDERATIONS

Hypovolemic shock may not alter physical examination findings if it is compensated, so additional tests (lactate, pH, venous oxygen saturation) may be required to identify tissue oxygen debt.

SUGGESTED READING

Magdesian KG: Acute blood loss. *Compend Contin Ed Vet Equine* 3(5):80–90, 2008.

Ross J, Dallap BL, Dolente BA, et al: Pharmacokinetics and pharmacodynamics of epsilon-aminocaproic acid in horses. *Am J Vet Res* 68(9):1016–1021, 2007.

Sellon DC, Wise LN: Disorders of the hematopoietic system. In Reed SM, Bayly WM, Sellon DC, editors: *Equine internal medicine*, ed 3, St Louis, 2008, Saunders Elsevier, pp 730–776.

Taylor EL, Sellon DC, Wardrop KJ, et al: Effects of intravenous administration of formaldehyde on platelet and coagulation variables in healthy horses. *Am J Vet Res* 61(10):1191–1194, 2000.

AUTHOR: AMELIA MUNSTERMAN

EDITORS: R. REID HANSON and **AMELIA MUNSTERMAN**

Hemorrhage, Postpartum

BASIC INFORMATION

DEFINITION

- Rupture of the middle uterine (most common), utero-ovarian, external iliac, vaginal, or adrenal artery near parturition
- Hemorrhage may be contained within the broad ligament or uterine wall, forming a hematoma, or may occur into the peritoneal cavity or uterine lumen.

SYNONYM(S)

Broad ligament hematoma, rupture of the uterine artery

EPIDEMIOLOGY

SPECIES, AGE, SEX

- Intact mares during the immediate postpartum period; may also occur prepartum
- More common in multiparous mares older than 10 years of age
- Postpartum hemorrhage affects 2% to 3% of broodmares and accounts for 40% of deaths in peripartum mares.

RISK FACTORS

- Aging
- Multiple pregnancies
- Uterine prolapse
- Uterine torsion

CLINICAL PRESENTATION

HISTORY, CHIEF COMPLAINT

- History of recent parturition
- Abdominal pain
- Cardiovascular shock
- Hemorrhagic vulvar discharge
- Weakness, depression
- Cold sweat
- Ataxia

PHYSICAL EXAM FINDINGS

- Tachycardia
- Tachypnea
- Sweating
- Muscle fasciculation
- Pale mucous membranes. Mucous membrane color may be pink during the acute phase.
- Delayed capillary refill time
- Weak pulse

ETIOLOGY AND PATHOPHYSIOLOGY

- Aged-related degenerative changes in the elastic and collagen fibers of the arterial walls may predispose to rupture, especially during stretching of the broad ligament and arteries during late gestation.
- Low serum copper concentrations in aged mares may result in vessel fragility.
- Displacement of the uterus to the left by the cecum may increase tension on the right vessels and account for the predisposition for right-side ruptures.
- Uterine prolapse or torsion may result in rupture of the middle uterine artery.
- Bleeding may occur into the peritoneal cavity or uterine lumen, often resulting in exsanguination. Hemorrhage may also dissect into the broad ligament or between the myometrium and perimetrium, resulting in hematoma without exsanguination, unless the broad ligament or perimetrium tear.
- Necrosis, thrombosis, and rupture of the external iliac artery may result from damage to the intima and media by parasites.

DIAGNOSIS

DIFFERENTIAL DIAGNOSIS

- Postpartum abdominal pain or depression
  - Toxic metritis
  - Uterine rupture
  - Intussusception of the uterine horn
  - Intestinal or mesenteric rupture or trauma
  - Colon torsion
  - Ileus
  - Diaphragmatic rupture
  - Bladder rupture
- Postpartum vulvar discharge
  - Soft tissue trauma of the birth canal
  - Normal lochia
  - Metritis

INITIAL DATABASE

- Complete blood count (CBC): Anemia and hypoproteinemia, hyperfibrinogenemia or hypofibrinogenemia. Clinicopathologic changes may not be present during the acute phase because of vascular compensation, splenic contraction, and relative loss of red blood cells and plasma.
- Transrectal palpation: Enlarged uterus or large, firm swelling within the broad ligament. Transrectal palpation may elicit pain.
- Vaginal speculum examination: Accumulation of blood in the cranial vagina
- Transrectal ultrasonography: Hematoma within the broad ligament or uterine wall
- Transabdominal ultrasonography: Swirling hyperechoic particles within the hypoechoic fluid consistent with hemoperitoneum

ADVANCED OR CONFIRMATORY TESTING

Abdominocentesis: Pink or red peritoneal fluid, increased total protein concentration and red blood cell count, phagocytized red blood cells consistent with hemoperitoneum

TREATMENT

THERAPEUTIC GOAL(S)

- Restore cardiovascular volume.
- Aid in hemostasis.
- Provide analgesia and sedation.
- Provide antimicrobial prophylaxis.

ACUTE GENERAL TREATMENT

- Restoration of cardiovascular volume
  - Resuscitation with hypertonic saline (7.5% NaCl solution): 2 to 4 mL/kg IV followed by 10 to 20 L of lactated Ringer's solution (LRS) over 2 to 4 hours.
  - Whole-blood transfusion from a cross-matched blood donor: 6 to 8 L at 30 mL/kg/h if estimated loss is 25% of blood volume or there is rapid uncontrollable hemorrhage
- Improvement of oxygen perfusion
- Intranasal oxygen insufflation: 5 to 10 L/min
- Pentoxifylline: 7.5 mg/kg PO q12h
- Hemostasis
  - Aminocaproic acid: Loading dose of 20 g diluted in 1 L of LRS IV given over 20 min followed by 10 g q12h for 36 to 48 hours
  - 10% formalin: 30 mL diluted in 1 L of isotonic fluids, IV q12–24h. The effect of formalin on coagulation parameters and bleeding times in horses is controversial.
  - Yunnan baiyao: 8 mg/kg PO q4h for 3 to 4 days
- Analgesia and sedation
  - Flunixin meglumine: 1.1 mg/kg q12h IV
  - Butorphanol tartrate: 0.02 to 0.04 mg/kg IV
  - Xylazine: 0.5 to 1.1 mg/kg IV q6–12h
  - Detomidine: 0.01 to 0.02 mg/kg IV or IM q6–12h
- Antimicrobial prophylaxis
  - Potassium penicillin: 22,000 IU/kg IV q6h and gentamicin 6.6 mg/kg IV q24h
  - Ceftiofur: 2.2 mg/kg IV q12h
  - Trimethoprim/sulfamethoxazole: 15 to 30 mg/kg PO q12h
- Maintain the mare in a dark, quiet environment to prevent increases in

blood pressure and disruption of the blood clot.

- Protect the foal from the mare's colic episodes. Do not separate the mare and foal to prevent agitation and further bleeding.

CHRONIC TREATMENT

Maintain strict stall confinement for 3 to 4 weeks.

POSSIBLE COMPLICATIONS

- Death
- Abscessation
- Peritonitis
- Endotoxemia secondary to abscessation
- Cardiac arrhythmias

RECOMMENDED MONITORING

- Monitor the CBC.
- Monitor hematoma for abscessation.
- Monitor for signs of colic or ileus that may result from release of inflammatory mediators that alter gastrointestinal activity or intestinal blood flow. Monitor fecal output and consistency and administer mineral oil (0.5–1 gallon) or bran mash if necessary.

PROGNOSIS AND OUTCOME

- Prognosis for survival is good for hemorrhage contained within the broad ligament because hemorrhage is usually self-limited, resulting in formation of a hematoma. Bleeding into the peritoneal cavity or uterine lumen carries a poor prognosis, and hemorrhage is often fatal.
- Reported survival rate is 84% with early diagnosis and aggressive medical therapy.
- A total of 49% of mares were reported to deliver one foal in subsequent pregnancies without further hemorrhage.

PEARLS & CONSIDERATIONS

COMMENTS

Blood volume replacement and therapeutic or diagnostic procedures may elevate blood pressure and may result in further bleeding.

CLIENT EDUCATION

- Postpartum hemorrhage may be life threatening.
- The veterinarian must be contacted immediately if a postpartum mare develops colic, weakness, or depression.

SUGGESTED READING

Arnold CE, Payne M, Thompson JA, et al: Periparturient hemorrhage in mares: 73 cases (1998–2005). *J Am Vet Med Assoc* 232:1345–1351, 2008.

Blanchard TL, MacPherson ML: Postparturient abnormalities. In Samper JC, Pycock JF, McKinnon, editors: *Current therapy in equine reproduction*, St Louis, 2007, Saunders Elsevier, pp 465–475.

AUTHOR: **MARIA S. FERRER**

EDITOR: **JUAN C. SAMPER**

Hemospermia

BASIC INFORMATION

DEFINITION

- The presence of blood (erythrocytes) in the ejaculate, either macroscopic (as evident on gross examination of red-tinged semen) or microscopic (occult hemospermia)
- Causes infertility by an unknown mechanism of the red blood cells on semen

SYNONYM(S)

Hematospermia

EPIDEMIOLOGY

SPECIES, AGE, SEX Occurs in stallions of any breed or age
RISK FACTORS Stallions that are bred frequently may be at increased risk.
ASSOCIATED CONDITIONS AND DISORDERS
- Urethritis
- Seminal vesiculitis
- Other diseases of the urogenital tract
- Hematuria

CLINICAL PRESENTATION

HISTORY, CHIEF COMPLAINT

- Red-tinged semen (if collected), or red fluid discharge from the mare's vulva or stallion's prepuce (if bred by natural cover)
- Bloody discharge from the penis after breeding (Figure 1)
- Blood on the collection dummy or phantom (Figure 2)
- Potentially slow or painful ejaculation when the stallion is bred or collected
- Potential observation of penile or preputial lesions

PHYSICAL EXAM FINDINGS

- Blood traces on the hind legs
- Presence of erythrocytes in semen (may not be grossly discolored if microscopic hemospermia is present [Figure 3])
- Stallions are usually clinically healthy with no systemic signs of illness.

ETIOLOGY AND PATHOPHYSIOLOGY

- Blood from lesions on the surface of the penis: Habronemiasis and squamous cell carcinoma are the most common.
- Blood from an inflammatory process in the urethra or seminal vesicles
- A urethral defect (urethral rent) results in hemospermia because of the increase in pressure in the corpus spongiosum penis during erection and ejaculation.

DIAGNOSIS

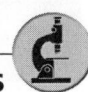

DIFFERENTIAL DIAGNOSIS

- Bacterial or viral urethritis: Ulcerated urethral epithelium may slough
- Lesions of the glans penis or urethral process
  - Lacerations
    - Trauma
    - From the mare's tail hairs during breeding
  - Squamous cell carcinoma or other neoplasms
  - Cutaneous habronemiasis
- Improperly used stallion rings
- Urethral defects or rents
- Inflammation or infection of accessory sex glands (especially the seminal vesicles)

INITIAL DATABASE

- Complete examination of the stallion's penis should be performed.
- Inspect the glans, urethral process, and prepuce for lacerations or lesions
- Examination of the urethra and accessory sex glands via videoendoscopy (1-m endoscope)
  - Commonly, a linear urethral rent 5 to 10 mm long is present caudodorsally on the convex surface

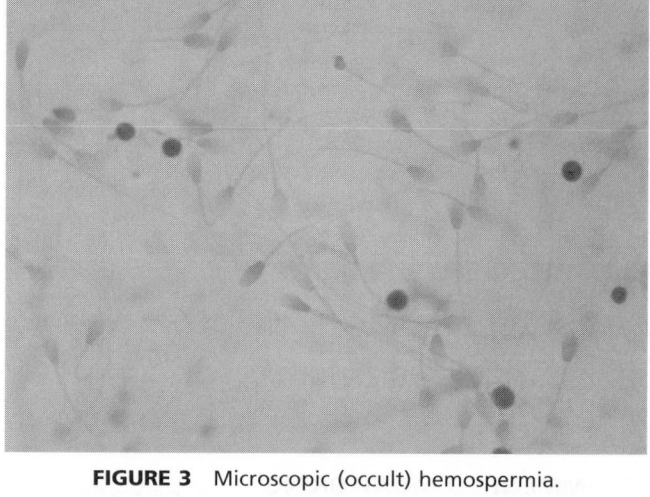

FIGURE 1 Bloody discharge from the urethral process of a stallion after semen collection.

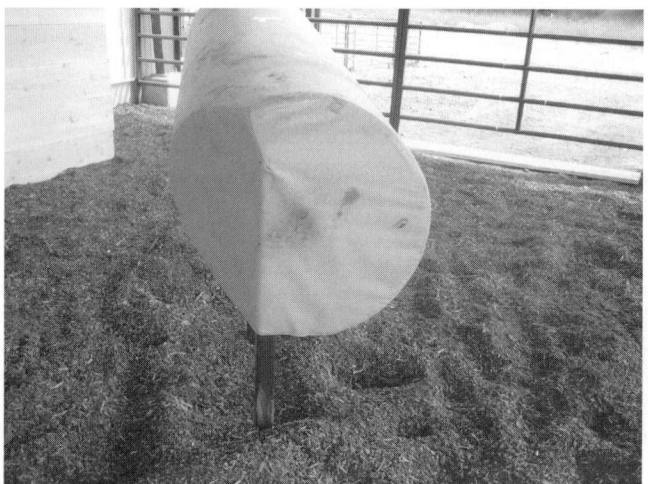

FIGURE 2 Bloody discharge on the collection dummy or phantom after collection.

FIGURE 3 Microscopic (occult) hemospermia.

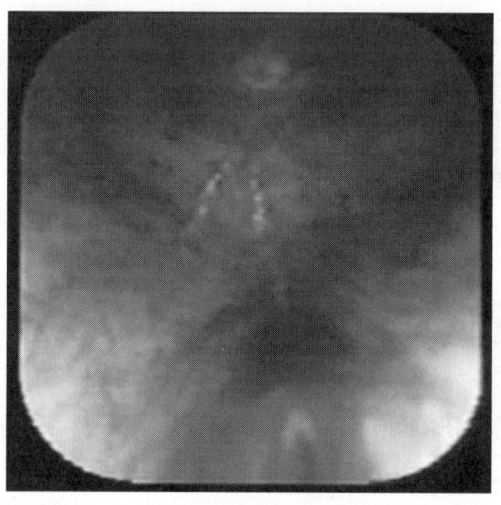

FIGURE 4 Endoscopic view of a urethral rent after collection.

of the urethra at the level of the ischial arch, which communicates with the corpus spongiosum penis (Figure 4).

○ Examination after collection may demonstrate bleeding from the rent.
  ■ Double-contrast radiography of the penis may demonstrate urethral strictures or luminal defects.
  ■ Cytologic samples obtained from the urethra after collection may demonstrate viral inclusion bodies or neoplastic cells.

TREATMENT

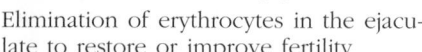

THERAPEUTIC GOAL(S)

Elimination of erythrocytes in the ejaculate to restore or improve fertility

ACUTE/CHRONIC GENERAL TREATMENT

• Sexual rest (required with all treatments)

• Systemic antiinflammatory medications
• Traumatic lesions may be treated by washing the penis and applying appropriate topical medications or ointments.
• Bacterial urethritis may be treated with antimicrobial therapy based on culture and sensitivity results of collected samples.
• If blood contamination is minimal, semen may be collected in extender and washed before use.
• Formalin IV has been used as a last resort, but bleeding recurred when treatment was stopped.
• Surgical treatment by temporary subischial urethrotomy
  ○ Relieves the buildup of pressure in the corpus spongiosum penis
  ○ ± Topical application of antiinflammatories or steroids into the urethrotomy site

○ Return to sexual function after treatment of a urethral rent with a buccal mucosal urethroplasty via subischial urethrotomy has been reported recently.

POSSIBLE COMPLICATIONS

• From urethrotomy: Postoperative hemorrhage or infection (incisional infection, cystitis, or orchitis); urethral fistula, diverticulum, or stricture formation; dysuria
• Loss of libido
• Ejaculatory disorders

RECOMMENDED MONITORING

• Examination via videoendoscopy is suggested before return to sexual function to evaluate the urethral mucosa integrity.
• Collection and evaluation of semen for residual hemospermia is recommended before breeding.

PROGNOSIS AND OUTCOME

- Variable because of low numbers of stallions treated and evaluated by these methods
- Subischial urethrotomy has returned some stallions to breeding but has not shown to be reliably effective in treating urethral rents.

- Penile lacerations and cutaneous habronemiasis carry better prognoses for return to sexual function.

SUGGESTED READING

Hackett ES, Bruemmer J, Hendrickson DA, McCue PM: Buccal mucosal urethroplasty for treatment of recurrent hemospermia in a stallion. *J Am Vet Med Assoc* 235(10):1212–1215, 2009.

Tibary A, Rodriguez J, Samper JC: Microbiology and diseases of semen. In Samper JC, editor: *Equine breeding management and artificial insemination*, St Louis, 2009, Elsevier, pp 99–112.

AUTHORS: **LISA K. PEARSON, JACOBO S. RODRIGUEZ**, and **AHMED TIBARY**

EDITOR: **JUAN C. SAMPER**

Hendra Virus

BASIC INFORMATION

DEFINITION

Exotic pneumotropic and neurotropic virus resulting in severe respiratory and neurologic signs and often death of infected horses

SYNONYM(S)

- Equine Morbillivirus
- Equine acute respiratory syndrome

EPIDEMIOLOGY

RISK FACTORS Mainly relate to bat exposure, including outdoor housing and feeding under trees and bats roosting in barns.

CONTAGION AND ZOONOSIS

- *Pteropus* fruit bats are natural hosts and are not affected by clinical disease.
- Transmission to horses is rare; the virus is not highly contagious between horses.
- Exposure to bat saliva, urine, aborted fetuses, and reproductive fluids are thought to result in transmission from bat to horse, possibly through contaminated food or water.
- Aerosol transmission to and between horses is not a primary method of spread; rather, the virus is possibly spread through human fomites.
- Disease in humans is rare, but Hendra virus is zoonotic, resulting in frequently fatal infection in humans exposed to infected equine tissues or bodily fluids.

GEOGRAPHY AND SEASONALITY All known outbreaks have occurred in Australia.

CLINICAL PRESENTATION

PHYSICAL EXAM FINDINGS

- High fever
- Tachypnea and tachycardia
- Respiratory distress with blood-tinged, foamy nasal and oral discharge
- Neurologic signs, including head pressing, ataxia, and tonic spasms of the neck and hind limb muscles

- Collapse
- Death within 36 hours in horses that fail to survive
- Incubation period is 6 to 10 days

ETIOLOGY AND PATHOPHYSIOLOGY

- Closely related to *Nipah* virus from Malaysia, only two members of the genus Henipavirus
- Enveloped, single-stranded RNA virus
- Pneumotropic and probably neurotropic
- Little is known about portal of entry, distribution and persistence of virus in body, and routes of excretion.
- The virus attacks vascular endothelial cells, resulting in pulmonary edema.
- The pathogenesis in neurologic tissues is likely similar.

DIAGNOSIS

DIFFERENTIAL DIAGNOSIS

- Acute African horse sickness
- Virulent equine influenza

INITIAL DATABASE

- Not many diagnostic tests are performed in most cases because efforts are focused on triage care.
- Diagnosis is generally made on necropsy.

ADVANCED OR CONFIRMATORY TESTING

- Characteristic immunofluorescence and immunoperoxidase staining of tissues histopathologically
- Virus isolation can be performed antemortem with blood, nasal swabs, urine, or tissues and can be more effectively isolated postmortem from the lung, liver, spleen, or brain.
- Polymerase chain reaction, electron microscopy, and immunohistochemistry can be used as well to detect organisms.
- Serum neutralization, enzyme-linked immunosorbent assay, and indirect fluorescent antibody tests can be used for serology.

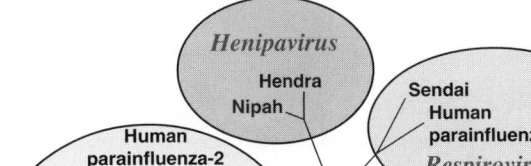

FIGURE 1 Phylogenic relation of Hendra virus to other members of the family Paramyxoviridae, based on analyses of predicted amino acid sequences of virus matrix proteins. (Courtesy Linfa Wang, CSIRO Livestock Industries' Animal Health Laboratory. From Sellon DC, Long MT: *Equine infectious diseases.* St Louis, 2007, Saunders Elsevier.)

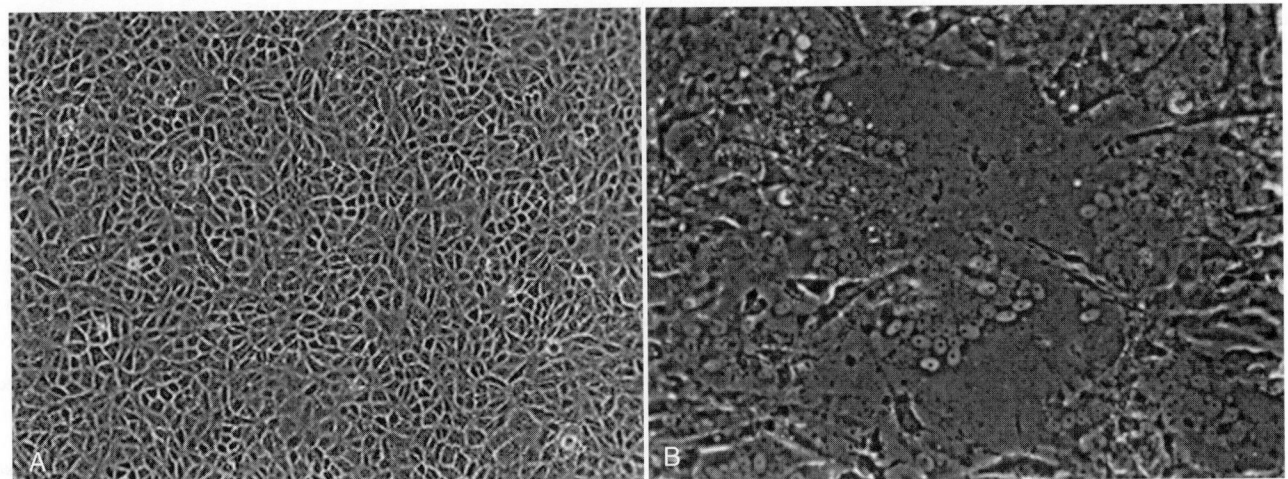

FIGURE 2 **A,** Normal Vero monolayer cell culture. **B,** Vero monolayer cell culture 24 hours after infection with Hendra virus. Note syncytium. (Courtesy Gary Crameric, CSIRO Livestock Industries' Australian Animal Health Laboratory. From Sellon DC, Long MT: *Equine infectious diseases.* St Louis, 2007, Saunders Elsevier.)

TREATMENT

THERAPEUTIC GOAL(S)

None. Treatment is not pursued after a diagnosis of Hendra virus infection is made because of the serious zoonotic potential.

ACUTE GENERAL TREATMENT

- No specific therapy
- Before diagnosis and subsequent euthanasia, horses are usually treated with supportive care.

PROGNOSIS AND OUTCOME

- There is a 70% fatality rate in reported outbreaks because of the virus itself.

- There is a 100% death rate because of euthanasia of surviving horses.

PEARLS & CONSIDERATIONS

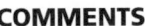

COMMENTS

- Because of the severity of disease and potential for zoonotic transmission, horses diagnosed with Hendra virus are euthanized if they do not die acutely from disease.
- It is unknown whether the virus would persist in recovered animals, resulting in a carrier state.
- Hendra virus is considered a Biocontainment Level 4 agent.

PREVENTION

- No vaccine is available.
- Prevent exposure to bats.

- Early diagnosis of potential cases and containment via euthanasia are recommended.
- Serologic surveillance of potentially exposed horses is also recommended.

SUGGESTED READING

The Center for Food Security and Public Health, Iowa State University: Hendra virus infection. Available at http://www.cfsph.iastate.edu/Factsheets/pdfs/hendra.pdf.

Eaton BT, Broder CC, Wang LF: Hendra and Nipah viruses: pathogenesis and therapeutics. *Curr Mol Med* 5:805–816, 2005.

Studdert MJ: Miscellaneous viral respiratory diseases. In Sellon DC, Long MT, edited: *Equine infectious diseases,* St Louis, 2007, Saunders Elsevier, pp 174–177.

AUTHOR: **SIDDRA HINES**

EDITORS: **MAUREEN LONG** and **DEBRA C. SELLON**

Hepatic Abscesses

BASIC INFORMATION

DEFINITION

Hepatic abscesses are chronic focal to multifocal areas of infection that are relatively uncommon in horses. They may develop as a sequela to bacterial invasion of the liver.

SYNONYM(S)

Liver abscess

EPIDEMIOLOGY
ASSOCIATED CONDITIONS AND DISORDERS

- Bacterial hepatitis
- Cholangitis
- Cholangiohepatitis

CLINICAL PRESENTATION
HISTORY, CHIEF COMPLAINT

- Signs of hepatic abscessation are typically vague and not indicative of primary hepatic disease.
- Weight loss from reduced appetite is often present.

PHYSICAL EXAM FINDINGS

- Physical examination of horses with hepatic abscessation generally reveals signs of chronic infection, such as poor body condition, lethargy, fever, and dull haircoat.

ETIOLOGY AND PATHOPHYSIOLOGY

- In foals, hepatic abscessation may develop as a sequela to bacteremia or ascending infection through the umbilical vein secondary to omphalophlebitis.
- In mature horses, bacteremia and septicemia are uncommon, so hepatic

abscesses are more like to develop secondary to ascending infection of the biliary tract or infection that originates in the intestinal tract or mesenteric lymph nodes and is carried to the liver via the portal blood.

DIAGNOSIS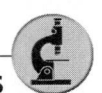

DIFFERENTIAL DIAGNOSIS

- Hepatic abscessation must be differentiated from any chronic infectious disease or chronic illness.
- Other causes of chronic hepatic disease that may have a similar clinical presentation include:
  - Hepatic neoplasia
  - Cholangitis or cholangiohepatitis
  - Cholelithiasis
  - Chronic active hepatitis
  - Chronic megalocytic hepatopathy

INITIAL DATABASE

- Complete blood count: Anemia of chronic disease, mature neutrophilia
- Fibrinogen concentration: Increased
- Serum total protein concentration: Increased from hyperglobulinemia
- Liver enzyme activities (ie, sorbitol dehydrogenase, gamma glutamyltransferase): Typically within normal limits

unless extensive hepatic abscessation is present
- Serum bile acid concentration: Typically within normal limits unless extensive hepatic abscessation is present

ADVANCED OR CONFIRMATORY TESTING

- Transabdominal ultrasonography of the liver may reveal focal changes in echogenicity in areas of abscessation.
- Ultrasound-guided aspiration of hepatic abscesses may reveal suppurative or septic purulent inflammation.

TREATMENT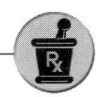

THERAPEUTIC GOAL

The primary goal of treatment is to eliminate the bacterial agent responsible for inciting the hepatic abscess.

ACUTE GENERAL TREATMENT

- Long-term antimicrobial therapy is warranted.
- When possible, antimicrobial therapy should be guided by culture results obtained from percutaneous aspiration or hepatic biopsy.

POSSIBLE COMPLICATIONS

Hepatic abscesses could rupture spontaneously or during attempts to aspirate or biopsy, causing septic peritonitis.

RECOMMENDED MONITORING

Antimicrobial therapy should be continued until resolution of clinical signs and laboratory indications of infection.

PROGNOSIS AND OUTCOME

- The prognosis is variable and depends on the duration and degree of abscessation.
- Extensive or widespread abscessation warrants a poor to guarded prognosis.

PEARLS & CONSIDERATIONS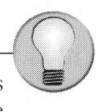

Common abdominal abscess isolates in horses include *Streptococcus equi* subsp. *equi, Streptococcus equi* subsp. *zooepidemicus,* and *Corynebacterium pseudotuberculosis.*

AUTHOR & EDITOR: **MICHELLE HENRY BARTON**

Hepatic Amyloidosis

BASIC INFORMATION

DEFINITION

A rare disorder of protein folding in which normally soluble proteins are deposited as insoluble fibrils that progressively disrupt tissue structure and impair function

EPIDEMIOLOGY

SPECIES, AGE, SEX Affected animals tend to be mature, although some may be relatively young (ie, 3–4 years of age).

ASSOCIATED CONDITIONS AND DISORDERS

- The condition may develop either locally or systemically; the liver is commonly affected in horses with systemic amyloidosis.
- Hepatic amyloidosis occurs after repeated or prolonged inflammatory stimulation and has been most frequently reported in horses used for hyperimmune serum production.
- Hepatic amyloidosis has also been described in horses with severe

strongylosis, peritonitis, chronic pleuropneumonia, tuberculosis, and neoplasia.

CLINICAL PRESENTATION

HISTORY, CHIEF COMPLAINT

- Hepatic amyloidosis typically occurs secondary to recurrent acute or chronic infections, inflammatory diseases, or neoplasia. History and primary complaints are therefore often related to the underlying disease.
- Chronic weight loss is common.
- Horses used for serum production reportedly show few, if any, clinical signs despite severe liver amyloid deposition.

PHYSICAL EXAM FINDINGS

- Clinical signs related to the underlying disease tend to dominate the clinical picture. Clinical signs directly related to amyloidosis depend on the organ distribution of the amyloid deposition and may be caused by either functional disturbances or mechanical alterations because of organ enlargement.

  - May be found dead after hepatic (or splenic) rupture without prior clinical signs
  - Poor body condition
  - Nephrotic syndrome, proteinuria, and hypoproteinemia are features of amyloidosis in many species and may occur in some horses used for serum production.

ETIOLOGY AND PATHOPHYSIOLOGY

- Amyloidosis may be systemic or localized and life threatening or merely an incidental finding. Extracellular amyloid deposition occurs as a result of protein misfolding, disrupting tissue structure and function.
- The amyloidoses are classified by the type of protein deposited; in human medicine, at least 23 different proteins have been implicated.
- AA- and AL-type amyloidosis are most commonly reported in equine cases.
- Both systemic and localized disease occur in horses.
- The protein in AA amyloidosis (secondary or reactive amyloidosis) is derived from serum amyloid A (SAA), which is synthesized by hepatocytes

in response to inflammatory stimulation.

- Systemic amyloidosis in horses usually involves AA amyloid.
- Sustained overproduction of SAA is required for development of AA amyloidosis; however, amyloidosis occurs only in a small proportion of patients with chronic inflammatory disorders.
- The protein in AL amyloidosis (primary or immunocytic amyloidosis) is derived from the variable region of immunoglobulin light chains.
- AL amyloidosis is the most common form in humans and is often associated with myeloma.
- AL amyloidosis in horses is usually localized and characterized by firm, circumscribed nodules in the nasal cavity and subcutis.

DIAGNOSIS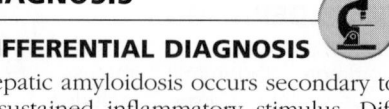

DIFFERENTIAL DIAGNOSIS

Hepatic amyloidosis occurs secondary to a sustained inflammatory stimulus. Differential diagnoses depend on the clinical signs of the underlying disease. Hepatic amyloidosis must be differentiated from other forms of chronic hepatic disease.

INITIAL DATABASE

- Complete blood count: Anemia, leukocytosis
- Fibrinogen concentration: Increased
- Gamma glutamyltransferase activity: Increased
- Serum bile acid concentration: May be normal to increased

- Serum total protein concentration: Increased because of hypergammaglobulinemia
- Albumin concentration: Decreased
- Urinalysis: Proteinuria if renal involvement
- Abdominocentesis
  - Hemoperitoneum in animals with a ruptured liver or spleen
  - Increased leukocyte counts and protein concentrations are expected when peritonitis is the underlying disease.
- Fecal egg counts: Strongylosis has been associated with hepatic amyloidosis.

ADVANCED OR CONFIRMATORY TESTING

- Liver biopsy
  - Amyloid appears as hyaline aggregates in hematoxylin and eosin–stained tissues.
  - Amyloid is detected as green birefringence of Congo Red–stained tissues viewed under polarized light.
- AA and AL amyloid can be differentiated by treatment of stained tissue sections with potassium permanganate.
  - Tissue containing AA amyloid loses its green birefringence.
  - Tissue containing AL amyloid continues to appear green.

TREATMENT

THERAPEUTIC GOAL(S)

Treatment should be directed toward the underlying disease and attempts made to

reduce inflammation. However, systemic amyloidosis with amyloid deposits in the viscera is usually fatal. Therapies are being developed for use in human medicine that prevent amyloid deposition or enhance its clearance.

ACUTE GENERAL TREATMENT

None is usually required because amyloidosis occurs secondary to chronic conditions. Animals presenting with signs of liver failure may require general supportive care until a diagnosis can be made.

PROGNOSIS AND OUTCOME

The prognosis is grave after significant amyloid accumulates within the viscera.

PEARLS & CONSIDERATIONS

Amyloidosis should be considered in animals with chronic inflammatory disease and signs of hepatic (or renal) dysfunction.

SUGGESTED READING

van Andel ACJ, Gruys E, Kroneman J, et al: Amyloid in the horse: a report of nine cases. *Equine Vet J* 20:277, 1998.

AUTHOR: **BRETT TENNENT-BROWN**

EDITOR: **MICHELLE HENRY BARTON**

Hepatic Encephalopathy

BASIC INFORMATION

DEFINITION

Hepatic encephalopathy occurs when there is significant loss of normal hepatic function to the degree that cerebral function is secondarily compromised. Hepatic encephalopathy is potentially reversible, depending on the underlying cause of liver disease.

SYNONYM(S)

Hepatoencephalopathy

EPIDEMIOLOGY

RISK FACTORS Hepatic encephalopathy may accompany either acute or chronic hepatic disease.

ASSOCIATED CONDITIONS AND DISORDERS Hepatic encephalopathy must be differentiated from other causes of acute or chronic cerebral disease.

CLINICAL PRESENTATION

HISTORY, CHIEF COMPLAINT

- Initial clinical signs may manifest only as subtle behavioral changes that are recognized by those familiar with the patient.
- Advancing clinical signs:
  - Depression and anorexia
  - Head pressing
  - Aimless circling or wandering
  - Ataxia
  - Persistent yawning
  - Excessive somnolence and lack of responsiveness (eg, standing for

hours with food in the mouth but not chewing)
  - Periods of aggressiveness or violent behavior (eg, excessive pawing, biting), interspersed with periods of stupor
  - Although atypical of hepatic encephalopathy, seizures may occur in the late stages.

PHYSICAL EXAM FINDINGS

- Other signs of hepatic disease may be present, including icterus, hepatic photosensitization, weight loss, and coagulopathy.
- A complete neurologic examination should be performed. Cranial nerve function is typically intact, although bilateral laryngeal paralysis may occur. In addition to the behavioral changes

listed above, ataxia and central blindness (lack of a menace response with normal pupillary light reflexes) may be present.

ETIOLOGY AND PATHOPHYSIOLOGY

The cause of hepatic encephalopathy is complex, incompletely understood, and likely multifactorial. Many mechanisms of altered cerebral function during hepatic insufficiency have been proposed, including:

- Acute astrocyte swelling, cytotoxic cerebral edema, and intracranial hypertension
- Gastrointestinal (GI)-derived neurotoxins that are incompletely cleared by the failing liver (eg, increased blood ammonia, mercaptans, short chain fatty acids, and phenol concentrations)
- Augmented activity of cerebral inhibitory neurotransmitter systems such as γ-aminobutyric acid, serotonin, and benzodiazepine (eg, glutamate) with concurrent depression of excitatory pathways
- Increased inflammatory cytokine expression and neurosteroid synthesis
- False neuroinhibitory transmitter accumulation (eg, phenylethanolamine, serotonin, octopamine) in the brain as a consequence to an increased ratio of aromatic amino acid (phenylalanine, tyrosine, tryptophan) to branch chain (valine, leucine, isoleucine) amino acids in the blood
- Impaired central nervous system metabolism secondary to energy depletion

DIAGNOSIS

DIFFERENTIAL DIAGNOSIS

Hepatic encephalopathy must be differentiated from other causes of acute and chronic cerebral disease or altered behavior, including:

- Head trauma
- Viral encephalopathies
- Leukoencephalomalacia
- Brain abscess or neoplasia
- Equine protozoal myeloencephalitis
- Parasitic larval migrans
- Fluphenazine administration
- Heavy metal toxicosis
- Hypocalcemia
- Uremic encephalopathy

INITIAL DATABASE

The diagnosis of hepatic encephalopathy is based on the presence of clinical signs of cerebral dysfunction in conjunction with laboratory diagnostic evidence of hepatic insufficiency.

- Serum bile acid concentration: Increased
- Liver-specific enzymes (gamma glutamyltransferase, sorbitol dehydro-

genase): Generally increased, but may be normal with end-stage fibrotic diseases of the liver
- Blood urea nitrogen (BUN) concentration: Decreased
- Serum total protein: Normal to increased in chronic hepatic disease caused by hyperglobulinemia
- Albumin: Normal to decreased
- Ammonia: Increased
- Clotting profile: Prothrombin time, activated partial thromboplastin time may be normal to increased

ADVANCED OR CONFIRMATORY TESTING

- Hepatic clearance of pharmaceuticals is prolonged
- Branched chain amino acid to aromatic amino acid ratio in the blood: Decreased
- Cerebrospinal fluid analysis: Normal
- Hepatic ultrasonography or liver biopsy: See Diagnostic Imaging of the Liver and Liver Biopsy in Section II).
- At necropsy, patients with hepatic encephalopathy may have increased numbers and size of astrocytes in the gray matter of the cerebrum (ie, Alzheimer type II changes).

TREATMENT

THERAPEUTIC GOAL(S)

The general therapeutic goals of hepatic encephalopathy are to stabilize the underlying liver disease when possible and to reestablish normal blood and brain concentrations of substances that alter neurofunction.

ACUTE GENERAL TREATMENT

- When sedation is necessary to control behavior, small doses of xylazine and detomidine should be used.
- Acute severe hepatic encephalopathy is often accompanied by cerebral edema; thus, the following treatments have been recommended:
  - Hypertonic saline
  - Mannitol: 0.5 to 1 g/kg body weight given slowly over 30 minutes
  - Vitamin E: 25 IU/kg/d
  - Dimethyl sulfoxide: 1 g/kg IV q2h diluted in fluids to 10%
- Dehydration and fluid needs may need to be addressed.
  - Even in normoglycemic patients, a continuous rate infusion of 5% dextrose (2 mL/kg/hr) can be beneficial, and if continued for more than 24 hours, 2.5% to 5% dextrose in half-strength saline or lactated Ringer's solution with supplemental potassium should be considered.
  - 0.9% saline may help enhance urinary clearance of ammonia.

- Bicarbonate replacement in acidotic patients should be given with caution because it may increase blood levels of ammonia.
- Treatments to decrease GI-derived neurotoxins, such as ammonia, include:
  - PO administration of mineral oil
  - Oral administration of antimicrobials, including neomycin (10–100 mg/kg PO q6h) and metronidazole (10–15 mg/kg PO q12h)
  - Lactulose: 333 mg/kg PO q8h
  - Administration of probiotics containing Lactobacillus acidophilus
- Antiinflammatory therapy to control cytokine production may be beneficial and could include the use of flunixin meglumine, pentoxifylline, and dimethyl sulfoxide.
- Benzodiazepine antagonists (flumazenil) and dopamine agonists (bromocriptine) have been used in human patients with hepatic encephalopathy.

CHRONIC TREATMENT

- Drugs that have been shown to reduce hepatic fibrosis in human patients include pentoxifylline, steroids, colchicine, and cyclosporine. Pentoxifylline can be safely given to horses at 8 to 16 mg/kg PO q8–24h, although its efficacy in controlling hepatic fibrosis in this species is unknown.
- Dietary management to reduce ammonia formation is targeted by feeding rations high in carbohydrate and low in protein but rich with branched chain amino acids. Examples include beet pulp, sweet feeds, sorghum, bran, milo, oats, or grass hay. Branched chain amino acids supplements are available from several commercial sources.

DRUG INTERACTIONS

- Diazepam is contraindicated because it may enhance the neuroinhibitory response.

POSSIBLE COMPLICATIONS

- Seizures or uncontrolled maniacal behavior
- Coma
- Altered blood levels of drugs that rely on hepatic metabolism

RECOMMENDED MONITORING

- Easy to monitor tests of hepatic function include blood concentrations of ammonia, BUN, and serum bile acids.

PROGNOSIS AND OUTCOME

- Patients with severe hepatic fibrosis, especially bridging hepatic fibrosis, have a poor to grave prognosis.

PEARLS & CONSIDERATIONS

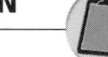

- The severity of hepatic encephalopathy correlates with the severity of hepatic insufficiency but does not correlate with

the reversibility of the underlying disease.

SUGGESTED READING

Ahboucha S, Butterworth R: The neurosteroid system: an emerging therapeutic target for hepatic encephalopathy. *Metab Brain Dis* 22:291, 2007.

Divers T: Therapy of liver failure. In Smith BP, editor: *Large animal internal medicine*, ed 4, St Louis, 2008, Mosby Elsevier, p 921.

King Han M, Hyzy R: Advances in critical care management of hepatic failure and insufficiency. *Crit Care Med* 34(suppl):S225, 2006.

Scarratt W, Warnick L: Effects of oral administration of lactulose in healthy horses. *J Equine Vet Sci* 18:405, 1998.

Tofteng F, Larsen F: Management of patients with fulminant hepatic failure and brain edema. *Metab Brain Dis* 19:207, 2004.

AUTHOR & EDITOR: **MICHELLE HENRY BARTON**

Hepatic Lipidosis and Hyperlipemia

BASIC INFORMATION

DEFINITION

- Hepatic lipidosis is a result of excess triglyceride deposition in the liver. The liver plays a critical role in lipid metabolism and is responsible for processing chylomicrons, volatile fatty acids, and free fatty acids (FFAs) when fat is mobilized from adipose tissue. When the rate of hepatic triglyceride formation exceeds the oxidation of fatty acids and release of very low-density lipoprotein (VLDL) into the peripheral circulation, hepatic lipidosis ensues.
- Hyperlipemia is characterized by visibly cloudy serum and serum triglyceride levels of 500 mg/dL or higher. Hyperlipidemia refers to serum triglyceride levels below 500 mg/dL. The serum remains clear, and it is not typically associated with fatty infiltration of the liver.

SYNONYMS

- Fatty liver disease
- Hyperlipemia syndrome

EPIDEMIOLOGY

GENETICS AND BREED PREDISPOSITION

- Ponies (especially Shetland and mare ponies), American Miniature horses, and donkeys are predisposed
- Occasionally seen in other breeds (Quarter Horses, Tennessee Walking Horses, Paso Finos) secondary to the development of a negative energy balance

RISK FACTORS

- Obesity
- Stress
- Pregnancy or hormonal imbalance
- Lactation
- History of weight loss or decreased caloric intake
- Negative energy balance

- An underlying illness of several days' duration
- Winter season or ingestion of poor-quality feed

GEOGRAPHY AND SEASONALITY

- Late gestation and early lactation during the winter months in conjunction with poor pasture availability in winter depending on geography
- No true geographic predilection

ASSOCIATED CONDITIONS AND DISORDERS

- Clinical signs of hepatic lipidosis can be indistinguishable from the clinical signs of liver disease or liver failure from other causes.
- Signs of the predisposing primary disease may overshadow other signs. The most commonly reported predisposing primary diseases include enterocolitis, endotoxemia, pituitary adenoma, parasitism, azotemia, and neonatal septicemia.

CLINICAL PRESENTATION

DISEASE FORMS/SUBTYPES

- Hyperlipidemia refers to an increased serum triglyceride concentration (typically <500 mg/dL) without the presence of lipemic (cloudy white) serum or liver disease. Hyperlipemia is characterized by cloudy serum and triglyceride concentrations of 500 mg/dL or higher. Prolonged hyperlipemia results in fatty infiltration of the liver and subsequent signs of liver disease.

HISTORY, CHIEF COMPLAINT

- Typically obese
- Recent history of stress or weight loss
- Commonly in late pregnancy or early lactation
- Owners typically report acute anorexia and depression.

PHYSICAL EXAM FINDINGS

- Combination of two or more of these signs is likely:
  - Icterus
  - Anorexia
  - Depression

  - Weakness
  - Mild colic
  - Diarrhea
  - Recumbency
  - Muscle weakness
  - Fever
  - Ataxia
  - Dependent edema
- Clinical signs of liver failure, such as hepatic encephalopathy, bleeding, and endotoxemia, may predominate in severe cases. Sudden death caused by hepatic rupture is reported rarely.

ETIOLOGY AND PATHOPHYSIOLOGY

- Negative energy balances that may occur during late gestation, early lactation, starvation, or secondary to another primary disease, may result in hyperlipemia caused by fatty acid mobilization.
- Glucose is made in the liver from fatty acids and amino acids and is stored as glycogen.
- When glycogen stores are depleted because of a negative energy balance, fatty acids are oxidized to provide energy.
- Hormone-sensitive lipase is activated, which converts adipose to FFAs, nonesterified fatty acids, and glycerol.
- Increased mobilization of FFAs results in FFA oxidation, increased triglyceride synthesis, and production of VLDLs (which contain triglycerides) for release into the peripheral circulation.
- The equine liver is efficient in synthesizing and exporting VLDLs into the peripheral circulation. Endothelial lipoprotein lipase is the enzyme responsible for removing VLDLs from the blood back into adipose tissue and is increased in horses with hyperlipemia.
- The overproduction of VLDLs by the liver is responsible for the hyperlipemia. Hepatic lipidosis results from fatty acid mobilization and triglyceride synthesis that exceeds the liver's rate of oxidation and VLDL secretion.

- Liver function is disrupted by excess triglyceride infiltration, and liver failure and hepatic rupture have been reported in severe cases.

DIAGNOSIS

DIFFERENTIAL DIAGNOSIS

Differential diagnoses include other causes of liver disease in horses and ponies
- Toxic hepatopathies
- Theiler's disease
- Cholangiohepatitis or cholelithiasis
- Chronic active hepatitis
- Pyrrolizidine alkaloid toxicosis
- Hepatic neoplasia
- Hepatic abscess

INITIAL DATABASE

- A complete blood count (CBC), serum chemistry profile with liver enzymes, triglyceride levels, and serum bile acid concentration are recommended for any obese pony, Miniature horse, or donkey with signs of depression, anorexia, icterus, and ataxia.
- Serum chemistry profile:
- CBC: May be normal or have abnormalities associated with underlying disease
- Serum chemistry profile
  - Blood glucose: Typically decreased but may be normal or increased
  - Gamma glutamyltransferase: Variably increased
  - Triglycerides: Above 500 mg/dL consistent with lipemia
  - Serum bilirubin: Variably increased
  - Serum bile acids: Increased if liver function is impaired
  - Metabolic acidosis is possible
  - Lipemia may falsely increase serum creatinine.
  - Blood ammonia: May be increased with liver failure
  - Albumin: May be decreased

ADVANCED OR CONFIRMATORY TESTING

- Diagnosis is confirmed by the presence of increased triglyceride levels and evidence of hepatic disease with increased liver enzymes and serum bile acids in addition to ultrasonography (see "Diagnostic Imaging of the Liver" in Section II) or histopathologic evidence of fatty infiltration of the liver.
- Liver biopsy with evidence of fatty infiltration confirms diagnosis.
- Bromsulphalein clearance may be prolonged.
- PO and IV glucose tolerance tests may reveal glucose intolerance caused by insulin insensitivity.

TREATMENT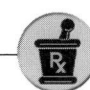

THERAPEUTIC GOALS

The goals of treatment include elimination of the negative energy balance and improving energy intake, treatment of liver disease or failure, treatment of concurrent disease, elimination of stress, inhibition of fat mobilization from adipose tissue, and increasing triglyceride uptake by peripheral tissues.

ACUTE GENERAL TREATMENT

- Supportive treatment should include a concentrate feed and high-quality pasture or hay, as well as treatment for liver failure (see the Treatment section in "Hepatic Encephalopathy" in this section).
- Every effort should be made to encourage voluntary enteral nutrition. Enteral nutrition can also be provided via nasogastric intubation of a feed slurry or an enteral diet such as Equine Critical Care Meals (MD's Choice, Inc., Louisville, TN).
- A continuous rate infusion (CRI) of 5% dextrose at a rate of 2 mL/kg/h should be administered to anorectic horses.
- Partial parenteral nutrition with 50% dextrose and 8.5% amino acids is recommended in horses in which enteral nutrition is not possible.
- Treat concurrent disease when appropriate.
- Consider early weaning of the foal if the mare is lactating to reduce energy demand.
- Provide supportive treatment for hepatic failure such as antiinflammatory drugs (flunixin meglumine, dimethyl sulfoxide, pentoxifylline), lactulose, and neomycin or other oral antibiotics that may help reduce the production of ammonia or other enteric toxins.
- Insulin therapy may help control hyperglycemia. Protamine zinc insulin has been suggested at 15 to 30 IU IM q12h for 3 days in combination with oral glucose (100 g) q12h. Insulin has also been used as a CRI at 0.02 to 0.2 U/kg/h. Regular blood glucose monitoring should be performed.
- Metformin (15–30 mg/kg PO q12h) may be used as an unproven but potentially helpful adjunctive therapy in ponies with insulin resistance and hepatic lipidosis.
- Heparin potentiates the activity of lipoprotein lipase, which enhances the rate of triglyceride removal from the blood. Lipoprotein lipase activity is already increased in affected horses, so heparin may not provide additional benefit. Suggested dosages of heparin range from 40 to 250 IU/kg BID.

CHRONIC TREATMENT

Ensure resolution of negative energy balance and provide high-quality nutrition to prevent relapse.

POSSIBLE COMPLICATIONS

- Permanent liver failure caused by fatty infiltration is a severe and life-threatening complication.
- Hepatic rupture has been reported in some cases.
- Ketosis rarely develops.

RECOMMENDED MONITORING

- Monitor blood glucose concentrations because some horses will have glucose intolerance, which may potentiate acidosis and result in hypokalemia.
- Monitor triglyceride levels, liver enzymes, and serum bile acids for response to treatment.
- If heparin therapy is used, monitor hemostasis.
- If liver failure is present, monitor signs of hepatic encephalopathy and blood ammonia levels.

PROGNOSIS AND OUTCOME

- Guarded to poor prognosis
- Treat primary illness if identified.
- Most Miniature horses with triglyceride levels below 1200 mg/dL survive.

PEARLS & CONSIDERATIONS

COMMENTS

Prevention through management and early recognition through client education can significantly reduce the incidence of this condition.

PREVENTION

Provide appropriate nutrition without inducing obesity, avoid or minimize stress, and provide good management and routine health care.

CLIENT EDUCATION

- Educate owners about the risk associated with obesity. It is important to provide good management and routine health care in conjunction with an appropriate diet.
- Improve owner awareness about anorexia and associated signs, especially during late gestation and early lactation, which will result in earlier recognition and treatment of disease.

SUGGESTED READING

Durham AE, Rendle DI, Newton JE: The effect of metformin on measurements of insulin sensitivity and beta cell response in 18 horses and ponies with insulin resistance. *Equine Vet J* 40(5):493, 2008.

Mogg TD, Palmer JE: Hyperlipidemia, hyperlipemia, and hepatic lipidosis in American

Miniature horses: 23 cases (1990–1994). *J Am Vet Med Assoc* 207:604, 1995.

Moore BR, Abood SK, Hinchcliff KW: Hyperlipemia in 9 miniature horses and miniature donkeys. *J Vet Intern Med* 8:376, 1994.

AUTHOR: **AMANDA MARTABANO HOUSE**

EDITOR: **MICHELLE HENRY BARTON**

Hepatitis, Bacterial

BASIC INFORMATION

DEFINITION

Primary bacterial hepatitis (inflammation of the liver caused by bacterial infection) and primary bacterial cholangiohepatitis (inflammation of the liver and biliary system) are infrequent causes of hepatic disease in adult horses.

EPIDEMIOLOGY

SPECIES, AGE, SEX
- Middle-aged to older horses
- Neonatal foals

ASSOCIATED CONDITIONS AND DISORDERS Secondary septic or nonseptic peritonitis may be present.

CLINICAL PRESENTATION

HISTORY, CHIEF COMPLAINT Depression, weakness, anorexia, colic, and weight loss in chronic cases

PHYSICAL EXAM FINDINGS
- Fever, weight loss, and variable icterus.
- Clinical signs of hepatoencephalopathy may be present.

ETIOLOGY AND PATHOPHYSIOLOGY
- The etiopathogenesis of bacterial hepatitis is uncertain. Retrograde bacterial infection from the small intestine is the probable cause in mature horses as a sequela to biliary stasis, cholelithiasis, chronic active hepatitis, intestinal obstruction, and proximal enteritis.
- The most common isolates associated with ascending bacterial hepatitis in mature horses are enteric organisms, including *Escherichia coli*, *Salmonella*, *Klebsiella*, *Citrobacter*, *Aeromonas*, and *Acinetobacter* spp.
- Hematogenous dissemination secondary to sepsis is the probable cause in neonatal foals. Bacterial sepsis in foals

may result in focal to multifocal bacterial hepatitis.

DIAGNOSIS

DIFFERENTIAL DIAGNOSIS
- Cholelithiasis
- Theiler's disease
- Tyzzer's disease
- Chronic active hepatitis

INITIAL DATABASE
- Leukocytosis, characterized primarily by a mature neutrophilia
- Hyperfibrinogenemia
- Sorbitol dehydrogenase (SDH), arginase, and gamma glutamyltransferase (GGT) activity: variable increases

ADVANCED OR CONFIRMATORY TESTING

Definitive diagnosis is based on histopathologic findings on liver biopsy (primarily neutrophilic infiltration with bacterial invasion) and bacterial growth on liver biopsy.

TREATMENT

THERAPEUTIC GOAL(S)

Control bacterial replication to prevent advanced hepatic damage and fibrosis.

ACUTE GENERAL TREATMENT
- Provide general and supportive care with IV balanced fluids.
- Nonsteroidal antiinflammatory drugs (flunixin meglumine) may be indicated.
- Antimicrobial therapy should be based on culture and sensitivity results and

should continue until resolution of clinical and laboratory abnormalities: procaine penicillin G 22,000 IU/kg IM q12h and gentamicin 6.6 mg/kg IM q24h; ceftiofur 2.2 to 4.4 mg/kg IM q12h; ampicillin 20 mg/kg IV q6–8h; chloramphenicol 50 mg/kg PO q6h; enrofloxacin 7.5 mg/kg PO q24h; trimethoprim-sulfa 20 to 30 mg/kg PO q12h.

RECOMMENDED MONITORING

Recheck complete blood cell count and serum biochemical indices of hepatobiliary disease before discontinuing antimicrobial therapy.

PROGNOSIS AND OUTCOME

The prognosis is good with appropriate antimicrobial and supportive medical therapy.

PEARLS & CONSIDERATIONS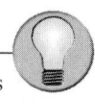

Primary bacterial hepatitis (Tyzzer's disease) is uncommon.

SUGGESTED READING

Peek SF, Divers TJ: Medical treatment of cholangiohepatitis and cholelithiasis in mature horses: 9 cases (1991–1998). *Equine Vet J* 32(4):301, 2000.

Savage CJ: Diseases of the liver. In Colahan PT, Merritt AM, Moore JM, et al, editors: *Equine medicine and surgery*, St Louis, 1999, Mosby, pp 816–833.

AUTHOR: **MONICA DIAS FIGUEIREDO**

EDITOR: **MICHELLE HENRY BARTON**

Hepatitis, Chronic Active

BASIC INFORMATION

DEFINITION

Chronic active hepatitis is a general term embracing any active, progressive liver disease characterized by a marked inflammatory response with concurrent evidence of longstanding disease (ie, fibrosis). The primary histopathologic feature of chronic active hepatitis is periportal infiltration with inflammatory cells accompanied by different stages of hepatocellular necrosis, biliary hyperplasia, and fibrosis.

EPIDEMIOLOGY

SPECIES, AGE, SEX Suppurative chronic active hepatitis has been reported in foals as young as 2 months; however, chronic active hepatitis, particularly the form characterized by mononuclear infiltrate, is more prevalent in adult horses (4–18 years).

CLINICAL PRESENTATION

DISEASE FORMS/SUBTYPES
- Most commonly subtle and gradual in onset.
- Two forms of chronic active hepatitis are described based on the predominant cell population within the liver inflammatory infiltrate:
  - Mononuclear cell infiltration.
  - Neutrophilic infiltration, indicative of a suppurative hepatitis. This type of hepatitis is frequently associated with biliary stasis and hyperplasia and is consistent with a histopathologic diagnosis of cholangitis or cholangiohepatitis (see also "Cholangiohepatitis, Chronic, and Biliary Fibrosis" in this section).

HISTORY, CHIEF COMPLAINT Owners may report depressed mentation, inappetence, weight loss, signs of mild to moderate abdominal discomfort, and loose stools.

PHYSICAL EXAM FINDINGS
- Vital signs may be normal or patient may be febrile
- Icterus
- Mild dehydration
- Moist exfoliative coronary band dermatitis (uncommon)
- Photosensitization (uncommon)

ETIOLOGY AND PATHOPHYSIOLOGY
Idiopathic; the etiology is often undetermined. Possible causes include:
- Autoimmune disease
- Viral infection
- Bacterial infection (hematogenous or ascending from the gastrointestinal tract)
- Toxic insult
- Adverse drug reaction
- Based on the distribution of the lesions predominantly in the area surrounding the portal triad, delivery of noxious agents (eg, bacteria, viruses, endotoxins, toxic agents, inflammatory mediators, or a combination of these) via the portal vein is hypothesized. The presence of inflammatory cells in the periportal area would then be explained by extravasation from the hepatic arterioles or lymphatic vessels in response to the primary insult.

DIAGNOSIS

DIFFERENTIAL DIAGNOSIS

- Toxic hepatopathy
- Theiler's disease
- Biliary obstruction secondary to acute or chronic colon displacement
- Cholelithiasis
- Bacteria hepatitis or cholangiohepatitis
- Hepatic neoplasia
- Amyloidosis
- Liver parasites

INITIAL DATABASE

- Packed cell volume: Normal or increased from hemoconcentration or erythrocytosis induced by liver disease
- Serum total protein concentration: Normal or increased (from dehydration or hyperglobulinemia)
- Fibrinogen concentration: Normal or increased
- Sorbitol dehydrogenase (SDH) activity: Increased; may be normal
- Aspartate aminotransferase (AST), gamma glutamyltransferase (GGT), alkaline phosphatase (ALP) activity: Increased
- Serum total bilirubin concentration: Increased; may be normal in rare cases
- Bile acids concentration: Normal to increased

ADVANCED OR CONFIRMATORY TESTING

- Plasma ammonia concentration may be increased.
- Clotting profile: Prothrombin time and activated partial thromboplastin time may be increased.
- Transabdominal ultrasonographic examination of the liver:
  - May be normal.
  - Liver size may be smaller or larger than normal.
  - Increased liver parenchyma echogenicity compared with adjacent parenchymatous organs (spleen).
- Ultrasound-guided liver biopsy:
  - Histopathology
    - Periportal infiltration
    - Mononuclear cells (histiocytes, lymphocytes and plasma cells)
    - Neutrophils (see also "Cholangiohepatitis, Chronic, and Biliary Fibrosis" in this section)
    - Hepatocellular degeneration or necrosis (or both)
    - Biliary hyperplasia
    - Fibrosis
  - Bacterial culture of liver tissue
    - Most commonly negative in the presence of mononuclear infiltrate
    - May be positive with suppurative inflammation (see also "Cholangiohepatitis, Chronic, and Biliary Fibrosis" in this section)
  - Toxicology screen of liver tissue

TREATMENT

THERAPEUTIC GOAL(S)

Treatment of the form of chronic active hepatitis characterized by mononuclear cell infiltrate is aimed at stopping ongoing inflammation and preventing fibrosis. In the presence of neutrophilic infiltrate and especially with a positive bacterial culture result, therapy is also aimed at treatment of bacterial hepatitis.

ACUTE GENERAL TREATMENT

- IV fluids if the horse is febrile and dehydrated
- Flunixin meglumine (1.1 mg/kg IV) to control signs of abdominal pain

CHRONIC TREATMENT

- Antimicrobial therapy (potentiated sulfonamides, ceftiofur, penicillin and gentamicin, enrofloxacin or ampicillin, alone or in association with metronidazole; chloramphenicol).
- Corticosteroids if the inflammatory infiltrate is represented by histiocytes, lymphocytes, and plasma cells and liver biopsy culture results are negative.
  - Dexamethasone: 0.05 to 0.1 mg/kg IV q24h for 3 to 5 days; decreased over the following 7 to 14 days
  - Oral prednisolone (1–2 mg/kg q24h) after initial dexamethasone therapy; may need to continue for weeks to months
- S-adenosylmethionine (SAMe): 5 g PO q24h; the bioavailability of crushed pills is questionable in horses.

- Prevention of hepatic fibrosis.
  - Pentoxifylline: 8 to 16 mg/kg PO q8–12h
  - Colchicine: 0.03 mg/kg PO q24h; there have been anecdotal reports of presumed toxicity
- Also see treatment for "Hepatic Encephalopathy" in this section.

POSSIBLE COMPLICATIONS

- Immune suppression caused by long-term steroid therapy
- Laminitis
- Diarrhea

RECOMMENDED MONITORING

- GGT, AST, ALP, serum bile acids
- Repeat liver biopsy

PROGNOSIS AND OUTCOME

- Good prognosis with early diagnosis and treatment of bacterial infection and suppurative hepatitis
- Guarded long-term prognosis of hepatitis characterized by mononuclear infiltrate and fibrosis

PEARLS & CONSIDERATIONS

Autoimmune hepatitis characterized by histiocytic and lymphoplasmacytic infiltrate is described in human and small animal medicine. Even if a similar pathogenesis is suspected in horses, the disease is not well described and understood in the equine species.

SUGGESTED READING

Carlson GP, Vivrette S: Chronic active hepatitis in horses. *Proceedings of the 7th ACVIM Forum*, San Diego, 1989.

Pearson EG: Liver disease in the mature horse. *Equine Vet Ed* 11(2):87, 1999.

AUTHOR: **ALESSANDRA PELLEGRINI-MASINI**

EDITOR: **MICHELLE HENRY BARTON**

Hepatopathy, Chronic Megalocytic

BASIC INFORMATION

DEFINITION

Chronic megalocytic hepatopathy is caused by ingestion of pyrrolizidine alkaloid–containing plants (*Senecio jacobaea, S. vulgaris, S. longilobus, S. riddellii, S. spetabilis, S. integerrimus, Amsinckia intermedia, Crotalaria sagittalis, C. spetabilis, Heliotropium europaeum, Echium plantagineum*), resulting in the delayed onset of chronic progressive liver failure.

SYNONYM(S)

Pyrrolizidine alkaloid toxicity

EPIDEMIOLOGY

RISK FACTORS

- Overgrazed pasture
- Hay harvested with pyrrolizidine alkaloid–containing plants

GEOGRAPHY AND SEASONALITY

- The disease occurs worldwide and is the most common cause of hepatic failure in horses in certain parts of the United States.
  - *S. jacobaea, S. vulgaris:* Pacific Coast
  - *A. intermedia:* West
  - *C. sagittalis, C. spetabilis, H. europaeum:* Southeast

ASSOCIATED CONDITIONS AND DISORDERS Clinical signs of chronic megalocytic hepatopathy may be indistinguishable from other chronic liver disorders.

CLINICAL PRESENTATION

DISEASE FORMS/SUBTYPES

- Chronic (most common): Insidious onset of signs that is usually delayed 1 to 3 months after ingestion of plants containing pyrrolizidine alkaloids.
- Despite a delay in development of signs from time of exposure, the onset of signs may be acute.
- If consumption of toxic plants is excessive, the onset of signs may be acute.

HISTORY, CHIEF COMPLAINT Owners may observe weakness, weight loss, lethargy, anorexia, head pressing, yawning, or depression. The horse may have a history of being fed pyrrolizidine alkaloid–contaminated hay or exposure to an overgrazed pasture.

PHYSICAL EXAM FINDINGS

- Icterus, photosensitivity dermatitis, weight loss, hepatic encephalopathy, petechiae (rarely).
- Diarrhea, edema, polydipsia, polyuria, hemolysis, and laryngeal hemiplegia may occur late in the disease.

ETIOLOGY AND PATHOPHYSIOLOGY

- Pyrrolizidine alkaloids are metabolized by hepatic microsomal enzymes to pyrrole derivatives.
- Pyrroles inhibit cellular replication and protein synthesis, resulting in cells that cannot divide and instead continue to grow (formation of megalocytes).
- Megalocytes are eventually replaced by fibrosis.

DIAGNOSIS

DIFFERENTIAL DIAGNOSIS

- Aflatoxicosis
- Clover toxicity
- Cholelithiasis
- Chronic active hepatitis
- Cholangiohepatitis
- Hepatic neoplasia

INITIAL DATABASE

- Complete blood count: Leukocytosis characterized by neutrophilia, left shift, hyperfibrinogenemia
- γ-glutamyltransferase (GGT) and alkaline phosphatase (ALP) activity: Increased
- Aspartate aminotransferase (AST) and sorbitol dehydrogenase (SDH) activity: Increased to normal
- Hyperglobulinemia
- Serum bile acids concentration: Increased
- Total and direct bilirubin concentrations: Increased
- Coagulation times: May be prolonged
- Plasma ammonia concentration: May be increased
- Urinalysis: Bilirubinuria

ADVANCED OR CONFIRMATORY TESTING

- Ultrasonography: Hepatic atrophy, distended bile ducts
- Liver biopsy: Periportal to extensive fibrosis, megalocytosis, biliary hyperplasia, bile stasis, hepatocellular necrosis

TREATMENT

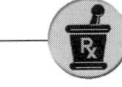

THERAPEUTIC GOAL(S)

Palliation

ACUTE GENERAL TREATMENT

- IV fluids may be required in animals that are febrile and dehydrated. Dextrose may be added for patients that are anorectic.
- Nonsteroidal antiinflammatory drugs (NSAIDs): flunixin meglumine

(1.1 mg/kg PO or IV q12h) or phenylbutazone (2.2 mg/kg PO q12h).
- Nutritional support (low-protein diet with a high content of branched-chain amino acids).
- If hepatic encephalopathy is present, see treatment for "Hepatic Encephalopathy" in this section.

CHRONIC TREATMENT

- Nutritional support, including removal from hay or pasture.
- S-adenosylmethionine (SAMe): 5 g PO q24h; the bioavailability of crushed pills is questionable in horses.
- Colchicine: 0.03 mg/kg PO q24h, although there have been anecdotal reports of toxicity.
- NSAIDs (flunixin meglumine and phenylbutazone), prednisolone (0.5–1.0 mg/kg PO q24h), dexamethasone (0.05–0.10 mg/kg PO q24h).
- Antifibrotics: Pentoxifylline (8–16 mg/kg PO q8–12h).

POSSIBLE COMPLICATIONS

- Hepatic encephalopathy
- Photosensitivity dermatitis

RECOMMENDED MONITORING

- Monitor GGT activity and serum bile acids concentrations every 2 to 3 weeks.
- Perform serial liver biopsies (q2–3mo).

PROGNOSIS AND OUTCOME

- Fair to grave, depending on the degree of megalocytosis and fibrosis.
- The presence of bridging fibrosis is considered invariably fatal.

PEARLS & CONSIDERATIONS

COMMENTS

- Frequently, the onset of clinical signs is delayed (1 month to 1 year after consumption).
- Consumption of 2% to 5% of body weight over 1 to 3 days may result in acute toxicity.

PREVENTION

Avoid contaminated hay and overgrazed pastures.

CLIENT EDUCATION

Remove the source of pyrrolizidine alkaloid (reseed pasture, provide a new source of hay).

SUGGESTED READING

Mendel VE, et al: Pyrrolizidine alkaloid-induced liver disease in horses: an early diagnosis. *Am J Vet Res* 49:572, 1988.

AUTHOR: **HEIDI BANSE**

EDITOR: **MICHELLE HENRY BARTON**

Herbicide Toxicosis

BASIC INFORMATION

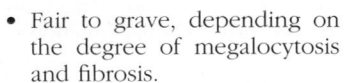

DEFINITION

- Condition resulting from ingestion of products used to destroy plants
- Most herbicides have been developed to be selective to plants and have low mammalian toxicity.
- However, arsenicals and paraquat can cause potentially serious toxicosis in horses if ingested. The use of these types of herbicides has greatly declined, but they still may be in use in some areas of the country.

SYNONYMS

- Arsenic-based herbicides include MSMA (monosodium methanearsonate); DSMA (disodium methanearsonate); arsenic trioxide; sodium arsenite; and arsenates of sodium, potassium, calcium, and lead.
- Bipyridyl (dipyridyl) herbicides include paraquat and diquat.
- Glyphosate (glyphosate-isopropylamine, glyphosate-isopropylammonium, glyphosate sesquiodium, glyphosate-trimesium) is an organophosphorus herbicide, but it has no anticholinesterase activity.
- Phenoxy-type herbicides include 2,4-D (2,4-dichlorophenoxyacetic acid), MCPA (2-methyl-4-chlorophenoxyacetic acid, MCPP (2-(4 chloro-2-methoxy) propionic acid), and dicamba (3,6-dichloro-2-methoxybenzoic acid).
- Pyridine herbicides include trichlopyr.
- Triazine herbicides include atrazine, simazine, and propazine.

EPIDEMIOLOGY

RISK FACTORS Horses grazing pastures adjacent to areas where herbicides are sprayed (eg, power lines, crop fields) may be exposed to overspray or to treated plants along fence lines.
GEOGRAPHY AND SEASONALITY More commonly used during times of rapid plant growth (eg, spring, summer); may also be used in fall as defoliants on crops

CLINICAL PRESENTATION

DISEASE FORMS/SUBTYPES

- Most herbicides, with the exceptions stated below, are of low mammalian toxicity and are unlikely to cause clinical problems if horses graze on treated plants.
- Most herbicides are gastrointestinal (GI) irritants and can cause inappetence, colic, and diarrhea if horses are exposed to large amounts of concentrated product (eg, ingested from container).
- Arsenic-based herbicides cause severe GI hemorrhage, resulting in severe colic, hypovolemia, prostration, and death.
- Paraquat is a caustic compound that causes dermal and alimentary tract erosion and ulceration and can cause rapidly progressive pulmonary fibrosis as well as renal failure.

HISTORY, CHIEF COMPLAINT History of grazing on recently treated plant material or having access to concentrated product
PHYSICAL EXAM FINDINGS

- Most herbicides: No specific findings are expected in cases of horses grazing treated pastures; if large quantities of concentrated product have been directly ingested, diarrhea or evidence of colic (sweating, agitation, tachycardia) may be seen.
- Arsenic-based herbicides: Severe abdominal discomfort, central nervous system depression, watery to bloody diarrhea, weakness, shock. Death may occur acutely, or signs may progress to include cardiac arrhythmias, pulmonary edema, and acute renal failure.
- Paraquat: Oral and/or esophageal ulceration, dermal ulceration, abdomi-

nal discomfort, diarrhea; within days, development of renal insufficiency (polyuria, polydipsia) and progressive respiratory insufficiency (dyspnea, cyanosis)

ETIOLOGY AND PATHOPHYSIOLOGY

- Arsenic-based herbicides: Corrosive effects on GI mucosa along with severe vasculitis of capillary beds results in severe GI hemorrhage, hypovolemia, and possibly pulmonary edema.
- Paraquat: Predominantly isolated to the lung, where production of oxygen-derived free radicals causes damage to alveolar epithelium with subsequent pulmonary fibrosis. The presence of oxygen accelerates the development of pulmonary lesions.

DIAGNOSIS

DIFFERENTIAL DIAGNOSIS

- Most herbicides: Other causes of mild GI irritation or discomfort
- Arsenic-based herbicides: Colitis X, salmonellosis, other causes of acute hemorrhagic gastroenteritis
- Paraquat: Other causes of alimentary ulceration or pulmonary dysfunction (eg, chronic obstructive pulmonary disease)

INITIAL DATABASE

- Most herbicides: Serum electrolytes if severe diarrhea is present
- Arsenic-based herbicides: Serum chemistry panel (renal values), complete blood count (CBC), acid-base status, urinalysis
- Paraquat: Serum chemistry (renal and liver values), CBC, and urinalysis

ADVANCED OR CONFIRMATORY TESTING

- Most herbicides: None
- Arsenic-based herbicides: Serum and urine arsenic levels are rarely diagnostic; elevated arsenic levels in the kidney and liver; elevated arsenic levels in hair (chronic exposures)
- Paraquat: Detection of paraquat in the blood or urine (first 30 hours); "classic" histopathologic lesions in lung tissue; detection of paraquat in lung tissue

TREATMENT

THERAPEUTIC GOAL(S)

- Most herbicides: Manage diarrhea and correct any electrolyte imbalances.
- Arsenic-based herbicides: Manage shock and pulmonary edema, correct

hypovolemia and acid-base imbalances, minimize renal injury, and manage pain.
- Paraquat: Prevent absorption, minimize renal injury, and manage pain and alimentary injury.

ACUTE GENERAL TREATMENT

- Asymptomatic
  - Most herbicides: Dilute with water; monitor for signs of GI discomfort.
  - Arsenic-based herbicides and paraquat: Cathartics (magnesium sulfate), activated charcoal via nasogastric tube, IV fluids (maintain hydration, protect renal function)
- Symptomatic
  - Most herbicides: Symptomatic treatment as needed for GI discomfort
  - Arsenic-based herbicides: IV fluids (monitor closely for pulmonary edema), pain medication, general supportive care (prevention of secondary infections, dietary alterations)
    - Chelation with dimercaprol (3 mg/kg IM q4h) has questionable efficacy in horses.
    - The GI tract must be free of arsenic before chelation or the chelator will pull more arsenic into the blood.
  - Paraquat: IV fluid diuresis (enhance elimination), GI protectants, pain medication, monitor blood gases, prevent secondary infections

CHRONIC TREATMENT

- Arsenic-based herbicides: Management of residual renal insufficiency, dietary alterations
- Paraquat: Management of residual renal or pulmonary insufficiency

DRUG INTERACTIONS

- Paraquat: Oxygen therapy is contraindicated because it accelerates free radical production and pulmonary fibrosis.

POSSIBLE COMPLICATIONS

- Arsenic-based herbicides: Permanent renal insufficiency
- Paraquat: Permanent pulmonary and/or renal insufficiency, esophageal strictures, gastric ulceration with secondary peritonitis

RECOMMENDED MONITORING

- Arsenic-based herbicides: Renal values, acid-base status, electrolytes
- Paraquat: Renal and liver values, acid-base status, electrolytes, oxygen saturation, pulmonary function

PROGNOSIS AND OUTCOME

- Most herbicides: Excellent prognosis because GI irritation is expected to be self-limiting
- Arsenic-based herbicides: Guarded to poor prognosis depending on the amount ingested and the severity of signs
- Paraquat: Prognosis is poor in horses developing signs after exposure.

PEARLS & CONSIDERATIONS

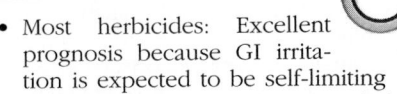

COMMENTS

- As they wilt, plants that have been treated with herbicides may become more attractive to horses, which can increase the likelihood that horses will ingest toxic plants that they would normally avoid. Therefore, many herbicide manufacturers recommend a "graze-out" period (usually 2–3 weeks) during which horses should not be allowed to graze on treated areas.

PREVENTION

- Keep containers of herbicides away from areas to which horses have access.
- Follow label directions regarding the use of herbicides in areas near grazing animals.
- Follow graze-out recommendations to prevent toxicosis from toxic plants in treated areas.

CLIENT EDUCATION

- Because of the past use of highly toxic herbicides, such as paraquat, horse owners frequently suspect herbicides as the cause of any illness that a horse may develop. However, with the advent of modern herbicides that target biochemical mechanisms unique to plants, the likelihood of herbicide-induced toxicosis is very low unless older herbicides such as arsenicals or paraquat are involved.

SUGGESTED READING

Ensley S: Arsenic. In Plumlee KH, editor: *Clinical veterinary toxicology*, St Louis, 2004, Mosby Elsevier, pp 193–195.

Gupta PK: Toxicity of herbicides. In Gupta PK, editor: *Veterinary toxicology: basic and clinical principles*, Boston, 2007, Academic Press, pp 567–586.

AUTHOR: SHARON GWALTNEY-BRANT

EDITOR: CYNTHIA L. GASKILL

Hernia, Diaphragmatic

BASIC INFORMATION

DEFINITION
Protrusion of an organ or tissue through a defect in the diaphragm

CLINICAL PRESENTATION
DISEASE FORMS/SUBTYPES
- Etiology: May be congenital or acquired
  - Congenital: Often small hernias with smooth, round edges
  - Acquired: Often larger hernias with torn edges and often originating at the dorsal body wall
- Location: Peritoneal pericardial or peritoneal pleural

HISTORY, CHIEF COMPLAINT
- Variable
  - May be an incidental finding at necropsy
  - May have low-grade, intermittent colic signs
  - May have acute severe episode of colic or respiratory distress

PHYSICAL EXAM FINDINGS
- Temperature is normal unless the patient is severely compromised.
- The patient often has tachycardia.
- The respiratory rate may be normal or may be markedly elevated; borborygmi are often audible in the thorax.
- The mucous membranes are variable from pink and moist to pale to toxic-appearing depending on the severity of compromise.
- Colic signs are variable from mild, intermittent pain to acute, severe abdominal crisis.
- Hydration is variable depending on the severity of systemic compromise.

ETIOLOGY AND PATHOPHYSIOLOGY
- Congenital diaphragmatic hernias result from failed fusion of the four embryonic components of the diaphragm.
- Acquired diaphragmatic hernias result from trauma.

DIAGNOSIS

DIFFERENTIAL DIAGNOSIS
- Mild, intermittent colic
  - Nonstrangulating large intestinal disease: Large colon displacement or sand colic
  - Nonstrangulating small intestinal lesion: Stricture
  - Nonstrangulating gastric lesion: Gastric impaction or gastric ulcers
  - Peritonitis

- Severe colic
  - Strangulating small intestinal lesion: Strangulating lipoma
  - Strangulating large intestinal lesion: Large colon volvulus
- Respiratory crisis
  - Acute pneumothorax
  - Pleural effusion
  - Pleuropneumonia
  - Hemothorax

INITIAL DATABASE
- Nasogastric intubation: Reflux production is variable depending on the area of intestine within the thorax; in general, reflux is present if there is strangulated small bowel within the thorax.
- Rectal examination: Frequently normal. If the intestine is obstructed, then the practitioner may feel distension of the oral segment (commonly the small intestine). An "empty" feeling within the abdomen may sometimes be appreciated because of displacement of abdominal contents.
- Complete blood count: Normal initially but demonstrates leukopenia or leukocytosis with time if the patient has an acute crisis.
- Peritoneal fluid: Frequently normal initially. Sometimes remains normal as strangulated bowel is sequestered in thorax but may become serosanguineous with elevated total protein and white blood cell counts.
- Transabdominal ultrasonography: Often normal unless there is strangulated bowel; may then see peritoneal effusion and distension of bowel oral to strangulated segment.
- Transthoracic ultrasonography: Can identify abdominal contents within the thorax. Can sometimes identify lack of diaphragmatic contour, especially if a ventral hernia is present.
- Radiography: May appreciate abdominal contents within the thorax or may just identify radiopacity at the ventral thorax.

TREATMENT

THERAPEUTIC GOALS
- Stabilize the patient.
- Remove the herniated bowel from the thorax with or without resection and anastomosis depending on whether the patient has a compromised bowel or not.
- Repair the diaphragmatic defect.

ACUTE GENERAL TREATMENT
After clinical signs become apparent, prevention of recurrence requires surgical intervention.
- Dorsal recumbency under general anesthesia using positive-pressure ventilation.
- Reduce herniated bowel with or without resection and anastomosis depending on whether the patient has compromised bowel. Tilting the horse can facilitate reduction.
- Attempt repair of defect.
  - Small defects (<5 cm) can be sutured with a large-diameter suture in a simple continuous pattern. Ventrally positioned defects are easier to repair this way.
  - Larger defects may require repair with synthetic mesh.
  - Dorsally positioned defects may require a thoracotomy for repair.
  - Some defects prove impossible to repair in dorsal recumbency.
- Evacuate pneumothorax.
  - Maximum inflation of the lungs during closure of the abdominal incision.
  - Place chest tube and Heimlich valve.

CHRONIC TREATMENT
- Postoperative treatment:
  - Management of pneumothorax
  - If the defect proved impossible to repair through ventral midline incision, other methods of repair are occasionally attempted.
- Routine postoperative care:
  - IV fluid therapy
  - IV antibiotics
  - IV antiinflammatory drugs and analgesics with or without antiendotoxic agents
  - Stall rest

POSSIBLE COMPLICATIONS
- Hernia repair breakdown and recurrence
- Pneumothorax
- Pleuropneumonia
- Peritonitis
- Endotoxemia
- Adhesions
- Ileus
- Jugular thrombophlebitis
- Diarrhea
- Pyrexia
- Incisional infection
- Recurrent colic

RECOMMENDED MONITORING
- Pain
- Respiratory rate and effort

- Mentation
- Fecal output

PROGNOSIS AND OUTCOME

- Horses undergoing diaphragmatic hernia repair have a guarded prognosis.

- Hernias are not always amenable to repair.
- Hernia repairs are at a high risk of dehiscence.
- Hernias can recur in another location.

SUGGESTED READING

Dabareiner RM, White NA: Surgical repair of a diaphragmatic hernia in a racehorse. *J Am Vet Med Assoc* 214:1517, 1999.

Edwards GB, Proudman CJ: Diseases of the small intestinal resulting in colic. In Mair TS, Divers T, Ducharme N, editors: *Manual of equine gastroenterology*, St Louis, 2002, Saunders Elsevier, pp 249–265.

Stick JA: Abdominal hernias. In Auer JA, Stick JA, editors: *Equine surgery*, ed 3, St Louis, 2006, Saunders Elsevier, pp 491–499.

AUTHOR: CERI SHERLOCK

EDITORS: TIM MAIR and CERI SHERLOCK

Hernia, Incisional

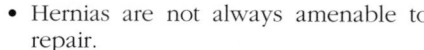

BASIC INFORMATION

DEFINITION

Protrusion of an organ or tissue through the ventral abdominal wall

SYNONYM(S)

- Ventral midline hernia
- Ventral abdominal hernia

EPIDEMIOLOGY

RISK FACTORS

- Ventral midline incisions such as for exploratory celiotomy or for umbilical herniorrhaphy
  - Incisional infection
  - Incisional trauma (especially in the recovery stall)
  - Poor tissue viability
  - Poor tissue apposition

CLINICAL PRESENTATION

HISTORY, CHIEF COMPLAINT Swelling and lack of normal definition of ventral abdominal midline

PHYSICAL EXAM FINDINGS

- Nonpainful, fluctuant swelling of ventral midline; may be one or multiple hernias and therefore swellings
- Occasionally, incisional infection is still present characterized by discharge, heat, pain on palpation, and edema.
- Horses are otherwise normally systemically stable.
  - Normal heart rate, temperature, respiratory rate, and mucous membranes
  - Normal mentation and appetite
  - Audible borborygmi and normal fecal output

ETIOLOGY AND PATHOPHYSIOLOGY Incisional hernias are associated with failure of normal healing of the linea alba.

DIAGNOSIS

DIFFERENTIAL DIAGNOSIS

- Incisional infection
- Incisional edema
- Incisional dehiscence

INITIAL DATABASE

- Complete blood count: Frequently normal
- Peritoneal fluid: Frequently normal initially
- Ultrasonography (transcutaneous of ventral midline): Body wall thickness decreased or absent

TREATMENT

THERAPEUTIC GOAL(S)

- Monitor hernia for deterioration: Enlargement, signs of incarceration, or signs of systemic compromise
- Facilitate optimal abdominal wall strength and cosmesis
  - Abdominal support and strengthening
  - Surgical repair

ACUTE GENERAL TREATMENT

- Conservative management: Eliminate any residual infection.
  - Facilitate ventral drainage
    - Prevent pooling of purulent material (express any pus from the incision twice daily).
    - Keep incisions clean.
    - Consider the use of a supportive belly band; however, this must be changed frequently to cleanse and facilitate drainage.
    - Perform culture for bacterial sensitivity.
    - Treat with appropriate antibiotics if nonresponsive.
  - Supportive belly bands may decrease tension on the body wall.
  - Commencing turnout and exercise may improve the strength of the body wall after sufficient time for healing has occurred.
- Surgical management: This is indicated if the hernia fails to heal or continues to enlarge after exercise has commenced.

CHRONIC TREATMENT

- Conservative management
  - Continue belly bands for support and continue exercise program.
  - Although not cosmetically perfect, many horses perform at or beyond their previous levels of performance with hernias.
- Surgical management can be considered if the hernia enlarges or there is a risk of strangulation or body wall failure. Herniorrhaphy should not be performed until all infection is resolved.
- Large defects may require prosthetic reconstruction with a synthetic mesh.

POSSIBLE COMPLICATIONS

- Repeat incisional hernia
- Local infection
- Peritonitis
- Endotoxemia
- Adhesions
- Jugular thrombophlebitis
- Diarrhea
- Pyrexia
- Incisional infection
- Recurrent colic

RECOMMENDED MONITORING

- Pain
- Hernia or incisional swelling, pain, or discharge
- Mentation
- Fecal output

PROGNOSIS AND OUTCOME

- Most incisional hernias are treated conservatively and only pose a cosmetic defect.

- There is a risk of incisional hernia recurrence after incisional herniorrhaphy.

PEARLS & CONSIDERATIONS

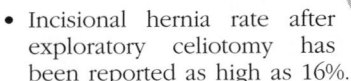

- Incisional hernia rate after exploratory celiotomy has been reported as high as 16%.

- Horses that develop incisional hernias normally demonstrate signs by 4 months after surgery.

SUGGESTED READING

Mair TS, Smith L: Survival and complication rates in 300 horses undergoing surgical treatment of colic. Part 3: Long-term complications and survival. *Equine Vet J* 37:310–314, 2005.

Orsini J: Small intestinal diseases associated with colic in the foal. In Mair TS, Divers T, Ducharme N, editors: *Manual of equine gastroenterology*, St Louis, 2002, Saunders Elsevier, pp 477–484.

Stick JA: Abdominal hernias. In Auer JA, Stick JA, editors: *Equine surgery*, ed 3, St Louis, 2006, Saunders Elsevier, pp 491–499.

AUTHOR: **CERI SHERLOCK**

EDITORS: **TIM MAIR** and **CERI SHERLOCK**

Hernia, Inguinal

BASIC INFORMATION

DEFINITION

- Protrusion of an organ or tissue through the inguinal ring into the inguinal canal
- Indirect hernia is the most common form of inguinal hernia in equines. The small intestine passes through the vaginal ring into the inguinal canal and can extend into the scrotum. It is a congenital condition in foals and an acquired condition in adults.
- Direct hernia is less common and involves the small intestine and occasionally the testicle passing through a rent in the peritoneum adjacent to the vaginal ring into the inguinal region and scrotum, exterior to the vaginal tunic.

SYNONYMS

- Scrotal hernia (although by definition, the organ or tissue has passed through the inguinal canal into the scrotum)
- Caudal abdominal hernias

EPIDEMIOLOGY

SPECIES, AGE, SEX

- Young colts
- Stallions
- Congenital inguinal or scrotal hernia: Seen shortly after birth
- Acquired inguinal hernia: Intact male older than 1 year; may occur in geldings but very uncommon

GENETICS AND BREED PREDISPOSITION

- Congenital: Standardbreds and heavier breeds (eg, Shires) may be more frequently affected.
- Acquired: Standardbreds, Tennessee Walking Horses, and American Saddlebreds are most commonly affected.

RISK FACTORS

- Intact males
- Straining in the foal
- Breeding and strenuous exercise
- Enlarged internal inguinal ring

CLINICAL PRESENTATION

DISEASE FORMS/SUBTYPES

- Foals
  - Congenital inguinal hernias
  - Seen in young colt foals
  - Often bilateral
    - Often indirect (contents pass through vaginal ring into vaginal tunic)
    - May involve rupture of the common vaginal tunic so contents escape subcutaneously
    - Rarely direct (contents pass through a weakness that creates a defect in the body wall
- Adults
  - Acquired hernias
  - Seen in mature stallions

HISTORY, CHIEF COMPLAINT

- Indirect congenital hernias in foals present with scrotal enlargement shortly after birth. Signs of colic are not common.
- Direct inguinal hernias usually present within the first 24 to 48 hours of parturition because of an increased abdominal pressure and are commonly accompanied with signs of abdominal discomfort.
- Acquired inguinal hernias in adult horses present with clinical signs consistent with moderate to severe colic.
- Swelling is present on the axial thigh if the hernia is direct or the common vaginal tunic is ruptured.
- Associated edema and skin excoriations may be caused by a subcutaneous position of the bowel.

PHYSICAL EXAM FINDINGS

- Inguinal hernias in foals are most commonly nonstrangulating and can be reduced, but inguinal hernias in adults are most commonly strangulating and cannot be reduced; physical examination findings reflect the systemic status.
- Congenital
  - Foals with indirect hernias usually present with normal physical findings.

  - Enlarged normothermic scrotum; scrotal herniation is usually reducible
  - Foals with direct hernias may present for signs of abdominal discomfort and scrotal enlargement. The scrotal enlargement is nonreducible and is confined to more of the subcutaneous space as well as the scrotum.
- Acquired
  - Moderate to severe abdominal pain
  - Tachycardia
  - Tachypnea
  - Normothermic
  - Pale, tacky mucous membranes with prolonged capillary refill time
  - Reduced or absent borborygmi
  - Scrotal palpation reveals swollen cool scrotum on the affected side. Early in the entrapment, scrotal palpation may be normal.

ETIOLOGY AND PATHOPHYSIOLOGY

- Inguinal hernias in foals are mostly congenital. An enlarged vaginal process is believed to be associated with an excessive enlargement of the gubernaculum during descent of the testicle, resulting in abnormal enlargement of the vaginal ring. They may be associated with increased intraabdominal pressure (ie, trauma or straining).
- Inguinal hernias in adults are acquired. They are associated with increased abdominal pressure during breeding, exercise, or trauma resulting in herniation of the small intestine through the vaginal ring.

DIAGNOSIS

DIFFERENTIAL DIAGNOSIS

- Other causes of strangulating obstruction of the small intestine
  - Small intestinal volvulus
  - Epiploic foramen entrapment
  - Gastrosplenic entrapment
- Strangulating lipoma
- Testicular thrombosis

- Orchitis
- Testicular seroma
- Scrotal hematoma
- Torsion of the spermatic cord
- Testicular neoplasia
- Umbilical hernia

INITIAL DATABASE

- Complete blood count: Variable depending on systemic compromise
- Peritoneal fluid: Normal initially but may become serosanguineous with an elevated protein content and white blood cell count with time if strangulated bowel present
- Rectal palpation (adults): Palpable structures entering the internal inguinal ring; most commonly small intestine with distended small intestine coursing to the ring
- Ultrasonography (transabdominal): Possibly small intestinal distension if involved in the inguinal hernia
- Ultrasonography (transcutaneous of inguinal and scrotal region): Intestines within scrotum ± subcutaneously. Edema of the testicle and spermatic cord are common because of vascular compromise. Peritoneal effusion is often seen.

TREATMENT

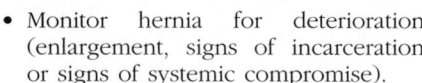

THERAPEUTIC GOAL(S)

- Monitor hernia for deterioration (enlargement, signs of incarceration or signs of systemic compromise).
- Remove any predispositions (eg, straining).
- Attain closure of the inguinal hernia.
  - Repeated manual reduction
  - Surgical repair
- Congenital
  - Manual reduction of scrotal hernia and maintenance until spontaneous permanent resolution
- Acquired
  - Correction of metabolic derangements
  - Pain management
  - Reduction of inguinal hernia
  - Castration of the affected testicle

ACUTE GENERAL TREATMENT

- Reducible hernias in foals
  - Confine to a stall.
  - Reduce hernia manually several times per day (sometimes easier in recumbency).
  - Occasionally compressive inguinal bandages (figure 8 pattern) are necessary in larger hernias.
  - If conservative therapy is not successful or the hernia becomes nonreducible, surgical intervention is required.
  - A routine inguinal approach is made and the hernia reduced.

Closed castration is recommended, and the external inguinal rings are closed.
  - Laparoscopic reduction and closure of the internal inguinal ring and testicular preservation have been reported.
- Nonreducible hernias in foals or adults
  - Surgical reduction ± resection of compromised bowel and herniorrhaphy: Dorsal recumbency under general anesthesia
  - Two approaches are usually required for successful reduction of the hernia, a ventral midline and inguinal approach.
  - Depending on the duration of the colic, after the entrapment is reduced and the affected loop is replaced back into the abdomen, allowing for reperfusion of the segment, intestinal viability may improve significantly, eliminating the need for resection and anastomosis. If intestinal viability does not return, resection of the segment is necessary. If the ileum is involved, a jejunocecostomy may be required.
  - Bilateral castration should be discussed with the owner because of the risk, although small, of herniation through the non-affected side. Hemicastration and preservation of the opposite testicle are often performed in breeding stallions.
- Partial or complete laparoscopic closure of the internal inguinal ring with or without testicular preservation has also been reported in adults.

CHRONIC TREATMENT

- Reducible hernias in foals: Continue manual reduction several times daily for 3 to 6 months or until there are signs of incarceration or enlargement or colic.
- Surgical herniorrhaphy and castration are recommended if the hernia is still present at 3 to 6 months.
- After herniorrhaphy
  - Castration is recommended. (Horses may otherwise reherniate and can herniate through the contralateral ring subsequently.)
  - Stall rest is required for 30 to 45 days.

POSSIBLE COMPLICATIONS

- Repeat herniation (incisional hernia)
- Local infection
- Peritonitis
- Endotoxemia
- Adhesions
- Reobstruction
- Jugular thrombophlebitis
- Diarrhea
- Pyrexia
- Incisional infection
- Recurrent colic

RECOMMENDED MONITORING

- Pain
- Hernia or incisional swelling, pain, or discharge
- Mentation
- Fecal output

PROGNOSIS AND OUTCOME

- Congenital inguinal hernias in foals may resolve spontaneously, and strangulation is rare.
- The prognosis for horses with strangulating lesions is variable and depends on the severity of compromise of the bowel.

PEARLS & CONSIDERATIONS

- The predisposition of foals for reducible nonstrangulating inguinal hernias is probably associated with the relatively short and wide inguinal ring compared with adult horses.
- Even if an inguinal hernia spontaneously corrects in a foal, care should be taken during castration because the horse is still at risk of evisceration subsequent to castration.
- An inguinal hernia should always be considered in intact males with colic, especially if predisposed by breed.
- Direct herniation is rare.
- The small intestine can often be felt rectally passing through the vaginal ring. Slight tension placed on the affected mesentery elicits a painful response.
- The condition may occur in geldings, but it is very rare.
- Congenital inguinal or scrotal hernias in neonates seldom cause strangulation and resolve spontaneously with conservative therapy by 3 to 6 months of age.

SUGGESTED READING

Fischer AT Jr, Vachon AM, Klein SR: Laparoscopic inguinal herniorrhaphy in two stallions. *J Am Vet Med Assoc* 207:1599–1601, 1995.

Orsini J: Small intestinal diseases associated with colic in the foal. In Mair TS, Divers T, Ducharme N, editors: *Manual of equine gastroenterology*, St Louis, 2002, Saunders Elsevier, pp 477–484.

Stick JA: Abdominal hernias. In Auer JA, Stick JA, editors: *Equine surgery*, ed 3, St Louis, 2006, Saunders Elsevier, pp 491–499.

AUTHORS: CERI SHERLOCK and **RANDY EGGLESTON**

EDITORS: TIM MAIR and **CERI SHERLOCK**

Hernia, Lateral Abdominal

BASIC INFORMATION

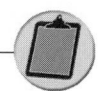

DEFINITION

Protrusion of an organ or tissue through a defect in the body wall

SYNONYM(S)

Body wall hernias

CLINICAL PRESENTATION

DISEASE FORMS/SUBTYPES

- Closed abdominal wall hernia
- Open abdominal wall hernia

HISTORY, CHIEF COMPLAINT

- May have a history of known trauma
- Horse demonstrates alteration of the normal contour of the body wall with or without a wound
- May have low-grade colic signs and appear distressed or reluctant to move

PHYSICAL EXAM FINDINGS

- Abnormal contour and swelling in the area of the hernia
  - Associated edema
  - Thin feeling to the body wall
  - The intestines may be palpable or visible subcutaneously, especially in foals
- Temperature generally normal
- May have normal heart rate or be tachycardic
- Respiratory rate may be normal or mildly elevated
- Mucous membranes are variable from pink and moist to pale and tacky
- Colic signs are variable; may be absent or demonstrate mild colic signs
- Hydration variable

ETIOLOGY AND PATHOPHYSIOLOGY

- Trauma (eg, hit by a car, impact with a solid object such as a fence post or a kick)
- May be associated with dystocia in foals

DIAGNOSIS

DIFFERENTIAL DIAGNOSIS

- Edema
- Local infection
- Prepubic tendon rupture
- Inguinal, incisional, or umbilical hernia

INITIAL DATABASE

- Complete blood count: Generally normal
- Peritoneal fluid: May demonstrate mild elevations in protein and white blood cell counts. Hemoabdomen may also be present associated with underlying trauma.
- Transabdominal ultrasonography: Bowel often normal unless it becomes herniated through the body wall defect; peritoneal effusion is frequently present; body wall defect visible with lack of definition of normal muscular layers and hemorrhage and edema associated with the trauma
- Hernia may be palpable rectally depending on its position.

TREATMENT

THERAPEUTIC GOAL(S)

- Stabilize the patient.
- Initiate wound management if applicable and prevent further contamination using a bandage.
- Surgical repair
  - Provide analgesia and antiinflammatory drugs.
  - Promote repair of the defect.
    - If it is a nonpenetrating injury, support the defect in the abdominal wall to allow fibrosis and scarring of the area.
    - Surgical repair is sometimes necessary but is preferentially performed after 60 days.

ACUTE GENERAL TREATMENT

- Penetrating wounds
  - Wound management, including antibiotics
  - Surgical closure to prevent evisceration and peritonitis
- Nonpenetrating wounds
  - Small defects
    - Local therapy to minimize swelling (eg, hydrotherapy)
    - Antiinflammatory drugs and analgesics
    - Supportive bandages
    - Stall rest

- Large defects: Surgical reconstruction may be indicated and may require synthetic mesh placement.

CHRONIC TREATMENT

Consider direct suture apposition after 60 days if residual body wall defects remain. This allows fibrosis of tissues, which therefore has improved suture-holding strength.

POSSIBLE COMPLICATIONS

- Hernia repair breakdown and recurrence
- Peritonitis
- Endotoxemia
- Adhesions
- Ileus
- Jugular thrombophlebitis
- Diarrhea
- Pyrexia
- Incisional infection
- Recurrent colic

RECOMMENDED MONITORING

- Pain
- Body contour
- Colic
- Mentation
- Local swelling, heat or pain on palpation

PROGNOSIS AND OUTCOME

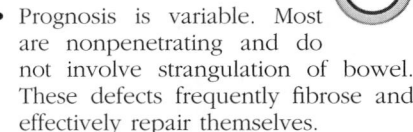

- Prognosis is variable. Most are nonpenetrating and do not involve strangulation of bowel. These defects frequently fibrose and effectively repair themselves.
- Penetrating defects have a high risk of peritonitis, adhesions, and local wound infection

SUGGESTED READING

Stick JA: Abdominal hernias. In Auer JA, Stick JA, editors: *Equine surgery*, ed 3, St Louis, 2006, Saunders Elsevier, pp 491–499.

AUTHOR: **CERI SHERLOCK**

EDITORS: **TIM MAIR** and **CERI SHERLOCK**

Hernia, Umbilical

BASIC INFORMATION

DEFINITION

Protrusion of an organ or tissue through a defect in the normal abdominal wall at the umbilicus

EPIDEMIOLOGY

SPECIES, AGE, SEX Affects foals
RISK FACTORS Females are more commonly affected.
ASSOCIATED CONDITIONS AND DISORDERS Umbilical cord infection

CLINICAL PRESENTATION

DISEASE FORMS/SUBTYPES
Classifications
- Size
- Shape
- Contents of the hernial sac
- Reducible or nonreducible

HISTORY, CHIEF COMPLAINT
- Swelling around the umbilicus: May be permanent or intermittent
- If a foal has an incarcerated, strangulated bowel, the foal will demonstrate inappetence, lethargy, and colic signs, and the hernia may have recently increased in size, becoming irreducible.

PHYSICAL EXAM FINDINGS
- Nonincarcerated hernia
  - Soft, reducible hernia
  - Most commonly normothermic
  - Normal heart rate
  - Normal mentation
  - Mucous membranes pale pink and moist
  - Normal borborygmi
  - Normal fecal output
  - Normal hydration
- Incarcerated or nonreducible hernia
  - May be firm
  - If painful and warm or edematous, often strangulated incarcerated hernia
  - May demonstrate colic signs (definitely if strangulated)
  - May demonstrate tachycardia (definitely if strangulated)
  - May be normothermic but often hyperthermic or hypothermic depending on systemic status
  - Often depressed and lethargic
  - Mucous membranes variable: May be pale pink and moist but progress to toxic with time
  - Often decreased or absent borborygmi
  - Normal or decreased fecal output
- Depending on complete occlusion of bowel or partial involvement in the

hernia (Richter's hernia): Variable hydration

ETIOLOGY AND PATHOPHYSIOLOGY

- Most are congenital
- May have a hereditary component
- May be associated with trauma to the umbilical cord at birth
- May be associated with neonatal excessive straining
- May be associated with umbilical cord infection

DIAGNOSIS

DIFFERENTIAL DIAGNOSIS

- Umbilical infection
- Patent urachus
- Local infection
- Inguinal hernia

INITIAL DATABASE

- Nonincarcerated
  - Complete blood count: Frequently normal
  - Peritoneal fluid: Normal
  - Palpation reveals a soft, reducible hernia with well defined hernial ring.
  - Ultrasonography demonstrates a defect in the body wall but normal motile intestines close by defect.
- Incarcerated
  - Leukopenia or leukocytosis common; occasionally normal
  - Peritoneal fluid has increasing total protein and white blood cell counts with time
  - Palpation reveals a firm, swollen, nonreducible hernia that is painful to palpation, especially if strangulated.
  - Ultrasonography demonstrates a defect in the body wall containing intestine, which frequently demonstrates thickened walls if strangulated.
  - Radiography may be helpful to identify contents of hernial sac.
  - Gas may be visible within loops of bowel.

TREATMENT

THERAPEUTIC GOAL(S)

- Monitor hernia for deterioration: Enlargement, signs of incarceration, or signs of systemic compromise
- Attain closure of the umbilical hernia.
  - Repeated reduction
  - Surgical repair

ACUTE GENERAL TREATMENT

- Reducible hernias smaller than 10 cm in diameter
  - Reduce the hernia manually.
  - Occasionally, compressive belly bandages can be worn and are tolerated by foals.
- Reducible hernias larger than 10 cm in diameter: Surgical herniorrhaphy
- Risks of strangulation high
- Nonreducible hernias with signs of incarceration: Surgical herniorrhaphy ± resection of compromised bowel

CHRONIC TREATMENT

- Reducible hernias smaller than 10 cm in diameter: Continue manual reduction at least daily for 4 months or until signs of incarceration or enlargement
- Most hernias smaller than 5 cm in diameter regress.
- Herniorrhaphy is recommended if the hernia still present at 4 months or deterioration of the hernia is noted.
- After herniorrhaphy
  - Belly band application may aid decrease in dead space at surgery site.
  - Stall rest is required for 30 to 45 days.

POSSIBLE COMPLICATIONS

- Repeat herniation (incisional hernia)
- Local infection
- Peritonitis
- Endotoxemia
- Adhesions
- Reobstruction
- Jugular thrombophlebitis
- Diarrhea
- Pyrexia
- Incisional infection
- Recurrent colic

RECOMMENDED MONITORING

- Pain
- Hernia or incisional swelling, pain, or discharge
- Mentation
- Fecal output

PROGNOSIS AND OUTCOME

- Hernias are predominantly a cosmetic defect and are rarely life threatening; however, incarceration of bowel within the hernia does become a life-threatening condition.
- Good prognosis if the hernia is smaller than 5 cm in diameter.

- Frequently close spontaneously as foal grows: Poor prognosis for spontaneous closure if the hernia is larger than 10 cm in diameter

PEARLS & CONSIDERATIONS

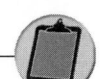

Umbilical hernias are the most common type of hernia in

horses. The estimated occurrence is 0.5% to 2% of foals.

SUGGESTED READING

Enzerink E, van Weeren PR, van der Velden MA: Closure of the abdominal wall at the umbilicus and the development of umbilical hernias in a group of foals from birth to 11 months of age. *Vet Rec* 147:37–39, 2000.

Orsini J: Small intestinal diseases associated with colic in the foal. In Mair TS, Divers T, Ducharme N, editors: *Manual of equine gastroenterology*, St Louis, 2002, Saunders Elsevier, pp 477–484.

Stick JA: Abdominal hernias. In Auer JA, Stick JA, editors: *Equine surgery*, ed 3, St Louis, 2006, Saunders Elsevier, pp 491–499.

AUTHOR: **CERI SHERLOCK**

EDITOR: **TIM MAIR**

Herpesvirus

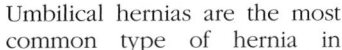

BASIC INFORMATION

DEFINITION

- Equine herpesviruses (EHVs) are ubiquitous enveloped DNA viruses that have a major economic and welfare impact on the horse industry worldwide.
- Nine EHVs have been characterized. Five (EHV-1 to EHV-5) infect domestic horses, and two (EHV-6 and EHV-9) are associated with infections in wild Equids, including asses and zebra.
- EHV-1 through EHV-5 may be further classified into viral subfamilies on the basis of their genetic sequence:
  - *α-Herpesviridae:* EHV-1, EHV-3, and EHV-4
  - *γ-Herpesviridae:* EHV-2 and EHV-5
- In domestic horses, EHV-1 is associated with respiratory disease, abortion, and neurologic disease.
- EHV-2 has not been convincingly associated with pathology in horses as a primary etiologic agent, but some evidence suggests that it may be associated with keratoconjunctivitis in young horses and superficial keratopathies in adult horses.
- EHV-3 causes coital exanthema, a venereal disease of stallions and mares (see "Venereal Diseases in the Stallion: Viruses," in this section).
- EHV-4 is associated primarily with respiratory tract disease in horses.
- EHV-5 is epidemiologically associated with pulmonary nodular fibrosis in adult horses.

SYNONYM(S)

- EHV-1
  - Equine rhinopneumonitis
  - Viral abortion
  - Neurologic herpes
  - Equine herpesvirus myeloencephalopathy (EHM)
- EHV-3: Coital exanthema
- EHV-4: Equine rhinopneumonitis
- EHV-5: Pulmonary nodular fibrosis

EPIDEMIOLOGY

SPECIES, AGE, SEX

- Most adult horses have serologic evidence of exposure to EHVs.
- The neurologic form of disease appears to be more common in adult horses.

RISK FACTORS

- Areas of high comingling of horses: Racetracks, show grounds, veterinary hospitals
- Stress or immunosuppression: Transport, hospitalization, training, showing, weaning, high doses of corticosteroids

GEOGRAPHY AND SEASONALITY

- Worldwide
- Highest incidence of EHV-1 neurologic disease in late winter, spring, and early summer with concomitant outbreaks of respiratory disease or abortion.

CLINICAL PRESENTATION

DISEASE FORMS/SUBTYPES

- Respiratory disease
  - Usually EHV-4, occasionally EHV-1
  - Typically causes a self-limiting upper respiratory disease
  - In neonates or immunocompromised young animals, may cause a severe viral pneumonitis with secondary bacterial pneumonia
- Abortion
  - Almost always EHV-1
  - EHV-4 with single cases rather than outbreaks (possibly indicating reactivation of latent infection)
- Neurologic disease: See "Myeloencephalitis, Equine Herpesvirus-1" in this section.
- Ocular disease
  - Recurrent conjunctivitis ± corneal ulceration may be caused by EHV-1 or EHV-2.
  - Uveitis has been described in association with EHV-1.
  - Keratitis has been described in association with EHV-2.

- Multinodular pulmonary fibrosis: EHV-5 has been associated with this disorder and may be a cofactor or primary etiologic agent.

HISTORY, CHIEF COMPLAINT

Horses may present with one or more of the following common complaints:
- Inappetence, fever, nasal discharge
- Mare in late gestation with sudden abortion or expulsion of placenta
- Multiple abortions on the premises
- Acute-onset neurologic deficits in one or more horses with some horses febrile
- Weak foal that is not thriving
- Persistent keratitis or keratoconjunctivitis
- Adult horse with weeks-long history of intermittent fever, weight loss, coughing, or tachypnea

PHYSICAL EXAM FINDINGS

- Respiratory disease
  - Depression, anorexia
  - Fever from 101° to 106° F that may be biphasic peaking at 24 to 48 hours after infection and again on days 6 to 7
  - Serous nasal discharge changing to mucopurulent
  - Conjunctivitis
  - Serous ocular discharge
  - Progressive lymphadenopathy of mandibular and retropharyngeal lymph nodes
  - Coughing may or may not be evident (less consistent than with equine influenza)
  - Occasional limb edema, diarrhea, colic
- Viral pneumonitis of neonates
  - Fever, marked depression
  - Tachypnea
  - Dyspnea, respiratory distress
  - Abnormal lung sounds
  - Petechia, icterus
- Abortion
  - Abortion in the last third of pregnancy; refractory to abortion if

infected less than 120 days' gestation

○ After abortion, mare may be normal or have respiratory disease or neurologic signs before abortion

○ Typically no premonitory signs, with rapid expulsion of placenta

○ After abortion, mares generally breed successfully and foal normally.

○ May result in birth of stillborn or very weak foals that die shortly after birth

○ Stallions may develop scrotal edema, loss of libido, reduction in sperm quality, and shedding of infectious virus in semen.

○ Foals may be stillborn or born weak and die

- Neurologic disease: See "Myeloencephalitis, Equine Herpesvirus-1" in this section.

- Infectious keratitis
  ○ Blepharospasm, serous epiphora
  ○ Chemosis, conjunctival hyperemia
  ○ Superficial punctuate or dendritic lesions
  ○ Recurrent cases may have corneal vascularization.

- Multinodular pulmonary fibrosis
  ○ Weight loss, poor body condition
  ○ Fever
  ○ Cough, nasal discharge
  ○ Tachypnea, respiratory disease

ETIOLOGY AND PATHOPHYSIOLOGY

- Principal reservoir of infection is latently infected horses.
  ○ An estimated 80% to 90% of horses are latently infected with EHV-1 or EHV-4 by 2 years of age.
  ○ Foals are exposed and may become latently infected as early as 1 to 2 weeks of age (from their dam or other adult horses).
  ○ Latently infected horses serve as a source of virus for spread to other foals.
  ○ Reactivation of latent virus may occur with any stressful situation, including transport, handling, rehousing, or weaning.
  ○ Reactivation of latent virus in adult horses often causes viral shedding without clinical signs.

- Environmental transmission is important during outbreaks and may occur by:
  ○ Aerosolization of virus in nasopharyngeal secretions of infected horses
  ○ Direct horse-to-horse contact
  ○ Exposure to aborted fetal and placental tissues and fluids
  ○ Exposure to fomites contaminated with respiratory or reproductive secretions

- For EHV-1 and EHV-4
  ○ The virus invades respiratory epithelium and incubates 1 to 10 days.

○ Onset of clinical signs (fever, nasal and ocular discharge) in 1 to 3 days

○ Shedding of virulent virus for 6 to 10 days after onset of fever.

○ Latent infection of virus in circulating CD8+ T lymphocytes, upper respiratory lymph nodes, and trigeminal ganglia (EHV-1 and EHV-4) or in lymphocytes and trigeminal ganglia (EHV-2 and EHV-5)

○ Reactivation of virus during periods of stress (eg, transport, hospitalization, illness) may result in symptomatic or asymptomatic nasal shedding of virus.

○ Natural infection of EHV-1 induces protective immunity for only a few weeks to a few months.

○ Abortion: EHV-1 infects endothelial cells in pregnant uterus to cause a vasculitis of small arteriolar branches in the glandular layer of endometrium at base of microcotyledons. Fetus may be aborted before transplacental spread of virus to fetus.

○ Neurologic disease: See "Myeloencephalitis, Equine Herpesvirus-1" in this section.

DIAGNOSIS

DIFFERENTIAL DIAGNOSIS

- Respiratory disease
  ○ Equine influenza
  ○ Equine viral arteritis
  ○ Equine adenovirus
- Neurologic disease: See "Myeloencephalitis, Equine Herpesvirus-1" in this section.
- Abortion
  ○ Equine viral arteritis
  ○ Leptospirosis
  ○ Bacterial placentitis
  ○ Nocardioform abortion
  ○ *Neorickettsia risticii*
  ○ *Chlamydia* spp.
  ○ *Mycoplasma* spp.
  ○ Mare reproductive loss syndrome
- Viral pneumonitis
  ○ Equine viral arteritis
  ○ Equine adenovirus
  ○ Equine influenza
- Infectious keratitis
  ○ Opportunistic bacteria or fungi with trauma
  ○ Other respiratory viruses (adenovirus, influenza, Borna virus)
- Conjunctivitis
  ○ Equine adenovirus
  ○ Equine viral arteritis
  ○ Bacterial agents (*Streptococcus equi* subsp. *equi*, *Moraxella* spp., *Chlamydia* spp., *Mycoplasma* spp.)
  ○ *Histoplasma farciminosus*
  ○ *Aspergillus* spp.
  ○ *Rhinosporidium seeberi*
  ○ Blastomycosis

○ Parasitic (*Thelazia* spp., *Onchocerca* spp., *Habronema* spp., *Trypanosoma* spp.)

- Uveitis
  ○ Equine influenza
  ○ Equine viral arteritis
  ○ Equine infectious anemia
  ○ Bacterial agents
  ○ Parasitic agents
  ○ Equine recurrent uveitis

INITIAL DATABASE

- EHV-1 and EHV-4
  ○ Leukopenia (transient; first 7–10 days)
  ○ Lymphopenia
- Viral pneumonitis
  ○ Diffuse bronchointerstitial pattern on thoracic radiographs
  ○ Toxic, neutropenic, lymphopenic, leukopenia
- Infectious keratitis:
  ○ Superficial and punctate lesions identified with rose Bengal stain of cornea
- Multinodular pulmonary fibrosis
  ○ Neutrophilic leukocytosis with hyperfibrinogenemia
  ○ Severe nodular interstitial pattern on thoracic radiographs
  ○ Discrete nodular lesions (1–7 cm) on thoracic ultrasound

ADVANCED OR CONFIRMATORY TESTING

- EHV-1 and EHV-4
  ○ Virus isolation using whole blood (EDTA, heparin) or swabs of nasopharyngeal secretions collected using a 6-inch polyester or Dacron swab. Collect within the first 24 to 48 hours after clinical onset.
  ○ Serology using paired sera (acute and convalescent) collected 10 to 21 days apart
    ▪ Most available tests cannot differentiate between EHV-1 and EHV-4.
    ▪ EHV IgG enzyme-linked immunosorbent assay differentiates between EHV-1 and EHV-4.
  ○ Real-time polymerase chain reaction (PCR) on whole blood, nasal swabs
    ▪ Test available to identify DNA mutation associated with "neuropathic" strains of EHV-1
  ○ Aborted fetus: Liver, lung, adrenal, and thymus samples are important.
    ▪ Histopathology, immunohistochemistry, PCR, virus isolation
  ○ Cerebrospinal fluid
    ▪ Xanthochromia, high protein (100–500 mg/dL), normal nucleated cell numbers.
  ○ Foals
    ▪ Postmortem findings: Severe diffuse interstitial pneumonia, hepa-

titis with viral inclusion bodies and bone marrow depletion
  - Histopathology, immunohistochemistry, PCR, virus isolation
- Coital exanthema: Virus isolation from lesions, inclusion bodies seen on histopathology, PCR
- Infectious keratitis
  - Corneal cytology
  - Culture and sensitivity
  - Histopathology
  - PCR for EHV-2 and EHV-5
- Multinodular pulmonary fibrosis
  - PCR assay for EHV-5
    - Bronchoalveolar lavage fluid
    - Lung biopsy sample
  - Transtracheal wash
    - Of the five reported cases, only one horse had *Enterobacter* spp. infection
    - Purulent inflammation with nondegenerate to degenerate neutrophils

TREATMENT

THERAPEUTIC GOAL(S)

- Provide symptomatic treatment.
- Establish biosecurity measures to minimize spread of infection, particularly with EHV-1 induced abortion and neurologic EHV-1.
- Confirm EHV-1 diagnosis with testing.

ACUTE GENERAL TREATMENT

- Respiratory disease
  - Nonsteroidal antiinflammatory drugs (NSAIDs) for high fever
  - Nursing care
  - Hydration and fluids if needed
  - Rest for at least 7 days after clinical signs
  - Maintain good air hygiene in stables with (minimal dust with low concentrations of allergens, bacteria, and irritants)
- Viral pneumonitis
  - Treatment for septic foal
    - Broad-spectrum antibiotics, IV plasma (see "Neonatal Sepsis" in this section)
    - NSAIDs
    - Nursing care
    - Nasal insufflation with O_2
  - Generally unrewarding because foals fail to survive
  - Consider antiviral therapy as described below
- Neurologic disease: See "Myeloencephalitis, Equine Herpesvirus-1" in this section.
- Infectious keratitis
  - Topical antivirals, four to 12 times per day for 3 to 5 days; then three to six times per day
    - Idoxuridine (0.1%)
    - Trifluridine (0.3%)

- Topical NSAIDs
  - 0.03% flurbiprofen
  - 0.1% diclofenac
- Avoid topical corticosteroids
- Oral L-lysine 10 to 30 g q24h
- Multinodular pulmonary fibrosis
  - Supportive treatment (IV fluids, nasal O_2, nasogastric feeding)
  - Broad-spectrum antimicrobials
  - Corticosteroids
    - Dexamethasone: 0.037 mg/kg IV q24h for several weeks, tapering
    - Prednisolone: 1 mg/kg PO q24h
  - Antiviral medications
  - NSAIDs
  - For pulmonary hypertension
    - Sildenafil
    - Furosemide
  - Inhaled medications
    - Fluticasone (2200 µg q12h)
    - Albuterol
    - Nebulized antibiotics

POSSIBLE COMPLICATIONS

Bacterial pneumonia or pleuropneumonia

RECOMMENDED MONITORING

- Guidelines for management of infectious disease outbreaks are available at the website of the American Association of Equine Practitioners (AAEP) (see Recommended Reading below) and include the following:
  - Monitor horses twice daily for increased rectal temperature. Segregate horses with fever from the general horse population.
  - Quarantine of horses for 28 days after the last known clinical case.
  - Affected horses should be tested with nasopharyngeal swabs to make sure they are no longer contagious.
  - Proper disinfection of trailers, equipment, and so on
  - Use of separate equipment for each horse
  - Efficient and open communication among attending veterinarian, premises' owners, and other parties working with the affected premises

PROGNOSIS AND OUTCOME

- The majority of respiratory infections are inapparent and self-limiting with clinical signs lasting for 24 hours up to 3 days.
- Foals born with EHV-1 infection are weak and fail to thrive despite treatment. Foals that survive for more than 2 or 3 days develop secondary bacterial pneumonia, and may survive for 10 to 14 days, but eventually die from respiratory disease and a complex

combination of other complications, including lymphoid depletion and profound leukopenia.
- Horses with neurologic disease manifest rapid progression of signs and then stabilize in a few days. Recumbency for more than 24 hours signifies a poor prognosis. Horses that remain standing usually improve and may recover completely within weeks to months. Control of urination returns typically before gait abnormalities (see "Myeloencephalitis, Equine Herpesvirus-1" in this section).
- Multinodular pulmonary fibrosis
  - Of the five horses reported, two horses survived and returned to previous level of activity after several months of therapy.
  - Horses that had evidence of pulmonary hypertension had a poor prognosis.

PEARLS & CONSIDERATIONS

COMMENTS

EHVs are endemic within the equine population. Control of EHV disease occurs by a combination of management and hygiene measures supplemented by vaccination.

PREVENTION

- Horses returning from areas of high exposure risk (eg, shows, breeding, hospitalization) should be housed separately from the general barn population for at least 21 days (ideally 28 days) and monitored for clinical signs.
- Mares that abort should be isolated for a minimum of 4 weeks and not mixed with pregnant mares for 56 days.
- Practice good hygiene measures and biosecurity on the farm.
  - Separate different age groups of horses; maintain small numbers of horses in each cohort.
  - Isolate pregnant mares from other horses.
  - Individually house mares in the last third of gestation.
  - Disinfect stalls, equipment, and so on before use by another horse.
  - Minimize visitor contact and traffic with animals.
  - Practice appropriate pest and vector control.
- Vaccination recommendations (see AAEP guidelines for vaccination)
  - Broodmares: Killed virus vaccines at 5, 7, and 9 months of gestation
  - Foals: Begin three-dose series of vaccinations at 4 to 6 months of age.
  - Young horses: Vaccinate against EHV-1 and EHV-4 to prevent respiratory disease.

- Booster for EHV-1 and EHV-4 every 6 months
  - In the face of a neurologic EHV-1 outbreak:
    - None of the current vaccines for EHV-1 have been labeled as protective against neurologic disease.
    - Horses showing clinical disease *should not* be vaccinated.
    - Exposed horses potentially harboring the virus should not be vaccinated.
    - Booster nonexposed horses at risk that must enter the premises if they have not been vaccinated within the previous 90 days.
- Further preventative measures
  - Immunomodulators: Zylexis (Parapox ovis) labeled for prevention of respiratory signs from EHV-1 and EHV-4

- Antivirals: Prophylactic use may be beneficial to reduce viral replication, viremia, and shedding in the face of a disease outbreak (especially neurologic disease); these drugs are costly.

CLIENT EDUCATION

- Establish guidelines for general husbandry and preventative measures such as outlined in the US Department of Agriculture brochure *Biosecurity: The Key to Keeping your Horses Healthy* available at http://www.aphis.usda.gov/animal_health/animal_dis_spec/horses/.
- Establish a contingency plan in the case of abortion for the proper handling of biologic tissues and measures to isolate the aborting mare from the rest of the herd.

SUGGESTED READING

American Association of Equine Practitioners: *Equine infectious disease outbreak: AAEP outbreak guidelines.* Available at http://www.aaep.org/control_guidelines.

American Association of Equine Practitioners: *Equine vaccination guidelines.* Available at http://www.aaep.org/vaccination_guidelines.htm.

Patel JR, et al: Equine herpesvirus 1 (EHV1) and 4 (EHV4) epidemiology, disease, and immunoprophylaxis: a brief review. *Vet J* 170:14–23, 2005.

Slater J: Equine herpesviruses. In Sellon DC, Long MT, editors: *Equine infectious diseases*, St Louis, 2007, Elsevier, pp 134–153.

Wong DM, Belgrave RL, Williams KJ, et al: Multinodular pulmonary fibrosis in five horses. *J Am Vet Med Assoc* 232:898–905, 2008

AUTHOR: **KATHY K. SEINO**

EDITORS: **DEBRA C. SELLON** and **MAUREEN T. LONG**

Histoplasmosis

BASIC INFORMATION

DEFINITION

- A systemic fungal infection of horses caused by the fungus *Histoplasma capsulatum* that may result in pulmonary disease, abdominal or gastrointestinal disease, placentitis and abortion, or disseminated disease

EPIDEMIOLOGY

SPECIES, AGE, SEX
- No known age, sex, or breed predilection

RISK FACTORS
- Immune compromise
- Residing in or traveling through endemic areas.

CONTAGION AND ZOONOSIS
- People in endemic regions are at risk of exposure and disease.
- Concurrent common source infection of humans and animals has been observed.
- There is no evidence of direct transmission of histoplasmosis from animals to humans.

GEOGRAPHY AND SEASONALITY
- In the United States, histoplasmosis is endemic in the Mississippi, Missouri, and Ohio River valleys; southwestern and eastern Ontario to Montreal, Ottawa; and the St. Lawrence River valley.

CLINICAL PRESENTATION

DISEASE FORMS/SUBTYPES
- Pulmonary disease is most common
- Abdominal or gastrointestinal disease
- Placentitis and abortion
- Disseminated disease

HISTORY, CHIEF COMPLAINT
- Weight loss
- Depression
- Dyspnea
- Edema
- Diarrhea
- Abortion, neonatal death

PHYSICAL EXAM FINDINGS
- Vary depending on the site of infection
- Fever, poor body condition, depression
- Dyspnea, increased respiratory rate, abnormal lung sounds
- Diarrhea, abdominal pain

ETIOLOGY AND PATHOPHYSIOLOGY
- In nature, *H. capsulatum*, a dimorphic ascomycete, exists as a filamentous fungus.
- At 37° C, microconidia germinate and form mycelia that are transformed into small, budding, oval yeasts.
- In nature, the organism is found in bat and bird guano, especially that of chickens and starlings.
- Infection occurs by inhalation of microconidia that germinate in vivo to the yeast form.
- Immune competent hosts can usually control the organism with a cell-mediated immune response.
- Many horses in endemic areas are seropositive with no evidence of disease.
- Exposure to a large inoculum may result in disease in immune competent hosts.

DIAGNOSIS

DIFFERENTIAL DIAGNOSIS
- Varies depending on the site of infection

INITIAL DATABASE
- Usually evidence of chronic infection and inflammation
- With gastrointestinal disease, panhypoproteinemia is often observed.

ADVANCED OR CONFIRMATORY TESTING
- Observation of organism in tissue samples stained with Gömöri methenamine silver or periodic acid-Schiff.
- Culture of the organism remains the gold standard for diagnosis.
- Serology: Immunodiffusion and complement fixation test results are usually positive but do not provide a definitive diagnosis.
- Antigen detection in blood, urine, and other body fluids may provide a diagnosis.
- Intradermal testing with histoplasmin is not diagnostically useful because of the large number of false-positive reactions.

TREATMENT

THERAPEUTIC GOAL(S)

- Eliminate infection.

ACUTE GENERAL TREATMENT

- Systemic antifungal therapy is recommended.
- Disease is rare, so there is minimal information on individual drug efficacy.
- Amphotericin B, itraconazole, or both may be used.

- Therapy may need to be continued for many weeks.

PROGNOSIS AND OUTCOME

Histoplasmosis is a rare disease in horses, and data are insufficient to draw conclusions about equine treatment. Treatment of affected horses has been infrequently attempted because of the severity of clinical signs, failure to make the diagnosis, expense of treatment, and concerns of a poor prognosis for recovery from fungal disease.

SUGGESTED READING

Kohn C: Miscellaneous fungal diseases. In Sellon DC, Long MT, editors: *Equine infectious diseases*, St Louis, 2007, Elsevier, pp 431–445.

AUTHOR & EDITOR: **DEBRA C. SELLON**

EDITOR: **MAUREEN T. LONG**

Hoary Alyssum Toxicosis

BASIC INFORMATION

DEFINITION

Characterized by limb edema and laminitis, hoary alyssum toxicity occurs primarily in horses grazing the plants in pastures or eating the plants when incorporated in hay.

SYNONYM(S)

Hoary alyssum (*Berteroa incana*), hoary false madwort

EPIDEMIOLOGY

SPECIES, AGE, SEX Horses are the only domestic animals affected by hoary alyssum.
RISK FACTORS The plants are toxic when green and remain toxic for months when dried in hay. Overgrazing favors the invasiveness of this weed.
GEOGRAPHY AND SEASONALITY *B. incana*, a member of the Brassicaceae family, is an annual, biennial, or perennial introduced weed that has become naturalized in most areas of North America. Stems are gray-green, hairy (hoary), 1 to 3 feet tall, with many branches near the top. Leaves are gray-green, hairy, alternate, oblong, narrow, 0.5 to 3 inches long, with smooth edges. Flowers are white with four deeply divided petals. Seed pods are hairy and oblong with short beaks on the end (Figure 1).

CLINICAL PRESENTATION

HISTORY, CHIEF COMPLAINT Edematous swelling of the legs, lameness and, in severe cases, laminitis
PHYSICAL EXAM FINDINGS Lameness caused by distal limb edema and laminitis is a typical sign of hoary alyssum poisoning. Experimentally horses fed hay containing 30% hoary alyssum develop pyrexia, an increased digital pulse, and limb edema within 24 hours. Severe lami-

nitis with rotation of the third phalanx may occur in severe cases. Red-colored urine (hemoglobinuria) as a result of red blood cell hemolysis and hemorrhagic diarrhea have been reported in pregnant mares fed alfalfa hay containing hoary alyssum. Late-term abortion is reported in pregnant mares. Death may occur in 1% to 2% of natural cases of hoary alyssum poisoning.
ETIOLOGY AND PATHOPHYSIOLOGY The toxin responsible for the limb edema and laminitis is not known.

DIAGNOSIS

DIFFERENTIAL DIAGNOSIS

- Laminitis secondary to grain overload, fever, sustained trauma to the feet
- Black walnut intoxication
- Congestive heart failure with peripheral edema
- Edema of the legs secondary to photosensitization affecting the white-skinned areas

INITIAL DATABASE

- Complete blood count: Hemolytic anemia.
- Serum biochemical analysis: Serum bilirubin, urea nitrogen, and creatinine elevated
- Urine analysis: Hemoglobinuria, proteinuria

ADVANCED OR CONFIRMATORY TESTING

Radiography to assess the severity of laminitis

TREATMENT

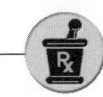

THERAPEUTIC GOAL(S)

Remove the source of hoary alyssum

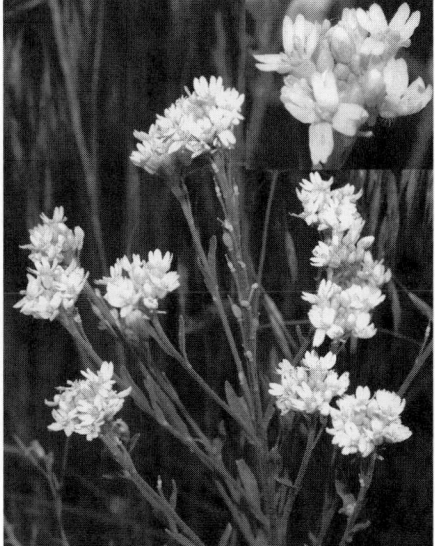

FIGURE 1 Hoary alyssum (*Berteroa incana*).

ACUTE GENERAL TREATMENT

- Antiinflammatory and analgesic therapy: Flunixin meglumine, or phenylbutazone
- Cold water hydrotherapy for the swollen legs
- Supportive therapy, including IV fluids and electrolytes is indicated in severe cases

CHRONIC TREATMENT

Appropriate hoof care to manage the chronic effects of laminitis

POSSIBLE COMPLICATIONS

- Rotation of the third phalanx in severely laminitic feet
- Abortion in late-term pregnant mares

PROGNOSIS AND OUTCOME

Early recognition and removing the horses from hoary alyssum immediately favors a rapid recovery.

PEARLS & CONSIDERATIONS

COMMENTS

Hoary alyssum is an aggressive invasive weed of hay meadows and should not be allowed to become established.

PREVENTION

Feed weed-free hay whenever possible.

CLIENT EDUCATION

- Educate clients so they can recognize hoary alyssum in pastures and hay.
- Application of herbicides (2,4-dichlorophenoxyacetic acid) according to label directions before the plants bloom is effective in controlling hoary alyssum. Preventing the plant from producing seed will stop the spread of hoary alyssum.

SUGGESTED READING

Geor RJ, Becker RL, Kanara EW, et al: Toxicosis in horses after ingestion of hoary alyssum. *J Am Vet Med Assoc* 201:63–67, 1992.

Hovda LR, Rose ML: Hoary alyssum (*Berteroa incana*) toxicity in a herd of broodmare horses. *Vet Hum Toxicol* 3539–3540, 1993.

Jacobs J, Mangold J: *Ecology and management of hoary alyssum (Berteroa incana (L.) DC.)*, 2008. Available at http://www.plant-materials.nrcs.usda.gov/pubs/mtpmstn8346.pdf.

AUTHOR: **ANTHONY P. KNIGHT**

EDITOR: **CYNTHIA L. GASKILL**

Hydronephrosis

BASIC INFORMATION

DEFINITION

Distension and dilation of the kidney and renal pelvis caused by obstruction of urine flow (Figure 1)

EPIDEMIOLOGY

SPECIES, AGE, SEX

- Males are predisposed to urolithiasis in general.
- Urolithiasis is typically seen in adult horses, with a mean age of 10 years.

RISK FACTORS

- Obstructive urinary tract disease of any cause
- Uroliths (calculi) are the most common cause of urinary tract obstruction, although neoplasia, trauma, or urinary tract displacement may also obstruct urine flow.

ASSOCIATED CONDITIONS AND DISORDERS

- Chronic renal failure
- Urolithiasis
- Neoplasia

CLINICAL PRESENTATION

DISEASE FORMS/SUBTYPES Complete or incomplete obstruction may occur, and signs may be acute or chronic.

HISTORY, CHIEF COMPLAINT

- Complete obstruction typically results in moderate to severe abdominal pain (colic).
- Incomplete obstruction typically results in mild, intermittent abdominal pain or no clinical signs.
- Many horses present for signs consistent with chronic renal failure (anorexia, lethargy, weight loss).

PHYSICAL EXAM FINDINGS The physical examination may be unremarkable, consistent with signs of abdominal pain (eg, tachycardia, tachypnea), or consistent with signs of renal failure (eg, poor hair coat and body condition, excessive dental tartar).

ETIOLOGY AND PATHOPHYSIOLOGY

- Urinary flow is obstructed, primarily via nephroliths or ureteroliths.
- Outflow obstruction causes a backflow of urine and increased pressure in the kidney, resulting in renal distension and dilatation of the renal pelvis.
- Postrenal azotemia and chronic renal failure occurs with occlusion of urinary outflow, backpressure in the collecting system, and resultant decreased renal blood flow.
- A retrospective study reported uroliths in the kidneys (22%; 53% bilaterally) and ureters (3%; 50% bilaterally) of affected horses. Approximately 9% of horses had urolithiasis in more than one location.

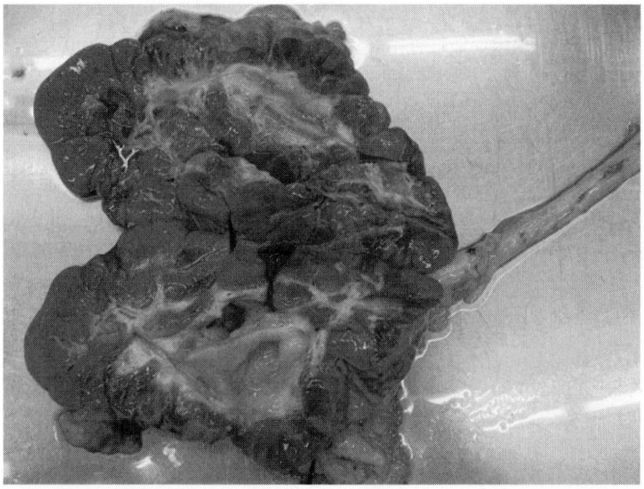

DIAGNOSIS

DIFFERENTIAL DIAGNOSIS

- Any urinary tract obstruction (urolithiasis)
- Gastrointestinal disease (if showing signs of abdominal pain)
- Hepatic or renal disease (if vague signs consistent with renal failure)

INITIAL DATABASE

- Complete blood count: Typically unremarkable unless there is an infectious process present
- Serum chemistries: May have elevated blood urea nitrogen (BUN) and creatinine concentrations if the obstruction is bilateral or chronic and has

FIGURE 1 A left kidney with hydronephrosis and hydroureter. The ureter was obstructed with numerous small ureteroliths.

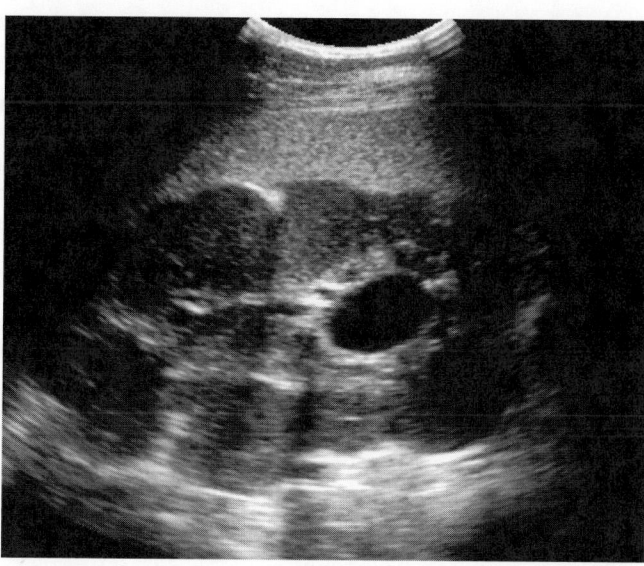

FIGURE 2 Ultrasound image of the kidney in Figure 1. The renal pelvis is dilated.

resulted in renal compromise or failure.

- Renal ultrasongraphy: Dilated ureter or renal pelvis. The affected kidney will likely be enlarged and dilated. Calculi may be present within the renal pelvis or ureter. Lesions may be unilateral or bilateral (Figure 2).
- Rectal examination: May be able to palpate an enlarged, dilated kidney or ureter

ADVANCED OR CONFIRMATORY TESTING

- Cystoscopy: Able to evaluate urine flow from both ureters. May be able to perform ureteroscopy if the ureter is dilated on the side of the affected kidney. May also observe the presence of calculi in the bladder or urethra as well as neoplasia or other sources of urinary tract obstruction.
- Urine culture: May be useful if there is an infectious component to the obstructive disease.
- Urinalysis: May reveal hematuria, proteinuria, and pyuria, especially in horses that also have cystic or urethral calculi. There may also be evidence of bacteriuria.

TREATMENT

THERAPEUTIC GOAL(S)

- Remove the source of obstruction.
- Prevent further obstruction.

ACUTE GENERAL TREATMENT

- Surgical removal of obstruction (typically nephrectomy): Nephrectomy should only be pursued if the disease is unilateral. Nephrostomy and ureterostomy have been rarely reported, with poor long-term outcomes. It is imperative that renal function is assessed before surgery because signs of chronic renal failure may not resolve after resolution of the obstruction.
- Medical treatment: Diuresis, antimicrobials, and dietary modification (low-calcium diet) have been used successfully in a few cases.

CHRONIC TREATMENT

- Attempt to prevent formation of additional uroliths that can cause urinary obstruction.
- Urinary acidification (efficacy is questionable in horses): Ammonium sulfate (175 mg/kg PO q12h), ammonium chloride (100 mg/kg PO q1–2h), or ascorbic acid (4 g PO q12h). Ascorbic acid has been reported to be more palatable.
- Increase water intake by adding salt to the diet (50–75 mg/day).
- Dietary modifications may be helpful, with the goal of reducing the intake of protein, calcium, phosphorous, and magnesium. This can be accomplished by feeding grass hay and avoiding legumes.

POSSIBLE COMPLICATIONS

Chronic renal failure is a common sequela to hydronephrosis.

RECOMMENDED MONITORING

Monitor BUN and creatinine concentrations as well as clinical condition.

PROGNOSIS AND OUTCOME

- Horses with signs of chronic renal failure have a poor prognosis.
- Nephrectomy has been associated with a good prognosis if the disease is unilateral and contralateral renal function is normal.
- Recurrence of urolithiasis is common in horses, so there remains a risk for future obstructive events.

PEARLS & CONSIDERATIONS

COMMENTS

The majority of hydronephrosis cases are diagnosed after the horse is already in chronic renal failure.

PREVENTION

Optimize renal health (judicious use of nephrotoxic drugs, maintenance of hydration) to minimize the risk of urolithiasis and obstructive urinary tract disease.

SUGGESTED READING

Duesterdieck-Zellmer K: Equine urolithiasis. *Vet Clin North Am Equine Pract* 23:613–629, 2007.
Macbeth B: Obstructive urolithiasis, unilateral hydronephrosis and probable nephrolithiasis in a 12-year-old Clydesdale gelding. *Can Vet J* 49:287–290, 2008.
Waldridge B: Disorders of the urinary system. In Reed S, Bayly WM, Sellon DC, editors: *Equine internal medicine*, ed 3, St Louis, 2010, Saunders, pp 1140–1247.

AUTHOR: KELLY L. CARLSON

EDITOR: BRYAN M. WALDRIDGE

Hymen, Persistent

BASIC INFORMATION

DEFINITION
The hymen is a sheet of tissue separating the vagina and the vestibular vault, just cranial to the urethral meatus.

SYNONYM(S)
Imperforate hymen

EPIDEMIOLOGY
SPECIES, AGE, SEX It may be identified in the maiden mare during routine vaginal examination.
GENETICS AND BREED PREDISPOSITION Persistent hymen is one of the most common congenital reproductive anomalies seen in mares.
ASSOCIATED CONDITIONS AND DISORDERS Conditions related to chromosomal or genetic defects such as vaginal hypoplasia and aplasia.

CLINICAL PRESENTATION
HISTORY, CHIEF COMPLAINT
- May manifest as a pink mass protruding from the vulva of a recumbent maiden female
- May manifest as infertility (failure of intrauterine semen deposition)
PHYSICAL EXAM FINDINGS Digital palpation of the persistent hymen (wrist deep in the vestibular vault)
ETIOLOGY AND PATHOPHYSIOLOGY A persistent or imperforate hymen results from the failure of this tissue to naturally break at the time of breeding or artificial insemination. Could also be considered a form of segmental aplasia as a result of an embryonic malunion of the paramesonephric (Müllerian) ducts and the ectodermal urogenital sinus.

DIAGNOSIS
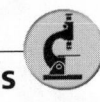

DIFFERENTIAL DIAGNOSIS
- Hypoplasia of the tubular reproductive tract at the level of the vestibular vaginal junction
- Vaginal mural adhesions
- Vaginal septum: This is a band of tissue that may be found running from the dorsal to ventral vaginal surfaces. A vaginal septum results from failure of proper fusion of the paramesonephric ducts.

INITIAL DATABASE
Visualization of the persistent hymen by vaginoscopic examination (presence of a blind-ending short vagina with no visible cervix)

ADVANCED OR CONFIRMATORY TESTING
Transrectal ultrasound examination of the reproductive tract may show the cranial portion of the vagina filled with fluid as a result of mucus accumulation.

TREATMENT

THERAPEUTIC GOAL
Perforate the hymen to allow future successful breeding

ACUTE GENERAL TREATMENT
- When identified in maiden mares during routine examination, the hymen can be broken with firm steady pressure and digital dilatation.
- Sometimes the persistent hymen may be so tough that it may need to be ruptured with a guarded scalpel blade or scissors, then enlarged by using the fingers and hand.
- Laser ablation or electrocautery fulguration may be useful when available.

POSSIBLE COMPLICATIONS
It is very important to identify and isolate the location of the urethra as to avoid any damage to it, specifically the dorsal wall, while working to transect the hymen.

PROGNOSIS AND OUTCOME

This condition has no adverse effect on fertility once corrected.

PEARLS & CONSIDERATIONS

Twice daily application of a soft emollient cream (such as udder balm), phenylephrine ointment, topical antibiotics, and/or steroid-impregnated ointments can help prevent mural adhesions.

SUGGESTED READING
Pycock J, Ricketts S: *Perineal and cervical abnormalities.* Proceedings of the 10th International Congress of World Equine Veterinary Association, 2008, pp 257–265
McCue P: The problem mare: management philosophy, diagnostic procedures, and therapeutic options. *J Equine Vet Sci* 28(11):619–626, 2008.
Steenholdt C: Infertility due to noninflammatory abnormalities of the tubular reproductive tract. In Youngquist R, Threlfall W, editors: *Current therapy in large animal theriogenology,* ed 2, St Louis, 2007, Saunders Elsevier, pp 383–387.

AUTHOR: **HERNÁN J. MONTILLA**

EDITOR: **JUAN C. SAMPER**

Hyperparathyroidism

BASIC INFORMATION

DEFINITION
A pathologic condition characterized by excessive secretion of parathyroid hormone (PTH) by the parathyroid glands, hypercalcemia, and bone loss. Hyperparathyroidism can be primary or secondary (nutritional).

SYNONYM(S)
Osteodystrophia fibrosa, equine osteoporosis

EPIDEMIOLOGY
SPECIES, AGE, SEX
- Hyperparathyroidism has been reported in horses of all ages.
- Clinical signs of hyperparathyroidism secondary to nutritional imbalances are more evident in young, growing animals.
- In nutritional hyperparathyroidism, many horses can be affected in one farm, but only one horse is affected in primary hyperparathyroidism.

GEOGRAPHY AND SEASONALITY

- There is no information on seasonality.
- There are no geographical differences for primary hyperparathyroidism.
- Nutritional secondary hyperparathyroidism remains a problem in developing countries, where appropriate nutritional management of horses is lacking.

CLINICAL PRESENTATION

DISEASE FORMS/SUBTYPES

- Hyperparathyroidism may be primary or secondary.
  - Primary hyperparathyroidism: An autonomous and excessive secretion of PTH from the parathyroid glands. The parathyroid glands in these horses are not responsive to calcium concentrations (refractory).
  - In secondary hyperparathyroidism, the inciting cause of excessive PTH secretion is not in the parathyroid gland but rather the result of unbalanced nutrition or renal disease.
  - Secondary hyperparathyroidism in horses is primarily nutritional (nutritional secondary hyperparathyroidism).
  - Renal secondary hyperparathyroidism has not been reported in horses.
- Another condition associated with abnormal calcium and phosphorus concentrations is humoral hypercalcemia of malignancy (HHM; pseudohyperparathyroidism).

HISTORY, CHIEF COMPLAINT

- Signs of hyperparathyroidism include weight loss, anorexia, soft tissue mineralization, lameness, angular deformities, pathological fractures, facial enlargement (osteodystrophia fibrosa), and polyuria and polydipsia.

PHYSICAL EXAM FINDINGS

- Horses with nutritional secondary hyperparathyroidism (also termed *big head, Miller's disease*) may have generalized swelling of the skull and narrowing of the nasal meatus, which may lead to upper airway stridor.
- Whereas facial changes or deformations are evident in young animals, lameness and decreased bone mass are the main findings in old horses.

ETIOLOGY AND PATHOPHYSIOLOGY

- Under physiological conditions, PTH is secreted by the chief cells of the parathyroid gland in response to hypocalcemia.
- PTH increases renal reabsorption of calcium, renal excretion of phosphorus, and bone resorption by osteoclasts.
- The cause of primary hyperparathyroidism in horses remains unknown because few cases have been documented.
- In nutritional secondary hyperparathyroidism, the parathyroid glands secrete PTH in response to excessive dietary phosphorus and oxalates or low dietary calcium.
- Dietary phosphate and oxalate bind calcium to decrease its absorption.
- Low calcium leads to hypocalcemia and PTH secretion.
- Excessive phosphorus in the diet also results in hyperphosphatemia, which stimulates PTH secretion. High phosphorus levels may precipitate calcium in the extracellular compartment, contributing to hypocalcemia and soft tissue mineralization.
- In renal hyperparathyroidism, hypovitaminosis D and hyperphosphatemia from renal dysfunction result in excessive PTH secretion. Unlike in small animals, renal secondary hyperparathyroidism has not been reported in horses.
- Of interest, horses with chronic renal disease also develop hypercalcemia, which is the result of decreased glomerular filtration and calcium retention (the equine kidney eliminates large amounts of calcium) because PTH concentrations in these horses are normal.
- In horses with pseudohyperparathyroidism (HHM) the clinical signs are the result of the malignancy rather than hypercalcemia. In HHM, there is excessive secretion of parathyroid hormone–related protein (PTHrP), which interacts with the PTH receptor to increase renal reabsorption of calcium and bone resorption, resulting in hypercalcemia.

DIAGNOSIS

DIFFERENTIAL DIAGNOSIS

- HHM
- Chronic renal failure
- Equine systemic granulomatous disease
- Hypervitaminosis D (plants, iatrogenic)
- Malignancies that secrete vitamin D

INITIAL DATABASE

- Measurement of serum PTH, ionized calcium, phosphorus concentrations, and serum and urine chemistry; determination of the fractional excretion of calcium and phosphorus; radiography; and measurement of plasma PTHrP concentrations
- Horses with primary hyperparathyroidism have hypercalcemia, hypophosphatemia, hyperphosphaturia, and increased serum PTH concentrations.
- Horses with secondary hyperparathyroidism have normocalcemia or hypercalcemia, normophosphatemia or hyperphosphatemia, hyperphosphaturia, and increased PTH concentrations.
- Plasma PTHrP concentrations are normal in both conditions.

- Markers of bone resorption have been determined in horses with bone diseases, but their use remains impractical.
- Radiography may be helpful in assessing bone density; mineralization of soft tissues, tendons, and ligaments; and fractures.
- Scintigraphy has been proposed for the diagnosis of primary hyperparathyroidism.

TREATMENT

ACUTE GENERAL TREATMENT

- There is no specific treatment for primary hyperparathyroidism.
- Surgical excision of the affected parathyroid gland may be performed. However, the variable location of the parathyroid glands may require scintigraphy to localize them.
- The use of glucocorticoids to decrease intestinal calcium absorption and to increase renal calcium elimination has been proposed.

CHRONIC TREATMENT

- Restrict access to pastures rich in oxalates and diets high in phosphorus.
- Animals in pastures rich in oxalates may require calcium supplementation (calcium carbonate, dicalcium phosphate).

PROGNOSIS AND OUTCOME

- Depends on clinical signs
- Growing animals with nutritional hyperparathyroidism may improve (6 months), but facial deformation may remain.
- Animals with soft tissue mineralization, particularly of the internal organs, have a poor prognosis.

PEARLS & CONSIDERATIONS

CLIENT EDUCATION

- The disease is incurable.
- Secondary infections are common.

SUGGESTED READING

Toribio RE: Disorders of calcium and phosphorus. In Reed SM, Bayly WM, Sellon DC, editors: *Equine internal medicine*, ed 3, St Louis, 2010, Saunders Elsevier, pp 1277–1291.

AUTHOR & EDITOR: **RAMIRO E. TORIBIO**

Hyperthermia

BASIC INFORMATION

DEFINITION

An increase in body temperature without an alteration in the body temperature set point

EPIDEMIOLOGY

Caused by an increase in heat production, impaired heat loss, or absorption of heat beyond the ability of the body to compensate

GENETICS AND BREED PREDISPOSITION

- Quarter Horses are genetically prone to malignant hyperthermia (MH).
- Draft horses are predisposed to anhydrosis, which can induce hyperthermia.

GEOGRAPHY AND SEASONALITY Hot, humid weather may predispose to heat stroke as well as anhydrosis.

CLINICAL PRESENTATION

DISEASE FORMS/SUBTYPES

- Heat stroke (Figure 1)
- Exercise- or seizure-related hyperthermia

- Anhydrosis
- MH
- Drug or toxin reaction
- Central nervous system (CNS) disorders

HISTORY, CHIEF COMPLAINT

- Depression
- Excessive sweating or unusual lack thereof
- Increased respiratory rate
- Seizures
- Weakness or collapse

PHYSICAL EXAM FINDINGS

- Elevated rectal temperature (>106° F)
- Altered mentation

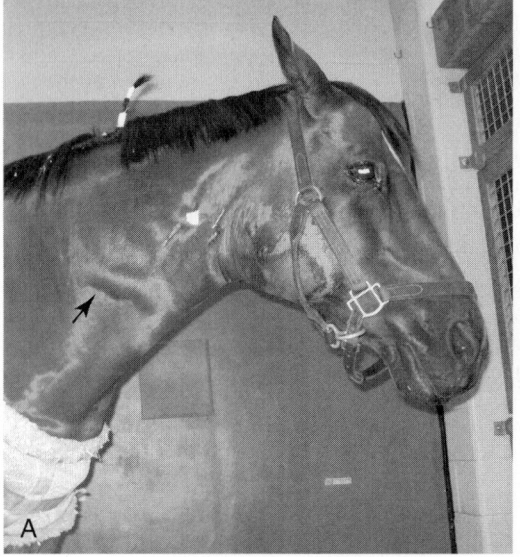
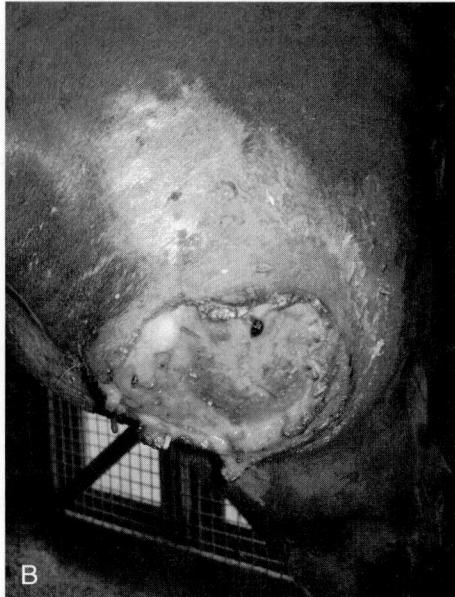
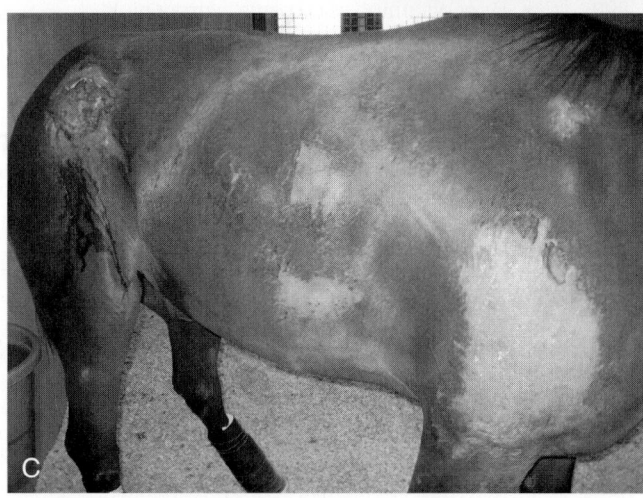

FIGURE 1 The consequences of heat stroke after becoming tangled in a fence in right lateral recumbency. **A** shows the acute edema of the neck (*arrow*) and localized swelling in the throatlatch. **B** (right mandible) and **C** (right flank) were taken 10 days later, where extensive tissue necrosis has occurred. Coagulation abnormalities were noted by increased bleeding times and right jugular thrombosis. Acute laminitis without rotation also developed.

- Hyperemic mucous membranes ± a toxic line
- Tachycardia
- Tachypnea
- Petechiation
- Myopathy
- Synchronous diaphragmatic flutter

ETIOLOGY AND PATHOPHYSIOLOGY

Depends on the initiating cause of hyperthermia:

- Heat stroke occurs when environmental factors elevate the body temperature above 107° F (41.5° C).
  - Sweating and dehydration may increase the risk because of electrolyte imbalances.
  - Vasoconstriction, reduced cardiac output, and decreased blood pressure initiate circulatory shock and may lead to disseminated intravascular coagulation (DIC), multiorgan failure, and death.
- Anhydrosis is caused by the loss of the ability to sweat.
  - Unknown etiology
  - Draft foals may be susceptible
  - Hot, humid climates predispose
- MH is caused in Quarter Horses by a mutation in exon 46 of the skeletal muscle ryanodine receptor gene, which alters calcium metabolism. Muscle hypermetabolism is triggered by halogenated inhalation anesthetics, depolarizing skeletal muscle relaxants, and stress.
- The antibiotic erythromycin increases the risk of hyperthermia, which may be triggered by exposure to direct sunlight. The causative mechanism has not been determined.
- Any condition that affects the hypothalamus (eg, hemorrhage, neoplasia, abscess) may prevent sweating and promote an excessive response to external cooling.

DIAGNOSIS

DIFFERENTIAL DIAGNOSIS

- Fever
  - An alteration in the body's hypothalamic set point for thermoregulation
  - Differentials include infectious, inflammatory, immunologic, and neoplastic diseases
  - All causes of fever induce a release of endogenous pyrogens, which stimulate the hypothalamus to increase heat production and conservation.

INITIAL DATABASE

- Physical examination
- Neurological examination
- Packed cell volume (PCV)
- Complete blood count
- Serum chemistry, including electrolytes

- Coagulation panel (activated partial thromboplastin time, prothrombin time, platelet count)
- Lactate
- Urinalysis

ADVANCED OR CONFIRMATORY TESTING

- Ephedrine or terbutaline challenge test for anhydrosis
  - Affected horses do not sweat
    - 0.1 mL SC 1:1000 epinephrine
    - 0.5 mg intradermal terbutaline
- Genetic testing for MH

TREATMENT

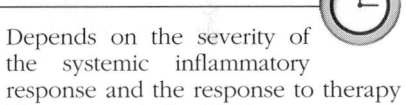

THERAPEUTIC GOALS

- Lower the core body temperature to an acceptable range.
- Treat the primary disease process.
- Prevent or treat unwanted sequelae, including coagulation disorders and renal insufficiency.

ACUTE GENERAL TREATMENT

- For hyperthermia caused by heat stroke, overexertion, anhydrosis, medications, toxins, or CNS disorders:
  - Remove the animal from high ambient temperature (if an instigating cause).
  - Cool the animal internally and externally.
    - Initiate internal cooling with room temperature IV fluids. Correct electrolyte abnormalities.
    - External cooling (misting and fans) may augment temperature reduction.
      - Avoid ice and large volumes of cold water externally because vasoconstriction may hinder heat loss. Room temperature water is better.
      - Alcohol may be used sparingly if water is not available or in high humidity. Large volumes of external alcohol and its fumes can be fatal.
      - Stop cooling when temperature reaches 103° F to prevent hypothermia.
  - Administer flunixin meglumine (1.1 mg/kg q12h IV) for antipyretic and antiendotoxin effects.
  - Plasma may be administered for clotting factors and an antiendotoxin effect.
  - Cerebral edema may be treated with hypertonic saline or mannitol. Use only 3% hypertonic (half strength) in endurance horses because of extreme cellular swelling.
  - Seizures may be controlled with IV diazepam (adults, 0.05–0.44 mg/kg; foals, 0.1–0.2 mg/kg) or IV phenobarbital (5–15 mg/kg slowly).

- MH: Treatment is often ineffective, but external cooling, mechanical ventilation, and room temperature fluid resuscitation should be attempted.
- For mild exercise-induced hyperthermia, inactivity or rest typically reduces the temperature to an acceptable range.

CHRONIC TREATMENT

- Treat the primary disease process.
- Provide a more temperate climate or air conditioning for horses with anhydrosis.

POSSIBLE COMPLICATIONS

- Disseminated intravascular coagulation
- Cerebral edema
- Renal failure with severe dehydration
- Laminitis may result from systemic inflammation

RECOMMENDED MONITORING

- PCV
- Total protein
- Coagulation profile
- Platelet count
- Renal parameters: Blood urea nitrogen and creatinine
- Muscle enzymes: Creatine kinase and aspartate aminotransferase

PROGNOSIS AND OUTCOME

- Depends on the severity of the systemic inflammatory response and the response to therapy
- The prognosis for MH is poor.

PEARLS & CONSIDERATIONS

PREVENTION

- Horses with the genetic potential for MH should not receive halogenated anesthetics.
- Prophylaxis: Dantrolene (a skeletal muscle relaxant; 4 mg/kg 30–60 minutes before anesthesia PO)
- Endurance horses and other high-level athletes should be closely monitored for signs of heat exhaustion and dehydration.

CLIENT EDUCATION

- Clients should be educated as to the genetic potential and clinical signs for progressive anhydrosis.
- The risks of MH caused by local and general anesthesia should always be presented to the client before the procedure.

SUGGESTED READING

Divers TJ: Shock and temperature related problems. In Orsini JA, Divers TJ, editors: *Equine emergencies treatment and proce-* *dures*, St Louis, 2008, Saunders Elsevier, pp 556–557.

Finno CJ, Spier SJ, Valberg SJ: Equine diseases caused by known genetic mutations. *Vet J* 179(3):336–347, 2009.

AUTHOR: **AMELIA MUNSTERMAN**

EDITORS: **R. REID HANSON** and **AMELIA MUNSTERMAN**

Hyperthyroidism

BASIC INFORMATION

- The equine thyroid glands are two firm lobes located in the dorsolateral aspect of the third to sixth tracheal rings.
- In most healthy horses, the thyroid glands are not visible but are palpable.
- The follicular cells of the thyroid gland secrete two thyroid hormones (THs), thyroxine (T4) and triiodothyronine (T3).
- The synthesis and secretion of THs is regulated by a negative feedback system that includes the hypothalamus, pituitary gland, and thyroid gland (hypothalamus-pituitary-thyroid axis)
- Hypothalamic neurons release thyrotropin-releasing hormone (TRH), which stimulates thyrotropes in the pituitary gland to secrete thyroid-stimulating hormone (TSH, thyrotropin), which in turn increases the synthesis and secretion of THs by the follicular cells of the thyroid gland.
- Most of the THs released into circulation is T4, which is converted to active T3 by deiodinases.
- Circulating THs are T4, T3, and reverse T3 (rT3).
- Free T3 is the most active hormone.
- THs circulate free and bound to proteins.
- THs are important in cell growth, differentiation, and energy metabolism.
- An increase in THs leads to a hypermetabolic state; a decrease results in the opposite.

DEFINITION

Hyperthyroidism is defined as a hypermetabolic state, the result of high concentrations of free THs (T3, T4).

EPIDEMIOLOGY

SPECIES, AGE, SEX Most cases occur in performance horses and in horses older than 20 years.

GEOGRAPHY AND SEASONALITY No evidence that hyperthyroidism is associated with geography or season.

CLINICAL PRESENTATION

HISTORY, CHIEF COMPLAINT

- Horses with hyperthyroidism have a history of hyperexcitability, weight loss, polyphagia, and polydipsia.
- Thyroid gland enlargement may be present, although this rarely occurs.
- Anhidrosis and hyperhidrosis have been reported.
- Hyperthyroidism has not been documented in foals.
- In adult horses, there is a history of weight loss.
- There may be unilateral thyroid enlargement.
- Hyperexcitability, tachycardia, tachypnea, tremors, sweating, alopecia, polydipsia, anhidrosis, hyperhidrosis, enophthalmos, and weight loss have been described in horses suspected of hyperthyroidism.

ETIOLOGY AND PATHOPHYSIOLOGY

- There are few documented cases of equine hyperthyroidism.
- The disease can be spontaneous, associated with malignancies (thyroid adenocarcinoma), or iatrogenic from iodide-containing compounds (Jod-Basedow phenomenon) or administration of THs (thyrotoxicosis).
- Autoimmune hyperthyroidism has not been documented in horses.
- Clinical signs result from high TH concentrations.
- Most thyroid adenomas are nonfunctional tumors.

DIAGNOSIS

DIFFERENTIAL DIAGNOSIS

- Thyroid adenocarcinomas
- Unilateral nonfunctional adenomas are common and associated with aging.
- Parafollicular cell (C cell) adenomas, which in general are nonfunctional tumors
- Masses in the laryngeal area

INITIAL DATABASE

- Clinical history and clinical signs
- Biopsy
- Serum TH concentrations are elevated
- Important: Normal TH values depend on each laboratory

- TSH stimulation test
- T3 suppression test: T4 concentrations do not decrease after the administration T3 in hyperthyroid horses.
- TH concentrations in newborn foals are up to 10 times the values of adult horses, which may lead to misdiagnosis.

TREATMENT

ACUTE GENERAL TREATMENT

- Remove access to iodide-containing compounds.
- Thyroidectomy of affected gland
- Potassium iodide (1 g/d PO)
- Glucocorticoids in horses with severe clinical signs
- There is limited information on the use of the antithyroid drugs such as propylthiouracil and methimazole in horses with hyperthyroidism.
- Propylthiouracil (1–4 mg/kg/d PO) has been used in horses to decrease thyroid function.

PROGNOSIS AND OUTCOME

- Good
- Signs improve with surgical or medical treatment.

PEARLS & CONSIDERATIONS

CLIENT EDUCATION

- The use of compounds containing iodide may lead to hyperthyroidism.

SUGGESTED READING

Beuhaus BA: Thyroid glands. In Smith BP, editor: *Large animal internal medicine*, ed 4, St Louis, 2009, Mosby Elsevier, pp 1347–1351.

Toribio RE: Thyroid gland. In Reed SM, Bayly WM, Sellon DC, editors: *Equine internal medicine*, ed 3, St Louis, 2010, Saunders Elsevier, pp 1251–1260.

AUTHOR & EDITOR: **RAMIRO E. TORIBIO**

Hypogammaglobulinemia, Transient

BASIC INFORMATION

DEFINITION

A syndrome characterized by the delayed onset of immunoglobulin synthesis in newborn foals

EPIDEMIOLOGY

GENETICS AND BREED PREDISPOSITION Has been described in Thoroughbred and Arabian foals but has not been proven to be genetic in origin

CLINICAL PRESENTATION

HISTORY, CHIEF COMPLAINT
- Affected foals appear normal at birth but develop infections as maternal immunoglobulin levels decline.
- Recurrent opportunistic infections, especially diarrhea, arthritis, or respiratory disease.

ETIOLOGY AND PATHOPHYSIOLOGY
- At birth, foals are protected by maternal antibodies acquired through colostrum. These antibodies provide effective protection for 1 to 3 months, although their levels decline gradually.
- As maternal antibodies decline, the foal begins to make its own immunoglobulins. Under normal circumstances, the decline of maternal antibodies occurs at the same time as autologous antibody production begins, so there is no gap in protection.
- In transient hypogammaglobulinemia, there is a delay in autologous immunoglobulin synthesis, leaving the foal temporarily unprotected and susceptible to opportunistic bacterial infections.

DIAGNOSIS

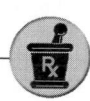

DIFFERENTIAL DIAGNOSIS
- Infections secondary to other primary immunodeficiencies such as severe combined immunodeficiency and agammaglobulinemia
- Failure of passive transfer

INITIAL DATABASE
- Complete blood count
- Serum chemistry profile
- Bacterial culture and sensitivity
- Serum immunoglobulin levels: At 2 to 4 months of age, all immunoglobulin classes and subclasses will be substantially below age-matched levels.

ADVANCED OR CONFIRMATORY TESTING
- Repeated serum immunoglobulin quantitation is required to document this condition and monitor the onset of immunoglobulin synthesis.
- Affected foals have normal blood lymphocytes, and T-cell function assays are normal.
- Lymphoid tissue structure is normal.

TREATMENT

THERAPEUTIC GOAL(S)
- Minimize opportunistic infections until the foal's immune system develops.
- Provide prompt immunologic treatment designed to remedy any immunologic deficit.
- Foals presenting with severe infections must be promptly addressed.

ACUTE GENERAL TREATMENT
- A total of 50 to 70 g of lyophilized equine immunoglobulin G (IgG) may be administered to increase serum IgG levels to greater than 400 mg/dL.
- If plasma transfusions are not given, then owners should be advised of the risks of infection and the foals maintained in an environment where exposure to potential pathogens is minimal.
- Frozen horse plasma is available commercially, although it may not contain antibodies against local pathogens.
- Plasma may be obtained from local donors. Blood should be collected aseptically with heparin or sodium citrate. The plasma is collected after the erythrocytes settle and is stored frozen until used. The plasma must be prechecked for antierythrocyte antibody and must be free of bacterial contamination. The transfusion should be given slowly while the foal is monitored for untoward reactions.
- All foals receiving plasma should have their IgG levels rechecked 12 to 24 hours later.
- Antibiotic treatment: A combination of a penicillin and an aminoglycoside is a good starting therapy. A suitable aminoglycoside, such as gentamicin (6.6–8.8 mg/kg IV or IM q24h) or amikacin (22–25 mg/kg IV or IM q24h), may be given.
- Other third-generation cephalosporins, such as cefotaxime (20–40 mg/kg IV or IM q6–8h), may also be used.
- Circulatory support: It is essential to maintain or restore effective circulating volume through aggressive IV fluid therapy. Administer fluids at the highest tolerated rate.
- Septicemic foals are hypoglycemic so dextrose should be provided.

CHRONIC TREATMENT
- Move the foal to as clean an environment as possible.
- Immunoglobulin preparations should be administered as required to maintain adequate blood levels.

RECOMMENDED MONITORING

Immunoglobulin levels must be monitored on a regular basis until they reach normal ranges.

PROGNOSIS AND OUTCOME

Prognosis is good provided bacterial and viral infections are well controlled.

PEARLS & CONSIDERATIONS

COMMENTS

The true prevalence of this disease is unclear. It may well be much more common than reported, and its severity and duration are highly variable.

PREVENTION

Because this disease is likely heritable, it is appropriate to discourage future breeding of the parent animals.

CLIENT EDUCATION

Provide advice on future breeding policies.

SUGGESTED READING

Baldwin JL, Cooper WL, Vanderwall DK, Erb HN: Prevalence (treatment days) and severity of illness in hypogammaglobulinemic and normogammaglobulinemic foals. *J Am Vet Med Assoc* 198:423–428, 1991.

Clabough DL, Clabough DL, Conboy HS, Roberts MC: Comparison of four screening techniques for the diagnosis of equine neonatal hypogammaglobulinemia. *J Am Vet Med Assoc* 194:1717–1720, 1989.

Davis DG, Schaefer DM, Hinchcliff KW, et al: Measurement of serum IgG in foals by radial immunodiffusion and automated turbidimetric immunoassay. *J Vet Intern Med* 19:93–96, 2005.

McGuire TC, Poppie MJ, Banks KL: Hypogammaglobulinemia predisposing to infection in foals. *J Am Vet Med Assoc* 166:71–75, 1975.

Riggs MW: Evaluation of foals for immune deficiency disorders. *Vet Clin North Am Equine Pract* 3:515–528, 1987.

AUTHOR & EDITOR: IAN TIZARD

Hypoparathyroidism

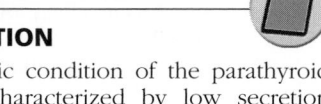

BASIC INFORMATION

DEFINITION
Pathologic condition of the parathyroid glands characterized by low secretion of parathyroid hormone (PTH), hypocalcemia, and hyperphosphatemia. Hypoparathyroidism can be primary or secondary.

SYNONYM(S)
Parathyroid gland dysfunction

CLINICAL PRESENTATION
DISEASE FORMS/SUBTYPES
- Hypoparathyroidism can be primary or secondary.
- Primary hypoparathyroidism: Few cases have been documented in horses. These horses have clinical signs consistent with hypocalcemia, including muscle tremors and fasciculations, synchronous diaphragmatic flutter (thumps), cardiac arrhythmias, hyperexcitability, seizures, ileus, and (in severe cases) death.
- In secondary hypoparathyroidism, parathyroid gland dysfunction is the consequence of a primary problem elsewhere, typically sepsis or hypomagnesemia.
- In sepsis, hypoparathyroidism may also be associated with high concentrations of inflammatory systemic mediators (interleukin-1 [IL-1]) that decrease parathyroid gland function in horses.
- In hypomagnesemia, hypoparathyroidism may be subclinical, and horses will not show improvement until magnesium is supplemented.

ETIOLOGY AND PATHOPHYSIOLOGY
- PTH is secreted by the chief cells of the parathyroid gland in response to hypocalcemia. PTH increases renal reabsorption of calcium and excretion of phosphorus. Thus, an appropriate response to hypocalcemia would be an increase in PTH concentrations.
- Horses with hypoparathyroidism have hypocalcemia and hyperphosphatemia and low or normal PTH concentrations. This is indicative of parathyroid gland dysfunction.
- The cause of primary hypoparathyroidism in horses remains unknown.

- Hypoparathyroidism secondary to sepsis occurs in horses.
- Inflammatory mediators such as IL-1 have been shown to decrease PTH secretion in horses.
- Hypomagnesemia is a frequent finding in critically ill horses.
- Magnesium is required for PTH secretion and PTH action.
- In hypomagnesemia, PTH concentrations are low until the magnesium status is restored.

DIAGNOSIS

DIFFERENTIAL DIAGNOSIS
- Acute renal failure
- Hypoproteinemia (pseudohypocalcemia)

INITIAL DATABASE
- Sepsis
- Clinical findings
- Measurement of serum PTH, ionized calcium, ionized magnesium, and phosphorus concentrations, serum and urine chemistry, and determination of the fractional excretion of calcium and phosphorus
- Horses with hypoparathyroidism have hypocalcemia, hyperphosphatemia, hypophosphaturia, and low serum PTH concentrations.
- Horses with hypocalcemia from acute renal failure may have hyperphosphatemia and elevated PTH concentrations.

TREATMENT

ACUTE GENERAL TREATMENT
- There is no specific treatment for primary hypoparathyroidism.
- Parenteral administration of calcium gluconate is the treatment of choice.
- Calcium gluconate 23% solution in crystalloid fluids (lactated Ringer's solution, 0.9% sodium chloride) can be administered safely to horses.
- Typical calcium gluconate rates are 50 to 100 mL/5 L of crystalloids. Horses with normal renal function can tolerate calcium gluconate rates of 200 mL/hr with no problem. This rate is rarely required.

- Determining serum ionized calcium concentrations helps to calculate the dose.
- Vitamin D supplementation should be considered, keeping in mind that this treatment may result in soft tissue mineralization.

CHRONIC TREATMENT
- Horses with recurrent hypocalcemia can be supplemented orally with calcium carbonate (100–200 g/d PO) or dicalcium phosphate.
- A number of horses may require frequent IV administration of calcium. These animals have a poor prognosis.

PROGNOSIS AND OUTCOME
- The prognosis depends on the clinical signs.
- In general, prognosis is poor because some horses may show improvement with medical treatment, but signs reoccur soon after discontinuation of calcium supplementation.
- Long-term supplementation with calcium carbonate or dicalcium phosphate may be necessary.

PEARLS & CONSIDERATIONS

CLIENT EDUCATION
A number of horses may require frequent IV administration of calcium. These animals have a poor prognosis.

SUGGESTED READING
Toribio RE: Disorders of calcium and phosphorus. In Reed SM, Bayly WM, Sellon DC, editors: *Equine internal medicine*, ed 3, St Louis, 2010, Saunders Elsevier, pp 1277–1291.

Toribio RE, Kohn CW, Capen CC, et al: Parathyroid hormone (PTH) secretion, PTH mRNA and calcium-sensing receptor mRNA expression in equine parathyroid cells, and effects of interleukin (IL)-1, IL-6, and tumor necrosis factor-alpha on equine parathyroid cell function. *J Mol Endocrinol* 31:609–620, 2003.

AUTHOR & EDITOR: RAMIRO E. TORIBIO

Hypothyroidism

BASIC INFORMATION

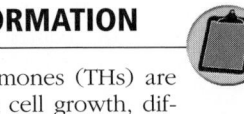

- Thyroid hormones (THs) are important in cell growth, differentiation, and energy metabolism.
- Development of the skeletal, nervous, and respiratory systems are highly dependent on THs.
- Low concentrations of THs do not mean hypothyroidism.
- Nonthyroidal diseases decrease THs but do not mean the horse has hypothyroidism; the horse may actually have nonthyroidal illness syndrome (euthyroid sick syndrome).
- Functional tests are required to assess thyroid gland function.

DEFINITION

- Hypothyroidism is defined as a deficiency of THs or a disruption of the hypothalamus-pituitary-thyroid axis.
- Hypothyroidism can be primary when there is thyroid gland disease or secondary to hypothalamic or pituitary dysfunction.

SYNONYM(S)

Thyroprivia

EPIDEMIOLOGY

SPECIES, AGE, SEX Most cases occur in newborn foals; rarely occurs in adult horses

GEOGRAPHY AND SEASONALITY

- Prevalence can be higher in iodide deficient areas and in regions with high concentrations of nitrates in the water or pasture.
- Congenital hypothyroidism is endemic in areas of western Canada and the United States.

CLINICAL PRESENTATION

HISTORY, CHIEF COMPLAINT

- Foals: Prematurity, weakness, incoordination, hypothermia, poor suckle reflex, musculoskeletal abnormalities (physeal dysgenesis, defective ossification of carpal and tarsal bones, extensor tendon rupture, flexural deformities), prognathism, goiter, respiratory distress, failure to thrive, and death. Thyroid enlargement may be present at birth (congenital goiter).
- Adults: Hair coat abnormalities, poor performance, infertility, lethargy, obesity, laminitis

ETIOLOGY AND PATHOPHYSIOLOGY

- In general, the cause of the problem is not identified

- Foals:
  - In fetuses and newborn foals, THs are required for the development and differentiation of various body systems, including the nervous, musculoskeletal, and pulmonary systems.
  - Neuronal differentiation and myelin synthesis are highly dependent on THs.
  - Chondrocyte and osteoblast proliferation and differentiation depend on THs.
  - Pulmonary maturation, including surfactant production, requires THs.
  - Deficient or excessive iodide intake by the mare may lead to hypothyroidism in a newborn foal.
  - Endophyte (*Neotyphodium coenophialum*)–infected fescue plants may decrease thyroid gland function in pregnant mares and their foals.
  - Hypothyroidism is associated with abnormal development of the growth plates and the carpal and tarsal bones, angular and flexural deformities, weakness, maladjustment, and respiratory failure.
  - Recovery in these foals is unlikely because many critical developmental stages are passed at birth.
- Adults:
  - Inadequate or excessive ingestion of iodide in the diet or topical treatments with iodide-containing compounds may lead to hypothyroidism (Wolff-Chaikoff effect).
  - TH deficiency in adults is associated with a hypometabolic state that results in obesity, lethargy, poor appetite, poor performance, hypothermia, anhidrosis, anemia, laminitis, hair loss, and infertility.

DIAGNOSIS

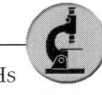

- Measurement of baseline THs have limited value.
- Thyroid stimulation tests are more appropriate for the diagnosis of hypothyroidism
- Foals: Elevated serum concentrations of THs are normal in foals (serum triiodothyronine [T3] concentrations in newborn foals are ≤10% of adult values), which can lead to misdiagnosis.
- Adults
  - Measurement of T3 and thyroxine (T4) concentrations
  - Response to thyroid-stimulating hormone (TSH) or thyrotropin-

releasing hormone (TRH) stimulation tests
- Animals with normal thyroid function should have a twofold increase in T3 at 2 hours and T4 at 4 hours after TSH or TRH administration.
- Factors affecting the diagnosis
  - Low TH concentrations have limited clinical value in horses because they can be decreased with various pathological conditions, but it does not imply hypothyroidism. This is known as the nonthyroidal illness syndrome (euthyroid sick syndrome).
  - Nutrition: Feed deprivation and anorexia decrease TH concentrations; high-carbohydrate and high-protein diets increase THs.
  - Stress decreases THs.
  - Exercise and cold weather increase THs.
  - Age: THs are several-fold higher in foals.
  - Drugs:
    - Dexamethasone: One dose can decrease THs for 5 days
    - Phenylbutazone: One dose can decrease THs for up to 10 days. This does not mean the horse has hypothyroidism.
  - These drugs are often used in equine practice; not knowing their effect on thyroid function can lead to misdiagnosis.

DIFFERENTIAL DIAGNOSIS

- Adults: Equine metabolic syndrome, Cushing's disease, obesity, laminitis, infertility
- Foals: Sudden death, prematurity or dysmaturity, developmental orthopedic diseases

TREATMENT

ACUTE GENERAL TREATMENT

- Adults
  - Iodinated casein: 5 g PO q24h
  - Levothyroxine sodium: 1 to 6 mg/ 100 kg PO q24h
  - T3: 1 mg/kg PO q24h
  - Thyroid extract: 2 mg/kg PO q24h
- Foals
  - Mares should have adequate access to iodide.
  - In endemic areas, mares should receive supplemental iodide.
  - The value of supplementing hypothyroid foals with THs is limited.

PROGNOSIS AND OUTCOME

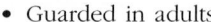

- Guarded in adults
- Poor in foals because many of the problems present are irreversible

PEARLS & CONSIDERATIONS

- In endemic areas, mares should receive supplemental iodide.

- Avoid excess or inadequate iodide in pregnant mares.
- Avoid nonthyroidal factors and consider supplementation.
- Remove access to goitrogenic plants such as *Brassica* spp. (turnips, cabbage, broccoli, cauliflower, kale, kohlrabi, black mustard), *Raphanus sativus* (radish), and *Thiaspi arvense* (stinkweed).

SUGGESTED READING

Beuhaus BA: Thyroid glands. In Smith BP, editor: *Large animal internal medicine*, ed 4, St Louis, 2009, Mosby Elsevier, pp 1347–1351.

Toribio RE: Thyroid gland. In Reed SM, Bayly WM, Sellon DC, editors: *Equine internal medicine*, ed 3. St Louis, 2010, Saunders Elsevier, pp 1251–1260.

AUTHOR & EDITOR: RAMIRO TORIBIO

Hypotrichosis
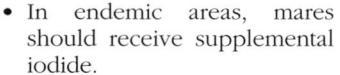

BASIC INFORMATION

DEFINITION
Less than the normal amount or density of hair

SYNONYM(S)
Hair follicle dystrophy

EPIDEMIOLOGY
GENETICS AND BREED PREDISPOSITION Arabians and Appaloosas are reportedly predisposed (the long hairs of the mane and tail are affected)

CLINICAL PRESENTATION
HISTORY, CHIEF COMPLAINT Thinning of the hair, mane, or tail

PHYSICAL EXAM FINDINGS Thinning or lack of hair, especially around eyes and muzzle, resulting in a scaly appearance of the skin; mane and tail density are decreased

ETIOLOGY AND PATHOPHYSIOLOGY Inherited

DIAGNOSIS
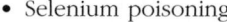

DIFFERENTIAL DIAGNOSIS
- Selenium poisoning
- Copper and iodine deficiency
- Chronic or recurring mild trauma (rubbing from equipment)

ADVANCED OR CONFIRMATORY TESTING
Histopathologic examination of skin biopsy shows a decrease in the number of hair follicles.

TREATMENT
No treatment is currently available.

SUGGESTED READING
Pascoe RRR, Knottenbelt DC: Non-infectious diseases. In Pascoe RRR, Knottenbelt DC, editors: *Manual of equine dermatology*, London, 1999, WB Saunders, pp 147–148.

AUTHOR: JENNIFER TAINTOR

EDITOR: DAVID A. WILSON

Hypoxemia

BASIC INFORMATION
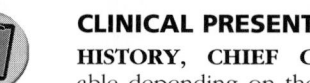

DEFINITION
A reduction in the oxygen tension in arterial blood that may lead to a reduction in oxygen at the tissue level, referred to as hypoxia

SYNONYM(S)
- Low PaO_2 level
- Low dissolved oxygen level

EPIDEMIOLOGY
SPECIES, AGE, SEX Hypoxemia may affect any age or breed and both sexes and is related to any condition that prevents adequate levels of arterial oxygen.

CLINICAL PRESENTATION
HISTORY, CHIEF COMPLAINT Variable depending on the cause of hypoxemia

PHYSICAL EXAM FINDINGS Variable depending on the cause of hypoxemia:
- Respiratory system: tachypnea, hypopnea, apnea, stridor, stertor, auscultation abnormalities
- Neurologic system: May note depression, ataxia, signs of central nervous system (CNS) involvement
- Musculoskeletal system: Muscle weakness, tremors, hyperreflexia, hyporeflexia

- Cardiovascular system: Tachycardia, murmur, poor peripheral pulses, increased capillary refill time

ETIOLOGY AND PATHOPHYSIOLOGY Hypoxemia is the result of diseases or conditions that:
- Reduce the ability of oxygen to diffuse across the alveoli
- Reduce perfusion of ventilated alveoli
- Reduce the ventilation of perfused alveoli
- Reduce the oxygen tension of inspired air
- Reduce the volume of inspired air

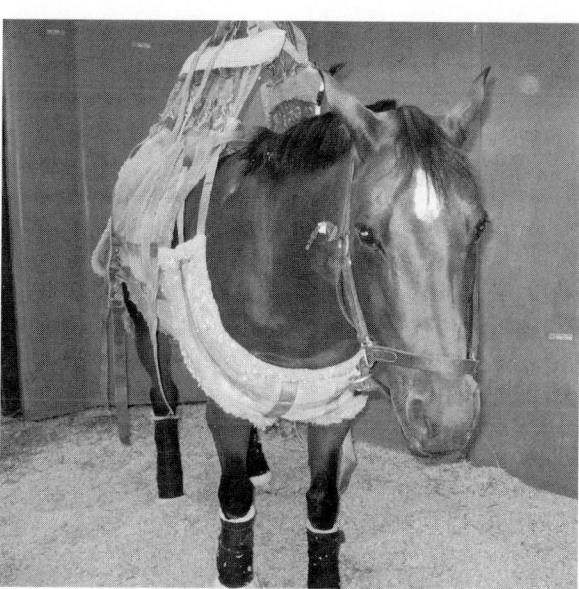

FIGURE 1 Hoisting a recumbent horse in a sling may help to improve oxygenation due to ventilation/perfusion mismatching caused by recumbency.

DIAGNOSIS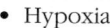

DIFFERENTIAL DIAGNOSIS

- Hypoxia
  - Iatrogenic (reduced inspired oxygen content): Anesthetic circuit malfunction
  - Environmental: High altitude
- Hypoventilation (ventilation/perfusion [V/Q] ratio <1)
  - Neurogenic: Anesthesia, head trauma, CNS neoplasia, edema or infection
  - Musculoskeletal: Botulism, tetanus, paralytic medications
  - Pulmonary: Pneumothorax, pleural effusion, flail chest
  - Mechanical; Upper airway obstruction, laryngeal hemiplegia
  - Iatrogenic: Anesthetic circuit malfunction, anesthetic overdose
- Reduced diffusion
  - Pulmonary disease: Pneumonia, pulmonary edema or fibrosis, recurrent airway obstruction, acute respiratory distress syndrome, or acute lung injury
- V/Q mismatch (V/Q ratio >1) (Figure 1)
  - Positional: Prolonged recumbency
- Vascular shunt
  - Pulmonary: Atelectasis, pneumonia, pulmonary edema
  - Cardiovascular: Tetralogy of Fallot, patent foramen ovale, patent ductus arteriosus

INITIAL DATABASE

- Arterial blood gas (ABG) analysis to identify reduced PaO_2 level

ADVANCED OR CONFIRMATORY TESTING

- Dependant on physical examination findings and suspected cause of hypoxemia:
  - Complete blood count
  - Serum chemistry
  - Thoracic ultrasonography and radiography
  - Neurologic examination, skull radiography, computed tomography, cerebrospinal fluid analysis
  - Echocardiography
  - Assessment of anesthetic circuit

TREATMENT

THERAPEUTIC GOALS

- Restore PaO_2 to normal levels
  - Pressure greater than 80 mm Hg in adults; may be lower in normal neonates because of a physiologic shunt fraction
  - PaO_2 increases from 53.9 to 84.3 mm Hg in the first 4 days of life.

ACUTE GENERAL TREATMENT

- Oxygen therapy: For hypoxia, hypoventilation, reduced diffusion, and V/Q mismatch

- May require additional ventilatory stimulation or mechanical ventilation
- Oxygen is not effective for shunting.
- Treat the primary cause.

CHRONIC TREATMENT

Depends on the initiating cause of hypoxemia

POSSIBLE COMPLICATIONS

PaO_2 does not determine the oxygen content of the blood, only dissolved oxygen; therefore, hemoglobin concentration and cardiac output must be accounted for to determine true tissue oxygen delivery.

RECOMMENDED MONITORING

- Serial ABG analysis
- Lactate
- Central venous oxygen levels

PROGNOSIS AND OUTCOME

Depends on the initiating cause of hypoxemia

PEARLS & CONSIDERATIONS

COMMENTS

Prolonged hypercapnia may blunt the horse's ability to respond to increase CO_2. These horses rely on hypoxia for respiratory drive. Oxygen administration may adversely affect ventilation by reducing this stimulus and cause further hypoventilation.

PREVENTION

Horses with predisposing factors or diseases should be monitored by serial ABG analysis.

SUGGESTED READING

Chevalier H, Divers TJ: Pulmonary dysfunction in adult horses in the intensive care unit. *Clin Tech Equine Pract* 2(2):165–177, 2003.

Prittie J: Optimal endpoints of resuscitation and early goal-directed therapy. *J Vet Emerg Crit Care* 16(4):329–339, 2006.

Wilkins PA: Disorders of foals. In Reed SM, Bayly WM, Sellon DC, editors: *Equine internal medicine*, ed 3, St Louis, 2010, Saunders Elsevier, pp 1311–1363.

AUTHOR: **AMELIA MUNSTERMAN**

EDITORS: **R. REID HANSON** and **AMELIA MUNSTERMAN**

Ileus

BASIC INFORMATION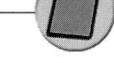

DEFINITION
Functional obstruction of abnormal gastrointestinal (GI) transit

SYNONYM(S)
Postoperative ileus, paralytic ileus

EPIDEMIOLOGY
RISK FACTORS
- Intestinal surgery: Postoperative ileus occurs predominantly after surgical correction of lesions involving the small intestine. Postoperative ileus may also be seen after correction of ascending colon lesions, primarily large colon volvulus. Traumatic handling of the intestine, intestinal distension, resection and anastomosis, and intestinal ischemia may contribute to ileus in these cases.
- Other conditions that have been associated with ileus include:
  - Anterior enteritis
  - Peritonitis
  - Electrolyte imbalances
  - Endotoxemia
  - General anesthesia
- Risk factors for postoperative ileus identified in one equine retrospective study were age older than 10 years, Arabian breed, packed cell volume (PCV) above 45%, high serum concentrations of protein and albumin, anesthesia longer than 2.5 hours, surgery longer than 2 hours, resection and anastomosis, and lesions in the small intestine. Performing a pelvic flexure enterotomy decreased the risk of postoperative ileus in this study.
- In another report PCV above 48%, high heart rate, elevated serum glucose, small intestinal lesions, and ischemic small intestine were identified as risk factors. The incidence of postoperative ileus in horses undergoing surgical treatment of colic has been reported to be between 21% and 18.4%.

ASSOCIATED CONDITIONS AND DISORDERS
- Intestinal diseases and surgery

CLINICAL PRESENTATION
HISTORY, CHIEF COMPLAINT
- The major signs associated with ileus are depression and anorexia.
- As the intestine distends, the horse demonstrates increasing signs of abdominal pain, such as pawing, flank watching, lying down, and rolling.

PHYSICAL EXAM FINDINGS
- Borborygmi are usually decreased or absent.
- The heart rate is elevated as a result of pain associated with the intestinal distension and hypovolemia.
- The mucous membranes become discolored, and capillary refill time is prolonged.
- Fecal production stops.

ETIOLOGY AND PATHOPHYSIOLOGY
- The muscle layers in the intestinal tract responsible for gross motility are contained in the muscularis externa layer, which is divided into an inner circular muscle and an outer longitudinal muscle and separated by the myenteric plexus. Coordination of activity of both of these muscle layers is necessary for normal progressive motility. Coordination of smooth muscle cell activity occurs at four levels:
  - GI smooth muscle cells demonstrate continual oscillations in membrane potential that initiate contractile activity.
  - Interstitial cells of Cajal are highly branched cells located in the myenteric and submucosal plexuses of the enteric nervous system (ENS) and are involved in the coordination of muscle activity.
  - The third level of control is the ENS. The ENS has been described as the third division of the autonomic nervous system (ANS) with the parasympathetic and sympathetic systems comprising the other two divisions. The cell bodies of neurons in the ENS are located within walls of the GI tract either in the myenteric or submucosal ganglia.
  - The next level of control is through extrinsic neural input from the sympathetic and parasympathetic divisions of the ANS.
- The precise cause of ileus is unknown, although evidence suggests that inflammation may play a central role.

DIAGNOSIS

DIFFERENTIAL DIAGNOSIS
- Other types of colic
- Mechanical intestinal obstruction (including impaction at the anastomosis after small intestinal resection)
- Peritonitis
- Equine grass sickness

INITIAL DATABASE
- Hemoconcentration is reflected by increases in the PCV and total protein.
- Decreases in plasma chloride and potassium are the most common electrolyte abnormalities seen, although sodium and chloride may also be low.
- As the severity of the intestinal distension increases, abdominal distension may become grossly visible.
- Rectal examination and ultrasonography aid in determining if the small or large intestine is involved.
- In foals, both abdominal radiography and ultrasonography can be helpful in assessing distension.
- Nasogastric decompression often retrieves 3 to 10 L of fluid.
- After nasogastric decompression, the horse usually shows some clinical improvement, such as decreased pain and decreased heart rate.
- Uses of intestinal obstruction

ADVANCED OR CONFIRMATORY TESTING
Confirmation of the presence of ileus and differentiation from other mechanical causes of intestinal distension can only be achieved by exploratory celiotomy.

TREATMENT

THERAPEUTIC GOAL(S)
- Maintain circulating blood volume and normal electrolyte balance.
- Stimulate return of normal intestinal motility.
- Relieve gastric distension to reduce the risk of gastric rupture.

ACUTE GENERAL TREATMENT
- Supportive therapy: Fluid, acid-base, and electrolyte therapy
- Antibiotics are indicated if there is compromised intestine or the possibility of bacterial contamination of the abdomen.
- Nasogastric intubation and decompression remains the primary method of treating postoperative ileus in horses. This may be achieved by repeated nasogastric intubation every 3 to 4 hours (or more frequently if indicated) or leaving an indwelling nasogastric tube in place.
- Management of pain and inflammation are also important. Phenylbutazone and flunixin meglumine have been shown to significantly attenuate the disruption of gastric, small intestine, and large colon motility associated with endotoxemia.
- Food and water should not be offered until intestinal motility has returned.

CHRONIC TREATMENT

- Pharmacologic modulation of intestinal motility is directed at either increasing excitatory cholinergic activity with the administration of the parasympathomimetic agents such as bethanechol or neostigmine or blocking inhibitory sympathetic hyperactivity with α-adrenergic blockers such as yohimbine and acepromazine.
  - Bethanechol: Bethanechol chloride is a muscarinic cholinergic agonist that stimulates acetylcholine receptors (M2 receptors) on GI smooth muscle, causing them to contract. It has been used in the treatment of certain GI motility dysfunctions such as postoperative ileus, gastric impactions, and cecal impactions. The recommended dosage is 0.025 mg/kg IV or SC q4–6h. The most common side effect of the drug is salivation, with abdominal cramping and diarrhea occurring less frequently.
  - Neostigmine: Neostigmine methylsulfate is a cholinesterase inhibitor that prolongs the activity of acetylcholine at the synaptic junction. In studies on normal horses, the effects of neostigmine (0.022 mg/kg IV) vary depending on the location of the GI tract examined. These results suggest that the drug would not be appropriate for gastric and small intestinal problems but may be beneficial for large intestine motility dysfunction. The dosage used clinically is 0.0044 mg/kg (2 mg per adult horse) SC or IM repeated in 20 to 60 minutes. If there is no response and the horse is not exhibiting any side effects, the dose can be increased by 2-mg increments to a total of 10 mg per treatment. The most common side effect is abdominal pain.
  - Acepromazine and yohimbine: Both of these drugs are α-adrenergic antagonists. Acepromazine administered at 0.01 mg/kg IM q4h is thought to reduce the severity of postoperative ileus in horses with small intestinal lesions. However, it may produce hypotension, so the horse should be well hydrated before the drug is administered. Yohimbine hydrochloride should not produce the hypotensive response seen with acepromazine.
  - Metoclopramide: Metoclopramide is a substituted benzamide whose primary prokinetic activity is through dopamine receptor antagonism with additional prokinetic activity through augmentation of acetylcholine release from intrinsic cholinergic nerves. In horses, the drug is commonly administered at a dose of 0.25 mg/kg diluted in 500 mL of saline infused over 30 to 60 minutes. Metoclopramide may cause extrapyramidal side effects such as excitement, restlessness, and sweating, as well as abdominal cramping.
  - Cisapride: Cisapride is a substituted benzamide that functions as an indirect cholinergic stimulant by selectively enhancing the release of acetylcholine from postganglionic neurons in the myenteric plexus. There have been conflicting reports on its efficacy for correcting motility dysfunction caused by endotoxins. Unfortunately, cisapride is now difficult to obtain because of its cardiotoxic effects.
  - Erythromycin: Erythromycin is a macrolide antibiotic that influences motility by acting on motilin receptors on GI smooth muscles. The recommended dosage is 2.2 mg/kg diluted in 1 L of saline and infused over 60 minutes q6h. A recent study suggested that a lower dose of 1.0 mg/kg is effective in stimulating both cecal and small intestinal propulsive activity. Alternatively, it may be administered as a continuous rate infusion of 0.1 mg/kg/h. There is evidence that erythromycin can downregulate motilin receptors, which may explain why the prokinetic effect can diminish with repeated treatments. There have been a few reports of severe colitis associated with its use, making some clinicians reluctant to use it.
  - Lidocaine: Lidocaine hydrochloride may act by (1) reducing the concentration of circulating catecholamines by suppressing the sympathoadrenal response, (2) suppressing the activity of the primary afferent neurons involved in reflex inhibition of gut motility, (3) stimulating smooth muscle directly, and (4) decreasing the inflammation in the bowel wall. The recommended protocol includes an initial loading bolus of 1.3 mg/kg IV administered slowly over 5 minutes followed by 0.05 mg/kg/min in saline or lactated Ringer's solution q24h. Side effects include muscle fasciculations, trembling, and ataxia.
  - Repeat celiotomy is advocated by some surgeons after 48 to 72 hours if intestinal motility has not returned. This allows decompression of the distended small intestine as well as checking the intestine for mechanical obstruction (eg, impaction at an anastomosis) or secondary ischemia.

POSSIBLE COMPLICATIONS

- Gastric rupture
- Endotoxemia
- Hypovolemia and dehydration

RECOMMENDED MONITORING

- During treatment, horses should be monitored for signs of dehydration, acid-base derangements, and electrolyte abnormalities.
- Heart rate, mucous membrane color, and signs of pain are monitored.
- Intestinal motility can be assessed by abdominal auscultation and abdominal ultrasonography.
- The volume of gastric reflux should be recorded.

PROGNOSIS AND OUTCOME

The prognosis is guarded. The chance of a good prognosis declines with the length of time that the ileus persists

PEARLS & CONSIDERATIONS

Postoperative ileus is a major postoperative complication after emergency celiotomy for the treatment of small intestinal obstruction.

SUGGESTED READING

Little D, Tomlinson JE, Blikslager AT: Postoperative neutrophilic inflammation in equine small intestine after manipulation and ischaemia. *Equine Vet J* 37:329–335, 2005.

Mair TS, Smith LJ: Survival and complication rates in 300 horses undergoing surgical treatment of colic. Part 2: Short-term complications. *Equine Vet J* 37:303–309, 2005.

Smith MA, Edwards GB, Dallap BL, et al: Evaluation of the clinical efficacy of prokinetic drugs in the management of postoperative ileus: can retrospective data help us? *Vet J* 170:230–236, 2005.

AUTHOR: TIM MAIR

EDITORS: TIM MAIR and CERI SHERLOCK

Immunodeficiency, Agammaglobulinemia

BASIC INFORMATION

DEFINITION

A rare primary immunodeficiency disease characterized by a lack of B cells and thus a failure to make any immunoglobulins

EPIDEMIOLOGY

- Observed only in males, so it may be an X-linked disorder
- Described in Thoroughbreds, Quarter horses, and Standardbreds

CLINICAL PRESENTATION

- Recurrent opportunistic bacterial infections, especially arthritis or respiratory disease
- Bacterial dermatitis and enteritis also reported
- Affected foals appear normal at birth but fail to thrive.
- Infections develop at 2 to 32 weeks of age as maternal immunity wanes.
- The foals become extremely anemic.
- Death occurs 4 to 8 weeks after maternal immunity wanes.

ETIOLOGY AND PATHOPHYSIOLOGY

- Foals remain healthy as long as they have protective levels of maternal antibodies.
- Infections develop as maternal antibodies wane and are not replaced by autologous antibodies.
- Although total lymphocyte numbers remain within the normal range, B cells are absent.
- The molecular basis of this disease is unknown but appears to be the result of a stem cell defect that results in a failure to produce any functional B cells.
- There may be a persistent low level of immunoglobulin production suggesting that a few B cells may develop.

DIAGNOSIS

DIFFERENTIAL DIAGNOSIS

- Severe combined immunodeficiency
- Other primary immunodeficiencies
- Transient hypogammaglobulinemia
- Failure of passive transfer
- Upper respiratory tract infections
- Chronic diarrhea
- Sepsis
- Bacteremia

INITIAL DATABASE

- Complete blood count
- Serum chemistry profile
- Bacterial culture and sensitivity

ADVANCED OR CONFIRMATORY TESTING

- Serum protein electrophoresis to evaluate immunoglobulin concentrations
- Repeated serum immunoglobulin quantitation to provide assurance that the animal is persistently agammaglobulinemic and that the hypogammaglobulinemia is not transient
- T-cell numbers are normal, but B cells are undetectable.

TREATMENT

THERAPEUTIC GOAL(S)

- Supportive care to control opportunistic infections is entirely appropriate until it is determined whether the agammaglobulinemia is persistent.
- Euthanasia is commonly the most humane option if persistent agammaglobulinemia is diagnosed

ACUTE GENERAL TREATMENT

- Immunologic support to minimize recurrence risks
- Immediate control and elimination of infection
- Circulatory support to correct any deficits in intravascular volume and to maintain organ perfusion
- If the foal is determined to lack immunoglobulins before the development of infections, then prompt immunologic treatment should be instituted designed to remedy any immunologic deficit. If, however, the foal presents with severe infections, then they must be promptly controlled.
- A total of 50 to 70 g of lyophilized equine immunoglobulin G (IgG) may be administered to increase serum IgG levels to greater than 800 mg/dL.
- If plasma transfusions are not given, then owners should be advised of the risks of infection and the foals maintained in an environment where exposure to potential pathogens is minimal.
- Ideally, the dose to be used can be calculated in order to attain an IgG level of at least 800 mg/dL.
- Frozen horse plasma is available commercially, although it may not contain antibodies against local pathogens.
- Plasma may be obtained from local donors. Blood should be collected aseptically with heparin or sodium citrate. The plasma is collected after the erythrocytes settle and is stored frozen until used. The plasma must be checked for antierythrocyte antibody and must be free of bacterial contamination. The transfusion should be

given slowly while the foal is monitored for untoward reactions.
- All foals receiving supplemental plasma should have their IgG levels rechecked 12 to 24 hours later.
- Antibiotic treatment: A combination of a penicillin and an aminoglycoside is a good starting therapy. A suitable aminoglycoside such as gentamicin (6.6–8.8 mg/kg IV or IM q24h) or amikacin (22–25 mg/kg IV or IM q24h) may be given.
- Other third-generation cephalosporins such as cefotaxime (20–40 mg/kg IV or IM q6–8h) may be used.
- Circulatory support: It is essential to maintain or restore effective circulating volume by aggressive IV fluid therapy. Administer fluids at the highest tolerated rate.
- Septicemic foals are hypoglycemic so dextrose should be provided.

POSSIBLE COMPLICATIONS

Complications of sepsis include disseminated intravascular coagulation, acute renal failure, pulmonary thromboembolism, acute respiratory distress syndrome, and intractable hypotension and cardiac arrest.

RECOMMENDED MONITORING

- Heart rate and pulse
- Respiratory rate, mentation, blood pressure as dictated by the case
- CBC, hematocrit, total protein and electrolytes, urine output
- During long-term aminoglycoside therapy, dehydration must be prevented and urinalysis and serum creatinine monitored once weekly.

PROGNOSIS AND OUTCOME

This disease is uniformly fatal but animals may survive for as long as 1 to 2 years. Given that these recurrent infections are usually bacterial in origin and may be controlled for a time by aggressive antibiotic therapy, prolonging their lives may be achievable but may not be the most appropriate course.

PEARLS & CONSIDERATIONS

COMMENTS

This is a rare disease with a poor prognosis.

PREVENTION

This is an inherited disease. The parents of affected foals may be considered to carry the relevant genes, so they should be excluded from breeding programs.

CLIENT EDUCATION

It is important to explain to the client that this is an inherited disease and that other foals from these parents may also be affected.

SUGGESTED READING

Banks KL, McGuire TC, Jerrells TR: Absence of B lymphocytes in a horse with primary agammaglobulinemia. *Clin Immunol Immunopathol* 5:282–290, 1976.

Deem DA, Traver DS, Thacker HL, et al: Agammaglobulinemia in a horse. *J Am Vet Med Assoc* 175:469–472, 1979.

Perryman LE: Primary immunodeficiencies of horses. *Vet Clin North Am Equine Pract* 16:105–116, vii, 2000.

Perryman LE, McGuire TC, Banks KL: Animal model of human disease. Infantile X-linked agammaglobulinemia. Agammaglobulinemia in horses. *Am J Pathol* 111:125–127, 1983.

Riggs MW: Evaluation of foals for immune deficiency disorders. *Vet Clin North Am Equine Pract* 3:515–528, 1987.

AUTHOR & EDITOR: IAN TIZARD

Immunodeficiency, Common Variable

BASIC INFORMATION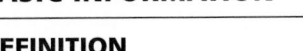

DEFINITION

A heterogeneous group of immunodeficiency diseases characterized by a failure of B cells to make antibodies. The B-cell deficiency is secondary to a defect in helper T cells.

EPIDEMIOLOGY

SPECIES, AGE, SEX
- Sporadic in occurrence and severity
- Usually in animals older than 3 years of age and hence distinctly different from the inherited primary immunodeficiencies

CLINICAL PRESENTATION

- Recurrent infections that are not responsive to medical treatment
- Bacterial meningitis may be a consistent feature.
- Severe liver disease may also be present.

ETIOLOGY AND PATHOPHYSIOLOGY
- Absence of B cells in lymphoid organs, blood, or bone marrow
- The underlying defect is only expressed when the immune system is stressed by infection.
- Also associated with a selective immunoglobulin M (IgM) deficiency
- Many develop a concurrent lymphosarcoma

DIAGNOSIS

DIFFERENTIAL DIAGNOSIS

- Naturally occurring bacterial meningitis or other infections
- Infections occurring after secondary immunodeficiencies induced by stresses such as transportation, malnutrition, or excessive work or exercise

INITIAL DATABASE

- Complete blood count (CBC), serum chemistry profile with culture and sensitivity, urinalysis, fibrinogen
- Serum protein electrophoresis to evaluate immunoglobulin concentrations
- Serum immunoglobulin quantitation is highly variable. Usually, however, one or more of the IgG subclasses is severely reduced. Some cases, for example, contain only trace levels of IgG and IgM, no detectable IgG3, and very low IgA levels.
- Sometimes individual IgG subclasses are deficient but IgA levels are normal.
- T-cell numbers are normal, but B cells are undetectable.
- Neutrophil function assays are normal.

ADVANCED OR CONFIRMATORY TESTING

Peripheral blood lymphocytes show depressed responses to mitogens compared with age-matched control horses.

TREATMENT

Because of the great variability in severity of this syndrome, treatment success and prognosis are unpredictable. Some animals may require minimal support. Others may require euthanasia.

THERAPEUTIC GOAL(S)

Reduce suffering and maintain quality of life by controlling opportunistic infections until the animal regains immune function or the immunodeficiency is considered irreversible.

ACUTE GENERAL TREATMENT

- A total of 50 to 70 g of lyophilized equine IgG may be administered to increase serum IgG levels to greater than 400 mg/dL.

- Frozen horse plasma is available commercially, although it may not contain antibodies against local pathogens.
- Plasma may be obtained from local donors. Blood should be collected aseptically with heparin or sodium citrate. The plasma is collected after the erythrocytes settle and is stored frozen until used. The plasma must be prechecked for antierythrocyte antibody and must be free of bacterial contamination. The transfusion should be given slowly while the horse is monitored for untoward reactions.
- Animals receiving plasma should have their IgG levels rechecked 12 to 24 hours later.
- Antibiotic treatment: A combination of a penicillin and an aminoglycoside is a good starting therapy. A suitable aminoglycoside such as gentamicin (6.6–8.8 mg/kg IV or IM q24h) or amikacin (22–25 mg/kg IV or IM q24h) may be used.
- Other third-generation cephalosporins such as cefotaxime (20–40 mg/kg IV or IM q6–8h) may be used
- Circulatory support: It is essential to maintain or restore effective circulating volume by aggressive IV fluid therapy. Administer fluids at the highest tolerated rate.
- Septicemic horses are hypoglycemic, so dextrose should be provided.
- Appropriate antifungal therapy should be provided.

CHRONIC TREATMENT

- Nonspecific supportive therapy
- Frequent monitoring with aggressive antimicrobial therapy when warranted

POSSIBLE COMPLICATIONS

- Overwhelming sepsis
- Recurrent, antibiotic resistant infections

RECOMMENDED MONITORING

- Appetite, activity level, temperature, and CBCs may permit early detection of infections.
- During long-term aminoglycoside therapy, dehydration must be prevented and urinalysis and serum creatinine monitored once weekly.

PROGNOSIS AND OUTCOME

As with all immunodeficiency diseases, the prognosis is guarded. However, common variable immunodeficiency (CVID), as its name suggests, is of variable severity. Some horses succumb rapidly. Some with mild disease may well survive in apparent health, especially if recurrent infections are promptly and aggressively treated.

PEARLS & CONSIDERATIONS

COMMENTS

Possibly much more common than realized. Consider CVID in all meningitis cases.

PREVENTION

Because this condition may be heritable, consider reviewing the horse's pedigree and altering breeding strategies to minimize the chance of other animals developing the disease.

CLIENT EDUCATION

Be cautious to pessimistic in the prognosis. Consider alterations in breeding strategies.

SUGGESTED READING

Flaminio MJ, LaCombe V, Kohn CW, et al: Common variable immunodeficiency in a horse. *J Am Vet Med Assoc* 221:1296–1302, 2002.

Flaminio MJ, Tallmadge RL, Salles-Gomes CO, et al: Common variable immunodeficiency in horses is characterized by B cell depletion in primary and secondary lymphoid tissues. *J Clin Immunol* 29(1):107–116, 2009.

Pelligrini-Masini A, Bentz AI, Johns IC, et al: Common variable immunodeficiency in three horses with presumptive bacterial meningitis. *J Am Vet Med Assoc* 227:114–122, 2005.

AUTHOR & EDITOR: **IAN TIZARD**

Immunodeficiency, Fell Pony Syndrome

BASIC INFORMATION

DEFINITION

An autosomal recessive syndrome consisting of anemia, peripheral, ganglionopathy, and immunodeficiency occurring in foals of the Fell Pony breed

EPIDEMIOLOGY

SPECIES, AGE, SEX Restricted to Fell Ponies, so it is assumed to be of genetic origin. It occurs in animals of both sexes and is believed to be autosomal in nature.

CLINICAL PRESENTATION

HISTORY, CHIEF COMPLAINT
- Recurrent opportunistic infections, especially diarrhea or respiratory disease
- Affected foals appear normal at birth but fail to thrive.
- Decreased suckling, cough
- Chewing motions
- Infections develop at 2 to 32 weeks of age as maternal immunity wanes.
- The foals become extremely anemic.
- Death usually occurs 4 to 8 weeks after maternal immunity wanes.

ETIOLOGY AND PATHOPHYSIOLOGY
- Foals develop severe normochromic to macrocytic anemia as a result of a failure to develop bone marrow erythroid stem cells.
- Affected animals lack germinal centers and plasma cells, suggesting a B-cell deficiency. B-cell numbers in affected foals are less than 10% of normal.
- CD4 and CD8 T-cell numbers are within the normal range but show reduced major histocompatibility class II expression.
- Immunoglobulin levels are relatively normal, but any immunoglobulin deficiency may be masked by maternal antibodies.
- Neutrophil counts are normal.

DIAGNOSIS

DIFFERENTIAL DIAGNOSIS

- Failure of passive transfer
- Other primary immunodeficiency syndromes
- Upper respiratory tract infections
- Chronic diarrhea
- Sepsis
- Bacteremia

INITIAL DATABASE

- Complete blood count (CBC) showing severe erythroid hypoplasia
- White blood cell counts: Normal or reflecting infection status
- Lymphopenia: Inconsistent
- Thrombocytopenia has been described.
- Blood immunoglobulin levels: Severely depressed
- Serum chemistry profile
- Blood culture and sensitivity, urinalysis

ADVANCED OR CONFIRMATORY TESTING

- Bone marrow aspirate to characterize the anemia
- Serum protein electrophoresis to evaluate immunoglobulin concentrations
- Serum immunoglobulin quantitation
- Flow cytometry shows that T-cell numbers are normal, but B cells are undetectable.
- Mitogenic responses to phytohemagglutinin and concanavalin A are normal.
- Mitogenic responses to bacterial lipopolysaccharide, a B-cell mitogen, are severely depressed.

TREATMENT

THERAPEUTIC GOAL(S)

Supportive care to treat opportunistic infections. Euthanasia is commonly the most humane option.

ACUTE GENERAL TREATMENT

- Immunologic support to minimize recurrence risks
- Immediate control and elimination of infection
- Circulatory support to correct any deficits in intravascular volume and to maintain organ perfusion
- If the foal lacks immunoglobulins before the development of sepsis or pneumonia, then prompt immunologic treatment should be instituted to address the immunologic deficit. If, however, the foal presents with severe infections, then these must be promptly controlled.
- A total of 50 to 70 g of lyophilized equine immunoglobulin G (IgG) may be administered to increase serum IgG levels to greater than 800 mg/dL.

- If plasma transfusions are not given, then owners should be advised of the risks of infection and the foals maintained in an environment where exposure to potential pathogens is minimal.
- Ideally, the dose to be used can be calculated to attain an IgG level of at least 800 mg/dL.
- Frozen horse plasma is available commercially, although it may not contain antibodies against local pathogens.
- Plasma may be obtained from local donors. Blood should be collected aseptically with heparin or sodium citrate. The plasma is collected after the erythrocytes settle and is stored frozen until used. The plasma must be checked for antierythrocyte antibody and must be free of bacterial contamination. The transfusion should be given slowly while the foal is monitored for untoward reactions.
- All foals receiving supplemental plasma should have their IgG levels rechecked 12 to 24 hours later.
- Antibiotic treatment: A combination of penicillin and an aminoglycoside is a good starting therapy. A suitable aminoglycoside such as gentamicin (6.6–8.8 mg/kg IV or IM q24h) or amikacin (22–25 mg/kg IV or IM q24h) may be used.
- Other third-generation cephalosporins such as cefotaxime (20–40 mg/kg IV or IM q6–8h) may be given.
- Circulatory support: It is essential to maintain or restore effective circulating volume with aggressive IV fluid therapy. Administer fluids at the highest tolerated rate.
- Septicemic foals are hypoglycemic, so dextrose should be provided.

CHRONIC TREATMENT

Inappropriate because of the poor prognosis

POSSIBLE COMPLICATIONS

- Sepsis and recurring infections
- Complications of sepsis include disseminated intravascular coagulation, multiorgan dysfunction syndrome, acute renal failure, pulmonary thromboembolism, acute respiratory distress syndrome, intractable hypotension, and cardiac arrest.

RECOMMENDED MONITORING

- Heart rate and pulse
- Respiratory rate, mentation, blood pressure as dictated by the case
- CBC, hematocrit, total protein and electrolytes, urine output
- During long-term aminoglycoside therapy, dehydration must be prevented and urinalysis and serum creatinine monitored once weekly.

PROGNOSIS AND OUTCOME

This disease is uniformly fatal. The foals usually die or are euthanized by 3 months of age as a result of infections with *Cryptosporidium* spp. or adenoviruses.

PEARLS & CONSIDERATIONS

COMMENTS

This is a rare disease with a poor prognosis.

PREVENTION

Given that this disease appears to affect only the Fell Pony breed, appropriate screening of potential breeding pairs and of pairs that have produced affected foals should be done.

CLIENT EDUCATION

It is important to explain to the client that this is an inherited disease and that other foals from these parents may also be affected. Advice should be provided on appropriate selection of breeding animals.

SUGGESTED READING

Bell SC, Savidge C, Taylor P, et al: An immunodeficiency in Fell Ponies: a preliminary study into cellular responses. *Equine Vet J* 33:687–692, 2001

Butler CM, Westermann CM, Koeman JP, et al: The Fell pony immunodeficiency syndrome also occurs in the Netherlands: a review and six cases. *Tijdschr Diergeneeskd* 131:114–118, 2006.

Gardner RB, Hart KA, Stokol T, et al: Fell Pony syndrome in a pony in North America. *J Vet Intern Med* 20:198–203, 2006.

Scholes SF, Holliman A, May PD, et al: A syndrome of anemia, immunodeficiency and peripheral ganglionopathy in Fell pony foals. *Vet Rec* 142:128–134, 1998.

Thomas GW, Bell SC, Carter SD: Immunoglobulin and peripheral B-lymphocyte concentrations in Fell pony foal syndrome. *Equine Vet J* 37:48–52, 2005.

Thomas GW, Bell SC, Phythian C, et al: Aid to the antemortem diagnosis of Fell pony foal syndrome by the analysis of B lymphocytes. *Vet Rec* 152:618–621, 2003.

AUTHOR & EDITOR: **IAN TIZARD**

Immunodeficiency, Selective Immunoglobulin M

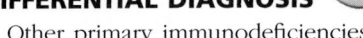

BASIC INFORMATION

DEFINITION

An immunodeficiency syndrome characterized by low or absent serum immunoglobulin M (IgM) with normal or elevated levels of other immunoglobulin classes

EPIDEMIOLOGY

SPECIES, AGE, SEX

- Probably of genetic origin and hence a primary immunodeficiency, but breeding studies have yielded inconclusive results
- Most often reported in Arabians and Quarter Horses but other breeds also affected

CLINICAL PRESENTATION

DISEASE FORMS/SUBTYPES

- Recurrent severe infections, especially diarrhea, arthritis, or respiratory disease leading to death before age 10 months
- Foals with a history of repeated infections that usually respond to aggressive antibiotic treatment. Infections recur after treatment has stopped. These foals do poorly and show stunted growth but may survive for several years.

ETIOLOGY AND PATHOPHYSIOLOGY

- Foals have unusually low levels of IgM. This may be because of decreased production or increased catabolism or because of excessive regulatory T-cell activity.
- Lymphocyte counts are usually within normal ranges, so there is no gross B- or T-cell deficit.

DIAGNOSIS

DIFFERENTIAL DIAGNOSIS

- Other primary immunodeficiencies
- Failure of passive transfer
- Delayed immunoglobulin synthesis
- Infections not associated with immunodeficiency, upper respiratory tract infections, chronic diarrhea, sepsis, arthritis, bacteremia

INITIAL DATABASE

- Complete blood count (CBC) and serum chemistry profile may reflect the ongoing infection and inflammation
- Bacterial culture and sensitivity

ADVANCED OR CONFIRMATORY TESTING

- Serum protein electrophoresis to evaluate immunoglobulin concentrations.
- Serum immunoglobulin quantitation.
- Serum IgM levels are more than two standard deviations below the age-specific normal IgM levels.
- Multiple IgM assays must be performed to confirm that the levels are persistently depressed.
- Other immunoglobulin classes are within normal limits or elevated for age.
- On necropsy lymphoid tissues are apparently normal. Evidence of bacterial infection, pneumonia, sepsis, and arthritis is present.

TREATMENT

THERAPEUTIC GOAL(S)

- Supportive care to treat opportunistic infections and to maintain quality of life until a definitive diagnosis is obtained. After it has been confirmed, euthanasia is commonly the most humane option.
- Immunologic support to minimize recurrence risks
- Immediate control and elimination of infection
- Circulatory support to correct any deficits in intravascular volume and to maintain organ perfusion
- If the foal is identified as lacking IgM before the development of sepsis or pneumonia, then prompt immunologic treatment should be instituted to address the immunologic deficit. If, however, the foal presents with severe infections, then these must be promptly controlled.
- A total of 50 to 70 g of lyophilized equine IgG may be administered to increase serum IgG levels to greater than 800 mg/dL.

- If plasma transfusions are not given, then owners should be advised of the risks of infection and the foals maintained in an environment where exposure to potential pathogens is minimal.
- Ideally, the dose to be used can be calculated to attain an IgG level of at least 800 mg/dL.
- Frozen horse plasma is available commercially, although it may not contain antibodies against local pathogens.
- Plasma may be obtained from local donors. Blood should be collected aseptically with heparin or sodium citrate. The plasma is collected after the erythrocytes settle and is stored frozen until used. The plasma must be checked for antierythrocyte antibody and must be free of bacterial contamination. The transfusion should be given slowly while the foal is monitored for untoward reactions.
- All foals receiving supplemental plasma should have their IgG levels rechecked 12 to 24 hours later.
- Antibiotic treatment: A combination of a penicillin and an aminoglycoside is a good starting therapy. A suitable aminoglycoside such as gentamicin (6.6–8.8 mg/kg IV or IM q24h) or amikacin (22–25 mg/kg IV or IM q24h) may be used.
- Other third-generation cephalosporins such as cefotaxime (20–40 mg/kg IV or IM q6–8h) may be given.
- Circulatory support: It is essential to maintain or restore effective circulating volume by aggressive IV fluid therapy. Administer fluids at the highest tolerated rate.
- Septicemic foals are hypoglycemic, so dextrose should be provided.

POSSIBLE COMPLICATIONS

Complications of sepsis include disseminated intravascular coagulation, acute renal failure, pulmonary thromboembolism, acute respiratory distress syndrome, intractable hypotension, and cardiac arrest.

RECOMMENDED MONITORING

- Heart rate and pulse
- Respiratory rate, mentation, blood pressure as dictated by the case

- CBC, hematocrit, total protein and electrolytes, urine output
- During long-term aminoglycoside therapy, dehydration must be prevented and urinalysis and serum creatinine monitored once weekly.

PROGNOSIS AND OUTCOME

Very poor to fatal

PEARLS & CONSIDERATIONS

COMMENTS

This is a rare disease with a poor prognosis.

PREVENTION

Given that this disease may be genetic in origin, appropriate screening of potential breeding pairs and of pairs that have produced affected foals should be considered seriously.

CLIENT EDUCATION

It is important to explain to the client that this is an inherited disease and that other foals from these parents may also be affected.

SUGGESTED READING

Boy MG, Zhang C, Antczak DF, et al: Unusual selective immunoglobulin deficiency in an Arabian foal. *J Vet Intern Med* 6:201–205, 1992.

Freestone JF, Shoemaker S, McClure JJ: Pulmonary abscessation, hepatoencephalopathy and IgM deficiency associated with *Rhodococcus equi* in a foal. *Aust Vet J* 66:343–344, 1989.

Perryman LE: Biochemical and functional characterization of lymphocytes from a horse with lymphosarcoma and IgM deficiency. *Comp Immunol Microbiol Infect Dis* 7:53–62, 1984.

Perryman LE: Primary immunodeficiencies of horses. *Vet Clin North Am Equine Pract* 16:105–116, 2000.

Weldon AD, Zhang C, Antczak DF, et al: Selective IgM deficiency and abnormal B-cell response in a foal. *J Am Vet Med Assoc* 201:1396–1398, 1992.

AUTHOR & EDITOR: IAN TIZARD

Immunodeficiency, Severe Combined

BASIC INFORMATION

DEFINITION

A genetic disorder resulting in absence of mature functional B and T lymphocytes

SYNONYM(S)

Combined immunodeficiency

EPIDEMIOLOGY

SPECIES, AGE, SEX
- Arabian foals and part-Arabian foals, but sporadic cases have been reported in breeds other than Arabians.
- Age at presentation is typically 1 to 2 months.

GENETICS AND BREED PREDISPOSITION
- Autosomal recessive inheritance in Arabians
- Only homozygous animals affected

CLINICAL PRESENTATION

HISTORY, CHIEF COMPLAINT
- Recurrent infection in foals ages 1 to 4 months
- Opportunistic infectious agents commonly isolated

PHYSICAL EXAM FINDINGS
- Clinical examination findings vary with the type of infection.
- Bronchopneumonia and diarrhea are common.

ETIOLOGY AND PATHOPHYSIOLOGY
- The severe combined immunodeficiency (SCID) trait results from a 5-base pair deletion.
- Affected foals are born without functional B and T lymphocytes, rendering them unable to produce either antibody-mediated or cell-mediated immune responses.
- Acquisition of maternal antibodies through colostrum ingestion provides initial immunity.

DIAGNOSIS

DIFFERENTIAL DIAGNOSIS

Because SCID results in chronic infection, primary infectious disease is a differential.

INITIAL DATABASE

Complete blood count: Persistent and severe lymphopenia (<1000 lymphocytes/μL)

ADVANCED OR CONFIRMATORY TESTING

Genetic testing (performed by VetGen, Ann Arbor, Mich.)

TREATMENT

THERAPEUTIC GOAL(S)

Treatment of causative agent of disease is recommended until a diagnosis of SCID is confirmed with genetic testing.

ACUTE GENERAL TREATMENT

- No treatment exists for SCID foals. Most do not survive beyond 5 months of age.
- Respiratory infections with adenovirus, *Rhodococcus equi*, or *Pneumocystis carinii* are common. Treatment for infectious disease should be initiated until results of genetic testing are available.

RECOMMENDED MONITORING

Lymphocyte count: Persistent lymphopenia is suggestive of SCID in Arabian foals.

PROGNOSIS AND OUTCOME

Grave; most foals do not survive beyond 5 months of age.

PEARLS & CONSIDERATIONS

COMMENTS

Persistent lymphopenia in an Arabian foal warrants genetic testing for SCID even if the foal appears healthy.

PREVENTION

Responsible breeding practices involve testing of both mares and stallions for the SCID gene and elimination of carriers from breeding programs.

SUGGESTED READING

Lunn P, Horohov D: Primary immunodeficiencies. In Reed S, Bayly W, Sellon D, editors: *Equine internal medicine*, ed 3, St Louis, 2010, Saunders Elsevier, pp 37–38.

AUTHOR: **PHOEBE A. SMITH**

EDITORS: **PHOEBE A. SMITH** and **ELIZABETH M. SANTSCHI**

Infertility, Chromosomal or Genetic

BASIC INFORMATION

DEFINITION

- The horse (*Equus caballus*) has 64 chromosomes—62 autosomal chromosomes and two sex chromosomes (XX-female and XY-male). Horses of all domestic breeds have the same number, size, and shape of chromosomes.
- Horses are affected by chromosomal abnormalities that cause congenital abnormalities, embryonic loss and infertility. Most chromosomal abnormalities reported in horses are associated with the sex chromosomes. However, abnormalities in autosomal chromosomes have also been reported.
- Common abnormalities include deletion or translocation of specific genes (testicular feminization, XTfmY; sex reversal, XXSxr or XYSxr), absence of a sex chromosome (Turner's syndrome, 63, X or 63, XO), and an extra copy of the X chromosome in males (XXY syndrome, 65,XXY). Moreover, some horses carry normal cells and cells with chromosome abnormalities, such as sex chromosome mosaics (63, X/64,XX).

SYNONYM(S)

Gonadal dysgenesis, Turner's syndrome, sex reversal, testicular feminization, trisomies, Klinefelter's syndrome, sex chromosome aneuploidy, sex chromosome mosaics

EPIDEMIOLOGY

SPECIES, AGE, SEX
- Chromosome abnormalities affect stallions primarily as sex chromosome

mosaicism or sex-reversal syndromes. In mares, the most common form of chromosome abnormality is 63,X (Turner's syndrome).

- Most abnormalities occur during gametogenesis, embryogenesis, or both. However, the majority of cases are only diagnosed later in life, usually after puberty when infertility is evident.
- A recent study conducted in Poland with 500 randomly selected mares and stallions of several breeds found that 2% of the overall population had a chromosome abnormality, and 3.7% of mares (n = 272) had chromosome abnormalities. A similar study conducted in the United States with 204 broodmares of different breeds found that fewer than 3% of animals had chromosome abnormalities.

CLINICAL PRESENTATION
DISEASE FORMS/SUBTYPES
- Gonadal dysgenesis: This condition is usually caused by absence of an X chromosome (63,X). However, mares affected with partial deletions of an X chromosome or mosaicism may also present with vestigial gonads. Affected mares are presented with chronic primary infertility, failure to cycle regularly or at all, small ovaries, and an underdeveloped reproductive tract. Usually, animals are small in size relative to the breed and may present angular limb deformities and poor overall conformation.
- Sex reversal: This condition is the result of a translocation of the SRY region from the Y chromosome into the X chromosome. Two main types of this condition are recognized: (1) animals with a mare-like phenotype and a male genotype (64, XYSry−), and (2) animals with a stallion-like phenotype and a female genotype (64, XXSry+). Sex-reversal horses have also been reported with karyotype of 64, XX and SRY negative; the etiology of this particular type of abnormality is unknown.
- Testicular feminization (XTfmY) or androgen insensitivity syndrome: This condition is caused by a mutation in the androgen receptor encoded by a gene in the X chromosome. XTfmY animals have the phenotype of females, with testes usually located in the abdomen or both testes and ovaries and absence of tubular genitalia (cervix and uterus). The vagina may end in a blind pocket. These animals are SRY positive, have stallion-like behavior, and have high levels of testosterone in the circulation.
- Trisomies of the sex chromosomes or Klinefelter syndrome (XXY): Affected animals are phenotypically males and

may present with normal sexual behavior; small, soft, or normal testes; azoospermia; and a small or normal penis.
- Autosomal chromosome disorders: There have been few reports of horse autosomal chromosome abnormalities; the abnormalities can be classified as deletions, translocations, and autosomal trisomies. Only four horses have been reported with autosomal deletions. Seven cases of autosomal trisomy have been reported in horses, all involving smaller chromosomes. It has been suggested that trisomy of larger chromosomes may be involved in early embryonic loss. Animals with abnormalities in autosomal chromosomes are presented with a history of subfertility. The diagnosis of autosomal translocations is rare in horses, probably because most horses have a normal phenotype and the subfertility may not be attributed to chromosomal abnormalities.

HISTORY, CHIEF COMPLAINT
- Animals are usually presented with a history of subfertility or infertility or abnormal sexual behavior (eg, stallion-like behavior in a mare). Mares are presented with a history of chronic infertility, anestrous, failure to cycle regularly, and sometimes persistent estrus, and some mares are reported to be small in size for their age and breed and have poor body conformation. Intersex animals are often presented for their ambiguous external genitalia.

PHYSICAL EXAM FINDINGS
- The clinical signs vary according to the chromosome abnormality. Reproductive examination often reveals small, inactive ovaries and a flaccid, small uterus and cervix. The external genitalia are feminine, but the vulva may be smaller than normal, and there is no clitoral hypertrophy. A sex-reversed animal may have ambiguous external genitalia and retained testicles.
- Findings in genital examinations of intersex animals include enlargement of the clitoris; increased anogenital distance; incomplete vaginal and or scrotal development; presence of subcutaneous, inguinal, or abdominal testes; and a small penis and prepuce, which are often associated with hypospadias. Internally, the gonadic structures vary from inactive testicular tissues to ovotestes.

ETIOLOGY AND PATHOPHYSIOLOGY
Chromosomal sex (either XX or XY) is determined at the time of fertilization, depending on whether the male gamete that fertilizes the X-bearing female gamete contains an X or a Y

chromosome. During normal early embryonic development, the chromosomal sex of the zygote determines the eventual gonadal sex. The presence of genetic information borne on the SRY region of the Y chromosome directs the XY embryo to become a male. In the presence of the SRY region, the indifferent gonad will develop into testicles: Leydig cells secrete testosterone, and Sertoli cells secrete anti-Müllerian hormone (AMH). As a result, the Müllerian (paramesonephric) ducts regress, the Wolffian (mesonephric) ducts form vasa deferentia and epididymides, and masculinization of the external genitalia occurs. In the absence of the Y chromosome (or SRY region), the indifferent gonad will develop into ovaries. The absence of testosterone results in regression of the Wolffian ducts, and the absence of AMH results in development of the Müllerian ducts into oviducts, a uterus, and a cervix. Thus female physical development is not attributable to the presence and influence of estrogens but to the absence or ineffectiveness of androgens. The inherent trend is for any fetus to develop female external genitals and general body form in the absence of the masculinizing effects of male hormones.

DIAGNOSIS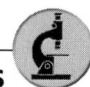

DIFFERENTIAL DIAGNOSIS
- Subnutrition
- Acyclic or anestrous
- Senility
- Retarded puberty

INITIAL DATABASE
- A cytogenetic analysis (karyotype) is the most useful tool to diagnose chromosome abnormalities.
- Blood samples must be collected into acid citrate dextrose or heparin and sent by overnight shipping to a laboratory specializing in animal karyotyping.
- An examination of peripheral blood smears for sex chromosome appendages, or drumsticks, on polymorphonuclear neutrophils (PMNs) may be used as a screening procedure to detect a reduced number of chromosomes. Drumsticks appear as lobes on the nucleus of PMNs and are present in approximately 10% of PMNs from normal mares but are absent in stallions and geldings. An examination of peripheral blood smears reveals an absence of drumsticks in XO mares.

ADVANCED OR CONFIRMATORY TESTING
Fluorescence in situ hybridization test

TREATMENT

THERAPEUTIC GOALS

- Eliminate stallion-like behavior.
- Remove intraabdominal testis or testes, which are prone to become neoplastic.

ACUTE GENERAL TREATMENT

Elective castration and removal of the testicle(s)

RECOMMENDED MONITORING

Animals presenting any of the signs described above should undergo a cytogenetic evaluation to determine if chromosomal abnormalities are present.

PROGNOSIS AND OUTCOME

- Favorable for life
- Reserved to poor for reproduction

PEARLS & CONSIDERATIONS

Recently, new laboratory techniques in cell culture, chromosome visualization, and chromosome banding have helped to improve our diagnostic capabilities for the different types of genetic infertilities. However, an accurate clinical examination constitutes the basis for deciding which animals need to be tested to avoid extra expenses

to the breeders as well as achieve a precise diagnosis.

SUGGESTED READING

Buoen LC, Zhang TQ, Weber AF, Ruth GR: SRY-negative, XX intersex horses: the need for pedigree studies to examine the mode of inheritance of the condition. *Equine Vet J* 32:78–81, 2000.

Lear TL: Cytogenetic evaluation. In Samper JC, Pycock JF, McKinnon AO, editors: *Current therapy in equine reproduction*, St Louis, 2007, Saunders Elsevier, pp 73–77.

Lear TL, Bailey E: Equine clinical cytogenetics: the past and future. *Cytogenet Genome Res* 120:42–49, 2008.

Power MM: Chromosomes of the horse. *Advan Vet Sci Comp Med* 34:131–167, 1990.

AUTHORS: **IGOR FREDERICO CANISSO** and **MARCO A. COUTINHO DA SILVA**

EDITOR: **JUAN C. SAMPER**

Inflammatory Airway Disease

BASIC INFORMATION

DEFINITION

- Inflammatory airway disease (IAD) is a respiratory disease of adult horses that is characterized by noninfectious inflammation of the small airways accompanied by airway hyperreactivity.
- It is not yet clear whether IAD is entirely a particulate-induced inflammation or if there is an allergic component to this disease.

SYNONYM(S)

- Small airway inflammatory disease
- Small airway disease
- Allergic airway disease

EPIDEMIOLOGY

SPECIES, AGE, SEX Equine adults
RISK FACTORS Stabling, a dusty environment, poor ventilation, high ambient endotoxin levels, high particulates of any kind
GEOGRAPHY AND SEASONALITY Seen more frequently in areas where horses are kept stabled and during months when horses are stabled

CLINICAL PRESENTATION

DISEASE FORMS/SUBTYPES

- Older horses may present with a more advanced form of disease that is more easily recognized as arising from the respiratory system.
- Younger horses may have much milder disease without distinct respiratory signs.

HISTORY, CHIEF COMPLAINT

- Horses may present with variable cough, nasal discharge, exercise intolerance, poor recovery from work, and mild tachypnea.
- Dressage horses may be reluctant to come onto the bit. Racehorses may have no specific airway signs but may exhibit poor performance.

PHYSICAL EXAM FINDINGS

- Affected animals are usually in good flesh.
- There is no evidence of increased respiratory effort at rest. The horse may have a mildly elevated respiratory rate, serous to mucoid nasal discharge, and cough or may have no distinct respiratory signs. Loud bronchovesicular sounds or mild wheezes and crackles on auscultation of the chest and mild fluid noises on auscultation of the trachea may be heard.
- Horses are afebrile.

ETIOLOGY AND PATHOPHYSIOLOGY

- The cause of IAD has not been fully elucidated. However, contributing factors include high environmental particulate and endotoxin levels and high levels of noxious gases, such as ammonia. It is unclear whether there is an allergic component to IAD.

DIAGNOSIS

DIFFERENTIAL DIAGNOSIS

- Noninfectious respiratory diseases such as recurrent airway obstruction, various forms of pulmonary fibrosis

(eg, silicosis or equine multinodular pulmonary fibrosis), toxicosis from inhaled gases, perilla mint
- Infectious lung disease such as septic bronchitis, bronchopneumonia, or viral pneumonia
- Exercise-induced pulmonary hemorrhage
- Toxicoses, including inhaled toxins (silicosis, various gases) as well as systemically ingested substances such as perilla mint
- Neoplastic disease, including primary tumors of the respiratory tract, or more commonly, distant metastases
- Static or dynamic upper airway obstructions

INITIAL DATABASE

- Complete blood count and serum chemistry profile show no abnormalities.
- Auscultation after using a rebreathing bag may show no abnormalities, or the horse may cough or have mild wheezes or crackles.
- Palpation of the larynx or trachea may elicit a cough.
- Arterial blood gas analysis is within normal limits at rest; however, horses have an early onset of hypoxemia and hypocapnia during exercise.
- Bronchoalveolar lavage is the preferred method of sampling and shows elevated levels of neutrophils (>5%), mast cells (>2%), or eosinophils (>0.1%) or a combination, along with variable amounts of mucus, without evidence of infection.

ADVANCED OR CONFIRMATORY TESTING

- Lung function testing is extremely helpful in characterizing the disease. Measures of airway resistance are often normal at baseline, but histamine bronchoprovocation reveals airway hyperreactivity ("twitchy airways").
- Endoscopy may or may not show excessive amounts of tracheal mucus.
- Radiography is not helpful in characterizing the disease but may show nonspecific mild interstitial or bronchial pattern.
- Ultrasonography is not helpful.

TREATMENT

THERAPEUTIC GOAL(S)

- Immediate goals involve dilating the small airways to achieve improved exercise tolerance.
- Longer term goals involve reduction of inflammation and control of contributing environmental factors.

ACUTE GENERAL TREATMENT

- Inhaled albuterol (metered dose inhaler [MDI]) using a spacer device (450–900 µg). Ipratropium via MDI may be used in addition for a more sustained effect.
- Treatment with corticosteroids (prednisolone 0.8 mg/kg PO q12h, tapering over a 4-week period).
- Environmental control to minimize dust and noxious gases is extremely important.

CHRONIC TREATMENT

Environmental control is critical to successful long-term treatment. Horses may require long-term treatment with inhaled corticosteroids such as fluticasone propionate or beclomethasone. Mast cell stabilizers such as sodium cromoglycate may be helpful with mast cell–mediated disease.

RECOMMENDED MONITORING

Patients should undergo radiographic (or less ideally, sonographic) monitoring until the disease is resolved.

PROGNOSIS AND OUTCOME

Prognosis for neutrophil-mediated IAD is good, provided environmental remediation takes place. Horses with mast cell–mediated IAD may be less responsive.

SUGGESTED READING

Couëtil LL, Hoffman AM, Hodgson J, et al: Inflammatory airway disease in horses: ACVIM Consensus Statement. *J Vet Intern Med* 21:356–361, 2007.

Bedenice D, Mazan MR, Hoffman AM: Association between cough and cytology of bronchoalveolar lavage fluid and pulmonary function in horses diagnosed with inflammatory airway disease. *J Vet Intern Med* 22(4):1022–1028, 2008.

AUTHOR & EDITOR: **MELISSA R. MAZAN**

Inflammatory Bowel Disease

BASIC INFORMATION

DEFINITION

Primary inflammatory disease of immune-mediated or idiopathic etiology affecting focal or diffuse portions of the small (and sometimes large) intestine and resulting in intestinal malabsorption

EPIDEMIOLOGY

SPECIES, AGE, SEX No age or sex predisposition, although most cases occur in adult horses

GENETICS AND BREED PREDISPOSITION

- Some studies report increased incidence in Standardbreds and Thoroughbreds, although this may represent regional equine populations rather than true breed predispositions.
- Granulomatous enteritis has been described in some related horses, suggesting a potential genetic predisposition, although this has not been definitively documented.

CLINICAL PRESENTATION

DISEASE FORMS/SUBTYPES

Inflammatory bowel disease (IBD) is characterized histopathologically by the predominant cell type in the inflammatory infiltrate.

- Granulomatous enteritis
- Lymphocytic-plasmacytic enteritis
- Multisystemic eosinophilic epitheliotropic disease (MEED)
- Eosinophilic enterocolitis
- Focal eosinophilic enteritis (see "Enteritis, Focal Eosinophilic" in this section)

HISTORY, CHIEF COMPLAINT

- Weight loss (usually with a good appetite) and intermittent, mild colic signs are the most common presentations.
- ± Skin lesions or diarrhea (most common in MEED or eosinophilic enterocolitis)

PHYSICAL EXAM FINDINGS

- Thin body condition
- Temperature, pulse, and respiratory rate are usually within normal limits.
- Ventral edema (caused by hypoproteinemia) is frequently present.
- A generalized, exudative, crusting dermatitis and ulcerative lesions on the coronary bands are often present in horses with MEED.
- Rectal examination
  - May be within normal limits, although focally or diffusely thickened small intestine is often appreciated

- Colonic and rectal mural thickening may also be evident with diffuse disease.
- In contrast, initial evaluation of horses with focal eosinophilic enteritis is identical to horses presenting for other causes of nonstrangulating small intestinal obstruction (see "Enteritis, Focal Eosinophilic" in this section).

ETIOLOGY AND PATHOPHYSIOLOGY

- The specific etiology of all types of IBD is unknown. Infectious, toxic, allergic, or autoimmune mechanisms have been postulated to play a role. IBD has been reported in horses after *Salmonella* or parasitic infections and in horses that may have ingested feed contaminated with aluminium.
- In most cases, though, by the time clinical signs are evident, the primary pathology appears to be immune mediated in nature, even though an initial toxic, dietary, or infectious insult may have initiated the pathology.
- In some cases, IBD may represent a chronic hypersensitivity reaction to unknown (likely dietary) antigens.
- Regardless of the inciting cause, intestinal inflammation results in dysfunction of the intestinal villous epithelial cells, resulting in malabsorption and maldigestion of nutrients and causing weight loss and hypoproteinemia.

With severe inflammation involving the submucosal vasculature, plasma protein is also lost.
- Partial intermittent small intestinal obstruction with hay and fibrous feed caused by small intestinal thickening is likely the cause of intermittent colic in IBD.
- In most cases of IBD, the predominant inflammatory infiltrates are found in the small intestine, although colonic involvement does occur, and some lesser degree of inflammation is usually evident on histopathologic evaluation of the entire intestinal tract in most affected horses.
- In MEED, inflammatory infiltrates are found in the skin, liver, pancreas, and large intestine in addition to the small intestine. The reason these locations are targeted is not known.

DIAGNOSIS

DIFFERENTIAL DIAGNOSIS
- Intestinal lymphosarcoma
- *Rhodococcus equi* enterocolitis or proliferative enteropathy (in foals and weanlings)

INITIAL DATABASE
- Complete blood count
  - Variable
  - Mild to moderate anemia is frequently observed.
  - Leukocytosis and hyperfibrinogenemia associated with chronic inflammation may be present but are not consistently seen.
  - Thrombocytopenia (caused by concurrent disseminated intravascular coagulation) is rarely reported.
- Serum biochemistry profile
  - Hypoproteinemia and hypoalbuminemia are frequently seen.
  - Globulin concentrations may be low, normal, or increased.
  - Liver function should be assessed by measuring serum hepatocellular enzyme activity and serum bile acid concentration to ensure that hypoproteinemia is not associated with liver failure.
- Transabdominal ultrasonography
  - Diffusely or focally increased small intestinal mural thickness (>5 mm) is usually but not always appreciated.
  - Concurrent colonic mural thickening (>5 mm) may also be appreciated.
- Peritoneal fluid analysis: Variable. In most cases, the peritoneal fluid is normal or has a mildly increased nucleated cell count and total protein concentration.
- Urinalysis should be performed to rule out renal protein loss.

- Fecal flotation for parasites should also be performed because intestinal inflammation may occur secondary to chronic parasite infestation.

ADVANCED OR CONFIRMATORY TESTING
- The D-glucose or D-xylose absorption test can confirm the presence of small intestinal malabsorptive disease but does not help differentiate between IBD and other intestinal infiltrative diseases such as lymphosarcoma.
- Rectal mucosal biopsy: In some cases of inflammatory or infiltrative intestinal disease, a diagnosis can be obtained via rectal mucosal biopsy. However, a normal rectal biopsy does not rule out inflammatory intestinal disease confined to the more proximal intestinal tract. In addition, many causes of intestinal inflammation result in nonspecific inflammation on rectal mucosal biopsy.
- Gastroduodenoscopy
  - Concurrent gastroesophageal ulceration is common in IBD.
  - Gastric and duodenal mucosal biopsies may be obtained endoscopically, although these are not always diagnostic for IBD because a full-thickness sample cannot be obtained.
- Exploratory celiotomy and intestinal biopsy
  - Intestinal biopsies may be obtained via laparotomy or laparoscopically from some locations.
  - Several sites (grossly normal and abnormal) should be biopsied, and samples should be evaluated histopathologically.

TREATMENT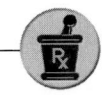

THERAPEUTIC GOAL(S)
Immunosuppressive or antiinflammatory therapy

ACUTE GENERAL TREATMENT
- Immunosuppressive therapy
  - The mainstay of treatment for IBD
  - Corticosteroids are used most frequently and may include:
    - Dexamethasone: 0.1 mg/kg IV, IM, or PO q24h
    - Prednisolone: 1 to 2 mg/kg PO q24h
- In general, parenteral therapy is preferred initially in severe cases because of limited intestinal absorption.
- If a good response to the above therapy is observed, with improvement in serum protein levels and weight gain, steroid therapy may be tapered slowly over 6 to 12 weeks, with a goal of reaching the lowest possible dosage that controls the horse's signs.

- Gastric ulcer prophylaxis with omeprazole: 1 to 2 mg/kg PO q24h
  - If corticosteroids are ineffective, azathioprine (2–3 mg/kg PO q24h) alone or in combination with corticosteroids may be effective, although this has not been well studied in horses.
  - Occasionally, horses respond well to immunosuppressive therapy and remain in remission after discontinuation of treatment. Most horses, though, either do not respond sufficiently or require lifelong immunosuppressive therapy.
- Dietary management
  - Hay and fibrous feed is poorly tolerated in most horses with IBD.
  - Maintenance on good-quality, short, clipped pasture and a well-balanced complete pelleted feed is ideal.
  - In other species, allergy testing and exclusion diets can be helpful in determining the role dietary antigens may play in IBD. In horses, designing an effective yet nutritionally balanced exclusion dietary regimen for horses is quite difficult and requires the input of a veterinary nutritionist and great motivation and expense on the part of the owner.
- Euthanasia is warranted in horses with severe disease that fail to respond to immunosuppressive and dietary therapy.

PROGNOSIS AND OUTCOME

Guarded to poor

PEARLS & CONSIDERATIONS

Intestinal biopsy of the affected intestinal segment is required to make a definitive diagnosis of IBD. Laparotomy allows the most thorough diagnostic evaluation of the intestinal tract, but it is associated with the greatest expense and morbidity.

SUGGESTED READING
Davis JL: Medical disorders of the small intestine: duodenitis-proximal jejunitis. In Smith BP, editor: *Large animal internal medicine*, St Louis, 2009, Mosby Elsevier, pp 725–728.
Sanchez LC: Diseases associated with malabsorption and maldigestion. In Reed SM, Bayly WM, Sellon DC, editors: *Equine internal medicine*, ed 3, St Louis, 2010, Saunders Elsevier, pp 850–856.

AUTHOR: **KELSEY A. HART**

EDITORS: **TIM MAIR** and **CERI SHERLOCK**

Influenza

BASIC INFORMATION

DEFINITION

Influenza virus A-Eq2 (H3N8) is an orthomyxovirus that is an important worldwide respiratory pathogen of horses.

SYNONYM(S)

Flu

EPIDEMIOLOGY

SPECIES, AGE, SEX

- Most common in younger horses (yearlings, ages 2–3 years)
- Rare in foals; however, 11 foals during a recent outbreak in Australia died of severe bronchointerstitial pneumonia as a result of equine influenza infection.

GENETICS AND BREED PREDISPOSITION

Affects all breeds. Disease may be more severe in donkeys and mules.

RISK FACTORS

- Areas of high comingling of horses (eg, racetracks, show grounds, veterinary hospitals)
- Immunosuppression (eg, traveling, hospitalization, training, showing)

CONTAGION AND ZOONOSIS

- Eurasian and American lineage strains of equine influenza virus (H3N8) have been isolated.
- There is no known zoonosis.
- Equine influenza A(H3N8) strains were found to be the causative agent of pathogenic respiratory disease outbreaks in dogs in 2004.

GEOGRAPHY AND SEASONALITY

- Not seen in New Zealand and Iceland.
- Australia had been influenza free until an outbreak in 2007. Strict quarantine and massive surveillance measures resulted in declaration of Australia as free of Equine influenza in December 2007.
- Most common in fall and winter.

CLINICAL PRESENTATION

HISTORY, CHIEF COMPLAINT

- Anorexia
- Fever that may be biphasic (48–96 hours after infection and at 7 days)
- Depression, lethargy, inappetence
- Nasal discharge
- Coughing

PHYSICAL EXAM FINDINGS

- High fever (≤106° F)
- Mild depression, inappetence
- Distal limb edema
- Serous nasal discharge becoming mucopurulent after 72 to 96 hours
- Slightly enlarged retropharyngeal lymph nodes
- Coughing (dry) that may persist for up to 21 days
- Tachypnea
- Arrhythmia (rare) cause of cardiomyopathy
- Muscle soreness
- Weight loss

ETIOLOGY AND PATHOPHYSIOLOGY

- Highly infectious virus transmission through aerosolized droplets
- Transmission through fomites probably also occurs.
- The virus is inhaled and attaches and multiplies in the respiratory epithelium with a short incubation period of 1 to 3 days.
- The virus causes epithelial cell death and desquamation, with predominant damage in the trachea and bronchial tree, resulting in disruption of mucociliary clearance critical for preventing secondary bacterial infection.
- A high concentration of virus is shed through nasal secretions.
- Fever and virus shedding 48 hours after exposure; shedding for 6 to 7 days
- Subclinical infection with shedding is possible.
- The virus survives on wet surfaces for 72 hours and dry surfaces for 48 hours.

DIAGNOSIS

DIFFERENTIAL DIAGNOSIS

- Equine herpesviruses 1 and 4
- Equine viral arteritis
- Equine rhinoviruses
- Bacterial pneumonia or pleuropneumonia
- Other respiratory pathogens

INITIAL DATABASE

- Complete blood count may reveal leukopenia caused by lymphopenia

ADVANCED OR CONFIRMATORY TESTING

- Virus isolation from nasopharyngeal secretions collected from the nasal passage using a 6-inch polyester or Dacron swab. Samples should be collected within first 24 to 48 hours after clinical onset.
- Serology using paired sera (acute and convalescent) collected 10 to 21 days apart. Common tests include hemagglutination inhibition, single radial hemolysis, fluorescent antibody, and enzyme-linked immunosorbent assay (ELISA).
- ELISA (eg, Directogen test, Becton Dickinson, Franklin Lakes, NJ) to detect viral antigen in nasopharyngeal secretions can be done stall side using a nasal swab sample.
- Reverse transcriptase polymerase chain reaction may be used to detect viral RNA in clinical samples.

TREATMENT

THERAPEUTIC GOALS

- Provide supportive and symptomatic treatment.
- Establish biosecurity measures to minimize the spread of infection.

ACUTE GENERAL TREATMENT

- Rest with minimal stress is the most important component of therapy. Damaged respiratory epithelium takes a minimum of 3 weeks to regenerate.
- Antipyretics (nonsteroidal antiinflammatory drugs [NSAIDs]) for high fever or significant myalgia
- Hydration and fluids if needed
- Nursing care
- Antiviral medication has not been evaluated in horses, but there have been some suggestions that amantadine at 10 mg/kg IV q8h or 5 mg/kg q4h (avoid in renal patients because central nervous system effects have been reported) or rimantadine at 30 mg/kg PO q12h may reduce the severity and duration of infection in horses.

POSSIBLE COMPLICATIONS

- Secondary bacterial infections
- Pleuropneumonia
- Reactive airway obstruction
- Myocarditis, myositis

RECOMMENDED MONITORING

- Monitor horses twice daily for increased rectal temperature. Segregate horses with fever from the general horse population.
- Monitor hydration status, especially if treating with NSAIDs.
- Quarantine horses for 21 days after the last known clinical signs resolve.

PROGNOSIS AND OUTCOME

- The majority of infections are self-limiting with clinical signs lasting for 24 hours to 3 days.
- High morbidity (60%–90%); less than 1% mortality rate

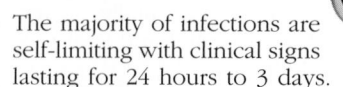

PEARLS & CONSIDERATIONS

COMMENTS

- Common cause of self-limiting respiratory disease in young horses
- Confirming the diagnosis with virus isolation is important for monitoring viral antigenic variation.
- Serologic confirmation of the diagnosis is most accurate if several sick and in-contact horses are simultaneously tested.
- It is important to use vaccines produced from current and clinically relevant strains of equine influenza.

PREVENTION

- Horses returning from areas of high exposure risk (eg, shows, breeding, hospitalization) should be housed apart from the general barn population for at least 14 days and monitored for clinical signs.
- Vaccines for Equine influenza that are currently available in the United States include
  - Inactivated virus intramuscular vaccines
    - A recombinant canarypox vector intramuscular vaccine
    - A modified-live virus (MLV) cold adapted intranasal equine influenza vaccine
- The American Association of Equine Practitioners recommends that mature performance, show, or pleasure horses at regular risk of exposure be revaccinated at 6-month intervals. Other adult horses could be vaccinated as infrequently as once a year.
- Pregnant mares that have been previously vaccinated should be vaccinated with an intramuscular product 30 days before foaling.
- Foals from vaccinated mares should be vaccinated once with the MLV intranasal vaccine or a primary series of three doses of IM vaccine beginning at 6 months of age. There should be 4 to 6 weeks between the first and second dose of IM vaccine; the third dose should be administered at 10 to 12 months of age.
- Vaccination of clinically normal horses in an outbreak situation may be beneficial. Horses with no known history of vaccination may benefit from a modified intranasal vaccine in which onset of protective immunity is within 7 days with a single dose.

CLIENT EDUCATION

- Emphasize the importance of rest for minimum of 3 weeks for affected horses (1 week of rest for every day of fever).
- Training and stress may increase the risk of secondary infections.

SUGGESTED READING

Crawford PC, Dubovi EJ, Castleman WL, et al: Transmission of equine influenza to dogs. *Science* 310:482–485, 2005.

Landolt GA, et al: Equine influenza infection. In Sellon DC, Long MT, editors: *Equine infectious diseases*, St Louis, 1997, Mosby, pp 124–134.

OIE Reference Laboratory for Equine Influenza. Available at http://www.ca.uky.edu/gluck/ServOIE.asp.

OIE terrestrial animal health code, ed 12, 2004. Available at http://www.oie.int/.

Patterson-Kane JC, Carrick JB, Axon JE, et al: The pathology of bronchointerstitial pneumonia in young foals associated with the first outbreak of equine influenza in Australia. *Equine Vet J* 40:199–203, 2008.

AUTHOR: KATHY K. SEINO

EDITORS: DEBRA C. SELLON and MAUREEN T. LONG

Insect Hypersensitivity

BASIC INFORMATION

DEFINITION

A hypersensitivity reaction to bites by various insects

SYNONYM(S)

Summer itch, summer "fungus," sweet itch, lichen tropicus, Queensland itch (Australia), Sommerekzem (Germany), Manochsvankorv (Sweden), Kasen (Japan)

EPIDEMIOLOGY

SPECIES, AGE, SEX

- Common in horses but may also be seen in other Equidae
- Signs may start at any age but more commonly start between 2 and 4 years of age and often become more severe as the horse ages.

GENETICS AND BREED PREDISPOSITION

- Several horse breeds appear to have a hereditary predisposition, including Icelandic, German Shire, Arabian, Connemara, Swiss Warmblood, Quarter Horse, and ponies.
- A genetic influence in the frequency of the disease has been found in Swiss Warmbloods.
- Breeding of affected horses is not recommended.

GEOGRAPHY AND SEASONALITY

Insect hypersensitivity in horses has a worldwide distribution. The disease is prevalent during the warm weather season or year round in more tropical regions.

ASSOCIATED CONDITIONS AND DISORDERS

Insect hypersensitivity is commonly seen in conjunction with atopic dermatitis (environmental allergies).

CLINICAL PRESENTATION

HISTORY, CHIEF COMPLAINT

Owners frequently notice increasing self-trauma (scratching, biting, and rubbing of the skin; hair loss; and loss of the mane and tail hair; excoriations) during insect season. Other horses on the same premises may be unaffected. The history often reveals similar problems in previous years at similar times of year.

PHYSICAL EXAM FINDINGS

- Skin lesions vary from mild with areas of broken-off hair only, papules, and crusts to complete alopecia and severe excoriation.
- The distribution of the lesions depends on where the involved insects are feeding and can affect any combination of locations, including the face, mane, ventrum, dorsal back, legs, and tail.
- "Classic" lesions of *Culicoides* hypersensitivity include "buzzed-off manes" and "rat tails."
- Chronic lesions may include lichenification and hyperpigmentation and skin fold development (rugae) at the base of mane and tail.
- Some severely affected horses may also show behavioral changes (restlessness and irritability) and even weight loss, making the horse unsuitable for riding in some cases.
- Affected horses may also develop secondary bacterial infection of the skin (folliculitis). Signs of this complication

range from erected hairs over small papules with or without crusts to deeper lesions with nodules and draining tracts in rare cases.

- Urticaria is an uncommon manifestation of insect hypersensitivity in horses.

ETIOLOGY AND PATHOPHYSIOLOGY

- Type I (immunoglobulin E–mediated) hypersensitivity reaction to saliva from various biting insects ± type IV (delayed or cell-mediated) hypersensitivity reaction.
- Insects found most commonly to be involved are *Culicoides* spp. (biting midges, "no-see-ums") but also by mosquitoes, black flies, horse flies, horn flies, stable flies, sand flies and, less commonly ants, wasps, and bees.

DIAGNOSIS

DIFFERENTIAL DIAGNOSIS

- Sarcoptic mange affecting the head, especially the ears, that has progressed to the whole body.
- Psoroptic mange affecting the mane, forelock, and tail.
- Chorioptic mange affecting the (lower) legs.
- Straw itch mites affecting areas on the horse that are exposed to hay and straw.
- Trombiculiasis (chiggers, harvest mites, red bugs), which is most common in the late summer and fall and affects mostly the legs and face.
- Migrating microfilarial stage *Onchocerca cervicalis* may cause similar lesions anywhere on the body but have been mostly eliminated since the introduction of ivermectin.
- Habronemiasis (summer sores) may cause a hypersensitivity reaction to aberrant intradermal migration of the larvae of the horses stomach worms.
- Lice infestation usually affects the neck and mane but may also affect the head, dorsum, flanks, fetlock, and tail or may be generalized in chronic cases.

INITIAL DATABASE

- Take a detailed history.
- Take skin scrapings of the lesions.
- Ivermectin trial (treatment every 2 weeks at least three times) of the affected horse and all in-contact horses.

ADVANCED OR CONFIRMATORY TESTING

- Intradermal testing for insect and environmental allergens (preferred over enzyme-linked immunosorbent assay [ELISA] testing).
- ELISA testing for insect and environmental allergens if skin testing is not available.

- Food trial (if symptoms are year round): Stop all supplements and grains and try to find a hay to which the horse has not been previously exposed.
- Complete blood count and serum chemistry profile: Usually normal (rarely shows eosinophilia).
- Skin biopsies for histopathology reveal a perivascular eosinophilic and lymphocytic dermatitis (this will only rule allergic dermatitis in or out, but not the type of hypersensitivity, ie, insect versus food versus environmental allergies).

TREATMENT

THERAPEUTIC GOALS

- It may not be possible to avoid insect bites completely, but clinical sign usually improve with treatment that lowers the exposure to insect bites and reduces the hypersensitivity reaction.
- An allergic reaction is only triggered if a certain threshold of allergen exposure is exceeded. This threshold varies for each individual animal.

ACUTE GENERAL TREATMENT

- Permethrin sprays (ideally 2% or higher in concentration applied q12–24h), spot-on products (at 45% applied once weekly), or both
- For pruritus: Prednisolone tablets mixed in the grain at 1 mg/kg q24h or dexamethasone liquid injectable given PO 0.05 to 0.1 mg/kg q24h
- Fly sheets (with or without permethrin impregnation) covering the affected areas of the horse

CHRONIC TREATMENT

- Elimination of standing water (including frequent dumping and cleaning of water buckets and troughs) to reduce breeding grounds for mosquitoes, *Culicoides* spp., and black flies.
- Stabling of the horse during peak feeding times:
  ○ *Culicoides* spp. and mosquitoes are active predominantly at dusk and dawn and in warm, humid weather.
  ○ Black flies, horse flies, stable flies, and horn flies are more active during the daylight.
- Use of mosquito dunks containing a bacterium that kills mosquito and black fly larvae in water sources.
- Installing large strong box fans in the barn and stall front because *Culicoides* spp. are weak fliers.
- Frequent manure removal or dragging pastures to break up manure pile because most flies use manure as breeding grounds.

- Use of feed-through fly control products containing insect growth regulators or chitin synthesis inhibitors to prevent larvae development in the manure pile.
- Allergen-specific immunotherapy, especially when environmental allergies are concurrently present.

PROGNOSIS AND OUTCOME

As with most allergic diseases, treatment is usually lifelong, and no cure should be expected. With the above treatments, regular use of the horse should be possible, and a good quality of life can be expected.

PEARLS & CONSIDERATIONS

COMMENTS

Treating horses with insect hypersensitivity usually requires a combination of the above treatments. One treatment alone will not likely resolve the clinical signs. Treatment protocols need to be tailored to the client's abilities.

PREVENTION

Strict insect control

CLIENT EDUCATION

The client needs be aware that long-term cure is unlikely, but the disease can be managed with a multimodal approach. This includes a combination of daily application of a high-percentage permethrin spray, fly sheets, elimination of standing water, use of fans, and so on. For most cases of equine insect hypersensitivity, these measures reduce the insect exposure enough to gain clinical control.

SUGGESTED READING

Knottenbelt DC: *Pascoe's principles & practice of equine dermatology*, St Louis, 1999, WB Saunders, pp 284–286.

Petersen A: Equine insect hypersensitivity. In Robinson NE, Sprayberry KA, editors: *Current therapy in equine medicine*, ed 6, St Louis, 2009, Saunders Elsevier, pp 678–680.

Rosenkrantz WS, Griffin CE, Esch RE, et al: Response in horses to intradermal challenge of insects and environmental allergens with specific immunotherapy. In Kwochka KW, et al, editors: *Advances in veterinary dermatology III*, Boston, 1998, Butterworth-Heinemann, pp 191–200.

AUTHOR: ANNETTE PETERSEN

EDITOR: DAVID A. WILSON

Insulin Resistance

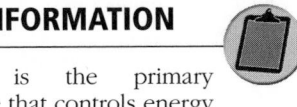

BASIC INFORMATION

- Insulin is the primary hormone that controls energy metabolism.
- The pancreatic β cells secrete insulin in response to glucose and glucagon.
- Insulin secretion is also regulated by sympathetic and parasympathetic systems: epinephrine (stress) inhibits and acetylcholine (food intake) stimulates insulin secretion.
- Somatostatin inhibits insulin secretion.
- Insulin regulates three major fuels: carbohydrates, proteins, and fats.
- The liver, skeletal muscle, and adipose tissue are the major targets for insulin.
  - Liver: Insulin decreases glycogen, gluconeogenesis, and ketogenesis, and stimulates glycogen and fatty acid synthesis.
  - Adipose tissue: Insulin decreases lipolysis and stimulates fatty acid uptake, synthesis, and esterification.
  - Skeletal muscle: Insulin decreases proteolysis and amino acid output and increases glucose and amino acid uptake, protein synthesis, and glycogen synthesis.
- Understanding insulin physiology is central to understanding the pathogenesis of equine pathological conditions such as hyperlipemia, pituitary pars intermedia dysfunction (Cushing's disease), equine metabolic syndrome (EMS), and polysaccharide storage myopathy.

DEFINITION

Insulin resistance (IR) is defined as a decreased response to endogenous or exogenous insulin

EPIDEMIOLOGY

SPECIES, AGE, SEX IR is more commonly reported in horses older than 7 years (metabolic syndrome, Cushing's disease), but it may be present in ponies at any age.

GENETICS AND BREED PREDISPOSITION

- There is a genetic predisposition: Saddlebreds, Morgans, Tennessee Walking Horses, Paso Finos, and Quarter Horses are predisposed to IR.
- IR is a common finding in ponies (genetics).

GEOGRAPHY AND SEASONALITY

- There is no evidence that IR is associated with geography or season per se.
- The condition is more often reported in developed countries, likely associated with the feeding habits of horses because IR in general is a condition of obese horses.

ASSOCIATED CONDITIONS AND DISORDERS

- See "Equine Metabolic Syndrome" in this section.
- Diabetes mellitus is a rare condition in horses.

CLINICAL PRESENTATION

HISTORY, CHIEF COMPLAINT

- IR has been reported in horses and ponies with pars intermedia dysfunction (Cushing's disease), EMS, obesity, hyperlipemia, diabetes mellitus, laminitis, granulosa cell tumors, and endotoxemia.
- Laminitis is a consistent clinical finding of IR.
- Often these horses are obese, although horses with poor body condition (Cushing's disease) can have IR.
- A "cresty neck" or "stallion-like" appearance in mares is suggestive of IR (see "Metabolic Syndrome" in this section).

PHYSICAL EXAM FINDINGS

- Obesity, fat redistribution (tailhead, prepuce, mammary gland, supraorbital fat pads, shoulder area) and laminitis in EMS
- Laminitis, delayed haircoat shedding, hirsutism, weight loss, and polyuria and polydipsia in horses with Cushing's disease
- Anorexia, diarrhea, arrhythmias, and icterus in ponies with hyperlipemia
- Infertility

ETIOLOGY AND PATHOPHYSIOLOGY

- Decreased number of insulin receptors or lack of receptor response upon insulin stimulation (nonfunctional receptors).
- This leads to insulin insensitivity or resistance.
- This results in hyperinsulinemia with normoglycemia (compensated IR) or with hyperglycemia (noncompensated IR).
- Glucocorticoids stimulate glycogen formation, gluconeogenesis, and proteolysis; induce IR; and increase glycemia.
- Glucocorticoids induce IR by decreasing the receptor response to insulin.
- Increased glucocorticoid concentrations are present in conditions such as metabolic syndrome, hyperlipemia, and Cushing's disease.
- Carbohydrate feeding to horses increases glucocorticoid release and has been associated with IR.
- Dexamethasone administration to healthy horses decreases insulin sensitivity.
- Growth hormone also induces IR in horses.

DIAGNOSIS

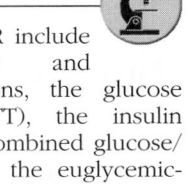

- Tests to diagnose IR include baseline glucose and insulin concentrations, the glucose tolerance test (GTT), the insulin tolerance test, the combined glucose/insulin test (CGIT), the euglycemic-hyperinsulinemic clamp (EHC), and the minimal model analysis of a frequently sampled IV glucose tolerance test (FSIGT).
- Baseline insulin concentrations should be less than 20 μU/mL.
- Insulin concentration above 30 μU/mL suggests IR.
- Whereas hyperglycemia with hyperinsulinemia suggests IR, hyperglycemia with hypoinsulinemia indicates insulin-dependent diabetes mellitus.
- Contrary to IR, there are few cases of diabetes mellitus documented in horses

DIFFERENTIAL DIAGNOSIS

- IR is an endocrine abnormality present in various pathological conditions.
- IR is present in horses with obesity, hypothyroidism, Cushing's disease, metabolic syndrome, and hyperlipemia.
- IR is the hallmark of EMS.
- Consider IR in horses with laminitis.
- Hyperglycemia may be the result of diabetes mellitus (rare in horses).

TREATMENT

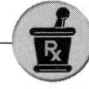

ACUTE GENERAL TREATMENT

- Address the primary problem.
- Start a weight loss plan.
- Increase physical activity.
- Consider levothyroxine sodium (1–6 mg/100 kg PO q24h)
- Levothyroxine is used to induce a hypermetabolic state, not because these horses have hypothyroidism.
- Do not feed carbohydrate-rich diets, except in ponies with hyperlipemia.

PROGNOSIS AND OUTCOME

Guarded to poor depending on disease

PEARLS & CONSIDERATIONS

- The excessive feeding of carbohydrate-rich diets and obesity may lead to IR and laminitis.

- A good management plan (deworming, vaccination) should be used in ponies to avoid hyperlipemia.
- Obese horses and ponies are prone to IR.

SUGGESTED READING

Eiler H, Frank N, Andrews F: Physiologic assessment of blood glucose homeostasis via combined intravenous glucose and insulin testing in horses. *Am J Vet Res* 66:1598–1604, 2005.

Frank N: Equine metabolic syndrome. In Smith BP, editor: *Large animal internal medicine*, ed 4. St Louis, 2009, Mosby Elsevier, pp 1352–1355.

McFarlane D: Pituitary and hypothalamus. In Smith BP, editor: *Large animal internal medicine*, ed 4. St Louis, 2009, Mosby Elsevier, pp 1339–1344.

Toribio RE, Frank N: Insulin resistance and equine metabolic syndrome. In Reed SM, Bayly WM, Sellon DC, editors: *Equine internal medicine*, ed 3, St Louis, 2010, Saunders Elsevier, pp 1270–1277.

AUTHOR & EDITOR: **RAMIRO E. TORIBIO**

Intracarotid Injection

BASIC INFORMATION

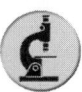

DEFINITION

Introduction of venous medications into the arterial system

EPIDEMIOLOGY

SPECIES, AGE, SEX Common in equine patients because of the high prevalence of IV medications administered
RISK FACTORS Reactions may occur with a number of medications, including sedatives, anesthetic agents, electrolyte solutions, and antibiotics.

CLINICAL PRESENTATION

HISTORY, CHIEF COMPLAINT History of recent IV injection followed by immediate clinical abnormalities (within 10 seconds of injection)
PHYSICAL EXAM FINDINGS
Neurologic deficits are common:
- Excitement
- Seizures
- Central blindness (lack of menace, normal pupillary light reflex)
- Abnormal postural reactions
- Lethargy
- Circling
- Collapse
- Coma
- Death

ETIOLOGY AND PATHOPHYSIOLOGY
- Introduction of a medication intended for IV use only into the carotid artery may result in ischemic cerebral necrosis.
- The forebrain (prosencephalon, including the thalamus, hypothalamus, and cerebrum) is most commonly affected because of delivery of the medication from the external carotid to the circle of Willis, resulting in infarction and cavitation.
- Damage occurs, from most to least severe, in the thalamus, midbrain,

cerebral cortices, hippocampus, corpus striatum, and cerebellum. However, the dose and type of medication injected may cause even more widespread cerebral damage.

DIAGNOSIS

DIFFERENTIAL DIAGNOSIS

- Drug reaction
- Head trauma
- Neoplasia
- Encephalitis
- Endotoxic shock

INITIAL DATABASE

- History
- Neurologic examination

ADVANCED OR CONFIRMATORY TESTING

- Cerebrospinal fluid analysis if neurologic disease is suspected
- Computed tomography or magnetic resonance imaging may show cavitary lesions in the prosencephalon.

TREATMENT

THERAPEUTIC GOALS

- Treat seizures.
- Provide cardiopulmonary support.
- Prevent or treat secondary trauma to the horse caused by seizures and loss of consciousness.
- Reduce cerebral edema and inflammation.

ACUTE GENERAL TREATMENT

- Sedation may be required to control the patient for therapy, but ensure that it is a venous injection.

- Anticonvulsants
  - Diazepam: Adults, 0.05 to 0.44 mg/kg IV; foals, 0.1 to 0.2 mg/kg IV
  - Phenobarbital: 5 to 15 mg/kg IV slowly
- Cardiovascular resuscitation
  - See "Shock Dose Fluid Administration" in Section II.
  - Mechanical ventilation
- Antiinflammatory medications
  - Flunixin meglumine (1.1 mg/kg q12h IV) for antiinflammatory and antiendotoxin effects
  - Hypertonic saline (adults, ≤4 mL/kg IV) for cerebral edema and shock
  - Mannitol (0.25–2.0 g/kg, infused over 30–45 min IV) for cerebral edema
  - Dimethylsulfoxide (0.5–1.0 g/kg in a 20% solution q8–12h IV) for edema and inflammation
- General wound and orthopedic trauma management; radiography when indicated

CHRONIC TREATMENT

May require continued seizure management

RECOMMENDED MONITORING

Repeated neurologic examinations are recommended to monitor recovery.

PROGNOSIS AND OUTCOME

- The severity of the reaction depends on the medication injected.
- Horses exhibit a wide range of individual variation in drug reaction and recovery.
- Most horses recover within hours to 1 week of injection.
- Neurologic deficits may be permanent.

PEARLS & CONSIDERATIONS

PREVENTION

- To administer an IV medication, place the needle in the vessel with the syringe unattached.
- An 18-gauge needle or larger is recommended. The pulsations or flow of arterial blood can be seen.
- The tip of the needle can also be palpated in the vein to confirm placement. If unsure of placement, a test dose of the medication may be administered.
- The horse should be monitored for immediate reaction.
- The safest method to prevent intracarotid injection is through a catheter or IM injection.

CLIENT EDUCATION

Any IV medication administered by a needle should be performed by a veterinarian to reduce the risk of intracarotid injection.

SUGGESTED READING

Christian RG, Mills JH, Kramer LL: Accidental intracarotid artery injection of promazine in the horse. *Can Vet J* 15(2):29–33, 1974.

Delahunta A, Glass EN: *Veterinary neuroanatomy and clinical neurology*, St Louis, 2009, Saunders Elsevier, p 425.

AUTHOR: **AMELIA MUNSTERMAN**

EDITORS: **R. REID HANSON** and **AMELIA MUNSTERMAN**

Ionophore Toxicosis

BASIC INFORMATION

DEFINITION

Ionophore toxicosis is caused by the feed additives lasalocid, monensin, narasin, salinomycin, or other ionophores.

SYNONYM(S)

Ionophore antibiotics

EPIDEMIOLOGY

RISK FACTORS Exposure to premixes or feeds designed for other species such as swine, cattle, or chickens
ASSOCIATED CONDITIONS AND DISORDERS Chronic heart damage resulting in congestive heart failure or cardiomyopathy

CLINICAL PRESENTATION

DISEASE FORMS/SUBTYPES
- Acute toxicosis
- Delayed heart failure

HISTORY, CHIEF COMPLAINT
- Acute: Horses with ionophore toxicosis may have clinical signs of anorexia, diarrhea, depression, dyspnea, weakness, ataxia, hypermetria, paresis, colic, sweating, groaning, recumbency, paddling, and death.
- Delayed signs: Horses that recover from acute intoxication may develop signs consistent with heart failure. Signs include chronic unthriftiness, poor performance, poor exercise tolerance, cardiac arrhythmias, and sudden death.

PHYSICAL EXAM FINDINGS
- Acute: Elevated heart rate, congested mucous membranes, tachypnea, cardiac arrhythmias, and myoglobinuria
- Chronic: Cardiac arrhythmias, edema, weight loss, exercise intolerance

ETIOLOGY AND PATHOPHYSIOLOGY Ionophores enhance movement of ions through membranes. Increased intracellular calcium is associated with degeneration and necrosis of skeletal and cardiac muscle.

DIAGNOSIS

DIFFERENTIAL DIAGNOSIS

Any myopathy, exertional myopathies, pasture myopathy, injection reactions, white snakeroot, rayless goldenrod, coffee senna, blister beetles, other causes of colic.

INITIAL DATABASE

- Myoglobinuria
- Elevated muscle enzymes
- Hyperglycemia

ADVANCED OR CONFIRMATORY TESTING

- Elevated serum cardiac troponin: Best to measure at 24 to 48 hours after exposure
- Analysis for ionophores in feeds or stomach contents
- Echocardiography and electrocardiography findings suggestive of cardiac abnormalities
- Histopathologic findings: Petechiation and pale skeletal or cardiac muscle; degeneration and necrosis of skeletal or cardiac muscle or both; and loss of striation and fiber swelling. Cardiac muscle lesions are generally more prominent than skeletal muscle lesions in horses.
- Animals that die peracutely may not have any histopathologic lesions evident.

TREATMENT

THERAPEUTIC GOALS

- Decontamination if possible
- Symptomatic treatment

ACUTE GENERAL TREATMENT

- Decontamination can be attempted soon after exposure. The efficacy of activated charcoal or mineral oil has not been specifically demonstrated for ionophore toxicosis in horses; however, these agents are generally not contraindicated and are commonly given within hours of exposure.
- Treatment of clinical signs is symptomatic and supportive. There is no antidote available for ionophore intoxication.
- Vitamin E therapy is often given to horses with ionophore toxicosis, although prevention of further muscle degeneration has not been demonstrated.

CHRONIC TREATMENT

Rest

DRUG INTERACTIONS

Some antibiotics can potentiate ionophore toxicity.

POSSIBLE COMPLICATIONS

Cardiac fibrosis resulting in congestive heart failure or cardiac arrhythmias

RECOMMENDED MONITORING

- Serum muscle enzymes
- Serum cardiac troponin
- Electrocardiology
- Cardiac ejection volume, cardiopulmonary flow index

PROGNOSIS AND OUTCOME

Prognosis varies depending on the dosage and treatment. Some horses die acutely with no chance of treatment. Other horses return to former performance after weeks to months of recovery. Some horses develop cardiac fibrosis and congestive heart failure that can hinder future performance and rarely results in sudden death months after initial exposure.

PEARLS & CONSIDERATIONS

COMMENTS

- For horses, the lowest reported toxic dosage of monensin incorporated into feed is 2 mg/kg of body weight and for lasalocid is 15 mg/kg of body weight.
- The presence of an ionophore in horse feed is not proof of toxicosis.

Safety studies of horses consuming cattle feeds that contained the maximum approved concentration of monensin (33 ppm) showed that this did not cause clinical signs of intoxication in horses.

- Ionophore toxicosis most commonly occurs when premixes or feed intended for poultry, swine, or cattle are ingested by horses from feed mixing errors or inadvertent carryover.
- Occasionally, carryover of ionophore-containing feeds in mills or bulk delivery trucks may occur.
- Exercise stress tests, echocardiography, and electrocardiography may be used to determine if an exposed horse can return to athletic use.

PREVENTION

Flush feed bins and trucks used to make or haul ionophore-containing feeds with other untreated grain before loading horse feed.

CLIENT EDUCATION

Do not feed horses premixes or feeds intended for other species.

SUGGESTED READING

Novilla MN: Ionophores. In Gupta RC, editor: *Veterinary toxicology*, New York, 2007, Elsevier, pp 1021–1036.

AUTHOR: **MIKE MURPHY**

EDITOR: **CYNTHIA L. GASKILL**

Ischemia-Reperfusion Injury

BASIC INFORMATION

DEFINITION

- Ischemia is the deficiency of blood flow to tissues or organs.
- Reperfusion is the restoration of blood flow of blood to a previously ischemic tissue or organ.

EPIDEMIOLOGY

SPECIES, AGE, SEX All equine species are affected, but the underlying causes of intestinal injury vary among different age groups.

ASSOCIATED CONDITIONS AND DISORDERS

- Intestinal injury: Strangulating lesions of both small and large intestines, ileus
- Shock: Hypovolemic or endotoxic
- Dehydration

CLINICAL PRESENTATION

HISTORY, CHIEF COMPLAINT

- Severe colic unresponsive to medical management
- Abdominal distension

PHYSICAL EXAM FINDINGS

- Tachycardia (>60 beats/min)
- Tachypnea (>40 beats/min)
- Prolonged capillary refill time (2–3 sec)
- Mucous membranes bright red to purple and tacky to the touch; a toxic line may be present
- Dehydration (enophthalmos, skin tenting)

ETIOLOGY AND PATHOPHYSIOLOGY

- Decreased blood flow to an area minimizes available oxygen for tissues.
- Decreased energy production in endothelial cells leads to cellular degeneration.
- Endothelial cell mitochondrial damage leads to production of cytokines that alert other cells (primarily neutrophils) to migrate to the affected area when perfusion is reestablished.
- The neutrophils that migrate from capillary beds cause the most prominent damage because of their inflammatory response (release of elastase, oxygen radicals, and proteases that attack collagen, ground substance, and cellular membranes).
- Because of the overwhelming inflammatory response during reperfusion, there may be a delayed onset or inhibition of the healing process.
- Areas that have been damaged by reperfusion can expand through inflammation from the initial injury site to surrounding viable tissue and cause irreversible damage.

DIAGNOSIS

DIFFERENTIAL DIAGNOSIS

Continued ischemia

INITIAL DATABASE

- Complete blood cell count: Depends on the underlying cause of intestinal issue
- Packed cell volume (PCV) and total protein (TP): Elevation of a PCV (>45%) as well as total protein (>7.5–8.0 g/dL) are indicative of hypovolemia as well as systemic compromise.
- Serum chemistry, including lactate: Electrolyte abnormalities may be appreciated along with elevation in serum lactate resulting from tissue ischemia causing acidosis.
- Abdominal ultrasonography
  - Multiple loops of distended, nonmotile small intestine (5–7 cm in diameter)
  - Edema present within the walls of the small or large intestine.
- Abdominocentesis: Elevation in white blood cell count (>10,000 cells/dL), elevation in protein (>2 g/dL)
- Rectal examination
  - Palpable loops of distended small intestine
  - Large colon displacement with gas distension

ADVANCED OR CONFIRMATORY TESTING

- Coagulation profiles to identify underlying disseminated intravascular coagulation (DIC)

TREATMENT

THERAPEUTIC GOALS

- Correct underlying surgical lesion
- Restore circulating blood volume to ensure appropriate perfusion to tissues

ACUTE GENERAL TREATMENT

- IV fluid therapy (See "Shock Dose Fluid Administration" in Section II)
- Antiinflammatory drugs: Flunixin meglumine, dimethylsulfoxide
- Systemic antibiotics
- Antiendotoxin therapy

POSSIBLE COMPLICATIONS

- Loss of gastrointestinal integrity with absorption of bacteria and bacterial toxins
- Loss of vascular tone

- DIC
- Sepsis
- Death

PROGNOSIS AND OUTCOME

Prognosis and outcome are case dependent based on the underlying lesion.

PEARLS & CONSIDERATIONS

Healing of the affected area has been correlated with the resolution of colic, obstruction, or strangulation. However, fibrosis and residual mucosal inflammation may increase the risk of future colic episodes.

SUGGESTED READING

White NA: Intestinal injury and healing in the horse. In Smith BP, editor: *Large animal internal medicine*, ed 4, St Louis, 2008, Elsevier, pp 702–711.

AUTHOR: **HEATHER DAVIS**

EDITORS: **R. REID HANSON** and **AMELIA MUNSTERMAN**

Ivermectin and Moxidectin Toxicosis

BASIC INFORMATION

DEFINITION

The macrocyclic lactones ivermectin and moxidectin are widely used parasiticides in equine medicine. Although they have a large margin of safety when used as directed, overdose causes central nervous system (CNS) toxicity that can be fatal.

EPIDEMIOLOGY

SPECIES, AGE, SEX Neonates, miniature donkeys, miniature horses, and underweight adult horses are at higher risk of overdose.

RISK FACTORS

- Drug administered: Toxicity is more frequent from the administration of moxidectin than ivermectin.
- Owner administration: Owners frequently do not follow the label directions, and the equine paste and gel formulations are easily overdosed in foals, miniature donkeys, miniature horses, and debilitated adult horses.

CLINICAL PRESENTATION

HISTORY, CHIEF COMPLAINT

- Oral overdose of ivermectin at 10 times the label dose or at three times the label dose for moxidectin
- IV administration of bovine formulations
- Onset of CNS signs is immediate after IV injection and within 8 to 12 hours of PO administration.
- Presence of clinical signs as described below if exposure is unknown

PHYSICAL EXAM FINDINGS

- Depression, ataxia, stupor, coma, mydriasis, blindness, tremors, hypersalivation, decreased respiratory rate, and drooping lower lip. In foals, the clinical signs are similar, but in addition, include a protruding tongue, vacant stare, and recumbency.
- Because ivermectin and moxidectin are γ-aminobutyric acid (GABA)

agonists, seizures are not seen with toxicity.

ETIOLOGY AND PATHOPHYSIOLOGY

- Equine formulations of moxidectin and ivermectin are dosed at 0.4 mg/kg body weight and 0.2 mg/kg body weight, respectively. Moxidectin is not labeled for use in foals younger than 4 months.
  - Over-the-counter pastes and gels contain enough drug to treat 520 to 600 kg of body weight, and owners frequently administer the entire syringe regardless of the horse's actual weight.
  - At label dosing, the peak plasma concentrations of moxidectin are approximately twice the concentrations of ivermectin.
- Moxidectin is 100 times more lipid soluble than ivermectin, so it distributes to a greater degree in fat and has a much longer plasma elimination half-life (23 days for moxidectin; 4 days for ivermectin).
  - In animals with low fat stores, such as debilitated adults and neonates, plasma concentrations of moxidectin are higher, so the neurotoxic dose is lower.
  - Because neonates have a less developed blood-brain barrier, they appear to be more sensitive to toxicosis.
- Toxicity results from the potentiation of GABA, an inhibitory neurotransmitter.
  - Ivermectin and moxidectin stimulate synaptic secretion of GABA and enhance postsynaptic GABA binding to its receptor site, resulting in open chloride channels and membrane hyperpolarization.
  - P-glycoprotein is the transporter protein of the blood-brain barrier that effluxes these drugs out of the brain, protecting it from GABA-ergic neurotoxicity.

- Moxidectin has less affinity than ivermectin for P-glycoprotein, which allows it to penetrate the brain more easily to cause neurotoxicity than ivermectin.

DIAGNOSIS

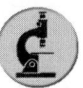

DIFFERENTIAL DIAGNOSIS

- CNS trauma or neoplasia
- Idiopathic Arabian epilepsy (postictal presentation only)
- Viral encephalitides
- Hepatic encephalopathy
- Locoweed toxicity
- Fluphenazine toxicity

INITIAL DATABASE

Routine complete blood count and serum chemistries are typically within normal limits.

ADVANCED OR CONFIRMATORY TESTING

- High-pressure liquid chromatography or enzyme-linked immunosorbent assays can be performed on the liver, brain, fat, gastrointestinal contents, and feces to confirm exposure.
- No specific gross or histopathologic lesions are associated with ivermectin or moxidectin toxicity in horses.

TREATMENT

THERAPEUTIC GOAL(S)

Most affected foals and horses recover with intensive supportive therapy.

ACUTE GENERAL TREATMENT

- Good nursing care and fluid therapy are usually sufficient therapy. Fluid therapy is supportive because macrocyclic lactones are predominantly excreted through bile into the feces, so diuresis does not facilitate elimination.

- Repeated doses of activated charcoal may limit further intestinal absorption and enhance elimination.
- If the horse is fractious, sedate with IV propofol by continuous rate infusion at the lowest dose that controls clinical signs without causing respiratory and cardiovascular depression.
- Sarmazenil (0.04 mg/kg IV q2h) is a competitive antagonist at the benzodiazepine binding site of the GABA receptor in the CNS. Administration may hasten clinical recovery.
- Physostigmine and picrotoxin have been used for transient relief of ivermectin intoxication symptoms in dogs.
  - Physostigmine is a cholinesterase inhibitor that causes neuronal hypopolarization by increasing postsynaptic sodium conduction. It may cause severe bradycardia, so pretreatment with glycopyrrolate should be considered.
  - Picrotoxin is a chloride channel blocking drug that blocks GABA-mediated postsynaptic hyperpolarization. It has a very narrow safety margin.

DRUG INTERACTIONS

- Do not treat affected foals or horses with benzodiazepines (eg, diazepam) or barbiturates because these drugs potentiate the toxicity of ivermectin and moxidectin and prolong the duration of neurotoxicity. Benzodiazepines increase the frequency of chloride channel opening in the presence of GABA, further hyperpolarizing membranes. Barbiturates increase the duration of GABA-mediated chloride channel opening.

POSSIBLE COMPLICATIONS

- Aspiration pneumonia
- Bladder rupture
- Death

PROGNOSIS AND OUTCOME

With good supportive care, most foals and horses recover within days and are clinically normal. Because of slower elimination, moxidectin toxicity lasts longer than ivermectin toxicity.

PEARLS & CONSIDERATIONS

COMMENTS

IV lipid solution is used in the management of toxicoses in humans from a variety of lipophilic compounds. It has recently been successfully used in the treatment of moxidectin toxicity in dogs. It is thought that the lipid compartment formed in the blood acts as a sink for lipophilic drugs, preventing them from acting on their target receptors.

PREVENTION

When used according to label directions and dosed according to accurate body weight, ivermectin and moxidectin are very safe products for horses.

CLIENT EDUCATION

Owners should carefully dose ivermectin and moxidectin according to actual body weight using a scale or calibrated weight tape. Deworming of neonatal foals is not recommended.

SUGGESTED READING

Gwaltney-Brant S, Dunayer E: The use of intravenous lipid solution in the treatment of moxidectin overdose in a dog. *Proceedings of the American Association of Veterinary Laboratory Diagnosticians*, Greensboro, NC, October 22–27, 2008, p118.

Lespine A, Martin S, Dupuy J, et al: Interaction of macrocyclic lactones with P-glycoprotein: structure-affinity relationship. *Eur J Pharm Sci* 30:84–94, 2007.

Möller JM, Feige K, Kästner SB, et al: The use of sarmazenil in the treatment of a moxidectin intoxication in a foal. *J Vet Intern Med* 19:348–349, 2005.

Pérez R, Cabezas I, García M, et al: Comparison of the pharmacokinetics of moxidectin (Equest) and ivermectin (Eqvalan) in horses. *J Vet Pharmacol Ther* 22:174–180, 1999.

AUTHOR: PATRICIA M. DOWLING

EDITOR: CYNTHIA L. GASKILL

Keratitis, Infectious

BASIC INFORMATION

DEFINITION

- Acute or chronic corneal ulcer with associated bacterial, fungal, or viral infection

SYNONYM(S)

- Infected corneal ulcers
- Fungal keratitis
- Bacterial keratitis

EPIDEMIOLOGY

RISK FACTORS

- Any type of ocular trauma
- Feeding hay from hay bags, nets, or balls

GEOGRAPHY AND SEASONALITY

- Infectious keratitis is more common in warm, humid environments.

CLINICAL PRESENTATION

DISEASE FORMS/SUBTYPES

- Bacterial keratitis (Figure 1)
- Fungal (mycotic) keratitis (Figure 2)
- Viral keratitis
- Other infectious keratopathies (parasitic)

HISTORY, CHIEF COMPLAINT

- Corneal ulceration with white to yellow cellular infiltrate, melting corneal ulceration, secondary uveitis

PHYSICAL EXAM FINDINGS

- A corneal ulcer is present when there is a break in the corneal epithelium. Clinically, this results in lacrimation, blepharospasm, photophobia, conjunctival hyperemia, corneal edema, and possibly miosis and aqueous flare. The diagnosis of a corneal ulcer is made based on these clinical signs and fluorescein staining of the cornea. Fluorescein stain will be retained by the underlying stroma and appear green in color.

- A corneal ulcer should be characterized regarding its size, depth, and the presence or absence of cellular infiltration. In addition, the anterior chamber is examined for anterior uveitis. It is essential with all corneal ulcers to attempt to establish the cause of the ulceration and eliminate it.
- The palpebral conjunctiva and bulbar surface of the nictitans are examined for the presence of a foreign body, the blink response and tear film are evaluated, and a complete history is obtained regarding trauma and previous medication. A history of previous topical corticosteroid therapy increases the likelihood of infectious, especially fungal, keratitis.

ETIOLOGY AND PATHOPHYSIOLOGY

After a break of the corneal epithelium, opportunistic microorganisms, such as bacteria or fungi, invade the corneal stroma. Cellular infiltrate occurs, and there is release of enzymes, resulting in destruction of the corneal stroma.

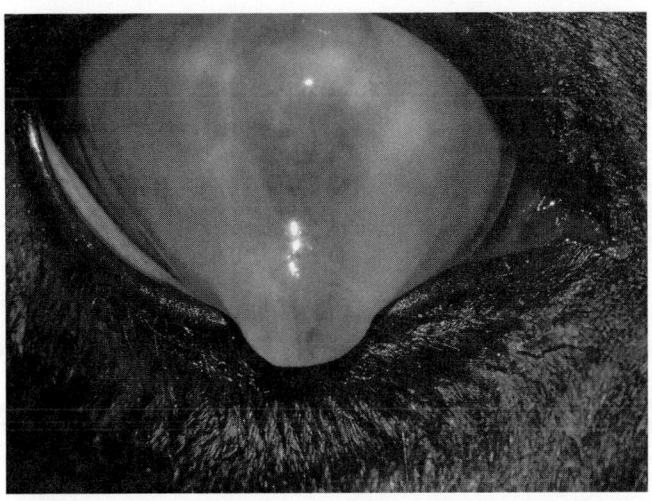

FIGURE 1 Bacterial corneal ulcer in a horse. These are typically called *melting corneal ulcers*.

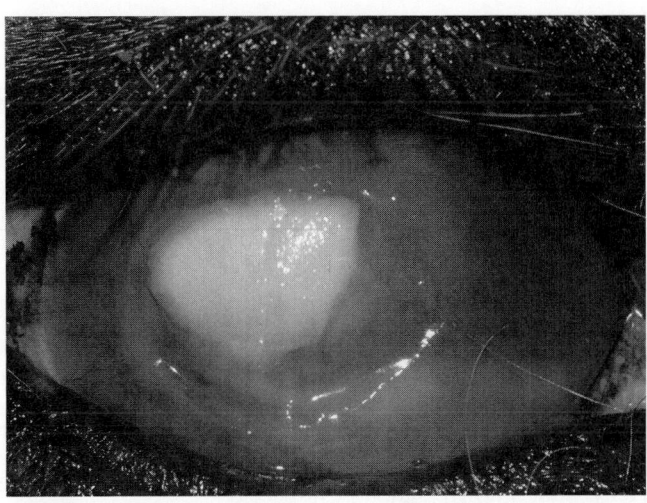

FIGURE 2 Mycotic corneal ulcer in a horse. The white plaque is typical of fungal keratitis.

DIAGNOSIS

DIFFERENTIAL DIAGNOSIS

Other causes of corneal ulceration should be ruled out before a diagnosis is made.
- Foreign body: Burdock bristles
- Ectopic cilia, distichiasis
- Infectious keratitis
- Viral keratitis
- Lagophthalmos (eg, facial nerve paralysis)
- Neurotrophic keratitis (lack of cranial nerve V innervation)
- Chronic trauma

INITIAL DATABASE

- A bacterial and fungal culture should be submitted from all corneal ulcers in the horse. Cultures should be obtained from the margin of the ulcer itself before instilling any therapeutic or diagnostic agents in the eye.
- After a culture has been obtained and the cornea has been fluorescein stained, topical anesthetic is applied, and a scraping is obtained from the ulcer for cytologic examination. The cells are placed on a glass slide and stained to examine for bacteria, fungal hyphae, and cell type. Gram, Giemsa, and Diff-Quik stains work well for examination.
- The presence of gram-negative rods indicates the possibility of an infection with *Pseudomonas* spp. The presence of fungal hyphae is pathognomonic for mycotic keratitis, with *Aspergillus* spp. being the most frequent corneal pathogen. Mixed bacterial and fungal infections are common.

ADVANCED OR CONFIRMATORY TESTING

- Cytologic evidence or isolation by culture of the microorganism is typi-

cally confirmatory of infectious keratitis.
- Polymerase chain reaction testing may be more sensitive and specific but is not widely available.

TREATMENT

THERAPEUTIC GOAL(S)

Treatment of infected corneal ulcers in horses is directed at eliminating the causative organism, minimizing corneal enzymatic destruction, and suppressing secondary uveitis.

ACUTE GENERAL TREATMENT

Treatment options reported in horses include:
- Medical therapy
  - Topical broad-spectrum antimicrobials (aggressive; every 2 hours)
  - Topical and systemic antifungals when indicated
  - Systemic nonsteroidal antiinflammatory drugs to control secondary uveitis
- Surgical therapy (if nonresponsive to medical therapy or pending perforation)
  - Conjunctival pedicle graft
  - Corneal and conjunctival graft

CHRONIC TREATMENT

If the lesions persists or if there is pending perforation (ie, depth of corneal ulcer >50% of the cornea), then surgical repair followed by antimicrobial treatment and treatment of secondary uveitis

POSSIBLE COMPLICATIONS

The most common complication is corneal perforation, leading to endophthalmitis, and possibly loss of the eye.

RECOMMENDED MONITORING

Examine daily until the cornea has healed.

PROGNOSIS AND OUTCOME

The prognosis for saving the eye is guarded.

PEARLS & CONSIDERATIONS

COMMENTS

- Infected corneal ulcers are very common in horses.
- They are frustrating to treat and generally take up to 4 to 6 weeks to heal.
- It is essential to have definitive culture and cytology results to specifically direct the antimicrobial therapy.

PREVENTION

- Minimizing ocular and corneal trauma may help prevent the development of infected corneal ulcers.
- Use of a quality fly mask is recommended.
- Feeding hay on the ground is recommended to minimize ocular trauma.

CLIENT EDUCATION

Client communication is essential so that expectations are not too high for quick healing of the corneal ulcer.

SUGGESTED READING

Andrew S, Willis M: Diseases of the cornea and sclera. In Gilger BC, editor: *Equine ophthalmology*, St Louis, 2005, Elsevier, pp 157–251.

AUTHOR & EDITOR: BRIAN C. GILGER

Keratitis, Noninfectious

BASIC INFORMATION

DEFINITION
Immune-mediated keratitis (IMMK) is one of the most common noninfectious corneal diseases in horses.

SYNONYM(S)
Chronic equine keratitis

EPIDEMIOLOGY
GENETICS AND BREED PREDISPOSITION None known, although suspected in IMMK

CLINICAL PRESENTATION
DISEASE FORMS/SUBTYPES Clinical features of IMMK are based on the depth of the corneal lesion, and four distinct levels have been described. These include epithelial, superficial stromal (45% of cases) (Figure 1), midstromal (27% of cases), and endothelial (23% of cases). With endothelial IMMK, there is commonly focal or diffuse corneal edema and pigment deposition on or at the endothelial surface. Unilateral presentation of IMMK is most common (85%).
HISTORY, CHIEF COMPLAINT Chronic corneal opacities with mild to moderate cellular infiltrate and vascularization without secondary uveitis or severe ocular discomfort and not associated with infectious agents have been described as IMMK.
PHYSICAL EXAM FINDINGS
- Diagnosis of IMMK is made if there is a progressive or chronic (>3 mo in duration), nonulcerative, recurrent corneal opacity with or without mild signs of keratitis with cellular infiltrate, corneal vascularization, and ocular discomfort (ie, mild epiphora, slight blepharospasm). Other characteristic features include a lack of secondary uveitis or severe discomfort, a lack of microorganisms, and clinical improvement with antiinflammatory medications.
- Superficial stromal keratitis appears as a diffuse, mild to moderate, yellow to white, cellular infiltrate with diffuse superficial vascularization. Mid or deep stromal cellular infiltrate is less common and appears as diffuse, yellow to white, cellular infiltrate with mild surrounding corneal edema and vascularization. Endotheliitis appears as cellular infiltrate at the endothelium with associated diffuse corneal edema.

ETIOLOGY AND PATHOPHYSIOLOGY The possible pathogenesis of IMMK in horses is that the immune system has recognized a self-antigen in the cornea (ie, molecular mimicry) or a foreign protein or organism antigen within the cornea. An underlying infectious agent may be either the inciting or perpetuating cause (or both) in many horses with IMMK. The microorganism may be directly inciting active inflammation or may have induced immunologic cross-reaction with self-antigen in the cornea. Immunologic cross-reaction with self-antigens has been well documented with leptospiral organisms or their DNA in the equine cornea. Further study is warranted to define the pathogenesis of IMMK.

DIAGNOSIS

DIFFERENTIAL DIAGNOSIS
- Infectious keratitis (corneal abscessation)
- Keratouveitis
- Corneal squamous cell carcinoma
- Eosinophilic keratitis
- Glaucoma

INITIAL DATABASE
- In cases of epithelial, superficial, or midstromal IMMK (see description below), ocular cytology and culture collection should be attempted to rule out infectious causes of the lesions.
- Complete ophthalmic examination
- Ocular ultraonsonography results should be normal.
- Intraocular pressure (tonometry)

ADVANCED OR CONFIRMATORY TESTING
If the diagnosis is still in doubt, a superficial keratectomy or biopsy should be considered.

TREATMENT

THERAPEUTIC GOAL(S)
Treatment for IMMK depends on the clinical characteristics and type of IMMK that is present. The goals are to control the immune response characteristic of the disease.

ACUTE GENERAL TREATMENT
- Epithelial, superficial stromal, and midstromal IMMK are initially treated with topical neomycin, polymyxin, and dexamethasone (q6h; Alcon Laboratories, Houston, TX) or topical neomycin, bacitracin, and polymyxin (q6h; Bausch & Lomb, Rochester, NY) (eg, after creation of an epithelial defect during diagnostic corneal scraping) with 0.2% cyclosporine topically (q12h; Merck, Whitehouse Station, NJ).
- Topical neomycin, polymyxin, and dexamethasone HCl (q6h) is added after reepithelialization of the corneal wound.
- After the lesion has resolved, neomycin, polymyxin, and dexamethasone are tapered and discontinued, and the topical cyclosporine is maintained at q24h.

CHRONIC TREATMENT
- If the lesions persist, then a superficial keratectomy with or without a conjunctival graft is recommended.
- Several horses have been tapered off all medications after corneal healing with a keratectomy and conjunctival graft.
- The deeper the lesion, the more slowly and incompletely one would expect resolution of the lesions with therapy.

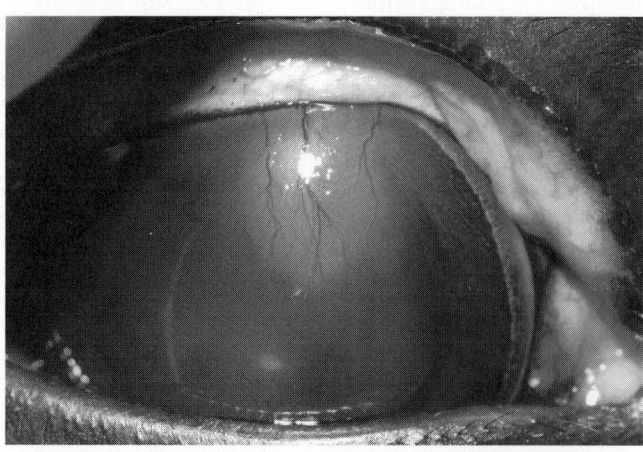

FIGURE 1 Superficial immune-mediated keratitis in a horse.

POSSIBLE COMPLICATIONS

The most common complication is the formation of infectious keratitis secondary to chronic topical steroid use.

RECOMMENDED MONITORING

Reexamine monthly until the disease is under control; then every 3 months.

PROGNOSIS AND OUTCOME

Prognosis is good for superficial lesions but poor for endothelial lesions.

PEARLS & CONSIDERATIONS

COMMENTS

- IMMK should be considered in horses with chronic, minimally painful corneal cloudiness.
- Infectious keratitis is more common, so be careful with use of topical corticosteroids, which will worsen infectious keratitis.

PREVENTION

Minimizing ocular and corneal trauma may help prevent the development of IMMK. Use of a quality fly mask is recommended.

CLIENT EDUCATION

IMMK can be controlled in most horses but not cured. The owner must be informed that persistent treatment to keep the eye clear may be required.

SUGGESTED READING

Gilger BC, Michau TM, Salmon JH: Immune-mediated keratitis in horses: 19 cases (1998–2004). *Vet Ophthalmol* 8:233–239, 2005.
Matthews AG: Nonulcerative keratopathies in the horse. *Equine Vet Educ* 12:271–278, 2000.

AUTHOR & EDITOR: **BRIAN C. GILGER**

Lameness of the Carpus

BASIC INFORMATION

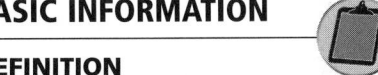

DEFINITION

The equine carpus, often referred to as the "knee," consists of three main joints. The most proximal joint, the radiocarpal (antebrachial) joint, is composed of the radius proximally and the proximal row of carpal bones distally. The middle carpal joint is located between the proximal and distal row of carpal bones. In 50% of horses, the first carpal bone is present in the distal row and is located medial and palmar to the second carpal bone. The fifth carpal bone is rare but can occasionally be found lateral to the fourth carpal bone. The carpometacarpal joint is composed of the distal row of carpal bones proximally and the second, third, and fourth metacarpal bones distally. The radiocarpal and middle carpal joints are high-motion joints and never communicate. The middle carpal joint and carpometacarpal joints always communicate, and the radiocarpal joint occasionally communicates with the carpal sheath.

SYNONYM(S)

Lameness of the knee

EPIDEMIOLOGY

SPECIES, AGE, SEX

- Injury to the carpus can occur at any age. Thoroughbred and Quarter Horse racehorses are predisposed to some of the injuries mentioned below, but they can happen to any breed.
- Angular limb deformity (ALD) is primarily seen in young foals and is associated with developmental orthopedic disease. It can be the result of asymmetric growth of the distal radial metaphysis or distal radial epiphysis, incomplete development of the cuboidal bones or proximal second and fourth metacarpal bones, or joint laxity. If left untreated, ALDs can result in permanent deformity and chronic, progressive lameness because of osteoarthritis (OA). ALDs can occasionally be seen in adult horses, but they are usually related to traumatic injury to the carpus.

RISK FACTORS Any athlete that undergoes highly repetitive loading, such as a racehorse, is predisposed to injury to the carpus.

ASSOCIATED CONDITIONS AND DISORDERS OA may be a primary issue or may be secondary to intracapsular conditions of the carpus.

CLINICAL PRESENTATION

HISTORY, CHIEF COMPLAINT

- Most commonly, horses present with a history of front limb lameness. Occasionally, the chief complaint is carpal joint effusion or the horse is "moving wide," and the owner may not appreciate a noticeable lameness.
- Horses with ALDs, whether they are foals or adult horses, present with a history of abnormal angulation to the front limbs. The angulation originates from the carpus. With traumatic injuries in the adult horse, lameness is often associated with the ALD. Lameness may not be appreciated in foals.

PHYSICAL EXAM FINDINGS

- On palpation, joint effusion in the radiocarpal joint or middle carpal joint may be evident. Effusion can be identified with the horse standing and is typically a reliable indicator of carpal synovitis. Pain is often elicited by pressing upward on the carpal bones during flexion in horses with chip or slab fractures of the carpal bones.
- Decreased range of motion of the carpus may be noted.
- A positive response to flexion of the carpus during a lameness examination also indicates that the carpus or the soft tissues around the carpus is the source of lameness. When asked to trot, the horse may try to minimize carpal flexion and will thus trot with the forelimbs abducted.

DIAGNOSIS

DIFFERENTIAL DIAGNOSIS

- Carpal bone fracture
- Carpal bone chip (osteochondral) fragment
- OA of the radiocarpal joint or middle carpal joint
- Subchondral bone sclerosis
- ALD
- Injury to intercarpal ligaments

INITIAL DATABASE

- The initial evaluation should include a thorough lameness evaluation, including flexion tests. If the carpus is suspected as the source of lameness, then a full series of carpal radiographs should be obtained. A minimum of six radiographic views should be obtained, including the dorsopalmar, lateromedial, dorsolateral-palmaromedial oblique, dorsomedial-palmarolateral oblique views, skyline view (dorsoproximal-dorsodistal) of distal row of carpal bones, and a flexed lateromedial view. If the concern is in the proximal row of carpal bones, a skyline view of the proximal row of carpal bones should be taken.

- Intraarticular anesthesia is often the definitive diagnosis for localizing the carpus as the source of lameness.

ADVANCED OR CONFIRMATORY TESTING

- Nuclear scintigraphy can be used to further localize carpal injury when radiograph results are negative or equivocal for any abnormalities. The sensitivity is high, but the specificity is low, so specific localization is unlikely. Nuclear scintigraphy can be useful to diagnose early stress-related subchondral bone injury or to quantify the importance of a lesion visualized with radiography.
- Arthroscopy can further qualify the source of lameness in the carpus. Arthroscopy may be a treatment option as well as a diagnostic tool. The degree of OA can be quantified by visualizing cartilage erosions or proliferative synovium. Tearing of an intercarpal ligament can be identified, and osteophytes can be localized and removed. Arthroscopy can be used to remove chip fragments or to aid in lag screw placement for slab fractures.

TREATMENT

THERAPEUTIC GOAL(S)

- Stabilize fractures
- Remove fragments
- Stimulate healing (microfractures)
- Assess the full extent of injury with arthroscopy
- Control synovitis

ACUTE GENERAL TREATMENT

Very rarely do injuries to the carpus require immediate treatment. Situations that require immediate treatment are often related to traumatic fractures that result in severe instability of the carpus. Most injuries to the carpus are subtle and may be present for a length of time before a diagnosis is made. After a definitive diagnosis has been made, treatment may revolve around removing the inciting cause, stabilization of fractures, or control of synovitis.

CHRONIC TREATMENT

- Synovitis related to OA can often be controlled with intraarticular medications such as hyaluronic acid and corticosteroids, autologous conditioned serum (ACS) or interleukin-1 receptor antagonist protein (IRAP) or polysulfated glycosaminoglycans. To obtain the full effect of intraarticular medications, it is important to first address the inciting cause of OA (ie, removal of osteochondral [chip] fragments). Treatment with extracorporeal shockwave therapy has also been useful for treatment of lameness related to the carpus.
- Often rest and nonsteroidal antiinflammatory drug therapy are the most

important aspects of a treatment regimen for horses with carpal injuries. Racehorses with subchondral bone sclerosis and osteophyte formation benefit from extended rest of 3 to 4 months.

PROGNOSIS AND OUTCOME

- Prognosis for injury to the carpus depends on a number of factors, including but not limited to the severity of clinical signs, severity of cartilage damage, duration of lameness, and level of competition.
- Horses in the early stages of mild to moderate disease can often be managed with a favorable prognosis.
- Advanced OA or severe disease warrants a guarded prognosis.

SUGGESTED READING

Bertone AL: The carpus. In Stashak TS, editor: *Adams' lameness in horses*. Philadelphia, 2002, Lippincott Williams & Wilkins, pp 830–863.

Diagnostic and surgical arthroscopy of the carpal joints. In McIlwraith CW, Nixon AJ, Wright IM, et al, editors: *Diagnostic and surgical arthroscopy in the horse*, ed 3, Edinburgh, 2005. Mosby Elsevier, pp 47–127.

Ross MW: Carpus. In Dyson SJ, Ross MW, editors: *Diagnosis and management of lameness in the horse*, Philadelphia, 2002, Saunders Elsevier, pp 376–394.

AUTHORS: KATIE S. AMEND and CHRIS KAWCAK

EDITOR: ANDRIS J. KANEPS

Lameness of the Elbow and Shoulder

BASIC INFORMATION

DEFINITION

Injuries and lameness associated with the upper forelimb, cubital joint, or scapulohumeral joint

EPIDEMIOLOGY

SPECIES, AGE, SEX Young horses are predisposed to osteochondrosis and cyst-like lesions. Osteoarthritis is usually found in mature horses. Traumatic injuries may occur in any age group.

CLINICAL PRESENTATION

HISTORY, CHIEF COMPLAINT

- Acute, severe lameness of the elbow or shoulder region may be associated

with a fall or crashing into a solid object. The horse will shift weight to the opposite limb and will often stand with the carpus slightly flexed.
- In motion, the horse may have a shortened anterior phase to the stride, especially if the biceps tendon or bicipital bursa is affected.
- Upper forelimb fractures usually result in non–weight-bearing lameness. If nerve injury has occurred, the primary complaint may be muscle atrophy over the shoulder, abduction of the shoulder during weight bearing, or dropped elbow.

PHYSICAL EXAM FINDINGS

- Mild upper forelimb lameness may be difficult to localize. Horses with fractures and luxations will not bear

weight on the affected limb, will have localized swelling, and often stand with the carpus partially flexed. If the olecranon is displaced or the radial nerve is damaged, the horse will have a dropped elbow.
- Manipulation of the fracture will cause significant pain and may have auscultable and palpable crepitus.
- Stress fractures or enostoses may have no outward signs whatsoever except for acute lameness.
- Soft tissue injuries may have only a shortened anterior phase to the stride because swelling of the affected tissue is often not observed.
- Nerve injuries may result in abaxial displacement of the shoulder at the walk ("Sweeney shoulder"), dropped

elbow, or muscle atrophy. Horses with septic arthritis will usually not bear weight on the affected limb.

DIAGNOSIS

DIFFERENTIAL DIAGNOSIS

- Osteoarthritis: Usually a mild but progressive lameness that is relieved with intraarticular anesthesia
- Fractures: Olecranon, proximal radius, humerus, scapula
- Luxations: Elbow luxations are usually associated with proximal fractures of the radius; shoulder luxations are very rare
- Osteochondrosis: Very uncommon in the elbow but is recognized infrequently in the shoulder, particularly the glenoid fossa
- Osseous cyst: May be found in the proximal radius and rarely in the distal humerus
- Stress fracture: Common in racehorses and may be found in the proximal caudal, distal cranial, or caudal aspects of the humerus
- Enostosis (stress reaction, bone islands): Usually only recognized after scintigraphy and high-detail radiography
- Collateral ligament desmitis of the elbow: Usually associated with trauma
- Bicipital bursitis: May be caused by blunt force trauma or strain of the overlying tendon
- Biceps tendinitis
- Nerve injury to the suprascapular nerve, brachial plexus, or radial nerve
- Septic arthritis

INITIAL DATABASE

- Lameness evaluation with complete palpation of the upper limb. Comparative palpation of the contralateral limb often provides a baseline to determine the significance of findings. Manipulative tests of the upper limb often do not assist localization.
- Diagnostic anesthesia should be used to rule out the lower limb and then intraarticular anesthesia of the upper limb synovial structures should be done to localize the lameness.
- Radiography of the affected area should always be performed.

ADVANCED OR CONFIRMATORY TESTING

- Nuclear scintigraphy should be performed if diagnostic anesthesia does not help localize the lameness and evaluation of radiographs does not lead to a diagnosis.
- Ultrasonography helps determine if soft tissue injury is a component of the lameness.

TREATMENT

THERAPEUTIC GOAL(S)

- Reduce inflammation to reduce pain.
- Identify and stabilize recognized fractures.
- Provide appropriate rest and rehabilitative exercise

ACUTE GENERAL TREATMENT

- Osteoarthritis: Nonsteroidal antiinflammatory drugs (NSAIDs), oral joint support such as glucosamine/chondroitin, injectable systemic joint support such as polysulfated glycosaminoglycans or hyaluronan, and intraarticular injection with hyaluronan and corticosteroids. If the patient is not responsive to the aforementioned treatments, injection with autologous conditioned plasma should be considered.
- Fractures: Displaced fractures should be repaired and stabilized. Horses with incomplete or some nondisplaced fractures may respond favorably to stall confinement. In many cases, the horse must be prevented from lying down by using a "high line." On a high line, the horse is attached by a short rope from the halter to a carabiner clipped to a wire that runs over the top of the stall. The wire usually is placed from one corner diagonally to the other well above the horse's head. The horse is tied short enough to prevent lying down but long enough to allow reaching strategically placed water, hay, and feed.
- Luxations: Acute displacements without attendant fractures may be reduced under general anesthesia. The horse must have an assisted recovery and should often be put on a high line.
- Osteochondrosis: Usually requires arthroscopic evaluation and debridement
- Osseous cyst: If accessible from the joint, it may be debrided under arthroscopic control. A periarticular approach under radiographic control for debridement or injection of corticosteroid should be done if not accessible arthroscopically. IV tiludronate has also been used to successfully treat bone cysts.
- Stress fracture: Stall rest and handwalking over approximately 3 months. Gradual return to work using a controlled exercise program after that time. Recurrence is unusual.
- Enostosis: As for stress fracture
- Collateral ligament desmitis of the elbow: Rest for 4 to 9 months with restriction of free exercise and progressively increasing controlled exercise. Consider facilitating healing by

injection of platelet-rich plasma, stem cells, or both.
- Bicipital bursitis: Injection with hyaluronan and corticosteroids
- Biceps tendinitis: As for collateral ligament desmitis
- Nerve injury: Suprascapular nerve entrapment or injury may be treated with surgery to notch the cranial aspect of the scapula and allow decompression of the nerve. Excessive notching may predispose the scapula to fracture. Radial nerve paresis without attendant fracture and trauma to the brachial plexus usually resolves with rest, NSAIDs, and parenteral corticosteroids alone or in combination. In acute nerve injury, dimethyl sulfoxide may be administered IV to reduce inflammation and swelling.
- Septic arthritis: Joint lavage, intraarticular and parenteral antibiotics, and NSAIDs

CHRONIC TREATMENT

Horses with osteoarthritis may require long-term supportive care as described for acute treatment.

POSSIBLE COMPLICATIONS

Any injuries involving the articular surfaces may result in osteoarthritis.

PROGNOSIS AND OUTCOME

- Osteoarthritis: The prognosis depends on the horse's response to treatment. This condition usually requires long-term management.
- Fractures: Horses with nondisplaced fractures without an articular component have a good prognosis for soundness. Horses with displaced fractures that require fixation usually have a guarded prognosis because of the difficulty in maintaining the stability of the fracture during healing, the possibility of infection, and the potential for laminitis in the contralateral limb.
- Luxations: Always a guarded prognosis and dependent on the ultimate level of joint stability and degree of osteoarthritis
- Osteochondrosis: Guarded prognosis for athletic soundness, particularly for large glenoid fossa lesions
- Osseous cyst: Often a guarded prognosis, even with surgical debridement
- Stress fracture: Good prognosis for full athletic use
- Enostosis: Usually a good prognosis for athletic function
- Collateral ligament desmitis of the elbow: Guarded prognosis for athletic

soundness, often complicated by osteoarthritis
- Bicipital bursitis: Often a favorable prognosis but may depend on response of concurrent tendinitis
- Biceps tendinitis: Favorable prognosis for acute injuries; poor for chronic injuries

- Nerve injury: Usually a slow, months-long convalescence that may result in complete recovery if the injury is mild
- Septic arthritis: Prognosis is favorable if treated aggressively early after occurrence

SUGGESTED READING

Dyson SJ: The elbow, brachium and shoulder. In Ross MW, Dyson SJ, editors: *Diagnosis and management of lameness in the horse*, Philadelphia, 2003, Saunders Elsevier, pp 399–416.

AUTHOR & EDITOR: **ANDRIS J. KANEPS**

Lameness of the Heel Region

BASIC INFORMATION

DEFINITION

Lameness caused by soreness originating at the palmar or plantar aspect of the foot

SYNONYM(S)

Palmar heel pain, navicular syndrome, heel soreness

EPIDEMIOLOGY

SPECIES, AGE, SEX
- Quarter Horse, Thoroughbred, and Warmblood breeds are most commonly affected.
- The average age at onset is 9 years (range, 3–18 years), but the average for Warmbloods is 7 years.

GENETICS AND BREED PREDISPOSITION Horses with small feet and a large body size are predisposed.

RISK FACTORS
- Predisposing factors include a long toe or an underrun heel; a long, sloping pastern; and small feet with a large body mass.
- Horses used for jumping or used frequently on hard footing are also predisposed.

CLINICAL PRESENTATION

DISEASE FORMS/SUBTYPES
- There are numerous causes of pain in the palmar aspect of the foot. These causes can be arbitrarily divided into conditions of the hoof wall and horn-producing tissues, conditions of the third phalanx, and conditions of the navicular region. Hoof problems include hoof wall defects, contusions of the hoof causing bruising or corn formation, abscess formation, and thrush or canker. Third phalanx lamenesses blocked out by palmar digital anesthesia include wing fractures, marginal fractures, solar fractures of the distal phalanx, and deep digital flexor insertional tenopathy.
- Conditions of the navicular region include distal interphalangeal synovi-tis, deep digital flexor tendinitis, des-mitis of the impar (distal navicular) ligament or collateral sesamoidean ligaments, navicular osteitis or osteopathy, and vascular disease.

HISTORY, CHIEF COMPLAINT Chronic, recurring forelimb lameness that is most evident on hard ground or when the horse is worked in circles

PHYSICAL EXAM FINDINGS The lameness is usually mild to moderate but may be intermittently severe. It usually affects the front feet and is bilateral in most cases. The onset is chronic and insidious, yet owners frequently complain of sudden onset of lameness. The gait is often short and choppy at a trot, and lameness is exacerbated in a circle.

ETIOLOGY AND PATHOPHYSIOLOGY Excessive stress on the structures of the heel results in wear and tear of the flexor surface of the navicular bone and associated soft tissue structures.

DIAGNOSIS

DIFFERENTIAL DIAGNOSIS
- Heel pain not associated with the navicular structures
- Bruising of the sole
- Fractures of the palmar aspect of the distal phalanx or the navicular bone
- Coffin joint arthrosis
- Pedal osteitis
- Digital sheath synovitis
- Tendinitis of the distal deep digital flexor tendon, superficial digital flexor tendon, or distal ligaments of the proximal sesamoid bones

INITIAL DATABASE
- Lameness examination
- Diagnostic local anesthesia (palmar digital nerve block)
- Contrast-enhanced computed tomography
- Radiography

ADVANCED OR CONFIRMATORY TESTING
- Intraarticular diagnostic anesthesia of the distal interphalangeal joint or navicular bursa
- Nuclear scintigraphy
- Magnetic resonance imaging
- Ultrasonography

TREATMENT

THERAPEUTIC GOAL(S)
- Correct hoof imbalance and provide corrective shoeing.
- Provide antiinflammatory treatment.
- Follow up to judge the effect of treatments.

ACUTE GENERAL TREATMENT
- Adjust hoof angles to reduce stress on heel structures (usually by raising the heels).
- Correct lateral-to-medial hoof imbalance.
- Ease breakover with rolled toe and shoe set back from the natural toe.
- Provide concussion protection with a full pad or rim pad.
- Administer nonsteroidal antiinflammatory drugs (NSAIDs) for 3 to 4 weeks.
- If lameness is severe, consider navicular bursa or distal interphalangeal joint injection with hyaluronan and corticosteroids.

CHRONIC TREATMENT
- Horses with navicular bone pain may be treated with the bisphosphonate drug tiludronate (Tildren; CEVA Sante Animal, Libourne, France). This medication is not currently approved by the Food and Drug Administration.
- If the horse has a limited response to initial therapy, consider advanced imaging with computed tomography or magnetic resonance to identify more clearly the specific cause of the pain.
- If the horse has a limited response to shoeing and NSAIDs, consider palmar digital neurectomy.

RECOMMENDED MONITORING

- Reevaluate hoof angles and shoeing 3 to 6 months after making the initial changes.
- Monitor the level of lameness as needed.

PROGNOSIS AND OUTCOME

- Shoeing alone is a very effective method for treating horses with heel pain and navicular syndrome.

- When lameness is not resolved, consider reevaluation of the shoeing protocol, direct medication of the navicular bursa, and advanced imaging.

PEARLS & CONSIDERATIONS

Maintaining good hoof balance is the most important preventive step.

SUGGESTED READING

Dyson S, Marks D: Foot pain and the elusive diagnosis. *Vet Clin North Am Equine* 19:531, 2003.

Kaneps AJ, Turner TA: Lameness of the foot. In Hinchcliff KW, Kaneps AJ, Geor RJ, editors: *Equine sports medicine and surgery*, New York, 2004, Saunders Elsevier.

AUTHOR & EDITOR: **ANDRIS J. KANEPS**

Lameness of the Hip and Pelvis

BASIC INFORMATION

DEFINITION

Lameness that originates in the hip and pelvis is uncommon in most horses.

CLINICAL PRESENTATION

HISTORY, CHIEF COMPLAINT

- Acute non–weight-bearing lameness or finding a horse down and unable to rise may indicate a fracture of the pelvis or proximal femur or coxofemoral luxation.
- Acute, severe lameness that resolves substantially with rest may indicate an ileal stress fracture or fracture of the tuber coxae.
- Progressive lameness that initially responds to nonsteroidal antiinflammatory drugs (NSAIDs) may be associated with osteoarthritis.

PHYSICAL EXAM FINDINGS

- Horses with coxofemoral luxation, fracture of the tuber coxa, and long-standing lameness have observable physical abnormalities such as a leg length discrepancy, displaced tuber coxa, and gluteal muscle atrophy, respectively. With most pelvic fractures, the horse will have no outward signs apart from severe lameness.

DIAGNOSIS

DIFFERENTIAL DIAGNOSIS

- Osteoarthritis of the coxofemoral joint
- Fractures: Proximal femur, capital femoral fracture (Salter-Harris type 1 fracture), ileal shaft, ileal wing, acetabulum, tuber ischium, tuber coxa ("knocked-down" hip)

- Stress fracture of the ileal wing: Commonly found in young racing Thoroughbreds but difficult to identify without scintigraphy
- Coxofemoral luxation: With or without fractures of the proximal femur or acetabulum
- Sacroiliac injuries (see "Sacroiliac Joint Disorders" in this section)
- Muscle injuries or myositis (see "Back Pain," "Nutritional Myopathy," "Polysaccharide Storage Myopathy," and "Rhabdomyolysis" in this section)

INITIAL DATABASE

- The complete lameness evaluation should include palpation and visualization of the pelvic musculature. Severe lameness of chronic duration will result in atrophy of the gluteal muscles on the affected side.
- Manipulation of the hind limbs to stress the hip joint (adduction of each hindlimb) may help localize the soreness.
- A rectal examination should be done if a pelvic fracture is suspected.
- The pelvis or hind limb should be manipulated and the horse walked during the rectal exam to determine if instability is palpable. Some pelvic fractures cannot be detected on rectal palpation.
- Radiography and ultrasonography should be done when appropriate. High-quality radiography of the pelvis and hip of adult horses is only possible under general anesthesia. Induction and recovery from anesthesia may displace pelvic fractures that could lacerate the internal pudendal vessels, resulting in fatal hemorrhage. Ultrasonography may be done externally and per rectum to determine the continuity

of the pelvic bones and sacrum and to evaluate the hip.

ADVANCED OR CONFIRMATORY TESTING

Nuclear scintigraphy of the lower back, pelvis, and upper hind limbs is often the best means to anatomically localize injuries in this area. This technique is done with the horse standing to minimize the risk to the horse from laceration of the pelvic vessels by fracture fragments.

TREATMENT

THERAPEUTIC GOAL(S)

- Reduce inflammation to reduce pain.
- Provide appropriate rest and rehabilitative exercise.

ACUTE GENERAL TREATMENT

- Osteoarthritis of the coxofemoral joint: The most immediate treatment is with NSAIDs. Injection of the coxofemoral joint is not easily accomplished, but intraarticular hyaluronan and corticosteroids may be administered.
- Fractures: Most fractures of the proximal femur and pelvis cannot readily be reduced and stabilized. Treatment for most fractures consists of stall rest for 3 to 6 months. A high line to prevent the horse from lying down may be useful for many pelvic fractures in which displacement may result in fatal hemorrhage.
- Stress fracture of the ileal wing: Rest and rehabilitative exercise often result in a return to work.
- Coxofemoral luxation: Usually not treated because of the grave prognosis for even pasture comfort.

CHRONIC TREATMENT

Osteoarthritis often requires long-term management with NSAIDs, oral or injectable joint support medications, and repeated intraarticular injections.

POSSIBLE COMPLICATIONS

Pelvic fractures of the ileal body or acetabulum may displace and lacerate the major vessels within the pelvis, resulting in fatal hemorrhage.

RECOMMENDED MONITORING

Response to rest and medication should be monitored with a follow-up lameness evaluation and imaging or rectal palpation as appropriate for the injury.

PROGNOSIS AND OUTCOME

- Osteoarthritis of the coxofemoral joint: Guarded for long-term soundness as an active high-level athlete but depends on response to treatment
- Fractures: Horses with fractures of the tuber coxa and tuber ischium and stress fractures of the ileum have a good prognosis for return to athletic use. Horses with fractures of the proximal femur and ileal body and wings with little displacement have a fair prognosis for pasture soundness. Horses with capital femoral and acetabulum fractures have a grave prognosis for soundness in adults. Acetabular fractures in foals with minimal displacement may have a fair to good prognosis for soundness.
- Stress fracture of the ileal wing: Good prognosis for return to athletic soundness
- Coxofemoral luxation: Grave prognosis for pasture soundness

SUGGESTED READING

Dyson SJ: Pelvic injuries in the non-racehorse. In Ross MW, Dyson SJ, editors: *Diagnosis and management of lameness in the horse,* Philadelphia, 2003, Saunders Elsevier, pp 491–508.

Pilsworth RC: Diagnosis and management of pelvic fractures in the Thoroughbred racehorse. In Ross MW, Dyson SJ, editors: *Diagnosis and management of lameness in the horse,* Philadelphia, 2003, Saunders Elsevier, pp 484–490.

AUTHOR & EDITOR: **ANDRIS J. KANEPS**

Lameness of the Stifle

BASIC INFORMATION

DEFINITION

Soreness that originates within the stifle and associated soft tissues that causes lameness

EPIDEMIOLOGY

SPECIES, AGE, SEX Horses from 6 months to 2 years of age may present with osteochondrosis of the stifle.
GENETICS AND BREED PREDISPOSITION Fast-growing, large-breed horses are predisposed to osteochondrosis (Warmbloods, Quarter Horses).
RISK FACTORS Horses that use a high degree of hindlimb impulsion, such as dressage, jumper, cutting or reining horses, may be more likely to experience stifle injury.

CLINICAL PRESENTATION

HISTORY, CHIEF COMPLAINT Horses with traumatic injuries present with acute, moderate to severe lameness often after a fall or encounter with a hard object such as a fence or wall. Horses with osteochondrosis may also have a history of acute lameness with turnout or exercise that may subside somewhat with restriction of activity. Complete upward fixation of the patella results in the horse dragging its limb behind its body because of the inability to flex the joint. Most horses with stifle injuries have effusion of the joints as a presenting complaint.
PHYSICAL EXAM FINDINGS Effusion, lameness, localized to the stifle with manipulative tests, and intraarticular anesthesia. With upward fixation of the patella, the horse may lock the stifle, making it unable to advance the limb.

DIAGNOSIS

DIFFERENTIAL DIAGNOSIS

- Osteoarthritis: Often associated with osteochondrosis or cystlike lesions, joint instability
- Soft tissue injury: Patellar ligament desmitis, intermittent or complete upward fixation of the patella, meniscal injury, meniscal ligament injury, collateral ligament desmitis, cruciate ligament desmitis, synovitis
- Developmental orthopedic disease: Osteochondrosis, cystlike lesions
- Trauma: Fractures or luxation of the patella, fracture of the intercondylar eminence of the proximal tibia, distal femur or proximal tibia, tibial crest fracture or avulsion
- Infection: Septic arthritis

INITIAL DATABASE

- Lameness examination with manipulative tests (full limb flexion, localized stifle flexion, cruciate ligament stress test, stress of the medial collateral ligament).
- Diagnostic anesthesia to localize the lameness. To completely desensitize the stifle, all three joints should be blocked.
- Radiography, ultrasonography, or both.

ADVANCED OR CONFIRMATORY TESTING

If the lameness is subtle or could not be localized with diagnostic anesthesia, nuclear scintigraphy may be indicated.

TREATMENT

THERAPEUTIC GOAL(S)

- Reduce pain and inflammation.
- Treat the inciting cause (eg, debride osteochondrosis lesions).
- Provide rehabilitative exercise to strengthen the hindlimbs and lower back.

ACUTE GENERAL TREATMENT

- Osteoarthritis: Nonsteroidal antiinflammatory drugs (NSAIDs), oral joint support such as glucosamine/chondroitin, injectable systemic joint support such as polysulfated glycosaminoglycans or hyaluronan, or intraarticular injection with hyaluronan and corticosteroids or polysulfated glycosaminoglycans. If not responsive to the aforementioned treatments, injection with autologous conditioned plasma should be considered.
- Soft tissue injuries: Rest, NSAIDs, extracorporeal shock wave therapy, diagnostic arthroscopy with possible debridement of meniscal and cruciate injuries
- Developmental orthopedic disease: Arthroscopic debridement of osteochondrosis lesions and cystlike lesions,

ultrasonographic or arthroscopically guided injection of corticosteroid in cystlike lesions, rest with follow-up radiography in young horses without significant lameness.

- Intermittent upward fixation of the patella: Build strength in the quadriceps muscles by backing for 5 to 10 minutes twice daily, working over ground poles, and walking up and down hills if the horse is capable of that type of work without excessive upward fixation. If not responsive to strengthening, consider medial patellar ligament splitting or transection. Horses with complete upward fixation may need medial patellar ligament transection to permit ambulation.
- Fractures: Small, nonarticular patellar fractures heal with fibrous union after rest. Larger articular or horizontal patellar fractures may be repaired with screws or wires but have a high incidence of fixation failure. Moderate-sized articular patellar fractures may be evaluated arthroscopically, and the fragments may be removed.
- Other fractures: Arthroscopic evaluation should be done for all articular fractures to determine the extent and condition of associated soft tissues. Extraarticular fractures of the tibia or femur may require internal fixation.

CHRONIC TREATMENT

Intraarticular injections of hyaluronan and (if appropriate) corticosteroids may help return the joint to a comfortable state.

POSSIBLE COMPLICATIONS

- Intraarticular injuries may result in secondary osteoarthritis.
- Soft tissue injuries may require prolonged time for healing (6–9 months).

RECOMMENDED MONITORING

Follow-up lameness evaluation and radiography is indicated to determine the condition of the joint(s).

PROGNOSIS AND OUTCOME

- Soft tissue injuries: Prognosis for soundness depends on the extent of injury because horses with mild to moderate injuries have a fair prognosis for soundness but those with extensive soft tissue injuries have a guarded prognosis.
- Osteochondrosis lesions that are debrided in horses younger than 2 years have a fair to good prognosis for soundness. Horses with cystlike lesions treated arthroscopically also have a good prognosis. Conservative treatment for either condition results in soundness about 50% of the time.
- Horses with patellar upward fixation usually respond favorably to rehabilitative exercise and to surgical treatment if it is necessary.
- Fractures that are not articular and heal with rest or fixation have a good prognosis for soundness. Intraarticular fractures with minimal joint disruption may also have a good prognosis, but injuries that result in osteoarthritis may require management of the arthritis.

PEARLS & CONSIDERATIONS

Localization of the lameness and detailed imaging are required to make a specific diagnosis.

SUGGESTED READING

Latimer F: Tarsus and stifle. In Hinchcliff KW, Kaneps AJ, Geor RJ, editors: *Equine sports medicine and surgery*, Philadelphia, 2004, Saunders Elsevier, pp 361–385.

Walmsley JP: The stifle. In Ross MW, Dyson SJ, editors: *Diagnosis and management of lameness in the horse*, Philadelphia, 2003, Saunders Elsevier, pp 455–470.

AUTHOR & EDITOR: ANDRIS J. KANEPS

Lameness of the Tarsus

BASIC INFORMATION

DEFINITION

Conditions of the tarsal bones or joints that result in lameness

SYNONYMS

Hock soreness, spavin

EPIDEMIOLOGY

SPECIES, AGE, SEX There is no species or sex predilection. Juvenile horses may present with developmental orthopedic disease or traumatic injuries. Mature horses may present with degenerative conditions such as osteoarthritis (OA) or traumatic injuries.

RISK FACTORS Premature birth or neonatal sepsis may predispose to incomplete mineralization of the cuboidal bones. Fast-growing young horses are predisposed to osteochondrosis. Mature horses with straight hindlimb conformation may be predisposed to OA.

CLINICAL PRESENTATION

HISTORY, CHIEF COMPLAINT

- Neonatal incomplete mineralization of the tarsal bones often results in abnormal conformation of the tarsus ("sickle hock"). The foal may be reluctant to stand.
- Trauma usually causes acute, moderate to severe lameness with accompanying soft tissue swelling or effusion.
- OA usually causes varying levels of stiffness and reluctance to change canter leads, jump, or drive forward using the hindlimbs.

PHYSICAL EXAM FINDINGS Varying degrees of lameness depending on the cause

DIAGNOSIS

DIFFERENTIAL DIAGNOSIS

- Neonatal: Incomplete mineralization of the cuboidal bones
- Mature: OA of the distal tarsal joints

- Any age: Trauma resulting in fracture; luxation; desmitis of collateral ligaments; osteomyelitis or septic arthritis involving the tarsal sheath, sustentaculum tali, or tuber calcis

INITIAL DATABASE

- General physical and lameness examinations, including flexion tests if appropriate
- Radiography

ADVANCED OR CONFIRMATORY TESTING

Diagnostic ultrasonography if soft tissue involvement is possible

TREATMENT

THERAPEUTIC GOAL(S)

- Reduce and manage pain.
- If trauma or incomplete mineralization is a cause, confine to a stall.
- Treat the inciting cause if trauma or infectious origin.

ACUTE GENERAL TREATMENT

- Nonsteroidal antiinflammatory drugs (NSAIDs) are very useful for most causes of tarsal pain.
- External coaptation with cast or bandage may be needed to provide more stability of the tarsus for luxations, incomplete mineralization, or fractures.
- Antibacterial medications should be administered if an open wound or infection is present.

CHRONIC TREATMENT

For OA, the hierarchy of treatment from minimal to most effective is (1) oral joint support supplements such as those containing glucosamine and chondroitin, (2) NSAIDs (parenteral or topical), (3) intraarticular medication such as hyaluronan and steroids, and (4) facilitated ankylosis of the affected joints.

RECOMMENDED MONITORING

- Lameness should be monitored until the problem resolves or the situation is at a manageable level.
- Radiographic evaluations should be made at appropriate intervals (often every 6 to 12 months).

PROGNOSIS AND OUTCOME

The outcome depends on the disease process. OA is usually manageable for most uses of the horse, fractures may heal with resultant OA that may require management, and incomplete mineralization of cuboidal bones may resolve without problems or result in juvenile OA caused by malformation of tarsal articulations.

SUGGESTED READING

Dabareiner RM, et al: The tarsus. In Ross MW, Dyson SJK, editors: *Diagnosis and management of lameness in the horse*, Philadelphia, 2003, Saunders Elsevier, pp 440–449.

AUTHOR & EDITOR: **ANDRIS J. KANEPS**

Laminitis, Acute

BASIC INFORMATION

DEFINITION

- A painful inflammatory condition of the hoof-lamellar interface (HLI) that causes lameness, abnormal hoof growth and appearance, and separation of the hoof from underlying dermal connective tissue.
- The affected HLI is permanently weakened and predisposed to recurrence.

SYNONYM(S)

Founder

GENETICS

- Pony breeds at greater risk than are horse breeds.
- Acute laminitis and sloughing of the hoof in foals is a component of junctional epidermolysis bullosa in the Belgian and American Saddlebred breeds.
- One report of laminitis in a foal resulting from inherited deficiency of the plectin protein (a critical cytoplasmic component of hemidesmosomes).

CLINICAL PRESENTATION

DISEASE FORMS/SUBTYPES

- Classification of laminitis categories
  - Acute laminitis: Hoof lamellar inflammation has been activated for the first time and is associated with pain.
  - Chronic laminitis:
    - The HLI has been compromised by the laminitic condition.
    - May or may not be associated with pain at any one time

  - Acute laminitis evolves into chronic laminitis at some arbitrary point.
  - There is evidence of abnormal hoof growth on physical examination.
  - Developmental laminitis
    - Period of time that transpires between the onset of an acute laminitis-provoking event and the first signs of acute laminitis (eg, endotoxemia associated with acute typhlocolitis)
    - HLI is compromised and at risk for structural failure (acute laminitis)
  - Endocrinopathic laminitis: Acute or chronic laminitis arising in the context of underlying hormonal influence such as hypercortisolism or insulin resistance
    - Pasture-associated laminitis: Acute or chronic laminitis arising in the context of grazing pasture grasses
    - Weight-bearing (contralateral limb) laminitis: Acute laminitis arising in an opposite limb as a complication of primary lameness in any limb

PHYSICAL EXAMINATION FINDINGS

- The clinical presentation of acute laminitis differs depending on which foot and in how many feet the disease develops.
- More common in adult horses than in foals (affected foals may have genetic disease).
- Most commonly presents as severe pain affecting both forelimbs.

- Pain-associated conjunctival membrane injection
- Tachycardia
- Tachypnea
- Characteristic apprehensive facial expression
- Reluctance to move
- Stiffness
- Subcutaneous edema of the distal limbs (because of reduced mobility)
- Affected feet are often warm
- Digital arterial pulses are very prominent ("bounding" pulses)
- Recumbency
- Reluctance to move or to stand up
- When forced to stand and bear weight, stiffness and a characteristic stance make it clear that acute laminitis has developed.
- Horses stop moving around in their environment.
- Tendency to "oscillate in situ" (attempting to seek a comfortable stance by transferring the center of gravity toward the pelvis and shifting the weight between both forelimbs).
- The pelvic limbs are drawn forward under the body and both forelimbs are extended out in front of the body.
- Horses walk in a manner such as to reduce weight bearing by the dorsal aspect (toe) of the forefeet, preferring to extend the forelimbs and bear greater weight at the heel.
- Walking movements are careful, slow, and deliberate, and the patient tends to bear increased weight in the pelvic limbs, giving rise to the descriptor "walking on eggshells."

- Systemic signs of pain such as sweating, trembling, muscle fasciculations, and rapid breathing
- Shaking of the affected limbs (especially affected pelvic limbs)
- Hoof pain is accentuated by turning sharply on a hard surface.
- Moving affected horses on hard surfaces may worsen laminitis and convert subtle signs of stiffness and lameness into a more severe and clinically prominent manifestation.
- Serosanguineous discharge at the coronary band (intracapsular necrosis)
- Sloughing of the affected hoof or hooves (exungulation)
- Unwillingness to bear weight on the opposite affected hoof (difficult to pick up the foot)
- "Resting" the opposite limb after one hoof has been picked up for examination and released
- The strength of the digital arterial pulses increases during the examination as a result of forcing the patient to bear weight.
- Coronary band develops a trough/shelf or depression
- Hemorrhage at the coronary band (coronary vessel rupture)
- Hoof testers yield a pain reaction at the toe (both false-positive and -negative reactions to hoof testers)
- Signs of preexisting laminitis may be evident, including prominent circumferential growth rings in the hoof wall, palmar or plantar divergence of growth rings, broadening of the white line zone, and the development of a "dropped" sole.
- Conservative paring of the sole may reveal flecks of hemorrhage as a result of either chronic or acute laminitis.
- Sudden or unanticipated "improvement" in the extent to which weight is borne by the primary limb during fracture management (implicative for laminitis in the contralateral limb)
- Laminitis may develop in one hoof when a sufficiently severe inflammatory process is present within the hoof for other reasons (eg, unresolved sole abscesses, nail or other foreign body penetrations, or exercise on hard surfaces ["road founder"]).

DIAGNOSIS

- Medical history
- Inspection and physical examination of all four feet
- Plain film radiography is essential for purposes of corroborating the diagnosis, characterizing the severity and extent of laminitis, and establishing the baseline appearance of the affected foot for purposes of monitoring

responses to treatment and making a prognosis.

RADIOGRAPHIC CHARACTERIZATION

- It is important to emphasize the value of a meticulous approach for the acquisition of valuable and meaningfully diagnostic radiographic images.
- Acquisition of helpful radiographic metrics necessitates excellent lateromedial projection technique.
- Zero hoof-to-film distance minimizes magnification and standardizes the resulting images for serial comparisons during treatment.
- Use a radiopaque marker at the dorsal aspect of the hoof (starting at the point at which the coronary band connects with the hoof wall).
- Specific components of the lateromedial view of the equine hoof that should be carefully scrutinized include:
  - The palmar/plantar angle of the third phalanx (angle of palmar margin of the third phalanx relative to the bearing surface of the hoof)
  - The hoof-lamellar (H-L) zone width (distance between the outer surface of the dorsal aspect of the hoof wall and the dorsal aspect of the third phalanx; usually measured at a point just distal to the pyramidal process and also at the distal tip of the third phalanx)
  - The distance between the extensor process and the coronary band (vertical distance between the dorsal limit of the pyramidal process and the point at which the haired skin stops at the coronary band)
  - The sole depth at the tip and at the wing of the third phalanx
  - Evidence of remodeling or fracture of the third phalanx (implicative for chronic laminitis)
- Reference measurements in healthy hooves
  - The palmar/plantar angle of the third phalanx should be positive and in the range of 3 to 5 degrees.
  - The H-L zone width should be between 15 and 19 mm depending on the size of the horse.
  - The vertical distance between the pyramidal process and the coronary band should not exceed approximately 14 mm.
  - Sole depths at the tip and at the wing of the third phalanx are generally given as 20 and 23 mm, respectively.
- Dorsopalmar/plantar views of the affected hoof are essential for identification of (uncommon) axial rotational displacements of the third phalanx and for complete characterization of bone pathology that develops in cases of chronic laminitis.

- Readers are directed to more extensive descriptions (see Suggested Reading) for more information.

DIFFERENTIAL DIAGNOSIS

- Any condition causing inflammation in the hoof (positive response to hoof testers, results of distal limb anesthesia, pronounced digital arterial pulse strength)
- Sole abscess
- Nail binding
- Foreign body perforation
- P3 fracture
- Navicular bone fracture
- Distal interphalangeal joint inflammation
- Deep solar bruising
- Some other conditions may be mistaken for acute laminitis by virtue of clinical signs associated with abnormal stance, reluctance to move, or protracted periods of recumbency.
  - Polysaccharide storage myopathy
  - Tetanus
  - Botulism
  - Equine motor neuron disease
  - Colic
  - Rhabdomyolysis
  - Vertebral trauma
  - Protozoal myelitis
  - Hyperkalemic periodic paralysis
  - Aortic or iliac thrombosis

INITIAL DATABASE

- Physical examination data (including vital signs)
- Radiographic images
- Hematology and plasma biochemical profile (primary inflammatory condition elsewhere in the body)
- Etiologic test protocols (eg, fecal microbiology)
- Endocrine testing

ADVANCED OR CONFIRMATORY TESTING

- Retrograde digital venography
- Computed tomography
- Magnetic resonance imaging

TREATMENT

GENERAL PRINCIPLES

- Treat underlying or predisposing primary conditions (examples include restoration of the circulation during management of typhlocolitis, administration of effective antimicrobial agents for the treatment of gram-negative pleuropneumonia, and the removal of placental remnants and irrigation of the uterus after placental retention in mares).
- Prevent access to ingested laminitis-inducing toxins and drugs (eg, corticosteroids).

- Expedient institution of effective emergency treatment for acute laminitis may both impede progression of the disease and serve to rescue the HLI.
- Be skeptical of many unfounded and unscientific treatment approaches.
- Clinical improvement could be a result of either the action of treatment or the natural progression of the disease.

LAMINITIS PREVENTION DURING THE DEVELOPMENTAL PHASE OF LAMINITIS

- The HLI is at risk during the developmental phase; institute laminitis prevention strategies.
- Restrict patient movements.
- Further injury to the HLI may be prevented with the provision of sole support in the form of deep bedding, Styrofoam pads; Lily pads; or a fast-setting, customized two-component silicone rubber insert against the sole.
- Sole support must not exert pressure between the sole and the point toward which the third phalanx might be displaced (just in front of the point of the frog).
- Consider application of foot casts (eg, plaster of Paris).
- Avoid very hard, inflexible surfaces such as concrete.
- Accommodate on deep sand, pea gravel, thick shavings, or peat moss.
- Additional strategies intended to promote stability of P3 include removing shoes (if worn) and simply providing a deeply littered bedding.
- Rasp the dorsal aspect of the toe to facilitate breakover.
- Special reusable tape-on shoes (Redden modified Ultimate shoes) may be used in conjunction with silicone putty applied over the palmar/plantar aspect of the sole or frog. (These shoes also provide heel elevation, if indicated, to reduce the tensile pull of the deep digital flexor tendon and a "rolled" toe that serves to move the point of breakover to a more palmar/plantar location, thus relieving forces on the dorsal aspect of the HLI.)
- Optimize circulation (blood volume and plasma colloidal oncotic pressure).
- Address endotoxemia as needed (eg, polymixin B).
- Administer nonsteroidal antiinflammatory drugs (NSAIDs) such as phenylbutazone.
- Continuous distal limb cryotherapy (3°–5° C) is well tolerated for up to 7 days and has been shown to be very safe and effective.
- Avoid dietary strategies that might promote hyperglycemia (eg, feeding grain).

TREATMENT OF ACUTE LAMINITIS

- Restrict patient movements.
- Do not discourage the patient from lying down.
- Provide deep, soft bedding to minimize the risk of decubital ulcers.
- Continuous distal limb cryotherapy may be helpful for the management of acute laminitis.
- Provide sole support (see previous section).
- Consider using a sling to reduce pressure in the HLI.

DRUGS USED FOR THE MANAGEMENT OF ACUTE LAMINITIS

- It is important to emphasize that scientifically validated drugs do not exist for the predictably successful prevention or treatment of laminitis.
- Drug strategies include analgesic drugs, drugs intended to promote blood flow, and antiinflammatory drugs.
- Strive to reduce pain (humane consideration; reduction of pain might promote blood flow).
- Note that reduction of pain may worsen damage in the HLI.
- NSAIDs such as phenylbutazone (2.2 mg/kg IV q12h), flunixin meglumine (1.1 mg/kg IV q12h), ketoprofen (2.2 mg/kg IV q24h), or firocoxib (0.1 mg/kg PO q24h) may be administered to reduce inflammation in the HLI and to improve comfort.
- Phenylbutazone is the most commonly used NSAID for management of laminitis.
- Use of firocoxib for the management of laminitis is untested.
- Use of other NSAIDs (eg, naproxen) in horses should be considered carefully because pharmacologic data are either not available or suggest that oral bioavailability may be unsatisfactory.
- Strategies that might minimize NSAID toxicosis should be considered because protracted administration of NSAIDs is associated with risk of gastrointestinal ulceration and renal papillary necrosis.
- Reduce the dependence on effective NSAID administration by using other drugs that have different pharmacologic mechanisms of (analgesic) action.
- Butorphanol tartrate: 0.03 to 0.05 mg/kg, IM q6h
- Dimethyl sulfoxide (DMSO): 0.5 to 1.0 g/kg mixed as a 10% solution in physiologic crystalloid
- Tramadol: 2 mg/kg PO q8–12h (Data supporting demonstrable analgesic effect and appropriate dose for horses are lacking; low bioavailability PO.)

- Gabapentin: 3 to 10 mg/kg PO q8h (data supporting demonstrable analgesic effect and appropriate dose for horses are lacking; low bioavailability PO; should be given at lower doses if there is hypoproteinemia because this is a protein-bound drug.)
- Ketamine hydrochloride: 0.25 to 0.5 mg/kg IM q8h (Use as a "rescue" analgesic on days when pain is worse to avoid giving more NSAIDs.)
- Pentoxifylline: 8 to 10 mg/kg PO q8–12h (Should be given at lower doses if there is hypoproteinemia because this is a protein-bound drug.)
- Acetyl-L-carnitine: 0.02 mg/kg PO q24h (Advocated for treatment of neuropathic pain; evidence for value to reduce diabetic peripheral neuropathy in humans.)
- Transdermal fentanyl patches seem to be ineffective for the management of laminitic pain. Compared with other species, extremely high serum concentrations of fentanyl are needed for significant antinociceptive action in horses. It is unlikely that application of fentanyl patches to the skin will accomplish these high serum concentrations and, if they work, it is likely that the patient would be affected with significant central nervous system excitation
- Misoprostol (5 µg/kg PO q12h) and omeprazole (2–4 mg/kg PO q24h) may be co-administered with NSAIDs to reduce the risk of ulceration of the gastrointestinal tract.
- When faced with severe pain in a hospitalized setting, further relief may be provided via an IV constant-rate infusion (CRI) of one or several other analgesic drugs. Selected drugs may include butorphanol tartrate, detomidine hydrochloride, xylazine hydrochloride, acepromazine, ketamine hydrochloride, and lidocaine hydrochloride.)
- Administration of morphine sulfate (0.1 mg/kg in 50 mL isotonic saline) via an epidural catheter
- Drugs that may inhibit activated matrix metalloproteinases in the HLI include oxytetracycline (7.5 mg/kg IV q12h) and pentoxifylline (8–10 mg/kg q12h)
- Drugs that have been advocated for the management of laminitis based on their purported ability to promote perfusion of the HLI include nitroglycerine, isoxsuprine hydrochloride, aspirin, heparin, and pentoxifylline. However, studies undertaken to demonstrate a benefit for HLI perfusion have yielded negative or conflicting results.

FARRIERY

- There are many approaches, but the best results occur when there is a good veterinarian–farrier team.

- There is no all-encompassing treatment that works best for all cases of laminitis.
- Planning should be based on the physical and radiographic appearance of the affected hoof.
- Nailing on a shoe may be detrimental to the stability of the HLI.
- Consider removal of shoes and provision of sole support.
- Overgrown hoof wall should be trimmed judiciously to promote breakover in the developmental or acute stages of laminitis.
- Application of permanent therapeutic shoes should be delayed until 4 to 6 weeks after the acute phase of laminitis has transitioned into the chronic phase and HLI stability has been established.
- Serial radiographic examinations are essential (assessment of response and progress).
- Commonly used farriery techniques that often meet the needs of the foundered patient include trimming back the toe to facilitate breakover and reduce (detrimental) loading stresses in the dorsal aspect of the HLI, provision of palmar/plantar support (heel wedge or elevation) to offset tension on the HLI resulting from the pull of the deep digital flexor tendon, resection of the aspects of the hoof capsule that have become undermined by necrosis and infection, and hoof wall resection or grooving of the coronary band to promote restoration of hoof wall growth.

EUTHANASIA

- Severe laminitis and specific physical findings may warrant consideration of euthanasia.
- Prognosis is unfavorable if signs of pain are refractory and unresponsive to analgesics.
- Sunken or collapsed coronary band (especially when evident throughout the circumference of the coronary band)
- Prolapse of the coronary band
- Complete physical separation of the hoof capsule from underlying connective tissues (exunguilation)
- Radiographic evidence of infection involving the third phalanx, air densities resulting from intracapsular separation during the acute phase of the disease, vertically oriented distal displacement ("sinking")
- A satisfactory outcome for the treatment of a case of laminitis characterized by solar attenuation (<15 mm) and a reduced (<2 degrees) or negative palmar/plantar angle of the third phalanx should be regarded as challenging.
- Severe reduction of hoof perfusion using retrograde digital venography or perfusion scintigraphy points to an unfavorable prognosis.

RISK FACTORS

- Idiosyncratic and genetic predisposition
- Evidence of preexisting chronic laminitis

- Ponies are at greater risk than horses.
- Any primary lameness
- Extensive unresolved intracapsular inflammation
- Endocrinologic risk factors (obesity, hypercortisolism, insulin resistance, pregnancy)
- Dietary risk factors include those associated with ingestion of specific plants (noted above)
- Feeding either forage (pasture or hay) or concentrates (grain) that contain high concentrations of simple sugars, starch, or oligofructans
- Standing or exercising on hard, inflexible surfaces (eg, concrete) for prolonged periods of time
- Medical conditions that are characterized by gastrointestinal ulceration or endotoxemia (systemic inflammation)

SUGGESTED READING

Floyd AE: Grading the laminitic horse. In Floyd AE, Mansmann RA, editors: *Equine podiatry*, St Louis, 2007, Saunders Elsevier, pp 320–327.

Moyer W, Schumacher J, Schumacher J, et al: Are drugs effective for horses with acute laminitis? *Proceedings of the 54th Annual Convention of the AAEP*, San Diego, 2008, pp 337–340.

Parks AH, O'Grady SE: Chronic laminitis. In Robinson NE, Sprayberry KA, editors: *Current therapy in equine medicine*, ed 6, St Louis, 2009, Saunders Elsevier, pp 550–560.

AUTHORS: **PHILIP J. JOHNSON** and **JOANNE KRAMER**

EDITOR: **PHILIP J. JOHNSON**

Laminitis, Chronic

BASIC INFORMATION

DEFINITION

- A painful inflammatory condition of the hoof-lamellar interface (HLI) that causes lameness, abnormal hoof growth and appearance, and separation of the hoof from underlying dermal connective tissue
- The HLI has been compromised by the laminitic condition.
- May or may not be associated with pain at any one time
- Acute laminitis evolves into chronic laminitis at some arbitrary point.
- There is evidence of abnormal hoof growth on physical examination.
- The development of chronic laminitis is an inescapable consequence of the acute laminitic condition, whatever the cause.

- When laminitic pain is diagnosed for the first time in a horse with hoof growth changes and radiographic abnormalities implicative for underlying chronic laminitis, the episode is usually referred to as subacute laminitis.
- Insidious-onset, chronic laminitis may result from underlying endocrinopathic influences such as insulin resistance or corticosteroid influence and is commonly identified in horses that have been grazing pastures ("pasture associated laminitis" [PAL]).
- Also classified depending on the clinical behavior of the condition over time
- Recurrent, exacerbative, or refractory (chronic) laminitis is characterized by repetitive and recurrent bouts of activated inflammation in the HLI that

cause progressive deterioration of the integrity of the hoof and persistent pain.
- Chronic subacute laminitis refers to the situation in which pathologic changes in the HLI are recognized by the abnormal manner with which the affected hoof has grown but tends not to be so readily associated with pain and lameness.

SYNONYM(S)

Founder

CLINICAL PRESENTATION

- Abnormal hoof growth is usually evident with or without pain (lameness).
- When present, lameness and hoof pain are similar to those described for

acute laminitis (see "Laminitis, Acute" in this section).

- When exercised on hard ground, chronically affected horses are likely to develop bilateral forelimb lameness, and the digital arterial pulses become transiently prominent.
- Visual inspection of the hoof reveals prominent circumferential growth lines, palmar/plantar divergence of the growth lines, bunching up of growth lines at the dorsal aspect of the hoof, slippering of the toe, broadening of the white line zone (especially at the toe), seedy toe, solar convexity, and heel contracture.
- Conservative paring of the solar aspect of the hoof often reveals flecks of hemorrhage.
- The chronically foundered hoof is prone to developing recurrent sole abscesses.
- Coronary band develops a trough/shelf or depression.

DIAGNOSIS

- May be diagnosed several days after the development of painful acute laminitis (see "Laminitis, Acute" in this section)
- May also be diagnosed based on observation of characteristic physical abnormalities observed on examination of the hoof (see above) in the absence of overt signs of pain or lameness
- The patient may develop bilateral lameness and increased prominence in the digital arterial pulse strength when exercised on hard ground surfaces.
- Confirmed by radiography
- Examine the patient for evidence of underlying predisposing endocrinopathy such as pituitary pars intermedia dysfunction (PPID) and equine metabolic syndrome (EMS).
- Endocrinologic tests performed on horses affected with laminitis may yield falsely positive results as a result of stress and pain (cortisol response and reduced insulin sensitivity).

RADIOGRAPHY

See section on hoof radiography in "Laminitis, Acute" in this section.

TREATMENT

GENERAL PRINCIPLES

- The two essential goals are pain management and restoration of the structural integrity of the hoof.

- The athletic capability of many affected horses will be reduced or nullified as a consequence of laminitis.
- Sometimes the prognosis for severe laminitis is unfavorable and warrants euthanasia.
- Emphasize to the owner that the prognosis may become clearer after some time has passed to allow the effects of treatment to be assessed and that treatment may be labor intensive and lengthy.
- Be cautious about enthusiastically encouraging horse owners to pursue treatment for severe laminitis without first discussing the fact that it might not be effective.
- Specific treatments for chronic laminitis are applied to the continuum of treatments started when acute laminitis first occurred.
- Treatments that must be addressed include both those pertaining to rehabilitation of the affected hoof and those that promote the general health of the patient.
- Treatment and management of chronic laminitis is usefully addressed under the following categories: rest and stall confinement, stabilization of P3, pain management, hoof trimming and farriery, surgical treatments, nutritional factors, endocrinopathic factors, and miscellaneous
- There are no validated reports for the predictably successful prevention or treatment of laminitis using drugs.
- Both rehabilitation of the affected hoof and the prognosis depend on new hoof growth. (The rate of new hoof growth along a chronically diseased HLI is slower than it is in the healthy horse.)
- When successful, the management of chronic laminitis typically requires at least 6 to 12 months of closely invested care.

REST AND STALL CONFINEMENT

- The patient's movement should be restricted (large stall confinement) to minimize further mechanical damage and to promote healing of the HLI.
- Premature exercise (eg, as soon as signs of hoof pain have abated) often causes further damage to the HLI (and pain).
- Allow time to establish stability in the HLI akin to the value of stabilization during bone fracture repair.
- Limited and strictly regulated hand-walking exercise should only be contemplated after evidence has been demonstrated that the HLI has stabilized (see below).

STABILIZE P3

- Although it is not possible to completely stabilize P3 in the same manner

that internal fixation techniques may be used to immobilize bone fractures, strategies aimed at promoting stability of P3 within the hoof capsule are helpful from the perspectives of both pain management and optimal healing (promoting reestablishment of the normal relationship between P3 and the hoof capsule).
- Effective stabilization of P3 inhibits further damage to the compromised HLI.
- Evaluation of the effectiveness of stability-promoting strategies includes observation of a reduction in pain (especially after pain medications such as phenylbutazone are withdrawn) and (objectively) the use of serially acquired hoof radiographs.
- Radiographic evidence of stability can be attributed to the effects of stability-promoting treatments as well as the effects of healing.
- Provision of stability is intended to relieve loading of the compromised aspects of the HLI (commonly at the dorsal aspect of the hoof) and redistribute loading to the more palmar/plantar aspects of the HLI and the ground-bearing surface of the hoof (sole and frog).
- Stability may also be promoted by reducing the turning force ("moment") acting on the dorsal HLI by the pull of the deep digital flexor tendon (DDFT) through the distal interphalangeal joint.
- Reduction of the distal interphalangeal joint moment is not recommended for horses affected by distal displacement of the (entire) third phalanx ("sinking").
- Stability promoting strategies include restriction of movement, removing the patient's shoes (standing on regular shoes tends to increase tension in the HLI), and simply providing a deeply littered bedding.
- The provision of sand or pea gravel for bedding is often helpful.
- Patients should not be discouraged from lying down.
- Support to the sole or frog may also be provided in the form of high-density styrofoam cut to the shape of the hoof and attached using tape.
- Other commonly used treatments include the application of Lily pads to the frog, silicone putty, and plaster of Paris casts applied to fill in the concavities of the sole.
- The dorsal aspect of the wall at the toe should be beveled using a rasp to facilitate breakover.
- Specially designed reusable tape-on shoes (Redden modified Ultimate shoes) can be used in conjunction with silicone putty applied over the palmar/plantar aspect of the sole or frog to provide heel elevation (if indi-

cated) to reduce the tensile pull of the DDFT and a "rolled" toe that serves to move the point of breakover to a more palmar/plantar location.

PAIN MANAGEMENT

- It is important from the perspective of humane consideration to reduce the systemic consequences of pain-associated stress and facilitate weight redistribution to reduce the risk of laminitis at other locations (increased loading).
- Analgesic treatments that were initiated for acute laminitis are generally continued into the chronic phase.
- Promoting stability of P3 within the hoof capsule is important from the perspective of reducing pain (see above).

HOOF TRIMMING AND FARRIERY

- Complete discussion of surgical farriery for chronic laminitis is beyond the scope of this chapter; readers are directed elsewhere (see Suggested Reading below).
- There is not a single shoeing method or approach that is uniformly effective for all cases of chronic laminitis.
- Before embarking on substantial trimming or the application of therapeutic shoes, sufficient time should have transpired after the acute phase of laminitis to allow for stabilization of the HLI (attenuation of the degradative processes and the facilitation of healing).
- Trimming and farriery should be considered approximately 4 to 8 weeks after onset of acute laminitis.
- "Normal farrier landmarks" for trimming and application of shoes are not applicable (position of P3 with respect to the hoof capsule has changed as a consequence of mechanical failure in the HLI).
- Optimal approach entails discussion between veterinarian and farrier and must be based on current hoof radiographs.
- Special shoes are not needed in all cases. Chronic laminitis may be managed by simply trimming the affected hoof (especially if solar depth is adequate).
- Targets for trimming include establish a normal angle of alignment between P3 and the ground surface, reduce the "breakover distance" (the distance between the hoof wall or shoe ground contact and the distal margin of P3), and maintain sole depth (in the healthy hoof, there normally exists a positive angle between the solar margin of P3 and the ground of 2 to 5 degrees).
- If adequate tissue healing and growth occur, the normal (parallel) relationship between the dorsal aspects of P3 and the hoof capsule should be reestablished (a relatively long-term objective that will not be achieved in all cases).
- Evaluate the thickness of the sole, especially in the dorsal part of the sole.
- Sole thickness is ideally 15 to 20 mm or greater at the dorsal aspect of the hoof near the tip of P3.
- If the solar depth is sufficient, the hoof may be trimmed with a single plane of flatness at the weight-bearing surface (if there is insufficient solar depth at the dorsal part of the sole, trimming will cause bruising, pain, and instability).
- If solar depth is insufficient, it must *not* be trimmed, and a special shoe, intended to support weight at the palmar aspect of the hoof and to relieve weight bearing at the dorsal aspect, should be helpful. (Trimming for purposes of establishing a normal angle of alignment between P3 and the ground surface can then only be undertaken at the palmar or plantar aspect of the hoof by creating two separate planes of flatness on the weight-bearing surface.)
- Trimming the palmar aspect of the hoof increases tension in the DDFT and may cause further pain. (Additional pain-reducing treatments such as temporary heel elevation, further nonsteroidal antiinflammatory drug [NSAID] administration, or solar padding may be indicated at this time.)
- Three important principles for selection of an appropriate shoe are position of the facilitated point of breakover, whether to provide support for the weight-bearing surfaces of the sole and the frog, and whether to elevate the heels.
- Moving back the point of breakover reduces stress in the dorsal aspect of the HLI and can be accomplished by several shoe design principles such as simply rolling or squaring the toe (taking care to preclude pressure at the sole), setting the shoe back to the more palmar aspect of the hoof, or using a curved or "rocker" shoe.
- Shoeing methods that promote weight-bearing support at the sole or frog include the use of a simple bar or heart bar, incorporation of pads, and insertion of a synthetic composite (eg, silicone putty) between a pad and the frog.
- Heel elevation reduces the pull of the DDFT, diminishes tension in the dorsal HLI, and is helpful for foundered horses that tend to walk by bearing weight on the toe first.
- Heel elevation may be accomplished using wedge pads or wedged shoes or through the application of rails.

- An especially practical approach that uses many of the principles discussed using a plywood-based wooden construct for shoeing foundered horses has been recently described (see Suggested Reading below).

SURGICAL

- Resection of part of the hoof wall is indicated when underlying connective tissue is infected. (Resection of parts of the dorsal hoof wall may minimize stress in the underlying HLI during breakover.)
- Resection of the hoof wall (to relieve the tourniquet effect of the hoof wall) has been advocated as a potential salvage procedure (in preference to euthanasia) for extreme cases (eg, sinking).
- Grooving of the coronary band may be considered as an alternative to extensive hoof wall resection; provision of a groove just below the coronary band serves to disconnect the (potential) new wall growth from the more distal wall. (This procedure may both stimulate new wall growth and promote better alignment between the new growth and P3.)
- Transection of the DDFT may be used to reduce tensile stress in the dorsal HLI (generally regarded as a salvage procedure because most treated horses will not return to athletic performance).

NUTRITIONAL FACTORS

- Dietary energy content should meet the needs of a physically inactive convalescent patient without being excessive and without causing starvation.
- The patient's rations must provide sufficient protein and should be appropriately balanced from the perspective of meeting mineral and vitamin requirements.
- Feeding should be undertaken on a continual or semi-continual basis.
- Discourage provision of intermittent glycemic meals (prevent glucose and insulin spiking).
- Dietary strategies should be aimed at reversing obesity (if present).
- Pasture grazing should be discouraged.
- Obtain laboratory analysis of forage and do not provide forage with a high nonstructural carbohydrate (NSC) content (>12% on a dry-matter basis).
- The NSC content of some hay may be reduced by soaking in water for 60 minutes.

ENDOCRINOPATHIC FACTORS

- Horses with PPID-associated chronic laminitis should be managed using orally administered low-dose pergolide, cyproheptadine, or trilostane.

- Metformin (15–20 mg/kg PO q6–8h) may be administered to EMS-affected horses to promote insulin sensitivity
- Thyroxine (Thyrol-L) may be administered to EMS-affected horses to promote insulin sensitivity and weight loss.

MISCELLANEOUS

- Supplementation with vitamins such as biotin may promote healing and strengthen the hoof tissues (poorly supported by the scientific literature).
- Antibiotic treatment (coupled with appropriate surgical drainage) should be considered if chronic laminitis has been complicated by infection (infection may arise in either or both P3 and the solar/HLI connective tissues).
- Consider IV regional digital perfusion of antibiotics.
- Intraosseous infusion of the distal phalanx as a delivery route targeting the HLI. (Infusion of a drug into P3 leads to effective and high concentrations of the drug within the HLI, facilitating use of expensive and powerful drugs for "topical" localized treatment with less concern for oral bioavailability or toxic systemic side effects.)

RECOMMENDED MONITORING

- Careful attention to the growth of the hoof
- Signs of pain may vary over time.
- Maintain records of the patient's pain or lameness. These observations will be keyed to use of analgesic drugs such as phenylbutazone.
- Photographic documentation (every 8 weeks) of the appearance of the surface of the hoof

- Radiographic records (every 2–6 months) of the appearance of P3 and its position with respect to the hoof capsule
- Records of body condition score and feeding program
- Monitoring for evidence of NSAID-induced gastrointestinal ulceration (colic, inappetence, decreased passage of feces, bruxism, hypoalbuminemia, and anemia) or renal disease (water consumption, urinalysis, and plasma creatinine concentration)

SPECIFIC FINDINGS SUGGESTIVE OF AN UNFAVORABLE PROGNOSIS

- Signs of pain that are refractory and unresponsive to analgesic medication
- Development of a sunken or collapsed coronary band (especially when this abnormality is evident throughout the circumference of the coronary band)
- Prolapse of the coronary band
- Complete physical separation of the hoof capsule from the underlying connective tissue (exungulation)
- Radiographic evidence of infection involving the third phalanx
- Radiographic demonstration of vertically oriented distal displacement ("sinking") is also implicative for an unfavorable prognosis.
- Although the severity of capsular rotation of the third phalanx has been traditionally regarded as useful for prognosis, a more useful marker for prognosis before embarking on the treatment of laminitis may be the thickness of the sole coupled with the angle of palmar margin of P3 rela-

tive to the weight-bearing surface of the hoof.
- Satisfactory outcome for the treatment of a case of laminitis characterized by solar attenuation (<15 mm) and a reduced (<2 degrees) or negative angle should be regarded as challenging.
- Either retrograde digital venography or perfusion scintigraphy may be used to demonstrate severe reduction of hoof perfusion (indicating an unfavorable prognosis).

EUTHANASIA

- Severe refractory, chronic laminitis may warrant consideration of euthanasia.

SUGGESTED READING

Nourian AR, Mills PC, Pollitt CC: Development of intraosseous infusion of the distal phalanx to access the foot lamellar circulation in the standing, conscious horse. *Vet J* 183(3):273–277, 2010.

O'Grady SE, Steward ML: The wooden shoe as an option for treating chronic laminitis. *Equine Vet Educ* 21(2):107–112, 2009.

Parks AH, O'Grady SE: Chronic laminitis. In Robinson NE, Sprayberry KA (eds). *Current therapy in equine medicine*, ed 6, St Louis, 2009, Saunders Elsevier, pp 550–560.

Santschi EM, Adams SB, Murphey ED: How to perform equine intravenous digital perfusion. *Proc Annual Convention of the AAEP*, 1998, pp 198–201.

Watts KA: Forage and pasture management for laminitic horses. *Clin Tech Equine Pract* 3:88–95, 2004.

AUTHORS: PHILIP J. JOHNSON and JOANNE KRAMER

EDITOR: PHILIP J. JOHNSON

Large Colon: Congenital Abnormalities

BASIC INFORMATION

DEFINITION

Abnormal development of the large colon resulting in alterations in the anatomy

EPIDEMIOLOGY

SPECIES, AGE, SEX

- Foals with atresia coli present within the first days of life.
- Information on other congenital abnormalities of the large colon is restricted to case reports, personal communications, and clinical experience; therefore accurate information on epidemiology is not available.

Because of the congenital cause of the problem, it is presumed that horses with defects that result in signs of abdominal disease will be relatively young at presentation. However, one case report described a 27-year-old mare, illustrating that horses of any age may be affected.

CLINICAL PRESENTATION

DISEASE FORMS/SUBTYPES Described malformations associated with signs of abdominal pain include atresia coli, diverticula, duplication cyst, and defects in the mesentery.

HISTORY, CHIEF COMPLAINT Clinical signs are variable depending on the abnormality.

- Foals with atresia coli present with acute, sometimes severe signs of colic and abdominal distension. Complete lack of fecal production is a hallmark clinical sign.
- The presence of a diverticulum may result in intermittent impaction or obstruction, resulting in signs of recurrent colic.
- In the case report describing a large duplication cyst, the affected horse had clinical signs of recurrent colic and a pendulous abdomen.
- Defects within the mesentery allow displacement or volvulus of the colon through the defect, resulting in signs of colic; there have been no reports of

strangulation of the segment of the intestine.

PHYSICAL EXAM FINDINGS Findings on physical examination during an episode of colic will be consistent with a nonstrangulating obstruction, including tachycardia, abdominal distension, decreased or absent borborygmi, and signs of dehydration.

ETIOLOGY AND PATHOPHYSIOLOGY

- The cause and heritability of these congenital defects is unknown because of the low number of cases reported.
- The defects may result in obstruction caused by alterations in the flow of ingesta or extraluminal obstruction associated with displacement or volvulus.

DIAGNOSIS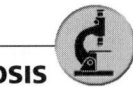

DIFFERENTIAL DIAGNOSIS

- Other causes of colic and lack of fecal production in foals: Meconium impaction, lethal white syndrome, and acute colitis.
- Other causes of mild to moderate abdominal pain: Simple or nonstrangulating obstructions of the gastrointestinal (GI) tract such as feed or sand impaction, enterolithiasis, large colon tympany, other large colon displacements, large intestinal intraluminal obstructions, small colon impactions, and ileal impactions.
- Other causes of large intestinal distension on examination per rectum: Feed or sand impaction, enterolithiasis, large colon tympany, other large colon displacements, large colon volvulus, and other intraluminal obstructions.

INITIAL DATABASE

- Atresia coli
  - ○ Foals with atresia coli have no meconium staining when their rectal temperature is taken and after repeat enemas.
  - ○ Contrast studies of the GI tract (barium swallow or enema) are diagnostic.
- Other congenital abnormalities
  - ○ Findings on examination per rectum vary depending on the defect. Distension of the large colon or cecum secondary to obstruction or impaction of the large colon is possible.
  - ○ Nasogastric reflux is unexpected.
  - ○ Bloodwork is expected to be normal or consistent with mild to moderate dehydration (prerenal azotemia, elevated packed cell volume, elevated total protein).
  - ○ Abdominal fluid analysis is expected to be within normal limits.

TREATMENT

THERAPEUTIC GOAL(S)

- Removal or repair of congenital defect
- Supportive care

ACUTE GENERAL TREATMENT

- Surgical exploration is required for diagnosis and repair of the defect.

- Personal communications on attempts to bypass atresia coli indicate that success may be limited because of concurrent disease and abnormalities in motility adjacent to the affected segment.
- Resection of the affected portion has been reported to be curative in cases of diverticula.
- Closure of the mesenteric defect has been reported to be curative in cases of mesenteric defects.

PROGNOSIS AND OUTCOME

If surgical correction is possible, prognosis appears good with the exception of atresia coli.

PEARLS & CONSIDERATIONS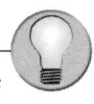

Congenital defects of the large colon are an uncommon cause of colic in horses.

SUGGESTED READING

Rakestraw PC, Hardy J: Large intestine. In Auer JA, Stick JA, editors: *Equine surgery*, ed 3, St Louis, 2006, Saunders Elsevier, pp 436–478.

AUTHOR: **KIRA L. EPSTEIN**

EDITORS: **TIM MAIR** and **CERI SHERLOCK**

Large Colon: Impaction (Feed)

BASIC INFORMATION

DEFINITION

Obstruction of the flow of ingesta, gas, or both in the large colon by dehydrated feed material

SYNONYM(S)

Feed impaction, impaction, pelvic flexure impaction

EPIDEMIOLOGY

SPECIES, AGE, SEX Appears most common in horses older than 1 year of age

GENETICS AND BREED PREDISPOSITION Clinical experience suggests that Miniature Horses may be predisposed.

RISK FACTORS Numerous risk factors have been suggested or identified, including:

- Change in activity: Increased stall time, change in exercise program, transport
- Diet: High-grain diet
- Stall vices: Cribbing and windsucking
- Concurrent disease: Hospitalization, recent lameness
- Parasites: More than 12 months since use of ivermectin or moxidectin
- Dental prophylaxis
- Medications: Amitraz, atropine, glycopyrrolate, morphine, general anesthesia, nonsteroidal antiinflammatory drugs (NSAIDs); the effect of NSAIDs on motility is poorly understood and controversial

GEOGRAPHY AND SEASONALITY Clinical experience suggests that changes in weather may predispose horses to the development of large colon impactions. Cold water associated with cold weather may decrease water consumption and increase the risk.

ASSOCIATED CONDITIONS AND DISORDERS Infiltrative inflammatory disease and neurologic dysfunction of the large colon associated with large colon impactions have been reported.

CLINICAL PRESENTATION

DISEASE FORMS/SUBTYPES

- Large colon impactions can be separated into primary and secondary subtypes. This entry focuses on primary impactions. However, large colon impaction may occur secondary to other conditions. Secondary impactions are associated with other large colon obstructions such as right dorsal displacement (impaction within the right dorsal colon), enteroliths, fecaliths, bezoars, and foreign bodies (see chapters on these conditions).

- Dehydration of feed material within the large colon is frequently associated with small intestinal obstructions (so-called "secondary impactions"). Although this is not a true impaction (ie, it does not obstruct the flow of ingesta), differentiation can be difficult.

HISTORY, CHIEF COMPLAINT

Horses with large intestinal impactions present with signs of mild to moderate abdominal pain (colic) and decreased to absent fecal production. Historical findings may indicate any of the risk factors identified in the epidemiology section.

PHYSICAL EXAM FINDINGS

- Horses with large intestinal impactions are generally cardiovascularly stable with signs of mild to moderate dehydration and mild elevation in heart rate (associated with pain).
- Other findings may include mild to moderate abdominal distension and decreased or absent borborygmi.

ETIOLOGY AND PATHOPHYSIOLOGY

- Risk factors described in the epidemiology section likely affect motility, particle size of feed material, and water content of ingesta.
- The most common intestinal sites for impaction are areas where the lumen size decreases. The pelvic flexure–left ventral colon is the most common site for impaction because the lumen dramatically narrows at the left dorsal colon. The right dorsal colon and transverse colon are other common sites because of narrowing as the ingesta passes into the transverse and small colons, respectively.

DIAGNOSIS

DIFFERENTIAL DIAGNOSIS

- Other causes of mild to moderate abdominal pain: Simple or nonstrangulating obstructions of the gastrointestinal (GI) tract such as sand impaction, enterolithiasis, large colon displacements, large intestinal intraluminal obstructions, tympany, small colon impactions, and ileal impactions
- Other causes of large intestinal distension on examination per rectum: Sand impaction, enterolithiasis, tympany, large colon displacements, and other intraluminal obstructions.
- Dehydration of feed within the large intestine may occur secondary to small intestinal obstruction.

INITIAL DATABASE

- Findings on examination per rectum depend on the location of the impaction. Pelvic flexure–left ventral colon impactions are frequently palpable. Whereas primary impactions are typically smooth and rounded, dehydrated feed secondary to small intestinal obstruction will have a corrugated surface.
- Impactions within the right dorsal colon or transverse colon are not palpable; instead, the resulting distension of the large colon and cecum is the primary palpable abnormality.
- Secondary impactions of the right dorsal colon associated with right dorsal displacement can be differentiated from pelvic flexure impactions based on the location of the ingesta-filled viscus. Secondary impactions of the right dorsal colon are caudal and lateral to the cecum and are generally more cranial in the abdomen than pelvic flexure impactions. Additionally, the end of the pelvic flexure should be identifiable in horses with pelvic flexure impactions.
- Nasogastric reflux is uncommon but may occur.
- Blood work may be normal or consistent with mild to moderate dehydration (prerenal azotemia, elevated packed cell volume, elevated total protein).
- Abdominal fluid analysis is generally within normal limits. Impaction of the large colon may predispose to enterocentesis.

TREATMENT

THERAPEUTIC GOAL(S)

- Hydration of the ingesta
- Pain management
- Appropriate monitoring to identify any progression of the disease resulting in intestinal or cardiovascular compromise

ACUTE GENERAL TREATMENT

- Withhold *all* feed
- Fluid therapy
  - Enteric isotonic or slightly hypotonic fluids: Experimentally, this is the most effective method of hydrating ingesta within the large colon. Balanced electrolyte solution prevents electrolyte disturbances associated with saline; 3 to 6 L every 2 to 4 hours or continuous administration at rate of 2 to 3 L/hr is recommended.
  - IV isotonic fluids: Replace fluid deficits associated with dehydration and allow fluid administration if nasogastric reflux is present. Provide overhydration to prevent dehydra-

tion with use of osmotic cathartics; at least two times maintenance (120 mL/kg/d) is recommended.

- Cathartics or laxatives: Hydrate ingesta or promote transit
  - Mineral oil: Lubricant and intestinal transit marker (12–24 hr after administration normally); 5 to 10 mL/kg is recommended.
  - Dioctyl sodium sulfosuccinate (DSS): Surfactant that allows water and fat to penetrate the fecal mass; the recommended dose is 16.5 to 55 mg/kg. It is important to stick to the recommended dose.
  - Osmotic cathartics such as $MgSO_4$ (0.5–1.0 g/kg) and polyethylene glycol 3350 (not well evaluated) draw water into the lumen of the intestine with an osmotic gradient.
- Analgesics are important to control pain during hydration and passage of the impaction. NSAIDs (primarily flunixin meglumine) are used most frequently because of the minimal affect on motility. The use of intermittent doses of an α_2 agonist with or without butorphanol may be necessary in severe impactions. Other analgesic options include lidocaine and butorphanol continuous rate infusions. It is important to monitor for any signs of systemic or GI deterioration while administering analgesics.
- Surgical treatment may be required if pain is unrelenting or systemic or GI deterioration occurs.

CHRONIC TREATMENT

- Treatment of recurrent impactions is not well documented.
- Methods of treatment may include:
  - Dietary modification: Some clinicians report success with low-residue diets such as complete pelleted feeds and fresh grass.
  - Stimulation of water consumption: Salt feed or hay, warm water in cold weather, electrolyte water.
  - Make any changes to daily routine (stall hours, diet, exercise) as gradually as possible.
  - In severe cases unresponsive to medical management, large colon resection may be recommended.

DRUG INTERACTIONS

- Combining DSS with mineral oil may result in systemic absorption of the mineral oil with unknown consequences.
- Combining DSS with $MgSO_4$ may increase the potential for systemic toxicity of the Mg.

POSSIBLE COMPLICATIONS

- Complications are uncommon with medical management but may include intestinal rupture and diarrhea.

- Complications that have been reported with surgical treatment include intestinal rupture, diarrhea, incisional complications, and septic peritonitis. Intestinal rupture during exteriorization of the colon may occur in up to 20% of cases.

RECOMMENDED MONITORING

- Monitoring for resolution of the impaction should include fecal output and repeat examination per rectum.
- During treatment, horses should be monitored for signs of unrelenting pain, nasogastric reflux, progressive abdominal distension, systemic deterioration (climbing heart rate, cardiovascular compromise), and GI deterioration (abdominocentesis may be useful).

PROGNOSIS AND OUTCOME

Overall, the prognosis for large colon impaction is very good. The prognosis appears better for horses that respond to medical management compared with horses that require surgical management.

PEARLS & CONSIDERATIONS

COMMENTS

- Consider large colon impaction as an important differential diagnosis in horses with signs of mild to moderate abdominal pain with consistent findings on examination per rectum.
- Mainstays of treatment include withholding feed, fluid therapy, cathartics, and analgesics.

PREVENTION

Avoiding risk factors is a key to prevention.

CLIENT EDUCATION

Education of clients about risk factors may decrease the incidence of colic caused by large colon impactions.

SUGGESTED READING

Dabareiner RM: Impaction of the ascending colon and cecum. In White NA, Moore JN, editors: *Current techniques in equine surgery and lameness*, Philadelphia, 1998, WB Saunders, pp 270–273.

Dabareiner RM, White NA: Large colon impaction in horses: 147 cases (1985–1991). *J Am Vet Med Assoc* 206:679–685, 1995.

Rakestraw PC, Hardy J: Large intestine. In Auer JA, Stick JA, editors: *Equine surgery*, ed 3, St Louis, 2006, Saunders Elsevier, pp 436–478.

AUTHOR: KIRA L. EPSTEIN

EDITORS: TIM MAIR and **CERI SHERLOCK**

Large Colon: Intraluminal Obstruction

BASIC INFORMATION

DEFINITION

Obstruction of the flow of ingesta, gas, or both associated with the presence of an ingested foreign body; a fecalith (concretion of feces); or a bezoar (concretion of plant material [phytobezoar], hair [trichobezoar], or combination [trichophytobezoar])

EPIDEMIOLOGY

SPECIES, AGE, SEX Foals and young adults may be predisposed.

GENETICS AND BREED PREDISPOSITION

- Fecaliths are the most common cause of surgical colic reported in Miniature Horses.
- Clinical experience suggests that Miniature Horse foals are also predisposed to trichophytobezoars.

RISK FACTORS

- Suggested risk factors for fecaliths include poor-quality roughage, poor dentition, and decreased water consumption.
- Although no studies are available describing risk factors for the development of obstruction with bezoars or foreign material, clinical experience suggests that foals that chew on their mare's tail may be predisposed to forming trichophytobezoars, and

access to foreign material and inadequate exercise may predispose horses to consuming foreign material.

CLINICAL PRESENTATION

HISTORY, CHIEF COMPLAINT Clinical signs are consistent with simple obstruction of the large or small colon, including mild to moderate abdominal pain (colic) and decreased or absent fecal production. Signalment and risk factors should be recognized.

PHYSICAL EXAM FINDINGS Horses with obstruction associated with fecaliths, bezoars, and foreign bodies have similar physical examination findings to horses with other simple obstructions of the large or small colon (see "Large Colon: Impaction" and "Small Colon: Impaction" in this section).

ETIOLOGY AND PATHOPHYSIOLOGY

- The development of fecaliths and bezoars is not well understood but may be associated with the accumulation and dehydration of feed and foreign material larger than the normal particulate size of properly chewed and digested feed material.
- Obstruction may occur in any part of the large intestine, including the large, transverse, and small colons. Obstruction of the small colon appears common with fecaliths in Miniature Horses.

DIAGNOSIS

DIFFERENTIAL DIAGNOSIS

- Other causes of mild to moderate abdominal pain: Simple or nonstrangulating obstructions of the gastrointestinal tract such as large colon impactions (feed and sand), enterolithiasis, large colon displacements, tympany, small colon impactions, and ileal impactions (see respective chapters)
- Other causes of large intestinal distension on examination per rectum: Tympany, large colon impactions (feed and sand), enterolithiasis, and large colon displacements (see respective chapters)

INITIAL DATABASE

- Findings on examination per rectum depend on the location of the impaction (see "Large Colon: Impaction" and "Small Colon: Impaction" in this section). Distension of the large colon and cecum are common with the addition of distension of the small colon if the fecalith or bezoar is within the small colon. It is uncommon to palpate the obstruction.
- Nasogastric reflux is uncommon but may occur
- Blood work may be normal or consistent with mild to moderate dehydration (prerenal azotemia, elevated

packed cell volume, elevated total protein).
- Abdominal fluid analysis is generally within normal limits.

TREATMENT

THERAPEUTIC GOAL(S)
Remove the obstruction

ACUTE GENERAL TREATMENT
- Surgical exploration and removal. If pressure necrosis is present, resection may be required.
- Perioperative supportive care as required

CHRONIC TREATMENT
Risk factors should be addressed to prevent recurrence. This should include appropriate dental care, providing plenty of fresh water, and providing plenty of good-quality roughage.

POSSIBLE COMPLICATIONS
- Postoperative complications may include diarrhea, inappetence, and impaction at the surgery site if damage to the intestinal wall has occurred that results in inflammation or fibrosis.

- Although not specifically reported, it is possible that pressure necrosis could occur at the site of obstruction. Clinical signs and diagnostic findings are similar to those described for pressure necrosis associated with enterolithiasis.

PROGNOSIS AND OUTCOME

Prognosis is likely excellent if surgical removal is pursued.

PEARLS & CONSIDERATIONS

COMMENTS
- Fecaliths and bezoars are important differential diagnoses in young Miniature Horses that present with signs of simple obstruction.
- Although uncommon, obstruction of the large intestine with a foreign body should be considered as a differential diagnosis in young horses.
- Surgical removal generally results in a good prognosis.

PREVENTION
Changes in management as described under Chronic Treatment may also serve as methods of prevention.

CLIENT EDUCATION
Client education may be useful in prevention.

SUGGESTED READING
Boles CL, Kohn CW: Fibrous foreign body impaction colic in young horses. *J Am Vet Med Assoc* 171(2):193, 1977.
Haupt JL, McAndrews AG, Chaney KP, et al: Surgical treatment of colic in the miniature horse: a retrospective study of 57 cases (1993–2006). *Equine Vet J* 40(4):364, 2008.
Hughes KJ, Dowling BA, Matthews SA, et al: Results of surgical treatment of colic in miniature breed horses: 11 cases. *Aust Vet J* 81(5):260, 2003.
McClure JT, Kobluk C, Voller K, et al: Fecalith impaction in four miniature foals. *J Am Vet Med Assoc* 200(2):205, 1992.

AUTHOR: **KIRA L. EPSTEIN**

EDITORS: **TIM MAIR** and **CERI SHERLOCK**

Large Colon: Intussusception

BASIC INFORMATION

DEFINITION
One segment of the colon telescoping (intussusceptum) into an adjacent segment of the colon (intussuscipiens)

SYNONYM
Colo-colic intussusception

EPIDEMIOLOGY
SPECIES, AGE, SEX As with other intussusceptions, younger horses (younger than age 3 years) appear predisposed.

CLINICAL PRESENTATION
HISTORY, CHIEF COMPLAINT
- Reported cases have had a history of mild, recurrent colic, and soft feces.
- Increased severity of colic signs occurs with progressive obstruction.
PHYSICAL EXAM FINDINGS Physical examination reveals mild tachycardia with variable decreased borborygmi and increased temperature.
ETIOLOGY AND PATHOPHYSIOLOGY
- As with other intussusceptions, hypermotility is believed to contribute to the

development of colo-colic intussusceptions.
- Although not reported for colo-colic intussusceptions, it is possible that an intussusception may occur in association with an intramural mass at the leading edge of the intussusceptum.
- Colo-colic intussusceptions have been reported in the left ventral and dorsal colons and the pelvic flexure.

DIAGNOSIS

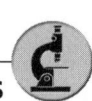

DIFFERENTIAL DIAGNOSIS
- Other causes of mild to moderate abdominal pain: Simple or nonstrangulating obstructions of the gastrointestinal tract such as feed or sand impaction, enterolithiasis, large colon tympany, other large colon displacements, large intestinal intraluminal obstructions, small colon impactions, and ileal impactions
- Other causes of large intestinal distension on examination per rectum: Feed or sand impaction, enterolithiasis, large colon tympany, other large colon

displacements, large colon volvulus, and other intraluminal obstructions
- Other causes of fever associated with recurrent mild colic: Peritonitis
- Other causes of colitis: salmonellosis and sand colitis or impaction

INITIAL DATABASE
- Distension of the large colon and cecum secondary to obstruction of the lumen by the intussusceptum is the most consistent finding on examination per rectum. The ability to palpate the intussusception is variable. If palpable, the intussusception will feel like a doughy mass.
- Nasogastric reflux is unexpected.
- Leukocytosis has been reported in cases of colo-colic intussusception. Hyperfibrinogenemia has also been reported.
- Increased abdominal fluid, nucleated cell count, and a variable increase in peritoneal fluid total protein have been reported.
- Although not performed in reported cases, it is possible that abdominal ultrasonography could provide a pre-

operative diagnosis. Intussusceptions in other regions have a bulls-eye pattern when imaged with ultrasonography. The ability to image the intussusception depends on its location adjacent to the body wall, accumulation of gas in surrounding segments of bowel, and luminal contents of the affected segment.

TREATMENT

THERAPEUTIC GOAL(S)

- Reduction or resection of the intussusception
- Supportive care

ACUTE GENERAL TREATMENT

Surgical treatment has been described in several case reports. The ability to reduce the intussusception has been variable. In cases in which reduction is possible and no ischemic damage has occurred, no further treatment is required. In cases in which reduction is not possible, resection of the region is successful.

PROGNOSIS AND OUTCOME

Based on the limited number of cases in the literature, the prognosis appears good with surgical treatment.

PEARLS & CONSIDERATIONS

Intussusception of the large colon is an uncommon cause of progressive, recurrent colic and fever in young horses.

SUGGESTED READING

Johnston JK, Freeman DE: Diseases and surgery of the large colon. *Vet Clin North Am Equine Pract* 13(2):317, 1997.
Sullins KE: Diseases of the large colon. In Colohan PT, Merritt AM, Moore JN, et al (eds). *Equine medicine and surgery*, St Louis, 1999, Mosby Elsevier, pp 741–768.

AUTHOR: **KIRA L. EPSTEIN**

EDITORS: **TIM MAIR** and **CERI SHERLOCK**

Large Colon: Left Dorsal Displacement

BASIC INFORMATION

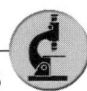

DEFINITION

- Displacement or entrapment of the large colon within the nephrosplenic space (between the spleen and the left kidney)
- Some clinicians include displacement of the large colon lateral to the spleen.

SYNONYM(S)

Nephrosplenic entrapment, renosplenic entrapment

EPIDEMIOLOGY

SPECIES, AGE, SEX

- No age predisposition has been reported, and left dorsal displacement of the large colon (LDDLC) has been reported in horses of all ages, including weanlings.
- Some studies have reported that geldings are predisposed, but other studies have reported no sex predisposition.

GENETICS AND BREED PREDISPOSITION Clinical experience suggests that larger breed horses are predisposed. There have been no reported cases of LDDLC in ponies or Miniature Horses.

RISK FACTORS A deep nephrosplenic space may predispose horses to LDDLC.

CLINICAL PRESENTATION

HISTORY, CHIEF COMPLAINT

- Clinical signs of LDDLC are variable depending on the tension on the nephrosplenic ligament, pull on the mesentery, distension of the large colon, and secondary gastric distension. Most affected horses show signs

of moderate pain, but severe pain may occur. Some horses may have chronic displacement with little gas distension and little to no signs of discomfort.
- Horses frequently have decreased to absent fecal production and may have abdominal distension. In some horses, the visible distension is confined to the area of the left paralumbar fossa.

PHYSICAL EXAM FINDINGS

- Because LDDLC is generally a nonstrangulating obstruction, affected horses are cardiovascularly stable.
- Physical examination findings may include tachycardia, abdominal distension, decreased or absent borborygmi, and signs of dehydration.
- As distension becomes more severe, compromise to the cardiovascular system and respiratory system are possible. With chronicity or severe distension, ischemia of the entrapped region of the left colons may occur, and clinical signs and physical examination will reflect the associated cardiovascular compromise.

ETIOLOGY AND PATHOPHYSIOLOGY

- It is likely that changes in motility or gas distension of the large colon result in abnormal migration of the pelvic flexure.
- The left large colon may migrate lateral to the spleen and dorsally until it reaches the nephrosplenic space or the pelvic flexure may migrate cranially and then back caudally to pass through the nephrosplenic space from cranial to caudal.
- Frequently, the left colon rotates 180 degrees such that the left dorsal colon is ventral to the left ventral colon.

DIAGNOSIS

DIFFERENTIAL DIAGNOSIS

- Other causes of moderate abdominal pain: Simple or nonstrangulating obstructions of the gastrointestinal tract such as feed or sand impaction, enterolithiasis, large colon tympany, other large colon displacements, large intestinal intraluminal obstructions, small colon impactions, and ileal impactions
- Other causes of large intestinal distension on examination per rectum: Feed or sand impaction, enterolithiasis, large colon tympany, other large colon displacements, large colon volvulus, and other intraluminal obstructions

INITIAL DATABASE

- Typical findings on examination per rectum are distended large colon caudal to the nephrosplenic space and compressed within the nephrosplenic space.
- Other findings may include gas distension (sometimes marked) of the cecum and ventromedial displacement of the spleen. Palpation of the nephrosplenic space may be difficult, especially with severe distension of the large colon and in large-breed horses. It is important to remember that with severe distension of the large colon from any cause (eg, impaction, enterolithiasis, tympany), the bands of the large colon may course toward the nephrosplenic space and mimic LDDLC.
- Nasogastric reflux is present in up to 43% of horses with LDDLC. This may

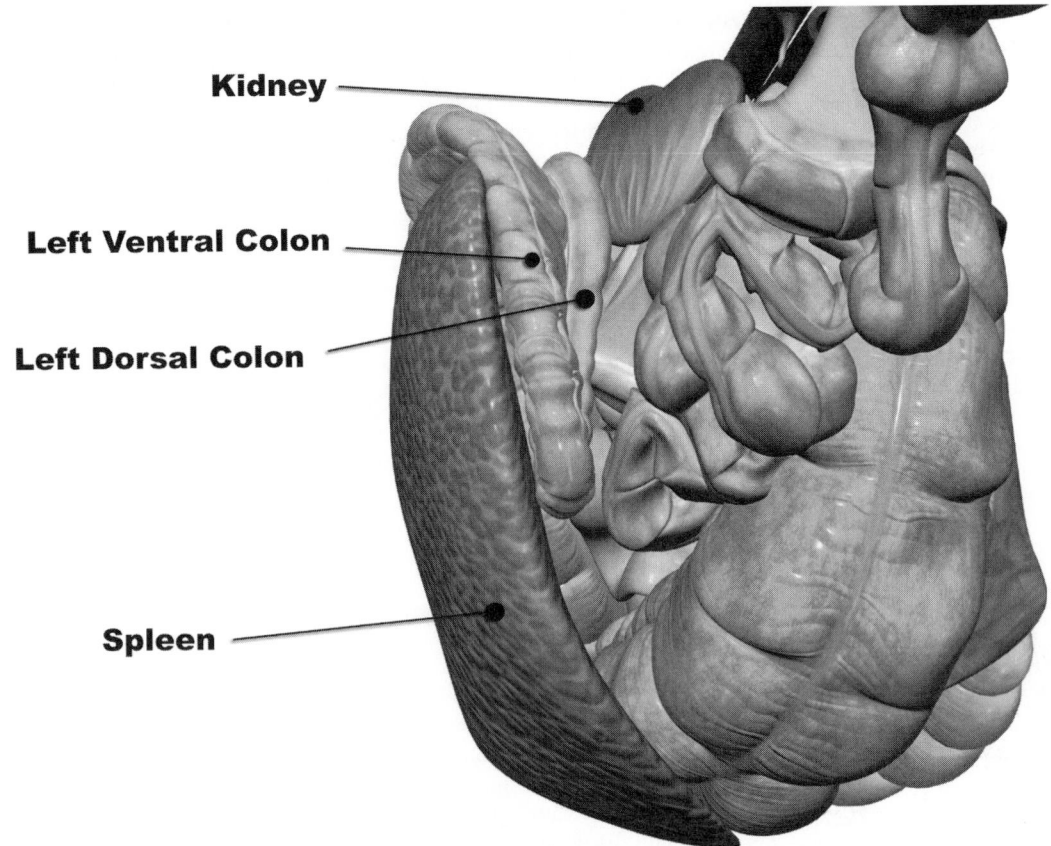

FIGURE 1   Diagram showing left dorsal displacement of the colon (caudal view). (From The Equine Colic CD 2007. The Glass Horse Project LLC and University of Georgia Research Foundation Inc. Used with permission.)

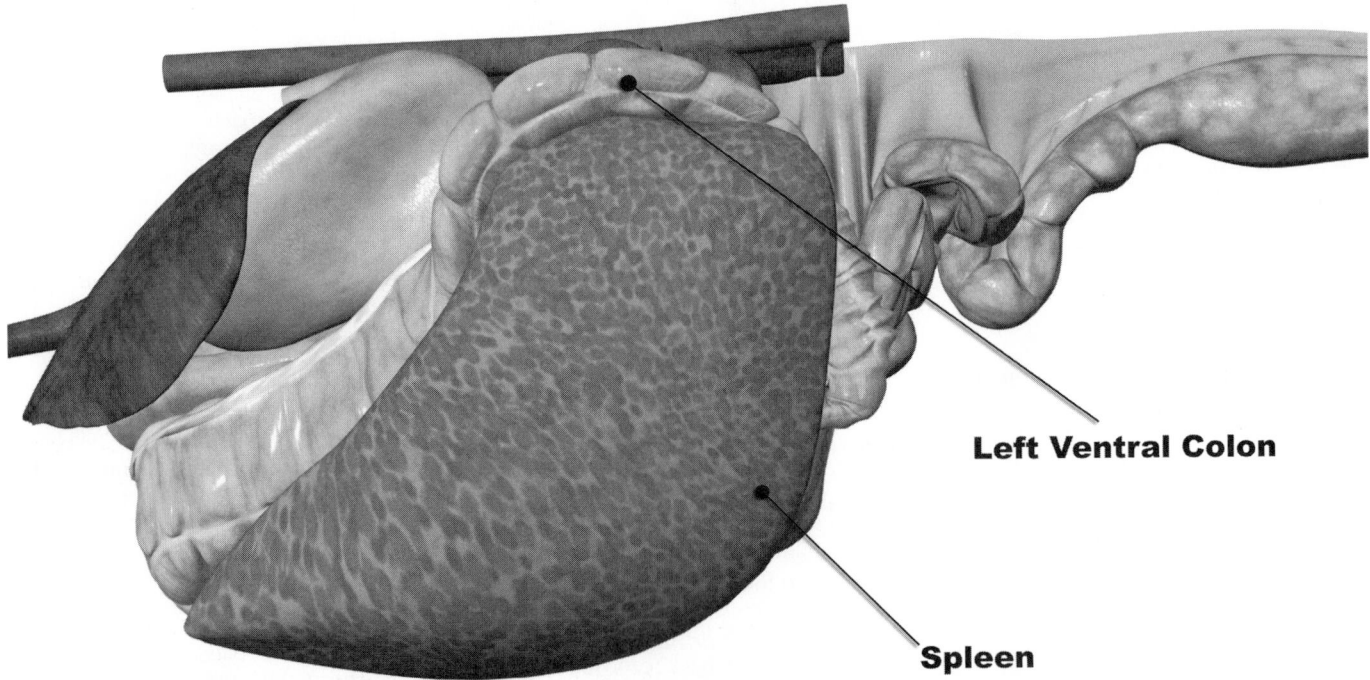

FIGURE 2   Diagram showing left dorsal displacement of the colon (left lateral view). (From The Equine Colic CD 2007. The Glass Horse Project LLC and University of Georgia Research Foundation Inc. Used with permission.)

be caused by pressure on the duodenum or tension on the mesentery associated with LDDLC.

- Blood work is frequently normal. Some clinicians believe that a relatively low PCV in the face of dehydration indicates sequestration of red blood cells within the spleen associated with LDDLC.
- Abdominocentesis may result in splenic blood (packed cell volume > peripheral blood) in up to 25% of horses with LDDLC.
- Ultrasonography (percutaneous): In horses with LDDLC, gas within the large colon will obscure the caudodorsal aspect of the spleen. The ability to image the kidney adjacent to the spleen does not appear as accurate as gas obscuring the caudodorsal aspect of the spleen. In some cases of LDDLC, it is possible to obtain an image of the kidney adjacent to the spleen, and in many cases of other sources of colic, it is not possible to obtain the same image.
- If ischemic damage has occurred, blood work and abdominal fluid may be altered.

TREATMENT

THERAPEUTIC GOAL(S)

- Correction of the displacement
- Supportive care

ACUTE GENERAL TREATMENT

- If pain and distension are not severe, medical management is frequently attempted, and good success rates have been reported. The two main methods for medical management are administration of phenylephrine and rolling the horse under general anesthesia.
  - The administration of phenylephrine at 3 to 6 μg/kg/min for 15 minutes results in splenic contraction and a dramatic decrease in the size of the spleen. During adminis-

tration, horses should be monitored for reflex bradycardia, and administration should be discontinued if bradycardia becomes severe. Horses are given phenylephrine and walked, jogged, or lunged to encourage the colon to come out of the nephrosplenic space.
  - Horses can be rolled under general anesthesia. They should be anesthetized, placed in right lateral recumbency, and rolled over their back into left lateral recumbency. While in dorsal recumbency, horses can be jostled to encourage the colon to come out of the nephrosplenic space. The administration of phenylephrine and manipulation per rectum in conjunction with rolling has also been described.
- Surgical exploration is recommended for horses that present with severe pain or that are unresponsive to attempts at medical management. Surgical exploration may also be recommended in horses with severe gas distension because of the potential for increased complications associated with medical management.

POSSIBLE COMPLICATIONS

- Recurrence rates ranging from 3% to 21% have been reported.
- Reported complications of medical management have included rupture and displacement or volvulus of the large colon.

RECOMMENDED MONITORING

If medical treatment is pursued, horses should be monitored for signs of unrelenting pain, nasogastric reflux, progressive abdominal distension, and systemic deterioration (climbing heart rate, cardiovascular compromise).

PROGNOSIS AND OUTCOME

Prognosis is good to excellent.

PEARLS & CONSIDERATIONS

COMMENTS

- Diagnosis of LDDLC is based on examination per rectum and ultrasonography.
- Medical management of horses with LDDLC can be very successful.
- Multiple methods of surgical prevention of recurrence are available.

PREVENTION

- In cases of recurrent LDDLC, surgical prevention of recurrence may be recommended.
- Multiple methods of laparoscopic and hand-assisted laparoscopic closure of the nephrosplenic space have been reported. Complications appear rare.
- Other methods of surgical prevention include closure of the nephrosplenic space via a rib resection, colopexy, and large colon resection. However, these procedures are not preferred because of an increased frequency and severity of complications associated with these procedures and longer lay-up time after surgery.

SUGGESTED READING

Johnston JK, Freeman DE: Diseases and surgery of the large colon. *Vet Clin North Am Equine Pract* 13(2):317, 1997.

Rakestraw PC, Hardy J: Large intestine. In Auer JA, Stick JA (eds). *Equine surgery*, ed 3, St Louis, 2006, Saunders Elsevier, pp 436–478.

Rocken M, Schubert C, Mosel G, et al: Indications, surgical technique, and long-term experience with laparoscopic closure of the nephrosplenic space in standing horses. *Vet Surg* 34:637, 2005.

Sullins KE: Diseases of the large colon. In Colohan PT, Merritt AM, Moore JN, et al (eds). *Equine medicine and surgery*, St Louis, 1999, Mosby, pp 741–768.

AUTHOR: **KIRA L. EPSTEIN**

EDITORS: **TIM MAIR** and **CERI SHERLOCK**

Large Colon: Nonstrangulating Infarction

BASIC INFORMATION

DEFINITION

Loss of blood supply to the colon not associated with strangulation

SYNONYM(S)

Mural infarction, thromboembolic colic

EPIDEMIOLOGY

RISK FACTORS

- High parasite load and inappropriate deworming programs may predispose to *Strongylus vulgaris* infestation.
- Coagulopathies associated with severe gastrointestinal (GI) disease and sepsis may predispose to thromboembolic disease.

CLINICAL PRESENTATION

DISEASE FORMS/SUBTYPES

- Verminous arteritis of the cranial mesenteric artery caused by *S. vulgaris* larval migration may present in acute or chronic forms.
- Conditions associated with systemic inflammatory response syndrome (SIRS) such as severe GI disease and

sepsis may result in coagulopathies and thromboembolic disease that may present as nonstrangulating infarction of the large colon.

HISTORY, CHIEF COMPLAINT The history and presenting complaints are variable depending on the cause of the nonstrangulating infarction. Whereas acute cases of verminous arteritis have rapid onset of colic, chronic cases have recurrent colic and weight loss. In cases associated with coagulopathies, the history will indicate the primary disease (see the various entries on colitis) with acute progression or development of signs of colic.

PHYSICAL EXAM FINDINGS

- Physical examination findings are variable depending on the cause of the nonstrangulating infarction, the degree of vascular compromise, and the amount of bowel affected.
- Variable tachycardia, tachypnea, and fever are associated with pain and endotoxemia.
- Other findings may include abdominal distension, decreased or absent borborygmi and alterations in fecal consistency and production.
- Endotoxemic shock may present with hyperemic or toxic mucous membranes, prolonged or decreased capillary refill time, poor pulse quality, cold extremities, and decreased jugular refill.

ETIOLOGY AND PATHOPHYSIOLOGY

- The pathophysiology of verminous arteritis is not well understood. Although some cases have obvious thrombosis, enlargement, aneurysm, or abscessation of the cranial mesenteric artery, other cases have no evidence of physical obstruction, and vasospasm has been proposed as the inciting cause of ischemia.
- Diseases associated with SIRS are frequently associated with coagulopathies caused by the procoagulant nature of many proinflammatory mediators. In horses with colitis, loss of antithrombin (a major anticoagulant protein) out of leaky vessels within the inflamed colon may also contribute to a procoagulant state.

DIAGNOSIS

DIFFERENTIAL DIAGNOSIS

- Other causes of colic: Feed or sand impaction, enterolithiasis, large colon tympany, other large colon displacements, large intestinal intraluminal obstructions, small colon impactions, ileal impactions, strangulating small

intestinal obstructions, large colon volvulus, and colitis.
- Other causes of endotoxemia: Colitis and large colon volvulus.
- Other causes of peritonitis: Idiopathic cases, GI rupture, and other strangulating GI lesions such as small intestinal or large colon volvulus.

INITIAL DATABASE

- Findings on examination per rectum are variable. Distension of the large colon and cecum is possible but not consistent. If venous occlusion has led to formation of edema and hemorrhage within the wall of the intestine, ischemic regions may be thickened on palpation if they can be accessed.
- Nasogastric reflux is unexpected.
- Findings on routine blood work vary with the cause of the infarction. Chronic parasitism may be associated with anemia, hypoalbuminemia (if associated with protein-losing enteropathy), or hyperglobulinemia (if associated with chronic inflammation). Endotoxemia is frequently accompanied by leukopenia caused by neutropenia with left shift. Horses with colitis often have hypoproteinemia and may have electrolyte abnormalities. Thromboembolic disease may affect multiple organ systems, and as a result, blood work may reveal evidence of insufficiencies (eg, azotemia with renal insufficiency).
- Abdominal fluid is frequently consistent with peritonitis with changes in color (serosanguineous), increased total nucleated cell count, and increased total protein concentration. However, normal peritoneal fluid analysis may occur even with severe ischemia to large portions of the large colon.
- If the ischemic region is edematous, abdominal ultrasonography may reveal a thickened, hypoechoic bowel wall.

TREATMENT

THERAPEUTIC GOAL(S)

- Remove ischemic bowel
- Treat the underlying cause
- Provide supportive care

ACUTE GENERAL TREATMENT

- Depending on the accessibility and size of the segment of affected bowel, surgical resection may or may not be possible.
- The underlying disease and degree of endotoxemia may make some affected animals poor surgical candidates.

- Supportive care required may include all or some of the following: fluid therapy, colloid support, and antiendotoxic treatment.

CHRONIC TREATMENT

A good deworming program should be started if verminous arteritis is the underlying cause.

PROGNOSIS AND OUTCOME

- Prognosis is variable based on the extent of the lesion and the severity of the underlying disease.
- Prognosis is best if the region affected is small and easy to resect. However, the infarction can progress to other segments after surgery.
- If the cranial mesenteric artery is palpably enlarged, has an aneurysm, or is associated with an abscess at the time of surgery, prognosis is guarded to poor.
- Clinical experience suggests that infarction associated with colitis has a poor prognosis.

PEARLS & CONSIDERATIONS

COMMENTS

- Nonstrangulating infarction of the large colon is an uncommon cause of colic in horses.
- Nonstrangulating infarction may be associated with verminous arteritis or coagulopathies secondary to inflammatory diseases, most commonly colitis.

PREVENTION

Appropriate deworming appears to have decreased the incidence of nonstrangulating infarction of the large colon associated with *S. vulgaris*.

SUGGESTED READING

Johnston JK, Freeman DE: Diseases and surgery of the large colon. *Vet Clin North Am Equine Pract* 13(2):317, 1997.

Rakestraw PC, Hardy J: Large intestine. In Auer JA, Stick JA (eds). *Equine surgery*, ed 3, St Louis, 2006, Saunders Elsevier, pp 436–478.

Sullins KE: Diseases of the large colon. In Colohan PT, Merritt AM, Moore JN, et al (eds). *Equine medicine and surgery*, St Louis, 1999, Mosby, pp 741–768.

AUTHOR: KIRA L. EPSTEIN

EDITORS: TIM MAIR and CERI SHERLOCK

Large Colon: Other Displacements

BASIC INFORMATION

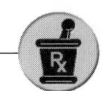

DEFINITION

- Displacement of the large colon (primarily the left dorsal and ventral colons)

CLINICAL PRESENTATION

DISEASE FORMS/SUBTYPES

- The most commonly reported malpositioning of the large colon aside from right dorsal displacement of the large colon (RDDLC) and left dorsal displacement of the large colon (LDDLC) is retroflexion or cranial flexion of the pelvic flexure.
- Other entrapments that have been reported include displacement through a rent in the mesoductus deferens, through a rent in the gastrosplenic ligament, through a rent in the diaphragm, and through the epiploic foramen.
- The author has also observed the sternal and diaphragmatic flexure displaced cranial to the stomach. Some clinicians include nonstrangulating large colon volvulus or torsion in this category. With the exception of entrapment in the epiploic foramen, these displacements generally result in nonstrangulating obstruction of the large colon.

HISTORY, CHIEF COMPLAINT

- Clinical signs of displacement of the large colon are variable depending on the degree of displacement and associated pull on the mesentery and distension of the large colon.
- Signs of colic range from chronic mild signs of pain to severe signs of colic.
- Other clinical signs may include decreased to absent fecal production and abdominal distension.

PHYSICAL EXAM FINDINGS

- Because malpositioning of the large colon generally results in nonstrangulating obstruction, affected horses are cardiovascularly stable.
- Physical examination findings may include tachycardia, abdominal distension, decreased or absent borborygmi, and signs of dehydration.
- As distension becomes more severe, compromise to the cardiovascular system and respiratory system are possible.
- If entrapment results in ischemia of the entrapped region of the colon, the clinical signs and physical examination

will reflect the associated cardiovascular compromise.

ETIOLOGY AND PATHOPHYSIOLOGY Similar to the more common displacements (RDDLC and LDDLC), it is likely that changes in motility or gas distension of the large colon result in abnormal migration of the pelvic flexure.

DIAGNOSIS

DIFFERENTIAL DIAGNOSIS

- Other causes of mild to moderate abdominal pain: Simple or nonstrangulating obstructions of the gastrointestinal tract such as feed or sand impaction, enterolithiasis, large colon tympany, right or left dorsal displacement of the large colon, large intestinal intraluminal obstructions, small colon impactions, and ileal impactions.
- Other causes of large intestinal distension on examination per rectum: feed or sand impaction, enterolithiasis, large colon tympany, right or left dorsal displacement of the large colon, large colon volvulus, and other intraluminal obstructions.

INITIAL DATABASE

- Findings on examination per rectum vary with the type of displacement and the degree of gas distension. Distension of the cecum and an inability to palpate the pelvic flexure are common findings. Distension of the large colon may also be palpable. It is important to remember that these findings are not specific for displacement and may result from other nonstrangulating obstruction of the large colon (eg, impaction, enterolithiasis, tympany).
- Nasogastric reflux may be associated with distension of the large colon adjacent to the duodenum resulting in gastric outflow obstruction.
- Bloodwork may be normal or consistent with mild to moderate dehydration (prerenal azotemia, elevated packed cell volume, elevated total protein).
- Abdominal fluid analysis is generally within normal limits.
- If ischemic damage has occurred, bloodwork and abdominal fluid may be altered.

TREATMENT

THERAPEUTIC GOAL(S)

- Correction of the displacement
- Supportive care

ACUTE GENERAL TREATMENT

- If pain and distension are not severe, medical management can be attempted. Horses can be held off feed, placed on IV fluids, and monitored for signs of progression or resolution. It is impossible to determine how successful medical management will be because definitive preoperative diagnosis is not possible. However, a percentage of horses may resolve with this therapy.
- Surgical exploration is recommended for horses that present with severe pain or that are unresponsive to attempts at medical management.

RECOMMENDED MONITORING

If medical treatment is pursued, horses should be monitored for signs of unrelenting pain, nasogastric reflux, progressive abdominal distension, and systemic deterioration (climbing heart rate, cardiovascular compromise).

PROGNOSIS AND OUTCOME

Prognosis is good to excellent for horses with nonstrangulating displacements of the large colon.

PEARLS & CONSIDERATIONS

COMMENTS

- Displacement of the large colon should be considered as a differential diagnosis in any horse presenting for colic with cecal and large colon distension.
- Definitive diagnosis requires surgical exploration.

PREVENTION

In cases of recurrent large colon displacement, surgical prevention of recurrence may be recommended. Methods of surgical prevention include colopexy and large colon resection. Both of these procedures have potentially life-threatening complications and are generally not recommended before the second or third episode of displacement confirmed at surgery.

SUGGESTED READING

Johnston JK, Freeman DE: Diseases and surgery of the large colon. *Vet Clin North Am Equine Pract* 13(2):317, 1997.
Sullins KE: Diseases of the large colon. In Colohan PT, Merritt AM, Moore JN, et al (eds). *Equine medicine and surgery*, St Louis, 1999, Mosby, pp 741–768.

AUTHOR: **KIRA L. EPSTEIN**

EDITOR: **TIM MAIR**

Large Colon: Right Dorsal Displacement

BASIC INFORMATION

DEFINITION

Right dorsal displacement of the large colon (RDDLC) is displacement of the large colon lateral to (to the right of) the cecum.

EPIDEMIOLOGY

GENETICS AND BREED PREDISPOSITION Clinical experience suggests that larger breed horses are predisposed, and ponies and miniature horses are uncommonly affected.

ASSOCIATED CONDITIONS AND DISORDERS RDDLC can be associated with impaction of the right dorsal colon (see "Large Colon Impaction" in this section) and a variable degree of rotation along the long axis (see "Large Colon Volvulus" in this section).

CLINICAL PRESENTATION

HISTORY, CHIEF COMPLAINT Clinical signs of RDDLC are variable depending on the degree of displacement and associated pull on the mesentery and distension of the large colon. Signs of colic may range from chronic mild signs of pain to severe signs of colic. Other clinical signs may include decreased to absent fecal production and abdominal distension.

PHYSICAL EXAM FINDINGS Horses with RDDLC are frequently cardiovascularly stable. Physical examination findings may include tachycardia, abdominal distension, decreased or absent borborygmi, and signs of dehydration. As distension becomes more severe, compromise to the cardiovascular system and respiratory system are possible.

ETIOLOGY AND PATHOPHYSIOLOGY

- It is likely that changes in motility or gas distension of the large colon result in abnormal migration of the pelvic flexure.
- Most commonly, the pelvic flexure migrates counterclockwise (viewed from the ventral aspect of the abdomen). Initially, the pelvic flexure moves cranially, then across the abdomen toward the right body wall,

then lateral to the cecum, then around the caudal aspect of the cecum, and finally again cranially to the level of the sternum.

- Less commonly, the pelvic flexure migrates clockwise (viewed from the ventral aspect of the abdomen). Initially, the pelvic flexure moves toward the right body wall caudal to the cecum and then migrates cranially to the right of the cecum to the level of the sternum.
- Variable degrees of rotation around the long axis (volvulus) are possible with RDDLC. The volvulus is generally nonstrangulating (see "Large Colon: Volvulus" in this section).

DIAGNOSIS

DIFFERENTIAL DIAGNOSIS

- Other causes of mild to moderate abdominal pain: Simple or nonstrangulating obstructions of the gastrointestinal tract such as feed or sand impaction, enterolithiasis, large colon tympany, other large colon displacements, large intestinal intraluminal obstructions, small colon impactions, and ileal impactions.
- Other causes of large intestinal distension on examination per rectum: Feed or sand impaction, enterolithiasis, large colon tympany, other large colon displacements, large colon volvulus, and other intraluminal obstructions.

INITIAL DATABASE

- Typical findings on examination per rectum are distended large colon with bands coursing transversely across the abdomen. The colon is caudal and lateral to the cecum, and it is generally not possible to palpate the ventral band of the cecum. It is also not possible to palpate the pelvic flexure. It is important to remember that with severe distension of the large colon from any cause (eg, impaction, enterolithiasis, tympany), the anatomy can be distorted, and findings on examination per rectum are similar, but a final diagnosis requires surgery.

- Nasogastric reflux may occur associated with distension of the large colon adjacent to the duodenum.
- Blood work may be normal or consistent with mild to moderate dehydration (prerenal azotemia, elevated packed cell volume, elevated total protein). Elevation of gamma-glutamyl transferase is believed to be associated with partial obstruction of the duodenum.
- Abdominal fluid analysis is generally within normal limits.

TREATMENT

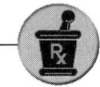

THERAPEUTIC GOAL(S)

- Correction of the displacement
- Supportive care

ACUTE GENERAL TREATMENT

- If pain and distension are not severe, medical management is frequently attempted. Horses are held off feed, placed on IV fluids, and monitored for signs of progression or resolution. It is impossible to determine how successful medical management is because preoperative diagnosis of RDDLC is impossible. However, a percentage of horses with findings consistent with RDDLC on physical examination and examination per rectum resolve with this therapy.
- Surgical exploration is recommended for horses that present with severe pain or that are unresponsive to attempts at medical management. Surgical exploration and correction is the only way to definitively diagnose and treat RDDLC.

POSSIBLE COMPLICATIONS

Redisplacement can occur and has been reported as early as 48 hours after surgical correction.

RECOMMENDED MONITORING

If medical treatment is pursued, the horse should be monitored for signs of unrelenting pain, nasogastric reflux, progressive abdominal distension, and systemic

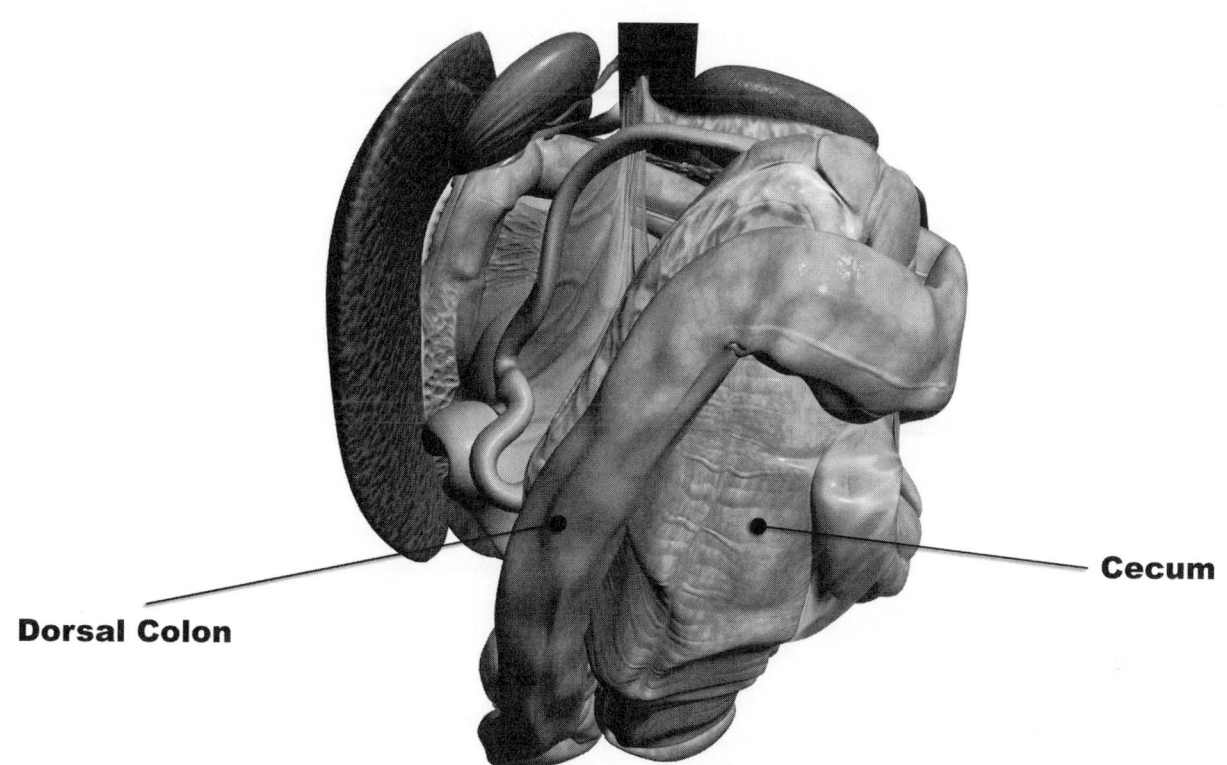

Cecum

Dorsal Colon

FIGURE 1 Right dorsal displacement of the colon (dorsal view). (From The Equine Colic CD. 2007. The Glass Horse Project LLC and University of Georgia Research Foundation Inc. Used with permission.)

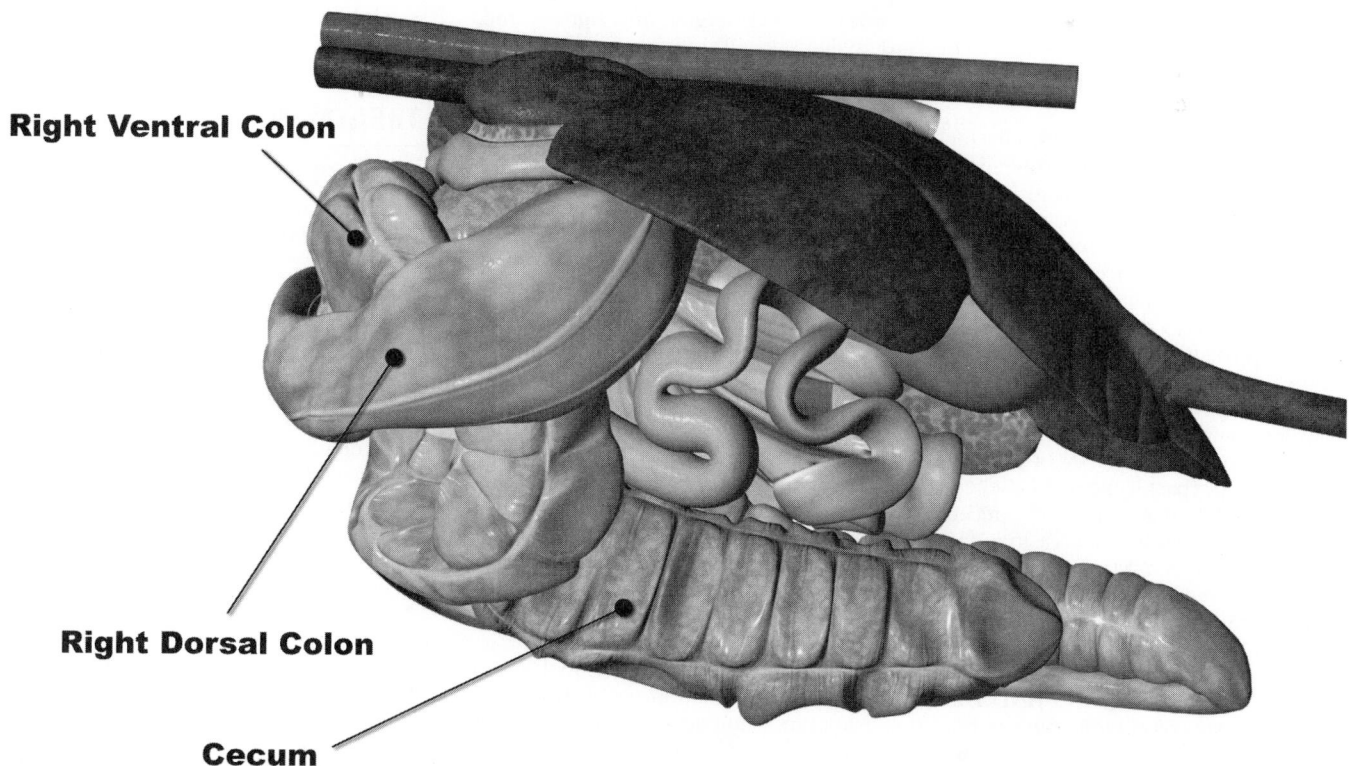

Right Ventral Colon

Right Dorsal Colon

Cecum

FIGURE 2 Right dorsal displacement of the colon (right lateral view). (From The Equine Colic CD. 2007. The Glass Horse Project LLC and University of Georgia Research Foundation Inc. Used with permission.)

deterioration (climbing heart rate, cardiovascular compromise).

PROGNOSIS AND OUTCOME

Prognosis is good to excellent.

PEARLS & CONSIDERATIONS

COMMENTS

- RDDLC should be considered as a differential diagnosis in any horse presenting for colic with large colon distension and tight bands traversing the abdomen on examination per rectum.
- Definitive diagnosis requires surgical exploration.

PREVENTION

In cases of recurrent RDDLC, surgical prevention of recurrence may be recommended. Methods of surgical prevention include colopexy and large colon resection. Both of these procedures have potentially life-threatening complications and are generally not recommended before the second or third episode of RDDLC confirmed at surgery.

SUGGESTED READING

Johnston JK, Freeman DE: Diseases and surgery of the large colon. *Vet Clin North Am Equine Pract* 13(2):317, 1997.

Rakestraw PC, Hardy J: Large intestine. In Auer JA, Stick JA (eds). *Equine surgery*, ed 3, St Louis, 2006, Saunders Elsevier, pp 436–478.

Sullins KE: Diseases of the large colon. In Colohan PT, Merritt AM, Moore JN, et al (eds). *Equine medicine and surgery*, St Louis, 1999, Mosby, pp 741–768.

AUTHOR: **KIRA L. EPSTEIN**

EDITORS: **TIM MAIR** and **CERI SHERLOCK**

Large Colon: Tympany

BASIC INFORMATION

DEFINITION

Accumulation of gas in the large colon secondary to excessive fermentation or functional obstruction (ileus)

SYNONYM(S)

Gas colic, spasmodic colic

EPIDEMIOLOGY

RISK FACTORS

- Changes to diets that are rapidly fermentable such as high-carbohydrate feeds (grain) and roughage with a high surface area (mowed grass) are commonly associated with tympany. In some horses, beet pulp appears to cause excessive gas production.
- There is an association between tapeworm infestation and tympany.
- Other factors that have been associated with simple obstruction and gas distension of the large colon (eg, impaction) include history of previous colic, recent (past 4 weeks) lameness, travel in the past 24 hours, recent change in exercise, increasing time spent stabled, crib biting or windsucking, increasing time since last dental examination, and longer than 12 months since deworming with ivermectin or moxidectin.

ASSOCIATED CONDITIONS AND DISORDERS Large colon tympany may predispose horses to displacement and volvulus of the large colon.

CLINICAL PRESENTATION

HISTORY, CHIEF COMPLAINT Horses with large colon tympany present with signs of abdominal pain (colic) and distension. Historical findings may indicate any of the risk factors identified in the epidemiology section.

PHYSICAL EXAM FINDINGS Horses with large colon tympany are generally cardiovascularly stable. They may have elevations of heart rate associated with pain, abdominal distension, decreased or absent borborygmi, and signs of mild dehydration. If distension becomes severe, compromise to the cardiovascular and respiratory systems can occur.

ETIOLOGY AND PATHOPHYSIOLOGY Risk factors described in the epidemiology section likely affect motility and bacterial flora within the large colon. These changes result in stasis, increased gas production, or both within the large colon, leading to distension and pain.

DIAGNOSIS

DIFFERENTIAL DIAGNOSIS

- Other causes of mild to moderate abdominal pain: Simple or nonstrangulating obstructions of the gastrointestinal (GI) tract such as feed or sand impaction, enterolithiasis, large colon displacements, large intestinal intraluminal obstructions, small colon impactions, and ileal impactions.
- Other causes of large intestinal distension on examination per rectum: Feed or sand impaction, enterolithiasis, large colon displacements, large colon volvulus, and other intraluminal obstructions

INITIAL DATABASE

- Examination per rectum reveals a variable degree, possibly severe, of gas distension of the large colon. Distension of the cecum may occur as the duration of the obstruction increases.
- Nasogastric reflux is uncommon.
- Blood work may be normal or consistent with mild dehydration (prerenal azotemia, elevated packed cell volume, elevated total protein).
- Abdominal fluid analysis within normal limits.

TREATMENT

THERAPEUTIC GOAL(S)

- Pain management
- Supportive care

ACUTE GENERAL TREATMENT

- Withhold feed.
- Most horses with large colon tympany have a good response to analgesics (flunixin meglumine, α_2 agonists, butorphanol). Analgesics minimize sympathetic inhibition of motility.
- Some clinicians recommend administration of mineral oil to decrease the absorption and speed the intestinal transit of the feed material responsible for the increase in gas production.
- Some horses may benefit from IV fluids to support the cardiovascular system and treat any dehydration.
- Trocharization of the large colon (right or left flank depending on distension) has been described for the treatment of horses with severe large colon tympany. Because of the potential for complications (peritonitis, abscess formation) and the difficulty in completely ruling out other more serious, causes of large colon distension, the

use of trocharization remains controversial. Before performing trocharization, the clinician should take into account the cardiovascular status of the horse and the potential for referral and surgery.
- Gentle exercise (eg, walking) may stimulate GI motility and the natural evacuation of gas.

CHRONIC TREATMENT
- As with large colon impactions, treatment of recurrent tympany is not well documented.
- Similar to large colon impactions, methods of treatment focus on avoiding risk factors and may include:
  ○ Avoiding feed that results in rapid production of gas
  ○ Making any changes to daily routine (stall hours, diet, exercise) as gradually as possible
  ○ Routine parasite and dental care
- In severe cases unresponsive to medical management, large colon resection may be recommended.

RECOMMENDED MONITORING
- During treatment, horses should be monitored for signs of unrelenting pain, nasogastric reflux, progressive abdominal distension, and systemic deterioration (climbing heart rate, cardiovascular compromise).
- Progression of signs may indicate an inability to resolve the gas distension medically or progression to a large colon displacement or volvulus. Surgical exploration may be required.

PROGNOSIS AND OUTCOME

The prognosis is excellent.

PEARLS & CONSIDERATIONS

COMMENTS
- Large colon tympany is one of the most common causes of colic caused by gas distension of the large colon.

- Lack of response to analgesics or systemic deterioration may indicate a more serious cause of colic.

PREVENTION
Avoiding risk factors is a key to prevention.

CLIENT EDUCATION
Education of clients about risk factors may decrease the incidence of colic caused by large colon tympany.

SUGGESTED READING
Rakestraw PC, Hardy J: Large intestine. In Auer JA, Stick JA (eds). *Equine surgery*, ed 3, St Louis, 2006, Saunders Elsevier, pp 436–478.
Sullins KE: Diseases of the large colon. In Colohan PT, Merritt AM, Moore JN, et al (eds). *Equine medicine and surgery*, St Louis, 1999, Mosby, pp 741–768.

AUTHOR: **KIRA L. EPSTEIN**

EDITORS: **TIM MAIR** and **CERI SHERLOCK**

Large Colon: Volvulus

BASIC INFORMATION

DEFINITION
Rotation of the colon around the mesenteric axis (which is also the long axis of the large colon)

SYNONYM(S)
Large colon torsion, "twisted gut"

EPIDEMIOLOGY
SPECIES, AGE, SEX
- Mares are overrepresented.
- Large colon volvulus is uncommon in immature horses.

RISK FACTORS
- Postpartum mares appear to be at increased risk.
- A recent diet change and recent introduction to lush pasture may also predispose horses to the development of large colon volvulus.

GEOGRAPHY AND SEASONALITY
Because postpartum mares are at increased risk, regions with a high density of broodmares and times of year when parturition is more frequent have an increased incidence.

CLINICAL PRESENTATION
DISEASE FORMS/SUBTYPES Large colon volvulus may be strangulating or

nonstrangulating. Volvulus of 270 degrees or more results in strangulation. The findings associated with strangulating volvulus are discussed here. Nonstrangulating volvulus results in findings similar to large colon displacements (see "Large Colon: Left Dorsal Displacement" and "Large Colon: Right Dorsal Displacement" in this section).

HISTORY, CHIEF COMPLAINT In almost all cases, horses present with a history of rapid onset of severe, intractable pain. In most cases, the episode of colic is acute; less frequently, horses have a history of mild or moderate colic for a longer duration that progresses rapidly.

PHYSICAL EXAM FINDINGS
- Physical examination findings depend on the duration and degree of colonic compromise and distension. Initially, because of the very acute nature of the disease, physical examination may reveal normal vital signs, decreased to absent borborygmi, and severe pain.
- As distension progresses, respiratory and cardiovascular collapse may result.
- As endotoxemia occurs, compromise to the cardiovascular system worsens. Physical examination reveals signs of

hypovolemic or endotoxemic (maldistributive) shock, including hyperemic or toxic mucous membranes, prolonged or decreased capillary refill time, poor pulse quality, cold extremities, and decreased jugular refill.

ETIOLOGY AND PATHOPHYSIOLOGY
- It is possible that, similar to large colon displacements, changes in motility or distension of the large colon result in abnormal migration of the colon.
- Because of the increased incidence in postpartum mares, some have suggested that a sudden increase in the volume available for the colon to occupy plays a role in the development of large colon volvulus.
- The most common location for large colon volvulus is at the level of the cecocolic ligament. Less frequently, volvulus may include the cecum or occur at the level of the sternal-diaphragmatic flexure.
- The direction of the large colon volvulus is almost always with the ventral colon rotating dorsomedially (counterclockwise when viewed from a ventral midline incision), but rotation in the other direction may also occur.

DIAGNOSIS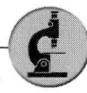

DIFFERENTIAL DIAGNOSIS

- Other causes of severe colic: Strangulating lesions of the small intestine such as small intestinal volvulus, epiploic foramen entrapment and strangulating lipoma, severe colitis
- Other causes of large intestinal distension on examination per rectum: Feed or sand impaction, enterolithiasis, large colon tympany, large colon displacements, and other intraluminal obstructions
- Other causes of endotoxemia: Colitis and nonstrangulating infarction of the large colon

INITIAL DATABASE

- Examination per rectum may be within normal limits in the acute stage. As the disease progresses, severe gas distension of the colon and cecum results.
- Nasogastric reflux is unlikely.
- Blood work varies depending on the degree of cardiovascular compromise and endotoxemia. Progressive increase in packed cell volume (PCV), decrease in total protein (TP), and leukopenia caused by neutropenia with a left shift indicate an increased severity of systemic compromise. Hyperlactatemia is associated with poor perfusion and ischemia of the strangulated region.
- Abdominal fluid is frequently normal even in cases with severe ischemic damage. An increase in TP is associated with a decreased prognosis.
- Thickening of the large colon wall may be evident on ultrasonography. However, the severity of pain generally makes ultrasound evaluation difficult and unnecessary.

TREATMENT

THERAPEUTIC GOALS

- Preoperative stabilization
- Correction of volvulus
- Determination of viability of the colon
- Supportive care

ACUTE GENERAL TREATMENT

- Preoperative stabilization generally requires rapid fluid resuscitation. Trocharization may decrease abdominal distension and can be performed based on clinician discretion.
- Correction of large colon volvulus requires surgery. The level of pain displayed by almost all horses with large colon volvulus makes the decision for surgery fairly obvious.
- During surgery, viability can be assessed, although accurate determination can be very difficult. Resection of the large colon is at the discretion of the surgeon.
- Supportive care required may include all or some of the following: fluid therapy, colloid support, antiendotoxic treatment, antimicrobials, and pain management.

POSSIBLE COMPLICATIONS

Recurrence of large colon volvulus may occur.

RECOMMENDED MONITORING

Intensive postoperative monitoring is generally required to manage horses with large colon volvulus.

PROGNOSIS AND OUTCOME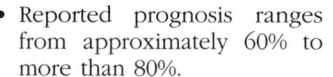

- Reported prognosis ranges from approximately 60% to more than 80%.

- Prognosis is related to the severity of compromise and amount of intestine affected. Early recognition and surgical treatment result in a better prognosis.
- Preoperative parameters associated with decreased prognosis include tachycardia (>80 beats/min), elevated PCV (>50%), fever (>102° F), and hyperlactatemia.

PEARLS & CONSIDERATIONS

COMMENTS

- Large colon volvulus should be considered in any horse with a rapid onset of uncontrollable signs of colic.
- Rapid detection and treatment are important to maximize the prognosis.

PREVENTION

Methods of surgical prevention include colopexy and large colon resection.

SUGGESTED READING

Ellis CM, Lynch TM, Slone DE, et al: Survival and complications after large colon resection and end-to-ed anastomosis for strangulating large colon volvulus in seventy-three horses. *Vet Surg* 37:786, 2008.

Johnston JK, Freeman DE: Diseases and surgery of the large colon. *Vet Clin North Am Equine Pract* 13(2):317, 1997.

Johnston K, Holcombe SJ, Hauptman JG: Plasma lactate as a predictor of colonic viability and survival after 360° volvulus of the ascending colon in horses. *Vet Surg* 36: 563, 2007.

Rakestraw PC, Hardy J: Large intestine. In Auer JA, Stick JA (eds). *Equine surgery*, ed 3, St Louis, 2006, Saunders Elsevier, pp 436–478.

Sullins KE: Diseases of the large colon. In Colohan PT, Merritt AM, Moore JN, et al (eds). *Equine medicine and surgery*, St Louis, 1999, Mosby, pp 741–768.

AUTHOR: **KIRA L. EPSTEIN**

EDITORS: **TIM MAIR** and **CERI SHERLOCK**

Laryngeal Hemiplegia

BASIC INFORMATION

DEFINITION

Chronic and progressive degenerative neuropathy of the recurrent laryngeal nerve (RLN) resulting in loss of motor function of the intrinsic muscles of the larynx, which leads to paresis or paralysis of the associated arytenoid cartilage

SYNONYM(S)

Recurrent laryngeal neuropathy, laryngeal paralysis, "roaring"

EPIDEMIOLOGY

GENETICS AND BREED PREDISPOSITION Large breeds are more commonly affected than small breeds and ponies. Familial correlation has been investigated with equivocal results. Height was also found to be associated with the inci-

dence of RLN. RLN probably has a phenotypic as well as inherited component.

RISK FACTORS

- In most cases, RLN is idiopathic without defined risk factors.
- Trauma or diseases associated with the neck or larynx can affect either side but are considered more likely associated if the dysfunction is on the right side of the horse. Trauma includes perivascular jugular vein or carotid

artery injection, surgery associated with the neck or larynx, and blunt or penetrating trauma to the neck.

- Diseases include guttural pouch mycosis and empyema, strangles abscessation, septic jugular thrombophlebitis, neoplasia of the neck, various central nervous system diseases, and toxicities.

ASSOCIATED CONDITIONS AND DISORDERS Vocal fold collapse

CLINICAL PRESENTATION

DISEASE FORMS/SUBTYPES

- Most commonly left laryngeal hemiplegia.
- Right laryngeal hemiplegia is uncommon and is usually associated with some type of trauma to the right RLN in the neck.

HISTORY, CHIEF COMPLAINT

- Respiratory noise on inspiration, exercise intolerance
- Clinical signs will not be demonstrated in horses that are not exercising

PHYSICAL EXAM FINDINGS On palpation of the throatlatch region, there is atrophy of the cricoarytenoideus dorsalis muscle on the affected side.

ETIOLOGY AND PATHOPHYSIOLOGY

- Idiopathic. The left nerve is thought to be affected more significantly because of its greater length relative to the right RLN.
- Chronic degenerative neuropathy of the RLN resulting in loss of the motor function of the intrinsic muscles of the larynx
- Distal axonopathy with demyelination and proliferation of Schwann cells, endoneurium, and perineurium in the RLN with most of the changes observed distally

DIAGNOSIS

DIFFERENTIAL DIAGNOSIS

- Arytenoid chondropathy
- Vocal fold collapse
- Axial deviation of the aryepiglottic fold
- Pharyngeal collapse

INITIAL DATABASE

- Physical examination: The muscular process of the affected side will be more prominent than the contralateral side as a result of the muscle atrophy caused by the neuropathy.

- Upper airway endoscopy: Incomplete abduction or motion of the affected arytenoid without a change in shape of the arytenoid is indicative of RLN.

ADVANCED OR CONFIRMATORY TESTING

- Treadmill endoscopy: Dynamic collapse of the arytenoid during exercise
- Ultrasound examination: An increased echogenicity of the cricoarytenoid lateralis on the affected side is reflective of RLN.

TREATMENT

THERAPEUTIC GOAL(S)

Stabilization of the arytenoid cartilage corniculate process so that it does not collapse axially during inhalation.

ACUTE GENERAL TREATMENT

- Ventriculocordectomy (unilateral or bilateral)
- Ventriculectomy
- Prosthetic laryngoplasty
- Partial arytenoidectomy
- Neuromuscular pedicle graft or laryngeal reinnervation

POSSIBLE COMPLICATIONS

- With prosthetic laryngoplasty: Chronic coughing, aspiration pneumonia, seroma, abscess, prosthesis failure
- With arytenoidectomy: Dyspnea, dysphagia, chronic coughing, aspiration pneumonia
- With ventriculectomy or ventriculocordectomy: Mucocele, granuloma

RECOMMENDED MONITORING

Follow-up endoscopy

PROGNOSIS AND OUTCOME

- Prognosis depends on the use of the horse and the surgical procedure performed.
- In racehorses, prosthetic laryngoplasty plus ventriculocordectomy is the treatment of choice. Success ranges from 48% to 71%.
- Partial arytenoidectomy, which can be used as a first choice surgery or for failed laryngoplasty has a 61% to 78% prognosis of return to racing. This surgery is primarily used for horses with arytenoid chondritis. Partial ary-

tenoidectomy apparently does not have the same success as laryngoplasty for treatment of RLN.

- Laryngeal reinnervation: Success ranges from 53% to 65%. It is important to note that it can take up to 12 months before a response is observed and the horse can return to training.
- In competition horses (nonracehorses), any of the above procedures can be performed. Ventriculocordectomy has been shown to be effective at reducing respiratory noise and improving performance both experimentally and clinically. This procedure is associated with fewer and less significant complications than the other laryngeal surgeries used to address RLN and may be considered as a primary treatment, particularly for those horses that have mild dysfunction.

PEARLS & CONSIDERATIONS

COMMENTS

- For show, sport, or performance horses, ventriculocordectomy alone may be considered as the primary treatment of choice. This procedure has the least complications and can be effective at reducing respiratory noise.
- Prosthetic laryngoplasty with ventriculocordectomy is the treatment of choice for racehorses because it improves upper airway mechanics and eliminates respiratory noise.

SUGGESTED READING

Davenport-Goodall, CLM, Parente EJ: Disorders of the larynx. In Parente EJ (ed). *The veterinary clinics of North America equine practice: respiratory disease*, Philadelphia, 2003, Saunders Elsevier, pp 159–187.

Dixon PM, McGorum BC, Railton DI, et al: Laryngeal paralysis: a study of 375 cases in a mixed-breed population of horses. *Equine Vet J* 33:452–458, 2001.

Stick JA: Larynx. In Auer JA, Stick JA (eds). *Equine surgery*, ed 3, St Louis, 2006, Elsevier, pp 566–590.

Witte TH, Mohammed H, Radcliffe O, et al: Racing performance after combined prosthetic laryngoplasty and ipsilateral ventriculocordectomy or partial arytenoidectomy: 135 Thoroughbred racehorses competing at less than 2400 m (1997-2007). *Equine Vet J* 41:70-75, 2009.

AUTHOR: JENNIFER A. BROWN

EDITOR: ERIC J. PARENTE

Lead Poisoning

BASIC INFORMATION

DEFINITION

Lead is a heavy metal that has been associated with poisonings around the world for thousands of years. It has been used in a variety of products, including but not limited to paints (before 1977 in the United States), shotgun pellets, car batteries, leaded gasoline and oil, pipes, and roofing material. Environmental contamination may occur near lead mining and smelting facilities; battery factories and battery recycling centers; and on a smaller scale, areas where lead paint has been used and then removed by sand blasting or high-pressure washing, and burn piles.

SYNONYM(S)

Lead toxicosis, plumbism

EPIDEMIOLOGY

SPECIES, AGE, SEX Young animals are at higher risk.
- Young animals absorb lead more efficiently from the gastrointestinal (GI) tract.
- Young animals are more prone to dietary indiscretion.

RISK FACTORS Dietary deficiencies of calcium, iron, zinc, or vitamin D may enhance lead absorption.

CONTAGION AND ZOONOSIS Lead is not an infectious agent and therefore is not contagious or zoonotic. However, if lead toxicosis is diagnosed in a domestic animal, people living in the area should be assessed for possible environmental exposure.

GEOGRAPHY AND SEASONALITY Worldwide distribution

CLINICAL PRESENTATION

DISEASE FORMS/SUBTYPES
- Acute lead poisoning
- Chronic lead poisoning (more common in horses)

HISTORY, CHIEF COMPLAINT
- The horse lives near a battery factory or a lead mine or smelter.
- The barn was built before 1977 (in the United States).
  - Paint may have recently been removed by power washing or sand blasting.
  - There may be evidence of chewing on painted wood.
- Clinical signs of acute lead poisoning
  - Seizures
  - Colic
  - Unexpected death

- Clinical signs of chronic lead poisoning include:
  - Depression
  - Ataxia
  - Weight loss
  - Change in voice, stridor
  - Muscle fasciculations
  - Dysphagia, drooping lips or ears

PHYSICAL EXAM FINDINGS
- Laryngeal paralysis
- Secondary aspiration pneumonia
- Peripheral neuropathy
- Facial nerve deficits
- Emaciation
- Metallic foreign body in GI tract on radiographs

ETIOLOGY AND PATHOPHYSIOLOGY

Lead causes its clinical effects by competing with calcium ions in bones, muscles, and nerves and at binding sites on proteins. Lead may affect zinc-containing enzymes. Lead also binds to sulfhydryl groups on enzymes.

DIAGNOSIS

DIFFERENTIAL DIAGNOSIS
- Rabies
- Other viral encephalitides
- Equine protozoal myeloencephalitis
- Hepatic encephalopathy
- Equine leukoencephalomalacia
- Equine nigropallidal encephalomalacia
- Equine motor neuron disease

INITIAL DATABASE
- Packed cell volume and blood smear
  - Anemia
  - Basophilic stippling of erythrocytes
  - Nucleated red blood cells

ADVANCED OR CONFIRMATORY TESTING
- Elevated blood lead concentrations
- Elevated liver or kidney lead concentrations
- Environmental lead testing to determine the source such as:
  - Paint chips
  - Soil
  - Water
  - Feed

TREATMENT

THERAPEUTIC GOAL(S)
- Provide symptomatic and supportive care.

- Remove lead from the GI tract.
- Remove free lead from the soft tissues (chelation).
- Remove lead from the horse's environment.

ACUTE GENERAL TREATMENT
- Stabilization as necessary
  - Seizure control
  - Treat cerebral edema if needed
- Symptomatic and supportive care
  - Fluid and electrolyte therapy
  - Maintain hydration during chelation therapy
  - Provide nutritional support
  - Treat aspiration pneumonia if needed
  - Provide thiamin (efficacy not known in horses)
- GI decontamination: Cathartics
  - Magnesium sulfate and sodium sulfate may decrease absorption
- Chelation: Calcium ethylenediamine-tetraacetic acid (EDTA)
  - 75 mg/kg diluted and divided over two doses per day for 3 to 5 days; slow IV infusion over 30 minutes
  - Dilute to 6.6% in normal saline or 5% dextrose
  - Follow initial treatment with 2 days of rest and another 5 days of treatment if needed

CHRONIC TREATMENT
Supportive care

DRUG INTERACTIONS
Calcium EDTA may bind nutritional minerals such as zinc, copper, iron, and calcium.

POSSIBLE COMPLICATIONS
- Do not substitute sodium EDTA for calcium EDTA; sodium EDTA will cause acute hypocalcemia.
- EDTA is nephrotoxic.
  - Maintain hydration
  - Monitor renal function
- EDTA may cause anorexia, diarrhea, or depression.
- EDTA may cause pain if injected subcutaneously or intramuscularly.
- EDTA may mobilize lead from the bone, causing an early increase in circulating lead.

RECOMMENDED MONITORING
- Monitor blood lead concentrations at least weekly through the treatment period.
- Monitor renal function if chelating with EDTA.

PROGNOSIS AND OUTCOME

- May be fatal without treatment
- Guarded if clinical signs are severe
- Good if clinical signs are relatively mild

PEARLS & CONSIDERATIONS

COMMENTS

- Toxicity
  - The acutely toxic dose for lead in horses is estimated to be 500 to 700 mg/kg.
  - The chronic toxic dose for lead in horses is estimated to be 1.7 to 7 mg/kg/d for several weeks.
    - 80 ppm lead (dry matter) in the diet is associated with toxicosis.

- Sources of calcium EDTA:
  - Contact human hospital pharmacies to obtain Food and Drug Administration–approved products (expensive).
  - Contact veterinary compounding pharmacies to obtain compounded products (less expensive). Consult a veterinary toxicologist for information on drug sources.

PREVENTION

- Prevent exposure to lead.
  - Have paint tested in old buildings and before moving animals in or remodeling.
  - Contaminated soil may need to be removed.
  - Remove point sources of lead (old batteries and trash such as roofing materials, oil, and gasoline) from pastures and hay fields.

CLIENT EDUCATION

- See Prevention.
- It is important to determine the source of lead to prevent further exposure to animals and humans.
- Blood lead concentrations from children and adults living in the same area of the horses may be needed to determine if they have been exposed.

SUGGESTED READING

Casteel SW: Metal toxicosis in horses. *Vet Clin North Am Equine Pract* 17:517–528, 2001.

Gwaltney-Brandt S: Lead. In Plumlee KH (ed). *Clinical veterinary toxicology.* St Louis, 2004, Mosby Elsevier, pp 204–210.

Thompson LJ: Lead. In Gupta RC (ed). *Veterinary toxicology basic and clinical principles.* New York, 2007, Academic Press, pp 438–441.

AUTHOR: **KARYN BISCHOFF**

EDITOR: **CYNTHIA L. GASKILL**

Lethal White Foal Syndrome

BASIC INFORMATION

DEFINITION

Congenital ileocecocolonic aganglionosis caused by a genetic mutation seen in some all-white overo-overo Paint Horse crosses

SYNONYM(S)

Enteric angiogliosis

EPIDEMIOLOGY

SPECIES, AGE, SEX

- Signs are present shortly after birth.
- Seen in all-white or predominantly white foals of either sex produced by overo-overo Paint Horse crosses when both parents are carriers of the mutated gene

GENETICS AND BREED PREDISPOSITION
Caused by an autosomal recessive mutation seen predominantly in American Paint Horses with an overo coat color pattern, although not all overo horses carry the mutated gene

CLINICAL PRESENTATION

HISTORY, CHIEF COMPLAINT

- Affected foals are usually full-term foals with no trouble standing and nursing after birth.
- Colic and meconium retention are noted shortly after birth, and progressive abdominal distension occurs with nursing.

PHYSICAL EXAM FINDINGS

- Affected foals are all-white or mostly white and have blue or pink eyes.
- With the exception of colic and abdominal distension, no other significant abnormalities are typically identified on general physical examination.
- Digital rectal examination may reveal the absence of meconium in the rectum.

ETIOLOGY AND PATHOPHYSIOLOGY

- Lethal white foal syndrome is caused by an autosomal recessive mutation in the endothelin receptor type B (*ENDRB*) gene.
- The *ENDRB* gene regulates migration and development of both melanocytes and neural crest cells in the developing fetus. When two copies of the mutated allele are present, melanocyte migration essentially fails, resulting in the white coat color, and neural crest migration is altered, resulting in failure of neuronal development in the ileum, cecum, and colon.
- The resulting intestinal aganglionosis results in a dysplastic, amotile hindgut. Signs of colic thus occur shortly after birth because of an inability of the gastric and jejunal contents to be expelled into the hindgut when the foal nurses.

DIAGNOSIS

DIFFERENTIAL DIAGNOSIS

- Meconium impaction
- Atresia coli

INITIAL DATABASE

- Complete blood count and serum biochemistry profile: Usually within normal limits.
- Abdominal imaging: Abdominal radiography and ultrasonography usually reveal mild to moderate gas distension of the small intestine.

ADVANCED OR CONFIRMATORY TESTING

- Histopathologic evaluation of the intestine showing lack of enteric ganglia is necessary for definitive diagnosis. However, presumptive diagnosis is often made based on parentage, coat color, and failure to respond to medical management for meconium impaction.
- If exploratory celiotomy is performed because of a failure to respond to medical therapy for meconium impaction, a presumptive diagnosis can be made based on identification of a small, dystrophic, pale ileum, cecum, and colon with more proximal intestinal distension.

TREATMENT

ACUTE GENERAL TREATMENT

- There is no effective treatment for lethal white foal syndrome.
- However, in suspect cases, medical therapy for meconium impaction (see "Meconium Impaction" in this section) should be initiated because not all white foals born to overo–overo crosses have this syndrome. If medical therapy is ineffective, then exploratory celiotomy or euthanasia is indicated.

PROGNOSIS AND OUTCOME

Grave

PEARLS & CONSIDERATIONS

COMMENTS

Not all foals with lethal white foal syndrome are all white, and not all all-white foals have lethal white foal syndrome.

PREVENTION

Genetic testing for the mutated *ENDRB* gene is available for potential carriers. Paint Horses used for breeding should be tested and crosses between two carriers avoided if possible because there is a 25% chance that a cross between carriers will result in a lethal white foal.

SUGGESTED READING

Santschi EM, Purdy AK, Valberg SJ, et al: Endothelin receptor-B polymorphism associated with lethal white foal syndrome in horses. *Mammalian Genome* 9:306–309, 1998.

Wilkins PA: Disorders of foals: lethal white syndrome. In Reed SM, Bayly WM, Sellon DC (eds). *Equine internal medicine*, ed 2, St Louis, 2001, Saunders Elsevier, pp 1346.

AUTHOR: **KELSEY A. HART**

EDITORS: **TIM MAIR** and **CERI SHERLOCK**

Listeriosis

BASIC INFORMATION

DEFINITION

A disease caused by a gram-positive bacterium that causes encephalitis, septicemia, conjunctivitis, and abortion in animals

SYNONYM(S)

Silage disease

EPIDEMIOLOGY

SPECIES, AGE, SEX

- Central nervous system (CNS) infections: No predilection
- Mares: Abortion
- Foals: Septicemia

RISK FACTORS

- Found in soil, water, vegetation, and silage. In horses, infection is highly associated with feeding of fermented feeds. Shed in feces of carrier animals, including horses. Shed in urine, uterine discharge, aborted fetal tissues, and milk. Abortions tend to occur in the winter months.
- Listeriosis infections are highly associated with horses located on farms where disease has occurred previously.

CONTAGION AND ZOONOSIS

- *Listeria monocytogenes* is considered a zoonotic agent. Clinical listeriosis in humans occurs most often in pregnant women and immunocompromised patients.
- Possible sources for human infections include exposure to contaminated soil and food or to human and animal carriers. Most human epidemics have been traced to food sources of animal origin. Horse meat used for human consumption has been contaminated with *L. monocytogenes*.
- Direct transmission from animals to humans is uncommon.

GEOGRAPHY AND SEASONALITY

- Bacteria can multiply efficiently in cold temperatures from 39° F to 113° F (4°–45° C).
- Grows best at high pH, especially when the pH is above 5.4
- Problem in Icelandic horses fed silage

ASSOCIATED CONDITIONS AND DISORDERS

- Immunodeficiency
- Pregnancy
- Ophthalmic corticosteroids

CLINICAL PRESENTATION

DISEASE FORMS/SUBTYPES

- Encephalitis
- Septicemia
- Keratitis and ophthalmitis
- Abortion

HISTORY, CHIEF COMPLAINT

- Encephalitis: Sudden onset of change in mentation or sudden death
- Septicemia: Weakness and severe depression
- Keratitis and ophthalmitis: Bilateral or unilateral blepharospasm
- Abortion: Late gestation in winter months

PHYSICAL EXAM FINDINGS

- Encephalitis: Characterized as a meningoencephalitis with the pathology in horses demonstrating a granulomatous encephalitis with microabscessation on histopathology. Animals may exhibit normal mentation with circling similar to ewes; however, severe mental depression is the most frequent presentation. Animals become unresponsive to external stimuli and usually die within 3 to 5 days.
- In Icelandic horses, many are febrile and inappetent, with diffuse diarrhea and death.
- Septicemia: Clinical signs include depression, anorexia, fever, diarrhea, and abdominal pain. Weakness, seizures, ataxia, jaundice, and respiratory distress have been reported as well.
- Conjunctivitis and keratitis: Range from purulent conjunctivitis to deep ulcerative keratitis and ophthalmitis
- Abortion: Sudden spontaneous abortion about 48 to 72 hours after infection in a dam. Fetuses are infected late in gestation and acquire septicemia. The fetus will be fairly fresh and is either dead at expulsion or dies shortly thereafter. Dams are usually normal and do not exhibit problems after abortion.

ETIOLOGY AND PATHOPHYSIOLOGY

- *L. monocytogenes* infection
- The organism usually enters through ingestion.
- Oral and pharyngeal abrasion allows infection.
- For encephalitis, bacteria likely travel transaxonally as they do in other species. In ewes, the trigeminal (V) and hypoglossal (XII) cranial nerves are considered the most likely routes for CNS invasion.

- Replication in the pons and medulla occurs.
- If bloodstream infection occurs, the gravid uterus is a site of localization.
- Direct infection of monocytes and macrophages occurs, and the organism evades the immune system and initiates an inflammatory cascade that is consistent with septic shock and leads to tissue necrosis.

DIAGNOSIS

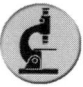

DIFFERENTIAL DIAGNOSIS

- Encephalitis
  - Rabies
  - Flavivirus encephalitis: West Nile virus, Japanese encephalitis virus, Kunjin virus
  - Alphavirus encephalitis: Eastern, Western, and Venezuelan equine encephalitis virus
  - Hepatoencephalopathy
  - Theiler's disease
  - *Halicephalobus gingivalis* infection
- Septicemia
  - Gram-negative sepsis in foals
  - Neonatal asphyxia
  - Equine herpesvirus-1 (EHV-1) Infection
- Abortion
  - Noninfectious late-term causes of abortion
  - EHV-1
  - Nocardioform abortion
  - *Neorickettsia risticii* infection
  - Ascending bacterial infections (*Streptococcus equi* subsp. *zooepidemicus* and *Actinobacillus equuli* most common)

INITIAL DATABASE

- Complete blood count: Leukopenia or leukocytosis consistent with bacterial infection
- Hyperfibrinogenemia
- Serum biochemical analysis: Elevated liver enzymes
- Cytologic examination of a direct smear from infected tissue or body fluids, corneal scrapings, or aborted tissue for the presence of gram-positive rods

ADVANCED OR CONFIRMATORY TESTING

- Microbiologic culture of feces, blood or affected organs, including the liver, spleen, and brain.
- Culture of feedstuffs, especially silage
- Polymerase chain reaction has also been described but has not been used in horses.
- Genotyping of isolates to confirm feed contamination with fecal isolates of horses has been performed.
- At necropsy, histopathology, culture, and immunohistochemistry are needed to confirm a diagnosis. It is difficult to culture organisms from the brain in neural listeriosis, so the laboratory must do cold enrichment.

TREATMENT

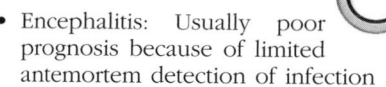

THERAPEUTIC GOAL(S)

Correct and timely identification to allow early intervention

ACUTE GENERAL TREATMENT

- *L. monocytogenes* is susceptible to many antibiotics, including penicillin. Very large loading dosages for systemic signs are recommended.
- However, isolates from a corneal scraping and from blood cultures from three foals were all resistant to ceftiofur.

PROGNOSIS AND OUTCOME

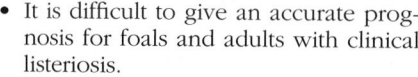

- Encephalitis: Usually poor prognosis because of limited antemortem detection of infection
- It is difficult to give an accurate prognosis for foals and adults with clinical listeriosis.
- Listerial keratitis has resolved after topical antibiotic therapy.

SUGGESTED READING

Gudmundsdottir KB, Svansson V, Aalbaek B, et al: *Listeria monocytogenes* in horses from Iceland. *Vet Rec* 155:456, 2004.
Hines MT: Listeriosis. Equine influenza infection. In Sellon DC, Long MT (eds). *Equine infectious diseases*, St Louis, 1997, Elsevier, pp 276–277.

AUTHOR: **MAUREEN T. LONG**

EDITORS: **DEBRA C. SELLON** and **MAUREEN T. LONG**

Liver: Parasitic Conditions

BASIC INFORMATION

DEFINITION

Parascaris equorum, Strongylus edentates, Strongylus equinus, and occasionally *Strongylus vulgaris* migrate through the liver during larval development; however, these parasites cause little permanent liver damage. *Fasciola* spp. and *Echinococcus equinus* may affect the liver more directly, although clinical disease with either is rare.

SYNONYM(S)

- Liver flukes
- Hydatid cysts

EPIDEMIOLOGY

SPECIES, AGE, SEX

- *P. equorum* is usually a problem in younger animals because adults develop effective immunity.
- *Strongylus* spp. may affect animals of any age.
- *Fasciola hepatica* is the most common liver fluke infecting large animals and may affect Equids of all ages.
- *E. equinus* infections in horses tend to involve older animals.

RISK FACTORS
Uncontrolled home slaughter and offal disposal are probably the main factors associated with persistence of *Echinococcus* infection.

CONTAGION AND ZOONOSIS
Although cystic echinococcosis is an important public health disease in many parts of the world, *E. equinus* does not appear to be infective to humans.

GEOGRAPHY AND SEASONALITY

- Fascioliasis in horses has been reported all over the world, and the disease may be more common in areas with high infection rates in cattle and sheep.
- The life cycle of the liver fluke depends on the availability of water and the presence of appropriate *Lymnaeid* snail hosts in grazing areas. Temperatures above 50° F (10° C) are necessary for completion of the life cycle.
- Most cases of equine echinococcosis in North America have occurred in animals imported from the United Kingdom.

CLINICAL PRESENTATION

HISTORY, CHIEF COMPLAINT

- *S. edentates, S. equinus,* and *P. equorum* infestations are most commonly characterized by nonspecific signs of weight loss or poor growth, rough hair coat, and poor performance. No clinical signs are associated with migration of these parasites through the liver.
- Vague signs of poor performance, loss of condition, and diarrhea have been described in horses living in areas with high *F. hepatica* infection rates in cattle.
- *E. equinus* infection is usually asymptomatic. When clinical signs do appear, they are usually related to pressure of the cyst on adjacent organs.

PHYSICAL EXAM FINDINGS In many cases, findings on physical examination are nonspecific, as described above. Few, if any, findings are referable to hepatic involvement.

ETIOLOGY AND PATHOPHYSIOLOGY

- Disease caused by *S. edentates, S. equinus,* or *P. equorum* infection is primarily attributable to the gastrointestinal (GI) effects of these parasites rather than direct effects on the liver.
- In other species, infection with *F. hepatica* may cause acute or chronic disease.
- Acute disease occurs after migration of immature flukes through the hepatic parenchyma.
- Chronic disease is caused by the effects of mature parasites within the bile ducts.
- Cystic echinococcosis (hydatid disease) in horses is caused by *E. equinus.*
- The life cycle is indirect; horses are intermediate hosts, and the carnivorous definitive host is usually canid.
- In the intermediate host, ingested larvae penetrate the intestinal wall and form hydatid cysts in various organs, most often in the liver and occasionally the lungs.
- Cystic echinococcosis is often an incidental finding in horses; if clinical signs occur, they are usually caused by pressure on adjacent organs.

DIAGNOSIS

DIFFERENTIAL DIAGNOSIS

- Few, if any, clinical signs are typically related to liver disease in these parasitic infections.
- Differential diagnoses are likely to include diseases causing weight loss, poor growth rates, and poor performance.

INITIAL DATABASE

- Complete blood count: Mild anemia and leukocytosis with or without eosinophilia
- Fibrinogen concentration: Normal to increased
- Serum or plasma biochemistry
  - Hypoalbuminemia, β-globulinemia, and increased immunoglobulin G(T) concentrations may be present.
  - There are typically no changes in the serum biochemistry related to liver dysfunction.

ADVANCED OR CONFIRMATORY TESTING

- Patent parasitic infections with nematodes may be detected by fecal examination using one of several qualitative or quantitative concentration techniques.
- Eggs are typically shed intermittently in animals with liver fluke infections.
- Hydatid cysts may be identified ultrasonographically in some cases.

TREATMENT

THERAPEUTIC GOAL(S)

- Hepatic migration of the GI nematodes through the liver is not accompanied by clinical signs, and there is no evidence of long-term injury to the liver. Therefore specific treatment is not indicated.
- Triclabendazole (12 mg/kg) has been used with apparent efficacy to control *F. hepatica* infection in horses (and donkeys). This is an off-license use of this anthelmintic, but it appears to be safe.
- Treatments for human cystic echinococcosis have included surgery and chemotherapy with benzimidazole compounds. More recently, percutaneous cyst puncture followed by aspiration injection of chemicals, and re-aspiration has been used. None of these therapies have been described in horses.

ACUTE GENERAL TREATMENT

Specific acute treatment is generally not required for patients with these conditions.

PROGNOSIS AND OUTCOME

These conditions result in little to no long-term effects on liver function.

PEARLS & CONSIDERATIONS

- Parasitic migration through the liver has little or no long-term effect on the liver because of its tremendous ability to regenerate.
- Horses appear to have pronounced resistance to establishment of infectious *Fasciola* spp., and the incidence of clinical disease in this species is very low compared with that of sheep, goats, and cattle.
- Hydatid cysts in horses are usually an incidental finding and do not appear to pose a human health threat.

SUGGESTED READING

Owen JM: Liver fluke infection in horses and ponies. *Equine Vet J* 9:29, 1977.
Varcasia A, Garippa G, Pipia AP, et al: Cystic echinococcosis in equids in Italy. *Parasitol Res* 102:815–818, 2008.

AUTHOR: BRETT TENNENT-BROWN

EDITOR: MICHELLE HENRY BARTON

Locoweed Toxicosis

BASIC INFORMATION

DEFINITION

- Locoweeds (*Astragalus* and *Oxytropis* species) are native plants of North America that can cause a variety of systemic effects, especially on the central nervous system (CNS) and reproductive system. They can also affect the heart, intestinal system, and lymphocytes of horses and other livestock species.
- In addition, some locoweed species are selenium accumulators.

SYNONYM(S)

Locoism, a term derived from the Spanish word *loco,* meaning "crazy," describes the abnormal neurologic signs in horses poisoned by locoweeds (milk vetches) of the *Astragalus* and *Oxytropis* species.

EPIDEMIOLOGY

SPECIES, AGE, SEX Horses, livestock, and wild ruminants are susceptible. Nursing young are most susceptible because the toxic alkaloid in locoweeds is passed through the milk.

RISK FACTORS

- Toxic at all growth stages, locoweeds are most palatable to horses in the spring when the plants are in flower. Some toxicity is retained in the dried plants.
- Although not truly addictive, horses find locoweeds palatable and may seek them out in preference to other forages, especially when the plants are in flower.

GEOGRAPHY AND SEASONALITY

- More than 350 native species of locoweeds belong to the *Astragalus* and *Oxytropis* genera in North America. Relatively few species are important toxicologically.
- Geographically, the toxic species of locoweed are concentrated in the intermountain and southwestern United States. Locoweeds are short-lived perennial legumes that reproduce from seeds that can remain viable in the soil for more than 50 years (Figures 1 and 2).

CLINICAL PRESENTATION

DISEASE FORMS/SUBTYPES Depending on the species of *Astragalus* and *Oxytropis*, three distinct toxins may be present: swainsonine, nitrotoxins, or selenium.

HISTORY, CHIEF COMPLAINT Changes in temperament, behavior, incoordination, and weight loss are typical presenting signs

ETIOLOGY AND PATHOPHYSIOLOGY

- Locoism results from the consumption of locoweeds infected with an endophyte (*Embellisia* spp.) that produces the indolizidine alkaloid swainsonine.
  - Swainsonine inhibits α-mannosidase, an enzyme critical in the metabolism of oligosaccharides.
  - Complex sugars accumulate in cells with resulting cellular dysfunction and death.
  - Locoism is a lysosomal storage disease affecting the CNS and many other cells.
  - Impaired lymphocyte function may cause decreased immune response.
  - Asymptomatic mares in the first trimester of pregnancy may produce foals with arthrogryposis.
  - Stallions grazing locoweed may develop temporary infertility similar to the sperm maturation defects seen in rams and bulls grazing locoweed.
  - Horses can be experimentally poisoned with as little as 1 lb/d of dried locoweed for 75 to 85 days.
  - The half-life of swainsonine in the body is 15 to 20 hours.
- Some species of *Astragalus* (milk vetches) contain nitrotoxins.
  - Ruminants are most commonly affected.
  - Nitrotoxins are hydrolyzed in the rumen to toxic 3-nitropropanol and 3-nitropropionic acid.
  - Nitrotoxins induce methemoglobinemia and neuropathy, leading to depression, weakness, ataxia, and death. Horses are rarely affected under natural conditions but are susceptible to the toxins.
- Some species of locoweed only grow in selenium-rich soils and are known as "selenium indicator" species. Their presence in the rangeland indicates selenium soils; therefore other forages and grasses will likely contain selenium that can cause chronic selenium poisoning in horses and other animals grazing the area (see "Selenium Toxicosis" in this section).

DIAGNOSIS

DIFFERENTIAL DIAGNOSIS

- Encephalitis: Rabies, West Nile virus, Eastern and Western equine encephalitis virus, equine Venezuelan encephalitis
- Equine herpesvirus
- Sage poisoning
- Pyrrolizidine alkaloid toxicity
- Bracken fern poisoning
- Chronic weight loss from malnutrition, poor teeth, parasites
- Other causes of arthrogryposis (eg, sorghum/sudan grass toxicosis, genetic causes)

INITIAL DATABASE

- Serum protein: Decreased
- Triiodothyronine (T3) and thyroxine (T4) levels: Decreased
- Aspartate aminotransferase: Elevated
- Alkaline phosphatase: Elevated
- Lactate dehydrogenase: Elevated
- Peripheral lymphocytes: Vacuolated cytoplasm in early toxicity

ADVANCED OR CONFIRMATORY TESTING

- Serum swainsonine levels: Obtain serum sample within 2 days of ingestion of locoweeds.
- Serum α-mannosidase activity: Decreased within 24 hours of eating a toxic dose of locoweed. Levels return to normal 6 days after locoweed consumption is stopped.

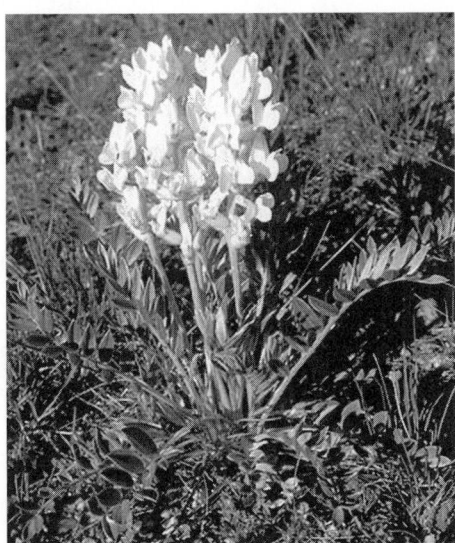

FIGURE 1 White locoweed (*Oxytropis sericea*).

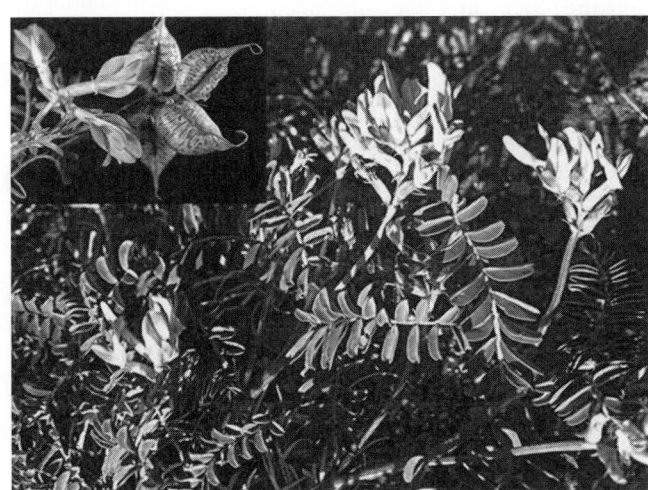

FIGURE 2 Spotted or blue locoweed (*Astragalus lentiginosus*).

- Histopathology: Cytoplasmic vacuoles in brain Purkinje cells, thyroid, lymphoid tissue, hepatocytes, renal tubules, placenta, and intestine after clinical signs are evident.

TREATMENT

THERAPEUTIC GOAL(S)

There is no specific treatment for locoism. Horses will show improvement over time but may never fully recover, especially from residual neurologic deficits.

ACUTE GENERAL TREATMENT

- Remove all locoweed from the animal's diet.
- Provide good-quality hay and concentrate ration.

POSSIBLE COMPLICATIONS

Horses will have compromised lymphocytes while eating locoweeds, which may affect their response to vaccines, and they may be prone to other infectious diseases.

PROGNOSIS AND OUTCOME

- Horses have a guarded to poor prognosis depending on the severity and chronicity of signs.
- Residual neurologic deficits may render horses unsafe to ride.

PEARLS & CONSIDERATIONS

COMMENTS

Locoweed poisoning is a long-standing problem in the western United States and should always be considered in the differential diagnosis of neurologic disease and weight loss in horses.

PREVENTION

- Recognition of locoweeds in a pasture facilitates pasture management to reduce grazing locoweeds.
- Remove horses when locoweed is blooming.

- Avoid overgrazing pasture.
- Selectively use herbicides.

CLIENT EDUCATION

Take inventory of plants in native pasture and rangeland.

SUGGESTED READING

Braun K, Romero J, Liddell C, et al: Production of swainsonine by fungal endophytes of locoweed. *Mycol Res* 107:980–988, 2003.

Knight AP: *Guide to poisonous plants.* Available at http://southcampus.colostate.edu/poisonous_plants.

Stegelmeier BL, James LF, Panter KE, et al: The pathogenesis and toxicokinetics of white locoweed (*Astragalus* and *Oxytropis* spp.) poisoning in livestock. *J Nat Toxins* 8:35–45, 1999.

Stegelmeier BL, James LF, Panter KE, et al: Serum swainsonine concentration and alpha-mannosidase activity in sheep and cattle ingesting *Oxytropis sericea* and *Astragalus lentiginosus* (locoweeds). *Am J Vet Res* 56:149–154, 1995.

AUTHOR: **ANTHONY P. KNIGHT**

EDITOR: **CYNTHIA L. GASKILL**

Lupus Complex

BASIC INFORMATION

DEFINITION

A multisystemic disease caused by the production of multiple autoantibodies, especially those directed against nucleic acids. It usually involves the skin and at least one other organ.

SYNONYM(S)

Systemic lupus erythematosus, SLE

EPIDEMIOLOGY

SPECIES, AGE, SEX Sporadic in onset but rare

CLINICAL PRESENTATION

DISEASE FORMS/SUBTYPES

- Generally presents as a generalized skin disease with alopecia, dermal ulceration, and crusting
- Antiglobulin-positive anemia
- Glomerulonephritis
- Nonseptic, nonerosive synovitis
- Lymphadenopathy

HISTORY, CHIEF COMPLAINT

- Extensive skin lesions
- Nonspecific lethargy and weakness

ETIOLOGY AND PATHOPHYSIOLOGY

- This is a complex syndrome that results from major dysregulation of the B-cell system.

- It leads to the production of multiple autoantibodies directed against nuclear, cytoplasmic, and cell membrane antigens.
- The pathognomonic antibodies are those directed against nucleic acids.

DIAGNOSIS

The diagnosis of lupus is difficult. As a syndrome, its diagnosis cannot be based on a single diagnostic test but rather on a collection of different lesions and exclusion of other causes

DIFFERENTIAL DIAGNOSIS

- Bacterial or fungal skin diseases
- Pemphigus complex

INITIAL DATABASE

- Complete blood count, including differential leukocyte count and platelet count
- Serum biochemical profile. Abnormalities may reflect chronic inflammation and evidence of glomerulonephritis such as azotemia and hypogammaglobulinemia
- Urinalysis showing possible proteinuria
- Skin cultures ruling out infectious cause

- Skin biopsy may reveal characteristic histologic pattern with inflammatory infiltrates at the dermal/epidermal junction. Also basement membrane degeneration typical of lupus
- If arthritis/synovitis is present, radiographs may show nonerosive joint swelling
- Serum antinuclear antibody titer: Sensitivity and specificity are unclear
- False-positive results occur in other species, in many cases because of drug use
- Variable laboratory standardization
- Lupus erythematosus cell tests are equivocal and rarely useful.

ADVANCED OR CONFIRMATORY TESTING

- Coombs test and rheumatoid factor: Usually negative
- Immunofluorescence testing of the skin biopsy may show the skin basement membrane contains immunoglobulin deposits (a lupus band).

TREATMENT

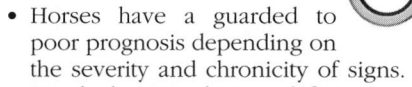

THERAPEUTIC GOAL(S)

Suppress the animal's excessive immune function so that damage to the skin, kidneys, and other organs is reversed.

ACUTE GENERAL TREATMENT

- Immunosuppressive treatment with steroids and immunosuppressive drugs has generally been unsuccessful, but experience is limited.
- Dexamethasone sodium phosphate solution (0.08 mg/kg PO q24h): After a response has been obtained, progressively decrease the dose to 0.02 mg/kg/d.
- Alternatively, prednisolone (1 mg/kg PO q24h)
- Azathioprine (3 mg/kg PO q24h) may be as effective as dexamethasone. After 30 days, half the daily dose for another 30 days.

CHRONIC TREATMENT

Dexamethasone or prednisolone until resolution of signs (2 weeks); then slow reduction of dose. Lifelong treatment may be required.

POSSIBLE COMPLICATIONS

- Secondary infections after immunosuppression
- Progressive renal damage
- Laminitis secondary to steroid treatment

PROGNOSIS AND OUTCOME

Limited experience suggests that the prognosis is poor.

PEARLS & CONSIDERATIONS

- The diagnosis of lupus is difficult and largely based on excluding other possibilities.
- Biopsy normal skin adjacent to ulcerated areas.

SUGGESTED READING

Gershwin LJ: Antinuclear antibodies in domestic animals. *Ann N Y Acad Sci* 1050:364–370, 2005.

Geor RJ, Clark EG, Haines DM, et al: Systemic lupus erythematosus in a filly. *J Am Vet Med Assoc* 197:1489–1492, 2005.

AUTHOR & EDITOR: **IAN TIZARD**

Lyme Disease

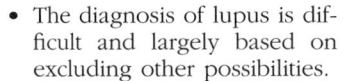

BASIC INFORMATION

DEFINITION

Infection with a tickborne, gram-negative helical spirochete, *Borrelia burgdorferi*, which causes disease resulting in equivocal signs of lameness or behavioral changes

SYNONYM(S)

Borreliosis

EPIDEMIOLOGY

- No known breed, age, or sex predilection
- Seroprevalence ranges from less than 1% to 68% in endemic regions.
- Highest seroprevalence in mid-Atlantic and northeastern states, Minnesota, and Wisconsin (30%–40% of ticks are infected with *B. burgdorferi*)
- Rare positive horses in the Rocky Mountain states, North and South Dakota, and Nebraska (only 1%–3% of tick vector population are infected with *B. burgdorferi*)
- Occurs primarily in the spring, summer, and fall, with peak incidence in June and July in most endemic climates
- Not directly zoonotic; unknown if horses serve as source of infection for ticks

CLINICAL PRESENTATION

- History of tick exposure or residing in a Lyme disease endemic area
- Nonspecific clinical signs
- Vague signs of lameness or stiffness (generally in more than one limb)
- Lethargy, depression, decreased performance
- May observe muscle pain, hyperesthesia, or behavioral changes
- Polysynovitis usually with minimal joint effusion
- Low-grade fever
- Distal limb edema
- Rare neurologic signs
- Rarely, anterior uveitis
- Possible muscle wasting and pain over thoracolumbar area with severe cases

ETIOLOGY AND PATHOPHYSIOLOGY

- The spirochete *B. burgdorferi* is the etiologic agent of Lyme disease.
- Prolonged attachment and feeding (>24 hours) of infected adult *Ixodes* spp. ticks transmits the organism.
- Invades the connective tissues, muscle, skin, and nerves and blood vessels near synovial membranes
- A lymphocytic plasmocytic reaction in tissue occurs in association with the organism.
- Unknown whether polysynovitis is the result of an immune-mediated reaction (immune complex deposition) or infection of the joint

DIAGNOSIS

DIFFERENTIAL DIAGNOSIS

- Arthritis: Trauma, osteoarthritis, other immune-mediated arthritis
- Neurologic signs: Equine herpes virus-1, equine protozoal encephalomyelitis, rabies, cervical vertebral malformation, cauda equine syndrome, West Nile virus, Eastern or Western equine encephalitis
- Distal limb edema: Purpura hemorrhagica, equine viral arteritis, equine infectious anemia, cellulitis, hypoproteinemia, *Anaplasma phagocytophilum* infection, or normal "stocking up"

INITIAL DATABASE

- Antemortem diagnosis is generally presumptive.
- Low-grade fever
- Complete blood count and serum chemistries: No significant findings
- Radiography to help rule out other causes of lameness
- Synovial fluid cytology to rule out sepsis; may have neutrophilic inflammation with Lyme disease
- Cannot visualize the pathognomonic erythema migrans rash that is diagnostic in humans

ADVANCED OR CONFIRMATORY TESTING

- Enzyme-linked immunosorbent assay (ELISA), C6 test, indirect fluorescent antibody test, and Western Blot available for serology
- Serology confirms exposure; ELISA titers above 110 U may provide stronger support for infection
- Histopathology: Lymphocytic plasmacytic infiltrate
- May perform polymerase chain reaction or immunohistochemistry on affected tissues to detect the organism

TREATMENT

THERAPEUTIC GOAL(S)
- Eradicate organisms from the host
- Treat symptomatically
- Often treated presumptively

ACUTE GENERAL TREATMENT
- Generally respond to treatment within 2 to 4 days
- Antimicrobial therapy: IV oxytetracycline (thought to be most effective) or PO doxycycline are usually recommended; may add metronidazole for possible cyst forms
- May also treat with enrofloxacin, ceftiofur, or procaine penicillin G
- Judicious nonsteroidal antiinflammatory therapy
- Cold hosing and leg wraps for distal limb swelling and polysynovitis
- Atropine may be required for uveitis
- Intraarticular corticosteroid administration is controversial

CHRONIC TREATMENT
Long-term treatment with antimicrobials is required (>1 month).

POSSIBLE COMPLICATIONS
- Chronic arthritis
- Laminitis
- Damage to the central nervous system
- Possible recurrent uveitis

PROGNOSIS AND OUTCOME

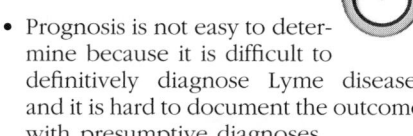

- Prognosis is not easy to determine because it is difficult to definitively diagnose Lyme disease, and it is hard to document the outcome with presumptive diagnoses.
- In other species, the prognosis is fair for survival, but in horses, it is likely to be guarded for return to athletic function.

PEARLS & CONSIDERATIONS

COMMENTS
- Horses may be an important sentinel animal for risk of Lyme disease for humans in a particular area.
- Infection may occur in conjunction with *Anaplasma phagocytophilum* because many ticks are co-infected with both organisms. This may contribute to the observed clinical signs and affect evaluation of response to treatment because *A. phagocytophi-*

lum is very susceptible to tetracyclines.
- Reliable experimental reproduction of Lyme disease in horses has proven to be difficult, limiting the success of Lyme disease research and characterization.

PREVENTION
- Prevent tick exposure or prolonged attachment. Canine tick sprays may be effective for tick repellent.
- Regular grooming and removal of attached ticks.
- Pursue appropriate antimicrobial treatment after exposure to *Ixodes* ticks.
- No vaccine is currently available.

SUGGESTED READING
Butler CM, Houwers DJ, Jongejan F, et al: *Borrelia burgdorferi* infections with special reference to horses. A review. Vet Q 27:146–156, 2005.
Divers TJ: Lyme disease. In Sellon DC, Long MT (eds) *Equine infectious diseases*, St Louis, 2008, Saunders Elsevier, pp 310–312.
Reed SM, Toribio R: Lyme disease in horses. In Reed SM, Bayly WM, Sellon DC, et al: *Equine internal medicine*, ed 3, St Louis, 2010, Saunders Elsevier, pp 644–646.

AUTHOR: SIDDRA HINES

EDITORS: **DEBRA C. SELLON** and **MAUREEN T. LONG**

Lymphangitis, Epizootic

BASIC INFORMATION

DEFINITION
Chronic ulcerative lymphangitis caused by infection with the fungus *Histoplasma capsulatum* var. *farciminosum*.

EPIDEMIOLOGY
SPECIES, AGE, SEX Horses, donkeys, and mules are susceptible.
CONTAGION AND ZOONOSIS Considered both contagious and zoonotic
GEOGRAPHY AND SEASONALITY
- Most common in Egypt, India, North Africa, the Middle East, southern Asia, southern Europe, and areas of Russia
- Endemic in countries that border the Mediterranean

CLINICAL PRESENTATION
DISEASE FORMS/SUBTYPES
- Cutaneous
- Ocular
- Respiratory

HISTORY, CHIEF COMPLAINT Ulcerative nodules with exudate and cording
PHYSICAL EXAM FINDINGS
- Cutaneous disease: Granulomatous, often ulcerated, masses in chains following lymphatic vessels. Lesions eventually heal and scar as others form. The forelimbs, neck, and head are most common sites.
- Ocular: Conjunctivitis; nodular enlargements over facial lymphatics and nasolacrimal lesions. Serous ocular discharge and swelling of the eyelids are observed with nodules on the conjunctiva or nictitans.
- Respiratory: Yellowish papules or nodules in the upper respiratory tract often near the external nares. Lesions may ulcerate and bleed. Pulmonary granulomata may cause fatal disease.
- Disseminated disease: Infrequent.
ETIOLOGY AND PATHOPHYSIOLOGY
- Caused by a dimorphic fungal organism.
- Direct inoculation of fungus through abraded skin or mucous membranes is

suspected as the primary mode of transmission.
- Fomites such as harness, mangers, water buckets, and flies may contribute to transmission.
- May be transmitted from stallions to mares during breeding.
- Lower respiratory tract disease may result from inhalation of organisms in dust.

DIAGNOSIS

DIFFERENTIAL DIAGNOSIS
- Ulcerative lymphangitis: *Corynebacterium pseudotuberculosis*
- Glanders: *Burkholderia mallei*
- Epizootic lymphangitis: *H. capsulatum* var. *farciminosum*

INITIAL DATABASE
Evidence of chronic infection and inflammation

ADVANCED OR CONFIRMATORY TESTING

- Culture of organism from body fluids or tissues is considered the gold standard for diagnosis.
- Cytologic observation of yeast forms in tissue exudates
- Serology: Tube agglutination and passive hemagglutination tests are suggestive of disease if the results are positive but may reflect only past exposure or asymptomatic infection.
- Intradermal testing with soluble antigen may have low specificity.

TREATMENT

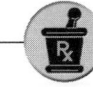

THERAPEUTIC GOAL(S)

Reportable disease in many countries with policy of slaughter for eradication

ACUTE GENERAL TREATMENT

In endemic areas where treatment is allowed, oral and IV iodide or amphotericin B may be used. Other antifungals may also be effective.

PROGNOSIS AND OUTCOME

Reportable disease with mandatory slaughter in many countries

PEARLS & CONSIDERATIONS

Mortality from cutaneous disease is uncommon, but an inability to work because of painful nodules can lead to significant economic loss.

SUGGESTED READING

Kohn C: Miscellaneous fungal infections. In Sellon DC, Long MT (eds). *Equine infectious diseases*, St Louis, 2007, Elsevier, pp 431–445.

AUTHOR: **DEBRA C. SELLON**

EDITORS: **DEBRA C. SELLON** and **MAUREEN T. LONG**

Lymphoma, Equine

BASIC INFORMATION

DEFINITION

Neoplasia of lymphoid origin

SYNONYM(S)

Lymphosarcoma; malignant lymphoma (*lymphoma* is currently the preferred term)

EPIDEMIOLOGY

SPECIES, AGE, SEX
- Most common form of hematopoietic neoplasia in horses
- The prevalence at postmortem examination is 2% to 5%.
- Most common in horses age 5 to 10 years but can occur in any age, including neonates

GENETICS AND BREED PREDISPOSITION Genetic causes may exist because rare reports exist of aborted feti affected by lymphoma.

ASSOCIATED CONDITIONS AND DISORDERS Paraneoplastic syndromes that have been reported include hypercalcemia, immune-mediated hemolysis, immune-mediated thrombocytopenia, hypereosinophilia, and polycythemia. A case of generalized pruritus and alopecia was also reported in a horse with lymphoma.

CLINICAL PRESENTATION

DISEASE FORMS/SUBTYPES Occurs in four anatomic forms based on the major site of tumor involvement (overlap between forms is common).
- Generalized: Regional lymph nodes are often affected with involvement of the thoracic and abdominal organs. Solitary tumors in various tissues also occur but less commonly. Clinical signs and diagnostic findings depend on the affected tissues. Chronic disease with often acute, severe terminal progression of clinical signs. Most commonly affects horses 5 to 10 years of age, but all ages are at risk.
- Alimentary: Most common in young horses ages 2 to 5 years. Presenting complaints include weight loss, ill thrift, intermittent colic, fever, and chronic diarrhea. Diagnosis can be made by cytologic analysis of peritoneal fluid in 35% to 50% of cases.
- Mediastinal: May cause dyspnea, cough, recurrent pleural effusion. Most commonly affects horses 5 to 10 years of age.
- Cutaneous: Generalized cutaneous or subcutaneous nodules with acute or chronic onset or progression. Lesions may be affected by hormone alterations (eg, pregnancy, estrous).

HISTORY, CHIEF COMPLAINT

- Progressive disease with acute onset of clinical signs related to dysfunction of the affected organs.
- Chronic weight loss is a common presenting complaint.
- Signs are generally nonspecific.

PHYSICAL EXAM FINDINGS

Poor body condition score, peripheral lymphadenomegaly, ventral edema; other findings consistent with the affected organ system

ETIOLOGY AND PATHOPHYSIOLOGY

- Lymphoma in horses is clinically and pathologically quite variable.
- Literature reports do not classify whether T- or B-cell tumors predominate.

DIAGNOSIS

DIFFERENTIAL DIAGNOSIS

- Generalized form: Chronic systemic infections, such as internal abscessation or bacterial pneumonia; other forms of metastatic neoplasia (adenocarcinoma, carcinoma)
- Alimentary form: Gastrointestinal parasites, inflammatory bowel disease, chronic bacterial enterocolitis
- Mediastinal form: Bacterial pneumonia or pulmonary abscessation, pleuropneumonia, metastasis of other forms of neoplasia (adenocarcinoma, carcinoma)
- Cutaneous form: Folliculitis, furunculosis, dermatophytosis, nodular necrobiosis, urticaria, amyloidosis

INITIAL DATABASE

- Perform complete blood count (CBC), serum chemistry profile, and urinalysis.
- Laboratory findings are variable. CBC often indicates nonspecific, chronic, inflammatory disease (neutrophilic leukocytosis, anemia, hyperfibrinogenemia, hyperglobulinemia). Lymphocyte count is often normal or low, but atypical or neoplastic cells may be observed on smear.

- Lymphocytic leukemia is rare but is typified by a marked lymphocytosis.
- Hypercalcemia is present in some cases. Decreased serum concentrations of immunoglobulin M have been reported but are not consistent.
- If thoracic or abdominal involvement is suspected, thoracic radiographs or ultrasonography and abdominal ultrasonography often allow visualization of the tumor and facilitate sample collection for cytology or histopathology.

ADVANCED OR CONFIRMATORY TESTING

- Biopsy of enlarged lymph node or abnormal tissue. Fine-needle aspirate of fluid or tissue can also be diagnostic if biopsy is not possible.
- Analysis of pleural or peritoneal fluid may reveal the presence of neoplastic cells in some cases.
- Removal of subcutaneous nodules for analysis is diagnostic for cutaneous form.
- Immunophenotyping (flow cytometry, immunohistochemistry) to confirm T- or B-cell origin.

TREATMENT

THERAPEUTIC GOALS

- Chemotherapy protocols have been used with reported success in the form of case reports only.
- The goal of therapy is complete remission or cessation of clinical signs while maintaining quality of life.

ACUTE GENERAL TREATMENT

- As with all chemotherapeutic agents, appropriate handling is essential for animal, client, and veterinarian safety. Consultation with or referral to a veterinary oncologist or internist is recommended.
- Chemotherapy regimens include a combination of cytotoxic and immunosuppressive drugs. Doses have been extrapolated from humans and small animals because no pharmacokinetic data have been published. The dosages provided below were taken from case reports and proceedings and were judged safe by the authors.
  - Thoracic lymphoma was treated in one mare with cytosine arabinoside (170 mg/m^2 IM twice at a 2-week interval), alternating with cyclophosphamide (142 mg/m^2 IV twice at a 2-week interval), and prednisolone (86 mg/m^2 PO) every 48 hours for the remainder of the horse's life. The horse remained in remission 8 months after therapy.
  - A protocol has been used with variable success that includes cytosine arabinoside ($200-300 \text{ mg/m}^2$ SC or IM once every 1–2 weeks), alternating with chlorambucil (20 mg/m^2 PO every 2 weeks), and prednisolone ($0.5-1.0 \text{ mg/lb}$ PO) q48h. Cyclophosphamide (200 mg/m^2 IV) every 2 to 3 weeks can be substituted for the oral chlorambucil. If the patient responds, remission is expected in 2 to 4 weeks. May add vincristine (0.5 mg/m^2 IV) once weekly if no response is seen.
  - Cytosine arabinoside and cyclophosphamide (dosages above) can also be used as single agents. L-asparaginase ($10,000-40,000 \text{ IU/m}^2$ IM) can also be used every 2 to 3 weeks as a single agent.
  - Doxorubicin at a dose of 70 mg/m^2 IV at 3-week intervals is also considered a safe, effective drug choice for systemic chemotherapy.
- Immunosuppressive doses of corticosteroids alone will often transiently decrease the size of the tumor or affected lymph nodes.
- With solitary tumors, complete surgical resection may be curative. Large colon and small intestine resection afforded several months of survival after discharge from the hospital in reports of two horses with intestinal lymphoma.
- Radiation has been used with success in solitary tumors, especially those of the nasal cavity (see "Radiation Therapy" in Section II).
- Cutaneous lymphoma has been treated successfully with corticosteroids, progestins, low-dose systemic chemotherapy, intralesional chemotherapy (with cisplatin), and immunomodulators.

CHRONIC TREATMENT

After remission, horses have been treated long term with prednisolone as mentioned above.

DRUG INTERACTIONS

- Before using chemotherapeutics, consultation with or referral to a veterinary oncologist or internist is recommended.
- Antioxidants such as vitamin E should be avoided in conjunction with doxorubicin.
- Digoxin has reported to interact with several chemotherapy agents (in humans).
- Vincristine should not be given with other drugs that require metabolism by cytochrome P450, including itraconazole.

POSSIBLE COMPLICATIONS

- Acute severe deterioration can occur with generalized disease. Depending on the tissues affected, acute organ failure often occurs.
- Reported reactions to chemotherapy include neutropenia with or without sepsis, thrombocytopenia, colic, laminitis, bone marrow suppression, focal dermatitis at the injection site, and delayed allergic reactions.

RECOMMENDED MONITORING

- CBC should be performed before every dose of chemotherapy.
- Progression of clinical signs is likely without treatment.
- Cutaneous lesions often wax and wane over time without therapy, especially with hormonal variations.

PROGNOSIS AND OUTCOME

Any form of lymphoma can, and usually does, progress despite therapy. There have only been a few reported cases of survival after aggressive therapy, so an accurate outcome and prognosis are difficult to estimate. Most horses present late in the course of disease, which may preclude treatment.

PEARLS & CONSIDERATIONS

COMMENTS

- Chemotherapy may successfully manage lymphoma to give good function and quality of life.
- Surgery is appropriate only for localized lesions that are functionally impairing the horse and can be completely resected. Even in those cases, surgery is unlikely to be curative.
- Careful physical examination and sampling for cytologic or histologic analysis is key for diagnosis.

CLIENT EDUCATION

- Treatment may result in comfortable survival with a good quality of life.
- Lymphoma is usually progressive and ultimately fatal.

SUGGESTED READING

McClure JT: Leukoproliferative disorders in horses. *Vet Clin North Am Equine Pract* 16:1, 2000.

Sellon DC, Wise LN: Disorders of the hematopoietic system. In Reed SM, Bayly WM, Sellon DC (eds). *Equine internal medicine*, St Louis, 2010, Saunders Elsevier, pp 730–776.

Couto CG: Lymphoma in the horse, *Proc 12th Annual Am College Vet Int Med* 12:865, 1994.

Tan RHH, Crisman MV, Clark SP, et al: Multicentric mastocytoma in a horse, *J Vet Intern Med* 21:340–343, 2007.

AUTHORS: L. NICKI WISE and **MELISSA T. HINES**

EDITOR: JEFFREY N. BRYAN

Malocclusions, Dental

BASIC INFORMATION

DEFINITION

Abnormal occlusal wear patterns involving the premolar and molar arcades

SYNONYM(S)

Hooks, ramps, waves, steps

EPIDEMIOLOGY

RISK FACTORS Age, dental trauma, orthodontic abnormalities, dental dysplasia

ASSOCIATED CONDITIONS AND DISORDERS Periodontal disease, endodontic disease, premature expiration and exfoliation

CLINICAL PRESENTATION

HISTORY, CHIEF COMPLAINT
- Most often, no complaint
- Occasionally, poor performance, weight loss, dysphagia, quidding, poor appetite

PHYSICAL EXAM FINDINGS
- Abnormal occlusal wear
- Occasionally, poor occlusal contact
- Occasionally, restricted lateral or rostrocaudal mandibular range of motion (ROM)

ETIOLOGY AND PATHOPHYSIOLOGY
- Unopposed teeth or portions thereof
- Abnormal enamel content or distribution
- Misaligned teeth
- Any abnormality in dental tissue or alignment or restriction of normal mandibular movement can lead to excessive wear in specific areas along the arcades. Compensatory shifts in mandibular position or ROM can lead to secondary malocclusions.

DIAGNOSIS

DIFFERENTIAL DIAGNOSIS

- Skeletal curve in dish-faced breeds or individuals can mimic a wave.
- Caudal molar set well into curve of Spee can mimic a hook or ramp.

INITIAL DATABASE

- Oral examination: Identification of malocclusions such as but not limited to:
  - Hooks: Excessive crown height of maxillary 6s or mandibular 11s where the vertical height of the excessive crown is greater than the horizontal length

- Ramps: Excessive crown height in which the horizontal length of the excessive crown is greater than the vertical height
- Waves: Gradual increase or decrease in crown heights along the length of the arcade involving two or more teeth
- Steps: Excessive crown height of a single tooth
- Knowledge of previous dental care
- Age
- Severity of malocclusion
- Amount of clinical crown

ADVANCED OR CONFIRMATORY TESTING

Intraoral radiographs may be necessary to assess severely compromised teeth.

TREATMENT

THERAPEUTIC GOAL(S)

- Reduction or correction of malocclusions to restore more normal masticatory biomechanics
- Promote normal wear patterns to prolong the useful life of individual teeth.

ACUTE GENERAL TREATMENT

- Small malocclusions can often be corrected fully at initial treatment by reducing abnormally tall crowns or portions thereof.
- More severe malocclusions or those involving large portions of the arcades should be corrected in stages over periods of months to years.

CHRONIC TREATMENT

- Severe malocclusions in mature or geriatric horses may not be curable. Treatment should be aimed at improving masticatory biomechanics, preventing pain, preserving compromised dental tissue, preventing disease, and maintaining functional occlusion.
- Regular treatment is necessary to maintain chronic cases in a functional state.

POSSIBLE COMPLICATIONS

- Aggressive corrections can cause damage to sensitive dental tissues, resulting in pain, dysphagia or inappetence, or endodontic disease.
- Iatrogenically induced soft tissue trauma may cause dysphagia.
- Overly aggressive or poorly executed corrections may result in a loss of

minimum functional occlusion, causing prolonged dysphagia.

RECOMMENDED MONITORING

- All horses should receive a comprehensive oral and dental examination at least once yearly.
- Patients with severe malocclusions may require examination and treatment every 6 to 9 months.

PROGNOSIS AND OUTCOME

- The vast majority of malocclusions are correctable. All are manageable.
- Early recognition usually leads to more successful outcomes.

PEARLS & CONSIDERATIONS

COMMENTS

- Frequent small corrections are usually the best approach for severe malocclusions.
- Operator expertise is a critical factor in successful outcomes.
- Consider referral to a more experienced colleague for advanced cases.
- Client education and expectation management is key for client compliance (ie, dental malocclusions do not develop overnight). Complete correction takes time and dedication to the goal.

PREVENTION

- All horses should have an oral examination before age 3 years (much earlier if an overjet or underjet is detected) and at least yearly thereafter.
- Malocclusions recognized at this age are typically small and very manageable or completely correctable.

CLIENT EDUCATION

- Prevention requires owner acceptance of the comprehensive dental examination as a fundamental health care necessity from an early age.
- Older horses or those with severe malocclusions may not be candidates for complete correction. Clients must be educated as to realistic outcomes and requirements for long-term management.

SUGGESTED READING

Equine Dental Seminars for Veterinarians: Available at http://www.digitalequus.com.
Klugh DO: *Principles of Equine Dentistry*, London, 2010, Thieme, pp 63–70, 81–90.

Rucker BA: Incisor and Molar occlusion: normal ranges and indications for incisor reduction. *Proc Am Assoc Equine Pract* 50:7–12, 2004.

AUTHOR: **MARY S. DELOREY**

EDITOR: **JAMES L. CARMALT**

Mast Cell Tumors

BASIC INFORMATION

DEFINITION

A tumor composed of a neoplastic population of mast cells

SYNONYM(S)

Mastocytoma, mastocytosis (indicates systemic involvement)

EPIDEMIOLOGY

SPECIES, AGE, SEX Ages of reported cases range from 9 months to 27 years of age (mean, 9.5 years). Males predominate in these cases.
GENETICS AND BREED PREDISPOSITION Arabians are overrepresented in the reported cases; however, these tumors have been identified in numerous other breeds, including Quarter Horses, Thoroughbreds, ponies, and donkeys.
ASSOCIATED CONDITIONS AND DISORDERS Peripheral eosinophilia

CLINICAL PRESENTATION

DISEASE FORMS/SUBTYPES
Appears in two forms:
- Most common as a solitary, soft tissue nodule occurring most frequently on the extremities, head, and neck and less commonly on the trunk. Isolated case reports have identified these tumors in such locations as the nares, nasopharynx, trachea, synovium, trabecular bone of P3, sclera, and nictitating membrane. The mass can be either soft or firm but is loosely attached to the underlying tissues except for those that occur on the distal limb that are hard and firmly attached. The mass generally appears as a subcutaneous nodule covered with skin, although the skin may be ulcerated or alopecic. Most often, the mass is slow growing or static in nature. The lesions are most often benign, although local invasion of surrounding tissues and metastatic disease with invasion of local lymph nodes has been reported.
- A congenital form of generalized mast cell tumor development was reported in a neonatal Quarter Horse foal. The foal developed numerous subcutaneous nodules over the trunk and limbs shortly after birth. The nodules began

as small subcutaneous masses but later enlarged and then ulcerated before spontaneous regression. The lesions reappeared cyclically during the horse's first year of life. This syndrome has been related to urticaria pigmentosa in humans.
HISTORY, CHIEF COMPLAINT Identification of a soft tissue mass (most likely on the head, neck, or limbs) possibly changing in size or appearance over time
PHYSICAL EXAM FINDINGS
- Generally unremarkable with the exception of the presenting complaint
- Horses with periocular tumors may have ophthalmic abnormalities.
- Tumors associated with a joint or bone may cause lameness in the affected limb; tumors in the respiratory tract may cause respiratory noise or epistaxis.
- Although rare, metastatic disease may cause evidence of systemic illness, including weight loss, lethargy, lymphadenopathy, and dyspnea.
ETIOLOGY AND PATHOPHYSIOLOGY
Unknown. Possible theories include a response to chronic inflammation, immune-mediated disease, or parasitic infestation. Mast cell tumors in horses are unique in their appearance, behavior, and histology compared with those of other domestic species.

DIAGNOSIS

DIFFERENTIAL DIAGNOSIS

Variable depending on the lesion's location and appearance: Nodular necrobiosis, abscess, cutaneous habronemiasis, enlarged lymph node, cutaneous lymphoma, sarcoid, fibroma, squamous cell carcinoma, or melanoma

INITIAL DATABASE

- Diagnosis of the mass can often be made on fine-needle aspiration and cytologic examination.
- A complete blood cell count and serum chemistry may reveal a peripheral eosinophilia, which is often associated with more aggressive forms.
- If located on the limb or adjacent to an osseous structure, radiographs are

recommended to examine the underlying bone. The tumors may appear calcified on radiographs.

ADVANCED OR CONFIRMATORY TESTING

Definitive diagnosis relies on biopsy, most often excisional biopsy. Given the relatively benign nature of the solitary mass, adjacent lymph node aspirates and further imaging studies to assess for metastasis are not warranted unless the physical examination and laboratory work reveal other abnormalities.

TREATMENT

THERAPEUTIC GOAL(S)

Removal of the tumor en bloc

ACUTE GENERAL TREATMENT

Complete surgical resection of the tumor with wide margins (2 to 3 cm) as described in small animal practice

CHRONIC TREATMENT

- If complete resection is not possible or if the tumor recurs despite surgical removal, debulking followed by radiation has been used with success.
- Systemic corticosteroid use and sublesional injections of triamcinolone have been reported with variable success as well.
- No other chemotherapy agents have been reported.

POSSIBLE COMPLICATIONS

Removal or manipulation of a tumor can cause systemic signs in the form of diffuse urticaria or local pruritus. The potential for clinical signs of systemic degranulation exists in horses but has not been reported. In small animals, these reactions may be mild and include local swelling, erythema, and pruritus or may be severe enough to cause hypotension and death.

RECOMMENDED MONITORING

With the potential for recurrence and infrequent metastasis, these tumors should be removed and the horse moni-

<![CDATA[**Mast Cell Tumors**   **Meconium Impaction** 353]]>

tored for recurrence or signs of systemic illness.

PROGNOSIS AND OUTCOME

Good with surgical removal

<![CDATA[DISEASES AND DISORDERS]]>

PEARLS & CONSIDERATIONS

Any new mass on a horse should be aspirated for cytologic examination to facilitate early diagnosis.

SUGGESTED READING

<![CDATA[Brown HM, Cuttino E, LeRoy BE: A subcutaneous mass on the neck of a horse. *Vet Clin Pathol* 36:109, 2007.
Rees C: Disorders of the skin. In Reed S, Bayly W (eds). *Equine internal medicine*, ed 3, St Louis, 2010, Elsevier, p 712.]]>

AUTHOR: **L. NICKI WISE**

EDITOR: **JEFFREY N. BRYAN**

Meconium Impaction

BASIC INFORMATION

DEFINITION
Retention of meconium in the distal gastrointestinal (GI) tract

EPIDEMIOLOGY
SPECIES, AGE, SEX
- All breeds of newborn foals may be affected.
- Colts may be overrepresented.

RISK FACTORS Weak foals and recumbent foals present an increased risk.

ASSOCIATED CONDITIONS AND DISORDERS Ruptured bladder

CLINICAL PRESENTATION
HISTORY, CHIEF COMPLAINT
- Tail flagging, restlessness, colic signs (lying in dorsal recumbency, looking at flank)
- Straining to defecate; must be distinguished from straining to urinate
- Abdominal distension

PHYSICAL EXAM FINDINGS
- Digital rectal palpation may reveal meconium in the proximal rectum.
- Abdominal distension results in tachypnea.
- Severe abdominal distension results in respiratory distress.
- Weak, recumbent foals and those with altered mentation often exhibit subtle signs such as mild, repeated abdominal press.

ETIOLOGY AND PATHOPHYSIOLOGY
Immature pacemaker cells in the neonatal foal's GI tract may contribute to meconium impactions in neonatal foals. Passing of meconium should begin by 2 hours of age and be completed by 48 hours. Intraluminal obstruction with meconium results in gaseous distension of the bowel orad to the impaction.

DIAGNOSIS

DIFFERENTIAL DIAGNOSIS
- Intestinal atresia
- Ruptured bladder
- Intestinal aganglionosis (see "Lethal White Foal Syndrome" in this section)
- All other causes of colic

INITIAL DATABASE
- Physical examination: Identify concurrent or contributory disease, if present.
- Digital rectal palpation for detection of meconium in proximal rectum: Lack of meconium in the rectum does not rule out meconium impaction proximal to the rectum.

ADVANCED OR CONFIRMATORY TESTING
- Contrast radiography: Barium enema administered via gravity flow through a 24-Fr Foley catheter (with bulb inflated) will outline intraluminal meconium; also useful to identify or rule out atresia coli and lethal white foal syndrome.
- Abdominal ultrasonography: Intraluminal echogenic masses visualized in the small or large colon are consistent with meconium; hypoechoic free fluid in the abdomen should prompt investigation of the urinary tract.

TREATMENT

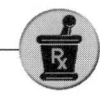

THERAPEUTIC GOAL(S)
- Remove impacted meconium
- Control pain
- Restore circulating volume if dehydrated
- Maintain an adequate glucose level

ACUTE GENERAL TREATMENT
- Enema: Warm, soapy water enema made with a non-irritating soap administered via a soft, flexible tube such as a Foley or stallion catheter. The tube is advanced gently until resistance is met; 500 mL to 1 L volume by gravity flow should be used to minimize trauma to rectum. Repeated enemas may be necessary if the initial enema does not resolve the impaction; however, repeated enemas result in irritation and swelling of the rectal mucosa and should therefore be used judiciously.
- Walking: It is often beneficial for the foal to walk around (by leading the dam) after the administration of an enema.
- Laxative: Mineral oil (2–3 mL/kg) may be administered via nasogastric tube if reflux is not present.
- Analgesia: Allows for relaxation of the bowel in straining foals; flunixin meglumine (0.5–1.1 mg/kg IV), butorphanol (0.02–0.04 mg/kg IV or IM).
- IV fluids: If dehydrated; isotonic crystalloids with 2.5% to 5% dextrose if the foal has not been nursing (slow bolus of 10–20 mL/kg).

CHRONIC TREATMENT
- If routine enemas are not successful at resolving the impaction, a retention enema with 4% acetylcysteine may be administered (see "Enema, Retention/ High" in Section II).
- Surgical intervention is required in very few cases.

POSSIBLE COMPLICATIONS
Ruptured bladder

RECOMMENDED MONITORING
- Monitor for continued straining after successful enemas; additional meconium may become retained, especially if the small colon and rectum are swollen from multiple enemas.
- Repeated episodes of forceful straining may cause the bladder to rupture; therefore monitor for signs of ruptured bladder (See "Uroperitoneum" in this section).

PROGNOSIS AND OUTCOME

- Foals with meconium impactions generally respond well to medical therapy; surgery is rarely required.
- After the impaction is resolved, normal GI function should return provided that concurrent or secondary disease is not present.

PEARLS & CONSIDERATIONS

- Meconium impactions are the most common cause of colic in neonatal foals.
- Over-the-counter enemas typically contain phosphate. Repeated use of these products may lead to severe electrolyte disturbances, especially hyperphosphatemia.

SUGGESTED READING

Bernard WV: Assessment of abdominal pain in foals. In *49th annual convention of the AAEP*. New Orleans, 2003, American Association of Equine Practitioners.

AUTHOR: **PHOEBE A. SMITH**

EDITORS: **ELIZABETH M. SANTSCHI** and **PHOEBE A. SMITH**

Megaesophagus

BASIC INFORMATION

DEFINITION

Chronic dilation (ectasia) and atony of the body of the esophagus

SYNONYM(S)

Esophageal ectasia

EPIDEMIOLOGY

SPECIES, AGE, SEX
- Congenital megaesophagus is seen in foals and young adult horses.
- Acquired megaesophagus may occur at any age.

ASSOCIATED CONDITIONS AND DISORDERS
- Gastroduodenal ulceration
- Botulism
- Equine grass sickness
- Fourth branchial arch defect

CLINICAL PRESENTATION

HISTORY, CHIEF COMPLAINT
- Clinical signs of esophageal dysphagia:
  - Hypersalivation
  - Regurgitation
  - Weight loss
  - Coughing associated with eating
  - Nasal discharge containing food material
- Onset of signs usually insidious

PHYSICAL EXAM FINDINGS
The findings of physical examination confirm the presenting signs, including dysphagia, hypersalivation, and nasal discharge containing food material. Distension of the cervical esophagus may be visible or palpable. The horse may be noted to eructate frequently.

ETIOLOGY AND PATHOPHYSIOLOGY
- Congenital megaesophagus may be inherited in a similar fashion to congenital megaesophagus in dogs. Some horses affected by fourth branchial arch defect may also have megaesophagus and achalasia of the upper esophageal sphincter.
- Acquired megaesophagus may be secondary to chronic or recurrent esophageal obstruction, esophageal obstruction by tumors and other masses, vascular ring anomalies, neurologic diseases (eg, equine protozoal myeloencephalitis, idiopathic vagal neuropathy), pleuropneumonia (and associated vagal neuropathy), equine grass sickness, botulism, or myasthenia gravis.
- Temporary iatrogenic megaesophagus may occur after sedation with α_2-adrenergic agonists, such as detomidine.

DIAGNOSIS

DIFFERENTIAL DIAGNOSIS
- Other causes of dysphagia (especially abnormalities of the pharyngeal and esophageal phases of deglutition): Pharyngeal paralysis, pharyngeal cysts, pharyngeal compression by strangles abscesses and guttural pouch empyema, subepiglottic cyst, fourth branchial arch defect, esophageal obstruction, esophageal stricture, esophageal rupture, and equine grass sickness
- Other obstructions of the esophagus: Intramural esophageal cysts, duplication cysts of the esophagus, esophageal neoplasia

INITIAL DATABASE
- The leukogram, hematology, and blood chemistry results are likely to be normal unless they reflect abnormalities associated with any underlying disease.
- Confirmation of megaesophagus is achieved by endoscopic examination (esophagoscopy) and radiography (positive or double-contrast esophagraphy). On endoscopic examination, the esophagus appears dilated, and there is an absence of peristaltic waves. Esophagitis and reflux esophagitis may be noted. Fluoroscopy and contrast radiography may be used to measure the transit time of a bolus from the cervical esophagus to the stomach. Contrast radiography also demonstrates pooling of contrast agent or dilation of the esophageal lumen. Contrast radiography is helpful to identify gastric outflow obstruction in foals.

ADVANCED OR CONFIRMATORY TESTING
- Esophageal manometry can be used to document esophageal pressures.
- Cerebrospinal fluid analysis may be useful to identify underlying neurologic disorders.
- Electromyography may be indicated to diagnose underlying neuromuscular diseases.

TREATMENT

THERAPEUTIC GOAL(S)
- Treat any underlying diseases
- Treat any secondary inhalation pneumonia
- Aid transit of food along the esophagus

ACUTE GENERAL TREATMENT
- Treat any underlying diseases.
- Treat any secondary inhalation pneumonia.
- Dietary modification may help esophageal transit of food boluses to the stomach. Feeding slurries of pellets and feeding from an elevated position may help.
- Metoclopramide or bethanechol may benefit patients with reflux esophagitis associated with megaesophagus by increasing lower esophageal tone and gastric emptying and reducing gastroesophageal reflux.

CHRONIC TREATMENT

Frequent small meals of slurries or fresh grass should be fed.

POSSIBLE COMPLICATIONS

- Inhalation pneumonia
- Weight loss

PROGNOSIS AND OUTCOME

Prognosis is poor in most cases.

PEARLS & CONSIDERATIONS

Megaesophagus should be considered in horses showing chronic signs of esophageal dysphagia.

SUGGESTED READING

Bowman KF, Vaughan JR, Quick CB, et al: Megaesophagus in a colt. *J Am Vet Med Assoc* 172:334, 1978.
Broekman LE, Kuiper D: Megaesophagus in the horse. A short review of the literature and 18 known cases. *Vet Q* 24:199, 2002.

Greet TR: Observations on the potential role of oesophageal radiography in the horse. *Equine Vet J* 14:73, 1982.
Sanchez LC: Esophageal diseases. In Reed SM, Bayly WM, Sellon DC (eds). *Equine internal medicine*, ed 3, St Louis, 2004, Saunders Elsevier, pp 830–838.
Murray MJ, Ball MM, Parker GA: Megaesophagus and aspiration pneumonia secondary to gastric ulceration in a foal. *J Am Vet Med Assoc* 192:381, 1988.
Stick JA, Derksen FJ, McNitt DL, et al: Equine esophageal pressure profile. *Am J Vet Res* 44:272, 1983.

AUTHOR: **TIM MAIR**

EDITORS: **TIM MAIR** and **CERI SHERLOCK**

Melanoma, Cutaneous

BASIC INFORMATION

DEFINITION

Neoplasm of dermal melanocytes or "nevus cells" within the basal layer of the epidermis

SYNONYM(S)

- Equine melanocytic disease
- Cutaneous melanoma

EPIDEMIOLOGY

SPECIES, AGE, SEX

- Occurs mostly in aging, gray and white horses, and mules.
- Bays, chestnut, and other colors are less frequently affected.
- More than 80% of gray horses older than 15 years develop melanoma.
- Some have suggested that all gray horses will develop melanoma over their lifetime.
- Case reports in non-gray horses, usually of the hoof, coronary band, and metacarpal/metatarsal area.
- The juvenile form may occur in horses of any coat color.
- Sex predisposition reported by some but not consistently.

GENETICS AND BREED PREDISPOSITION

- Most common in Lipizzaners, Arabians, and Quarter Horses.
- Arabians are thought to be predisposed because they progressively change color with age; they are usually white by 9 years of age.

RISK FACTORS

- The gray phenotype appears to be a disturbance in melanin metabolism, which stimulates the formation of melanoblasts or increased activity, resulting in overproduction of melanin in the dermis.

- Autosomal dominant trait associated with high incidence of melanoma and vitiligo-like depigmentation (cis-acting regulatory mutation)

GEOGRAPHY AND SEASONALITY

Generally accepted to be more common in sunnier latitudes

CLINICAL PRESENTATION

DISEASE FORMS/SUBTYPES Four distinct clinical syndromes:

- Melanocytic nevus
  - Average age of presentation is 5 years (range, 2 months to 16 years)
  - Approximately 50% of all melanotic tumors in horses
  - Considered benign
  - Gray and non-gray horses
  - Discrete, small, superficial tumors that involve the superficial dermal layer with variable pigmentation and occasional mitotic figures noted on histopathology
  - Studies suggest an Arabian overrepresentation and a female predisposition
- Dermal melanoma
  - Average age of presentation is 13 years (range, 2–19 years)
  - Discrete masses that occur in mature, middle-aged gray horses at various locations (see Physical Exam)
  - Located in the deep dermis and characterized by small, homogenous, indistinct, round tumor cells with condensed chromatin and dense cytoplasmic pigmentation
  - More aggressive forms appear to occur in atypical locations (limbs) and at a younger age
- Dermal melanomatosis
  - Average age of presentation is 17 years (range, 7–29 years); multiple sites or coalescence

  - Older gray horses, frequently in typical locations (tail base, perineum, and genitalia)
  - Histologically similar to dermal melanoma but more confluent
  - High metastatic rate
  - Surgical excision usually not feasible
- Anaplastic melanoma
  - Average age of presentation is 20 years and not exclusively in gray horses
  - May occur more commonly in other colors (chestnut)
  - Extremely pleomorphic, epithelioid cells with poor pigmentation, widespread single-cell invasion of the dermis and numerous mitotic figures noted on histopathology

HISTORY, CHIEF COMPLAINT

- Usually related to size and location of tumor burden
- Physical obstruction of the anal sphincter, penis, prepuce, or vulvar commissure may occur, which may result in dyschezia, dysuria, and difficulty with coitus and parturition.
- Metastatic melanoma: May present for weight loss, colic, epistaxis, ataxia, and respiratory distress
- 43% have peripheral edema from lymphatic obstruction
- Clinical progression: Three forms:
  - Slow growth over a number of years without metastasis
  - Benign growth transforms into malignant lesion and metastasizes
  - Malignant from inception and readily metastasizes

PHYSICAL EXAM FINDINGS

- Occurs mostly on areas of glabrous skin
- Slow-growing, locally invasive masses
- Primary affected sites include the ventral tail, perineum, lips, periocular

region, parotid gland, and external genitalia.
- Progression frequently results in metastasis through direct extension, lymphatics, or blood.
- Necropsy reveals typical metastasis to autonomic nervous system, lungs, lymph nodes, bone, adrenals, eye, skin, intima of the heart, and blood vessels.

ETIOLOGY AND PATHOPHYSIOLOGY
- In Arabians, thought to result from destruction of normal melanocytes through an autoimmune or cytotoxic process
- Consequence of disturbance in melanin metabolism that leads to formation of melanoblasts or increased activity of resident melanoblasts, resulting in overproduction of melanin in a focal area
- In time, hyperplastic melanoblasts undergo malignant transformation (may take up to 20 years).
- Increased ultraviolet light exposure may play a role.
- The STX17 duplication leads to proliferation of dermal melanocytes, thus predisposing to melanoma development.

DIAGNOSIS

DIFFERENTIAL DIAGNOSIS
- Melanoma should be considered in any gray horse older than 10 years of age presenting for virtually any clinical condition.
- Other dermal neoplasms: Equine cutaneous mastocytosis, squamous cell papillomas (viral papillomatosis), cutaneous lymphoma, mycosis fungoides

INITIAL DATABASE
- Diagnosis is usually based on the physical appearance of the neoplasm (firm, flat, solitary or multiple cutaneous masses that give skin a cobblestone or verrucous appearance and are usually hyperpigmented) and histopathology.
- Diagnostic tests that are useful in detecting metastatic disease include rectal palpation, ultrasonography, biopsy or fine-needle aspirate of suspect internal metastasis, and cytology of peritoneal fluid.

ADVANCED OR CONFIRMATORY TESTING
- Histopathology may predict clinical behavior.
- Melanocytic nevi should not progress, but malignant transformation may occur in dermal melanoma or melanomatosis.

TREATMENT

THERAPEUTIC GOAL(S)
- A uniform standard therapy for melanoma does not exist.
- The goal of therapy is to manage local and metastatic disease.

ACUTE GENERAL TREATMENT
Relieve immediate obstructive lesions through surgery if possible.

CHRONIC TREATMENT
- Surgical removal of affected tissues is usually curative. Around the anus or tail, surgery is contraindicated because complete removal is not possible and may stimulate more rapid growth of neoplastic tissue.
- Surgery
  - Removal of all affected tissues with wide margins is usually curative for melanocytic nevi and solitary dermal melanomas. Necessary margins for cure have not been established, so as aggressive a surgery as possible is recommended.
  - If wide margins are not achieved, the tumors tend to recur at the surgical site.
  - Multiple surgeries may be necessary over time, and the client should be warned at the outset.
  - Laser ablation has been suggested as an adjunct to achieve complete excision.
- Bacillus Calmette-Guérin
  - Attenuated strain of *Mycobacterium bovis*.
  - Injection into the tumor causes inflammatory response in melanocytic tumors.
  - Not usually effective at stimulating tumor regression.
- Radiotherapy
  - Effective for local management in other species
  - Not yet evaluated in horses
- Cryonecrosis
  - May be used in conjunction with surgery, especially for large, difficult to remove tumors
  - Tend to regrow into sites of previous treatment (may increase the risk of aggressive regrowth)
- Chemotherapy: Intralesional cisplatin is successful with small lesions (<2-3 cm)
  - More effective when a vasoconstrictive agent (epinephrine chloride solution) is added to the formulation.
  - Four intratumoral injection sessions at 2-week intervals. Cisplatin beads

surgically implanted after surgical debulking yielded the best result.
- Immunotherapy
  - Cimetidine (a biologic response modifier with antitumor activity and H2 receptor antagonism)
    - Effect through inhibiting suppressor T cells and enhancing cell-mediated immunity
    - Induction dosage: 4 mg/kg PO q8h, then 2.5 mg/kg q12h for maintenance therapy
    - If favorable response is not seen in 3 months, discontinue therapy
  - Interferon-α has become more popular, but evaluation has not been performed.
  - Whole-cell vaccine
    - 2 cm³ of excised melanoma in Hank's balanced salt solution with 10% fetal calf serum (shipped overnight on ice)
    - Injected into the patient every 14 days for 12 weeks and then every 6 weeks
    - The efficacy of the vaccine is variable and depends on an individual horse's immune response.

POSSIBLE COMPLICATIONS
- Recurrence may be more aggressive than the original lesion.
- Care should be taken in handling cisplatin and all urine excreted for at least 72 hours after cisplatin administration to avoid human exposure.

RECOMMENDED PREVENTION/ MONITORING
Sunscreen has been advocated for horses that are poorly pigmented and cannot be stabled during sunny weather.

PROGNOSIS AND OUTCOME
- Tumor size is considered prognostic in humans and may be prognostic in horses with discrete melanocytic tumors.
- Signalment should help guide; aggressive dermal melanoma in younger horse in an atypical location warrants further investigation.
- High metastatic rate with dermal melanomatosis and anaplastic forms.
- Small tumors often do not cause clinical signs and could be considered a cosmetic blemish.
- May remain benign for as long as 10 to 20 years.
- Survival time depends on the level of disease at diagnosis, location of tumor burden, and surgical resectability.

PEARLS & CONSIDERATIONS

COMMENTS

Melanoma should be considered in any gray horse older than 10 years of age presenting for virtually any clinical condition.

PREVENTION

Protect at-risk horses from the sun with shade or sunscreen.

CLIENT EDUCATION

- More than 80% of gray horses older than 15 years develop melanoma.
- Multiple surgeries may be necessary over time.

SUGGESTED READING

Johnson PJ: Dermatologic tumors (excluding sarcoids). In *Vet Clin North Am Equine Pract* 14(3):625–658, viii, 1998.

Rowe EL, Sullins KE: Excision as treatment of dermal melanomatosis: 11 cases (1994–2000). *J Am Vet Med Assoc* 225(1):94, 2004.
Valentine BA: Equine melanocytic tumors: a retrospective study of 53 horses (1988–1991). *J Vet Intern Med* 9(5):291, 1995.

AUTHORS: **CHELSEA D. TRIPP** and **JEFFREY N. BRYAN**

EDITOR: **JEFFREY N. BRYAN**

Metabolic Syndrome, Equine

BASIC INFORMATION

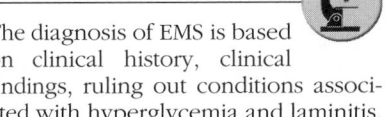

- Endocrinopathy of energy metabolism in horses
- Associated with insulin resistance (IR) and laminitis (see "Insulin Resistance" in this section)

DEFINITION

- Equine metabolic syndrome (EMS) is a recently described endocrine pathologic condition of obese horses that is associated with IR, laminitis, and fat redistribution.
- IR is the hallmark of EMS.

EPIDEMIOLOGY

SPECIES, AGE, SEX EMS is more commonly reported in middle-aged horses, but unlike Cushing's disease, younger animals can develop EMS.

GENETICS AND BREED PREDISPOSITION

- There is a genetic predisposition to IR and EMS in Saddlebreds, Morgans, Tennessee Walking Horses, Paso Finos, Quarter Horses, and ponies.
- Ponies have the highest prevalence of IR.
- The predisposition to IR and EMS relates to these breeds being prone to obesity.
- These animals require fewer calories to maintain body weight or become obese ("easy keepers").
- There is no evidence that EMS is directly associated with geography or season.
- There appears to be an indirect association with geography that relates to quality of pasture.

RISK FACTORS

- EMS is associated with excessive feeding of carbohydrates and thus is more often reported in developed countries.
- Lack of physical activity contributes to EMS.

CLINICAL PRESENTATION

- Obesity, fat redistribution (tailhead, neck, prepuce, mammary gland, shoulder area, supraorbital fat pads), and laminitis are the clinical features of EMS (and IR).
- A "cresty neck" or "stallion-like" appearance in mares is suggestive of EMS.
- Mares may have a history of infertility.
- Unlike horses with Cushing's disease, horses with EMS have a normal hair coat and shed their coats in the summer.

HISTORY, CHIEF COMPLAINT

- The most common presenting complaint of horses with EMS is laminitis.
- These horses are easy keepers and obese and spend more time grazing.
- A "cresty neck" from fat redistribution is typical of these horses.
- Infertility is a complaint in mares.

ETIOLOGY AND PATHOPHYSIOLOGY

- IR is the key pathophysiologic process that leads to EMS (see "Insulin Resistance" in this section).
- Having fewer insulin receptors or inappropriate receptor response upon insulin stimulation results in IR.
- Depending on the stage of IR, horses with EMS may have hyperinsulinemia with normoglycemia (compensated IR) or with hyperglycemia (noncompensated IR).
- Glucocorticoids appear to be central in the pathogenesis of IR and EMS.
  - Glucocorticoids induce IR by decreasing the receptors response to insulin.
  - Glucocorticoid concentrations are often elevated in horses fed hypercaloric diets.
- Dexamethasone administration in healthy horses induces IR.
- It has been proposed that conversion of inactive cortisone to active cortisol by 11β-hydroxysteroid dehydrogenase

in adipocytes may play a role in the pathogenesis of EMS.
- The mechanisms responsible for fat redistribution (regional adiposity) appear to be a combination of IR and increased cortisol concentrations.
- IR leads to less glucose uptake and hyperglycemia, vascular dysfunction and inflammation, vasoconstriction, and increased vascular resistance.
- Laminitis is believed to result from decreased laminar blood flow, decreased endothelial glucose uptake, vascular dysfunction and inflammation, and a pro-oxidative state from insulin insensitivity.
- Insulin mediates vasodilation via nitric oxide.

DIAGNOSIS

- The diagnosis of EMS is based on clinical history, clinical findings, ruling out conditions associated with hyperglycemia and laminitis, and testing for IR.
- Tests for IR include baseline glucose and insulin concentrations, the glucose tolerance test (GTT), the combined glucose/insulin test (CGIT), the euglycemic-hyperinsulinemic clamp (EHC), and the minimal model analysis of a frequently sampled IV glucose tolerance test (FSIGT).
  - Of these, the GTT are CGIT are the most commonly performed.
  - Baseline insulin concentrations should be less than 20 μIU/mL.
  - Insulin level above 30 μIU/mL suggests IR and is consistent with EMS.
- Normoglycemia with hyperinsulinemia (compensated IR) or hyperglycemia with hyperinsulinemia (noncompensated IR) suggests EMS.
- Hyperglycemia with normal or low insulin concentrations indicates diabetes mellitus.

- Low thyroid hormone concentrations are frequent findings, but their significance is unclear.
- Liver enzymes can be elevated in some horses with EMS, suggesting hepatic fatty infiltration.
- GTT: See Section II, Procedures and Techniques.
  - A delayed return in glucose concentrations to baseline (>3 hours) suggests IR (EMS).
- CGIT: See Section II, Procedures and Techniques.
  - Glucose concentrations do not decrease below baseline before 90 minutes in horses with IR and EMS.
  - Glucose concentrations above baseline at 45 minutes are consistent with IR and EMS

DIFFERENTIAL DIAGNOSIS

- Obesity, conditions associated with laminitis (Cushing's disease), hypothyroidism.
- Hyperglycemia may be the result of diabetes mellitus.

TREATMENT

ACUTE GENERAL TREATMENT

- Start a weight loss plan.
- Increase physical activity.

- Do not feed carbohydrate-rich diets.
- Limit access to carbohydrate-rich pastures.
- Consider levothyroxine sodium (1–6 mg/100/kg PO q24h) to induce a hypermetabolic state.
- Trilostane, an inhibitor of steroid synthesis, has been used with variable results.
- Metformin, a drug that increases insulin sensitivity, has also been used in horses with IR with promising results.

PROGNOSIS AND OUTCOME

Guarded, depending on response to treatment and owner compliance

PEARLS & CONSIDERATIONS

- The excessive feeding of carbohydrate-rich diets and obesity leads to IR and EMS.

- Lack of recognition between appropriate body condition and obesity is a contributing factor in EMS.
- Do not feed grain to horses that can maintain body condition on pasture.
- Increase physical activity in obese and "easy keeper" horses.

SUGGESTED READING

Durham AE, Rendle DI, Newton JE: The effect of metformin on measurements of insulin sensitivity and beta cell response in 18 horses and ponies with insulin resistance. *Equine Vet J* 40:493–500, 2008.

Frank N: Equine metabolic syndrome. In Smith BP (ed). *Large animal internal medicine*, ed 4, St Louis, 2009, Mosby Elsevier, pp 1352–1355.

Frank N: Insulin resistance and equine metabolic syndrome. In Reed SM, Bayly WM, Sellon DC (eds). *Equine Internal Medicine*, ed 3, St Louis, 2010, Elsevier, pp 1270–1277.

McFarlane D: Pituitary and hypothalamus. In Smith BP (ed). *Large animal internal medicine*, ed 4, St Louis, 2009, Mosby Elsevier, pp 1339–1344.

McGowan CM, Neiger R: Efficacy of trilostane for the treatment of equine Cushing's syndrome. *Equine Vet J* 35:414–418, 2003.

AUTHOR & EDITOR: RAMIRO E. TORIBIO

Metacarpal Disease, Dorsal

BASIC INFORMATION

DEFINITION

Dorsal metacarpal disease (DMD) includes two conditions: dorsal metacarpal periostitis ("bucked shins") and dorsal cortical stress fractures of the third metacarpus (MC-III).

SYNONYM(S)

DMD is also known as *bucked shins complex*. The periostitis is sometimes referred to as *sore shins*. The stress fractures are commonly referred to as *saucer fractures*.

EPIDEMIOLOGY

SPECIES, AGE, SEX DMD affects young flat-racing horses. Bucked shins are classically seen in 2- and 3-year-old racehorses in early training. Dorsal cortical stress fractures of MC-III are typically seen in a slightly older population (3 to 5 years and sometimes older).

GENETICS AND BREED PREDISPOSITION Thoroughbred racehorses, racing Quarter Horses, and racing Arabians

RISK FACTORS DMD is seen more frequently in horses training on a dirt surface (vs. grass). Training regimens that have disproportionately high mileage at a gallop and an inappropriately low proportion of high-speed work favor the development of DMD.

GEOGRAPHY AND SEASONALITY The incidence of DMD is comparatively higher in Thoroughbred racehorses in the United States than in Europe. Differences in racing surfaces likely account for much of this discrepancy, with the majority of horses trained on grass in Europe and on dirt in the United States.

CLINICAL PRESENTATION

HISTORY, CHIEF COMPLAINT

- Horses with bucked shins present with an acute onset of bilateral soft tissue swelling, heat, and sensitivity over the dorsal aspect of the metacarpi, with an

associated lameness or stiffness. Very often this occurs after the first race or first speed work (a "breeze") at near-racing distances. Some horses have a more gradual onset of these signs, with exacerbation after a race or breeze.

- Horses with an acute dorsal cortical stress fracture of MC-III typically exhibit moderate to severe lameness after a high-speed work (breeze) or race.

PHYSICAL EXAM FINDINGS

- In the acute stage, horses with bucked shins exhibit variable degrees of soft tissue swelling, heat, and sensitivity on palpation over the dorsal diaphyses of MC-III. When viewing the metacarpi from the lateral aspect, a distinct dorsal convexity is often seen. Firm pressure in this location often elicits a painful response. Lameness ranges from grade 1 to 3 (American Association of Equine Practitioners scale). These horses exhibit a bilateral stiff or choppy forelimb gait at a trot (sometimes mimicking a foot or carpal lameness). When one metacarpus is more severely affected than the other, a distinct head nod may be recognized. After a short period of rest and antiinflammatory treatment, there is generally considerable improvement.

- In horses with acute stress fractures, soft tissue swelling and signs of inflammation are commonly more focal and overlie a corresponding bony knot or periosteal irregularity (hard swelling or exostosis) along the dorsal or dorsolateral diaphysis of MC-III. Firm pressure at the fracture site consistently elicits a painful response and often exacerbates lameness. Acutely, lameness is moderate to severe (typically grade 3 to 4). With a brief period of rest (a few days to a few weeks), horses generally walk comfortably but remain lame at a trot in-hand (grade 2 to 3). Horses with chronic fractures may exhibit only mild lameness at a trot in-hand.

ETIOLOGY AND PATHOPHYSIOLOGY

- Both components of DMD are the result of maladaptive remodeling associated with repetitive strain of the metacarpus.
- Stress fractures are fatigue fractures resulting from accumulated high-strain cyclic loading.
- The majority of horses with dorsal cortical stress fractures of MC-III have experienced clinical bucked shins in the 6 to 12 months before fracture.
- In the United States, the majority of these fractures involve the left forelimb; this is attributed to the counterclockwise direction of racing.

DIAGNOSIS

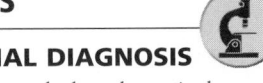

DIFFERENTIAL DIAGNOSIS

Bucked shins and dorsal cortical stress fractures of MC-III are each a differential diagnosis for the other.

INITIAL DATABASE

- Physical and lameness examinations (diagnostic analgesia is usually not necessary in acute cases)
- Radiography (Figure 1)

ADVANCED OR CONFIRMATORY TESTING

Nuclear scintigraphy may be helpful in differentiating a true stress fracture (focal increased radioisotope uptake [IRIU]) from bucked shins (diffuse IRIU) in cases in which radiographs are negative or equivocal.

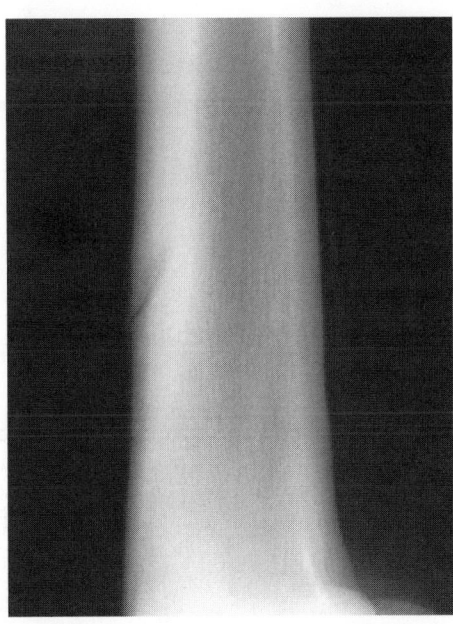

FIGURE 1 Lateral radiograph of the left metacarpus of a horse with a dorsal cortical stress fracture of the third metacarpus (MC-III). The fracture exhibits the most common configuration, propagating in a distodorsal-to-proximopalmar direction.

TREATMENT

THERAPEUTIC GOAL(S)

- Bucked shins
  - Reduce acute inflammation
  - Decrease or eliminate further excessive cyclic strains on MC-III and shift the balance from net bone resorption to net bone apposition
- Dorsal cortical stress fractures: promote fracture healing

ACUTE GENERAL TREATMENT

- Bucked shins
  - Local and systemic antiinflammatory therapy initially (cold therapy, poultice, bandage, nonsteroidal antiinflammatory drugs)
  - Stall rest until soft tissue swelling and pain on palpation have subsided
  - Controlled exercise: handwalking 2 to 4 weeks in mild cases; handwalking and paddock turnout for 1 to 4 months in more severe or chronic or recurrent cases
- Dorsal cortical stress fractures: stall rest and antiinflammatory therapy (as above)

CHRONIC TREATMENT

- Bucked shins
  - Modification of the training protocol to promote adaptive remodeling of the dorsal cortices of MC-III.

- In general, this involves increasing the frequency of high-strain cyclic compressive loading (high-speed exercise or breezes) and decreasing the total distance worked at a gallop.
  - The distances of high-speed work are increased in a slow, incremental manner to allow adaptation.
- Dorsal cortical stress fractures
  - Controlled exercise for 3 to 4 months may be sufficient for healing in some cases.
  - Most horses are best treated surgically to minimize healing time and maximize the likelihood of complete healing (ie, minimize fracture recurrence).
  - Surgical options include osteostixis (cortical drilling), neutral screw placement (unicortical screw), or a combination (Figure 2).
  - Screws are removed in 2 to 3 months, and training can generally resume by 3 to 4 months.

POSSIBLE COMPLICATIONS

In rare cases, a dorsal cortical stress fracture may propagate to a complete, catastrophic fracture of MC-III.

RECOMMENDED MONITORING

Complete fracture healing should be confirmed radiographically before training is resumed.

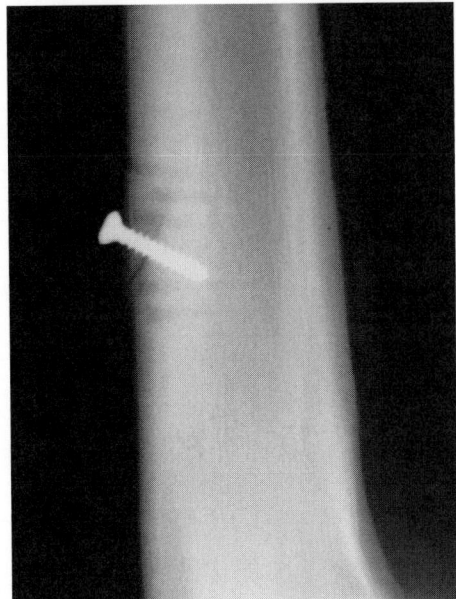

FIGURE 2 Postoperative lateral radiograph of the fracture shown in Figure 1. This horse was treated with a combination of osteostixis (note drill holes) and unicortical screw placement. (The screw was countersunk; the gap is artifactual.)

PREVENTION

Early detection of shin soreness and early intervention should decrease the incidence of both conditions. Chronic or recurrent bucked shins or stress fractures of MC-III can most often be attributed to premature resumption of training or failure to modify the training protocol in young horses.

SUGGESTED READING

Bassage LH: Metacarpus/metatarsus. In Hinchcliff KW, Kaneps AJ, Geor RJ (eds). *Equine sports medicine and surgery*, London, 2004, Saunders Elsevier, pp 319–348.

Dallap BL, Bramlage LR, Embertson RM: Results of screw fixation combined with cortical drilling for treatment of dorsal cortical stress fractures of the third metacarpal bone in 56 Thoroughbred racehorses. *Equine Vet J* 31:252–257, 1999.

Nunamaker DM: The bucked shins complex. In Ross MW, Dyson SJ (eds). *Diagnosis and management of lameness in the horse*, St Louis, 2003, Saunders Elsevier, pp 847–853.

AUTHOR: **LANCE H. BASSAGE II**

EDITOR: **ANDRIS J. KANEPS**

PROGNOSIS AND OUTCOME

The prognosis for both components of DMD is very good to excellent if identified early and appropriate treatment is instituted.

PEARLS & CONSIDERATIONS

COMMENTS

Bucked shins are usually bilateral, and stress fractures are typically unilateral.

Milkweed Toxicosis

BASIC INFORMATION

DEFINITION

Milkweeds are native plants of North America comprising about 150 species capable of causing cardiotoxicity or neurotoxicity in horses and other animals. The toxicity of milkweeds varies with the species. Generally, the narrow-leafed species are more toxic than the broad-leafed species.

SYNONYM(S)

Many plant species contain a milky sap, but the term *milkweed* generally refers to plants of the genus *Asclepias*. Other common names for milkweeds include *butterfly weed*, *pleurisy root*, and *silkweed*.

EPIDEMIOLOGY

GEOGRAPHY AND SEASONALITY
Milkweeds are found throughout North America but especially in the southern and western states (Figures 1 and 2). Some species of milkweed are invasive, forming spreading colonies. Most are perennials. Milkweeds have a milky sap, broad or narrow leaves, single or branched stems that may be prostrate or erect, and terminal clusters of flowers ranging from white to pink to orange in color. Characteristic pods filled with seeds with silky hairs that aid in wind distribution form in late summer.

CLINICAL PRESENTATION

DISEASE FORMS/SUBTYPES Milkweeds are either cardiotoxic or neurotoxic depending on the species. The cardiotoxic species generally have broad, heavily textured leaves that are rarely palatable to animals unless they are without good forage. Examples of the cardiotoxic species are *Asclepias speciosa*, *Asclepias eriocarpa*, and *Asclepias labriformis*. The neurotoxic species generally have narrow (grasslike) leaves and tend to be quite palatable green or dried. Some neurotoxic species also contain cardiotoxins. Examples of the neurotoxic species include *Asclepias subverticillata*, *Asclepias fascicularis*, *Asclepias pumila*, and *Asclepias incarnata*.

HISTORY, CHIEF COMPLAINT Animals eating the broad-leafed milkweeds exhibit cardiotoxic and gastrointestinal signs. Neurotoxic milkweeds cause neurologic signs, including weakness, ataxia, muscle tremors, recumbency, and tetanic seizures.

PHYSICAL EXAM FINDINGS
- Cardiotoxic milkweeds induce primarily a gastrointestinal syndrome characterized by signs of colic, including teeth grinding, reluctance to stand, and diarrhea. Rarely are cardiac dysrhythmias detected. Death may occur suddenly without signs of convulsions.
- Horses that have eaten as little as 1 kg of the neurotoxic species of milkweed show signs of colic, weakness, and

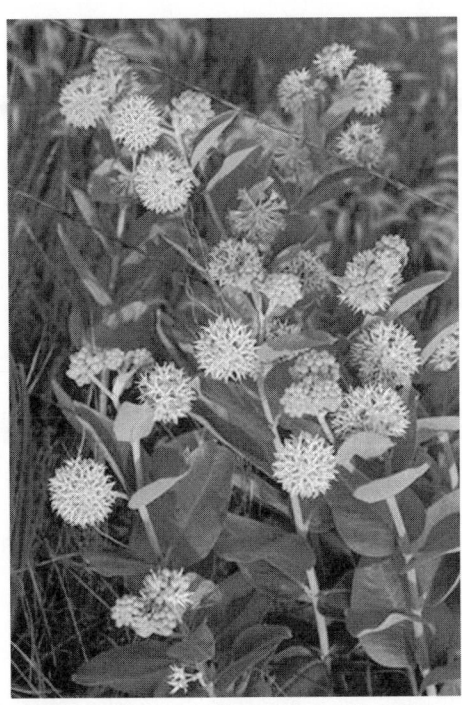

FIGURE 1 Showy milkweed (*Asclepias speciosa*).

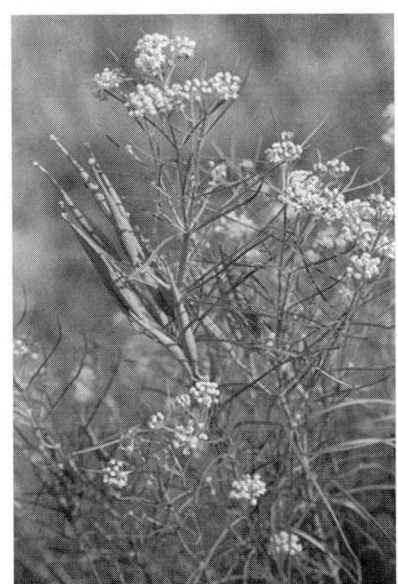

FIGURE 2 Whorled milkweed (*Asclepias subverticillata*).

incoordination progressing to recumbency and tetanic seizures. Clonic seizures with paddling of the legs may develop. Death may follow the seizures or the horse may recover.

ETIOLOGY AND PATHOPHYSIOLOGY

- Steroidal glycosides known as *cardenolides* are present in the broad-leafed milkweeds.
- Cardenolides are highest in the sap and early plant growth.
- Neurotoxic milkweeds contain poorly defined glycosides.
- The specific sites of action of the cardenolides and neurotoxic glycosides are poorly understood.
- Milkweeds are potentially toxic at any time, even when dried in hay.

DIAGNOSIS

DIFFERENTIAL DIAGNOSIS

- Ionophore toxicity
- Oleander (*Nerium oleander*) toxicity
- Foxglove (*Digitalis* spp.) toxicity
- Viral encephalitis, rabies, Eastern and Western equine encephalitis
- Other causes of CNS signs, such as viral, bacterial, and parasitic infections

INITIAL DATABASE

- Hematocrit: Reflects dehydration.
- No specific serum biochemical or CBC analysis abnormalities are characteristic of milkweed poisoning.

ADVANCED OR CONFIRMATORY TESTING

- A field test for detecting cardenolides in the milkweed latex is available.
- The stomach contents may yield detectable cardenolides.
- No gross lesions are detectable at necropsy.

TREATMENT

THERAPEUTIC GOAL(S)

Manage symptoms as necessary.

ACUTE GENERAL TREATMENT

- No specific antidote is available.
- Use of activated charcoal should be considered when the milkweed has been consumed in the previous few hours.
- General supportive treatment such as IV polyionic fluids should be provided.
- Animals with seizures should be sedated with diazepam.

PROGNOSIS AND OUTCOME

The prognosis depends on the quantity of the toxic milkweeds consumed. Animals observed with clinical signs have a better prognosis because lethal doses usually cause acute death.

PEARLS & CONSIDERATIONS

COMMENTS

Milkweed poisoning is only likely to occur when horses are deprived of adequate nutrition and are hungry. Hay should always be carefully inspected before it is fed to horses because the narrow-leafed milkweeds remain toxic even when dried.

PREVENTION

- Feed weed-free hay.
- Selective herbicides can be used to control invasive perennial species.

CLIENT EDUCATION

Recognition and removal of milkweed species in the environment can do much to prevent milkweed poisoning.

SUGGESTED READING

Burrows GE, Tyrl RJ: Asclepiadaceae. In Burrows GE, Tyrl RJ (eds). *Toxic plants of North America*, Ames, IA, 2001, Iowa State University Press, pp 125–135.
Sady MB, Seiber JN: Field test for screening milkweed latex for cardenolides. *J Natural Products* 54:1105–1107, 1991.

AUTHOR: **ANTHONY P. KNIGHT**

EDITOR: **CYNTHIA L. GASKILL**

Mitral/Tricuspid Regurgitation, Acquired

BASIC INFORMATION

DEFINITION

- Mitral valve regurgitation is the most important valvular condition affecting athletic performance in horses. It may be caused by dysfunction of any part of the mitral valve apparatus, including the valve annulus, leaflets, chordae tendineae, or papillary muscles.
- The etiology remains unclear. Degenerative myxomatous changes as well as cellular infiltration with lymphocytes, histiocytes, and fibroblasts in the valves leading to general or nodular thickening are often reported. In addition, physical training may result in regurgitation because of training-induced myocardial hypertrophy. This may expand the valvular annulus, leading to valvular incompetence, but in these cases, the valves may also be affected pathologically.
- Whereas mitral regurgitation may affect athletic performance, tricuspid valve regurgitation rarely gives rise to clinical signs in horses.

SYNONYM(S)

- Mitral or tricuspid insufficiency
- Mitral or tricuspid valve disease
- Atrioventricular (AV) valve regurgitation or insufficiency

EPIDEMIOLOGY

SPECIES, AGE, SEX Horses of all ages and both sexes can be affected, but degenerative changes are most frequently seen in middle-aged or older horses.
GENETICS AND BREED PREDISPOSITION There is no genetic predisposition, but the prevalence appears higher in Standardbreds and Thoroughbreds compared with the general horse population.
ASSOCIATED CONDITIONS AND DISORDERS Depends on the severity of the regurgitation

CLINICAL PRESENTATION

DISEASE FORMS/SUBTYPES

- Mitral or tricuspid regurgitation incidentally diagnosed in clinically normal horses
- Mitral (or very rarely tricuspid) regurgitation causing clinical signs of reduced performance or in severe cases signs of heart failure

HISTORY, CHIEF COMPLAINT

- With mild regurgitation, there are no clinical signs. This may also be the case with even severe tricuspid regurgitation.

- If regurgitation is more severe, there may be signs of poor performance (eg, increased respiratory effort after or during work, reduced exercise tolerance).

PHYSICAL EXAM FINDINGS

- A systolic cardiac murmur will be heard at the apical area of the left hemi-thorax (mitral regurgitation) or right hemi-thorax (tricuspid regurgitation). The intensity of the murmur is not always an accurate guide to the severity of the disease. However, in general, loud murmurs occurring throughout systole are more often associated with significant disease than quiet murmurs of shorter duration, particularly if a palpable thrill accompanies the loud murmur.
- Depending on the severity of the regurgitation, one or more of the following signs may be observed:
  ○ Resting tachycardia
  ○ Resting tachypnea
  ○ Cough
  ○ Distension or pulsation of the jugular veins
  ○ Dependent edema (primarily ventral, not limb)
  ○ Increased respiratory sounds
  ○ Cardiac arrhythmia (eg, atrial fibrillation or atrial premature complexes [APCs])
  ○ Nasal froth caused by pulmonary edema (only in cases of severe heart failure)
  ○ Prolonged capillary refill time (only in cases of severe heart failure)
  ○ Weight loss

ETIOLOGY AND PATHOPHYSIOLOGY

- Initiating factors leading to degenerative changes of the valvular apparatus are unknown.
- An insidious onset of mitral regurgitation can generally be completely compensated for years without clinical signs.
- Compensatory mechanisms include atrial and ventricular dilatation; eccentric hypertrophy; and increased resting HR, contractility of the ventricles, and lymphatic drainage.
- For a minor proportion of horses with mitral regurgitation, the valvular regurgitation can no longer be compensated, leading to signs of left-sided heart failure with pulmonary edema. Initially, this may only manifest during high demand such as more strenuous exercise, but as the disease progresses, compensatory mechanisms fail, and tachycardia, coughing, and frothy fluid at the nostrils are observed when the

horse is at rest. Eventually, signs of right-sided heart failure may appear, including edema and distension of the jugular veins.
- Rarely, acute mitral regurgitation develops (eg, secondary to rupture of major chorda tendineae), and in these situations, pulmonary pressures increase abruptly with development of pulmonary edema. Shortly thereafter, signs of right-sided heart failure develop with dependent edema and distension of the jugular veins.
- Severe mitral regurgitation is the most common cause of heart failure in horses.
- The mitral valve and the aortic valve are the most common locations for bacterial endocarditis (see "Endocarditis, Infective" in this section); however, the disease is not commonly encountered.
- Tricuspid regurgitation rarely causes clinical signs. If the regurgitation is severe, signs of right-sided heart failure may develop with jugular distension, jugular pulsation, and dependent edema.
- Murmurs of tricuspid, mitral, and aortic regurgitation are often detected in Standardbred and Thoroughbred racehorses. They may develop in response to training, and the prevalence may increase with age and training. However, the regurgitations are generally mild and remain constant over time, with no negative effect on racing performance documented.

DIAGNOSIS

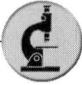

DIFFERENTIAL DIAGNOSIS

- Functional murmur (systolic flow murmur, systolic ejection murmur). Large stroke volume and large diameters of the great vessels induce turbulent blood flow in the aortic and pulmonary artery roots in early systole, which leads to early or mid-systolic murmurs heard at the basal area that are of no clinical significance.
- Physiologic murmurs caused by systemic diseases such as colic, anemia, septicemia, or endotoxemia.
- Endocarditis.
- Ventricular septal defect (VSD). This is an important differential diagnosis for tricuspid regurgitation. Typically, the murmur associated with VSD is lower on the chest wall toward the sternum. In addition, a systolic murmur over the pulmonary valve on the left hemi-

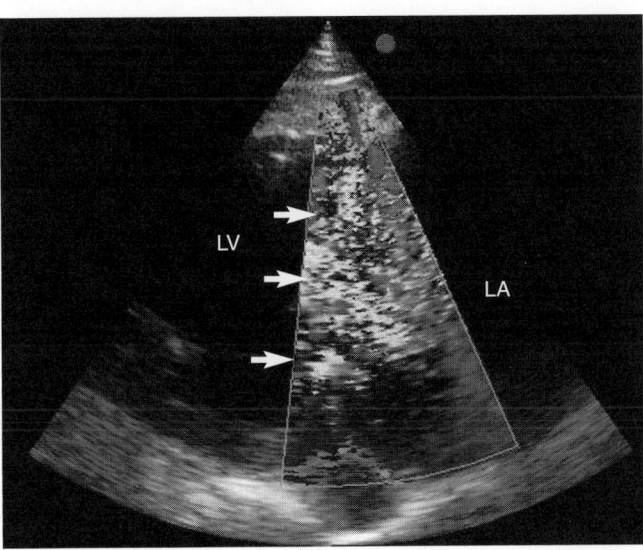

FIGURE 1 Long-axis color flow Doppler echocardiogram of the left atrium and ventricle obtained from the left cardiac window showing severe mitral regurgitation (*arrows*). LA, left atrium LV, left ventricle.

thorax is often heard because of relative pulmonic stenosis.

INITIAL DATABASE

- Definitive diagnosis of mitral or tricuspid regurgitation requires echocardiographic examination with the regurgitant jet visualized by Doppler echocardiography (Figure 1).
- The severity of the disease can be assessed by echocardiography. Generally, extensive nodular changes on the valve and ruptured chordae tendineae indicate more severe pathology. In addition, the dimensions of the left ventricle, left atrium, and pulmonary artery are of significant importance when evaluating mitral regurgitation. The size of the regurgitant jet can be estimated by Doppler echocardiography. However, the size of the jet is influenced by a variety of factors and should always be compared with the size of the cardiac chambers as well the contractility of the myocardium.
- Electrocardiography (ECG) for diagnosing arrhythmias such as atrial fibrillation and atrial premature complexes
- Complete blood cell counts and serum biochemistry results are usually unremarkable.

ADVANCED OR CONFIRMATORY TESTING

To assess the significance of the valvular regurgitation during exercise, exercising ECG is of great value. If possible, exercise testing on a treadmill is preferable because arterial oxygen measurements can be obtained continuously during exercise. Stress echocardiography immediately after exercise may be helpful to assess myocardial function.

TREATMENT

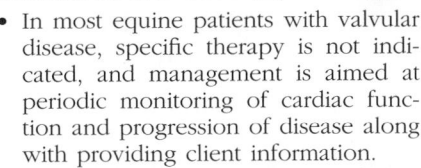

THERAPEUTIC GOAL(S)

- In most equine patients with valvular disease, specific therapy is not indicated, and management is aimed at periodic monitoring of cardiac function and progression of disease along with providing client information.
- Supportive therapy is indicated if heart failure is present. Treatment of horses in heart failure is primarily recommended to make the horse more comfortable. This is most often used for some breeding horses and horses to which the owner is very emotionally attached and wishes to try any treatment to prolong lifespan.

ACUTE GENERAL TREATMENT

- Supportive treatment of patient in heart failure includes diuretics to reduce congestion (furosemide 1–2 mg/kg IV q12h) in combination with a vasodilator such as an angiotensin-converting enzyme (ACE) inhibitor (eg, enalapril 0.5 mg/kg IV q24h) (see "Cardiac Failure" in this section).
- If severe tachycardia is present, digoxin can be given at a dose of 0.0022 mg/kg IV q12h or 0.011 mg/kg PO q24h. For more treatment details, see "Cardiac Failure" in this section.

CHRONIC TREATMENT

As for acute treatment (see "Cardiac Failure" in this section), with drugs and doses tailored to the individual horse's clinical signs

POSSIBLE COMPLICATIONS

- Reoccurrence of heart failure or no effect of treatment
- Tachyarrhythmias
- Syncope or ataxia

RECOMMENDED MONITORING

- Clinical exam findings such as attitude, appetite, weight, respiratory rate and effort, heart rate, and exercise tolerance should be monitored by the owner regularly. Any changes should prompt a veterinary reexamination.
- Periodic ECGs and echocardiograms to assess progression of regurgitation or heart failure.

PROGNOSIS AND OUTCOME

- For mitral regurgitation, a good prognosis can be given if the regurgitant jet is small, no structural changes of the valve are identified, and the size of the cardiac chambers and myocardial function are within normal values. However, the progression can be unpredictable, so the significance of mitral regurgitation for future athletic use is difficult to predict at the time of initial examination. Serial examinations to gauge changes over time will help to predict more long-range progression.
- For tricuspid regurgitation, the prognosis is generally good, although severe cases may lead to right-sided heart failure.

PEARLS & CONSIDERATIONS

CLIENT EDUCATION

- The owner should be informed of common signs of heart failure to recognize them if they develop and should be in the habit of checking the horse regularly.
- Athletic performance may be negatively affected by valvular insufficiency; therefore, a reduction of activity level may be needed.
- Because of the unpredictable nature of the progression of mitral regurgitation, this is regarded as a preexisting condition by most insurance companies and may thus be subject to exclusion from the insurance policy. In addition, the resale value of the horse may be affected because future buyers may be discouraged. Therefore, the sale prices of horses are often reduced in cases of diagnosed valvular regurgitation greater than insignificant or mild.

SUGGESTED READING

Buhl R, Ersbøll AK, Eriksen L, Koch J: Use of color Doppler echocardiography to assess the development of valvular regurgitation in Standardbred Trotters. *J Am Vet Med Assoc* 227:1630, 2005.

Else RW, Holmes JR: Cardiac pathology in the horse. Microscopic pathology. *Equine Vet J* 4:57–62, 1972.

Gehlen H, Vieht JC, Stadler P: Effects of the ACE inhibitor quinapril on Echocardiographic variables in horses with mitral valve insufficiency. *J Vet Med A Physiol Pathol Clin Med* 50:460–465, 2003.

Marr CM: Cardiac murmurs: Acquired valvular disease. In Marr CM (ed). *Cardiology of the horse*, London, 1999, WB Saunders, pp 232–255.

Reef VB, Bain FT, Spencer PA: Severe mitral regurgitation in horses: clinical, echocardiographic and pathological findings. *Equine Vet J* 30:18–27, 1998.

AUTHOR: **RIKKE BUHL**

EDITOR: **MARY M. DURANDO**

Motor Neuron Disease, Equine

BASIC INFORMATION

DEFINITION

An acquired destruction of lower motor neurons in the brainstem and spinal cord of affected horses leading to clinical signs characterized by postural weakness and muscle atrophy

SYNONYM(S)

Equine motor neuron disease (EMND) resembles progressive muscular atrophy (a form of amyotrophic lateral sclerosis [ALS], or Lou Gehrig's disease) seen in humans. However, only lower motor neurons are affected with EMND in contrast to upper and lower motor neurons with ALS.

EPIDEMIOLOGY

SPECIES, AGE, SEX Age: Older horses are at a higher risk than young animals (range, 2–23 years). Peak incidence occurs at 16 years of age and then declines.

GENETICS AND BREED PREDISPOSITION

- Breed: Quarter Horses appear to be more likely to develop the disease. Appaloosas, Standardbreds, and Thoroughbreds are also reported.
- Genetic factors: A mutation affecting vitamin E metabolism occurs in other species with similar conditions.

RISK FACTORS

- Unknown and likely multifactorial mechanism of acquiring disease.
- A depleted vitamin E status is strongly incriminated as a causal factor in the disease. Affected animals have lower levels than normal control subjects on the same premises.
- The vast majority of cases have limited or no access to grass.
- Concentrate feeding with poor-quality hay: Pelleted ration or supplement feeding lacking vitamin E
- Stall confinement
- Pica: Wood
- Coprophagia

- Malabsorption: Concurrent enteric or hepatic disease
- Iron and copper supplementation

GEOGRAPHY AND SEASONALITY

- United States: New England states have highest incidence, decreasing toward the west and south.
- Also reported in Canada, British Isles, Europe, Japan, and South America.
- Sporadic occurrence of isolated cases. Outbreaks have been reported.

CLINICAL PRESENTATION

HISTORY, CHIEF COMPLAINT

- In early cases, weight and muscle loss despite a normal to increased appetite.
- Muscle tremors, sweating, and increased periods of recumbency are seen.
- Tends to stabilize or improve 1 or 2 months after the onset of signs. Muscle tremors and periods of recumbency tend to become less frequent.
- Progression of signs after a period of stabilization does occur.
- Body weight may return to prediseased levels as the horse accumulates fat.
- A subclinical syndrome has been recognized; however, the athletic ability is permanently impaired to varying degrees.

PHYSICAL EXAM FINDINGS

- Marked muscle wasting is common, especially of the antigravity muscles (triceps, quadriceps, gluteals). May precede neurologic signs by up to 1 month.
- Horse prefers to stand with the legs gathered beneath them.
- Trembling is exacerbated by standing the horse in a fixed location, with constant shifting of weight from one hindlimb to the other occurring. The horse is more comfortable when walking.
- Unable to engage stay apparatus
- An abnormally low head carriage and short stride length are common.
- No ataxia or loss of proprioception is noted (compare with equine degenerative myeloencephalopathy [EDM]).

- The tail head appears raised (dorsal coccygeal muscle wasting), and excessive sweating is seen in more than half of the patients.

ETIOLOGY AND PATHOPHYSIOLOGY

- The precise cause of EMND is not known.
- Impaired vitamin E metabolism: Absorption or retention may be affected in horses with malabsorptive disease.
- Pro-oxidant factor excess: Elevated iron and copper levels in some affected horses.
- Antioxidant activity deficient in the central nervous system: Similar to EDM.
- Loss of highly oxidative type I muscle fibers: Characteristic antigravity muscle wasting and weakness.
- Endothelial lipopigment: Spinal cord capillaries indicative of oxidative damage.

DIAGNOSIS

DIFFERENTIAL DIAGNOSIS

- Botulism
- Organophosphate, lead, and other toxicities
- Myositis or myopathy
- Malabsorptive disorders
- Laminitis
- Protozoal myeloencephalitis
- Neglect

INITIAL DATABASE

- No definitive premortem diagnostic test exists.
- Serum chemistry: Signs of myopathy (elevated creatinine kinase, aspartate aminotransferase) but not specific for EMND.
- Plasma glucose concentrations are normal in all horses, but the mean peak value after an oral glucose absorption test may be low.
- Plasma vitamin E concentrations: Significantly lower than in normal control subjects; collect serial samples throughout the day and pool samples to level diurnal variability.

ADVANCED OR CONFIRMATORY TESTING

- Needle electromyographic studies: Consistently abnormal; suggestive of denervation. Prolonged insertional activity, fibrillation potentials and positive sharp waves are frequently recorded in cervical, facial, triceps, quadriceps, and tail head musculature.
- Ophthalmic examination: Varying degrees of a mosaic pattern of dark brown to yellow brown pigment (ceroid lipofuscin) deposited in the pigmented retinal epithelium of 30% of cases; no visual deficits noted.
- Glucose tolerance test, xylose absorption: Low peak absorption may occur.
- CSF: Cytology normal; protein and IgG levels may be increased.
- Muscle biopsy: Atrophy of predominantly type I fibers.
- Nerve biopsy: Ventral branch of spinal accessory nerve; Wallerian degeneration of axons and Schwann cell proliferation is diagnostic; loss of myelination occurs in chronic cases.
- Necropsy: Gross evaluation of peripheral nerves and central nervous tissue are unremarkable.
- Histopathology: Definitive diagnosis. Loss of neurons in ventral horns of the spinal cord (lower motor neuron); degeneration of brainstem cranial nerve nuclei (except III, IV, and VI); ceroid lipofuscin in the retinal epithelium and spinal cord capillaries; angular degeneration of type I muscle fibers; widespread signs of muscle degeneration (denervation atrophy).

TREATMENT

THERAPEUTIC GOAL(S)

Avoid further deterioration in affected horses.

ACUTE GENERAL TREATMENT

- Oral vitamin E supplementation: Appears to have improved the clinical syndrome in a few cases (6000–10,000 IU q24h).
- Antioxidants: Dimethyl sulfoxide may be of benefit initially.
- Antiinflammatory drugs: Corticosteroids may be helpful in acute onset cases.

PROGNOSIS AND OUTCOME

- Grave prognosis for affected animals.
- Progressive deterioration and euthanasia in large percentage of horses (40%) regardless of treatment.
- A similar percentage may stabilize and improve with treatment and management changes in the short to medium term. Recrudescence of disease leads to unremitting progression of disease.
- A minority survive medium term with permanent muscle wasting deficits.

PEARLS & CONSIDERATIONS

COMMENTS

Incidence has decreased with greater awareness of need for vitamin E supplementation in grain-based concentrate rations.

PREVENTION

Vitamin E supplementation (2000 IU q24h) for horses with limited pasture or green hay access for a prolonged period

CLIENT EDUCATION

Neuronal cell death is irreversible.

SUGGESTED READING

MacKay R: Neurodegenerative disorders. In Furr M, Reed S (eds). *Equine neurology*, Ames, IA, 2008, Blackwell Publishing, pp 235–256.

Mayhew IG: Nutritional diseases. In Mayhew IG (ed). *Large animal neurology*, ed 2, Ames, IA, 2009, Wiley Blackwell, pp 360–373.

Nout YS: Equine motor neuron disease. In Reed S, Bayly W, Sellon D (eds). *Equine internal medicine*, ed 3, St Louis, 2010, Saunders Elsevier, pp 634–637.

AUTHOR: **PETER R. MORRESEY**

EDITOR: **STEPHEN M. REED**

Multiple Organ Dysfunction Syndrome

BASIC INFORMATION

DEFINITION

Multiple organ dysfunction syndrome (MODS) typically occurs because of unchecked systemic inflammation as seen in the systemic inflammatory response syndrome (SIRS) or sepsis.

EPIDEMIOLOGY

SPECIES, AGE, SEX Any age or breed may be at risk for MODS because of trauma, infection, or inflammation that remains untreated or unresolved.

CLINICAL PRESENTATION

HISTORY, CHIEF COMPLAINT Horses with a history of critical illness or traumatic injury with a systemic inflammatory response are at risk for the development of MODS.

PHYSICAL EXAM FINDINGS Physical examination findings are variable and specific to the organ system involved but may include:

- Depression, lethargy
- Injected mucous membranes, increased capillary refill time
- Tachycardia or bradycardia, poor pulse quality, cool extremities
- Tachypnea
- Decreased borborygmi, decreased fecal output, colic
- Fever or hypothermia

ETIOLOGY AND PATHOPHYSIOLOGY

- Primary MODS is organ dysfunction caused by an initial disease or infectious process resulting in injury to an organ system.
- Secondary MODS is organ dysfunction caused by the systemic inflammatory response syndrome or sepsis (see "Systemic Inflammatory Response Syndrome" in this section).
- Organ systems commonly affected include:
  - Central nervous system
  - Respiratory system
  - Renal or urinary system
  - Cardiovascular system
  - Coagulation system
  - Gastrointestinal system
  - Musculoskeletal system
  - Hepatobiliary system

DIAGNOSIS

DIFFERENTIAL DIAGNOSIS

Insult or injury to an organ system caused by infection or inflammation may occur without organ failure, which indicates sepsis or SIRS but not MODS.

INITIAL DATABASE

- Packed cell volume
- Total protein

- Complete blood count and differential
- Serum chemistry
- Blood lactate
- Blood pressure
- Blood gas
- Coagulation profile
- Urinalysis

ADVANCED OR CONFIRMATORY TESTING

Relates to the specific system involved:
- Central nervous system: Neurologic exam, cerebrospinal fluid analysis
- Respiratory: Thoracic ultrasonography, radiography, transtracheal wash
- Renal: Analysis of fractional excretion of electrolytes, renal biopsy, cystoscopy
- Cardiovascular: Echocardiography, cardiac output monitoring, electrocardiography
- Coagulation system: Additional coagulation tests (D-dimer, protein C, thromboelastography)
- Gastrointestinal: Glucose absorption testing, fecal cultures, fecal egg count, biopsy
- Musculoskeletal: Pedal venogram

TREATMENT

THERAPEUTIC GOAL(S)

- Identify organ failure early.
- Treat the initiating cause of systemic inflammation or primary cause of organ dysfunction.
- Provide supportive care and optimize tissue perfusion.

ACUTE GENERAL TREATMENT

- Therapy is based on the organ systems that are failing; however, general supportive care is indicated as for SIRS.
- Early goal-directed therapy may reduce the risk of tissue hypoxia and shock (see "Shock, Hypovolemic" in this section).
- Fluid therapy
  - Shock-dose fluid administration (see "Shock-Dose Fluid Administration" in Section II) when indicated
  - Maintenance fluids to maintain tissue perfusion without causing tissue edema (see "Dehydration" in this section)
- Inotropes and vasopressors for cardiovascular support (see "Shock, Hypovolemic" in this section)
- Oxygen therapy mechanical ventilation based on response and blood gas analysis

- Antimicrobial therapy: Broad spectrum initially, narrowed by culture results of the local infectious process
- Antiendotoxin therapy
  - Hyperimmune plasma (against *Salmonella typhimurium,* or J5 *Escherichia coli*)
    - Antibodies bind and clear endotoxin using the innate immune system.
    - Dose: 1.5 mL/kg J5 serum diluted twofold in crystalloid solution.
    - Results are conflicting, and therapy may increase endotoxic effects.
    - Drawbacks include high financial cost and risk of adverse immune reactions.
  - Polymixin B
    - Binds to circulating endotoxin and prevents interaction with its receptors
    - Dose: 6000 U/kg diluted to 500 mL IV q8–12h
    - Risk of nephrotoxicity in dehydrated horses
  - Nonsteroidal antiinflammatory medications
    - Block the production of eicosanoids and reduces inflammation
    - Flunixin meglumine appears most beneficial in ameliorating clinical signs (1.1 mg/kg, IV q12h).
    - The antiendotoxin dose (0.25 mg/kg, IV q8h) reduces inflammatory mediators, but does not eliminate signs of endotoxemia.
- Closely monitor serum glucose; may reduce mortality and inflammation (noted in human medicine). Insulin may be supplied (0.1–1 IU/kg/h) to maintain normoglycemia.
- Low-dose corticosteroid therapy may be beneficial for patients with critical illness related to corticosteroid insufficiency.
  - Identified by low serum cortisol and lack of response to exogenous adrenocorticotropin
  - May require low-dose prednisolone or hydrocortisone
  - Risk of laminitis with corticosteroid therapy should be considered
- Treat coagulopathies (see "Disseminated Intravascular Coagulation" in this section)
- Surgically debride septic foci
- Antioxidant therapy
  - Dimethylsulfoxide IV
  - Vitamin E IM

- Gastrointestinal protectants
  - Glutamine may provide supportive nutrition to enterocytes to maintain gastrointestinal barrier.
  - Antiulcer medications are commonly prescribed because of the risk of ulcers with anorexia.
    - Omeprazole is preferred.
    - Ranitidine may be effective in foals (1.5 mg/kg IV q8h).
    - May increase risk of infection because of loss of protective gastric acid

RECOMMENDED MONITORING

- Vital parameters should be monitored closely for change.
- The initial database should be repeated at intervals based on initial findings and new results.

PROGNOSIS AND OUTCOME

- Guarded prognosis
- In humans, as the number of organs involved increases, the mortality rate also increases up to 100% mortality with four organ systems involved.

PEARLS & CONSIDERATIONS

COMMENTS

- Horses with systemic inflammation or a septic process should be monitored closely for changes in any physical parameter and for any sign of impending organ failure.
- Those with one organ failure should be monitored closely for a new system failure, which may greatly reduce prognosis.

PREVENTION

Horses with sepsis or SIRS should be treated aggressively to prevent failure of any organ system.

SUGGESTED READING

Johnson V, Gaynor A, Chan DL, et al: Multiple organ dysfunction syndrome in humans and dogs. *J Vet Emerg Crit Care* 14(3):158–166, 2004.

Roy MF: Sepsis in adults and foals. *Vet Clin North Am Equine Pract* 20:41–61, 2004.

AUTHOR: **AMELIA MUNSTERMAN**

EDITORS: **R. REID HANSON** and **AMELIA MUNSTERMAN**

Mushroom Toxicosis

BASIC INFORMATION

DEFINITION

Clinical condition caused by ingestion of any of a variety of toxic mushrooms. The toxic syndrome produced depends on mushroom type and amount ingested.

SYNONYM(S)

- Gastrointestinal (GI) irritant mushrooms: Large variety of species
- Isoxazole mushrooms: *Amanita gemmata*, *Amanita muscaria*, *Amanita smithiana*, *Amanita strobiliformis*, and *Tricholoma muscarium*
- Muscarinic mushrooms: *Inocybe* spp., *Clitocybe* spp.
- Hallucinogenic mushrooms: *Psilocybe* spp., *Panaeolus* spp.
- Hepatotoxic mushrooms: See "Amanitin Toxicosis" in this section

EPIDEMIOLOGY

SPECIES, AGE, SEX

- All mammalian species are susceptible.
- Reports of nonhepatotoxic mushroom exposures in horses are very rare, so few signs are reported. However, exposure to toxic mushrooms is expected to cause similar signs in horses as in other species.

GEOGRAPHY AND SEASONALITY

- GI: Wide distribution throughout North America; large range of fruiting seasons
- Isoxazoles: Throughout the eastern United States and the Pacific Northwest; coniferous and deciduous forests; fruits in spring and early summer and then again in fall
- Muscarinic: Wide distribution; forests or fields; fruits in fall or early winter in temperate areas and year round in warm, moist climates
- Hallucinogenic: Wide distribution, especially in the Pacific Northwest and Gulf Coast; lawns, gardens, roadsides, open woods; cultivated in homes for recreational use

ASSOCIATED CONDITIONS AND DISORDERS

- GI: Acute, self-limiting GI distress
- Isoxazole: Acute inebriation followed by coma; generally self-limiting
- Muscarinic: Acute muscarinic signs
- Hallucinogenic: Acute central nervous system (CNS) signs, generally self-limiting

CLINICAL PRESENTATION

HISTORY, CHIEF COMPLAINT

- History of exposure to mushrooms; presence of mushrooms in pasture; presence of mushroom parts in mouth and stomach contents
- GI: Abdominal discomfort, diarrhea within 4 hours of exposure
- Isoxazole: Abdominal discomfort, ataxia, and disorientation progressing to sleep or coma within 4 hours of ingestion
- Muscarinic: Hypersalivation, abdominal discomfort, diarrhea, lacrimation, and bradycardia within 4 hours of ingestion
- Hallucinogenic: Disorientation, dysphoria, ataxia, agitation, and hyperesthesia within 30 minutes to 2 hours of ingestion

PHYSICAL EXAM FINDINGS

- GI: Dehydration possible; abdominal discomfort and diarrhea
- Isoxazole: As described above; seizures may occur rarely
- Muscarinic: As described above; moist lung sounds
- Hallucinogenic: As described above; seizures may occur rarely

ETIOLOGY AND PATHOPHYSIOLOGY

- GI: Several mechanisms proposed, including hypersensitivity, local irritation, induced enzyme deficiencies
- Isoxazole: Muscimol mimics γ-aminobutyric acid (GABA), resulting in sedation; ibotenic acid acts on glutamate receptors to cause CNS stimulation; combined effects result in hyperesthesia, sedation, intermittent agitation, and "hallucinations" (reported in humans)
- Muscarinic: Bind muscarinic acetylcholine receptors in parasympathetic nervous system; prolonged duration because of lack of degradation; does not inhibit acetylcholinesterase
- Hallucinogenic: Stimulate serotonin and norepinephrine receptors in the CNS and peripheral nervous system

DIAGNOSIS

DIFFERENTIAL DIAGNOSIS

- GI, isoxazole: Primary and secondary colic, GI foreign body
- Isoxazole, hallucinogenic: Encephalitis, hepatic encephalopathy, locoism, equine leukoencephalomalacia
- Muscarinic: Slaframine, organophosphorous and carbamate pesticide toxicosis

INITIAL DATABASE

Complete blood count, serum biochemistry profile

ADVANCED OR CONFIRMATORY TESTING

- Isoxazole: Muscimol can be detected in urine, but this analysis can have a long turnaround time
- GI, isoxazole, hallucinogenic, and muscarinic: No specific necropsy lesions expected

TREATMENT

THERAPEUTIC GOAL(S)

- Manage life-threatening conditions
- Manage clinical signs
- Decontaminate the patient
- Provide supportive care as needed

ACUTE GENERAL TREATMENT

- Manage life-threatening conditions.
  - Control seizures (isoxazole, hallucinogenic mushrooms)
    - Diazepam: 0.05 to 0.4 mg/kg slow IV for foals, 25 to 50 mg total dose slow IV for adults; repeat as needed
    - Barbiturates, gas anesthetics may be required if diazepam is ineffective
  - Excessive bronchial secretions and bradycardia (muscarinic mushrooms)
    - Atropine: 0.01 to 0.02 mg/kg IV
- Manage clinical signs
  - Flunixin meglumine (1.1 mg/kg IV as needed) for abdominal discomfort
  - Xylazine (1.1 mg/kg IV) or detomidine (20–40 μg/kg IV) for agitation, hyperesthesia
  - Cyproheptadine (0.3–0.6 mg/kg PO or per rectum) for dysphoria associated with hallucinogenic mushrooms. Note: This has been used successfully in small animal patients, but efficacy in horses is unknown.
- Decontamination: Activated charcoal (1–4 g/kg) via stomach tube; repeat in 8 hours if signs are still present.
- Supportive care
  - Thermoregulation
  - Confinement for dysphoric, disoriented horses to prevent accidental injury. A quiet, dark, padded environment is preferred.

RECOMMENDED MONITORING

Hydration, electrolytes if severe diarrhea

PROGNOSIS AND OUTCOME

Generally good prognosis with supportive care

PEARLS & CONSIDERATIONS

- Because of the difficulty in differentiating between toxic and nontoxic mushrooms, any inges-tion of unidentified mushrooms by horses should merit decontamination (activated charcoal) and monitoring.
- Identification of mushrooms is best done by a mycologist; local college biology departments or museums are potential sources of expertise. The use of keys or photos, in the attempted identification of mushrooms should be avoided because these can be extremely unreliable in the hands of inexperienced individuals.
- Only two case reports of nonhepato-toxic mushroom toxicosis were found in the literature; both of these involved hallucinogenic mushroom ingestions, and the animals made full recoveries.

SUGGESTED READING

Jones J: "Magic mushroom" poisoning in a colt. *Vet Rec* 127:603, 1990.
Tegzes JH, Puschner B: Toxic mushrooms. *Vet Clin Small Anim Pract* 32:297–407, 2002.

AUTHOR: **SHARON GWALTNEY-BRANT**

EDITOR: **CYNTHIA L. GASKILL**

Myeloencephalitis, Equine Herpesvirus-1

BASIC INFORMATION

DEFINITION

An uncommon manifestation of infection with equine herpesvirus-1 (EHV-1; an α-herpesvirus), resulting in a diffuse and multifocal neurologic disease caused by widespread vasculitis, thrombosis, and ischemic necrosis of neural tissue

SYNONYM(S)

- Equine herpesvirus myeloencephalop-athy
- Equine rhinopneumonitis
- Neurologic herpesvirus

EPIDEMIOLOGY

SPECIES, AGE, SEX

- Females are more commonly affected.
- Foals rarely show neurologic disease during outbreaks in adults.
- Horses younger than 3 years are less likely to develop the condition.

GENETICS AND BREED PREDISPOSI-TION Ponies and smaller breeds are less likely to develop the condition.

RISK FACTORS

- Crowding
- Contact with transient or sale horses
- Presence of latently infected horses in the herd

CONTAGION AND ZOONOSIS

- Sporadic cases or multiple horses over a prolonged period within a limited area.
- Recrudescence of latent infection important in spread of disease, which may occur in close populations of horses.
- Infection is by inhalation or ingestion of infective aerosol of virus. The disease may also spread by direct contact with infected discharges (saliva, ocular, nasal and abortion products) of shedding horses.

GEOGRAPHY AND SEASONALITY

- Ubiquitous virus in worldwide horse population; however, disease reports outside North America are uncommon.
- Seasonality: Peak incidence is in the late fall, winter, and early summer.

CLINICAL PRESENTATION

HISTORY, CHIEF COMPLAINT

- Acute onset of fever, ataxia, or acute recumbency about 1 week after expo-sure to the virus. Signs may stabilize early in clinical course.
- Recent fever, respiratory disease, or abortion may have occurred on the property.
- Multiple horses may be affected on a single property: Ataxia, paresis, and urinary incontinence.

PHYSICAL EXAM FINDINGS

- Symmetrical pelvic limb ataxia and paresis.
- Limb edema is frequently seen.
- Urinary bladder paralysis and over-flow incontinence often occurs.
- Sensory deficits are sometimes present in the trunk, perineum.
- Occasional cranial signs: Depression; diffuse face, jaw, tongue, and pharyn-geal weakness.

ETIOLOGY AND PATHOPHYSIOLOGY

- The virus crosses respiratory epithe-lium. Local replication is in the regional lymph nodes followed by mononu-clear cell-associated viremia.
- The virus is thought to invade the endothelium of the central nervous system (CNS).
- Vasculitis and associated ischemic necrosis of gray and particularly white matter is widespread.
- The pathogenesis of disease is sus-pected to be the direct effects of a neurotropic strain of EHV-1 associated with an immune-mediated Arthus-type reaction in the vessel walls.
- The duration and magnitude of viremia determine the occurrence of myeloen-cephalitis.
- Disease outbreak may be caused by one or both of the following: recru-descence of neuropathogenic EHV-1 strain or mutation to virulent biotype and shedding of a formerly low-risk variant.

DIAGNOSIS

DIFFERENTIAL DIAGNOSIS

- Equine protozoal myeloencephalitis (EPM)
- Arboviral diseases (Eastern equine encephalitis, Western equine encepha-litis, Venezuelan equine encephalitis, West Nile virus)
- Cervical vertebral malformation
- Trauma: Brain, spinal cord
- Botulism
- Equine degenerative myeloencepha-lopathy
- Rabies
- Toxicities
- Focal spinal cord lesions: Abscess and aberrant parasite migration

INITIAL DATABASE

Rule out other conditions based on phys-ical and neurologic examinations.

ADVANCED OR CONFIRMATORY TESTING

- Viral isolation or polymerase chain reaction: Nasal swabs, tracheal fluids, and blood buffy coat. Sample both affected and in-contact horses to increase the chance of detection.
- Cerebrospinal fluid (CSF): Best obtained from the lumbosacral site; xanthochromia and elevated protein but usually very few cells are seen.

- EHV-1 serum (and possibly CSF) titers: Helpful in making a diagnosis on a herd basis, but in individual animals, interpretation can be problematic. Collect acute and convalescent serum (2- to 3-week interval) to demonstrate a fourfold increase in antibody. High acute titers may be confirmatory.
- Histopathology: Widespread focal hemorrhage throughout the CNS; vasculitis, congestion, and ischemic necrosis of neural tissue; axonal swelling and malacia of gray and white matter.
- Immunofluorescent antibody testing: Brain and spinal cord.

TREATMENT

THERAPEUTIC GOAL(S)

- Strictly isolate suspected cases until the condition is ruled out.
- Antiinflammatory drugs may help ameliorate neurologic signs.
- Broad-spectrum antibiotic therapy is indicated to manage bacterial pulmonary superinfection and possible cystitis from chronic urinary bladder catheterization.
- Antiviral drugs may be of use.
- Provide supportive care.

ACUTE GENERAL TREATMENT

- Antiinflammatory drugs: Nonsteroidal antiinflammatory drugs; flunixin meglumine (1 mg/kg q12h)
- Dimethyl sulfoxide: 0.5 to 1.0 g/kg IV q12–24h; must be diluted to a 10% solution or less in an isotonic balanced electrolyte solution
- Corticosteroids (controversial): Dexamethasone (0.05–0.1 mg/kg PO, IV, or IM q12h tapering down over 3 days) or prednisolone (1–2 mg/kg IV or PO q24h)
- Antimicrobials: Trimethoprim-sulfonamide (2.2 mg/kg IM or IV q12–24h), ceftiofur (15–30 mg/kg IM or IV q12–24h)
- Acyclovir: 20 mg/kg PO q8h for 5 days; variable absorption and plasma levels
- Valacyclovir: 30 mg/kg PO q8h for 2 days, then 20 mg/kg PO q12h

- Supportive therapies: IV fluids; enteral or parenteral nutrition
- Bladder catheterization, manual evacuation of feces
- Leg wraps, head protectants
- Encourage the horse to stand if able; a sling is useful as an aid to standing but not as complete support

CHRONIC TREATMENT

- Adult horses are unable to tolerate prolonged periods of recumbency. It is essential to reposition the horse every 4 to 6 hours to minimize decubital ulcers over bony prominences.
- Great care must be taken when a sling is used because although some horses learn to use the sling to assist standing, urination, and defecation, some resort to using the sling as complete support, resulting in significant respiratory impairment and pressure sores.

POSSIBLE COMPLICATIONS

- Aspiration pneumonia
- Decubital ulceration
- Corneal ulceration
- Cystitis
- Constipation

PROGNOSIS AND OUTCOME

- Ambulatory horses usually improve over a few days to a few months and often return to normal.
- Recumbent horses have recovered completely with dedicated nursing care; however, secondary complications may be severe with prolonged recumbency, necessitating euthanasia.
- Residual neurologic deficits may occur.

PEARLS & CONSIDERATIONS

COMMENTS

- Prevention is difficult because the majority of horses are latently infected with virus.

- Vaccination aims to decrease nasal shedding of virus.
- In the face of an outbreak, diagnose early, prevent spread, and treat clinical cases.

PREVENTION

- Modified-live and inactivated vaccines are available for protection against respiratory and abortion strains, although they have not been proven protective against the neurologic syndrome.
- New arrivals: Isolate for at least 3 weeks. Ensure that their vaccination status is current.
- Minimize comingling of resident horses with recent arrivals.
- Minimize management practices, nutritional plane, and concurrent diseases as stressors.
- Outbreak: Efficacy of vaccination in the face of outbreak is unknown. May be deleterious because of immune-mediated pathogenesis of disease. However, no reports exist of deleterious effects of vaccination in this situation.
- Neuropathic strains may spread in aerosol up to 10 m.
- Isolate the facility for 28 days after last clinical case onset.

CLIENT EDUCATION

Preexisting EHV-1 serum neutralization titers are not protective.

SUGGESTED READING

Friday PA, Scarratt WK, Elvinger F, et al: Ataxia and paresis with equine herpesvirus type 1 infection in a herd of riding school horses. *J Vet Intern Med* 14:197–201, 2000.

Goehring L: Viral diseases of the nervous system. In Furr M, Reed S (eds). *Equine neurology*, Ames, IA, 2008, Blackwell Publishing, pp 169–186.

Lunn DP, et al: Equine herpesvirus-1 consensus statement. *J Vet Intern Med* 23:450, 2009.

Wilson WD, Pusterla N: Equine herpesvirus 1 myeloencephalopathy. In Reed S, Bayly W, Sellon D (eds). *Equine internal medicine*, ed 3, St Louis, 2010, Saunders Elsevier, pp 615–622.

AUTHOR: **PETER R. MORRESEY**

EDITOR: **STEPHEN M. REED**

Myeloencephalopathy, Equine Degenerative

BASIC INFORMATION

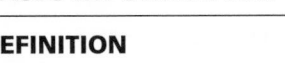

DEFINITION

Progressive, symmetrical neurologic condition with prominent ataxia and

weakness resulting from widespread degeneration of the spinal cord and brainstem

SYNONYM(S)

Neuroaxonal dystrophy of Morgan horses is a related condition with similar, but more localized, degenerative histologic changes.

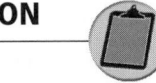

EPIDEMIOLOGY

SPECIES, AGE, SEX
- Domestic and captive Equids
- Onset from 1 month to several years of age; most cases, younger than 6 months of age

GENETICS AND BREED PREDISPOSITION
- Most breeds of domestic horses have been affected.
- Familial or hereditary basis suspected: Arabian, Appaloosa, Thoroughbred, Standardbred, Paso Fino and Morgan horses, and exotic Equidae (zebra, Przewalskii's horse).

RISK FACTORS
- Prolonged exposure to dry dirt lots with no grass.
- Feeding of heated, pelleted feed and sun-baked forages with very low vitamin E content (<5 U/kg dry matter).
- A familial tendency has been observed, suggesting vitamin E deficiency has a greater effect in genetically predisposed animals.
- Some chronically affected animals have been found to have normal serum vitamin E concentrations because of subsequent pasture exposure.
- Use of insecticide and exposure to wood preservative has been identified (with others) as risk factors in equine degenerative myeloencephalopathy (EDM), although a causal relationship has not been established.

GEOGRAPHY AND SEASONALITY
- United States: Northeastern states predominantly, but the occurrence is widespread
- British Isles and Europe

CLINICAL PRESENTATION

HISTORY, CHIEF COMPLAINT
- Signs are first seen in suckling and weanling foals younger than 6 months.
- Signs are usually insidious in onset and slowly progressive. However, an acute onset of severe ataxia and weakness in the pelvis or all four limbs may occur.
- Clinical signs occasionally progress to recumbency, although most frequently the clinical signs plateau with maturity of the horse and chronicity of the condition.

PHYSICAL EXAM FINDINGS
- Neurologic examination reveals upper motor neuron and general proprioceptive deficits: symmetrical ataxia, and weakness and hypometria affecting all limbs but often worse in the pelvic limbs (compare with equine motor neuron disease).
- Severely affected patients may assume a "dog-sitting" posture.
- Marked hyporeflexia or areflexia involving the thoracolaryngeal (slap),

local cervical, and cutaneous trunci reflexes may occur without loss of sensation or regional muscle atrophy.

ETIOLOGY AND PATHOPHYSIOLOGY
- Neuroaxonal dystrophy: Spinal cord and brainstem. Sensory, proprioceptive, and neuronal fiber degeneration within ascending and descending spinal cord pathways. Most prominent in the thoracolumbar region.
- High oxygen demand, high metabolic rate, and high content of polyunsaturated fats within the central nervous system (CNS) make it susceptible to oxidative damage from abundant free radical production.
- Neurotransmitter metabolism is another source of oxygen-derived free radicals.
- EDM is thought to be caused by a relative lack of antioxidant molecules (including vitamin E).

DIAGNOSIS

DIFFERENTIAL DIAGNOSIS
- Cervical vertebral malformation.
- Equine protozoal myeloencephalitis (EPM)

INITIAL DATABASE
- Routine blood tests, cervical radiography, cerebrospinal fluid (CSF), and electromyography do not aid diagnosis. Reports of increased CSF creatine kinase enzyme activity exist.
- Early in the course of the disease, young affected animals and unaffected foals on the same farm may have reduced serum vitamin E concentrations; however, mature animals with chronic disease may have normal levels if they have access to fresh green forage.

ADVANCED OR CONFIRMATORY TESTING
- Necropsy: Gross evaluation is unremarkable.
- Histopathology: Symmetrical neuronal fiber degeneration throughout the spinal cord, especially the medial and ventral parts of ventral funiculi and spinocerebellar tracts. Demyelination is prominent. Astrocytosis, astrogliosis, vacuolation, and axonal swelling are noted. Accumulation of endothelial lipopigment in the CNS occurs.

TREATMENT

THERAPEUTIC GOAL(S)
- Stabilize the horse's clinical signs.
- Cure is unlikely; treatment is of doubtful benefit.

ACUTE GENERAL TREATMENT
- Vitamin E supplementation: Affected horses may stabilize with 6000 to 10,000 U/d. Treatment should be continued until the patient is 3 years old.
- There is an improved probability of success if treatment initiated at the first signs of disease.

PROGNOSIS AND OUTCOME

- The disease is progressive; however, signs may stabilize with treatment.
- After it is evident, clinical signs do not resolve.
- Euthanasia is the likely outcome.

PEARLS & CONSIDERATIONS

COMMENTS
- An earlier onset indicates a more severe disease process and a more rapid progression.
- A later onset of signs suggests less severe disease and a slower progression.

PREVENTION
- Vitamin E supplementation: Lack of pasture, insecticide or wood preservative exposure, processed feeds, and familial disposition are risk factors, suggesting that supplementation in these situations may be protective. The incidence in foals on affected properties has been shown to be reduced with supplementation of 1500 U/d of vitamin E.
- Supplementation of groups of horses in which there has been a high prevalence of the disease with adequate vitamin E (≥2000 IU q24h) has been associated with cessation of new cases.
- Maintain vitamin E dietary intake of 500 to 1000 IU/kg of dry weight of feed.

SUGGESTED READING
MacKay R: Neurodegenerative diseases. In Furr M, Reed S (eds). *Equine neurology.* Ames, IA, 2008, Blackwell, pp 169–186.

Nout YS: Equine degenerative myeloencephalopathy. In Reed S, Bayly W, Sellon D (eds). *Equine internal medicine*, ed 3, St Louis, 2010, pp 606–609.

Mayhew IG: Nutritional diseases. In Mayhew IG (ed). *Large animal neurology*, ed 2, Ames, IA, 2009, Wiley Blackwell, pp 225–293.

AUTHOR: **PETER R. MORRESEY**

EDITOR: **STEPHEN M. REED**

Myocarditis

BASIC INFORMATION

DEFINITION

Any disease process causing active inflammation of the heart muscle. Myocarditis is an uncommon sequela that may occur secondary to a variety of causes.

EPIDEMIOLOGY

RISK FACTORS

- Myocarditis may result from an extension of infection or inflammation associated with other sources. Risk factors include:
  - Recent infection (bacterial, viral, or parasitic) of the respiratory tract
  - Systemic inflammation, such as bacteremia or septicemia
  - Pericardial disease or endocardial disease
- Exposure to various toxins, including ionophore antimicrobials (eg, monensin, lasalocid, salinomycin), heavy metals, various cardiotoxic plants (eg, gossypol, *Cassia occidentalis*, *Philaria* spp., yew, oleander, white snakeroot, foxglove, lily of the valley, rhododendron), cantharidin toxicosis, recent snakebite envenomation
- Nutritional imbalances, including vitamin E and selenium deficiency (neuromuscular degeneration), copper deficiency, excess molybdenum, excess sulfates
- Hyperthermia or heat stroke

GEOGRAPHY AND SEASONALITY

- Sporadic
- Myocarditis associated with vitamin E or selenium deficiency is usually seen in horses younger than 1 year old and in geographic locations with low soil selenium (northeast, eastern seaboard, northwest United States).
- Snakebite envenomation is more common in certain areas of the country (southwest, southeast) and more likely when snakes are active in the spring and summer.
- Cantharidin exposure is more likely with the consumption of alfalfa hay harvested in the southwest (Texas, Oklahoma), particularly later cuttings or certain processing methods such as crimping of hay during cutting.

ASSOCIATED CONDITIONS AND DISORDERS

- Arrhythmias are commonly associated with myocarditis. Chronic myocarditis may lead to cardiomyopathy.
- In addition, clinical signs associated with the primary disease process might be present. These may include

evidence of recent infection, snakebite, or clinical signs associated with the toxic effects of the ingested plant or toxin (weakness, colic, diarrhea, renal disease).

CLINICAL PRESENTATION

DISEASE FORMS/SUBTYPES In other species, three phases (acute, subacute and chronic) have been recognized. This has not been well characterized in horses.

HISTORY, CHIEF COMPLAINT

- Historical findings and presenting complaints may either be specific to the cardiovascular system or vague and associated with the causative factor.
- Exercise intolerance or poor performance
- Syncope or sudden death
- Fever, lethargy, inappetence, respiratory abnormalities (tachypnea, dyspnea), distress, colic, colitis, lameness, ataxia

PHYSICAL EXAM FINDINGS

- Tachycardia, arrhythmias, gallop rhythm
- Cardiac murmurs
- Tachypnea, dyspnea, nostril flare, cough
- Myalgia, reluctance to move
- Weak systemic pulses, jugular pulses, jugular distension, syncope
- Nonspecific signs associated with primary disease process, including fever, anorexia, weakness, colic, diarrhea, nasal discharge

ETIOLOGY AND PATHOPHYSIOLOGY

- Inflammation of the myocardium may be caused by:
  - Bacterial infection: Staphylococcus aureus, Streptococcus equi, Clostridium chauvoei, Mycobacterium spp.
  - Viral infection: Equine infectious anemia, equine viral arteritis, equine influenza, African horse sickness, equine herpesvirus-1 (EHV-1)
  - Parasitic infection: Strongylosis, onchocerciasis, babesiosis
  - Bacteremia, septicemia, or the spread of contiguous disease from the pericardium or endocardium
  - Other infiltrative or inflammatory diseases
- Exposure to various toxins, including ionophore antimicrobials (eg, monensin, lasalocid, salinomycin), heavy metals, various cardiotoxic plants (eg, gossypol, *C. occidentalis*, *Philaria* spp., yew, oleander, white snakeroot, foxglove, lily of the valley, rhododendron), cantharidin toxicosis, recent snakebite envenomation.

- Nutritional imbalances: Vitamin E and selenium deficiency (neuromuscular degeneration), copper deficiency, excess molybdenum, excess sulfates.
- Hyperthermia or heat stroke.
- Inflammation associated with infection or infiltrative diseases may lead to conduction disturbances, chamber dilatation, and decreased systolic function.
- The pathophysiology of the individual etiology (toxins, nutritional imbalances) is associated with the specific mechanism of action of each toxic principle.

DIAGNOSIS

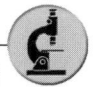

DIFFERENTIAL DIAGNOSIS

- For exercise intolerance, lethargy, weakness: Abnormalities in respiratory or musculoskeletal systems; neuromuscular diseases
- For arrhythmias: Systemic diseases, electrolyte abnormalities, primary valvular or congenital heart diseases with chamber enlargement
- For heart failure: Primary valvular or pericardial diseases, congenital heart diseases
- For respiratory signs: Primary pulmonary or pleural diseases

INITIAL DATABASE

- Complete blood count: Normal or changes consistent with inflammation or infection (leukocytosis, neutrophilia, lymphopenia, anemia of chronic disease, hyperfibrinogenemia, hyperproteinemia).
- Chemistry panel: Changes consistent with passive congestion from right-sided heart failure (increased liver enzymes) or changes consistent with organ dysfunction caused by decreased cardiac output (azotemia). Electrolyte abnormalities concurrent with the primary disease process (eg, hypocalcemia with cantharidin toxicosis). Elevated lactate concentration in association with poor systemic perfusion. Elevations in creatine kinase may be seen secondary to neuromuscular degeneration (selenium deficiency) or cantharidin exposure.
- Urinalysis: Hemoglobinuria is consistent with certain toxicities or nutritional myodegeneration. Hematuria may be seen with snakebite, cantharidin toxicosis.
- Electrocardiogram (ECG): May be normal or show any arrhythmia

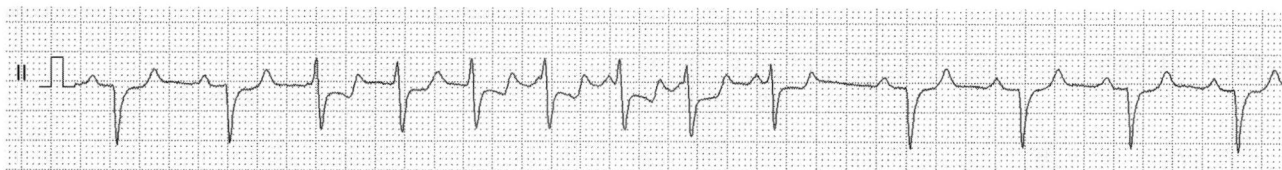

FIGURE 1 Base-apex electrocardiogram from a horse with idiopathic myocarditis showing underlying sinus tachycardia (heart rate, 83 beats/min) and a paroxysm of ventricular tachycardia. Amplitude, 5 mm/mV; paper speed, 25 mm/sec.

(premature atrial contractions, premature ventricular contractions, supraventricular tachycardia, ventricular tachycardia, atrial fibrillation) (Figure 1)

- 24-hour ECG (Holter) monitoring: More accurately identifies the occurrence and prevalence of arrhythmias than a single rhythm strip.
- Cardiac troponin I: Likely elevated in cases of myocarditis associated with myocardial necrosis.
- Echocardiogram: May be normal or show evidence of myocardial inflammation such as thick or thin myocardial walls, heteroechogenicity of myocardial walls, or reduced systolic and diastolic function.

ADVANCED OR CONFIRMATORY TESTING

- Culture and antimicrobial sensitivity testing of blood, pericardial fluid, tracheal wash fluid, or pleural fluid as indicated (bacterial infections)
- Pursuit of viral etiology such as:
  - Serology (equine viral arteritis, equine influenza, EHV-1).
  - Polymerase chain reaction (EHV-1).
  - Antibody binding assays such as enzyme-linked immunosorbent assay (equine influenza)
  - Agar-gel immunodiffusion (AGID) test (Coggins test) for equine infectious anemia
  - Virus isolation
- Evaluation of pasture for exposure to toxic plants and feed for ionophore antimicrobials such as monensin.
- Evaluation of gastric contents or body fluids for oleandrin and serum digoxin concentrations (cardiac glycoside containing plants). If the patient is not receiving digoxin therapy, should have no detectable concentrations.
- Evaluation of urine or gastric contents for cantharidin.
- Pursuit of potential nutritional imbalances such as selenium deficiency (blood concentrations).
- Pursuit of heavy metal exposure.
- Endomyocardial biopsy with histopathologic evaluation is the gold standard for diagnosis in human medicine, however, because of its invasive nature, it is currently not performed in clinical equine practice.

TREATMENT

THERAPEUTIC GOAL(S)

Normalize cardiac function by reducing arrhythmias, providing inotropic support, and treating heart failure while ultimately correcting or controlling the underlying disease process.

ACUTE GENERAL TREATMENT

- Arrhythmias: Treat with antiarrhythmic drugs (AADs) as dictated by the arrhythmias documented on the ECG. Use AADs for arrhythmias that are hemodynamically significant (ie, causing clinical signs attributable to the arrhythmia) or are likely to progress to fatal arrhythmias.
- Congestive heart failure: Treat with furosemide (1–2 mg/kg IV as needed) and intranasal oxygen; minimize stress (see "Cardiac Failure" in this section).
- Systolic failure: Administer positive inotropes (eg, dobutamine 1–5 µg/kg/min IV) and vasodilators (eg, hydralazine 0.5–1.5 mg/kg PO) (see "Cardiac Failure" in this section).
- Suspected recent feed intoxication or toxic plant ingestion: Remove all suspected contaminated feed; remove horse from pasture. Administer activated charcoal, mineral oil, or both via nasogastric intubation.
- Suspected monensin intoxication: Administer high levels of vitamin E and selenium to stabilize cell membranes.
- Suspected cardiac glycoside toxicosis (eg, oleander ingestion): Digoxin should not be used to control heart rate or rhythm. May consider administering antidigoxin immune antibodies (Digibind), although this is likely prohibitively expensive in an adult horse.
- Antimicrobial therapy as warranted for specific disease (see appropriate infectious disease chapter for recommendations).
- Provide appropriate supportive care for the underlying disease (eg, crystalloid or colloid fluid therapy, electrolyte replacement, nonsteroidal antiinflammatory drugs, nutritional support).
- Address mineral deficiencies (eg, provide selenium supplementation and vitamin E if needed).

CHRONIC TREATMENT

- Arrhythmias: AADs can be given orally if necessary to treat persistent arrhythmias.
- Standard treatment for congestive heart failure (see "Cardiac Failure" in this section).
- After an active infection has been ruled out, treatment with corticosteroids is indicated to decrease inflammatory or immune-mediated responses.
- Strict stall rest until clinical and echocardiographic signs of myocarditis completely resolve.

DRUG INTERACTIONS

- Digoxin should not be used in cases of monensin intoxication or in exposure to plants containing cardiac glycosides (eg, oleander, foxglove) because they cause an increase in intracellular calcium; this may enhance myocardial cell death, leading to arrhythmias.
- Corticosteroids should only be used after active infections are ruled out.

POSSIBLE COMPLICATIONS

- Any AAD can be proarrhythmic and have other cardiovascular side effects such as hypotension.
- Until the disease has fully resolved, sudden cardiac death in horses is always possible during treatment for myocarditis.
- Chronic myocarditis can progress to dilated cardiomyopathy.

RECOMMENDED MONITORING

- Acute monitoring
  - Arrhythmias: Continuous ECG monitoring using radiotelemetry, particularly if treating arrhythmias
  - Monitoring clinical signs such as heart rate, respiratory rate, and respiratory effort
  - Serum lactate concentrations may be used as an indicator of tissue perfusion.
  - Blood pressure monitoring (direct or indirect) may be performed.
- Chronic monitoring:
  - Monitoring heart rate, respiratory rate, and respiratory effort should continue at home after the horse is discharged from the hospital. Any

change in status should prompt a repeat complete cardiovascular examination.

- ○ Cardiac troponin I is relatively labile and can therefore reflect changes from day to day in the degree of myocardial cell injury or necrosis.
- ○ Monitoring as needed for the primary disease process.
- ○ Therapeutic drug levels and standard monitoring of chronic cardiac drug therapy (see "Cardiac Failure" in this section).
- ○ Periodic echocardiograms to assess resolution of disease. These should be repeated every 3 to 6 months after the horse is discharged from the hospital until return to normal function.
- ○ Periodic 24-hour ECG (Holter) monitoring.
- ○ Exercising ECG to determine whether exercise-induced arrhythmias are present and to assess the safety of use as a riding horse (after clinical disease has resolved and before being used as a riding horse).
- ○ Monitoring exercise tolerance after the horse is no longer on stall rest.

PROGNOSIS AND OUTCOME

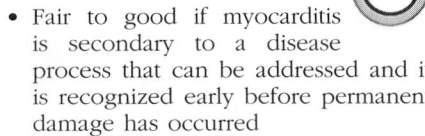

- Fair to good if myocarditis is secondary to a disease process that can be addressed and it is recognized early before permanent damage has occurred
- Guarded to poor if cardiomyopathy and heart failure occurs

PEARLS & CONSIDERATIONS

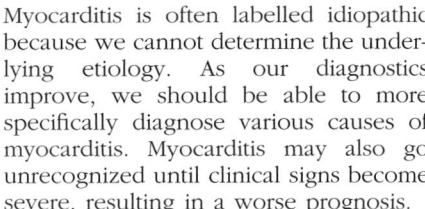

COMMENTS

Myocarditis is often labelled idiopathic because we cannot determine the underlying etiology. As our diagnostics improve, we should be able to more specifically diagnose various causes of myocarditis. Myocarditis may also go unrecognized until clinical signs become severe, resulting in a worse prognosis.

PREVENTION

- Maintenance of a good vaccination and deworming program to decrease the risk of predisposing viral infections and parasitic infestations.

- Monensin intoxication: Use a reputable feed supplier, preferably one that does not mix equine feed in the same location as poultry or cattle feed.
- Plant intoxications: Know the content of pastures on which horses are kept.
- Selenium deficient areas: Have soil tested and supplement if needed for the area.

CLIENT EDUCATION

If owners note nonspecific signs within a few weeks of a respiratory tract infection, consultation with a veterinarian should be sought.

SUGGESTED READING

Martin BB, Reef VB, Parente EJ, et al: Causes of poor performance of horses during training, racing, or showing: 348 cases (1992–1996). *J Am Vet Med Assoc* 216:554–558, 2000.

Reef VB: A monensin outbreak in horses in the eastern United States: pathogenesis, clinical signs, and epidemiology. *Proceedings of the eighth annual Veterinary Medicine Forum* 126–128, 1990.

AUTHOR: **SOPHY A. JESTY**

EDITOR: **MARY M. DURANDO**

Myonecrosis, Clostridial

BASIC INFORMATION

DEFINITION

An acute, life-threatening disease of horses caused by infection of muscle with any of a variety of *Clostridium* spp. that elaborate dermonecrotizing and vasoactive toxins, leading to gas production, extensive tissue damage, and life-threatening systemic toxemia

SYNONYM(S)

- Clostridial myositis or cellulitis
- Malignant edema
- Gas gangrene

EPIDEMIOLOGY

RISK FACTORS

- Puncture wound or intramuscular injection.
- The most frequently incriminated pharmacologic agent is flunixin meglumine.
- The most common injection site is the cervical musculature.

CLINICAL PRESENTATION

HISTORY, CHIEF COMPLAINT

- Onset of signs within 48 hours of injection of a pharmacologic or biologic agent in the affected area of the body.
- Incriminated medications include nonsteroidal antiinflammatory drugs, antihistamines, multivitamins, antipyretics, dewormers, vaccines, diuretics, and synthetic prostaglandins.
- Depression, lethargy, and inappetence are chief signs.
- Swelling and crepitus of the affected area.

PHYSICAL EXAM FINDINGS

- Rapidly progressive soft tissue swelling with subcutaneous and deeper soft tissue emphysema
- Fever
- Tachycardia
- Tachypnea
- Depression
- Toxic mucous membranes with prolonged capillary refill time
- Occasionally, signs of a hemolytic crisis: hemoglobinuria, icterus
- Possible signs consistent with multiorgan failure

ETIOLOGY AND PATHOPHYSIOLOGY

- Most commonly, the etiologic agent is *Clostridium perfringens*.
- *Clostridium septicum*, *Clostridium chauvoei*, *Clostridium novyi*, and others are occasionally incriminated.
- Infection may originate from introduction of surface bacteria into soft tissue at the time of injection.
- Alternatively, dormant spores may be present in the muscle and convert to vegetative form when anaerobic conditions develop secondary to injection-site inflammation.
- α-Toxins from *C. perfringens* are dermonecrotic and considered critical in development of the disease.
- Toxins lead to systemic toxemia, cardiovascular collapse, and multiorgan dysfunction.

DIAGNOSIS

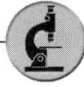

DIFFERENTIAL DIAGNOSIS

Any soft tissue infection or injection site inflammation or abscess

INITIAL DATABASE

- Complete blood count findings consistent with toxemia and dehydration:
  - Neutropenia, left shift with toxic changes
  - Increased packed cell volume, total solids
  - Moderate to marked anemia if hemolysis is occurring
- Serum biochemical profile to assess organ function
  - Azotemia common
  - Marked increase in serum creatine kinase activity
- Ultrasonography to identify affected areas in deeper tissues

ADVANCED OR CONFIRMATORY TESTING

- Gram stain of aspirates from affected subcutaneous areas reveals large numbers of gram-positive rods.

- Anaerobic culture of fluid aspirates for definitive diagnosis.

TREATMENT

THERAPEUTIC GOAL(S)

- Eliminate the infection.
- Provide supportive treatment for systemic toxemia and multiorgan failure.

ACUTE GENERAL TREATMENT

- A combination of aggressive medical and surgical treatment is required.
- High-dose antimicrobial therapy such as potassium penicillin at 88,000 IU/kg q2h (minimum, 22,000 IU/kg q6h).
- Oral metronidazole (25 mg/kg q6h) should be administered if the use of oral medication is possible.
- Oxytetracycline is an alternative IV antimicrobial agent (6.6 mg/kg IV q12–24h).

- Fenestrate affected soft tissues by aggressive incising areas of subcutaneous emphysema, extending incisions into deeper tissues and adjoining areas of healthy tissue.
- Local infusions of penicillin at the margins of infected tissue may be of benefit.
- Intensive fluid, electrolyte, and cardiovascular support should be provided in the acute stages of disease.

CHRONIC TREATMENT

- Horses that survive acute disease may have significant soft tissue and skin sloughing over the next days to weeks.
- Long-term wound care is required.
- Many patients may require weeks to months for granulation and second-intention skin healing to be complete.

POSSIBLE COMPLICATIONS

Extensive tissue sloughing is common.

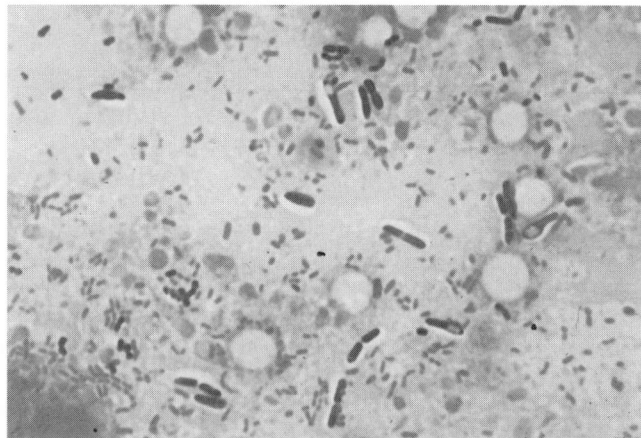

FIGURE 1 Gram stain of aspirate from subcutaneous tissues of horse with acute clostridial myonecrosis. Notice the numerous, large, gram-positive rods. (From Sellon DC, Long MT: *Equine infectious diseases.* St Louis, 2007, Saunders.)

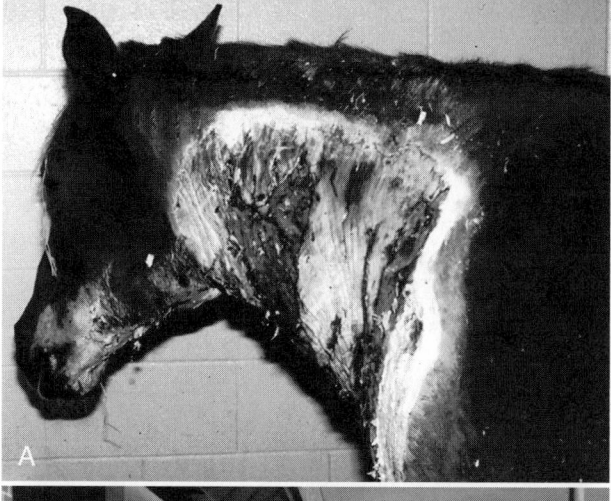

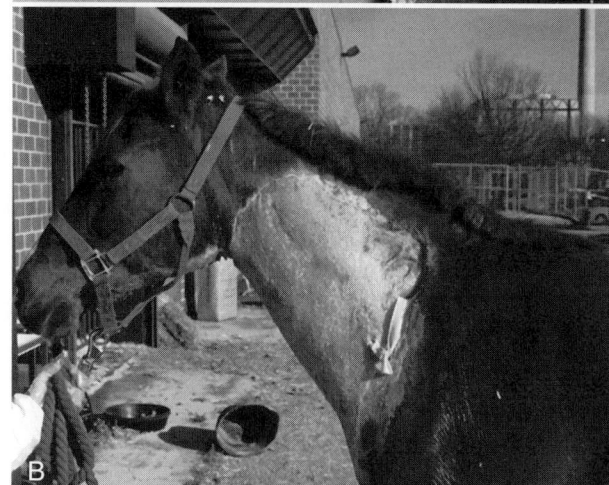

FIGURE 3 **A,** Mature Quarter Horse gelding showing skin and muscle sloughing 2 weeks after surgical fenestration of an area of clostridial myonecrosis in the cervical region. **B,** The same horse approximately 30 days after surgical fenestration showing near-complete granulation bed in prior area of clostridial myonecrosis. (From Sellon DC, Long MT: *Equine infectious diseases.* St Louis, 2007, Saunders.)

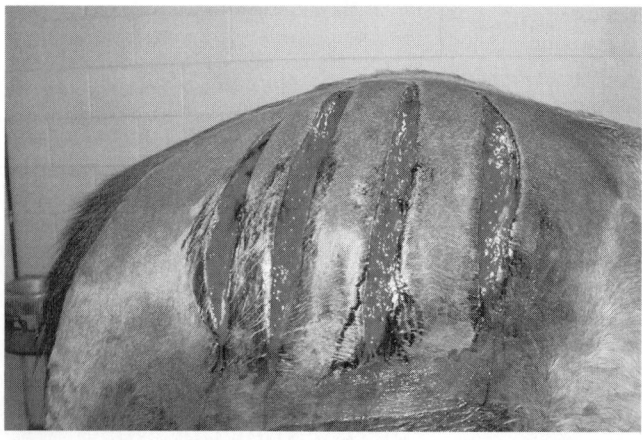

FIGURE 2 Fasciotomy/myotomy incisions in gluteal region of 2-year-old Quarter Horse filly that developed clostridial myonecrosis secondary to vaccination at the site. (Courtesy Dr. Susan Semrad. From Sellon DC, Long MT: *Equine infectious diseases.* St Louis, 2007, Saunders.)

RECOMMENDED MONITORING

- Monitor the patient's cardiovascular status; hypotension, tachycardia, and shock are common in the acute stages.
- Monitor electrolyte, acid-base, and fluid balance.
- Monitor renal function. Multiorgan failure, toxemia, and pigmenturia from damaged muscle may result in acute renal insufficiency.
- Frequently reevaluate site of infection and extend surgical fenestrations as needed.

PROGNOSIS AND OUTCOME

- The prognosis varies depending on the species of *Clostridium* involved.
- Horses with *C. perfringens* infection have a survival rate of 80% if treated aggressively.

- Horses with *C. septicum* or *C. chauvoei* infections have a significantly poorer prognosis.
- Some horses may heal with pigmentation changes and significant cicatrix formation.
- Most horses that die will succumb in the first few days of infection.

PEARLS & CONSIDERATIONS

COMMENTS

- Although there is no protective effect demonstrated from skin disinfection, hair clipping, or disinfection of the top of multidose vials before IM injection, proper injection technique for all IM injections is recommended.
- When administering potentially irritant substances, particularly flunixin meglumine, it may be advisable to encourage use of the larger, better

vascularized, caudal thigh musculature rather than the cervical musculature.

CLIENT EDUCATION

Clients should be encouraged to report all injection-site reactions to their veterinarian as soon as they are noticed and to monitor closely for changes in condition suggestive of clostridial infection.

SUGGESTED READING

Jeanes LV, Magdesian KG, Madigan JE: Clostridial myonecrosis in horses. *Comp Contin Educ Pract Vet* 23:577, 2001.
Peek SF: Clostridial myonecrosis. In Sellon DC, Long MT (eds). *Equine infectious diseases*, St Louis, 2007, Saunders Elsevier, pp 367–369.
Peek SF, Semrad SD, Perkins GA: Clostridial myonecrosis in horses (37 cases 1985–2000). *Equine Vet J* 35:86, 2003.

AUTHOR: **DEBRA C. SELLON**

EDITORS: **DEBRA C. SELLON** and **MAUREEN T. LONG**

Nasal Polyps

BASIC INFORMATION

DEFINITION

Fibrous, inflammatory growths arising from the nasal (septal or conchal) mucosa. They are often pedunculated and may contain cystic cavities.

SYNONYM(S)

Sinonasal polyps, inflammatory polyps

EPIDEMIOLOGY

SPECIES, AGE, SEX Most commonly diagnosed in older horses
ASSOCIATED CONDITIONS AND DISORDERS Progressive ethmoid hematomas have been described as hemorrhagic nasal polyps, and they share histologic similarities with true nasal polyps.

CLINICAL PRESENTATION

DISEASE FORMS/SUBTYPES

- Polyps can develop as firm, fibrous masses on long stalks or consist of a fibrous capsule surrounding a single or polycystic, fluid-filled cavity. They are most often unilateral and occur as singular or multiple masses.
- Polyps can also originate from paranasal sinus mucosa or far less likely from the pulpal tissues (hyperplastic pulpitis) of the upper cheek teeth and extend into the nasal passage on pedicles.

HISTORY, CHIEF COMPLAINT

- Owners may notice a nasal discharge, reduced airflow at the nares, and abnormal respiratory noise developing and worsening over a prolonged period of time.
- The nasal discharge may be malodorous and can be mucoid to purulent. Head shaking may be a reported concern.
- The onset of clinical signs can be insidious, and lesions may be present weeks to years before veterinary attention is sought.

PHYSICAL EXAM FINDINGS Malodorous nasal discharge (mucoid to purulent); reduced nasal airflow; increased respiratory noise localized to the nasal passage; enlarged submandibular lymph nodes; external facial swelling (uncommon); white, pink, or yellow mass visible at the external nares

ETIOLOGY AND PATHOPHYSIOLOGY

- Probably an inflammatory origin (maybe allergies) with the inciting cause not determined.
- Inflamed nasal or sinus mucosal epithelial glands become occluded, leading to their enlargement, dilatation, and rupture.
- Leaking glandular fluid may cause ongoing inflammation and the development of a granulomatous reaction with cystic cavities.

- Slowly growing masses gradually occlude the nasal passage and expand rostrally, caudally, or both.

DIAGNOSIS

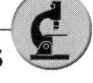

DIFFERENTIAL DIAGNOSIS

- Progressive ethmoid hematoma
- Granuloma
- Paranasal sinus cyst extending into the nasal passage
- Fungal rhinitis
- Sinonasal neoplasia
- Nasal epidermal inclusion cyst (atheroma)
- Amyloidosis

INITIAL DATABASE

- Complete blood count and chemistry panel: Expected to be normal; not indicated.
- Rhinoscopy: Smooth-walled; white, pink, or yellow; bulbous structure occluding and distorting the nasal passage and septal and conchal tissues. Lesions are located a variable distance from the external nares; a pedunculated attachment to the nasal mucosa is often visualized. If the nasal polyp originates from the sinus mucosa, increased drainage at the nasomaxillary opening can be expected if it can be visualized.

- Radiography: A nonspecific soft tissue mass effect obliterating the nasal meati, nasal septum deviation, paranasal air-fluid interface, may be bony changes associated with the mass, increased periapical opacity.

ADVANCED OR CONFIRMATORY TESTING

- Sinoscopy: May confirm a secondary sinusitis and the origin of a sinus-based polyp; useful for biopsying mass.
- Computed tomography provides the most detailed imaging of polyps and their exact anatomic location and structures involved; however, it is usually not required.
- Histopathology of removed tissue confirms the diagnosis: Granulation tissue, myxomatous connective tissue, inflammatory cells, secretory epithelium lining cystic cavities, inflamed epithelial glands.

TREATMENT

THERAPEUTIC GOAL(S)

- Complete removal of the polyp is required to restore normal air flow and function of the nasal passage and prevent recurrence.
- Resolve any concurrent secondary paranasal sinusitis.

ACUTE GENERAL TREATMENT

- Rarely, a horse may require an emergency tracheotomy to provide comfortable airflow and allow manipulations of the nasal passage without undue respiratory distress.
- Surgical removal of the polyp
  - Endoscopically guided wire or electrocautery snaring and extraction of pedunculated polyps; varying degrees of bleeding at the site of mucosal attachment should be expected.
  - Transendoscopic laser ablation of small polyps or laser excision of

  pedunculated polyps and ablation of the mucosal base.
  - Incising the nostril and alar cartilage can improve exposure and access to a rostrally located large polyp.
  - Sinusotomy may be required for removal of polyps known to arise in the paranasal sinus.
  - Polyps of dental origin may require specific tooth extraction.
- Treatment of a secondary paranasal sinusitis: Systemic broad-spectrum antimicrobials or culture and sensitivity-guided antimicrobial therapy and sinus lavage for 7 to 10 days.

CHRONIC TREATMENT

Follow-up laser ablation of residual tissue may be indicated at 2 to 4 weeks.

POSSIBLE COMPLICATIONS

- Inexperienced use of lasers may result in adjacent normal tissue destruction, leading to nasal passage disfiguration, increased scarring, and possibly granulation tissue formation that requires subsequent management to remove.
- Hemorrhage may be severe in some cases.
- Sinusotomy and dental extractions have associated complications.

RECOMMENDED MONITORING

- After any removal procedure, reexamination via endoscopy is recommended at 2 weeks and then subsequently at 2 months and 6 months if no further treatment is required.
- Additional procedures may be required at 2 weeks to remove residual tissue. Reexamination should be as described above after no signs of abnormal tissue remain.
- Nasal discharge should resolve within 2 weeks if all polypoid tissue is removed. Monitoring for this is important to detect ongoing disease or disease recurrence in the future.
- Airflow and airway noise are also monitored for any abnormal signs to suggest recurrence or new disease.

PROGNOSIS AND OUTCOME

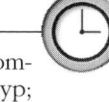

Excellent prognosis with complete removal of the polyp; recurrence is rare in these cases

PEARLS & CONSIDERATIONS

COMMENTS

- A very infrequently encountered cause of nasal discharge and airflow obstruction in horses
- Careful assessment may be required to differentiate among ethmoid hematomas, nasal tumors, or expansile paranasal sinus cysts.
- Laser excision and ablation of polyps is the preferred treatment if available because of reduced hemorrhage and complete removal of tissue.

CLIENT EDUCATION

- Occurrence of polyps appears to be sporadic and of unknown cause.
- Polyps are locally benign, expanding masses.
- At the first sign of abnormal nasal discharge, reduction in nasal airflow, or increase in airway respiratory sounds, consult a veterinarian.

SUGGESTED READING

Tate LP: Application of lasers in equine upper respiratory surgery. *Vet Clin North Am Equine Pract* 7:165–195, 1991.

Tremaine WH, Dixon PM: A long-term study of 277 cases of equine sinonasal disease. Part 1: details of horses, historical, clinical and ancillary diagnostic findings. *Equine Vet J* 33:274–282, 2001.

Tremaine WH, Dixon PM: A long-term study of 277 cases of equine sinonasal disease. Part 2: treatments and results of treatments. *Equine Vet J* 33:283–289, 2001.

Watt BC, Beck BE: Removal of a nasal polyp in a standing horse. *Can Vet J* 38:108–109, 1997.

AUTHOR: MATHEW P. GERARD

EDITOR: ERIC J. PARENTE

Neck Pain (Cervical Dysfunction)

BASIC INFORMATION

DEFINITION

Abnormal cervical function characterized by soft tissue, bony, or articular pain; muscle hypertonicity; or neck stiffness.

Severe cases include neurologic deficits of ataxia, spasticity, or weakness.

SYNONYM(S)

- Cervical hyperesthesia
- Cervical hyperpathia
- Neck stiffness
- Cervical osteoarthritis

- Cervical vertebral compressive myelopathy

EPIDEMIOLOGY

SPECIES, AGE, SEX

- Cervical vertebral compressive myelopathy has an increased prevalence in young horses (<4 yr).

- Young horses have an increased susceptibility for vertebral column trauma.
- Males have increased risk for developmental orthopedic disease (DOD) and cervical vertebral compressive myelopathy.

GENETICS AND BREED PREDISPOSITION

- Genetic predisposition for cervical vertebral compressive myelopathy in Thoroughbreds, Tennessee Walking Horses, and Warmbloods
- Familial predisposition for equine degenerative myelopathy in Standardbreds and Appaloosas
- Breed predisposition for enthesopathy of the nuchal ligament in Warmbloods

RISK FACTORS

- Trauma
- Vertebral malformations
- Nutritional factors linked to osteochondrosis development include overfeeding (high protein and carbohydrates), calcium-phosphorous imbalance, copper or manganese deficiency, and zinc excess.
- Cervical vertebral instability or chronic microtrauma
- Abnormal biomechanical forces associated with the ill-fitting or improper use of draw reins or other restraint or training devices
- Exposure to environmental oxidants and vitamin E deficiency

CONTAGION AND ZOONOSIS Cranial and caudal nuchal bursitis (poll evil) and diskospondylitis have zoonotic potentials if caused by *Brucella abortus* infections.

ASSOCIATED CONDITIONS AND DISORDERS Forelimb lameness caused by brachial plexus injury or avulsion

CLINICAL PRESENTATION

DISEASE FORMS/SUBTYPES

- Congenital: Occipitoatlantoaxial malformation (OAAM) in Arabians
- Developmental: Osteochondrosis of articular processes, vertebral canal stenosis
- Degenerative: Osteoarthritis of cervical synovial articulations
- Traumatic: Cervical fractures, penetrating wounds
- Infectious (neurologic): Equine protozoal myelitis (EPM)
- Infectious (osseous): Discospondylitis, vertebral osteomyelitis
- Inflammatory: Intramuscular vaccine reactions
- Nutritional: High-protein and high-carbohydrate diets, vitamin E deficiency
- Neoplasia: Cervical vertebral myeloma
- Vascular: Thrombophlebitis of the external jugular vein
- Iatrogenic: Improper fit or use of training devices used for restraining head and neck position

HISTORY, CHIEF COMPLAINT

- History of having the head or neck caught in a fence
- History of a fall or running into a solid obstacle or jump
- Abnormal conformation or head and neck carriage
- Neck pain or stiffness
- Neck held in a fixed or guarded position
- Inability to raise or lower the head and neck
- History of recent intramuscular injection
- Pronounced heat or soft tissue swelling
- Head shyness or resentful of palpation of the poll region
- History of pulling back in the crossties or flipping over
- Unwillingness to work on the bit
- Difficulty or resistance in turning in one direction
- Weakness or ataxia
- History of recent respiratory infections or abortions on the farm

PHYSICAL EXAM FINDINGS

- Abnormal head and neck posture
- Pain elicited on palpation of the cervical musculature
- Localized heat or soft tissue swelling
- Local muscle atrophy or regional lack of cervical muscle development
- Cervical muscle hypertonicity, fasciculations, or fibrosis
- Neck stiffness
- Resentment of poll flexion or extension
- Pain elicited on manipulation of the head or neck
- Audible or palpable crepitus with induced neck motion
- Lateral bending joint range of motion (ROM) asymmetry
- Loss of local skin sensation along the lateral neck
- Focal or patchy neck sweating (caused by focal sympathetic degeneration)
- Base-wide stance at rest
- Ataxia, spasticity, or weakness (pelvic limbs more affected than the thoracic limbs)
- Stumbling, toe dragging, circumduction of the pelvic limbs, or truncal sway
- Delayed response to proprioceptive challenges or abnormal limb positioning

ETIOLOGY AND PATHOPHYSIOLOGY Numerous tissues may be the source of neck pain or stiffness

- Soft tissue
  - Trauma: Lacerations; penetrating wounds; Contusions caused by bites or kicks
  - Infection: Myositis, abscessation
  - Inflammation: Intramuscular vaccine reaction, enthesopathy of the nuchal

ligament, cranial or caudal nuchal bursitis (poll evil)
  - Metabolic: Polysaccharide storage myopathy (PSSM)
  - Vascular: Thrombophlebitis of the external jugular vein
- Vertebral column
  - Congenital: OAAM, torticollis caused by in utero malpositioning
  - Developmental: Cervical vertebral malformation causing constant or intermittent spinal cord compression
  - Degeneration: Osteoarthritis, intervertebral disk degeneration
  - Trauma: Atlantoaxial subluxation, vertebral fractures
  - Infection: Discospondylitis
  - Nutritional: High-protein and high-carbohydrate diet, calcium–phosphorus imbalance, copper deficiency, vitamin E or selenium deficiency
  - Neoplasia: Cervical vertebral myeloma
- Neurologic
  - Trauma: Cervical spinal cord compression
  - Developmental: Vertebral canal stenosis
  - Acquired: Vertebral instability
  - Infection: Equine herpesvirus type 1 (EHV-1) myelitis, verminous encephalomyelitis
  - Nutritional: Exposure to environmental oxidants, vitamin E deficiency
  - Space-occupying mass: Articular process osteophytosis and ligamentum flava hypertrophy

DIAGNOSIS

DIFFERENTIAL DIAGNOSIS

Neck pain or dysfunction is a nonspecific clinical sign. Diagnosis is based on exclusion of soft tissue, orthopedic, and neurologic disorders of the cervical region.

- Cervical soft tissues
  - Enthesopathy of the nuchal ligament
  - Penetrating wound or laceration
  - Traumatic muscle injury
  - Intramuscular vaccine reactions or abscessation
  - PSSM
  - Recurrent exertional rhabdomyolysis
  - Thrombophlebitis of the external jugular vein
  - Perivascular injection of irritating substance (eg, phenylbutazone)
- Cervical vertebral column
  - Vertebral malformations: OAAM, ankylosis
  - C1-C2 subluxation: Agenesis of dens, luxated dens, or fractured dens

○ Vertebral malalignment: Instability, subluxation, or luxation
○ Osteochondrosis of the articular processes
○ Osteoarthritis of the cervical synovial articulations
○ Joint capsule and ligamentum flavum proliferation
○ Synovial cysts
○ Intervertebral disk degeneration
○ Vertebral fractures
○ Discospondylitis
○ Vertebral osteomyelitis
• Cervical spinal cord and peripheral nerves
○ Cervical vertebral compressive myelopathy: Continuous or intermittent
○ Spinal nerve compression at the cervical intervertebral foramen
○ Brachial plexus injury or avulsion
○ Bacterial or fungal meningitis
○ EPM
○ EHV-1 myelitis
○ Equine degenerative myelopathy
○ West Nile virus encephalitis
○ Verminous encephalomyelitis
○ Rabies
• Other regional disorders
○ Forelimb lameness
○ DOD causing physitis, osteochondrosis, and flexural limb deformities

INITIAL DATABASE

• Inspection of neck conformation, posture, muscle symmetry and development, and motor control
• Gait evaluation
• Lameness examination
• Neurologic examination
• Soft tissue and bony palpation
• Active and passive segmental cervical joint ROM
• Cervical radiography

ADVANCED OR CONFIRMATORY TESTING

• Ultrasonography of soft tissues and articular processes
• Ultrasound-guided intraarticular injection of the cervical synovial articulations
• Doppler ultrasonography of the external jugular vein
• Cervical myelography with neutral and flexed views to confirm spinal cord compression
• Cerebrospinal fluid analysis
• Nuclear scintigraphy
• Computed tomography
• Thermography
• Pressure algometry to assess mechanical nociceptive thresholds
• Electromyography to confirm myopathy or neuropathy
• Serology and virus isolation
• Serum vitamin E levels

• Therapeutic trial with high dosage of nonsteroidal antiinflammatory drug (NSAID) for 7 to 10 days

TREATMENT

THERAPEUTIC GOAL(S)

• Immobilize vertebral fractures or soft tissue instabilities
• Prevent secondary spinal cord injuries
• Reduce pain and inflammation
• Remove any source of infection
• Reduce muscle hypertonicity
• Restore normal neurologic function
• Promote full joint range of cervical motion in flexion-extension, lateral bending, and axial rotation
• Increase muscle mass and symmetry

ACUTE GENERAL TREATMENT

• Antiinflammatories: NSAIDs, corticosteroids, dimethyl sulfoxide (DMSO)
• Cryotherapy to minimize heat, swelling, or pain
• Stall confinement or exercise restriction to prevent reinjury and promote healing
• Neck brace or fiberglass neck cast to provide temporary stabilization of nondisplaced cervical fractures or soft tissue instability
• Surgical exploration or debridement of puncture wounds or draining tracts
• Surgical drainage of intramuscular or osseous abscess
• Spinal surgery to provide vertebral stabilization or decompression of the spinal cord
• Intraarticular corticosteroid injections
• Muscle relaxants
• Antibiotic therapy based on culture and sensitivity testing
• Antiprotozoal, antihelmintics, or antiviral medications, as indicated
• Antioxidant supplementation with vitamin E (IM initially; then PO long term)
• Chondroprotective agents
• Electroacupuncture or mesotherapy to reduce pain and muscle hypertonicity
• Electrical muscle stimulation to normalize muscle tone and maintain or stimulate development
• Elevation of water and feed to normal head height if the horse is not able to lower the head and neck
• Controlled handwalking

CHRONIC TREATMENT

• Active and passive neck stretching exercises to restore joint mobility
• Acupuncture to reduce pain
• Chiropractic treatment to increase segmental mobility
• Massage therapy
• Physical therapy and rehabilitation

• Moist heat therapy to reduce pain and muscle hypertonicity
• Extracorporeal shock-wave therapy
• Ground pole and Cavalletti exercises to stimulate proprioception and neuromuscular control
• Warm-up or flexibility exercises: "Long and low" on lunge line, circles, figure-8's, and serpentine movements
• Lunge in a chambon
• Active retraction stretches of the thoracic limb

DRUG INTERACTIONS

• Complications associated with long-term phenylbutazone use in horses include gastritis and right dorsal colitis.
• Gastric ulceration and renal failure
• NSAIDs should not be used in conjunction with corticosteroids

POSSIBLE COMPLICATIONS

• Adverse reaction to antiinflammatory medications.
• Neurologic complications associated with spinal surgery.
• Assess underlying predisposition and total dosage of corticosteroids to reduce the risk of corticosteroid-induced laminitis.

RECOMMENDED MONITORING

• Soft tissue palpation for resolution of cervical pain and muscle hypertonicity
• Repeat physical and chiropractic examination to assess the response to therapy or rehabilitation
• Repeat neurologic examinations to assess ataxia or paresis

PROGNOSIS AND OUTCOME

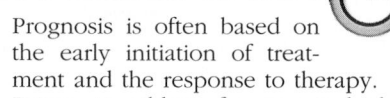

• Prognosis is often based on the early initiation of treatment and the response to therapy.
• Return to athletic function is highly variable depending on the specific etiology and the severity of the underlying disease process.
• Depends on severity and duration of neurologic deficits and intended use.

PEARLS & CONSIDERATIONS

COMMENTS

• Active and passive neck ROM exercises are useful for identifying affected vertebral levels and laterality of the cervical dysfunction.
• If appropriate and timely therapeutic responses are not noted with conservative care, then advanced diagnostics are warranted.

PREVENTION

- Restricted protein and carbohydrate diet in foals (<1 year) with potential for rapid growth
- Provide quick releases or break-away fasteners to reduce the risk of pulling back and flipping over backward in cross-ties.
- Importance of maintaining neck flexibility and ROM exercises
- DNA testing and selective breeding to noncarriers of genetic-based diseases

CLIENT EDUCATION

- Monitor signs of pain, muscle hypotonicity, and stiffness.
- Avoid riding exercise in any horse with neurologic deficits.

SUGGESTED READING

Barber SM: Management of neck and head injuries. *Vet Clin North Am Equine Pract* 21:191–215, 2005.

Clayton HM, Townsend HG: Kinematics of the cervical spine of the adult horse. *Equine Vet J* 21:189–192, 1989.

Dyson SJ: The cervical spine and soft tissues of the neck. In Ross MW, Dyson SJ, editors: *Diagnosis and management of lameness in the horse*, St Louis, 2003, Elsevier, pp 522–531.

AUTHOR: **KEVIN K. HAUSSLER**

EDITOR: **ANDRIS J. KANEPS**

Nematodiasis, Cerebrospinal

BASIC INFORMATION

DEFINITION

A central nervous system (CNS) dysfunction resulting from aberrant migration of nematode or larval parasites

SYNONYM(S)

- Aberrant parasite migration
- Meningeal worm
- Parasitic encephalomyelitis
- Verminous myelitis or encephalitis

EPIDEMIOLOGY

RISK FACTORS

- Exposure to white-tailed deer, which are commonly affected with the meningeal worm (*Parelaphostrongylus tenuis*)
- Immunocompromise, chronic, debilitating disease or prolonged recumbency (*Halicephalobus deletrix*)

CONTAGION AND ZOONOSIS

- Infections take place in incidental hosts or if aberrant parasite migration occurs in definitive hosts.
- Transmammary transmission of *H. deletrix* from a mare to her foal has been reported.

ASSOCIATED CONDITIONS AND DISORDERS

- Acquired scoliosis has been associated with *P. tenuis* infection.
- Horses affected with *H. deletrix* often have concurrent renal disease and osteolysis and granulomatous lesions involving the gingiva, mandible, or maxilla. Infections may also involve the udder, prepuce, lymph nodes, heart, stomach, lung, eye, or liver.
- Aberrant migration of *Strongylus vulgaris* may be more likely in horses with very poor deworming history and evidence of large strongyle migration, such as cranial mesenteric endarteritis.

CLINICAL PRESENTATION

HISTORY, CHIEF COMPLAINT

- Acquired scoliosis
- Ataxia (often asymmetrical)
- Blindness
- Cranial nerve deficits (dysphagia, head tilt, circling)
- Depression
- Granulomatous inflammation of the mouth, mandible, or maxilla
- Paresis
- Recumbency
- Seizures
- Weight loss
- Most cases are acute and rapidly progressive but may have an insidious onset

PHYSICAL EXAM FINDINGS

- Ataxia, paresis, or both (often asymmetrical)
- Behavioral changes
- Cranial nerve deficits: Blindness, circling, dysphagia, head tilt
- Granulomas of the mouth or nasal cavity
- Scoliosis: Cervical muscle flaccidity and cutaneous hypalgesia on the convex side of neck; ataxia ipsilateral or more severe on the convex side of scoliosis

ETIOLOGY AND PATHOPHYSIOLOGY

- Clinical signs result from migration of parasites through the CNS, direct damage to neural tissue, and the resultant inflammatory response.
- *Draschia megastoma*
- *H. deletrix*
- *Hypoderma* spp.
- *P. tenuis*
- *Setaria* spp.
- *Strongylus equinus*
- *S. vulgaris*

DIAGNOSIS

DIFFERENTIAL DIAGNOSIS

- Cervical vertebral malformation
- Equine degenerative myelopathy
- Equine herpesvirus-1 myelopathy
- Equine protozoal myeloencephalitis
- Leukoencephalomalacia
- Meningitis
- Neoplasia
- Temporohyoid osteoarthropathy
- Trauma
- Viral encephalitides (Eastern equine encephalitis, Western equine encephalitis, Venezuelan equine encephalitis, rabies, West Nile virus)

INITIAL DATABASE

- Complete blood count
- Serum chemistries
- Neurologic examination

ADVANCED OR CONFIRMATORY TESTING

- Radiographs of the skull, cervical spine, or both
- Cerebrospinal fluid (CSF) analysis and cytology: Xanthochromia, pleocytosis, and elevated protein concentration
- Magnetic resonance imaging
- Biopsy of granulomas may reveal *H. deletrix* nematodes.
- Postmortem examination, histopathology, and microscopic parasite morphology are most useful for a definitive diagnosis.

TREATMENT

THERAPEUTIC GOAL(S)

- Kill migrating parasites.
- Control and reduce CNS inflammation.
- Provide supportive care until the horse's neurologic function improves.

ACUTE GENERAL TREATMENT

- Fenbendazole: 50 mg/kg PO q24h for 5 days
- Ivermectin: 0.2 mg/kg PO; some authors recommend treatment q24h for 5 days
- Moxidectin: 0.4 mg/kg PO; has improved lipid solubility compared

with ivermectin and may better cross the blood-brain barrier
- Corticosteroids: Dexamethasone (0.05–0.2 mg/kg IV q12–24h) or methylprednisolone sodium succinate (1.0–2.5 mg/kg IV q6h); the dose and interval depend on the severity of clinical signs
- Flunixin meglumine: 1.1 mg/kg IV q12–24h
- Dimethyl sulfoxide: 0.5 to 1.0 g/kg IV q12–24h; must be diluted to a 10% solution or less in an isotonic balanced electrolyte solution
- IV fluids in recumbent, dehydrated, or dysphagic horses

CHRONIC TREATMENT

- Flunixin meglumine (0.5–1.1 mg/kg PO q12–24h), phenylbutazone (1–2 mg/kg PO q12–24h), prednisolone (0.5–1.0 mg/kg PO q12–24h), or dexamethasone (0.05–0.2 mg/kg PO q12–24h) as needed for CNS inflammation.
- Diethylcarbamazine (20–50 mg/kg PO q24h for ≤10 days) has been recommended for killing microfilaria or migrating larval parasites.
- Horses that are unable to stand or get up on their own need to be placed into a sling periodically.

POSSIBLE COMPLICATIONS

Ivermectin and moxidectin do not normally cross the blood-brain barrier. Clinical signs of avermectin toxicity are

possible if the blood-brain barrier has been significantly damaged by migrating parasites.

RECOMMENDED MONITORING

- Periodic repeat neurologic examinations to assess response to therapy
- Packed cell volume, total protein, blood urea nitrogen, and creatinine concentrations to monitor hydration and renal function with possible nephrotoxic drugs

PROGNOSIS AND OUTCOME

- The overall prognosis for complete recovery is guarded to poor. Most cases are rapidly progressive after clinical signs begin.
- Horses that are recumbent or unable to stand or support themselves in a sling for longer than 2 to 3 days are unlikely to recover.
- Horses that survive may have permanent neurologic deficits or scoliosis.

PEARLS & CONSIDERATIONS

COMMENTS

Cerebrospinal fluid pleocytosis and eosinophilia are reportedly inconsistent

findings. However, CSF eosinophilia along with consistent clinical signs is strongly suggestive of cerebrospinal nematodiasis.

PREVENTION

- Ivermectin and moxidectin are highly effective against *S. vulgaris*.
- Regular deworming may reduce numbers of migrating larvae in the host, environmental exposure to parasite eggs, and overall parasite burden.
- Avoiding possible ingestion of terrestrial snails and slugs on pasture and grazing with white-tailed deer may decrease the risk of *P. tenuis* infection.
- Because most cases involve incidental infections or aberrant parasite migration, no preventive strategy is likely to be efficacious or beneficial.

SUGGESTED READING

Johnson AL, de Lahunta A, Divers TJ: Acquired scoliosis in equids: case series and proposed pathogenesis, In *Proc Am Assoc Equine Pract*, 54:192–197, 2008.
Lester G: Parasitic encephalomyelitis in horses. *Compend Contin Educ Prac Vet* 14:1624, 1992.

AUTHOR: **BRYAN M. WALDRIDGE**

EDITOR: **STEPHEN M. REED**

Neonatal Colic

BASIC INFORMATION

DEFINITION

Colic is the descriptive term used for abdominal pain and can have many causes.

EPIDEMIOLOGY

SPECIES, AGE, SEX There is no gender predisposition for most forms of neonatal colic. Meconium impactions are suggested to occur more commonly in colts because of their smaller pelvic opening diameter.
GENETICS AND BREED PREDISPOSITION For most causes of neonatal colic, there is no genetic or breed predilection. Overo lethal white syndrome (OLWS) occurs in breeds that commonly carry the mutation, including American Paint Horses, Miniature Horses, Pintos, and less commonly Quarter Horses.
RISK FACTORS For colic caused by enteritis, unsanitary farm conditions and

failure of passive transfer are contributory.
CONTAGION AND ZOONOSIS Infectious causes of enteritis include infection with *Salmonella* spp., *Campylobacter* spp., *Escherichia coli*, and *Clostridium* spp.
ASSOCIATED CONDITIONS AND DISORDERS Failure of passive transfer, peritonitis, pneumonia, enteritis

CLINICAL PRESENTATION

DISEASE FORMS/SUBTYPES Neonatal colic can be caused by congenital abnormalities for which there is no treatment (atresia coli, OLWS); medical causes such as enteritis and meconium impactions; and causes that require surgery such as small intestinal volvulus, hernias, and (rarely) meconium impactions refractory to medical treatment.
HISTORY, CHIEF COMPLAINT Failure to nurse, lethargy, recumbency, failure to pass feces, fever, rolling on back, abdominal distension

PHYSICAL EXAM FINDINGS Variable depending on condition and severity. Elevated (>100 beats/min) heart rate, reduced borborygmi, and abdominal bloating are common. If enteritis is a component of the colic episode, fever (>102° F), dehydration, and clinical signs of endotoxemia are present. Digital palpation may reveal meconium impactions or a lack of any fecal output (atresia coli, OLWS).
ETIOLOGY AND PATHOPHYSIOLOGY
- Atresia coli is the result of incomplete formation of the intestinal tract, but the cause is unknown.
- OLWS is caused by a genetic mutation resulting in abnormal autonomic innervation of the intestinal tract.
- Meconium impactions are caused by large amounts or very sticky and tenacious meconium.
- Enteritis often has an infectious component.

DIAGNOSIS

DIFFERENTIAL DIAGNOSIS

- Uroperitoneum
- Enteritis
- Sepsis

INITIAL DATABASE

- Complete blood count, serum chemistry, serum immunoglobulin G concentration
- Physical examination, including digital examination, enema, and nasogastric intubation
- Percutaneous abdominal ultrasonography

ADVANCED OR CONFIRMATORY TESTING

- Abdominal radiography, which may include positive contrast material
- Rectal endoscopy for suspected cases of atresia coli
- Abdominocentesis
- Exploratory laparotomy

TREATMENT

THERAPEUTIC GOAL(S)

- Determination of the cause of colic
- Alleviation of pain
- Surgical correction of the cause if necessary

ACUTE GENERAL TREATMENT

- Exploratory laparotomy if pain cannot be controlled
- Medical therapy for ileus and enteritis, including IV fluid therapy, feeding restrictions, and intestinal protectants

CHRONIC TREATMENT

Most neonatal colic episodes are acute and do not require long-term therapy. One exception is gastric ulcer syndrome, which is treated with drugs to increase gastric pH such as omeprazole and cimetidine. Sucralfate can also be used to provide local ulcer therapy.

POSSIBLE COMPLICATIONS

Abdominal adhesions may result from either medical or surgical colic treatment if there is sufficient peritoneal inflammation.

PROGNOSIS AND OUTCOME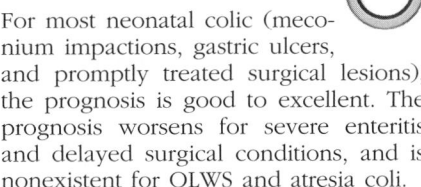

For most neonatal colic (meconium impactions, gastric ulcers, and promptly treated surgical lesions), the prognosis is good to excellent. The prognosis worsens for severe enteritis and delayed surgical conditions, and is nonexistent for OLWS and atresia coli.

PEARLS & CONSIDERATIONS

COMMENTS

- Medical therapy is much preferred for meconium impactions because of the risk of small colon adhesions when treated surgically.
- Functional and mechanical ileus can be difficult to discriminate between, and early laparotomy is preferred if a mechanical cause is suspected.

PREVENTION

- Consumption of sufficient colostrum is important for its laxative effects and should be ensured.
- Avoiding breeding carriers of the mutation responsible for OLWS will eliminate this condition.
- Good management, including hygiene and isolation of potentially infectious animals, will reduce the incidence of infectious enteritis, which can lead to ileus, diarrhea, and small intestinal surgical lesions.

SUGGESTED READING

Cohen ND, Chaffin MK: Assessment and initial management of colic in foals. *Compend Contin Educ Pract Vet* 17:93–102, 1995.
Santschi EM, Slone DE, Embertson RM, et al: Colic surgery in 206 juvenile thoroughbreds: survival and racing results. *Equine Vet J Suppl* June(32):32–36, 2000.

AUTHOR: **ELIZABETH M. SANTSCHI**

EDITORS: **PHOEBE A. SMITH** and **ELIZABETH M. SANTSCHI**

Neonatal Flexural Deformities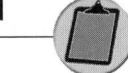

BASIC INFORMATION

DEFINITION

Neonatal flexural deformities are abnormalities of limb posture that result in abnormal extension or flexion of limbs. A rare, severe, and uniformly fatal condition known as arthrogryposis results in deformities in many joints of the axial as well as appendicular skeleton.

SYNONYM(S)

Contracted tendons, calf knees, arthrogryposis

EPIDEMIOLOGY

SPECIES, AGE, SEX Age: Congenital
RISK FACTORS
- Speculative risk factors: Lack of fetal movement or reduced uterine space (flexural) and prematurity or dysmaturity (extensor).
- For arthrogryposis, ingestion of toxic plants such as locoweed or hybrid Sudan grass. Congenital hypothyroidism due to ingestion of nitrates may also result in flexural deformities.

ASSOCIATED CONDITIONS AND DISORDERS

- Because congenital flexural deformities may result in dystocia, asphyxia and its systemic effects often occur after a difficult delivery. Failure of passive transfer may occur in foals having difficulty standing to nurse and may lead to septic complications.
- Strain or rupture of the extensor tendons at the carpus is common in foals with forelimb flexural deformities, and crushing of the tarsal bones is commonly associated in foals with hindlimb extension deformities.
- Radial nerve injury rarely occurs with forelimb flexural deformities and may be the result of dystocia.
- Foals with arthrogryposis often have multiple abnormalities and either are born dead or die soon after birth.

CLINICAL PRESENTATION

DISEASE FORMS/SUBTYPES

- Arthrogryposis is a rare, severe, diffuse, and untreatable form of congenital flexural deformity and will not be further discussed here. Congenital hypothyroidism is discussed in "Hypothyroidism" in this section. More common flexural and extensor deformities generally occur in either the forelimbs or the hindlimbs and can be unilateral or more commonly bilateral.

- Flexural deformities in the forelimb most commonly involve the carpus and result in flexion of all joints distal to the carpus. Flexural deformities in the hindlimb generally involve only the fetlock and exhibit coffin joint extension.
- A rare form of flexural deformity in the hindlimbs involves only the tarsus.
- Both forelimb and hindlimb flexural deformities vary in severity from mild deformities that do not hinder ambulation to severe deformities that cannot be corrected.
- Extensor deformities in the forelimb result in hyperextension of the carpus and distal joints and in the hindlimb result in hock and stifle flexion and digital extension.

HISTORY, CHIEF COMPLAINT Inability to stand, difficulty in ambulation, abnormal limb posture

PHYSICAL EXAM FINDINGS
- Flexural deformities: Inability to manipulate the limb into normal extension, swellings of the lateral digital extensor tendon sheath in the forelimbs
- Extensor deformities: Excessive extension of the joints, lack of tension in the palmar or plantar soft tissues, reduced gluteal muscle mass

ETIOLOGY AND PATHOPHYSIOLOGY
- Flexural deformities: Speculated to be a lack of fetal movement or reduced uterine space, restricting movement
- Extensor deformities: Speculated to be the result of relative immaturity of the musculoskeletal system

DIAGNOSIS

DIFFERENTIAL DIAGNOSIS
- Congenital neurologic conditions, including vertebral abnormalities
- Septicemia

INITIAL DATABASE
- Physical examination is sufficient to diagnose flexural and extensor deformities; however, a determination of the serum immunoglobulin G concentration is appropriate to ensure passive transfer of immunoglobulins.
- If prematurity or dysmaturity is suspected, dorsopalmar radiography of the carpi and lateral-medial radiography of the tarsi can ascertain cuboidal bone maturity.

TREATMENT

THERAPEUTIC GOAL(S)
- Flexural deformities
  - Relax the palmar or plantar soft tissues.

- Properly align the limb to allow body weight to stretch the palmar or plantar soft tissues.
  - Provide analgesia to promote weight-bearing.
- Extensor deformities
  - Properly align hyperextended joints.
  - Allow exercise to strengthen tissues but not to cause damage.

ACUTE GENERAL TREATMENT
The severity of the deformity dictates the level of treatment.
- Flexural deformities
  - Mild: Limb posture abnormal but can bear weight without assistance; usually no definitive treatment is necessary. Exercise should be cautiously provided to avoid pain. Cautious use of nonsteroidal anti-inflammatory drugs (NSAIDs) may be beneficial. Firm support bandages can be used to extend and protect the dorsal surface of the fetlock.
  - Moderate: Cannot bear weight unassisted; limb cannot be manually straightened. Oxytetracycline (50 mg/kg IV q24h) and limb splints (12-h limit daily) to load palmar or plantar soft tissues. Phenylbutazone (2–4 mg/kg IV q24h) or flunixin meglumine (1 mg/kg IV q24h) for analgesia. Application of acrylic toe extensions may be used to extend the digit.
  - Severe: Carpal flexion angles of 90 degrees and fetlock joints with no range of motion, tarsal flexion. Treatment as indicated for moderate deformities can be attempted but is difficult to achieve and rarely successful. Surgery to cut palmar or plantar soft tissues can be attempted but is also often unsuccessful. Euthanasia for humane reasons is a realistic option for foals with severe flexural deformities.
- Extensor deformities
  - Mild: Hyperextension of the digit; usually self-limiting. Trimming of rounded heels, quarters, and bars may promote a flat foot placement. Exercise should be cautiously provided to avoid pain and direct trauma to the limb. A light bandage may be applied to the heel bulbs to limit abrasions.
  - Moderate: Fetlock dropped but pastern above horizontal. Similar therapy to the mild cases with the addition of heel extensions to promote flat foot placement and limit hyperextension of limb; especially important if the cuboidal bones are immature.
  - Severe: Fetlock palmar or plantar surface on the ground; carpal joints

hyperextended. Some form of coaptation is necessary to avoid crushing of bones because of abnormal loading. Exercise is necessary to promote musculotendinous strength but can cause permanent skeletal deformities. These foals are very difficult to manage successfully, and euthanasia may be appropriate.

CHRONIC TREATMENT
- Most flexural and extensor deformities improve within 1 week, so long-term therapy is unnecessary. However, because these limbs are not normal even if they have assumed an apparently normal posture, exercise should be cautiously reintroduced to allow tissues to adapt. The horse should be kept in a large double stall for the first 10 days and then in a very small paddock or round pen for the next 10 days before free exercise is allowed.
- Foals with very active dams should initially have limited time in the pasture after free exercise commences.
- For neglected moderate flexural deformities of the forelimb fetlock, inferior check ligament desmotomy may be performed with reasonable success expectations.

POSSIBLE COMPLICATIONS
- Most complications are traumatic in nature and are related to abnormal limb loading, coaptation injuries, or overexercise.
- Injuries seen include proximal sesamoid fractures, extensor tendon ruptures, crushed tarsal bones, damage to heel bulbs, and cast or bandage sores.
- Septic complications occur secondary to failure of passive transfer caused by an inability to nurse. Gastric ulceration may be the result of stress or treatment with NSAIDs.

PROGNOSIS AND OUTCOME
- Foals with mild to moderate flexural and extensor deformities have an excellent prognosis if treated immediately.
- Foals with severe deformities have a guarded to poor prognosis depending on the severity of the deformity.

PEARLS & CONSIDERATIONS
- Foals have extremely thin skin and are very susceptible to sores from coaptation. Splints and casts should be cautiously applied and removed when any sign of discomfort

referable to the coaptation is noted. When splints are used to provide strong posture correction, they should be placed on limbs for 12 hours and then removed for 12 hours.
- The dose of oxytetracycline used to relax the soft tissues is very high and

may be contraindicated in foals with renal compromise. In normal foals, its use once daily has been safe and effective, and it may be used several days consecutively. Its use may result in excessive relaxation, so the position of all limbs should be monitored.

SUGGESTED READING

Adams SB, Santschi EM: Congenital equine flexural deformities. *Proc Am Assoc Equine Pract* 46:117–125, 2000.

AUTHOR: **ELIZABETH M. SANTSCHI**

EDITORS: **PHOEBE A. SMITH** and **ELIZABETH M. SANTSCHI**

Neonatal Isoerythrolysis

BASIC INFORMATION

DEFINITION

Hemolytic anemia of newborn foals caused by alloantibodies directed against the foal's red blood cells (RBCs).

SYNONYM(S)

- Jaundiced foal syndrome
- Isoimmune hemolytic anemia
- Alloimmune hemolytic anemia

EPIDEMIOLOGY

SPECIES, AGE, SEX Newborn foals are affected, with clinical signs appearing at 1 to 8 days.
GENETICS AND BREED PREDISPOSITION Any breed may be affected, but Thoroughbreds, Standardbreds, and American Paint Horses are overrepresented. There is a higher incidence in mule foals than in horse foals because of a unique blood group antigen called "donkey factor."
RISK FACTORS
- Dams previously administered blood transfusions or other equine biologic agents
- Mares are exposed to fetal RBCs with each pregnancy; thus multiparous mares produce foals at higher risk than primiparous mares.

CLINICAL PRESENTATION

DISEASE FORMS/SUBTYPES
- Subclinical
- Peracute

HISTORY, CHIEF COMPLAINT
- Foal normal at birth, stood and nursed, acute or insidious onset of weakness, tachypnea, icterus. Presentation of clinical signs typically occurs 2 to 5 days after birth.
- Peracute cases may collapse 8 to 36 hours after nursing.

PHYSICAL EXAM FINDINGS
- Weakness, lethargy, tachypnea, tachycardia, pale or icteric mucous membranes, pigmenturia, cardiovascular collapse.
- Fever is variable.

- Death may occur before icterus develops in peracute cases.
- Mild cases result in subclinical disease.

ETIOLOGY AND PATHOPHYSIOLOGY

- NI occurs when a fetus inherits the RBC antigens of the stallion and the mare is negative for these RBC antigens. She develops alloantibodies to the offending RBC antigen of the foal through exposure by prior pregnancy, blood transfusion, or transplacental contamination with fetal blood earlier in the current pregnancy. At birth, the foal ingests colostrum containing the alloantibodies. The alloantibodies then bind to the RBCs of the foal, resulting in agglutination, lysis, or both.
- The most common factors (antigens) involved in neonatal isoerythrolysis (NI) are Qa and Aa; mares without Qa and Aa factors are at an increased risk of producing NI-causing antibodies.

DIAGNOSIS

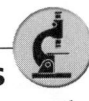

DIFFERENTIAL DIAGNOSIS

- Disseminated intravascular coagulation
- Hemolysis secondary to septicemia
- Transfusion reaction

INITIAL DATABASE

- Packed cell volume (PCV) and total solids (TS): PCV will be low with normal total solids.
- Jaundiced foal agglutination (JFA) assay: Serial dilutions of the mare's colostrum are centrifuged in the presence of the foal's RBCs. A positive reaction is indicated by clumping of RBCs at the bottom of the tube at dilutions of 1:16 or greater.
- Lactate above 5 mmol/L; not specific for NI.

ADVANCED OR CONFIRMATORY TESTING

- Hemolytic cross-match test
- Coomb's test: Not specific for NI

TREATMENT

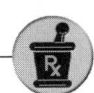

THERAPEUTIC GOAL(S)

- Prevent further ingestion of alloantibodies in colostrum in foals less than 18 hours of age.
- Maintain adequate oxygen-carrying RBC mass.

ACUTE GENERAL TREATMENT

- Mild cases (mild tachypnea, still nursing, and ambulatory): Muzzle if younger than 18 hours old and give alternate source of colostrum or plasma if IgG is below 400 mg/dL; monitor for increase in severity of clinical signs; minimize exercise and stress.
- Moderate (weak, tachycardic and tachypneic) and severe cases (recumbent): Blood transfusion is indicated. Twice-washed RBCs from the dam, a cross-matched donor whose RBCs do not react with the foal's serum, or a known Qa- and Aa-negative donor are ideal choices. If typed donors and cross-matching are not possible, the donors least likely to contain Aa and Qa antibodies are geldings of Standardbred, Quarter Horse, or Morgan breeds.
- The volume of blood needed for transfusion can be calculated as Body weight (kg) × 150 mL/kg × (PCV desired − PCV observed)/PCV of donor.
- Milk out the mare while the foal is muzzled to ensure colostrum is removed from the mammary gland and to maintain milk production.

POSSIBLE COMPLICATIONS

- Hypoxic-ischemic damage to organs
- Seizures in severe cases
- Kernicterus (deposition of unconjugated bilirubin and neuronal necrosis of certain areas of the brain)

RECOMMENDED MONITORING

Monitor affected foals closely during and after transfusion. Transfused RBCs remain in circulation for approximately 3 to 9 days, allowing for oxygen delivery until the bone marrow responds adequately.

PROGNOSIS AND OUTCOME

Prognosis depends largely on the quantity of alloantibodies absorbed, the affinity of the antibody for the RBC antigen, and the time before initiation of treatment. In uncomplicated cases, the prognosis is generally good. Survival rates have been reported as 73% for all NI cases.

PEARLS & CONSIDERATIONS

COMMENTS

- Relying on PCV to dictate necessity for transfusion is difficult because plasma volume affects PCV, and oxygen carrying-capacity may not be accurately reflected by this number. Clinical signs of hypoxemia are best used to determine the need for transfusion.
- In cases requiring muzzling of the foal, continue to strip out the dam's udder to encourage milk production.

PREVENTION

- Screen mares for RBC antibodies against the major blood group antigens.

- Crossmatch antibody screened mares with stallions.
- JFA test should be done before the foal nurses in matings of unknown blood types or in mares delivering NI foals previously.
- Muzzle a foal for 18 to 24 hours born to a dam known to produce NI foals and administer alternate colostrum source or feed milk from another dam and administer IV plasma to provide immunoglobulins.

SUGGESTED READING

Whiting JL, David JB: Neonatal isoerythrolysis. *Compend Contin Educ Pract Vet* 22:968, 2000.

AUTHOR: **PHOEBE A. SMITH**

EDITORS: **PHOEBE A. SMITH** and **ELIZABETH M. SANTSCHI**

Neonatal Sepsis

BASIC INFORMATION

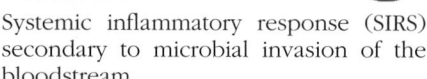

DEFINITION

Systemic inflammatory response (SIRS) secondary to microbial invasion of the bloodstream

SYNONYM(S)

Septicemia, blood poisoning

RISK FACTORS

- Prenatal: Dystocia, premature placental separation, placentitis, colic, other maternal illness
- Postnatal: Umbilical, gastrointestinal (GI), or respiratory infection; environmental conditions; altered gestation length

ASSOCIATED CONDITIONS AND DISORDERS Septic shock, multiple organ dysfunction syndrome (MODS)

CLINICAL PRESENTATION

HISTORY, CHIEF COMPLAINT Lethargy, decreased or poor affinity for the dam, weak suckle reflex, decreased nursing

PHYSICAL EXAM FINDINGS
- Dehydration: Sunken eyes, tacky mucous membranes, sluggish jugular fill, cool extremities
- Lethargy, weakness
- Hypothermia or hyperthermia
- Tachycardia or tachypnea (absence of these does not rule out sepsis)
- Mucous membranes: Injected, hyperemic with bounding pulse (hyperdynamic phase); pale and slow capillary refill time with weak pulse (hypodynamic phase)

- Localized signs of infection may be present: Diarrhea, reflux, ileus, dyspnea, uveitis, seizures, joint effusion, edema overlying joint or physis, omphalophlebitis, patent urachus

ETIOLOGY AND PATHOPHYSIOLOGY
- Microbes invade the immunologically naïve foal via the respiratory, GI, umbilicus, or skin; gain access to the bloodstream; and cause the release of inflammatory mediators. These increase microvascular permeability, creating a reduced effective circulating volume.
- Hypotension results from reduced systemic vascular resistance and arterial and venous dilatation. Induction of excess nitric oxide via endogenous pathways is responsible for these changes.
- Stimulation of the coagulation cascade and reduction of endogenous anticoagulants such as protein C and antithrombin may occur, leading to coagulopathies.
- Progression of sepsis results in reduced tissue perfusion; decreased oxygen delivery to tissues; and, ultimately, MODS and possibly death.

DIAGNOSIS

DIFFERENTIAL DIAGNOSIS

Hypoxic-ischemic encephalopathy, (also called neonatal maladjustment syndrome or dummy foal): Foals may appear weak and depressed with poor affinity for the dam with both hypoxic-ischemic encephalopathy and neonatal sepsis.

INITIAL DATABASE

- Complete blood count: Leukopenia or leukocytosis; leukopenia characterized by neutropenia is most common; left shift and toxic neutrophils are common; thrombocytopenia is common in early disseminated intravascular coagulation (DIC)
- Blood lactate: Elevated in hypoperfusion and in sepsis; normal lactate in a 1- to 2-day-old foal is 2 to 5 mmol/L
- Arterial blood gas: Acidemia (respiratory, metabolic, or mixed), hypoxemia (PaO$_2$ <80 mm Hg), severe hypoxemia (PaO$_2$ <60 mm Hg), and hypercapnia (PaCO$_2$ >65 mm Hg) indicate ventilatory insufficiency
- Blood glucose: Low because of a lack of intake and dysregulation in sepsis
- Serum chemistry panel: Azotemia, hyperbilirubinemia common
- Blood culture: Gold standard for definitive diagnosis of sepsis; results available in 48 to 72 hours; negative blood culture results do not rule out sepsis
- Sepsis score calculation: Developed to aid in predicting septicemia before return of blood culture results; compiled physical examination and laboratory data are used

ADVANCED OR CONFIRMATORY TESTING

- Indirect blood pressure: Low blood pressure occurs with septic shock (mean arterial pressure <65 mm Hg).
- Pulse oximetry (SpO$_2$): Estimates oxygen saturation (SpO$_2$ of 95% cor-

relates with PaO_2 of 80 mm Hg, and SpO_2 of 80% correlates with PaO_2 of 39 mm Hg); hypoxemia is common.

- Central venous pressure (CVP): Provides an estimate of preload and right heart function; elevations occur with iatrogenic fluid overload and right heart failure; trends are more significant than absolute numbers; estimated normal CVP for neonatal foals is 3 to 12 cm H_2O.
- Urine output: An indicator of renal blood flow; urine production should be at least 66% of fluid intake; indwelling urinary catheters can be used in recumbent neonates.
- Urine specific gravity: Normal neonatal foal urine is hyposthenuric (<1.008); dehydration results in concentrated urine in functioning kidneys.
- Umbilical ultrasonography: To measure umbilical structures for evidence of infection and initially for baseline values
- Thoracic and abdominal ultrasonography: To investigate both cavities for evidence of infection (pneumonia, peritonitis)
- Body weight: Serial measurements (daily or twice daily) help to estimate fluid balance and nutritional status.

TREATMENT

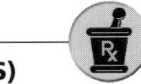

THERAPEUTIC GOAL(S)

- Eradicate infection and prevent secondary localized infection (septic physitis, arthritis, pneumonia)
- Maintain organ perfusion
- Maintain adequate nutrition

ACUTE GENERAL TREATMENT

- Antibiotic therapy
  - Broad-spectrum coverage should be initiated in all septic foals; coverage can be altered if results of blood culture and sensitivity indicate.
  - Avoid aminoglycosides in azotemic foals (consider a cephalosporin in azotemic foals); the minimum course of therapy recommended is 2 weeks; if localized signs of infec-

tion occur, a minimum of 4 weeks therapy is recommended.
  - Gram-negative isolates are more common than gram-positive isolates; more gram-negative isolates in septic foals are sensitive to amikacin than to gentamicin. Common regimens include penicillin (potassium penicillin 22,000 IU/kg IV q6h) and amikacin (22–25 mg/kg IV q24h) or a third-generation cephalosporin (cefotaxime 40 mg/kg IV q6h) with or without amikacin. Fluoroquinolones are associated with arthropathies in foals and should be reserved for cases with documented resistance to other antimicrobial agents and with owner consent.
- Nutrition
  - If too weak to nurse effectively, feeding via an indwelling nasogastric tube is recommended provided the GI tract tolerates feeding. Close monitoring of tube position and checking for reflux are essential.
  - Begin feeding with small volumes of 100 mL of milk to ensure that feeding will be tolerated; increase the volume slowly to achieve 20% body weight per day (divided into hourly or every 2-hour feedings).
  - If greater than 6 to 10 mL of reflux present, do not feed and investigate GI tract ultrasonographically; foals not tolerating enteral feeding require parenteral nutrition.
- Cardiovascular support
  - Fluid therapy is critical in foals with dehydration, acid-base derangements, and hypotension; IV crystalloids (lactated Ringer's solution, Normosol) supplemented with 2.5% to 10% dextrose are commonly used for emergency resuscitation.
  - After normovolemia has been established, most foals require an average of 100 mL/kg/d of IV crystalloids to maintain adequate hydration.

POSSIBLE COMPLICATIONS

- Short term: Acute renal failure, DIC, acute respiratory distress syndrome, intractable hypotension leading to cardiac arrest

- Long term: Localization of bacteria to joint, physis, diaphysis, brain, lung, eye, or other organ

RECOMMENDED MONITORING

- Vital parameters every 2 to 4 hours
- Blood gases, lactate, electrolytes as needed
- Urine production
- Body weight
- Joints, eyes, limbs for evidence of localized infection

PROGNOSIS AND OUTCOME

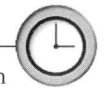

- Short-term survival has been reported to be 35% to 72%.
- Development of septic arthritis or physitis reduces the prognosis for long-term survival and future athleticism but is a viable option for committed clients.

PEARLS & CONSIDERATIONS

COMMENTS

- Early diagnosis and aggressive therapy provide the best opportunity for survival.
- Treatment and monitoring are intensive, so referral to a 24-hour hospital is common.

PREVENTION

Diagnose and treat failure of passive transfer early. This does not ensure that sepsis will not occur, but it decreases the likelihood.

SUGGESTED READING

Corley KTT: Evaluation of a score used to predict sepsis in foals. *J Vet Emerg Crit Care* 21:2, 2005.
Sanchez C: Neonatal sepsis. In Sanchez C (ed). *Neonatal medicine and surgery*, Philadelphia, 2005, Saunders Elsevier, pp 273–294.

AUTHOR: **PHOEBE A. SMITH**

EDITORS: **ELIZABETH M. SANTSCHI** and **PHOEBE A. SMITH**

Neonatal Septic Arthritis and Osteomyelitis

BASIC INFORMATION

DEFINITION

Orthopedic infection in neonates caused by hematogenous delivery of bacteria to joints and growth centers

SYNONYM(S)

Navel ill

EPIDEMIOLOGY

RISK FACTORS Failure of passive transfer; other septic processes, including septicemia, pneumonia, gastroenteritis, and omphalophlebitis

CONTAGION AND ZOONOSIS Enteritis from infectious causes such as *Salmonella* spp., rotavirus, and *Clostridium difficile*

ASSOCIATED CONDITIONS AND DISORDERS Failure of passive transfer; other septic processes, including septicemia, pneumonia, gastroenteritis, and omphalophlebitis

CLINICAL PRESENTATION

DISEASE FORMS/SUBTYPES Osteomyelitis has been classified by location, but these descriptive classifications are only relevant to treatment and outcome when discriminating between articular and nonarticular infections.

HISTORY, CHIEF COMPLAINT The foal's history may include dystocia, failure of passive transfer, and diarrhea. The chief complaint is usually lameness but may be stiffness, swollen joints, or recumbency.

PHYSICAL EXAM FINDINGS Lameness, limb swelling (especially around growth plates), joint effusion

ETIOLOGY AND PATHOPHYSIOLOGY
- Bacteria cause the infections and reach the musculoskeletal system because of a failure of normal barriers to infection such as mucosal barriers and the immune system.
- Most commonly, bacteria causing orthopedic infection are gram negative, but gram-positive and mixed infections do occur. Anaerobic bacteria are uncommon. Cultures of synovial fluid and affected bone should be performed to identify the organism(s) involved.

DIAGNOSIS

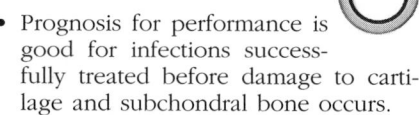

DIFFERENTIAL DIAGNOSIS

Immune-mediated synovitis

INITIAL DATABASE

- Complete blood count, serum chemistry, and immunoglobulin G concentration
- Radiography may be useful in determining if bone infection exists, but it takes several days after infection to show definitive radiographic changes.
- Cytologic examination of joint fluid can confirm if infection is present.
- Blood cell counts greater than 10,000 white blood cells/dL that are predominantly polymorphonuclear leukocytes indicate infection is likely.

ADVANCED OR CONFIRMATORY TESTING

- Aerobic and anaerobic bacterial culture of joint fluid, blood, or physeal aspirate may reveal causative bacteria.
- Cross-sectional imaging modalities such as computed tomography and magnetic resonance imaging may reveal bone destruction before it is radiographically apparent.

TREATMENT

THERAPEUTIC GOAL(S)

Immediate elimination of the causative organism to limit damage to critical structures

ACUTE GENERAL TREATMENT

- Administration of supplemental IV plasma to deliver immunoglobulins, complement, and other beneficial factors
- IV administration of broad-spectrum bactericidal antimicrobials
- Physical removal of bacteria and products of inflammation in joints and growth plates
- Regional treatment (intraarticular injection, regional IV perfusion, intralesional injection) of infected foci with antimicrobial drugs if possible

CHRONIC TREATMENT

- Implantation of beads containing antimicrobials
- Long-term (≥4 weeks) administration of oral antimicrobial agents

POSSIBLE COMPLICATIONS

The greatest complication is damage to structures critical to ambulation such as articular cartilage, subchondral bone, tendons, and tendon sheaths.

PROGNOSIS AND OUTCOME

- Prognosis for performance is good for infections successfully treated before damage to cartilage and subchondral bone occurs.
- Prognosis is worse when several locations are involved and when any joint surface is degraded.

PEARLS & CONSIDERATIONS

COMMENTS

- Aggressive therapy is indicated as soon as septic arthritis is suspected and at a minimum includes joint lavage and systemic antimicrobial therapy.
- Local therapy with antimicrobials should also be considered and may be delivered by intraarticular injection, regional IV perfusion, local injection, or implantation of antimicrobial-containing beads.

CLIENT EDUCATION

- Ensuring passive transfer of immunoglobulins and clean husbandry are important.
- Early identification of lameness is critical if infection occurs.

SUGGESTED READING

Hance SR, Schneider RK, Embertson RM, et al: Lesions of the caudal aspect of the femoral condyles in foals: 20 cases (1980-1990). *J Am Vet Med Assoc* 202:637–646, 1993.

Neil KM, Axon JE, Todhunter PG, et al: Septic osteitis of the distal phalanx in foals: 22 cases (1995–2002). *J Am Vet Med Assoc* 230:1683–1690, 2003.

Steel CM, Hunt AR, Adams PL, et al: Factors associated with prognosis for survival and athletic use in foals with septic arthritis: 93 cases (1987–1994). *J Am Vet Med Assoc* 215:973–977, 1995.

AUTHOR: ELIZABETH M. SANTSCHI

EDITORS: ELIZABETH M. SANTSCHI and PHOEBE A. SMITH

Neoplasia, Abdominal

BASIC INFORMATION

DEFINITION

Neoplasia of the abdominal (peritoneal) cavity

EPIDEMIOLOGY

SPECIES, AGE, SEX More likely in older horses

CLINICAL PRESENTATION

HISTORY, CHIEF COMPLAINT Typical signs associated with abdominal neoplasia include:

- Chronic weight loss
- Poor appetite
- Abdominal discomfort; chronic or recurrent colic
- Lethargy and exercise intolerance
- Ascites or edema may occur in some cases

Acute colic caused by intestinal strangulation may occur with mesenteric lipomas, which are frequently pedunculated.

PHYSICAL EXAM FINDINGS

- The physical examination findings confirm the presenting signs, which are weight loss with or without signs of abdominal pain. Persistent or intermittent pyrexia may occur with advanced neoplasia.
- Physical examination of the horse is often unrewarding but is essential, together with a thorough history, to eliminate other more common causes of weight loss such as:
  - Inadequate or unsuitable feeding
  - Dental or swallowing disorders
  - Excessive exercise or energy demands
  - Parasitism

ETIOLOGY AND PATHOPHYSIOLOGY

- The most common neoplasm of the abdominal cavity is mesenteric lipoma, which is common in older horses and especially ponies (>15 years). However, it is often clinically insignificant. When significant, the lipoma may produce signs only related to its physical properties, namely as a space-occupying mass causing a simple intestinal obstruction (caused by compression of the intestine), or more commonly as a pedunculated mass causing an acute strangulating intestinal obstruction.
- Other primary tumors originating in the peritoneal cavity are rare. Mesothelioma is a rare tumor of the mesothelial surfaces. It is most commonly reported in the thoracic cavity, although there have been a few reported cases in which the tumor appeared to develop within the peritoneal cavity.
- There have been isolated reports of omental leiomyoma and mesenteric myofibroblastoma in horses.
- Many other tumors may metastasize to the abdominal cavity. These include lymphoma (lymphosarcoma), squamous cell carcinoma, leiomyoma or leiomyosarcoma (gastrointestinal stromal tumors), adenocarcinoma, melanoma, testicular seminoma, teratoma, transitional cell carcinoma, hepatoblastoma, adrenocortical carcinoma, metastatic granulosa cell tumor, myxosarcoma, and hemangiosarcoma.
- Pheochromocytoma has been associated with acute colic in a small number of horses.

DIAGNOSIS

DIFFERENTIAL DIAGNOSIS

Other causes of chronic weight loss and chronic or recurrent colic

INITIAL DATABASE

- The diagnostic evaluation should consist of a complete physical examination, including rectal examination, routine bloodwork (complete blood count, serum chemistry panel), urinalysis, and peritoneal fluid analysis.
- Many horses with abdominal neoplasia have anemia (as a result of chronic disease or blood loss), leukocytosis (as a result of chronic inflammation), and hyperfibrinogenemia. In a small number of cases of lymphoma, abnormal lymphocytes may be present in the peripheral blood.
- Immune-mediated anemia or thrombocytopenia may occur secondary to neoplasia, especially lymphoma.
- Some affected horses have hypoalbuminemia and hypoproteinemia caused by malabsorption, bowel inflammation, and protein exudation, but other horses have hyperglobulinemia (as a result of chronic inflammation).
- Increased concentrations of the intestinal fraction of the alkaline phosphatase enzyme (IAP) may also indicate the presence of intestinal disease.
- Hypercalcemia has been reported in association with both lymphoma and gastric carcinoma.
- Rectal examination is essential in the investigation of any horse with suspected abdominal neoplasia. Although normal findings may be present in many animals, an increased volume of peritoneal fluid, distension of the intestine, or an abnormal tissue mass or masses increase the index of suspicion of abdominal neoplasia and allow further directed investigations to be selected.
- Peritoneal fluid varies from normal to an exudate. Neoplastic cells from a primary abdominal neoplasm (eg, mesothelioma or lymphoma) are occasionally observed in a sample of peritoneal fluid. In one study comparing the diagnostic features of cases of abdominal neoplasia and abdominal abscesses, peritoneal fluid was classified as an exudate in 12 of 15 horses with intraabdominal abscesses and 14 of 25 horses with intraabdominal neoplasms. Cytologic examination of peritoneal fluid yielded an accurate diagnosis in 11 of 25 horses with neoplasia and in three of 15 horses with abscesses. A mean number of 1.45 cytologic analyses per horse was needed to diagnose neoplasms in the 11 horses in which the analysis was successful in definitively diagnosing the condition.
- In some cases, peritoneal fluid is serosanguineous or frankly hemorrhagic.
- In cases of malignant melanoma of the peritoneal cavity, the peritoneal fluid may be discolored black.
- Neoplastic cells may also be identified in samples of pleural fluid if a pleural effusion is present.
- Pheochromocytoma should be considered in older horses with signs of abdominal pain, sweating, muscle fasciculations, ataxia, azotemia, and intraperitoneal hemorrhage. Identification by per rectum palpation of retroperitoneal swelling in the dorsal aspect of the abdomen also should alert the diagnostician to the possibility of a ruptured pheochromocytoma.

ADVANCED OR CONFIRMATORY TESTING

- Ultrasonography, laparoscopy, and laparotomy may be used to further evaluate the patient.
- Percutaneous or per rectum ultrasonography may provide information about the volume and character of the peritoneal fluid. Intestinal distension may be recognized together with abnormal bowel wall thickening and abnormal tissue masses. Ultrasonography also allows guided collection of fluid or tissue samples for further evaluation.

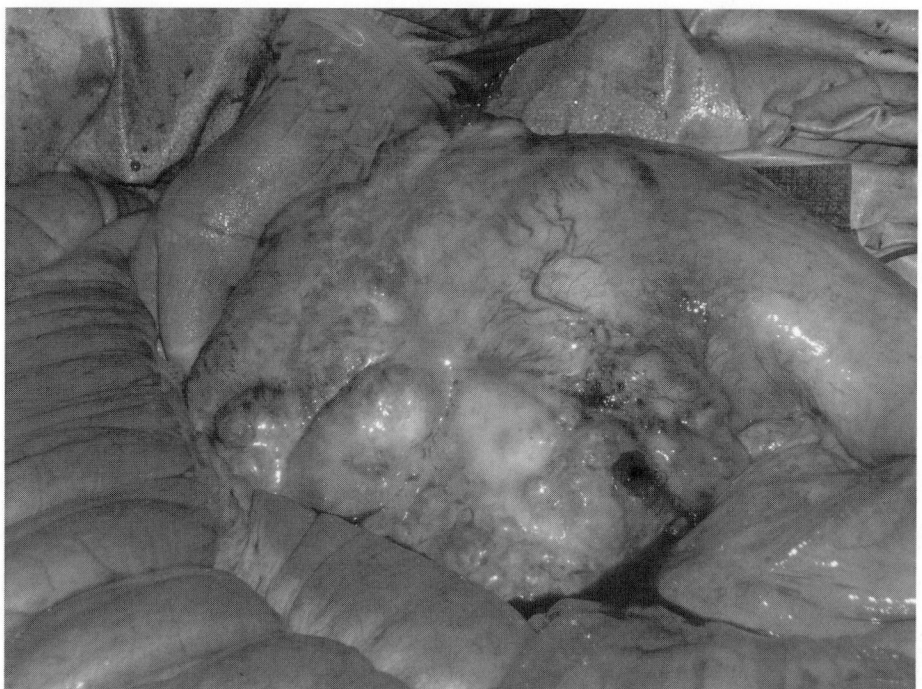

FIGURE 1 Mesenteric carcinoma identified at exploratory laparotomy.

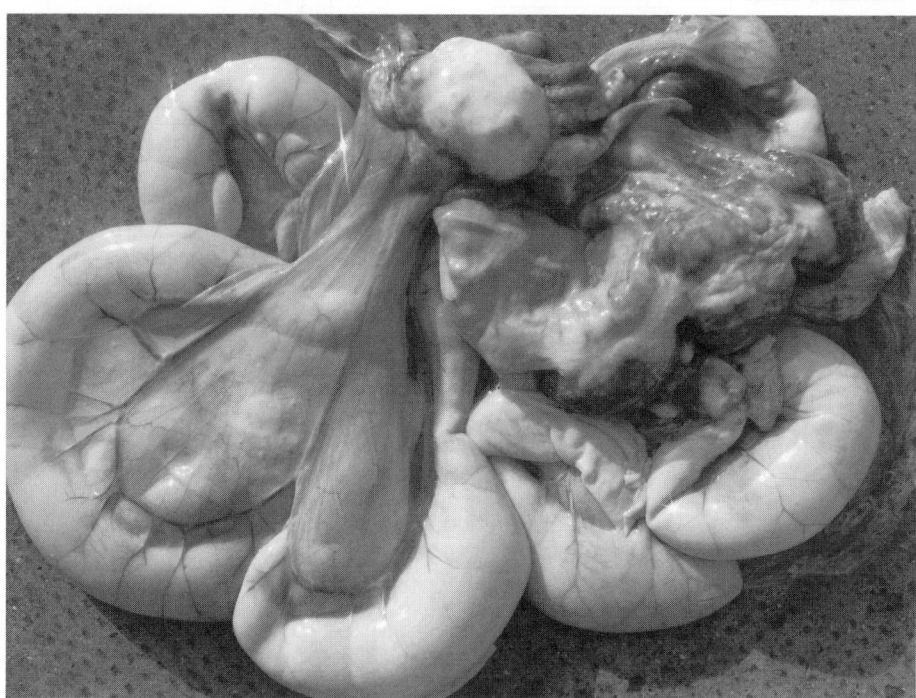

FIGURE 2 Mesenteric lymphoma masses identified at postmortem examination.

- Laparoscopy or exploratory laparotomy may be used to identify and biopsy tumor deposits in the abdominal cavity.
- Pleuroscopy (thoracoscopy) allows examination of the thoracic cavity in cases with evidence of spread of tumor to the thorax.
- Serum immunoglobulin (Ig) M is low in some cases of lymphoma; some also have low IgG and IgA levels.

TREATMENT

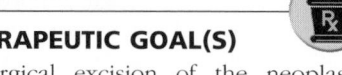

THERAPEUTIC GOAL(S)

- Surgical excision of the neoplastic mass if possible
- Chemotherapeutic treatment of the neoplasia if possible

ACUTE GENERAL TREATMENT

- Early surgical removal of mesenteric lipomas causing intestinal obstruction is frequently successful.
- Systemic corticosteroids, although not curative, may have a short-term beneficial effect on horses with lymphoma and may help treat secondary immune-mediated anemia and thrombocytopenia that may occur in association with lymphoma.

- Surgical removal of solitary neoplastic masses can be curative. Care should be taken that all the neoplastic tissue is removed during surgery, but this may be difficult because the limits of the neoplastic tissue may not be grossly visible.

CHRONIC TREATMENT

The systemic use of antineoplastic agents for the treatment of abdominal tumors in horses has received little attention and has unproven long-term efficacy. However, multiple drug protocols are available for palliative chemotherapy of multicentric lymphoma.

- The following is a suggested multiple agent induction protocol for horses with lymphoma:
  - Cytosine arabinoside: 200 to 300 mg/m^2 SC or IM once every 1 to 2 weeks
  - Chlorambucil: 20 mg/m^2 PO once every 2 weeks
  - Prednisone: 1.1 to 2.32 mg/kg PO every other day
- Alternatively, 200 mg/m^2 IV cyclophosphamide once every 2 to 3 weeks may be substituted for chlorambucil. Antineoplastic agents are typically given on alternating weeks but have been given on the same day without apparent ill effects. A response to this induction therapy should occur within 2 to 4 weeks. If no response is observed, adding vincristine (0.5 mg/m^2 IV once a week) has been recommended.
- Horses in remission should be maintained on the induction protocol for a total of 2 to 3 months before being switched to a maintenance protocol. The first cycle of maintenance therapy increases the treatment interval for each antineoplastic agent by 1 week. Prednisone is continued for the duration of therapy (but may be gradually reduced in dose). If the horse remains in remission after 2 to 3 months on the first cycle, the second cycle is begun by adding 1 more week to the treatment intervals of each agent. Several cycles of maintenance therapy may be given. Signs of toxicity, including bone marrow suppression and gastrointestinal irritation, have been rarely recognized using this protocol.
- Other protocols include:
  - Single-agent L-asparaginase: 10,000 to 40,000 IU/ m^2 IM once every 2 to 3 weeks
  - Single-agent cyclophosphamide: given as described above
  - Combinations of either cytosine arabinoside or cyclophosphamide with prednisone

RECOMMENDED MONITORING

During treatment, horses should be monitored for signs of pain, dehydration, and weight loss.

PROGNOSIS AND OUTCOME

- In most cases, the prognosis is poor.
- If a focal neoplasm that is amenable to surgical excision is present, then curative treatment may be possible.

PEARLS & CONSIDERATIONS

COMMENTS

- Abdominal neoplasia should be considered in all horses demonstrating signs of weight loss and chronic or recurrent colic.
- In all cases of neoplasia, the quality of life, economic issues, prognosis, and owner expectations must be carefully considered and discussed before any treatment is attempted.

SUGGESTED READING

Edwards GB, Proudman CJ: An analysis of 75 cases of intestinal obstruction caused by pedunculated lipomas. *Equine Vet J* 26:18, 1994.

Elce Y: Neoplastic disease of the gastrointestinal tract. In Robinson NE, Sprayberry KA (eds). *Current therapy in equine medicine*, ed 6, St Louis, 2009, Saunders Elsevier, pp 448–450.

Gift LJ, Gaughan EM, Schoning P: Metastatic granulosa cell tumor in a mare. *J Am Vet Med Assoc* 200:1525, 1992.

Hikita M, Ishikawa Y, Shibahara T, et al: Mesenteric myofibroblastoma in a horse. *Vet Rec* 154:795–796, 2004.

Hillyer MH: The use of ultrasound in the diagnosis of abdominal tumors in the horse. *Equine Vet Educ* 6:273, 1994.

Johnson PJ, Goetz TE, Foreman JH, et al: Pheochromocytoma in two horses. *J Am Vet Med Assoc* 206:837–841, 1995.

Johnson PJ, Wilson DA, Turk JR, et al: Disseminated leiomyomatosis in a horse. *J Am Vet Med Assoc* 205:725, 1994.

Mair TS, Hillyer MH: Clinical features of lymphosarcoma in the horse. *Equine Vet Educ* 4:108, 1992.

Schaudien D, Müller JM, Baumgärtner W: Omental leiomyoma in a male adult horse. *Vet Pathol* 44:722–726, 2007.

Stoica G, Cohen N, Mendes O, et al: Use of immunohistochemical marker calretinin in the diagnosis of a diffuse metastatic mesothelioma in an equine. *J Vet Diagn Invest* 16:240–243, 2004.

Tarrant J, Stokol T, Bartol J, et al: Diagnosis of malignant melanoma in a horse from cytology of body cavity fluid and blood. *Equine Vet J* 33:531–534, 2001.

Zicker SC, Wilson WD, Medearis I: Differentiation between intra-abdominal neoplasms and abscesses in horses, using clinical and laboratory data: 40 cases (1973–1988). *J Am Vet Med Assoc* 196:1130–1134, 1990.

AUTHOR & EDITOR: TIM MAIR

Neoplasia, Esophageal

BASIC INFORMATION

DEFINITION

Neoplasia of the esophagus

EPIDEMIOLOGY

SPECIES, AGE, SEX More likely in older horses

CLINICAL PRESENTATION

HISTORY, CHIEF COMPLAINT

- Clinical signs of recurrent esophageal obstruction.

- Weight loss.
- Inappetence or anorexia may be present in advanced cases.
- Recurrent colic (often associated with feeding) may be seen in some cases, especially if the patient has neoplastic involvement of the stomach as well as the esophagus.
- There may be a fetid odor around the mouth or nares.

PHYSICAL EXAM FINDINGS

- The findings on physical examination confirm the presenting signs, which include repeated bouts of esophageal dysphagia, hypersalivation, nasal discharge of saliva and food, retching, and bruxism.
- Persistent or intermittent pyrexia may occur with advanced neoplasia.

ETIOLOGY AND PATHOPHYSIOLOGY

- Squamous cell carcinoma is the most commonly reported neoplasm affecting the esophagus. In addition, extension of gastric squamous cell carcinoma into the distal esophagus may occur.
- In one reported case, squamous cell carcinoma developed within an esophageal diverticulum.

- Leiomyosarcoma has also been reported in association with gastric neoplasia.
- Exuberant granulation tissue in the esophagus without evidence of neoplasia has been reported in one horse.

DIAGNOSIS

DIFFERENTIAL DIAGNOSIS

Other causes of dysphagia (especially abnormalities of the pharyngeal and esophageal phases of deglutition), including pharyngeal paralysis, pharyngeal cysts, pharyngeal compression by strangles abscesses and guttural pouch empyema, subepiglottic cyst, fourth branchial arch defect, esophageal obstruction, megaesophagus, esophageal stricture, intramural esophageal cysts, esophageal rupture, and equine grass sickness.

INITIAL DATABASE

- The leukogram and hematology results are likely to be normal unless there is dehydration from chronic esophagitis or changes secondary to neoplasia elsewhere.
- Esophagoscopy reveals a mass obstructing the esophageal lumen. Biopsy of the mass may be possible via the endoscope. Squamous cell carcinoma typically has an ulcerated, cobblestone, or florid appearance.
- Contrast (or double-contrast) radiography is useful to confirm the position and extent of a filling defect in the esophagus.
- Gastroscopy, thoracic radiography, and a complete physical examination should be performed to identify the presence of neoplasia in other sites.

ADVANCED OR CONFIRMATORY TESTING

Pleuroscopy (thoracoscopy) allows examination of the thoracic portion of the esophagus and may permit surgical biopsy of esophageal tumors located in this region.

TREATMENT

THERAPEUTIC GOAL(S)

- Surgical excision of the neoplastic mass if possible
- Chemotherapeutic treatment of the neoplasia if possible

ACUTE GENERAL TREATMENT

- Transendoscopic excision and ablation of granulation tissue in the esophagus using a neodymium: yttrium-aluminum-garnet laser has been described. A similar treatment modality may be applicable to focal neoplasms in the esophagus.
- There have been no reports of chemotherapy or radiotherapy for the treatment of esophageal neoplasia, although these forms of treatment could be considered in appropriate cases.

CHRONIC TREATMENT

- Frequent small meals of moistened pellets or fresh grass should be fed.
- Piroxicam (0.2 mg/kg PO q24h) for squamous cell carcinoma.

POSSIBLE COMPLICATIONS

Complications include esophageal stricture and esophageal impaction.

RECOMMENDED MONITORING

During treatment, horses should be monitored for signs of dehydration and weight loss.

PROGNOSIS AND OUTCOME

- In most cases, the prognosis is poor.

PEARLS & CONSIDERATIONS

COMMENTS

- Esophageal neoplasia is rare but should be considered in horses presenting with recurrent esophageal obstruction.
- In all cases of neoplasia, the quality of life, economic issues, prognosis, and owner expectations must be carefully considered and discussed before any treatment is attempted.

SUGGESTED READING

Boy MG, Palmer JE, Heyer G, et al: Gastric leiomyosarcoma in a horse. *J Am Vet Med Assoc* 200:1363, 1992.

Campbell-Beggs CL, Kiper ML, MacAllister C, et al: Use of esophagoscopy in the diagnosis of esophageal squamous cell carcinoma in a horse. *J Am Vet Med Assoc* 202:617, 1993.

Erkert RS, MacAllister CG, Higbee R, et al: Use of neodymium-aluminium-garnet laser to remove granulation tissue from the esophagus of a horse. *J Am Vet Med Assoc* 221:403, 2002.

Ford TS, Vaala WE, Sweeney CR, et al: Pleuroscopic diagnosis of gastroesophageal squamous cell carcinoma in a horse. *J Am Vet Med Assoc* 190:1556, 1987.

Sanchez LC: Esophageal diseases. In Reed SM, Bayly WM, Sellon DC (eds). *Equine internal medicine*, ed 3, St Louis, 2010, Saunders, pp 830–838.

Moore JN, Kintner LD: Recurrent esophageal obstruction due to squamous cell carcinoma in a horse. *Cornell Vet* 66:590, 1976.

Roberts MC, Kelly WR: Squamous cell carcinoma of the lower cervical oesophagus in a pony. *Equine Vet J* 11:199, 1979.

AUTHOR & EDITOR: **TIM MAIR**

Neoplasia, Gastric

BASIC INFORMATION

DEFINITION

Neoplasia of the stomach

EPIDEMIOLOGY

SPECIES, AGE, SEX More likely in older horses

RISK FACTORS Because gastric neoplasias are so uncommon in horses, contributing factors are not known.

CLINICAL PRESENTATION

HISTORY, CHIEF COMPLAINT Typical signs associated with gastric squamous cell carcinoma include:

- Chronic weight loss
- Poor appetite
- Abdominal discomfort
- Lethargy
- Ascites or edema may occur in some cases. If the esophagus is involved,

dysphagia or ptyalism will be the predominant sign. Gastric squamous cell carcinoma involving the cardia may also result in dysphagia. Involvement at other sites in the stomach may result in signs of obstruction to outflow (colic) or weight loss.

- In some cases, tachypnea is a prominent sign, either because of metastasis to the thoracic cavity or pressure on the diaphragm from the tumor.

- Recurrent colic, especially colic associated with feeding, may occur.

PHYSICAL EXAM FINDINGS The findings of physical examination confirm the presenting signs, which include weight loss with or without signs of esophageal dysphagia. Persistent or intermittent pyrexia may occur with advanced neoplasia.

ETIOLOGY AND PATHOPHYSIOLOGY

- Squamous cell carcinoma is the most commonly reported neoplasm affecting the stomach.
- The rate of growth and aggressiveness of gastric squamous cell carcinoma in horses is variable. In some horses, the tumor remains localized within the stomach, but in others, the tumors may extend through the stomach wall and spread to other abdominal viscera or metastasize to other locations in the body.
- Leiomyosarcoma (gastrointestinal stromal tumors), adenocarcinoma, and lymphoma have also been reported in the equine stomach in many cases in association with neoplasia elsewhere in the body.
- Amyloid deposition in the stomach wall has been recorded secondary to myeloma (in association with amyloid deposition in other organs).
- Gastric hyperplastic polyp has been recorded in one horse.

DIAGNOSIS

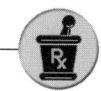

DIFFERENTIAL DIAGNOSIS

- Other causes of dysphagia (especially abnormalities of the pharyngeal and esophageal phases of deglutition), including pharyngeal paralysis, pharyngeal cysts, pharyngeal compression by strangles abscesses and guttural pouch empyema, subepiglottic cyst, fourth branchial arch defect, esophageal obstruction, megaesophagus, esophageal stricture, intramural esophageal cysts, esophageal rupture, and equine grass sickness.
- Other causes of chronic weight loss.
- Other causes of recurrent colic.

INITIAL DATABASE

- The diagnostic evaluation should consist of a complete physical examination, including rectal examination, routine blood work (complete blood count, serum chemistry panel), urinalysis, and peritoneal fluid analysis.
- Many horses with squamous cell carcinoma have anemia, leukocytosis, and hyperfibrinogenemia. Some have hypoproteinemia because of bowel inflammation and protein exudation; other horses have hyperglobulinemia.

- Gastroscopy reveals a mass within the stomach protruding from the mucosa. Biopsy of the mass may be possible via the endoscope. Squamous cell carcinoma originates from the squamous mucosa and typically has the appearance of an ulcerated, cobblestone, or florid mass.
- Peritoneal fluid varies from normal, if the tumor is confined within the stomach, to an exudate if the tumor has spread. Neoplastic cells from a primary gastric squamous cell carcinoma are occasionally observed in a sample of peritoneal fluid and are large, poorly differentiated epithelial cells with a bluish, ground-glass–appearing cytoplasm (Wright's stain).
- Neoplastic cells may also be identified in samples of pleural fluid if a pleural effusion is present.

ADVANCED OR CONFIRMATORY TESTING

- Ultrasonography, laparoscopy, and laparotomy may be used to further evaluate the patient.
- Abdominal ultrasonography (transcutaneous) may be used to determine whether there is excessive abdominal fluid and possibly to identify a mass associated with the stomach wall. Occasionally, gastric squamous cell carcinoma will metastasize to the spleen or liver, which may be seen by ultrasonography.
- Laparoscopy or exploratory laparotomy may be used to identify and biopsy tumor deposits in the abdominal cavity.
- If gastric squamous cell carcinoma is suspected, cytology of aspirated stomach contents may reveal large, poorly differentiated squamous carcinoma cells.
- Pleuroscopy (thoracoscopy) allows examination of the thoracic portion of the esophagus and may permit surgical biopsy of esophageal tumors located in this region.

TREATMENT

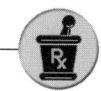

THERAPEUTIC GOAL(S)

- Surgical excision of the neoplastic mass if possible
- Chemotherapeutic treatment of the neoplasia if possible

ACUTE GENERAL TREATMENT

- Transendoscopic excision and ablation of small focal neoplastic masses in the stomach may be possible; however, in most cases, the tumor will be too large or extensive by the time the diagnosis is reached.

- There have been no reports of chemotherapy for treatment of gastric neoplasia, although this form of treatment could be considered in appropriate cases.
- Intralesional injection of cisplatin can be successful for cutaneous squamous cell carcinoma and could be done through an endoscope to treat gastric squamous cell carcinoma.

CHRONIC TREATMENT

- Frequent small meals of moistened pellets or fresh grass should be fed.
- Piroxicam (0.2 mg/kg PO q24h) for squamous cell carcinoma.

RECOMMENDED MONITORING

During treatment, horses should be monitored for signs of dehydration and weight loss.

PROGNOSIS AND OUTCOME

- In most cases, the prognosis is poor.
- If a focal neoplasm amenable to laser ablation is present, then curative treatment may be possible.

PEARLS & CONSIDERATIONS

- Gastric squamous cell carcinoma and other forms of gastric neoplasia are rare, and by the time disease is recognized, treatment is rarely possible.
- In all cases of neoplasia, the quality of life, economic issues, prognosis, and owner expectations must be carefully considered and discussed before any treatment is attempted.

SUGGESTED READING

Del Piero F, Summers BA, Cummings JF, et al: Gastrointestinal stromal tumors in equids. *Vet Pathol* 38:689, 2001.

Ford TS, Vaala WE, Sweeney CR, et al: Pleuroscopic diagnosis of gastroesophageal squamous cell carcinoma in a horse. *J Am Vet Med Assoc* 190:1556, 1987.

McKenzie EC, Mills JN, Bolton JR: Gastric squamous cell carcinoma in three horses. *Aust Vet J* 75:480, 1997.

Morse CC, Richardson DW: Gastric hyperplastic polyp in a horse. *J Comp Pathol* 99:337, 1988.

Murray MJ: Diseases of the stomach. In Mair T, Divers T, Ducharme N (eds). *Manual of equine gastroenterology*, London, 2002, Saunders, pp 241–248.

Olsen SN: Squamous cell carcinoma of the equine stomach: a report of five cases. *Vet Rec* 131:170, 1992.

Tenant B, Keirn DR, White KK, et al: Six cases of squamous cell carcinoma of the stomach of the horse. *Equine Vet J* 14:238, 1982.

Wester PW, Franken P, Hani HJ: Squamous cell carcinoma of the equine stomach. A report of seven cases. *Tijdschr Diergeneeskd* 15:105, 1980.

Wrigley RH, Gay CC, Lording P, et al: Pleural effusion associated with squamous cell carcinoma of the stomach of a horse. *Equine Vet J* 13:99, 1981.

AUTHOR & EDITOR: **TIM MAIR**

Neoplasia, Hepatic

BASIC INFORMATION

DEFINITION

The liver may be affected by primary hepatic or metastatic neoplasms.

EPIDEMIOLOGY

SPECIES, AGE, SEX
- Hepatic neoplasia has been recorded in a number of breeds, and there does not appear to be a gender predisposition.
- Hepatocellular carcinomas and hepatoblastomas affect animals younger than 3 years of age.
- Cholangiocarcinomas occur more commonly in older horses.

RISK FACTORS Hepatic neoplasia is rare in horses.

CLINICAL PRESENTATION

DISEASE FORMS/SUBTYPES Primary hepatic neoplasms that have been reported in horses include cholangiocarcinoma, hepatocellular carcinoma, and hepatoblastoma. Of these, cholangiocarcinoma is the most common. Lymphomas and other tumor types may occasionally metastasize to the liver.

HISTORY, CHIEF COMPLAINT Presenting complaints commonly include weight loss and inappetence. Depression, lethargy, intermittent fever, and mild signs of colic are frequently reported historically.

PHYSICAL EXAM FINDINGS
- Clinical signs are typically nonspecific and rarely evident until tumor growth is advanced.
- Findings on physical examination often include poor body condition, depression, weakness, and fever.
- Mild intermittent signs of abdominal discomfort are commonly reported, and young animals may present with abdominal distension.
- Horses with severe liver dysfunction may demonstrate signs of hepatic encephalopathy.
- In some cases of hepatic neoplasia, horses present with signs suggestive of thoracic disease as a result of pulmonary metastases or pleural effusion, which may occur in the absence of metastatic lung disease.

ETIOLOGY AND PATHOPHYSIOLOGY

- Predisposing factors or conditions causing hepatic neoplasia in horses are unknown and remain speculative in light of the low number of cases.
- Colic may be caused by distension of the hepatic capsule or indicate a primary gastrointestinal neoplasia with hepatic metastases.
- Pleural effusion may occur as a consequence of direct pulmonary involvement (ie, metastasis). Other suggested mechanisms include lymphatic obstruction, increased venous hydrostatic pressure, and erythrocytosis.
- Erythrocytosis is well documented in some horses with liver disease and neoplasia. The mechanism is unknown; extramedullary hemopoiesis and tumor production of erythropoietin (or an erythropoietin-like substance) has been suggested.

DIAGNOSIS

DIFFERENTIAL DIAGNOSIS

- The differential list for hepatic neoplasia should include more common causes of chronic liver disease, weight loss, and chronic low-grade colic.
- Causes of pleuropneumonia should be included in the differential list for horses presenting with signs of respiratory disease.

INITIAL DATABASE

- Complete blood count: Normal to anemia of chronic disease and leukocytosis
- Fibrinogen concentration: Normal to increased
- Hepatic specific enzymes: May be normal to mildly increased
- Serum bile acid concentration: May be normal to mildly increased
- Abdominocentesis indicated in horses with signs of colic or excessive peritoneal fluid

ADVANCED OR CONFIRMATORY TESTING

- Peritoneal or pleural effusions may occasionally reveal neoplastic cells, confirming the diagnosis.
- Ultrasonographic examination of the liver may support a diagnosis of neoplasia.
- Definitive diagnosis requires histopathologic examination of biopsy samples.

TREATMENT

THERAPEUTIC GOAL(S)

Unfortunately, tumor growth is usually advanced at the time of diagnosis, and treatment is palliative at best. Chemotherapeutic regimens for some neoplastic conditions have been described for horses, but there is little evidence of their efficacy, and expense precludes their use in many cases.

ACUTE GENERAL TREATMENT

- Supportive, symptomatic therapy may be required in some cases to allow definitive antemortem diagnosis.
- Hypoglycemia should be treated with IV dextrose administration.

PROGNOSIS AND OUTCOME

Prognosis is uniformly poor for most neoplastic conditions in horses.

PEARLS & CONSIDERATIONS

Because hepatic neoplasia is rare, diagnostic efforts are often directed elsewhere initially. It is not uncommon to make a final diagnosis at postmortem.

SUGGESTED READING

Axon JE, Russell CM, Begg AP, et al: Erythrocytosis and pleural effusion associated with a hepatoblastoma in a thoroughbred yearling. *Aust Vet J* 86:329–333, 2008.

Mueller POE, Morris DD, Carmichael KP, et al: Antemortem diagnosis of cholangiocellular carcinoma in a horse. *J Am Vet Med Assoc* 201:899–901, 1992.

Schnabel LV, Njaa BL, Gold JR, et al: Primary alimentary lymphoma with metastasis to the liver causing encephalopathy in a horse. *J Vet Intern Med* 20:204–206, 2006.

AUTHOR: **BRETT TENNENT-BROWN**

EDITOR: **MICHELLE HENRY BARTON**

Neoplasia, Intestinal

BASIC INFORMATION

DEFINITION
Neoplasia of the intestine

EPIDEMIOLOGY
SPECIES, AGE, SEX More common in older horses
RISK FACTORS Contributing factors are not known. Previous reports of equine pathology studies suggest an estimated incidence of gastrointestinal (GI) neoplasia of less than 0.1% in routine postmortem examinations and about 5% of horses with clinical signs of abdominal disease (excluding mesenteric lipoma).

CLINICAL PRESENTATION
HISTORY, CHIEF COMPLAINT
- Typical signs associated with intestinal neoplasia include:
  - Chronic weight loss
  - Poor appetite
  - Abdominal discomfort or recurrent colic
  - Lethargy and exercise intolerance
  - Ascites or edema in some cases
  - Diarrhea in some cases
- Acute colic caused by intestinal strangulation may occur with mesenteric lipomas, which are frequently pedunculated. Other solitary neoplasms may initiate intestinal intussusception, with the development of acute colic.

PHYSICAL EXAM FINDINGS
- The findings of physical examination confirm the presenting signs, including weight loss with or without signs of abdominal pain and diarrhea. Persistent or intermittent pyrexia may occur with advanced neoplasia.
- Physical examination of the horse is often unrewarding but is essential, together with a thorough history, to eliminate other more common causes of weight loss such as:
  - Inadequate or unsuitable feeding
  - Dental or swallowing disorders
  - Excessive exercise or energy demands
  - Parasitism

ETIOLOGY AND PATHOPHYSIOLOGY
- Intestinal neoplasms are usually classified according to their cell type and site of origin. Primary neoplasms are most common, although metastases to the intestine from other sites may also occur.
- The most common neoplasm of the intestinal tract is the mesenteric lipoma, which is common in older horses and especially ponies (>15 years). However, it is often clinically insignificant. When significant, the lipoma may produce signs only related to its physical properties, namely as a space-occupying mass causing a simple intestinal obstruction (caused by compression of the intestine) or more commonly as a pedunculated mass causing an acute strangulating intestinal obstruction.
- Excluding lipomas, lymphoma (lymphosarcoma), leiomyoma and leiomyosarcoma (GI stromal tumors), and adenocarcinoma are the most commonly reported neoplasms affecting the GI tract.
- Lymphoma may affect any age of horse, not infrequently young adults.
- Lymphoma may take the form of discrete masses affecting the intestine and its associated mesentery (usually associated with signs of recurrent colic), or a diffuse infiltrate in the intestinal wall (especially the small intestine), resulting in progressive weight loss associated with malabsorption syndrome. There may be diarrhea if the tumor infiltrates the large intestine wall.
- Amyloid deposition in the intestinal wall has been recorded secondary to myeloma (in association with amyloid deposition in other organs).
- Occasionally, inflammatory hyperplastic polyps cause signs similar to those of neoplasms.

DIAGNOSIS

DIFFERENTIAL DIAGNOSIS
Other causes of chronic weight loss, chronic or recurrent colic, or diarrhea

INITIAL DATABASE
- The diagnostic evaluation should consist of a complete physical examination, including rectal examination, routine blood work (complete blood count, serum chemistry panel), urinalysis, and peritoneal fluid analysis.
- Many horses with intestinal neoplasia have anemia (as a result of chronic disease or blood loss), leukocytosis (as a result of chronic inflammation), and hyperfibrinogenemia. In cases of intestinal lymphoma, rarely abnormal lymphocytes may be present in the peripheral blood.
- Immune-mediated anemia or thrombocytopenia may occur secondary to intestinal neoplasia, especially lymphoma.
- Some affected horses have hypoalbuminemia and hypoproteinemia because of malabsorption, bowel inflammation, and protein exudation; other horses have hyperglobulinemia (as a result of chronic inflammation).
- Increased concentrations of the intestinal fraction of the alkaline phosphatase enzyme (IAP) may also indicate the presence of intestinal disease.
- Hypercalcemia has been reported in association with both lymphoma and gastric carcinoma.
- Gastroscopy and duodenoscopy may reveal a mass or masses within the stomach or duodenum only if the neoplasms have involved that region of the GI tract. Biopsy of the mass may be possible via the endoscope.
- Rectal examination is essential in the investigation of any case with suspected GI neoplasia. Although normal findings may be present in many animals, an increased volume of peritoneal fluid, distension of the intestine, or an abnormal tissue mass or masses increase the index of suspicion of intestinal disease and allow further directed investigations to be selected.
- Peritoneal fluid varies from normal, if the tumor is confined to the intestinal wall, to an exudate if the tumor has spread. Neoplastic cells from a primary intestinal neoplasm (eg, lymphoma) are occasionally observed in a sample of peritoneal fluid.
- Neoplastic cells may also be identified in samples of pleural fluid if pleural effusion is present.

ADVANCED OR CONFIRMATORY TESTING
- Ultrasonography, laparoscopy, and laparotomy may be used to further evaluate the patient.

- Percutaneous or per rectum ultrasonography may provide information about the volume and character of the peritoneal fluid. Intestinal distension may be recognized together with abnormal bowel wall thickening and abnormal tissue masses. Ultrasonography also allows guided collection of fluid or tissue samples for further evaluation.
- Laparoscopy or exploratory laparotomy may be used to identify and biopsy tumor deposits in the abdominal cavity. Full-thickness bowel wall biopsies may be necessary to diagnose diffuse alimentary lymphoma. (The intestine may look grossly normal with lymphoma infiltration.)
- Pleuroscopy (thoracoscopy) allows examination of the thoracic cavity when there is evidence of tumor spread to the thorax.
- Glucose or xylose absorption tests are useful to demonstrate a state of malabsorption from the small intestine, which may occur with a diffuse intestinal lymphoma. Although not diagnostic, a reduced sugar uptake curve is highly suggestive of an infiltrative condition of the small intestine.
- Histopathologic examination of a rectal biopsy may be helpful if the horse has diarrhea.
- Serum immunoglobulin M (IgM) is low in some cases of lymphoma; some also have low IgG and IgA levels.

TREATMENT

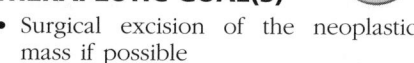

THERAPEUTIC GOAL(S)

- Surgical excision of the neoplastic mass if possible
- Chemotherapeutic treatment of the neoplasia if possible

ACUTE GENERAL TREATMENT

- Early surgical removal of mesenteric lipomas that are causing intestinal obstruction is frequently successful.
- Systemic corticosteroids, although not curative, may have a short-term beneficial effect in horses with intestinal lymphoma, and these drugs may help to treat secondary immune-mediated anemia and thrombocytopenia that may occur in association with lymphoma.
- Surgical treatment by removal of solitary lymphoma, adenocarcinoma, leiomyoma or sarcoma, and neurofibroma may be curative. Care should be taken that all neoplastic tissue is removed during surgery, but this may be difficult, especially in horses with lymphoma, in which the limits of the neoplastic tissue may not be grossly visible.

CHRONIC TREATMENT

- The systemic use of antineoplastic agents for the treatment of GI tumors in horses has received little attention and has unproven long-term efficacy. However, multiple drug protocols are available for palliative chemotherapy of multicentric lymphoma. The following is a suggested multiple-agent induction protocol for horses with lymphoma.
  - Cytosine arabinoside: 200 to 300 mg/m^2 SC or IM once every 1 to 2 weeks
  - Chlorambucil: 20 mg/m^2 PO once every 2 weeks
  - Prednisone: 1.1 to 2.32 mg/kg PO every other day
- Alternatively, cyclophosphamide 200 mg/m^2 IV once every 2 to 3 weeks can be substituted for chlorambucil. Antineoplastic agents are typically given on alternating weeks but have been given on the same day without apparent ill effects. A response to this induction therapy should occur within 2 to 4 weeks. If no response is observed, adding vincristine (0.5 mg/m^2 IV once a week) has been recommended.
- Horses in remission should be maintained on the induction protocol for 2 to 3 months before switching to a maintenance protocol. The first cycle of maintenance therapy increases the treatment interval for each antineoplastic agent by 1 week. Prednisone is continued for the duration of therapy (but can be gradually reduced in dose). If the horse remains in remission after 2 to 3 months on the first cycle, the second cycle is begun by adding 1 more week to the treatment intervals of each agent. Several cycles of maintenance therapy can be given. Signs of toxicity, including bone marrow suppression and GI irritation, have been rarely recognized using this protocol.
- Other protocols include:
  - Single-agent L-asparaginase: 10,000 to 40,000 IU/m^2 IMV once every 2 to 3 weeks
  - Single-agent cyclophosphamide (give as described above)
  - Combinations of either cytosine arabinoside or cyclophosphamide with prednisone

RECOMMENDED MONITORING

During treatment, horses should be monitored for signs of pain, dehydration, and weight loss.

PROGNOSIS AND OUTCOME

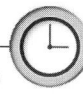

- In most cases, the prognosis is poor.
- If a focal neoplasm that is amenable to surgical excision is present, then curative treatment may be possible.

PEARLS & CONSIDERATIONS

COMMENTS

- Intestinal neoplasia should be considered in all horses demonstrating signs of weight loss and recurrent colic.
- In all cases of neoplasia, the quality of life, economic issues, prognosis, and owner expectations must be carefully considered and discussed before any treatment is attempted.

SUGGESTED READING

Dabareiner RM, Sullins KE, Goodrich LR: Large colon resection for treatment of lymphosarcoma in two horses. *J Am Vet Med Assoc* 208:895, 1996.

Del Piero F, Summers BA, Cummings JF, et al: Gastrointestinal stromal tumors in equids. *Vet Pathol* 38:689, 2001.

Edwards GB, Proudman CJ: An analysis of 75 cases of intestinal obstruction caused by pedunculated lipomas. *Equine Vet J* 26:18, 1994.

Elce Y: Neoplastic disease of the gastrointestinal tract. In Robinson NE, Sprayberry KA (eds). *Current therapy in equine medicine.* ed 6, St Louis, 2009, Saunders (Elsevier), pp 448–450.

Hillyer M: Gastrointestinal neoplasia. In Mair T, Divers T, Ducharme N (eds). *Manual of equine gastroenterology,* London, 2002, Saunders, pp 334–338.

Hillyer MH: The use of ultrasound in the diagnosis of abdominal tumours in the horse, *Equine Vet Educ* 6:273, 1994.

Mair TS, Hillyer MH: Clinical features of lymphosarcoma in the horse. *Equine Vet Educ* 4:108, 1992.

Mair TS, Hillyer MH, Taylor FGR, et al: Small intestinal malabsorption in the horse: an assessment of the oral glucose tolerance test. *Equine Vet J* 23:344, 1991.

Savage CJ: Lymphoproliferative and myeloproliferative disorders. *Vet Clinics North Am Equine Pract* 14:563, 1998.

Taylor SD, Pusterla N, Vaughan B, et al: Intestinal neoplasia in horses. *J Vet Intern Med* 20:1429, 2006.

Zicker SC, Wilson WD, Medearis I: Differentiation between intra-abdominal neoplasms and abscesses in horses, using clinical and laboratory data: 40 cases (1973–1988). *J Am Vet Med Assoc* 196:1130, 1990.

AUTHOR: TIM MAIR

EDITORS: TIM MAIR and **CERI SHERLOCK**

Neoplasia, Nasal and Paranasal

BASIC INFORMATION

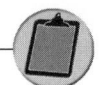

DEFINITION

Tumors of the nasal passage and paranasal sinuses are uncommon and include a wide range of tumor types, reflecting the diverse tissues present in the head. Squamous cell carcinoma (SCC) is the most commonly diagnosed sinonasal tumor. Paranasal tumors are more common than nasal tumors. Most tumors are unilateral in occurrence.

SYNONYM(S)

Sinonasal neoplasia

EPIDEMIOLOGY

SPECIES, AGE, SEX Surface and glandular epithelial tumors are more common in teenage and older horses. Young and immature horses are more likely to be diagnosed with fibro-osseous and bone tumors.

ASSOCIATED CONDITIONS AND DISORDERS

- Secondary paranasal sinusitis is common with primary neoplasia of the sinuses because of disruption of normal sinus drainage mechanisms and the presence of necrotic tissue and secondary bacterial infection.
- Paranasal sinus cysts commonly present with similar clinical signs of nasal discharge and external facial swelling.

CLINICAL PRESENTATION

DISEASE FORMS/SUBTYPES SCC, adenoma, adenocarcinoma, lymphoma, chondrosarcoma, fibroma, fibrosarcoma, osteoma (hamartoma), osteosarcoma, fibro-osseous tumors (fibrous dysplasia and ossifying fibroma), undifferentiated carcinomas and sarcomas, tumors of dental origin (eg, ameloblastoma), hemangioma, melanoma, mast cell tumor

HISTORY, CHIEF COMPLAINT

- Most sinonasal tumors are slowly growing with an insidious onset of clinical signs. Horses typically have a history of developing nasal discharge (mucoid to purulent; maybe bloody) that persists and perhaps has a foul odor.
- The presence of an expanding external facial swelling is also a common presenting complaint.
- An increased respiratory noise and reduced nasal airflow may be reported.
- Some horses may be presented for head shaking.

- Clinical signs may advance over weeks to months before veterinary attention is sought.

PHYSICAL EXAM FINDINGS Nasal discharge: Malodorous, mucoid to purulent, and often bloody; unilateral or bilateral; reduced nasal airflow; increased respiratory noise localized to the nasal passage; dyspnea; external facial swelling (frontal and maxillary regions) is common with advanced disease; enlarged submandibular lymph nodes; epiphora; exophthalmos; ocular discharge; neurologic deficits; halitosis; dysphagia; inappetence.

ETIOLOGY AND PATHOPHYSIOLOGY

- SCC and bone tumors are more common in the maxillary sinus. Glandular epithelial tumors (eg, adenocarcinoma) are more likely to arise from the frontal and ethmoidal sinuses.
- The frontal and ethmoidal sinuses have a greater density of mucosal glands, which may account for the increased incidence of glandular epithelial tumors in these locations compared with other sinus regions.
- Distant metastasis is rare; in addition to locally invasive and destructive growth, carcinomas frequently spread to other sites in the head (nasopharynx, oropharynx, periorbital, cranium, guttural pouch), resulting in diverse clinical signs.
- Osteomas are benign, generally well-circumscribed masses and are not infiltrative.

DIAGNOSIS

DIFFERENTIAL DIAGNOSIS

- Paranasal sinus cyst, possibly extending into nasal passage
- Sinonasal polyp
- Ethmoid hematoma
- Fungal rhinitis or sinusitis
- Granuloma
- Nasal epidermal inclusion cyst (atheroma)
- Amyloidosis
- Infection with *Halicephalobus gingivalis* (a saprophytic nematode)

INITIAL DATABASE

- Complete blood count and chemistry panel: May see increased fibrinogen and mature leukocytosis if significant secondary bacterial infection is present; decreased red blood cell indices occur with anemia of chronic disease and in the presence of hemangioma.

- Upper airway endoscopy: Distorted, compressed nasal passage; variable-sized mass in the nasal passage; abnormal discharge at the nasomaxillary opening.
- Radiographs: Soft tissue, bony, or heterogenous mass effect in the paranasal sinuses, nasal passages, or both; air-fluid interface in the paranasal sinuses may be apparent with secondary sinusitis or blood accumulation from a bleeding tumor; deviated nasal septum; displaced cheek teeth; lysis and distortion of facial bones; soft tissue swelling; gas opacities in soft tissues.
- Contrast paranasal sinusography is helpful to delineate masses but is rarely used.

ADVANCED OR CONFIRMATORY TESTING

- Sinoscopy: Presence of mass and fluid in the paranasal sinuses; may obtain a biopsy specimen.
- Fine-needle aspirate of enlarged submandibular lymph nodes most commonly reveals inflammatory changes secondary to infection and tumor necrosis rather than metastatic tumor cells.
- Computed tomography provides the most detailed imaging of the location and extent of the tumor and assists with any intended surgical or radiation therapy planning.
- Head scintigraphy may help identify subclinical, early tumor development but is not indicated in the typical case of advanced disease.
- Histopathology is required for definitive diagnosis and should be performed before any therapeutic options are considered; some tumors are very difficult to classify.

TREATMENT

THERAPEUTIC GOAL(S)

- If possible, treatment is targeted at improving the horse's quality of life and preventing further destruction or invasion by the tumor. For many horses, effective treatment of advanced tumor growth in the head, diagnosed months after its onset, is impractical and unwarranted, and humane euthanasia is often chosen for these animals.
- For a minority of tumors, complete removal is possible and curative.

ACUTE GENERAL TREATMENT

- Rarely, a horse may require an emergency tracheotomy if it is presented

with severe airflow reduction and obvious respiratory distress.
- Cytoreductive surgery of invasive tumors is significantly complicated by inaccessibility and hemorrhage.
- Sinusotomy and complete excision are practical for osteomas of the paranasal sinuses.
- A localized tumor of the nasal septum may be amenable to complete removal by nasal septum resection.
- Palliative or therapeutic radiotherapy is a strong consideration for radiosensitive tumors, particularly lymphoma and SCC.
- Laser ablation and cryotherapy are considerations for early-onset, small tumors.
- Nonsteroidal antiinflammatory drugs and antimicrobials contribute to horse comfort and limit secondary bacterial infections.

CHRONIC TREATMENT

Palliative radiation treatments may be used periodically in an ongoing therapeutic plan.

POSSIBLE COMPLICATIONS

Side effects of radiation therapy include development of white hair, hair loss, scaly skin, superficial skin necrosis, increased nasal drainage, temporary local lymphadenopathy, and bone remodeling.

RECOMMENDED MONITORING

- After any palliative or therapeutic measures, it is prudent to monitor for recurrence or persistence of initial clinical signs.

- Radiographic and endoscopic evaluation of the head may be indicated every 4 to 6 months after apparent tumor removal or regression.

PROGNOSIS AND OUTCOME

- Poor to guarded prognosis for advanced, invasive tumors; most horses are euthanized at diagnosis or when the quality of life is considered unacceptable.
- Guarded to fair prognosis for radiosensitive tumors that are accessible for radiotherapy.
- Good to excellent prognosis for benign, noninfiltrative tumors (eg, osteoma) that can be surgically removed in their entirety.

PEARLS & CONSIDERATIONS

COMMENTS

- Each horse should be considered on an individual basis with regard to possible treatment and outcome.
- Early diagnosis remains uncommon because tumors can expand considerably within the sinus space before clinical signs are readily apparent.
- Radiation therapy is becoming more frequently used and available and should always be considered.
- Accurate diagnosis is critical before any treatment plan is developed.

PREVENTION

- There are no known current preventive measures.
- Vaccination against certain tumors (eg, melanoma) may become the mainstay of future preventive management programs.

CLIENT EDUCATION

- At the first sign of abnormal nasal discharge, notable reduction in airflow, increase in airway respiratory sounds, foul odor to the breath, or external facial swelling, consult a veterinarian.
- Early diagnosis increases the chance of successful treatment.
- Geriatric horses are at increased risk of developing tumors and should receive thorough physical examinations at least twice a year.

SUGGESTED READING

Head KW, Dixon PM: Equine nasal and paranasal sinus tumours. Part 1: review of the literature and tumour classification. *Vet J* 157:261–278, 1999.
Head KW, Dixon PM: Equine nasal and paranasal sinus tumours. Part 2: a contribution of 28 case reports. *Vet J* 157:279–294, 1999.
Henson FMD, Dobson JM: Use of radiation therapy in the treatment of equine neoplasia. *Equine Vet Educ AE* 6:405–408, 2004.
Tremaine WH, Dixon PM: A long-term study of 277 cases of equine sinonasal disease. Part 1: details of horses, historical, clinical and ancillary diagnostic findings. *Equine Vet J* 33:274–282, 2001.

AUTHOR: MATHEW P. GERARD

EDITOR: ERIC J. PARENTE

Neoplasia, Urinary Tract

BASIC INFORMATION

DEFINITION

Epithelial tumors of the equine urinary tract include papilloma, adenoma, and carcinoma. Tumors are further classified as adenocarcinoma, transitional cell carcinoma (TCC), squamous cell carcinoma (SCC), and undifferentiated carcinomas.
- Renal cell carcinoma (RCC; adenocarcinoma) is the most common renal tumor and usually arises from the epithelium of the proximal convoluted tubules.
- Nephroblastoma is an embryonal tumor that develops from primitive nephrogenic tissue or dysplastic tissue from the uroepithelium of the renal pelvis or ureter.

- SCC is the most common bladder tumor in horses followed by TCC and leiomyosarcomas.
- Metastatic disease from lymphosarcoma, hemangiosarcoma, melanoma, adenocarcinoma, or adenoma can invade any region of the urinary tract.

EPIDEMIOLOGY

SPECIES, AGE, SEX
Nephroblastoma occurs in young horses; other tumors tend to occur in older animals

ASSOCIATED CONDITIONS AND DISORDERS
- RCCs frequently metastasize to the lungs, liver, and other tissues. Metastasis is common with hemangiosarcoma, melanomas, and TCC of the

bladder and kidney. Lymphosarcoma is often multicentric.
- A paraneoplastic process leading to severe hypoglycemia has been reported in two cases of equine RCC, probably caused by production of an insulin-like factor, an abnormal variant of insulin-like growth factor II, or less likely from excessive glucose utilization by the tumor.

CLINICAL PRESENTATION

DISEASE FORMS/SUBTYPES
- RCC (adenocarcinoma)
- Nephroblastoma
- TCC
- SCC
- Metastatic disease from lymphosarcoma, hemangiosarcoma, melanoma, adenocarcinoma, or adenoma

HISTORY, CHIEF COMPLAINT
- Renal neoplasia
  - Hematuria
  - Weight loss
  - Chronic colic
  - Poor performance
  - Depression
  - Anorexia
  - Sudden death caused by hemorrhage from the neoplasm
- Bladder neoplasia
  - Hematuria
  - Weight loss
  - Stranguria
  - Pollakiuria
  - Depression
  - Anorexia
  - Unthriftiness

PHYSICAL EXAM FINDINGS
- Enlargement of the left or even the right kidney detected by rectal palpation in some cases of renal neoplasia. Pain may be evident on palpation of the mass per rectum or percutaneously through the flank.
- Bladder tumors can frequently be palpated rectally.

ETIOLOGY AND PATHOPHYSIOLOGY
- Nephroblastoma occurs in young horses.
- In other species, increased exposure to insecticides has been linked to bladder neoplasia.
- Chronic urinary tract infections may predispose to neoplasia in some cases.
- In horses, an underlying cause of urinary tract neoplasia is rarely determined.

DIAGNOSIS

DIFFERENTIAL DIAGNOSIS
- RCC (adenocarcinoma) is the most common primary renal tumor in horses followed by nephroblastoma. Whereas RCC tends to occur in older horses, nephroblastoma often occurs in young horses.
- Multiple myeloma involving the kidney has been reported, which resulted in hypercalcemia and elevated serum parathyroid hormone–related protein concentration.
- A young horse with a RCC has been reported to have increased production of insulin-like growth factor and secondary hypoglycemia.
- Mucinous hyperplasia of the renal pelvis and proximal urethral uroepithelium or a ureteropelvic polyp can result in renal masses that are not truly neoplastic but may result in obstruction of the kidney or ureter and hydronephrosis.
- The most common bladder tumor is SCC followed by TCC, which occur in middle-aged to older horses.

- Fibromatous polyps of the bladder may occur in young horses.
- Metastatic lymphosarcoma, hemangiosarcoma, adenoma, and melanoma can also involve the kidneys and rarely the bladder.
- Differential diagnoses for renal masses include abscesses, pyelonephritis, renal calculi, polycystic kidneys, and aberrant nematode migration.
- Cystitis or cystic calculi may cause stranguria and pollakiuria. Bladder paresis may lead to inadequate bladder emptying, urine stasis, and accumulation of sabulous concentrations ventrally in the bladder. Neoplasia may predispose to cystitis or cystic calculi and should be ruled out by careful cystoscopy.

INITIAL DATABASE
- Complete blood count is usually normal. Mild to moderate anemia associated with gross hematuria is possible, and anemia of chronic disease is common. Neutrophilia and thrombocytopenia occur occasionally.
- Serum biochemistry profile is usually normal. Decreased iron and increased fibrinogen concentrations secondary to inflammation are possible. Azotemia rarely occurs with renal neoplasia because the contralateral kidney maintains normal renal function. Hypoglycemia and hypoalbuminemia have been reported on occasion.
- Urinalysis: Hematuria and associated proteinuria are common. Neoplastic cells are more likely to be observed with bladder rather than renal tumors. Secondary cystitis with increased urine leukocytes and bacteriuria are possible, in which case a quantitative urine culture should then be performed (>10,000 CFU/mL is significant).
- Abdominocentesis is often abnormal, with nonspecific increases in white blood cell count and total protein concentration. Occasional neoplastic cells are observed.
- Transabdominal ultrasonography can be used to detect all but very small renal tumors. Biopsy of renal masses under ultrasonographic guidance can be used to obtain a definitive diagnosis.
- Transrectal ultrasonography can be used to image most bladder tumors, which can be viewed directly using cystoscopy. It is important to retroflex the endoscope to view the trigone region and bladder neck. Biopsy specimens can usually be obtained during cystoscopy.
- Thoracic radiography may detect pulmonary metastases.
- Abdominal ultrasonography may detect intraabdominal metastases.

ADVANCED OR CONFIRMATORY TESTING
Histopathology or cytology of biopsy specimens collected from the kidney or bladder can be used to obtain a definitive diagnosis.

TREATMENT

THERAPEUTIC GOAL(S)
- For unilateral renal neoplasia detected before metastasis, the treatment of choice is unilateral nephrectomy. Careful assessment should be done to ensure normal function of the contralateral kidney and to look for metastatic disease (thoracic radiography and abdominal and thoracic ultrasonography) before surgery. Nephrectomy is best performed in the standing horse. Laparoscopic visualization of the abdomen looking for metastatic disease is recommended. Nephrectomy can be performed via a flank incision or via hand-assisted laparoscopy.
- Bladder tumors have been treated with surgical excision via a caudal ventral midline laparotomy in mares and via a parainguinal approach in male horses.
- Topical therapy using intracystically instilled 5-fluorouracil or triethylenethiophosphoramide has been attempted to treat bladder tumors.
- Some horses with SCCs and TCCs have responded to piroxicam (nonselective cyclooxygenase inhibitor) in horses and other species. Such treatment is recommended after surgical resection.
- No reports of systemic chemotherapy for urogenital neoplasia have yet been published in horses.

ACUTE GENERAL TREATMENT
Secondary cystitis may be treated with antibiotics according to bacterial culture and sensitivity results.

CHRONIC TREATMENT
Long-term treatment with piroxicam (0.2–0.3 mg/kg PO q24h) should be monitored with sequential assessment of urine specific gravity, serum creatinine, and albumin concentrations because of the risk of possible renal damage or right dorsal colitis.

POSSIBLE COMPLICATIONS
- Renal neoplasia may erode into the vasculature and result in hemoabdomen and even sudden death from exsanguination.
- Bladder, urethral, renal, or ureteral neoplasia may result in uroabdomen or uroperitoneum if there is severe tissue destruction of the urinary tract.

RECOMMENDED MONITORING

- Signs of metastatic disease include weight loss, inappetence, depression, exercise intolerance, respiratory distress, or lameness.
- Elevations in liver enzymes or alkaline phosphatase may be used as indicators of hepatic or osseous metastatic disease.
- Periodic rectal examination and abdominal and thoracic ultrasonography may be warranted.
- Quality of life should be assessed and euthanasia recommended before the development of severe discomfort, chronic pain, or cachexia.

PROGNOSIS AND OUTCOME

- Generally, the prognosis is poor for all forms of urinary tract neoplasia in horses.
- Nephroblastomas are generally confined to the kidney and may be amenable to nephrectomy with a fair prognosis.
- As chemotherapeutic protocols become more widely used in equine practice, prognosis may improve. Unfortunately, diagnosis is often late in the disease process. Most tumors of the urinary tract are either locally aggressive with the tendency for transmural spread or highly metastatic. Early diagnosis, ideally as an incidental finding, provides the best opportunity for successful outcome for these conditions, which generally have a very poor prognosis.

PEARLS & CONSIDERATIONS

COMMENTS

- Renal tumors are rare in horses (~1% of all equine tumors), and bladder tumors are uncommon.
- Adenocarcinomas are the most common renal tumor in horses and usually arise from the epithelium of the proximal convoluted tubules.
- SCCs are the most common bladder tumor in horses followed by TCCs.
- Primary and metastatic tumors of the kidney or bladder are frequently fatal.

CLIENT EDUCATION

Euthanasia is often performed at the initial diagnosis because tumors may be extensive and interfere with other organs. Early diagnosis may allow for surgical resection or chemotherapy.

SUGGESTED READING

Barrell E, Hendrickson DA: Tumours of the equine bladder: what makes treatment of these cases so difficult? *Equine Vet Educ* 21:267, 2009.

Wise LN, Bryan JN, Sellon DC, et al: A retrospective analysis of renal carcinoma in the horse. *J Vet Intern Med* 23:913–918, 2009.

AUTHOR: **ALLISON J. STEWART**

EDITOR: **BRYAN M. WALDRIDGE**

Nephrolithiasis

BASIC INFORMATION

DEFINITION

A stone (urolith) within the kidney

SYNONYM(S)

- Renal calculi
- Stag-horn calculi

EPIDEMIOLOGY

SPECIES, AGE, SEX

Males, especially intact males, are reportedly more commonly affected.

GENETICS AND BREED PREDISPOSITION

Nephrolithiasis has been reported with increased frequency in Thoroughbred racehorses.

RISK FACTORS

Nonsteroidal antiinflammatory drug (NSAID) administration and subsequent subclinical renal medullary crest necrosis may be a risk factor.

ASSOCIATED CONDITIONS AND DISORDERS

- Urolithiasis
- Hematuria
- Hydronephrosis
- Chronic renal failure

CLINICAL PRESENTATION

DISEASE FORMS/SUBTYPES Unilateral or bilateral nephrolithiasis

HISTORY, CHIEF COMPLAINT

- Similar to chronic renal failure: Weight loss, anorexia, depression
- Colic
- Hematuria

PHYSICAL EXAM FINDINGS

- Weight loss
- Enlarged kidney (left) palpated during evaluation per rectum

ETIOLOGY AND PATHOPHYSIOLOGY

- Nephroliths begin as a nidus of damaged tissue (fibrosis, inflammation, or infection).
- Nephroliths are typically composed of calcium carbonate crystals but may also be composed of calcium phosphate.

DIAGNOSIS

DIFFERENTIAL DIAGNOSIS

- Chronic renal failure
- Ureterolithiasis
- Pyelonephritis
- Neoplasia
- Cystic calculi
- Chronic gastrointestinal pain (colic)

INITIAL DATABASE

- Complete blood count and fibrinogen concentration.
- Serum chemistries reveal azotemia (especially if bilateral disease).
- Urinalysis reveals macroscopic or microscopic hematuria.

ADVANCED OR CONFIRMATORY TESTING

- Ultrasound examination of the affected kidney may show changes in echogenicity or acoustic shadowing suggestive of nephrolithiasis.
- Endoscopic evaluation of the urinary tract may reveal the origin of hematuria from one or both ureteral openings.
- Quantitative urine culture if pyelonephritis is suspected

TREATMENT

THERAPEUTIC GOAL(S)

- Supportive care of renal function (IV fluids, antibiotics, analgesics)
- Removal of the nephrolith via nephrectomy (if unilateral)

ACUTE GENERAL TREATMENT

- Support renal perfusion and urine production with IV fluids if the urinary tract is unobstructed.
- Analgesia as needed (avoid NSAIDs if azotemia is present)
- Broad-spectrum antibiotics if nephrectomy will be attempted

- Nephrectomy if stones are unilateral and the contralateral kidney is normal.

RECOMMENDED MONITORING

- Regular monitoring of blood urea nitrogen and creatinine concentrations to assess renal function, especially if a kidney has been removed. Horses with bilateral nephrolithiasis should be monitored for decreasing renal function and worsening renal failure.
- The horse should be carefully monitored for normal urination and any signs of urinary obstruction.

PROGNOSIS AND OUTCOME

- Usually good if a nephrectomy can be performed and the contralateral kidney is normal

- Poor to grave if nephroliths are bilateral and renal function is decreased (azotemia)

PEARLS & CONSIDERATIONS

COMMENTS

- A retrospective study reported uroliths in the kidneys of 15 of 68 (22%) horses with urolithiasis, and more than 50% of these cases were bilateral. Approximately 9% of horses had uroliths in more than one location.
- Nephrolithiasis should be ruled out in horses with clinicopathologic indications of renal failure, chronic weight loss, and colic.

PREVENTION

Careful use and monitoring of kidney function with long-term or high doses of NSAIDs

CLIENT EDUCATION

Consult with a veterinarian before administration of NSAIDs.

SUGGESTED READING

Divers TJ: Urolithiasis and obstructive disease: disease of the renal system. In Smith BP (ed). *Large animal internal medicine*, ed 4, St Louis, 2009, Mosby Elsevier, pp 938–942.
Laverty S, Pascoe JR, Ling GV, et al: Urolithiasis in 68 horses. *Vet Surg* 21:56, 1992.

AUTHOR: JENNIFER TAINTOR

EDITOR: BRYAN M. WALDRIDGE

Nephrotic Syndrome

BASIC INFORMATION

DEFINITION

A syndrome of hypoproteinemia, proteinuria, and edema formation caused by damaged glomerular basement membranes

SYNONYM(S)

Nephrosis

EPIDEMIOLOGY

RISK FACTORS
Hyperimmunized horses
ASSOCIATED CONDITIONS AND DISORDERS
- Amyloidosis
- Aortoiliac thrombosis
- Chronic antigenic stimulation or inflammatory disease
- Equine infectious anemia
- Immune mediated disease
- Purpura hemorrhagica or *Streptococcus equi* subsp. *equi* infection

CLINICAL PRESENTATION

HISTORY, CHIEF COMPLAINT
- Weight loss
- Ventral edema
- Polyuria
- Polydipsia
PHYSICAL EXAM FINDINGS
- Abdominal distension
- Ascites
- Generalized or ventral midline edema

- Poor body condition
- Pleural or peritoneal effusion
ETIOLOGY AND PATHOPHYSIOLOGY
- Nephrotic syndrome can be the end stage outcome of glomerulonephritis.
- Severe glomerular damage affects the filtration pore size and membrane charge of the glomerulus and results in proteinuria.

DIAGNOSIS

DIFFERENTIAL DIAGNOSIS

- Acute renal failure
- Chronic renal failure
- Diabetes insipidus
- Heart failure
- Pituitary pars intermedia dysfunction
- Psychogenic water drinking
- Purpura hemorrhagica

INITIAL DATABASE

- Complete blood count
- Serum chemistries
- Urinalysis

ADVANCED OR CONFIRMATORY TESTING

- Renal ultrasound examination: The kidneys may appear small and shrunken.
- Renal biopsy: Specialized immunohistochemistry or electron microscopy

may be needed to identify the cause and severity of disease.
- *S. equi* subsp. *equi* M (SeM) protein titer: Very high titers are found with purpura hemorrhagica (immune complex hypersensitivity) secondary to *S. equi* infection.
- Ultrasound examination may also reveal thoracic or abdominal effusion (or both).

TREATMENT

THERAPEUTIC GOAL(S)

- Reduce edema formation
- Reduce azotemia
- Maintain hydration

ACUTE GENERAL TREATMENT

- Treatment of any possible predisposing conditions
- IV fluids (60 mL/kg q24h) with electrolytes if needed for dehydration

CHRONIC TREATMENT

- Provide palliative, symptomatic therapy
- Restrict dietary salt intake
- Avoid excessive dietary protein (adult horses at maintenance require only 7% dietary protein)
- Feed a low-protein and low-calcium diet as recommended for patients with chronic renal failure (avoid legumes)

RECOMMENDED MONITORING

Periodic determination of blood urea nitrogen, creatinine, and total protein concentrations

PROGNOSIS AND OUTCOME

Poor

PEARLS & CONSIDERATIONS

- Pleural and abdominal effusion appears to be less common in horses with nephrotic syndrome than for other animals.
- Nephrotic syndrome likely indicates that end-stage kidney disease is present.

SUGGESTED READING

Bernard WV: Inflammatory, infectious, and immune diseases. In Colahan PT, Merritt AM, Moore JM, et al (eds). *Equine medicine and surgery*, ed 5, St Louis, 1998, Mosby, pp 1770–1772.

AUTHOR & EDITOR: **BRYAN M. WALDRIDGE**

Neurotoxic Plant (Miscellaneous) Toxicosis

BASIC INFORMATION

DEFINITION

Plants with the potential to cause neurologic poisoning in horses

SYNONYM(S)

- Buckeye, horse chestnut, red buckeye (*Aesculus* spp.)
- Carolina jessamine, woodbine, false jasmine (*Gelsemium sempervirens*)
- Carolina allspice, sweet shrub (*Calycanthus floridus*)
- Golden chain tree, bean tree (*Laburnum anagyroides*)
- Scotch broom, broom (*Cytisus scoparius*)

EPIDEMIOLOGY

GEOGRAPHY AND SEASONALITY

- Buckeye: Six *Aesculus* spp. native to North America; small to large trees with large palmate leaves and distinctive brown fruits
- Carolina jessamine: Woody evergreen, perennial vines with trumpet-shaped yellow flowers
- Carolina allspice: Perennial, branching shrubs with opposite leaves and maroon-brown colored aromatic flowers of the southeastern states
- Golden chain tree: Perennial, deciduous, small trees with palmate, compound leaves, numerous pendulous inflorescences with pea-like yellow flowers and seed pods
- Scotch broom: A nonnative, perennial, shrub or small tree with ribbed branches, palmate leaves, and yellow pea-like flowers and seed pods

CLINICAL PRESENTATION

HISTORY, CHIEF COMPLAINT

- Incoordination
- Weakness
- Ataxia

PHYSICAL EXAM FINDINGS

- Buckeye: Incoordination, weakness, staggering gait, hypermetria, sawhorse stance, muscle spasms, gastroenteritis, colic
- Carolina jessamine: Incoordination, weakness, muscle convulsions, respiratory paralysis
- Carolina allspice: Muscle fasciculations, hypersensitivity, incoordination, recumbency, tetanic seizures, extensor rigidity
- Golden chain tree: Short-duration weakness, muscle tremors, incoordination, colic
- Scotch broom: Excitement, ataxia, incoordination, colic

ETIOLOGY AND PATHOPHYSIOLOGY

- Buckeye: Numerous triterpenoid saponins are found in new leaves and seeds.
- Carolina jessamine: Gelsemine and other alkaloids in all parts of the plant cause paralysis.
- Carolina allspice: Calycanthine and other alkaloids are potent stimulants of the nervous system, acting like strychnine.
- Golden chain tree: Quinolizidine cystine–like alkaloids are nicotinic receptor agonists causing ganglionic blockade similar to curare. Seeds are most toxic. Anagyrine in the seeds may be teratogenic.
- Scotch broom: Several quinolizidine alkaloids are similar to those in *Laburnum* spp. with similar activity on nicotinic receptors. Anagyrine in the seeds may be teratogenic.

DIAGNOSIS

DIFFERENTIAL DIAGNOSIS

- Encephalitis: Rabies, West Nile virus, eastern and western equine encephalitis virus
- Equine herpes virus
- Equine leukoencephalomalacia
- Sage poisoning
- Pyrrolizidine alkaloid toxicity
- Bracken fern and horsetail poisoning
- Strychnine poisoning

INITIAL DATABASE

No specific clinical pathologic findings with any of these plants

ADVANCED OR CONFIRMATORY TESTING

- Postmortem finding are generally nonspecific.
- Stomach contents should be submitted for plant identification.
- Golden chain tree and Scotch broom can cause skeletal myopathy histologically.

TREATMENT

THERAPEUTIC GOAL(S)

- Decontamination and administration of activated charcoal if recent ingestion
- Symptomatic and supportive care

ACUTE GENERAL TREATMENT

- Buckeye poisoning is self-limiting after ingestion of the plant ceases.
- Carolina jessamine: There is no specific antidote, and treatment should be symptomatic.
- Carolina allspice: Diazepam or pentobarbital to control seizures; dark and quiet environment
- Golden chain tree: Supportive treatment as necessary
- Scotch broom: Supportive treatment as necessary

PROGNOSIS AND OUTCOME

- Buckeye poisoning is rarely fatal.
- Carolina jessamine poisoning carries a guarded prognosis after clinical signs appear.
- Carolina allspice has a guarded prognosis after seizures occur.

- Golden chain tree and Scotch broom poisonings are usually of short duration unless consumption of the seeds continues.

PEARLS & CONSIDERATIONS

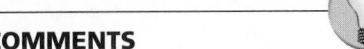

COMMENTS

Although horses have rarely been poisoned by these plants and published case reports are rare or nonexistent, the plants should still be considered potentially hazardous to horses.

PREVENTION

Do not plant any of these plants in or around horse pastures or corrals where horses have access to them.

SUGGESTED READING

Burrows GE, Tyrl RJ: Laburnum. In *Toxic plants of North America*, Ames, IA, 2001, Iowa State Press, pp 562–564.

Bradley RE, Jones TJ: Strychnine-like toxicity of *Calycanthus*. *Southwest Vet* 14:71–73, 1963.

Keeler RF, Baker DC: Myopathy in cattle induced by alkaloid extracts from *Thermopsis montana, Laburnum anagyroides*, and *Lupinus* spp. *J Comp Pathol* 103:169–182, 1990.

Zhang Z, Li S, Zhang S, Gorenstein D: Triterpenoid saponins from the fruits of *Aesculus pavia*. *Phytochemistry* 67:784–794, 2006.

AUTHOR: **ANTHONY P. KNIGHT**

EDITOR: **CYNTHIA L. GASKILL**

Nightshade Toxicosis

BASIC INFORMATION

DEFINITION

Nightshades are a large, diverse group of plants in the family Solanaceae that contain a variety of toxic alkaloids with profound effects on the nervous system and digestive tract. A few species, such as day- and night-blooming jessamine, cause excess calcification of the tissues.

SYNONYM(S)

- Black nightshade, poison berry, yerba mora (*Solanum nigrum*)
- Common or American nightshade (*Solanum americanum*)
- Silverleaf nightshade, desert nightshade, western or white horse nettle (*Solanum elaeagnifolium*)
- Horse or bull nettle, Carolina horse nettle, Sodom apple (*Solanum carolinense*)
- Hairy nightshade (*Solanum physalifolium*)
- Jimson weed, Datura, sacred Datura, thorn apple, Indian apple, tolguacha (*Datura* spp.)
- Tomato (*Lycopersicon esculentum*)
- Day or wild jessamine, day cestrum, Chinese inkberry (*Cestrum diurnum*)
- Night-blooming jessamine, huele de noche (*C. nocturnum*)

EPIDEMIOLOGY

RISK FACTORS

- Weedy hay containing dried nightshade species
- Grain contaminated with *Datura* seeds
- Horses given access to green tomato and potato vines

GEOGRAPHY AND SEASONALITY

- The nightshades, including *Datura* spp., are frost sensitive and tend to be annuals except in milder climates. There are at least 70 species of native and introduced *Solanum* spp. in North America.

- The common nightshades range from herbaceous, small, weedy, erect shrubs to small trees with alternate or opposite, hairy or smooth leaves, some with prominent spines, and with five-lobed, white to purple flowers that form round, fleshy berries or fruits that are usually green and turn yellow or black when mature (Figures 1 to 3).

CLINICAL PRESENTATION

HISTORY, CHIEF COMPLAINT

- Clinical signs of colic within hours of eating the nightshade plants.
- Depending on the quantity of nightshade eaten, severe colic, recumbency, and seizures may develop.

PHYSICAL EXAM FINDINGS

Nightshades cause variable signs of colic because of intestinal stasis and gas accumulation. Gastric dilatation and death may occur.

ETIOLOGY AND PATHOPHYSIOLOGY

- Members of the Solanaceae family contain a variety of toxic compounds; the two that most often affect animals are glycoalkaloids and tropane alkaloids.
- Glycoalkaloids, common in the *Solanum* spp., are gastrointestinal (GI) irritants and are neurotoxic.
- Horses that have been eating silverleaf nightshade and are treated with ivermectin develop severe depression and die, apparently because of increased permeability of the blood-brain barrier to ivermectin.
- Tropane alkaloids found in *Datura* spp. are competitive antagonists of acetylcholine, causing dilated pupils,

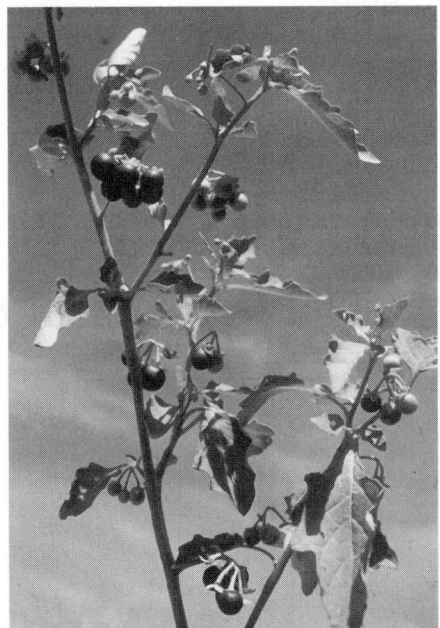

FIGURE 1 American nightshade (*Solanum americanum*).

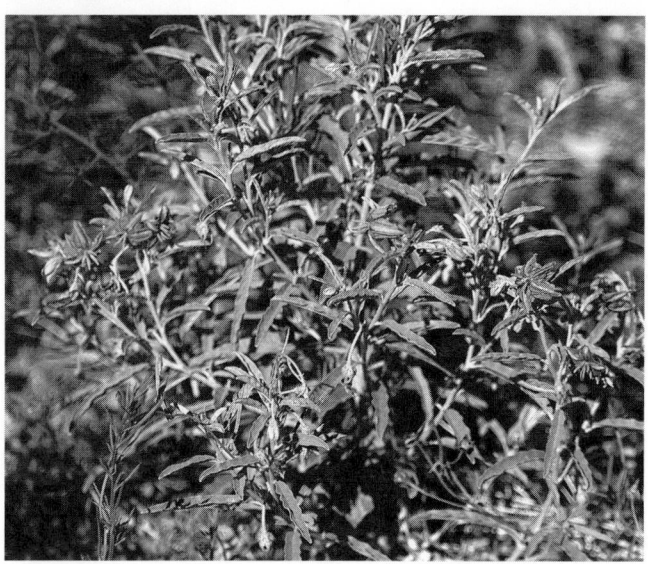

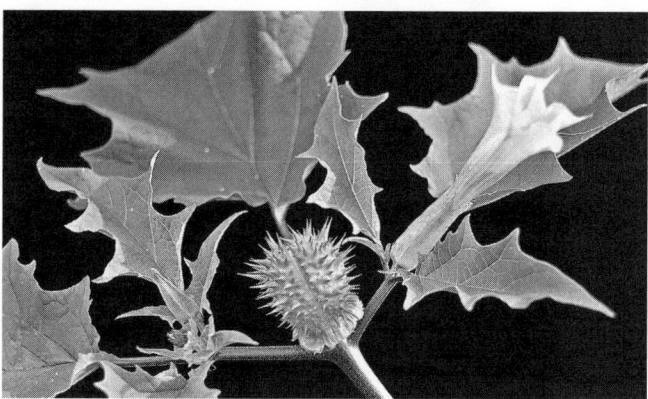

FIGURE 3 Jimson weed (*Datura stramonium*).

FIGURE 2 Silverleaf nightshade (*Solanum elaeagnifolium*).

intestinal atony, decreased salivation, tachycardia, and tachypnea typical of the effects of atropine.
- Grain contaminated with *Datura* seeds (~600 seeds/kg of grain) cause poisoning in horses.
- Day- and night-blooming jessamines (*Cestrum* spp.) have a different effect and cause excess calcification of the tissues, leading to weight loss, lameness, and debilitation.

DIAGNOSIS

DIFFERENTIAL DIAGNOSIS
- Colic from other causes
- Calcification of tissues: Cholecalciferol or vitamin D toxicosis

INITIAL DATABASE
Hematocrit and serum biochemistry changes may be minimal initially.

ADVANCED OR CONFIRMATORY TESTING
- Stomach contents and urine can be analyzed for tropane alkaloids.
- Plants in stomach contents or feed sources can be identified both visually and microscopically.
- Postmortem lesions may show GI reddening or gaseous distension.

TREATMENT

THERAPEUTIC GOAL(S)
Decontaminate patient and provide symptomatic care

ACUTE GENERAL TREATMENT
- Place a nasogastric tube if gastric dilation is suspected.
- Adsorption of toxins with activated charcoal as early in the course of poisoning as possible
- Control seizures with diazepam.
- Do not use phenothiazine tranquilizers because of their anticholinergic effects.
- Cholinergics such as physostigmine may be useful.
- Supportive treatment should include IV fluids when dehydration and shock are evident.

RECOMMENDED MONITORING
Serum electrolytes and hematocrit to manage colic progress

PROGNOSIS AND OUTCOME

Horses recover in 1 or 2 days unless they have consumed large amounts of the nightshade.

PEARLS & CONSIDERATIONS

COMMENTS
- Nightshades are common weeds in pastures in some areas and are more often a problem for ruminants than for horses. Exposures in horses most commonly occur from ingestion of hay heavily contaminated with nightshade leaves and fruits or ingestion of tomato or potato vines.
- Poor-quality grain contaminated with *Datura* seeds is a significant cause for concern.

PREVENTION
Recognize the common nightshades and control them with appropriate herbicides or mowing.

CLIENT EDUCATION
- Inspect hay and grain for nightshade leaves, stems, berries, and seeds.
- Ensure horses have adequate and good-quality feeds and forages to prevent hungry horses from eating excessive amounts of weeds.

SUGGESTED READING
Burrows GE, Tyrl RJ: Solanaceae. In Burrows GE, Tyrl RJ (eds). *Toxic plants of North America*, Ames, IA, 2001, Iowa State University Press, pp 1104–1148.
Garland T, Bailey EM, Reagor JC: Probable interaction between *Solanum elaeagnifolium* and ivermectin in horses. In Garland T, Barr AC (eds). *Toxic plants and other natural toxicants*, New York, 1998, CAB International, pp 423–427.
Schulman ML, Bolton LA: Datura seed intoxication in two horses. *J S Afr Vet Assoc* 69:27–29, 1998.

AUTHOR: **ANTHONY P. KNIGHT**

EDITOR: **CYNTHIA L. GASKILL**

Nocardiosis

BASIC INFORMATION

DEFINITION

A bacterial disease caused by opportunistic saprophytes of *Nocardia* spp. resulting in suppurative to granulomatous tissue reactions in a localized or disseminated manner

EPIDEMIOLOGY

SPECIES, AGE, SEX
- No known breed or sex predilection
- Present in most environments as part of the normal soil microflora; found worldwide
- Prevalence of 0.009% in equine patients

RISK FACTORS
- Considered an opportunistic pathogen, infecting immunosuppressed individuals
- Primarily associated with severe combined immunodeficiency syndrome in Arabian foals and pituitary pars intermedia dysfunction (PPID) as immunosuppressive conditions
- Infection occurs via inhalation or direct inoculation through a wound.

CONTAGION AND ZOONOSIS
- Not contagious
- Infectious to humans but not transmitted directly from horses to humans

CLINICAL PRESENTATION

DISEASE FORMS/SUBTYPES May be localized or disseminated:
- Pulmonary
- Disseminated
- Localized cutaneous
- Nocardia-induced mycetoma
- Abortion

HISTORY, CHIEF COMPLAINT Normally a chronic course of disease but can present acutely and be rapidly progressive

PHYSICAL EXAM FINDINGS
- Pulmonary nocardiosis: Increased respiratory rate and effort, cough, nasal discharge; may be acute or chronic; may result in pneumonia, abscess formation, or pleuritis.
- Disseminated nocardiosis: Widespread abscess formation in multiple organs; may occur secondary to pulmonary disease. In humans, most commonly affects the central nervous system, eyes, kidneys, joints, bone, heart, and skin or subcutaneous tissues.
- Localized cutaneous nocardiosis: Occasionally occurs without systemic lesions, usually after direct inoculation

of the organism via trauma. Results in cellulitis or pyoderma, often becoming a circumscribed abscess. These lesions may ulcerate and have thick, odorless purulent discharge.
- Nocardia-induced mycetomas: Subcutaneous infection usually resulting from a traumatic injury. Generally starts with a painless nodule that chronically progresses in size and eventually becomes purulent and necrotic. Granulomatous inflammation surrounds the lesion, and secondary nodules and drainage tracts occur. Exudate may contain sandlike particles.
- Abortion: Rare; lesions are observed in the aborted fetuses within the lung and liver as well as in the placenta.

ETIOLOGY AND PATHOPHYSIOLOGY
- *Nocardia* spp. bacteria are aerobic gram-positive actinomycetes that are saprophytic, non–spore-forming, and partially acid fast.
- Most infections are caused by members of the *Nocardia asteroides* complex; however, *Nocardia brasiliensis* has also been isolated.
- Infection cannot be eliminated by macrophages and neutrophils alone; protective responses appear to be T-cell mediated.
- L-form variants can survive dormant within macrophages and lead to occasional relapses.

DIAGNOSIS

DIFFERENTIAL DIAGNOSIS
- Other causes of bacterial pneumonia, including *Streptococcus* spp., *Actinobacillus* spp., *Pasteurella* spp., *Klebsiella pneumoniae*, *Rhodococcus equi*, *Escherichia coli*, *Staphylococcus aureus*, *Bordetella bronchiseptica*, *Bacteroides fragilis*, *Peptostreptococcus anaerobius*, and *Fusobacterium* spp.
- Fungal pneumonia
- Pulmonary parasite migration
- Other causes of mycetomas include fungal (*Curvularia geniculata*, *Pseudallescheria boydii*) and other bacteria (*Actinobacillus* spp., *Actinomyces* spp.)
- Cutaneous lesions may resemble those caused by *Staphylococcus* and *Streptococcus* spp. or cutaneous neoplasia such as sarcoids or squamous cell carcinoma.
- Other causes of abortion include bacterial or fungal placentitis, leptospirosis, and equine herpesvirus-1.

INITIAL DATABASE
- Results of complete blood count and serum chemistry are not specific and may reflect an inflammatory process as well as evidence of immunosuppression (lymphopenia, neutrophilia with left shift and toxic changes, hyperfibrinogenemia, and hyperglobulinemia or hypoglobulinemia).
- Gram-stained samples reveal gram-positive rod- to coccoid-shaped branching filaments. Acid-fast staining can confirm the partially acid-fast nature of most isolates.
- Culture can be performed, but refrigeration of samples should be avoided.

ADVANCED OR CONFIRMATORY TESTING
- Serology: Not routinely used because patients usually do not develop a significant antibody response.
- Speciation of *Nocardia* isolates is performed by polymerase chain reaction (PCR); a semi-nested PCR method is under investigation that could help detect L forms of *Nocardia* that are especially difficult to identify with culture.

TREATMENT

THERAPEUTIC GOAL(S)

Elimination of pathogenic organisms with antimicrobial therapy and surgical drainage of lesions

ACUTE GENERAL TREATMENT
- If possible, abscesses and exudative lesions should be drained, debrided, and lavaged.
- Proliferative granulomatous lesions may need to be resected.
- Antimicrobial susceptibility testing should be performed, but often in vitro results do not correlate well with clinical efficacy in these cases.
- The general recommendation for antibiotic therapy is the use of a trimethoprim-sulfonamide, ideally in combination with amikacin.
- Other antibiotics that have been used include amoxicillin-clavulanate, third-generation cephalosporins, newer macrolides, imipenem, and other aminoglycosides.

CHRONIC TREATMENT
- Although clinical improvement may be observed 5 to 10 days after institution of therapy, long-term treatment with antibiotics (ie, 6–12 months) may be required to prevent relapses.

- PPID can be managed with pergolide, which helps to limit the clinical manifestations of disease, including immunosuppression.

PROGNOSIS AND OUTCOME

- The prognosis is based primarily on host factors, specifically the severity of compromise to the immune system and the site and extent of the lesions.
- Pulmonary and disseminated nocardiosis carry a poor prognosis because of severe debilitation, but lesions limited to the skin have a good prognosis.

PEARLS & CONSIDERATIONS

COMMENTS

Nocardioform placentitis is a condition not actually caused by *Nocardia* spp. but rather *Crossiella equi* or *Cellulosimicrobium cellulans*, organisms unrelated to *Nocardia*.

PREVENTION

No method of prevention exists other than trying to prevent immunosuppression if possible (ie, by managing horses with PPID with pergolide).

SUGGESTED READING

Arguedas MG: Miscellaneous gram-positive bacterial infections—nocardiosis. In Sellon DC, Long MT (eds). *Equine infectious diseases*, St Louis, 2006, Saunders Elsevier, pp 269–273.

Biberstein EL, Jang SS, Hirsh DC: *Nocardia asteroides* infection in horses: a review. *J Am Vet Med Assoc* 186:273–277, 1985.

AUTHOR: **SIDDRA HINES**

EDITORS: **DEBRA C. SELLON** and **MAUREEN T. LONG**

Nonsteroidal Antiinflammatory Drug Toxicosis

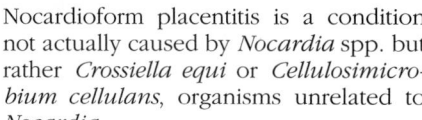

BASIC INFORMATION

DEFINITION

- Adverse effects of the nonsteroidal antiinflammatory drugs (NSAIDs) are caused by cyclooxygenase (COX) inhibition in tissues where prostaglandins are beneficial and protective.
- Renal papillary necrosis (medullary crest necrosis), oral and gastrointestinal (GI) ulceration, and right dorsal colitis are common signs of NSAID toxicity in horses.
- Platelet aggregation is classically inhibited by NSAIDs that prevent thromboxane production via the COX-1 pathway.

EPIDEMIOLOGY

SPECIES, AGE, SEX Neonates and geriatrics are more at risk.
RISK FACTORS Renal insufficiency, dehydration, concurrent use of both phenylbutazone and flunixin meglumine, concurrent nephrotoxic drug therapy (eg, aminoglycosides), and history of previous NSAID toxicity

CLINICAL PRESENTATION
HISTORY, CHIEF COMPLAINT

- NSAID administered
  - NSAIDs approved for use in horses include aspirin, flunixin meglumine (Banamine, generics), ketoprofen (Ketofen, Anafen), diclofenac (topical, Surpass), phenylbutazone (generics), firocoxib (Equioxx), meclofenamic acid (Arquel), and vedaprofen (Quadrisol, Canada and Europe).
  - The highest incidence of toxicity is associated with phenylbutazone administration.
- Amount administered: Phenylbutazone may cause toxicity when administered according to the label dose. Other NSAIDs usually require an overdose to cause toxicity.

PHYSICAL EXAM FINDINGS

- Colic
- Anorexia
- Poor body condition
- Diarrhea
- Oral mucosal erosions, odontoprisis, sialism
- Regurgitation of milk and pain after nursing in foals
- Oliguria

ETIOLOGY AND PATHOPHYSIOLOGY

- Nephrotoxicity: NSAIDs typically have little effect on renal function in normal adult animals, but they decrease renal blood flow and glomerular filtration rate in patients with congestive heart failure, those that are hypotensive or hypovolemic (especially during anesthesia and surgery), and those that have chronic renal disease. Renal papillary necrosis is a severe dose-dependent toxicity most commonly associated with phenylbutazone. Although attributed to impaired renal blood flow, other mechanisms such as direct nephrotoxicity of the drug or its metabolites may be involved.
- GI toxicity: Reduced prostaglandin (PG) concentrations in the large colon may decrease colonic blood flow, resulting in mucosal atrophy, protein loss, ulceration, and inflammation.

DIAGNOSIS

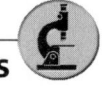

DIFFERENTIAL DIAGNOSIS

- Stress-induced gastric ulceration
- Inflammatory bowel disease
- Other toxin-induced renal failure (eg, cantharidin)

INITIAL DATABASE

- In asymptomatic horses, consider obtaining baseline renal and hepatic function tests.
- In symptomatic horses, monitor:
  - Complete blood count and serum chemistries for anemia, neutrophilia or neutropenia, hypoproteinemia, hypoalbuminemia, hypocalcemia, and elevated liver enzymes
  - Arterial blood gases for metabolic acidosis
  - Renal function tests for azotemia, increased urine γ-glutamyl transferase (GGT), and increased urine GGT/urine creatinine ratio

ADVANCED OR CONFIRMATORY TESTING

- Nuclear scintigraphy with ^{99m}Tc-HMPAO labeled white blood cells or ^{99m}Tc-albumin are noninvasive methods for detecting right dorsal colitis caused by NSAID toxicity.
- Ultrasonography of the kidneys may show a medullary rim sign (a distinct curvilinear hyperechoic band parallel to the corticomedullary junction). This is thought to result from dystrophic calcification of the outer zone of the medulla parallel to the corticomedullary junction.

- Postmortem findings
  - Most common gross lesions
    - Oral erosions or ulcers
    - Gastric and duodenal ulcers
    - Right dorsal colon ulceration
  - Less frequent gross lesions
    - Renal crest necrosis
    - Focal to diffuse hepatic pallor
  - Histopathologic lesions
    - Mucosal atrophy to erosion and ulceration in the GI tract
    - Accumulation of plasma cells, lymphocytes, and macrophages in the lamina propria and submucosa
    - Moderate to severe villous atrophy and epithelial necrosis and mucosal inflammation
    - Renal proximal convoluted tubular degeneration
    - Chronic, active cholangiohepatitis

TREATMENT

THERAPEUTIC GOAL(S)

- Treatment of NSAID GI toxicity is intensive and mainly symptomatic.
- Patients with significant toxicity that develop severe acidosis may require supportive treatment with IV sodium bicarbonate.

ACUTE GENERAL TREATMENT

- Activated charcoal may bind and limit absorption of NSAIDs from the GI tract.
- Sodium bicarbonate is indicated for the treatment of recalcitrant acidosis (pH <7).
- Hypoproteinemia: Plasma infusion.
- Dehydration and electrolyte losses: Commercially available IV fluids.
- Sepsis: Broad-spectrum antimicrobial therapy.
- Pain: Further NSAID therapy must be avoided. Use a continuous butorphanol infusion at 13 μg/kg/h IV (diluted in lactated Ringer's solution) for colic pain control.
- Anti-ulcer medications may be beneficial and speed recovery.
  - Proton pump inhibitors (PPIs) appear to be the most effective therapies for both gastric ulcer prevention and treatment. Omeprazole (Gastrogard) paste should be administered at 4 mg/kg PO q24h for 4 weeks.
  - Histamine H2-receptor antagonists (cimetidine, ranitidine, famotidine) decrease gastric acid secretion but have a shorter duration of effect than PPIs and must be dosed more frequently. Oral bioavailability in horses is very low, so large doses are required.
  - Sucralfate may provide some protection against NSAID-induced gastric ulceration.
  - Antacids (aluminum hydroxide, magnesium oxide or hydroxide, and calcium carbonate) increase gastric pH but have a short duration of action and must be administered very frequently to be effective.

CHRONIC TREATMENT

- Corn oil supplementation may be an effective and inexpensive way to increase the protective properties of equine glandular gastric mucosa. When supplemented with 45 mL q24h of corn oil, ponies had significantly decreased acid output and significantly increased PGE2 and sodium outputs compared with those measured before corn oil supplementation.
- The ideal dietary management of horses with right dorsal colitis is unknown. Some veterinarians recommend feeding no roughage and only pelleted feeds, but others recommend feeding a high-roughage diet to stimulate production of specific short-chain volatile fatty acids (VFAs), which have been associated with intestinal mucosal protection in experimentally induced colitis. If hay is fed, alfalfa induces significantly higher pH and VFA concentrations in gastric juice than brome grass hay.

DRUG INTERACTIONS

- Concurrent administration of an aminoglycoside (eg, gentamicin) may increase the toxicity of both the aminoglycoside and the NSAID.
- Omeprazole in humans is metabolized by polymorphically expressed cytochrome P450, with populations of extensive, moderate and poor metabolizers. It is not known if equine metabolism of omeprazole is polymorphic. Omeprazole and cimetidine are known to inhibit the hepatic metabolism of other drugs metabolized by the cytochrome P450 system, but there are no reports of specific adverse drug interactions.
- All drugs that alter gastric acid pH have the potential to interfere with the normal absorption of other orally administered drugs.
- Antacids should not be administered concurrently with fluoroquinolones or tetracyclines because of binding to calcium and aluminum, reducing absorption.
- Sucralfate disassociates in the acidic environment of the stomach to sucrose octasulfate and aluminum hydroxide. If administered after other antiulcer drugs have increased the gastric acid pH, its activity will be reduced. If it is administered before the histamine H2-receptor antagonists, they adsorb to the aluminum hydroxide, and their absorption is reduced.

POSSIBLE COMPLICATIONS

- Surgical removal of damaged sections of stomach or colon may be necessary in some cases.
- Duodenal ulcers, duodenal strictures with gastric outflow obstruction, erosive esophagitis, and gastric rupture occur infrequently.

RECOMMENDED MONITORING

- Clinical signs
- Plasma protein concentrations

PROGNOSIS AND OUTCOME

Recovery is usually slow, and in severe cases, the prognosis is guarded. Alternative pain drugs must be used in horses that demonstrate sensitivity to NSAIDs.

PEARLS & CONSIDERATIONS

PREVENTION

Use the lowest effective dose and the longest possible dosing intervals for any NSAID in horses. Avoid phenylbutazone in high-risk foals and horses. Consider prophylactic use of omeprazole and feeding corn oil to high-risk patients.

CLIENT EDUCATION

Caution clients to not administer NSAIDs to horses without veterinary supervision. Horses receiving NSAIDs must have adequate water intake.

SUGGESTED READING

Cargile JL, Burrow JA, Kim I, et al: Effect of dietary corn oil supplementation on equine gastric fluid acid, sodium, and prostaglandin E2 content before and during pentagastrin infusion. *J Vet Intern Med* 18:545–549, 2004.

Cohen ND, Carter GK, Mealey RH, Taylor TS: Medical management of right dorsal colitis in 5 horses: a retrospective study (1987–1993). *J Vet Intern Med* 9:272–276, 1995.

Reed SK, Messer NT, Tessman RK, et al: Effects of phenylbutazone alone or in combination with flunixin meglumine on blood protein concentrations in horses. *Am J Vet Res* 67:398–402, 2006.

McConnico RS, Morgan TW, Williams CC, et al: Pathophysiologic effects of phenylbutazone on the right dorsal colon in horses. *Am J Vet Res* 69:1496–1505, 2008.

AUTHOR: **PATRICIA M. DOWLING**

EDITOR: **CYNTHIA L. GASKILL**

Nutritional Myopathy

BASIC INFORMATION

DEFINITION
An acute to chronic myodegenerative disease of skeletal and cardiac muscle assumed to be caused by a dietary deficiency in selenium, vitamin E, or both

SYNONYM(S)
White muscle disease, nutritional muscular dystrophy

EPIDEMIOLOGY
SPECIES, AGE, SEX
- Horses and probably donkeys and mules may be affected.
- Foals seem to be more susceptible than adults.

GEOGRAPHY AND SEASONALITY
Nutritional myopathies are found more often in areas of selenium deficient soils, including the Pacific Northwest; Great Lakes area; northeast and southeast Gulf Coast areas of North America; and parts of Europe, New Zealand, Australia, and Asia.

ASSOCIATED CONDITIONS AND DIS-ORDERS Aspiration pneumonia, malnutrition and steatitis, impaired immune function

CLINICAL PRESENTATION
DISEASE FORMS/SUBTYPES The type of disease depends on the muscle group affected and the horse's age.
- Acute disease: Cardiovascular collapse, sudden death
- Subacute disease in foals: Muscle weakness or dysphagia
- Chronic disease in adults: Dysphagia, weakness, muscle atrophy

HISTORY, CHIEF COMPLAINT Vary with muscle group affected and age
- Sudden death or recumbency
- Inability to eat
- Weakness or stiffness

PHYSICAL EXAM FINDINGS Vary with muscle group affected
- Cardiac muscle: Tachycardia, tachypnea, dyspnea, irregular heartbeat, unable to rise, sudden death
- Masseter muscles: Trismus, bruxism, weight loss, dysphagia, atrophy of muscles
- Lingual or pharyngeal muscles: Dysphagia, weight loss, aspiration pneumonia, quidding
- Muscles of locomotion: Weakness, stiffness, difficulty rising, weight loss, painful muscles, neck pain, trembling

ETIOLOGY AND PATHOPHYSIOLOGY
Most cases are caused by a dietary deficiency in selenium and sometimes vitamin E. Muscle cell membranes may be destroyed by oxidative free radicals, which disrupts the integrity of the muscle cell. Selenium and vitamin E are antioxidants that can prevent this. Selenium destroys some of the peroxides that have been formed. Vitamin E is a lipid-soluble antioxidant that is active within the cell membrane. Lack of these antioxidants along with other factors may lead to muscle degeneration.

DIAGNOSIS

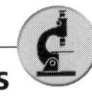

DIFFERENTIAL DIAGNOSIS
- Other cardiovascular disease
- Temporomandibular joint disease
- Toxicities caused by gossypol, ionophores, yew, oleander, and other cardiotoxic plants
- Exertional rhabdomyolysis
- Tetanus

INITIAL DATABASE
- Creatine kinase (CK) is usually increased to above 5000 IU/L except in chronic cases in which the muscle has already undergone fibrosis. CK has a short half-life, so levels may decrease over time if the degeneration stops and may be of prognostic value.
- Aspartate aminotransferase (AST) has a longer half-life and remains elevated longer.
- Lactate dehydrogenase (LDH) may also be elevated but is derived from tissues other than muscle, as is AST.
- Hyperkalemia may be present in foals along with hyponatremia and hypochloremia.
- Myoglobinuria may be present in foals.

ADVANCED OR CONFIRMATORY TESTING
- Whole-blood selenium, glutathione peroxidase, or serum selenium.
- Muscle biopsy and histopathology to identify hyalin degeneration or fibrosis of muscle.
- Serum vitamin E.
- Liver selenium concentration may be determined on tissue taken by biopsy or at postmortem. Normal liver concentrations should be 1.05 to 3.5 μg/g dry matter.

TREATMENT

THERAPEUTIC GOAL(S)
Prevent continued muscle degeneration and allow for regeneration of affected skeletal muscle.

ACUTE GENERAL TREATMENT
- Limit exertion that might promote cardiac failure.
- Provide selenium supplement to stop further degeneration.
- Treatment of horses with the acute form with cardiac failure is not often successful.

CHRONIC TREATMENT   0.06
- Give injectable selenium at ~~8~~ mg/kg body weight IM or SC.
- Warning: Selenium is a trace mineral with a narrow range of safety. There have been recent cases in which a large number of horses were killed by an overdose of selenium.
- Vitamin E as DL-α tocopherol can be added to the treatment, but the concentration in most combination products is not sufficient to increase blood levels because vitamin E is present only as a preservative.
- Provide supportive care such as providing rehydration and nutrition if the animal is unable to swallow.

POSSIBLE COMPLICATIONS
- Aspiration pneumonia may occur in foals unable to swallow.
- Malnutrition may occur in horses unable to open their mouths or swallow.

PROGNOSIS AND OUTCOME

Guarded for any case; grave for cardiac cases and chronic cases with muscle fibrosis

PEARLS & CONSIDERATIONS

COMMENTS
Proving that a deficiency in selenium or vitamin E caused the degeneration may be difficult. Whole-blood selenium (which is preferred) or whole-blood glutathione peroxidase indicates the selenium status at the time the red blood

cells were formed weeks to months before the appearance of clinical signs. Serum selenium indicates the selenium status at present and not necessarily at the time the degeneration started to occur. The serum or liver vitamin E concentration is related to the current dietary intake and not necessarily the amount available at the time the muscle was degenerating. Vitamin E levels in the serum also fluctuate throughout the day and vary with the season and diet.

PREVENTION

Prevention is achieved by supplementation of selenium and vitamin E, especially in selenium-deficient areas. Under current US regulations, the maximum selenium concentration of rations is 0.3 ppm, and the maximum concentration of mineral mixtures is 120 ppm. However, this may not be enough to prevent the condition in certain selenium-deficient areas. Oral supplementation of horses at 1 mg/d of selenium will increase blood levels to concentrations not associated with nutritional myodegeneration.

SUGGESTED READING

Dill SG, Rebhun WC: White muscle disease in foals. *Compend Contin Educ Pract Vet* 7(suppl):S627–S636, 1985.

Lofstedt J: White muscle disease in foals. *Vet Clin North Am Equine Pract* 13:165–185, 1997.

Pearson E, Snyder S, Saulez M: Masseter myodegeneration as a cause of trismus or dysphagia in adult horses. *Vet Rec* 156:642–646, 2005.

Mass J: Nutritional and toxic rhabdomyolysis. In Smith BP (ed). *Large animal internal medicine*, ed 4, St Louis, 2009, Mosby Elsevier, pp 1405–1408.

AUTHOR: **ERWIN G. PEARSON**

EDITOR: **ANDRIS J. KANEPS**

Oak Toxicosis

BASIC INFORMATION

DEFINITION

Oaks (*Quercus* spp.) in North America include approximately 85 native and introduced species and 100 named hybrids that occur as hardwood trees and woody perennial shrubs. In horses, oak toxicity is characterized primarily by gastrointestinal (GI) disease.

EPIDEMIOLOGY

SPECIES, AGE, SEX
- All horses are potentially susceptible with some individual variability.
- Compared with cattle, horses are less likely to exhibit renal effects.

RISK FACTORS
- Buds, twigs, leaves, and acorns are all potentially harmful.
- Most toxic ingestions involve young, immature leaves and freshly fallen acorns, although horses must typically consume very large quantities for 4 to 5 days or more to develop GI or renal disease.

GEOGRAPHY AND SEASONALITY
Oaks are found nearly worldwide in a wide variety of habitats. Toxicosis most commonly occurs after spring storms when animals have access to young leaves or in autumn when acorns begin to fall.

CLINICAL PRESENTATION

DISEASE FORMS/SUBTYPES
- GI disease (most common form in horses)
- Kidney disease
- Hepatotoxicity

HISTORY, CHIEF COMPLAINT The primary signs observed in horses are GI, most commonly presenting as varying degrees of colic and diarrhea.

PHYSICAL EXAM FINDINGS
- Mildly affected horses will be depressed with reduced peristalsis and constipation.
- More severe cases may have tenesmus and hemorrhagic diarrhea. Hemoglobinuria, hematuria, and icterus may also be observed.

ETIOLOGY AND PATHOPHYSIOLOGY
- Immature oak leaves and freshly fallen acorns contain the highest concentrations of condensed and hydrolyzable tannins.
- Condensed tannins are resistant to hydrolysis and tend to pass through the GI tract unchanged without causing significant disease problems.
- Hydrolyzable tannins are hydrolyzed in the gut to their constituent phenolics and sugars. These tannins or their polyphenolic products have an irritant astringent effect on the small intestinal mucosa, favoring absorption.
- If absorbed in large quantities, tannin metabolites reach increased levels in the kidneys and can result in the destruction of renal tubular cells.
- Liver involvement may also be seen in horses when the capacity to conjugate phenolics is exceeded.

DIAGNOSIS

DIFFERENTIAL DIAGNOSIS
- Other causes of GI disease or colic
- Kidney failure: Oxalate-containing plants
- Other hepatotoxins

INITIAL DATABASE

Abnormalities reported in one fatal case of equine acorn poisoning included dehydration, a mildly elevated serum creatine kinase concentration, hypoproteinemia, and hyperglycemia, along with decreased serum calcium and chloride and elevated phosphorus activity. The urine contained protein, blood, and hemoglobin casts. Prothrombin time, activated partial thromboplastin, and fibrin degradation products were increased.

ADVANCED OR CONFIRMATORY TESTING

- The most prominent necropsy lesions in horses are hemorrhagic enteritis and severe edema affecting the mesentery, cecum, and colon.
- Acorns have reportedly caused bowel obstruction, gastric rupture, and acute peritonitis.
- Acorn husks may be evident in the manure or GI contents.
- Histologically, renal tubular necrosis and hepatocellular degeneration may be observed.

TREATMENT

THERAPEUTIC GOAL(S)
- Treatment of GI disease
- Treatment of renal disease if present

ACUTE GENERAL TREATMENT

Symptomatic and supportive care should include IV electrolyte solutions for rehydration and support of renal function as well as pain relief.

PROGNOSIS AND OUTCOME

Prognosis depends on the severity of the GI disease

PEARLS & CONSIDERATIONS

- Most animals will not readily forage on oak leaves and acorns if other good-quality feed sources are available. Poisoning is most likely in the spring and fall when immature leaves and acorns are most likely to be easily accessible.
- Goats can be used to effectively control oak plants because they are unaffected by the tannins in oaks.

SUGGESTED READING

Burrows GE, Tyrl RJ (eds). *Toxic plants of North America*, Ames, IA, 2001, Iowa State University Press, pp 685–700.

Knight AP, Walter RG: *A guide to plant poisoning of animals in North America*, Jackson, WY, 2001, Teton NewMedia, pp 263–277.
Plumlee KH: Tannic acid. In Plumlee KH (ed). *Clinical veterinary toxicology*, St Louis, 2004, Mosby Elsevier, pp 346–348.

AUTHOR: **LISA A. MURPHY**

EDITOR: **CYNTHIA L. GASKILL**

Obstructive Disease of the Urinary Tract

BASIC INFORMATION

DEFINITION

Occlusion or impediment of urinary flow by a urolith or soft tissue obstruction

EPIDEMIOLOGY

SPECIES, AGE, SEX Males are more likely to develop urethral obstruction.

RISK FACTORS
- Urinary tract mucosal trauma (eg, dystocia, breeding injuries, surgery)
- Urine stasis or retention
- High dietary minerals or calcium (legumes)
- Administration of nephrotoxic drugs, especially nonsteroidal antiinflammatory drugs (NSAIDs)

ASSOCIATED CONDITIONS AND DISORDERS
- Urolithiasis
- Neoplasia
- Pyelonephritis
- Previous urethrostomy
- Stallion breeding injuries

CLINICAL PRESENTATION

HISTORY, CHIEF COMPLAINT
- Abdominal pain
- Stranguria or dysuria
- Pollakiuria
- Hematuria
- Apparent urinary incontinence
- Abdominal distension
- Preputial swelling
- Poor body condition

PHYSICAL EXAM FINDINGS
- Balanoposthitis
- Preputial swelling, heat, and pain
- Occasionally, a urolith may be palpable in the urethra.
- Spasm of the urethra over the urethrolith
- Rectal palpation may reveal a swollen kidney(s), and the ureter(s) may also be palpable. The bladder may be enlarged with urethral occlusion.

ETIOLOGY AND PATHOPHYSIOLOGY
- Uroliths occasionally occlude the ureter, urethra, or renal pelvis.
- Urethral obstruction occurs most commonly in males when uroliths lodge at the ischial arch, where the urethra narrows.
- Scarring or mucosal proliferation can sometimes be a sequela of urinary tract surgery (urethrotomy) or trauma and result in obstruction.
- Postrenal azotemia occurs with occlusion of urinary outflow, backpressure in the collecting system, and resultant decreased renal blood flow.
- Extrusion through the floor of the vagina or prolapse and eversion of the bladder may occur in mares when straining during foaling or colic.
- Breeding injuries in stallions may cause hematomas from cavernous penile tissues that result in urethral obstruction.

DIAGNOSIS

DIFFERENTIAL DIAGNOSIS
- Urolithiasis
- Estral behavior in females
- Neoplasia or granuloma of the urinary tract
- Acute abdominal pain (colic)

INITIAL DATABASE
- Complete blood count and fibrinogen concentration.
- Serum chemistries (blood urea nitrogen [BUN], creatinine, and electrolyte concentrations).
- Urinalysis
- Rectal palpation may reveal urolithiasis, an enlarged bladder, or palpable ureters
- Ultrasonography (transabdominal renal and transrectal of the bladder): Should show hydronephrosis, hydro-ureter, or an enlarged urinary bladder. Peritoneal effusion or fluid accumulation along the ureters or urethra indicates probable urinary tract rupture.

ADVANCED OR CONFIRMATORY TESTING
- The inability to completely pass a urinary catheter indicates urethral obstruction.
- Urethroscopy and cystoscopy: Ureteroscopy is difficult with most endoscopes, but urine may be observed exiting from the ureteral openings in the caudodorsal trigone of the bladder.
- Urine culture
- Intravenous pyelography, magnetic resonance imaging, or computed tomography in foals.

TREATMENT

THERAPEUTIC GOAL(S)
- Relieve urinary tract obstruction
- Resolve azotemia and any electrolyte abnormalities that may be present

ACUTE GENERAL TREATMENT
- Surgical removal of urinary tract obstruction
- Relieve spasm of the ureter or urethra
  - Acepromazine: 0.02 to 0.04 mg/kg IV q8h
  - Phenazopyridine: 4 mg/kg PO q8h
- Broad-spectrum antibiotics, especially those that are eliminated in the urine (penicillins, aminoglycosides, potentiated sulfonamides, cephalosporins)
- IV fluids (60 mL/kg q24h in adult horses) after the obstruction has been relieved to maintain urination and diuresis
- NSAIDs in non-azotemic and normally hydrated patients

RECOMMENDED MONITORING

- Urine output
- Serial BUN, creatinine, and electrolyte concentrations
- Repeated ultrasound examinations to determine if suspected urinary tract obstruction is causing leakage or accumulation of urine

PROGNOSIS AND OUTCOME

- Prognosis is good with resolution of urinary tract obstruction, especially if the urethra is occluded.
- Horses with obstructive lesions of the urinary tract may have chronic renal failure.

PEARLS & CONSIDERATIONS

COMMENTS

- Early recognition and treatment of urinary tract obstruction greatly improve prognosis and response to therapy.
- A retrospective study of urolithiasis in horses reported uroliths in the kidneys (22%), urethra (16%), and ureters (3%) of affected horses. Approximately 9% of horses had urolithiasis at more than one location.
- Obstruction of the urinary tract is an uncommon cause of abdominal pain.

PREVENTION

- Judicious use of potentially nephrotoxic drugs
- Avoidance of high mineral diets, especially calcium (legumes)

SUGGESTED READING

Laverty S, Pascoe JR, Ling GV, et al: Urolithiasis in 68 horses. *Vet Surg* 21:56, 1992.
Schott HC: Obstructive disease of the urinary tract. In Reed SM, Bayly WM, Sellon DC (eds). *Equine internal medicine*, ed 3, St Louis, 2010, Saunders Elsevier, pp 1201–1209.

AUTHOR & EDITOR: **BRYAN M. WALDRIDGE**

Oral Soft Tissue Trauma: Hard and Soft Palate

BASIC INFORMATION

DEFINITION

Traumatic injuries to the hard or soft palate

EPIDEMIOLOGY

ASSOCIATED CONDITIONS AND DISORDERS

- Severe head trauma
- Mandibular and maxillary fractures
- Associated fractures of the cheek teeth
- Oronasal fistulae

CLINICAL PRESENTATION

HISTORY, CHIEF COMPLAINT

- History of severe trauma
- The chief complaint may revolve around associated ataxia, dysphagia, or noise at exercise

PHYSICAL EXAM FINDINGS

- Obvious facial depression or facial deformity
- Feed material at the nares
- Evidence of dysphagia
- Mucosal lesions suggesting an underlying osseous pathology on oral examination
- Gross instability of the rostral portion of the head

ETIOLOGY AND PATHOPHYSIOLOGY

- Hard palate
  - Congenital abnormalities such as cleft palate
  - Traumatic injuries
- Soft palate
  - Congenital abnormalities such as cleft palate

  - Iatrogenic injuries: Complication of aryepiglottic fold surgery via the nose

DIAGNOSIS

INITIAL DATABASE

- Complete oral examination, including sedation, full-mouth speculum, and mirror with light source
- Manual examination (assuming the hand is small enough) and oropharyngeal endoscopy
- Radiography
- Endoscopy of the nasal passages and nasopharynx

ADVANCED OR CONFIRMATORY TESTING

Computed tomography

TREATMENT

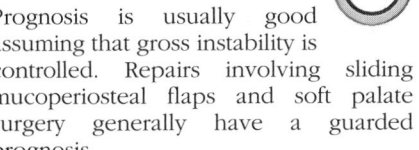

THERAPEUTIC GOAL(S)

- Close oronasal fistulae
- Attempt repair of hard palate defect (sliding mucoperiosteal flap)
- Attempt closure of soft palate defect to return horse to being an obligate nasal breather

ACUTE GENERAL TREATMENT

- Sedation
- Complete initial database to obtain presurgical information
- General anesthesia and surgery if warranted, indicated, or financially viable

POSSIBLE COMPLICATIONS

Wound breakdown in the face of infection

RECOMMENDED MONITORING

Recheck endoscopy in 2 weeks.

PROGNOSIS AND OUTCOME

Prognosis is usually good assuming that gross instability is controlled. Repairs involving sliding mucoperiosteal flaps and soft palate surgery generally have a guarded prognosis.

PEARLS & CONSIDERATIONS

COMMENTS

Closure of the soft palate in at least two layers will significantly improve the likelihood of surgical success.

CLIENT EDUCATION

Congenital cleft palates present an ethical dilemma for equine surgeons because of the proposed heritable component.

SUGGESTED READING

Dixon PM, Gerard MP: Oral cavity and salivary glands. In Auer JA, Stick JA (eds). *Equine surgery*, ed 3, St Louis, 2006, Saunders Elsevier, pp 321–351.

Ducharme NG: Pharynx. In Auer JA, Stick JA (eds). *Equine surgery*, ed 3, St Louis, 2006, Saunders Elsevier, pp 544–565.

Greet TRC: The management of oral trauma. In Baker GJ, Easley J (eds). *Equine dentistry*, ed 2, St Louis, 2005, Saunders Elsevier, pp 79–86.

AUTHOR & EDITOR: **JAMES L. CARMALT**

Oral Soft Tissue Trauma: Lips and Cheeks

BASIC INFORMATION

DEFINITION

Traumatic injuries to the lips and cheeks associated with wire, bit, or other foreign bodies. Additionally, direct trauma in the form of a kick or bite may also cause significant damage.

CLINICAL PRESENTATION

HISTORY, CHIEF COMPLAINT Trauma evidenced by bleeding, dysphagia, or protrusion of the tongue. In some cases, the traumatic episode was witnessed by the owner or caretaker; in most cases, however, it is not.

PHYSICAL EXAM FINDINGS Areas of partial- or full-thickness mucosal ulceration with underlying damage to musculature, vasculature, and in some cases osseous pathology

DIAGNOSIS

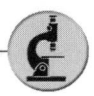

INITIAL DATABASE

- Complete oral examination
- Radiographs to determine whether there is a fracture of the underlying bone (including intraoral projections)

ADVANCED OR CONFIRMATORY TESTING

Sialogram if there is a possibility of involvement of the parotid duct or other salivary structure

TREATMENT

THERAPEUTIC GOAL(S)

To reoppose damaged tissue to effect healing

ACUTE GENERAL TREATMENT

- Sedation and appropriate nerve blocks to desensitize the region
- Close examination and debridement of gross debris and blood clots
- Determine if suturing is necessary or if the wound will heal satisfactorily by second intention
- Suture in three layers if possible (oral mucosa, muscle and fascial tissue, and skin)

POSSIBLE COMPLICATIONS

Wound breakdown in the face of infection (oral cavity) and continual bathing of the region by saliva

RECOMMENDED MONITORING

Recheck in 2 weeks

PROGNOSIS AND OUTCOME

Usually good. The relatively high blood supply to the face and oral cavity make surgical intervention relatively uncommon (assuming that gross anatomic distortion and injury have not occurred).

PEARLS & CONSIDERATIONS

COMMENTS

Sutured lips (especially at the commissure of the mouth) have to withstand significant tension and the forces of prehension and mastication. The placement of stented tension sutures (near-far-far-near or vertical mattress) can improve the likelihood of surgical success.

CLIENT EDUCATION

Horses with lip injuries should not be bitted for 2 to 3 weeks after surgical intervention, especially in cases with commissure wounds where the presence of the bit will irritate the sutures and underlying healing tissue. Failure may ensue.

SUGGESTED READING

Greet TRC: The management of oral trauma. In Baker GJ, Easley J (eds). *Equine dentistry*, ed 2, New York, 2005, Saunders Elsevier, pp 79–86.

AUTHOR & EDITOR: **JAMES L. CARMALT**

Oral Soft Tissue Trauma: Salivary Glands and Ducts

BASIC INFORMATION

DEFINITION

Injuries involving either the salivary glands or their associated ducts

SYNONYM(S)

Sialocele

EPIDEMIOLOGY

RISK FACTORS Trauma

ASSOCIATED CONDITIONS AND DISORDERS

- Mandibular and maxillary fractures
- Associated fractures of the cheek teeth
- Trauma

CLINICAL PRESENTATION

HISTORY, CHIEF COMPLAINT

- Trauma
- Visible tissue defect
- Fistula present

ETIOLOGY AND PATHOPHYSIOLOGY Trauma to the parotid duct (because it is relatively superficial) or the

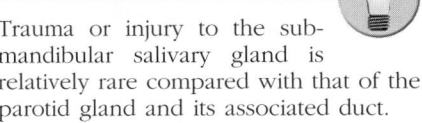

duct as it crosses the ventral mandible may result in luminal transection. If second intention healing fails, a salivary cutaneous fistula may develop.

DIAGNOSIS

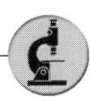

INITIAL DATABASE

- Complete oral examination (including sedation, full-mouth speculum, and mirror with light source)
- Radiography (if necessary)

ADVANCED OR CONFIRMATORY TESTING

Salivary duct cannulation if necessary

TREATMENT

THERAPEUTIC GOAL(S)

Reoppose the damaged duct such that fistulae do not occur.

ACUTE GENERAL TREATMENT

- Sedation
- Close examination and debridement of gross debris and blood clots
- Determination if the wound will heal satisfactorily by second intention or if skin suturing alone is sufficient

CHRONIC TREATMENT

Surgical intervention if conservative management is inadequate

POSSIBLE COMPLICATIONS

- Wound breakdown
- Salivary cutaneous fistula

PROGNOSIS AND OUTCOME

Usually good with conservative management. Prognosis good with surgical repair in the event that conservative therapy is unsuccessful. If surgical therapy is unsuccessful, then continued saliva drainage, especially during eating, is a greater aesthetic problem than it is a functional problem.

PEARLS & CONSIDERATIONS

Trauma or injury to the sub-mandibular salivary gland is relatively rare compared with that of the parotid gland and its associated duct.

SUGGESTED READING

Greet TRC: The management of oral trauma. In Baker GJ, Easley J (eds). *Equine dentistry*, ed 2, St Louis, 2005, Saunders Elsevier, pp 79–86.

Dixon PM, Gerard MP: Oral cavity and salivary glands. In Auer JA, Stick JA (eds). *Equine surgery*, ed 3, St Louis, 2006, Saunders Elsevier, pp 321–351.

AUTHOR & EDITOR: JAMES L. CARMALT

Oral Soft Tissue Trauma: Tongue and Oral Mucosa

BASIC INFORMATION

DEFINITION

Traumatic injuries to the tongue and oral mucosa associated with wire, bits, or other foreign bodies. Additionally direct trauma in the form of a kick, bite, or misadventure may also cause significant damage.

EPIDEMIOLOGY

ASSOCIATED CONDITIONS AND DISORDERS

- Avulsion injuries to the incisors
- Mandibular and maxillary fractures
- Associated fractures of the cheek teeth

CLINICAL PRESENTATION

DISEASE FORMS/SUBTYPES Tongue lacerations (partial or full thickness)

HISTORY, CHIEF COMPLAINT
- Trauma or bit-related history
- Presenting complaint of bleeding, dysphagia, or protrusion of the tongue

PHYSICAL EXAM FINDINGS
- Partial- or full-thickness laceration of the tongue
- Presence of foreign bodies within the mouth or jammed across the hard palate

DIAGNOSIS

INITIAL DATABASE

Radiography (if necessary)

TREATMENT

THERAPEUTIC GOAL(S)

Reoppose damaged lingual tissue or perform a partial glossectomy

ACUTE GENERAL TREATMENT

- Sedation appropriate nerve blocks to desensitize region (see "Anesthesia, Local Diagnostic" in Section II)
- Close examination and debridement of gross debris and blood clots
- Determination if suturing is necessary or if the wound will heal satisfactorily by second intention
- Induction of general anesthesia if suturing is necessary
- Suture in three layers if possible
  - Ventral mucosa (thin and poor holding capability)
  - Lingual musculature (one or two layers; this will address the bulk of the tension)
  - Dorsal mucosa (thick and has good suture retention characteristics; use a combination of simple interrupted and vertical mattress sutures).

- Oral mucosa injuries tend to heal well by second intention, assuming that the inciting causes (foreign bodies and fracture fragments) are removed.

POSSIBLE COMPLICATIONS

- Wound breakdown in the face of infection (oral cavity) and continual bathing of the region by saliva
- Necrosis of the tip of the tongue associated with vascular compromise

RECOMMENDED MONITORING

Recheck in 2 weeks

PROGNOSIS AND OUTCOME

Usually good. The relatively high blood supply to the face and oral cavity allow for good healing, assuming that tension can be addressed.

PEARLS & CONSIDERATIONS

COMMENTS

The placement of tension sutures (near-far-far-near or vertical mattress) will significantly improve the likelihood of surgical success.

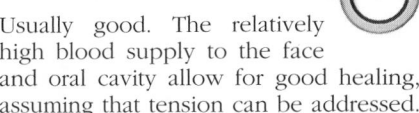

CLIENT EDUCATION

Horses with tongue injuries should not be bitted for 2 to 3 weeks after surgical intervention or failure may ensue.

SUGGESTED READING

Dixon PM, Gerard MP: Oral cavity and salivary glands. In Auer JA, Stick JA (eds). *Equine surgery*, ed 3, New York, 2006, Saunders Elsevier, pp 321–351.

Greet TRC: The management of oral trauma. In Baker GJ, Easley J (eds). *Equine dentistry*, ed 2, New York, 2005, Saunders Elsevier, pp 79–86.

AUTHOR & EDITOR: **JAMES L. CARMALT**

Oral Tumors of Bone Origin

BASIC INFORMATION

DEFINITION

Tumors having their origin within bone elements

SYNONYM(S)

- Osseous tumors
- Osteogenic tumors

EPIDEMIOLOGY

ASSOCIATED CONDITIONS AND DISORDERS Dental displacements, facial swelling

CLINICAL PRESENTATION

DISEASE FORMS/SUBTYPES
- Osteoma
- Osteosarcoma
- Fibroma (ossifying fibroma)

HISTORY, CHIEF COMPLAINT
- Facial swelling (usually painless).
- Abnormalities of mastication caused by swelling and dental displacement may occur, as can severe dyspnea if the nasal passages have been compromised.

PHYSICAL EXAM FINDINGS Firm, nonpainful, non-ulcerated (usually) masses. May be visible externally characterized by facial deformity. In some cases, the masses are contained within the lips until they expand beyond the margins (fibroma) or may not be seen without endoscopy of the nasal passages (osteoma)

ETIOLOGY AND PATHOPHYSIOLOGY
- Osteoma: Slowly growing, well-differentiated lamellar bone that may

enclose fat or marrow. They are non-malignant, but they still cause problems by distorting nasal passages and causing facial distortion.
- Osteosarcoma: Rare, painful, aggressive swelling of the mandible (usually). Classical "star burst" appearance of trabecular bone.

DIAGNOSIS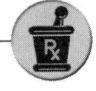

DIFFERENTIAL DIAGNOSIS

- Tumors of dental origin (eg, amelo-blastoma or odontoma).
- Extreme periosteal reaction to trauma, fracture, or infection (osteomyelitis). These usually have evidence of trauma, drainage, or odor.
- Periapical infection.

INITIAL DATABASE

- Complete oral examination
- Facial palpation
- Radiographic examination (including intraoral projections if necessary)

ADVANCED OR CONFIRMATORY TESTING

- Oral endoscopy (if mass is situated caudal to the interdental space)
- Biopsy
- Computed tomography

TREATMENT

THERAPEUTIC GOAL(S)

- Restoration of normal prehension and mastication

- Resolution of associated dyspnea
- Resolution of facial deformity
- Removal of benign, slowly infiltrative growths

ACUTE GENERAL TREATMENT

General anesthesia and surgical removal or debridement (radiation therapy)

CHRONIC TREATMENT

Hemimandibulectomy may be the only method of complete mass removal.

POSSIBLE COMPLICATIONS

Incomplete removal of neoplastic mass

PROGNOSIS AND OUTCOME

- Osteoma: Good, assuming complete removal
- Osteosarcoma: Poor
- Ossifying fibroma: Good
- Fibroma: Good

SUGGESTED READING

Dixon PM, Gerard MP: Oral cavity and salivary glands. In Auer JA, Stick JA (eds). *Equine surgery*, ed 3, St Louis, 2006, Saunders Elsevier, pp 321–351.
Knottenbelt DC, Kelly DF: Oral and dental tumors. In Baker GJ, Easley J (eds). *Equine dentistry*, ed 2, St Louis, 2005, Saunders Elsevier, pp 127–148.

AUTHOR & EDITOR: **JAMES L. CARMALT**

Oral Tumors of Dental Tissue Origin

BASIC INFORMATION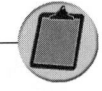

DEFINITION

Tumors having their origin within dental elements: enamel, dentine, or cementum

SYNONYM(S)

Dental tumors, odontogenic tumors, ameloblastoma, odontoma, cementoma

EPIDEMIOLOGY

SPECIES, AGE, SEX Odontomas tend to develop before age 3 years; cementomas and ameloblastomas have a wide range of age at onset.

ASSOCIATED CONDITIONS AND DISORDERS Dental displacements, facial swelling

CLINICAL PRESENTATION

DISEASE FORMS/SUBTYPES

- Ameloblastoma
- Odontoma
- Cementoma

HISTORY, CHIEF COMPLAINT Facial swelling (usually painless). In some cases, fistulation to the overlying skin may occur. Abnormalities of mastication caused by swelling and dental displacement may occur, as can severe dyspnea if the nasal passages have been compromised.

PHYSICAL EXAM FINDINGS Firm, nonpainful, non-ulcerated (usually) masses visible externally characterized by facial deformity

ETIOLOGY AND PATHOPHYSIOLOGY

- Ameloblastoma: Tumors of the odontogenic epithelium that by definition do not contain any dental elements
- (Complex or compound) odontoma: A well-differentiated mass of odontogenic mesenchymal tissue containing varying amounts of enamel, dentine, and cementum
  - Complex odontomas have all dental elements in a chaotic structure.
  - Compound odontomas have all dental elements but are more organized.
- Cementoma: Dysplastic tissue of mesenchymal, not epithelial, elements and as such lacks enamel and dentine.

DIAGNOSIS

DIFFERENTIAL DIAGNOSIS

- Tumors of osseous origin (eg, osteoma or osteosarcoma)
- Extreme periosteal reaction to trauma, fracture, or infection (osteomyelitis) These usually have evidence of trauma, drainage, or odor.
- Periapical infection.

INITIAL DATABASE

- Complete oral examination
- Facial palpation
- Radiographic examination (including intraoral projections if necessary)

ADVANCED OR CONFIRMATORY TESTING

- Oral endoscopy (if mass is situated caudal to the interdental space)
- Biopsy
- Computed tomography

TREATMENT

THERAPEUTIC GOAL(S)

- Restoration of normal prehension and mastication
- Resolution of associated dyspnea
- Resolution of facial deformity
- Removal of benign, slowly infiltrative growths

ACUTE GENERAL TREATMENT

General anesthesia with surgical removal or debridement (radiation therapy)

CHRONIC TREATMENT

Hemi-mandibulectomy may be the only method of complete mass removal.

POSSIBLE COMPLICATIONS

Incomplete removal of neoplastic mass

RECOMMENDED MONITORING

These benign masses should not recur if surgical removal is complete.

PROGNOSIS AND OUTCOME

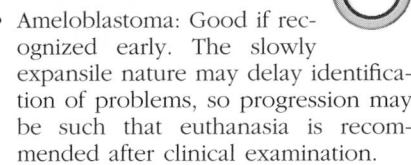

- Ameloblastoma: Good if recognized early. The slowly expansile nature may delay identification of problems, so progression may be such that euthanasia is recommended after clinical examination.
- Odontoma: Fair to good. A second surgery may be necessary.
- Cementoma: Excellent.

SUGGESTED READING

Dixon PM, Gerard MP: Oral cavity and salivary glands. In Auer JA, Stick JA (eds). *Equine surgery*, ed 3, St Louis, 2006, Saunders Elsevier, pp 321–351.

Knottenbelt DC, Kelly DF: Oral and dental tumors. In Baker GJ, Easley J (eds). *Equine dentistry*, ed 2, St Louis, 2005, Saunders Elsevier, pp 127–148.

AUTHOR & EDITOR: JAMES L. CARMALT

Oral Tumors of Soft Tissue Origin

BASIC INFORMATION

DEFINITION

Tumors having their origin within soft tissue elements

SYNONYM(S)

Soft tissue tumors

EPIDEMIOLOGY

ASSOCIATED CONDITIONS AND DISORDERS Dental displacements, facial swelling, halitosis, ptyalism

CLINICAL PRESENTATION

DISEASE FORMS/SUBTYPES

- Squamous cell carcinoma
- Melanoma

HISTORY, CHIEF COMPLAINT Halitosis, ptyalism, dysphagia, dysmastication, quidding, anorexia, and weight loss

PHYSICAL EXAM FINDINGS Ulcerated masses within the oral cavity that may or may not involve underlying bone. May not be visible externally characterized by facial deformity.

ETIOLOGY AND PATHOPHYSIOLOGY

- Squamous cell carcinoma: A malignant neoplastic mass with origins in the squamous epithelium; of soft tissue origin but is highly aggressive and can invade bone and surrounding structures
- Melanoma: Typically benign tumors of melanocytes; slow growth rate; minimal invasion of adjacent structures, but it does occur; classically associated with the parotid salivary glands and gray horses

DIAGNOSIS

DIFFERENTIAL DIAGNOSIS

- Squamous cell carcinoma: Other invasive tumors of the head (eg, sarcoid, myxomatous tumors, fibrosarcoma)
- Melanoma: Sarcoid, mast cell tumor

INITIAL DATABASE

- Complete oral examination
- Facial palpation
- Radiographic examination (including intraoral projections if necessary) to assess bone involvement
- Upper airway endoscopy

ADVANCED OR CONFIRMATORY TESTING

- Oral endoscopy (if mass is situated caudal to the interdental space)
- Biopsy

TREATMENT

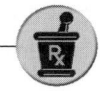

THERAPEUTIC GOAL(S)

- Complete removal and treatment of neoplastic tissue
- Restoration of normal prehension and mastication

ACUTE GENERAL TREATMENT

General anesthesia with surgical removal or debridement (radiation therapy)

CHRONIC TREATMENT

Hemimandibulectomy may be the only method of complete mass removal.

POSSIBLE COMPLICATIONS

- Incomplete removal of neoplastic masses

- Inability to improve quality of life
- Possible euthanasia if treatment is not successful

PROGNOSIS AND OUTCOME

- Squamous cell carcinoma: Metastasis, extensive local infiltration by neoplastic tissue combined with anatomic and physiologic constraints posed by the oral cavity, nasal passages, and paranasal sinus system in the horse often render prognosis guarded to poor despite intervention.

- Melanomatosis: Good to excellent. A large number of horses have melanomas that do not result in significant problems. Expansion of the masses over time may lead to long-term concerns.

SUGGESTED READING

Dixon PM, Gerard MP: Oral cavity and salivary glands. In Auer JA, Stick JA (eds). *Equine surgery*, ed 3, St Louis, 2006, Saunders Elsevier, pp 321–351.

Knottenbelt DC, Kelly DF: Oral and dental tumors. In Baker GJ, Easley J (eds). *Equine dentistry*, ed 2, St Louis, 2005, Saunders Elsevier, pp 127–148.

AUTHOR & EDITOR: **JAMES L. CARMALT**

Organophosphate and Carbamate Toxicosis

BASIC INFORMATION

DEFINITION

Organophosphates and carbamates are cholinesterase-inhibiting chemicals. Organophosphates include dichlorvos, ronnel, diazinon, chlorpyrifos, and phosmet, and carbamates include carbaryl, aldicarb, methomyl, and carbofuran. Many other organophosphates and carbamates exist.

SYNONYM(S)

Organophosphates have been called organic phosphates, phosphorus insecticides, and nerve gas relatives.

EPIDEMIOLOGY

SPECIES, AGE, SEX Organophosphates and carbamates inhibit the enzyme cholinesterase, which is used by the nervous system of all mammals. All animals are affected, so there is no species, age, or sex predilection.

RISK FACTORS Farm animals are at a higher risk because of the common use of these chemicals in a farm setting.

GEOGRAPHY AND SEASONALITY The organophosphates and carbamates are used as insecticides, so more of the compounds are used in the warmer months, but exposure can occur year round. Rural areas can be more at risk than urban environments.

CLINICAL PRESENTATION

DISEASE FORMS/SUBTYPES There is great variation in the types of clinical signs observed from an excessive dose of either of these groups of compounds.

Many times these compounds are so potent that animals will be found dead with no previous signs of illness.

HISTORY, CHIEF COMPLAINT Acute death may be the chief complaint. The history often indicates exposure to these two classes of chemicals because insecticides were being used or animals gained access to these chemicals inadvertently.

PHYSICAL EXAM FINDINGS

- The clinical signs observed are associated with muscarinic, nicotinic, and central nervous system (CNS) stimulation.
- Muscarinic receptor–associated effects include salivation, lacrimation, urination, diarrhea, miosis (pinpoint pupils), and lung edema.
- Bradycardia, bronchoconstriction, and bronchorrhea may also be observed.
- Nicotinic receptor–associated effects are related to the stimulation of autonomic ganglia and skeletal muscles. The clinical signs of nicotinic stimulation include muscle twitching, tremors, and seizures.
- CNS stimulation can cause depression, hyperactivity, and seizures.

ETIOLOGY AND PATHOPHYSIOLOGY

- Organophosphates and carbamates inhibit the enzyme acetylcholinesterase, which is within nerve tissue and at neuromuscular junctions. Acetylcholinesterase destroys the neurotransmitter acetylcholine.
- When the acetylcholine concentrations increase in nerve tissue or at the neuromuscular junction, the acetylcholine receptors become overstimulated.

- The cholinergic system is widely distributed within the CNS and peripheral nervous system. There is a wide range in clinical signs when the cholinergic system is upregulated.

DIAGNOSIS

DIFFERENTIAL DIAGNOSIS

Differential diagnosis includes exposure to stimulants and compounds with mixed effects on the CNS such as:

- Lead
- Mercury
- Carbon disulfide
- Ivermectin
- Ionophores
- Plant toxins such as fumonisins, yellow star thistle poisoning, marijuana, and sleepy grass, as well as others

INITIAL DATABASE

- A history of exposure to an organophosphate or carbamate insecticide within 24 hours before the onset of clinical signs is usually enough to begin treatment with atropine.
- Usually there is not enough time to measure acetylcholinesterase values in whole blood before initiation of treatment. Response to treatment with atropine helps confirm an excess exposure to an organophosphate or carbamate.
- Many times an animal will exhibit clinical signs compatible with an organophosphate or carbamate toxicosis but the history is not complete, and there is no time to evaluate acetylcholinesterase activity. In these

cases, a test dose of atropine can be used to rule in or rule out organophosphate or carbamate toxicosis. After a low dose of atropine (0.02 mg/kg IV), if an organophosphate or carbamate toxicosis has not occurred, the pupils will dilate, salivation will stop within 15 minutes, and the heart rate will increase dramatically. If none of the clinical signs decrease in severity, this indicates a probable organophosphate or carbamate toxicosis, and a therapeutic dose of atropine can be used.

ADVANCED OR CONFIRMATORY TESTING

- Measurement of acetylcholinesterase activity in whole blood or the brain will help rule in or out exposure to organophosphates or carbamates.
- Stomach content, hair, grain, hay, or suspected baits can be analyzed for the presence of organophosphates or carbamates.
- There are no specific micropathologic lesions associated with these compounds because death is rapid.

TREATMENT

THERAPEUTIC GOAL(S)

Activate acetylcholinesterase in the body, remove the organophosphate or carbamate and provide symptomatic care.

ACUTE GENERAL TREATMENT

- Initial treatment for exposure to excessive amounts of organophosphates and carbamates is to administer atropine. The recommended dosage of atropine is somewhat controversial, and no one standard dosage is accepted by all. The dosage of atropine for treatment of organophosphates and carbamates is higher than the dosage used for other conditions because the drug must outcompete acetylcholinesterase that has accumulated at receptor sites.
  - One suggested regimen is to administer atropine at a dosage of 0.2 mg/kg, dosing 25% of the dose IV with the remainder given IM or SC. However, this can potentially result in ileus, causing serious complications in horses.

- Another method of administration designed to avoid ileus involves diluting the calculated dosage of atropine in saline and administering the diluted solution slowly IV while auscultating the abdomen. The suggested dose range is 0.02 to 0.2 mg/kg given to effect with the endpoint of treatment based on improvement of respiratory signs. Administration should be stopped before any decrease in gastrointestinal (GI) motility occurs. Treating until salivation stops can potentially result in atropine toxicity. Also remember that atropine will not reverse nicotinic signs, so muscle tremors will not diminish with atropine treatment.
  - Repeated doses of atropine may be given every few hours if needed to effect.
- Oximes such as 2-PAM (protopam chloride or pralidoxime chloride) may be used as ancillary therapy for organophosphate exposure but not carbamate exposure. 2-PAM can be dosed at 20 mg/kg given IV and repeated at 4- to 6-hour intervals.
- As soon as the horse is stabilized, activated charcoal should also be used at a dose of 250 g in foals and 750 g in adults. This amount of activated charcoal should be suspended in water to make a slurry. Up to 4 L of water can be used in adults. The water should be warm and the mixture administered with a stomach tube. The mixture should be left in the stomach for 20 to 30 minutes, and then a laxative can be given to move this mixture out of the GI tract.
- Gastric lavage can be used but is more problematic.
- Dermally exposed animals should be washed with soap and water.

DRUG INTERACTIONS

Morphine, physostigmine, phenothiazine tranquilizers, pyridostigmine, neostigmine, and succinyl chloride can interfere with cholinesterase activity and should be avoided.

POSSIBLE COMPLICATIONS

Ileus may occur after treatment with atropine.

RECOMMENDED MONITORING

The degree of salivation, pupillary size, respiratory signs, intestinal motility, and heart rate can all be monitored to evaluate treatment success.

PROGNOSIS AND OUTCOME

Early treatment is effective and the prognosis is good. Some organophosphates and carbamates are so potent that treatment has to be within minutes to hours to be effective. Treatment may be needed for up to 48 hours postexposure with supportive care needed for days.

PEARLS & CONSIDERATIONS

COMMENTS

Atropine will not reverse the clinical signs associated with nicotinic stimulation.

PREVENTION

Use caution when applying insecticides. Keep all chemicals safely stored away from animals and remove chemicals from barns and sheds where animal can gain access.

CLIENT EDUCATION

Remind clients that repeated applications of organophosphate or carbamate insecticides for fly control can potentially be problematic.

SUGGESTED READING

Blodgett DJ: Organophosphate and carbamate insecticides. In Peterson ME, Talcott PA (eds). *Small animal toxicology*, St Louis, 2006, Elsevier, pp 941–955.

Meerdink GL: Anticholinesterase Insecticides. In Plumlee KH (ed). *Clinical veterinary toxicology*, St Louis, 2004, Mosby Elsevier, pp 178–180.

Plumb DC: Veterinary drug handbook, Ames, IA, 2002, Iowa State University Press.

AUTHOR: STEVE ENSLEY

EDITOR: CYNTHIA L. GASKILL

Osteoarthritis

BASIC INFORMATION

DEFINITION

A process involving the inflammation of joint tissues leading to the loss of articular hyaline cartilage matrix

SYNONYM(S)

Degenerative joint disease, osteoarthrosis, ringbone (in the pastern), osselets (in the fetlock), spavin (in the hock)

EPIDEMIOLOGY

SPECIES, AGE, SEX

- Although osteoarthritis (OA) has been reported in wild horses and may be a feature of old age, most OA seen in horses occurs in younger animals and is posttraumatic.
- Occupational activities predispose certain joints, such as fetlocks, hocks, and carpi in racehorses; hocks in Quarter Horses and show horses; and stifles in show horses.

GENETICS AND BREED PREDISPOSITION Transmitted conformational features may predispose a horse to developing OA.

RISK FACTORS Inappropriate conformation for the occupation, excessive exercise regimes, intraarticular osteochondral fragmentation or other articular trauma, osteochondrosis

ASSOCIATED CONDITIONS AND DISORDERS Any disease leading to joint inflammation (eg, osteochondrosis)

CLINICAL PRESENTATION

DISEASE FORMS/SUBTYPES

- Acute, subacute, and chronic
- Occasionally immune mediated

HISTORY, CHIEF COMPLAINT Lameness, pain on flexion or palpation; stiffness often improves with exercise

PHYSICAL EXAM FINDINGS Synovial effusion, pain on joint manipulation, increase heat in area, lameness

ETIOLOGY AND PATHOPHYSIOLOGY Intraarticular sepsis or repeated trauma evokes an inflammatory process characterized by cellular activity responsible for the production of enzymes and inflammatory mediators leading to destruction of articular cartilage matrix compromising the biomechanical properties of the joint and thus its function.

DIAGNOSIS

DIFFERENTIAL DIAGNOSIS

Because arthritis may also be a symptom, it is important to rule out the primary diagnosis (eg, osteochondral fragmentation, osteochondrosis).

INITIAL DATABASE

Lameness exam, flexion tests, and radiography

ADVANCED OR CONFIRMATORY TESTING

Synovial fluid cytology and biomarkers, magnetic resonance imaging, histopathology on postmortem specimens

TREATMENT

THERAPEUTIC GOAL(S)

- Facilitate joint mobility and break the inflammatory cycle.
- Provide the needed conditions for cartilage to repair, which includes blood supply, removing the inciting cause, and rest.

ACUTE GENERAL TREATMENT

Aggressive antiinflammatory therapy (eg, systemic nonsteroidal antiinflammatory drugs [NSAIDs], intraarticular corticosteroids, cold and massage combination, rest, support), joint lavage, autologous conditioned serum (ACS), aggressive antibiotic therapy if infectious cause

CHRONIC TREATMENT

Exercise modification, mobility exercises, weight control, joint support medication (eg, hyaluronan, polysulfated glycosaminoglycans, ACS), arthrodesis of selected joints

DRUG INTERACTIONS

Intraarticular corticosteroids and ACS

POSSIBLE COMPLICATIONS

Renal papillary necrosis and gastrointestinal (GI) disorders such as GI ulcerations, gastritis, and dorsal colitis from excessive NSAID use, and overall stiffness from prolonged rest. Excessive use of intraarticular methylprednisolone may lead to accelerated cartilage degeneration.

RECOMMENDED MONITORING

- Radiography every 6 to 12 months
- Lameness exam every 6 to 8 weeks

PROGNOSIS AND OUTCOME

Depending on stage of disease; poor to fair

PEARLS & CONSIDERATIONS

COMMENTS

The early diagnosis of OA remains elusive and the process is usually at an advanced stage by the time it is detectable radiographically. It is important to treat joint inflammation aggressively and allow the tissues the necessary time to repair before inflicting more damage.

PREVENTION

Selection of horses with the appropriate conformation, appropriate conditioning and exercise regimens (avoid obesity)

CLIENT EDUCATION

Detect early stages by recognizing lameness, heat, and joint pain. OA in the degenerative state is not curable but is manageable in many occasions.

SUGGESTED READING

Cruz AM, Hurtig MB: Multiple pathways to osteoarthritis and articular fractures: is subchondral bone the culprit? *Vet Clin North Am Equine Pract* 24(1):101–116, 2008.

Goodrich LR, Nixon AJ: Medical treatment of osteoarthritis in the horse—a review. *Vet J* 171(1):51–69, 2006.

AUTHOR: ANTONIO M. CRUZ

EDITOR: ANDRIS J. KANEPS

Osteoarthritis, Infectious (Septic)

BASIC INFORMATION

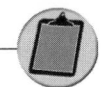

DEFINITION

Rapid onset of joint heat, swelling, and lameness caused by an infectious agent in the joint

SYNONYM(S)

Septic arthritis, septic joint, infected joint

EPIDEMIOLOGY

RISK FACTORS Foals with failure of passive transfer, recent joint injection, recent joint surgery, wounds
ASSOCIATED CONDITIONS AND DISORDERS Joint disease such as fractures or osteoarthritis

CLINICAL PRESENTATION

DISEASE FORMS/SUBTYPES Acute bacterial infection, chronic infection, fungal infection, mycobacterium
HISTORY, CHIEF COMPLAINT Frequently a history of injection or puncture; the chief complaint is joint swelling and lameness
PHYSICAL EXAM FINDINGS In adults, the physical examination is usually normal with the exception of the affected limb. The limb is often warm and edematous with joint effusion. Lameness is often marked and may be non–weight bearing. Wounds or injection sites may drain. In foals, multiple joints and bone may be simultaneously affected. Foals may be systemically ill with septicemia and foci of infection such as the umbilicus, pneumonia, or diarrhea.
ETIOLOGY AND PATHOPHYSIOLOGY
- Septicemia is the primary cause in foals. Bacteria that gain access to the bloodstream selectively settle in the interstitium of the synovium because of the extensive capillary network, high surface area, and slow blood flow. Foals with failure of passive transfer cannot control the infection, rapidly deteriorate, and frequently have multiple sites affected.
- Subchondral bone is also frequently affected, and osteomyelitis is present in 50% of foals with infectious arthritis.
- In adults, a source of contamination (inoculation) is usually present, such as a joint injection, joint surgery, or puncture wound.
- Bacteria gain access and, particularly in damaged tissue, begin to establish infection and proliferate. Initial contamination progresses to infection (defined as 1×10^6 bacteria per gram of tissue) within 12 to 24 hours. Organisms vary in virulence, and some

bacteria can rapidly progress to severe infection.

DIAGNOSIS

DIFFERENTIAL DIAGNOSIS

- Fracture
- Periarticular infection
- Abscess

INITIAL DATABASE

- Physical examination
- Lameness examination
- Radiography
- Synovial fluid analysis
- Gram stain
- Bacterial culture

ADVANCED OR CONFIRMATORY TESTING

- Synovial fluid fungal or mycoplasma culture
- Synovial biopsy for histology or culture
- Contrast arthrogram
- Computed tomography for bone lesions
- Arthroscopy for direct visual joint inspection can aid the diagnosis and causative agent

TREATMENT

THERAPEUTIC GOAL(S)

- Eliminate the joint infection.
- Suppress the joint inflammation.
- Prevent cartilage injury.

ACUTE GENERAL TREATMENT

- Systemic broad spectrum antimicrobials
- Local antimicrobials (often direct injection at the time of arthrocentesis)
- Antiinflammatory and pain medication
- Joint lavage with appropriate volumes of balanced polyionic fluids
- Physical therapy to reduce swelling and potentially support the joint

CHRONIC TREATMENT

- Sustained systemic and local antibiotics selected based on culture results
- Arthroscopic surgery to debride and lavage the joint
- Antiinflammatory and pain medication to balance limb use
- Pressure and support bandages

DRUG INTERACTIONS

- Enrofloxacin can be chondrotoxic and may not be the best first choice for intraarticular use or systemically for mares with nursing foals.

- Recognize that in foals receiving antimicrobials at multiple sites (eg, multiple joints) the toxic systemic dosage may be unintentionally exceeded.

POSSIBLE COMPLICATIONS

- Osteomyelitis if infection localizes in bone
- Chronic synovitis or osteoarthritis secondary to joint tissue and cartilage injury
- Continued joint infection in cases of antimicrobial resistance, inadequate lavage, or inadequate clearance of fibrin

RECOMMENDED MONITORING

- Daily joint treatment initially to sustain local antimicrobial concentrations and lavage
- Repeat synovial cytology within 3 days to assess progress
- Repeat synovial fluid analyses at key time points, such as before transitioning from systemic to oral antibiotics or when terminating antimicrobial treatment or if lameness worsens
- If osteomyelitis was present, repeat radiographs at key time points as noted above. Importantly, radiographic appearance lags behind clinical progress.

PROGNOSIS AND OUTCOME

- Good for adult horses
- Fair for foals with adequate immunoglobulin
- Guarded for foals sick with septicemia, failure of passive transfer, progressive osteomyelitis, or with multiple joints affected

PEARLS & CONSIDERATIONS

COMMENTS

- Most joint infections can be successfully treated with methodical and aggressive treatment.
- Cost is frequently the limiting factor in treatment.

PREVENTION

- Ensure a clean foaling environment and excellent foaling management.
- Rapid treatment of intraarticular wounds.
- Scrupulous aseptic technique for intraarticular injections

CLIENT EDUCATION

- Foaling management (antiseptic treatment of the navel, screening immunoglobulin levels)
- Quick and early veterinary inspection of wounds over joints or joint swelling after injections or surgeries

SUGGESTED READING

Bertone AL: Infectious arthritis. In Dyson SJ, Ross MW (eds). *Diagnosis and management of lameness in horses.* Philadelphia, 2003, Saunders Elsevier, pp 598–606.

Bertone AL, Davis DM, Cox HU, et al: Arthrotomy versus arthroscopy and partial synovectomy for treatment of experimentally induced infectious arthritis in horses. *Am J Vet Res* 53:585, 1992.

Holcombe SJ, Schneider RK, Bramlage LR, et al: Use of antibiotic-impregnated polymethylmethacrylate in horses with open or infected fractures or joints: 19 cases (1987–1995). *J Am Vet Med Assoc* 211:889, 1997.

Lloyd KCK, Stover SM, Pascoe JR, et al: Synovial fluid pH, cytologic characteristics and gentamicin concentration after intra-articular administration of the drug in an experimental model of infectious arthritis in horses. *Am J Vet Res* 51:1363, 1990.

Meagher DT, Latimer FG, Sutter WW, et al: Evaluation of a balloon constant rate infusion system for treatment of septic arthritis, septic tenosynovitis, and contaminated synovial wounds: 23 cases (2002–2005). *J Am Vet Med Assoc* 228(12): 1930, 2006.

Whitehair KJ, Bowersock TL, Blevins WE, et al: Regional limb perfusion for antibiotic treatment of experimentally induced septic arthritis. *Vet Surg* 21:367, 1992.

Wright IM, Smith MR, Humphrey DJ, et al: Endoscopic surgery in the treatment of contaminated and injected synovial cavities. *Equine Vet J* 35:613, 2003.

AUTHOR: **ALICIA L. BERTONE**

EDITOR: **ANDRIS J. KANEPS**

Osteoarthritis, Proximal Interphalangeal Joint (Ringbone)

BASIC INFORMATION

DEFINITION

A progressive and permanent deterioration of the articular cartilage of the proximal interphalangeal (PIP) joint accompanied by changes in the bone and soft tissue of the joint, including subchondral bone sclerosis and marginal osteophyte formation.

SYNONYM(S)

- High ringbone
- Osteoarthritis

EPIDEMIOLOGY

SPECIES, AGE, SEX Increasing prevalence with age
RISK FACTORS

- Poor conformation (short upright pasterns)
- Selective excessive weight bearing because of contralateral limb injury
- Osteochondrosis or subchondral cystic lesions
- Athletic activity that requires quick stops and hard turns

CLINICAL PRESENTATION

HISTORY, CHIEF COMPLAINT Mild to severe lameness
PHYSICAL EXAM FINDINGS

- Variable enlargement of the pastern region; heat and pain on palpation
- Lameness that is exacerbated at the trot by circling, joint flexion tests, or work on a slope
- Limited range of motion

ETIOLOGY AND PATHOPHYSIOLOGY

- See "Osteoarthritis" in this section
- Osteochondrosis in young horses
- Trauma
- Selective weight bearing

- Septic arthritis
- Conformational defects
- Each of the above lead to damage of the articular cartilage and joint inflammation.
- A catabolic imbalance results with chondrocytes unable to replace degraded extracellular matrix.

DIAGNOSIS

DIFFERENTIAL DIAGNOSIS

- Palmar heel pain
- Navicular syndrome
- Chronic laminitis

INITIAL DATABASE

- Clinical examination localizing joint pain
- Lameness that resolves after PIP joint anesthesia or a palmar/plantar digital anesthesia
- Complete radiographic evaluation of the PIP joint
- When confirmed, radiographs should be taken of the contralateral limb.

TREATMENT

THERAPEUTIC GOAL(S)

- Pain alleviation
- Improved function
- Limiting disease progression

ACUTE GENERAL TREATMENT

- See "Osteoarthritis" in this section
- Conservative management: Decreased exercise, corrective shoeing
- Antiinflammatory treatments
  - Phenylbutazone: 2.2 mg/kg PO q24h or before performance on days of performance

  - Adequan (polysulphated glycosaminoglycans) injections (intramuscular) weekly for 4 to 6 weeks
  - Methylprednisolone: 20 to 40 mg intraarticularly
  - Triamcinolone: 4 to 6 mg intraarticularly
- Surgical treatment: Arthrodesis of the PIP joint
  - Surgical options include lag screw compression.
  - Dynamic compression plating

CHRONIC TREATMENT

- Nonsteroidal antiinflammatory drugs
- Joint arthrodesis

PROGNOSIS AND OUTCOME

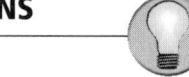

Fair to favorable, particularly for condition involving the hindlimbs

PEARLS & CONSIDERATIONS

COMMENTS

- Intraarticular corticosteroid injections are often a short-term fix with diminishing returns.
- Horses can often be managed for prolonged periods with judicious use of phenylbutazone.
- Horses with recalcitrant lameness are treated with surgical fusion of the PIP joint.

SUGGESTED READING

Nixon AJ: Phalanges and the metacarpophalangeal and metatarsophalangeal joints.

In Auer JA, Stick JA (eds). *Equine surgery*, ed 3, Philadelphia, 2006, Saunders Elsevier, pp 1221–1222.

Stashak TS: The pastern. In Stashak TS, editor: *Adams lameness in horses*, ed 5, Philadelphia, 2002, Lippincott Williams & Wilkins, pp 733–741.

AUTHOR: **KELLY FARNSWORTH**

EDITOR: **ANDRIS J. KANEPS**

Osteochondrosis

BASIC INFORMATION

DEFINITION

- General term used to describe a disorder of bone and cartilage of an unspecified etiology
- Developmental disorder of endochondral ossification
- Osteochondritis dissecans (OCD) is used to describe developmental or traumatic lesions of articular cartilage and subchondral bone
- Typically, it is identified as a detached fragment or flap of abnormal cartilage or cartilage and bone from the surrounding tissue
- Subchondral bone cysts (SBCs) are another manifestation of osteochondrosis, which can also be developmental or acquired.

SYNONYM(S)

Although the term OCD is not truly a synonym of osteochondrosis, it is thought of as one by many.

EPIDEMIOLOGY

SPECIES, AGE AND SEX May occur at any age, although OCD mostly becomes clinically apparent in patients from neonate to 3 years of age.

GENETICS AND BREED PREDISPOSITION

- Although certain genetic lines have been shown to have a high heritability of osteochondrosis lesions, a specific genetic defect responsible for alteration of endochondral ossification has not yet been identified.
- Any breed can be affected, but it is common or overrepresented in Standardbred, Thoroughbred, and Warmblood breeds.

RISK FACTORS

- Growth rate: Rapid growth because of high-energy diets
- Dietary factors
  - A high carbohydrate load may lead to a disruption of chondrocyte metabolism.
  - Extremely low serum Cu^{2+} levels or excessive amounts of Zn^{2+} may lead to abnormal collagen cross-linking.

- Genetics
  - Highly suspected in certain breeding lines, although a specific genetic defect has not been identified.
  - Heritability of a predisposition for fast growth and larger skeletal size might be the most important factor.
- Trauma
  - Trauma alone may not be the sole primary factor, but in susceptible cartilage, it may be the necessary contributing factor.
  - There seem to be time-dependent windows of vulnerability to trauma for growth cartilages in specific locations.

ASSOCIATED CONDITIONS AND DISORDERS

- Lameness
- Osteoarthritis
- Neurologic deficits (cervical lesions)

CLINICAL PRESENTATION

DISEASE FORMS/SUBTYPES

- Osteochondrosis shows very different clinical signs and physical findings based on the location.
- OCDs are bilateral in 45% to 60% of affected horses.
- Tarsus
  - Dorsal, distal, intermediate ridge of the tibia (DIRT)*
  - Lateral trochlear ridge of the talus
  - Medial malleolus of the tibia
  - Medial trochlear ridge of the talus
- Stifle
  - Lateral trochlear ridge of the femur*
  - SBC of the medial femoral condyle*
  - Other locations within the stifle possible, albeit relatively rare
- Fetlock Joint
  - Distal, dorsal MC-3/MT-3 (along the proximal to distal aspect of the mid-sagittal ridge and the adjacent region of the medial or lateral condyles)*
  - Proximal palmar/plantar eminence (tubercle) of P-1*
  - SBCs of the distal MC-3/MT-3 and proximal P-1
  - Osteochondral fragments of proximal, dorsal P-1 (different from traumatic osteochondral fragments)

- Shoulder
  - Humeral head: OCD and SBC
  - SBC of the glenoid fossa
- Cervical vertebral articular facets: One of the recognized causes of cervical vertebral instability or stenosis in young horses ("wobblers" disease)
- Other locations
  - Distal P-1; proximal and distal P-2; proximal and distal radius; distal humerus; proximal tibia: These are rare and usually present themselves as SBCs.

HISTORY, CHIEF COMPLAINT

- Tarsus
  - Joint effusion: Mild to severe
  - No lameness in horses not in training
  - Mild lameness may be present in horses under training.
- Stifle
  - OCD of the lateral trochlear ridge of the femur
    - Effusion of the femoropatellar joint ranging from mild to severe
  - SBC of the medial femoral condyle
    - No or mild effusion
    - Lameness from mild to severe
- Fetlock: Mild to moderate lameness
- Shoulder: Mild to severe lameness in pasture
- Cervical facets
  - Neck stiffness
  - Poor performance

PHYSICAL EXAM FINDINGS

- Tarsus
  - Mild to severe effusion of the tarsocrural joint
  - Lameness absent or mild in severity
- Stifle
  - Joint effusion ranging from absent to severe
  - Lameness ranging from mild to severe and worse with SBCs of the medial femoral condyle
  - Muscle atrophy (unilateral lesions)
  - Undermuscled (bilateral lesions)
- Fetlock: Joint effusion and the degree of lameness ranging from absent to moderate
- Shoulder
  - Shortened cranial phase of the stride and may scuff the toe
  - Often some degree of appreciable muscle atrophy over the shoulder

---

*Identifies the most common locations for OCDs, SBCs, or both.

- Cervical facets: Neck stiffness, difficulty or unwillingness to bend the neck to certain direction, or poor performance (horses in training)

ETIOLOGY AND PATHOPHYSIOLOGY

- Osteochondrosis is a failure of normal endochondral ossification, resulting in thickening and retention of the hypertrophic zone of the growth cartilage.
- Histologically, osteochondrosis is characterized by persistence of chondrocytes in the mid to late hypertrophic zone with failure of vascular invasion and subsequent osteogenesis.
- These lesions may be precipitated by abnormal chondrocyte structure or function, abnormal extracellular matrix production, or a vascular disorder.
- Whereas high-motion areas may subject the articular surface to shear forces predisposing to OCD "flaps," SBCs tend to be located in areas of maximal compressive loads.
- Trauma leading to subchondral bone microfracture and necrosis followed by cystic resorption and collapse of overlying articular cartilage may also be part of the pathogenesis of SBCs.
- Full-thickness, linear defects in the articular cartilage at the points of maximal weight bearing may lead to SBC development.

DIAGNOSIS

DIFFERENTIAL DIAGNOSIS

- Nonseptic synovitis
- Septic synovitis
- Osteomyelitis
- Equine protozoal myelitis
- Traumatic fractures

INITIAL DATABASE

- Radiography: Important to image the contralateral joint
- Ultrasonography
  - Evaluation of osteochondrosis at the level of the cervical articular facets
  - Other locations such as the tarsocrural joint (medial malleolus of the tibia)

ADVANCED OR CONFIRMATORY TESTING

- Nuclear scintigraphy: Often false-negative results because of minimal radionuclide uptake
- Computed tomography or magnetic resonance imaging
  - In rare cases, occult SBCs might only be identified with these modalities
  - Synovial fluid analysis and culture
  - Used to differentiate osteochondrosis from septic arthritis in young foals

TREATMENT

THERAPEUTIC GOAL(S)

- Reduce or eliminate joint effusion
- Avoid the development of lameness
- Reduce or eliminate the level of lameness present
- Return to previous level of athletic soundness
- Improve quality of life

ACUTE GENERAL TREATMENT

- Conservative management
  - Young foals (<6–8 months): Exercise restriction for an average of 6 to 10 months; antiinflammatory medications (nonsteroidal antiinflammatory drugs [NSAIDs]); diet modification (reduce energy, balance minerals, correct protein excesses)
  - In mature patients with clinical manifestation of the condition, conservative management may not be effective.
- Surgical management
  - Tarsal lesions
    - Removal of the lesion(s) arthroscopically
    - Allows for a thorough evaluation of the articular surfaces
  - Stifle lesions
    - Arthroscopy remains the treatment of choice for most clinicians dealing with both OCD and SBC lesions in the stifle.
    - When managing SBCs, techniques such as mosaicoplasty, joint resurfacing using metallic implants, injection of corticosteroids (triamcinolone) directly into the SBCs under arthroscopic guidance, and infiltration of nucleated cells (stem cells) with growth factors (platelet-rich plasma) and fibrin in the SBCs after arthroscopic debridement have been used with positive results.
    - Packing of the cysts with cancellous bone grafts is seldom used because it may lead to secondary cyst formation.
  - Fetlock lesions
    - Arthroscopic removal is the treatment of choice for lesions of the dorsal aspect of MC3/MT3 and at the level of the palmar/plantar eminences of P-1.
    - For nonarticular lesions off the palmar/plantar eminence of P-1, a routine open approach is used centered over the fragment.
  - Shoulder lesions: Although certain areas of the glenoid can be very difficult to reach, exploration of the joint using arthroscopy can be very

valuable, both from a diagnostic and therapeutic standpoint.
  - Cervical facet lesions: Ventral cervical vertebral stabilization using a stainless steel basket filled with cancellous bone has been effective at reducing or eliminating clinical signs in affected horses.
  - SBCs in locations not reachable arthroscopically such as in the fetlock or pastern joints: The cyst may be debrided using an extraarticular approach with subsequent packing of the cyst with cancellous bone.

CHRONIC TREATMENT

- Stall confinement and exercise restriction postoperatively will vary depending on the severity of the lesion and its location.
  - In general, 2 weeks of strict stall rest followed by 4 to 8 weeks of stall rest with handwalking exercise. After this time and after radiographic imaging of the surgical site, limited turnout in a small paddock for 4 to 6 weeks is added followed by another 4 to 6 weeks of regular paddock turnout.
  - Horses with SBC lesions typically require 6 to 12 months of rest and controlled exercise before initiating or returning to regular training exercise.
- The use of NSAIDs such as phenylbutazone (2.2–4.4 mg/kg PO or IV q12–24h), firocoxib (Equioxx; 0.1 mg/kg PO q24h), or flunixin meglumine (1.1 mg/kg PO or IV q12–24h) will provide antiinflammatory relief to affected horses treated both medically and surgically.
- Joint treatment with corticosteroids and hyaluronic acid, alone or in combination, may provide a palliative effect on clinical cases but will not eliminate the condition.

DRUG INTERACTIONS

- Fluoroquinolones (Baytril) should not be used in neonates because they have been shown to have the potential for developing significant osteochondrosis.

POSSIBLE COMPLICATIONS

- Lameness.
- NSAIDs can be both ulcerogenic and nephrotoxic, especially in young patients.

RECOMMENDED MONITORING

- Radiography
  - Provides an objective assessment of the progression of the condition
  - In horses that have OCDs or SBCs managed surgically, radiographs should be taken immediately after

surgery. Depending on the severity of the condition, follow-up radiographs are recommended at least 2 and 6 months after surgery.
- Lameness examination
  - Should be performed on a regular basis in horses treated conservatively to assess their response to treatment
  - In horses treated surgically, it should be performed after the patient is ready to begin controlled exercise, which can be anywhere from 3 to 12 months.

PROGNOSIS AND OUTCOME

- Tarsus
  - The prognosis for horses with OCD in this joint is quite favorable in most cases, particularly when single lesions are removed before clinical signs of lameness develop.
  - Even horses with radiographically extensive lesions typically carry a fairly good prognosis.
  - Lesions of the lateral trochlear ridge of the talus involving the majority of the articular surface have the least favorable prognosis for racing soundness.
  - Although distention of the joint capsule often improves postoperatively, some horses with marked, chronic effusion before surgery will always carry a slight increase in effusion relative to the unaffected side.
- Stifle
  - The prognosis for horses with OCD of the lateral trochlear ridge of the femur is generally fair to good but directly depends on the size of the lesion.
  - In general, the prognosis becomes less favorable in horses with more extensive disease, in those with

bilateral disease, and in horses with patellar involvement.
- In horses with SBCs of the medial femoral condyle, the prognosis is fair to good when managed surgically in young horses with clinical signs of lameness.
- Older horses (ages 7–10 years) with SBCs tend to do relatively worse compared with young horses after arthroscopic surgical debridement, although this appears to be changing with the advent of new techniques and therapies (see Acute General Treatment above).
- Fetlock
  - In cases of OCD in racehorses, the prognosis is fair to good (depending on the degree of pathology and secondary degenerative changes) and very good to excellent in non-racehorses.
  - For nonarticular lesions off the palmar/plantar eminence of P-1, the prognosis is guarded.
  - Horses with SBCs have a similar prognosis to those with SBCs of the medial femoral condyle of the femur.
- Shoulder: The prognosis is generally guarded at best for hard athletic use even after surgical management.
- Cervical vertebral facets: In horses showing clinical signs, the prognosis is guarded after ventral stabilization.
- The prognosis for horses showing clinical signs of osteochondrosis in other joints varies depending on its location, size of the lesion, and amount of concurrent degenerative changes present.

PEARLS & CONSIDERATIONS

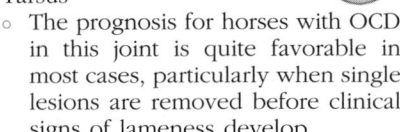

COMMENTS
- Foals and yearlings should not be fed in groups because the more dominant individuals will consume more, leading

to excessive energy (carbohydrate and protein) intake.
- Decrease or eliminate high-energy hay such as alfalfa and high-energy concentrate (eg, 14% protein) in young horses (weanlings to 2-year-olds) that are either at risk or identified as developing osteochondrosis.

PREVENTION
- Diet modification
- Use caution when selecting for certain breeding lines

CLIENT EDUCATION
- Should be aimed at avoiding feeding high-energy feeds, which can lead to excessive rapid growth and secondary osteochondrosis development.
- Breeders should monitor sires and mares suspect of yielding offspring with osteochondrosis.

SUGGESTED READING

Douglas J: Pathogenesis of osteochondrosis. In Ross MW, Dyson SJ (eds). *Diagnosis and management of lameness in the horse*, St Louis, 2003, Saunders Elsevier, pp 534–543.

Relave F, Meulyzer M, Alexander K, et al: Comparison of radiography and ultrasonography to detect osteochondrosis lesions in the tarsocrural joint: a prospective study. *Equine Vet J* 41(1):34–40, 2009.

Van Weeren PR: Osteochondrosis. In Auer JA, Stick JA (eds). *Equine surgery*, ed 3, Philadelphia, 2006, Saunders Elsevier, pp 1166–1177.

Von Rechenberg B, Auer JA: Subchondral cystic lesions. In Auer JA, Stick JA (eds). *Equine surgery*, ed 3, St Louis, 2006, Saunders Elsevier, pp 1178–1183.

Wallis TW, Goodrich LR, McIlwraith CW, et al: Arthroscopic injection of corticosteroids into the fibrous tissue of subchondral cystic lesions of the medial femoral condyle in horses: a retrospective study of 52 cases (2001–2006). *Equine Vet J* 40(5):461–467, 2008.

AUTHOR: **JOSÉ M. GARCÍA-LÓPEZ**

EDITOR: **ANDRIS J. KANEPS**

Ovarian Enlargement, Physiologic

DEFINITION
Increase in ovarian size caused by physiologic changes in ovarian cells or architecture

SYNONYM(S)
Multiple ovarian follicles, anovulatory follicles, hemorrhagic anovulatory follicle (HAF), autumn follicle, supplementary or accessory corpora lutea, ovarian hematoma

EPIDEMIOLOGY
SPECIES, AGE, SEX
- Unilateral or bilateral enlargement of ovaries might be the result of physiologic or pathological conditions.

- Physiologically, ovarian size varies considerably depending on the season of the year, age, and pregnancy.
- Generally, a young maiden mare's ovaries are about 2 to 4 cm long and 2 to 3 cm wide during the winter anestrous and increase to 5 to 8 cm by 3 to 4 cm in the spring.
- Older broodmares' ovaries are usually larger; during the anestrous period,

they are about 3 to 6 cm long and 4 to 5 cm wide, and during the breeding season, the ovaries vary from 6 to 12 cm long and 6 to 9 cm wide.

GENETICS AND BREED PREDISPOSITION

- Physiologic enlargement of the ovaries may occur in mares of any breed.
- Spontaneous multiple ovulations appear to be higher in some breeds such as Thoroughbred mares. A retrospective study reported a more than 30% incidence of multiple ovulations (double and triple) in this breed.
- Multiple ovulations are more frequent in older mares, with an incidence of 22% in young mares (2–4 years old) and 51% in older mares (17–19 years old). Because of the relative large size of the equine preovulatory follicle (35–70 mm), the presence of multiple preovulatory follicles results in significant enlargement of the ovaries.
- Large Equine breeds tend to develop larger ovulatory follicles (≤55–70 mm) compared with pony breeds (≤35–45 mm); consequently, large horse breeds with multiple ovulatory follicles develop larger ovaries.

RISKS FACTORS

Prostaglandin F-2α may predispose mares to develop HAFs or multiple ovulations. However, in the authors' opinion, the use of prostaglandin F-2α or its analogues to induce luteolysis during mid-diestrus is safe and results in a subsequent fertile estrus. The authors have not experienced an increase in the incidence of anovulatory follicles in mares receiving prostaglandin F-2α. Further studies are necessary to confirm the role of exogenous prostaglandin F-2α on the development of HAFs.

GEOGRAPHY AND SEASONALITY

Both geography and seasonality affect the occurrence and duration of the transitional period in mares.

- In equatorial regions, mares tend to cycle year round if good nutrition is provided.
- In the Northern hemisphere, mares exposed to natural daylight cycle regularly from April to September.
- In general, spring and autumn transitional periods last approximately 40 to 60 days and occur immediately before and after the period with regular estrous cycles.
- Mares in the Southern hemisphere cycle from October to April and have transitional periods as described above.

CLINICAL PRESENTATION

DISEASE FORMS/SUBTYPES

- Anovulatory follicles: Luteinized, nonluteinized, or hemorrhagic
- Accessory corpora lutea during first trimester of gestation

HISTORY, CHIEF COMPLAINT

- A detailed reproductive history, including changes in behavior, estrous cycle characteristics, sexual behavior, and the last observed estrus, should be obtained.
- During the transitional period, mares may be presented with the complaint of persistent estrus, a history of reduced performance, and intolerance of riding.
- Mares in early gestation can be presented with a history of stallion-like behavior or exhibit estrus signs. In addition, if mating was missed by the owner, mares may be presented with a history of anestrous.

PHYSICAL EXAM FINDINGS

- During palpation per rectum, the ovary (or ovaries) will be enlarged; the size varies from a softball size to a basketball size.
- Transrectal ultrasonography is the method of choice to identify ovarian structures and to determine the cause of enlarged ovaries.
- Anovulatory follicles are usually as large as or larger than preovulatory sizes. The appearance of the follicular wall and its contents can vary.
- In luteinized follicles, the walls of the follicles have increased echogenicity and thickness, as opposed to a thin and less echogenic wall of nonluteinized follicles.
- Follicular fluid may contain hyperechoic particles (red blood cells), strands (fibrin), or both.
- In pregnant mares, the ovaries will contain multiple follicular structures that may undergo normal ovulation or luteinization. Therefore, the appearance of some of these structures may be indistinguishable from the luteinized anovulatory follicles. However, the fetus can be observed within the uterus.

ETIOLOGY AND PATHOPHYSIOLOGY

- Ovarian enlargement during transitional period
  - All Equine breeds present with ovarian enlargement during the transitional period.
  - During the spring and fall transitional period, the presence of multiple follicles larger than 25 mm can cause a significant enlargement of the ovaries.
  - The occurrence of large anovulatory follicles is also common during this period.
  - Transition periods are characterized by waves of follicular development and regression without ovulation, which may last 2 to 3 months.
  - These follicles reach preovulatory size but are thought to be steroidogenic incompetent, resulting in lack of sufficient pituitary gonadotropin

stimulation to induce ovulation, and most follicles regress within a few days.

- Anovulatory follicles
  - May continue to grow, reaching 5 to 15 cm in diameter.
  - May persist for 4 to 8 weeks and result in persistent estrous or prolonged interovulatory interval.
  - Most undergo partial luteinization with time, and progesterone levels may be elevated above baseline.
  - Most regress spontaneously in 1 to 4 weeks.
- HAFs
  - May occur at any time during the breeding season, although this is a more common occurrence during the autumn transition compared with the spring transition
  - Occur more often in elderly mares (ie, >20 years)
  - Tend to occur repeatedly in the same mare
- In pregnant mares, Equine chorionic gonadotropin is secreted by the endometrial cups starting around day 35 of gestation and results in the growth of multiple follicles in the ovaries. Most follicles undergo ovulation to form accessory corpora lutea; however, some follicles undergo luteinization without ovulation and can have the appearance of HAFs.

DIAGNOSIS

- Rectal palpation
- Ultrasonography
- Hormonal assays (progesterone, inhibin, and testosterone)
- Sequential assessments might be useful in determining changes in the size of the ovaries as well as dynamic changes of structures.

DIFFERENTIAL DIAGNOSIS

- Granulosa or theca cell tumor (by far the most common pathologic cause of ovarian enlargement in mares)
- Paraovarian cysts
- Ovulation fossa inclusion cysts
- Dysgerminoma
- Teratoma
- Cystadenoma or adenocarcinoma
- Ovarian hematoma
- Ovarian torsion
- Superovulation
- Ovarian abscess (less common)

INITIAL DATABASE

- Unremarkable findings in the body systems except the reproductive tract with enlarged ovary or ovaries
- Progesterone levels may be elevated above baseline if luteinization of the anovulatory follicle has occurred or the animal is pregnant. Testosterone

concentrations may also be elevated during the first third of gestation, reaching peak concentrations at approximately 200 days of gestation. Mares with granulosa cell tumor likely have elevated inhibin levels (>2 ng/mL).

ADVANCED CONFIRMATORY TESTING

- Ultrasonography
- Hormonal assays to rule out granulosa theca cell tumor

TREATMENT

THERAPEUTIC GOALS

- Ovulation or luteinization
- Shorten transitional period
- Stop estrus signs

ACUTE GENERAL TREATMENT

- Daily oral administration of altrenogest (0.044 mg/kg or 1 mL per 50 kg of body weight) and other progestagens for 14 days can be used to discontinue persistent estrus behavior during the transition period and to hasten the first ovulation of the year.
- Luteinization or ovulation of anovulatory follicles can be induced by administration of 1.5 mg of deslorelin (gonadotropin-releasing hormone analogue) intramuscularly.
- After luteinization or ovulation of the anovulatory follicle has been achieved, administration of dinoprost (10 mg IM) or cloprostenol (250 µg IM) may be used to induce luteolysis and return to estrus.

PROGNOSIS AND OUTCOME

Favorable

PEARLS & CONSIDERATIONS

COMMENTS

Diagnosis of an ovarian enlargement may be a normal finding during routine reproductive examination or may be instigated by specific clinical signs, such as reproductive behavior changes and colic. It is important that the veterinarian be aware of the physiologic possibilities and be able to differentiate those from pathologic conditions to establish the correct diagnosis and treatment as well to avoid unnecessary surgical removal of normal ovaries.

PREVENTION

There are multiple causes and predisposing factors to the development of HAFs. Chronic stress has been shown to negatively affect gonadotropin secretion, particularly luteinizing hormone, which may result in lack of ovulation and persistence of anovulatory follicle(s). Therefore, it may be beneficial to reduce chronic stress in mares with a high incidence of HAFs.

CLIENT EDUCATION

Inexperienced breeders must be educated to recognize normal estrus behavior and be informed that many mares will display annual transitional periods that are often associated with prolonged estrus.

SUGGESTED READING

Cuervo-Arango J, Newcombe JR: The effect of hormone treatments (hCG and cloprostenol) and season on the incidence of hemorrhagic anovulatory follicles in the mare: a field study. *Theriogenology* 72:1262–1267, 2009.

Ginther OJ, Gastal EL, Gastal MO, et al: Incidence, endocrinology, vascularity and morphology of hemorrhagic anovulatory follicles in mares. *J Equine Vet Sci* 2009; 27:130–139.

McCue PM: Ovulation failure. In Samper JC, Pycock JF, McKinnon AO (eds). *Current therapy in equine reproduction*, St Louis, 2007, Saunders Elsevier, pp 83–86.

Morel MC, Newcombe JR, Swindlehurst JC: The effect of age on multiple ovulation rates, multiple pregnancy rates and embryonic vesicle diameter in the mare. *Theriogenology* 63:2482–2493, 2005.

Pinto CRF, Paccamonti DL: Mare reproductive pathology In Reed SM, Bayly WM, Sellon DC (eds). *Equine internal medicine*, ed 3, St Louis, 2010, Saunders Elsevier, pp 1016–1024.

AUTHORS: **IGOR FREDERICO CANISSO** and **MARCO ANTONIO COUTINO DA SILVA**

EDITOR: **JUAN C. SAMPER**

Oviductal Pathology

BASIC INFORMATION

DEFINITION

Changes related to the normal function and appearance of the oviduct. May take the form of oviductal obstruction caused by plugs, inflammation, complete obstruction caused by hydrosalpinx, and infundibular adhesions.

SYNONYM(S)

Oviductal obstruction, adhesions, hydrosalpinx

EPIDEMIOLOGY

SPECIES, AGE, SEX Older mares with histories of poor reproductive performance or chronic infections

GENETICS AND BREED PREDISPOSITION Pony and Norwegian Fjord mares have fewer lesions than other European breeds.

RISK FACTORS Infundibular lesions tend to be more common in older mares (>10 years). Perimetritis tends to be associated with infundibular lesions. Endometritis is associated with salpingitis.

CONTAGION AND ZOONOSIS No specific organism has been associated with inflammation other than the association with endometritis.

GEOGRAPHY AND SEASONALITY Does not appear to be associated with mare cyclicity (anestrus vs. normal cyclicity)

ASSOCIATED CONDITIONS AND DISORDERS May be associated with endometritis and perimetritis

CLINICAL PRESENTATION

HISTORY, CHIEF COMPLAINT The clinical significance is virtually unknown because of the inability to clinically examine the oviduct. Hydrosalpinx may present as a mare with a persistent follicle that is in fact the dilated oviduct. Repeated ovulations from one ovary without pregnancy in a mare with no other risk factors could suggest oviductal blockage.

PHYSICAL EXAM FINDINGS Hydrosalpinx can present as a "persistent follicle."

ETIOLOGY AND PATHOPHYSIOLOGY Chronic infections or pyometra possibly result in the migration of bacteria into the oviductal lumen. The type of organism and the mechanism by which bacteria could enter the oviduct are unknown or purely speculative. Pressure form the uterine side, bacterial transport by sperm, or entrance of bacteria from the infundibular site could be possibilities.

DIAGNOSIS

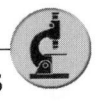

DIFFERENTIAL DIAGNOSIS

All other causes of infertility in horses

INITIAL DATABASE

Thorough history including all breedings, the side of ovulation, and the resulting pregnancy from each ovulation

ADVANCED OR CONFIRMATORY TESTING

Recent advances have used laparoscopy to facilitate placement of fluorescent beads of different colors in each oviduct and flushing the uterus 24 and 48 hours later to determine the passage of the beads. If the beads do not pass, it is suggestive of oviductal blockage.

TREATMENT

- Laparoscopic placement of 0.5 mL of a gel containing 0.2 mg of prostaglandin E2 on the serosal surface of the oviduct
- Surgery to flush the oviduct from the infundibulum to the uterus or the uterotubal junction to the infundibulum

THERAPEUTIC GOAL(S)

Removal of oviductal plugs

POSSIBLE COMPLICATIONS

- Surgical complications include rupture of the oviduct if the obstruction does not pass, particularly if the flushing is toward the uterus.
- There are likely fewer complications with the prostaglandin E2.

PROGNOSIS AND OUTCOME

There is reported success with the above techniques. It is advisable to determine the endometrial health (endometrial biopsy, culture, cytology) before the procedure is performed.

PEARLS & CONSIDERATIONS

The oviduct is difficult to evaluate because of it size, but blockage should be considered in aged mares, particularly those that appear to get pregnant when they ovulate only from one side. Oviductal plugs are more common in older mares, but so are other reproductive pathologies.

SUGGESTED READING

Allen WR, Wilsher S, Morris L, et al: Laparoscopic application of PGE(2) to re-establish oviducal patency and fertility in infertile mares: a preliminary study. *Equine Vet J* 38:454–459, 2006.

Bennett SD: Diagnosis of oviductal disorders and diagnostic techniques. In Samper JC, Pycock JP, McKinnon AO (eds). *Current therapy in equine reproduction*, St Louis, 2007, Elsevier pp 78–82.

Bennett SD, Griffin RL, Rhoads WS: Surgical evaluation of oviduct disease and patency in the mare. *Proc Am Assoc Equine Pract* 347–349, 2002.

Henry M, Vandeplassche M: Pathology of the oviduct [in German], *Vlaams Dier Tijd* 50:301–325, 1981.

Ley WB, Bowen JM, Purswell BJ, et al: Modified technique to evaluate uterine tubal patency in the mare. *Proc Am Assoc Equine Pract* 44:56–59, 1998.

Vandeplassche M, Henry M: Salpingitis in the mare. *Proc Am Assoc Equine Pract* 23:123–131, 1977.

Zent WW, Lui IKM, Spirito MA: Oviduct flushing as a treatment for fertility in the mare. *Equine Vet J Suppl* 15:47–48, 1993.

AUTHOR: **CHARLES C. LOVE**

EDITOR: **JUAN C. SAMPER**

Pancreatic Disease, Chronic

BASIC INFORMATION

DEFINITION

Neoplasia of the pancreas and chronic pancreatitis

SYNONYM(S)

Chronic pancreatic necrosis

EPIDEMIOLOGY

SPECIES, AGE, SEX More likely in older horses

CLINICAL PRESENTATION

HISTORY, CHIEF COMPLAINT

- Clinical signs of chronic pancreatic disease include:
  - Chronic weight loss
  - Depression
  - Inappetence
  - Intermittent colic
  - Persistent or recurrent pyrexia
  - Jaundice
- If the horse has concurrent insulin-dependent diabetes mellitus (IDDM), polyuria and polydipsia may also be present.

- Rarely, horses with pancreatitis may also have panniculitis.
- Hematuria was recorded in one horse with pancreatic adenocarcinoma.
- Pancreatic adenocarcinoma may metastasize to other parts of the body, such as the chest cavity, resulting in signs of tachypnea or dyspnea.

PHYSICAL EXAM FINDINGS The findings of physical examination confirm the presenting signs. There are no specific pathognomic signs that indicate pancreatic disease.

ETIOLOGY AND PATHOPHYSIOLOGY

- The pancreas is a compound gland that has important exocrine and endocrine functions. Digestion in the small intestine is partly dependent on pancreatic secretions but also on biliary secretions and mucosal enzymes. The volume of pancreatic fluid secreted by a 100-kg pony is approximately 10 to 12 L/day. Pancreatic juice contains bicarbonate ions, amylase, lipase, and peptidases. The islets of Langerhans secrete insulin, gastrin, and glucagon but account for only about 2% of the pancreas' total weight.

- Adult horses and ponies may develop signs of exocrine pancreatic insufficiency, with or without associated IDDM, after destruction of the pancreas by diseases such as neoplasia (pancreatic adenocarcinoma) and chronic pancreatic necrosis.
- Chronic eosinophilic pancreatitis has been reported and is assumed to be caused by parasite (*Strongylus equinus, Strongylus edentatus*) migration through the gland.

DIAGNOSIS

DIFFERENTIAL DIAGNOSIS

Other causes of progressive weight loss, other causes of recurrent colic, and other causes of chronic or recurrent pyrexia

INITIAL DATABASE

- Clinical pathologic abnormalities are inconsistent but may include:
  - Increased serum amylase
  - Increased serum lipase
  - Increased peritoneal fluid amylase
  - Hypoalbuminemia

- ○ Hypocalcemia
- ○ Hyperglycemia
- ○ Glucosuria
- ○ Hypertriglyceridemia
- ○ Increased serum gamma glutamyl transferase, aspartate transferase, and alkaline phosphatase
- ○ Hyperbilirubinemia
- Examination of peritoneal fluid may reveal evidence of peritonitis (total nucleated cell count >5.0 × 10⁹ cells/L; total protein concentration >40 g/L). In horses with chronic eosinophilic pancreatitis, there may be an increase in numbers of eosinophils in the peritoneal fluid.
- Results of rectal examination are likely to be normal, although the horse may demonstrate nonspecific pain caused by peritoneal inflammation.

ADVANCED OR CONFIRMATORY TESTING

- Fractional excretion of amylase may be increased. The fractional excretion of amylase (FEam) is calculated by the following formula:

$$\frac{\text{Urine amylase}}{\text{Serum amylase}} \times \frac{\text{Serum creatinine}}{\text{Urine creatinine}} \times 100$$
$$= \text{FEam}$$

FEam in normal horses is less than 1%.
- Abdominal ultrasonography should be performed to establish if metastatic neoplasia is present.
- Laparoscopic examination may show an enlarged pancreas, which may be amenable to laparoscopic biopsy.

TREATMENT

THERAPEUTIC GOAL(S)

Symptomatic treatment only is likely possible.

ACUTE GENERAL TREATMENT

There have been no reports of successful treatment for horses with chronic pancreatic disease or neoplasia.

POSSIBLE COMPLICATION

Diabetes mellitus

PROGNOSIS AND OUTCOME

- In most cases, the prognosis is very poor.

- If a focal neoplasm that is amenable to surgical excision is present, then curative treatment may be possible.

PEARLS & CONSIDERATIONS

Chronic pancreatic disease and pancreatic neoplasia are rare causes of chronic weight loss in horses.

SUGGESTED READING

Carrick JB, Morris DD, Harmon BG, et al: Haematuria and weight loss in a mare with pancreatic adenocarcinoma. *Cornell Vet* 82:91, 1992.

Church S, West HJ, Baker JR: Two cases of pancreatic adenocarcinoma in horses. *Equine Vet J* 19(1):77, 1987.

East LM, Savage CJ: Abdominal neoplasia. *Vet Clin North Am* 14:478, 1998.

Rendle DI, Hewetson M, Barron R, et al: Tachypnoea and pleural effusion in a mare with metastatic pancreatic adenocarcinoma. *Vet Rec* 159:356, 2006.

Waitt LH, Cebra CK, Tornquist SJ, et al: Panniculitis in a horse with peripancreatitis and pancreatic fibrosis. *J Vet Diagn Invest* 18:405, 2006.

AUTHOR: TIM MAIR

EDITORS: TIM MAIR and CERI SHERLOCK

Pancreatitis, Acute

BASIC INFORMATION

DEFINITION

Acute inflammation of the pancreas

EPIDEMIOLOGY

SPECIES, AGE, SEX All ages but more likely in older horses

CLINICAL PRESENTATION

HISTORY, CHIEF COMPLAINT The clinical signs of acute pancreatitis include:
- Severe abdominal pain
- Tachypnea
- Sweating

PHYSICAL EXAM FINDINGS The findings of physical examination confirm the presenting signs.
- The horse may show signs of hypovolemic shock (eg, tachycardia, cool extremities, congested mucous membranes, prolonged capillary refill time).
- Passage of a nasogastric tube may yield significant gastric reflux.
- There are no specific pathognomic signs that indicate pancreatic disease.

ETIOLOGY AND PATHOPHYSIOLOGY

- The pancreas is a compound gland that has important exocrine and endocrine functions. Digestion in the small intestine is partly dependent on pancreatic secretions but also on biliary secretions and mucosal enzymes. The volume of pancreatic fluid secreted by a 100-kg pony is approximately 10 to 12 L/day. Pancreatic juice contains bicarbonate ions, amylase, lipase, and peptidases. The islets of Langerhans secrete insulin, gastrin, and glucagon but account for only about 2% of the pancreas' total weight.
- Acute pancreatitis is a rare cause of severe abdominal pain in horses. The cause is uncertain, and antemortem diagnosis is rarely made because the clinical signs mimic other gastrointestinal diseases producing acute colic (especially small intestinal strangulating obstructions and anterior enteritis). The pancreas is not easily visualized during routine surgical exploration of the abdomen and may be overlooked at necropsy, especially if gastric rupture has occurred.

- Acute pancreatitis may occur in association with adenovirus infection in Arabian foals affected by combined immunodeficiency syndrome (CID). Infection of the pancreatic duct by *Cryptosporidium* spp. may also occur in foals affected by CID.
- Pancreatitis is also sometimes found in association with hyperlipemia. It has been speculated that excess lipid is deposited in and around the pancreas in hyperlipemia. This lipid is subsequently hydrolyzed by pancreatic lipase and released as free fatty acids. Free (unbound to albumin) fatty acids are cytotoxic, and when the albumin-binding capacity is exceeded, pancreatic vascular injury occurs, resulting in necrotizing pancreatitis.

DIAGNOSIS

DIFFERENTIAL DIAGNOSIS

Other causes of acute colic

INITIAL DATABASE

- Clinical pathologic abnormalities are nonspecific and reflect hypovolemia (elevated packed cell volume, elevated total serum protein concentration).

- Some cases may have hyperlipemia.
- Peritoneal fluid may be normal, serosanguineous, or frankly hemorrhagic.
- Abdominal sounds may be reduced or absent.
- Results of rectal examination are likely to be normal, although the horse may demonstrate nonspecific pain because of peritoneal inflammation.

ADVANCED OR CONFIRMATORY TESTING

Fractional excretion of amylase may be increased. The fractional secretion of amylase (FEam) is calculated by the following formula:

$$\frac{\text{Urine amylase}}{\text{Serum amylase}} \times \frac{\text{Serum creatinine}}{\text{Urine creatinine}} \times 100$$

$$= \text{FEam}$$

FEam in normal horses is less than 1%.

TREATMENT

THERAPEUTIC GOAL(S)

There is no specific treatment. Symptomatic treatment is possible but likely ineffective.

ACUTE GENERAL TREATMENT

- There have been no reports of specific treatment for acute pancreatitis in horses.
- Treatment is aimed at analgesia and restoration of normal circulating blood volume.

POSSIBLE COMPLICATION

Diabetes mellitus

PROGNOSIS AND OUTCOME

- In most cases, the prognosis is very poor.

- In many cases, acute pancreatitis is diagnosed after death.

PEARLS & CONSIDERATIONS

Acute pancreatitis is a rare cause of acute colic in horses.

SUGGESTED READING

Lilley CW, Beeman GM: Gastric dilatation associated with acute necrotizing pancreatitis. *Equine Pract* 3:8, 1981.

McClure JJ: Acute pancreatitis. In Robinson NE, editor: *Current therapy in equine medicine*, ed 2, Philadelphia, 1987, WB Saunders, pp 46–47.

Parry BW, Crisman MV: Serum and peritoneal fluid amylase and lipase reference values in horses. *Equine Vet J* 23:390, 1991.

AUTHOR: TIM MAIR

EDITORS: TIM MAIR and CERI SHERLOCK

Papillomatosis, Cutaneous

BASIC INFORMATION

DEFINITION

Common benign, viral-induced epithelial growths with dry, horny surfaces

SYNONYM(S)

- Warts
- Verrucae
- Grass warts
- Ear papillomas
- Aural plaque
- Papillary acanthoma
- Hyperplastic dermatitis of the ear

EPIDEMIOLOGY

SPECIES, AGE, SEX

- Warts occur mostly in young animals (generally horses <3 years).
- Ear papillomas can affect horses of any age but rarely animals younger than 1 year.

RISK FACTORS Exposure to affected horses

CONTAGION AND ZOONOSIS Viral-induced warts are contagious to other horses.

ASSOCIATED CONDITIONS AND DISORDERS The lesions, formerly called *congenital warts*, now termed *hamartomatous lesions* or *epithelial nevus*, are not viral-induced lesions.

CLINICAL PRESENTATION

DISEASE FORMS/SUBTYPES Two forms of viral papilloma are recognized:

- Equine viral papillomatosis (warts, verrucae, grass warts)
- Ear papillomas (aural plaque, papillary acanthoma, hyperplastic dermatitis of the ear)

HISTORY, CHIEF COMPLAINT Insidious onset of very small papules progressing to larger and larger wartlike lesions

PHYSICAL EXAM FINDINGS

- Warts begin as small, 1- to 2-mm diameter, raised, smooth, shiny, gray papules and then undergo rapid growth and increase number of lesions, up to 2 cm in diameter, broad-based pedunculated gray to pink, hyperkeratotic lesions.
- Ear papillomas begin as small 1- to 2 mm in diameter, raised, depigmented, shiny papules on the lateral surface of the pinna, often bilaterally symmetrical; the lesions enlarge and coalesce to become up to 3 cm in diameter, white, hyperkeratotic plaques.

ETIOLOGY AND PATHOPHYSIOLOGY

- Equine viral papillomatosis are caused by host-specific papovavirus that infects the basal cell layer of the epithelium, leading to formation of small gray to pink, vegetative-type growths.
- Contagious

DIAGNOSIS

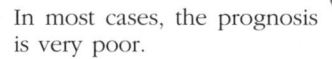

DIFFERENTIAL DIAGNOSIS

- Verrucous (wartlike form) or the occult form of equine sarcoid
- Squamous cell carcinoma
- Molluscum contagiosum (caused by molluscipox virus, suggested anthropozoonosis)

INITIAL DATABASE

- Distinctive characteristic appearance and distribution are strongly suggestive of cutaneous papillomas.
- A further diagnostic workup is rarely pursued or indicated.

ADVANCED OR CONFIRMATORY TESTING

- Histopathologic evaluation of biopsy specimen
- Immunohistochemistry and detection of viral antigens within the lesion
- Electron microscopy and identification of hexagonal viral particles

TREATMENT

THERAPEUTIC GOAL(S)

- Therapy is rarely pursued.
- Lesions may be removed for aesthetic reasons.

ACUTE GENERAL TREATMENT

- Viral papillomatosis typically resolves spontaneously within 3 months.
- Ear papillomas rarely regress spontaneously, and no therapy has been reported to be effective.
- Lesions may be removed by surgical excision or cryosurgery.
- Topical agents might be used when surgical treatment:
  - Podophyllin
  - Trifluoroacetic acid
  - Tincture of benzoin
  - Imiquimod
- Intralesional injection of cisplatin or interleukin-2
- Immunostimulant therapy, including intralesional or IV injection of *Propionibacterium acnes*
- Autogenous wart vaccines have been used and reported to be effective

CHRONIC TREATMENT

Horses chronically affected with viral papillomatosis should be suspected of being immunosuppressed.

POSSIBLE COMPLICATIONS

Topical treatments that lead to inflammatory reaction may result in permanent depigmentation.

PROGNOSIS AND OUTCOME

- Usually good
- Spontaneous regression is likely to occur within 1 year.

PEARLS & CONSIDERATIONS

COMMENTS

Viral-induced warts occur in several species, most commonly in cattle followed by horses and small ruminants.

PREVENTION

- Virus can be transmitted by direct contact between animals or indirectly via fomites.
- Isolate affected animals.
- Avoid sharing of halters, brushes, and other equipment.

SUGGESTED READING

Scott DW, Miller WH Jr: Epithelial neoplasms—papillomas. In *Equine dermatology*, St Louis, 2003, Saunders Elsevier, pp 700–707.
White SD: Viral diseases—papillomas; aural plaques. In Smith BP, editor: *Large animal internal medicine*, ed 4, St Louis, 2009, Mosby Elsevier, pp 1316–1318.

AUTHOR: **LAIS R.R. COSTA**

EDITOR: **DAVID A. WILSON**

Paraphimosis

BASIC INFORMATION

DEFINITION

The inability to retract the penis into the prepuce

SYNONYM(S)

Penile paralysis, penile prolapse

EPIDEMIOLOGY

SPECIES, AGE, SEX Equine in general, any age, gelding or stallion. Stallions may be overrepresented because paraphimosis is often related to breeding accidents.
RISK FACTORS Breeding accidents, phenothiazine-derived tranquilizers (acepromazine), weight loss
GEOGRAPHY AND SEASONALITY Summer associated if *Habronema muscae* larvae colonize the penis or associated structures

CLINICAL PRESENTATION

HISTORY, CHIEF COMPLAINT Large amounts of penile swelling and an inability to retract the penis into the sheath or prepuce
PHYSICAL EXAM FINDINGS Physical examination findings depend on the cause of paraphimosis. There may be signs of trauma. This condition is also seen in debilitated horses that have had significant weight loss (body condition score of 1 to 2). Despite the initial cause, the penis is usually edematous.

ETIOLOGY AND PATHOPHYSIOLOGY

- When the penis remains exposed for any length of time, the venous and lymphatic drainage is impaired, causing edema within the penis and prepuce.
- The preputial ring becomes constricted, and the edema increases the penile weight, making it more pendulous and difficult to retract.
- The exposed tissue becomes irritated and friable.
- Damaged tissue becomes excoriated and infected, resulting in fibrosis.
- Weight of tissue may lead to internal pudendal nerve damage, leading to paralysis.

DIAGNOSIS

DIFFERENTIAL DIAGNOSIS

- Priapism
- Penile paralysis

INITIAL DATABASE

Complete blood count and serum chemistry are typically within normal limits.

ADVANCED OR CONFIRMATORY TESTING

Ultrasonography of the penis may be helpful to rule out hematoma, seroma, or abscess.

TREATMENT

THERAPEUTIC GOAL(S)

- The penis should be returned to the prepuce as soon as possible to eliminate further swelling and prevent damage to the tissue.
- If penile replacement is not possible, the penis should be elevated using a sling or bandage to keep it against the body wall.
- Keep penis lubricated with antibacterial emollient.

ACUTE GENERAL TREATMENT

- The penis should be cleaned thoroughly to allow adequate examination and assessment of the damage.
- Emollients such as silver sulfadiazine or an antibiotic ointment should be applied to the penis, massaging the tissue from the tip to the base to provide lubrication, decrease the incidence of adhesions, and remove edema.

- If the penile swelling is too severe, an elastic bandage (Esmarch) can be applied, starting at the tip to push edema from the tissue. The bandage should be left in place for 10 to 15 minutes. Sedation may be required. After the bandage has been removed, an attempt should be made to replace the penis into the prepuce. Bandage application may be repeated if necessary.
- Fluid accumulation may be drained using a large-gauge needle (14–16 gauge) or stab incision in the ventral aspect of the pocket. Aseptic technique should be maintained to avoid abscessation. Removal of fibrin or blood clots may be performed using sterile forceps or hemostats.
- After the penis has been replaced within the prepuce and sheath, a purse-string suture can be placed around the sheath, leaving a small orifice to allow the drainage of urine.
- As an alternative to the purse-string suture, a mesh sling may be made using breathable fabric suspended by rubber tubing around the horse's flank and lateral to the scrotum. A narrow-necked plastic bottle may also be used by removing the bottom of the bottle. The penis is placed inside the top half of the padded bottle, inserted into the sheath, and secured with rubber tubing.
- Placing roll cotton around the penis and supporting it close to the ventral body wall using an abdominal wrap or Elastikon bandage is an acceptable alternative.

- Nonsteroidal antiinflammatory drugs should be administered to reduce inflammation and alleviate pain.
- Broad-spectrum antibiotics are indicated if the exposed tissue is devitalized.

CHRONIC TREATMENT

If medical management fails, penile amputation may be necessary.

POSSIBLE COMPLICATIONS

- Failure to replace the penis will result in pudendal nerve damage and penile paralysis.
- Adhesions of the penis to the prepuce may result in phimosis.

RECOMMENDED MONITORING

- Daily examination and lubrication of the penis reduces the incidence of adhesions.
- Initially, the animal may have a relapse after a short period of time; when this occurs, the penis should be replaced and treatment continued.
- When the horse can maintain the penis within the sheath, treatment can be discontinued.

PROGNOSIS AND OUTCOME

- Good in the case of breeding accidents if treatment is instituted promptly
- Fair in the case of cachexia
- Poor in cases of pudendal nerve damage

- The longer the penis remains exposed and edematous, the lower the prognosis for return to function.

PEARLS & CONSIDERATIONS

COMMENTS

- A combination of treatments may be instituted to reduce inflammation and keep the penis within the sheath.
- Medical management may require 7 to 10 days before any improvement is seen.
- Thirty days of rest from all sexual activity is essential.

PREVENTION

- Healthy breeding management
- Judicious use of phenothiazine derivatives

CLIENT EDUCATION

- Immediate aggressive treatment yields a better prognosis.
- Sperm viability is affected because of local heat and swelling.

SUGGESTED READING

Brinsko SP, Blanchard TL, Varner DD, et al: How to treat paraphimosis. *Proc Am Assoc Equine Pract* 53:580–582, 2007.
Gaughan EM, Van Harreveld PD: Trauma to the penis. In Samper JC, Pycock JF, McKinnon AO, editors: *Current therapy in equine reproduction*, St Louis, 2007, Saunders Elsevier, pp 227–230.

AUTHOR: **AIME K. JOHNSON**

EDITOR: **JUAN C. SAMPER**

Parturition, Premature Signs

BASIC INFORMATION

DEFINITION

- Premonitory signs of premature parturition are often not recognized in mares. Unrecognized premature parturition often results in a dead foal, either because of prepartum fetal death or postpartum death of an immature foal.
- Clinical signs that may occur are precocious mammary development and vulvar discharge. They are most often seen in cases of primary or secondary placental insufficiency.

SYNONYM(S)

Precocious mammary development, premature lactation, vulvar discharge, premature labor, placental insufficiency

EPIDEMIOLOGY

SPECIES, AGE, SEX Occurs in mares
GENETICS AND BREED PREDISPOSITION Some breeds and lines within breeds have a higher likelihood of double ovulation and twinning.
RISK FACTORS
- Twin pregnancy
- Placental disease, including infectious placentitis
GEOGRAPHY AND SEASONALITY Nocardioform placentitis is rare outside of Kentucky but has been described in Florida, Europe, and South Africa. Clinical

signs of premature parturition are most often observed in late-pregnant mares (7–11 months of gestation).
ASSOCIATED CONDITIONS AND DISORDERS
- Twin pregnancy
- Ascending bacterial placentitis
- Nocardioform placentitis

CLINICAL PRESENTATION

HISTORY, CHIEF COMPLAINT
- Most commonly, mares have no predictive signs, and the presenting complaint is abortion, stillbirth, or premature delivery of a live foal.
- Mares with twin pregnancies or placentitis may have premonitory signs, including precocious mammary development or milk production 2 or more

weeks before the expected parturition (most common) or mucopurulent vulvar discharge.

PHYSICAL EXAM FINDINGS

- Systemic health parameters of the mare are typically within normal limits.
- Precocious mammary development may take two forms—premature glandular development with a "full bag" or streaming milk loss from the teat more than 2 to 3 weeks before the expected due date.
- Vulvar discharge may be copious or scant and intermittent. It may be seen only as dried mucoid material in the tail or on the hindquarters of the mare.

ETIOLOGY AND PATHOPHYSIOLOGY

- Vulvar discharge is a product of an inflammatory or infectious process cranial to the cervix, which results in softening of the cervix and expulsion of inflammatory products into the vagina. This condition may be found in mares with ascending bacterial placentitis but is not seen in mares with twin pregnancies or nocardioform placentitis. Lesions are seen ventrally in the uterus with nocardioform placentitis and do not generally extend to the cervix. This organism is believed to reach the uterus hematogenously.
- The physiology of peripartum mammary development is poorly understood in mares but is believed to be induced by fetal hormonal changes resulting from stressors before foaling. Premature mammary development is seen in conditions that cause chronic placental insufficiency. These conditions may also be associated with premature fetal maturation.

DIAGNOSIS

DIFFERENTIAL DIAGNOSIS

- Twin pregnancy
- Ascending bacterial placentitis
- Nocardioform placentitis

INITIAL DATABASE

- The complete blood count and serum chemistry panel are usually normal but may be indicated to determine other organ involvement.
- The electrolyte content of the milk may be useful to predict the timing of parturition in mares in some cases. It may be less reliable in mares with placental disease than in normally foaling mares.
- A progesterone assay (estimating total progestagens of fetoplacental origin) or estrogen assay may be useful to predict the timing of parturition or the severity of disease in some cases.
- Transrectal palpation and ultrasonography should be performed to confirm

the presence of a fetus or to confirm the complete evacuation of the uterus in a mare that presents after abortion.

ADVANCED OR CONFIRMATORY TESTING

- Transrectal palpation and ultrasound to evaluate the combined thickness of the uterus and placenta (CTUP), fetal fluid characteristics, and fetal parameters
- Transabdominal ultrasonography of the fetus may be used to obtain a fetal heart rate and measures for a fetal biometric profile.
- Transabdominal ultrasonography of the uterus and placenta may be used to evaluate the CTUP ventrally and aid in the diagnosis of nocardioform placentitis before parturition.
- A speculum examination of the vagina may provide additional information and allow the collection of sample for bacterial culture.
- Bacterial culture of cervical or vaginal discharge may be useful to guide antibiotic selection before or after parturition.

TREATMENT

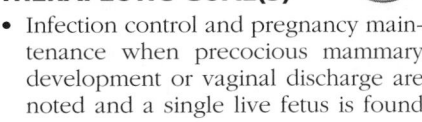

THERAPEUTIC GOAL(S)

- Infection control and pregnancy maintenance when precocious mammary development or vaginal discharge are noted and a single live fetus is found on examination
- Reduction of maternal morbidity and mortality caused by secondary complications associated with delivery of a compromised or dead foal
- Infection control and enhancement of uterine clearance in mares after premature delivery

ACUTE GENERAL TREATMENT

- Pregnancy maintenance
  - Prepartum treatment is attempted in cases of placentitis when the foal is known to be alive. Treatment should be multimodal and address the causative agent as well as the inflammatory processes. Whenever possible, antibiotic treatment should be directed by a culture; however, immediate broad-spectrum antibiotic therapy is warranted before results are available.
  - Broad-spectrum antibacterial treatment (ie, trimethoprim-sulfamethoxazole [25–30 mg/kg PO q12h] or potassium penicillin G [22000 U/kg IV q6h] and gentamicin [6.6 mg/kg IV q24h])
  - Antiinflammatory therapy (flunixin meglumine [1.1 mg/kg IV q12h] or pentoxifylline [8.5 mg/kg PO q12h])

  - Tocolytic therapy (altrenogest, 0.088 mg/kg PO q24h)
- Pregnancy termination: Twin pregnancy is highly unlikely to result in healthy, viable offspring and is associated with a significant risk of morbidity and mortality to the dam. Termination of a twin pregnancy or singleton pregnancy with a severely compromised or dead fetus may be preferable in some cases (see "Parturition, Induction" in Section II).
- Foaling assistance: Mares with compromised or dead fetuses are at increased risk for dystocia and periparturient disease. They should be considered high-risk patients. Foaling should be attended, and the mare should be observed closely for signs of dystocia.
- Postpartum treatment of the mare
  - Postpartum treatment should be directed at elimination of any infectious agent from the uterus and improving uterine clearance and involution.
  - Broad-spectrum antibacterial treatment (ie, trimethoprim-sulfamethoxazole 25–30 mg/kg q12h) may be warranted in known cases of placentitis.
  - Large-volume uterine lavage with sterile or nonsterile saline may promote uterine clearance and involution.
  - Oxytocin (5–40 IU IM q4–8h) is the most common ecbolic agent used in postpartum mares.

CHRONIC TREATMENT

Current evidence suggests that treatment should be continued until delivery.

POSSIBLE COMPLICATIONS

- Fetal death
- Dystocia
- Retained fetal membranes (RFMs)
- Retention of a dead fetus is a rare complication of therapy with altrenogest but warrants monitoring of treated mares.

RECOMMENDED MONITORING

- Mares with premature mammary development or vulvar discharge should be examined thoroughly and treated based on the identified condition. Pregnant treated mares should be examined frequently (minimum once weekly) because of their increased risk for dystocia, RFMs, and neonatal disease.
- Postpartum mares should be evaluated within 24 hours of foaling to confirm passage of the fetal membranes, systemic health, and adequate milk production.

- Neonatal foals should be examined within 24 hours of foaling to ensure adequate passive transfer of maternal antibodies and general well-being.
- Necropsy examination should be done on placentas and dead fetuses.

PROGNOSIS AND OUTCOME

- The prognosis for neonatal survival in all complications of equine pregnancy is guarded to grave.
- The prognosis for future fertility of the mare is good with appropriate postpartum care unless secondary complications occur.

PEARLS & CONSIDERATIONS

COMMENTS

Signs of premature parturition may be subtle and should be considered urgent indicators of fetal distress. Client education and routine pregnancy monitoring may minimize the occurrence or effects of these conditions.

PREVENTION

- Ultrasound-aided pregnancy examination in early gestation has dramatically reduced the prevalence of pregnancy loss caused by twins. Multiple methods are described to eliminate one co-twin at various stages in the first half of pregnancy.
- Repeated ultrasonographic examination and measurement of CTUP in late

pregnancy may enhance early diagnosis and treatment of placentitis and prevent premature delivery or abortion.

SUGGESTED READING

Macpherson ML, Bailey CS: A clinical approach to managing the mare with placentitis. *Theriogenology* 70:435, 2008.

Macpherson ML, Hayna JT, Troedsson MHT: Premature lactation in mares. In Samper JC, Pycock JF, McKinnon AO, editors: *Current therapy in equine reproduction*, St Louis, 2007, Saunders Elsevier, pp 435–440.

Wolfsdorf KE: Management of postfixation twins in mares. *Vet Clin Equine* 22:713–725, 2006.

AUTHOR: C. SCOTT BAILEY

EDITOR: JUAN C. SAMPER

Pediculosis

BASIC INFORMATION

DEFINITION

Pediculosis can be caused by either biting lice (*Damalinia equi*) or sucking lice (*Haematopinus asini*). Lice are highly host-specific obligate parasites.

SYNONYM(S)

Lice

EPIDEMIOLOGY

RISK FACTORS Groups of horses that are congregated in small or confined spaces are more likely to be affected. Animals in poor body condition and with inadequate nutrition are also more susceptible.

CONTAGION AND ZOONOSIS Animals can become infected by either direct or indirect contact.

GEOGRAPHY AND SEASONALITY Horses worldwide can be affected, with the majority showing clinical signs mostly in the winter months.

ASSOCIATED CONDITIONS AND DISORDERS Overcrowding, malnutrition, and other debilitating diseases can predispose animals to be affected by lice.

CLINICAL PRESENTATION

DISEASE FORMS/SUBTYPES Whereas biting lice (*D. equi*) prefer to live on the dorsum of the back and on the sides of the neck, sucking lice (*H. asini*) are frequently found on the mane, tail, and limbs, especially in the fetlock area.

HISTORY, CHIEF COMPLAINT The primary complaint in severely affected animals is loss of body condition with the presence of patchy alopecia that is typically the result of pruritus. In the majority of cases, the pruritus may be mild to moderate.

PHYSICAL EXAM FINDINGS Clinical signs depend on the severity and site of infestation. Pruritus is typically mild to moderate, but in severe infestation cases, pruritus will be significant and can lead to multiple areas of alopecia. Evidence of anemia can be found even with moderate sucking lice infestations.

ETIOLOGY AND PATHOPHYSIOLOGY

- Biting lice (*D. equi*) typically feed on exfoliated epithelium and skin debris.
- Sucking lice (*H. asini*) typically feed on blood and tissue fluid.

DIAGNOSIS

DIFFERENTIAL DIAGNOSIS

- Chorioptic mange
- Psoroptic mange
- *Culicoides* hypersensitivity
- *Oxyuris equi*
- Dermatophilosis
- Trombiculosis
- Poultry mite infestation
- Ringworm
- Seborrheic skin disease
- Scalding
- Shedding

INITIAL DATABASE

- Visual examination of the patient to determine the presence of nits or lice and microscopic examination to identify the species involved.
- In severe cases, skin biopsies may be obtained to differentiate from other diseases. These biopsies will reveal varying degrees of superficial perivascular to interstitial dermatitis with multiple eosinophils.
- Occasionally, epidermal necrosis, edema, leukocytic exocytosis, and intra-epidermal microabscesses may be seen.

TREATMENT

THERAPEUTIC GOAL(S)

- Eliminate both adult and louse eggs present on the animal
- Prevent infestation of other horses in the same environment

ACUTE GENERAL TREATMENT

Use of systemic ivermectin products is effective against *H. asini,* and the use of organophosphates, fipronil, topical "pour-on" ivermectin or permethrins is effective against *D. equi.* Treatment of affected and all other horses at risk is recommended.

CHRONIC TREATMENT

Treatment of both affected and at risk animals at 2-week intervals is recommended against both types of louse.

Animals need to be treated two to three times to break the life cycle of the parasite because topical treatments do not destroy the eggs, which hatch within 7 to 10 days. A total of three treatments is commonly used to eliminate both adults and eggs.

PROGNOSIS AND OUTCOME

Excellent prognosis after treatment has been established and both adults and eggs have been eradicated

PEARLS & CONSIDERATIONS

COMMENTS

All horses that have been exposed should be treated at the same time as the affected horse to prevent transmission from affected to healthy horses.

PREVENTION

Even though lice will not survive for long after they are off the host, it is important to clean and disinfect any potential fomites, such as blankets, halters, and brushes.

CLIENT EDUCATION

To prevent contamination with lice, do not share any brushes or equipment that can potentially transmit the organisms.

SUGGESTED READING

Pilsworth RC, Knottenbelt DC: Louse infestation. *Equine Vet Ed* 228–230, 2004.
White SD: Parasitic skin diseases. In Smith BP, editor: *Large animal internal medicine*, ed 4, St Louis, 2009, Mosby Elsevier, pp 1320–1321.

AUTHOR: **ALFREDO SANCHEZ LONDOÑO**

EDITOR: **DAVID A. WILSON**

Pemphigus

BASIC INFORMATION

DEFINITION

Most common autoimmune skin disease of horses. Even though it is the most common autoimmune skin disease, it accounts only for a very small percentage (<2%) of the dermatologic cases seen. The term *pemphigus* is derived from the Greek word for *blister* and is used to describe vesiculobullous disorders in the skin or mucous membranes.

EPIDEMIOLOGY

SPECIES, AGE, SEX
- Both males and females have been affected.
- The majority of affected horses are older than 5 years, but occasionally it can affect horses younger than 1 year. The age of onset of the disease is very important for prognosis because younger horses appear to be less severely affected by the disease; they tend to respond better to treatment and can spontaneously regress.
- No relationship to drug use seen in horses.

GENETICS AND BREED PREDISPOSITION Quarter Horses, Appaloosas, and Thoroughbreds seem to be overrepresented.

GEOGRAPHY AND SEASONALITY No obvious seasonal pattern, but a hint of summer recurrence

CLINICAL PRESENTATION

DISEASE FORMS/SUBTYPES
- Pemphigus foliaceous (PF), the most common of these autoimmune skin diseases
- Pemphigus vulgaris (very rare)
- Drug-induced pemphigus
- Paraneoplastic pemphigus

HISTORY, CHIEF COMPLAINT
- Presence of vesicles or pustules in the early stages, typically located over non-haired skin adjacent to mucocutaneous junctions, such as the nostrils, eyelids, or lips. These lesions can progress rapidly and develop to multifocal areas of crusting.
- Urticaria (transient, persistent, or recurrent), may be the only clinical sign and may be present for weeks before any pustules or vesicles are seen.
- Pustules are rarely seen.
- Vesicles rupture readily.
- Fever, anorexia, lethargy, and weakness are seen in up to 50% of cases.

PHYSICAL EXAM FINDINGS
- Ventral and limb edema with crusting are the most frequently recognized clinical signs. The primary lesions are pustules, which are transient and are very fragile. These pustules rupture shortly after formation, resulting in erosions, epidermal collarettes, scales, and crusts.
- Even though PF affects mucocutaneous junctions, the mucous membranes are very rarely involved.
- In severely affected horses, the entire body can be affected, and the horse may also have fever, depression, and anorexia. Horses are typically nonpruritic but can be very painful.

ETIOLOGY AND PATHOPHYSIOLOGY
- Factors that precipitate development of PF in horses are unknown.
- The main characteristic of PF is the production of autoantibodies that attack a cell adhesion protein called *desmoglein-3,* resulting in acantholysis, which leads to formation of intraepidermal clefts and vesicles.

- It has been proposed that allergen loads (pollens and insects) or the use of preventive medications such as dewormers, vaccinations, or supplements can precipitate the disease.

DIAGNOSIS

DIFFERENTIAL DIAGNOSIS

- Dermatophytosis
- Dermatophilosis
- Systemic granulomatous disease
- Seborrhea
- Epitheliotropic lymphoma
- Drug reaction
- Multisystemic eosinophilic epitheliotropic disease
- Bacterial folliculitis
- Sarcoidosis
- Lupus complex

INITIAL DATABASE

- A complete blood count may show a low-grade anemia and a mildly elevated white blood cell count.
- The location of the lesions in the limbs and ventral midline edema and the presence of vesicles or pustules can favor a clinical suspicion of PF, but further diagnostics are required to confirm the diagnosis.

ADVANCED OR CONFIRMATORY TESTING

- Skin biopsies, ideally three to four, of the affected areas for histopathologic evaluation are the most reliable diagnostic test. The most common finding is acantholytic keratinocytes, neutrophils, and eosinophils in the crusts. When obtaining these biopsies, it is important to not surgically scrub the biopsy site to prevent disruption of the

affected tissue and to ideally keep the crust attached to the underlying tissue.
- When intact pustules are present, an impression smear may be helpful to identify large numbers of acantholytic keratinocytes, which is compatible with PF but is not a confirmatory diagnosis.
- Special staining for fungi should also be submitted in all samples taken for biopsy, because dermatophytosis lesions that cause ringworm may cause microscopic lesions similar to those seen in PF.
- Direct immunofluorescent examination may show immunoglobulins deposited on the intercellular cement in a typical "chicken wire" pattern.

TREATMENT

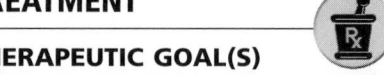

THERAPEUTIC GOAL(S)
- Decrease progression of clinical signs and eruption of new vesicles and pustules.
- Prevent development of severe disease that can cause secondary bacterial infections.
- Induce sufficient immunosuppression to cause remission of lesions with minimal side effects.

ACUTE GENERAL TREATMENT
- Corticosteroids are the treatment of choice, and dexamethasone is the first choice. The initial dose is 0.02 to 0.1 mg/kg IM; then maintenance at 0.01 to 0.02 mg/kg q48–72h IM. The dose can be gradually reduced after new lesions stop developing.
- Prednisolone can also be used, starting at a dose of 1.5 to 2.5 mg/kg/d for 7 to 10 days and then tapering over several weeks to a maintenance dose of 0.1 to 0.5 mg/kg q48h.

- Gold salts can also be used in treatment of PF. The most common one used is aurothioglucose given IM, initially once a week at a dose of 1 mg/kg of body weight. Treatment with gold salts can take up to 6 weeks for it to be effective. Corticosteroids can be used concurrently with gold salts.
- Azathioprine (3 mg/kg/d PO) may be as effective as dexamethasone. After 30 days, halve the daily dose for another 30 days.

CHRONIC TREATMENT
- It may be necessary to establish a maintenance dose of alternate-day prednisone or prednisolone at 0.5 mg/kg.
- In horses at risk of steroid-induced laminitis or horses that do not respond to glucocorticoid therapy, cyclophosphamide, chlorambucil, or cyclosporine may be of assistance.
- Consider treatment with prophylactic antibiotics.
- Some horses may require lifelong treatment.

POSSIBLE COMPLICATIONS
With the use of dexamethasone for a long period of time, it is important to consider the risk of development of laminitis.

RECOMMENDED MONITORING
Animals on immunosuppressants require regular checking of complete blood count every 2 to 3 weeks.

PROGNOSIS AND OUTCOME

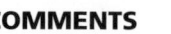

- The disease in young horses has an excellent response to initial treatment and may not require

any further treatment after it is in remission.
- Older horses have a less favorable prognosis because even with initial response to therapy and going into remission, the horse will require lifelong maintenance therapy, which can be very expensive.
- Individual responses are highly variable.
- In one study, 38% of horses were euthanized either for lack of response or for steroid-induced laminitis.

PEARLS & CONSIDERATIONS

COMMENTS
- Younger horses have the best prognosis, and it is worth treating them because the response is usually excellent and does not require any further therapy after they are in remission.
- If possible, eliminate the inciting factor, and as long as the animal is showing adequate response, medications can be tapered and eventually discontinued.

SUGGESTED READING
Olivry T: A review of autoimmune skin diseases in domestic animals: 1—superficial pemphigus. *Vet Dermatol* 17:291–305, 2006.
Stannard AA: Immunologic diseases. *Vet Dermatol* 11:163–178, 2000.
White SD: Immune mediated skin disorders. In Smith BP, editor: *Large animal internal medicine*, ed 4, St Louis, 2009, Mosby Elsevier, pp 1306–1307.
Zabel S, Mueller RS, Fieseler KV, et al: Review of 15 cases of pemphigus foliaceus in horses and a survey of the literature. *Vet Rec* 157:505–509, 2005.

AUTHOR: **ALFREDO SANCHEZ LONDOÑO** and **IAN TIZARD**

EDITOR: **DAVID A. WILSON**

Perennial Ryegrass Staggers

BASIC INFORMATION

DEFINITION
Mycotoxicosis associated with the ingestion of endophyte (*Neotyphodium lolii*)-infected perennial ryegrass (*Lolium perenne*)

SYNONYM(S)
Stagger syndrome

EPIDEMIOLOGY

GEOGRAPHY AND SEASONALITY
Perennial ryegrass is a hardy, popular grass grown for forage and seed production in many parts of the United States. Toxicoses may result from grazing contaminated pastures or ingesting contaminated hay.

CLINICAL PRESENTATION

DISEASE FORMS/SUBTYPES Clinical signs are neurologic in nature.

HISTORY, CHIEF COMPLAINT Abrupt onset of staggering, with a high percentage of animals in the group affected
PHYSICAL EXAM FINDINGS
- Fine muscle tremors of the head and neck
- Ataxic, uncoordinated jerky gait, primarily affecting the forelimbs and then the hind limbs
- Signs become worse when the animal is forced to move

ETIOLOGY AND PATHOPHYSIOLOGY
- The endophyte, *N. lolii*, is found within the lower leaf sheaths and seeds.
- The toxic substance produced by the endophyte are called lolitrems.
- Lolitrems are thought to affect the Purkinje cells and may impair inhibitory pathways in the nervous system, especially those mediated by γ-aminobutyric acid or glycine.

DIAGNOSIS

DIFFERENTIAL DIAGNOSIS
Other stagger syndromes include:
- Dallis grass staggers, Paspalum staggers
- Bermuda grass staggers
- Annual ryegrass staggers
- Phalaris staggers
- Penitrem A intoxication

INITIAL DATABASE
No specific abnormalities

ADVANCED OR CONFIRMATORY TESTING
The suspect forage material can be analyzed for the presence of the endophyte or more commonly for the presence of lolitrem.

TREATMENT

THERAPEUTIC GOAL(S)
Reduce exposure to the contaminated feed and control the tremors

ACUTE GENERAL TREATMENT
- Remove the contaminated feed material from the diet
- Allow animals to rest and relax; protect them from self-induced injuries

PROGNOSIS AND OUTCOME

- Morbidity is high, but mortality is low and generally confined to self-induced injuries.

- Most animals recover within 48 hours; some require a few weeks to return to normal.

PEARLS & CONSIDERATIONS

PREVENTION
Prevent access to endophyte-infected perennial ryegrass.

CLIENT EDUCATION
Purchase endophyte-free grass or test suspect feed for the presence of the toxin.

SUGGESTED READING
Burrows GE, Tyrl RJ: Lolium L. In Burrows GE, Tyrl RJ, editors: *Toxic plants of North America*, Ames, IA, 2001, Iowa State University, pp 906–913.

AUTHOR: **PATRICIA A. TALCOTT**

EDITOR: **CYNTHIA L. GASKILL**

Pericardial Disease

BASIC INFORMATION

DEFINITION
Diseases involving the visceral or parietal pericardial layers. There is usually some degree of inflammation of the pericardium (pericarditis), which can be associated with infectious agents, spread of contiguous disease from the lungs or pleura, congestive heart failure, sepsis, immune-mediated disease, trauma, or neoplasia.

SYNONYM(S)
- Pericarditis
- Pericardial effusion
- Cardiac tamponade

EPIDEMIOLOGY
RISK FACTORS
- Recent respiratory tract infection
- Trauma
- Septicemia or bacteremia
- Exposure to Eastern tent caterpillars (mare reproductive loss syndrome)

CONTAGION AND ZOONOSIS Many respiratory tract viruses are contagious between horses; however, there is no significant zoonotic potential for pericarditis.

GEOGRAPHY AND SEASONALITY
- Mostly sporadic
- Mare reproductive loss syndrome was seen in and around Kentucky in the spring and summer of 2001.

ASSOCIATED CONDITIONS AND DISORDERS
- Respiratory tract infections
- Sepsis
- Mare reproductive loss syndrome

CLINICAL PRESENTATION
DISEASE FORMS/SUBTYPES
- Acute
- Chronic
- Effusive
- Constrictive

HISTORY, CHIEF COMPLAINT
- History of a respiratory tract infection
- Cardiac or respiratory concerns (tachypnea, dyspnea, tachycardia, distended jugular veins)
- Nonspecific signs (exercise intolerance, fever, lethargy, reluctance to move, inappetence, weight loss, and colic)

PHYSICAL EXAM FINDINGS
- If cardiac tamponade is present, common physical examination abnormalities include those consistent with right-sided heart failure (tachycardia, jugular and other peripheral venous distension, ventral edema), poor pulses or pulsus paradoxus, variably abnormal mucous membranes (pale, injected, cyanotic), and muffled heart sounds.
- A gallop rhythm might be heard in cases of constrictive pericarditis.
- Pericardial friction rubs can be heard in cases of fibrinous pericarditis.
- Nonspecific signs in cases that may not have cardiac tamponade include fever, lethargy, tachypnea or dyspnea, and quiet lung sounds ventrally.

ETIOLOGY AND PATHOPHYSIOLOGY
- Inflammation of the pericardium may be caused by infectious agents, spread of contiguous disease from the lungs or pleura, congestive heart failure, sepsis, immune-mediated disease, trauma, or neoplasia.
- This leads to fluid accumulation within the pericardial space (effusive pericarditis) or fibrosis of the pericardial membranes (constrictive pericarditis).
- Restriction to cardiac filling occurs, which predominantly affects the right heart.
- Right-sided congestive heart failure and forward failure may occur; the latter also leads to left-sided forward failure (see "Cardiac Failure" in this section).

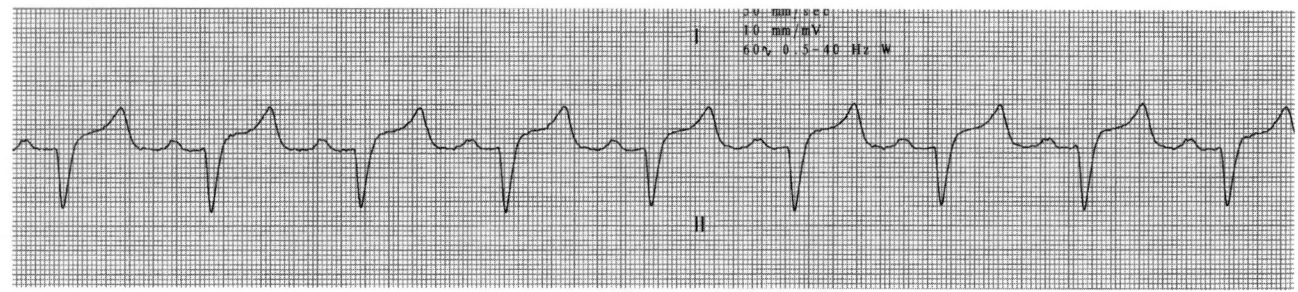

FIGURE 1 Base-apex electrocardiogram from a horse with significant pericardial effusion. Note the sinus tachycardia (heart rate, 93 beats/min) and electrical alternans; the latter has high specificity for pericardial effusion. Amplitude, 10 mm/mV; paper speed, 50 mm/sec.

DIAGNOSIS

DIFFERENTIAL DIAGNOSIS

- Right-sided heart failure: Primary myocardial, valvular, or congenital heart disease; cranial mediastinal mass
- Respiratory signs: Pulmonary or pleural disease
- Tachycardia: Primary arrhythmia such as ventricular tachycardia or supraventricular tachycardia
- Fever, anorexia, depression, weight loss: Other systemic illnesses
- Reluctance to move: Laminitis, pleuritis, colic

INITIAL DATABASE

- Complete blood count: Changes consistent with infection or inflammation or with a stress leukogram (leukocytosis, neutrophilia, lymphopenia, anemia of chronic disease, hyperfibrinogenemia)
- Chemistry panel: Changes consistent with third spacing of fluids (hypoalbuminemia, hyponatremia), congestion from right-sided heart failure (increased liver enzymes), or organ dysfunction caused by decreased cardiac output (azotemia)
- Electrocardiography (ECG): Sinus tachycardia (compensatory) and low-amplitude QRS complexes. Electrical alternans can be seen (Figure 1), although the sensitivity of this diagnostic test is low.
- Thoracic radiography: Not sensitive for a specific diagnosis of pericarditis but can show an enlarged cardiac silhouette with effusive pericarditis. Useful to assess pulmonary involvement and concurrent pneumonia or pleuropneumonia.

ADVANCED OR CONFIRMATORY TESTING

- Echocardiography: Pericardial effusion with or without excess fibrin in the pericardial space, evidence of cardiac tamponade (right atrial and ventricular diastolic collapse, respiratory variation in cardiac filling, including right-sided

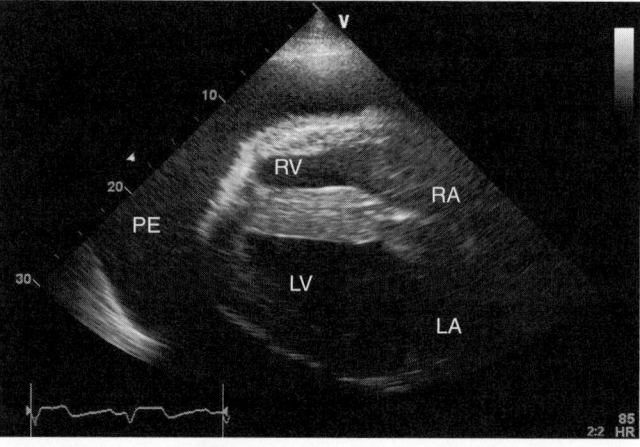

FIGURE 2 Right-sided parasternal longitudinal four-chamber echocardiographic view from a horse with pericardial effusion (*PE*). Note the large volume of hypoechoic fluid surrounding the heart and the layer of fibrin on the epicardium. This scan was acquired at 1.7 MHz and a depth of 30 cm.

increase and left-sided decrease with inspiration, volume-depleted, or "small," heart), or a thick and echoic pericardium (Figure 2)
- Pericardiocentesis: Yields fluid for analysis, including total and differential cell count and cytologic evaluation and protein concentration. Fluid should also be submitted for bacterial culture (aerobic and anaerobic) and antimicrobial susceptibility testing and viral and mycobacterial isolation (equine influenza, equine herpesvirus type 1 [EHV1], equine viral arteritis [EVA], *Mycobacterium* spp.).
- Serum titers: For upper respiratory viruses; can be assessed at the time of diagnosis and convalescent samples taken 3 to 4 weeks later (equine influenza virus, EHV-1, EVA).
- If concurrent respiratory disease is evident, cytologic analysis and bacterial and viral culture from pleural fluid and transtracheal wash fluid is important.
- Cardiac troponin I: Might be increased with myocardial involvement
- Central venous and cardiac catheterization can yield the following information:

  ○ Central venous and right atrial pressures will be significantly elevated in cases of cardiac tamponade.
  ○ On central venous or right atrial pressure tracings, the patterns of the x and y descents can differentiate effusive pericarditis (blunted y descent with prominent x descent) from constrictive pericarditis (prominent y descent followed by an abrupt rise to an increased end-diastolic pressure—the "dip and plateau").
  ○ Kussmaul's sign: Venous pressure increases rather than decreases with inspiration; this is very consistent with constrictive pericarditis.
  ○ Cardiac catheterization might show increased and equal end-diastolic pressures in the right atrium, right ventricle, and pulmonary artery.

TREATMENT

THERAPEUTIC GOAL(S)

Restore normal cardiac filling (and thereby reverse right-sided congestive heart failure and left-sided forward failure) by eliminating the pressure exerted by pericardial fluid or fibrosis.

ACUTE GENERAL TREATMENT

- Pericardial drainage and lavage in cases of effusive pericarditis (see "Pericardiocentesis" in this section).
  - If possible, pericardiocentesis should be performed with a large-bore catheter, which can be left indwelling if indicated.
  - Drainage should be complete, and lavage can be performed with 5 L of warmed isotonic fluids.
  - 1 L of fluids (with or without anti-microbials, depending on the index of suspicion for septic pericarditis) should be left in the pericardial space until the next drainage.
- Antimicrobials (intrapericardial and systemic) should be administered until septic pericarditis has been ruled out. Antimicrobials that can be instilled into the pericardial space include sodium penicillin, gentamicin, ceftiofur, ampicillin, and ticarcillin. Potassium penicillin should be avoided. Systemic antimicrobials should be broad spectrum.
- Supportive care
  - Replacement of fluids IV during or after pericardiocentesis to ensure adequate blood volume for reperfusion.
  - Nonsteroidal antiinflammatory drugs (NSAIDs) as analgesic and antiinflammatory agents.
- Note that furosemide is contraindicated in cases of cardiac tamponade; diuretics do not mobilize pericardial fluid rapidly enough to be useful and decrease preload, which is required to promote cardiac filling.

CHRONIC TREATMENT

- Pericardial drainage and lavage: The process of pericardial drainage followed by lavage with 5 L of warmed isotonic fluids should be repeated twice daily until the accumulation of fluid within the pericardial space between treatments is less than 1 L (this should be confirmed with ultrasonography) or until the tube dislodges (often 2 to 4 days in either case).
- Corticosteroids: Antiinflammatory doses of corticosteroids can be considered after septic pericarditis has been ruled out. This treatment is aimed at reducing the immune-mediated sequelae and inflammation associated with viral infections and idiopathic pericarditis.
- Other reported therapies include heparin, colchicine, pentoxifylline, and vitamin E.

- If constrictive pericarditis develops, surgical pericardiectomy or pericardial stripping is required.

DRUG INTERACTIONS

- If instilling penicillin into the pericardial space, it should be sodium penicillin rather than potassium penicillin because the latter can increase the likelihood of cardiac arrhythmias.
- The coincident use of NSAIDs and corticosteroids should be carefully considered.

POSSIBLE COMPLICATIONS

- Immediate complications associated with pericardiocentesis include arrhythmias and cardiac puncture with subsequent blood loss into the pericardial space.
- Later complications of pericardiocentesis include the risk of introducing air (pneumopericardium) or bacterial infection (septic pericarditis) into the pericardial space via an indwelling catheter.
- Fluid shifts associated with draining pericardial fluid very rapidly can lead to hemodynamic consequences (significant hypotension).

RECOMMENDED MONITORING

- IV access should be established before pericardiocentesis.
- Continuous ECG monitoring should be used throughout the procedure.
- After it is in place, the pericardial tube should be closely monitored until it is removed.
- Ideally, daily echocardiographic examinations should be performed to assess tube placement, the volume and character of residual fluid after draining, and cardiac function. They should be continued after catheter removal to ensure that significant fluid does not re-accumulate.
- After the horse is at home, horses should be monitored for a reoccurrence of pericardial effusion via heart rate, heart sounds, pulse quality, and jugular vein distension. Any changes should prompt an immediate veterinary reexamination.

PROGNOSIS AND OUTCOME

- Good for horses with viral, immune-mediated, or idiopathic pericarditis

- Fair to guarded for horses with septic or traumatic pericarditis and for constrictive pericarditis
- Poor for horses with neoplastic pericarditis and constrictive pericarditis with a large amount of mature fibrous tissue

PEARLS & CONSIDERATIONS

COMMENTS

- The classic triad of clinical signs (Beck's triad) in cases of cardiac tamponade includes muffled heart sounds, venous distension, and weak arterial pulses.
- Pericardiocentesis is the most important therapeutic procedure in cases of cardiac tamponade.
- Equine pericarditis is often categorized as idiopathic because we cannot identify the underlying etiology. As our diagnostics continue to improve, we may be able to specifically diagnose (and therefore specifically treat) more cases of pericarditis in horses.

PREVENTION

To date, there is no known preventive strategy for equine pericarditis with the exception of maintaining a good vaccination program to limit predisposing respiratory infections and limiting exposure to Eastern tent caterpillars during high-risk years.

CLIENT EDUCATION

An optimal outcome requires early recognition; if any nonspecific signs are noted within a few weeks of a respiratory tract infection, consultation with a veterinarian should be sought.

SUGGESTED READING

LeWinter MM: Pericardial diseases. In Libby P, Bonow RO, Mann DL, et al, editors: *Heart disease: a textbook of cardiovascular medicine,* ed 8, Philadelphia, 2008, Saunders Elsevier, pp 1829–1855.

Slovis NM: Clinical observations of the pericarditis syndrome. In *Proceedings of First Workshop Mare Reproductive Loss Syndrome,* 2002, pp 18–20.

Worth LT, Reef VB: Pericarditis in horses: 18 cases (1986–1995), *J Am Vet Med Assoc* 212:248–253, 1998.

AUTHOR: **SOPHY A. JESTY**

EDITOR: **MARY M. DURANDO**

Perineal Conformation

BASIC INFORMATION

DEFINITION

The perineum is the body wall surrounding the pelvic outlet, anal canal, and urogenital passage. The vulva is composed of the labia and clitoris. Normal conformation is required for normal reproductive health. The vulvar lips should meet evenly to form a tight mucosal seal, and two thirds of the vulvar cleft should lie below the pelvic floor. The vulvar lips should be vertical with no more than a 10-degree slope from cranial to caudal.

SYNONYM(S)

Vulvar anatomy, angle of declination (slope to vulvar lips)

EPIDEMIOLOGY

SPECIES, AGE, SEX

- All Equids used for breeding should be assessed for normal perineal conformation.
- An increase in age results in elongation of the vulvar opening and an increase in slope caused by ligament and muscle relaxation.
- An increase in parity may result in stretching and trauma to the reproductive structures.

GENETICS AND BREED PREDISPOSITION

- Thoroughbreds and American Saddlebreds have an increased likelihood to have more angulation to the vulva.
- Quarter Horses and Standardbreds are more likely to have vertical orientation to the vulva.

RISK FACTORS

- Repeated vulvoplasty results in vulvar trauma and scarring, often requiring vulvoplasty in subsequent breeding seasons.
- Dystocia or natural cover leading to perineal trauma.
- Trauma to the perineum may result in permanent vulvar pathology.
- Underweight resulting in decreased intrapelvic fat.
- Flat croup or elevated tail results in more vulvar angulation.
- Neoplasia altering the apposition of the vulvar labia.

GEOGRAPHY AND SEASONALITY

- Mares under the influence of estrogen will have decreased vulvar tone.
- Mares under the influence of progesterone will have increased vulvar tone.

ASSOCIATED CONDITIONS AND DISORDERS

Poor perineal conformation may lead to subfertility or infertility associated with pneumovagina, urovagina, fecal contamination with subsequent endometritis, cervicitis, or placentitis. The most common neoplasias of the external genitalia are squamous cell carcinoma, melanoma, and papillomas. Trauma may occur during parturition, resulting in various degrees of perineal lacerations.

CLINICAL PRESENTATION

HISTORY, CHIEF COMPLAINT

- Abnormal conformation
  - Unsuccessful breeding attempts
  - Vulvar discharge
  - Vulvar air aspiration during riding or when working
  - Discharge present on base of tail
  - Pre- or postbreeding endometritis
  - Early embryonic death
- Neoplasia
  - Vulvar discharge
  - Swollen vulva
  - Perineal or vulvar mass(es)
  - Ulcerations on vulva

PHYSICAL EXAM FINDINGS

- More than one-third of the vulvar cleft dorsal to the pelvic floor
- Greater than 10-degree slope of the vulvar lips from cranial to caudal
- Urine pooling on vaginal speculum examination
- Positive windsucker test result: Aspiration of air into the vagina upon separation of the vulvar lips
- Vulvar discharge present on vulvar lips or ventral base of the tail
- Disruption of normal vulvar mucosal seal
- Caslick's index greater than 150: Taken by multiplying the length (in centimeters) of the vulvar opening above the pelvic floor by the angle of declination of the vulva
- Presence of air or fluid on ultrasonographic examination of the uterus

ETIOLOGY AND PATHOPHYSIOLOGY

- Poor perineal conformation may be a result of genetics, trauma, age-related weakening of the muscular and neurologic control, or development of neoplasia.
- Compromise of the normal vulvar seal eliminates the first barrier between the external environment and the uterus, allowing contaminants access.
- Vaginal contamination may lead to ascending infection or inflammation, resulting in vaginitis, cervicitis, endometritis, or placentitis.

DIAGNOSIS

DIFFERENTIAL DIAGNOSIS

- Perineal lacerations
- Rectovaginal fistulas
- Perineal abscess
- Perineal neoplasia or tumor
- Hematoma
- Varicosity
- Urovagina
- Vestibular trauma postfoaling

INITIAL DATABASE

- External perineal conformation examination, including evaluation of the vulvar seal, angle of the vulva, and location of the pelvic brim, and calculation of Caslick's index (Length of vulva (cm) × Angle of declination)
- Windsucker test
- Internal examination, including palpation of the internal genitalia per rectum, manual vaginal examination, vaginal speculum, and ultrasonography per rectum of the reproductive tract and associated soft tissue

ADVANCED OR CONFIRMATORY TESTING

- Uterine culture and sensitivity
- Uterine biopsy
- Vaginoscopy using an endoscope
- Biopsy of soft tissue mass
- Ultrasonography of soft tissue mass

TREATMENT

THERAPEUTIC GOAL(S)

- Correction of abnormal conformation to reestablish a protective barrier at the level of the vulva
- Elimination of internal contamination or inflammation

ACUTE GENERAL TREATMENT

- Abnormal conformation
  - Caslick's vulvoplasty
  - Placement of staples for temporary vulvoplasty
  - Treatment of secondary infection or inflammation
- Trauma
  - Nonsteroidal antiinflammatory drugs
  - Antibiotics
  - Ointments (eg, Vaseline, silver sulfadiazine) applied to the external ulceration to prevent tail abrasion
- Neoplasia
  - Cryosurgical removal (melanomas or papillomas)

- ○ Intralesional cisplatin (melanoma)
- ○ Oral cimetidine (melanoma)
- ○ Surgical excision followed by topical 5-fluoruracil (squamous cell carcinoma)
- ○ Benign neglect (nonmalignant melanoma or papillomas)

CHRONIC TREATMENT

- Episioplasty (deep Caslick's index, Gadd technique, or perineal body reconstruction)
- Perineal body transection (Pouret's perineal reconstruction)
- Caudal relocation of the transverse Fold (Monin urethroplasty)
- Urethral extension (Brown, Shires, McKinnon, or combined McKinnon and Brown techniques)

POSSIBLE COMPLICATIONS

- Inadequate vulvar seal
- Formation of excessive scar tissue
- Rectovaginal or urethrovaginal fistulas
- Nerve damage

RECOMMENDED MONITORING

- Normal postsurgical monitoring for excessive inflammation and development of infection at the surgical site
- Monitor for development of fistulation

PROGNOSIS AND OUTCOME

- Good reproductive prognosis if able to reestablish external barrier and eliminate infection pending uterine culture or cytology and biopsy results
- May require repeated vulvoplasty or reconstructive surgical correction depending on the degree of alteration of the normal vulvar seal

PEARLS & CONSIDERATIONS

COMMENTS

- Normal perineal conformation is imperative for good reproductive health.
- Elimination of mares with abnormal conformation from breeding stock will help decrease the number of mares needing vulvoplasty treatment caused by genetic factors.
- Correction of abnormal conformation is required to reestablish good reproductive health.

PREVENTION

- Quick correction of dystocia
- Proper surgical technique when performing routine vulvoplasty

CLIENT EDUCATION

Clients should understand the importance of normal perineal conformation in the prevention of ascending infection or inflammation, leading to poor reproductive health.

SUGGESTED READING

Caslick EA: The vulva and vulvo-vaginal orifice and its relation to genital health of the Thoroughbred mare, *Cornell Vet* 27: 178–187, 1937.

Easley J: External perineal conformation. In McKinnon AO, Voss JL, editors: *Equine reproduction, 1993*, Philadelphia, 1993, Lea & Febiger, pp 20–24.

Miller CD: Infectious and neoplastic conditions of the vulva and perineum. In Samper JP, Pycock JF, McKinnon AO, editors: *Current therapy in equine reproduction*, St Louis, 2007, Saunders Elsevier, pp 161–165.

Pascoe RR: Observations on the length and angle of declination of the vulva and its relation to fertility in the mare, *J Reprod Fertil Suppl* 27:299–305, 1979.

Woodie B: Vulva, vestibule, vagina, and cervix. In Auer JA, Stick JA, editors: *Equine surgery*, St Louis, 2006, Elsevier, pp 835–855.

AUTHORS: LEEAH R. CHEW and **JOHN J. DASCANIO**

EDITOR: JUAN C. SAMPER

Perineal Injury

BASIC INFORMATION

DEFINITION

Traumatic wound(s) to the perineal and perianal area

SYNONYMS

- Perineal lacerations (first, second, and third degree)
- Rectovestibular fistulas (rectovaginal fistulas)

EPIDEMIOLOGY

SPECIES, AGE, SEX Brood mares
RISK FACTORS

- Primiparous mares
- Highly strung mares
- Unassisted foaling

CLINICAL PRESENTATION

DISEASE FORMS/SUBTPES

- First-degree perineal injury: Lesions involve only the mucosa of the vestibule and the skin at the dorsal commissure of the vulva.

- Second-degree perineal injury: Lesions involve the vestibular mucosa and submucosa as well as continuing into the musculature of the perineal body (including the constrictor vulvae muscle). The rectum and anal sphincter remain intact.
- Third-degree perineal injury: Lesions penetrate into the rectum through disruption of the rectovestibular shelf. These lesions also continue through the perineal body and anal sphincter and therefore cause a common rectal and vestibular opening.
- Rectovestibular fistula: Lesions penetrate into the rectum through disruption of the rectovestibular shelf; however, the perineal body and anal sphincter remain intact.

HISTORY, CHIEF COMPLAINT

- Foaling; normally unassisted foaling
- Visible lesions in the perianal area: Tearing of perianal tissues, swelling of perianal tissues distorting anatomy, hemorrhage or complete loss of

normal anatomy with formation of a common rectal and vestibulovulval opening

- Pain on defecation
- Fecal retention in vestibule
- Sucking sound from vestibular area

PHYSICAL EXAM FINDINGS

- Heart rate may be normal or may be elevated.
- Temperature is most frequently normal.
- The mucous membranes are often pale pink and moist.
- May have no colic signs or may demonstrate mild colic signs secondary to constipation and decreased fecal output.
- Swelling, hemorrhage, and pain on palpation of perineal area.
- Distortion of the perineal area.

ETIOLOGY AND PATHOPHYSIOLOGY

- Although perineal injuries can be rarely associated with malicious behavior, self–trauma, or breeding injuries, most are associated with foaling.

- Increased risk if there is a persistent hymen or a prominent vestibulovaginal sphincter in mares that are foaling for the first time.
- Passage of the foal's foot through the vestibule can be hindered by a prominent dorsal transverse fold of the vestibulovaginal junction. If the mare contracts to expel the fetus, the foal's foot can be forced into the roof of the vestibule causing injury.

DIAGNOSIS

DIFFERENTIAL DIAGNOSIS

- Colic caused by a gastrointestinal (GI) complication of parturition such as entrapment or damage to GI structures (most commonly the small colon)
- Vestibular bruising
- Vestibular hematomas
- Excessive vulvar stretching

INITIAL DATABASE

- Complete blood count: Leukopenia or leukocytosis common; occasionally normal
- Vaginal examination: Compromise of the perianal area varies depending on the degree of the perianal injury
- First- and second-degree injuries isolated to the reproductive tract
- Third-degree injuries also involve the rectum
- Rectal evaluation
  - As for the vaginal examination, compromise of the perianal area is variable depending on the degree of the perianal injury.
  - Fecal retention may be palpable within the small colon.

TREATMENT

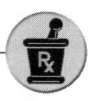

THERAPEUTIC GOAL(S)

Restore normal perineal conformation

ACUTE GENERAL TREATMENT

- First-degree injury
  - Tetanus prophylaxis
  - Local wound care
  - Possibly including a Caslick procedure
  - Antiinflammatories (flunixin meglumine, 1.1 mg/kg IV q12h)
  - Laxative diet
- Second-degree injury
  - Tetanus prophylaxis
  - Local wound care

  - Including a Caslick procedure
  - Antiinflammatories (flunixin meglumine, 1.1 mg/kg IV q12h)
  - Laxative diet
- Third-degree injury or rectovestibular fistula
  - Tetanus prophylaxis
  - Local wound care
  - Antiinflammatories (flunixin meglumine, 1.1 mg/kgIV q12h)
  - Laxative diet

CHRONIC TREATMENT

- First- and second-degree injury: Removal of the Caslick and a prebreeding examination.
- Third-degree injury: Only consider surgical repair after local wound care and debridement.
  - Four to 6 weeks minimum between injury and repair.
  - Delaying repair until the foal is weaned prevents the necessity for a healthy foal to enter the hospital.
  - Fecal consistency must be soft before repair (fresh grass, pelleted feeds, mineral oil ± magnesium sulphate).
  - Repair can be achieved as a one- or two-stage procedure under standing sedation and local epidural anesthesia.
    - One-stage repair: Repair of the rectovaginal shelf and perineal body occur concurrently; however, this can predispose to obstipation, causing repair failure.
    - Two-stage repair: Repair of the rectovaginal shelf occurs followed by repair of the perineal body 3 to 4 weeks later.
  - Maintain soft fecal consistency for 2 to 3 weeks postoperatively.
  - A prebreeding examination is recommended before breeding because of the uterine contamination subsequent to the perineal injury; however, most mares "clear" their uteri after repair.
  - Breeding should preferably be delayed for 8 to 12 weeks after repair.
- Rectovestibular fistulas
  - Only consider surgical repair after local wound care and debridement.
    - Three to 4 weeks minimum between injury and repair
    - Delaying repair until the foal is weaned prevents the necessity for a healthy foal to enter the hospital.

  - Fecal consistency must be soft before repair (fresh grass, pelleted feeds, mineral oil ± magnesium sulphate).
  - A third-degree perineal injury can be created and closed as above under standing sedation and caudal epidural.
  - Alternatively, a vaginal mucosal pedicle graft can be used to close the defect.
  - After care is as for third-degree perineal injuries.

POSSIBLE COMPLICATIONS

- Repair breakdown
- Pneumovagina
- Obstipation
- Straining: Prolapse of viscera (eg, the bladder)
- Uterine contamination: Decreased conception
- Suture line abscessation
- Stricture formation
- Recurrence

RECOMMENDED MONITORING

- Pain
- Fecal output and consistency and any blood on feces or in urine
- Colic
- Prebreeding examinations

PROGNOSIS AND OUTCOME

- First-degree injuries have a good prognosis.
- Second-degree injuries: Mares will develop a sunken perineum and be predisposed to pneumovagina and urovagina if the perineal body is not reconstructed with a Caslick procedure.
- Third-degree injuries
  - Good fertility rates after repair
  - Possibility of recurrence with subsequent parturition

SUGGESTED READING

Schweizer CM: Colic in the parturient mare. In Mair TS, Divers T, Ducharme N, editors: *Manual of equine gastroenterology*, St Louis, 2002, Saunders Elsevier, pp 357–363.

Woodie B: Vulva, vestibule, vagina and cervix. In Auer JA, Stick JA, editors: *Equine surgery*, ed 3, St Louis, 2006, Saunders Elsevier, pp 853–864.

AUTHOR: CERI SHERLOCK

EDITORS: TIM MAIR and CERI SHERLOCK

Peritonitis

BASIC INFORMATION

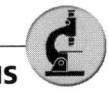

DEFINITION

Focal or generalized inflammation of the peritoneal cavity

CLINICAL PRESENTATION

HISTORY, CHIEF COMPLAINT
- Inappetence
- Depression
- Colic
- Fever

PHYSICAL EXAM FINDINGS
- Fever
- Variable tachycardia and tachypnea
- Depression
- Variable signs of abdominal pain (often mild)
- Decreased gastrointestinal (GI) borborygmi
- Variable signs of endotoxemia (injected, hyperemic to purple mucous membranes; prolonged capillary refill time; cool extremities)
- Ventral edema may be present.
- Rectal examination is usually within normal limits, although the presence of intestinal distension or an intraabdominal mass may be noted if peritonitis is secondary to intestinal obstruction or an intraabdominal abscess.

ETIOLOGY AND PATHOPHYSIOLOGY

- Peritonitis is classified as aseptic or septic and can be focal or diffuse.
- Some degree of aseptic peritonitis occurs after abdominal surgery (and routine castration) caused by inflammation induced by invasion of the peritoneal cavity and intestinal handling. This usually resolves without specific therapy.
- Uroperitoneum caused by bladder or ureteral rupture can also induce peritoneal inflammation and result in aseptic peritonitis.
- There are a variety of causes of septic (bacterial) peritonitis, including:
  - Inflammatory or obstructive intestinal disease, resulting in disruption of the intestinal mucosal barrier and translocation of enteric bacteria
  - Perforation of the GI tract caused by ulceration or obstructive disease
  - Peritonitis due to intestinal rupture results in endotoxic or septic shock, leading to rapid systemic compromise and death within 2 to 24 hours
- Systemic bacterial infection
  - *Actinobacillus* spp. frequently causes peritonitis in the absence of infection in other body systems in adult horses.
  - *Streptococcus equi, Rhodococcus equi,* and *Corynebacterium pseudotuberculosis* may cause intraabdominal abscessation with or without associated peritonitis.
- Iatrogenic after enterocentesis during attempted abdominocentesis or after celiotomy
- Penetrating intestinal foreign body (rare)

DIAGNOSIS

DIFFERENTIAL DIAGNOSIS

Enterocolitis

INITIAL DATABASE

- Passage of a nasogastric tube: Gastric reflux (>2–4 L) is occasionally observed in severe, acute peritonitis caused by intestinal ileus but is not consistently observed.
- Complete blood count: Leukocyte count is variable but usually abnormal.
  - Leukopenia (neutropenia) and toxic changes in neutrophils are typical in acute, septic peritonitis cases.
  - Leukocytosis characterized by a mature neutrophilia and hyperfibrinogenemia are seen in more chronic septic peritonitis and those with intraabdominal abscesses.
- Serum biochemistry profile: No consistent abnormalities; variable azotemia and electrolyte or acid-base derangements may be present depending on the severity of endotoxemia and the underlying disease.
- Peritoneal fluid analysis
  - Peritoneal fluid is often grossly cloudy and yellow to orange to pink in color. A foul odor suggests intestinal perforation or anaerobic infection.
  - Increased total protein concentration (>2 g/dL) and increased nucleated cell count (15,000 to >500,000 cells/μL)
  - Cytologic evaluation reveals a predominance of neutrophils. Free or phagocytosed bacteria are frequently but not always seen. The presence of plant material and a mixed population of extracellular bacteria is consistent with GI rupture.
  - A sample should be submitted for aerobic and anaerobic bacterial culture, although culture results are occasionally negative even in septic peritonitis.

- Transabdominal ultrasonography
  - Variable findings. Should be performed to evaluate for the presence of an intraabdominal abscess or other abnormalities but can be within normal limits
  - An increased amount of variably echogenic free peritoneal fluid is often but not always appreciated.
- Exploratory celiotomy: Indicated in cases with recurrent peritonitis or those in which intestinal perforation or strangulating obstruction is suspected

TREATMENT

THERAPEUTIC GOAL(S)

- Treat the primary disease or underlying cause.
- Broad-spectrum antimicrobial therapy
- Supportive care to manage abdominal pain, hypovolemia, dehydration, and metabolic derangements as indicated

ACUTE GENERAL TREATMENT

- Broad-spectrum antimicrobial therapy: Initial therapy should be aggressive and include the following:
  - Potassium penicillin (22,000–44,000 IU/kg IV q6h) or ampicillin (22 mg/kg IV q8h) and gentamicin (6.6 mg/kg IV q24h) or enrofloxacin (5 mg/kg IV q24h) and metronidazole (15–20 mg/kg PO or PR q6–8h).
  - Initial antimicrobial therapy may ultimately be tailored according to culture results.
- Flunixin meglumine
  - 0.5 to 1.1 mg/kg IV q12h for 1 to 3 days for analgesic and antiinflammatory effects
  - May be continued at 0.25 mg/kg IV q6–8h for continued antiinflammatory effects for an additional 3 to 5 days
- Additional antiendotoxic therapy is indicated in horses with clinical signs associated with endotoxemia and may include:
  - Polymixin-B (2000–6000 IU/kg IV q12h)
  - Endoserum (1–2 mL/kg diluted in 3–5 L IV fluids once) or equine plasma (regular or from horses hyperimmunized against endotoxin, 2–4 L IV slowly once)
- Supportive care
  - Initial fluid resuscitation may include isotonic crystalloids (25–50 mL/kg IV bolus), hypertonic saline (2–4 mL/kg IV once) or hetastarch (5–10 mL/kg IV bolus once)

○ Should be followed by balanced polyionic crystalloid IV fluids at 100 to 200 mL/kg/d until rehydration is established and then at 50 to 100 mL/kg/d for maintenance as needed

○ Laminitis prophylaxis with frog supports, deep bedding, and maintenance in ice boots for 1 to 2 days may be initiated in horses with signs of severe endotoxemia.

• Surgical treatment and abdominal lavage

○ Although horses with primary peritonitis are usually managed medically, exploratory celiotomy is indicated after stabilization if peritonitis secondary to a surgical lesion is suspected.

○ Surgical placement of an abdominal drain or serial abdominal lavage may be indicated in cases with severe septic peritonitis.

• Severe, acute peritonitis caused by GI rupture carries a grave prognosis because of overwhelming abdominal contamination and septic shock. Thus, humane euthanasia is indicated in horses exhibiting severe systemic compromise with peritoneal fluid analysis consistent with GI rupture. Exploratory celiotomy can be performed to confirm GI rupture but may be precluded by humane considerations.

CHRONIC TREATMENT

Appropriate duration of antimicrobial therapy depends on the underlying cause, severity of disease, and causative organism.

• A 7- to 14-day course of therapy is often effective in uncomplicated primary peritonitis or cases secondary to enterocentesis.

• Long-term parenteral or oral antimicrobial therapy may be indicated in horses with intraabdominal abscessation or severe peritonitis.

• Serial peritoneal fluid analysis should be performed to assess the response to treatment and guide the duration of therapy.

POSSIBLE COMPLICATIONS

• Intraabdominal adhesions
• Laminitis

PROGNOSIS AND OUTCOME

• Good for primary peritonitis and horses that exhibit a rapid response to medical therapy.

• Guarded to grave if peritonitis occurs secondary to intestinal perforation or severe intestinal inflammatory disease.

PEARLS & CONSIDERATIONS

• Peritonitis should be considered as a differential diagnosis in any horse with mild colic, depression, and fever.

• The absence of cytologic evidence of bacteria on peritoneal fluid analysis and negative bacteria culture results does not definitely rule out septic peritonitis. An appropriate course of antimicrobial therapy should thus be administered if the peritoneal fluid nucleated cell count is moderately to severely increased.

SUGGESTED READING

Mueller POE, Moore JN, Diver TJ: Peritonitis, In Orsini JA, Divers TJ, editors: *Equine emergencies: treatments and procedures*, ed 3, St Louis, 2008, Saunders Elsevier, pp 154–155.

AUTHOR: **KELSEY A. HART**

EDITORS: **TIM MAIR** and **CERI SHERLOCK**

Persistent Right Aortic Arch

BASIC INFORMATION

DEFINITION

Rare congenital abnormality in which the right fourth aortic arch becomes the definitive aorta instead of the left aortic arch. The esophagus becomes constricted by the ligamentum arteriosum as it extends between the anomalous right aorta and the left pulmonary artery.

SYNONYM(S)

• Vascular ring anomaly
• Vascular compression of the esophagus

EPIDEMIOLOGY

SPECIES, AGE, SEX Foals, weanlings, and yearlings

CLINICAL PRESENTATION

HISTORY, CHIEF COMPLAINT Clinical signs of persistent right aortic arch are the result of esophageal dysphagia: Excessive salivation, retching (repeated flexion and extension of the neck), coughing, and discharge of milk or food and saliva from the nostrils. Affected foals are usually stunted and fail to thrive. Secondary inhalation pneumonia may result in chronic cough and purulent nasal discharge.

PHYSICAL EXAM FINDINGS

• In addition to the presenting signs, there may be a palpable swelling of the cervical esophagus (megaesophagus).

• Examination of the chest may reveal evidence of inhalation pneumonia.

ETIOLOGY AND PATHOPHYSIOLOGY

Congenital abnormality in which the right fourth aortic arch becomes the definitive aorta instead of the left aortic arch. The esophagus becomes constricted by the ligamentum arteriosum as it extends between the anomalous right aorta and the left pulmonary artery. Occasionally, other vascular ring anomalies may cause similar signs.

DIAGNOSIS

DIFFERENTIAL DIAGNOSIS

• Other causes of dysphagia in foals, especially gastrointestinal ulcer disease and cleft palate
• Megaesophagus

INITIAL DATABASE

• The leukogram and hematology results are likely to be normal unless there is dehydration from chronic dysphagia or inhalation pneumonia (in which case there is likely to be leucocytosis and neutrophilia).

• Confirmation of esophageal compression can be made by endoscopic examination. The esophagus appears dilated proximal to the obstruction. There is evidence of esophagitis.

• Radiography (contrast esophagraphy) reveals dilatation of the distal cervical esophagus and cranial thoracic esophagus proximal to the obstruction at the heart base.

ADVANCED OR CONFIRMATORY TESTING

Radiographic assessment of the lungs should be performed to identify inhalation pneumonia.

TREATMENT

THERAPEUTIC GOAL(S)

- Surgical correction
- Medical treatment of inhalation pneumonia

ACUTE GENERAL TREATMENT

Surgical correction should be undertaken as soon as possible after the diagnosis has been reached. A thoracotomy is performed, and the ligamentum arteriosum and any other constricting bands around the esophagus are resected.

RECOMMENDED MONITORING

During treatment, horses should be monitored for signs of dehydration, weight loss, signs of infection (especially pneumonia), or surgical dehiscence.

PROGNOSIS AND OUTCOME

The prognosis is poor with conservative or medical treatment but fair with surgical treatment.

PEARLS & CONSIDERATIONS

Attempted surgical treatment should be undertaken as early as possible to minimize the effects of inhalation pneumonia and stunted growth.

SUGGESTED READING

Butt TD, MacDonald DG, Crawford WH, et al: Persistent right aortic arch in a yearling horse, *Can Vet J* 39:714, 1998.
Sanchez LC: Esophageal diseases. In Reed SM, Bayly WM, Sellon DC, editors: *Equine internal medicine*, ed 3, St Louis, 2010, Saunders Elsevier, pp 800–838.
Smith TR: Unusual vascular ring anomaly in a foal. *Can Vet J* 45:1016, 2004.
van der Linde-Sipman JS, Goedegebuure SA, Kroneman J: Persistent right aortic arch associated with a left ductus arteriosus and interventricular septal defect in a horse. *Tijdschr Diergeneeskd* 104(suppl 4):189, 1979.

AUTHOR: **TIM MAIR**

EDITORS: **TIM MAIR** and **CERI SHERLOCK**

Petroleum Product Toxicosis

BASIC INFORMATION

DEFINITION

Petroleum is a complex mixture of hydrocarbons that can be in a gaseous (sweet gas or sour gas with hydrogen sulfide, ethane, methane, propane), liquid (crude and refined oils) or solid form (bitumen, asphalt). Exposure to petroleum mixtures can be from ingestion, inhalation, or ocular or dermal contact and can cause adverse effects primarily in the gastrointestinal (GI), respiratory, and nervous systems. Refined petroleum products (eg, gasoline, kerosene, diesel, petroleum naphtha and distillates) may contain additional toxic compounds, including heavy metals, surfactants-emulsifiers, anti-wear additives, and antioxidants.

EPIDEMIOLOGY

RISK FACTORS

- Accidental releases from petroleum facilities or pipelines could result in petroleum contamination of soil, forage, water, and air. Iatrogenic dermal exposures may occur if horses are pastured in fields with "cattle oilers" or "back rubbers" containing pesticides and petroleum distillates. Oral exposures may result from "folk remedy" dosing with petroleum products.
- Petroleum products with lower viscosity, defined as resistance to flow, and higher volatility or ability to vaporize are more likely to produce inhalation or aspiration into the lungs and pneumonia. These products include naphtha, kerosene, gasoline, diesel fuel, fuel oil No. 2, and paint thinners.
- The toxicity of petroleum hydrocarbons is quite variable. Low-viscosity, volatile hydrocarbons can cause aspiration pneumonia at a very low dose; clinical signs and death can be acute. In other cases with exposure to longer chain hydrocarbons, chronic ill thrift may be the predominant sign.

CLINICAL PRESENTATION

DISEASE FORMS/SUBTYPES Depending on the route of exposure, clinical signs may be primarily:
- GI
- Neurologic (petroleum products with lighter chain hydrocarbons and aromatic hydrocarbons)
- Respiratory

HISTORY, CHIEF COMPLAINT
- Oral exposures may result in anorexia, weight loss, diarrhea or constipation, lethargy, unthriftiness, depression, ataxia, laminitis, seizures and hyperactivity, and death. Aspiration pneumonia may lead to chronic pneumonia and pleural adhesions. Animals may show damage to the hepatic and renal systems. Abortions and impaired reproduction have been reported in ruminants.
- Inhalation exposure may cause coughing, rhinitis, dyspnea, pneumonia, anorexia, unthriftiness, lethargy, depression, and death.
- Ocular and dermal exposures may lead to inflammation, blisters, and ulcerations of epithelium.

PHYSICAL EXAM FINDINGS
- Hyperthermia
- Dehydration
- Dyspnea, coughing, salivating, and bronchospasms
- Lethargy and depression
- Seizures and hyperactivity
- Ataxia and incoordination
- Diarrhea, bloody diarrhea, and colic
- Cachexia
- Pneumonia, particularly of the ventral portions of the lungs
- Cardiac arrhythmias
- Ocular inflammation and ulcers
- Dermal inflammation, blisters, and ulceration
- May observe petroleum around the perianal region or tail
- May smell petroleum hydrocarbons on the breath, from the skin, and in urine and feces
- Death

ETIOLOGY AND PATHOPHYSIOLOGY
- Many hydrocarbons are readily absorbed after oral and percutaneous exposures and can be distributed to all major organ systems. Respiration is an important route of elimination of volatile hydrocarbons, regardless of the route of exposure. Volatile hydrocarbons may displace alveolar oxygen and produce acute cyanosis.

- The potential for aspiration pneumonia and pulmonary damage from oral exposure can be life threatening. Petroleum hydrocarbons act on the lipid membranes of cells in contact with the hydrocarbon and cause swelling and necrosis. This can lead to lung edema, bronchospasms, hemorrhage, thrombosis, emphysema, and secondary bacterial pneumonia.
- Less volatile petroleum products may remain in the GI tract for a period of time and cause GI irritation.
- A limited amount of metabolism occurs in the liver and kidney. Some hydrocarbons are excreted in bile and urine.
- Nervous system signs are related to the direct interaction between the petroleum hydrocarbon and the neuronal membranes. These clinical signs can appear acutely.
- Cardiac arrhythmias are thought to result from hydrocarbons sensitizing the myocardium to endogenous catecholamines.

DIAGNOSIS

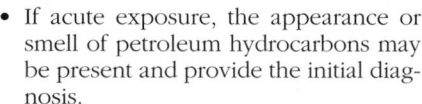

DIFFERENTIAL DIAGNOSIS

- If acute exposure, the appearance or smell of petroleum hydrocarbons may be present and provide the initial diagnosis.
- Viral or bacterial pneumonia
- Sodium ion toxicity
- Nutritional deficiencies, parasitism

INITIAL DATABASE

Monitor the complete blood count and serum biochemistry profile for hemoconcentration, elevated blood urea nitrogen, and increased liver enzyme activities. An initial leukopenia may be followed within 48 to 72 hours later by a relative increase in neutrophils.

ADVANCED OR CONFIRMATORY TESTING

- Petroleum hydrocarbons may be seen grossly and smelled in the GI tract. Lesions may include ulcers and areas of inflammation and hemorrhage.
- Pathologic changes in the lungs include hemorrhage, pulmonary consolidation, emphysema, atelectasis, bronchopneumonia, alveolitis, necrosis, and sometimes the appearance of visible oil.
- Pathologic changes in the liver include swelling, fatty change, and centrilobular congestion.
- Lesions in the kidneys caused by petroleum toxicosis may include tubu-lonephrosis, renal vascular thrombi, and tubular epithelial necrosis.

TREATMENT

THERAPEUTIC GOAL(S)

Remove animals from the source of exposure. Keep the animal quiet and in an area where clinical signs can be monitored. Watch for respiratory signs, which should be treated immediately.

ACUTE GENERAL TREATMENT

- Activated charcoal or mineral oil is of limited value in binding or diluting petroleum hydrocarbons after an oral exposure.
- Treat aspiration pneumonia; use antibiotics to prevent secondary bacterial infections. Oxygen therapy may be required.
- With dermal exposure to petroleum hydrocarbons, wash the affected area with a nonsolvent, mild detergent and use copious amounts of warm water. In horses with ocular exposure, wash the eyes with saline for 10 to 15 minutes.
- Provide adequate nutrition and fluids and electrolytes in supportive care.

POSSIBLE COMPLICATIONS

- Aspiration pneumonia
- Chronic pneumonia
- Chronic weight loss

PROGNOSIS AND OUTCOME

Horses appear to be more discriminating than ruminants regarding ingestion of petroleum-contaminated feeds and water. Petroleum toxicosis in horses is rarely reported.

PEARLS & CONSIDERATIONS

COMMENTS

- Petroleum exposures in animals often develop into legal cases. Document the evidence (exposure situation and clinical signs) in writing and with photographs and videos. Place environmental samples in clean glass containers and seal them with air-tight lids. During a postmortem examination, take samples from a variety of organs (liver, kidney, fat, brain, bone marrow, GI tract, soiled skin); place the samples in clean glass containers, aluminum foil, or resealable plastic bags; and freeze them. Contact an analytical laboratory capable of analyzing the source petroleum hydrocarbons and petroleum hydrocarbons in GI contents and tissues; compare the characteristic chromatographic "fingerprints" of petroleum hydrocarbons.

- A wide variety of chemicals and toxic substances are found with and used in production of petroleum. In oil and gas well production, drilling fluids or mud containing water-based fluids with bentonite clay, barium, and potassium and sodium compounds and non–aqueous-based drilling fluids with diesel and emulsifiers can be used along with acids, salts, solvents, biocides, defoaming agents, heavy metals, lubricants, and corrosion inhibitors. Toxic emissions from gas flaring may release polyaromatic hydrocarbons, natural gases, combustion products, and sulfur compounds, including hydrogen sulfide, carbon disulfide, carbonyl sulfide, and sulfur dioxide. Animals can be exposed to methanol used to prevent freezing of water in pipes, diethylene and triethylene glycols to remove water from natural gas, greases containing lithium or lead, production water that can be high in sodium ions, buried sumps containing drilling fluids and other petroleum wastes, and pipeline spills containing petroleum products or waste materials. The petroleum-related compounds can pose numerous and varied hazards and clinical effects if animals are exposed. The clinician needs to have a thorough history and timeline of an exposure and may need to contact a veterinary toxicologist to assist in exposure assessment and clinical interpretation.

PREVENTION

If hydrocarbon releases occur from petroleum facilities, move the animals to locations away from petroleum contamination of water sources and feedstuffs and out of the path of gaseous plumes.

SUGGESTED READING

Coppock RW, Christian RG: Petroleum. In Gupta RC, editor: *Veterinary toxicology*, New York, 2007, Elsevier, pp 615–639.

Raisbeck, MF, Dailey RN: Petroleum hydrocarbons. In Peterson ME, Talcott PA, editors: *Small animal toxicology*, ed 2, St Louis, 2006, Saunders Elsevier, pp 986–995.

AUTHOR: **MICHELLE S. MOSTROM**

EDITOR: **CYNTHIA L. GASKILL**

Pharyngeal Collapse, Dynamic

BASIC INFORMATION

DEFINITION

Dynamic pharyngeal collapse occurs when the dorsal or lateral walls of the pharynx or portions of the rostral soft palate collapse into the airway on inspiration during exercise.

SYNONYM(S)

Pharyngeal collapse, dorsal pharyngeal collapse

EPIDEMIOLOGY

SPECIES, AGE, SEX
- Primarily noted in horses in training
- Males have a higher incidence

GENETICS AND BREED PREDISPOSITION Noted mostly in racing breeds such as Thoroughbreds and Standardbreds but seen in all breeds and uses

RISK FACTORS Pharyngitis, upper airway inflammation

ASSOCIATED CONDITIONS AND DISORDERS Dorsal displacement of the soft palate, palatal instability

CLINICAL PRESENTATION

HISTORY, CHIEF COMPLAINT Horses present with exercise intolerance, poor performance, or respiratory noise.

PHYSICAL EXAM FINDINGS
- None at rest
- Nasal occlusion during endoscopic examination may suggest the diagnosis.
- Definitive diagnosis is made with high-speed treadmill endoscopic examination.

ETIOLOGY AND PATHOPHYSIOLOGY
- Neuropathy of the nerves controlling the muscles of the pharynx
- Dysmaturity

DIAGNOSIS

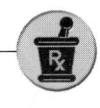

DIFFERENTIAL DIAGNOSIS

- Dorsal displacement of the soft palate
- Axial deviation of the aryepiglottic folds
- Laryngeal paresis

INITIAL DATABASE

Resting endoscopy with nasal occlusion

ADVANCED OR CONFIRMATORY TESTING

Treadmill endoscopy during exercise

TREATMENT

THERAPEUTIC GOAL(S)

Decrease inflammation that may contribute to nerve dysfunction

ACUTE GENERAL TREATMENT

- Rest; removal from training
- Throat spray (usually combination of corticosteroids, glycerine, and dimethyl sulfoxide [DMSO])
- Systemic administration of prednisolone or dexamethasone
- Decrease exposure to allergens in the environment: Hay or bedding dusts and molds

CHRONIC TREATMENT

None. Acute general treatment may be repeated if there is a lack of response.

POSSIBLE COMPLICATIONS

- Lack of response to treatment
- Medication reactions

RECOMMENDED MONITORING

Repeat endoscopy

PROGNOSIS AND OUTCOME

Guarded

PEARLS & CONSIDERATIONS

COMMENTS

Anecdotally, laser cautery of the collapsing tissues has been used to stiffen the area and prevent collapse. No scientific evaluation of this procedure has been done, but it reportedly has had some success.

PREVENTION

Because the direct cause has not been identified, preventive measures cannot be recommended.

SUGGESTED READING

Boyle AG, Martin BB Jr, Davidson EJ, et al: Dynamic pharyngeal collapse in racehorses. *Equine Vet J Suppl* 36:546–550, 2006.
Ducharme NG: Pharynx. In Auer JA, Stick JA, editors: *Equine surgery*, St Louis, 2006, Saunders Elsevier, pp 544–565.
Sullivan EK, Parente EJ: Disorders of the pharynx, *Vet Clin North Am Equine Pract Respir Dis* 159–167, 2003.

AUTHOR: **JENNIFER A. BROWN**

EDITOR: **ERIC J. PARENTE**

Phimosis

BASIC INFORMATION

DEFINITION

An inability to exteriorize the penis from the sheath. This may be a congenital or acquired condition.

EPIDEMIOLOGY

SPECIES, AGE, SEX Equine, any age, gelding or stallion. Congenital conditions are most often diagnosed in younger animals.

CLINICAL PRESENTATION

HISTORY, CHIEF COMPLAINT An inability to exteriorize the penis from the sheath either during urination or sexual arousal. There may be a history of recent injury either by blunt trauma (kick) or abrasion (laceration). If the phimosis is caused by a mass, the onset of clinical signs may be gradual.

PHYSICAL EXAM FINDINGS Phimosis and possibly preputial scalding

ETIOLOGY AND PATHOPHYSIOLOGY
- Phimosis is normal in young foals. The internal prepuce can be exteriorized, but the penis is adhered to the internal portion of the prepuce. These adhesions resolve by 4 to 6 weeks of age.
- Acquired phimosis is usually secondary to a space-occupying lesion or mass or the result of acute or chronic

posthitis leading to adhesion or preputial ring stricture formation.

DIAGNOSIS

DIFFERENTIAL DIAGNOSIS
- Penile hypoplasia
- Penile retroversion
- Penile dysgenesis

INITIAL DATABASE
Complete blood count and serum chemistry are usually within normal limits.

ADVANCED OR CONFIRMATORY TESTING
Ultrasonography of the prepuce or sheath may rule out the presence of a mass.

TREATMENT

THERAPEUTIC GOAL(S)
Determine the cause of phimosis and treat the underlying condition

ACUTE GENERAL TREATMENT
- If sedation is required, care must be taken because phenothiazine derivatives have been linked to paraphimosis. Blocking the dorsal nerves of the penis as they cross the ischium provides excellent relaxation.
- Gentle traction of the penis is necessary to determine the cause of phimosis.
- If adhesions are present:
  ○ If possible, break down the adhesions manually. Local anesthesia may be necessary.
  ○ General anesthesia should be implemented if the adhesions are extensive. Affected areas may be

surgically removed (see Suggested Reading below for surgical options).
  ○ After the breakdown of adhesions, application of an emollient such as silver sulfadiazine cream or an antibiotic ointment should be applied daily to prevent recurrence.
- If preputial edema is preventing exteriorization of the penis: Cold hydrotherapy, diuretics, nonsteroidal antiinflammatory drugs, exercise, and massage are helpful in relieving the edema.
- If a mass is present:
  ○ Surgical debulking and biopsy of the mass are recommended for accurate diagnosis. Surgical options are chosen based on the severity and location of the lesion and include mass removal and partial or complete resection of the penis and prepuce.
  ○ Surgery may be combined with nonsurgical therapy (cryotherapy, topical chemotherapy, and radiation).

CHRONIC TREATMENT
If medical management fails, penile amputation may be necessary.

POSSIBLE COMPLICATIONS
Urine scalding secondary to uncorrected phimosis

RECOMMENDED MONITORING
Daily examination and lubrication of the penis minimize the formation of adhesions.

PROGNOSIS AND OUTCOME

- The prognosis depends on the severity, location, and type of lesion present.

- If the adhesions are not extensive, the stallion may be returned to full function.
- Biopsy results determine the prognosis of a mass.

PEARLS & CONSIDERATIONS

COMMENTS
Squamous cell carcinoma, melanoma, sarcoid, hemangioma, mastocytoma, and habronemiasis are the most common neoplastic diseases observed in equine male genitalia.

PREVENTION
- Aggressive treatment of posthitis will prevent adhesion formation.
- Frequent examination of external genitalia, especially in breeding stallions, will lead to earlier diagnoses of neoplasias.

CLIENT EDUCATION
Space-occupying lesions and masses frequently recur despite therapy.

SUGGESTED READING
Gaughan EM, Van Harreveld PD: Penile infections. In Samper JC, Pycock JF, McKinnon AO, editors: *Current therapy in equine reproduction*, St Louis, 2007, Saunders Elsevier, pp 222–226.
Schumacher J: Penis and prepuce. In Auer JA, Stick JA, editors: *Equine surgery*, St Louis, 2006, Saunders Elsevier, pp 811–835.

AUTHOR: **AIME K. JOHNSON**

EDITOR: **JUAN C. SAMPER**

Photosensitization

BASIC INFORMATION

DEFINITION
- Photosensitization is a light-induced dermatitis caused by increased sensitivity and reactivity of the skin to sunlight because of the presence of photodynamic agents or chromophores in both the skin and the circulation. These photodynamic agents are responsible for absorbing energy from light and transferring it to the body

cells. Melanin in the skin is responsible for limiting photosensitivity reaction to the light pigmented or white areas of the body.
- Sunburn is different than photosensitization because sunburn is a primary direct damage to the epidermis caused by intense ultraviolet radiation. Sunburn most frequently affects the light-colored areas of the body that are at a maximum exposure to sun rays, such as the muzzle and face areas.

SYNONYM(S)
Photodermatitis, photo-induced dermatoses

EPIDEMIOLOGY
SPECIES, AGE, SEX Adult horses are most frequently affected.
RISK FACTORS
- Exposure to and ingestion of photodynamic plants such as buckwheat, St. John's wort (*Hypericum perforatum*), perennial rye grass, and burr trefoil

that will be directly absorbed into the bloodstream.

- When hepatic damage is present and it is unable to conjugate phylloery-thrin, a porphyrin derivative produced by microbial degradation of chloro-phyll in the gut, accumulates in the blood and tissues. In the superficial skin layers, phylloerythrin absorbs ultraviolet radiation of the sun. Energy from the activated phylloerythrin mol-ecule is then transferred to adjacent cells, causing chronic inflammation and subsequent necrosis.

GEOGRAPHY AND SEASONALITY Seen in all areas, but more cases can be identified in areas where horses get more exposure to sunlight. Commonly seen in the summer months from June to August.

ASSOCIATED CONDITIONS AND DIS-ORDERS Horses with liver disease can have a higher risk of being affected by the disease.

CLINICAL PRESENTATION

DISEASE FORMS/SUBTYPES

- Photosensitization in horses occurs by two mechanisms. The first is through compounds and plants that cause primary photosensitization. In this type of photosensitization, the photo-dynamic agent is ingested in the pre-formed dynamic state or is produced as a result of metabolic processing. Primary photosensitization is most commonly caused by ingestion of pho-todynamic plants, such as buckwheat, St. John's wort, perennial rye grass and burr trefoil. Other agents that have been identified in primary photosensi-tization are photosensitizing chemicals including tetracyclines, chlorthiazides, acriflavines, rose bengal, methylene blue, and sulfonamides.
- The second mechanism is hepatoge-nous and occurs when the liver cannot conjugate phylloerythrin, a porphyrin derivative produced by microbial deg-radation of chlorophyll in the gut, causing it to accumulate in the blood-stream and tissues. In the superficial layers of the skin, phylloerythrin absorbs ultraviolet radiation of the sun. Energy from the activated phyl-loerythrin molecule is then transferred to adjacent cells, causing chronic inflammation and necrosis. The hepa-togenous form is the most commonly identified for photosensitization in horses. Hepatic damage may be caused by multiple factors such as toxic plants, hepatotoxic chemicals, mycotoxins, infections, and neoplasia. Of particular importance are plants containing pyrrolizidine alkaloids, *Senecio* spp., *Amsinckia* spp., *Crota-laria* spp., unknown agents in burning bush (*Kochia* spp.), toxins produced by blue-green algae and equine serum

or antiserum. Other agents that can cause sensitizations by mechanisms that are yet unclear include oats, clover, vetch, alfalfa, and *Dermatophi-lus* spp.

HISTORY, CHIEF COMPLAINT White or lightly pigmented areas of the body affected by ulceration or vesicle forma-tion after exposure to photodynamic agents or possible liver disease are typi-cally involved in the history of affected horses.

PHYSICAL EXAM FINDINGS Lesions are most commonly present in the white or lightly pigmented areas. The affected area will initially be erythematous, swollen, and painful. As the condition progresses, serum exudation, skin necro-sis and ulceration, and in severe cases sloughing will be present. If hepatic disease is present, related clinical signs such as icterus, weight loss, or hepato-encephalopathy can also be present.

ETIOLOGY AND PATHOPHYSIOLOGY

- Primary photosensitization: Exposure to photodynamic plants (buckwheat, St. John's wort, perennial rye grass and burr trefoil) or to photosensitizing chemicals (tetracyclines, chlorthia-zides, acriflavines, rose bengal, methy-lene blue, and sulphonamides)
- Hepatogenous photosensitization: Plants containing pyrrolizidine alka-loids, *Senecio* spp., *Amsinckia* spp., *Crotalaria* spp., unknown agents in burning bush (*Kochia* spp.), toxins produced by blue-green algae, and serum or antiserum

DIAGNOSIS

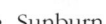

DIFFERENTIAL DIAGNOSIS

- Sunburn
- Dermatophytosis
- Dermatophilosis

INITIAL DATABASE

- Affected unpigmented areas of the skin should be considered suspicious.
- Liver enzyme assay.
- Hepatic function tests.

ADVANCED OR CONFIRMATORY TESTING

- Biopsy is typically unrewarding be-cause it confirms chronic inflammation with necrotic tissue.
- Evaluation of pasture to identify any potential photodynamic plants or toxins and complete history of medi-cations being administered.

TREATMENT

THERAPEUTIC GOAL(S)

Prevent further damage of the affected areas by removing the animal from the

photodynamic agent and removing from the sunlight.

ACUTE GENERAL TREATMENT

- Remove the animal from the source of photodynamic agents, which can in-volve changing pastures or feed or eliminating or changing any medica-tions or supplements the animal may be receiving.
- Remove animal from sunlight and maintain it indoors for 1 to 2 weeks until resolution of the lesions is achieved.
- Application of topical creams and oint-ments containing moisturizing agents and corticosteroids to help decrease inflammation and maintain surround-ing healthy skin well moisturized and hydrated.

CHRONIC TREATMENT

If liver disease is identified, the treatment can be aimed at trying to preserve liver function.

PROGNOSIS AND OUTCOME

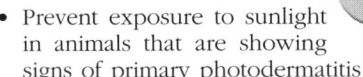

- The prognosis for primary photosensitization is typically good, and most of the lesions will resolve after the animal is removed from the source of exposure and maintained away from sunlight.
- The prognosis for hepatogenous pho-tosensitization is guarded, and treat-ment of skin lesions can be expensive and not resolve after multiple weeks and incurring significant expense to try to maintain liver function.

PEARLS & CONSIDERATIONS

- Prevent exposure to sunlight in animals that are showing signs of primary photodermatitis.
- The presence of lesions in lightly colored or white areas of skin is typi-cally consistent with photosensitiza-tion, especially if different areas of the body are affected.

SUGGESTED READING

Pilsworth RC, Knottenbelt D: Photosensitisa-tion and sunburn. *Equine Vet Educ* 19(1):32–33, 2007.

Stannard AA: Miscellaneous. *Vet Dermatol* 11:217–223, 2000.

White SD. Parasitic Skin Diseases. In Smith BP, editors: *Large animal internal medicine*, ed 4, St Louis, 2009, Mosby Elsevier, pp 1321–1322.

AUTHOR: **ALFREDO SANCHEZ LONDOÑO**

EDITOR: **DAVID A. WILSON**

Piroplasmosis

BASIC INFORMATION

DEFINITION

Tickborne hemoprotozoan disease of horses, mules, and donkeys caused by *Babesia equi* and *Babesia caballi*; characterized by signs of acute hemolytic anemia commonly followed by an inapparent carrier status.

SYNONYM(S)

Equine babesiosis

EPIDEMIOLOGY

SPECIES, AGE, SEX No predilection for sex, breed, or age, although horses in endemic countries become infected by 1 year of age.

RISK FACTORS
- Travel to endemic countries
- Exposure to horses or ticks from endemic countries
- Splenectomy

CONTAGION AND ZOONOSIS
- Tickborne disease, transmitted primarily by *Ixodid* ticks but also by species of *Rhipicephalus*, *Dermacentor*, *Boophilus*, and *Hyalomma*.
- Not a zoonotic concern; no reports of human infection with the equine species of *Babesia*.

GEOGRAPHY AND SEASONALITY
- Endemic in all countries in the world except Australia, Canada, England, Ireland, Japan, and the United States, although sporadic outbreaks from these countries have been reported. Recent outbreaks of disease in the United States threaten its classification as free of piroplasmosis.
- Occurrence of disease related only to presence of the appropriate tick vectors and the necessary climate for survival of the vector.
- Before 2009, only sporadic cases were identified in states with tropical climates, such as Florida and Texas. However, an outbreak involving more than 250 horses occurred in late 2009 involving Texas and New Mexico. Competent vectors were recovered, but the United States remains officially free of piroplasmosis.

CLINICAL PRESENTATION

DISEASE FORMS/SUBTYPES
- Clinical signs generally more severe for *B. equi* than *B. caballi*.
- Inapparent carrier:
  - Most common form because infected horses commonly become carriers.

  - Not related to natural resolution versus drug-induced recovery from acute disease.
  - Low level of parasitemia and no clinical signs, although has been reported to reduce athletic performance as compared with uninfected individuals.
  - Pregnant carrier mares can have late term abortions or stillbirths as a result of in utero infection.
  - This form of the disease creates substantial economic impact on the import and export of horses around the world.
- Peracute form
  - Observed in neonates infected in utero, in naive adults exposed to a large number of infected ticks, or in horses infected after strenuous exercise
  - Poor prognosis
  - Neonates exhibit progressive weakness, fever, anemia, and icterus; signs are consistent with neonatal isoerythrolysis.
  - In adults, the capillaries and small vessels become occluded, and clinical signs are related to the affected organ system. Sudden death has been reported.
- Acute form: Clinical signs occur after incubation period of 12 to 19 days for *B. equi* and 10 to 30 days for *B. caballi*.
- Subacute form: Clinical signs are similar to acute form yet less progressive and more insidious in onset
- Chronic: Nonspecific clinical signs (of weight loss, depression, inappetence) consistent with other chronic inflammatory conditions or equine infectious anemia

HISTORY, CHIEF COMPLAINT History of travel to endemic country or exposure to horses that have traveled. Vague clinical signs of depression, inappetence, prolonged recumbency, fever.

PHYSICAL EXAM FINDINGS
- Fever (in excess of 104° F)
- Anemia
- Icterus
- Hemoglobinuria
- Dehydration
- Tachycardia
- Tachypnea
- Sweating
- Limb edema

ETIOLOGY AND PATHOPHYSIOLOGY
- Tick transmits parasite via its saliva as it feeds on the horse.
- The parasite enters circulation and invades red blood cells (RBCs) and lymphocytes.

- Red blood cells rupture, and signs of hemolysis result.
- After rupture, parasites enter new RBCs and continue to replicate.
- The horse is now infective for other ticks.
- Depending on the species, the parasite can be transmitted through the tick's life cycle as well.

DIAGNOSIS

DIFFERENTIAL DIAGNOSIS

For acute form (fever, hemolytic anemia, and icterus)
- Equine infectious anemia
- *Anaplasma phagocytophilum*
- Red maple leaf toxicity
- Purpura hemorrhagicum
- Immune-mediated hemolytic anemia
- Drug toxicity
- African horse sickness
- Dourine
- Surra

INITIAL DATABASE

Acute form:
- Decreased packed cell volume (~20%), RBC count, and hemoglobin
- Platelet count may also be decreased.
- Neutropenia and lymphopenia may be observed.
- Hyperbilirubinemia and prolonged clotting times may occur.
- Hemoglobinuria may occur in severe cases.

ADVANCED OR CONFIRMATORY TESTING

- Serologic testing is most commonly recommended for definitive diagnosis
  - Complement fixation test
  - Indirect immunofluorescent antibody test
  - Enzyme-linked immunosorbent assay (ELISA)
- Other available diagnostic tests
  - Polymerase chain reaction
  - Visualization of organisms via microscopy on a peripheral blood smear during the acute phase of parasitemia
- Before transport of horses in or out of non-endemic nations, one must contact the authorities regarding appropriate sampling and testing of horses.
- All currently available diagnostic tests have advantages and limitations.
- Currently, the US Department of Agriculture requires all horses entering the United States from endemic countries to test negative using the competitive ELISA.

TREATMENT

ACUTE GENERAL TREATMENT

- *B. caballi*
  - Treatment of choice is imidocarb dipropionate (2.2 mg/kg IM q24h) for two treatments for alleviation of clinical signs only.
  - Mild adverse effects include salivation, colic, and alterations in gastrointestinal (GI) motility; severe toxicity, including liver and renal failure, can be fatal.
  - Other therapies include diminazene (11 mg/kg IM q24h) for two treatments and amicarbalide (10 mg/kg IM) for one dose only.
- *B. equi*
  - Treatment of choice is imidocarb dipropionate (4 mg/kg IM q72h) for four treatments.
  - Horses must be monitored closely for signs of toxicity, including local injection site reactions, salivation, colic, alterations in GI motility, liver disease, renal disease, and death.
- For neonatal foals, information regarding the safety and efficacy of these drugs is lacking.
- Donkeys may be especially sensitive to adverse effects of imidocarb.

CHRONIC TREATMENT

- Horses chronically infected with *B. caballi* can be cleared with imidocarb (4 mg/kg IM q72h) for four treatments.
- No successful treatment for the eradication of the carrier state of *B. equi* has been reported, but the aforementioned dose is under investigation.

DRUG INTERACTIONS

For imidocarb: None documented, but the use of any cholinergic drugs may mimic the signs of toxicity.

POSSIBLE COMPLICATIONS

Some horses affected with *B. equi* may not respond to one treatment regimen. Can repeat but should wait 30 days. Imidocarb is eliminated in the milk, but toxicity to nursing foals is unclear.

RECOMMENDED MONITORING

With treatment, monitor carefully for signs of toxicity.

PROGNOSIS AND OUTCOME

- Native horses (from endemic countries) have good prognosis for recovery from acute disease (~90%–95%).
- Mortality rates can be as high as 50% for naive horses.
- Infected neonates have a poor prognosis.

PEARLS & CONSIDERATIONS

PREVENTION

- No vaccine is available.
- Appropriate testing and quarantine of imported and exported horses as ordered by the specific country is essential.

CLIENT EDUCATION

Regulations for horses entering the United States may be found at http://www.aphis.usda.gov, and international information may be reviewed at http://www.oie.int.

SUGGESTED READING

Rothschild CM, Knowles DP: Equine piroplasmosis. In Sellon DC, Long MT, editors: *Equine infectious diseases*, St Louis, 2007, Saunders Elsevier, pp 465–473.

AUTHOR: **L. NICKI WISE**

EDITORS: **MAUREEN LONG** and **DEBRA C. SELLON**

Pleuropneumonia

BASIC INFORMATION

DEFINITION

Inflammation or infection (or both) of the pleural surfaces associated with bacterial pneumonia

EPIDEMIOLOGY

RISK FACTORS Risk factors for the development of pleuropneumonia are the same as those associated with the development of pneumonia (see "Bronchopneumonia" in this section) and include any disease or situation that compromises the respiratory defenses or increases the risk of aspiration.

- Compromised respiratory defenses
  - Concurrent respiratory viral infection (equine influenza, equine herpesvirus-1, -2, and -4; equine arteritis virus; equine rhinovirus A and B)
  - Strenuous exercise
  - Long-distance transport
  - Mechanical ventilation (general anesthesia)
- Increased risk of aspiration: Laryngeal or pharyngeal dysfunction
  - Primary neuropathy of cranial nerves IX and X (equine protozoal myeloencephalitis, botulism, *Streptococcus equi* infection, guttural pouch mycosis)
  - Primary myopathy of pharyngeal, laryngeal, or esophageal musculature (vitamin E and selenium deficiencies, megaesophagus)
  - Physical limitation of laryngeal function after prosthetic laryngoplasty
  - Esophageal obstruction (choke)

ASSOCIATED CONDITIONS AND DISORDERS Pneumonia, pleuritis, lung abscesses

CLINICAL PRESENTATION

HISTORY, CHIEF COMPLAINT In acute stages, the chief complaint may or may not be related to respiratory tract disease. The history may include recent long-distance transportation or exposure to horses with respiratory viruses.

- May include vague history of fever, depression, and inappetence
- Exercise intolerance
- History referable to associated pneumonia may include
  - Cough
  - Weight loss
  - Mucopurulent nasal discharge

PHYSICAL EXAM FINDINGS Physical exam findings depend on the severity and chronicity of the disease. Some findings can be confused with colic, laminitis, or rhabdomyolysis.

- Crackles and wheezes (focal or diffuse): Lung sounds should be assessed both before and after application of a rebreathing bag (if no respiratory distress is present) because the deep breaths achieved after rebreathing can be invaluable in more accurately ausculting the presence and degree of abnormal lung sounds.
- Abnormal lung sounds are often ausculted only in the dorsal lung field because the presence of pleural fluid

will attenuate these sounds in the ventral lung field.

- Thoracic percussion may be useful to delineate the dorsal limit of pleural effusion (percussion is dull in areas with pleural effusion).
- Fever
- Depression
- Guarded cough
- Painful, stilted gait (reluctance to move) associated with pleurodynia (pleural pain)
- Mucopurulent to fetid nasal discharge
- Weight loss
- Plaque of sternal edema (nonspecific)

ETIOLOGY AND PATHOPHYSIOLOGY

- Progression of bacterial pneumonia (see "Bronchopneumonia" in this section)
- Parenchymal inflammation increases capillary permeability and allows translocation of protein, cells, and bacteria into the pleural space.
- The first stage of pleuropneumonia is accumulation of a sterile exudate, which will quickly evolve to become septic if not treated aggressively with appropriate antimicrobial therapy.
- The second stage of pleuropneumonia is fibrinopurulent, with the deposition of fibrinous sheets that cover the surfaces of the pleural cavity, causing loculation and eventually the formation of an inelastic pleural peel that severely compromises lung function.
- Bacteria most commonly isolated from pleural effusions include *Streptococcus* spp., *Pasteurella* spp., *Actinobacillus* spp., *Escherichia coli*, *Bacteroides* spp., *Peptostreptococcus* spp., *Fusobacterium* spp., and *Clostridium* spp.

DIAGNOSIS

DIFFERENTIAL DIAGNOSIS

- Other systemic diseases causing fever, depression, and inappetence: Enterocolitis, ehrlichiosis, Potomac horse fever, encephalides viruses
- Other respiratory diseases: Fungal pneumonia, interstitial pneumonia, recurrent airway obstruction
- Diseases causing reluctance to move: Laminitis, rhabdomyolysis, colic
- Other causes of pleural effusion: Hemothorax, thoracic trauma, neoplasia, pericarditis, congestive heart failure

INITIAL DATABASE

- Complete blood count: Leukocytosis and neutrophilia (with or without left shift) may be present, although neutropenia may be present in cases of severe gram-negative bacterial pneumonia (associated with the effects of endotoxin). Hyperfibrinogenemia, hyperglobulinemia, and anemia of

chronic disease are compatible with chronic bacterial pneumonia.
- Serum biochemistry profile: Usually normal
- Thoracic ultrasound examination: Optimal diagnostic tool for the diagnosis of pleuropneumonia through identification of pleural effusion and fibrin tags
- Thoracic radiographs: Alveolar and interstitial patterns in dependent areas of the lung

ADVANCED OR CONFIRMATORY TESTING

- Tracheal wash: Degenerative neutrophils, intracellular bacteria
- Tracheal wash culture: Isolation of pathogenic bacteria
- Arterial blood gas analysis: Hypoxemia may be present and is generally indicative of a more severe lower airway disease.
- Thoracocentesis: Generally above 10,000 cells/µL with greater than 70% neutrophils, including degenerative neutrophils; bacteria may or may not be evident
- Culture of pleural effusion fluid: Isolation of pathogenic bacteria

TREATMENT

THERAPEUTIC GOAL(S)

- Removal of excessive pleural fluid to ensure adequate respiratory capacity and reduce bacteria and inflammatory cells in the pleural space
- Elimination of pathogenic bacteria through the use of broad-spectrum antimicrobial drugs
- Antiinflammatory treatments to reduce the effects of excessive inflammation within the pleural spaces

ACUTE GENERAL TREATMENT

- Removal of excessive pleural fluid
  - Ultrasound guidance allows the clinician to assess the amount and location of pleural fluid, as well as the presence of loculations that may limit how much fluid can be removed.
  - In general, chest tubes should be inserted aseptically through the seventh to eighth intercostal space dorsal to the costochondral junction (cannula or chest tube).
  - To allow continued drainage, chest tubes may be left in place using a purse-string suture. To ensure that the tube remains sterile and to avoid creating a pneumothorax, a Heimlich valve or nonlubricated condom with the tip cut off should be attached to the end of the tube.
  - Pleural lavage through indwelling chest tubes (5–10 L of warm sterile

saline) may be required to break up pockets of loculation and remove fibrinous debris. Note that coughing or drainage of lavage fluid from the nose suggests the presence of a bronchopleural fistula, and lavage should be discontinued.
- Broad-spectrum antimicrobial therapy until culture results are available and antimicrobial therapy can be tailored. Any combination should at least initially cover both aerobic and anaerobic bacteria.
  - For more severely affected animals, use IV antibiotic combinations such as potassium penicillin (22,000 IU/kg IV q6h) or ceftiofur (4.4 mg/kg IV q12h) and an aminoglycoside (gentamicin is the most cost effective in adults, 6.6 mg/kg IV q24h) or fluoroquinolone (enrofloxacin 5–10 mg/kg IV q24h).
  - Note that gentamicin does not penetrate well into purulent excretions; therefore, some clinicians prefer enrofloxacin over gentamicin for initial treatment of pleuropneumonia in adult Equids. However, enrofloxacin should not be used alone for treatment of pleuropneumonia because this drug has limited activity against *Streptococcus* spp. and anaerobes.
  - Metronidazole can also be added to increase anaerobic coverage (15 mg/kg PO q6h), especially against the penicillin-resistant *Bacteroids fragilis*.
  - Chloramphenicol (50 mg/kg PO q12h) has excellent broad-spectrum coverage against many gram-positive and -negative as well as anaerobic bacteria. It can be given orally, but care must be taken by personnel administering the drug because it can cause fatal aplastic anemia in humans.
- Nonsteroidal antiinflammatory drugs (NSAIDs) such as flunixin meglumine can be given for pain (0.5–1.1 mg/kg IV or PO q12h) and for antiendotoxic effects (0.25 mg/kg IV or PO q6h). Additional analgesia (butorphanol, fentanyl) may be necessary for horses with severe pleurodynia.
- Maintain adequate hydration; this is especially important if aminoglycosides or NSAIDs are used in treatment. IV fluids may be necessary if the animal is depressed and not drinking sufficiently.
- Nasal insufflation of oxygen, bronchodilation (eg, inhaled albuterol 600–720 µg q6–8h) and measures to prevent laminitis (icing feet, foot support, deep bedding) may be required.
- Provide palatable food choices to maintain appetite.

CHRONIC TREATMENT

- Antibiotic treatment should be continued for 2 to 4 months until clinical signs, ultrasound, clinical pathology, and radiographic abnormalities have returned to normal.
- Exercise should be severely restricted until clinical signs have resolved (ie, the horse is eating well and has no evidence of respiratory difficulty) and then limited to handwalking until clinical signs, ultrasound, clinical pathology, and radiographic abnormalities have completely resolved.

POSSIBLE COMPLICATIONS

- Pneumothorax may occur secondary to anaerobic gas-producing organisms in the pleural space or from bronchopleural fistulae.
- Mechanical debridement of excessive fibrinous material from the pleural space (via lavage or thoracotomy) may be necessary if excessive loculation prevents adequate removal and resolution of pleural effusion.
- Laminitis may occur secondary to the effects of endotoxemia and should be aggressively monitored and treated.
- Other possible complications include pleural abscesses, cranial thoracic masses, pericarditis, and bronchopleural fistulas.

RECOMMENDED MONITORING

- Clinical signs: Animals should be carefully monitored for improvement in respiratory signs, ease of movement, appetite, and resolution of fever within 72 hours. Lack of improvement in this time period may indicate the necessity of an antibiotic change.
- Thoracic ultrasound results should be evaluated every 2 to 4 days to document pleural effusion. Both thoracic percussion and ultrasonography can be used to monitor the height of fluid within the pleural cavity and determine the need for fluid drainage and

more invasive techniques to reduce fibrinous adhesions within the pleural space.
- Thoracic radiographs should be reevaluated 7 to 10 days after the initiation of treatment and may lag behind clinical signs by 2 to 3 days.
- Repeat arterial blood gas analysis: For severe pneumonia, repeated analysis of gas exchange may provide information about the response to treatment.
- Complete serum chemistry

PROGNOSIS AND OUTCOME

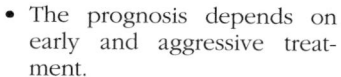

- The prognosis depends on early and aggressive treatment.
- The prognosis declines as complications such as pleural adhesions, mediastinal abscessation, pulmonary necrosis, bronchopleural fistulae, constrictive pericarditis, and laminitis develop.
- Studies of racing Thoroughbreds after resolution of pleuropneumonia indicate that 61% return to racing, with 56% winning at least one race.

PEARLS & CONSIDERATIONS

COMMENTS

- Pleuropneumonia occurs most commonly as a sequela to pneumonia or pulmonary abscessation, which can be determined using the diagnostic tests listed above.
- The prognosis depends on early aggressive treatment.
- Clients should be informed that pleuropneumonia can carry a variable prognosis depending on the chronicity of disease, response to treatment, and development of complications.

PREVENTION

Preventive measures involve reducing the occurrence of risk factors.

- Avoid long-distance transport, especially with head restraint. Studies have shown that simple measures such as increased rest stops and trailer cleaning can result in respiratory insult during long-distance transport.
- Adequate immunization against respiratory viral diseases (equine herpes viruses, equine influenza) that can predispose animals to the development of secondary bacterial pneumonia
- Adequate dental care in older horses to avoid esophageal obstruction

CLIENT EDUCATION

Clients should be informed of possible risk factors and advised on appropriate measures to avoid recurrence.

SUGGESTED READING

Ainsworth D, Cheetham J: Disorders of the respiratory system. In Reed S, Bayly W, Sellon D, editors: *Equine internal medicine*, ed 3, St Louis, 2010, Saunders Elsevier, pp 290–371.

Giguere S: Bacterial pneumonia and pleuropneumonia in adult horses. In Smith B, editor: *Large animal internal medicine*, ed 4, St Louis, 2009, Mosby Elsevier, pp 500–510.

Racklyeft DJ, Raidal S, Love DN: Towards an understanding of equine pleuropneumonia: factors relevant for control, *Aust Vet J* 78:334, 2000.

Riadal S: Equine pleuropneumonia, *Br Vet J* 151:233, 1995.

Seltzer KL, Byars TD: Prognosis for return to racing after recovery from infectious pleuropneumonia in Thoroughbred racehorses: 70 cases (1984–1989), *J Am Vet Med Assoc* 208:1300, 1996.

Sweeney C: Pleuropneumonia. In Robinson NE, editor: *Current therapy in equine medicine V*, St Louis, 2003, Saunders Elsevier, pp 421–424.

AUTHOR: **JULIA A. PAXSON**

EDITOR: **MELISSA R. MAZAN**

Pneumocystis

BASIC INFORMATION

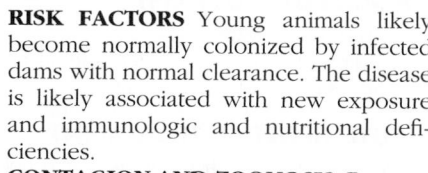

SYNONYM(S)

PcP (*Pneumocystis carinii* pneumonia)

EPIDEMIOLOGY

GENETICS AND BREED PREDISPOSITION Associated with Arabian horses secondary to congenital immunodeficiency

RISK FACTORS Young animals likely become normally colonized by infected dams with normal clearance. The disease is likely associated with new exposure and immunologic and nutritional deficiencies.

CONTAGION AND ZOONOSIS Because of the recent identification of a host adapted species of pneumocystis, its

classification as a zoonosis is questioned. However, because the organism is capable of infecting humans, personal protection consisting of gloves, boots, gowns, and possibly masks are recommended when performing necropsy, handling respiratory secretions, or performing invasive pulmonary techniques to minimize inadvertent exposure.

ASSOCIATED CONDITIONS AND DISORDERS

- In foals, severe combined immunodeficiency (SCID) of Arabian foals, any acquired combined immunodeficiency state of horses
- Associated changes in liver and lung of older horses consistent with chronic pyrrolizidine exposure

CLINICAL PRESENTATION

DISEASE FORMS/SUBTYPES Interstitial pneumonia

HISTORY, CHIEF COMPLAINT Persistent fevers and dyspnea in both foals and adult horses

PHYSICAL EXAM FINDINGS

- The onset of pneumocystitis is insidious, with foals presenting in moderate to low body condition and other systemic signs such as anorexia and depression. These foals usually have intermittent fevers and nasal discharge that may initially respond to antibiotics. Foals become increasingly dyspneic, with developing persistent fevers, tachycardia, and tachypnea. On auscultation, foals have bilateral crackles and moist rales in the trachea. Eventually, an abdominal breathing pattern ensues, and foals exhibit signs of respiratory compromise and hypoxia (low arterial oxygenation and overextraction) and eventually become nonresponsive. These foals frequently develop infections of other body systems (joint ill and diarrhea), which may also ultimately result in their demise.
- The primary condition in which pneumocystis has been described in foals (4 months to 1 year of age) and adults that are not affected with SCID is severe, atypical interstitial pneumonia. Animals are presented in acute respiratory distress with exceptional abdominal effort. Usually, these animals are persistently febrile. Horses may or may not have lymphadenopathy. A dry, harsh cough is common, and wheezes and crackles are audible over both thoracic cavities. Therapy is unrewarding, and horses often die within 1 week. Sudden collapse and death have also been described. Whether or not there is an acquired or other sort of immune deficiency is variable; however, where investigated, most of these horses have either normal lymphocyte or CD4+ T cells.

ETIOLOGY AND PATHOPHYSIOLOGY

- *Pneumocystis carinii* subsp. *equi*
- Exact pathogenesis is not known
- Overwhelming infection on the surface of cells lining alveoli
- Alveoli secrete high levels of a proteinaceous fluid.
- Severe oxygen impairment

- Tissue hypoxia and death in SCID foals
- Chronic interstitial pneumonia, weight loss, and eventual death in non-SCID foals

DIAGNOSIS

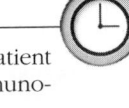

DIFFERENTIAL DIAGNOSIS

- Interstitial pneumonia of herpesvirus etiology
- Interstitial pneumonia of foals of unknown etiology
- Aspiration pneumonia caused by esophageal problems in foals
- Allergic alveolitis
- Bacterial bronchointerstitial pneumonia
- Thoracic pain from trauma
- Hemothorax
- Collapsing trachea of miniature horses

INITIAL DATABASE

- Complete blood count identifying severe lymphopenia (<1000 cells/dL) in SCID foals
- Fibrinogen: >300 mg/dL
- Thoracic radiographs: Severe interstitial pattern
- Arterial blood gas: Decreased PaO_2 and increased $PaCO_2$

ADVANCED OR CONFIRMATORY TESTING

- Bronchoalveolar lavage (BAL): Identification of fungal elements (negative staining round organisms) within and around collections of macrophages and giant cells; high amounts of extracellular pink staining proteinaceous fluid in nonwashed samples
- Gomori's methenamine silver (GMS) stain demonstrates oval to crescent-shaped organisms in areas of negative staining.
- Postmortem histology: Alveolar changes consist of proliferation of the alveolar epithelia consistent with type II pneumocyte hyperplasia. Within the alveoli, accumulation of pink or acidophilus acellular fluid. "Cysts with parenthesis-like bodies" is the criterion for diagnosis.

TREATMENT

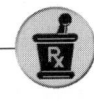

THERAPEUTIC GOAL(S)

- SCID: Not curable.
- Older foals and adults: Clearance if no underlying cause is present

ACUTE GENERAL TREATMENT

- Potentiated sulfonamides (trimethoprim-sulfamethoxazole 30 mg/kg PO q12h for 30 days)
- Dapsone, a sulfone antimicrobial that also inhibits folic acid, has also been

used treat *P. carinii* infection a foal (3 mg/kg PO q24h)
- Supportive care: Nasal insufflation with oxygen
- Supportive care: Furosemide (0.5–1.0 mg/kg IM q8–12h) for treatment of alveolar edema
- Supportive care: Fluid and nutritional support as needed

CHRONIC TREATMENT

For prolongation of life past 30 days or failure to clear organism, additional month-long rounds of potentiated sulfonamides

POSSIBLE COMPLICATIONS

- Long-term high doses of sulfonamides may lead to anemia caused by folic acid inhibition; weekly or bimonthly CBC is recommended in horses treated past 30 days.
- Infectious diarrhea secondary to antimicrobial use in horses.

RECOMMENDED MONITORING

- Radiographs every week to 10 days
- Repeat BAL every 2 to 4 weeks

PROGNOSIS AND OUTCOME

- Poor outcome if the patient has an underlying immunodeficiency
- Poor outcome if the patient has an underlying severe nutritional deficiency
- Reports of recovery in horses or foals with normal immune system

PEARLS & CONSIDERATIONS

COMMENTS

Identification of oval to crescent-shaped organisms after GMS staining of BAL fluid in areas that were originally negatively stained is indicative of pneumocystis.

PREVENTION

- Because of the sporadic nature of pneumocystitis and pneumocystosis, preventive strategies have not been developed. The cause of underlying pulmonary fibrosis is actually not known, although viral infection has been suggested as a cause. Thus immunoprophylaxis of foals, horses, and broodmares against respiratory pathogens should be performed to minimize herd respiratory disease.
- Control of dust and ammonia within the environment also contribute to overall respiratory health.

- Exposure to some toxins, such as plants containing pyrrolizidine alkaloids, should be minimized.

CLIENT EDUCATION

Proper breeding of Arabian horses and Arabian-cross horses

SUGGESTED READING

Clark-Price SC, Cox JH, Baroe JT, Davis EG: Use of Dapsone in the treatment of Pneumocystis carinii pneumonia in a foal, *J Am Vet Med Assoc* 224:404, 2004.
Perryman LE, McGuire TC, Crawford IB: Maintenance of foals with combined immunodeficiency: causes and control of secondary infections, *Am J Vet Res* 39:1043, 1978.
Whitwell K: Pneumocystis carinii infection in foals in the UK, *Vet Rec* 131:19, 1992.

AUTHOR: **MAUREEN T. LONG**

EDITORS: **DEBRA C. SELLON** and **MAUREEN T. LONG**

Pneumonia, Fungal

BASIC INFORMATION

DEFINITION

Lower respiratory tract infection caused by pathogenic fungus

EPIDEMIOLOGY

GENETICS AND BREED PREDISPOSITION

- Arabians with severe combined immunodeficiency syndrome (SCIDS), especially pneumocystosis and aspergillosis
- Przewalskii horses possibly more susceptible to coccidiomycosis

RISK FACTORS Primary fungal pneumonia is uncommon. Instead, fungal pneumonia usually occurs secondary to conditions in which fungal growth is favored:

- Unfavorable housing conditions where horses are exposed to high numbers of fungal organisms
- Concurrent bacterial infection that interferes with normal respiratory tract clearance mechanisms and favors invasion of fungal organisms
- Concurrent administration of antibiotics that interfere with normal flora
- Immune-suppressive conditions (genetic, neoplastic, endocrinologic, or iatrogenic through the administration of immune-suppressive drugs such as glucocorticoids) that result in quantitative granulocyte abnormalities and favor invasion of fungal organisms

GEOGRAPHY AND SEASONALITY

- *Histoplasma capsulatum, Blastomyces dermatitidis*: Endemic to the Mississippi and Ohio River basins
- *Coccidioides immitis*: Endemic to the arid West and Southwest United States
- *Cryptococcus neoformans*: Widespread

ASSOCIATED CONDITIONS AND DISORDERS

- *Pneumocystis carinii*: Opportunistic; associated with immune-suppressive state. Seen in foals with SCIDS and *Rhodococcus equi* and other causes of chronic debilitation
- *Aspergillus* spp.: Opportunistic; often secondary to gastrointestinal tract compromise and fungal invasion secondary to enterocolitis or other causes of immune suppression (Cushing's disease, SCIDS)

CLINICAL PRESENTATION

DISEASE FORMS/SUBTYPES

- Primary pathogenic fungal pneumonia
- Secondary opportunistic fungal pneumonia

HISTORY, CHIEF COMPLAINT As with other forms of pneumonia, horses with fungal pneumonia may be presented for a variety of complaints, including inappetence, weight loss, exercise intolerance, and respiratory signs. The patient history includes suboptimal housing conditions, other primary disease processes, or prior use of antimicrobial medications or immune-suppressive medications (glucocorticoids).

PHYSICAL EXAM FINDINGS

- Primary pathogenic fungal pneumonia (blastomycosis, histoplasmosis, cryptococcidiosis, coccidiomycosis)
  - Cough
  - Inappetence
  - Weight loss
  - Exercise intolerance
  - Nasal discharge
  - Tachypnea
- Secondary opportunistic fungal pneumonia (pneumocystosis, aspergillosis)
  - Signs compatible with underlying primary disease
  - May be severe, vague, or absent respiratory signs
  - Variable fever
- With both primary and secondary fungal pneumonia, other body systems may be affected (liver, bone, peritoneal, skin, reproductive, and intestinal lesions)

ETIOLOGY AND PATHOPHYSIOLOGY

- Primary fungal pneumonia is uncommon. Instead, fungal pneumonia usually occurs secondary to conditions in which fungal growth is favored (see risk factors above).
- Primary pathogenic fungi such as *B. dermatitides, H. capsulatum, C. immitis*, and *C. neoformans* may infect immunologically normal horses, although affected animals often have other concurrent systemic illnesses.
- Secondary opportunistic fungi such as *Aspergillus* spp., *Candida* spp., *Fusarium* spp., *Emmonsia crescens* and *P. carinii* cause infection in animals with underlying immune compromise or severe underlying infection associated with reduced neutrophil function.

DIAGNOSIS

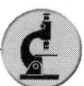

DIFFERENTIAL DIAGNOSIS

- Noninfectious lower airway diseases such as recurrent airway obstruction and idiopathic pulmonary fibrosis (silicosis)
- Bacterial pneumonia (see "Bronchopneumonia" in this section)
- Pulmonary neoplasia
- Respiratory parasites
- Granulomatous disease complex
- Other causes of systemic disease resulting in weight loss and inappetence

INITIAL DATABASE

- Complete blood count (CBC): Often an inflammatory leukogram (leukocytosis, neutrophilia, hyperfibrinogenemia)
- Serum biochemistry profile: Usually normal
- Thoracic radiography: Although diffuse miliary patterns are sometimes present, discrete areas of opacity throughout the lung are more common and may be complicated by concurrent bacterial pneumonia with more diffuse alveolar or interstitial radiographic patterns.

ADVANCED OR CONFIRMATORY TESTING

- Tracheal wash: Degenerative neutrophils, fungal elements, and bacteria. Note that fungal elements may be present in the tracheal washes of normal horses. The presence of a significant inflammatory reaction and intracellular fungal hyphae is more convincing of fungal pneumonia, although it is important to remember that phagocytosis of extracellular fungal hyphae may occur if processing of the sample is delayed.

- Tracheal wash culture: To rule out concurrent bacterial infection.
- Lung biopsy: A sensitive diagnostic tool but with some risk associated with pulmonary bleeding after accidental biopsy of pulmonary vessels.
- Serologic detection: May be useful for primary pathologic fungal infections; however, titers of opportunistic fungi such as *Aspergillosis* spp. may be present in normal, healthy horses.
- Further tests (eg, tests for SCIDS, Cushing's disease) may be required to investigate concurrent primary disease processes or causes of immune suppression.

TREATMENT

THERAPEUTIC GOAL(S)
- Correction of underlying primary disease processes
- Long-term antifungal therapy
- Supportive care

ACUTE GENERAL TREATMENT
- Choice of antifungal treatments depends on the fungus involved.
  - Histoplasmosis, aspergillosis, cryptococcidiosis: Amphotericin B (0.1–0.5 mg/kg administered IV in 5% dextrose over 30 min three times a week). Note that administration of amphotericin is associated with

several adverse effects, including nephrotoxicity, phlebitis, anemia, cardiac arrhythmias, hepatic and renal dysfunction, and hypersensitivity reactions and should be used with caution
  - Coccidiomycosis, blastomycosis, histoplasmosis, aspergillosis: Itraconazole (2.5 mg/kg PO q12h or 5 mg/kg PO q24h).
- Supportive care depends on the severity of respiratory and systemic signs.
  - Maintain adequate hydration. IV fluids may be necessary if the animal is depressed and not drinking sufficiently.
  - Intranasal oxygen, bronchodilators (eg, inhaled albuterol, 600–720 μg puffs q4–6h).
  - Provide palatable food choices to maintain the patient's appetite.

CHRONIC TREATMENT
- Treatment with antifungal medications may be required for 1 to 3 months depending on the patient's response to treatment.

RECOMMENDED MONITORING
Thoracic radiography should be repeated at regular intervals to assess the patient's response to treatment. However, radiographs lag behind resolution of clinical signs, and residual scarring of parenchymal tissue may cause permanent changes in thoracic radiographic patterns.

PROGNOSIS AND OUTCOME

- Variable; depends on the type of fungus involved, exis-

tence and resolution of any underlying primary disease process, and response of the fungal pneumonia to treatment with antifungal agents
- Note that the presence of secondary fungal pneumonia (eg, *Aspergillosis* spp.) with concurrent systemic disease (eg, gastrointestinal disease) usually indicates severe immune compromise and a more guarded prognosis.

PEARLS & CONSIDERATIONS

- Fungal pneumonia is uncommon and is associated with conditions that predispose the horse to invasion by fungal organisms.
- Special attention should be paid to identification of predisposing factors and underlying primary disease processes.

SUGGESTED READING
Ainsworth D, Cheetham J: Disorders of the respiratory system. In Reed S, Bayly W, Sellon D, editors: *Equine internal medicine*, ed 3, St Louis, 2010, Saunders Elsevier, pp 290–371.

Stewart A: Fungal infections of the equine respiratory tract. In Smith B, editor: *Large animal internal medicine*, ed 4, St Louis, 2009, Mosby Elsevier, pp 522–533.

Sweeney C, Habecker P: *Pulmonary aspergillosis* in horses: 29 cases (1974–1997), *J Am Vet Med Assoc* 214:808, 1999.

AUTHOR: **JULIA A. PAXSON**

EDITOR: **MELISSA R. MAZAN**

Pneumonia, Interstitial Foal

BASIC INFORMATION

DEFINITION
Sporadic, rapidly progressive bronchointerstitial pneumonia that may lead to sudden death from fulminant respiratory failure

SYNONYM(S)
Acute severe bronchointerstitial pneumonia

EPIDEMIOLOGY
SPECIES, AGE, SEX Foals between 1 and 6 months of age

CLINICAL PRESENTATION

HISTORY, CHIEF COMPLAINT Acute onset of respiratory distress and tachypnea. Affected animals may die suddenly or be found dead.

PHYSICAL EXAM FINDINGS Fever, tachypnea, respiratory distress (usually severe)

ETIOLOGY AND PATHOPHYSIOLOGY
- Typically, sporadic cases with only one foal in the herd affected; however, clusters of cases have been observed.
- The definitive underlying cause is unknown. Suspected causes include viral infection, *Pneumocystis carinii* infection, heat stroke, exposure to

environmental toxin, or gram-negative bacterial infection.
- Recent cases of acute bronchointerstitial pneumonia in foals after an influenza outbreak in Australia suggest a connection with this viral infection.
- Respiratory distress may be associated in some foals with erythromycin administration.

DIAGNOSIS

INITIAL DATABASE
- Arterial blood gas: Hypoxemia, hypercapnia, respiratory acidosis typically present

- Transtracheal wash (only if patient stability allows)
- Complete blood count with fibrinogen: Hyperfibrinogenemia and neutrophilic leukocytosis typically present
- Thoracic radiography
  - Caudodorsal interstitial and bronchointerstitial pulmonary opacities
  - Coalescing alveolar nodular pattern, air bronchograms in advanced cases

ADVANCED OR CONFIRMATORY TESTING

Histopathologic lesions
- Severe diffuse necrotizing bronchiolitis
- Alveolar septal necrosis
- Neutrophilic alveolitis

TREATMENT

THERAPEUTIC GOAL(S)

Symptomatic treatment and supportive care

ACUTE GENERAL TREATMENT

- Broad-spectrum antimicrobials
- Antiinflammatory medication (flunixin meglumine)
- Bronchodilation
- Nasal oxygen therapy
- Modified environment (cool if in hot ambient temperatures)
- Inhaled corticosteroids may be of use in limiting adverse parenchymal remodeling

POSSIBLE COMPLICATIONS

- Sudden death.
- Horses with hypoxemia are often nonresponsive to supplemental oxygen therapy.
- Blood gas for patient response to oxygen therapy.

PROGNOSIS AND OUTCOME

- Very guarded to grave prognosis.

- Sequelae in surviving foals may include bronchiolar and alveolar epithelial hyperplasia, alveolar type II cell hyperplasia, and hyaline membrane formation.

PEARLS & CONSIDERATIONS

Sudden onset, rapid progression, and very high mortality rate

SUGGESTED READING

Bedenice D: Pneumonia in foals. In Smith BP, editor: *Large animal internal medicine*, ed 4, St Louis, 2009, Mosby Elsevier, p 521.
Patterson-Kane JC, Carrick JB, Axon JE, et al: The pathology of bronchointerstitial pneumonia in young foals associated with the first outbreak of equine influenza in Australia, *Equine Vet J* 40:199–203, 2008.

AUTHOR: **KARA M. LASCOLA**

EDITOR: **MELISSA R. MAZAN**

Pneumonia, Neonatal

BASIC INFORMATION

DEFINITION

Inflammatory disease of the lungs characterized in neonates most commonly as infectious in nature

EPIDEMIOLOGY

SPECIES, AGE, SEX Neonates of any age
RISK FACTORS
- Failure of passive transfer
- Weak suckle reflex
- Dysphagia
- Cleft palate

ASSOCIATED CONDITIONS AND DISORDERS Cleft palate
CLINICAL PRESENTATION
- History, chief complaint
- Milk from nose after nursing, coughing while nursing
- Lethargy, tachypnea, nasal discharge

PHYSICAL EXAM FINDINGS
- Fever (>102.5° F), increased respiratory rate and effort, wheezes, squeaks on thoracic auscultation, or decreased lung sounds for the degree of effort exerted
- Absence of abnormal lung sounds does not rule out pneumonia.

ETIOLOGY AND PATHOPHYSIOLOGY

- Aspiration pneumonia (bacterial): Common in weak, premature, and hypoxic-ischemic encephalopathic foals; also common in bottle-fed foals; meconium aspiration can occur during dystocia; cleft palate anomaly will result in dysphagia and aspiration pneumonia.
- Hematogenous pneumonia (bacterial): A form of localized infection that occurs secondary to sepsis
- Viral pneumonia: equine herpesvirus type 1 (EHV-1), EHV-4, equine influenza, and equine viral arteritis occur less commonly than bacterial pneumonia.

DIAGNOSIS

DIFFERENTIAL DIAGNOSIS

- Cardiac anomaly
- Acute respiratory distress syndrome

INITIAL DATABASE

- Complete blood count: Leukocytosis and hyperfibrinoginemia are common; leukopenia may be present in septic foals.

- Ultrasonography of the thorax: Evidence of consolidation, cavitary lesions
- Radiography of the thorax: Bronchointerstitial to alveolar patterns; dense caudoventral lung field infiltrates suggests aspiration; diffuse lesions suggest a hematogenous origin
- Blood cultures should be performed in suspected sepsis cases.

ADVANCED OR CONFIRMATORY TESTING

- Arterial blood gas analysis: Used to assess respiratory function
- Endoscopy of the oral pharynx is indicated in dysphagic foals.
- Contrast esophography may be performed if the pharynx is normal.

TREATMENT

THERAPEUTIC GOAL(S)

- Treat infection.
- Maintain adequate arterial oxygen tension.

ACUTE GENERAL TREATMENT

- Broad-spectrum antibiotics: penicillin (22,000 IU/kg IV q6h) and amikacin (22–25 mg/kg IV q24h) or a cephalosporin (ceftazidime 40 mg/kg IM or IV q6h or ceftiofur 2.2–10 mg/kg IV q6–12h); blood cultures and sensitivity results may dictate a change in the therapeutic plan.
- Intranasal oxygen: Insufflation as needed (2–8 L/min) for hypoxemia

CHRONIC TREATMENT

Mechanical ventilation may be indicated in foals with hypoxemia and hypercapnia.

RECOMMENDED MONITORING

Repeat ultrasonography and radiography every 5 to 7 days to monitor progress.

PROGNOSIS AND OUTCOME

Aggressive therapy usually yields a favorable prognosis. Long-term complications have not been documented. Foals with cleft palate have a guarded prognosis.

PEARLS & CONSIDERATIONS

COMMENTS

- Weak foals with aspiration pneumonia may require muzzling and feeding via a nasogastric tube until a stronger suckle develops.

- Idiopathic dysphagia may occur in healthy foals. It is the author's experience that most of these foals "outgrow" this apparent weakness of the pharynx within 7 to 14 days.
- Clefts in the caudal palate cannot always be palpated digitally.

PREVENTION

Minimize bottle-feeding practices.

SUGGESTED READING

Wilkins PA: Lower respiratory problems of neonates. In Parente EJ, editor: *Respiratory disease*, Philadelphia, 2003, Saunders Elsevier, pp 19–34.

AUTHOR: **PHOEBE A. SMITH**

EDITORS: **ELIZABETH M. SANTSCHI** and **PHOEBE A. SMITH**

Pneumonia, Parasitic

BASIC INFORMATION

DEFINITION

Parasitic pneumonia in horses has two syndromes, primary lungworm infection (*Dictyocaulus arnfieldi*) and parasite migration through the lung.

EPIDEMIOLOGY

SPECIES, AGE, SEX

- Equine lungworm (*D. arnfieldi*): Donkeys are thought to be the natural host. The prevalence of infection is reported at 68% to 80% in donkeys, 2% to 11% in horses, and 29% in mules.
- Pulmonary parasite migration: Usually affects foals and weanlings.

GENETICS AND BREED PREDISPOSITION
No genetic or breed predisposition for either syndrome has been identified.

RISK FACTORS

- Equine lungworm: Housing with infected donkeys or mules increases potential exposure.
- Pulmonary parasite migration: Inadequate deworming, crowding, and poor sanitation all predispose to parasite infections.

CONTAGION AND ZOONOSIS

- Equine lungworm: Infections in donkeys and mules are patent and often asymptomatic, serving as reservoirs of infection. Horse-to-horse transmission is also thought to be possible.

- Pulmonary parasite migration: Disease occurs through ingestion of contaminated feces.

GEOGRAPHY AND SEASONALITY
Similar to any parasitic infection, transmission is less likely during cold weather.

ASSOCIATED CONDITIONS AND DISORDERS

- Secondary bacterial pneumonia may occur with both syndromes.
- Intestinal parasitism may be seen along with pulmonary parasite migration.

CLINICAL PRESENTATION

HISTORY, CHIEF COMPLAINT

- History
  - Cohabitation with donkeys or mules (lungworm infection).
  - History of insufficient anthelmintic therapy
- Chief complaint
  - Respiratory signs (cough, nasal discharge, increased respiratory effort)
  - Weight loss
  - Pneumonia unresponsive to antibiotics

PHYSICAL EXAM FINDINGS

- Cough
- Nasal discharge
- Abnormal tracheal auscultation
- Abnormal lung auscultation (crackles and wheezes)
- Increased expiratory effort
- Poor body condition (associated with intestinal parasite involvement)

ETIOLOGY AND PATHOPHYSIOLOGY

- Equine lungworm
  - *D. arnfieldi* larvae are the causative agent.

- Infections in donkeys and mules are patent and often asymptomatic, serving as reservoirs for infection of horses.
- Horse-to-horse transmission is also thought to be possible.
- Lungworm infections in horses are generally not patent.
- *Pilobolus* fungi in feces may facilitate the spread of the parasite.
- Pulmonary parasite migration:
  - *Parascaris equorum* and *Strongyloides* larvae both migrate through the lung en route to the intestinal tract.
  - Aberrant pulmonary migration of stages of *Habronema* spp., *Draschia megastoma*, and *Strongylus spp.* can also occur.
  - Prior sensitization may worsen the inflammatory response.

DIAGNOSIS

DIFFERENTIAL DIAGNOSIS

Diseases that exhibit symptomatic and diagnostic similarities include:

- Bacterial, viral, or fungal pneumonia
- Inflammatory airway disease (IAD)
- Recurrent airway obstruction (RAO, "heaves")

INITIAL DATABASE

- Complete blood count
  - Variable findings
  - Leukocytosis characterized by a mature neutrophilia
  - Hyperfibrinogenemia
  - Peripheral eosinophilia

- Serum chemistry
  - Hyperglobulinemia
  - Elevated hepatic enzymes (due to parasite migration)
- Thoracic radiography
  - Bronchointerstitial pattern
  - Evidence of granulomas or abscesses possible

ADVANCED OR CONFIRMATORY TESTING

- Tracheal aspirate
  - Eosinophilia
  - Neutrophilia (especially with secondary bacterial pneumonia)
  - *D. arnfieldi* larvae
- Because infection is rarely patent in horses, unlikely to see L1 stages in Baerman's method: Culture should be performed to rule out bacterial infection.
- Bronchoscopy
  - Lymphoid hyperplasia (pharyngeal)
  - Visualization of lungworm
- Modified Baermann or fecal float
  - Usefully only in patent infections
  - Low diagnostic yield

TREATMENT

THERAPEUTIC GOAL(S)

- Treat parasitic infection and any secondary bacterial infection
- Provide supportive care during acute phase

- Stop contact with infected donkeys and mules

ACUTE GENERAL TREATMENT

- Anthelmintics
  - Ivermectin (200 μg/kg)
  - Moxidectin (0.4 mg/kg, adult horses only): Effective in treating lungworm infections in donkeys
  - Fenbendazole (5 mg/kg and then 10 mg/kg for 5 days): Recommended for foals with *P. equorum* infections; less effective against lungworms
- Supportive care
  - Oxygen therapy if necessary
  - Laxative administration to prevent ascarid impactions in foals after therapy
  - Inhaled bronchodilators
  - Inhaled corticosteroids: Not recommended if secondary bacterial or viral infection is suspected
  - Broad-spectrum antibiotic therapy if secondary bacterial pneumonia is suspected

POSSIBLE COMPLICATIONS

- Increased pulmonary inflammation as parasite is killed
- Ascarid impactions after anthelmintic therapy

RECOMMENDED MONITORING

Monitor for signs of respiratory distress and gastrointestinal signs.

PROGNOSIS AND OUTCOME

The prognosis for treated properly patients is excellent.

PEARLS & CONSIDERATIONS

Any donkeys or mules in contact with horses infected with lungworms should be treated or contact with those animals should cease.

SUGGESTED READING

Ainsworth DM, Cheetham J: Disorders of the respiratory system: lungworms. In Reed SM, Bayly WM, Sellon DC, editors: *Equine internal medicine*, ed 3, St Louis, 2010, Saunders, pp 338–339.

Davis EG: Respiratory infections: parasitic pneumonia. In Sellon DC, Long MT, editors: *Equine infectious diseases*, St Louis, 2006, Saunders Elsevier, pp 12–13.

Landolt GA, Lunn DP: Equine respiratory viruses. In Smith BP, editor: *Large animal internal medicine*, ed 4, St Louis, 2009, Mosby Elsevier, pp 542–550.

Klei TR: Internal parasite infections: respiratory system. In Reed SM, Bayly WM, Sellon DC, editors: *Equine internal medicine*, ed 3, St Louis, 2010, Saunders Elsevier, pp 79–80.

AUTHOR: **ALISHA M. GRUNTMAN**

EDITOR: **MELISSA R. MAZAN**

Pneumonia, Viral

BASIC INFORMATION

DEFINITION

Lower respiratory tract infection associated with equine influenza virus, equine herpes viruses (EHV), equine arteritis virus (EAV), equine rhinitis virus (ERV), equine adenovirus, or Hendra virus (HeV)

EPIDEMIOLOGY

SPECIES, AGE, SEX

- Equine influenza virus: Affects horses, donkeys, and mules; less common in young foals. Outbreaks are usually associated with horses gathered and housed in close proximity with one another. The incubation period is about 2 days with viral shedding lasting 6 to 7 days (experimentally).
- EHV-1 and EHV-4: Latent infections are believed to occur early in life with

stress or immunosuppression leading to disease recrudescence. The virus is present in the respiratory tract within 12 to 24 hours of recrudescence, with viral shedding typically lasting 4 to 7 days (possible for >14 days) and viremia possibly persisting for 21 days. Infection occurs through inhalation secondary to close contact. Respiratory outbreaks are uncommon in patients older than 2 years.

- EHV-2: Infection is often associated with foals and young horses and has been implicated in chronic lymphoid hyperplasia. A humoral immune response is thought to clear the virus with age.
- EAV: Stallions are persistent carriers (testosterone dependent) and transmit the virus via the venereal route, both through live-cover and infected semen. Respiratory viral shedding in exposed

mares can then lead to horizontal spread of the virus for 7 to 16 days.

- Equine adenovirus: Adult horses may act as a reservoir for infection, although it plays an uncertain role in adult respiratory disease. Adenovirus may cause pneumonia in foals, with fatalities seen in foals with immunodeficiency syndromes. Transmission can occur through direct contact or via fomites. Adenoviruses may persist in the environment for 1 year at 4° C.
- ERV: Equine rhinitis A virus (ERAV) has been shown to infect multiple species, including humans. Horses are believed to be predominately infected as 2-year-olds. Contact with other horses or entrance into large groups of horses increases the risk of exposure. The incidence of ERAV infection increases in the late winter and spring. Persistent shedding has been shown 12 months after an acute infection.

- Hendra virus: Several Equine outbreaks have occurred in Australia since 1994. HeV can cause naturally occurring clinical disease in both humans and horses. Close contact with infected animals appears to be necessary for the transmission of infection. In experimental cases, the incubation period is 6 to 12 days with animals succumbing to the illness within 36 hours of the onset of clinical signs.

RISK FACTORS
- Increased stress
- Immunosuppression (eg, corticosteroid administration, concurrent illness)
- Poor housing ventilation
- Waning maternal antibodies
- Congregated horses or horses housed in close proximity to one another

CONTAGION AND ZOONOSIS
- Respiratory viruses are generally highly contagious to other Equids, with HeV having the least transmission potential.
- ERV and HeV have zoonotic potential, with HeV resulting in several human fatalities.

ASSOCIATED CONDITIONS AND DISORDERS
- Secondary bacterial pneumonia is a potentially serious complication.
- Neurologic signs are possible with EHV-1 and HeV.

CLINICAL PRESENTATION
HISTORY, CHIEF COMPLAINT
- Important history information
  - Recent participation in a sporting event (eg, race, show)
  - Return of a barn-mate from a sporting event
  - Introduction of a new horse into the barn
  - Other horses infected and rapidity of spread
- Chief complaint
  - Clear nasal discharge
  - High fever (often >103.5° F)
  - Dry cough

PHYSICAL EXAM FINDINGS
- Equine influenza virus
  - Clinical signs: Pyrexia, nasal discharge, and cough
    - Nasal discharge may progress from serous to mucopurulent in 3 to 4 days.
    - Signs usually resolve within 7 to 14 days.
    - Cough may persist for up to 3 weeks.
  - Secondary complications: Bacterial pneumonia, myositis, myocarditis, and limb edema
- EHV-1 and EHV-4
  - Clinical signs: Pyrexia, cough, nasal discharge, conjunctivitis, subman-

dibular lymphadenopathy, and vasculitis or edema.
  - Pyrexia peaks at 1 to 2 days and again at 4 to 8 days.
  - Nasal discharge progresses to mucopurulent by days 5 to 7.
  - Signs are often worse with EHV-1 versus EHV-4.
  - Respiratory distress and death are possible in 1- to 2-year-olds.
  - Foals infected in utero with EHV-1 appear normal at birth but quickly progress to profound respiratory distress.
- EHV-2
  - Clinical signs: Poorly defined; possible keratoconjunctivitis, pharyngitis, and lymphoid hyperplasia
    - Associated with outbreaks of pneumonia in 2- to 3-month-old foals
  - Secondary complications: Bacterial pneumonia in heavily infected foals
- EAV
  - Clinical signs: Pyrexia (105° F for 1–5 days), nasal discharge, and cough
    - Subclinical to severe disease depending on age, immune status, and viral virulence
    - Edema (secondary to vasculitis), diarrhea, stiffness, icterus, and papular eruptions along the upper lip are also possible
    - Abortion if infected any time from 2 to 10 months of gestation
    - Infected neonates and debilitated or immunosuppressed adults exhibit severe respiratory signs and often rapid death
- Equine adenovirus
  - Clinical signs: Serous nasal discharge (experimental infections in yearlings)
    - Foals: Pyrexia, tachypnea, cough, ocular and nasal discharge (experimental infections)
    - Immunocompromised foals progressively decline despite intensive care.
- ERV
  - Clinical signs: Pyrexia, lymphadenitis, nasal discharge, cough, and pharyngitis (experimental infections). Laryngitis and bronchitis are possible.
- Hendra virus:
  - Clinical signs: Acute pyrexia and respiratory signs
    - Rapid progression of disease (death may occur within 36 hours).
    - Ataxia, head pressing, and recumbency are possible.
    - Frothy nasal discharge and tachycardia often accompany death.

ETIOLOGY AND PATHOPHYSIOLOGY
- Equine influenza virus
  - Inhalation; then viral attachment and respiratory epithelial cell entrance
  - Viral replication and release from the cell with respiratory tract spread
  - Loss of the ciliated respiratory epithelium through induced apoptosis
  - Mucociliary clearance is impaired, predisposing to opportunistic infections.
  - Complete resolution of the epithelial damage takes at least 21 days.
- EHV-1
  - Primary infection occurs in the respiratory epithelium and leads to erosions and viral shedding.
  - Infection of the respiratory tract lymph nodes leads to viremia.
  - Viremia is responsible for infection of the uterus and other tissues.
  - Abortion and neurologic signs are the result of vasculitis.
  - Latency occurs in the lymphoreticular system and trigeminal ganglion.
- EHV-4 and EHV-2: Pathogenesis not defined; possibly similar to EHV-1
- EAV
  - With respiratory infection, the virus invades the respiratory epithelium, reaching lymph nodes within 48 hours.
  - The virus localizes in blood vessels by days 6 to 8, leading to hemorrhage and edema.
  - The virus is eliminated by day 28 except in carrier stallions.
- Equine adenovirus: Pathogenesis not defined
- ERV: Pathogenesis not defined
- Hendra virus
  - Experimentally, horses can be infected via parenteral and oronasal challenge.
  - Virus isolated from the buccal cavity, brain, spleen, lungs, bronchial lymph nodes, blood, kidneys, and urine

DIAGNOSIS
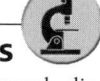

DIFFERENTIAL DIAGNOSIS
- Respiratory signs: Cough, nasal discharge
  - Bacterial pneumonia
  - Bacterial pleuropneumonia
  - Aspiration pneumonia
  - Recurrent airway obstruction (RAO; heaves), inflammatory airway disease (IAD)
  - Pharyngitis
  - *Streptococcus equi* subsp. *equi* infection (strangles)
  - Esophageal obstruction (choke)
  - Sinus infection or disease

- Pharyngeal or laryngeal abnormalities
- Guttural pouch infection
- Respiratory tract foreign body
- Lungworm infection
- Parasite migration
- Fever (104°–106° F)
  - More common
    - *S. equi* infection (strangles)
    - Salmonellosis
    - Equine granulocytic ehrlichiosis (*Anaplasma phagocytophila* infection)
    - Equine monocytic ehrlichiosis (Potomac horse fever)
  - Less common
    - Enterocolitis or proximal duodenitis-jejunitis
    - Bacterial pneumonia or pleuropneumonia
    - Peritonitis

INITIAL DATABASE

- Complete blood count
  - May be within normal limits
  - Abnormal findings tend to be nonspecific.
    - Mild leukopenia, anemia, or thrombocytopenia
    - Monocytosis
  - Leukocytosis and hyperfibrinogenemia are stronger evidence for a bacterial pneumonia
- Serum chemistry: Changes are nonspecific.
- Thoracic radiography and ultrasonography
  - Rule out aspiration and pleuropneumonia
  - Severe changes suggestive of bacterial involvement

ADVANCED OR CONFIRMATORY TESTING

- Polymerase chain reaction of nasopharyngeal swab
  - Ease of sampling and rapid turnaround

- Appropriate for
  - Equine influenza virus
  - EHV (can submit whole blood and tissue)
  - EAV (can submit whole blood, tissue, or semen)
  - Equine adenovirus
  - ERV
- Serology
  - A fourfold increase in antibody titer is usually considered diagnostic.
  - Requires paired samples 4 weeks apart.
  - Appropriate for
    - Equine influenza virus (may be insensitive)
    - EHV (can also submit whole blood and tissue)
    - EAV (change from seronegative to positive also diagnostic)
    - Equine adenovirus
    - ERV
- Hendra virus: Commercial testing is not readily available.

TREATMENT

THERAPEUTIC GOAL(S)

- Supportive care is primary.
- House in a clean, well-ventilated, low-stress area.

ACUTE GENERAL TREATMENT

- Nonsteroidal antiinflammatory drugs to control fever and inflammation
- Antiviral therapy has been used to treat influenza and EHV-1.

PROGNOSIS AND OUTCOME

The prognosis for viral infections in healthy adult animals is generally good, with the exception of HeV.

PEARLS & CONSIDERATIONS

COMMENTS

- EAV: Document negative status in stallions before vaccination. Test before vaccination. If test results are positive, test semen for shedding. Most common in Standardbreds.
- EHV-5
  - Associated with multinodular pulmonary fibrosis
  - Clinical signs: Pyrexia, weight loss, tachycardia, tachypnea, dyspnea, and nasal discharge
  - Radiographic change: Severe nodular interstitial pattern
  - Therapy: Corticosteroids ± acyclovir

PREVENTION

- Vaccination against respiratory viruses may decrease the spread and severity of disease.
- Isolate new horses and horses returning to the barn.

SUGGESTED READING

Ainsworth DM, Cheetham J: Disorders of the respiratory system: viral infections. In Reed SM, Bayly WM, Sellon DC, editors: *Equine internal medicine*, ed 3, St Louis, 2010, Saunders Elsevier, pp 311–321.

Landolt GA, Lunn DP: Equine respiratory viruses. In Smith BP, editor: *Large animal internal medicine*, ed 4, St Louis, 2009, Mosby Elsevier, pp 542–550.

Wong DM, Belgrave RL, Williams KJ, et al: Multinodular pulmonary fibrosis in 5 horses. *J Am Vet Med Assoc* 232(6):898–905, 2008.

AUTHOR: **ALISHA M. GRUNTMAN**

EDITOR: **MELISSA R. MAZAN**

Pneumothorax

BASIC INFORMATION

DEFINITION

Accumulation of air or gas within the pleural space

EPIDEMIOLOGY

RISK FACTORS Thoracic trauma, severe parenchymal disease (pleuropneumonia)

ASSOCIATED CONDITIONS AND DISORDERS Hemothorax, pleuropneumonia

CLINICAL PRESENTATION

DISEASE FORMS/SUBTYPES

- Open pneumothorax: Communication between pleural space and air secondary to defect in the thoracic wall
- Closed pneumothorax: Air accumulation within the pleural space secondary to a defect in the pulmonary parenchyma
- Tension pneumothorax: Buildup of trapped air causes increased pleural pressures and severe lung atelectasis or collapse

HISTORY, CHIEF COMPLAINT

- The patient history is variable depending on the underlying cause but frequently includes trauma.

- The chief complaint often includes respiratory distress or difficulty.

PHYSICAL EXAM FINDINGS
- Restlessness or agitation
- Dyspnea, tachypnea
- Cyanosis occasionally apparent
- Open thoracic wound may be present
- Subcutaneous emphysema over the dorsal thorax
- Absence of breath sounds dorsally, with tympany or hyperresonance over pneumothorax on auscultation of lung fields

ETIOLOGY AND PATHOPHYSIOLOGY
Causes:
- Traumatic: Blunt or penetrating trauma to the thoracic wall or lung parenchyma, esophageal rupture, tracheal puncture or laceration
- Severe pleuropneumonia or other lung parenchymal disease
- Iatrogenic: Transtracheal aspiration, lung biopsy, tube thoracostomy
- Maximal exercise
- Ruptured emphysematous lung bullae

DIAGNOSIS

DIFFERENTIAL DIAGNOSIS
- Primary differential for horse with dyspnea, thoracic wound or history of thoracic trauma, and subcutaneous emphysema
- Hemothorax (with history of trauma)

INITIAL DATABASE
- Thoracic radiography: Presence of pleural surfaces and absence of pulmonary vasculature caudodorsally.
- Thoracic ultrasonography: Subcutaneous emphysema often obscures the image. Pneumothorax with pleural effusion is easier to detect. Air artifact reverberations, "comet tail" artifacts, lack of pleural excursions, and "curtain image" artifact may be observed.
- Aspiration of air from thorax
- Arterial blood gas: May see hypoxemia.

TREATMENT

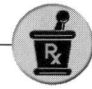

THERAPEUTIC GOAL(S)
- Address underlying cause
- Provide supportive care
- Improve ventilation

ACUTE GENERAL TREATMENT
- Mild: Rest and close monitoring.
- Severe: Removal of air if closed pneumothorax (teat cannula or thoracostomy tube). In long-standing cases, air must be removed gradually.
- Occlusion of open wound if present surgical exploration.
- Nasal insufflation of oxygen (15 L/min) if hypoxemia (PaO_2 <80 mm Hg, %O_2sat <90%). Nasal oxygen therapy may also improve the rate of reabsorption of air.

CHRONIC TREATMENT
- Indwelling thoracostomy tube with Heimlich chest drainage valve if continuous leak
- Broad-spectrum antibiotics

POSSIBLE COMPLICATIONS
- Reexpansion pulmonary edema secondary to rapid correction of pneumothorax in long-standing cases
- Tension pneumothorax

RECOMMENDED MONITORING
- Signs of dyspnea
- Evidence of continual buildup of air
- PaO_2 and %O_2sat values

PROGNOSIS AND OUTCOME

- Uncomplicated pneumothorax: Good prognosis
- Pneumothorax secondary to pleuropneumonia or parenchymal disease: Poor prognosis
- Pneumothorax secondary to esophageal rupture; Very poor to grave prognosis

PEARLS & CONSIDERATIONS

Often, but not always, bilateral because of incomplete mediastinum

SUGGESTED READING
Axon JE: Thoracic trauma. In Smith BP, editor: *Large animal internal medicine*, ed 4, St Louis, 2009, Mosby Elsevier, pp 551–554.
Boy MG, Sweeney CR: Pneumothorax in horses: 40 cases (1980–1997). *J Am Vet Med Assoc* 216:1955, 2000.
Wilkins PA: Lower airway diseases of the adult horse. *Vet Clin Equine* 19:101, 2003.

AUTHOR: **KARA M. LASCOLA**

EDITOR: **MELISSA R. MAZAN**

Polyarthritis and Polysynovitis

BASIC INFORMATION

DEFINITION
Inflammation of multiple joints

SYNONYM(S)
- Nonerosive polyarthritis
- Idiopathic immune-mediated polysynovitis

EPIDEMIOLOGY
SPECIES, AGE, SEX A sporadic disease (or group of diseases) with either no obvious epidemiologic associations or secondary to lupus or chest infections

ASSOCIATED CONDITIONS AND DISORDERS
- Lupus erythematosus–like syndrome
- May be associated with infections in the respiratory or digestive tracts or with concomitant tumors

CLINICAL PRESENTATION
DISEASE FORMS/SUBTYPES
- Noninfectious polyarthritis
- Polyarthritis in foals in association with a lupuslike syndrome
- Polyarthritis in foals in association with a thoracic lesion, gastroenteritis, or a tumor

HISTORY, CHIEF COMPLAINT
- Difficulty walking; disease of sudden onset
- Multiple swollen joints involving all four limbs
- Fever
- Weakness and lethargy
- Inappetence

PHYSICAL EXAM FINDINGS
- Joint pain and swelling
- Fever
- Synovial sheaths, including tendon sheaths and bursae, may be affected.
- Many of these animals have a lesion within the thorax, especially with *Rhodococcus equi* pneumonia.
- Some may have gastroenteritis; others have a neoplasm.

ETIOLOGY AND PATHOPHYSIOLOGY

- Probably immune mediated, but its cause is unknown.
- Many of these cases are associated with a focus of infection elsewhere in the body.
- This reactive arthritis may be associated with coincident gastrointestinal (GI), pulmonary, or neoplastic disease.
- It is possible that immune complexes originating in the lungs or other inflammatory foci may lodge in the synovia to trigger the synovitis.
- The polyarthritis usually resolves as the primary lesion resolves.

DIAGNOSIS

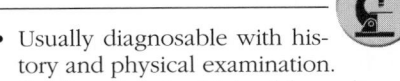

- Usually diagnosable with history and physical examination.
- Confirmation is obtained by radiography and arthrocentesis with joint fluid analysis.

DIFFERENTIAL DIAGNOSIS

- Other causes of arthritis
- Infectious arthritis
- Neurologic disease
- Muscular disease

INITIAL DATABASE

- Complete blood count, serum chemistry profile, urinalysis.
- Anemia and leukocytosis commonly occur in idiopathic polyarthritis. They simply reflect the occurrence of chronic inflammation.
- Serum chemistry profile may show hyperfibrinogenemia and hyperglobulinemia as well as problems in other organs.
- Proteinuria may indicate glomerulonephritis or amyloidosis.
- Radiography to determine whether the arthritis is erosive or nonerosive.

ADVANCED OR CONFIRMATORY TESTING

- Two or more joints should be sampled by arthrocentesis.
- Grossly, the joint fluid is plentiful and possibly turbid as a result of the presence of neutrophils.
- Cytologic examination helps differentiate sterile from bacterial arthritis.
- Culture: Synovial fluid culture results are usually negative.
- Thoracic radiography and abdominal ultrasonography to evaluate possible pulmonary or GI disease.
- Synovial biopsies show lymphocyte and plasma cell infiltration with some immunoglobulin deposits
- Negative test results for rheumatoid factor, antinuclear antibody, and lupus erythematosus cells

TREATMENT

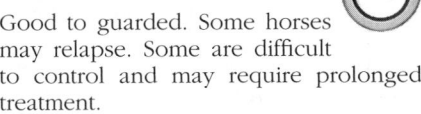

THERAPEUTIC GOAL(S)

- Resolution of clinical signs
- Reduction in synovial inflammation as shown by a reduction in synovial neutrophil counts
- Elimination of any predisposing pulmonary, GI, and neoplastic disease

ACUTE GENERAL TREATMENT

- The condition usually resolves on anti-inflammatory and immunosuppressive therapy.
- Dexamethasone sodium phosphate solution (0.08 mg/kg PO q24h) orally once daily. After a response is obtained progressively, may decrease the dose to 0.02 mg/kg/d.
- Alternatively, 1 mg/kg/d PO prednisolone.
- Azathioprine 3 mg/kg/d PO may be as effective as dexamethasone. After 30 days, half the daily dose for another 30 days.

CHRONIC TREATMENT

Dexamethasone or prednisolone until resolution of signs (2 weeks); then slow reduction of dose. Lifelong treatment may be required.

POSSIBLE COMPLICATIONS

- Secondary infections after immunosuppression
- Laminitis secondary to steroid treatment

RECOMMENDED MONITORING

Monitor the complete blood count in immunosuppressed animals.

PROGNOSIS AND OUTCOME

Good to guarded. Some horses may relapse. Some are difficult to control and may require prolonged treatment.

PEARLS & CONSIDERATIONS

COMMENTS

Suspect polyarthritis in a febrile animal unable to walk even in the absence of joint swelling.

CLIENT EDUCATION

Monitoring is required when animals are immunosuppressed.

SUGGESTED READING

Pusterla N, Pratt, SM, Magdesian KG, et al: Idiopathic immune-mediated polysynovitis in three horses. *Vet Rec* 159:13–15, 2006.

AUTHOR & EDITOR: **IAN TIZZARD**

Polycystic Kidney Disease

BASIC INFORMATION

DEFINITION

Polycystic kidney disease is characterized by the development of multiple fluid-filled cysts within the kidneys, resulting in a reduction of functional renal mass.

EPIDEMIOLOGY

SPECIES, AGE, SEX The age of presentation in reported cases is 9 to 15 years.

GENETICS AND BREED PREDISPOSITION No breed predilection. Although it has not been shown to be inherited in horses, this disease is autosomal dominant (adult form) or autosomal recessive (juvenile form) in humans and autosomal dominant in long-haired and flat-faced cats.

RISK FACTORS Breeding affected animals

ASSOCIATED CONDITIONS AND DISORDERS Chronic renal failure

CLINICAL PRESENTATION

HISTORY, CHIEF COMPLAINT

- Similar to other forms of chronic renal failure, weight loss, depression, lethargy, and anorexia
- Hematuria

PHYSICAL EXAM FINDINGS

- Weight loss
- Examination of the left kidney per rectum may reveal enlargement.

ETIOLOGY AND PATHOPHYSIOLOGY

- It is unknown if polycystic kidney disease in horses is an inherited condition as seen in other species.
- Cystic lesions most likely are congenital and increase in size over time, resulting in compression of surrounding renal parenchyma and eventually leading to chronic renal failure.

DIAGNOSIS

DIFFERENTIAL DIAGNOSIS

- Chronic renal failure
- Hydronephrosis
- Obstructive disease of the urinary tract
- Renal neoplasia

INITIAL DATABASE

- Complete blood count and fibrinogen concentration
- Serum chemistries
  - Azotemia (severity is reflected by the chronicity of the condition)
  - Hypercalcemia
- Ultrasonographic examination of the kidneys may show multiple hypoechoic cystic structures.

ADVANCED OR CONFIRMATORY TESTING

- Renal biopsy
- Gross and histopathologic examination of the kidneys

TREATMENT

THERAPEUTIC GOAL(S)

Palliative therapy only

ACUTE GENERAL TREATMENT

None; most cases are not recognized until the horse has reached end-stage kidney disease.

RECOMMENDED MONITORING

- Horses that are not euthanatized should have periodic measurement of urine specific gravity and blood urea nitrogen and creatinine concentrations.
- Repeat ultrasound examinations will reveal progression of cysts and potentially the presence of remaining normal kidney architecture.

PROGNOSIS AND OUTCOME

Grave. Polycystic kidney disease leads to chronic renal failure and death.

PEARLS & CONSIDERATIONS

COMMENTS

Clinical signs are usually not observed until cysts have enlarged to the point of compressing adjacent renal tissue and resulting in chronic renal failure.

PREVENTION

Affected animals should not be used for breeding because of the genetic predisposition in other species.

SUGGESTED READING

Aguilera-Tejero E, Estepa JC, López I, et al: Polycystic kidneys as a cause of chronic renal failure and secondary hypoparathyroidism in a horse. *Equine Vet J* 32:167–169, 2000.

Ramsey G, Rothwell TL, Gibson KT, et al: Polycystic kidneys in an adult horse. *Equine Vet J* 19:243–244, 1987.

AUTHOR: **JENNIFER TAINTOR**

EDITOR: **BRYAN M. WALDRIDGE**

Polyneuritis

BASIC INFORMATION

DEFINITION

Neurologic disease of horses characterized by inflammation and damage to multiple spinal nerve roots and especially affecting the cauda equina and cranial nerves (CNs) but all spinal nerve roots to some degree.

SYNONYM(S)

- Neuritis of the cauda equina
- Polyneuritis equi

EPIDEMIOLOGY

SPECIES, AGE, SEX

- No breed or gender predilection
- Mainly occurs in adult horses

CLINICAL PRESENTATION

HISTORY, CHIEF COMPLAINT

- Initial hyperesthesia provoking rubbing and chewing around the tail head
- Pain and resulting apprehension on handling

- Progress to hypoesthesia or anesthesia in the rump
- Progressive paresis of the tail, bladder, rectum, and anal sphincter
- Impotence caused by incomplete erection
- Hindlimb weakness and ataxia

PHYSICAL EXAM FINDINGS

- Tail paralysis
- Atonic distended anus
- Fecal retention or incontinence
- Urinary incontinence; the bladder is atonic, distended, and easily expressed manually
- Overflow incontinence may cause vaginal hyperemia, perineal scalding, and thigh scalding.
- The penis may be relaxed and protruding with decreased sensation.
- Hindlimb weakness and ataxia
- Stiff gait; degeneration atrophy of muscles
- CN involvement: Signs commonly involve the fifth and seventh CNs, but the eighth, ninth, tenth, and twelfth may also be involved. This may be

associated with facial and trigeminal paralysis.
- Although sacral and lumbar involvement is usually bilateral, the CN involvement is often unilateral.

ETIOLOGY AND PATHOPHYSIOLOGY

- Chronic granulomatous inflammation develops in the region of the extradural nerve roots.
- The affected nerves are thickened and discolored. They show a loss of myelinated axons; infiltration by macrophages, lymphocytes, giant cells, and plasma cells; and deposition of fibrous material in the perineurium.
- In severe cases, the nerve trunks may be almost totally destroyed.
- Affected horses have circulating antibodies to a peripheral myelin protein called P2.
- This may be an autoimmune disease because it resembles experimental allergic neuritis in rats and coonhound paralysis in dogs.
- Equine adenovirus-1 has been isolated from polyneuritis lesions.

DIAGNOSIS

DIFFERENTIAL DIAGNOSIS

- Sacral or coccygeal trauma
- Herpes myeloencephalopathy
- Equine protozoal myeloencephalitis
- Rabies
- Equine motor neuron disease
- Sorghum intoxication

ADVANCED OR CONFIRMATORY TESTING

- The cerebrospinal fluid (CSF) may contain elevated leukocytes with more than 100 neutrophils and monocytes/µL.
- CSF protein is moderately to markedly elevated.
- Electromyographic abnormalities resulting from denervation of affected muscles may be seen.

TREATMENT

THERAPEUTIC GOAL(S)

This is a slowly progressive disease, and animals may be maintained for a period with supportive care. However, euthanasia is eventually required.

ACUTE GENERAL TREATMENT

- Because of the severe nerve damage, immunosuppressive or antiinflammatory therapy is rarely successful.
- Corticosteroid therapy in the early stages may be beneficial, but objective data are lacking.

CHRONIC TREATMENT

- General supportive care, including fluid therapy.
- Manual evacuation of bladder and bowel may be required.

POSSIBLE COMPLICATIONS

Severe local infections may occur as a result of urinary and fecal incontinence.

RECOMMENDED MONITORING

If euthanasia is not indicated immediately, the patient should be monitored at regular intervals to ensure that it is humane to continue to maintain supportive therapy.

PROGNOSIS AND OUTCOME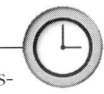

The disease is slowly progressive and apparently irreversible.

Gradual deterioration will eventually make euthanasia the appropriate choice.

PEARLS & CONSIDERATIONS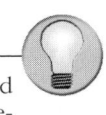

The client should be advised that this is a progressive, irreversible disease.

SUGGESTED READING

Edington N, Wright JA, Patel JR, et al: Equine adenovirus 1 isolated from cauda equina neuritis. *Res Vet Sci* 37:252–254, 1984.

Hahn CN: Polyneuritis equi: the role of T-lymphocytes and importance of differential clinical signs. *Equine Vet J* 40:100, 2008.

van Galen G, Cassart D, Sandersen C, et al: The composition of the inflammatory infiltrate in three cases of polyneuritis equi. *Equine Vet J* 40:185–188, 2008.

Wright JA, Fordyce P, Edington N: Neuritis of the cauda equina in the horse. *J Comp Pathol* 97:667–675, 1987.

Yvorchuk-St Jean K: Neuritis of the cauda equina. *Vet Clin North Am Equine Pract* 3:421–427, 1987.

AUTHOR & EDITOR: IAN TIZARD

Polysaccharide Storage Myopathy

BASIC INFORMATION

DEFINITION

An inherited metabolic myopathy

SYNONYM(S)

Equine polysaccharide storage myopathy is referred to by several acronyms, depending on the researcher and laboratory (eg, EPSM, PSSM, EPSSM).

EPIDEMIOLOGY

SPECIES, AGE, SEX
- Horses, ponies, and mules may be affected.
- Clinical signs can appear at any age.

GENETICS AND BREED PREDISPOSITION Quarter Horse, Paint Horse, Appaloosa, and Draft Horse–related breeds are at highest risk, but it may occur in any breed.

RISK FACTORS Breed, diet (high in starch and sugar), limited exercise

ASSOCIATED CONDITIONS AND DISORDERS
- Exertional rhabdomyolysis, shivers, and other abnormal hindlimb mechanical lameness
- Muscle atrophy

- Poor performance
- Back pain

CLINICAL PRESENTATION

DISEASE FORMS/SUBTYPES The severe form is associated with single nucleotide polymorphism in the skeletal muscle glycogen synthase 1 (*GYS1*) gene.

HISTORY, CHIEF COMPLAINT Exertional rhabdomyolysis, muscle atrophy, poor performance, muscle cramping or pain, back pain, unexplained hindlimb gait abnormality

PHYSICAL EXAM FINDINGS Tight, painful muscles or muscle atrophy; myoglobinuria associated with severe rhabdomyolysis; may be normal

ETIOLOGY AND PATHOPHYSIOLOGY
- Autosomal dominant inheritance of an as yet poorly defined metabolic defect. *GYS1* mutation does not explain all EPSM cases and does not adequately explain the clinical signs.
- Increased insulin sensitivity is reported in affected Quarter Horses but not in affected Belgian Draft Horses and therefore is not likely to be an underlying cause.

DIAGNOSIS

DIFFERENTIAL DIAGNOSIS

- Other causes of rhabdomyolysis (glycogen branching enzyme defect in Quarter Horse foals)
- Selenium deficiency
- Ionophore or plant intoxication
- Pasture-associated rhabdomyolysis
- Other mechanical lameness
- Equine motor neuron disease in horses with generalized muscle atrophy
- Hyperkalemic periodic paralysis (HYPP) in Quarter Horses
- Lyme disease
- Abnormal gait caused by neurologic disease

INITIAL DATABASE

- Serum creatine kinase (CK) before and 4 to 6 hours after exercise. CK above 350 IU is suspicious of exercise-induced muscle injury. Increase in CK is most likely in horses with a history of exertional rhabdomyolysis and is uncommon in horses with other manifestations and in affected draft breeds.
- Increase in serum aspartate aminotransferase (AST) or lactate

dehydrogenase are also possible in affected horses.

ADVANCED OR CONFIRMATORY TESTING

- Muscle biopsy (semimembranosus or semitendinosus)
- DNA test for *GYS1* polymorphism in predisposed breeds (see http://www.cvm.umn.edu/umec/lab/Advances_in_PSSM.html)

TREATMENT

THERAPEUTIC GOAL(S)

- Acute rhabdomyolysis: Maintain hydration to protect the kidneys from myoglobin-induced injury; pain relief
- Chronic: Reduce dietary starch and sugar, increase dietary fat, and provide as much turnout and regular exercise as possible

ACUTE GENERAL TREATMENT

- For severe rhabdomyolysis:
  - IV fluids
  - Acepromazine: 10 mg IM q6h
  - Nonsteroidal antiinflammatory medication (flunixin meglumine 1.1 mg/kg IV q8–12h)
  - Phenylbutazone: 2.2 mg/kg IV or PO q12–24h
- Provide at least turnout exercise as soon as the horse is moving more comfortably

CHRONIC TREATMENT

- Diet change to one that provides approximately 20% to 25% of calories from fat and less than 15% of calories from starch and sugar. This equates to approximately 1 lb fat per 1000 lb horse per day added to a feed that is as low in starch and sugar as the horse will accept with added fat.
- Provide as much turnout exercise and regular exercise as possible.

POSSIBLE COMPLICATIONS

Renal failure caused by myoglobinuric nephrosis after rhabdomyolysis; recumbency with inability to rise

RECOMMENDED MONITORING

For horses with exercise-induced increase in CK: Repeat blood testing starting 3 to 4 months after diet change. Re-biopsy of muscle is not useful.

PROGNOSIS AND OUTCOME

- Good to excellent for most horses.
- Clinical problems in horses homozygous for the *GYS1* mutation or those with mutations of the skeletal muscle ryandine receptor (RYR1) as well as of the *GYS1* gene may be more difficult to control.

PEARLS & CONSIDERATIONS

COMMENTS

Most failures can be attributed to not enough fat in the diet or not enough exercise. To date, no feeds provide the correct ratio of fat calories to starch and sugar calories without added digestible oil or high fat supplement.

PREVENTION

Weaning foals of high-risk breeds onto a high-fat and high-fiber and low-starch and low-sugar diet should minimize the occurrence of clinical disease. Many horses with polysaccharide storage myopathy are very high-performing horses at various disciplines, suggesting that selective breeding to reduce the problem may be very difficult and perhaps even undesirable.

CLIENT EDUCATION

Breeding affected horses should be considered only if the horse responds well to diet change and exercise therapy. Owners must be informed that there is a 50% risk of offspring being similarly affected.

SUGGESTED READING

Valberg SJ: Polysaccharide storage myopathy. *Proc Am Assoc Equine Pract* 52:373–380, 2006.

Valentine BA: Diagnosis and treatment of equine polysaccharide storage myopathy. *J Equine Vet Sci* 25:52–61, 2005.

Valentine BA: Equine polysaccharide storage myopathy. *Equine Vet Educ* 15:254–262, 2003.

AUTHOR: **BETH A. VALENTINE**

EDITOR: **ANDRIS J. KANEPS**

Polyuria and Polydipsia

BASIC INFORMATION

DEFINITION

Inappropriately increased water intake and urination

EPIDEMIOLOGY

GENETICS AND BREED PREDISPOSITION Nephrogenic diabetes insipidus (DI) has been reported in colts, two of which were full siblings.

RISK FACTORS Horses kept stalled for most of the time and meal fed are most likely to develop psychogenic water drinking.

ASSOCIATED CONDITIONS AND DISORDERS

- DI
- Pituitary pars intermedia dysfunction (PPID)
- Equine metabolic syndrome (EMS)
- Acute or chronic renal failure
- Endotoxemia or sepsis

CLINICAL PRESENTATION

HISTORY, CHIEF COMPLAINT Excessive drinking and urination

PHYSICAL EXAM FINDINGS

- No abnormal findings (psychogenic water drinking)
- Dehydration, increased skin turgor, and dry mucous membranes (renal failure, DI)
- Abnormal fat deposits (EMS)
- Hirsutism, weight loss, or hyperhidrosis (PPID)
- Laminitis (PPID or EMS)

ETIOLOGY AND PATHOPHYSIOLOGY

- Psychogenic water drinking is essentially a stable vice. Horses that are kept in stalls and not allowed to graze or have constant access to forage will drink water out of boredom.
- Central DI occurs because of hypothalamic or pituitary dysfunction and decreased antidiuretic hormone (ADH, or arginine vasopressin) production.
- Nephrogenic DI occurs when medullary collecting ducts cannot conserve water in response to ADH.
- Acquired nephrogenic DI may occur with trauma, vascular abnormalities, encephalitis, neoplasia, or pressure from an enlarged pituitary gland in PPID.

- Corticosteroids and α_2-agonist drugs can antagonize the effects of ADH and result in polyuria.

DIAGNOSIS

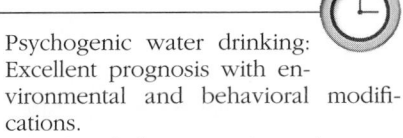

DIFFERENTIAL DIAGNOSIS

- Psychogenic water drinking
- DI
- PPID
- EMS
- Excessive or psychogenic salt ingestion
- Acute or chronic renal failure
- Iatrogenic polyuria: Administration of α_2-agonists, corticosteroids, or excessive fluid administration

INITIAL DATABASE

- Complete blood count
- Serum chemistries
- Urinalysis, especially urine specific gravity

ADVANCED OR CONFIRMATORY TESTING

- Water deprivation test: This should only be performed in nonazotemic horses. The horse should be weighed and its bladder emptied at the start of the test. Water is withheld and urine specific gravity is measured q6–12h. Water deprivation should stop if the horse loses 5% or more of its body weight or becomes azotemic or dehydrated. Practically, the test can stop whenever urine specific gravity is 1.025 or above.
- Modified water deprivation test: Some horses with polyuria and polydipsia lose concentrating ability because of medullary wash out. Water intake is restricted to 40 mL/kg/d for 3 to 4 days to restore renal osmotic gradients before performing the water deprivation test.

- Hickey-Hare test: Hypertonic (2.5%) saline is infused at 0.25 mL/min/kg for 45 minutes. Normal horses will have a reduced volume of concentrated urine after hypertonic saline administration.
- Exogenous vasopressin infusion: 2.5 mU/kg in 5% dextrose IV continuous rate infusion over 60 minutes or 0.5 U/kg IM. Urine specific gravity in normal horses should be 1.020 or above 60 to 90 minutes after administration. Horses with nephrogenic DI cannot concentrate urine after exogenous vasopressin.
- Desmopressin acetate: Human nasal spray can be diluted into sterile water (0.05 μg/kg IV). Normal horses with experimentally induced diuresis concentrate urine above 1.020 within 2 to 7 hours after administration. Horses with nephrogenic DI are not expected to concentrate urine after administration of desmopressin acetate.
- Endocrine testing: Measure ADH, adrenocorticotropic hormone, cortisol, insulin, and thyroid hormone concentrations. Dexamethasone suppression or thyrotropin-releasing hormone response test will diagnose PPID and help differentiate PPID from EMS.
- Blood glucose concentration: Hyperglycemia may be present with PPID, EMS, or recent administration of an α_2-agonist sedative.

TREATMENT

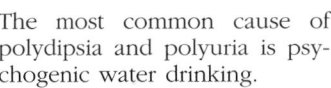

THERAPEUTIC GOAL(S)

Reestablish normal water intake and urination.

ACUTE GENERAL TREATMENT

- Ensure that affected animals remain hydrated until the cause can be determined
- Avoid or compensate for any iatrogenic causes of ADH antagonism

CHRONIC TREATMENT

- One case of nephrogenic DI improved clinically with salt restriction (only what was contained in feed) and limited but regular access to water.
- ADH replacement therapy may be attempted for patients with central DI.

PROGNOSIS AND OUTCOME

- Psychogenic water drinking: Excellent prognosis with environmental and behavioral modifications.
- DI: Guarded prognosis; colts may remain underweight for their age.
- PPID: Prognosis is generally good to guarded with appropriate therapy and podiatry.
- Equine metabolic syndrome: Prognosis is generally good to guarded with dietary restriction, exercise, farriery, and pharmacologic therapy (if needed).

PEARLS & CONSIDERATIONS

The most common cause of polydipsia and polyuria is psychogenic water drinking.

SUGGESTED READING

Brashier M: Polydipsia and polyuria in a weanling colt caused by nephrogenic diabetes insipidus. *Vet Clin North Am Equine Pract* 22:219–227, 2006.
McKenzie EC: Polyuria and polydipsia in horses. *Vet Clin North Am Equine Pract* 23:641–653, 2007.

AUTHOR & EDITOR: **BRYAN M. WALDRIDGE**

Poor Libido

BASIC INFORMATION

DEFINITION

The word *libido* from Latin means *desire* or *lust*. Poor libido is defined as slow or lack of sexual interest or arousal.

SYNONYM(S)

Inadequate sexual interest and arousal, poor sex drive

EPIDEMIOLOGY

SPECIES, AGE, SEX Stallions of breeding age
GENETICS AND BREED PREDISPOSITION

- Genetic predisposition has been postulated but not confirmed.
- Jacks (donkey males) display slower sexual desire than stallions.
- Draft breed horses seem to be more predisposed.

RISK FACTORS

- Inexperience
- Poor training or handling
- Negative experiences
- Housing conditions (proximity to other breeding stallions)
- Specific aversions or mare preferences (color, size, breed, age, lactation status)
- Hormonal treatments (progesterone, immunization against gonadotropin-releasing hormone [GnRH])

GEOGRAPHY AND SEASONALITY

- Libido is reduced during the non-breeding season.
- Libido is reduced by high temperature and humidity.

ASSOCIATED CONDITIONS AND DISORDERS

- Severe systemic diseases: Loss of libido may be one of the first symptoms of illness.
- Poor body condition.
- Exhaustion.

CLINICAL PRESENTATION

HISTORY, CHIEF COMPLAINT

- History of recent systemic disease
- Recently introduced to the breeding shed or retired from competition
- Increased latency to show interest in estrus mares and achieve erection (>2 min)
- Stallion stands quietly when presented to a mare in estrus.

PHYSICAL EXAM FINDINGS

- Poor body condition may be involved.
- Most stallions are otherwise clinically normal.

ETIOLOGY AND PATHOPHYSIOLOGY

- The cause is often multifactorial and is difficult to define unless there are physical problems or age-associated changes.
- The pathophysiology is often considered to involve either a reduction in testosterone or a complex chain of behavioral responses to specific conditions.
- Most of these cases are exacerbated by human intervention.
- Overt use of progesterone during training or performance to calm a stallion.
- Use of anti-GnRH vaccine.

DIAGNOSIS

INITIAL DATABASE

- Complete examination of the genitalia (including endoscopic and ultrasonographic imaging).
- Testosterone level may be helpful.

TREATMENT

THERAPEUTIC GOAL(S)

- To enhance sexual drive by behavioral modification, reduce anxiety, and increase the testosterone level
- Eliminate anxiety by behavioral therapy and anxiolytic medication
- Eliminate the predisposing or risk factors

ACUTE GENERAL TREATMENT

- Enhance sexual arousal in the presence of an estrous mare.
- GnRH 50 µg SC 1 to 2 hours before breeding
- Diazepam: 0.05 mg/kg slow IV

CHRONIC TREATMENT

Behavioral therapy
- Prolonged teasing under optimal conditions for the stallion (familiar environment, no distraction by other stallions)
- Exposure to mares initially with minimal interference
- Use mares in natural estrus (not ovariectomized estrogen-treated mares)
- Encouragement and positive reinforcement

DRUG INTERACTIONS

Overuse of testosterone or anabolic steroids

POSSIBLE COMPLICATIONS

Stallions may be become aggressive toward mares if not handled properly.

RECOMMENDED MONITORING

- Maintain a breeding schedule for maximum arousal
- Maintain the same breeding routine
- Avoid changes in handlers and breeding routine

PROGNOSIS AND OUTCOME

Very good in the majority of stallions without physical problems

PEARLS & CONSIDERATIONS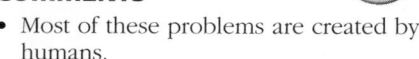

COMMENTS

- Most of these problems are created by humans.
- Knowledge of normal behavior of stallions in free mating as well as in-hand mating situations is paramount in understanding sexual behavioral alterations.
- Judicious use of disciplinary action is very important particularly in stallions that are used for breeding and still performing.

PREVENTION

- Proper handling during the introduction to breeding shed
- Avoid excessive discipline during performance.

CLIENT EDUCATION

- Stallion handling is a skill that requires a thorough understanding of stallion behavior and proper use of discipline.
  - Avoid excessive jingling on the lead shank or chain.
  - Avoid punishing stallions for mounting without erection.
  - Avoid overcorrection or explosive discipline during training.
- Avoid rough or excessive discipline of stallions during performance.
  - Use judicious behavioral modification techniques to train stallions.
  - Avoid use of devices to prevent erection and masturbation.
  - Avoid use of drugs to manage normal sexual drive.

SUGGESTED READING

McDonnell SM: Stallion sexual behavior. In Samper JC, editor: *Equine breeding management and artificial insemination*, St Louis, 2009, Saunders Elsevier, pp 41–46.

Tibary A: Stallion reproductive behavior. In Samper JC, Pycock JF, McKinnon AO, editors: *Current therapy in equine reproduction*, St Louis, 2007, Saunders Elsevier, pp 174–184.

AUTHORS: **JACOBO S. RODRIGUEZ, LISA K. PEARSON,** and **AHMED TIBARY**

EDITOR: **JUAN C. SAMPER**

Portosystemic Shunt

BASIC INFORMATION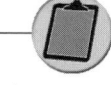

DEFINITION

Portosystemic shunts are vascular anomalies that cause blood from the portal circulation to bypass the liver and flow into the systemic circulation, allowing metabolic byproducts that are normally removed and detoxified by the liver to accumulate in the circulation. Portosystemic shunts can be either intrahepatic or extrahepatic and congenital or acquired.

EPIDEMIOLOGY

SPECIES, AGE, SEX Although rare, congenital extrahepatic shunts are most commonly reported in foals younger than 6 months.

ASSOCIATED CONDITIONS AND DISORDERS Clinical signs of a portosystemic shunt may be indistinguishable from other liver diseases causing hepatic encephalopathy.

CLINICAL PRESENTATION

DISEASE FORMS/SUBTYPES Portosystemic shunts may be congenital or acquired and intrahepatic or extrahepatic.

HISTORY, CHIEF COMPLAINT Nonspecific clinical signs include vague to obvious intermittent to persistent neurologic deficits (blindness, depression, head pressing, ataxia), decreased appetite, failure to thrive, colic, icterus, and fever.

PHYSICAL EXAM FINDINGS Physical examination findings are nonspecific and include neurologic deficits associated with hepatic encephalopathy (variable to profound depression, cerebral blindness, ataxia), fever, icterus, poor body condition, and abdominal pain.

ETIOLOGY AND PATHOPHYSIOLOGY

- Clinical signs and clinicopathologic abnormalities are the result of altered blood flow from the portal vein around or through the liver resulting in accumulation of metabolic by-products, such as ammonia, that circumvent detoxification by the liver and thus accumulate in the systemic circulation.
- Aberrant hepatic blood flow may also contribute to hepatic atrophy.

DIAGNOSIS

DIFFERENTIAL DIAGNOSIS

- Any liver disease causing signs of hepatic encephalopathy
- Biliary obstruction in foals secondary to duodenal stricture
- Biliary atresia
- Liver abscesses

- Cirrhosis
- Cholangiohepatitis
- Cholangitis
- Hepatic neoplasia (metastatic lymphoma)
- Other diseases causing weight loss

INITIAL DATABASE

- Complete blood count with fibrinogen: Typically normal
- Liver-specific enzyme activity: Normal to slightly increased
- Serum albumin and glucose concentrations: Normal to decreased
- Blood urea nitrogen concentration: Decreased
- Serum bile acid concentration: Increased
- Plasma ammonia concentration: Increased
- Cerebrospinal fluid analysis: Normal

ADVANCED OR CONFIRMATORY TESTING

- Ultrasound examination of the liver and abdomen: May reveal reduced hepatic size and tortuous perihepatic or intrahepatic vascular supply
- Liver biopsy: Hepatocellular atrophy and necrosis, fibrosis, biliary hyperplasia, prominent vessels in the portal triads
- Operative mesenteric portography to document vascular supply to the liver (see "Diagnostic Imaging of the Liver" in Section II)
- Nuclear hepatic scintigraphy (see "Diagnostic Imaging of the Liver" in Section II)

TREATMENT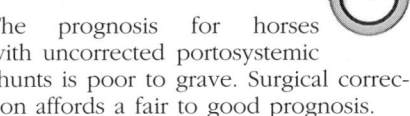

THERAPEUTIC GOAL(S)

The primary therapeutic goal is to surgically reestablish normal blood flow to the liver.

ACUTE GENERAL TREATMENT

- The only curative therapeutic option is surgical intervention to correct the shunt.

- See the supportive treatment information under "Hepatic Encephalopathy" in this section.
- Lactulose to decrease ammonia production and absorption in the gastrointestinal tract
- Broad-spectrum antimicrobial medications for treatment and prevention of septicemia
- Antifibrotic medications (pentoxifylline or colchicine) to prevent or slow the progression of hepatic fibrosis
- Antiinflammatory medications to decrease systemic inflammation

CHRONIC TREATMENT

- Similar to acute therapy
- Surgical correction

POSSIBLE COMPLICATIONS

- Inability to correct the shunt at surgery
- Failure of medications to relieve clinical signs

PROGNOSIS AND OUTCOME

The prognosis for horses with uncorrected portosystemic shunts is poor to grave. Surgical correction affords a fair to good prognosis.

PEARLS & CONSIDERATIONS

Portosystemic shunts are rare in horses, and limited information is available on successful treatment.

SUGGESTED READING

Buonanno AM, Carlson GP, Kantrowitz B: Clinical and diagnostic features of portosystemic shunt in a foal. *J Am Vet Med Assoc* 192:387–389, 1988.
Lindsay WA, Ryder JK, Beck KA, et al: Hepatic encephalopathy caused by a portosystemic shunt in a foal. *Vet Med* 83(8):798, 1988.

AUTHOR: **ERIN S. GROOVER**

EDITOR: **MICHELLE HENRY BARTON**

Potomac Horse Fever

BASIC INFORMATION

DEFINITION

Colitis or diarrhea caused by *Neorickettsia risticii*

EPIDEMIOLOGY

GEOGRAPHY AND SEASONALITY

- Originally reported in the Potomac River Valley.
- Cases have now been described in most states, though they occur most

frequently in the northeast, mid-Atlantic, and western parts of the country.

- Housing near (within ~5 miles of) a river in endemic regions is correlated with an increased incidence of Potomac horse fever (PHF).

CLINICAL PRESENTATION

HISTORY, CHIEF COMPLAINT

- Inappetence, colic, fever and diarrhea as for other causes of colitis (see "Colitis/Diarrhea, Acute" in this section).
- Occasionally, a transient fever is noted 7 to 14 days before signs of colitis develop shortly after infection, although this is often missed by the owner.
- Some horses present for acute laminitis in the absence of diarrhea.

PHYSICAL EXAM FINDINGS

- As for other causes of colitis (see "Colitis/Diarrhea, Acute" in this section).
- Laminitis seems to occur earlier in the course of disease with PHF than other causes of colitis and may be present at the time of initial evaluation.

ETIOLOGY AND PATHOPHYSIOLOGY

- *N. risticii* is an intracellular gram-negative coccus.
- The etiopathogenesis of PHF has not been fully elucidated, but current evidence suggests that the vector for *N. risticii* transmission is a trematode (helminth), with freshwater operculate snails or aquatic insects such as caddis flies likely intermediate hosts.
- The reservoir for *N. risticii* in the environment is also unknown, although many small mammals and birds may carry the infected trematode.
- The exact mode of transmission to horses is unknown, but infection is presumed to occur via ingestion of infected snails or insects or ingestion of water containing infected trematodes released in secretions from freshwater snails.
- After it has been ingested, *N. risticii* infects monocytes, thus evading the host's immune response.
- The organism also has a predilection for large colon epithelial cells, resulting in loss of microvilli and active reduction of electrolyte and fluid transport. This results in diarrhea and electrolyte, fluid, and protein loss as for other causes of colitis (see "Colitis/Diarrhea, Acute" in this section).
- Laminitis occurs in 30% to 40% of horses with PHF, although specific reasons for this increased incidence compared with other causes of equine colitis are not known.

DIAGNOSIS

DIFFERENTIAL DIAGNOSIS

Other causes of colitis (see "Colitis/Diarrhea, Acute" in this section).

INITIAL DATABASE

- In general, as for other causes of colitis (see "Colitis/Diarrhea, Acute" in this section).
- Hypoproteinemia and hypoalbuminemia are a fairly consistent finding and are often dramatic in horses with PHF.

ADVANCED OR CONFIRMATORY TESTING

- Polymerase chain reaction (PCR)
  - Done on EDTA-anticoagulated whole blood to detect *N. risticii* in leukocytes
  - Recently available but appears to be sensitive and specific in clinical cases of PHF
- Serology (immunofluorescent antibody or enzyme-linked immunosorbent assay)
  - Requires documentation of a more than fourfold increase in titer between acute and convalescent sera.
  - Problematic because some horses have already seroconverted when clinical disease is first apparent, and failure to seroconvert does not rule out disease. In addition, horses in endemic areas or vaccinated horses may have high serum titers in the absence of clinical disease.
  - Thus PCR is preferable to serology for diagnosis in clinical cases.
- Testing for other causes of colitis is also warranted as detailed in "Colitis/Diarrhea, Acute" in this section.

TREATMENT

THERAPEUTIC GOAL(S)

- Supportive care
- Specific antimicrobial therapy

ACUTE GENERAL TREATMENT

- Fluid and colloidal support, antiinflammatory and antiendotoxic therapy, and other supportive care as for other causes of colitis (see "Colitis/Diarrhea, Acute" in this section).

- Specific antimicrobial therapy: Oxytetracycline (6.6–11 mg/kg IV diluted q12h for 5–7 days)
- Clinical signs typically improve dramatically within 24 to 72 hours of initiating antimicrobial therapy, although some horses relapse several weeks after discontinuing therapy.
- Oral doxycycline may also be effective, although its absorption may be altered in gastrointestinal disease. Thus IV oxytetracycline is preferable. (Note: Doxycycline should not be given intravenously to horses.)

POSSIBLE COMPLICATIONS

- Laminitis (in 30%–40% of cases)
- As for other causes of colitis (see "Colitis/Diarrhea, Acute" in this section)

PROGNOSIS AND OUTCOME

- Fair to good with aggressive and early therapy
- Guarded with concurrent laminitis

PEARLS & CONSIDERATIONS

COMMENTS

PHF should be strongly suspected in horses in endemic areas with dramatic hypoproteinemia or in those that founder early on in the course of diarrheal disease. However, salmonellosis can present identically and should also be considered as a possible differential diagnosis.

PREVENTION

Annual vaccination (in the early spring and midsummer) should be considered in endemic areas.

SUGGESTED READING

Jones SJ: Medical disorders of the large intestine: acute diarrhea. In Smith BP, editor: *Large animal internal medicine*, ed 4, St Louis, 2009, Mosby Elsevier, pp 743–745.

AUTHOR: **KELSEY A. HART**

EDITORS: **TIM MAIR** and **CERI SHERLOCK**

Prematurity and Dysmaturity

BASIC INFORMATION

DEFINITION

Foals born with physical and physiologic abnormalities consistent with incomplete development of multiple organ systems. Gestation length varies significantly among mares, with an average of 320 to 360 days.

EPIDEMIOLOGY

ASSOCIATED CONDITIONS AND DISORDERS

- Hypoxemia
- Neonatal maladjustment syndrome (perinatal asphyxia, hypoxic ischemic encephalopathy)
- Incomplete ossification of cuboidal bones
- Pulmonary insufficiency

CLINICAL PRESENTATION

HISTORY, CHIEF COMPLAINT

- Low birth weight
- Floppy or droopy ears
- Haircoat: Short, soft, and silky (prematurity) or long and coarse (dysmature)
- Gestation shorter than 320 days or longer than 360 days or significantly different from the dam's normal gestational length

PHYSICAL EXAM FINDINGS

- Weak foal
- Flexor tendon laxity
- Respiration: Hypoventilation, periods of apnea, erratic respiratory rhythms, or tachypnea
- Suckle reflex: Absent, weak, or normal for short duration followed by progressive weakness
- Generalized muscle weakness: Unable to stand, stands only with assistance, or stands with hyperextension of fetlocks
- Hypothermia

ETIOLOGY AND PATHOPHYSIOLOGY

- Maternal illness or stress
- Infectious placentitis
- Placental insufficiency
- Idiopathic
- Chemical induction of parturition (prematurity)
- Twinning

DIAGNOSIS

DIFFERENTIAL DIAGNOSIS

- Congenital hypothyroidism
- Sepsis

INITIAL DATABASE

- Complete blood count (CBC): Normal or leukopenic with neutropenia; neutrophil:lymphocyte ratio less than 1:1
- White blood cells present are cytologically normal; a left shift or toxic neutrophils suggest sepsis
- Radiographs of cuboidal bones may reveal incomplete ossification.

TREATMENT

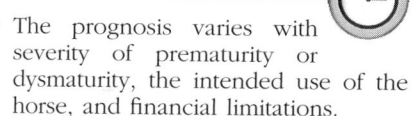

THERAPEUTIC GOAL(S)

- Glucose homeostasis
- Body temperature regulation
- Provision of nutrition
- Adequate transfer of passive immunity
- Cardiovascular support
- Respiratory support
- Protection of musculoskeletal system
- Prevention of infection

ACUTE GENERAL TREATMENT

- Pulmonary
  - Maintain sternal recumbency
  - Intranasal oxygen delivered at 5 to 10 L/min
  - Mechanical ventilation if warranted
- Nutrition
  - IV glucose as 2.5% to 10% solution in balanced crystalloid
  - Dam's milk or foal milk replacer at 15% to 20% body weight/day divided into 12 feedings if the gastrointestinal tract tolerates
  - Indwelling nasogastric tube for feeding if weak
- Antimicrobials
  - Perform blood cultures if sepsis is suspected.
  - Broad-spectrum antibiotics: 22,000 IU/kg potassium penicillin IV slowly q6h plus an aminoglycoside (gentamicin 8.8 mg/kg IV q24h or amikacin 22 mg/kg IV q24h); use a cephalosporin if azotemic (ceftiofur 2.2–10 mg/kg IV or IM q6–12h)
- Supportive care
  - Heating pads, heat lamps, warmed saline bags or bottles, blankets
  - Lubricate the corneas with artificial tears.
  - If the cuboidal bones are incompletely ossified, confine to a small pen to minimize crushing.

POSSIBLE COMPLICATIONS

- Aspiration pneumonia
- Pulmonary insufficiency

- Sepsis
- Cuboidal bone crush

RECOMMENDED MONITORING

- Markedly premature or dysmature foals require intensive medical care.
  - Glucose, lactate, and electrolyte values
  - Ventilation parameters
  - Mean arterial pressure
  - Pulse oximetry
  - Central venous pressure
  - Urine output
  - Fecal output
  - Weight gain
- Less severely affected premature or dysmature foals can be managed less intensively.
  - Cuboidal bone ossification
  - Weight gain
  - Distal limb tendon strength

PROGNOSIS AND OUTCOME

- The prognosis varies with severity of prematurity or dysmaturity, the intended use of the horse, and financial limitations.
- Pulmonary insufficiency is the most significant life-limiting factor affecting short-term prognosis.
- Long-term prognosis is affected by incompletely ossified cuboidal bones and potential for juvenile arthritis secondary to cuboidal bone crushing.

PEARLS & CONSIDERATIONS

COMMENTS

- Bottle feeding often results in aspiration pneumonia in weak foals.
- Failure of passive transfer is common because of both maternal and foal factors.
- Milk replacer brands contain different calorie and electrolyte concentrations. Therefore, monitor the foals's electrolytes while feeding the replacer.
- Diarrhea is common with milk replacer feeding. Goat's milk may be used in combination with or instead of milk replacer to decrease the likelihood of diarrhea.

CLIENT EDUCATION

Intensive critical care for severely affected foals is expensive.

SUGGESTED READING
Lester G: Maturity of the neonatal foal. In Sanchez C, editor: *Neonatal medicine and surgery*, St Louis, 2005, Saunders Elsevier, pp 333–355.

AUTHOR: **PHOEBE A. SMITH**

EDITORS: **ELIZABETH M. SANTSCHI** and **PHOEBE A SMITH**

Prepubic Tendon Rupture

BASIC INFORMATION

DEFINITION
Severe desmitis or complete breakdown of the prepubic tendon

SYNONYM(S)
Prepubic hernia

EPIDEMIOLOGY
SPECIES, AGE, SEX
- Brood mares, especially those in late-term pregnancy
- Older mares

GENETICS AND BREED PREDISPOSITION Draft breeds

RISK FACTORS
- Hydroallantosis
- Hydramnios
- Twin pregnancy
- Fetal giants

CLINICAL PRESENTATION
HISTORY, CHIEF COMPLAINT
- History of pregnancy
- Horse demonstrates alteration of the normal contour of the ventral body wall
- Ventral edema often present
- May have mild to moderate colic signs and appear distressed or reluctant to move

PHYSICAL EXAM FINDINGS
- Abnormal ventral abdominal wall contour
- Associated edema
- Temperature generally normal
- May have normal heart rate or be tachycardic
- Respiratory rate may be normal or mildly elevated
- Mucous membranes are variable from pink and moist to pale and tacky
- Colic signs variable; may be absent or demonstrate mild to moderate colic signs
- Hydration variable
- The pelvis may appear tilted cranially and ventrally.
- The mammary gland may appear more cranial and ventrally placed and may appear stretched.
- The tail head may be raised.
- The horse may adopt a "saw horse" stance.
- External palpation is often obscured by associated edema.

ETIOLOGY AND PATHOPHYSIOLOGY
Rupture of the strong, thick, fibrous prepubic tendon that normally attaches the rectus abdominus, oblique abdominus, gracilis, and pectineus muscles to the cranial border of the pelvis

DIAGNOSIS

DIFFERENTIAL DIAGNOSIS
- Edema
- Ventral abdominal wall hernia (transverse abdominal muscles, oblique abdominal muscles, rectus abdominus)
- Fetal hydrops

INITIAL DATABASE
- Complete blood count: Generally normal
- Peritoneal fluid: May demonstrate mild elevations in protein and white blood cell counts
- Transabdominal ultrasonography: Disruption of the tendon fibers immediately cranial to the pubis. Herniation of gastrointestinal contents may also be apparent. Some horses also have concurrent body wall tears characterized by tears within the muscle fibers and associated hematomas.
- Transrectal palpation: Normally obscured by the presence of a large fetus

TREATMENT

THERAPEUTIC GOAL(S)
- Stabilize the patient.
- Provide analgesia and antiinflammatories.
- If more than 315 days of gestation, promote fetal maturation and parturition.
- If less than 315 days of gestation, stabilize and support the mare if possible.
- If intractable pain or systemic deterioration, perform exploratory celiotomy and cesarean section.

ACUTE GENERAL TREATMENT
- Conservative treatments
  - Stall rest
  - Administer antiinflammatories (ie, nonsteroidal antiinflammatory drugs).
  - Provide abdominal support through a belly bandage.
  - Feed a low-bulk feed to decrease volume and weight of ingesta.
  - Treat as high-risk mare and observe and assist foaling.
- Surgical treatment
  - Perform exploratory celiotomy and cesarean section
- If more than 315 days of gestation
  - Give 100 mg of dexamethasone daily for 3 days to aid fetal maturity.

POSSIBLE COMPLICATIONS
- Laminitis
- Retained placenta
- Septic metritis
- Shock
- Dystocia
- Peritonitis
- Endotoxemia
- Gastrointestinal herniation
- Adhesions
- Ileus
- Jugular thrombophlebitis
- Diarrhea
- Pyrexia
- Incisional infection
- Recurrent colic

RECOMMENDED MONITORING
- Parturition
- Pain
- Body contour
- Colic
- Mentation
- Local swelling, heat, or pain on palpation

PROGNOSIS AND OUTCOME

- Prognosis is variable.
  - Rupture may cause hemorrhage, shock, and death in some mares.

○ Stabilized mares can raise foals.
○ Further breeding is not recommended.
○ Some mares with ruptured prepubic tendons have been used reproductively as embryo donor mares.

PEARLS & CONSIDERATIONS

Assisted delivery at parturition should be provided in any horse whose body wall is compromised.

SUGGESTED READING

Mair TS: Ventral body wall hernias and prepubic tendon rupture. In Mair TS, Divers T, Ducharme N, editors: *Manual of equine gastroenterology*, St Louis, 2002, Saunders Elsevier, pp 321–322.

Orsini JA, Divers, TJ: Gastrointestinal system. In *Equine emergencies: treatment and procedures*, St Louis, 2008, Saunders Elsevier, pp 153.

Ross J, Palmer JE, Wilkins PA: Body wall tears during late pregnancy in mares: 13 cases (1995–2006). *J Am Vet Med Assoc* 232:257–261, 2008.

AUTHOR: **CERI SHERLOCK**

EDITORS: **TIM MAIR** and **CERI SHERLOCK**

Priapism

BASIC INFORMATION

DEFINITION

Priapism is persistent erection with no evidence of sexual arousal.

SYNONYM(S)

Persistent erection

EPIDEMIOLOGY

SPECIES, AGE, SEX Reported in geldings but is far more common in stallions.
RISK FACTORS Administration of phenothiazine-derivative tranquilizers has been shown to lead to priapism and paraphimosis.

CLINICAL PRESENTATION

HISTORY, CHIEF COMPLAINT Penile prolapse with a partial or full erection
PHYSICAL EXAM FINDINGS The prolapsed penis is engorged and partially or completely erect. For this reason, attempts to replace it into the sheath are unsuccessful.

ETIOLOGY AND PATHOPHYSIOLOGY

- Persistent engorgement of the corpus cavernosum penis, most likely caused by disturbances of blood flow
- Lack of detumescence increases carbon dioxide tension within the tissue, leading to a change in blood viscosity and occlusion of the venous outflow.
- The occlusion causes tissue swelling and impairs venous outflow.
- Fibrosis of the cavernous trabeculae follows, causing permanent problems with erection.
- If erection lasts more than a few hours, penile and preputial swelling lead to penile necrosis.

DIAGNOSIS

DIFFERENTIAL DIAGNOSIS

- Paraphimosis: The penis is generally flaccid and cannot be retracted because of injury or disease.
- Penile paralysis: The penis is flaccid secondary to nerve damage.

INITIAL DATABASE

The complete blood count and serum chemistry are usually within normal limits.

ADVANCED OR CONFIRMATORY TESTING

Ultrasonography of the penis may be helpful in determining the extent of thrombosis within the corpus cavernosum. If thrombosis is present, the corpus cavernosum is more hyperechoic than normal.

TREATMENT

THERAPEUTIC GOAL(S)

- The penis should be returned to the prepuce to minimize tissue damage.
- If replacing the penis is impossible, it should be held using a sling or bandage.
- Keep the penis lubricated with antibacterial emollient.

ACUTE GENERAL TREATMENT

- The penis should be cleaned thoroughly to allow adequate examination and assessment of the damage.
- The treatment option depends on the severity and duration of the condition.
- Medical treatment alone is rarely successful but may be attempted in the acute stage and aims to remove blood from the penis.
  ○ Penile massage may help reduce edema and engorgement.
  ○ Intracavernosal injection with 10 mg of phenylephrine diluted in 10 cc of saline (inject 5 cc on each side) may allow the penis to return to the sheath temporarily.
  ○ Inserting a 12-gauge needle into the corpus cavernosum proximal to the glans penis and infusing heparinized saline under pressure will remove the sludged blood. Placing large-bore needles into the corpus cavernosum 10 cm caudal to the base of the scrotum allows drainage. The tissue should be flushed until fresh blood is seen and the penis relaxes. If venous blood is occluded, the procedure will fail because of persistent arterial flow.
  ○ A shunt between the corpus cavernosum penis and the corpus spongiosum penis should be considered if medical management fails.
  ○ Treatment with benztropine mesylate (8 mg IV) has been reported to be successful when treating priapism caused by phenothiazine tranquilization, but scientific data are scarce.
- An antibacterial emollient should be applied to the penis, massaging proximally from the tip to remove edema.
- After the penis has been replaced within the prepuce and sheath, a purse-string suture can be placed around the orifice of the sheath. A small area should be left open to allow the drainage of urine.
- As an alternative to the purse-string suture, a mesh sling may be made using breathable fabric suspended by rubber tubing around the horse's flank and lateral to the scrotum. A narrow-necked plastic bottle may also be used by removing the bottom of the bottle. The penis is placed inside the top half of the padded bottle, inserted into the sheath, and secured with rubber tubing.

- Placing roll cotton around the penis and supporting it close to the ventral body wall using an abdominal wrap or Elastikon bandage is an acceptable alternative.
- Nonsteroidal antiinflammatory drugs should be administered to reduce inflammation and alleviate pain.
- Broad-spectrum antibiotics are indicated if the exposed tissue is devitalized.

CHRONIC TREATMENT

- If the above management fails, penile amputation may be necessary.
- Sexual rest until complete healing occurs is vital.

DRUG INTERACTIONS

Phenylephrine use may cause hypertension and bradycardia.

POSSIBLE COMPLICATIONS

- If the priapism is not resolved, pudendal nerve damage may result in penile paralysis.
- If a surgical shunt is necessary, the stallion may exhibit erection failure caused by either the damaged erectile tissue or the shunt itself.

RECOMMENDED MONITORING

Daily progress should be monitored.

PROGNOSIS AND OUTCOME

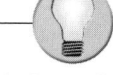

- Rest from all sexual activity is essential.
- Some stallions require assistance with intromission or collection after an episode of priapism.
- The prognosis for return to reproductive function is poor.

PEARLS & CONSIDERATIONS

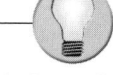

PREVENTION

Judicious use of phenothiazines is recommended.

CLIENT EDUCATION

Immediate aggressive treatment yields a better prognosis than if treatment is delayed.

SUGGESTED READING

Gaughan EM, Van Harreveld PD: Trauma to the penis. In Samper JC, Pycock JF, McKinnon AO, editors: *Current therapy in equine reproduction*, St Louis, 2007, Saunders Elsevier, pp 227–230.

Varner DD: Diseases of the penis. In Varner DD, Schumacher J, Blanchard TL, et al, editors: *Diseases and management of breeding stallions*, Goleta, CA, 1991, American Veterinary Publications, pp 279–290.

AUTHOR: **AIME K. JOHNSON**

EDITOR: **JUAN C. SAMPER**

Proliferative Enteropathy

BASIC INFORMATION

DEFINITION

Small intestinal mucosal inflammation and hyperplasia associated with *Lawsonia intracellularis* infection

SYNONYM(S)

- Proliferative ileitis
- Proliferative enteritis

EPIDEMIOLOGY

SPECIES, AGE, SEX Occurs predominantly in weanlings and yearlings; very rare in adult horses

CONTAGION AND ZOONOSIS May occur in individual animals in a farm or in a herd outbreak

GEOGRAPHY AND SEASONALITY Seen predominantly in the autumn and winter (although this may reflect the age of susceptible horses rather than a true seasonality because of the typical northern equine breeding season)

CLINICAL PRESENTATION

HISTORY, CHIEF COMPLAINT

- Progressive depression, lethargy, inappetence, mild colic, weight loss, and intermittent diarrhea are the most common clinical complaints.
- One or several foals on a farm may be affected.

PHYSICAL EXAM FINDINGS

- Depression.
- Poor body condition and rough hair coat. Affected foals are often smaller than herdmates but may have a "pot-bellied" appearance.
- Fever is not consistently present.
- Variable tachycardia and tachypnea
- Ventral edema (caused by hypoproteinemia) is very common.
- Diarrhea may be present but is not universally observed.
- Gastric reflux is not a characteristic feature.
- Concurrent respiratory signs or dermatitis are occasionally seen because of debilitation.

ETIOLOGY AND PATHOPHYSIOLOGY

- L. *intracellularis* is an intracellular gram-negative rod. It has long been known as the cause of a similar syndrome in pigs. It is shed in the feces of infected animals, but the duration of time it remains infectious in the environment and the source of exposure for affected horses are not known. Exposure to pigs is not required for equine disease.
- The organism invades the crypt cells in the ileum and stimulates mitotic division, resulting in hyperplasia.
- Eventually, marked mucosal thickening and loss of intestinal villi occur, limiting intestinal absorptive capacity and resulting in weight loss and hypoproteinemia.
- With more severe disease, lesions may involve the remainder of the small intestine and occasionally the colon.

DIAGNOSIS

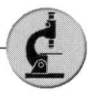

DIFFERENTIAL DIAGNOSIS

- Rhodococcus equi enterocolitis
- Gastroduodenal ulcer disease
- Cyathostominosis in older foals

INITIAL DATABASE

- Complete blood count
  - Leukocytosis characterized by a mature neutrophilia or lymphocytosis is frequently seen, although a normal or decreased leukocyte count may also be found.
  - Hyperfibrinogenemia and mild anemia are sometimes present.
- Serum biochemistry profile
  - Marked hypoproteinemia and hypoalbuminemia is a consistent finding.
  - Variable electrolyte derangements may be seen but are not consistent.
- Transabdominal ultrasonography: Increased small intestinal mural thickness (>5 mm; often >10 mm) is common.

- Peritoneal fluid analysis
  - May be grossly and cytologically normal but most often exhibits a mildly to moderately increased nucleated cell count and total protein concentration
  - More severe peritonitis with greatly increased nucleated cell counts is occasionally observed in foals with severe proliferative enteropathy and is likely attributable to translocation of intestinal bacteria in ulcerated areas.

ADVANCED OR CONFIRMATORY TESTING

- Serology (indirect fluorescent antibody test)
  - Titers above 1:30 are consistent with infection.
  - Most, but not all, foals have seroconverted by the time clinical signs are evident, although the seroprevalence in unaffected foals is not well established at present.
- Polymerase chain reaction (PCR)
  - Can be done on feces or intestinal tissue
  - Positive results confirm infection, although some false-negative results do occur.
- Performing both serology and PCR provides the greatest likelihood of obtaining an accurate diagnosis in clinical cases.
- Pathologic findings
  - Lesions are usually concentrated in the ileum and distal jejunum, although they may be more diffuse.
  - Mucosal thickening and corrugation with ulceration and mural edema are seen grossly.
  - Histopathologic findings include a variable mucosal inflammatory infiltrate with crypt hyperplasia and villous blunting or fusion.
  - Intracellular organisms are visible with silver staining in crypt cells.

TREATMENT

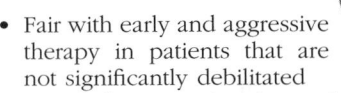

THERAPEUTIC GOAL(S)

- Supportive care: Fluid and colloidal support, nutritional support
- Antimicrobial therapy

ACUTE GENERAL TREATMENT

- IV fluid therapy
  - Colloidal support with equine plasma (20–40 mL/kg IV) or hydroxyethyl starch (5–10 mL/kg IV bolus q24–48h or 1 mL/kg/h IV continuous rate infusion) is usually necessary to treat hypoproteinemia. Repeat plasma transfusions are often needed due to ongoing enteric protein loss.
  - Isotonic balanced polyionic crystalloid fluids (eg, Normosol-R or Plasmalyte) at 50 to 100 mL/kg/d depending on the degree of dehydration and electrolyte derangements.
- Antimicrobial therapy: Several different antimicrobial classes are reportedly effective.
  - Erythromycin (25–30 mg/kg PO q6–8h) and rifampin (5–10 mg/kg PO q12h)
  - Oxytetracycline (6.6 mg/kg IV diluted q12h)
  - Doxycycline (10 mg/kg PO q12h), although its oral bioavailability may be limited in severe intestinal disease
  - Chloramphenicol (30–50 mg/kg PO q8h):
  - Appropriate duration of therapy is vital. Antimicrobials should be continued at least until resolution of clinical signs, clinicopathologic abnormalities, and ultrasonographic abnormalities. This is typically at least 3 weeks and may be more than 6 weeks in severe cases.
- Antiinflammatory and analgesic therapy: Flunixin meglumine (0.5–

1.1 mg/kg IV q12–24h for colic and fever or 0.25 mg/kg IV q8h for antiinflammatory effects). Nonsteroidal antiinflammatory drugs use should be conservative and of short duration in foals to minimize gastrointestinal and renal side effects.
- Gastroprotectants may be indicated in foals that are persistently inappetent (see "Gastric Ulceration in Foals" in this section).
- Diet and nutritional support: Adequate nutritional support is vital. If the foal will not eat well, parenteral nutrition should be considered.

PROGNOSIS AND OUTCOME

- Fair with early and aggressive therapy in patients that are not significantly debilitated
- Guarded to poor in advanced disease or if concurrent peritonitis is present

PEARLS & CONSIDERATIONS

As for *R. equi*, host-pathogen-environment interactions are likely responsible for the development of clinical disease in some foals and not in others.

SUGGESTED READING

David JB: Diarrheal diseases. In Orsini JA, Divers TJ, editors: *Equine emergencies: treatment and procedures*, St Louis, 2008, Saunders Elsevier, pp 159–165.

Davis JL: Medical disorders of the small intestine: proliferative enteropathy. In Smith BP, editor: *Large animal internal medicine*, ed 4, St Louis, 2009, Mosby Elsevier, pp 728–729.

AUTHOR: KELSEY A. HART

EDITORS: TIM MAIR and **CERI SHERLOCK**

Propylene Glycol Toxicosis

BASIC INFORMATION

DEFINITION

Condition caused by intoxication with propylene glycol (PG) characterized by neurologic disturbances

EPIDEMIOLOGY

RISK FACTORS Most reported cases of PG toxicosis in horses are associated with accidental administration via stomach tube (PG mistaken for mineral oil). The reported toxic dose of PG for horses is 6.0 mL/kg.

CLINICAL PRESENTATION

DISEASE FORMS/SUBTYPES Acute neurologic dysfunction, lactic acidosis, diarrhea

HISTORY, CHIEF COMPLAINT Acute onset (10–30 minutes) of central nervous system (CNS) depression and ataxia with progression to profound CNS depression and possible death

PHYSICAL EXAM FINDINGS
- Hypersalivation, diaphoresis, ataxia, CNS depression, tachypnea, fetid odor to feces and breath
- Cyanosis, colic, seizures, coma, and diarrhea have also been reported.

ETIOLOGY AND PATHOPHYSIOLOGY PG is metabolized via alcohol dehydrogenase to acetate, lactate, and pyruvate, resulting in systemic lactic acidosis. No primary renal injury occurs.

DIAGNOSIS

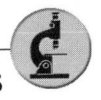

DIFFERENTIAL DIAGNOSIS

Other causes of acute onset of neurologic dysfunction: Viral and bacterial encephalidities, fumonisin, hepatic encephalopathy, ethylene glycol

INITIAL DATABASE

Baseline serum chemistry panel, blood gases: Expect changes consistent with metabolic acidosis

ADVANCED OR CONFIRMATORY TESTING

No specific gross or histologic lesions are expected.

TREATMENT

THERAPEUTIC GOAL(S)

Manage acidosis, provide supportive care, and enhance elimination.

ACUTE GENERAL TREATMENT

- IV fluid diuresis at twice maintenance rate (8.0 mL/kg/h IV) to enhance elimination of PG and metabolites
- Administration of sodium bicarbonate IV as needed based on blood gas results
- Provide quiet, padded environment with minimal sensory stimuli.

RECOMMENDED MONITORING

Acid–base status, oxygen saturation

PROGNOSIS AND OUTCOME

With appropriate aggressive therapy, the prognosis is usually favorable.

PEARLS & CONSIDERATIONS

COMMENTS

Although some sources suggest the use of activated charcoal to adsorb glycols, the current consensus is that activated charcoal is a poor adsorbent for small molecules such as these and is of little benefit in PG exposures.

PREVENTION

- Careful labeling of mineral oil and PG containers to prevent accidental administration of PG to horses
- Food dyes can be added to PG to assist in differentiation from mineral oil.

SUGGESTED READING

Bailey EM, Garland T: Management of toxicoses. In Robinson NE, editor: *Current therapy in equine medicine*, ed 3, Philadelphia, 1992, WB Saunders, pp 346–352.

Dorman DC, Haschek WM: Fatal propylene glycol toxicosis in a horse. *J Am Vet Med Assoc* 198:1643, 1991.

McClanahan S, Hunter J, Murphy M, et al: Propylene glycol toxicosis in a mare. *Vet Hum Toxicol* 40:294, 1998.

AUTHOR: **SHARON GWALTNEY-BRANT**

EDITOR: **CYNTHIA L. GASKILL**

Protein-Losing Nephropathy

BASIC INFORMATION

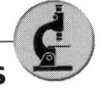

DEFINITION

A disease of protein loss via the kidney caused by an increase in glomerular permeability

EPIDEMIOLOGY

RISK FACTORS Systemic disease usually precedes the development of protein-losing nephropathy.
ASSOCIATED CONDITIONS AND DISORDERS
- Glomerulonephritis
- Thrombosis caused by renal loss of antithrombin III
- When clinical signs become apparent, renal failure often develops

CLINICAL PRESENTATION

DISEASE FORMS/SUBTYPES May be subclinical or clinical
HISTORY, CHIEF COMPLAINT
- Weight loss
- ± Ventral edema
- ± Anorexia
- ± Lethargy
PHYSICAL EXAM FINDINGS
- Poor body condition or weight loss
- ± Ventral edema

ETIOLOGY AND PATHOPHYSIOLOGY

Damage to the glomerular membrane allows proteins to leak from systemic circulation into the renal tubules. The protein cannot be reabsorbed, so it is lost via the urine.

DIAGNOSIS

DIFFERENTIAL DIAGNOSIS

- Glomerulonephritis (renal protein loss)
- Amyloidosis (renal protein loss)
- Protein-losing enteropathy (gastrointestinal protein loss)
- Hepatic disease (ill thrift, hypoproteinemia; decreased production of protein)
- Urinary tract infection (bacteriuria or pyuria)

INITIAL DATABASE

- Serum chemistries: Low total protein and albumin concentrations; may have elevated blood urea nitrogen and creatinine concentrations depending on the degree of renal insufficiency
- Urinalysis: Proteinuria alone is indicative of glomerular protein loss. The presence of red blood cells, leukocytes, and bacteria in addition to protein is suggestive of urinary tract infection.
- Rectal palpation: The left kidney may be small if the patient has advanced renal disease.
- Renal ultrasonography: May see loss of corticomedullary contrast if the patient has advanced renal disease

ADVANCED OR CONFIRMATORY TESTING

- A urine protein:creatinine ratio above 2:1 indicates glomerular protein loss.
- Sulfosalicylic acid precipitation is a sensitive test for urinary protein concentration. Urine dipsticks usually read trace protein because of the alkalinity of equine urine.
- Antithrombin III concentrations decreased in plasma and increased in urine.
- Renal biopsy and histopathology confirms glomerulonephritis. Specialized immunohistochemistry or electron microscopy may be needed to identify the cause and severity of disease.
- Systemic blood pressure may be elevated.
- Glucose or D-xylose absorption test to rule out protein-losing enteropathy
- Additional diagnostics to determine underlying disease may be beneficial.

TREATMENT

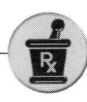

THERAPEUTIC GOAL(S)

- Address the underlying disease, if present.
- Address hypercoagulability.
- Address hypertension.
- Reduce dietary protein intake.

ACUTE GENERAL TREATMENT

- Treat any underlying disease process.
- Reduce dietary protein: 1.3 g of crude protein/kg/day is the lower end of protein requirement for horses. This can be accomplished by feeding 6.4 kg of grass hay and 2 kg of 12% protein senior-type feed per day.
- Hypercoagulability: Low-dose aspirin therapy (4–12 mg/kg PO q24–48h)
- Hypertension: Angiotensin converting enzyme (ACE) inhibitors, such as enalapril (2 mg/kg PO q12h), may be useful if not cost prohibitive. Acepromazine (0.02 mg/kg PO q8–12h) is inferior to ACE inhibitors but may be useful to reduce blood pressure.
- Immunosuppressive therapy: Only if indicated for underlying disease. Cor-

ticosteroids are known to increase glomerular filtration rate, stimulate glomerular hypertrophy, and enhance matrix production in humans. They can also increase the risk of infection, thrombosis, and azotemia.

CHRONIC TREATMENT

Same as for acute treatment

POSSIBLE COMPLICATIONS

None with protein restriction. Treatments for underlying disease process (immunosuppressive therapy) may have complications.

RECOMMENDED MONITORING

Monitor the degree of proteinuria as well as azotemia and the horse's clinical condition.

PROGNOSIS AND OUTCOME

- The prognosis for long-term survival is poor, even with treatment.

- Horses with chronic low-grade azotemia may still be useful for breeding or light riding.

PEARLS & CONSIDERATIONS

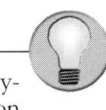

- Glomerulonephritis and amyloidosis are the most common causes of protein loss in the urine.
- Trace protein result using urine dipsticks is an often normal finding because of the alkalinity of equine urine interfering with the reagent.

SUGGESTED READING

Brunker J: Protein-losing nephropathy. *Compend Contin Educ Pract Vet* 27:686–694, 2005.

Toribio R: Essentials of equine renal and urinary tract physiology. *Vet Clin North Am Equine Pract* 23:533–561, 2007.

AUTHOR: **KELLY L. CARLSON**

EDITOR: **BRYAN M. WALDRIDGE**

Pulmonary Fibrosis, Multinodular

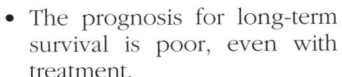

BASIC INFORMATION

DEFINITION

Multinodular pulmonary fibrosis (MPF) is a respiratory disease of adult horses that is characterized by interstitial and nodular pulmonary infiltrates of collagen and inflammatory cells. It has been associated with equine herpesvirus-5 (EHV-5).

EPIDEMIOLOGY

SPECIES, AGE, SEX Affects adults
CONTAGION AND ZOONOSIS
- Despite the association with EHV-5, there have been no clusters of MPF reported, suggesting that it is minimally to noncontagious.
- EHV-5 is not known to be zoonotic.

CLINICAL PRESENTATION

HISTORY, CHIEF COMPLAINT Horses with MPF typically have a history of respiratory distress, tachypnea, cough, increased rectal temperature, and chronic weight loss with hyporexia.
PHYSICAL EXAM FINDINGS
- Affected animals are usually thin and have an increased respiratory rate (20–30 breaths/min), mild to moderate tachycardia, and rectal temperatures up to 105° F.

- Thoracic auscultation may reveal either loud bronchovesicular sounds or widely dispersed crackles and wheezes.

ETIOLOGY AND PATHOPHYSIOLOGY
The cause of MPF has not been fully elucidated. However, EHV-5 was obtained from the bronchoalveolar (BAL) fluid or biopsies of all cases included in a recently published series and is found only rarely in unaffected horses. Despite this strong association, a causative relationship has not yet been established.

DIAGNOSIS

DIFFERENTIAL DIAGNOSIS

- Infectious lung disease such as bacterial, viral, or fungal pneumonia. In addition to bacterial pleuropneumonia, these include diseases such as EHV-1 and -4, blastomycosis, coccidiomycosis, histoplasmosis, cryptococcosis, and aspergillosis
- Inflammatory disease such as recurrent airway obstruction ("heaves")
- Toxicoses, including inhaled toxins (silicosis, various gases) as well as systemically ingested substances such as perilla mint

- Neoplastic disease, including primary tumors of the respiratory tract or, more commonly, distant metastases
- Other forms of idiopathic pulmonary fibrosis

INITIAL DATABASE

- The complete blood count usually demonstrates a moderate neutrophilic leukocytosis with hyperfibrinogenemia. Significant (<1000/µL) lymphopenia and mild anemia are often seen.
- Arterial blood gas analysis reveals hypoxemia consistent with the severity of the disease.
- Airway sampling (bronchoalveolar lavage or transtracheal aspirate) shows nonspecific degenerate or nondegenerate neutrophilic inflammation and mucus. Bacterial and fungal cultures are unremarkable but may reveal the presence of secondary bacterial infection.

ADVANCED OR CONFIRMATORY TESTING

- Radiography is extremely helpful in characterizing the disease and reveals diffuse nodular interstitial disease. With this result in hand, the differential diagnoses are typically narrowed to fungal, neoplastic, or idiopathic pulmonary fibrosis.

- Ultrasonography is nonspecific and may show pleural roughening or small nodules contiguous with the surface of the lung. Dense consolidation and abscessation of the ventral lung fields (as would be seen with pleuropneumonia) are absent.
- Lung biopsy can prove to be useful in differentiating between MPF and other potential diagnoses. Histopathology is characterized by interstitial collagen deposition, neutrophil and macrophage accumulation within the alveoli, and type II pneumocyte hyperplasia. Occasional alveolar macrophages may contain intranuclear inclusion bodies believed to be associated with EHV-5.
- Polymerase chain reaction for EHV-5 may be performed on BAL fluid or lung biopsy samples; a positive result is highly suggestive of MPF.
- On postmortem examination, the lungs show multiple 1- to 10-cm firm, white or tan nodules that may be discrete or coalescing. The lungs do not collapse upon opening the thorax.

TREATMENT

THERAPEUTIC GOAL(S)

- Immediate goals include stabilizing the patient by ensuring adequate oxygenation.

- Longer term goals involve reduction of inflammation and antiviral therapy to treat the suspected cause of MPF.

ACUTE GENERAL TREATMENT

- Intranasal oxygen at 15 L/min should be provided if the patient appears distressed, and a goal of maintaining arterial oxygen tension at >60 mm Hg is desirable.
- Therapy with acyclovir (15–20 mg/kg PO q4–8h or 10 mg/kg IV q12h) and prednisolone (1 mg/kg PO q24h) have been used successfully in some cases.
- Secondary bacterial bronchitis or pneumonia are possible comorbidities and should be treated based on culture results with the appropriate antimicrobial regimen.

RECOMMENDED MONITORING

Patients should undergo radiographic (or less ideally, sonographic) monitoring until the disease is resolved.

PROGNOSIS AND OUTCOME

- Prognosis for MPF is fair, with two of five horses from a published report surviving and returning to their previous level of work.

The remaining horses were euthanized because of poor response to treatment.

- Because response to therapy is often slow, treatment should ideally be continued for at least 6 weeks before considering further treatment futile.

PEARLS & CONSIDERATIONS

Interstitial pneumonia of donkeys has recently been linked to asinine herpesvirus (AHV)-2 and -5. The exact role of gamma Herpesviridae in equids is still unclear.

SUGGESTED READING

Williams KJ, Maes R, Del Piero F, et al: Equine multinodular pulmonary fibrosis: a newly recognized herpesvirus associated fibrotic lung disease. *Vet Pathol* 44(6):849–862, 2007.

Wilkins PA: Equine multinodular pulmonary fibrosis: new, emerging or simply recently described? *Equine Vet Educ* 20(9):477–479, 2008.

Wong DM, Belgrave RL, Williams KJ, et al: Multinodular pulmonary fibrosis in five horses. *J Am Vet Med Assoc* 232(6):898–905, 2008.

AUTHOR: **ROSE NOLEN-WALSTON**

EDITOR: **MELISSA R. MAZAN**

Pulmonary Hypertension

BASIC INFORMATION

DEFINITION

Elevated systolic, mean, and diastolic pulmonary artery (PA) pressures

SYNONYM(S)

Pulmonary artery hypertension

EPIDEMIOLOGY

RISK FACTORS

- Significant left-sided cardiac disease
- Severe pulmonary disease

GEOGRAPHY AND SEASONALITY Pulmonary hypertension (PH) has been associated with horses and ponies residing at high altitudes.

ASSOCIATED CONDITIONS AND DISORDERS

- Severe pneumonia; acute respiratory distress syndrome (ARDS)
- Severe recurrent airway obstruction (RAO)

- Severe left-sided cardiac disease
- Strenuous exercise

CLINICAL PRESENTATION

DISEASE FORMS/SUBTYPES

- Primary PH
  - A primary vascular disorder
  - Persistent fetal circulation (persistent PH of the newborn)
- Secondary PH
  - As a result of cardiac disease
  - As a result of pulmonary disease
- PH associated with strenuous exercise

HISTORY, CHIEF COMPLAINT

- Variable, depending on the underlying cause and chronicity
- May have exercise intolerance, elevated resting respiratory rate, dyspnea, cough
- May have syncope or collapse
- May have weight loss
- May have ventral edema

PHYSICAL EXAM FINDINGS

- Depend on the underlying cause
- May have signs associated with heart failure or severe respiratory compromise (eg, tachypnea, dyspnea, cough, nasal froth, crackles or wheezes on thoracic auscultation, tachycardia, venous distension, jugular venous pulse, arrhythmias, cardiac murmurs, weight loss, ventral edema)
- Other signs associated with primary disease process (eg, fever, depression).

ETIOLOGY AND PATHOPHYSIOLOGY

- Primary PH is not well-documented in horses.
  - The cause and mechanism are unknown in horses but may include structural and perhaps biochemical derangements of the pulmonary circulation.
  - Histopathology shows characteristic lesions in pulmonary vasculature in

the absence of significant pulmonary or cardiac disease.
- Persistence of fetal circulation
  - Abnormalities of transition from fetal pulmonary circulation (high resistance, low flow) to postnatal pulmonary circulation (low resistance, high flow)
  - Fetal and neonatal circulations normally have a heightened sensitivity to various stimuli, causing vasoconstriction and vascular smooth muscle proliferation or hypertrophy. Many factors may exacerbate this, including certain drugs, chronic in utero hypoxia or fetal distress, pulmonary disease, congenital cardiac anomalies causing increased pulmonary arterial flow, systolic dysfunction, hypoplastic lungs secondary to congenital diaphragmatic hernia, or genetics.
- Secondary PH is most commonly a complication of cardiac or pulmonary disease. Primary mechanisms:
  - Increased left atrial pressure (left-sided cardiac disease) causing increased pulmonary venous, capillary, and arterial pressures
    - May result from a variety of diseases but most commonly in horses is associated with severe mitral valve regurgitation, cardiomyopathy, or congestive heart failure (CHF; left ventricular failure)
  - Increased pulmonary vascular resistance (pulmonary diseases, high altitude) causing elevated PA pressures
    - Pulmonary diseases such as severe RAO, ARDS, or advanced pulmonary fibrosis; hypoxia associated with high altitude; and obstructive vascular diseases (pulmonary thromboembolism) may increase pulmonary vascular pressures.
    - Endotoxemia may also result in increased pulmonary vascular resistance and elevated PA pressures.
  - Increased pulmonary blood flow causing vascular remodeling. This may occur with congenital cardiac diseases that have large left-to-right shunts.

DIAGNOSIS

DIFFERENTIAL DIAGNOSIS

- It may be difficult to distinguish clinical signs of PH from those of the disease causing the PH.
- For clinical signs related to the respiratory tract (eg, tachypnea, dyspnea or distress, exercise intolerance, cough):

Respiratory diseases such as RAO, ARDS, pneumonia, and pleuropneumonia
- For clinical signs referable to the cardiovascular system (eg, tachycardia, arrhythmia, jugular distension or pulses, murmurs, exercise intolerance, collapse, ventral edema): Cardiac diseases such as severe mitral regurgitation, severe aortic regurgitation, severe tricuspid regurgitation (TR), CHF, cardiomyopathy, and pericarditis

INITIAL DATABASE

- Pursuit of diagnostics for pulmonary disease (eg, thoracic ultrasound, thoracic radiographs, tracheal wash, bronchoalveolar lavage)
- Echocardiography to assess cardiac contribution to disease (eg, large left atrium, severe mitral regurgitation, decreased left ventricular systolic function, structural defects), or the effect of PH on cardiac function (right ventricular dilatation or hypertrophy, abnormal septal wall motion, right atrial enlargement)
- Electrocardiography to document arrhythmias
- Arterial blood gas: May show hypoxemia, ± hypercapnia or hypocapnia
- Complete blood count: May be normal or show changes associated with primary disease process
- Chemistry panel: May be normal or show changes associated with primary disease process

ADVANCED OR CONFIRMATORY TESTING

- The gold standard for diagnosis of PH is PA catheterization. However, this is invasive, and the equipment is not readily available except in university settings and at some referral practices. PA catheterization gives systolic, diastolic, and mean PA pressures. In addition, pulmonary capillary wedge pressures can be obtained to estimate pulmonary venous and left atrial pressures (and thus confirm cardiac contribution).
- Because of the invasive nature of right heart catheterization, echocardiographic estimation of PA pressures has become common in human and small animal medicine.
  - The most commonly used measurement is to determine the velocity of tricuspid regurgitation using Doppler echocardiography and apply the modified Bernoulli equation:
    - $\Delta P = 4v^2$, where ΔP is the pressure gradient between the two chambers (right atrial and right ventricular) and v is the velocity of the regurgitant jet. This gives the systolic pressure of the right

ventricle if the right atrial pressure is known or (more commonly) estimated. In the absence of pulmonic stenosis, the systolic right ventricular pressure is approximately equal to the systolic PA pressure.
- The echocardiographic parameters used in other species have not been validated in horses. One disadvantage to use of Doppler estimation is the difficulty in aligning the cursor parallel to the TR jet in horses. This results in underestimation of the velocity of the regurgitant blood flow and consequently underestimation of systolic PA pressure. In addition, not all horses with PH have TR.
- The size of the PA relative to the aorta has been used to subjectively assess elevations in pressures; a PA diameter larger than aortic root diameter is suggestive of moderate to severely elevated PA pressures (Figure 1).

TREATMENT

THERAPEUTIC GOAL(S)

Treatment is aimed at reducing PA pressures, particularly if showing signs of right-sided heart failure and correcting or managing the underlying cause.

ACUTE GENERAL TREATMENT

- Oxygen therapy
- Specific treatment of underlying disease process causing PH (see "Airway Obstruction, Recurrent," "Cardiac Failure," "Cardiomyopathy," "Mitral/Tricuspid Regurgitation, Acquired," and "Endocarditis, Infective" in this section.)
- Inhaled nitric oxide (NO) decreases PA pressures acutely and can be used in intensive care cases; however, it is not readily available, must be supplied continuously if used alone because of extremely short half-life, and medical grade is exceedingly expensive.
- Sildenafil, a type 5 phosphodiesterase inhibitor, has been used in horses to decrease PA pressures. However, pharmacokinetics and appropriate dosing have not been evaluated in horses, and dosing regimens are extrapolated from humans and dogs. No controlled studies have evaluated the efficacy in horses.
- Antiarrhythmics to control tachyarrhythmias that are life threatening or have the potential to deteriorate (sustained heart rate >100–120 beats/min, hemodynamically significant dysrhythmias, multiform ventricular tachycardia, R on T phenomenon) (see "Ventricular Premature Complex/Ventricular Tachycardia" in this section).

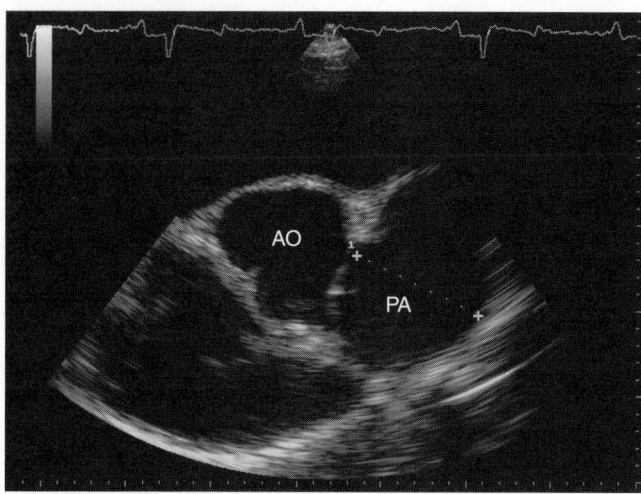

FIGURE 1 Right parasternal short axis view of the aorta and pulmonary artery. Note the diameter of the pulmonary artery (PA) is larger than the diameter of the aorta, suggestive of PH. This echocardiogram and PA pressures were obtained in a horse with recurrent airway obstruction in crisis that had a mean PA pressure of 82 mm Hg. (Photo courtesy Mary Durando.)

CHRONIC TREATMENT

- Treatment needed to control underlying disease should be continued. Specific treatment directed at controlling PH has not been adequately investigated in horses, and options are limited.
- Sildenafil administration can be continued; however, cost will likely prohibit long-term use in adult horses.

POSSIBLE COMPLICATIONS

- Right ventricular failure
- Rupture of PA if it becomes extremely enlarged
- Atrial fibrillation if right atrium becomes enlarged
- Complications associated with primary disease process

RECOMMENDED MONITORING

- Clinical examination parameters such as attitude, appetite, lethargy or exercise intolerance, respiratory rate and effort, nostril flare, heart rate, and weight should be monitored by the owner. Any changes should prompt a veterinary examination.
- Periodic echocardiograms to monitor either right heart function, size of PA, or underlying disease if secondary to cardiac disease are essential.

- If arrhythmias suspected, an electrocardiogram or 24-hour Holter monitor should be obtained.
- Monitor resolution of primary disease process.

PROGNOSIS AND OUTCOME

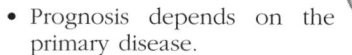

- Prognosis depends on the primary disease.
- Most cardiac diseases that cause PH cannot be resolved, and treatment aims are to improve quality of life and prolong life in the short term (usually <6 months to 1 year). Prognosis is guarded to poor for PH secondary to structural cardiac diseases that are advanced and irreversible. These horses are often euthanized because of poor prognosis. If PH is secondary to reversible cardiac disease, the prognosis may be fair.
- Horses with advanced cardiac disease and PH are at risk for sudden death.
- PH associated with respiratory diseases such as RAO have a good prognosis, providing RAO can be kept in remission using good management practices (environmental control and medical therapy such as antiinflammatory agents and bronchodilators).

- PH secondary to ARDS has a fair to poor prognosis, depending on response of ARDS to therapy.
- Horses with advanced pulmonary fibrosis and pulmonary thromboembolism have a poor prognosis.

PEARLS & CONSIDERATIONS

COMMENTS

- Most cases of PH are fairly advanced by the time they are diagnosed, worsening the prognosis.
- It is often difficult to differentiate PH from the primary cause, and diagnosis requires a strong index of suspicion. Therefore, horses with severe respiratory or cardiac disease and signs of right heart failure (distended jugular veins, ventral edema, ± pleural effusion, ± ascites) should be evaluated for PH.

PREVENTION

None, other than to control primary disease and reduce its severity

CLIENT EDUCATION

Horses with PH secondary to cardiac disease are not safe to ride and should never be ridden. They are at risk for collapse because of ventricular arrhythmia or sudden death due to PA rupture.

SUGGESTED READING

Dixon PM: Pulmonary artery pressures in normal horses and in horses affected with chronic obstructive pulmonary disease. *Equine Vet J* 10:195, 1978.

Greene HM, Wickler SJ, Anderson TP, et al: High-altitude effects on respiratory gases, acid-base balance and pulmonary artery pressure in equids. *Equine Vet J Suppl* 30:71–76, 1999.

Lester GD, DeMarco VG, Norman WM: Effect of inhaled nitric oxide on experimentally induced pulmonary hypertension in neonatal foals. *Am J Vet Res* 60:1207, 1999.

Miller PJ, Holmes JR: Observations on seven cases of mitral insufficiency in the horse. *Equine Vet J* 17:181–190, 1985.

Reef VB, Bain FT, Spencer PA, et al: Severe mitral regurgitation in horses: clinical, echocardiographic and pathologic findings. *Equine Vet J* 30:18, 1998.

AUTHORS: ERIC BIRKS and MARY M. DURANDO

EDITOR: MARY DURANDO

Purpura Hemorrhagica

BASIC INFORMATION

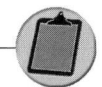

DEFINITION

A hemorrhagic and edematous disease that develops after infection or vaccination against *Streptococcus equi* subsp. *equi*; believed to be allergic in origin

SYNONYM(S)

Hypersensitivity vasculitis

EPIDEMIOLOGY

SPECIES, AGE, SEX

- An uncommon sporadic disease of horses associated with upper respiratory tract infections
- Develops in horses producing high antibody levels against *S. equi* subsp. *equi* in the presence of *S. equi* subsp. *equi* antigen
- Rarely occurs with infections with *Streptococcus equi* subsp. *zooepidemicus*, equine influenza virus, *Rhodococcus equi*, *Corynebacterium pseudotuberculosis*, and equine herpesvirus type 1
- In some cases, it develops in the absence of any obvious infection.
- May develop in a sensitized horse that is exposed to *S. equi* subsp. *equi*–infected animals.

CLINICAL PRESENTATION

DISEASE FORMS/SUBTYPES

- Two to four weeks after an acute *S. equi* subsp. *equi* infection (or vaccination against *S. equi* subsp. *equi*), horses develop extensive, well-demarcated cutaneous edema (urticaria) on the head, ventral abdomen, and extremities.
- Extensive limb edema is usual.
- The edema is not usually painful and pits with gentle pressure.
- Affected horses are depressed and reluctant to move.
- Mucosal petechial or ecchymotic hemorrhages appear in the mucosa and subcutaneous tissues such as the mouth and nasal cavities as well as under the conjunctiva.
- Affected horses are anorexic and depressed.
- Horses may have a high fever.
- The skin of the limbs may slough.

ETIOLOGY AND PATHOPHYSIOLOGY

- Immune complexes containing *S. equi* subsp. *equi* antigens (M-protein or R-protein) are generated in the bloodstream of affected animals.
- These immune complexes are deposited in the walls of capillaries, where they cause an acute vasculitis, as well as a type I Membranoproliferative glomerulonephritis with resulting proteinuria and azoturia.

DIAGNOSIS

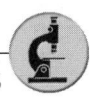

DIFFERENTIAL DIAGNOSIS

- Equine viral arteritis
- Equine herpesvirus infection
- Equine granulocytic ehrlichiosis
- Congestive heart failure
- Angioneurotic edema
- Equine infectious anemia
- Thrombocytopenia

INITIAL DATABASE

- Temperature normal or slightly elevated
- Heart rate raised (90–100 beats/min)
- Complete blood count shows mild anemia (packed cell volume >20%)
- Neutrophilia
- Elevated fibrinogen
- Platelets normal
- May have elevated creatine kinase

ADVANCED OR CONFIRMATORY TESTING

A skin biopsy shows the characteristic leukocytoclastic vasculitis.

TREATMENT

THERAPEUTIC GOAL(S)

- Remove the antigenic stimulus.
- Reduce the immune response.
- Reduce vascular inflammation.

ACUTE GENERAL TREATMENT

- Administer fluids by nasogastric tube or IV to depressed or dehydrated animals.
- Tracheotomy
- Antiinflammatory drugs
  - Flunixin meglumine (1.1 mg/kg PO or IV q12h).
  - Alternatively Phenylbutazone (2.2 mg/kg orally or IV q12h).
- Dexamethasone (0.08 mg/kg IV or IM once daily given in the morning). Administer sufficient amount to reduce edema. When the edema begins to resolve, corticosteroid doses should be gradually reduced over 7 to 21 days provided signs do not recur.
- Alternatively, prednisolone (1 mg/kg) IM or IV q24h
- Horses with streptococcal infection should receive penicillin (22,000 IU/kg of procaine penicillin IM q12h). Alternatively, potassium penicillin G may be given (22,000 IU/kg IV q6h) for at least 2 weeks.
- Bandage edematous limbs, provide aggressive hydrotherapy, and provide fluid replacement.

CHRONIC TREATMENT

- Some horses require more than 4 weeks of corticosteroid therapy.
- Relapses may occur despite treatment.

POSSIBLE COMPLICATIONS

- Pharyngeal edema leading to dyspnea. Emergency tracheotomy is required.
- Skin sloughing, cellulitis, pneumonia, diarrhea

PROGNOSIS AND OUTCOME

Prognosis is fair with aggressive early treatment and supportive care.

PEARLS & CONSIDERATIONS

Avoid exposure of sensitized horses to *S. equi* subsp. *equi* antigen.

SUGGESTED READING

Galan JE, Timoney JF: Immune complexes in purpura hemorrhagica of the horse contain IgA and M antigen of *Streptococcus equi*. *J Immunol* 135:3134–3137, 1985.

Heath SE, Geor RJ, Tabel H, et al: Unusual patterns of serum antibodies to *Streptococcus equi* in two horses with purpura hemorrhagica. *J Vet Intern Med* 5:263–267, 1991.

Kaese HJ, Valberg SJ, Hayden DW, et al: Infarctive purpura hemorrhagica in five horses. *J Am Vet Med Assoc* 226:1893–1898, 2005.

Pusterla N, Watson JL, Affolter VK, et al: Purpura haemorrhagica in 53 horses. *Vet Rec* 153:118–121, 2003.

AUTHOR & EDITOR: IAN TIZZARD

Pyelonephritis

BASIC INFORMATION

DEFINITION

A suppurative bacterial infection of the renal pelvis and parenchyma

EPIDEMIOLOGY

RISK FACTORS Pyelonephritis is often a consequence of an ascending urinary tract infection (UTI) secondary to urine stasis (bladder paralysis, pregnancy, urolithiasis, or urethral stricture). Although rare, hematogenous infection is also possible.

CONTAGION AND ZOONOSIS *Leptospira interrogans* can be a zoonotic pathogen with mucosal exposure to infective urine and may occur as a herd outbreak. Other conditions associated with equine leptospirosis include abortion and uveitis.

ASSOCIATED CONDITIONS AND DISORDERS
- Bladder paralysis
- Urolithiasis
- Urethral stricture
- Pregnancy
- Bacteremia

CLINICAL PRESENTATION

HISTORY, CHIEF COMPLAINT Similar to other causes of chronic renal disease, common complaints include weight loss, lethargy, depression, and anorexia. Other complaints or history may include hematuria (sometimes profuse), polydipsia, polyuria, dysuria, pollakiuria, and stranguria.

PHYSICAL EXAM FINDINGS Physical examination findings include but are not limited to fever, weight loss, depression, hematuria, or pyuria. Examination of the renal and urinary system per rectum may find abnormalities or enlargement of the ureters or left kidney.

ETIOLOGY AND PATHOPHYSIOLOGY
- Bladder distension as a result of urine stasis leads to laxity of the natural physical barrier created by the ureteral orifices. This results in vesiculoureteral reflux, which allows for ascending UTI to develop.
- Because the kidney is a highly vascular organ, hematogenous infection may occur in bacteremic or septicemic animals.
- Common bacterial isolates include *Escherichia coli*, *Proteus mirabilis*, *Corynebacterium* spp., *Enterobacter* spp., *Klebsiella* spp., *Pseudomonas* spp., *Staphylococcus* spp., *Streptococcus* spp., *Actinobacillus* spp., and *Salmonella* spp.

- Hematogenous infection most often involves *L. interrogans*, *Actinobacillus equuli*, and *Salmonella* spp.

DIAGNOSIS

DIFFERENTIAL DIAGNOSIS
- Chronic renal failure
- Chronic interstitial nephritis
- Renal neoplasia
- Urolithiasis
- Bacterial cystitis
- Verminous nephritis (*Halicephalobus gingivalis* infection)

INITIAL DATABASE
- Urinalysis may find pyuria or hematuria.
- Complete blood count (CBC) may show leukocytosis and hyperfibrinogenemia. Anemia may be present if gross hematuria is observed or caused by chronic disease.
- Serum biochemistries may show azotemia or acid-base disturbances.
- Ultrasonographic examination of the kidney may show increased renal echogenicity, abnormal renal outline, loss of corticomedullary distinction, dilatation of the renal pelvis, and echogenic debris in the renal pelvis. In some horses, ultrasound examination may reveal focal hypoechoic to hyperechoic wedge-shaped defects believed to be renal infarcts.

ADVANCED OR CONFIRMATORY TESTING
- Cystoscopic examination may reveal pyuria or hematuria originating from the ureter(s) or dilatation of the ureteral orifice.
- Endoscopic collection of urine from the affected ureter for bacterial culture and antimicrobial sensitivity testing
- Renal biopsy for histopathologic examination and bacterial culture
- Quantitative bacterial culture of urine and antimicrobial sensitivity testing

TREATMENT

THERAPEUTIC GOAL(S)

Eliminate the infection through a protracted course of antimicrobial therapy.

ACUTE GENERAL TREATMENT
- Broad-spectrum antibiotics, especially those that are eliminated in the urine (penicillins, aminoglycosides, potentiated sulfonamides, cephalosporins, and fluoroquinolones)
- IV fluids in azotemic or dehydrated animals

CHRONIC TREATMENT
- A prolonged course (often several months) of antimicrobial therapy based on culture and sensitivity testing is frequently necessary to clear the infection.
- Supportive therapy for treatment of acid-base disturbances
- Blood transfusion as necessary for treatment of anemia secondary to hematuria
- Surgical removal of the infected kidney and ureter (if the contralateral kidney has been found to be normal)

RECOMMENDED MONITORING
- CBC for improvement of leukocytosis and hyperfibrinogenemia
- Cystoscopy for collection of urine from the affected ureter and kidney for culture to determine if the infection has resolved

PROGNOSIS AND OUTCOME
- Prognosis is often poor because of failure to diagnose pyelonephritis early in the course of disease.
- The recurrence rate is high.

PEARLS & CONSIDERATIONS
- Pyelonephritis is typically a unilateral disease, but it may be bilateral. With unilateral involvement, the contralateral kidney usually maintains adequate renal function.
- Because of its subtle onset, pyelonephritis is often not recognized until it has become chronic.
- Most horses require several months of antibiotic therapy.

SUGGESTED READING

Divers TJ: Chronic renal failure: disease of the renal system. In Smith BP, editor: *Large animal internal medicine*, ed 4, St Louis, 2009, Mosby Elsevier, pp 930–935.

Schumacher J: Hematuria and pigmenturia in horses. *Vet Clin Equine* 23:655, 2007.

AUTHOR: JENNIFER TAINTOR

EDITOR: BRYAN M. WALDRIDGE

Pyloric Stenosis

BASIC INFORMATION

DEFINITION

Impaired gastric emptying caused by pyloric sphincter dysfunction or pyloric or duodenal stricture

SYNONYM(S)

- Pyloric stenosis
- Functional gastric outflow obstruction ("pseudoobstruction")

EPIDEMIOLOGY

SPECIES, AGE, SEX

- Idiopathic pyloric smooth muscle hypertrophy (pyloric stenosis) occurs predominantly in foals and weanlings.
- Pyloric sphincter dysfunction or pyloric stricture secondary to severe gastric ulceration also occurs predominantly in young horses with gastroduodenal ulcer disease but is occasionally seen in older horses with severe gastric ulceration.
- No apparent breed or sex predisposition has been described.

ASSOCIATED CONDITIONS AND DISORDERS

- Secondary gastroesophageal reflux may occur, resulting in esophagitis or esophageal ulceration.
- Gastric impaction.

CLINICAL PRESENTATION

HISTORY, CHIEF COMPLAINT

- Colic (usually mild and recurrent but may be acute)
- Inappetence
- ± Weight loss
- ± Spontaneous nasal reflux of gastric contents
- ± Signs associated with gastroesophageal ulceration (bruxism, hypersalivation, colic associated with eating; see "Gastric Ulceration" in this section)

PHYSICAL EXAM FINDINGS

- May be within normal limits or poor body condition, dehydration, or variable tachycardia (because of pain associated with gastric distension) may be present.
- Large-volume gastric reflux is usually obtained on passage of a nasogastric tube, although reflux may not be present if a concurrent gastric impaction is present.

ETIOLOGY AND PATHOPHYSIOLOGY

- The inciting cause of pyloric smooth muscle hypertrophy in foals with idiopathic pyloric stenosis is unknown. It is presumed to be a developmental abnormality that may be present from birth, or muscle hypertrophy may develop from abnormal pyloric myoelectrical activity in early life.
- Functional impairment of gastric outflow ("pseudoobstruction") occasionally occurs when pyloric myoelectric function is disrupted by mural inflammation associated with gastric ulceration.
- Chronic or severe gastroduodenal ulceration may result in fibrosis and subsequent pyloric or duodenal stricture.

DIAGNOSIS

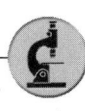

DIFFERENTIAL DIAGNOSIS

- Mechanical gastric outflow obstruction secondary to proximal small intestinal obstruction
- Functional gastric outflow obstruction caused by proximal small intestinal ileus, associated with proximal duodenitis or jejunitis, postoperative ileus, or equine grass sickness

INITIAL DATABASE

- Complete blood count: Usually within reference intervals.
- Serum biochemistry profile: A hypochloremic metabolic alkalosis is typically present because of gastric sequestration of hydrochloric acid.
- Transabdominal ultrasonography: Caudal displacement of the gastric contour beyond the left fifteenth intercostal space consistent with gastric distension may be noted.
- However, the sonographic location of the gastric contour varies dramatically and occasionally extends to this location in the absence of gastric distension.

ADVANCED OR CONFIRMATORY TESTING

- Gastroscopy
  - Active ulceration and mucosal inflammation is usually present in the region of the pylorus but may be absent in foals with idiopathic pyloric muscular hypertrophy.
  - The pyloric sphincter appears small and is not observed to open and close normally.
  - Biopsy samples may be taken of the pyloric region to differentiate between fibrosis and idiopathic muscular hypertrophy, although it is difficult to obtain representative pyloric mural biopsy samples endoscopically.

- Contrast radiography: Serial abdominal radiographs immediately after administration of barium (30%, 5 mL/kg via a nasogastric tube) and then q20–30 min for 2 to 6 hours reveal delayed gastric emptying and may be helpful in locating a duodenal stricture.
- Exploratory celiotomy
  - The pyloric wall is thickened and firm, and the pyloric luminal diameter is narrow on palpation. Moderate to severe gastric distension with fluid or feed is usually present.
  - Diagnostic pyloric biopsy samples may be more easily obtained than via gastroscopy, but surgical access to this region for safe biopsy is often limited in horses. Alternatively, biopsy samples may be obtained via laparoscopy, although definitive diagnosis of pyloric stenosis requires pyloric palpation and thus cannot be confirmed by this method.

TREATMENT

THERAPEUTIC GOAL(S)

- Support gastric mucosal healing and prevent further ulceration and scarring
- Promote gastric emptying

ACUTE GENERAL TREATMENT

- Medical therapy
  - Bethanechol: 0.02 to 0.04 mg/kg SC q8h or 0.22 to 0.45 mg/kg PO q8h
  - May result in significant abdominal discomfort in some horses, especially in those with severe pyloric stenosis or stricture
- Gastric ulcer treatment
  - Indicated if concurrent gastroduodenal or esophageal ulceration is present
  - May include proton pump inhibitors, histamine H2-receptor antagonists, and mucosal protectants (see "Gastric Ulceration" in this section)
- Diet modifications
  - Eliminate hay and maintain on a low-bulk complete pelleted feed.
  - Some horses can tolerate pasture if the grass is kept clipped short.

CHRONIC TREATMENT

- If the above medical therapy is unsuccessful, surgical therapy is indicated.
  - Pyloromyotomy has been successful in some cases of primary muscular hypertrophy.

○ In patients with severe fibrosis and marked stenosis, pyloric bypass (gastrojejunostomy) is indicated.
- The surgical procedure is technically challenging because of limited surgical access to the pylorus in the horse.
- In addition, the patient requires intensive postoperative therapy because normal, coordinated gastroenteric motility patterns take weeks to be established at the anastomosis site.
- Thus this is most often a "last resort" and carries a guarded to poor prognosis for successful long-term outcome.
- Medical therapy as above should be continued in the perioperative period to promote motility and treat or prevent gastric ulceration.

PROGNOSIS AND OUTCOME

- Pseudoobstruction: Good prognosis with prompt and aggressive medical management of gastric ulceration
- Pyloric stenosis or stricture: Guarded to poor prognosis because medical therapy is often unsuccessful and surgical management carries significant risks

PEARLS & CONSIDERATIONS

In the absence of severe pyloric ulceration, definitive gastro-scopic diagnosis of pyloric stenosis or stricture is difficult. Exploratory celiotomy is indicated in most cases if recurrent colic and gastric reflux persist to confirm pyloric stenosis and rule out a more distal intestinal obstruction.

SUGGESTED READING

Murray MJ: Stomach diseases of the foal. In Mair T, Divers T, Ducharme N, editors: *Manual of equine gastroenterology*, London, 2002, Saunders Elsevier, pp 469–476.

AUTHOR: **KELSEY A. HART**

EDITOR: **TIM MAIR** and **CERI SHERLOCK**

Pyoderma, Staphylococcal

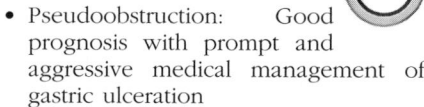

BASIC INFORMATION

DEFINITION
Common bacterial skin infection of horses caused by coagulase-positive *Staphylococcus aureus*

EPIDEMIOLOGY
SPECIES, AGE, SEX Horses of all ages and both sexes can be affected.
GENETICS AND BREED PREDISPOSITION Seen in all breeds, but has been more commonly reported in thin-skinned horses such as Thoroughbreds, Standardbreds, and Quarter Horses
RISK FACTORS
- Trauma to the skin and any kind of stress have been thought to be involved in the development of the condition.
- Excessive sweating in combination with friction from saddle pads and the saddle can create lesions that get infected with the organism.
- Excessive tail rubbing contributes to presence of lesion in this area.
CONTAGION AND ZOONOSIS Use of contaminated brushes, blankets, and tack between affected and healthy horses can occasionally cause the spread of *S. aureus*.
GEOGRAPHY AND SEASONALITY Frequently seen in the spring and summer when hair coat changes are occurring and also seen after clipping
ASSOCIATED CONDITIONS AND DISORDERS In severe cases, horses can develop systemic disease, which needs to be treated accordingly.

CLINICAL PRESENTATION
HISTORY, CHIEF COMPLAINT The primary complaint is the presence of papules centered around a hair follicle, which can be extremely painful to the horse, making it very difficult to palpate the affected area or place tack on the horse.
PHYSICAL EXAM FINDINGS The affected areas can be extremely painful to palpation, and the horse may require sedation to be adequately evaluated if multiple lesions are present. Exudation is not a common finding but can occasionally be present, causing clumping or matting of the hair coat.
ETIOLOGY AND PATHOPHYSIOLOGY *S. aureus* infection. Multiple papules or pustules, especially over the saddle area but can be found anywhere in the body. The lesions form crusts with hair incorporated and may coalesce to form large edematous nodules and plaques.

DIAGNOSIS

DIFFERENTIAL DIAGNOSIS
- *Corynebacterium* folliculitis
- Streptococcal folliculitis
- *Pemphigus foliaceous*
- Dermatophilosis
- Dermatophytosis
- Demodicosis
- Onchocerciasis
- When tail lesions are present, differential diagnoses to consider include:
  ○ Pinworms
  ○ Mange
  ○ Pediculosis
  ○ Insect hypersensitivity
  ○ Food allergies
  ○ Behavioral problems

INITIAL DATABASE
- Complete history and physical examination are important to rule out other potential diseases.
- Cytology and culture of the material taken from under one of the freshly removed crusts. It is important that this is performed under sedation or analgesia because these lesions can be extremely painful.

ADVANCED OR CONFIRMATORY TESTING
Growth of coagulase-positive *S. aureus* from the lesions is confirmatory of the disease.

TREATMENT

THERAPEUTIC GOAL(S)
- Eliminate lesions and provide analgesia to the affected area.
- Prevent potential transmission of the organism to other horses through use of contaminated brushes, blankets, or tack.

ACUTE GENERAL TREATMENT
- Nonsteroidal antiinflammatory drugs to provide analgesia.
- Clip affected areas and clean with an antiseptic shampoo such as chlorhexidine. Sedation may be required initially to achieve this.

- Antibiotics. Treatment should be based on culture and sensitivity, but empirical treatment for most routine cases is usually attempted using trimethoprim-sulfa (30 mg/kg PO q12h for 2–6 weeks). In severe infections, secondary bacterial proliferation may necessitate the use of procaine penicillin G (22000 IU/kg IM q12h for at least 2 weeks) or doxycycline (10 mg/kg PO q12h for at least 2 weeks).
- Use of warm compresses to speed up rupture of the lesions can be beneficial.

PROGNOSIS AND OUTCOME

- Recovery can be prolonged if lesions are severe, but prognosis is usually very good.

- Use of sedation and analgesics is very important to alleviate the signs in affected horses, especially if lesions are very severe or multiple areas are affected.
- The horse should be allowed to completely recover from the lesions before blankets, pads, or saddles are used because they can delay recovery.

PEARLS & CONSIDERATIONS

- Adequate grooming and bathing of horses after exercise reduce the risk of infections.

- Disinfection of all brushes, blankets, pads, and tack is recommended to decrease the risk of transmission to other horses.

SUGGESTED READING

Pilsworth RC, Knottenbelt D: *Staphylococcal pyoderma* and furunculosis. *Equine Vet Educ* March 88–89, 2007.

White SD: Bacterial diseases. In Smith BP, editor: *Large animal internal medicine.* ed 4, St Louis, 2009, Saunders Elsevier, pp 1313–1314.

AUTHOR: **ALFREDO SANCHEZ LONDOÑO**

EDITOR: **DAVID A. WILSON**

Pyometra

BASIC INFORMATION

DEFINITION

Accumulation of purulent material within the uterine lumen

EPIDEMIOLOGY

SPECIES, AGE, SEX Equine females of breeding age
RISK FACTORS
- Any condition that causes cervical closure and physically impedes uterine drainage.
- Although not always a factor, it is well-accepted that previous significant trauma to the cervix (eg, during foaling) that creates fibrous tissue and causes cervical adhesions may result in subsequent closure of the cervix and development of pyometra.
- Other causes of cervical closure include progestin therapy or creation of a tortuous cervical canal caused by the presence of neoplasia. Chronic infection with fungal organisms and *Pseudomonas aeruginosa* infection have also been implicated.

CLINICAL PRESENTATION

HISTORY, CHIEF COMPLAINT Typically an incidental finding when the mare is examined for pregnancy or other reasons. Unlike other species, pyometra in mares generally does not cause systemic illness.
PHYSICAL EXAM FINDINGS The external physical examination is usually unremarkable. Transrectal palpation reveals a closed cervix and an enlarged uterus. Careful palpation and ultrasonography should be used to differentiate this uterine enlargement from a pregnancy. Purulent fluid has a distinct appearance on ultrasonographic examination, and no fetus will be palpable. Because the cervix is typically closed upon presentation and diagnosis, no uterine discharge is noted.

ETIOLOGY AND PATHOPHYSIOLOGY

- Previous cervical trauma, such as a tear during foaling, predisposes mares to cervical adhesions.
- Cervical adhesions may cause the cervix to seal and lead to fluid accumulation within the uterine lumen. If infection is present at the time of cervical closure, this fluid becomes purulent and continues to accumulate with no opportunity for outflow.
- Alternatively, mares with residual endometritis that are inadvertently given progestin therapy (eg, altrenogest, progesterone) are at risk for developing a prolonged endometritis because of cervical closure and may develop pyometra over time.

DIAGNOSIS

DIFFERENTIAL DIAGNOSIS

- Pregnancy
- Contagious equine metritis (CEM)
- It is important to differentiate this disease from CEM. Mares with CEM typically present with copious mucopurulent discharge from the reproductive tract and have a history that includes breeding within the past 14 days. Although the presentation of these two conditions is very different, CEM should be mentioned here as a cause of purulent discharge from the reproductive tract because it is a reportable disease of great significance to the equine industry (see "Contagious Equine Metritis" in this section).

INITIAL DATABASE

The complete blood count and serum chemistry are usually within normal limits.

ADVANCED OR CONFIRMATORY TESTING

- Performing culture and sensitivity testing of uterine contents aids in treatment.
- If mare has a mucopurulent vaginal discharge with a history of recent breeding (<14 days), it is important to rule out CEM as a causative agent with appropriate cultures and media.

TREATMENT

THERAPEUTIC GOAL(S)

- Create a patent cervix
- Evacuate uterine fluid
- Lyse corpora lutea if present
- Treat infection, if present

ACUTE GENERAL TREATMENT

- Digital manipulation and manual dilatation of the cervix to establish drainage; allow to drain completely
- Catheterization of cervix for large-volume uterine lavage using either lactated Ringer's solution or sterile saline until fluid recovery is clear. Continue uterine lavage once daily until recovery becomes clear.
- Administration of ecbolic agents to stimulate uterine contractions, aid in evacuation of contents, and destroy any luteal tissue present. Prostaglandins may be administered as often as q8h for the first 2 to 3 days of treatment; then the frequency can be decreased at the veterinarian's discretion based on effective fluid clearance and the mare's tolerance of the medication. Effective prostaglandin treatments are as follows:
  - Cloprostenol (Estrumate) can be administered at a dose of 250 µg IM *or*
  - Dinoprost tromethamine (Lutalyse) can be administered at a dose of 5 mg IM
- Oxytocin may also be used as an effective ecbolic agent during treatment and is often well tolerated.
- Topical application of prostaglandin E2 (misoprostol) to the cervix may aid in cervical relaxation, depending on the underlying cause.
- Infusion of intrauterine antibiotics according to culture and sensitivity testing for a period of 3 to 5 days, depending on the pathogen.

CHRONIC TREATMENT

- After this course of appropriate acute therapy, the mare should be allowed to proceed through a normal estrous cycle to assess the integrity of the cervix and degree of fluid accumulation present during the subsequent diestral phase.
- In addition to assessing cervical integrity, uterine biopsy should be performed during a subsequent cycle as a helpful prognostic indicator for future fertility.

- Ovariohysterectomy has been reported by some authors as effective management of chronic pyometra cases (see Suggested Reading). This surgery is not without risk, so an educated decision must be reached by both the client and veterinarian before recommending this procedure.

POSSIBLE COMPLICATIONS

Be well aware of prostaglandin side effects before use and monitor the mare for tolerance of the chosen medication.

RECOMMENDED MONITORING

- Daily progress should be monitored during acute treatment with regard to clearance of uterine fluid.
- See Chronic Treatment above for indications of prognosis for fertility.
- If the owner elects to attempt future breedings, transrectal palpation and ultrasonography should be performed during estrus and 14 and 28 days after ovulation to confirm that a viable pregnancy has been established rather than excessive fluid accumulation.

PROGNOSIS AND OUTCOME

The prognosis for return to reproductive function ranges from fair to poor, depending largely on the chronicity of the condition and the predisposing factor(s). Prognostic indicators of future fertility include the degree of cervical integrity achieved on subsequent estrous cycles as well as uterine biopsy grade after treatment.

PEARLS & CONSIDERATIONS

COMMENTS

In a mare with pyometra, always perform a complete reproductive examination and look for a potential underlying cause (eg, previous cervical injury). Although this may not always be the case, it is a very helpful prognostic indicator of future fertility. Mares that do have

evidence of significant cervical trauma often never achieve cervical competence and have a poorer prognosis for their ability to establish and maintain a pregnancy.

PREVENTION

For valuable mares, institute postfoaling examinations for early detection of trauma to the cervix and vaginal vault after parturition. If the owner elects not to rebreed after foaling, consider having the mare examined at weekly intervals for a period of 14 to 28 days to ensure that gross uterine involution is proceeding normally and there is no excessive fluid accumulation or evidence of uterine infection. Postpartum uterine evaluation is especially important in mares that do not have a nursing foal (eg, stillborn foals, fetotomy).

CLIENT EDUCATION

- Postpartum examinations are especially important if the mare has any difficulty with delivery.
- After breeding, it is important to have a veterinarian confirm pregnancy rather than relying on the mare's non-return to estrus as an indicator of pregnancy.
- Mares that have had pyometra in the past should be monitored and managed very closely during future breeding attempts.

SUGGESTED READING

Freeman DE, Rötting AK, Köllman M: Ovariohysterectomy in mares: 17 cases (1988–2007), *Proc Am Assoc Equine Pract* 53:370–373, 2007.

Pycock JF: Therapy for mares with uterine fluid. In Samper JC, Pycock JF, McKinnon AO, editors: *Current therapy in equine reproduction*, St Louis, 2007, Elsevier, pp 93–104.

Swerczek TW, Caudle AB: Bacterial causes of subfertility and abortion in the mare. In Youngquist RS, Threlfall WR, editors: *Current therapy in large animal theriogenology*, St Louis, 2007, Elsevier, pp 168–175.

AUTHOR: **ROBYN R. WILBORN**

EDITOR: **JUAN C. SAMPER**

Pyospermia

BASIC INFORMATION

DEFINITION

The presence of neutrophils, pus, or both in the semen, which can cause decreased fertility or infertility; usually a result of seminal vesiculitis

SYNONYM(S)

Leukospermia

EPIDEMIOLOGY

SPECIES, AGE, SEX Occurs in stallions of any breed or age
CONTAGION AND ZOONOSIS Common agents of seminal vesiculitis, ampul-

litis, epididymitis, and urethritis include *Pseudomonas aeruginosa*, *Klebsiella pneumoniae*, *Streptococcus* spp., *Staphylococcus* spp., and *Brucella abortus*. Other agents have been reported in small numbers. Infections of the external genitalia may be caused by the opportunistic organisms; *P. aeruginosa*, *K. pneumoniae*, *Streptococcus equi* subsp. *zooepidemicus*. Equine viral arteritis (EVA) may rarely cause ampullitis and leukospermia.

ASSOCIATED CONDITIONS AND DISORDERS
- Seminal vesiculitis (vesicular gland adenitis)
- Epididymitis
- Ampullitis
- Urethritis
- EVA (rarely)
- Infection of the external genitalia

CLINICAL PRESENTATION
HISTORY, CHIEF COMPLAIN
- Semen evaluation
  - Abnormal color of ejaculate
  - Abnormal appearance of ejaculated semen: Heterogenous; presence of sediment
  - Poor semen motility and morphology
  - Poor preservation for shipping
  - Presence of neutrophils
- Ejaculatory disorders (painful ejaculation or incomplete ejaculation)
- Abnormal posturing after breeding or collection of semen
- Pain (acute epididymitis and vesicular gland adenitis)
- Infertility: Bred mares return to estrus or develop endometritis via venereal transmission of bacteria.

PHYSICAL EXAM FINDINGS
- Presence of pus or neutrophils on semen evaluation
- Stallions are usually clinically healthy with no systemic signs of illness.
- If seminal vesiculitis is acute in nature, stallions may experience pain when breeding or on transrectal palpation of affected glands.
- Acute epididymitis may be accompanied by fever and pain.
- Diagnosis requires complete evaluation of the reproductive system, including testicular palpation and ultrasonography, transrectal evaluation of the vesicular glands, and videoendoscopic evaluation of the urethra and vesicular glands.

ETIOLOGY AND PATHOPHYSIOLOGY
- Routes of infection of all internal structures (ampullae, seminal vesicles, epididymis, urethra) include ascending from the urethra; descending from the upper genital tract or urinary tract; lymphogenous or hematogenous spread; and direct infection from surrounding tissues.

- All seminal vesiculitis in stallions is infectious.
- Urethritis may be bacterial or viral, although viral urethritis rarely is a cause of leukospermia.
- Infections of the external reproductive organs, including the glans penis or prepuce, often as a sequela to disruption of the normal commensal flora, allowing for opportunistic infection, such as after rigorous repeated washing of the penis.

DIAGNOSIS

DIFFERENTIAL DIAGNOSIS
- Seminal vesiculitis (vesicular gland adenitis)
- Urethritis
- Epididymitis
- Ampullitis
- Any other site of inflammation or infection along the urogenital tract, including the external genitalia (prepuce, glans penis)

INITIAL DATABASE
- Examination of collected semen (gross and microscopic)
  - Abnormal color of ejaculate
  - Presence of neutrophils, bacteria, purulent material
  - Decreased to absent spermatozoa motility
  - Abnormal spermatozoal morphology
  - Agglutination or precipitation of spermatozoa
- Examination of the stallion
  - Chronically infected stallions are usually clinically healthy with no signs of systemic illness.
  - Acutely infected stallions may demonstrate pain when breeding or col-

lecting or on transrectal palpation of affected glands or structures and rarely during micturition or defecation.
  - Transrectal palpation may not be rewarding unless the horse is acutely infected.
  - Transrectal ultrasonography may demonstrate debris or fluid within the vesicular gland with a distended lumen or thickened glandular walls.
  - Inspection of external structures
- Culture of various anatomic locations to determine where the neutrophils in the semen are coming from
  - Swabs from the penis, urethral process, semen, preejaculatory and postejaculatory urethral samples
  - Culture and cytology of vesicular gland secretions (indicated if transrectal ultrasonography or video endoscopy demonstrates signs of seminal vesiculitis)
- Stimulate the stallion sexually for 15 minutes (tease to a receptive mare).
- Wash the penis and sterilely introduce a stallion urinary catheter or 1-m video endoscope to the colliculus seminalis (the opening of the seminal vesicles into the urethra) (Figure 1). If using a catheter, transrectal palpation may be used to help assist in placement.
- Transrectal ultrasonography is used to massage the glands and express secretions, which are collected sterilely with a catheter or aspirated through the endoscope (Figure 2). Alternatively, a biopsy instrument can be introduced through the endoscope directly into the gland and samples obtained.
- Care must be taken with the endoscope not to traumatize the tissues.
- Semen and serum submission for EVA testing, if indicated

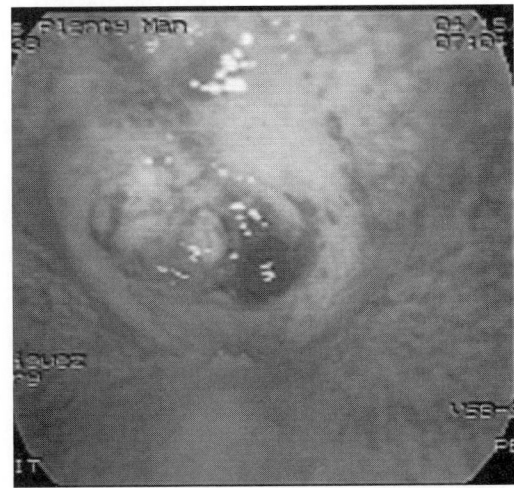

FIGURE 1 The colliculus seminalis (opening to the seminal vesicle) in a stallion with seminal vesiculitis. Note the inflammation and tissue irritation.

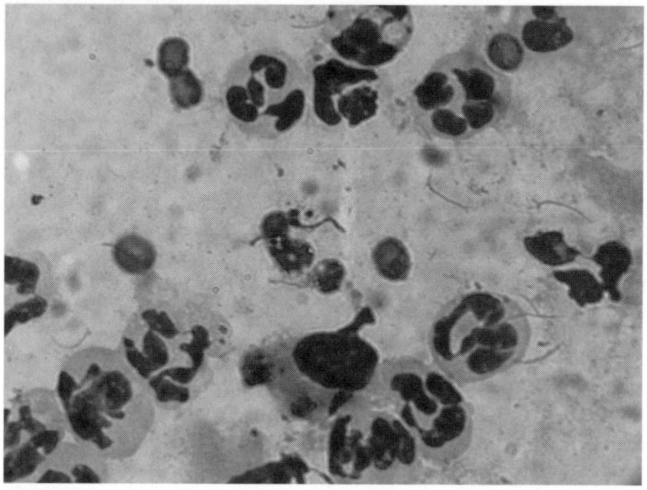

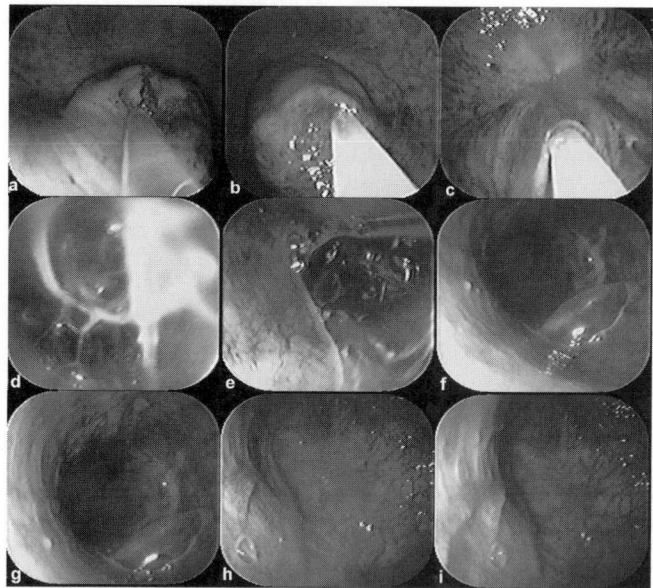

FIGURE 2 Cytology of collected secretions from the seminal vesicles of a stallion with seminal vesiculitis.

FIGURE 3 Endoscopic lavage and antibiotic infusion of the seminal vesicles in a stallion with seminal vesiculitis.

TREATMENT

THERAPEUTIC GOAL(S)

Elimination of inflammatory cells and debris in the ejaculate to restore or improve fertility; identification of and treatment to resolve the infection

ACUTE GENERAL TREATMENT

- Administration of systemic nonsteroidal antiinflammatory drugs
- Systemic antibiotics based on sensitivity report
  ○ Challenging because most antibiotics do not reach therapeutic levels in these tissues
  ○ Must be lipid soluble
  ○ Best options: Trimethoprim-sulfonamide or enrofloxacin if cultured organisms are susceptible
- If an external infection is diagnosed
  ○ Cleansing of the affected area
  ○ Appropriate use of topical antibiotic preparations or ointments
  ○ Sexual rest until lesions are healed
- If seminal vesiculitis is diagnosed
  ○ Lavage and local infusion of antibiotics into the affected gland (Figure 3)
    ▪ Under endoscopic guidance
    ▪ Reports of ampicillin and ticarcillin used for this purpose at systemic dosages
    ▪ Use in combination with systemic antibiotics

  ○ Surgical treatment
    ▪ Seminal vesiculectomy
    ▪ Not performed commonly
    ▪ High rate of complications
    ▪ Unknown effect on future fertility
  ○ Sexual rest until infection is cleared
- Implementation of minimum contamination breeding techniques
  ○ Collection of semen into antibiotic-infused extender
  ○ If live cover, can infuse extender directly into the mare's uterus before breeding
  ○ Postbreeding uterine lavage

POSSIBLE COMPLICATIONS

Trauma from endoscopic examination or catheter placement; surgical complications (eg, infection, hemorrhage, dysuria, inability to maintain or sustain erection); inability to clear the infection

RECOMMENDED MONITORING

Frequent monitoring of affected stallions is recommended.

PROGNOSIS AND OUTCOME

- Fair to guarded. Seminal vesiculitis is an uncommon disease that usually presents as a chronic infection. Unless the infection responds to therapy, the stallion may remain persistently infected. Fertility may be improved with use of minimum contamination breeding techniques but is not guaranteed.
- The prognosis of infections of other anatomic structures depends on the structure and nature of the disease.

PEARLS & CONSIDERATIONS

PREVENTION

Maintain proper hygiene during breeding and collection

CLIENT EDUCATION

- Maintain proper hygiene during breeding, especially live cover, to decrease the possibility of venereal transmission of organisms
- Perform regular breeding soundness examinations of affected stallions

SUGGESTED READING

Tibary A, Rodriguez J, Samper JC: Microbiology and diseases of semen. In Samper JC, editor: *Equine breeding management and artificial insemination*, St Louis, 2009, Elsevier, pp 99–112.

AUTHORS: **LISA K. PEARSON, JACOBO S. RODRIGUEZ,** and **AHMED TIBARY**

EDITOR: **JUAN C. SAMPER**

Pythiosis

BASIC INFORMATION

DEFINITION

Deep, invasive, and rapidly progressive subcutaneous oomycotic infection caused *Pythium insidiosum*

- Equine pythiosis: Ulcerative cutaneous granulomas often affecting the distal limbs.
- Deep or disseminated infection may invade the bone, tendon sheath, joints, lungs, and gastrointestinal tract.

SYNONYM(S)

- Swamp cancer
- Florida horse leeches
- Gulf Coast fungus
- Phycomycosis

EPIDEMIOLOGY

RISK FACTORS

- Prolonged contact with lake, pond, swamp, or flood water
- Minor wounds

CONTAGION AND ZOONOSIS Motile zoospores present in warm stagnant water have tropism to damaged animal and human tissues. After the oomycete contaminates wounds, it invades tissues. There is no direct contagion or zoonotic potential.

GEOGRAPHY AND SEASONALITY

- Pythiosis occurs in tropical and subtropical areas, including Australia, Brazil, Costa Rica, India, and Thailand. In the United States, pythiosis occurs in states along the Gulf of Mexico.
- Most cases occur during warmer and wetter months of the year, especially the summer.

ASSOCIATED CONDITIONS AND DISORDERS Dogs can also develop cutaneous pythiosis, as well as gastrointestinal lesions.

CLINICAL PRESENTATION

HISTORY, CHIEF COMPLAINT Insidious onset of cutaneous granulomas, often fast-growing lesions

PHYSICAL EXAM FINDINGS

- *P. insidiosum* generally infects the wounds in the distal portions of the body, including the limbs below the carpus and hock, ventral abdomen (Figure 1), and ventral thorax (areas more likely to be in contact with stagnant water), as well as the lips, nostrils, face, external genitalia, neck, and trunk.
  - Cutaneous granulomas may involve or spread to the muzzle and lips.
  - Lesions are usually single and large nodular eroded to ulcerative granu-

lomas associated with moderate to severe pruritus and oozing of serosanguineous discharge (Figure 2).
  - Severe pruritus, which often leads to self-mutilation
  - If excised, tissue has a thickened fibrotic dermis (pink) and contains scattered areas of red surrounding a yellow-tan, gritty, central necrotic core ("leeches" or "kunkers"). Kunkers range from 2 to 10 mm, which is larger than those seen with zygomycosis.
  - Malodorous (associated with tissue necrosis)
  - Lesions involving the limbs are accompanied by lymphangitis with severe edema or swelling (Figure 3)
  - The infection is locally invasive (spreading from the subcutaneous to lymphatics and deeper tissues (eg, bones, tendon sheaths, joints).
  - Osseous involvement generally occurs in chronic lesions (>2 months' duration).
  - Metastasis (spreading to lungs) may occur (Figure 4).
  - Gastrointestinal lesions may occur.
- Lesions are often heavily contaminated by bacteria (especially gram-negative organisms).

ETIOLOGY AND PATHOPHYSIOLOGY

- *P. insidiosum* is an aquatic oomycete requiring organic substrate, such as decaying vegetation, and warm environmental temperatures for maintenance of the life cycle.
- Infections are thought to develop secondary to wound inoculations.

- Motile zoospores have chemotaxis toward damaged animal tissues. When they are near the host tissue, zoospores lose flagella, encyst onto the tissue, and develop germ tubes that invade tissues.
- After inoculation, invasion of the dermis results in pyogranulomatous inflammation.
- Lesions progress and increase in size very rapidly.

DIAGNOSIS

DIFFERENTIAL DIAGNOSIS

- Exuberant granulation tissue
- Cutaneous habronemiasis
- Foreign body granuloma
- Zygomycosis
- Ulcerated neoplasia such as sarcoid or squamous cell carcinoma
- Cutaneous nocardiosis (generally distal limb)
- Bacterial pseudomycetoma or botryomycosis (limb, lips, head, mammary area, scrotum)
- Cutaneous actinomycosis (generally head and neck)
- Phaeohyphomycoses and eumycotic mycetomas

INITIAL DATABASE

Abnormalities in the complete blood count are often reported

- Anemia (either microcytic, hypochromic or normocytic, normochromic)
- Moderate leukocytosis associated with neutrophilia and eosinophilia

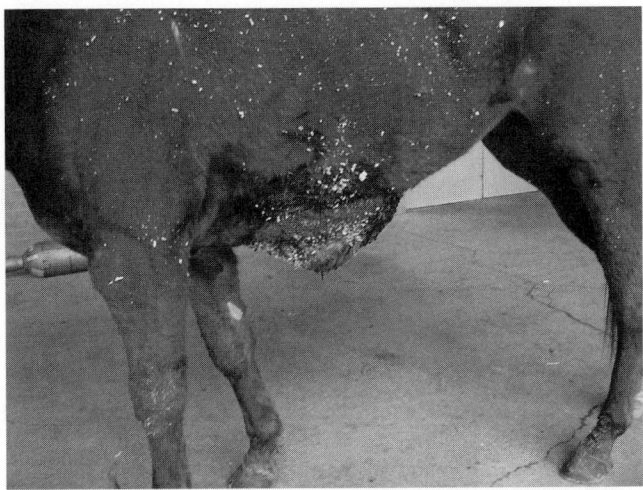

FIGURE 1 Quarter Horse mare with large ulcerative granulomatous lesion on the ventral abdomen. This lesion was caused by *Pythium insidiosum* infection.

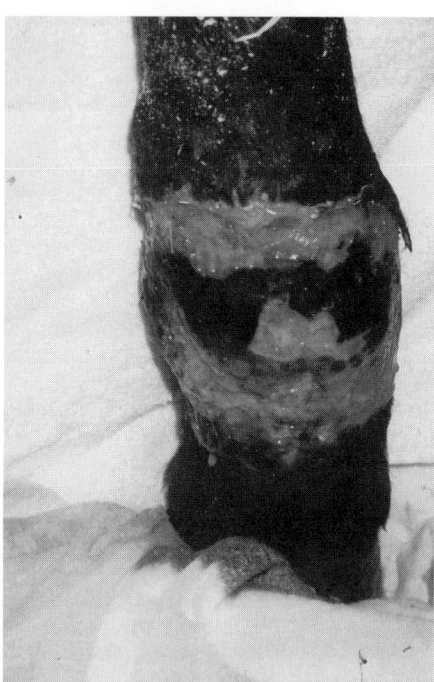

FIGURE 2 Quarter Horse mare with ulcerative granuloma (caused by *Pythium insidiosum* infection) on the palmar aspect of the pastern. The lesion contains thickened fibrotic dermis (pink) and areas of red granulation tissue surrounding a yellow-tan, gritty, central necrotic ("kunkers").

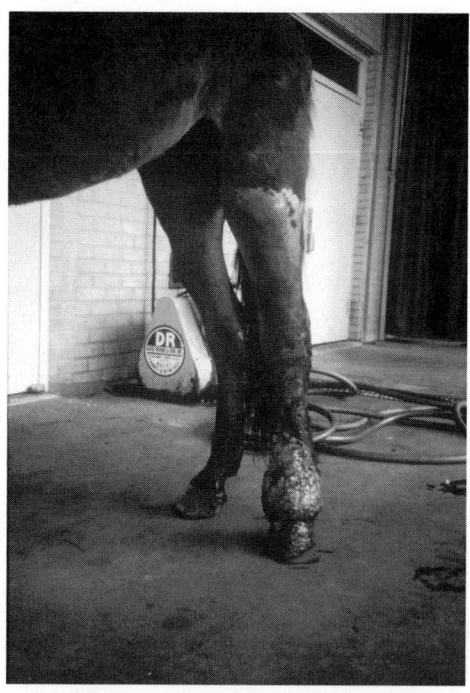

FIGURE 3 Bay Quarter Horse filly with severe lymphangitis, limb edema, and a large ulcerative granulomatous lesion (caused by *Pythium insidiosum* infection) on the left hindlimb.

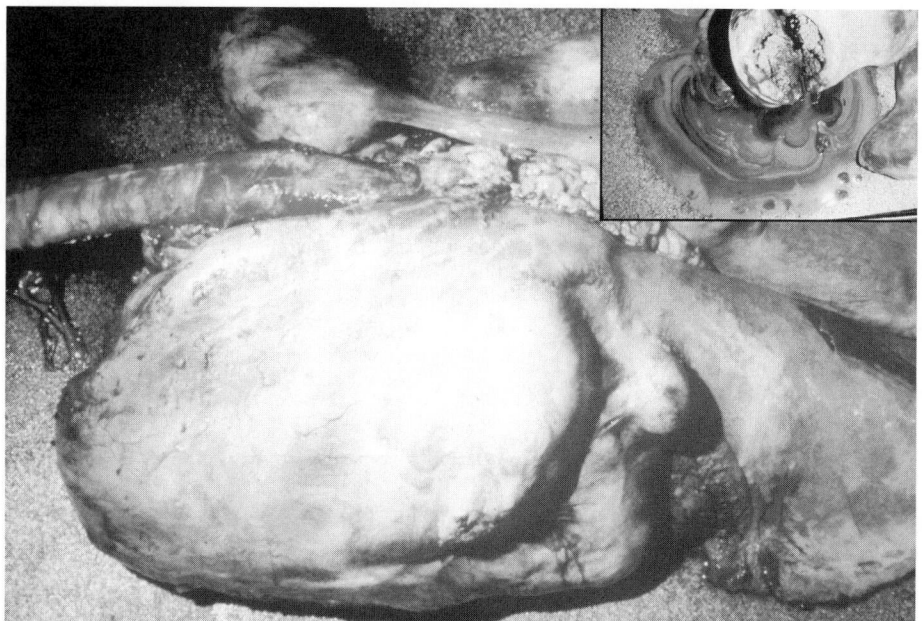

FIGURE 4 Pulmonary metastasis in a severe case of equine pythiosis (*Pythium insidiosum* infection). Most lung lobes were affected, especially the cranial portions. The *inset* depicts one of the pulmonary abscesses after section. (Courtesy Dr. E.P. Goad.)

ADVANCED OR CONFIRMATORY TESTING

- Cytologic evaluation of aspirate or direct smear: Pyogranulomatous to granulomatous inflammation with numerous eosinophils and only occasionally hyphae are visualized
- Definitive diagnosis requires demonstration of the organism by histopathology evaluation or fungal culture of a biopsy specimen.
  - Thickened fibrotic dermis with diffuse to nodular, pyogranulomatous to granulomatous inflammation containing numerous eosinophils; hyphae are often poorly stained and may appear as clear spaces
  - Scattered areas with a central core of necrotic tissue, which often contain hyphal forms, or "hyphal ghosts" (clear spaces) surrounded by eosinophilic infiltrate of the Splendore-Hoeppli phenomenon
    - Hyphae become evident in tissue sections stained with Giemsa stain (but not with periodic acid-Schiff).
    - Histologic findings of pythiosis resemble those of zygomycosis

(basidiobolomycosis and conidiobolomycosis); however, the hyphae in zygomycosis are larger.

- Indirect immunoperoxidase technique (formalin-fixed specimens) allows for specific and rapid confirmatory test for pythiosis.
  - Culture of either biopsy specimen or "kunkers" in blood or Sabouraud's dextrose agar at 25° to 37° C yield rapid growth of *Pythium* spp. The specimen should not be refrigerated or transported on ice.
- Polymerase chain reaction in frozen skin samples or samples kept in 95% ethanol is a reliable test.

TREATMENT

THERAPEUTIC GOAL(S)

- Attempt to eliminate organisms using both surgical and medical management.
- Treatment should be instituted as soon as possible because of rapid progression of the infection.
  - The longer the duration, the poorer the prognosis.
  - The location of lesions greatly influences the prognosis.

ACUTE AND CHRONIC GENERAL TREATMENT

- Combination of surgical excision, chemotherapy, and immunotherapy
- Surgical excision
  - Ideally, radical excision with removal of 2-cm margins surrounding the lesion.
  - Recurrence may occur in 30% of cases even if radical excision is done.
  - The location of the lesions greatly influences the ability for surgical excision.
    - Lesions in the trunk can be removed.
    - Lesions in limbs are less likely to be successfully excised.
    - Repeated surgeries are necessary.
- Drug therapy
  - Because the organism is not a true fungi, it lacks the cell wall characteristic such that antifungal agents (eg, amphotericin B and azoles) are not very effective.
  - Systemic antifungal agents are recommended in conjunction with other modes of therapy. The true impact of systemic antifungal agents in the treatment of pythiosis is unknown.

- Organic iodides such as ethylene diamine dihydroiodide at 1 to 2 mg/kg PO q12–24h for 7 days; then reduce to 0.5 to 1.0 mg/kg q24h for the remainder of the treatment
- Inorganic iodides
  - Sodium iodide: 10 to 40 mg/kg/d as 20% solution given IV slowly for 2 to 5 days; then oral iodide for the remainder of the treatment
  - Potassium iodide: 20 to 40 mg/kg/d PO (mixed with molasses and given by syringe or given with a small amount of feed or grain)
- Azoles (ketoconazole), flucytosine, and amphotericin B given systemically do not appear to greatly improve outcome.
  - Topical antifungals are recommended. Amphotericin B or ketoconazole (dissolved in water and dimethyl sulfoxide (DMSO), possibly in conjunction with iodophors.
- Immunotherapy with *Pythium* vaccines has been effective for the treatment of equine pythiosis and is therefore recommended.
  - A number of vaccine preparations have been used with considerable success
    - Crude, killed, whole-cell hyphal extract
    - Cell-mass antigen
    - Soluble-concentrated antigen
    - Vaccines are not commercially available and must be prepared for individual patients
- Concurrent systemic antibiotic therapy to control secondary bacterial infection is recommended.

POSSIBLE COMPLICATIONS

- Premature discontinuation of therapy may lead to relapse.
- Iodides have an unpleasant taste and might cause nausea (requiring molasses to mask it).
- For oral inorganic iodides, potassium iodide is often preferred.
- Tolerance to iodides is variable, and some horses show signs of iodism (see "Zygomycosis" in this section).
- Sodium iodide is very hydroscopic.
- Because amphotericin B is generally applied topically for the treatment of pythiosis, the risk of nephrotoxicity is greatly diminished.

RECOMMENDED MONITORING

- Monitor closely for the appearance of new foci of infection.

- Repeated surgeries are necessary and indicated as soon as new foci of infection are suspected because recurrence can happen in 30% of cases.

PROGNOSIS AND OUTCOME

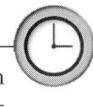

- The prognosis depends on the size, location, and duration of the lesion.
  - Chronic lesions (>1 to 2 months in duration) have a poorer prognosis.
  - If untreated, infection is 100% fatal.
- Treatment is difficult (especially if lesions affect limbs) and expensive. Severely affected horses are often euthanized.

PEARLS & CONSIDERATIONS

COMMENTS

Combination of treatments, including radical surgical excision and topical chemotherapy in conjunction with immunotherapy, should be instituted as soon as possible (early treatment has much more favorable prognosis).

CLIENT EDUCATION

- In contrast with subcutaneous dermatomycoses, which carry a fair to guarded prognosis, pythiosis carries a guarded to poor prognosis.
- Prognosis is worse if complete surgical excision cannot be achieved.
- Immediate and aggressive treatment is necessary.
- Treatment can be lengthy and expensive. Recurrence may occur in up to 30% of cases.

SUGGESTED READING

Biomedical Laboratory Diagnostics, College of Natural Sciences, Michigan State University, (Leonel Mendoza): *Pythium insidiosum*. Available at http://bld.msu.edu/mendoza.html.

Scott DW, Miller WH Jr: Antifungal therapy. In *Equine dermatology*, St Louis, 2003, Saunders Elsevier, pp 306-313.

Scott DW, Miller WH Jr: Fungal skin diseases—subcutaneous mycosis—pythiosis. In *Equine dermatology*, St Louis, 2003, Saunders Elsevier, pp 287–293.

White SD: Diseases of the skin—fungal diseases. In Smith BP, editor: *Large animal internal medicine*, ed 4, St Louis, 2009, Saunders Elsevier, p 1320.

AUTHOR: **LAIS R.R. COSTA**

EDITOR: **DAVID A. WILSON**

Rabies

BASIC INFORMATION

DEFINITION
Rabies virus is an enveloped RNA virus that induces lethal polioencephalomyelitis and ganglionitis in infected animals.

EPIDEMIOLOGY
SPECIES, AGE, SEX Younger horses are more commonly affected.
RISK FACTORS
- Unvaccinated horses (although vaccine may not be 100% effective)
- 24-hour access to pasture
- Residence in endemic area

CONTAGION AND ZOONOSIS Spread through bite wounds of infected animals, including dogs, foxes, raccoons, skunks, and bats
GEOGRAPHY AND SEASONALITY Endemic worldwide with few exceptions

CLINICAL PRESENTATION
DISEASE FORMS/SUBTYPES
- Paralytic rabies: Spinal form
- Dumb rabies: Brainstem form
- Furious rabies: Cerebral form

HISTORY, CHIEF COMPLAINT Colic and lameness are commonly reported.
PHYSICAL EXAM FINDINGS
- Wide variations in disease presentation and clinical signs are associated with phase 2 (see below).
- The spinal cord is most commonly affected followed by the brainstem and then the cerebrum.
- Paralytic rabies: Lameness, weight shifting, knuckling of one or both fetlocks, ascending ataxia, paresis progressing to paralysis, hyperesthesia or self-mutilation of an extremity. Recumbent in 3 to 5 days; normal eating and drinking.
- Dumb rabies: Depression, anorexia, head tilt, circling, ataxia, dementia, excess salivation, facial and pharyngeal paralysis, blindness, flaccid tail and anus, urine dribbling, self-mutilation
- Furious rabies: Convulsions, aggression, hydrophobia, photophobia, tenesmus, circling, hyperesthesia, self-mutilation
- Other signs reported: Blindness, head pressing, inability to drink or dysphagia, anorexia, constipation, paraphimosis in males, gastrointestinal signs, genitourinary signs
- Two forms of the disease may be present at one time.
- Incubation period is 9 days to 1 year.
- Clinical signs progress until death 5 to 10 days after onset of clinical signs.

ETIOLOGY AND PATHOPHYSIOLOGY
- Saliva containing the virus is inoculated into the skin after a bite wound from an infected animal.
- Phase 1 (days to weeks): Ascending or centripetal phase: Transmission of virus to the central nervous system (CNS) after a short period of multiplication in the local muscle cells. The virus then binds to nicotinic acetylcholine receptors at the neuromuscular junction and travels toward the CNS.
- Phase 2 (≤7 days): Viral replication in the CNS; ascending transmission from the spinal cord to the brainstem
- Phase 3: Centrifugal transmission from the brain to tissues and organs, including the salivary glands and nasal secretions

DIAGNOSIS

DIFFERENTIAL DIAGNOSIS
- Spinal cord signs leading to pelvic injuries other diseases affecting the spinal cord, such as neoplasia and abscess formation
- Severe depression to coma leading to encephalitis, toxic CNS diseases
- Hepatoencephalopathy
- West Nile virus
- Equine protozoal myeloencephalitis
- Botulism
- Lead poisoning
- Cauda equine neuritis
- Meningitis
- Space-occupying mass
- Trauma to the brain or spinal cord

INITIAL DATABASE
- The complete blood count, serum chemistries, and cerebrospinal fluid (CSF) analysis are all nondiagnostic.
- The CSF may show mild to moderate lymphocytic pleocytosis with a mild increase in protein and mild xanthochromia.

ADVANCED OR CONFIRMATORY TESTING
- No antemortem test is available.
- Clinical signs that do not progress over 5 days are not consistent with rabies.
- Histopathology: "Negri bodies" are seen in fewer than 50% of fluorescent antibody test positive samples. Diffuse perivascular cuffing with leukocytes in meninges and neural parenchyma, neuronal degeneration and neuronophagia, gliosis, and malacia of the gray matter of the spinal cord may be seen.
- Definitive diagnosis: Fluorescent antibody virus neutralization test on the brain or spinal cord

TREATMENT

THERAPEUTIC GOAL(S)
Inevitably progresses to death

ACUTE GENERAL TREATMENT
Supportive treatment has no effect on survival time, and some do not condone treatment because of public health concerns.

RECOMMENDED MONITORING
Serial neurologic examinations to confirm progression of the disease ruling out other neurologic diseases, although human exposure must be limited

PROGNOSIS AND OUTCOME

100% fatal disease in horses

PEARLS & CONSIDERATIONS

COMMENTS
- Unvaccinated infected horses should be euthanized or quarantined and observed for 6 months.
- Horses vaccinated within 1 year of exposure with a vaccine approved for equine use should be revaccinated and observed for 45 days after infection.

PREVENTION
- Yearly vaccination: Peak antibody titer is reached 28 days after primary vaccination.
- Proper protective equipment should always be worn when rabies is a differential diagnosis.
- Proper shipment of specimens to diagnostic laboratory

SUGGESTED READING
Goehring L: Viral diseases of the nervous system. In Furr M, Reed S, editors: *Equine neurology*, Ames, IA, 2008, Blackwell, pp 172–175.

Green SL, Smith LL, Vernau W, et al: Rabies in horses: 21 cases (1970–1990). *J Am Vet Med Assoc* 200:1133, 1992.

Sommardahl CS: Rabies. In Reed SM, Bayly WM, Sellon DC, editors: *Equine internal medicine*, ed 3, St Louis, 2010, Elsevier, pp 633–634.

Wilkins PA, Del Piero F: Rabies. In Sellon D, Long M, editors: *Equine infectious diseases*, St Louis, 2007, Saunders Elsevier, pp 185–191.

AUTHOR: **CAMERON M. CHILDERS**

EDITOR: **STEPHEN M. REED**

Rectal Prolapse

BASIC INFORMATION

DEFINITION
Protrusion of the rectum through the anus

EPIDEMIOLOGY
SPECIES, AGE, SEX Affects females
RISK FACTORS Conditions that cause tenesmus, including diarrhea, constipation, dystocia, urinary tract obstruction, colic, rectal tumor, rectal foreign body, or parasitism

CLINICAL PRESENTATION
DISEASE FORMS/SUBTYPES A grading system is used to classify prolapse.
- Type 1: Only the mucosa protrudes.
- Type 2: All or part of the ampulla recti protrudes.
- Type 3: All or part of the ampulla recti protrudes, and the peritoneal portion of the rectum or small colon is intussuscepted but does not protrude through the anus.
- Type 4: The peritoneal portion of the rectum or small colon is intussuscepted and protrudes through the anus.

HISTORY, CHIEF COMPLAINT
- Protrusion of light to dark pink to dark red to black mucosa circumferentially through the anus
- Colic may also be apparent.

PHYSICAL EXAM FINDINGS
- Temperature is variable depending on severity of compromise; rectal prolapse may hinder the ability to get an accurate temperature reading.
- Tachycardia is often present.
- Horses with type 1 or 2 prolapse may have normal mentation, but increasing duration and severity causes depression and lethargy.
- Mucous membranes are variable depending on severity of compromise; they are often pale pink and moist.
- Colic signs are variable; abdominal distension is variable; both are progressive in types 3 and 4 prolapse.

ETIOLOGY AND PATHOPHYSIOLOGY
Most commonly secondary to increased tenesmus

DIAGNOSIS

DIFFERENTIAL DIAGNOSIS
- Rectal intussusception
- Vaginal prolapse
- Uterine prolapse
- Cystic prolapse

INITIAL DATABASE
- Complete blood count: Leukopenia or leukocytosis common; occasionally normal
- Rectal evaluation: Establish if rectal prolapse or intussusception
- Prolapse: Continuum between anal sphincter and rectal mucosa
  - Intussusception: Defect between rectal mucosa and intussusceptum (ie, grade IV prolapse)
- Peritoneal fluid: Normal in types 1 and 2; variable increases in total protein and white blood cell counts seen in types 3 and 4.
- Transabdominal ultrasound: May see peritoneal effusion in horses with type 3 or 4 prolapse

TREATMENT

THERAPEUTIC GOAL(S)
- Provide systemic and local analgesia and antiinflammatory drugs
- Remove the primary cause of prolapse
- Reduce prolapse
- Prevent recurrence

ACUTE GENERAL TREATMENT
- Type 1 and 2 prolapse
  - Facilitate reduction
    - Apply topical glycerine, sugar, magnesium sulphate, or lidocaine to reduce edema.
    - Consider caudal epidural anesthesia 0.22 mg/kg of lidocaine.
    - Manually replace rectal prolapse.
  - Place a purse string around the anus with umbilical tape. Open the purse string every 2 to 3 hours to allow fecal passage.
- Type 3 or 4 prolapse
  - If viable tissue, can reduce prolapse.
    - Continued blood in feces is suggestive of necrosis of tissues.

- Perform serial abdominocentesis to monitor for peritonitis.
  - May require resection of nonviable tissue (colorectostomy)
    - Often easier to perform via a transrectal approach than exploratory celiotomy because of poor exposure of the aboral intestine. Consider leaving prolapsed for shipping if nonviable to prevent peritonitis.
    - Laparoscopic evaluation of reduced prolapse can help assess viability of bowel and mesentery.
    - Severe cases with marked vascular disruption may require a colostomy.

CHRONIC TREATMENT
- Type 1 or 2 prolapse
  - Analgesia (flunixin meglumine for 3–5 days)
  - Broad-spectrum antibiotics (trimethoprim-sulfonamide for 7–10 days)
  - Withhold feed for 12 to 24 hours
  - Maintain rectal purse string for 48 hours
  - Stool softeners and laxative diet (mineral oil for 10–14 days)
- Type 3 or 4 prolapse
  - Analgesia (flunixin meglumine for 3–5 days)
  - Stool softeners (mineral oil for 10–14 days)
  - Repeat abdominocentesis to evaluate for peritonitis
  - It may be necessary to manually evacuate feces if rectal impaction is present

POSSIBLE COMPLICATIONS
- Peritonitis
- Endotoxemia
- Laminitis
- Adhesions
- Perirectal abscesses
- Colic
- Diarrhea
- Recurrence of prolapse
- Structure formation
- Jugular thrombophlebitis

RECOMMENDED MONITORING
- Pain
- Fecal output and consistency and any blood on feces

- Signs of endotoxemia
- Colic

PROGNOSIS AND OUTCOME

- Prognosis is favorable for prolapse type 1 or 2.
- Prognosis is worsened in prolapse type 3 or 4 because vascular and mesenteric disruption is more common.

PEARLS & CONSIDERATIONS

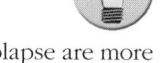

COMMENTS

- Types 1 and 2 rectal prolapse are more common than types 3 and 4.
- If more than 30 cm of prolapse is outside of the rectum, the vascular supply is compromised.

PREVENTION

Early prevention of tenesmus because this appears to be the most common underlying cause

SUGGESTED READING

Freeman D: Rectum and anus. In Auer JA, Stick JA, editors: *Equine Surgery*, St Louis, 2006, Saunders Elsevier, pp 479–491.

Schumacher J: Disease of the small colon and rectum. In Mair TS, Divers T, Ducharme N, editors: *Manual of equine gastroenterology*, St Louis, 2002, Saunders Elsevier, pp 299–315.

Turner TA: Rectal prolapse. In Robinson NE, editors: *Current therapy in equine medicine*, St Louis, 1987, WB Saunders.

AUTHOR: CERI SHERLOCK

EDITORS: TIM MAIR and **CERI SHERLOCK**

Rectal Tear

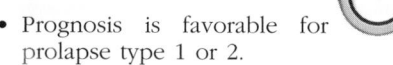

BASIC INFORMATION

DEFINITION

Partial- or full-thickness tear through the wall of the rectum (or occasionally the small colon)

EPIDEMIOLOGY

SPECIES, AGE, SEX
- Small horses or ponies
- Young horses
- Stallions and geldings

GENETICS AND BREED PREDISPOSITION
- Arabians
- Fractious horses

RISK FACTORS
- Palpation per rectum (examination for colic or breeding examinations)
- Enema administration

CLINICAL PRESENTATION

DISEASE FORMS/SUBTYPES Grading system used to classify tears:
- Grade 1: Only the mucosa and submucosa are torn.
- Grade 2: The muscularis is torn, but the mucosa and submucosa remain intact.
- Grade 3a: The mucosa, submucosa, and muscularis are torn, but the serosa remains intact.
- Grade 3b: The mucosa, submucosa, and muscularis are torn dorsally, and the mesorectum remains intact.
- Grade 4: Full-thickness tear

HISTORY, CHIEF COMPLAINT
- Shortly after a rectal examination, breeding, or an enema
- Colic
- Tenesmus
- Depression
- Sweating
- Reluctance to move

PHYSICAL EXAM FINDINGS
- Temperature variable depending on severity of compromise
- Possibly tachycardia depending on the severity
- Depression, lethargy, and colic signs
- Mucous membranes variable depending on the severity; pale pink and moist to toxic and purple
- Possibly abdominal distension and secondary ileus
- Possibly reduced fecal output, tenesmus, and blood-tinged feces
- Clinical hydration variable

ETIOLOGY AND PATHOPHYSIOLOGY
- Most commonly secondary to increase in rectal pressure
  - Rectal examination
  - Breeding injury
  - Foaling injury
  - Enema administration
  - Rarely fecal retention
- Neurogenic
- Obstructive (perineal or rectal melanomas)
- Spontaneous rupture is rare.
  - Ischemic necrosis after caudal mesenteric thrombosis
  - Rupture of a mural hematoma in the small colon

DIAGNOSIS

DIFFERENTIAL DIAGNOSIS

Depends on the severity or grade of the tear
- Small colon impaction
- Small colon strangulating disease (eg, lipoma, volvulus, or intussusception)
- Small colon nonstrangulating obstructive disease (eg, enterolith or fecalith)
- Gastric rupture
- Cecal rupture
- Rupture of other gastrointestinal viscus

INITIAL DATABASE

- Complete blood count: Leukopenia or leukocytosis are common; occasionally normal
- Bare arm rectal examination with the horse sedated and restrained and under the effects of medications to prevent further straining (see initial treatment): Identify blood on retraction of the arm and palpate the defect.
- Peritoneal fluid: Normal in grades 1 and 2, variable increases in total protein (TP) and white blood cell counts seen in grades 3a and 3b, marked elevations in TP and white blood cell counts and gross fecal contamination seen in grade 4 tears.
- Transabdominal ultrasonography: May see peritoneal effusion in horses with grade 3a, 3b, and 4 tears and may see gas artifacts caused by pneumoperitoneum in horses with grade 4 tears

TREATMENT

THERAPEUTIC GOAL(S)

- Grade 1 and 2 tears
  - Prevent progression of the tear
  - Facilitate healing
    - Stool softeners
    - ± Antiinflammatories ± antibiotics
- Grade 3a or 3b tears
  - Prevent progression of the tear
  - Facilitate healing
    - Medical management
      □ Fecal softeners
      □ Fecal evacuation
    - Surgical management
      □ Primary closure: Intraluminally or through exploratory celiotomy
      □ Fecal diversion techniques: Temporary indwelling rectal liner or colostomy

- Grade 4 tears normally result in gross fecal contamination of the peritoneal cavity, so euthanasia is justified. In rare cases when gross fecal contamination has not occurred, treatment is as for grade 3 tears.

ACUTE GENERAL TREATMENT

- Evaluation and prevention of progression
  - Sedate the horse
  - Administer parasympatholytic (Buscopan at 0.3 mg/kg)
  - Consider caudal epidural anesthesia with 0.22 mg/kg of lidocaine
  - Evacuate feces
  - Perform bare arm rectal evaluation
- Grade 1 tears
  - Analgesia (flunixin meglumine)
  - Broad-spectrum antibiotics (trimethoprim sulfonamide)
  - Stool softeners (mineral oil)
  - Tetanus prophylaxis
- Grade 2 tears
  - Analgesia (flunixin meglumine)
  - Stool softeners (mineral oil)
- Grade 3 tears
  - Consider packing with a Betadine-soaked rectal tampon (cotton wool in a stockinette) from the anus to cranial to the tear and holding in place with purse string for shipping.
  - Analgesia (flunixin meglumine)
  - Broad-spectrum antibiotics (potassium penicillin, gentamicin and metronidazole)
  - Tetanus prophylaxis
  - Consider baseline abdominocentesis
- Grade 4
  - Euthanasia if fecal contamination of the peritoneal cavity
  - As for grade 3 if no gross fecal contamination

CHRONIC TREATMENT

- Grade 1 tears
  - Analgesia (flunixin meglumine for 3–5 days)
  - Broad spectrum antibiotics (trimethoprim sulfonamide for 7–10 days)
  - Stool softeners (mineral oil for 10–14 days)

- Do not perform rectal palpation for 3 to 4 weeks unless clinically indicated.
- Grade 2 tears
  - Analgesia (flunixin meglumine for 3–5 days)
  - Stool softeners (mineral oil for 10–14 days)
  - Do not perform a rectal examination for 3 to 4 weeks unless clinically indicated.
- Grade 3
  - Continued broad-spectrum antibiotics
  - Continued analgesia
  - Antiendotoxic therapy as necessary
  - Medical management
    - Fecal softening
    - Fecal evacuation
  - Surgical management
    - Primary closure: Intraluminally or through exploratory celiotomy
    - Fecal diversion techniques
    - Temporary indwelling rectal liner
    - Colostomy
  - Do not perform rectal palpation for 3 to 4 weeks unless clinically indicated.

POSSIBLE COMPLICATIONS

- Peritonitis
- Endotoxemia
- Laminitis
- Adhesions
- Progression of rectal tear
- Jugular thrombophlebitis
- Diarrhea
- Pyrexia
- Perirectal abscesses

RECOMMENDED MONITORING

- Pain
- Fecal output and consistency
- Signs of endotoxemia
- Colic

PROGNOSIS AND OUTCOME

- Prognosis is excellent for grades 1 and 2.

- Prognosis is fair to poor for grade 3 tears. Horses with grade 3 tears in the rectum caudal to the peritoneal reflection have a better prognosis than with tears that enter the peritoneal cavity. Horses with grade 3b tears have a slightly better prognosis than those with grade 3a tears
- Horses with grade 4 tears have a grave prognosis.

PEARLS & CONSIDERATIONS

COMMENTS

- Iatrogenic rectal tears that occur during rectal palpation are a leading cause of malpractice claims.
- Attaining client consent before the procedure is advisable, and it is essential to implement prophylactic measures in an attempt to reduce the risks of rectal tears.

PREVENTION

- Adequate restraint
- Adequate relaxation
  - Sedation
  - Parasympatholytic agents
  - Intrarectal lidocaine
  - Caudal epidural with lidocaine

SUGGESTED READING

Freeman DE: Rectum and anus. In Auer JA, Stick JA, editors: *Equine surgery*, St Louis, 2006, Saunders Elsevier, pp 479–491.

Schumacher J: Disease of the small colon and rectum. In Mair TS, Divers T, Ducharme N, editors: *Manual of equine gastroenterology*, St Louis, 2002, Saunders Elsevier, pp 299–315.

Sherlock CE, Peroni JP: Management of rectal tears. In Robinson NE, Sprayberry KA, editors: *Current therapy in equine medicine*, St Louis, 2008, Saunders Elsevier, pp 451–455.

AUTHOR: **CERI SHERLOCK**

EDITORS: **TIM MAIR** and **CERI SHERLOCK**

Red Maple Leaf Toxicosis

BASIC INFORMATION

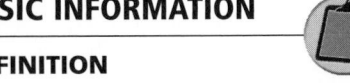

DEFINITION

The leaves (wilted or dried) from the native red maple (*Acer rubrum*) tree are known to cause oxidative damage to equine erythrocytes that may result in intravascular or extravascular hemolysis, Heinz body formation, and/or methemoglobinemia.

SYNONYM(S)

Swamp maple, soft maple, scarlet maple, Carolina maple

EPIDEMIOLOGY

RISK FACTORS Intoxication is more common in late summer and fall because of consumption of wilted or dried leaves. Branches that are downed in a storm may also be a problem.

GEOGRAPHY AND SEASONALITY Red maple trees grow extensively throughout the entire eastern part of North America. The trees are of medium size with 2- to 4-inch long leaves consisting of three to five lobes with serrated margins (Figures 1 and 2).

ASSOCIATED CONDITIONS AND DISORDERS Leaves from other maples (sugar maple and silver maple) may result in clinical signs similar to red maple toxicosis. Analysis of Norway maple leaves indicates that poisoning caused by the ingestion of leaves from this ornamental tree is much less likely.

CLINICAL PRESENTATION

HISTORY, CHIEF COMPLAINT

- History of ingestion or the presence of maple leaves in the pasture with appropriate clinical signs.

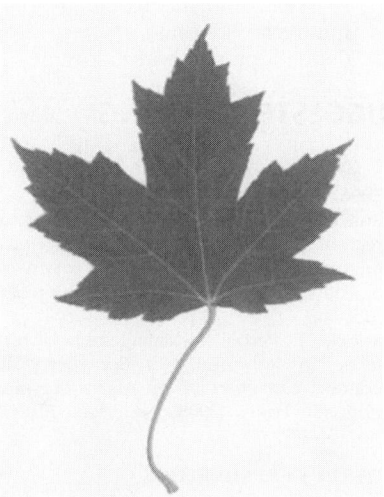

FIGURE 1 Red maple leaf.

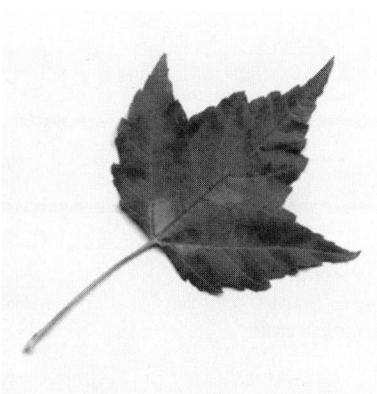

FIGURE 2 Red maple leaf.

- Clinical signs of red maple toxicosis vary depending on the severity and time course for hemolysis, degree of methemoglobinemia, efficacy of tissue perfusion, and severity of hypoxia.

PHYSICAL EXAM FINDINGS

- Signs associated with methemoglobinemia and hemolytic anemia.
- Rarely, peracute death from severe methemoglobinemia and tissue anoxia may be the only sign.
- More commonly, depression and anorexia develop on the first day, followed by:
  ○ Icterus
  ○ Cyanosis
  ○ Depression
  ○ Dehydration
  ○ Hemoglobinemia with decreased packed cell volume (PCV)
  ○ Polypnea
  ○ Tachycardia

ETIOLOGY AND PATHOPHYSIOLOGY

- The peak incidence of poisoning occurs in the fall, when horses have access to dried or wilted leaves.
- Affected animals may display clinical signs within 12 to 48 hours, and death often occurs within 3 to 6 days of intoxication.
- The toxin has not been identified, but is believed to be an oxidant because of its effect on red blood cells (RBCs).
- Gallic acid has been found to be involved in the development of methemoglobinemia, but an unidentified factor plays a significant part in hemolysis.
- As little as 1.5 g/kg of dried red maple leaves has been shown to cause fatal illness in a pony.

DIAGNOSIS

DIFFERENTIAL DIAGNOSIS

- Autoimmune hemolytic anemia
- Ehrlichiosis
- Equine infectious anemia
- Leptospirosis
- Disorders caused by other plants or chemicals (eg, nitrate, onions, *Brassica* spp. toxicosis)
- Piroplasmosis
- Babesiosis

INITIAL DATABASE

- Complete blood count: May show anemia (which may be quite marked), Heinz body formation, poikilocytosis, spherocytosis, increased RBC fragility, anisocytosis, and increased RBC indexes.
- Serum chemistry profile: Azotemia (increased serum urea and creatinine); elevated creatine kinase and aspartate aminotransferase; elevated gamma glutamyl transpeptidase, alkaline phosphatase, and gamma lactate dehydrogenase; increased total, conjugated, and unconjugated bilirubin; hyperglycemia; hypercalcemia and metabolic acidosis.
- Urinalysis: The urine is often dark red to black, with hematuria, hemoglobinuria, methemoglobinuria, proteinuria, bilirubinuria, and occasional casts.
- Horses with red maple toxicosis–induced acute renal failure may be oliguric, isosthenuric, or anuric.

ADVANCED OR CONFIRMATORY TESTING

- Elevated methemoglobin levels
- Microscopy of material in the mouth or gastric contents may identify margins and structure of leaves
- No specific test is available, so it is important to rule out other causes of hemolytic anemia and be aware of potential exposure.

TREATMENT

THERAPEUTIC GOAL(S)

- There is no specific antidote for red maple toxicosis.
- Remove leaves and branches from areas where horses are kept.
- Blood transfusion may be indicated if the PCV decreases to less than 10%.
- Therapy is largely supportive with fluid therapy to prevent renal failure.

ACUTE GENERAL TREATMENT

- Administer fluid therapy and maintain perfusion to the kidneys.
- Prevent shock.
- Correct dehydration and electrolyte abnormalities.
- Manage methemoglobinemia.
- Administer ascorbic acid (to reduce methemoglobin to hemoglobin).
- Administer activated charcoal.
- Oxyglobin (purified bovine hemoglobin) has been used successfully.
- Perform a blood transfusion.
- Administer ascorbic acid.
- Do not administer methylene blue; doing so may induce additional Heinz body formation and will not reduce methemoglobin.

POSSIBLE COMPLICATIONS

- Colic signs may develop secondarily to enteric ischemia, impaired mobility, and cecal impaction.
- Renal dysfunction caused by anoxia or hemoglobinuria may develop.

RECOMMENDED MONITORING

- Monitor for laminitis caused by severe systemic inflammation, hypoxia, and poor perfusion.
- Monitor routine clinical pathology data for renal damage (biochemistry, urinalysis, and hematology).

PROGNOSIS AND OUTCOME

- The mortality rates associated with natural and experimentally induced red maple toxicosis range from 60% to 70%.
- In one retrospective study, there were no clinicopathologic variables upon admission that accurately predicted survival. Acute renal failure is presumed to be caused by inadequate renal perfusion or oxygenation and hemoglobinuria. Even with aggressive treatment, the prognosis for these patients may be guarded.

PEARLS & CONSIDERATIONS

COMMENTS

Prevention is the key and is accomplished simply by preventing exposure of horses to the wilted leaves of red maple trees. Red maple leaves should not be incorporated into bales of hay meant for equine consumption. If storms occur, pastures should be examined for debris from maple trees, and leaves and branches should be removed.

PREVENTION

Remove all wilted maple leaves from areas where horses are kept.

CLIENT EDUCATION

Ingestion of dried or wilted maple leaves may result in hemolytic anemia and/or methemoglobinemia crisis in horses. The mortality rate can be quite high, and the best treatment for red maple toxicosis is prevention of exposure.

SUGGESTED READING

Alward A: Red maple toxicosis in horses. *Proc 26th ACVIM* 215–216, 2008.

Divers TJ, George LW, George JW: Hemolytic anemia in horses after the ingestion of red maple leaves. *J Am Vet Med Assoc* 180: 300–302, 1982.

Merola V, Volmer PA: Red maple. In Plumlee KH, editor: *Clinical veterinary toxicology*, St Louis, 2003, Mosby Elsevier, pp 437–438.

AUTHOR: **BRENT HOFF**

EDITOR: **CYNTHIA L. GASKILL**

Renal Dysplasia

BASIC INFORMATION

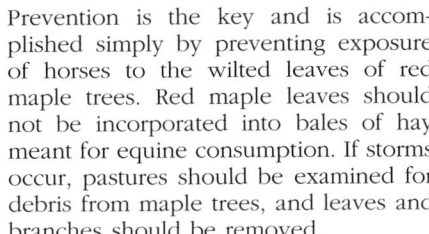

DEFINITION

Renal dysplasia is abnormal metanephric differentiation of the kidney(s). The kidneys experience embryonic arrest at some time before birth. Histologically, there is abnormal development of the renal vasculature, tubules, collecting ducts, or urine drainage structures.

SYNONYM(S)

Renal dysgenesis

EPIDEMIOLOGY

SPECIES, AGE, SEX Reported in other species such as dogs, cats, cattle, and humans. Renal dysplasia may not become clinically apparent until renal failure occurs, especially if unilateral. Bilaterally affected horses tend to manifest clinical signs at an earlier age.

GENETICS AND BREED PREDISPOSITION Although there is a known hereditary and breed (familial) predilection in dogs and cats, this association remains unclear in horses.

RISK FACTORS

- Possible genetic or hereditary factors may play a role.
- There is some evidence that aminoglycosides, corticosteroids, and angiotensin-converting enzyme (ACE) inhibitors used during pregnancy may lead to renal dysplasia of the fetus.

ASSOCIATED CONDITIONS AND DISORDERS Renal hypoplasia, renal agenesis or aplasia

CLINICAL PRESENTATION

HISTORY, CHIEF COMPLAINT Depression, anorexia, lethargy, weight loss or poor weight gain, salt craving, polydipsia, polyuria, ± uremia (oral ulcerations and dental tartar)

PHYSICAL EXAM FINDINGS Depression, ± mild tachycardia, ± mucous membrane pallor, poor body condition, dental tartar

ETIOLOGY AND PATHOPHYSIOLOGY

- Disorganized development of renal tissue caused by anomalous differentiation, intrauterine ureteral obstruction, fetal viral infection, or teratogens
- Occurs in utero when the ureteric bud fails to combine properly with the metanephric blastema because this is a necessary union for normal nephrogenesis. Normally, the metanephric blastema forms the proximal components of the nephron from the glomerulus to the distal convoluted tubule and the ureteric bud arises from the mesonephric duct and forms the distal components of the nephron, including the collecting ducts, calyces, and pelvis. The metanephric blastema is generally believed to differentiate into the renal parenchyma under the influence of the ampulla of the ureteric bud. Therefore, in cases of dysplasia, the ureteric bud arises from an abnormal position on the mesonephric duct. Although a kidney is formed and it may still produce urine, the resulting structure is dysplastic and does not retain normal function.

- Bilateral dysplasia generally leads to renal failure.

DIAGNOSIS

DIFFERENTIAL DIAGNOSIS

- Acute or chronic renal failure
- Psychogenic water consumption
- Osmotic diuresis (diabetes mellitus or psychogenic salt consumption)
- inappropriate free water loss (nephrogenic or neurogenic diabetes insipidus or pituitary pars intermedia dysfunction)
- pyelonephritis
- cystitis
- anatomical or congenital renal disorder (agenesis, hypoplasia, ectopic ureters, or renal cyst)

INITIAL DATABASE

- Complete blood count: Anemia
- Serum chemistries: Azotemia (increased blood urea nitrogen [BUN] and creatinine concentrations), hypercalcemia, hyponatremia, hypochloremia, hyperkalemia, ± hypophosphatemia
- Urinalysis: Isosthenuria
- Renal ultrasound examination: Normal to small-sized kidneys with poorly demarcated corticomedullary junction and increased echogenicity
  - Dysplastic kidneys are typically normal in size unless they are accompanied by concurrent renal hypoplasia or if the horse lives for a prolonged period of time before the development of renal failure.

ADVANCED OR CONFIRMATORY TESTING

- Definitive diagnosis is made via ultrasound-guided renal biopsy. Histopathology reveals immature, variably sized, and decreased numbers of glomeruli; primitive hypoplastic, dilated tubules; hypoplastic vasa recta; and an indistinct corticomedullary junction. Diffuse interstitial fibrosis may be present in the cortex and medulla.
- Scintigraphy: A glomerular filtration rate scan using technetium-labeled diethylenetriaminepentaacetic acid (DTPA) and a renal morphology scan using technetium-labeled dimercaptosuccinic acid (DMSA) can be performed to help determine the prognosis if the renal biopsy is inconclusive.
- Computed tomography of the abdomen (with positive contrast agent) in foals can be helpful to localize urinary tract pathology.
- Increased urine γ-glutamyl transpeptidase:creatinine ratio (>25 IU/g)
- Increased urinary fractional excretion of sodium and chloride.
- Abdominocentesis to rule out uroperitoneum; measurement of peritoneal fluid to serum creatinine concentration ratio (normal, <2)

TREATMENT

THERAPEUTIC GOAL(S)

- The ultimate goals are to maintain hydration, electrolyte balance, acid-base balance, and nutrition and to reverse azotemia.
- Maintain hydration and provide fresh water and electrolyte water.
- Supplement salt to promote water intake and diuresis.
- Provide a diet low in calcium and protein.
- Maintain a normotensive state.

ACUTE GENERAL TREATMENT

- Management of renal failure through supportive care: Rehydration (IV crystalloids 0.9% NaCl or Normosol-R), replenish electrolytes, reverse azotemia, and provide nutritional support.
- If oliguric renal failure is present: Furosemide (1 mg/kg IV q2–6h) and vasopressor therapy (dopamine 3–5 μg/kg/min IV continuous rate infusion to increase renal blood flow and urine output) if indicated.
- Mannitol (0.25–1.0 g/kg IV) can also be administered to increase renal blood flow and urine output.

CHRONIC TREATMENT

Dietary modification: Lowered calcium and protein (avoid legumes and feed grass hay only); increased salt (if animal is hyponatremic and hypochloremic) and water intake

DRUG INTERACTIONS

In cases of renal failure, avoid the use of nephrotoxic drugs such as aminoglycosides and nonsteroidal antiinflammatory drugs. These drugs should be used sparingly and only after careful consideration in cases of unilateral renal dysplasia.

RECOMMENDED MONITORING

- Monitor packed cell volume (PCV), total protein, BUN, creatinine, and electrolyte concentrations and urinalysis.
- Monitor noninvasive blood pressure while the patient is maintained on continuous-rate infusion of dopamine to avoid hypertension.
- Monitor body weight and condition.
- Useful advanced monitoring tools: Central venous pressure (CVP) to assess hydration status. Maintain CVP below 8 to 10 cm H_2O. If CVP is increased and the horse is euvolemic, then furosemide is indicated (1 mg/kg IV). Monitor noninvasive blood pressure via tail cuff. Treat hypertension with acepromazine, ACE inhibitors (enalapril), and diuretics (furosemide).

- Complications from renal biopsy include severe, life-threatening hemorrhage. Monitor heart rate, mucous membrane color, PCV, total protein, and lactate concentrations. Repeat renal ultrasound examinations after biopsy can be helpful to identify hemorrhage before the onset of clinical signs.

PROGNOSIS AND OUTCOME

Good if the dysplasia is unilateral; grave if bilateral

PEARLS & CONSIDERATIONS

COMMENTS

- Renal dysplasia is a congenital condition that may not become apparent until later in life when renal failure occurs, especially if only one kidney is affected.
- Euthanasia is warranted if bilateral renal dysplasia is present or if renal failure does not respond to medical management.

PREVENTION

Although the exact etiopathophysiology is unknown, renal dysplasia has been shown to have a familial incidence in some breeds of dogs. Therefore it is recommended to avoid breeding affected animals.

SUGGESTED READING

Chaney KP: Congenital anomalies of the equine urinary tract. *Vet Clin North Am Equine Pract* 23:3, 2007.

Gull T, Schmitz DG, Bahr A, et al: Renal hypoplasia and dysplasia in an American miniature foal. *Vet Rec* 149:199–203, 2001.

Plummer PJ: Congenital renal dysplasia in a 7-month-old quarter horse colt. *Vet Clin North Am Equine Pract* 22:1, 2006.

AUTHOR: **KELLY L. KALF**

EDITOR: **BRYAN M. WALDRIDGE**

Renal Failure, Acute

BASIC INFORMATION

DEFINITION

Sudden decrease in glomerular filtration and urinary excretion of waste products

EPIDEMIOLOGY

RISK FACTORS

- Dehydration
- Administration of nephrotoxic drugs (nonsteroidal antiinflammatory drugs [NSAIDs], aminoglycosides, polymyxin B, tetracyclines)

- Pigmenturia (hemoglobinuria and myoglobinuria)

ASSOCIATED CONDITIONS AND DISORDERS

- Colic
- Dehydration
- Diarrhea

- Heart failure
- Hemolysis
- Rhabdomyolysis

CLINICAL PRESENTATION
DISEASE FORMS/SUBTYPES
- Prerenal azotemia
- Postrenal azotemia

HISTORY, CHIEF COMPLAINT
- Anorexia
- Treatment with nephrotoxic drugs
- Depression, lethargy
- Hemolysis, rhabdomyolysis (pigmentary nephropathy)
- Oliguria (but urine production may be normal to polyuric)
- Urinary tract obstruction or disruption (urolithiasis, ruptured bladder)
- The predominant clinical signs are usually attributable to another primary problem that caused dehydration.

PHYSICAL EXAM FINDINGS
- Dehydration: Increased skin turgor, sunken eyes
- Dry or tacky mucous membranes
- Depression or obtundation

ETIOLOGY AND PATHOPHYSIOLOGY
- Dehydration: Administration of nephrotoxic drugs.
- Dehydrated animals depend on renal production of prostaglandins to maintain renal perfusion. Because most NSAIDs used in horses are nonselective cyclooxygenase inhibitors, their use in dehydrated animals blocks the kidneys' ability to increase its blood flow.
- Pigmentary nephropathy results when myoglobin or hemoglobin polymerizes and occludes renal tubules.
- Aminoglycosides are freely filtered at the glomerulus and are actively taken up by proximal tubular epithelial cells. Toxicity may involve lysosomal disruption and leakage of proteolytic enzymes.
- Postrenal azotemia occurs with occlusion of urinary outflow, backpressure in the collecting system, and resultant decreased renal blood flow.

DIAGNOSIS

DIFFERENTIAL DIAGNOSIS
- Urinary tract obstruction or rupture
- Chronic renal failure

INITIAL DATABASE
- Complete blood count (hematocrit)
- Serum chemistries (total protein, blood urea nitrogen [BUN], creatinine concentrations)

ADVANCED OR CONFIRMATORY TESTING
- Urinalysis (specific gravity, tubular casts, increased protein)
- Fractional excretion of electrolytes
- Urinary gamma glutamyltransferase: creatinine ratio
- Ultrasound examination of the kidneys and urinary tract
- Rectal palpation of the left kidney

TREATMENT

THERAPEUTIC GOAL(S)
- Restore circulating plasma volume and blood pressure.
- Promote normal urine production.
- Return BUN and creatinine concentrations to normal ranges.
- Treat any predisposing conditions that may have led to acute renal failure.

ACUTE GENERAL TREATMENT
- IV fluid replacement with balanced electrolyte solutions
  - Fluid deficit (liters) = Body weight (kg) × Estimated % dehydration
  - To stimulate diuresis, IV fluids at 1.5 to 2.0 times maintenance requirements
- Calcium gluconate (20 mg Ca/kg IV q12h) reduced experimental gentamicin-induced acute renal failure.
- If the horse remains oliguric or anuric after appropriate fluid therapy, then further therapy to increase renal blood flow is indicated.
- Mannitol (20% solution; 1 g/kg IV) may also be administered as an osmotic diuretic if the horse is producing some urine.

DRUG INTERACTIONS
Avoid nephrotoxic drugs until the horse is hydrated

POSSIBLE COMPLICATIONS
- Chronic renal failure and permanently increased renal indexes
- Oliguria or anuria
- Ascites, anasarca

RECOMMENDED MONITORING
- Creatinine and BUN concentrations at least every 48 hours
- Therapeutic drug monitoring of aminoglycosides
- Water intake
- Urine output
- Urinalysis, especially specific gravity and the presence of tubular casts

PROGNOSIS AND OUTCOME

- Generally good with appropriate therapy
- A favorable response is an approximate 50% decrease in BUN and creatinine concentrations within 24 hours of beginning therapy.
- Horses that do not urinate appropriately or remain oliguric or anuric or need additional therapy (vasopressors or diuretics) to produce urine have a poorer prognosis.

PEARLS & CONSIDERATIONS

COMMENTS
- Most acute renal failure is reversible with IV fluid replacement.
- The use of diuretics to stimulate urination should be avoided unless the horse does not urinate after appropriate fluid therapy.
- Potentially nephrotoxic drugs should be avoided as much as possible in dehydrated patients or at least until the fluid deficit has been replaced.

PREVENTION
- Routine (approximately q48h) measurement of serum BUN and creatinine concentrations in at-risk patients
- Therapeutic drug monitoring of potentially nephrotoxic drugs (amikacin, gentamicin)
- Once-daily administration of aminoglycosides
- Adjust dosages of potential nephrotoxic drugs in patients that lose weight during treatment.
- Experimentally, horses fed only alfalfa hay had less gentamicin-induced nephrotoxicity than horses fed only oats. It is possible that increased calcium in alfalfa or dietary differences in gastrointestinal to extracellular fluid fluxes may account for this difference.

CLIENT EDUCATION
- Be certain to administer appropriate doses of NSAIDs and use them only as needed in horses that are not dehydrated.
- Monitor appetite, water intake, and urine production in horses treated with NSAIDs and other potentially nephrotoxic drugs.

SUGGESTED READING
Bayly WM: Acute renal failure. In Reed SM, Bayly WM, Sellon DC, editors: *Equine internal medicine*, ed 3, St Louis, 2010, Saunders Elsevier, pp 1176–1182.

Divers TJ: Urine production, renal function, and drug monitoring in the equine intensive-care unit. *Clin Tech Equine Pract* 2:188, 2003.

AUTHOR & EDITOR: BRYAN M. WALDRIDGE

Renal Failure, Chronic

BASIC INFORMATION

DEFINITION

A progressive loss of renal function that affects the kidneys' ability to concentrate urine, remove bloodborne nitrogenous wastes, and maintain appropriate fluid and electrolyte balance. Endocrine function of the kidneys is also affected.

SYNONYM(S)

- Chronic kidney disease
- CRF

EPIDEMIOLOGY

SPECIES, AGE, SEX

- One-third of all cases have been reported in horses younger than 6 years, suggesting a congenital problem if it occurs the absence of an inciting event.
- One study showed a predominance of male horses; however, this may be skewed by the presence of elite stallions.

GENETICS AND BREED PREDISPOSITION Thoroughbreds, Standardbreds, and Clydesdales were most often affected in one study; however, multiple breeds may be affected.

RISK FACTORS Congenital renal abnormalities

ASSOCIATED CONDITIONS AND DISORDERS

- Anemia
- Hypoproteinemia
- Hypercalcemia
- Polyuria and polydipsia
- Nephrotic syndrome

CLINICAL PRESENTATION

HISTORY, CHIEF COMPLAINT

- The onset may be insidious and occur over a long period
  Horses usually present with advanced disease
  Weight loss
  Lethargy
  Anorexia
  Polydipsia
  Polyuria
- Previous illness leading to prolonged hypovolemia: Colitis
- Use of nephrotoxic drugs: Aminoglycosides, nonsteroidal antiinflammatory drugs (NSAIDs), amphotericin B, and oxytetracycline

PHYSICAL EXAM FINDINGS

- Weight loss
- Intermittent fever
- Rough hair coat
- Edema of the distal limbs and ventrum
- Oral cavity ulceration
- Dental tartar formation
- Gingivitis

ETIOLOGY AND PATHOPHYSIOLOGY

- Congenital anomalies may be responsible: Polycystic kidneys, renal agenesis, or renal hypoplasia. Acquired disease secondary to glomerular or tubular insult is a more common cause of CRF in horses.
- Glomerulonephritis rarely progresses to CRF. Vascular and tubular changes occur resulting from ischemia, infection, toxic insults, and immune-mediated damage. Permeability changes at the glomerular basement membrane result in proteinuria and hematuria. Histologic changes determining the genesis of glomerular injury are not useful prognostically.
- Chronic interstitial nephritis is considered to result from acute tubular nephrosis. Precipitating insults include ischemia, nephrotoxic drugs, heavy metals, septic processes, endotoxemia, ascending infection, pyelonephritis, ureterolithiasis, nephrolithiasis, hemolysis, and rhabdomyolysis. Histologic changes include tubular damage and interstitial inflammatory cell (lymphocyte, monocyte, and plasma cell) infiltrate. Fibrosis is also present, differentiating this condition from acute tubular and interstitial disease.
- Amyloidosis is a rare cause of CRF as a result of hyperimmunization for antibody production or chronic antigenic stimulation.
- Neoplasia: Usually unilateral disease only.
- End-stage kidney disease: Prominent fibrosis and loss of appropriate renal architecture. The kidneys are grossly irregular and shrunken.

DIAGNOSIS

DIFFERENTIAL DIAGNOSIS

- Renal agenesis, hypoplasia
- Pyelonephritis
- Protein-losing enteropathy
- Neoplasia: Primary renal neoplasms are rare; may have renal involvement secondary to systemic disease (lymphoma)
- Cardiac cachexia
- Hepatic failure

INITIAL DATABASE

- Complete blood count: Nonregenerative anemia
- Serum chemistries
  - Elevated creatinine and blood urea nitrogen (BUN) concentrations. The BUN/creatinine ratio is often greater than 10:1
  - Hypoproteinemia, hypoalbuminemia, hyponatremia, hyperkalemia, hypochloremia, and hypophosphatemia. Hypercalcemia is caused by decreased urinary excretion secondary to tubular dysfunction and loss
  - Metabolic acidosis may develop in terminal stages.
- Urinalysis: Persistent isosthenuria (1.008–1.015) with concurrent azotemia and compatible clinical signs. Hematuria and proteinuria are not found unless concurrent glomerular injury is present.
- Rectal palpation: Irregular shrunken left kidney. If urolithiasis, nephritis, or neoplasia is present, the ureters and kidney may be enlarged.
- Ultrasonography: Decreased renal mass, irregular renal margins, loss of appropriate renal architecture, loss of distinct corticomedullary junction, nephrolithiasis, or hydronephrosis.

ADVANCED OR CONFIRMATORY TESTING

- Creatinine clearance may be increased because of renal tubular creatinine secretion into urine in the early stages of CRF, leading to an overestimation of GFR.
- Urinary gamma-glutamyl transpeptidase:creatinine ratio: Elevated values (>25) indicate tubular damage but are of uncertain utility.
- Fractional electrolyte excretion values: Increased electrolyte loss in the urine, especially sodium, because of a lack of tubular resorption.
- Renal biopsy with ultrasound guidance. Because lesions may not be uniformly distributed throughout the kidney, normal tissue may be recovered in cases with widespread pathology. The causative agent or process may no longer be discernible in advanced cases with degenerative glomerular, tubular, and interstitial changes.

TREATMENT

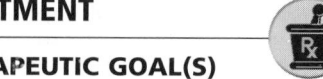

THERAPEUTIC GOAL(S)

- Treatment is largely palliative.
- Manage any inciting or concurrent disease process (immune-mediated disease, pyelonephritis).

ACUTE GENERAL TREATMENT

If an acute exacerbation of chronic disease occurs:
- Establish diuresis to counter azotemia. Cautious administration of IV fluids to prevent worsening hypoproteinemia and edema
- Manage infection (pyelonephritis), if present
- Resolve obstructive conditions: Ureterolithiasis, nephrolithiasis, and urethral obstruction

CHRONIC TREATMENT

- Ensure adequate hydration
- Ensure adequate nutritional intake and maintain bodyweight
- Discontinue nephrotoxic drug administration: Aminoglycosides, NSAIDs, amphotericin B, oxytetracycline
- Decrease dietary protein (grass hay, avoid legumes) and salt

RECOMMENDED MONITORING

- Serum BUN, creatinine, and electrolyte concentrations
- Hematocrit and total protein concentration
- Urine specific gravity
- Creatinine clearance to monitor progression of CRF in individual horses

- Water intake
- Body weight and condition

PROGNOSIS AND OUTCOME

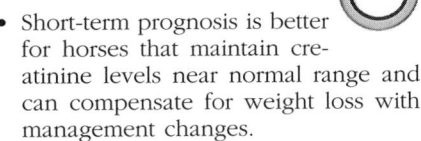

- Short-term prognosis is better for horses that maintain creatinine levels near normal range and can compensate for weight loss with management changes.
- Compensatory hypertrophy of nephrons and increased single nephron glomerular filtration rate can occur in the short term.
- Chronic and progressive disease with continual loss of renal functional mass; therefore long-term prognosis is poor.

PEARLS & CONSIDERATIONS

COMMENTS

- Avoid overzealous fluid administration during the initial treatment period because peripheral and pulmonary edema may result if albumin levels are diminished.

- Control azotemia: Avoid high-protein feeds with provision of grass hay, fat, and carbohydrate feeds.
- Control hypercalcemia: Minimize intake of alfalfa hay.
- Maintain feed intake even if less desirable feeds (as above) must be used.

CLIENT EDUCATION

- CRF is an incurable condition. Considerable loss ($\leq 75\%$) of renal function has occurred before the condition becomes clinically evident.
- Loss of kidney mass is irreversible.
- Long-term management is exacting but may markedly improve the quality and quantity of life for the affected horse.

SUGGESTED READING

Finco DR: Kidney function. In Kaneko JJ, Harvey JW, Bruss ML, editors: *Clinical biochemistry of domestic animals*, ed 5, San Diego, 1997, Academic Press, pp 441–484.

Schott HC II: Renal physiology. In Reed S, Bayly WM, Sellon DC, editors: *Equine internal medicine*, ed 3, St Louis, 2010, Saunders Elsevier, pp 1150–1161.

AUTHOR: PETER R. MORRESEY

EDITOR: BRYAN M. WALDRIDGE

Renal Tubular Acidosis

BASIC INFORMATION

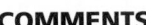

DEFINITION

Renal tubular acidosis (RTA) is a group of disorders affecting the renal tubular cells that result in hyperchloremic metabolic acidosis with a normal anion gap.

EPIDEMIOLOGY

ASSOCIATED CONDITIONS AND DISORDERS

- Hyperchloremic metabolic acidosis with a normal anion gap
- Weight loss, unthriftiness

CLINICAL PRESENTATION

DISEASE FORMS/SUBTYPES

- Type I: Distal or classic RTA (H^+ retention)
- Type II: Proximal RTA (HCO_3 wasting)

HISTORY, CHIEF COMPLAINT

- Depression
- Poor performance
- Anorexia
- Weight loss
- Unthriftiness
- Dull hair coat

- Weakness
- Colic
- Ataxia
- Polyuria or polydipsia

PHYSICAL EXAM FINDINGS

- Mild dehydration
- Mild abdominal distension
- Muscular weakness
- Tachypnea
- Tachycardia

ETIOLOGY AND PATHOPHYSIOLOGY

- Etiology: Underlying cause is usually undetermined, but is generally acquired
  - Renal tubular toxins: Heavy metals, ethylene glycol, drugs (gentamicin, cephalosporins, tetracyclines, salicylate)
  - Neoplasia
  - Hypoparathyroidism
  - Pyelonephritis
  - Ischemia-induced renal failure
  - Hypoaldosteronism or aldosterone resistance
- Pathophysiology
  - Type I (distal or classic RTA) is caused by an inability of the distal

tubule cells to secrete H^+ or to produce acidic urine. There is excessive K^+ secretion and severe hypokalemia.
  - Type II (proximal RTA) is caused by a failure of HCO_3^- resorption in the proximal tubule with subsequent loss of HCO_3^- into urine. The proximal tubule is the site where the majority of filtered HCO_3^- is reabsorbed via Na^+ and H^+ exchange and the breakdown of carbonic acid to carbon dioxide and water under the influence of carbonic anhydrase. Hydrogen ions are usually secreted when HCO_3^- ion is reabsorbed. Failure to reabsorb HCO_3^- results in excessive urinary losses, basic urine pH, and systemic acidosis.
  - Hyperchloremia develops because of renal conservation of chloride to maintain electroneutrality consequent to HCO_3^- loss.
  - Hypokalemia occurs in a proportion of cases secondary to anorexia or accelerated K^+ secretion.

DIAGNOSIS

DIFFERENTIAL DIAGNOSIS

- Hyperchloremic metabolic acidosis: Diarrhea, Fanconi syndrome, dilutional acidosis, medications (carbonic anhydrase inhibitors, ammonium chloride).
- The most common causes of metabolic acidosis are associated with an increased anion gap such as lactic acidosis and hypovolemic shock. Ingestion of exogenous anions (ethylene glycol, salicylate, or methanol) is a rare cause of metabolic acidosis. Hyperchloremic metabolic acidosis with a normal anion gap is associated with loss of HCO_3^- from diarrhea or renal causes such as RTA.

INITIAL DATABASE

- Complete blood count: Usually normal
- Serum biochemistry profile: Hyperchloremia, decreased bicarbonate or TCO_2, mild hyperbilirubinemia (attributed to anorexia), occasional hyponatremia, hypokalemia, and azotemia
- Urinalysis: Alkaline urine in the face of marked metabolic acidosis; isosthenuria is common; bacteriuria and increased white blood cells are possible, in which case a quantitative urine culture should then be performed (>10,000 CFU/mL is significant)

ADVANCED OR CONFIRMATORY TESTING

- Blood gas: Metabolic acidosis with normal anion gap, low $PvCO_2$ caused by compensatory respiratory alkalosis.
- Renal ultrasonography may show underlying renal disease or nonspecific hyperechoic kidneys.
- Renal biopsy and histopathology may determine the underlying cause of RTA.

TREATMENT

THERAPEUTIC GOAL(S)

- Resolution of acidosis and prevention of hypokalemia
- Correction of any predisposing causes

ACUTE GENERAL TREATMENT

- Aggressive $NaHCO_3$ therapy is recommended in the initial treatment of horses with RTA. The administration of large amounts of IV isotonic (1.3%) HCO_3^- during the initial correction of acidosis results in more rapid recovery and shorter hospitalization. Although frequent monitoring of serum pH and bicarbonate concentration is recommended, no complications have been observed with the rapid correction of acidosis in reported cases of RTA.
- IV polyionic fluids (60–120 mL/kg/d) are recommended in clinically dehydrated or azotemic horses.
- Formulas to determine the amount of HCO_3^- required generally provide insufficient HCO_3^- to compensate for massive urinary losses. Frequently large amounts (3000–9000 mEq) are required each day.
- A starting formula to calculate the amount of HCO_3^- required (mEq) per day is: Body weight (kg) × HCO_3^- deficit (mEq) × 0.6
- There is 12 mEq of HCO_3^- in every gram of $NaHCO_3$ powder or baking soda. Initially administer half of the calculated dosage; then administer one-third of the calculated dosage every 8 hours. This amount should be administered for 24 to 48 hours, and if no significant change in serum bicarbonate concentration occurs, then the amount can be increased. Often two to four times the calculated amount is initially required. The serum HCO_3^- concentration should be measured every 24 to 72 hours to adjust the dose.
- If bacteriuria and increased urinary white blood cells are present, then antibiotic therapy is indicated.

CHRONIC TREATMENT

Generally, HCO_3^- therapy can be reduced after acidemia is corrected. Continued bicarbonate therapy is often required for weeks to months because of underlying renal tubular losses. Frequently, RTA resolves spontaneously, at which time therapy can be discontinued.

POSSIBLE COMPLICATIONS

- It is important to remember that bicarbonaturia increases urinary potassium loss and alters the distribution of potassium between intracellular and extracellular fluid. Development or exacerbation of hypokalemia is likely to occur if supplemental potassium is not provided with concurrent HCO_3^- administration.
- Because potassium is an intracellular ion, total body potassium is difficult to estimate. Potassium chloride (KCl: 30 g = 510 mEq PO q12h) can be given empirically, but dose tailoring (based on frequent monitoring) is recommended.

RECOMMENDED MONITORING

- Serum pH, HCO_3^-, potassium, and creatinine concentrations.
- If bacteriuria is present, repeat urinalysis 1 week after completion of antibiotic therapy.

PROGNOSIS AND OUTCOME

- Bicarbonate therapy has been successful in more than 90% of cases and is generally required for days to months. Some animals require lifelong HCO_3^- supplementation.
- Relapses of RTA are common and are observed in approximately 30% of cases, with clinical signs returning from a few days to years after discontinuation of HCO_3^- therapy.
- Rarely, underlying problems are severe.

PEARLS & CONSIDERATIONS

COMMENTS

- Differentiation of type I from type II is difficult in horses, academic in nature, and not usually required for treatment.
- At the time of diagnosis, horses sometimes require aggressive fluid therapy and large dosages of HCO_3^- with supplemental potassium.
- Individually tailored maintenance therapy with HCO_3^- in accordance with repeated blood work (initially every few days, then every 2 weeks, and then monthly) results in rapid resolution of clinical signs.
- Maintenance therapy is relatively inexpensive, but repeated blood work is recommended as RTA usually spontaneously resolves.
- The combination of hypokalemia and acidosis is unusual. The classical situation in metabolic acidosis is the combination of hyperkalemia and acidosis caused by intracellular buffering of H^+ and the reciprocal role of K^+ and H^+ in the maintenance of extracellular fluid electroneutrality.

CLIENT EDUCATION

Return of clinical signs should prompt veterinary examination, blood work, and HCO_3^- therapy as required.

SUGGESTED READING

Arroyo LG, Stämpfli HR: Equine renal tubular acidosis. *Vet Clin North Am Equine Pract* 23:631, 2007.

Bayly WM: Acute renal failure. In Reed SM, Bayly WM, Sellon BC, et al, editors: *Equine internal medicine*, ed 3, St Louis, 2010, Saunders Elsevier, pp 1218–1221.

AUTHOR: **ALLISON J. STEWART**

EDITOR: **BRYAN M. WALDRIDGE**

Retained Fetal Membranes

BASIC INFORMATION

DEFINITION

Failure to expel all or part of the fetal membranes within 3 hours of delivery of a foal

SYNONYM(S)

Retained placenta, retained afterbirth

EPIDEMIOLOGY

SPECIES, AGE, SEX
- Intact female horses
- Breeding age
- Mares older than 15 years may have a higher incidence.

GENETICS AND BREED PREDISPOSITION
- The incidence is 2% to 10%. The incidence is reportedly lower in miniature mares (1.6%) and higher in Friesian mares (54%).
- A positive correlation between the incidence of retained fetal membranes (RFMs) and the inbreeding coefficient of the foal has been reported in Friesian mares.

RISK FACTORS
- Dystocia, fetotomy, cesarean section
- Abortion
- Consumption of endophyte-infected tall fescue (placental edema)
- Hydrops
- Placentitis
- Endometritis
- Overuse of large doses of oxytocin immediately postpartum
- Hypocalcemia (draft horses)
- Uterine tear
- Previous history of RFM
- Systemic infections or debilitating conditions

ASSOCIATED CONDITIONS AND DISORDERS
- Metabolic disorders
- Eclampsia

CLINICAL PRESENTATION

DISEASE FORMS/SUBTYPES Retention can be complete or partial if only a portion of the fetal membranes remain in the uterus.

HISTORY, CHIEF COMPLAINT
- History of parturition 3 hours before presentation.
- Presence of fetal membranes protruding from the vulva.
- Tear or missing portion of the chorioallantois.
- Mares with unnoticed partial retention may present with signs of toxic metritis.

PHYSICAL EXAM FINDINGS
- Presence of fetal membranes protruding from the vulva. The degree of protrusion can vary.
- RFMs may be present without being externally visible if they remain entirely within the uterine cavity or if only a portion of chorioallantois is retained.
- Straining and mild colic associated with uterine contractions are infrequently present.
- Metritis, endotoxemia, septicemia, or laminitis may occur as a complication of RFMs (see "Toxic Metritis" in this section).

ETIOLOGY AND PATHOPHYSIOLOGY
- Pathologic adhesions between the chorion and endometrium resulting from endometritis or placentitis
- Conditions associated with tissue inflammation or edema: Dystocia, fetotomy, cesarean section, fescue toxicosis
- Mechanical and hormonal imbalances: Low blood concentrations of total calcium, selenium, or oxytocin
- Debilitating conditions: Senility, fatigue, poor body condition or poor environment
- May need to include eversion of the tip of the uterine horn

DIAGNOSIS

INITIAL DATABASE
- Complete blood count and serum biochemistry profile: No specific changes unless metritis, septicemia, or endotoxemia develop as a complication (see "Toxic Metritis" in this section).
- Transrectal ultrasonography: Tags of hyperechoic fetal membranes within the uterine lumen
- Manual transcervical examination of the uterine lumen: Portions of the chorioallantois attached to the endometrium
- Examination of expelled fetal membranes: Presence of a tear or missing portion of the chorioallantois

ADVANCED OR CONFIRMATORY TESTING

Combined transabdominal ultrasonography and uterine flushing may show floating placental tags in a partially retained placenta.

TREATMENT

THERAPEUTIC GOAL(S)
- Induce nontraumatic expulsion of the fetal membranes.
- Prevent complications.

ACUTE GENERAL TREATMENT
- Oxytocin 20 IU IM or IV or 50 IU diluted in 500 mL of saline or calcium-magnesium-borogluconate solution administered over 1 hour. Repeat every 2 hours until the fetal membranes are expelled.
- Start treatment with systemic antibiotics if retained for more than 6 hours to prevent toxic metritis.
- Uterine lavage may help remove portions of RFMs and decrease bacterial load.
- If the chorioallantois is intact, redistension of the chorioallantoic cavity (Burn's technique) with fluids may be attempted.
- Administer tetanus prophylaxis.
- Spasmolytic if placenta is retained because of uterine spasm or partial eversion of the tip of the horn.
- Calcium borogluconate may be needed for some mares (draft horses).

CHRONIC TREATMENT

Daily or twice-daily uterine lavage if the placenta is not delivered in its entirety

POSSIBLE COMPLICATIONS
- Toxic metritis and laminitis
- Uterine prolapsed if aggressive manual removal is attempted

RECOMMENDED MONITORING
- Monitor once or twice daily for signs of metritis, septicemia, endotoxemia, or laminitis (see "Toxic Metritis" in this section).
- Perform a follow-up reproductive examination to determine the appropriate uterine involution and clearance of bacteria.

PROGNOSIS AND OUTCOME

If treated promptly and complications do not develop, prognosis for life is excellent, and reproductive parameters are not affected by RFMs.

PEARLS & CONSIDERATIONS

COMMENTS

- Life-threatening complications can arise secondary to RFMs in mares. This condition should always be regarded as an emergency, and treatment should be initiated if fetal membranes are not expelled by 3 hours of delivery of the foal.
- Routine examination of expelled fetal membranes in all foaling mares can help identify mares with partial retention and initiate treatment promptly.

PREVENTION

- Administer oxytocin within 2 hours postpartum to mares with predisposing factors
- Pastures with fescue
- Dietary supplementation with selenium

CLIENT EDUCATION

- Life-threatening complications may arise secondary to RFMs in mares. This condition should always be regarded as an emergency.
- Examine the fetal membranes immediately after expulsion to determine completeness.

- The veterinarian must be contacted if the mare fails to expel all or part of the fetal membranes by 3 hours after delivery of the foal.

SUGGESTED READING

Blanchard TL, MacPherson ML: Postparturient abnormalities. In Samper JC, Pycock JF, McKinnon AO, editors: *Current therapy in equine reproduction*, St Louis, 2007, Saunders Elsevier, pp 465–475.

Threlfall WR: Retained fetal membranes. In Youngquist RS, Threlfall WR, editors: *Current therapy in large animal theriogenology*, ed 2, St Louis, 2007, Saunders Elsevier, pp 23–36.

AUTHOR: **MARIA S. FERRER**

EDITOR: **JUAN C. SAMPER**

Rhabdomyolysis

BASIC INFORMATION

DEFINITION

Necrosis of skeletal muscle fibers. Rhabdomyolysis in horses occurs associated with exercise and in nonexercising horses on pasture.

SYNONYM(S)

- General synonyms: Degenerative myopathy, myonecrosis. Rhabdomyolysis is not inflammatory; therefore the term "myositis" does not apply.
- Exercise-associated rhabdomyolysis: Exertional rhabdomyolysis, tying up, Monday morning disease, myoglobinuria, azoturia, blackwater, setfast, chronic intermittent rhabdomyolysis, recurrent exertional rhabdomyolysis (RER).
- Nonexercising horses: Atypical myoglobinuria, pasture-associated rhabdomyolysis.

EPIDEMIOLOGY

SPECIES, AGE, SEX
- Horses, ponies, and mules
- Possible increased risk in females

GENETICS AND BREED PREDISPOSITION Dominant inheritance confirmed in Thoroughbreds with RER and in horses with polysaccharide storage myopathy

RISK FACTORS
- The primary risk factor is underlying inherited myopathy. Severe electrolyte disturbance (eg, hypokalemia), selenium deficiency, lack of exercise, anxiety, and high-starch and high-sugar diets increase likelihood of rhabdomyolysis in predisposed horses. Hypokalemia alone may cause rhab-

domyolysis, but this is poorly documented.
- Hypothyroidism, vitamin E deficiency, and lactic acidosis are not primary causes of rhabdomyolysis in horses. Severe selenium deficiency may result in severe acute rhabdomyolysis targeting masticatory muscles in adult horses (nutritional myopathy) but does not cause RER.

ASSOCIATED CONDITIONS AND DISORDERS Polysaccharide storage myopathy, RER

CLINICAL PRESENTATION

DISEASE FORMS/SUBTYPES
- Polysaccharide storage myopathy: Most common in Quarter Horse, Paint, Appaloosa, Arabian, Morgan, Warmblood, Saddlebred, Standardbred, and Draft-related horses and ponies but can occur in any breed (including Thoroughbreds)
- RER: Described in Thoroughbreds with evidence of a calcium handling defect; not confirmed in other breeds

HISTORY, CHIEF COMPLAINT Variable. Severe cases can exhibit reluctance to move, stretched-out stance, sweating, hard or swollen muscles, muscle pain on palpation, recumbency, and red-brown urine. Less severe cases may have performance, gait, stamina, or attitude problems under saddle or in harness.

PHYSICAL EXAM FINDINGS
- Muscles may be hard, swollen, or painful, especially the back and gluteal muscles. Back pain or stiff gait, particularly of pelvic limbs, may be evident.
- Severely affected horses may be recumbent.

- Physical findings may also be normal.

ETIOLOGY AND PATHOPHYSIOLOGY
- Polysaccharide storage myopathy: Linked to abnormal carbohydrate metabolism and an alteration in the skeletal muscle glycogen synthase 1 (*GYS1*) gene, but exact pathophysiology is not known.
- RER: Possible sarcoplasmic reticulum calcium handling defect, but exact pathophysiology is not known.
- Pasture-associated rhabdomyolysis: Possible as yet unidentified plant toxin, but rhabdomyolysis can also occur while on pasture in horses that are severely selenium deficient, in horses exposed to known myotoxins (eg, ionophores, *Cassia occidentalis*), and in horses with underlying myopathy (polysaccharide storage myopathy or RER).

DIAGNOSIS

DIFFERENTIAL DIAGNOSIS

Colic, laminitis. For recumbent horses, also consider botulism and central nervous system disease.

INITIAL DATABASE

- Serum creatine kinase (CK) and aspartate aminotransferase (AST): Ideally, blood should be drawn 4 to 6 hours after the onset of clinical signs. CK peaks at 4 to 6 hours after muscle injury, with a very short half-life (~6–9 hours). AST peaks much later, approximately 24 to 48 hours after injury, with a long half-life (~24–48 hours).

- CK and AST analysis in blood drawn 4 to 6 hours after exercise often reveals subclinical rhabdomyolysis in predisposed horses.
- Vitamin E and selenium analyses are useful to rule out antioxidant deficiency as a contributing factor.
- Environment: Rule out ionophore or toxic plant exposure.

ADVANCED OR CONFIRMATORY TESTING

- Semimembranosus, semitendinosus, or gluteal muscle biopsy evaluation for underlying myopathy (polysaccharide storage myopathy or RER)
- Genetic testing for *GYS1* mutation for polysaccharide storage myopathy: Minnesota Neuromuscular Disease Laboratory (http://www.cvm.umn. edu/umec/lab/home.html). Can be performed on whole blood or pulled mane or tail hairs. A positive test result is very specific, but a negative test result does not rule out polysaccharide storage myopathy.

TREATMENT

THERAPEUTIC GOAL(S)

- Relieve pain and anxiety
- Maintain hydration and electrolyte status
- Maintain renal function
- Limit muscle cell injury

ACUTE GENERAL TREATMENT

- Relieve pain: Nonsteroidal antiinflammatory drug such as phenylbutazone (2.2 mg/kg IV or PO q12h) or flunixin meglumine (0.25 mg/kg IV, IM, or PO q8–12h).
- Relieve anxiety: Acepromazine (0.02 mg/kg IV or IM q6h).
- Maintain hydration, electrolyte status, and renal function: IV fluids may be needed in severe cases. Preferred fluid is 0.9% NaCl with 20 to 40 mEq KCl/L.
- Limit muscle injury: Stall rest, but only until horse is moving comfortably again. Treatment with vitamin E and selenium may reduce secondary oxi-

dative injury. Prolonged stall rest is contraindicated for horses with polysaccharide storage myopathy or RER.
- For recumbent or severely weak horses: 2 cups of vegetable oil PO q24h or IV lipid emulsion, 0.2 g/kg).

CHRONIC TREATMENT

- Diet change: Reduce starch and sugar intake to minimal levels; gradually introduce and increase dietary fat. Best results are achieved in most cases with 0.45 kg of fat (2 cups of vegetable oil or equivalent in other fat sources) per 450 kg/d. Supplement with daily vitamin E (≥1000 IU per 450 kg) and, if needed, selenium (1 mg per 450 kg).
- Exercise: Provide as much time out of a stall and as much regular exercise as possible.
- Environment: Provide as stress free an environment as possible.
- Drug therapy: Some horses improve with 4 mg/kg of dantrolene PO, but best results are obtained when horses are fasted before treatment.

DRUG INTERACTIONS

Feed will interfere with dantrolene absorption.

POSSIBLE COMPLICATIONS

Renal failure caused by myoglobin-induced nephropathy; recumbency leading to respiratory failure with severe rhabdomyolysis; death caused by respiratory muscle necrosis.

RECOMMENDED MONITORING

- Repeat serum CK and AST 4 to 6 hours after exercise after at least 3 months of dietary and exercise therapy.
- Repeat muscle biopsy is not useful.

PROGNOSIS AND OUTCOME

Excellent for nonrecumbent horses. Guarded for recumbent horses and for horses that develop renal dysfunction.

PEARLS & CONSIDERATIONS

COMMENTS

- Any horse that develops rhabdomyolysis, even once, should be evaluated for underlying myopathy, especially polysaccharide storage myopathy.
- For horses on dietary therapy: Fat adaptation requires 3 to 4 months, and clinical signs of muscle dysfunction may still occur during this time.
- If rhabdomyolysis occurs in a horse that has been on dietary therapy for 4 months or more, carefully evaluate the diet to ensure that there is adequate fat intake and an adequate reduction in starch and sugar intake and husbandry to confirm sufficient provision of exercise.

PREVENTION

Diet (high fat and fiber and low starch and sugar) and exercise

CLIENT EDUCATION

- Horses with rhabdomyolysis most often have an underlying condition, and husbandry is the key to successful prevention.
- Careful consideration before breeding severely affected horses is warranted.

SUGGESTED READING

Beech J: Equine muscle disorders 1: chronic intermittent rhabdomyolysis. *Equine Vet Educ* 12:163–167, 2000.

McKenzie EC, Valberg SJ, Godden SM, et al: Effect of dietary starch, fat, and bicarbonate content on exercise responses and serum creatine kinase activity in equine recurrent exertional rhabdomyolysis. *J Vet Intern Med* 17:693–701, 2003.

Valentine BA, Hintz HF, Freels KM, et al: Dietary control of exertional rhabdomyolysis in horses. *J Am Vet Med Assoc* 212: 1588–1593, 1998.

AUTHOR: BETH A. VALENTINE

EDITOR: ANDRIS J. KANEPS

Rhinitis Virus

BASIC INFORMATION

DEFINITION

Common upper respiratory tract virus that is seldom diagnosed as a specific cause of respiratory disease in horses but may contribute to overall pathology

SYNONYMS

Equine rhinovirus

EPIDEMIOLOGY

SPECIES, AGE, SEX More common in younger horses

RISK FACTORS

- Four serotypes have been identified: Equine rhinitis A virus (ERAV), equine rhinitis B virus type 1 (ERBV1), equine rhinitis B virus type 2 (ERBV2), and equine rhinitis B virus type 3 (ERBV3)

- Seroprevalence of 73% in horses younger than 3 years and 90% in horses 4 years of age or older
- Horses are most commonly infected with rhinovirus after entering training and therefore are usually seronegative until about 1 to 2 years of age.
- ERAV is the most common isolate.

CONTAGION AND ZOONOSIS
- Spread by contact with nasal secretions and aerosol transmission, including aerosolization of urine.
- Human infection has been demonstrated experimentally; however, there have been no reports of naturally occurring clinical disease, so the risk is considered to be minimal.
- Clinical significance is debatable; equine rhinitis virus is rarely diagnosed as a specific cause of respiratory disease. This may be because of a lack of widely available diagnostic tests.

CLINICAL PRESENTATION

PHYSICAL EXAM FINDINGS
- Disease is often subclinical, and the severity of clinical signs is highly variable.
- Acute fever, nasal discharge, and coughing.
- Pharyngitis and laryngitis.
- Submandibular lymphadenitis.

ETIOLOGY AND PATHOPHYSIOLOGY
- ERAV is closely related to foot-and-mouth disease virus because they are the only two members of the genus *Aphthovirus*; ERAB viruses belong to the genus *Erbovirus*.

- Replicates in nasal epithelial cells; viremia occurs but is quickly controlled by antibody production.
- ERAV shed in urine for a prolonged period (at least 146 days).

DIAGNOSIS

DIFFERENTIAL DIAGNOSIS
- Equine influenza
- Equine herpesvirus type-1 and -4
- Equine viral arteritis
- *Streptococcus equi* subsp. *zooepidemicus*
- *Streptococcus equi* subsp. *equi*

INITIAL DATABASE
- Moderate hyperfibrinogenemia
- Moderate increase in neutrophil/lymphocyte ratio

ADVANCED OR CONFIRMATORY TESTING
- Serology: Demonstration of increasing serum neutralizing antibody titer with two samples collected 2 weeks apart
- Isolation in cell cultures often difficult
- Reverse transcriptase polymerase chain reaction for both ERAV and ERBV1 and ERBV2

TREATMENT

THERAPEUTIC GOALS
Supportive care and symptomatic treatment

ACUTE GENERAL TREATMENT
- No specific antiviral therapy
- Supportive and symptomatic therapy, including judicious use of nonsteroidal antiinflammatory drugs

PROGNOSIS AND OUTCOME

- Recovery usually occurs within 7 days.
- Prognosis is good, and no residual clinical effects are observed.
- Prolonged shedding in urine occurs with ERAV, generally without any clinical signs of disease.

PEARLS & CONSIDERATIONS

- No vaccine exists.
- Minimizing environmental stress and population density may help to decrease risk of developing disease.

SUGGESTED READING
Black WD, Wilcox RS, Stevenson RA: Prevalence of serum neutralizing antibody to equine rhinitis A virus (ERAV), equine rhinitis B virus 1 (ERBV1) and ERBV2. *Vet Microbiol* 119:65–71, 2007.
Studdert MJ: Miscellaneous viral respiratory diseases. In Sellon DC, Long MT, editors: *Equine infectious diseases*, St Louis, 2007, Elsevier, pp 177–180.

AUTHOR: **SIDDRA HINES**

EDITORS: **DEBRA C. SELLON** and **MAUREEN T. LONG**

Rhodococcus Enterocolitis

BASIC INFORMATION

DEFINITION
Diarrhea caused by gastrointestinal (GI) infection with *Rhodococcus equi*

EPIDEMIOLOGY
SPECIES, AGE, SEX Foals from 1 to 9 months of age

CLINICAL PRESENTATION

HISTORY, CHIEF COMPLAINT
- Depression, lethargy, inappetence, weight loss, and diarrhea of days' to weeks' duration are the most common complaints.
- Concurrent respiratory signs may be present but are not always observed.

- One or several foals on a farm may be affected with diarrhea or respiratory signs.

PHYSICAL EXAM FINDINGS
- Depression
- Pyrexia is common but not always observed
- Variable dehydration and evidence of endotoxemia and hypovolemia
- Hypermotile, "fluidy" GI borborygmi and diarrhea
- Evidence of involvement of the other organ systems may be noted
  ○ Tachypnea, increased respiratory effort, nasal discharge, cough, and adventitious lung sounds on thoracic auscultation with concurrent pneumonia
  ○ Lameness with concurrent septic physitis, arthritis, or osteomyelitis

  ○ Joint effusion in multiple joints with concurrent polysynovitis
  ○ Hypopyon, blepharospasm, miosis, and lacrimation with concurrent uveitis

ETIOLOGY AND PATHOPHYSIOLOGY
- *R. equi* is an intracellular gram-positive coccobacillus. The organism is ubiquitous in the soil. It primarily causes suppurative bronchopneumonia and pulmonary abscessation in foals but can also affect other body systems.
- Exposure to *R. equi* may occur through inhalation or ingestion of organisms from the soil or from the feces of adult horses or foals.
- Host-environment-pathogen interactions are key for the development of clinical *R. equi* infection in some foals and avoidance of clinical disease in

others because most foals are exposed to *R. equi*, but not all develop clinical disease.

- Intestinal lesions associated with *R. equi* are characterized by multifocal ulcerative enterocolitis with lesions predominantly located in the Peyer's patches.
- Concurrent granulomatous inflammation in mesenteric and colonic lymph nodes is common, and large mesenteric abscesses may develop.

DIAGNOSIS

DIFFERENTIAL DIAGNOSIS

- Salmonellosis
- Clostridial diarrhea
- Proliferative enteropathy (*Lawsonia intracellularis*)
- Rotavirus
- Gastroduodenal ulcer disease
- ± Cyathostominosis in older foals
- See "Salmonellosis," "Diarrhea of the Neonatal Foal," "Diarrhea, Clostridial," "Proliferative Enteropathy," "Gastric Ulceration in Foals," and "Cyathostominosis" in this section

INITIAL DATABASE

- Complete blood count
  - Leukocytosis is characterized by a mature neutrophilia and hyperfibrinogenemia.
  - The hematocrit varies with hydration status but can be misleadingly low because of concurrent anemia, which is often present.
- Serum biochemistry profile: Variable electrolyte derangements and hypoproteinemia may be seen but less frequently than with other causes of colitis.
- Transabdominal ultrasonography
  - Multifocal, often encapsulated, regions of colonic mural thickening (>4–5 mm) are frequently observed.
  - Multifocal hyperechoic or cavitary fluid-filled lesions consistent with mesenteric lymphadenopathy or abscessation may also be seen.
  - Fluid contents in the colon or cecum and increased hypoechoic free peritoneal fluid is often appreciated.
- Peritoneal fluid analysis
  - May be grossly and cytologically normal but most often exhibits a mildly to moderately increased nucleated cell count and total protein concentration.
  - May be submitted for polymerase chain reaction to detect *R. equi* DNA, although this is not sensitive for *R. equi* enterocolitis because bacterial organisms are typically confined within abscesses and the intestinal lumen.

ADVANCED OR CONFIRMATORY TESTING

- If *R. equi* enterocolitis is suspected, thoracic imaging and transtracheal wash should be performed to evaluate for concurrent pulmonary disease, which is present in the majority of cases. If *R. equi* pneumonia is identified, a presumptive diagnosis of concurrent *R. equi* enterocolitis can be made. However, absence of *R. equi* pneumonia does not rule out *R. equi* enterocolitis.
- Fecal culture demonstrating heavy growth of virulent (Vap-A positive) *R. equi* is supportive of *R. equi* enterocolitis in a foal with the above clinical signs, although some foals shed virulent *R. equi* in their feces in the absence of clinical disease.
- Serology for *R. equi*: Low sensitivity and specificity; not useful.

TREATMENT

THERAPEUTIC GOAL(S)

- Antimicrobial therapy
- Supportive care: Fluid support, antiinflammatory therapy, nutritional support

ACUTE GENERAL TREATMENT

- Antimicrobial therapy
  - Erythromycin (25–30 mg/kg PO q6–8h) *or* clarithromycin (7.5 mg/kg PO q12h) *or* azithromycin (10 mg/kg PO q24h for 5–10 days; then q48h) *with* rifampin (5–10 mg/kg PO q12h).
  - Doxycycline (10 mg/kg PO q12h) in combination with rifampin as above may also be effective for organisms resistant to macrolides.
  - Appropriate duration of therapy is key. Antimicrobials should be continued at least until resolution of clinical signs, clinicopathologic abnormalities, and radiographic or ultrasonographic abnormalities. This may be 6 to 12 weeks in severe cases.
- IV fluid therapy
  - Isotonic balanced polyionic crystalloid fluids (eg, Normosol-R or Plasmalyte) at 50 to 150 mL/kg/d, depending on the degree of dehydration and ongoing losses in diarrhea.
  - Supplementation with potassium chloride (10–40 mEq/L; rate not to exceed 0.5 mEq/kg/h), 23% calcium gluconate (1–2 mL/kg/d) or magnesium sulfate (20–25 g/450 kg body weight per day) is often necessary to correct electrolyte derangements.
  - Administration of sodium bicarbonate may be necessary with severe metabolic acidosis (pH <7.1; serum

bicarbonate concentration <15 mmol/L), but correction of dehydration often sufficiently corrects metabolic acidosis without the need for additional bicarbonate supplementation.
  - Colloidal support with equine plasma (20–40 mL/kg IV) or hydroxyethyl starch (5–10 mL/kg IV bolus q24–48h or 1 mL/kg/h IV continuous rate infusion) is indicated in hypoproteinemic patients.
- Antiinflammatory and analgesic therapy: Flunixin meglumine 0.5–1.1 mg/kg IV q12–24h for colic and fever or 0.25 mg/kg IV q8h for antiinflammatory effects. Nonsteroidal antiinflammatory drug use should be conservative and of short duration in foals to minimize GI and renal side effects.
- Gastroprotectants in foals that are persistently inappetent (see "Gastric Ulceration in Foals" in this section)
- Diet and nutritional support: Adequate nutritional support is vital. If the foal will not eat well, parenteral nutrition should be considered.

CHRONIC TREATMENT

Surgical excision, drainage, or marsupialization may be required in foals with large intraabdominal abscesses.

PROGNOSIS AND OUTCOME

As opposed to uncomplicated *R. equi* pneumonia, the prognosis for foals with isolated or concurrent *R. equi* enterocolitis is guarded. If intraabdominal abscessation or concurrent osteomyelitis is present, the prognosis is usually poor.

PEARLS & CONSIDERATIONS

It is important to note that *R. equi* enterocolitis may occur in the absence of respiratory disease and may only occur in one foal on a farm. Thus, it should not be overlooked as a differential diagnosis in a foal with diarrhea.

SUGGESTED READING

David JB: Diarrheal diseases. In Orsini JA, Divers TJ, editors: *Equine emergencies: treatment and procedures*, St Louis, 2008, Saunders Elsevier, pp 159–165.
Giguere S: *Rhodococcus equi* infections. In Smith BP, editor: *Large animal internal medicine*, ed 4, St Louis, 2009, Mosby Elsevier, pp 510–520.

AUTHOR: **KELSEY A. HART**

EDITORS: **TIM MAIR** and **CERI SHERLOCK**

Rhododendron Toxicosis

BASIC INFORMATION

DEFINITION

Members of the family Ericaceae, including *Rhododendron*, *Kalmia* (Laurel), *Pieris*, and *Leucothoe* (Fetter bush) are toxic to humans and livestock. The genus *Rhododendron* includes the deciduous azaleas. Horses are susceptible to poisoning, although it has been rarely reported.

SYNONYM(S)

Grayanotoxin or andromedotoxin poisoning

EPIDEMIOLOGY

RISK FACTORS Many of the Ericaceae retain their leaves in winter and so may be attractive to animals at any time.

GEOGRAPHY AND SEASONALITY Native to many parts of the temperate world where soils are acidic, rhododendrons, laurels, fetter bush, pieris, and other members of the family are small to large, branching shrubs with alternate, simple leaves and single or clusters of showy flowers (Figures 1 and 2). There are about 1000 species of *Rhododendron* with innumerable hybrids that are very popular showy ornamentals.

CLINICAL PRESENTATION

HISTORY, CHIEF COMPLAINT Anorexia, depression, and excessive salivation occur within a few hours of plant ingestion.

PHYSICAL EXAM FINDINGS
* Anorexia, excessive salivation, colic, and respiratory irregularity
* In more severe cases hypotension, cardiac irregularity, and bradycardia

ETIOLOGY AND PATHOPHYSIOLOGY
* Members of the Ericaceae contain numerous diterpenoids called grayanotoxins.
* Toxins are in all parts of the plants, including the nectar.
* Grayanotoxins attach to sodium channels, preventing their inactivation and prolonging depolarization and excitation of cells.
* The compromised sodium channels allow calcium influx into the cells that has a positive inotropic effect similar to digitalis at low doses.
* Vagal overstimulation causes hypotension and bradycardia.
* Impaired cardiac conductivity leads to dysrhythmias and heart block.

DIAGNOSIS

DIFFERENTIAL DIAGNOSIS
* Ionophore toxicity
* Oleander poisoning
* Yew poisoning

INITIAL DATABASE

Complete blood count and serum biochemistries: Generally normal initially

ADVANCED OR CONFIRMATORY TESTING
* Electrocardiography: Sinoatrial and atrioventricular block, bradycardia.
* Gross pathologic findings, such as pulmonary edema, are generally nonspecific.
* *Rhododendron* leaves are often present in the stomach.
* Stomach contents should be submitted for grayanotoxin analysis.

TREATMENT

THERAPEUTIC GOAL(S)
* There is no specific antidote.
* Provide supportive therapy when appropriate.

ACUTE GENERAL TREATMENT
* Activated charcoal via nasogastric tube if the plants have been eaten within the past 2 to 4 hours
* Analgesics for colic pain
* Atropine may be helpful in countering vagal effects.
* Sodium channel blockers may be helpful.

PROGNOSIS AND OUTCOME
* Acute signs last up to 24 hours, with some weakness and neurologic signs lasting 2 to 3 days.
* Horses are unlikely to consume a lethal dose, but the outcome depends on quantity of plant consumed, the time of year (more toxic in winter months), and the toxicity of the particular species involved.

PEARLS & CONSIDERATIONS

PREVENTION

Do not plant rhododendrons or other Ericaceae in or around horse pastures.

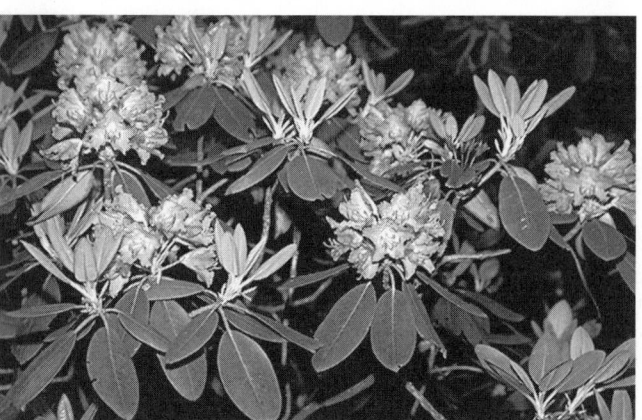

FIGURE 1 *Rhododendron.*

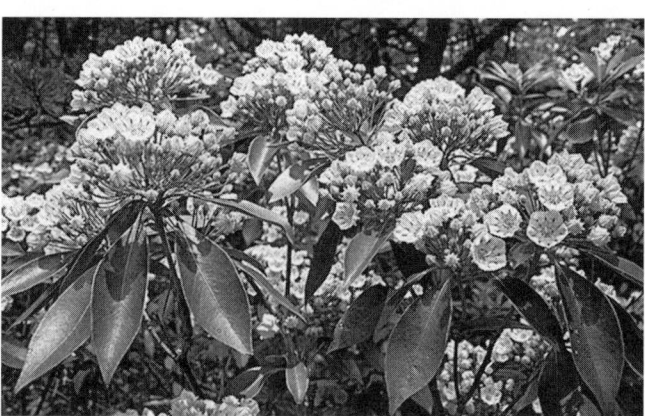

FIGURE 2 Laurel (*Kalmia* spp.).

CLIENT EDUCATION

Recognition and removal of rhododendrons and other Ericaceae will help prevent poisoning.

SUGGESTED READING

Burrows GE, Tyrl RJ: Ericaceae. In Burrows GE, Tyrl RJ, editors: *Toxic plants of North America*, Ames, IA, 2001, Iowa State University, pp 439–457.

AUTHOR: **ANTHONY P. KNIGHT**

EDITOR: **CYNTHIA L. GASKILL**

Rodenticide Toxicosis, Anticoagulant

BASIC INFORMATION

DEFINITION

Anticoagulant rodenticides are compounds that contain a coumarin or indandione group and act by inhibiting vitamin K recycling, thereby causing coagulopathy. Warfarin, a once common prototypical rodenticide, has a short half-life in the body. Newer anticoagulant rodenticides are more common and have prolonged half-lives.

SYNONYM(S)

Warfarin, brodifacoum, bromadiolone, difenacoum, chlorophacinone, diphacinone, pindone, or difethialone toxicosis

EPIDEMIOLOGY

SPECIES, AGE, SEX

- Anticoagulant rodenticide poisoning is not common in horses.
- Younger, more curious animals may be more likely to ingest rodenticides.
- Smaller individuals may be more likely to ingest a high enough dose to produce clinical signs.

RISK FACTORS

- Improper use of anticoagulant rodenticides around horses
- Storage of anticoagulant rodenticides in places horses can access

CLINICAL PRESENTATION

DISEASE FORMS/SUBTYPES

- Anticoagulant rodenticides cause coagulopathy.
- Presentation varies based on site of hemorrhage.

HISTORY, CHIEF COMPLAINT Signs vary depending on the site of hemorrhage but may include:

- Anemia
- Depression
- Anorexia
- Superficial swellings (hematomata)
- Evidence of excessive external bleeding
- Abdominal distension
- Dyspnea
- Central nervous system signs
- Lameness

PHYSICAL EXAM FINDINGS

- Pale mucous membranes
- Increased hemorrhage during phlebotomy or nasogastric tube placement
- Superficial hematomata
- Hemorrhage either externally or internally

ETIOLOGY AND PATHOPHYSIOLOGY

- Anticoagulant compounds inhibit vitamin K_1 epoxide reductase enzyme.
- Prevent recycling of vitamin K_1, needed for manufacture of clotting factors II, VII, IX, and X
- Cause depletion of clotting factors and coagulopathy
- Toxic dose varies for different anticoagulant rodenticides and has not been determined for all compounds.
  - 0.125 mg of brodifacoum/kg body weight was associated with severe toxicosis in some horses but minimal clinical signs in others.
  - 50 to 100 mg is the estimated lethal dose of brodifacoum for a mature horse.
  - 1 to 2 kg of brodifacoum bait (0.005% brodifacoum) would be expected to cause toxicosis in a mature horse.

DIAGNOSIS

DIFFERENTIAL DIAGNOSIS

Anticoagulant rodenticide poisoning may mimic a variety of diseases depending on the site of hemorrhage. Other causes of coagulopathy include:

- Disseminated intravascular coagulation
- Congenital coagulopathies
- Thrombocytopenia or thrombocytopathy
- Moldy sweet clover poisoning (caused by dicoumarol)

INITIAL DATABASE

- Clotting tests: Prolonged clotting times (prothrombin time [PT], partial thromboplastin time [PTT], activated coagulation time). PTT increases before PT in horses.
- Packed cell volume: May be decreased.
- Complete blood count: May show decreased red blood cells and platelets.

- Fecal occult blood test may show the presence of blood.
- Urinalysis may show the presence of blood.
- Needle aspirate of fluid in body cavities or swellings can determine if hemorrhage is present.

ADVANCED OR CONFIRMATORY TESTING

Laboratory analysis of serum, plasma or blood (antemortem), or tissue (liver) postmortem for the presence of anticoagulant compounds

TREATMENT

THERAPEUTIC GOAL(S)

Replace coagulation factors, stop hemorrhage, and replenish vitamin K_1

ACUTE GENERAL TREATMENT

- Stabilization and supportive care for clinically affected horses
  - Administer plasma or whole blood to replace clotting factors in an actively bleeding patient.
  - Whole blood is preferable for severely anemic patients.
- Early decontamination for recently exposed but asymptomatic horses
  - Within hours of ingestion
  - Not useful if clinical signs are apparent
  - Activated charcoal and sorbitol or other cathartic by nasogastric tube
  - Alternately, mineral oil via nasogastric tube

CHRONIC TREATMENT

- Vitamin K therapy
  - 0.5 to 2.5 mg/kg vitamin K_1 (phytonadione) SC or PO
  - Vitamin K_1 is fat soluble and is well absorbed by the gastrointestinal tract. Mixing with a digestible fatty substance (eg, vegetable oil) increases absorption.
  - Do not give orally if mineral oil has been administered.
  - Oral vitamin K_1 products can be obtained from veterinary compounding companies.
  - Treatment for warfarin should continue for at least 1 week.

○ Treatment for brodifacoum and other anticoagulant compounds with long half-lives should continue for 3 to 5 weeks.

• Keep horses confined; avoid exercise or stress to prevent injury and hemorrhage.

• Alfalfa hay increases dietary vitamin K for exposed horses.

DRUG INTERACTIONS

Various drugs such as nonsteroidal antiinflammatory drugs increase the bioavailability and clinical effects of anticoagulants.

POSSIBLE COMPLICATIONS

• Hemorrhage at injection sites.
• Vitamin K_1 may cause an anaphylactoid reaction if given IV.
• Vitamin K_3 (menadione) is known to cause renal failure in horses and is contraindicated.

RECOMMENDED MONITORING

• Check clotting times at 2 and 5 days after cessation of vitamin K_1 therapy.
• If clotting times increase, reinitiate vitamin K_1 therapy.

PROGNOSIS AND OUTCOME

• The prognosis is excellent if treatment is initiated before coagulopathy.
• Prognosis is guarded for animals that present with marked hemorrhage and anemia.
• Hemorrhage into the thorax or cranium can be rapidly lethal.

PEARLS & CONSIDERATIONS

COMMENTS

• Clinical signs of anticoagulant rodenticide toxicosis do not occur until 2 to 5 days after ingestion.
• Most anticoagulant rodenticide baits contain 0.005% to 0.05% of the active ingredient.
• Activated coagulation time is a rapid test that can be done in the field.
• Information on use of the PIVKA (proteins induced by vitamin K antagonist) test (Thrombotest) in horses is lacking.

PREVENTION

Keep all anticoagulant rodenticide products out of reach of horses.

CLIENT EDUCATION

• Appropriate use of small amounts of bait around horses is unlikely to cause poisoning in horses. Most poisonings occur when animals have access to large quantities of stored bait.
• Small animals (cats and dogs) are more likely to be affected by anticoagulant rodenticide poisoning.
• Owners should be aware that rodenticide baits sometimes contain ingredients and flavorings that are attractive to horses.

SUGGESTED READING

Ayala IM, Rodríguez MJ, Martos N, et al: Fatal brodifacoum poisoning in a pony. *Can Vet J* 48:627–629, 2007.

Boermans HJ, Johnstone I, Black WD, Murphy M: Clinical signs, laboratory changes and toxicokinetics of brodifacoum in the horse. *Can J Vet Res* 55:21–27, 1991.

McConnico RS, Copedge K, Bischoff KL: Brodifacoum toxicosis in two horses. *J Am Vet Med Assoc* 211:882–886, 1997.

Murphy MJ: Anticoagulant rodenticides. In Gupta RC, editor: *Veterinary toxicology: basic and clinical principles*, New York, 2007, Academic Press, pp 525–547.

AUTHOR: KARYN BISCHOFF

EDITOR: CYNTHIA L. GASKILL

Rotavirus

BASIC INFORMATION

DEFINITION

Acute viral diarrheal disease of foals

EPIDEMIOLOGY

SPECIES, AGE, SEX Occurs only in foals; most common at 3 to 4 months of age but can range from 2 days to 5 months

RISK FACTORS Foals from large breeding farms (increased foal population) seem to be at higher risk than other foals.

CONTAGION AND ZOONOSIS

• The virus particles passed in the feces of an affected foal are highly contagious.
• Particles can survive in the environment for up to 9 months.
• Most mares of affected foals are seropositive, but no fecal shedding of the virus occurs.
• Rotavirus is not a zoonotic disease.

GEOGRAPHY AND SEASONALITY

• Worldwide distribution, especially in countries with concentrated horse-breeding regions

• Seasonality related to foaling season only

ASSOCIATED CONDITIONS AND DISORDERS Electrolyte imbalances, acid-base abnormalities, and dehydration related to diarrhea

CLINICAL PRESENTATION

DISEASE FORMS/SUBTYPES Only one form exists, but the severity depends on the age and immune status of the foal, the magnitude of the viral exposure, and the virulence of the virus.

HISTORY, CHIEF COMPLAINT Lethargy, decreased suckling, diarrhea

PHYSICAL EXAM FINDINGS

• Varying fluidity of feces from "cow pie" to watery
• Can observe signs of weakness and prolonged recumbency
• Varying degrees of dehydration, electrolyte imbalances, and acid-base abnormalities
• Some foals exhibit signs of mild colic.

ETIOLOGY AND PATHOPHYSIOLOGY

• Rotaviruses are stable at any pH from 3 to 7, and they are resistant to many

widely used disinfectants, including bleach, iodophors, and quaternary ammonium compounds.

• Foals exposed to manure of infected foals acquire infection via fecal-oral transmission.
• When the virus enters the gastrointestinal tract, it multiplies in the cells of the villous tips of the small intestine.
• Villous atrophy and maldigestion or malabsorption result in diarrhea.
• The intestinal crypt cells are not affected, so they continue to multiply, which generally makes the disease self-limiting.

DIAGNOSIS

DIFFERENTIAL DIAGNOSIS

• May occur with other pathogens, although uncommon.
• Must consider enterocolitis caused by infection with *Clostridium* spp., *Salmonella* spp., *Coronavirus* spp., *Strongyloides westeri*, or *Cryptosporidium* spp. or nutritional causes such as

the use of milk replacer, ingestion of sand, or (rarely) lactose intolerance.
- Sepsis and asphyxial injury may also manifest as diarrhea.

INITIAL DATABASE
- May be unremarkable with mild cases.
- With moderate to severe diarrhea, foals are often hyponatremic, hypochloremic, hypokalemic, and acidotic.
- May observe polycythemia with dehydration, but otherwise the hemogram is unremarkable.

ADVANCED OR CONFIRMATORY TESTING
- Although electron microscopy is considered the gold standard, this method is expensive and time consuming.
- Diagnosis is commonly performed via fecal latex agglutination test (Virogen Rotatest; Wampole Laboratories, Princeton, NJ), which is considered to be both sensitive and specific.
- Numerous other molecular techniques exist for isolation of rotavirus.

TREATMENT

THERAPEUTIC GOAL(S)
- Supportive care is the cornerstone of therapy.

- Hygiene is important to minimize spread of the disease.

ACUTE GENERAL TREATMENT
- Supportive care with maintenance of fluid and electrolyte balances.
- With severe cases, especially those at risk for development of septicemia, broad-spectrum antibiotics can be used.
- Prophylactic antiulcer medications are recommended.
- Effort should be made to practice good hygiene to keep infected foals clean to prevent complications associated with perianal skin scalding and infection.

POSSIBLE COMPLICATIONS
- Perianal and hindlimb skin infections and scald may occur with inadequate hygiene. Prolonged recumbency may predispose foals to development of pneumonia and skin lesions.
- With the highly infective nature of the disease, outbreaks are possible.

RECOMMENDED MONITORING
- Monitoring for signs of colic, changes in fecal consistency, prolonged recumbency, or decreased suckling is recommended.
- Serial blood work can be helpful in monitoring changes in hydration, electrolytes, or acid-base status.

PROGNOSIS AND OUTCOME

Mortality rates are low even though morbidity is high. Foals younger than 14 days are at the highest risk of death.

PEARLS & CONSIDERATIONS

- An inactivated equine rotavirus vaccine (Fort Dodge Animal Health, Fort Dodge, IA) is recommended to reduce the incidence and severity of disease in high-risk foals at breeding operations. The vaccine is administered intramuscularly to mares at the eighth, ninth, and tenth months of gestation to increase the amount of antibodies in the colostrum.
- Good hygiene and husbandry practices are essential for prevention of the disease.

SUGGESTED READING
Dwyer RM: Equine rotavirus. In Sellon DC, Long MT, editors: *Equine infectious diseases*, St Louis, 2007, Saunders Elsevier, pp 181–183.

AUTHOR: **L. NICKI WISE**

EDITORS: **MAUREEN LONG** and **DEBRA C. SELLON**

Sacroiliac Joint Disorders

BASIC INFORMATION

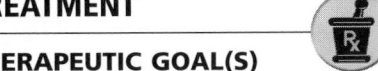

DEFINITION
Sacroiliac joint disorders include osseous, articular, and ligamentous injuries of the sacroiliac joint and immediate surrounding structures.

SYNONYM(S)
- Sacroiliac joint pain
- Sacroiliac osteoarthritis
- Sacroiliac desmitis
- Pelvic asymmetry
- Sacroiliac subluxation

EPIDEMIOLOGY
SPECIES, AGE, SEX
- Sacroiliac joint pain tends to occur more in older, taller, and heavier horses.
- Degenerative changes occur with increasing age.

GENETICS AND BREED PREDISPOSITION Warmbloods are more commonly affected.
RISK FACTORS
- Trauma
- Overuse injuries
- Back pain or thoracolumbar dysfunction
- Pelvic limb lameness
- Improper training or exercise programs
- Increased risk in horses used for dressage and show jumping
ASSOCIATED CONDITIONS AND DISORDERS
- Poor performance
- Lack of pelvic limb impulsion
- Pelvic limb lameness

CLINICAL PRESENTATION
DISEASE FORMS/SUBTYPES Two types of primary sacroiliac joint pathology

- Sacroiliac osteoarthritis
- Sacroiliac desmitis
HISTORY, CHIEF COMPLAINT
- Behavioral changes during ridden exercise
- Muscular or bony pelvic asymmetry
- History of falling backwards and landing on the croup region
- History of insidious onset and progression of clinical signs
- Lack of pelvic limb impulsion or loss of movement
- Intermittent pelvic limb lameness
- Not able to stand for the farrier
- Difficulty in working on the bit
- Difficulty in lateral movements such as shoulder-in and half-pass
- Reduced performance or unwillingness to work
- Unwilling to work under saddle
- Refusing jumps
PHYSICAL EXAM FINDINGS
- Asymmetry in the croup musculature or bony pelvis

- Asymmetric left-right tuber coxae position
- Asymmetric tuber sacrale position relative to the second sacral dorsal spinous process
- Variable pain over the tuber sacrale or surrounding region
- Pain on compression of the tuber sacrale
- Lumbar longissimus, middle gluteal, and proximal biceps femoris muscle atrophy, pain, or hypertonicity
- Lateral motion asymmetry of the sacral apex during joint mobilization
- Restricted or painful response to ventral displacement of the tuber coxae
- Pain, crepitus, or instability produced during repeated lateral translation of the pelvis or ventral displacement of the tuber coxae
- Concurrent thoracolumbar pain or stiffness
- Inconsistent or a shifting weight-bearing posture on the pelvic limbs
- Inability to stand squarely on both pelvic limbs
- Reluctance to stand on one pelvic limb when the other pelvic limb is elevated or flexed
- Reduced pelvic limb impulsion when trotted in hand
- Stiffness or inability to turn in a tight circle
- Stiffness and reduced pelvic limb impulsion
- Clinical signs worse when ridden or progress with continued exercise

ETIOLOGY AND PATHOPHYSIOLOGY Numerous tissues may be the source of sacroiliac pain or dysfunction
- Soft tissue
  - Trauma: Middle gluteal or biceps femoris myositis
  - Inflammation: Dorsal sacroiliac ligament desmitis
  - Infection: Abscessation
  - Metabolic: Polysaccharide storage myopathy, hyperkalemic periodic paralysis
  - Vascular: Aortoiliac thrombosis
- Orthopedic
  - Congenital: Lumbosacral malformation or transitional vertebrae
  - Trauma: Ilial wing or sacral fractures
  - Degeneration: Sacroiliac osteoarthritis
  - Infection: Pelvic or sacral osteomyelitis
- Neurologic
  - Trauma: Sacral nerve root compression
  - Inflammation: Cauda equina neuritis
  - Infectious: Equine protozoal myeloencephalitis
  - Nutritional: Vitamin E deficiency

- Neoplasia (space occupying mass): Malignant melanoma
- Iatrogenic: Alcohol tail block

DIAGNOSIS

DIFFERENTIAL DIAGNOSIS
Sacroiliac pain or dysfunction is a nonspecific clinical sign. Definitive diagnosis is often based on exclusion of other soft tissue, orthopedic, and neurologic disorders of the croup and upper pelvic limb.
- Pelvic soft tissues
  - Middle gluteal or biceps femoris muscle strain or atrophy
  - Exercise-related myopathies
  - Dorsal sacroiliac ligament desmitis
  - Sacroiliac joint subluxation or luxation
  - Trochanteric bursitis
  - Aortoiliac thrombosis
- Bony pelvis and sacrum
  - Left-right bony asymmetry of tuber sacrale and tuber coxae
  - Hunters' or jumpers' bump
  - Sacroiliac joint enthesophytes
  - Sacroiliac osteoarthritis
  - Sacroiliac joint ankylosis
  - Pelvic stress fractures
  - Pelvic fractures
  - Sacral or caudal vertebrae fractures
  - Lumbosacral osteoarthritis
  - Transitional lumbosacral vertebrae
  - Coxofemoral osteoarthritis
  - Coxofemoral dislocation
- Cauda equina and sacral nerve roots
  - Sacral spinal nerve root compression
  - Cauda equina neuritis
  - Equine motor neuron disease
  - Malignant melanoma
  - *Sorghum* spp. toxicosis (Sudan grass)
- Other regional disorders
  - Pelvic limb lameness
  - Bilateral proximal suspensory desmitis
  - Bilateral tarsal osteoarthritis
  - Impingement of lumbar dorsal spinous processes

INITIAL DATABASE
- Inspection of muscular or bony asymmetry of the croup region
- Lack of pelvic muscle development or altered muscle tone
- Inspection of abnormal tail carriage and motion
- Assessment of tail tone and perineal reflex to assess neurologic status
- Gait evaluation
- Neurologic examination
- Lameness examination and response to pelvic limb flexion tests
- Diagnostic anesthesia of the entire pelvic limb to rule out sources of pelvic limb lameness

- Firm palpation of the pelvic bony prominences for pain response
- Rocking pelvis side to side to assess bony instability or crepitus
- Detailed soft tissue palpation of the pelvic region to localize pain
- Active and passive lumbosacral, sacroiliac, and coxofemoral joint range of motion to assess flexibility
- Response to axial traction applied to the tail to assess neuromuscular coupling
- Rectal palpation to assess pelvic integrity, sacral fractures, and branches of the terminal aorta
- Evaluation of ridden exercise or athletic activity to assess if exercise exacerbates clinical signs
- Protraction, retraction, adduction, and abduction of the pelvic limbs to assess flexibility

ADVANCED OR CONFIRMATORY TESTING
- Serum creatine kinase and aspartate aminotransferase levels before and after 4-hour exercise
- Percutaneous ultrasonography of the dorsal sacroiliac ligaments, tubera sacralia, and dorsal surface of the iliac wings
- Diagnostic periarticular sacroiliac joint injection
- Nuclear scintigraphy of the pelvic region
- Transrectal ultrasonography of the ventral sacroiliac joint margins and terminal aorta
- Pelvic radiographs under general anesthesia to identify pelvic fractures
- Lateral sacral radiography in the standing horse to identify sacrocaudal fractures
- Pressure algometry to assess mechanical nociceptive thresholds of local bony and soft tissue landmarks
- Muscle biopsy of the sacrocaudalis dorsalis lateralis muscle to confirm equine motor neuron disease

TREATMENT

THERAPEUTIC GOAL(S)
- Eliminate or reduce the source of pain and inflammation so that affected horses can resume regular training programs
- Treat concurrent pelvic limb lameness
- Promote sacroiliac joint motion
- Strengthen the epaxial, gluteal, and proximal thigh musculature
- Improve neuromuscular coupling at the lumbosacral junction
- Prevent progression of sacroiliac osteoarthritis or desmitis
- Develop effective therapeutic exercises and training programs to promote flexibility, motor control, and strength

- Restore athletic and performance capabilities

ACUTE GENERAL TREATMENT

- Temporary reduction in the intensity, duration, or frequency of exercise or the training program
- Do not stop exercise; continue exercise to help maintain muscular fitness
- Controlled handwalking to reduce pain and maintain sacroiliac joint motion
- Passive mobilization of the sacroiliac joint to reduce pain and maintain joint motion
- Cryotherapy to reduce local heat, swelling, or pain
- Antiinflammatory drugs: Nonsteroidal antiinflammatory drugs (NSAIDs), corticosteroids, dimethyl sulfoxide
- Periarticular corticosteroid injections for sacroiliac osteoarthritis
- Periligamentous corticosteroid injections for sacroiliac desmitis
- Electroacupuncture to reduce pain and muscle hypertonicity
- Electric muscle stimulation to reduce pain and stimulate motor control
- Slow and prolonged warm-up periods

CHRONIC TREATMENT

- Turnout as much as possible to stimulate joint motion
- Exercise modification to limit strenuous exercise
- Active and passive stretching exercises to restore pelvic and sacroiliac joint mobility
- Stimulate somatic reflexes to induce active elevation of the back and lumbosacral flexion
- Therapeutic exercises to increase proprioceptive stimulation and core stabilization of the lumbosacral region
- Exercises to stimulate collection or a bascule posture: Stimulate somatic reflex to elevate the back, work on a lunge line, or ridden exercise
- Collection exercises: Stimulate tail reflex to elevate back, work on lunge line, or ridden
- Lunging or ridden exercise on inclines or hills to strengthen the pelvic musculature and stimulate motor control
- Local moist heat therapy to reduce pain and muscle hypertonicity
- Acupuncture to reduce pain and muscle hypertonicity

- Joint mobilization or manipulation (chiropractic treatment) to restore lumbosacral and sacroiliac joint motion
- Physical therapy and rehabilitation to stimulate motor control
- Extracorporeal shock-wave therapy to reduce pain
- Dietary modifications of increasing fat and reducing carbohydrate intake to help manage polysaccharide storage myopathies
- Pelvic limb protraction and retraction, mobilization, and active stretching to increase pelvic limb flexibility
- Prolotherapy with sclerosis agents to fibrose and strengthen sacroiliac ligaments and joint capsule

DRUG INTERACTIONS

- Complications associated with long-term phenylbutazone use in horses include gastritis and right dorsal colitis.
- NSAIDs should not be used in conjunction with corticosteroids.

POSSIBLE COMPLICATIONS

- Progressive sacroiliac osteoarthritis or desmitis
- Chronic poor performance or pelvic limb lameness

RECOMMENDED MONITORING

- Monitor signs of pain, muscle hypertonicity, and stiffness
- Periodic clinical examination to assess performance and compensatory lameness
- Pelvic limb lameness examinations

PROGNOSIS AND OUTCOME

- Increased risk for persistent poor performance and upper pelvic limb lameness in horses with sacroiliac osteoarthritis
- Long-term follow-up suggests that the prognosis for horses with sacroiliac joint injury is poor for return to the previous level of activity.
- Some horses may have an improvement in performance or lameness but will not be able to return to normal athletic activities because of recurring low-grade lameness.

PEARLS & CONSIDERATIONS

COMMENTS

- Definitive diagnosis is crucial to long-term management of horses with sacroiliac joint disorders.
- Many horses respond temporarily to regional corticosteroid injections; however, problems related to poor performance often recur unless the primary injury is identified and treated.
- Active and passive lumbosacral and sacroiliac range of motion is useful for assessing the presence and quality of neuromuscular coupling and motor control.

PREVENTION

- Limit trauma and overuse injuries to the pelvic limbs
- Provide daily low levels of exercise and turnout as much as possible

CLIENT EDUCATION

- Sacroiliac joint pain is often a long-term management issue.
- If an appropriate therapeutic response is not noted with conservative care, then additional diagnostics are warranted.

SUGGESTED READING

Dyson SJ: Pelvic injuries in the non-racehorse. In Ross MW, Dyson SJ, editors: *Diagnosis and management of lameness in the horse*, St Louis, 2003, Saunders Elsevier, pp 491–500.

Dyson S, Murray R: Pain associated with the sacroiliac joint region: A clinical study of 74 horses. *Equine Vet J* 35:240–245, 2003.

Engeli E, Haussler KK, Erb HN: Development and validation of a periarticular injection technique of the sacroiliac joint in horses. *Equine Vet J* 36:324–330, 2004.

Engeli E, Yeager AE, Erb HN, et al: Ultrasonographic technique and normal anatomy of the sacroiliac region in horses. *Vet Radiol Ultrasound* 47:391–403, 2006.

Goff L, Jeffcott LB, Jasiewicz J, et al: Structural and biomechanical aspects of equine sacroiliac joint function and their relationship to clinical disease. *Vet J* 176:281–293, 2008.

Haussler KK: Diagnosis and management of sacroiliac joint injuries. In Ross MW, Dyson S, editors: *Diagnosis and management of lameness in the horse*, Philadelphia, 2003, Saunders Elsevier, pp 501–508.

AUTHOR: **KEVIN K. HAUSSLER**

EDITOR: **ANDRIS J. KANEPS**

Sagebrush Toxicosis

BASIC INFORMATION

DEFINITION

Sagebrush poisoning, or *sage sickness*, refers to the neurologic disorder in horses caused by intoxication by *Artemisia* spp.

SYNONYM(S)

Sagebrush, sage, sagewort, wormwood, sand sage, budsage, and big sagebrush

RISK FACTORS

Overgrazed rangeland and snow cover of other forages predispose horses to eating large quantities of sagebrush. Horses unaccustomed to browsing on sage are most likely to be affected.

GEOGRAPHY AND SEASONALITY

There are some 68 native species of *Artemisia* prevalent in the drier western regions of North America. Some are annuals, and many are woody perennial plants that become dominant species in western rangelands. Considerable variation occurs among the species, with some being low growing while others are woody shrubs 4 to 6 feet in height. Leaves are alternate, simple, with varying shape, hairy, and often with a distinctive sage smell. Numerous flower spikes are produced with small, inconspicuous individual flowers.

CLINICAL PRESENTATION

HISTORY, CHIEF COMPLAINT Horses on overgrazed pastures where sagebrush predominates and is the sole food source for several days can develop neurologic signs. Signs include unpredictable behavior, nervousness, incoordination, walking in circles, and depression.
PHYSICAL EXAM FINDINGS Anorexia, depression, abnormal behavior similar to that encountered in locoweed poisoning, incoordination, and circling are suggestive of sagebrush toxicity. Characteristically, affected horses will have "sage halitosis," and even the feces may smell of sage.

ETIOLOGY AND PATHOPHYSIOLOGY

- *Artemisia* spp. contain a variety of sesquiterpene lactones and aromatic monoterpenes such as thujone and camphor that are irritants to the gastrointestinal tract and have neurotoxic properties.
- Horses need to eat large quantities of sagebrush for several days to become intoxicated.

DIAGNOSIS

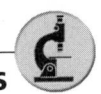

DIFFERENTIAL DIAGNOSIS

- Locoweed poisoning
- Encephalitis: Rabies, West Nile virus, Eastern and Western equine encephalitis virus
- Equine herpes virus
- Pyrrolizidine alkaloid toxicity
- Bracken fern poisoning
- Narrow-leaved milkweed poisoning

INITIAL DATABASE

Hematology and serum biochemical profile: Normal

ADVANCED OR CONFIRMATORY TESTING

Horses with severe chronic sagebrush poisoning may show histologic evidence of nonspecific oxidative injury to the neurons.

TREATMENT

THERAPEUTIC GOAL(S)

There is no specific treatment.

ACUTE GENERAL TREATMENT

- Remove "saged" horses from the source of the sagebrush
- Provide a normal balanced ration
- Provide supportive therapy as needed

PROGNOSIS AND OUTCOME

Horses generally recover from sagebrush poisoning after a few weeks on a well-balanced diet.

PEARLS & CONSIDERATIONS

COMMENTS

Poisoning generally results when naive horses are placed in a situation where they have little to eat but sagebrush. Horses will adapt to browsing on sagebrush over time and are not likely to develop toxicity unless sagebrush is the exclusive forage available.

PREVENTION

Provision of good hay at times when pasture or range forages are low or when snow covers the grass, leaving only sagebrush for the horses to browse on, reduces the likelihood of sage poisoning. Overgrazing can result in some sages such as fringed sage or sagewort (*Artemisia frigida*) becoming invasive weeds to the point of becoming a monoculture.

CLIENT EDUCATION

Recognition of *Artemisia* spp. and management of pasture and range conditions to avoid overgrazing help prevent sagebrush poisoning.

SUGGESTED READING

Burrows GE, Tyrl RJ: Artemisia. In Burrows GE, Tyrl RJ, editors: *Toxic plants of North America*, Ames, IA, 2001, Iowa State University, pp 1150–1153.

Cedarleaf, JD, Welch BL, Brotherson JD: Seasonal variation in monoterpenoids in big sagebrush (*Artemisia tridentata*). *J Range Manage* 36:492–494, 1983.

AUTHOR: **ANTHONY P. KNIGHT**

EDITOR: **CYNTHIA L. GASKILL**

Salmonellosis

BASIC INFORMATION

DEFINITION
Colitis or diarrhea caused by *Salmonella* spp. infection

EPIDEMIOLOGY
RISK FACTORS
- Increased horse density, such as equine referral hospitals or large breeding farms
- Treatment with antimicrobials
- Colic, other illness, or recent surgery
- Transportation
- Hot weather

CONTAGION AND ZOONOSIS
- There are a large number of *Salmonella* serovars and serotypes, many of which have been associated with equine disease. The most commonly isolated include *Salmonella typhimurium, Salmonella newport, Salmonella anatum,* and *Salmonella agona.*
- Horses are not typically *Salmonella* carriers because there are no equine-specific host adapted strains (other than *Salmonella abortus equi,* which has been eradicated from the United States and does not typically cause diarrhea).
- However, infected horses shed large numbers of organisms in their feces and can do so for weeks to months without developing clinical disease.
- Salmonellosis may occur in individual horses without any known risk factors or may occur in outbreaks at equine hospitals or large farms.
- Horses can be infected with *Salmonella* serovars that may also affect humans, although direct transmission from a horse to human is rare. Very young, very old, and immunocompromised individuals are at the greatest risk.

CLINICAL PRESENTATION
DISEASE FORMS/SUBTYPES
- Four main clinical presentations
  - Asymptomatic infection (organism is still shed in feces)
  - Mild colitis (fever, depression, and leukopenia without diarrhea)
  - Acute or peracute colitis with diarrhea
  - Septicemia with or without diarrhea (foals, see "Neonatal Sepsis" in this section)
- Several other less common associated clinical presentations:
  - Small colon impaction (see "Small Colon: Impaction" in this section)
  - Colic, fever, and gastric reflux (see "Proximal Enteritis" in this section)
  - Chronic diarrhea

HISTORY, CHIEF COMPLAINT
Inappetence, colic, fever, and diarrhea are most common, as for other causes of colitis (see "Colitis/Diarrhea, Acute, in Adult Horses" in this section)

PHYSICAL EXAM FINDINGS
- As for other causes of colitis (see "Colitis/Diarrhea, Acute, in Adult Horses" in this section).
- It is common to see fever and depression in the absence of diarrhea in mild cases.

ETIOLOGY AND PATHOPHYSIOLOGY
- *Salmonella* is an intracellular gram-negative rod-shaped bacterium.
- Transmission occurs via the fecal-oral route.
- Ingested organisms bind intestinal epithelial cells and are then taken up by the cells via endocytosis and deposited in the intestinal submucosa. There, their presence activates cellular receptors, recruiting neutrophils and producing a massive local inflammatory response.
- This results in inflammation and necrosis of intestinal villi and epithelial cells, damaging the mucosal barrier, resulting in systemic exposure to bacterial toxins and loss of fluid, electrolytes, and plasma proteins into the intestinal lumen as for other causes of colitis (see "Colitis/Diarrhea, Acute, in Adult Horses" in this section).
- *Salmonella* organisms also stimulate intraluminal chloride secretion, thus producing a secretory diarrhea with loss of chloride, sodium, and water into the feces.

DIAGNOSIS

DIFFERENTIAL DIAGNOSIS
Other causes of colitis (see "Colitis/Diarrhea, Acute, in Adult Horses" in this section)

INITIAL DATABASE
- In general, as for other causes of colitis (see "Colitis/Diarrhea, Acute, in Adult Horses" in this section).
- Hypoproteinemia and hypoalbuminemia are variable but can be dramatic in salmonellosis.

ADVANCED OR CONFIRMATORY TESTING
- Fecal culture
  - Requires selective media and culture techniques
  - Serial samples (three to five) should be collected approximately 24 hours apart because *Salmonella* organisms can be shed intermittently.
  - Very watery fecal material may be less likely to yield positive cultures. If salmonellosis is strongly suspected, culture should be repeated on more formed feces.
- Fecal polymerase chain reaction (PCR)
  - Very sensitive and specific for the presence of the organism in the feces.
  - Again, serial samples (three to five) should be tested.
  - However, some normal horses may have transient positive results on PCR but negative culture results if they are exposed to but clear the organism. Thus samples yielding positive PCR results should be subsequently cultured to determine the likelihood of transmission from that horse.
- Testing for other causes of colitis is also warranted, as detailed in "Colitis/Diarrhea, Acute, in Adult Horses" in this section

TREATMENT

THERAPEUTIC GOAL(S)
- Supportive care
- ± Antimicrobial therapy (controversial)

ACUTE GENERAL TREATMENT
- Fluid and colloidal support, antiinflammatory and antiendotoxic therapy, and other supportive care as for other causes of colitis (see "Colitis and Diarrhea, Acute, in Adult Horses" in this section).
- Administration of antimicrobials is controversial.
  - Foals with confirmed or suspected *Salmonella* septicemia should *always* be treated with antimicrobials.
  - However, in most adult horses with salmonellosis, antimicrobial therapy does not appear to alter the clinical progression or prognosis and may slow the reestablishment of normal enteric bacterial flora.
  - Conversely, in adult horses with severe and protracted acute colitis or chronic diarrhea caused by salmonellosis, antimicrobial therapy may result in clinical improvement. Fluoroquinolones (enrofloxacin, 5 mg/kg IV or 7.5 mg/kg PO q24h)

are likely to be the most effective at supporting clearance of intracellular *Salmonella* organisms from the intestinal tract given their excellent penetration into tissues and cells.

- Isolation of infected horses from other susceptible horses is vital to reduce the spread of disease at a veterinary clinic or farm.

POSSIBLE COMPLICATIONS

- Laminitis, thrombophlebitis, colonic infarction as for other causes of colitis
- Chronic diarrhea caused by colonic fibrosis or chronic infection
- Bacteremia or disseminated *Salmonella* infection (uncommon in adults)

RECOMMENDED MONITORING

- Serial fecal samples should be collected and tested by culture or PCR 2 to 3 weeks after resolution of clinical disease to ensure the horse is no longer shedding the organisms. The horse should be isolated until three serial PCRs or five serial culture results are negative. Some horses shed *Sal-*

monella for months and should be managed accordingly.

- Environmental cultures should be obtained after disinfection of stalls and treatment areas after a horse has been released from isolation to ensure that the organism has also been eradicated from the environment.

PROGNOSIS AND OUTCOME

- Fair with aggressive and early therapy
- Guarded with severe and protracted diarrhea, concurrent laminitis, or if poor response to therapy after 10 to 14 days because colonic damage may be too severe

PEARLS & CONSIDERATIONS

- Salmonellosis should be considered as a differential diag-

nosis in any horse with fever, leukopenia, or diarrhea.

- The development of multidrug-resistant *Salmonella* organisms is a significant concern, especially given the difficulty in eliminating these organisms from the environment and the potential for nosocomial infections among horses at equine referral hospitals or large farms. Antibiograms should be determined for all horses with positive fecal culture results to monitor for the development of antimicrobial resistance in regional *Salmonella* strains.

SUGGESTED READING

Jones SJ: Medical disorders of the large intestine: acute diarrhea. In Smith BP, editor: *Large animal internal medicine*, ed 4, St Louis, 2009, Mosby Elsevier, pp 743–744.

AUTHOR: **KELSEY A. HART**

EDITORS: **TIM MAIR** and **CERI SHERLOCK**

Sand Enteropathy

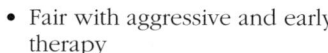

BASIC INFORMATION

DEFINITION

Colitis and/or diarrhea that occurs as a result of sand accumulation in the ventral or dorsal colon (or both)

EPIDEMIOLOGY

GEOGRAPHY AND SEASONALITY
Occurs most frequently in coastal regions, where horses may be pastured on sandy soils, but may also occur in horses turned out in sandy arenas or in some horses that actively ingest soil or gravel.

CLINICAL PRESENTATION

HISTORY, CHIEF COMPLAINT
- Horses with sand enteropathy most often present with mild recurrent colic, inappetence, and chronic or intermittent diarrhea (see "Diarrhea, Chronic" in this section).
- Acute inappetence, colic, fever, and diarrhea may also occur, as for other causes of colitis (see "Colitis/Diarrhea, Acute, in Adult Horses" in this section).

PHYSICAL EXAM FINDINGS
- As for other causes of colitis (see "Colitis/Diarrhea, Acute, in Adult Horses" in this section), although the diarrhea and clinical signs of endotox-

emia and hypovolemia are usually less severe.

- Occasionally, it is possible to auscultate sand moving in the ventral colon along the ventrum, which has been described as sounding like ocean waves crashing on a beach, although this is by no means a consistent finding.
- If concurrent large colonic obstruction with sand is present, gross abdominal distension and moderate to severe signs of colic are often present, and large colonic gas distension may be noted on rectal examination (see "Sand Impaction" in this section).

ETIOLOGY AND PATHOPHYSIOLOGY
- Small amounts of sand or soil are ingested during grazing or feeding of hay or grain in sandy environments. Alternatively, some (often young or bored) horses actively ingest sand or dirt when turned out.
- However, why sand accumulation only occurs in some horses in sandy regions is not understood. Individual dietary, anatomic, and colonic motility factors likely play roles.
- Because of its increased density, large amounts of sand settle in the ventral colon. The presence of a large amount of sand, when coupled with

normal colonic peristalsis, can irritate the colonic mucosa and damage the colonic mucosal barrier.

- This results in systemic exposure to bacterial toxins and diarrhea as for other causes of colitis (see "Colitis/Diarrhea, Acute, in Adult Horses" and "Diarrhea, Chronic" in this section).
- Colonic obstruction, particularly at the transverse colon, may also occur with sand ingestion and accumulation (See "Sand Impaction" in this section).

DIAGNOSIS

DIFFERENTIAL DIAGNOSIS

Other causes of colitis or chronic diarrhea (see "Colitis/Diarrhea, Acute, in Adult Horses" and "Diarrhea, Chronic" in this section)

INITIAL DATABASE

- As for other causes of colitis (see "Colitis/Diarrhea, Acute, in Adult Horses" in this section).
- With significant sand accumulation, an inability to visualize colonic haustra in the ventral abdomen with transabdominal ultrasonography is often seen, although this is not diagnostic for sand accumulation.

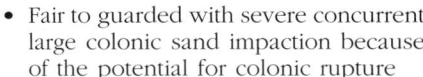

- Attempted abdominocentesis in horses with significant sand accumulation and related ventral colonic distension often results in enterocentesis, so this procedure should be carried out with caution or avoided in horses with a strong suspicion of sand enteropathy or sand impaction.

ADVANCED OR CONFIRMATORY TESTING

- Abdominal radiography
  - Diagnostic for sand accumulation or enteropathy.
  - Sand appears as mineral opacity in the ventral colon and can be visualized with abdominal radiography even in adult horses.
  - Many horses have some sand in their ventral colon, but a small amount of sand accumulation is likely not clinically significant.
- Fecal sedimentation for sand
  - Feces are suspended in water in a rectal sleeve and hung vertically for 10 to 20 minutes. If the feces contain a large amount of sand, the more dense sand will settle out into the fingers of the sleeve.
  - However, many horses with clinically significant sand accumulation are not actively passing sand in their feces, so the absence of sand on fecal sedimentation does not rule out sand enteropathy.

TREATMENT

THERAPEUTIC GOAL(S)

- Provide supportive care
- Aid in expulsion or removal of colonic sand

ACUTE GENERAL TREATMENT

- Fluid and colloidal support, antiinflammatory and antiendotoxic therapy, and other supportive care as indicated as for other causes of colitis (see "Colitis/Diarrhea, Acute, in Adult Horses" in this section)

- Laxative therapy
  - Administration of psyllium mucilage (10–16 oz/450 kg horse via nasogastric tube in 2–3 L of water; adjust accordingly for foals and ponies) once daily for 5 to 7 days is effective in facilitating clearance of sand from the colon in many cases.
  - Concurrent administration of other laxatives such as mineral oil or magnesium sulfate during this 5- to 7-day period may also facilitate sand removal. Administration of psyllium every morning and administration of mineral oil or magnesium sulfate every evening (or vice versa) has been effective in promoting clearance of even large amounts of sand in horses in our clinic.
  - During this treatment, horses should be maintained on a low-bulk diet such as pelleted complete feed to decrease fecal volume and minimize the risk of concurrent colonic impaction.
  - Repeat radiography after laxative therapy can be used to assess the success of this treatment regimen.
- If laxative therapy is unsuccessful and the horse continues to show signs of colic or diarrhea or if signs consistent with colonic obstruction occur, laparotomy and removal of the sand via a pelvic flexure enterotomy may be required.

POSSIBLE COMPLICATIONS

Colonic rupture

RECOMMENDED MONITORING

Repeat radiographs after laxative therapy can be used to assess the success of this treatment regimen. If treatment is effective, a large amount of sand may be grossly visible in the feces during and after treatment.

PROGNOSIS AND OUTCOME

- Good with response to medical or laxative therapy

- Fair to guarded with severe concurrent large colonic sand impaction because of the potential for colonic rupture

PEARLS & CONSIDERATIONS

COMMENTS

Aggressive laxative therapy is required for medical management of horses with sand enteropathy and is not successful in all cases.

PREVENTION

- Good dietary and pasture management can help prevent sand enteropathy.
  - In sandy areas, horses should be fed in raised buckets and feeders off of the ground, with rubber mats placed around feeding areas to minimize sand ingestion.
  - For horses that have recurrent sand impactions on pasture or those that actively ingest sand, a pasture companion, access to free-choice hay, or a grazing muzzle may decrease sand ingestion.
- Psyllium administration: Many psyllium products on the market claim to aid in the prevention of colonic sand accumulation in horses. These products typically involve feeding a small amount of psyllium daily and a larger amount for several days each month. Although these products appear to be safe, the efficacy of such protocols has not been evaluated critically.

SUGGESTED READING

Keppie NJ, Rosenstein DS, Holcombe SJ, et al: Objective radiographic assessment of abdominal sand accumulation in horses. *Vet Radiol Ultrasound* 49(2):122–128, 2008.

AUTHOR: **KELSEY A. HART**

EDITORS: **TIM MAIR** and **CERI SHERLOCK**

Sand Impaction

BASIC INFORMATION

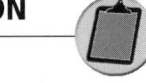

DEFINITION

Accumulation of sand or gravel within the intestine producing irritation and potentially obstructing the flow of ingesta or gas

SYNONYM(S)

Sand accumulation, sand colic, sand colitis

EPIDEMIOLOGY

SPECIES, AGE, SEX Most common in horses older than 1 year, but reported in horses of all ages, including foals
GENETICS AND BREED PREDISPOSITION Some suggest that Miniature horses are predisposed.

RISK FACTORS Reported risk factors include inadequate access to roughage and access to sand or mineral composition of the soil.

GEOGRAPHY AND SEASONALITY Regions with sandy soil such as California, Florida, Michigan, and coastal U.S. states have increased incidence.

ASSOCIATED CONDITIONS AND DISORDERS Sand impaction has been reported in combination with large colon displacements and volvulus (25%–54%). It has been suggested that this is a result of a change in motility associated with sand accumulation.

CLINICAL PRESENTATION

HISTORY, CHIEF COMPLAINT Clinical signs of sand impaction are variable depending on the degree of inflammation and obstruction. Owners may report signs of colic, diarrhea, and weight loss.

PHYSICAL EXAM FINDINGS

- Horses with sand impaction have similar physical examination findings to horses with other simple obstructions of the large colon (see "Large Colon: Impaction" in this section) or large colon displacements (see "Large Colon: Left Dorsal Displacements" and "Large Colon: Other Displacements" in this section) or volvulus (see "Large Colon: Volvulus" in this section) if present in combination.
- In addition, horses with sand impactions may show variable signs of endotoxemia and inflammation associated with irritation and compromise of the mucosa. Elevations in temperature, heart rate, and respiratory rate and changes in mucous membrane color and capillary refill time are consistent with endotoxemia.

ETIOLOGY AND PATHOPHYSIOLOGY

- Sand accumulation can result in irritation or inflammation of the mucosa, obstruction of the flow of ingesta, and alterations in motility.
- The most common sites for sand impaction are the right dorsal colon followed by the transverse colon followed by the left dorsal colon. However, impaction can occur throughout the large colon and in the small colon and ileocecal junction as well.

DIAGNOSIS

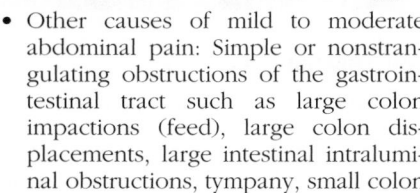

DIFFERENTIAL DIAGNOSIS

- Other causes of mild to moderate abdominal pain: Simple or nonstrangulating obstructions of the gastrointestinal tract such as large colon impactions (feed), large colon displacements, large intestinal intraluminal obstructions, tympany, small colon impactions, and ileal impactions (see respective entries in this section).
- Other causes of large intestinal distension on examination per rectum: Large colon impactions (feed), tympany, large colon displacements, and other intraluminal obstructions (see respective entries in this section).
- Other causes of diarrhea and weight loss: Chronic salmonellosis, parasitism, and inflammatory bowel disease.

INITIAL DATABASE

- Auscultation of the ventral abdomen (particularly cranioventral) may reveal the sound of the ocean or sand in a paper bag.
- Feces may contain sand detected by adding water to several fecal balls in a rectal sleeve and allowing the sand to sediment out. Additionally, the mucosa of the rectum may be covered in sand, producing a gritty texture.
- Findings on examination per rectum will depend on the location of the impaction (see "Large Colon: Impactions" in this section) and if concurrent displacement or volvulus is present (see "Large Colon: Displacements" and "Large Colon: Volvulus" in this section). Most commonly, distension of the large colon and cecum are the primary abnormalities detected on examination per rectum.
- Nasogastric reflux is uncommon but can occur.
- Blood work may be normal or consistent with mild to moderate dehydration (prerenal azotemia, elevated packed cell volume, elevated total protein). If mucosal compromise or inflammation is present, the leukogram may reveal a leukopenia with or without a left shift, and hypoproteinemia may occur.
- Abdominal fluid analysis is generally within normal limits unless the intestinal wall has been compromised. Sand impaction may predispose to enterocentesis and sand within the abdominal fluid or may be palpated during abdominocentesis.
- Abdominal radiographs reveal radiodense material within the cranioventral abdomen. Radiographs are helpful for quantifying and monitoring sand impactions.
- Abdominal ultrasonography may reveal increased contact of the ventral colon with the ventral body wall, decreased haustra, and decreased motility. Ultrasound evaluation is subjective, and variable accuracy has been reported. It may be most useful for monitoring after the diagnosis of sand impaction has been made.

TREATMENT

THERAPEUTIC GOAL(S)

- Removal of the sand
- Pain management
- Appropriate monitoring to identify any progression of the disease resulting in intestinal or cardiovascular compromise

ACUTE GENERAL TREATMENT

- Withhold feed and remove from source of sand.
- Rehydration or overhydration with enteral and IV fluids (see "Large Intestine: Impaction" in this section for details)
- Cathartics or laxatives
  - Mineral oil alone does not appear effective for treatment of sand impaction because it seems to glide around the impaction (see "Large Intestine: Impaction" in this section).
  - $MgSO_4$ has been used in conjunction with mineral oil and psyllium (see "Large Intestine: Impaction" in this section).
  - Psyllium formulations (8–12 oz/dose) are commonly administered as a bulk laxative in cases of sand impaction. Reports of success are variable.
- Analgesic administration similar to that used for treatment of large intestinal impactions
- Surgical treatment may be required if pain is unrelenting or systemic or gastrointestinal deterioration occurs.

CHRONIC TREATMENT

- Recurrence is possible and changes in management are frequently recommended to prevent further sand accumulation.
- Recommended changes in feed management include provision of adequate roughage, especially when pastures are depleted; feeding off of the ground in hay racks and feed troughs; and placing mats on the ground below areas of feeding to prevent sand accumulation when horses eat feed that has fallen.
- The administration of psyllium products by a variety of methods has been advocated for prevention of sand accumulation. The relative effectiveness of the various methods is unknown. Many protocols have periods during which no psyllium is administered to prevent increases in bacteria that digest the psyllium, decreasing the efficacy of the treatment.

POSSIBLE COMPLICATIONS

- Complications include diarrhea, intestinal rupture, peritonitis, and weight loss.
- Because of the weight of the sand and the irritation of the mucosa associated with sand impaction, the colon may be predisposed to rupture during exteriorization of the colon at surgery.

RECOMMENDED MONITORING

- Monitoring for resolution of the impaction should include fecal output and repeat radiography, ultrasonography, or both. If the impaction is palpable on examination per rectum, this can be repeated as well.
- During treatment, horses should be monitored for signs of unrelenting pain, nasogastric reflux, progressive abdominal distension, systemic deterioration (climbing heart rate, cardiovascular compromise), and gastrointestinal deterioration (abdominocentesis may be useful).

PROGNOSIS AND OUTCOME

- Prognosis appears good.
- Reports on surgical treatment have shown 92% discharge from hospital and 60% survival to 12 months.

PEARLS & CONSIDERATIONS

COMMENTS

- Sand impaction should be considered as a differential diagnosis in cases that present with signs of nonstrangulating obstruction of the large intestine as well as colitis.
- Radiographs are likely the most useful method of quantifying and monitoring the sand accumulation.
- Psyllium is frequently used as a laxative in cases of sand impaction.

PREVENTION

Changes in management and administration of psyllium as described in chronic treatment are also recommended as methods of prevention.

CLIENT EDUCATION

Client education is an important step in prevention.

SUGGESTED READING

Johnston JK, Freeman DE: Diseases and surgery of the large colon. *Vet Clin North Am Equine Pract* 13(2):317, 1997.
Ragle CA, Meagher DM, Lacroix CA, et al: Surgical treatment of sand colic. Results in 40 horses. *Vet Surg* 18:48, 1989.
Rakestraw PC, Hardy J: Large intestine. In Auer JA, Stick JA, editors: *Equine surgery*, ed 3, St Louis, 2006, Saunders Elsevier, pp 436–478.
Specht TE, Colahan PT: Surgical treatment of sand colic in equids: 48 cases (1978–1985). *J Am Vet Med Assoc* 193:1560, 1988.

AUTHOR: **KIRA L. EPSTEIN**

EDITORS: **TIM MAIR** and **CERI SHERLOCK**

Sarcoids

BASIC INFORMATION

DEFINITION

Cutaneous tumor of fibroblastic origin

SYNONYM(S)

Older literature may refer to invasive fibromas, fibrosarcomas, or fibropapillomas.

EPIDEMIOLOGY

SPECIES, AGE, SEX

- Equids: Reported in horses, donkeys, mules, and zebras
- Any age; 3 to 6 years most common

GENETICS AND BREED PREDISPOSITION

- Overall prevalence 0.5% to 2%; may be higher in some populations; most common skin neoplasm of horses.
- Although all breeds of horses are susceptible, some breed predispositions have been recognized. In the United States, sarcoids are relatively more common in Quarter Horses, Appaloosas, and Arabians and less common in Standardbreds.
- Genetic predispositions have been associated with specific equine leukocyte antigens.
- No apparent association with coat color.

CONTAGION AND ZOONOSIS

- Linked to bovine papilloma virus (BPV) type 1 and less commonly type 2
- Mechanism of infection with BPV currently unclear

CLINICAL PRESENTATION

DISEASE FORMS/SUBTYPES

- Six subtypes of sarcoids based on clinical appearance and biologic behavior
  - Occult: Mild cutaneous scaling and alopecia; most benign form; often remains quiescent with little change in appearance or growth
  - Verrucous (warty): Raised, scaly, lichenified appearance with hair loss and epidermal thickening; also typically very benign
  - Nodular: Freely movable, raised masses with normal or ulcerated skin
  - Fibroblastic: Proliferative ulcerated masses (may look similar to exuberant granulation tissue)
  - Mixed: Components of different subtypes
  - Malevolent: Infiltrate locally along fascial planes and vessels and grow rapidly; high recurrence rate; most aggressive form
- All subtypes are capable of transforming to more malignant variants.

- A simplified classified system has been proposed based on tumor behavior
  - Indolent
  - Invasive

HISTORY, CHIEF COMPLAINT Cutaneous lesions

PHYSICAL EXAM FINDINGS

- Appearance varies with subtype.
- Lesions are typically firm and annular. They may be any size and are often poorly circumscribed. The appearance of the overlying skin is highly variable, ranging from normal to alopecic to ulcerated.
- Site predilection: Lesions can develop anywhere on the body, but some sites are more common.
  - Face, including muzzle, ears, and periocular region
  - Distal limbs
  - Neck, ventral abdomen
  - Areas of previous injury or scarring
- Sarcoids on the distal limb and periorbital region may have a worse prognosis than sarcoids at other sites.

ETIOLOGY AND PATHOPHYSIOLOGY

- Malignant transformation of cells may result from genetic and exogenous factors.
- BPV DNA has been found in nearly all equine sarcoid tissues examined.
  - The exact role of BPV infection in sarcoid is currently unknown.

○ Oncogenesis is associated with the presence of virus and expression of transforming genes.
• Behavior: Generally classified as benign but often locally invasive with a tendency to recur
    ○ Behavior varies with subtype
    ○ Does not metastasize to distant organs; regional metastasis is extremely rare and is usually associated with unsuccessful treatment

DIAGNOSIS

DIFFERENTIAL DIAGNOSIS

• Appropriate differential diagnoses vary with the type of sarcoid.
• Potential differential diagnoses include papilloma, squamous cell carcinoma, exuberant granulation tissue, habronemiasis, infectious granuloma, dermatophytosis, dermatophilosis, staphylococcal folliculitis, onchocerciasis, dermal neoplasm (especially melanocytic neoplasms and mast cell tumors), and eosinophilic granuloma.

INITIAL DATABASE

Routine laboratory evaluation results are generally normal.

ADVANCED OR CONFIRMATORY TESTING

• Definitive diagnosis by biopsy: Fibroblastic proliferation with associated epidermal hyperplasia and dermoepidermal activity; variable dermal configuration and histologic appearance can make pathologic diagnosis difficult.
• Identification of BPV DNA by polymerase chain reaction on skin swabs and scrapings can be useful in the diagnosis of sarcoids (Lucy Whittier Molecular and Diagnostic Core Facility, UC Davis College of Veterinary Medicine, Davis, CA).

TREATMENT

THERAPEUTIC GOAL(S)

• Prevent or control invasion
• Eliminate primary mass

ACUTE GENERAL TREATMENT

• Large number of treatment options
    ○ Variable success
    ○ Factors to consider in developing a treatment protocol include tumor site, size, number of lesions, behavior, previous therapy, clinician experience, and availability of modalities.
• Monitoring is critical because of the chance of recurrence; retreatment is often necessary regardless of the protocol used.
• Some cases remain quiescent without treatment. Spontaneous regression also occurs.
• Common treatment options (often therapies are combined, eg, surgical excision followed by cryotherapy)
    ○ Surgical excision
        ▪ Most often used to debulk tumors followed by other adjunctive therapy
        ▪ Generally try to include 0.5 to 1.0 cm of normal tissue at the margin
        ▪ More likely to recur if outer surgical margin contains BPV DNA
    ○ Laser therapy: Ablation with a carbon dioxide laser; often combined with additional therapy (surgical debulking, intralesional chemotherapy, other)
    ○ Cryotherapy
        ▪ Cryotherapy with liquid nitrogen: Most often used as adjunctive therapy after debulking
        ▪ Lesions generally frozen two or three times to −20° to −30° C with complete thawing to room temperature between each freeze
    ○ Immunotherapy
        ▪ Mycobacterial cell wall extract immunomodulation (bacille Calmette-Guérin and related products: eg, Regressin-V, Bioniche Animal Health, Athens, Ga; Ribigen-E, Ribi ImmunoChem Research Inc., Hamilton, MT). Typically, intralesional injections are done every 2 to 3 weeks for an average of four treatments. Inflammation and necrosis are common after injection.
        ▪ Other: Systemic immunotherapy with *Propionibacterium acnes* (EqStim, Neogen Corporation, Lansing, MI); autogenous vaccines
    ○ Imiquimod (Aldara; 3M, Saint Paul, MN; 5% cream)
        ▪ Applied topically three times a week for up to 32 weeks
        ▪ Total of 80% showed a greater than 75% reduction in size; total resolution was seen in 60%
    ○ Chemotherapy
        ▪ Intralesional cisplatin
            □ Injection of cisplatin in oil emulsion: 1 mg cisplatin/cm^3 tumor mass (can add 1:1000 epinephrine at a 1:10 final volume to cause vasoconstriction and prolong tumor cell exposure). Generally, four treatments at 2-week intervals recommended; may be difficult to inject. May be used after debulking. A total of 87%

resolution rate has been seen at 1 year.
    ▪ Cisplatin-containing biodegradable beads (Royer Biomedical, Inc., Frederick, MD; 3-mm beads, 7% cisplatin by weight)
        □ Generally recommend debulking before implantation of bead(s) if tumor is larger than 1.5 cm
        □ Beads are implanted at approximately 1.5-cm intervals; incision is closed to hold bead(s) in place
        □ Treat with nonsteroidal antiinflammatory drugs for approximately 3 days; short-term antibiotic treatment depending on the lesion
        □ May repeat at 30-day intervals if needed
        □ A 91% resolution rate at 2-year follow-up with mean of 2.4 treatments (range, 1–8 treatments)
    ○ 5-fluorouracil (5-FU): Both topical cream and intralesional 5-FU have been used with reported success
    ○ Irradiation
        ▪ Brachytherapy: Continuous delivery of a radiation dose via implantable radioactive implants; has demonstrated efficacy, but use is limited by regulations regarding radiation
        ▪ Radiation treatment via a linear accelerator may be effective
    ○ Bloodroot (*Sanguinaria canadensis*) extract products (Animex, NIES, Las Vegas, NV; XXTERRA, Larson Laboratories, Fort Collins, CO): For topical use
    ○ Other treatments less commonly described
        ▪ AW-3-LUDES and AW-4-LUDES: Proprietary topical preparations containing heavy metals and anti-mitotic compounds
        ▪ Interleukin-2: May be combined with cisplatin
        ▪ Hyperthermia
        ▪ Photodynamic therapy

POSSIBLE COMPLICATIONS

• Progressive tumor growth and transformation to more malignant subtype after treatment or injury
• Inflammation and necrosis after some treatments.
• Occasionally, systemic signs such as lethargy and pyrexia after treatment. Anaphylaxis has been reported after immunomodulatory therapy
• Scarring and depigmentation are possible.

RECOMMENDED MONITORING

Monitor for tumor regrowth.

PROGNOSIS AND OUTCOME

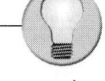

- The relative efficacy of different treatment strategies has been difficult to evaluate. Most studies are based on cases seen at referral hospitals, which may not be representative of sarcoids in general. Data are lacking for many treatments.
- There is no treatment which is 100% effective. Recurrence is relatively common (20%–30% in most studies).

PEARLS & CONSIDERATIONS

COMMENTS

- Sarcoids are seldom life threatening but may cause significant esthetic and performance-limiting problems.
- Follow-up is essential to successful treatment.

CLIENT EDUCATION

- Sarcoids vary widely in their appearance and behavior.
- Because recurrence is common regardless of the treatment strategy, continued monitoring is important for a successful outcome.

SUGGESTED READING

Carr EA: New developments in diagnosis and treatment of equine sarcoid. In Robinson NE, Sprayberry KA, editors: *Current therapy in equine medicine*, ed 6, St Louis, 2009, Saunders Elsevier, pp 698–702.

Hewes CA, Sullins KE: Use of cisplatin-containing biodegradable beads for treatment of cutaneous neoplasia in equidae: 59 cases (2000–2004). *J Am Vet Med Assoc* 229:1617–1622, 2006.

Nogueira SA, Torres SM, Malone ED, et al: Efficacy of imiquimod 5% cream in the treatment of equine sarcoids: a pilot study. *Vet Dermatol* 17:259–265, 2006.

Scott DW, Miller WH: Mesenchymal neoplasms. In *Equine dermatology*, St Louis, 2003, Saunders Elsevier, pp 719–731.

AUTHOR: **MELISSA T. HINES**

EDITOR: **JEFFREY N. BRYAN**

Scrotal Enlargement

BASIC INFORMATION

DEFINITION

Condition affecting the scrotum or its contents (or both) that results in a visible increase in size of the scrotum

EPIDEMIOLOGY

SPECIES, AGE, SEX Intact male horses of any age

GENETICS AND BREED PREDISPOSITION

- Any breed
- Inguinal hernias are more common in Standardbred, Tennessee Walking, and American Saddlebred horses.
- Congenital inguinal hernias are hereditary and are associated with a congenitally enlarged vaginal ring.

RISK FACTORS

- Breeding activity with scrotal trauma.
- Congenitally enlarged vaginal ring with inguinal hernia.
- Some sports (show jumping) may predispose intact stallions (personal observation).

ASSOCIATED CONDITIONS AND DISORDERS

- Orchitis, epididymitis
- Hydrocele
- Testicular torsion

CLINICAL PRESENTATION

HISTORY, CHIEF COMPLAINT

- Variable depending on the cause of the enlargement; see Differential Diagnosis below
- Unilateral or bilateral increase in scrotal size of acute or insidious onset
- History of recent breeding or trauma
- Pain (colic, reluctance to walk or breed)
- Fever, anorexia, lethargy
- Subfertility or infertility

PHYSICAL EXAM FINDINGS

- Variable depending on the cause of the enlargement
- Scrotal skin lesions or necrosis
- Scrotal and preputial edema
- Elevated scrotal or body temperature
- Tachycardia and tachypnea
- Depression and inappetence
- Palpably enlarged testes, epididymides, or spermatic cord

ETIOLOGY AND PATHOPHYSIOLOGY

Scrotal trauma is the most common cause of scrotal enlargement. Trauma occurs most frequently during breeding or jumping accidents and results in scrotal edema, orchitis, periorchitis, hydrocele, or hematocele.

DIAGNOSIS

DIFFERENTIAL DIAGNOSIS

- Inguinal hernia (congenital, acquired)
- Torsion of the spermatic cord
- Orchitis, epididymitis, periorchitis
  - Nonseptic
    - Traumatic
    - Autoimmune
  - Infectious
    - Ascending, hematogenous, extension of local infections
    - Bacterial (*Streptococcus equi*, subsp. *zooepidemicus*, *Corynebacterium* spp., *Proteus mirabilis*, *Corynebacterium pseudotuberculosis*, *Streptococcus equi*, subsp. *equi*, *Pseudomonas mallei*, *Salmonella abortus equi*, *Klebsiella pneumonia*)
    - Viral (equine arteritis virus, equine infectious anemia, equine influenza)
    - Parasitic (migration of *Strongylus edentatus*)
- Hydrocele
  - Idiopathic: Extremes in ambient temperature and humidity
  - Reactive
    - Testicular neoplasia
    - Scrotal trauma
    - Orchitis, epididymitis, periorchitis
  - Impaired venous or lymphatic drainage
    - Restricted exercise
    - Inguinal hernia
    - Torsion of the spermatic cord
  - Extension from peritoneal conditions: Ascites, peritonitis
- Pyocele
  - Ruptured testicular or scrotal abscess
  - Peritonitis
  - Scrotal puncture wound
- Hematocele
  - Scrotal trauma
  - Hemoperitoneum
- Varicocele
- Testicular neoplasia: Seminoma, teratoma or carcinoma, Leydig cell tumor, Sertoli cell tumor, embryonic carcinoma, mixed sex cord–stromal, mixed germ cell–sex cord–stromal, leiomyosarcoma

- Scrotal edema: Equine viral arteritis, equine infectious anemia, hypoproteinemia
- Scrotal dermatitis
- Scrotal cutaneous neoplasia: Lymphoma, squamous cell carcinoma, sarcoid, melanoma
- Habronemiasis: Associated with pain, fever, anorexia, lethargy, or clinicopathologic changes

INITIAL DATABASE

- Complete blood count: Leukocytosis with neutrophilia and hyperfibrinogenemia.
- Semen evaluation: Oligozoospermia, teratozoospermia, and asthenozoospermia. Leukospermia is possible with orchitis and epididymitis.
- Bacterial culture of ejaculated semen or biopsy specimen may aid in identification of the causative organism with orchitis and epididymitis.
- Scrotal ultrasonography
  - Loops of intestine within the scrotum with inguinal hernia
  - Hypoechoic or anechoic fluid surrounding the testes with hydrocele or pyocele
  - Free-floating echogenic particles that swirl if the scrotum is balloted with hematocele; after the hematoma becomes organized, the presence of hyperechoic fibrin strands within the hypoechoic or anechoic fluid
  - Heterogeneous echotexture of the testicular parenchyma with testicular neoplasia
  - Mottled-gray heterogenic image of the testicular parenchyma with orchitis
  - Irregular borders, heterogeneous image with hypoechoic pockets or dilated epididymal ducts with epididymitis
  - Increased thickness of the vaginal tunics with periorchitis
- Transabdominal ultrasonography
  - Free intraperitoneal anechoic fluid with ascites or peritonitis
  - Swirling hyperechoic particles within the hypoechoic fluid with hemoperitoneum

ADVANCED OR CONFIRMATORY TESTING

- Fine-needle aspiration of the contents of the vaginal cavity for diagnosis of hematocele and hydrocele
- Ultrasound-guided fine-needle aspiration and cytology of testicular lesions for diagnosis of testicular abscess or neoplasia

- Testicular biopsy for diagnosis of testicular inflammatory or neoplastic conditions
- Abdominocentesis for diagnosis of peritonitis, ascites, or hemoperitoneum
- Serology for equine viral arteritis and equine infectious anemia
- Surgical exploration

TREATMENT

THERAPEUTIC GOAL(S)

- Remove the inciting cause
- Minimize inflammation
- Prevent or control bacterial contamination
- Preserve function of the affected or contralateral (or both) testis
- Provide supportive treatment if systemic signs are present

ACUTE GENERAL TREATMENT

- Surgical procedures
  - Surgical reduction of acquired inguinal hernia
  - Unilateral orchidectomy
  - Surgical evacuation of blood from the vaginal cavity, debridement of fibrinous adhesions, and repair of the rent in the tunica albuginea with hematocele
- Control of inflammation and edema
  - Flunixin meglumine: 1.1 mg/kg IV or PO q12h
  - Phenylbutazone: 2 to 4 mg/kg IV or PO q12h
  - Furosemide: 0.5 to 1 mg/kg IV
  - Hydrotherapy with cold water for 20 minutes q2h
  - Controlled exercise
- Control of bacterial growth
  - Trimethoprim and sulfadiazine: 15 to 30 mg/kg PO q12h
  - Chloramphenicol: 40 to 60 mg/kg PO q6–8h
  - Continue therapy for 3 to 4 weeks
  - Adjust antibiotics based on the results of the culture and sensitivity test, if available
- Tetanus prophylaxis with trauma
- Sexual rest

POSSIBLE COMPLICATIONS

- Subfertility or infertility
- Ascending peritonitis or abscessation with septic orchitis, periorchitis, pyocele, or hematocele
- Descending ampullitis or seminal vesiculitis with septic orchitis or epididymitis
- Incarceration of inguinal hernia
- Metastasis with malignant testicular neoplasia

RECOMMENDED MONITORING

Semen collection and evaluation more than 60 days after clinical or surgical resolution to evaluate testicular function

PROGNOSIS AND OUTCOME

- Prognosis for life is usually good depending on the cause and provided medical attention is given immediately.
- Prognosis for fertility is guarded.
- The remaining testis may undergo compensatory hyperplasia after unilateral orchidectomy.

PEARLS & CONSIDERATIONS

COMMENTS

- Acute and painful scrotal enlargement should be considered an emergency.
- Fertility may be irreversibly affected because of testicular degeneration or production of antisperm antibodies.

PREVENTION

- Semen collection over a phantom and artificial insemination or proper mare restraint during mating to prevent breeding injuries
- Adequate parasite control and vaccination programs

CLIENT EDUCATION

- A veterinarian should be contacted immediately if acute and painful scrotal enlargement develops.
- Fertility may be irreversibly impaired because of testicular degeneration or production of antisperm antibodies.
- Given that inguinal hernias can be hereditary, use of affected stallions for breeding purposes should be discouraged.

SUGGESTED READING

Schumacher J, Varner DD: Surgical correction of abnormalities affecting the reproductive organs of stallions. In Youngquist RS, Threlfall WR, editors: *Current therapy in large animal theriogenology*, ed 2, St Louis, 2007, Saunders Elsevier, pp 23–36.

Turner RMO: Testicular abnormalities. In Samper JC, editor: *Equine breeding management and artificial insemination*, Philadelphia, 2000, WB Saunders, pp 195–204.

AUTHOR: **MARIA S. FERRER**

EDITOR: **JUAN C. SAMPER**

Seborrhea

BASIC INFORMATION

DEFINITION
Seborrhea is a chronic skin condition characterized by abnormal cornification or keratinization that causes excessive greasiness and scaling of the skin and haircoat. Seborrhea is a secondary manifestation of primary disease.

EPIDEMIOLOGY
ASSOCIATED CONDITIONS AND DISORDERS
- Systemic diseases such as intestinal malabsorption, liver disease, mineral and vitamin deficiencies or imbalances, toxicosis, neoplasia, or endocrine diseases can predispose horses to develop secondary seborrhea. Ectoparasites, bacterial or fungal diseases, and immune-mediated skin conditions are other underlying causes of seborrhea.
- Primary seborrhea is rare in horses, and its cause is unknown.

CLINICAL PRESENTATION
DISEASE FORMS/SUBTYPES
- Seborrhea sicca (dry)
- Seborrhea oleosa (greasy)
- Seborrheic dermatitis (patchy dermatitis)

HISTORY, CHIEF COMPLAINT The common complaint is dry, greasy skin or patchy dermatitis that is initially nonpruritic but can become pruritic later on if the seborrhea worsens or lesions are infected with *Staphylococcus* or *Malassezia* spp. Most of the lesions are present on the neck and trunk area.

PHYSICAL EXAM FINDINGS Physical examination is typically within normal limits unless there is some severe systemic disease that is affecting the animal at the time of examination for the skin condition.

ETIOLOGY AND PATHOPHYSIOLOGY
- Seborrhea sicca: Dryness of the skin and haircoat
- Seborrhea oleosa: Excessive greasiness of both the skin and haircoat
- Seborrheic dermatitis: Evidence of scaling and greasiness with local or diffuse inflammation

DIAGNOSIS

DIFFERENTIAL DIAGNOSIS
- Dermatophytosis
- Staphylococci skin infection
- Ectoparasites
- Endoparasites
- Vitamin or mineral imbalance
- Intestinal malabsorption
- Depressed immunologic system
- Drug reaction
- Neoplasia

INITIAL DATABASE
- Typical clinical signs
- Investigate underlying disease by obtaining a complete history, including a complete nutrition evaluation and physical examination

ADVANCED OR CONFIRMATORY TESTING
Biopsies are helpful in ruling out other causes.

TREATMENT

THERAPEUTIC GOAL(S)
Treat the underlying disease

ACUTE GENERAL TREATMENT
- Topical treatment with products containing benzoyl peroxide, coal tar, and sulphur and salicylic acid in combination with moisturizers is required multiple times a week. Depending on the severity of lesions, the horse may need to initially be bathed on a daily, biweekly, or weekly basis.
- The product should be lathered well and allowed to stand for at least 15 minutes and then completely rinsed off.
- Evaluate for possible secondary bacterial infection and presence of yeast. If at all present, appropriate antibacterial or antifungal treatment will need to be instituted.

PROGNOSIS AND OUTCOME
Accurate diagnosis and appropriate treatment typically provide a favorable prognosis.

SUGGESTED READING
Stannard AA: Disorders of cornification. *Vet Dermatol* 11:187–189, 2000.
White SD: Parasitic skin diseases. In Smith BP, editor: *Large animal internal medicine*, ed 4, St Louis, 2009, Saunders Elsevier, pp 1320–1321.

AUTHOR: **ALFREDO SANCHEZ LONDOÑO**

EDITOR: **DAVID A. WILSON**

Selenosis

BASIC INFORMATION

DEFINITION
Selenium poisoning is most commonly associated with excessive supplementation but may also result from naturally contaminated forages and feedstuffs.

SYNONYM(S)
- Alkali disease
- Selenium toxicosis

EPIDEMIOLOGY
SPECIES, AGE, SEX Horses are generally more susceptible than other common herbivores (ruminants).
RISK FACTORS Vitamin E and/or selenium deficiency potentiate the acutely toxic effects of selenium.
GEOGRAPHY AND SEASONALITY
- Poisonous vegetation is usually limited to certain geologic strata, most of which exist in the northern Great Plains and Intermountain West. Although accumulator plant species can bioconcentrate tens of thousands of parts per million, they are so unpalatable that poisoning usually involves common grains and forages such as alfalfa, which accumulate considerably less.
- Iatrogenic poisoning can occur anytime or anywhere.

CLINICAL PRESENTATION

DISEASE FORMS/SUBTYPES

- Acute selenosis
- Chronic selenosis, sometimes called *alkali disease*

HISTORY, CHIEF COMPLAINT

- Acute poisoning: Sudden death with no premonitory signs
- Smaller doses produce a gastrointestinal syndrome characterized by anorexia, colic and diarrhea, and cardiovascular damage resulting in shock, muscular weakness, and ataxia, followed by death.
- Chronic poisoning is characterized by epithelial lesions: Hair and hoof loss

PHYSICAL EXAM FINDINGS

- Acute poisoning: Initially, intoxicated animals become lethargic and lose interest in eating. Horses often become colicky and exhibit diarrhea, especially if the route of exposure was oral. The affected animal's breath may have a garlicky odor. Poisoned animals often exhibit a weak, wobbly gait as a result of generalized weakness and shock. Blood pressure is reported to decrease even before clinical signs become evident, and ventricular arrhythmias have been reported in experimentally poisoned animals. Heart rate and respiration are elevated, but the pulse is weak and thready and the peripheral circulation is compromised (slow capillary refill, cold extremities). Dyspnea, as a result of pulmonary edema, is a prominent finding, and poisoned animals may be cyanotic. Auscultation of the thorax reveals moist rales. Fever, polyuria, and hemolytic anemia have been reported but are not always present. Although blindness is still mentioned in a few texts, affected animals are not blind unless there is some complicating factor such as salt or lead intoxication. Death from circulatory or respiratory failure usually occurs within a day or two of exposure.
- Chronic poisoning: Usually results from sustained exposure to seleniferous grains or forages but may also be caused by overfeeding selenium supplements. The characteristic signs of chronic selenosis in cattle, sheep, horses, and swine involve bilaterally symmetric alopecia, especially of the mane and tail, and dystrophic hoof growth. The earliest signs of chronic poisoning are lameness, erythema, and swelling of the coronary bands, which subside quickly. These are followed in a few days to weeks by development of a circumferential crack parallel and just distal to the coronet. Ultimately, the hoof separates from the underlying new growth.

ETIOLOGY AND PATHOPHYSIOLOGY

- Excess selenium is metabolized to an electrophilic moiety that attacks tissue macromolecules and promotes oxidation, resulting in cell death.
- The distribution of such damage varies somewhat according to the chemical form of selenium, with selenomethionine from "natural" sources showing greater predilection for the skin and hooves than inorganic forms.
- The dietary threshold for chronic poisoning from forage or hay (data gleaned from field cases) is 10 to 20 ppm in most instances.
- Parenteral selenite or selenate may be hazardous after a single dose as small as 0.2 mg/kg.

DIAGNOSIS

DIFFERENTIAL DIAGNOSIS

- Acute poisoning may be mistaken for poisoning with other heavy metals that cause gastroenteritis and organ damage, such as arsenic or mercury.
- The hair and hoof lesions of chronic poisoning are fairly unique but may be confused in the early stages with laminitis.

INITIAL DATABASE

- Blood or liver selenium concentrations.
- Hair and hoof selenium concentrations may be useful if samples are taken from areas that were actively growing during exposure.
- Dietary selenium testing may be useful in identifying the source of poisoning but is less reliable than tissue testing in establishing a diagnosis.

ADVANCED OR CONFIRMATORY TESTING

Histopathology of affected skin or hooves may reveal characteristic keratin lesions in cases of chronic poisoning.

TREATMENT

THERAPEUTIC GOAL(S)

The toxic effects of selenium are the result of oxidative damage. Thus, in addition to supportive therapy and low selenium feedstuffs to restore normal homeostasis, antioxidants such as vitamin E are indicated.

CHRONIC TREATMENT

The hoof lesions of chronic selenosis usually resolve with corrective shoeing and supportive care.

PROGNOSIS AND OUTCOME

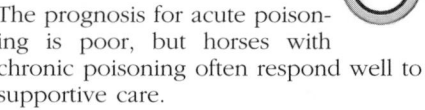

The prognosis for acute poisoning is poor, but horses with chronic poisoning often respond well to supportive care.

PEARLS & CONSIDERATIONS

COMMENTS

Because of the relatively rapid turnover in serum selenium, whole blood is a better sample to confirm exposure after the animal has been removed from the source of selenium.

PREVENTION

Ultimately, all selenium poisoning is the result of mismanagement. Whether from pasturing animals on seleniferous pastures, mixing errors in the feed mill, or exuberant use of nutritional supplements, a horse cannot poison itself without human help. Prevention consists of knowing what is in the horse's diet and keeping the intake of all trace element concentrations within acceptable limits.

SUGGESTED READING

O'Toole D, Raisbeck MF: Magic numbers, elusive lesions: comparative pathology and toxicology of selenosis in waterfowl and mammalian species. In Frankenberger WT, Engberg RA, editors: *Environmental chemistry of selenium*, New York, 1998, Marcel Dekker, pp 355–395.

AUTHOR: MERL F. RAISBECK

EDITOR: CYNTHIA GASKILL

Self-Mutilation

BASIC INFORMATION

DEFINITION

Self-mutilation is a broad term used to describe a complex group of behaviors often resulting in self-inflicted tissue damage or body harm.

SYNONYM(S)

- Self-injurious behavior
- Self-aggression
- Self-harm
- Self-injury
- Autotomy

EPIDEMIOLOGY

SPECIES, AGE, SEX Most commonly postpubertal stallions; however, the authors have seen similar behavioral problems in mares and geldings.
GENETICS AND BREED PREDISPOSITION Suspected but not fully documented
RISK FACTORS
- Painful conditions
- Inadequate sociosexual environment (presence of other stallions, smell of stallions)
- Housing and nutritional factors
GEOGRAPHY AND SEASONALITY Aggressive behavior may be exacerbated during the breeding season.
ASSOCIATED CONDITIONS AND DISORDERS Type I self-mutilation behaviors are often associated with painful conditions of the urogenital or gastrointestinal system, skin allergies, or parasite infestations.

CLINICAL PRESENTATION

DISEASE FORMS/SUBTYPES Three types of self-mutilation behavior:
- Type I: Often associated with chronic painful conditions
- Type II: A self-directed, intermale aggression triggered by factors simulating challenge by other stallions
- Type III: A more quiet, stereotypical, repetitive, compulsive behavior that is often rhythmic
HISTORY, CHIEF COMPLAINT
- Abnormal behavior including abnormal posture; biting of the abdomen, flank, groin, shoulders, chest; stomping, kicking, rubbing, and lunging into objects
- Behavior may be set off by specific conditions
- History of recent management changes
- History of castration or genital diseases.

- Chief complaints are undesirable behavior and concern about welfare, health, and value of the animal.
- Presence of obvious traumatic lesions on the body.

PHYSICAL EXAM FINDINGS

- Observation reveals typical behaviors: Flank biting, kicking, striking out, squealing, grunting.
- The primary findings on physical examination are lesions resulting from these behaviors, including lesions on the flank, genital area, chest, and limbs.
- Type I self-mutilation is often associated with symptoms of
  - Diseases of the reproductive organs: Inguinal cryptorchidism or retraction of testis in inguinal position, testicular cord torsion, phimosis, habronemiasis, squamous cell carcinoma, priapism, scrotal or testicular lesions, seminal vesiculitis
  - Diseases of the urinary tract: Cystitis, urethritis, uroliths, nephroliths
  - Disorders causing visceral pain: Impactions, adhesions, gastric ulcers, epiploic foramen entrapment, jejunal abscesses
  - Other conditions: Skin allergies, pruritus, parasite infestation

ETIOLOGY AND PATHOPHYSIOLOGY

- The cause is often multifactorial and is difficult to define unless there are physical problems or age-associated changes.
- Type II self-mutilation is often triggered by the perception of the challenge by another stallion either directly (presence of stallion in a confined area) or indirectly (presence of smell from feces, genital secretion. or even vocalization of other stallions). This behavior is believed to be an overt response to normal intermale aggression that is part of the social hierarchy. This abnormal behavior may develop over several weeks or months.
- Type III self-mutilation with a fixed pattern of biting is often displayed in anticipation of a barn routine such as grain feeding time.

DIAGNOSIS

DIFFERENTIAL DIAGNOSIS

- It is important to differentiate between the different types.
- Eliminate any physical cause of pain that may trigger type I self-mutilation.

INITIAL DATABASE

- Laboratory work is often not rewarding.
- Most important is a well-documented behavioral study using video observation without too much human interference.
- Analysis of time budget

ADVANCED OR CONFIRMATORY TESTING

Response to behavioral therapy or medication

TREATMENT

THERAPEUTIC GOAL(S)

- Reduce the major contributing factors
- Treat conditions associated with type I self-mutilation
- Protect the targeted area of the body
- Eliminate overt aggressiveness toward self by behavioral therapy or medical hormonal alterations

ACUTE GENERAL TREATMENT

- Physical restraint to protect from injury (however, these rarely work to eliminate the behavior)
  - Grazing muzzles
  - Neck cradles
  - Side poles, hobbles
  - Short tethers
- Protection of exposed areas (wraps, boots)
- Behavioral modification through changes in daily routine (time budget) is often praised as the most effective method and includes
  - Increase exercise
  - Provide distraction such as pasture with mares
  - Provide companionship (goat or miniature horse)
  - Eliminate all grain and concentrate (stallions on grass or grass hay spend most of their time eating)
- Masking odors from other stallions
- Elimination or reduction of testosterone secretion
  - Castration
  - Immunization against gonadotropin-releasing hormone (GnRH)
  - Progestagen therapy (Altrenogest 0.088 mg/kg PO q24h)
- Medication (sedatives)
  - Long-acting tranquilizers
    - Fluphenazine: 0.05 to 0.1 mg/kg IM q21 days
    - Reserpine: 2.5 mg/450 kg IM q30 days or PO q24h

○ Tricyclic antidepressants
  ▪ Imipramine: 1 to 3 mg/kg PO q24h
  ▪ Clomipramine 0.5 to 1 mg/kg PO q24h
○ Supplementation with L-tryptophan: 1 to 6 g/horse PO q24h

DRUG INTERACTIONS

Long-acting tranquilizers, particularly reserpine, produce prolonged penile relaxation and have been associated with penile paralysis.

POSSIBLE COMPLICATIONS

- Severe injuries
- Danger to other horses and humans
- Infertility in the stallion if progesterone or GnRH immunization is used

RECOMMENDED MONITORING

- Avoid changes in handlers and breeding routine

- Make sure that the stallion's time budget distracts him from self-mutilation
- Provide exercise

PROGNOSIS AND OUTCOME

- Prognosis is good with type I.
- Type II and type III require more effort.
- None of the techniques is 100% efficacious.

PEARLS & CONSIDERATIONS

COMMENTS

- Most of these problems are created by handlers.
- Behavioral modification by punishment is often discouraged.

PREVENTION

- Proper management
- Good socialization of horses early in life to help prevent these problems

CLIENT EDUCATION

- Treatment of these behavioral problems may take time.
- If treatment is unsuccessful, humane euthanasia should be considered.

SUGGESTED READING

Grimmett A, Sillence MN: Calmatives for the excitable horse: a review of L-tryptophan. *Vet J* 170:24–32, 2005.
McDonnell SM: Practical review of self-mutilation in horses. *Anim Reprod Sci* 107:219–228, 2008.
Tibary A: Stallion reproductive behavior. In Samper JC, Pycock, JF, McKinnon AO, editors: *Current therapy in equine reproduction*, St Louis, 2007, Saunders Elsevier, pp 174–184.

AUTHORS: **LISA K. PEARSON, JACOBO S. RODRIGUEZ,** and **AHMED TIBARY**

EDITOR: **JUAN C. SAMPER**

Serum Hepatitis

BASIC INFORMATION

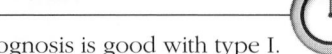

DEFINITION

Acute hepatic failure after administration of an equine serum product such as tetanus immune globulin

SYNONYM(S)

- Idiopathic acute hepatic disease
- Theiler's disease
- Postvaccinal hepatitis
- Acute liver atrophy

EPIDEMIOLOGY

SPECIES, AGE, SEX Primarily adult horses; mares are affected more often than stallions

RISK FACTORS

- Most commonly observed after animals receive tetanus immune globulin.
- Associated with the use of any equine serum product; morbidity may be as high as 18%.
- Disease occurs after an "incubation period" of 40 to 70 days.
- Periparturient lactating mares are at greatest risk.
- Tends to occur during summer months.

CLINICAL PRESENTATION

DISEASE FORMS/SUBTYPES Signs of acute liver failure

HISTORY, CHIEF COMPLAINT

- Depression
- Jaundice
- Inappetence
- Pica
- Photoactive dermatitis
- Hepatic encephalopathy
- Depression, anorexia, and icterus are evident in mild cases.
- Signs of hepatoencephalopathy include restlessness, excitement, compulsive walking, head pressing, seizures, apparent blindness, tremors, and ataxia.

ETIOLOGY AND PATHOPHYSIOLOGY

- The cause is unknown.
- One unproven cause is a virus similar to human hepatitis B. This is especially the case in horses that have not received tetanus antitoxin previously.
- Others have suggested that it is a form of immune complex hypersensitivity.

DIAGNOSIS

DIFFERENTIAL DIAGNOSIS

- Acute aflatoxicosis
- Rubratoxicosis
- Pyrrolizidine alkaloid intoxication
- Dioxin intoxication

INITIAL DATABASE

- Serum biochemical profile focusing on liver function tests.
- High serum levels of unconjugated and total bilirubin and serum bile acids.
- High serum gamma-glutamyl transpeptidase, sorbitol dehydrogenase, aspartate aminotransferase, lactate dehydrogenase, and alkaline phosphatase indicate hepatic necrosis.
- Leukocytosis with neutrophilia and mild lymphopenia is common.
- Hypoglycemia (<2 mmol/L) and hyperammonemia (>150 μmol/L) may be severe.
- Clotting time may be prolonged.

ADVANCED OR CONFIRMATORY TESTING

Hepatic biopsy showing widespread centrilobular and midzonal necrosis. There may be a mild inflammatory infiltrate in the portal area.

TREATMENT

THERAPEUTIC GOAL(S)

- Support liver function and control abnormal behavior.
- Correct metabolic and acid-base abnormalities.

- Reduce plasma ammonium concentration.
- Prevent horses with hepatic encephalopathy from injuring themselves.

ACUTE GENERAL TREATMENT

- Continuous IV administration of 5% dextrose and isotonic electrolytes to correct hypoglycemia and dehydration
- Metabolic acidosis can be corrected by infusion of sodium bicarbonate.
- If spontaneous bleeding is occurring, then plasma transfusion may replace clotting factors.
- Hyperammonemia may be treated by providing neomycin (20 mg/kg PO q6h for four doses) or lactulose (0.25 mL/kg PO q8h) to decrease intestinal absorption of ammonia.
- Sedation with xylazine or similar may be necessary to prevent the animal from injuring itself.
- Glucocorticoid treatment is controversial.

PROGNOSIS AND OUTCOME

Poor, with a case fatality rate of between 50% and 90%

PEARLS & CONSIDERATIONS

PREVENTION

- Given that this disease occurs most often in parturient or lactating mares, prudence suggests that tetanus immune globulin should not be administered around this time.
- If the disease occurs in one member of a herd, prudence suggests testing liver function in other herd members because they may have inapparent or subclinical disease.

CLIENT EDUCATION

Discussion on the advisability of further use of equine serum products

SUGGESTED READING

Aleman M, Nieto JE, Carr EA, Carlson GP: Serum hepatitis associated with commercial plasma transfusion in horses. *J Vet Intern Med* 19:120–122, 2005.

Guglick MA, MacAllister CG, Ely RW, Edwards WC: Hepatic disease associated with administration of tetanus antitoxin in eight horses. *J Am Vet Med Assoc* 206:1737–1740, 1995.

Hjerpe CA: Serum hepatitis in the horse. *J Am Vet Med Assoc* 144:734–740, 1964.

Messer NT 4th, Johnson PJ: Serum hepatitis in two brood mares. *J Am Vet Med Assoc* 204:1790–1792, 1994.

Panciera RJ: Serum hepatitis in the horse. *J Am Vet Med Assoc* 155:408–410, 1969.

AUTHOR and EDITOR: **IAN TIZARD**

Shivers

BASIC INFORMATION

DEFINITION

A mechanical lameness most often involving the pelvic limbs that appears to be caused by involuntary muscular spasms

SYNONYM(S)

Shivering, shiverer, shivers syndrome

EPIDEMIOLOGY

SPECIES, AGE, SEX

- Horses; rare in ponies. Not reported in donkeys and very rarely in mules.
- Onset is usually at an early age but can begin at any age.

GENETICS AND BREED PREDISPOSITION Likely inherited. Most common in Draft breeds and also common in Warmblood breeds. Occasionally occurs in other horse breeds.

ASSOCIATED CONDITIONS AND DISORDERS

- May be associated with polysaccharide storage myopathy (PSSM).
- Signs may begin after other illness or trauma.

CLINICAL PRESENTATION

DISEASE FORMS/SUBTYPES Affected limbs exhibit episodic hyperflexion, typically prolonged, that appears to be involuntary and associated with muscle spasms. During episodes, the tail may also elevate and exhibit fine tremoring, and the head may elevate slightly, with apparent "stretching" of the neck and rapid eye blinking. Horses with severe advanced cases can also exhibit forelimb and total-body spasms.

HISTORY, CHIEF COMPLAINT Abnormal gait invoked by backing and turning in tight circles. Signs are also common in the first walk stride after standing, in the last walk stride before halting, and when lifting hind limbs for hoof care. The abnormality is not present at gaits other than the walk. Affected horses may also hyperflex the pelvic limbs while standing.

PHYSICAL EXAM FINDINGS May be normal or may be associated with symmetric atrophy of pelvic limb musculature or of total body musculature. Muscle weakness occurs in advanced cases.

ETIOLOGY AND PATHOPHYSIOLOGY PSSM may be a cause of shivers, but this is controversial.

DIAGNOSIS

DIFFERENTIAL DIAGNOSIS

- Abnormal gait (ataxia) caused by spinal cord disease
- Horses with shivers are *not* ataxic, although the gait abnormality and hindlimb weakness may be mistaken for ataxia.

INITIAL DATABASE

- Neurologic examination to rule out neurologic disease
- Serum creatine kinase (CK) and aspartate aminotransferase (AST) 4 to 6 hours after exercise. Serum CK and AST levels are usually normal but may be slightly increased.

ADVANCED OR CONFIRMATORY TESTING

- Semimembranosus or semitendinosus muscle biopsy for PSSM.
- Genetic testing for *GYS1* mutation (Neuromuscular Disease Laboratory, University of Minnesota; http://www.cvm.umn.edu/umec/lab/Advances_in_PSSM.html) for type 1 PSSM.

TREATMENT

THERAPEUTIC GOAL(S)

Relieve muscle spasms and improve muscle strength or bulk.

CHRONIC TREATMENT

- High-fat, low-starch, and low-sugar diet (see "Polysaccharide Storage Myopathy" in this section) and as much exercise conditioning and time out of a stall as possible
- Massage and stretching exercises may also be beneficial, but further studies of these treatments are needed.

RECOMMENDED MONITORING

Monitor severity of signs at intervals as the disease is progressive (see below).

PROGNOSIS AND OUTCOME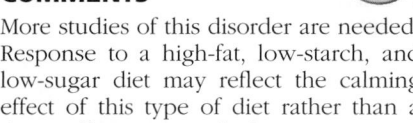

- Shivers is a progressive disease, although the rate of progression is not predictable. Progression will eventually result in profound disability, death caused by persistent recumbency, or the need for euthanasia.
- With diet change and exercise, most horses improve, although almost all will still show some signs of shivers, especially during times of stress, after confinement, or when there are other problems (eg, hoof abscess, degenerative joint disease) in an affected limb. Some horses do not respond to diet

and exercise, but this therapy may slow disease progression.

PEARLS & CONSIDERATIONS

COMMENTS

More studies of this disorder are needed. Response to a high-fat, low-starch, and low-sugar diet may reflect the calming effect of this type of diet rather than a direct effect on muscle function.

PREVENTION

Do not breed affected horses, especially those with severe disease and those that do not respond to diet and exercise therapy.

CLIENT EDUCATION

Proper husbandry (diet, turnout, exercise) are critical to management of

shivers. Discuss heritability in breeding animals.

SUGGESTED READING

Baird JD, Firshman AM, Valberg SJ, et al: Shivers (shivering) in the horse: a review. *Proc Am Assoc Equine Pract* 52:359–364, 2006.

Firshman AM, Baird JD, Valberg SJ: Prevalences and clinical signs of polysaccharide storage myopathy and shivers in Belgian Draft Horses. *J Am Vet Med Assoc* 227:1958–1964, 2005.

Shivers, Neuromuscular Disease Laboratory, University of Minnesota. Available at http://www.cvm.umn.edu/umec/lab/shivers.html.

Valentine BA, de Lahunta A, Divers TJ, et al: Clinical and pathologic findings in two draft horses with progressive muscle atrophy, neuromuscular weakness, and abnormal gait characteristic of shivers syndrome. *J Am Vet Med Assoc* 215:1661–1665, 1999.

AUTHOR: **BETH A. VALENTINE**

EDITOR: **ANDRIS J. KANEPS**

Shock, Hypovolemic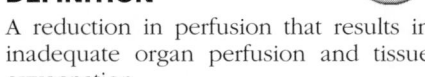

BASIC INFORMATION

DEFINITION

A reduction in perfusion that results in inadequate organ perfusion and tissue oxygenation

CLINICAL PRESENTATION

DISEASE FORMS/SUBTYPES

- Hemorrhagic
- Maldistributive (sepsis, endotoxemia)
- Traumatic

HISTORY, CHIEF COMPLAINT

- Ataxia, collapse
- History of observed trauma
- Weak, inappetent foals, often after dystocia
- History of overt hemorrhage or recent foaling
- Anorexia, colic, or signs of abdominal pain
- Increased respiratory rate or labored breathing

PHYSICAL EXAM FINDINGS Physical examination findings may be normal in early, compensated shock.

- Depression, stupor
- Tachycardia, bright-red mucous membranes (progressing to purple), poor pulse quality, physiologic murmurs
- Tachypnea, crackles, pleural friction rubs
- Reduced gastrointestinal borborygmi
- Hyperthermia or hypothermia

ETIOLOGY AND PATHOPHYSIOLOGY

- Etiology
  - Severe hemorrhage (guttural pouch mycosis, uterine artery rupture, trauma)
  - Sepsis (neonatal septicemia, enterocolitis, metritis, pleuritis)
  - Gastrointestinal accidents (large colon volvulus, gastric rupture) (Figure 1)
  - Hyperthermia (endurance rides, long distance hauling)
- Pathophysiology
  - Reduced tissue perfusion caused by a decrease in circulating volume

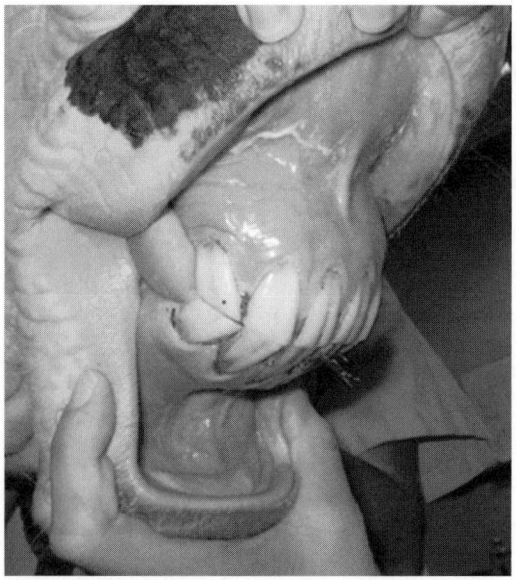

FIGURE 1 Hyperemic mucous membranes in a horse with a gastric rupture demonstrating hypovolemic shock caused by dehydration, systemic inflammation, and endotoxemia.

decreases the delivery of oxygen to tissues.

- Decreased circulating volume may result from loss of fluid (hemorrhage) or a relative decrease in volume (sepsis and endothelial disruption, causing vascular leak syndrome).
- Local hypoxia results in the conversion to anaerobic metabolism for energy production, with metabolic acids (lactate) as a byproduct.
- Severe blood loss (>40% of circulating volume) or hypovolemia with severe hypotension (mean pressures, 30–40 mm Hg) may lead to irreversible shock and death caused by:
  - Cellular dysfunction and death from free radical production
  - Activation of the inflammatory and coagulation cascades
  - Endothelial disruption permitting endotoxemia and bacterial translocation

DIAGNOSIS

DIFFERENTIAL DIAGNOSIS

- Cardiogenic
- Hypoxic
- Anaphylactic
- Neurogenic

INITIAL DATABASE

Hematocrit and hemoglobin may be normal in early hemorrhagic conditions.
- Complete blood count
- Packed cell volume (PCV) and total protein
- Serum chemistry
- Blood pressure
- Colloid oncotic pressure
- Serum lactate
- Coagulation profile

ADVANCED OR CONFIRMATORY TESTING

- Central venous pressure: Negative values may indicate hypovolemia (reference range, 2–15 cm H_2O)
- Ultrasonography of the abdomen or thorax (for specific infections, suspected rupture, or hemorrhage)
- Abdominocentesis or thoracocentesis to identify free fluid
- Coagulation profiles to monitor for disseminated intravascular coagulation (DIC)
- Endoscopy to identify guttural pouch mycosis
- Cortisol levels and response to an adrenocorticotropic hormone stimulation test to monitor appropriate endocrine response
- Cardiac output monitoring: Lithium dilution, echocardiography

TREATMENT

THERAPEUTIC GOAL(S)

Restore tissue perfusion and oxygenation

ACUTE GENERAL TREATMENT

- Cardiovascular support
  - Volume replacement
    - Shock-dose crystalloid fluids
    - Hypotensive resuscitation recommended in uncontrolled hemorrhage
      - Maintains hemostasis at the site of hemorrhage; does not dilute coagulation factors
      - Administer fluids at a 1 to 2:1 ratio to volume of blood lost.
      - Maintain a mean blood pressure of 60 mm Hg.
      - May also delay fluid administration until hemorrhage stopped if vasopressor support is provided
    - Colloids are recommended to prolong fluid effects and as therapy for vascular leakage.
    - Plasma (>1 L) may provide coagulation factors, fibronectin to reduce endotoxemia, and antiinflammatory protein C.
  - Positive ionotropes are recommended if volume resuscitation is inadequate.
    - Central venous pressure should be 3 to 12 cm H_2O in foals and up to 24 cm H_2O in adults
    - Dobutamine (2–15 µg/kg/min IV)
    - Dopamine (2–15 µg/kg/min IV)
  - Vasopressors only if fluids and ionotropes are unsuccessful or for delayed resuscitation
    - Norepinephrine (0.5 µg/kg/min IV)
    - Vasopressin (0.3–1 µg/kg/min IV): High doses of vasopressors may reduce splanchnic perfusion
- Oxygen supplementation (5–15 L/min)
  - Indicated with low PaO_2 (<70 mm Hg), PvO_2 (<35 mm Hg), and high lactate (>4 mmol/L)
  - Supplementation for low hemoglobin concentrations may be detrimental; induces temporary vasoconstriction
- Control of hemorrhage and PCV
  - Surgical hemostasis
  - Therapy for DIC
  - Hemoglobin replacement: Recommended for hemoglobin concentration below 7 g/dL, PCV below 15%, and lactate above 4 mmol/L
    - Blood transfusion
    - Autotransfusion of blood in body cavities
    - Hemoglobin-based fluids

- Oxyglobin (5–30 mL/kg, <10 mL/kg/h)
- Side effects include increased vascular resistance, formation of free radicals, methemoglobinemia, and fluid overload

DRUG INTERACTIONS

Calcium-containing crystalloid solutions may interfere with citrated blood transfusions.

POSSIBLE COMPLICATIONS

- Hypovolemia may lead to development of the systemic inflammatory response syndrome and multiorgan dysfunction (renal, pulmonary, cerebral, cardiac or hepatic dysfunction).
- Interstitial edema may result from overaggressive fluid therapy or endothelial compromise, which may inhibit oxygen diffusion into tissues.
- Conservative fluid management is required for congestive heart failure.
- May require earlier transfusions to support oxygenation.
- Maintain cerebral perfusion pressure with head trauma without fluid overload
  - Hypertonic saline
  - Mannitol

RECOMMENDED MONITORING

Repeat physical examinations, arterial blood pressure, central venous pressure, lactate, arterial and venous blood gas, urine output, colloid oncotic pressure, cardiac output

PROGNOSIS AND OUTCOME

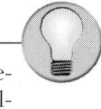

Depend on the success of treatment of the primary cause and rapid resolution of hypovolemic shock through normalization of physical parameters

PEARLS & CONSIDERATIONS

Goal-directed early management is key to reducing mortality from shock with goals of:
- Mean arterial pressure of 60 to 70 mm Hg
- Normal urine production
- Pink mucous membranes with a capillary refill of less than 3 seconds
- Warm extremities
- Normal central venous pressures
- Normalization of arterial and venous oxygen
- Blood lactate below 2 mmol/L
- Normalization of blood glucose

SUGGESTED READING

Driessen B, Brainard B: Fluid therapy for the traumatized patient. *J Vet Emerg Crit Care* 16(4):276–299, 2006.

Divers TJ: Shock and systemic inflammatory response syndrome. In Orsini JA, Divers TJ, editors: *Equine emergencies: treatment and procedures*, St Louis, 2008, Saunders Elsevier, pp 544–552.

Magdesian KG, Fielding CL, Rhodes DM, et al: Changes in central venous pressure and blood lactate concentration in response to acute blood loss in horses. *J Am Vet Med Assoc* 229(9):1458–1462, 2006.

AUTHOR: **AMELIA MUNSTERMAN**

EDITORS: **R. REID HANSON** and **AMELIA MUNSTERMAN**

Sinoatrial Block and Sinus Arrest

BASIC INFORMATION

DEFINITION

Failure of the sinus node to generate an impulse (sinus arrest) or failure of the generated pulse to "exit" the sinus node and depolarize the atria (sinoatrial block or sinus [exit] block)

EPIDEMIOLOGY

RISK FACTORS
- High vagal tone
- May occur in the immediate postexercise period

ASSOCIATED CONDITIONS AND DISORDERS Other vagally induced arrhythmias such as sinus bradycardia, sinus arrhythmia, first- or second-degree atrioventricular (AV) block

CLINICAL PRESENTATION

DISEASE FORMS/SUBTYPES
- Sinoatrial block
- Sinus arrest

HISTORY, CHIEF COMPLAINT
- Usually no complaints
- Drug administration
- On rare occasions associated with reduced performance, weakness, or syncope
- May suddenly (only) occur in the immediate postexercise period

PHYSICAL EXAM FINDINGS
- Often no clinical signs
- Pauses equal to or longer than twice the P-P interval during cardiac auscultation with absence of an atrial sound (Figure 1)
- Occasionally associated with weakness or syncope

ETIOLOGY AND PATHOPHYSIOLOGY
- High vagal tone
  - Physiologic
  - Vagal stimulation by surgery or a neoplastic process
  - Drugs
- Atrial myocardial lesions (fibrosis, cardiomyopathy)
- Electrolyte disorders

DIAGNOSIS

DIFFERENTIAL DIAGNOSIS
- Second-degree AV block: The atrial sound (S4) can be heard during the pause
- Sinus arrhythmia: Waxing and waning of heart rate
- Atrial fibrillation: Irregularly irregular rhythm

INITIAL DATABASE
- Cardiac auscultation
- Electrocardiogram (ECG) to make the diagnosis
  - A sudden pause without a P wave occurs during a normal to slow heart rate.
  - The duration of the pause is equal to (sinoatrial block) or longer than (sinus arrest) two normal P-P intervals.
  - Junctional or ventricular escape rhythms may occur during the pause.
  - The underlying rhythm is regular or may present slight variations in P-P intervals.
- The arrhythmia should disappear upon stress, exercise, or vagolytic drug administration (eg, atropine).
- Evaluate for electrolyte imbalances.

ADVANCED OR CONFIRMATORY TESTING
- Determine the presence of neoplastic processes along the vagal nerve.
- Exercise ECG
  - To check whether the arrhythmia disappears with exercise
  - To check if the arrhythmia occurs immediately postexercise
- Long-term ECG monitoring with permanent video monitoring of the animal if associated with syncope

TREATMENT

THERAPEUTIC GOAL(S)
- None if asymptomatic
- Treat the underlying cause
- Increase the heart rate

ACUTE GENERAL TREATMENT
- None if asymptomatic
- Treat the underlying cause such as electrolyte disorders
- Terminate drug administration that results in bradycardia and sinus block or arrest
- In case of syncope: Administer a vagolytic (0.005–0.01 mg/kg atropine IV or 0.005–0.01 mg/kg glycopyrrolate IV) or sympathomimetic (isoproterenol 0.1–0.2 μg/kg/min) drug

CHRONIC TREATMENT
- Treat the underlying cause such as a neoplastic process affecting the vagal nerve
- Permanent pacemaker implantation if associated with syncope

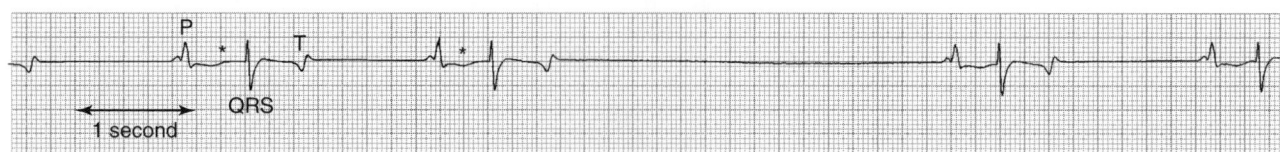

FIGURE 1 Sinus exit block in a healthy horse, appearing as a pause that is twice the normal P-P interval. P, QRS, and T-wave morphology are normal. Some P-Q intervals (*asterisk*) exceed 500 msec, indicating first-degree AV block. Both arrhythmias were caused by a high vagal tone and disappeared during exercise.

RECOMMENDED MONITORING

If symptomatic:
- Monitor heart rate and rhythm periodically
- Monitor exercise tolerance

PROGNOSIS AND OUTCOME

- Excellent if asymptomatic
- Depends on the underlying cause and the ability to successfully treat

SUGGESTED READING

Gasthuys F, Parmentier D, Goossens L, De Moor A: A preliminary study on the effects of atropine sulphate on bradycardia and heart blocks during romifidine sedation in the horse. *Vet Res Commun* 14:489–502, 1990.

McGuirk SM, Muir WW: Diagnosis and treatment of cardiac arrhythmias. *Vet Clin North Am Equine Pract* 1:353–370, 1985.

Reef VB: Arrhythmias. In Marr CM, editor: *Cardiology of the horse*, London, 1999, WB Saunders, pp 179–209.

van Loon G, Fonteyne W, Rottiers H, et al: Implantation of a dual-chamber, rate-adaptive pacemaker in a horse with suspected sick sinus syndrome. *Vet Rec* 151:541–545, 2002.

van Loon G, Laevens H, Deprez P: Temporary transvenous atrial pacing in horses: threshold determination. *Equine Vet J* 33:290–295, 2001.

AUTHOR: **GUNTHER VAN LOON**

EDITOR: **MARY M. DURANDO**

Sinonasal Cysts

BASIC INFORMATION

DEFINITION

Paranasal sinus cysts are benign, expansile masses originating from the paranasal sinuses. They consist of two separate clinical entities, developmental and acquired. Developmental cysts occur in young horses and are usually of dental origin. Acquired cysts are of unknown cause but may share a common pathogenesis with ethmoid hematoma.

EPIDEMIOLOGY

SPECIES, AGE, SEX Developmental sinus cysts typically affect horses younger than 3 years. There is no known breed or sex predilection. A variety of breeds have been diagnosed with congenital sinus cysts, including miniature and full-size horses. Acquired sinus cysts are most frequently diagnosed in horses ranging from 10 to 20 years of age.

ASSOCIATED CONDITIONS AND DISORDERS Horses with sinus cysts are typically affected with concurrent sinus empyema.

CLINICAL PRESENTATION

HISTORY, CHIEF COMPLAINT
- The most common clinical history for paranasal cysts is facial distortion and/or mucopurulent nasal discharge nonresponsive to antimicrobial therapy. Horses initially respond to antimicrobial therapy with a return to nasal discharge after antimicrobial therapy has been discontinued.
- Horses with occlusion of the nasal passage with a cystic mass may present with upper respiratory tract noise and decreased air flow on the affected side. Additional clinical signs associated with sinus cysts include a soft, fluctuant mass located under the skin; exophthalmos; and epiphora.

PHYSICAL EXAM FINDINGS Abnormal physical examination findings associated with sinus cysts include unilateral or bilateral mucopurulent nasal discharge; upper respiratory noise; decreased airflow from the affected nasal passage; facial bone distortion; a soft, fluctuant mass located under the skin; exophthalmos; and epiphora.

ETIOLOGY AND PATHOPHYSIOLOGY
- Developmental sinus cysts originate from abnormal dentigerous structures.
- In some instances, abnormally formed teeth can be identified after radiographic imaging of the skull.
- Acquired sinus cysts may form secondary to chronic submucosal hemorrhage.
- Some investigators believe these cysts share a common pathogenesis with ethmoid hematoma.
- Regardless of the origin, sinus cysts result in clinical signs after secondary sinusitis or sinus empyema. Large cystic structures can impede normal drainage from the maxillary or frontal sinuses. Secondary sinusitis is most likely the direct result of the prevention of normal drainage from the paranasal sinuses.
- Large, expansive cysts can also obstruct the nasal passage and lead to distortion of the facial bones and other clinical signs. Additional clinical signs of sinus cysts include exophthalmos and epiphora.

DIAGNOSIS

DIFFERENTIAL DIAGNOSIS
- Primary and secondary sinusitis
- Ethmoid hematoma (without epistaxis)
- Neoplasia
- Fungal sinusitis

INITIAL DATABASE
- Endoscopy: Endoscopic findings compatible with sinus cysts include one or more of the following: narrowing or complete blockage of the nasal passage; visible smooth, thin-walled cystlike structures; and mucopurulent discharge
- Skull radiography: A minimum of four radiographic views of the paranasal sinuses should be obtained—the dorsoventral, lateral, and left and right oblique views of the frontal and maxillary sinuses. Radiographic abnormalities associated with sinus cysts include fluid lines, the presence of a smooth mass in the absence of bone destruction, increased opacification of the affected sinus, and abnormally shaped cheek teeth in some cases.
- Oral examination: Should be performed to rule out dental abnormalities that may also lead to secondary sinusitis
- Complete blood count (CBC) and fibrinogen: Most horses with sinus cysts have normal CBC and fibrinogen levels.
- Sinocentesis: This technique is performed in the standing horse. A 3- to 5-mm Steinmann pin inserted into a Jacob's pin chuck can be used to create an opening into the frontal or maxillary sinus. A 14- to 18-gauge needle or teat cannula is inserted into the affected sinus (as determined by radiography), and a fluid aspirate is obtained. Horses affected with sinus cysts have a characteristic yellow, clear to mucinous fluid located within the cyst. This finding is pathognomonic for this condition.

ADVANCED OR CONFIRMATORY TESTING
- Computed tomography (CT): CT is available in referral centers and can be

very useful in determining the origin and location(s) of the cystic structures.

- Sinoscopy: This surgical technique can be useful in confirming the preoperative diagnosis, collecting tissue or fluid samples for biopsy or cytology, and preoperative planning but can result in complications if a flap sinusotomy is pursued later.
- Histopathology of biopsy samples or after surgical removal: Histopathology should be performed on all cases suspected of sinus cysts to confirm the diagnosis. Although the histologic diagnosis may be of an ethmoid hematoma, the cysts removed from clinically affected horses do not have the gross appearance of an ethmoid hematoma.

TREATMENT

THERAPEUTIC GOAL(S)

Surgical removal of the cystic structure and the establishment of drainage from the affected paranasal sinus is the primary therapeutic goal.

ACUTE GENERAL TREATMENT

- Preoperative antimicrobials (procaine penicillin G, 22,000 IU/kg IM q12h, or potassium penicillin G, 22,000 IU/kg IV q6h), and antiinflammatories (phenylbutazone, 2.2–4.4 mg/kg PO or IV q12h, or flunixin meglumine, 1.1 mg/kg IV q12h)
- To combat the effects of potential blood loss, horses can be preloaded with fluids delivered via a large-bore catheter. Blood transfusions are rarely needed.
- Osteoplastic bone flap to access the cystic structure: The cystic lining is

manually removed from the interior of the affected sinus. After the cystic lining has been completely removed, a new fistula can be surgically created between the affected sinus and the nasal passage. If required, nasal turbinates and concha can be removed to ensure an adequately sized opening. Creating a large fistula between the sinus and nasal passage can limit the chance of recurrent sinus empyema and facilitate postoperative monitoring of the affected sinus with endoscopy.

POSSIBLE COMPLICATIONS

- Blood loss after surgical removal may require a whole blood transfusion. Fortunately, this is rarely needed.
- The removal of abnormally shaped or formed cheek teeth can require surgical management of the opening between the sinus and oral cavity. Closure of the alveolus is important to prevent the formation of sino-oral fistula.

RECOMMENDED MONITORING

Horses should be monitored with endoscopy at intervals ranging from 6 months to 1 year to ensure satisfactory healing of the sinus after surgical removal of the cyst.

PROGNOSIS AND OUTCOME

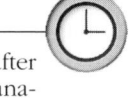

- The prognosis for horses after surgical removal of a paranasal sinus cyst is good.
- Complications after surgical removal are rare.
- Cosmetic issues with healing of the osteoplastic flap rarely occur.

PEARLS & CONSIDERATIONS

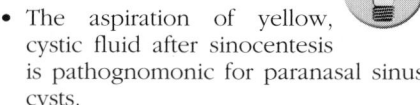

- The aspiration of yellow, cystic fluid after sinocentesis is pathognomonic for paranasal sinus cysts.
- Owners should be encouraged to pursue surgical resolution because the prognosis after surgery is favorable.
- Surgeons should not be afraid to create a new, large opening between the affected sinus and the nasal passage. The author has recognized no complications after this procedure. The benefits of excellent drainage and ease of postoperative endoscopy far outweigh any potential for problems associated with creation of the new opening.

SUGGESTED READING

Beard WL, Robertson JT, Leeth B: Bilateral congenital cysts in the frontal sinuses of a horse. *J Am Vet Med Assoc* 196:453–454, 1990.

Cannon JH, Grant BD, Sande RD: Diagnosis and surgical treatment of cystlike lesions of the equine paranasal sinuses. *J Am Vet Med Assoc* 169:610–613, 1976.

Lane JG, Longstaffe JA, Gibbs C: Equine paranasal sinus cysts: a report of 15 cases. *Equine Vet J* 19:537–544, 1987.

Sanders-Shamis M, Robertson JT: Congenital sinus cyst in a foal. *J Am Vet Med Assoc* 190:1011–1012, 1987.

Woodford NS, Lane JG: Long-term retrospective study of 52 horses with sinonasal cysts. *Equine Vet J* 38:198–202, 2006.

AUTHOR: **JAN F. HAWKINS**

EDITOR: **ERIC J. PARENTE**

Sinus Arrhythmia

BASIC INFORMATION

DEFINITION

A cyclic irregularity in sinus rhythm with a waxing and waning of heart rate. P, QRS, and T waves have a normal morphology and relation, but there is a cyclic increase and decrease in P-P interval. Many cases present a sudden prolongation of the P-P interval followed by a progressive shortening of the P-P interval after which the cycle is repeated again.

SYNONYM(S)

Sinus dysrhythmia

EPIDEMIOLOGY

GENETICS AND BREED PREDISPOSITION Occurs more frequently in horses than in ponies

RISK FACTORS Occurs most frequently in the postexercise period, when the heart rate drops to between 120 and 50 beats/min

ASSOCIATED CONDITIONS AND DISORDERS Other vagally induced arrhythmias such as first- and second-degree atrioventricular (AV) block

CLINICAL PRESENTATION

HISTORY, CHIEF COMPLAINT

- Usually no complaints; an incidental finding
- Occurs typically after exercise or stress, when an elevated heart rate returns to normal

PHYSICAL EXAM FINDINGS

- Waxing and waning of heart rate on auscultation (can be very obvious)
- No other abnormalities

ETIOLOGY AND PATHOPHYSIOLOGY

- This physiologic arrhythmia occurs because of (an increasing) vagal tone.

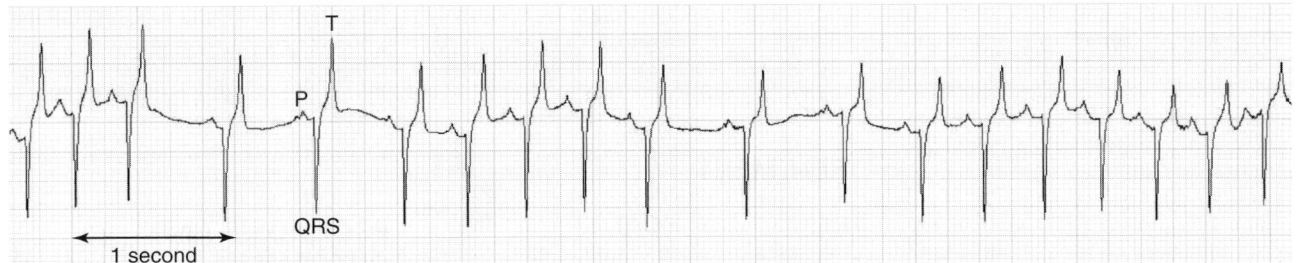

FIGURE 1 Sinus arrhythmia in a healthy horse recorded during recovery from exercise. A sudden P-P interval prolongation occurs, followed by a progressive P-P shortening. Subsequently, a long P-P interval occurs and the cycle is repeated.

- Most frequently found during the recovery phase after exercise, when the heart rate decreases. It usually occurs when the heart rate is between 120 and 50 beats/min.
- May also be found at rest, when the heart rate is low.

DIAGNOSIS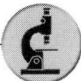

DIFFERENTIAL DIAGNOSIS

- Isolated atrial premature beats: One or more P waves occur earlier than expected while the underlying rhythm is regular.
- Atrial fibrillation (AF): Cardiac rhythm in animals with AF is more irregular than in those with sinus arrhythmia. In addition, AF remains irregular at rest, but sinus arrhythmia usually becomes regular when the heart rate returns to normal.
- Sinus exit block and second-degree AV block may occasionally be confused with sinus arrhythmia during auscultation after exercise because of

a rapid decrease in heart rate and the longer diastolic period.
- Sinus arrest: Appears as sudden pause, greater than two R-R intervals.
- Electrocardiography (ECG) is required to make a final diagnosis.

INITIAL DATABASE

- ECG
  - Normal morphology of P wave, QRS complex, and T wave. Slight variations in P-wave morphology are occasionally seen.
  - Normal relation between P, QRS, and T wave within a cardiac cycle.
  - P-P intervals vary, usually in a cyclic way, resulting in a cyclic increase and decrease in heart rate (accordionlike). Many cases present with a sudden prolongation of the P-P interval followed by a progressive shortening of the P-P interval after which the cycle is repeated again.
- Stress, exercise, or administration of a vagolytic agent should terminate the arrhythmia.
- An exercise ECG is useful to show the condition immediately after exercise.

TREATMENT

THERAPEUTIC GOAL(S)

Sinus arrhythmia is a physiologic phenomenon that does not require therapy.

ACUTE GENERAL TREATMENT

No treatment is necessary because the arrhythmia is physiologic.

PROGNOSIS AND OUTCOME

Excellent

SUGGESTED READING

Bonagura JD, Reef VB, Schwarzwald CC: Cardiovascular diseases. In Reed SM, Bayly WM, Sellon DC, editors: *Equine internal medicine*, ed 3, St Louis, 2010, Saunders Elsevier, pp 372–487.
McGuirk SM, Muir WW: Diagnosis and treatment of cardiac arrhythmias. *Vet Clin North Am Equine Pract* 1:353–370, 1985.

AUTHOR: GUNTHER VAN LOON

EDITOR: MARY M. DURANDO

Sinus Bradycardia

BASIC INFORMATION

DEFINITION

A sinus rhythm with a heart rate of less than 24 beats/min

EPIDEMIOLOGY

RISK FACTORS High vagal tone
ASSOCIATED CONDITIONS AND DISORDERS Other arrhythmias associated with a high vagal tone such as sinus arrhythmia, sinoatrial block, first- or second-degree atrioventricular (AV) block

CLINICAL PRESENTATION

DISEASE FORMS/SUBTYPES

- Physiologic form caused by the horse's vagal tone: Asymptomatic, and bradycardia disappears with stress or exercise
- Pathologic form caused by underlying disease: May or may not be associated with clinical signs

HISTORY, CHIEF COMPLAINT

- Usually incidental finding; asymptomatic
- Administration of drugs
- Poor performance, exercise intolerance

- Head trauma (increased intracranial pressure [ICP])
- Systemic disease
- Syncope

PHYSICAL EXAM FINDINGS

- Normal, alert animal or depression and weakness if bradycardia is severe
- Slow heart rate (<24 beats/min), which can be regular or irregular (if associated with other vagally induced arrhythmias)
- Signs of head trauma
- Hypothermia

ETIOLOGY AND PATHOPHYSIOLOGY

- High vagal tone (caused by eye pressure during ophthalmic surgery, increased ICP, hypothermia)

- Systemic disease
- Electrolyte disturbances (calcium, magnesium, and especially potassium). Foals with urinary bladder rupture and hyperkalemia are at an increased risk of developing bradycardia during anesthesia.
- Sinoatrial node disease
- Administration of drugs (digoxin, verapamil, diltiazem, sedatives, and anesthetics)
- Hypothyroidism

DIAGNOSIS

Diagnosis is made by electrocardiography. Further tests (blood examination, echocardiography, are necessary to look for underlying disease.

DIFFERENTIAL DIAGNOSIS

- Sinus block, sinus arrest
- Second-degree AV block
- Third-degree AV block

INITIAL DATABASE

- Electrocardiography (ECG) to make a definitive diagnosis
  - Normal morphology of P wave, QRS complex and T wave
  - Normal relation between P, QRS, and T wave within the cardiac cycle
  - P-P interval is prolonged, resulting in a slow heart rate (<24 beats/min).
- Long-term ECG monitoring with permanent video monitoring of the animal, especially when associated with syncope
- Blood analysis, serum biochemistry (electrolyte disturbance, systemic disease)
- Neurologic examination

ADVANCED OR CONFIRMATORY TESTING

- Echocardiography to look for cardiac (atrial myocardial) disease
- Stress test with continuous ECG monitoring to investigate chronotropic competence. This can be done by excitation, atropine administration, or a standard exercise test.
- Thyroid function tests

- In case of suspected intracranial disease: Cerebrospinal fluid analysis, computed tomography, magnetic resonance imaging

TREATMENT

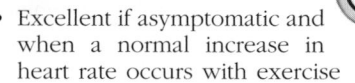

THERAPEUTIC GOAL(S)

- No treatment if asymptomatic
- Increase heart rate

ACUTE GENERAL TREATMENT

- Usually no treatment (ie, when the arrhythmia is asymptomatic).
- Treat electrolyte disturbances.
- Treat underlying disease.
- Terminate administration of drugs that cause bradycardia.
- If associated with severe clinical signs (eg, syncope, collapse): Administer vagolytic drug (atropine 0.01 mg/kg IV); if no increase in heart rate occurs, administer sympathomimetic drug (isoproterenol constant rate infusion at 0.1–0.2 µg/kg/min) or catecholamines (dobutamine, dopamine, epinephrine).
- If no reaction to medical treatment, transvenous temporary pacing can be performed.

CHRONIC TREATMENT

- Administration of clenbuterol or theophylline might be attempted.
- Transvenous implantation of a permanent pacemaker. In cases with normal chronotropic competence during exercise, a single-chamber ventricular pacemaker is technically the easiest model to implant and is sufficient to prevent clinical signs.

POSSIBLE COMPLICATIONS

- Side effects of theophylline
- Side effects of atropine (especially gastrointestinal complications)
- Complications of pacemaker implantation
- Foals with urinary bladder rupture and hyperkalemia undergoing surgery are at increased risk of developing sinus bradycardia as well as cardiac arrest or ventricular fibrillation during anesthesia.

RECOMMENDED MONITORING

- None if asymptomatic
- Repeated long-term ECG monitoring to observe effect of treatment and evolution of the bradycardia
- Follow-up of pacemaker function

PROGNOSIS AND OUTCOME

- Excellent if asymptomatic and when a normal increase in heart rate occurs with exercise
- When secondary to other disease: Depends on the prognosis of the underlying disease
- Good with pacemaker implantation

PEARLS & CONSIDERATIONS

The environment of a horse with syncope should be adapted to minimize trauma to the animal (wall and floor protection). Owners need to be aware of the danger of a collapsing horse. Because of these dangers, the recommendation should be that these animals never be ridden.

SUGGESTED READING

Bonagura JD, Reef VB, Schwarzwald CC: Cardiovascular diseases. In Reed SM, Bayly WM, Sellon DC, editors: Equine internal medicine, ed 3, St Louis, 2010, Saunders Elsevier, pp 372–487.

Reef VB: Arrhythmias. In Marr CM, editor: Cardiology of the horse, London, 1999, WB Saunders, pp 179–209.

Schwarzwald CC, Bonagura JD, Luis-Fuentes V: Effects of diltiazem on hemodynamic variables and ventricular function in healthy horses. J Vet Intern Med 19:703–711, 2005.

van Loon G, Fonteyne W, Rottiers H, et al: Dual chamber pacemaker implantation via the cephalic vein in healthy equids. J Vet Intern Med 15:564–571, 2001.

van Loon G, Laevens H, Deprez P: Temporary transvenous atrial pacing in horses: threshold determination. Equine Vet J 33:290–295, 2001.

AUTHOR: **GUNTHER VAN LOON**

EDITOR: **MARY M. DURANDO**

Sinus Tachycardia

BASIC INFORMATION

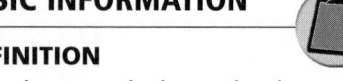

DEFINITION

A regular sinus rhythm with a heart rate above 50 to 60 beats/min (normal ranges

may vary among breeds, and fit, athletic horses have a lower normal heart rate range)

CLINICAL PRESENTATION

DISEASE FORMS/SUBTYPES

- Primary sinus tachycardia: Caused by stress, pain, or physical exercise

- Secondary sinus tachycardia: Response to underlying disease or drugs

HISTORY, CHIEF COMPLAINT
- Known episodes of stress, pain, or physical exercise
- Concurrent disease causing fever, hypovolemia, anemia, hypoxemia, hypotension, and catecholamine release (eg, pheochromocytoma)
- Administration of vagolytic (atropine), sympathomimetic or phosphodiesterase inhibitory (theophylline) drugs

PHYSICAL EXAM FINDINGS
- Tachycardia (heart rate >50–60 beats/min)
- Signs associated with underlying disease such as
  - Fever
  - Increased capillary refill time and weak pulse (hypotension, hypovolemia)
  - Pale or cyanotic mucous membranes (anemia, hypoxemia)
  - Signs of heart failure

ETIOLOGY AND PATHOPHYSIOLOGY
- Occurs in an otherwise healthy animal as a response to stress, fear, or exercise caused by a change in vagal and sympathetic tone
- Occurs because of an increased sympathetic tone as a response to fever, hypovolemia (shock, blood loss), anemia, hypoxemia, hypotension, or catecholamine release (pheochromocytoma)
- Occurs as a compensatory mechanism in case of heart failure
- Occurs in response to drug administration
- Hyperthyroidism
- Intoxication

DIAGNOSIS

Diagnosis is made by electrocardiography (ECG). Further tests are necessary to look for underlying disease.

DIFFERENTIAL DIAGNOSIS
- Atrial tachycardia: Based on an ambulatory ECG alone, it may be impossible to differentiate between sinus tachycardia and atrial tachycardia because both may appear identical on ECG.
- Ventricular tachycardia: QRS complexes with abnormal morphology and duration not associated with preceding P wave.

INITIAL DATABASE
- ECG for making a diagnosis
  - Normal morphology of P wave, QRS complex, and T wave.
  - Normal relation between P, QRS, and T wave within a cardiac cycle.
  - PP interval is shortened, resulting in a high heart rate (>50–60 beats/min).
  - At higher rates, the P wave may be buried in the preceding T wave.
  - Sinus tachycardia and atrial tachycardia may have a similar appearance on the ECG.
- Capillary refill time, facial pulse, presence of ventral edema, jugular pulsation, and signs of heart failure
- Cardiac auscultation to check for cardiac murmur (heart failure)
- Packed cell volume and total protein to check for hypovolemia and anemia
- White blood cell count, fibrinogen, and protein electrophoresis to check for infection or inflammation
- Biochemistry to check for electrolyte imbalances
- Echocardiography to diagnose reduced cardiac output, heart failure, or cause of hypotension
- Blood pressure monitoring (direct or indirect) to assess hypotension

ADVANCED OR CONFIRMATORY TESTING
- Arterial blood gas analysis to check for hypoxemia
- Determine catecholamines to check for pheochromocytoma

TREATMENT

THERAPEUTIC GOAL(S)
Attempts to reduce heart rate should not be made when sinus tachycardia occurs as a compensatory mechanism to hypotension, anemia, hypovolemia, and hypoxemia. Treat the underlying disease in these cases.

ACUTE GENERAL TREATMENT
- No treatment when caused by exercise or temporary stress
- Avoid stressors or fear; put the horse in a calming environment
- Analgesia and treatment of the cause of pain
- IV fluids (hypotension, hypovolemia)
- Intranasal oxygen (hypoxemia, anemia)
- Blood transfusion (anemia)
- Terminate drug administration that results in tachycardia
- Treat fever (nonsteroidal antiinflammatory drugs, antimicrobials)
- Treat heart failure (digoxin, furosemide, angiotensin-converting enzyme inhibitors)

CHRONIC TREATMENT
Treat heart failure or other underlying disease

PROGNOSIS AND OUTCOME

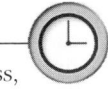

- Excellent in case of stress, fear, or exercise
- Otherwise, depends on underlying cause

PEARLS & CONSIDERATIONS

The horse should be rested and kept in a quiet environment until normalization of the arrhythmia and resolution of underlying problem.

SUGGESTED READING
Bonagura JD, Reef VB, Schwarzwald CC: Cardiovascular diseases. In Reed SM, Bayly WM, Sellon DC, editors: *Equine internal medicine*, ed 3, St Louis, 2010, Saunders Elsevier, pp 372–487.

AUTHOR: **GUNTHER VAN LOON**

EDITOR: **MARY M. DURANDO**

Sinusitis, Primary

BASIC INFORMATION

DEFINITION
An inflammatory process of the paranasal sinus system caused by bacterial upper respiratory tract infection

EPIDEMIOLOGY

SPECIES, AGE, SEX Primary sinusitis can affect horses of all ages with a reported higher incidence in 6- to 8-year-old animals.

RISK FACTORS
- Viral infections of the upper airway can cause swelling of the respiratory mucosal lining of the paranasal sinuses that is severe enough to occlude the nasomaxillary opening and therefore

prevent drainage of mucus from the sinus system into the nasal cavity. The accumulation of discharge within the sinuses can cause sinusitis and is more commonly observed in young horses.

- Horses with a compromised immune system (eg, Cushing's disease) also appear to be more prone to develop sinusitis.

ASSOCIATED CONDITIONS AND DISORDERS

- In chronic cases, the disease process may progress to bone involvement (osteitis) and become a therapeutic challenge.
- Some cases of primary sinusitis may be difficult to distinguish from secondary sinusitis (see "Sinusitis, Secondary" in this section).

CLINICAL PRESENTATION

DISEASE FORMS/SUBTYPES

- Horses present with different degrees of pathology. Horses with mild and early diagnosed forms may respond well to treatment with the appropriate antimicrobial medication alone.
- Horses with more severe or more chronic sinusitis require more aggressive therapy ranging from repeated lavage to sinotomy and surgical debridement.

HISTORY, CHIEF COMPLAINT Purulent or mucopurulent nasal discharge is the major presenting complaint in primary sinusitis. Only rarely is the nasal discharge bilateral. The owner may notice the nasal discharge during or after exercising the horse or while the animal holds its head down or even at rest with a normal head position.

PHYSICAL EXAM FINDINGS

- Unilateral nasal discharge is most commonly observed. In primary sinusitis, facial swelling is rare and, if present, may not be noticed by the owner. About 20% of cases with primary sinusitis have epiphora caused by interference with the nasolacrimal duct.
- If the ventral concha is affected, a partial nasal obstruction with subsequent respiratory noise may be detectable. The presence of discharge within the maxillary or frontoconchal sinuses changes the character of sound upon percussion of the respective regions. In about two-thirds of primary sinusitis cases, the submandibular lymph nodes are enlarged.

ETIOLOGY AND PATHOPHYSIOLOGY Commonly isolated microorganisms are *Streptococcus equi* subsp. *equi*, *Streptococcus equi* subsp. *zooepidemicus*, and *Staphylococcus* spp.

DIAGNOSIS

DIFFERENTIAL DIAGNOSIS

- Secondary sinusitis: Dental diseases, sinus cysts, sinus neoplasia, progressive ethmoid hematoma
- Other diseases with nasal discharge: Guttural pouch empyema, bronchitis

INITIAL DATABASE

- Purulent or mucopurulent nasal discharge
- Facial swelling
- Epiphora
- Endoscopy (discharge draining from the nasomaxillary opening)
- Radiography (fluid lines, gas-fluid interfaces within the sinuses, opacity in the region of the ventral concha)
- Bacterial culture

ADVANCED OR CONFIRMATORY TESTING

- Cross-sectional imaging techniques, such as computed tomography (CT) and magnetic resonance imaging (MRI), may be helpful in ruling out other causes of sinusitis.
- Scintigraphy has proven to be useful in distinguishing primary from secondary sinusitis.
- Direct sinoscopy via trephine holes if radiography or endoscopy is inconclusive

TREATMENT

THERAPEUTIC GOAL(S)

Eradication of causative bacteria and subsequent resolution of the clinical symptoms

ACUTE GENERAL TREATMENT

- In mild and early diagnosed cases, appropriate antimicrobial agents based on bacterial culture and sensitivity testing may be successful. Usually 4 to 6 weeks of treatment is required to prevent recurrence.
- In more advanced forms of sinusitis, antimicrobial treatment alone may not be sufficient and must be accompanied by removing the mucopurulent discharge from the sinus involved by lavage. Sinus lavage can be done via trephine holes most commonly created into the frontal sinus with warm 0.9% saline solution. This treatment can be repeated twice daily and may be necessary until the draining fluid clears up.
- In more chronic cases, an indwelling catheter (Foley) can be implanted into the frontal sinus or less common into the maxillary sinus for repeated lavage over a prolonged period of time.

- In refractory cases, a more aggressive surgical approach may become necessary to remove inspissated pus or infected soft tissue that cannot be drained out via lavage. Therefore, a sinusotomy (bone flap technique) provides access to the affected sinus and permits removal of necrotic tissue and inspissated pus and can be used to establish drainage into the nasal cavity. This can be done with the horse standing or with the horse under general anesthesia.

POSSIBLE COMPLICATIONS

Successful treatment, especially of horses with chronic sinusitis, can be complicated by progression of the bacterial infection into deeper structures such as bone leading to osteitis with bone necrosis and abscess formation. The removal of inspissated pus from the ventral concha almost always requires surgical opening of the concha and may be complicated by bleeding and prolonged aftercare.

RECOMMENDED MONITORING

- Clinical signs of sinusitis such as nasal discharge
- Repeated radiographic or endoscopic examination

PROGNOSIS AND OUTCOME

With appropriate treatment, the prognosis is good. One study showed a successful long-term outcome of 84%.

PEARLS & CONSIDERATIONS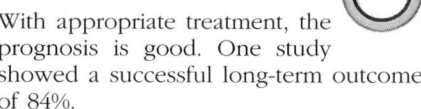

COMMENTS

- In some cases, it is difficult to distinguish primary from secondary sinusitis. Antimicrobial therapy alone may only be successful in very mild cases of sinusitis or when the diagnosis could be made quickly after the onset of symptoms.
- Treatment of more severe cases can be time and cost intensive.
- Expensive and more invasive diagnostic tools such as CT or MRI may have to be used to rule out subtle causes of secondary sinusitis.

PREVENTION

Horses with Cushing disease should be treated accordingly (see "Cushing's Disease" in this section).

SUGGESTED READING

Barakzai S, Tremaine H, Dixon P: Use of scintigraphy for diagnosis of equine paranasal sinus disorders. *Vet Surg* 35:94–101, 2006.

Tremaine WH, Dixon PM: A long-term study of 277 cases of equine sinonasal disease.

Part 1: details of horses, historical, clinical and ancillary diagnostic findings. *Equine Vet J* 33:274–282, 2001.

Tremaine WH, Dixon PM: A long-term study of 277 cases of equine sinonasal disease.

Part 2: treatments and results of treatments. *Equine Vet J* 33:283–289, 2001.

AUTHOR: **KARSTEN VELDE**

EDITOR: **ERIC J. PARENTE**

Sinusitis, Secondary

BASIC INFORMATION

DEFINITION

Secondary sinusitis is an inflammatory disease process localized to the paranasal sinus system in response to a variety of different primary pathologies, including:

- Dental diseases (dental sinusitis)
- Sinus cysts
- Sinus neoplasia
- Progressive ethmoid hematoma
- Trauma to the paranasal sinus system
- Mycotic sinusitis

EPIDEMIOLOGY

SPECIES, AGE, SEX The age distribution of secondary sinusitis depends on the underlying disease process but can span a wide range. Whereas dental sinusitis is less common in horses younger than 4 years of age, sinus neoplasia has been found in foals. The mean age with which horses are presented with secondary sinusitis ranges between 7 and 14 years.

RISK FACTORS

- As with primary sinusitis, horses with a compromised immune system (Cushing's disease) appear to be more prone to developing dental sinusitis.
- Because dental sinusitis is the most common form of secondary sinusitis, any dental pathology involving the fourth premolar through the third molar in the maxilla (108–111, 208–211 according to the Triadan system) may lead to secondary sinusitis.

ASSOCIATED CONDITIONS AND DISORDERS

- Space-occupying processes such as neoplasia, sinus cysts, and progressive ethmoid hematoma may lead to obstruction of one or both (if bilateral) nasal passages. Consequently, these animals exhibit abnormal respiratory noises. In rare cases of severe airway obstruction, a tracheotomy may become necessary. The space-occupying processes may not only compromise airflow but are also responsible for the considerably higher incidence of facial distortion and swelling in secondary compared with primary sinusitis. The expansion of neoplasia, sinus cysts, or progressive ethmoid hematomas may also cause pressure necrosis of various tissues within the sinus system or nasal cavity.

- Tooth root infections and abscesses may progress to the surrounding bone, causing osteitis.

- Disease processes that are localized in close proximity to the cribriform lamina, such as progressive ethmoid hematoma or trauma, may cause neurologic symptoms and may even lead to life-threatening meningitis.

CLINICAL PRESENTATION

DISEASE FORMS/SUBTYPES Secondary sinusitis is the common feature of the above-mentioned underlying pathologic processes; however, each original process leading to secondary sinusitis must be recognized as a distinct disease that requires specific treatment.

HISTORY, CHIEF COMPLAINT Owners may observe nasal discharge of different quantity and variable character ranging from purulent or mucopurulent and malodorous (dental sinusitis) to bloody or blood tinged in progressive ethmoid hematomas. Facial swelling is more likely present in secondary than in primary sinusitis cases. Other clinical signs the owners may observe are epiphora and abnormal respiratory noises. In some cases of dental sinusitis, the primary dental pathology may cause an abnormal chewing pattern or result in a prolonged time period the horse needs to finish a meal.

PHYSICAL EXAM FINDINGS

- Unilateral nasal discharge is most commonly observed followed by facial swelling. The character of the nasal discharge may give a hint to the underlying pathology. Facial swelling frequently accompanies secondary sinusitis caused by sinus neoplasia, sinus cyst, and dental sinusitis in decreasing order. When the disease involves the maxillary sinus, epiphora is more likely.

- Horses with sinonasal growths (neoplasia, cysts, and progressive ethmoid hematoma) can have a partial nasal airflow obstruction, leading to abnormal respiratory noises. Lymphadenopathy of the ipsilateral mandibular lymph nodes is more common in neoplasia, mycotic sinusitis, and dental sinusitis than in cases with progressive ethmoid hematoma.

ETIOLOGY AND PATHOPHYSIOLOGY

- Depends highly on the underlying pathology

- Commonly isolated microorganisms are *Streptococcus equi* subsp. *equi*, *Streptococcus equi,* subsp. *zooepidemicus,* and *Staphylococcus* spp., similar to primary sinusitis.

- Direct infection of the sinus system: Ascending pathway in dental sinusitis or direct penetrating wounds in traumatic sinusitis.

- Indirect infection of the sinus system: Sinus cysts, neoplasia, polyps, and progressive ethmoid hematomas may cause indirect infection by diminishing the mucociliary clearance of the respiratory mucosa with subsequent decreased local immunity.

DIAGNOSIS

DIFFERENTIAL DIAGNOSIS

- Primary sinusitis
- Other diseases with nasal discharge (guttural pouch empyema, bronchitis)
- Other diseases causing epistaxis (guttural pouch mycosis, exercise-induced pulmonary hemorrhage)

INITIAL DATABASE

- Purulent or mucopurulent or blood-tinged nasal discharge
- Facial swelling
- Epiphora
- Endoscopy: Discharge draining from the nasomaxillary opening or direct visualization of a possible sinonasal growth (progressive ethmoid hematoma, neoplasia, cyst, polyp)
- Radiography: Fluid lines, gas-fluid interfaces within the sinuses, opacity in the region of the ventral concha, increased soft tissue density (cysts, neoplasia, progressive ethmoid hematoma) or pathology associated with the tooth roots of the four last cheek

teeth (radiolucency and peripheral sclerosis of alveolar bone surrounding the dental apices, widened periodontal space, diastemata, supernumerary or displaced teeth)
- Bacterial culture (in chronic cases, the etiologic significance may be questionable)
- Oral examination to assess potential defects or fractures that could result in ascending infection

ADVANCED OR CONFIRMATORY TESTING

- Cross-sectional imaging techniques such as computed tomography (CT) or magnetic resonance imaging (MRI) are helpful in diagnosing the causes for the secondary sinusitis and showing the extent of the lesion in multiple dimensions and are often used for pre-operative planning.
- Scintigraphy has proven to be useful in distinguishing primary from secondary sinusitis and showed an excellent sensitivity in dental sinusitis cases.
- Direct sinoscopy via trephine holes should be considered if radiography and endoscopy are inconclusive
- Histopathology of biopsy specimens of a sinus mass will confirm the diagnosis.

TREATMENT

THERAPEUTIC GOAL(S)

Eradication of underlying pathology causing secondary sinusitis and subsequent resolution of clinical symptoms

ACUTE GENERAL TREATMENT

- Surgical intervention performed either on a standing sedated horse or under general anesthesia is required in most cases of secondary sinusitis to remove the underlying pathology. A variety of surgical procedures is available, and the appropriate treatment must be selected according to the causative pathologic process.
- Surgical procedures under general anesthesia
  - Dorsofrontal or maxillary bone flaps (cheek teeth repulsion, removal of

sinus cysts, neoplasia and progressive ethmoid hematomas)
  - Reconstruction of wounds after trauma
- Surgical procedures on the standing, sedated horse
  - Dorsofrontal or maxillary bone flaps (cheek teeth repulsion, removal of sinus cysts, neoplasia, and progressive ethmoid hematomas in selected cases)
  - Transendoscopic laser ablation (progressive ethmoid hematoma, sinus cysts, sinus polyps)
  - Transendoscopic formalin injection (progressive ethmoid hematoma)
  - Tooth extraction
  - Reconstruction of traumatic wounds in selected cases
  - Sinoscopy-guided removal of bony fragments
- Sinus lavage via indwelling catheters (Foley)
- Antimicrobial therapy
- Antiinflammatory therapy

POSSIBLE COMPLICATIONS

- Bone necrosis
- Abscess formation
- Extensive hemorrhage
- Incomplete resolution or recurrence of the underlying pathology (progressive ethmoid hematoma, neoplasia)
- Formation of fistulating (or fistulous) tracts
- Exostosis
- Chronic sinusitis unresponsive to treatment

RECOMMENDED MONITORING

- Clinical signs of secondary sinusitis such as nasal discharge or facial swelling
- Repeated radiographic or endoscopic examination, including oral endoscopy for monitoring of granulating dental alveolus after tooth removal

PROGNOSIS AND OUTCOME

Prognosis depends on the underlying pathology and ranges from less than 20% in sinus neo-

plasia to more than 80% in cases with sinus cysts. Full remission of the clinical symptoms in horses with dental sinusitis and traumatic sinusitis is reported to be seen in 70% to 80%, but only about one third of cases with progressive ethmoid hematoma have a successful outcome.

PEARLS & CONSIDERATIONS

COMMENTS

- In some cases, it is difficult to distinguish primary from secondary sinusitis. Clinical examination, oral endoscopy, and radiography alone may not allow a definitive diagnosis of dental sinusitis in up to 25% of cases.
- Treatment of more severe cases can require a long period of treatment and be costly. Repeated surgical interventions may be necessary in progressive ethmoid hematomas and some cases of dental sinusitis.
- Expensive and more invasive diagnostic tools such as CT or MRI may have to be used to detect subtle causes for secondary sinusitis.

PREVENTION

- Horses with Cushing's disease should be treated accordingly.
- Routine dental care may help to detect dental pathology early enough to prevent secondary dental sinusitis.

SUGGESTED READING

Barakzai S, Tremaine H, Dixon P: Use of scintigraphy for diagnosis of equine paranasal sinus disorders. *Vet Surg* 35:94–101, 2006.

Freeman DE: Sinus disease. *Vet Clin Pract Equine North Am* 19:209–243, 2003.

Tremaine WH, Dixon PM: A long-term study of 277 cases of equine sinonasal disease. Part 1: details of horses, historical, clinical and ancillary diagnostic findings. *Equine Vet J* 33:274–282, 2001.

Tremaine WH, Dixon PM: A long-term study of 277 cases of equine sinonasal disease. Part 2: treatments and results of treatments. *Equine Vet J* 33:283–289, 2001.

AUTHOR: KARSTEN VELDE

EDITOR: ERIC J. PARENTE

Slaframine Toxicosis

BASIC INFORMATION

DEFINITION
Slaframine is a mycotoxin produced by *Rhizoctonia leguminicola*, a fungus that infects legume plants. Chronic and acute toxicosis is caused by ingestion of contaminated feedstuffs.

SYNONYM(S)
Slobber factor, slobber syndrome, black patch disease

EPIDEMIOLOGY
GENETICS AND BREED PREDISPOSITION Guinea pigs are most sensitive, followed by horses, bovines, other ruminants, pigs, cats, dogs, rats, and chickens.
RISK FACTORS Risk of slaframine intoxication increases as the amount of legume forage increases in the diet.
GEOGRAPHY AND SEASONALITY Growth of *Rhizoctonia leguminicola* is most prevalent in second-cutting hay or clover associated with cool, wet weather. Hay may retain toxin for as long as 2 years. The disease is seedborn with sclerotia and mycelia of the fungus, which can overwinter. This fungus is known to occur in red clover, white clover, soybeans, kudzu, cow peas, blue lupine, alsike clover, alfalfa, *Korean lespedeza*, black medic, cicer milkvetch, and sanfoin. The fungus is usually only present on other legumes when red clover is near.

CLINICAL PRESENTATION
HISTORY, CHIEF COMPLAINT Excessive salivation is usually the first sign of slaframine exposure. Clinical signs usually develop after 1 hour of contaminated feed ingestion.
PHYSICAL EXAM FINDINGS Clinical signs:
- Excessive or profuse salivation
- Feed refusal
- Diarrhea
- Bloating
- Colic
- Lacrimation
- Lethargy
- Anorexia
- Polyuria
- Stiff joints
- Decreased milk production
- Rare occurrence of death
- No changes in heart rate, blood pressure, or respiration

ETIOLOGY AND PATHOPHYSIOLOGY
- Slaframine is a parasympathomimetic and acts on the cholinergic nervous system.
- Bioactivation of slaframine in the liver to an active metabolite results in clinical symptoms, most notably salivation. The action of active metabolite involves muscarinic receptors.
- Atropine has been shown to reduce symptoms in severe cases but otherwise does not alleviate clinical signs unless given before exposure.
- Slaframine is not a cholinesterase inhibitor.
- Slaframine affects the salivary and pancreas exocrine glands, causing viscous salivation and an increase in digestive enzymes, respectively.
- Reduced feed intake, decreased milk production, and decreased body weight are probably linked to loss of fluids.
- In most cases, exposure results in mild symptoms with no harmful effects.
- In severe cases, which are rare, excessive salivation and emphysematous lungs may result in suffocation, leading to death.
- Only one case of abortion has been reported in a mare, but there are no experimental data to substantiate this report.

DIAGNOSIS

DIFFERENTIAL DIAGNOSIS
- Other causes of excessive salivation include infectious, neoplastic, traumatic, and inflammatory disorders of the mouth, esophagus, gastrointestinal, and neurologic systems as well as various toxicologic causes, including plants, insects, chemicals, drugs, and pesticides.
- Rabies should always be ruled out for any animal with excessive salivation.

INITIAL DATABASE
Examine hay or feed to look for mold. *R. leguminicola* appears black or dark brown with concentric zonation on leaf or stem.

ADVANCED OR CONFIRMATORY TESTING
Analysis of feed for slaframine by gas chromatography/mass spectrometry

TREATMENT

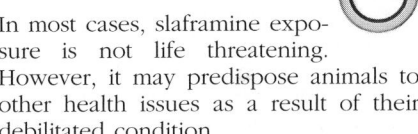

ACUTE GENERAL TREATMENT
- Remove the feed source causing problem. Cessation of clinical signs generally occurs at least 24 hours after feed removal.
- Supportive fluid treatment if needed
- In severe cases, treatment with atropine may be indicated.

PROGNOSIS AND OUTCOME
In most cases, slaframine exposure is not life threatening. However, it may predispose animals to other health issues as a result of their debilitated condition.

PEARLS & CONSIDERATIONS

PREVENTION
Examine forage for signs of mold contamination. If mold is evident on legume forage, a trial feeding to one or two animals may be prudent to avoid potential exposure of a large number of animals to slaframine. Remove feed or remove animals from pasture if clinical signs become evident.

CLIENT EDUCATION
There is a potential risk of slaframine exposure when feeding clover and other legumes.

SUGGESTED READING
Aust SD: Occurrence and clinical manifestations of lupinosis and slaframine toxicosis. In Richards JL, Thurston JR, editors: *Diagnosis of mycotoxicoses*, Boston, 1986, Martinus Nijhoff Publishers, pp 81–90.

Broquist HP, Snyder JJ: Rhizoctonia toxin. In Kadis S, CieglerA, Ajl SJ, editors: *Microbial toxins, vol VII*, New York, 1971, Academic Press, pp 319–333.

Hagler WM Jr, Croom WJ Jr: Slaframine occurrence, chemistry, and physiological activity. In Cheeke PR, editor: *Toxicants of plant origin*, Boca Raton, FL, 1989, CRC Press, pp 257–279.

AUTHOR: **PAULA M. IMERMAN**

EDITOR: **CYNTHIA L. GASKILL**

Small Colon: Impaction

BASIC INFORMATION

DEFINITION
Physical obstruction of the small colon with feces

SYNONYM(S)
Fecal impaction

EPIDEMIOLOGY
SPECIES, AGE, SEX Young horses and elderly (>15 years) horses are predisposed.
GENETICS AND BREED PREDISPOSITION
- Miniature horses, ponies
- Females predisposed

RISK FACTORS
- Ingestion of bedding or poor-quality hay, poor dentition, inadequate hydration, parasitic damage, or motility issues
- Inflammatory bowel disease

CONTAGION AND ZOONOSIS *Salmonella*-positive fecal cultures in 43% of surgically treated horses
GEOGRAPHY AND SEASONALITY Fall and winter
ASSOCIATED CONDITIONS AND DISORDERS Colitis, which may be a primary or secondary disease to the small colon impaction

CLINICAL PRESENTATION
HISTORY, CHIEF COMPLAINT
- Loose manure or diarrhea
- Decreased fecal output
- Colic
- Straining to defecate
- Tympany; gas distension
- Decreased appetite
- Lethargy

PHYSICAL EXAM FINDINGS
- Hyperthermic, normothermic, or hypothermic if severely compromised
- Mild to moderate tachycardia
- Depressed and lethargic
- Mucous membranes variable: May be pale pink and moist but progress to toxic with time
- Colic signs
- Decreased or absent borborygmi
- Abdominal distension, secondary ileus
- Absence of or scant loose feces
- Variable hydration

ETIOLOGY AND PATHOPHYSIOLOGY Impaction with dehydrated feces that have not formed fecal balls
- Idiopathic
- *Salmonella* infection
- Poor dentition occasionally implicated

DIAGNOSIS

DIFFERENTIAL DIAGNOSIS
- Small colon nonstrangulating lesions (early stages)
  - Small colon enterolith
  - Small colon fecalith
  - Small colon bezoar
  - Small colon phytoconglobate
  - Small colon foreign body
  - Small colon neoplasia
- Small colon strangulating lesion (later stages)
  - Small colon lipoma
  - Small colon intussusception
  - Small colon volvulus
  - Small colon herniation

INITIAL DATABASE
- Complete blood count: Leukopenia or leukocytosis common, left shift common, occasionally normal
- Rectal examination: Diagnostic in 75% to 83% of cases
  - Small colon impactions present as cylindrical, firm, sausage-shaped areas in the small colon. Normal tenial bands can be identified, but no haustrations or fecal balls are palpated.
  - Distended large colon (secondary)
  - Occasionally distended small intestine (secondary)
- Peritoneal fluid
  - Normal initially
  - Increased protein and white blood cell count, and serosanguineous appearance with time
- Transabdominal ultrasonography: Gas-distended large colon

ADVANCED OR CONFIRMATORY TESTING
- Fecal *Salmonella* polymerase chain reaction
- Check teeth

TREATMENT

THERAPEUTIC GOAL(S)
- Maintain hydration to maintain adequate organ system perfusion
- Provide analgesia
- Assist with passage of physical obstruction

ACUTE GENERAL TREATMENT
- Withhold feed
- Analgesics
  - Flunixin meglumine: 1.1 mg/kg IV
  - Detomidine (0.01 mg/kg IV) and butorphanol (0.01 mg/kg IV) for sedation if required
- Fluid therapy
  - Crystalloids: Volume dependent on hydration status and rate of ongoing losses (4–6 mL/kg/h)
  - Oral fluids and laxatives (if no reflux)
    - Water (2 to 4 L q2–6h) via nasogastric tube
    - Mineral oil (5 to 10 mL/kg q12h)
    - $MgSO_4$ maximum of 1 g/kg 24 hours for 2 to 3 days
    - Dioctyl sodium sulfosuccinate (DSS) (50 mg/kg in 6 L of water). Magnesium toxicity is more likely if administering both $MgSO_4$ and DSS.
- Enemas: Use with caution because of the risk of perforation; often unrewarding
- Exploratory celiotomy in dorsal recumbency with severe gas distension, or reflux or if unresponsive to analgesia
  - Enema and extraluminal breakdown of small colon impaction or small colon colotomy
  - Empty large colon to reduce passage of feces through small colon in the immediate postoperative period
- If surgical intervention is not an option, may try additional analgesics and mechanisms to relax the small colon
  - Butylscopolamine (0.3 mg/kg IV)
  - Morphine epidurals (0.1 mg/kg QS to 10 mL) if no butorphanol administered
  - Lidocaine constant-rate infusions (CRIs) (1.3 mg/kg loading dose over 10 minutes; then 0.05 mg/kg/min)
  - Ketamine CRIs (0.4–1.2 mg/kg/h)
- Consider adjunct antiendotoxic therapy
  - *Salmonella typhimurium* antiserum
  - Polymixin B (2000–6000 IU/kg IV)

CHRONIC TREATMENT
- After resolution: Nutrition
- Low-residue diet to prevent excessive trauma in small colon for 5 to 7 days

DRUG INTERACTIONS
Use of $MgSO_4$ and DSS concurrently increases the chances of magnesium toxicity

POSSIBLE COMPLICATIONS
- Peritonitis
- Endotoxemia
- Laminitis
- Adhesions
- Reobstruction
- Jugular thrombophlebitis

- Diarrhea
- Pyrexia
- Incisional infection
- Incisional hernia
- Recurrent colic

RECOMMENDED MONITORING

- Pain
- Distension
- Fecal output
- Reflux
- Packed cell volume and total solids

PROGNOSIS AND OUTCOME

Prognosis is directly affected by the severity of disease and the associated complications.

- 72% to 100% survival after medical therapy
- 47% to 95% survival after surgical therapy

PEARLS & CONSIDERATIONS

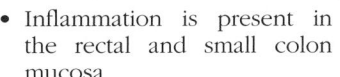

- Inflammation is present in the rectal and small colon mucosa.
  - The mucosa may feel rough and gritty or edematous.
  - The rectal mucosa is more likely to bleed than normal mucosa.
- A total of 43% of horses with surgically corrected small colon impactions are positive for *Salmonella* spp. on fecal culture; therefore, always sample feces for at least 3 consecutive days. Initiate isolation protocol until proven otherwise.

SUGGESTED READING

Rakestraw PC, Hardy J: Large intestine. In Auer JA, Stick JA, editors: *Equine surgery,* ed 3, St Louis, 2006, Saunders Elsevier, pp 436–478.

Peroni, JF: Disorders of the small colon. In White NA, Moore JN, Mair TS, editors: *The equine acute abdomen,* ed 2, Jackson, WY, 2008, Teton NewMedia, pp 650–658.

Schumacher J: Disease of the small colon and rectum. In Mair TS, Divers T, Ducharme N, editors: *Manual of equine gastroenterology,* St Louis, 2002, Saunders Elsevier, pp 299–315.

AUTHOR: CERI SHERLOCK

EDITORS: TIM MAIR and **CERI SHERLOCK**

Small Colon: Intestinal Atresia

BASIC INFORMATION

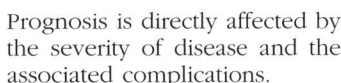

DEFINITION

Complete and abnormal congenital occlusion of the foal intestine

SYNONYM(S)

Atresia ani, atresia recti, atresia coli (large colon, transverse colon, or small colon)

EPIDEMIOLOGY

SPECIES, AGE, SEX Affects foals
GENETICS AND BREED PREDISPOSITION Rare condition
ASSOCIATED CONDITIONS AND DISORDERS Condition has been associated with other congenital abnormalities, such as renal agenesis, dysplasia or hypoplasia, absence of a tail, micro-ophthalmia, rectourethral fistula, cerebral gliomata, cerebellar dysplasia, hydrocephalus, dermal hemangioma, ventricular septal defect, common truncus arteriosus, or schistosomas reflexus.

CLINICAL PRESENTATION

DISEASE FORMS/SUBTYPES

- Type 1: Atresia or membranous atresia
  - Diaphragm or membrane occludes the intestine
- Type 2: Atresia or cord atresia
  - Proximal and distal blind ends are joined by a cord of connective tissue with or without a mesentery
- Type 3: Atresia or blind end atresia
  - Proximal and distal blind segments are completely separated with no mesentery

HISTORY, CHIEF COMPLAINT The condition normally becomes apparent a few hours after birth

- Colic
- Depression
- Tympany
- Absence of feces
- No response to enemas
- Tenesmus
- Tail flagging

PHYSICAL EXAM FINDINGS

- Temperature variable
- Often tachycardic
- Sometimes depressed and lethargic
- Mucous membranes variable: may be pale pink and moist but most commonly hyperemic and tacky
- Colic signs
- Absence of meconium passage or perianal staining
- Variable hydration

ETIOLOGY AND PATHOPHYSIOLOGY

- Unknown
- Possible association with a simple recessive gene
- Possible developmental arrest
- Possible vascular compromise to the fetal gut

DIAGNOSIS

DIFFERENTIAL DIAGNOSIS

- Small colon intussusception
- Meconium impaction

INITIAL DATABASE

- Complete blood count
  - Leukopenia or leukocytosis common, occasionally normal

- Digital rectal examination
  - Identify a blind-ending tube
- Proctoscopy
  - Blind-ending tube
- Radiography and barium contrast study
  - Gas distended intestine oral to the atresia; passage of contrast material oral to atresic intestine prevented
- Peritoneal fluid
  - Normal initially
- Transabdominal ultrasound
  - Gas-distended large colon
  - Occasionally small intestinal distension

ADVANCED OR CONFIRMATORY TESTING

When deciding whether to treat, the presence of other congenital lesions must be determined.

TREATMENT

THERAPEUTIC GOAL(S)

- Maintain hydration to maintain adequate organ system perfusion
- Provide analgesia
- Verify that no other congenital lesions are present
- Correct abnormal segment of bowel if possible

ACUTE GENERAL TREATMENT

- Analgesics
  - Flunixin meglumine 1.1 mg/kg IV

- Fluid therapy
  - Boluses of 20 to 90 mL/kg crystalloids given over 20 to 30 minutes until hypovolemia is resolved and urine is produced.
  - Maintenance rate of crystalloids depends on rate of ongoing losses (2–6 mL/kg/h).
- Atresia ani
  - If foal has type 1 atresia, remove a circular disk of membrane and avoid the anal sphincter. Suture the rectal wall to the skin in a simple interrupted pattern.
  - Atresia of the distal rectum requires more extensive dissection.
- Atresia recti
  - Deeper dissection is necessary to perform a similar procedure as for atresia ani.
- Atresia coli
  - Perform exploratory celiotomy with the foal in dorsal recumbency.
  - Administer broad-spectrum antibiotics.
  - Perform end-to-end anastomosis of colon.
    - Empty large colon to reduce passage of feces through anastomosis in the immediate postoperative period.
    - If the affected segment cannot be exteriorized, perform colostomy or transrectal exteriorization and colorectostomy.

CHRONIC TREATMENT

After resolution
- Balanced nutrition
- Low-residue diet to prevent excessive trauma in small colon for 5 to 7 days

POSSIBLE COMPLICATIONS

- Adhesions
- Fecal incontinence
- Peritonitis
- Endotoxemia
- Laminitis
- Reobstruction
- Jugular thrombophlebitis
- Diarrhea
- Pyrexia
- Incisional infection
- Incisional hernia
- Recurrent colic

RECOMMENDED MONITORING

- Pain
- Distension
- Fecal output
- Reflux
- Packed cell volume and total solids

PROGNOSIS AND OUTCOME

- If no other congenital abnormalities are present, the prognosis for type 1 atresia ani is favorable; however, fecal incontinence may persist.

- The prognosis is poor for atresia coli.
- The prognosis is grave for Overo Paint foals with aganglionosis.

PEARLS & CONSIDERATIONS

- Foals with atresia ani and rectovaginal fistulas may not show clinical signs of gastrointestinal obstruction.
- Overo white foals may have a recessive lethal syndrome: Ileocolonic agangliogenesis. This condition causes stenotic colons with thin muscular walls and few myenteric plexuses that cause megacolon and death (see "Lethal White Foal Syndrome" in this section).

SUGGESTED READING

Freeman D: Rectum and anus. In Auer JA, Stick JA, editors: *Equine surgery*, ed 3, St Louis, 2006, Saunders Elsevier, pp 479–491.

Nappert G, et al: Atresia coli in 7 foals (1964–1990). *Equine Vet J* 13:57, 1992.

Schumacher J: Disease of the small colon and rectum. In Mair TS, Divers T, Ducharme N. editors: *Manual of equine gastroenterology*, Philadelphia, 2002, WB Saunders, pp 299–315.

AUTHOR: CERI SHERLOCK

EDITORS: TIM MAIR and CERI SHERLOCK

Small Colon: Intramural Hematoma

BASIC INFORMATION

DEFINITION

Physical obstruction of the small colon caused by intramural or submucosal hematoma

EPIDEMIOLOGY

SPECIES, AGE, SEX Old horses appear predisposed; however, the rare occurrence of the disorder makes this difficult to verify.

CLINICAL PRESENTATION

HISTORY, CHIEF COMPLAINT
- Colic signs
- Tympany, gas distension of the large colon
- Decreased fecal output
- Decreased appetite

PHYSICAL EXAM FINDINGS
- Most horses are normothermic initially but may become hyperthermic

or hypothermic with increasing duration.
- Most horses are mildly to markedly tachycardic.
- Mucous membranes normal initially but may become tacky with a prolonged capillary refill time.
- Horses may have abdominal distension and secondary ileus.
- The fecal output is decreased, and there may be hemorrhage or clotted blood on recently passed feces.

ETIOLOGY AND PATHOPHYSIOLOGY
- Hemorrhage within the wall of the small colon occludes the intestinal lumen. Hemorrhage may also track along the intestine wall.
- The vascular disturbance that caused the hemorrhage may be severe enough to cause ischemic necrosis of the small colon. This can lead to septic peritonitis, endotoxemia, and death.
- Histology to identify the underlying cause has been unrewarding.

DIAGNOSIS

DIFFERENTIAL DIAGNOSIS

- Rectal tear
- Small colon enterolith
- Small colon fecalith
- Small colon phytoconglobate
- Small colon bezoar
- Small colon impaction
- Small colon foreign body

INITIAL DATABASE

- Complete blood count: Usually normal
- Rectal examination
  - Distended large colon may be present
  - May or may not feel obstruction of the small colon with pain on palpation
- Solid mass
  - May feel small colon distension
  - Often see clotted blood on retraction of hand

- Peritoneal fluid: Normal initially
- Abdominal ultrasonography: Gas-distended large colon

TREATMENT

THERAPEUTIC GOAL(S)

- Maintain hydration.
- Maintain adequate organ system perfusion.
- Stabilize the patient for surgical intervention.
- Perform surgical resection and anastomosis of the small colon. If the area cannot be resected, a colostomy may be necessary.

ACUTE GENERAL TREATMENT

- Analgesics: Flunixin meglumine (1.1 mg/kg IV)
- Fluid therapy: Crystalloids
- Volume depends on the patient's hydration status and rate of ongoing losses (2–6 mL/kg/h).
- Exploratory celiotomy in dorsal recumbency should be performed if the patient is unresponsive to analgesia or the diagnosis is confirmed. The small colon should be exteriorized and end-to-end anastomosis performed.

- Perform colostomy if resection not possible. Always empty the large colon to reduce passage of feces through the small colon in the immediate postoperative period.

CHRONIC TREATMENT

- Postoperatively: Balanced nutrition
- Low-residue diet to prevent excessive trauma in small colon for 5 to 7 days

POSSIBLE COMPLICATIONS

- Peritonitis
- Endotoxemia
- Laminitis
- Adhesions
- Reobstruction
- Jugular thrombophlebitis
- Diarrhea
- Pyrexia
- Incisional infection
- Incisional hernia
- Recurrent colic

RECOMMENDED MONITORING

- Pain
- Distension
- Fecal output
- Packed cell volume and total solids

PROGNOSIS AND OUTCOME

Prognosis is affected by the severity and location of disease. If complete resection is possible and transmural necrosis and septic peritonitis have not commenced, the prognosis is good.

PEARLS & CONSIDERATIONS

This disease is rare.

SUGGESTED READING

Pearson H, Waterman AE: Submucosal haematoma as a cause of obstruction of the small colon in the horse: a review of four cases. *Equine Vet J* 18:340, 1986.

Rakestraw PC, Hardy J: Large intestine. In Auer JA, Stick JA, editors: *Equine surgery*, ed 3, St Louis, 2006, Saunders Elsevier, pp 436–478.

Schumacher J: Disease of the small colon and rectum. In Mair TS, Divers T, Ducharme N, editors: *Manual of equine gastroenterology*, St Louis, 2002, Saunders Elsevier, pp 299–315.

AUTHOR: CERI SHERLOCK

EDITORS: TIM MAIR and CERI SHERLOCK

Small Colon: Intussusception

BASIC INFORMATION

DEFINITION

Physical obstruction of the small colon caused by telescoping of the small colon into itself

EPIDEMIOLOGY

SPECIES, AGE, SEX In the absence of rectal prolapse, seen rarely in foals and in broodmares

CLINICAL PRESENTATION

HISTORY, CHIEF COMPLAINT

- Colic
- Decreased fecal output
- Blood staining of feces
- Tympany, gas distension

PHYSICAL EXAM FINDINGS

- Temperature variable depending on severity of compromise
- Often tachycardic
- Sometimes depressed and lethargic
- Mucous membranes variable; most commonly injected and tacky
- Colic signs
- Abdominal distension and secondary ileus

- Decreased fecal output
- Variable hydration

ETIOLOGY AND PATHOPHYSIOLOGY When small colon telescopes into itself, it can cause intraluminal obstruction as well as strangulation of mesenteric vessels.

DIAGNOSIS

DIFFERENTIAL DIAGNOSIS

- Small colon lipoma
- Small colon volvulus
- Small colon enterolith
- Small colon fecalith
- Small colon bezoar
- Small colon impaction
- Small colon phytoconglobate
- Small colon foreign body
- Small colon neoplasia

INITIAL DATABASE

- Complete blood count: Leukopenia or leukocytosis common; occasionally normal

- Rectal examination
  - Possibly difficult to enter abdomen because of straining or physical obstruction in small colon
  - Digital palpation between the intussusceptum and the rectal wall until a blind end is reached confirms the diagnosis of an intussusception
  - Distended large colon (secondary)
  - Occasionally, distended small intestine (secondary)
- Increased peritoneal fluid protein and white blood cell count, serosanguinous appearance with time
- Transabdominal ultrasonography
  - Gas-distended large colon
  - Occasionally, small intestinal distension

TREATMENT

THERAPEUTIC GOAL(S)

- Maintain hydration to maintain adequate organ system perfusion
- Provide analgesia

- Reduce intussusception and resect nonviable bowel

ACUTE GENERAL TREATMENT

- Analgesics
  ○ Flunixin meglumine: 1.1 mg/kg IV
  ○ Detomidine (0.01 mg/kg IV) and butorphanol (0.01 mg/kg IV) for sedation if required
- Fluid therapy
  ○ Crystalloids
  ○ Volume dependent on hydration status and rate of ongoing losses (4–6 mL/kg/h)
- Exploratory celiotomy in dorsal recumbency if unresponsive to analgesia
  ○ Administer broad-spectrum antibiotics
  ○ Reduce intussusception
  ○ Perform end-to-end anastomosis of small colon if required
  ○ Empty large colon to reduce passage of feces through small colon in the immediate postoperative period
- Colostomies are sometime required depending on location and length of affected segment.
- Transrectal colorectostomy has also been described in a caudally located intussusception.

CHRONIC TREATMENT

- After resolution: Balanced nutrition
- Low-residue diet to prevent excessive trauma in small colon for 5 to 7 days

POSSIBLE COMPLICATIONS

- Peritonitis
- Endotoxemia
- Laminitis
- Adhesions
- Reobstruction
- Jugular thrombophlebitis
- Diarrhea
- Pyrexia
- Incisional infection
- Incisional hernia
- Recurrent colic

RECOMMENDED MONITORING

- Pain
- Distension
- Fecal output
- Reflux
- Packed cell volume and total solids

PROGNOSIS AND OUTCOME

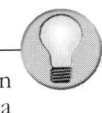

Prognosis is variable and is directly affected by the length and location of affected intestine, the severity of disease, and the associated complications.

PEARLS & CONSIDERATIONS

Small colon intussusception most commonly presents as a rectal prolapse.

SUGGESTED READING

Peroni JF: Disorders of the small colon. In White NA, Moore JN, Mair TS, editors: *The equine acute abdomen*, ed 2, Jackson, WY, 2008, Teton NewMedia, pp 650–658.

Rakestraw PC, Hardy J: Large intestine. In Auer JA, Stick JA, editors: *Equine surgery*, ed 3, St Louis, 2006, Saunders Elsevier, pp 436–478.

Schumacher J: Disease of the small colon and rectum. In Mair TS, Divers T, Ducharme N, editors: *Manual of equine gastroenterology*, St Louis, 2002, Saunders Elsevier, pp 299–315.

AUTHOR: **CERI SHERLOCK**

EDITORS: **TIM MAIR** and **CERI SHERLOCK**

Small Colon: Mesocolic Rupture

BASIC INFORMATION

DEFINITION

Tearing of the mesocolon leading to compromise of the vasculature to the small colon

EPIDEMIOLOGY

SPECIES, AGE, SEX Commonly occurs in brood mares because it is often a foaling complication. Middle-aged and pluriparous mares typically are affected.

RISK FACTORS
- Foaling
- Type III or IV rectal prolapse

CLINICAL PRESENTATION

HISTORY, CHIEF COMPLAINT
- Colic signs normally start in the first 24 hours after parturition. These may be very mild or severe.
- Decreased fecal output
- Progressive inappetence and lethargy

PHYSICAL EXAM FINDINGS
- Normothermic, hyperthermic, or hypothermic if severely compromised.
- Often tachycardic

- Sometimes depressed and lethargic
- Mucous membranes are variable depending on the stage of the disease; they may be pale pink but progressively become toxic.
- Decreased to absent borborygmi

ETIOLOGY AND PATHOPHYSIOLOGY
- Tearing of the mesocolon may occur through trauma from the foal's leg, especially during the first stages of labor.
- Tearing of the mesocolon may also occur when more than 30 cm of the rectum and small colon prolapses through the anus. This may also occur associated with foaling.

DIAGNOSIS

DIFFERENTIAL DIAGNOSIS

- Intramural hematoma
- Other causes of colic in postparturient mares
  ○ Mesenteric rent in another area of the intestine
  ○ Uterine artery rupture

INITIAL DATABASE

- Complete blood count: Normal initially; leukopenia or leukocytosis may be present later
- Rectal examination
  ○ Possibly difficult to enter abdomen because of straining and pain
  ○ Findings variable: Small colon and distended large colon may feel normal or impacted
- Peritoneal fluid
  ○ Increased protein and white blood cell count, serosanguineous appearance with time
  ○ Hemoabdomen may also be present.
- Transabdominal ultrasonography
  ○ Peritoneal effusion common
  ○ Large colon gas distension possible
  ○ Occasionally, secondary small intestinal distension present

ADVANCED OR CONFIRMATORY TESTING

Laparoscopy may be useful to identify and assess the severity of the mesocolic rupture.

TREATMENT

THERAPEUTIC GOAL(S)

- Maintain hydration to maintain adequate organ system perfusion
- Provide analgesia
- Resection of compromised area and perform end-to-end anastomosis

ACUTE GENERAL TREATMENT

- Withhold feed
- Analgesics
  - Flunixin meglumine (1.1 mg/kg IV)
  - Detomidine (0.01 mg/kg IV) and butorphanol (0.01 mg/kg IV) for sedation if required
- Fluid therapy
  - Crystalloids
  - Volume dependent on hydration status and rate of ongoing losses (4–6 mL/kg/h)
- Exploratory celiotomy in dorsal recumbency if unresponsive to analgesia
  - Administer broad-spectrum antibiotics.
  - Perform end-to-end anastomosis of small colon.
  - Empty large colon to reduce passage of feces through small colon in the immediate postoperative period

- Colostomies sometimes required depending on the location and length of affected segment

CHRONIC TREATMENT

- After resolution: Balanced nutrition
- Low-residue diet to prevent excessive trauma in small colon for 5 to 7 days

POSSIBLE COMPLICATIONS

- Peritonitis
- Endotoxemia
- Laminitis
- Adhesions
- Reobstruction
- Jugular thrombophlebitis
- Diarrhea
- Pyrexia
- Incisional infection
- Incisional hernia
- Recurrent colic

RECOMMENDED MONITORING

- Pain
- Distension
- Fecal output
- Reflux
- Packed cell volume and total solids

PROGNOSIS AND OUTCOME

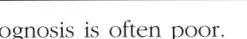

Prognosis is often poor.
- Signs of colic in postpartum mares are often attributed to uterine involution, so surgical intervention is delayed.
- The extent of the tear may preclude surgical repair.

SUGGESTED READING

Dart AJ, Pascoe JR, Snyder JR: Mesenteric tears of the descending (small) colon as a postpartum complication in two mares. *J Am Vet Med Assoc* 199:1612, 1991.

Peroni, JF: Disorders of the small colon. In White NA, Moore JN, Mair TS, editors: *The equine acute abdomen*, ed 2, Jackson, WY, 2008, Teton NewMedia, pp 650–658.

Rakestraw PC, Hardy J: Large intestine. In Auer JA, Stick JA, editors: *Equine surgery*, ed 3, St Louis, 2006, Saunders Elsevier, pp 436–478.

Schumacher J: Disease of the small colon and rectum. In Mair TS, Divers T, Ducharme N, editors: *Manual of equine gastroenterology*, St Louis, 2002, Saunders Elsevier, pp 299–315.

AUTHOR: **CERI SHERLOCK**

EDITORS: **TIM MAIR** and **CERI SHERLOCK**

Small Colon: Nonstrangulating Infarction

BASIC INFORMATION

DEFINITION

Segmental infarction of the small colon

EPIDEMIOLOGY

RISK FACTORS Verminous arteritis; however, small colon vascular supply is from the caudal mesenteric artery, which is rarely affected by occlusive verminous arteritis.

CLINICAL PRESENTATION

HISTORY, CHIEF COMPLAINT
- Colic
- Decreased fecal output
- Tympany, gas distension

PHYSICAL EXAM FINDINGS
- Temperature variable depending on severity of compromise
- Often tachycardic
- Sometimes depressed and lethargic
- Mucous membranes variable; commonly injected and tacky
- Abdominal distension and secondary ileus
- Variable hydration

ETIOLOGY AND PATHOPHYSIOLOGY

- There is often no evidence of arteritis at necropsy; however, occlusive vascular disease is seen.
- Segmental infarction of area of small colon

DIAGNOSIS

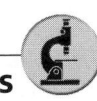

DIFFERENTIAL DIAGNOSIS

- Small colon strangulating disease (eg, lipoma, volvulus, intussusception)
- Small colon enterolith
- Small colon fecalith
- Small colon bezoar
- Small colon impaction
- Small colon phytoconglobate
- Small colon foreign body
- Small colon neoplasia
- Small colon lipoma

INITIAL DATABASE

- Complete blood count: Leukopenia or leukocytosis common; occasionally normal
- Rectal examination
  - Possibly difficult to enter abdomen because of straining

- Possibly secondarily distended large colon or small intestine
- Peritoneal fluid: Increased protein and white blood cell count, serosanguineous appearance with time
- Transabdominal ultrasonography: Occasionally gas-distended large colon and small intestinal distension

TREATMENT

THERAPEUTIC GOAL(S)

- Maintain hydration to maintain adequate organ system perfusion
- Provide analgesia
- Resect nonviable bowel

ACUTE GENERAL TREATMENT

- Analgesics
  - Flunixin meglumine (1.1 mg/kg IV)
  - Detomidine (0.01 mg/kg IV) and butorphanol (0.01 mg/kg IV) for sedation if required
- Fluid therapy
  - Crystalloids
  - Volume dependent on hydration status and rate of ongoing losses (4–6 mL/kg/h)

- Exploratory celiotomy in dorsal recumbency if unresponsive to analgesia
  - Administer broad-spectrum antibiotics
  - Perform end-to-end anastomosis of small colon to resect infarcted area
  - Empty large colon to reduce passage of feces through small colon in the immediate postoperative period
- If the affected area cannot be exteriorized, colostomy or transrectal colorectostomy may be necessary

CHRONIC TREATMENT

- After resolution: Balanced nutrition
- Low-residue diet to prevent excessive trauma in small colon for 5 to 7 days

POSSIBLE COMPLICATIONS

- Peritonitis
- Endotoxemia
- Laminitis

- Adhesions
- Reobstruction
- Jugular thrombophlebitis
- Diarrhea
- Pyrexia
- Incisional infection
- Incisional hernia
- Recurrent colic

RECOMMENDED MONITORING

- Pain
- Distension
- Fecal output
- Reflux
- Packed cell volume and total solids

PROGNOSIS AND OUTCOME

Prognosis is directly affected by the severity of disease, the loca-

tion of the lesion, and the associated complications.

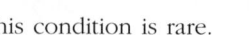

PEARLS & CONSIDERATIONS

This condition is rare.

SUGGESTED READING

Peroni JF: Disorders of the small colon. In White NA, Moore JN, Mair TS, editors: *The equine acute abdomen*, ed 3, Jackson, WY, 2008, Teton NewMedia, pp 650–658.

Schumacher J: Disease of the small colon and rectum. In Mair TS, Divers T, Ducharme N, editors: *Manual of equine gastroenterology*, St Louis, 2002, Saunders Elsevier, pp 299–315.

AUTHOR: **CERI SHERLOCK**

EDITORS: **TIM MAIR** and **CERI SHERLOCK**

Small Colon: Strangulating Lipoma

BASIC INFORMATION

DEFINITION

Physical obstruction of the small colon caused by external compression when it becomes entwined with a pedunculated lipoma

EPIDEMIOLOGY

SPECIES, AGE, SEX

- This condition is rarely seen in horses younger than 9 years; it is mainly seen in horses older than 15 years.
- Geldings appear more predisposed than mares or stallions.

GENETICS AND BREED PREDISPOSITION Ponies, Quarter Horses, and Morgans have been reported to be at an increased risk.

RISK FACTORS Fat horses

CLINICAL PRESENTATION

HISTORY, CHIEF COMPLAINT

- Colic signs
- Decreased or absent fecal output
- Tympany, gas distension

PHYSICAL EXAM FINDINGS

- Normothermic but hyperthermic or hypothermic if severely compromised
- Often tachycardic
- Sometimes depressed and lethargic
- Mucous membranes are variable; most commonly, they are injected or toxic and tacky
- Abdominal distension

ETIOLOGY AND PATHOPHYSIOLOGY

Mesenteric lipoma normally on a stalk wraps around segment of small colon

- Extraluminal obstruction
- Strangulation of mesenteric vessels

DIAGNOSIS

DIFFERENTIAL DIAGNOSIS

- Small colon enterolith
- Small colon fecalith
- Small colon bezoar
- Small colon impaction
- Small colon phytoconglobate
- Small colon foreign body
- Small colon intramural hematoma
- Small colon neoplasia
- Small colon intussusception
- Small colon volvulus

INITIAL DATABASE

- Complete blood count: Leukopenia or leukocytosis common; occasionally normal
- Rectal examination
  - Possibly difficult to enter abdomen because of straining or physical obstruction of small colon
  - Distended large colon (secondary)
  - Occasionally, distended small intestine (secondary)
  - Rarely, a taut fibrous band constricting the small colon can be palpated.
- Peritoneal fluid: Increased protein and white blood cell count, serosanguineous appearance with time
- Transabdominal ultrasonography
  - Gas-distended large colon
  - Occasionally, small intestinal distension

TREATMENT

THERAPEUTIC GOAL(S)

- Maintain hydration to maintain adequate organ system perfusion
- Provide analgesia
- Reduce strangulating lesion and resect nonviable bowel

ACUTE GENERAL TREATMENT

- Analgesics
  - Flunixin meglumine (1.1 mg/kg IV)
  - Detomidine (0.01 mg/kg IV) and butorphanol (0.01 mg/kg IV) for sedation if required
- Fluid therapy
  - Crystalloids
  - Volume dependent on hydration status and rate of ongoing losses (4–6 mL/kg/h)
- Exploratory celiotomy in dorsal recumbency if unresponsive to analgesia
  - Administer broad-spectrum antibiotics
  - Reduce strangulation
  - Perform end-to-end anastomosis of small colon
  - Empty large colon to reduce passage of feces through small colon in the immediate postoperative period

CHRONIC TREATMENT

- After resolution: Nutrition
- Low-residue diet to prevent excessive trauma in small colon for 5 to 7 days

POSSIBLE COMPLICATIONS

- Peritonitis
- Endotoxemia
- Laminitis
- Adhesions
- Reobstruction
- Jugular thrombophlebitis
- Diarrhea
- Pyrexia
- Incisional infection
- Incisional hernia
- Recurrent colic

RECOMMENDED MONITORING

- Pain
- Distension
- Fecal output
- Reflux
- Packed cell volume and total solids

PROGNOSIS AND OUTCOME

Prognosis is directly affected by the location of the lesion and the severity of the systemic consequences of the disease.

- Horses with intestine that cannot be safely resected have a poor prognosis.
- Horses with marked endotoxemia secondary to the strangulating lesion have a poor prognosis.

PEARLS & CONSIDERATIONS

- Small colon strangulating lipomas are less common than small intestinal strangulating lipomas because the small colon mesentery is shorter and is usually infiltrated with fat.

- About 7% of strangulating pedunculated lipomas affect the small colon, and about 93% affect the small intestine.

SUGGESTED READING

Edwards GB: Diseases and surgery of the small colon. *Vet Clin North Am Equine Pract* 13:359, 1997.

Peroni, JF: Disorders of the small colon. In White NA, Moore JN, Mair TS, editors: *The equine acute abdomen*, ed 2, Jackson, WY, 2008, Teton NewMedia, pp 650–658.

Rakestraw PC, Hardy J: Large intestine. In Auer JA, Stick JA, editors: *Equine surgery*, ed 3, St Louis, 2006, Saunders Elsevier, pp 436–478.

Schumacher J: Disease of the small colon and rectum. In Mair TS, Divers T, Ducharme N, editors: *Manual of equine gastroenterology*, St Louis, 2002, Saunders Elsevier, pp 299–315.

AUTHOR: **CERI SHERLOCK**

EDITORS: **TIM MAIR** and **CERI SHERLOCK**

Small Colon: Volvulus

BASIC INFORMATION

DEFINITION

Abnormal twisting of intestine around its mesentery, resulting in physical obstruction of the intestinal lumen and likely impaired blood flow to the intestine

EPIDEMIOLOGY

RISK FACTORS Adhesions and abscesses

CLINICAL PRESENTATION

HISTORY, CHIEF COMPLAINT

- Colic
- Decreased fecal output
- Tympany, gas distension

PHYSICAL EXAM FINDINGS

- Temperature variable depending on the severity of compromise
- Often tachycardic
- Sometimes depressed and lethargic
- Mucous membranes variable; most commonly injected and tacky
- Colic signs
- Abdominal distension and secondary ileus
- Decreased fecal output
- Variable dehydration

ETIOLOGY AND PATHOPHYSIOLOGY

Mesenteric lipoma normally on a stalk wraps around segment of small colon

- Extraluminal obstruction
- Strangulation of mesenteric vessels

DIAGNOSIS

DIFFERENTIAL DIAGNOSIS

- Small colon enterolith
- Small colon fecalith
- Small colon bezoar
- Small colon impaction
- Small colon phytoconglobate
- Small colon foreign body
- Small colon neoplasia
- Small colon intussusception

INITIAL DATABASE

- Complete blood count: Leukopenia or leukocytosis common; occasionally normal
- Rectal examination
  - Possibly difficult to enter abdomen because of straining or physical obstruction in small colon
  - Distended large colon (secondary)
  - Occasionally distended small intestine (secondary)
- Peritoneal fluid: Increased protein and white blood cell count, serosanguineous appearance with time
- Transabdominal ultrasonography
  - Gas-distended large colon
  - Occasionally, small intestinal distension

TREATMENT

THERAPEUTIC GOAL(S)

- Maintain hydration to maintain adequate organ system perfusion
- Provide analgesia
- Reduce strangulating lesion and resect nonviable bowel

ACUTE GENERAL TREATMENT

- Analgesics
  - Flunixin meglumine (1.1 mg/kg IV)
  - Detomidine (0.01 mg/kg IV) and butorphanol (0.01 mg/kg IV) for sedation if required
- Fluid therapy
  - Crystalloids
  - Volume dependent on hydration status and rate of ongoing losses (4–6 mL/kg/h)
- Exploratory celiotomy in dorsal recumbency if unresponsive to analgesia
  - Administer broad-spectrum antibiotics
  - Reduce volvulus
  - Perform end-to-end anastomosis of small colon if nonviable intestine
  - Empty large colon to reduce passage of feces through small colon in the immediate postoperative period

CHRONIC TREATMENT

- After resolution: Balanced nutrition
- Low-residue diet to prevent excessive trauma in small colon for 5 to 7 days

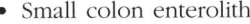

POSSIBLE COMPLICATIONS

- Peritonitis
- Endotoxemia
- Laminitis
- Adhesions
- Reobstruction
- Jugular thrombophlebitis
- Diarrhea
- Pyrexia
- Incisional infection
- Incisional hernia
- Recurrent colic

RECOMMENDED MONITORING

- Pain
- Distension
- Fecal output
- Reflux
- Packed cell volume and total solids

PROGNOSIS AND OUTCOME

Prognosis is directly affected by severity of disease, the location of the lesion, and the associated complications.

PEARLS & CONSIDERATIONS

This is a very rare condition associated with the relatively short length of the small colon that is anatomically fixed at either end and has a short and fatty mesentery.

SUGGESTED READING

Kirker-Head C, Steckel R: Volvulus of the small colon in a horse. *Mod Vet Pract* 69:14, 1988.

Peroni JF: Disorders of the small colon. In White NA, Moore JN, Mair TS, editors: *The equine acute abdomen*, ed 2, Jackson, WY, 2008, Teton NewMedia, pp 650–658.

Rakestraw PC, Hardy J: Large intestine. In Auer JA, Stick JA, editors: *Equine surgery*, ed 3, St Louis, 2006, Saunders Elsevier, pp 436–478.

Schumacher J: Disease of the small colon and rectum. In Mair TS, Divers T, Ducharme N, editors: *Manual of equine gastroenterology*, St Louis, 2002, Saunders Elsevier, pp 299–315.

AUTHOR: **CERI SHERLOCK**

EDITORS: **TIM MAIR** and **CERI SHERLOCK**

Small Intestine: Ascarid Impaction

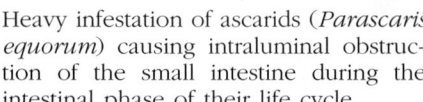

BASIC INFORMATION

DEFINITION

Heavy infestation of ascarids (*Parascaris equorum*) causing intraluminal obstruction of the small intestine during the intestinal phase of their life cycle

EPIDEMIOLOGY

SPECIES, AGE, SEX

- Young horses (foals, weanlings, yearlings).
- The prevalence of infection in horses younger than 1 year is 31% to 61%; in those older than 1 year, it is 25%.
- The median age of foals diagnosed with ascarid impaction is 5 months (range, 4–24 months).

RISK FACTORS

- Poor parasite control
- Infected pastures
- Deworming infected foals with paralytic dewormer causing immobilization and death of the parasite, potentially causing parasite impaction (no evidence to say rapid killing of the parasites contribute to impactions vs. slow onset death)
  - Macrocyclic lactones: Ivermectin
  - Pyrimidines: Pyrantel pamoate
  - Piperazine
  - Affected foals have no deworming history or had been dewormed 2 to 3 months previously (54% of affected foals had been dewormed within 6 days of onset of clinical signs)
- No prenatal or transmammary transfer of parasites

GEOGRAPHY AND SEASONALITY

Autumn: Foals are infected in the spring shortly after foaling. Foals are of the age and the parasite size and burden are such that the impactions are seen in the fall (prepatent period, 79–110 days).

ASSOCIATED CONDITIONS AND DISORDERS Parasitism

CLINICAL PRESENTATION

HISTORY, CHIEF COMPLAINT

- Foals are generally lethargic, inappetent, and show poor weight gain.
- May also present with nasal discharge and coughing.
- Colic signs may range from mild to severe.
- History of recent (1–6 days) deworming is likely.

PHYSICAL EXAM FINDINGS Physical examination findings consistent with abdominal discomfort (colic)

- Heart rate: Normal to tachycardic (60–120 beats/min)
- Respiratory rate: Normal to tachypneic (24–60 breaths/min)
- Rectal temperature: May have mild pyrexia (>38.5° C)
- Reduced or absent borborygmi
- Progressive signs of dehydration
  - Pale, tacky mucous membranes
  - Prolonged capillary refill time
  - Injected sclera
- Abdominal palpation: May be normal to exhibiting resentment on palpation with or without abdominal distension

ETIOLOGY AND PATHOPHYSIOLOGY

- *P. equorum* infection
- Direct life cycle. Free-living stage (development of the infective second-stage larva in the egg) ranges from 9 to 14 days depending on environmental conditions. Egg development is arrested during the winter period (eggs can survive for several years outside the host). Temperatures above 39° C (102° F) destroy the eggs unless protected from desiccation in organic matter.
- Ingested eggs containing the second-stage larvae hatch in the small intestine and penetrate the intestinal wall to enter the portal blood vessels. Larvae migrate to the liver within 48 hours of ingestion and can be seen in the lung by day 14. Larvae are coughed up and swallowed, where they continue development in the duodenum and proximal jejunum. Mature worms reach a length of 10 to 50 cm and a diameter of 3 to 5 mm in 6 to 12 weeks.
- Rapid increase in size and over burden cause impaction of intestinal lumen.
- Deworming with a paralytic anthelmintic potentially causes immobilization and death of parasite-causing impaction.
- There is some suggestion that release of potent allergens may cause subsequent intestinal damage and necrotizing enteritis and peritonitis (report of intradermal injection of *P. equorum* somatic extract causing severe systemic response and colic).

DIAGNOSIS

DIFFERENTIAL DIAGNOSIS

Other causes of colic in weanling foals

- Gastric ulceration
- Enteritis

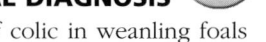

- Strangulating obstruction
- Other forms of intestinal obstruction
- Hernia
- Intussusception
- Abdominal abscess

INITIAL DATABASE

- Nasogastric reflux is variable depending on the degree of obstruction and may or may not contain ascarids.
- Abdominocentesis is very commonly abnormal with the appearance of the fluid ranging from serosanguineous to yellow and hazy. Both total protein and nucleated cell count are usually elevated, ranging from 2.6 to 6.0 g/dL and 3.0 to 87.4×10^3 cells/mL, respectively.
- Complete blood count and chemistry profile are commonly normal. Abnormalities are consistent with mild to moderate dehydration. May show stress leukogram. Eosinophilia is uncommon.

ADVANCED OR CONFIRMATORY TESTING

- Abdominal radiographs: May help distinguish between small intestinal and large colon disease. Will usually see gas- or fluid-distended small intestine.
- Abdominal ultrasonography: Multiple loops of distended small intestine located throughout the abdomen. May often identify parasites ultrasonographically.

TREATMENT

THERAPEUTIC GOAL(S)

- Pain management
- Surgical removal of the impaction

ACUTE GENERAL TREATMENT

- Gastric decompression
- Significant metabolic derangements are not common. If present, correction needs to be addressed in combination with rehydration and fluid therapy.
- Depending on the age of the foal and duration of the colic, partial or total parenteral nutrition should be considered.
- Fluid replacement: Balanced polyionic fluids (ie, lactated Ringer's solution)
  - Maintenance fluids: 50 to 60 mL/kg/d
  - Deficit replacement: Percentage dehydration based on physical examination findings
    - 200 kg × 60 mL/kg = 12.0 L/d (maintenance)
      - 200 kg × 0.08 = 16 L (deficit)
      - Administer calculated deficit over the first 1 to 2 hours
      - Administer remaining replacement volume over 12- to 24-hour period

- Use oral with great caution because of obstruction of the small intestine
- Pain management
  - Flunixin meglumine: 0.5 to 1.1 mg/kg IV
  - Xylazine: 0.4 to 0.6 mg/kg IV
  - Detomidine: 0.006 to 0.02 mg/kg IV
  - Butorphanol: 0.02 to 0.06 mg/kg IV (use in combination with xylazine or detomidine)
- Foals may respond favorably to medical management if parasite burden is not overwhelming
- Exploratory celiotomy
  - Ventral midline approach
  - Distal jejunum and ileum are the most common sites of impaction. Other less common sites include the cecum, other portions of the jejunum, and the pelvic flexure.
  - In mild cases, extraluminal massage may resolve the impaction.
  - Enterotomy is commonly required to resolve the impaction.
  - If devitalized segment of intestine is associated with the impaction, resection and anastomosis must be performed.
  - It is rarely possible to remove all the adult parasites from the entire intestinal tract.
  - Secondary lesions, including small intestinal volvulus and intussusception, may also be found at the time of surgery.

CHRONIC TREATMENT

Parasite control

POSSIBLE COMPLICATIONS

- Colic
- Endotoxemia
- Adhesions
- Diffuse severe enteritis
- Focal necrotizing enteritis
- Intestinal perforation
- Incisional complications
- Pneumonia

RECOMMENDED MONITORING

- Cardiovascular status
- Rectal temperature
- Postoperative ileus
- Recurrence of colic
- Abdominal incision
- Slow return to oral intake

PROGNOSIS AND OUTCOME

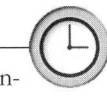

- Prognosis for medical management is good.
- Short-term prognosis (discharge from the hospital) for surgical patients is fair to poor (50%–79%) based on retrospectives studies; long-term survival is guarded (10%–33%).

PEARLS & CONSIDERATIONS

COMMENTS

- Long-term survival of these foals is not good. Proposed reasons for the low survival rate are subsequent damage to the intestinal wall from toxins and allergens released by the parasite after death and corresponding hypersensitivity reaction and inflammation.
- Appropriate parasite control is paramount to preventing this disease.
- Although not proven, numerous studies have shown an association between the use of paralytic anthelmintics and ascarid impactions (macrocyclic lactones [ivermectin, pyrimidines], pyrantel pamoate, and piperazine).

PREVENTION

- Parasite control
- Numerous studies have shown an increasing number of cases of *P. equorum* resistance to ivermectin; practitioners can no longer assume that routine use of anthelmintics will control this parasite.
- Multiple anthelmintic resistance is threatening *Parascaris* spp. control.
- Debate as to whether to deworm with fast-acting (paralytic) anthelmintic drug versus slow-acting anthelmintic.
- Frequent fecal monitoring starting at 3 to 4 months of age should be an integral component of the parasite control program.
- Environmental control
  - Pasture management
  - Stall management
- Initiate parasite control program at 6 to 8 weeks of age
  - Deworm at 6-week intervals until 6 months of age. Foals develop age-dependent immunity by 6 months of age.
    - Fenbendazole: 10 mg/kg PO for 5 consecutive days
    - Pyrantel pamoate: 6.6 mg/kg PO
    - Ivermectin: 0.2 mg/kg PO
    - Moxidectin: 0.4 mg/kg PO (not in foals <4 months)
- If heavy burden is suspected, deworming with fenbendazole at 5 mg/kg (half the normal dose) is recommended. Follow 1 week later with 10 mg/kg (full dose).
- Ivermectin and moxidectin are becoming less and less effective because of resistance.

CLIENT EDUCATION

- Pasture management
- Manure removal or harrowing of pastures
- Pasture rotation

SUGGESTED READING

Freeman DE: Diseases of the small intestine. In White NA, Moore JN, Mair TS, editors: *The equine acute abdomen*, ed 2, Jackson, WY, 2008, Teton NewMedia, pp 594–616.

Hearn PD, Peregrine AS: Identification of foals infected with *Parascaris equorum* apparently resistant to ivermectin. *J Am Vet Med Assoc* 223:482, 2003.

Knottenbelt D: Neonatal syndromes. In Knottenbelt D, Holdstock N, Madigan JE, editors: *Equine neonatology medicine and surgery*, St Louis, 2004, Saunders Elsevier, pp 235–247.

Lyons ET, Tolliver SC, Rathgeber RA, et al: Parasite field study in central Kentucky on thoroughbred foals (born in 2004) treated with pyrantel tartrate daily and other parasiticides periodically. *Parasitol Res* 100:473, 2007.

Southwood LL, Baxter GM, Bennett GD, et al: Ascarid impaction in young horses. *Compend Contin Educ Vet* 20:100, 1998.

Southwood LL, Ragle CA, Snyder JR, et al: Surgical treatment of ascarid impactions in horses and foals. *Proc Am Assoc Equine Pract* 1996:258–261.

AUTHOR: **RANDY EGGLESTON**

EDITORS: **TIM MAIR** and **CERI SHERLOCK**

Small Intestine: Diaphragmatic Hernia

BASIC INFORMATION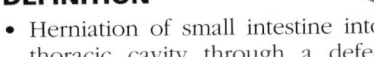

DEFINITION

- Herniation of small intestine into the thoracic cavity through a defect in the diaphragm.
- May be congenital in origin or acquired.
- Acquired diaphragmatic hernias are seen in foals secondary to rib fractures (ribs 3–8) sustained during parturition.
- The most common cause of acquired diaphragmatic hernias in the adult horse is trauma.
  - Traumatic dystocia
  - Direct trauma such as a kick or substantial fall or collision with solid object
- Herniation through the diaphragm can also include the stomach, ascending colon, liver, and spleen.

EPIDEMIOLOGY

SPECIES, AGE, SEX

- Acquired hernia in a foal is seen immediately after parturition.
- In an adult horse, the problem is seen in association with a traumatic incident.
- Congenital diaphragmatic hernias may be seen at any age.

RISK FACTORS Trauma

CLINICAL PRESENTATION

HISTORY, CHIEF COMPLAINT

- Usually associated with traumatic incident
- May present with signs of respiratory distress, abdominal discomfort, or both

PHYSICAL EXAM FINDINGS

- Respiratory distress
  - Tachypnea
  - Dyspnea
  - Auscultation of the thoracic cavity may reveal reduced, absent, or muffled lung sounds.
  - Percussion of the thoracic cavity may produce a dull resonance.

- Borborygmi may be heard within the thoracic cavity, but this is nonspecific.
- Abdominal pain: Depending on the size of the defect, the colic signs may be intermittent or persistent and may be mild to severe.
- Tachycardia: Heart sound may be dramatically louder on one side than the other.

ETIOLOGY AND PATHOPHYSIOLOGY

- Congenital: Incomplete formation of the diaphragm. Small congenital defects are usually found in the abaxial dorsal portion of the diaphragm.
- Acquired: Associated with increased abdominal pressure during parturition or a traumatic incident.
- Herniation through small defects causes strangulation and ischemic necrosis of the affected small intestine. Herniation through large defects may cause partial obstruction and respiratory distress because of an inability to expand the lungs normally.

DIAGNOSIS

DIFFERENTIAL DIAGNOSIS

Other causes of strangulating obstruction of the small intestine
- Small intestinal volvulus
- Epiploic foramen entrapment
- Gastrosplenic entrapment
- Strangulating lipoma

INITIAL DATABASE

- Rectal examination may or may not reveal abnormalities. May palpate distended small intestine.
- Nasogastric reflux (NGR) is seen as the disease progresses. NGR may be variable based on the size of the defect and the degree of obstruction.
- Abdominocentesis may or may not be abnormal and may significantly underestimate the degree of intestinal injury. With small defects, the affected segment of small intestine becomes

sequestered within the thoracic cavity, causing confusion in interpretation of the results of abdominocentesis.
- Complete blood count and chemistry profile are normal early in the disease process. As the colic progresses, changes consistent with dehydration and endotoxemia occur rapidly. A mild metabolic acidosis may also be present.
- Blood gas analysis may indicate respiratory compromise and hypoxemia.
- If the suspicion of diaphragmatic hernia is high based on the history and physical examination findings, thoracocentesis may be performed. This procedure should be done with caution because puncture of the intestine is a risk.

ADVANCED OR CONFIRMATORY TESTING

- Thoracic radiographs may be very useful in identifying the presence of intestinal contents within the thoracic cavity.
- Abdominal and thoracic ultrasonography is useful in identifying intestinal contents within the thoracic cavity and potentially visualization of the diaphragmatic defect. Identification of other abdominal viscera within the chest may also be possible and helpful in preoperative planning.
- Diaphragmatic hernias may be difficult to diagnose, and a definitive diagnosis may be made at the time of exploratory celiotomy.

TREATMENT

THERAPEUTIC GOAL(S)

- Rehydration
- Correction of metabolic and respiratory derangements
- Pain management
- Reduction of the entrapped intestine and repair of the defect

ACUTE GENERAL TREATMENT

- Rehydration and correction of metabolic derangements
  - Balanced polyionic fluids (ie, lactated Ringer's solution, Normosol-R)
  - Replacement fluid volume = Body weight (BW) (kg) × % dehydration
    - 500 kg × 0.08 = 40 L deficit
  - Maintenance fluid volume = BW (kg) × 50 to 60 mL/kg/d
    - 500 kg × 50 mL/kg/d = 25 L/d
  - Replacement fluid administration: 10 to 20 mL/kg/h
    - 500 kg × 10 to 20 mL/kg/h = 5 to 10 L/h until deficit volume is replaced
    - Maintenance rate after deficit replacement = 2 to 4 mL/kg/h
      - 500 kg × 2 to 4 mL/kg/h = 1 to 2 L/h
- Respiratory support: Supplemental nasal oxygen
- Pain management
  - Xylazine: 0.3 to 0.5 mg/kg IV
  - Butorphanol: 0.01 to 0.04 mg/kg IV (use in combination with xylazine or detomidine)
  - Nonsteroidal antiinflammatory drugs: Flunixin meglumine (1.1 mg/kg IV)
- Preoperative antibiotics
- Exploratory celiotomy
  - The abdominal incision usually needs to be extended to the xiphoid process and depending on the size and accessibility of the defect extended laterally. The horse can also be tilted, resulting in caudal displacement of the abdominal contents.
  - Small mature defects usually need to be enlarged to allow for reduction of the entrapment.
  - Resection and anastomosis of the incarcerated bowel is usually required, particularly with small defects.
  - Small defects can be repaired with a sutured primary closure. Larger defects are repaired with a synthetic mesh (Marlex, Proxplast, polyethylene).
  - Very large defects are difficult to repair, and the prognosis for a successful repair is grave.
  - Blind repair of small inaccessible dorsal defects with sutured or stapled mesh has been reported.
  - Laparoscopic-assisted repair in the laterally recumbent or standing patient has also been reported.
  - If the entrapment can be reduced but the defect is unable to be repaired, the horse can be recovered in hopes that adhesion of adjacent abdominal viscera or omental tissue occurs, resulting in sealing of the defect. The potential risk for recurrence is high.

POSSIBLE COMPLICATIONS

- Septic pleuritis
- Implant failure
- Complications associated with resection and anastomosis
- Recurrence
- Complication rate is lower in foals because of accessibility of the diaphragm and size of the foal

PROGNOSIS AND OUTCOME

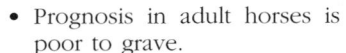

- Prognosis in adult horses is poor to grave.
- Prognosis in foals is also poor, but the chances for successful repair are better than in adult horses.

PEARLS & CONSIDERATIONS

- Diaphragmatic hernia should be suspected in foals or adults that have a history of a traumatic incident associated with the onset of clinical signs, especially if clinical signs include respiratory abnormalities.
- Respiratory signs are not always present.
- Thoracic radiographs and ultrasonography are very helpful in obtaining a diagnosis of diaphragmatic hernia.

SUGGESTED READING

Freeman DE: Small intestine. In Auer JA, Stick JA, editors: *Equine surgery*, ed 3, St Louis, 2006, Saunders Elsevier, pp 420–421.

Freeman DE: Diseases of the small intestine. In White NA, Moore JN, Mair TS, editors: *The equine acute abdomen*, ed 2, Jackson, WY, 2008, Teton NewMedia, pp 594–616.

Kelmer G, Kramer J, Wilson DA: Diaphragmatic hernia: etiology, clinical presentation, and diagnosis. *Compend Contin Educ Equine* Jan/Feb:28–36, 2008.

Kelmer G, Kramer J, Wilson DA: Diaphragmatic hernia: treatment, complications, and prognosis. *Compend Contin Educ Equine* Jan/Feb:37–46, 2008.

Mueller POE, Moore JN: Gastrointestinal emergencies and other causes of colic. In Orsini JA, Divers TJ, editors: *Equine emergencies treatment and procedures*, St Louis, 2008, Saunders Elsevier, pp 129–130.

Seahorn JL, Seahorn TL: Fluid therapy in horses with gastrointestinal disease. *Vet Clin North Am Equine Pract* 19(3):665–679, 2003.

AUTHOR: **RANDY EGGLESTON**

EDITORS: **TIM MAIR** and **CERI SHERLOCK**

Small Intestine: Epiploic Foramen Entrapment

BASIC INFORMATION

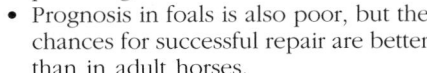

DEFINITION

- The epiploic foramen (foramen of Winslow) is bordered by the caudate liver lobe, forming the dorsal and craniodorsal border, the portal vein forming the cranioventral border, and the gastropancreatic fold forming the ventral border. The epiploic foramen is the entrance to the omental bursa.
- The small intestine can traverse the foramen and become entrapped, causing obstruction.

- The ileum is involved in 70% of cases with jejunal involvement in 40% to 60% of cases. The length of intestine involved is variable (8 cm–18 m) and increases with time. Multiple independent loops passing through the foramen can also be seen.

EPIDEMIOLOGY

SPECIES, AGE, SEX

- Once thought to be a disease of aged horses caused by a potential enlargement of the foramen with age; recent studies failed to support this theory.
- Males tend to be more frequently affected.

GENETICS AND BREED PREDISPOSITION A number of studies have shown a propensity for Thoroughbreds and Thoroughbred crosses to be at higher risk for epiploic entrapment.

RISK FACTORS Recent studies show a strong association with horses that crib bite and wind suck.

GEOGRAPHY AND SEASONALITY The majority of cases are seen between November and March.

CLINICAL PRESENTATION

HISTORY, CHIEF COMPLAINT Colic. A total of 48% to 68% of cases have a history of cribbing or wind sucking behavior. Clinical signs of colic can be highly variable. Early in the entrapment, the obstruction may be partial, resulting in intermittent gas and fluid accumulation and abdominal discomfort.

PHYSICAL EXAM FINDINGS

- Moderate to severe abdominal pain. Initially responsive to analgesics; response diminishes as disease progresses.
- Tachycardia
- Normothermic
- Cardiovascular status diminishes with progression of the disease. Signs of dehydration occur rapidly.
- As the disease progresses, horses may become depressed and show progressive signs of endotoxemia.
- Reduced or absent borborygmi

ETIOLOGY AND PATHOPHYSIOLOGY

- Entrapment of small intestine through the epiploic foramen. The ileum is involved in the majority of cases, either alone or in combination with jejunum.
- Progressive ischemia and necrosis of small intestine requiring resection and anastomosis.

DIAGNOSIS

DIFFERENTIAL DIAGNOSIS

Other causes of strangulating obstruction of the small intestine
- Small intestinal volvulus
- Gastrosplenic entrapment
- Strangulating lipoma
- Strangulation through mesenteric defect

INITIAL DATABASE

- Rectal examination early in disease often reveals no palpable small intestine because of the cranial location of the foramen. As the disease progresses, loops of distended small intestine become palpable. In the author's experience, it is common to feel a concentration of distended small intestine "suspended" in the upper right quadrant of the abdomen.
- Nasogastric reflux (NGR) is seen as the disease progresses. NGR may be absent early in the disease. Pain relief may not be seen after decompression.
- Abdominocentesis is useful in distinguishing between a simple obstruction and strangulating obstruction. Peritoneal protein and nucleated cell count are often normal early in the disease process. As the colic progresses, peritoneal protein elevates. Only in late disease with increased intestinal injury does the peritoneal nucleated cell count increase. Fluid is often serosanguineous. Results of abdominocentesis may underestimate the true severity of the disease.

- Complete blood count and chemistry profile are normal early in the disease process. As the colic progresses, changes consistent with dehydration and endotoxemia occur rapidly. A mild metabolic acidosis may also be present.

ADVANCED OR CONFIRMATORY TESTING

Abdominal ultrasonography: Multiple loops of distended small intestine located in the right ventral paralumbar fossa followed by the caudal ventral abdomen. Motility is slow to absent, and mural thickening is seen as the disease progresses.

TREATMENT

THERAPEUTIC GOAL(S)

- Surgical emergency
- Rehydrate
- Pain management
- Surgical reduction of entrapment

ACUTE GENERAL TREATMENT

- Rehydration
- Balanced polyionic fluids (ie, lactated Ringer's solution, Normosol-R)
  - Replacement fluid volume = Body weight (BW) (kg) × % dehydration
    - 500 kg × 0.08 = 40 L deficit
  - Maintenance fluid volume = BW (kg) × 50 to 60 mL/kg/d
    - 500 kg × 50 mL/kg/d = 25 L/d
  - Replacement fluid administration: 10 to 20 mL/kg/h
    - 500 kg × 10 to 20 mL/kg/h = 5 to 10 L/h until deficit volume is replaced
    - Maintenance rate after deficit replacement = 2 to 4 mL/kg/h
      - 500 kg × 2 to 4 mL/kg/h = 1 to 2 L/h
- Pain management
  - Xylazine: 0.3 to 0.5 mg/kg IV
  - Detomidine: 0.006 to 0.02 mg/kg IV
  - Butorphanol: 0.01 to 0.04 mg/kg IV (use in combination with xylazine or detomidine)
  - Nonsteroidal antiinflammatory drugs: Flunixin meglumine (1.1 mg/kg IV)
- Preoperative antibiotics
- Exploratory celiotomy
  - The goal of surgery is to release the strangulation and assess intestinal viability.
  - Reduction can be complicated because of an inability to visualize the strangulation.
  - The small intestine can pass through the foramen in either a left-to-right or right-to-left direction; the left-to-right direction is much more common with accumulation of intestine between the right body

wall and the right colons and cecum.
  - Small intestinal resection is often necessary.

CHRONIC TREATMENT

Provided the horse recovers through the immediate postoperative period, long-term treatment is not needed.

POSSIBLE COMPLICATIONS

- Ileus
- Intraabdominal adhesions
- Complications at the anastomosis site

RECOMMENDED MONITORING

During the postoperative period
- Cardiovascular status
- Nasogastric reflux
- Recurring signs of colic
- Incisional complications
- Slow return to oral intake

PROGNOSIS AND OUTCOME

- The prognosis depends on the duration and severity of the disease.
- Prognosis is good for horses not requiring resection of small intestine.
- Prognosis for horses requiring resection and anastomosis is fair provided postoperative complications (eg, ileus, endotoxemia) are minimal. In the face of prolonged complications, prognosis decreases.
- Prognosis worsens slightly with ileocecostomies and jejunocecostomies.
- Long-term prognosis for small intestinal strangulating disease is reported to be 40% to 70%.

PEARLS & CONSIDERATIONS

Based on evidence of an association between epiploic foreman entrapments and cribbing, management of behavioral vices is recommended.

SUGGESTED READING

Archer DC, Freeman DE, Doyle AJ, et al: Association between cribbing and entrapment of the small intestine in the epiploic foramen in horses: 68 cases (1991–2002). *J Am Vet Med Assoc* 224:562–564, 2004.

Archer DC, Pinchbeck GL, French NP, et al: Risk factors for epiploic foramen entrapment colic in a UK horse population: a prospective case-control study. *Equine Vet J* 40:405, 2008.

Archer DC, Proudman CJ, Pinchbeck G, et al: Entrapment of the small intestine in the epiploic foramen in horses: a retrospective analysis of 71 cases recorded between 1991 and 2001. *Vet Rec* 155:793–797, 2004.

Freeman DE: Small intestine. In Auer JA, Stick JA, editors: *Equine surgery*, ed 3, St Louis, 2006, Saunders Elsevier, pp 413–414.

Freeman DE, Schaeffer DJ: Short-term survival after surgery for epiploic foramen entrapment compared with other strangulating diseases of the small intestine in horses. *Equine Vet J* 37:292–295, 2005.

Freeman, DE: Diseases of the small intestine. In White NA, Moore JN, Mair TS, editors: *The equine acute abdomen*, ed 2, Jackson, WY, 2008, Teton NewMedia, pp 594–616.

Mueller POE, Moore JN: Gastrointestinal emergencies and other causes of colic. In Orsini JA, Divers TJ, editors: *Equine emergencies treatment and procedures*, St Louis, 2008, Saunders Elsevier, pp 125–126.

Seahorn JL, Seahorn TL: Fluid therapy in horses with gastrointestinal disease. *Vet Clin North Am Equine Pract* 19(3):665–679, 2003.

AUTHOR: **RANDY EGGLESTON**

EDITORS: **TIM MAIR** and **CERI SHERLOCK**

Small Intestine: Ileal Impaction

BASIC INFORMATION

DEFINITION
Impaction of the distal-most segment of the small intestine (ileum) extending from the ileocecal papilla orally for varying lengths

EPIDEMIOLOGY
SPECIES, AGE, SEX
- Reported in very young and older foals
- More common in adult horses

RISK FACTORS
- Associated with feeding coastal Bermuda hay (CBH)
- Parasitism: *Anoplocephala perfoliata* (tapeworms), *Strongylus vulgaris* (less common)
- Poor water intake

GEOGRAPHY AND SEASONALITY
- Particularly common in southeast United States
- Summer through late fall (June to November)

ASSOCIATED CONDITIONS AND DISORDERS
- Parasitism
  - Association between tapeworm infestation and ileal impactions has been made in the United States and Europe. These parasites attach to the intestinal mucosa at the ileocecal junction, causing mucosal inflammation, edema, and ulceration. Extent of injury is proportional to the number of parasites attached (>100 tapeworms)
  - *S. vulgaris* infestation may cause changes in motility and blood supply to the ileum. Uncommon because of current deworming practices.
- Ileal hypertrophy

CLINICAL PRESENTATION
HISTORY, CHIEF COMPLAINT
Clinical signs are consistent with abdominal discomfort or colic. Early in the disease, pain is caused by spasmodic contraction of the ileum around the impaction. Systemic compromise is not seen at this stage. As the disease progresses, signs of colic worsen caused by the progressive distension of the small intestine with gas and sequestered fluids. Systemic signs of dehydration also start to appear. If not treated, intestinal or gastric rupture may occur. Important historical information usually includes an abrupt change in feeding practices, such as
- Change from different type of grass hay or alfalfa to CBH over an inadequate period of time
- Horse has been on CBH but recently fed a new cutting of hay.
- On a different grass or alfalfa hay and had recent unexpected exposure to CBH

PHYSICAL EXAM FINDINGS
Physical examination findings consistent with abdominal discomfort (colic)
- Tachycardia
- Tachypnea
- Normothermic
- Reduced or absent borborygmi
- Progressive signs of dehydration
- Pale, tacky mucous membranes
- Prolonged capillary refill time
- Injected sclera

ETIOLOGY AND PATHOPHYSIOLOGY
- Abrupt change in feeding practices, particularly to CBH from other grass hay or legume hay. Lignin and crude fiber content increases as hay matures as with tall stands or in late summer and early fall.
- Tapeworm infestation causes mucosal injury, resulting in changes in intestinal motility and reduction in size of the ileocecal papilla.
- Ileal hypertrophy causes changes in intestinal motility and variable reduction in size of the ileal lumen.

DIAGNOSIS

DIFFERENTIAL DIAGNOSIS
Other causes of simple obstruction of the small intestine
- Inflammatory disease
- Intussusception
- Ascarid impaction (young animals)
- Ileal hypertrophy (older animals)
- Nonstrangulating infarction

INITIAL DATABASE
- Rectal examination is the most informative physical test performed. The impacted ileum can be palpated in approximately 25% of cases. Depending on the duration of colic, there is a variable amount of small intestinal distension. The distended loops are usually consistent in size, mural thickness, and compressibility.
- Nasogastric reflux (NGR) is variable because of the distal location of the impaction. NGR may be absent in initial 10 to 12 hours of the colic episode.
- Abdominocentesis is useful in distinguishing between a simple obstruction and strangulating obstruction. Peritoneal protein and nucleated cell count are often normal early in the disease process. As the colic progresses, the peritoneal protein elevates. Only in late disease with increased intestinal injury does the peritoneal nucleated cell count increase.
- Complete blood count and chemistry profile are normal early in the disease process. As the colic persists, changes consistent with dehydration occur. A mild metabolic acidosis may also be present.

ADVANCED OR CONFIRMATORY TESTING
Abdominal ultrasonography: Multiple loops of distended small intestine located in the caudal ventral abdomen. The size of the loops is fairly consistent; little or no motility is present, and mural thickening is minimal (normal <3 mm).

TREATMENT

THERAPEUTIC GOAL(S)
- Correction of metabolic derangements
- Pain management
- Resolution of ileal impaction

ACUTE GENERAL TREATMENT

- The initial approach to treating ileal impactions has recently shifted toward medical management. If suspicion of ileal impaction is strong based on physical and diagnostic evaluation and the horse is systemically stable, aggressive medical management should be attempted.
- Nasogastric intubation
- Fluid replacement: Balanced polyionic fluids (ie, lactated Ringer's solution)
  - Maintenance fluids: 50 to 60 mL/kg/d
  - 500 kg × 55 mL/kg = 27.5 L/d (maintenance)
  - Deficit replacement: Percentage dehydration based on physical examination findings
    - 500 kg × 0.08 = 40 L (deficit)
    - Administer calculated deficit over the first 1 to 2 hours. Remaining replacement volume should be administered over a 12- to 24-hour period.
  - Oral fluids should be used with great caution because of complete obstruction of the small intestine.
- Pain management
  - Flunixin meglumine: 1.1 mg/kg IV
  - Xylazine: 0.4 to 0.6 mg/kg IV
  - Detomidine: 0.006 to 0.02 mg/kg IV
  - Butorphanol: 0.02 to 0.06 mg/kg IV (use in combination with xylazine or detomidine)
    - Constant rate infusion (CRI): 13.0 µg/kg/h
  - Lidocaine: 1.3 mg/kg as bolus given over 5 minutes followed by CRI at 0.05 mg/kg/min. Acts to stimulate gastrointestinal motility and has analgesic effects. Monitor patient closely at onset of CRI for signs of toxicity, including muscle fasciculation, piloerection, weakness, and recumbency. Signs disappear quickly after discontinuance of CRI.
  - Butylscopolamine (Busconpan): 0.3 mg/kg IV. Can cause ileus if overdosed or used for a prolonged period. Can cause a transient increase in heart rate (≤30 min), making it difficult to use heart rate as a monitoring parameter.
- The majority of cases that respond favorably to medical management will do so within the first 12 to 24 hours of therapy. Surgical intervention should be pursued if there is a lack of response to medical management. Failure of medical management would include
  - Persistent nonresponsive abdominal discomfort
  - Deterioration of cardiovascular status
  - Persistent nasogastric reflux
  - Persistent or worsening small intestinal distension on rectal palpation
- Exploratory celiotomy
  - Extraluminal massage and breakdown of the impaction
  - Infusion of a combination of sterile fluid, sodium carboxymethylcellulose, and lidocaine into the lumen of the ileum, oral to the impaction, can facilitate reduction of the impaction.
  - Impaction is broken down into small pieces and worked orally, allowing for intermixing with infused fluid. After the entire impaction has been broken down, attempts are made to slowly work the material aborally into the cecum.
  - If the impaction is extensive and excessive manipulation of the intestine is required, jejunal enterotomy and evacuation of the impaction can be performed.
  - In rare cases if concurrent disease is present (eg, ileal hypertrophy or significant vascular compromise to the ileum), incomplete bypass, or resection and complete bypass may be necessary.

POSSIBLE COMPLICATIONS

Potential complications after medical management are uncommon, and recurrence is rarely seen, although feed changes are recommended to reduce the risk of recurrence. Complications after surgical reduction are those consistent with exploratory celiotomy for small intestinal disease. The risk and incidence of complications is highly dependent on procedures performed at the time of reduction.

- Postoperative ileus
- Intraabdominal adhesions
- Peritonitis
- Recurrence of colic

RECOMMENDED MONITORING

Feeding changes are made regardless of medical or surgical treatment, including feeding alternative grass hays or alfalfa hay. Postoperative monitoring for closed reduction of the impaction includes management of postoperative ileus if present, a slow return to feeding, and routine management of the abdominal incision. Monitoring for open reduction of the impaction is similar unless complications arise because of bypass procedures.

PROGNOSIS AND OUTCOME

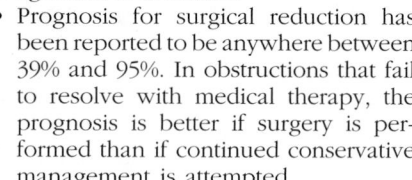

- Prognosis for medical management is favorable.
- Prognosis for surgical reduction has been reported to be anywhere between 39% and 95%. In obstructions that fail to resolve with medical therapy, the prognosis is better if surgery is performed than if continued conservative management is attempted.

PEARLS & CONSIDERATIONS

Prevention involves proper feeding management.

SUGGESTED READING

Freeman DE: Small intestine. In Auer JA, Stick JA, editors: *Equine surgery*, ed 3, St Louis, 2006, Saunders Elsevier, pp 408–409.

Hanson RR: Ileal impaction. In Robinson NE, editor: *Current therapy in equine medicine*, ed 5, St Louis, 2003, Saunders Elsevier, pp 127–130.

Hanson RR, Wright JC, Schumacher J, et al: Surgical reduction of ileal impactions in the horse: 28 cases. *Vet Surg* 27:555–560, 1998.

Little D, Blikslager AT: Factors associated with development of ileal impaction in horses with surgical colic: 78 cases (1986–2000). *Equine Vet J* 34:464, 2002.

Mueller POE, Moore JN: Gastrointestinal emergencies and other causes of colic. In Orsini JA, Divers TJ, editors: *Equine emergencies treatment and procedures*, St Louis, 2008, Saunders Elsevier, pp 130–132.

Proudman CJ, French NP, Trees AJ: Tapeworm infection is a significant risk factor for spasmodic colic and ileal impaction colic in the horse. *Equine Vet J* 30:194–199, 1998.

AUTHOR: **RANDY EGGLESTON**

EDITORS: **TIM MAIR** and **CERI SHERLOCK**

Small Intestine: Intussusception

BASIC INFORMATION

DEFINITION

Invagination of a segment of small intestine (intussusceptum) into the lumen of the adjacent small intestine (intussuscipiens) or viscus (cecum)

SYNONYM(S)

- Jejunojejunal intussusception
- Jejunoileal intussusception
- Ileoileal intussusception
- Ileocecal intussusception

EPIDEMIOLOGY

SPECIES, AGE, SEX Most common in horses between 3 months and 3 years of age

RISK FACTORS
- Heavy ascarid burden
- Tapeworm (*Anoplocephala perfoliata*) infestation
- Abrupt feed changes

ASSOCIATED CONDITIONS AND DISORDERS
- Enteritis: Segmental changes in motility
- Mesenteric arteritis
- Focal pedunculated mucosal masses such as a papilloma, leiomyoma, granuloma, or carcinoid may initiate the formation of an intussusception. In the author's experience, mural leiomyomas have been commonly indentified.
- Other reported predisposing causes of small intestinal intussusceptions include transverse enterotomies, functional end-to-end anastomoses, and end-to-end anastomoses.

CLINICAL PRESENTATION

HISTORY, CHIEF COMPLAINT
- Clinical signs may be variable. Short intussusceptions causing incomplete obstruction may present with intermittent bouts of colic, particularly in the postprandial period; reduced appetite; reduced fecal production; weight loss; and a generalized unthriftiness. Affected horses may also experience intermittent fevers.
- Longer intussusceptions often cause complete obstruction and present with signs consistent with an acute small intestinal obstruction.

PHYSICAL EXAM FINDINGS
- Chronic intermittent colic
  - Mild postprandial colic
  - Anorexia
  - Intermittent fevers
  - Weight loss
  - Reduced fecal production
  - Generalized unthriftiness
  - Clinical signs may persist for weeks to months.
- Acute colic
  - Moderate to severe abdominal discomfort
  - Tachycardia
  - Tachypnea
  - Normothermic
  - Reduced or absent borborygmi
  - Progressive signs of dehydration

ETIOLOGY AND PATHOPHYSIOLOGY

- Conditions causing segmental changes in intestinal motility
  - Enteritis, particularly in foals
  - Rapid feed changes
- Jejunojejunal and ileocecal intussusceptions have been associated with heavy ascarid and tapeworm infestations, respectively.
- Aggressive anthelmintic treatment in young horses
- Mural or intraluminal pedunculated masses can have a "ball valve" effect at the leading edge of the intussusception, causing the invagination of the small intestine; this condition is seen most commonly in adult horses.

DIAGNOSIS

DIFFERENTIAL DIAGNOSIS

Other causes of partial or complete obstruction of the small intestine

INITIAL DATABASE

- Rectal examination in adult horses is consistent with other causes of small intestinal obstruction. In chronic cases, the proximal loops of distended small intestine may be greatly distended with thickening of the walls caused by the slow, chronic, persistent distension of the intestine.
- Nasogastric reflux (NGR) is variable based on the degree of obstruction and the progression of the obstruction. With ileocecal intussusceptions, NGR may not develop if the obstruction is partial.
- Abdominocentesis is useful in distinguishing between a partial obstruction and complete obstruction leading to devitalization of the intestine. However, because of the isolation of the devitalized intussusceptum within the intussuscipiens, the abdominocentesis may underestimate the severity of the disease. Peritoneal protein and nucleated cell count increase with the progression of the disease.
- Complete blood count and chemistry profile are normal early in the disease

process. As the colic persists, changes consistent with dehydration occur. Electrolyte abnormalities and signs of endotoxemia may also be seen in cases involving intestinal devitalization.

ADVANCED OR CONFIRMATORY TESTING

Abdominal ultrasonography is often effective in diagnosing intussusceptions in foals. The characteristic "bull's eye" lesion is formed by the thickened intussusceptum and the thinner wall of the intussuscipiens. In adult horses, ultrasonography shows multiple loops of distended small intestine. In chronic cases, the proximal intestine may be greatly distended, more so than with other causes of obstruction, with thickened walls and some degree of motility.

TREATMENT

THERAPEUTIC GOAL(S)

- Correction of metabolic derangements
- Pain management
- Reduction of intussusception

ACUTE GENERAL TREATMENT

- Gastric decompression in acute cases
- Balanced polyionic fluids
- Fluid replacement: Balanced polyionic fluids (ie, lactated Ringer's solution)
  - Maintenance fluids: 50 to 60 mL/kg/d
  - 500 kg × 55 mL/kg = 27.5 L/d (maintenance)
  - Deficit replacement: Percentage dehydration based on physical examination findings
    - 500 kg × 0.08 (% dehydration) = 40 L (deficit)
    - Administer calculated deficit over the first 1 to 2 hours. Remaining replacement volume should be administered over a 12- to 24-hour period.
- Pain management
  - Flunixin meglumine: 1.1 mg/kg IV
  - Xylazine: 0.4 to 0.6 mg/kg IV
  - Detomidine: 0.006 to 0.02 mg/kg IV
  - Butorphanol: 0.02 to 0.06 mg/kg IV (use in combination with xylazine or detomidine)
    - Constant rate infusion (CRI): 13.0 μg/kg/h
- After the horse is stable, exploratory celiotomy is required to reduce the intussusception.
- In many cases, the intussusception can be manually reduced, allowing for

evaluation of the affected segment of intestine. Although the intestine may be viable, because of the damage to the adjacent mesentery and the potential for progressive damage, resection and anastomosis should be considered.

- In cases in which the intussusception cannot be manually reduced, an en bloc resection of the affected intestine is performed with the appropriate anastomosis.
- Nonreducible ileocecal intussusceptions often require special techniques to reduce the intussusception or bypass the affected intestine (typhlotomy, ileocecostomy, jejunocecostomy).
- In horses that present for low-grade intermittent colic, weight loss, intermittent fever, and generalized unthriftiness and intussusception is suspected, exploratory surgery is indicated.

CHRONIC TREATMENT

- In cases of chronic ileocecal intussusception, some horses can have a prolonged recovery and show slow weight gain and at times mild intermittent colic.
- Because of the suspicion of *A. perfoliata* involvement in cases of ileocecal

intussusception, horses should be dewormed appropriately postoperatively (pyrantel pamoate and praziquantel).

POSSIBLE COMPLICATIONS

Complications depend on the surgical procedures performed at the time of surgery.
- Postoperative ileus
- Intraabdominal adhesions
- Peritonitis
- Recurrence of colic

RECOMMENDED MONITORING

During the postoperative period
- Hydration status
- Nasogastric reflux
- Recurring signs of colic
- Incisional complications
- Slow return to oral intake

PROGNOSIS AND OUTCOME

- Prognosis for simple surgical reduction of intussusception is good.
- In chronic cases or those requiring resection and anastomosis, the prognosis is the same as horses experienc-

ing other small intestinal strangulating obstructions.
- Prognosis worsens slightly with ileocecostomies and jejunocecostomies.

PEARLS & CONSIDERATIONS

Practice a good parasite control program.

SUGGESTED READING

Bryant JE, Gaughan EM: Abdominal surgery in neonatal foals. *Vet Clin North Am Equine Pract* 21:2, 2005.

Freeman DE: Surgery of the small intestine. *Vet Clin North Am Equine Pract* 13:2, 1997.

Freeman DE: Small intestine. In Auer JA, Stick JA, editors: *Equine surgery*, ed 3, St Louis, 2006, Saunders Elsevier, pp 415–417.

Freeman DE: Diseases of the small intestine. In White NA, Moore JN, Mair TS, editors: *The equine acute abdomen*, ed 2, Jackson, WY, 2008, Teton NewMedia, pp 594–616.

Mueller POE, Moore JN: Gastrointestinal emergencies and other causes of colic. In Orsini JA, Divers TJ, editors: *Equine emergencies treatment and procedures*, St Louis, 2008, Saunders Elsevier, pp 123–124.

AUTHOR: RANDY EGGLESTON

EDITORS: TIM MAIR and CERI SHERLOCK

Small Intestine: Mesenteric Hernia

BASIC INFORMATION

DEFINITION

Passage of small intestine through a defect in the mesentery

SYNONYM(S)

- Gastrosplenic ligament entrapment
- Mesenteric rent
- Broad ligament incarceration
- Mesocolon incarceration
- Meckel's diverticulum incarceration
- Mesodiverticular band incarceration

EPIDEMIOLOGY

SPECIES, AGE, SEX Females are said to be predisposed because of foaling accidents or aggressive movement of the foal in utero.

RISK FACTORS
- Pregnancy
- Parturition
- Previous abdominal surgery
- Failure of vitelline and associated mesenteric structures to atrophy naturally during embryonic development

CLINICAL PRESENTATION

HISTORY, CHIEF COMPLAINT

- Colic. Clinical signs are consistent with small intestinal strangulating lesion (see "Small Intestine: Epiploic Foramen Entrapment" and "Small Intestine: Inguinal Hernia" in this section).
- History of late-term pregnancy or recent parturition is very important in these cases.

PHYSICAL EXAM FINDINGS

- Moderate to severe abdominal pain
- Tachycardia
- Normothermic
- Pale tacky mucous membranes with prolonged capillary refill time
- Reduced or absent borborygmi

ETIOLOGY AND PATHOPHYSIOLOGY

- Mesenteric defects may be congenital in origin or acquired from trauma or previous surgery.
- Late-term pregnancy or traumatic parturition may cause tearing of the mesocolon and potential incarceration of the small intestine.
- Trauma to the mesocolon may also cause avulsion of the blood supply to

the small colon, resulting in ischemic necrosis of the small colon.
- The gastrosplenic ligament is the mesenteric attachment between the left part of the greater curvature of the stomach and the hilus of the spleen. Trauma is the suspected cause of defects to this ligament.
- Jejunal mesentery is most commonly involved in small intestinal mesenteric defects. Defects can also be found in the mesentery of the duodenum and ileum.
- Mesenteric defects in the broad ligament are less common.
- Failure of the vitelline artery or duct and its associated mesentery to atrophy during embryonic development forms a mesodiverticular band. These remnants extend from the mesentery to the antimesenteric surface of the distal jejunum. Small intestine may herniate through defects in these structures.
- Although less common, defects may also be found in the mesentery of the large colon and cecum.

DIAGNOSIS

DIFFERENTIAL DIAGNOSIS

Other causes of strangulating obstruction of the small intestine
- Small intestinal volvulus
- Epiploic foramen entrapment
- Strangulating lipoma
- Inguinal hernia
- Diaphragmatic hernia

INITIAL DATABASE

- Rectal examination reveals small intestinal distension. Distension may not be palpable early in the disease. Because of the location of the lesion, distension may be felt late with gastrosplenic entrapments. The small intestine passes through the ligament in a caudal-to-cranial direction, leaving the affected small intestine lateral to the stomach and cranial to the spleen.
- Nasogastric reflux (NGR) is seen as the disease progresses. NGR may be absent early in the disease.
- Abdominocentesis is useful in distinguishing between a simple obstruction and strangulating obstruction. Peritoneal protein and nucleated cell count are often normal early in the disease process. As the colic progresses, the peritoneal protein will elevate. Only in late disease with increased intestinal injury will peritoneal nucleated cell count increase.
- Complete blood count and chemistry profile are normal early in the disease process. As the colic progresses, changes consistent with dehydration and endotoxemia occur. A mild metabolic acidosis may also be present.

ADVANCED OR CONFIRMATORY TESTING

- Abdominal ultrasonography: Multiple loops of distended small intestine can be identified. The size of the loops varies depending on the location of the lesion and the stage of the disease. Mural thickening can be seen within the incarcerated portion of the intestine (normal <3 mm).
- Gastrosplenic entrapments of the small intestine may be concentrated in the left cranial quadrant of the abdomen.

TREATMENT

THERAPEUTIC GOAL(S)

- Correction of metabolic derangements
- Pain management

- Surgical emergency
  - Reduction of the strangulation
  - Repair of the mesenteric defect

ACUTE GENERAL TREATMENT

- Supportive therapy is initiated in preparation for emergency celiotomy
- Gastric decompression
- Rehydration and correction of metabolic derangements
  - Balanced polyionic fluids (ie, lactated Ringer's solution, Normosol-R)
  - Replacement fluid volume = Body weight (BW) (kg) × % dehydration
    - 500 kg × 0.08 = 40 L deficit
  - Maintenance fluid volume = BW (kg) × 50 to 60 mL/kg/d
    - 500 kg × 50 mL/kg/d = 25 L/d
  - Replacement fluid administration: 10 to 20 mL/kg/h
    - 500 kg × 10 to 20 mL/kg/h = 5 to 10 L/h until deficit volume is replaced
    - Maintenance rate after deficit replacement = 2 to 4 mL/kg/h
      - 500 kg × 2 to 4 mL/kg/h = 1 to 2 L/h
- Pain management
  - Xylazine: 0.3 to 0.5 mg/kg IV
  - Detomidine: 0.006 to 0.02 mg/kg IV
  - Butorphanol: 0.01 to 0.04 mg/kg IV (use in combination with xylazine or detomidine)
  - Nonsteroidal antiinflammatory drugs: Flunixin meglumine (1.1 mg/kg IV)
- Exploratory celiotomy
  - Reduction of entrapment. Defect may require manual enlargement to remove the small intestine.
  - Resection and anastomosis are often necessary.
  - If accessible, the mesenteric defect should be repaired. In the case of gastrosplenic entrapments, the defect is left open.
  - Successful repair of mesenteric defects via standing laparoscopic surgery has been reported.

CHRONIC TREATMENT

Provided no postoperative complications are seen, long-term therapy is not necessary.

POSSIBLE COMPLICATIONS

- Ileus
- Incisional complications
- Complications at the anastomosis
- Intraabdominal adhesions
- Recurrence

RECOMMENDED MONITORING

During the postoperative period
- Cardiovascular status
- Nasogastric reflux
- Recurring signs of colic
- Incisional complications
- Slow return to oral intake

PROGNOSIS AND OUTCOME

- The prognosis depends on the duration and severity of the disease.
- Prognosis is good for horses not requiring resection of small intestine.
- Prognosis for horses requiring resection and anastomosis is fair provided preoperative complications (eg, ileus, endotoxemia) are minimal. In the face of prolonged complications, the prognosis decreases.
- The long-term prognosis for small intestinal strangulating disease is reported to be 40% to 70%.

PEARLS & CONSIDERATIONS

- Herniation through mesenteric defects is uncommon.
- Incarceration of small intestine through mesenteric defects should be considered in late-term pregnant or postparturient mares with signs of colic consistent with strangulating small intestinal disease.
- Exploratory surgery is often required for a definitive diagnosis.

SUGGESTED READING

Edwards GB, Proudman CJ: Diseases of the small intestine resulting in colic. In Mair TS, Divers T, Ducharme N, editors: *Manual of equine gastroenterology*, St Louis, 2002, Saunders Elsevier, pp 260–261.

Freeman DE: Small intestine. In Auer JA, Stick JA, editors: *Equine surgery*, ed 3, St Louis, 2006, Saunders Elsevier, pp 417–421.

Mueller POE, Moore JN: Gastrointestinal emergencies and other causes of colic. In Orsini JA, Divers TJ, editors: *Equine emergencies treatment and procedures*, St Louis, 2008, Saunders Elsevier, pp 126–128.

AUTHOR: **RANDY EGGLESTON**

EDITORS: **TIM MAIR** and **CERI SHERLOCK**

Small Intestine: Strangulating Lipoma

BASIC INFORMATION

DEFINITION
Smooth-walled, benign fat tumor of variable size. Suspended by mesenteric fibrovascular pedicle of variable length. The lipoma wraps around a loop of small intestine and its mesentery, causing strangulation of the affected segment. May also affect the descending and ascending colons as well as the cecum.

EPIDEMIOLOGY
SPECIES, AGE, SEX Disease of older horses, with a mean age of 14 to 19.2 years. Castrated males are at higher risk than females and intact males.
GENETICS AND BREED PREDISPOSITION Ponies, Arabians, Saddlebreds, and Quarter Horses are reported to be at higher risk than Thoroughbreds.
RISK FACTORS
- Once thought to be associated with obesity. Retrospective studies fail to support this notion.
- The increased incidence seen in aged geldings suggests an alteration in fat deposition caused by endocrine abnormalities such as insulin resistance, Cushing's disease, and metabolic syndrome.

CLINICAL PRESENTATION
HISTORY, CHIEF COMPLAINT Colic. Clinical signs of colic may be highly variable; usually reported as having an acute onset of abdominal pain that is persistent.
PHYSICAL EXAM FINDINGS
- Moderate to severe abdominal pain. Initially responsive to analgesics; response diminishes as disease progresses.
- Tachycardia (60–80 beats/min).
- Normothermic
- Cardiovascular status diminishes with progression of disease. Signs of dehydration occur rapidly.
- As disease progresses, horses may become depressed and show progressive signs of endotoxemia.
  - Tachycardia
  - Tachypnea
  - Congested mucous membranes
  - Prolonged capillary refill time
- Reduced or absent borborygmi
ETIOLOGY AND PATHOPHYSIOLOGY Strangulation of small intestine and its mesentery by pedunculated lipoma

DIAGNOSIS
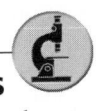

DIFFERENTIAL DIAGNOSIS
- Other causes of strangulating obstruction of the small intestine
  - Epiploic foramen entrapment
  - Small intestinal volvulus
  - Gastrosplenic entrapment
  - Strangulation through mesenteric defect
  - Diaphragmatic hernia
- Strangulating lipoma should always be the top rule-out disorder in horses older than 15 years with signs consistent with strangulating small intestinal lesion.
- Late in the disease as the abdominal discomfort lessens and depression and endotoxemia become more apparent, a strangulating lesion may be confused with inflammatory disease such as duodenitis–proximal jejunitis.

INITIAL DATABASE
- Rectal examination reveals multiple loops of distended small intestine. As the disease progresses, the size and number of loops increase. Late in the disease, it may be possible to palpate thickened turgid small intestine consistent with mural congestion and devitalization. In rare cases, the lipoma may be palpated rectally.
- Nasogastric reflux (NGR) is seen as the disease progresses. NGR may be absent early in the disease. Pain relief may not be seen after decompression. Late in the disease when the horse appears less painful and depressed, NGR persists because of complete obstruction.
- Abdominocentesis is useful in distinguishing between a simple obstruction and strangulating obstruction. Peritoneal protein and nucleated cell count are often normal early in the disease process. As the colic progresses, the peritoneal protein elevates. Only in late disease with increased intestinal injury does the peritoneal nucleated cell count increase. Fluid is often serosanguineous. Results of abdominocentesis may underestimate the true severity of the disease.
- Complete blood count and chemistry profile are normal early in the disease process. As the colic progresses, changes consistent with dehydration and endotoxemia occur rapidly. A mild metabolic acidosis may also be present.

ADVANCED OR CONFIRMATORY TESTING
Abdominal ultrasonography: Multiple loops of distended small intestine located in the caudal ventral abdomen. Motility is slow to absent, and mural thickening is seen as the disease progresses.

TREATMENT

THERAPEUTIC GOAL(S)
- Surgical emergency
- Rehydrate and correct metabolic derangements
- Pain management
- Surgical reduction of strangulation

ACUTE GENERAL TREATMENT
- Rehydration
  - Balanced polyionic fluids (ie, lactated Ringer's solution, Normosol-R)
  - Replacement fluid volume = Body weight (BW) (kg) × % dehydration
    - 500 kg × 0.08 = 40 L deficit
  - Maintenance fluid volume = BW (kg) × 50 to 60 mL/kg/d
    - 500 kg × 50 mL/kg/d = 25 L/d
  - Replacement fluid administration: 10 to 20 mL/kg/h
    - 500 kg × 10 to 20 mL/kg/h = 5 to 10 L/h until deficit volume is replaced
    - Maintenance rate after deficit replacement = 2 to 4 mL/kg/h
      - 500 kg × 2 to 4 mL/kg/h = 1 to 2 L/h
- Pain management
  - Xylazine: 0.3 to 0.5 mg/kg IV
  - Detomidine: 0.006 to 0.02 mg/kg IV
  - Butorphanol: 0.01 to 0.04 mg/kg IV (use in combination with xylazine or detomidine)
  - Nonsteroidal antiinflammatory drugs: Flunixin meglumine (1.1 mg/kg IV)
- Preoperative antibiotics
- Exploratory celiotomy
- Goal of surgery: Release the strangulation and assess intestinal viability
  - Reduction can be complicated because of an inability to visualize the strangulation. Often the lipoma must be manually dislodged from its pedicle blindly. Rarely can the pedicle be "un-tied" because of the size of the lipoma and the length of the pedicle.
  - If surgery is performed early, affected intestine may survive after release of the strangulation. Most

commonly, resection and anastomosis are required.

- Jejunojejunostomy
- Jejunoileostomy
- Jejunocecostomy
- Colocolostomy

○ It is common to find multiple incidental lipomas, which should be removed at the time of surgery.

CHRONIC TREATMENT

Provided the horse recovers through the immediate postoperative period, long-term treatment is not needed.

POSSIBLE COMPLICATIONS

- Ileus
- Abdominal pain
- Incisional complications
- Intraabdominal adhesions
- Complications at the anastomosis site
- Complications are more common among horses requiring resection and anastomosis.

RECOMMENDED MONITORING

During the postoperative period
- Cardiovascular status
- Nasogastric reflux
- Recurring signs of colic
- Incisional complications
- Slow return to oral intake

PROGNOSIS AND OUTCOME

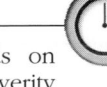

- The prognosis depends on the duration and severity of the disease.
- Prognosis is good for horses not requiring resection of small intestine.
- Prognosis for horses requiring resection and anastomosis is fair provided postoperative complications (eg, ileus, endotoxemia) are minimal. In the face of prolonged complications, the prognosis decreases.
- Prognosis worsens slightly with ileocecostomies and jejunocecostomies.
- Short-term survival for horses with strangulating lipoma disease is 43% to 65%. Long-term survival is reported to be between 26% and 75%.

PEARLS & CONSIDERATIONS

COMMENTS

Strangulating lipoma should be the top rule-out disorder in aged horses (older than 14 years) with signs of colic consistent with strangulating small intestinal disease.

PREVENTION

- Dietary management
- If metabolic disease is suspected, appropriate management is recom-

mended to reduce the risk of abnormal fat deposition.

SUGGESTED READING

Blikslager AT, Bowman KF, Haven ML, et al: Pedunculated lipomas as a cause of intestinal obstruction in horses: 17 cases (1983–1990). *J Am Vet Med Assoc* 201:1249–1252, 1992.

Edwards GB, Proudman CJ: An analysis of 75 cases of intestinal obstruction caused by pedunculated lipomas. *Equine Vet J* 26:18, 1994.

Freeman DE: Small intestine. In Auer JA, Stick JA, editors: *Equine surgery*, ed 3, St Louis, 2006, Saunders Elsevier, pp 415.

Freeman DE: Diseases of the small intestine. In White NA, Moore JN, Mair TS, editors: *The equine acute abdomen*, ed 2, Jackson, WY, 2008, Teton NewMedia, pp 594–616.

Garcia-Seco E, Wilson DA, Kramer J, et al: Prevalence and risk factors associated with outcome of surgical removal of pedunculated lipomas in horses: 102 cases (1987–2002). *J Am Vet Med Assoc* 226:1529–1537, 2005.

Mueller POE, Moore JN: Gastrointestinal emergencies and other causes of colic. In Orsini JA, Divers TJ, editors: *Equine emergencies treatment and procedures*, St Louis, 2008, Saunders Elsevier, p 130.

Seahorn JL, Seahorn TL: Fluid therapy in horses with gastrointestinal disease. *Vet Clin North Am Equine Pract* 19(3):665–679, 2003.

AUTHOR: RANDY EGGLESTON

EDITORS: TIM MAIR and CERI SHERLOCK

Small Intestine: Volvulus

BASIC INFORMATION

DEFINITION

- Rotation of a segment of jejunum, ileum, or both about its mesentery of 180 degrees or greater. May occur as a primary lesion or secondary to a preexisting lesion such as a strangulating lipoma, inguinal hernia, mesodiverticular band, Meckel's diverticulum, mesenteric rents, or adhesions. May also be seen after colic surgery most likely caused by postoperative ileus.
- Volvulus nodosus, seen less commonly, is described as the torsion of a segement of small intestine forming a mesenteric pouch in which additional small intestine can become entangled, forming an intestinal "knot." It is seen most commonly in foals.

EPIDEMIOLOGY

SPECIES, AGE, SEX Small intestinal volvulus seen primarily in foals between 2 and 7 months of age. It accounts for 15% to 19% of surgical colic cases in foals. A recent study examining horses with primary small intestinal volvulus found no effect of age.

RISK FACTORS Secondary small intestinal volvulus associated with conditions causing alteration in normal peristalsis or function of the small intestine (strangulating lipoma, inguinal hernia, mesodiverticular band, Meckel's diverticulum, mesenteric rents, adhesions, and postoperative ileus)

ASSOCIATED CONDITIONS AND DISORDERS Secondary small intestinal volvulus associated with conditions causing alteration in normal peristalsis or function of the small intestine (strangulating lipoma, inguinal hernia, mesodiverticular

band, Meckel's diverticulum, mesenteric rents, adhesions, and postoperative ileus)

CLINICAL PRESENTATION

HISTORY, CHIEF COMPLAINT

- Colic. Clinical signs consistent with acute small intestinal strangulation. Foals may exhibit signs of severe abdominal pain with intermittent periods of depression.
- Affected adult horses may have a history of previous abdominal surgery.

PHYSICAL EXAM FINDINGS

- Moderate to severe abdominal pain that is initially responsive to analgesics; response diminishes as the disease progresses.
- Foals commonly exhibit moderate to severe abdominal distension.
- Tachycardia (60–80 beats/min). Heart rate can be normal to greater than 100 beats/min.
- Normothermic

- Cardiovascular status diminishes with progression of disease. Signs of dehydration occur rapidly.
- As the disease progresses, horses may become depressed and show progressive signs of endotoxemia.
  - Tachycardia
  - Tachypnea
  - Congested mucous membranes
  - Prolonged capillary refill time
  - Reduced or absent borborygmi

ETIOLOGY AND PATHOPHYSIOLOGY

Strangulation of small intestine and its mesentery, causing ischemia and progressive necrosis

DIAGNOSIS

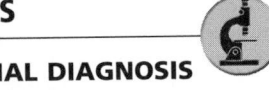

DIFFERENTIAL DIAGNOSIS

- Other causes of strangulating obstruction of the small intestine
  - Epiploic foramen entrapment
  - Gastrosplenic entrapment
  - Strangulation through mesenteric defect
  - Diaphragmatic hernia
  - Intussusception
  - Strangulating lipoma
- Late in the disease as the abdominal discomfort lessens and depression and endotoxemia become more apparent, strangulating lesions may be confused with inflammatory disease such as duodenitis-proximal jejunitis.

INITIAL DATABASE

- Rectal examination reveals multiple loops of distended small intestine. As the disease progresses, the size and number of loops increase. Late in the disease, it may be possible to palpate thickened turgid small intestine consistent with mural congestion and devitalization.
- Nasogastric reflux (NGR) will be seen as the disease progresses. NGR may be absent early in the disease. Pain relief may not be seen after decompression. Late in the disease when the horse appears less painful and depressed, NGR persists because of complete obstruction.
- Abdominocentesis is useful in distinguishing between a simple obstruction and strangulating obstruction. Peritoneal protein and nucleated cell count are often normal early in the disease process. As the colic progresses, the peritoneal protein level elevates. Only in late disease with increased intestinal injury does the peritoneal nucleated cell count increase. Fluid is often serosanguineous. Results of abdominocentesis may underestimate the true severity of the disease.
- Complete blood count and chemistry profile are normal early in the disease

process. As the colic progresses, changes consistent with dehydration and endotoxemia occur rapidly. A mild metabolic acidosis may also be present.

ADVANCED OR CONFIRMATORY TESTING

- Abdominal ultrasonography: Multiple loops of distended small intestine located in the caudal ventral abdomen. Motility is slow to absent, and mural thickening is seen as the disease progresses.
- Abdominal radiography can be useful in foals. A diffuse gas pattern is seen throughout the small intestine.

TREATMENT

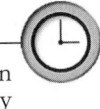

THERAPEUTIC GOAL(S)

- Surgical emergency
- Gastric decompression
- Rehydrate
- Pain management
- Surgical reduction of strangulation
  - If surgery is performed early, affected intestine may survive after release of the strangulation.
  - Resection and anastomosis are often required.

ACUTE GENERAL TREATMENT

- Rehydration
  - Balanced polyionic fluids (ie, lactated Ringer's solution, Normosol-R)
  - Replacement fluid volume = Body weight (BW) (kg) × % dehydration
    - 500 kg × 0.08 = 40 L deficit
  - Maintenance fluid volume = BW (kg) × 50 to 60 mL/kg/d
    - 500 kg × 50 mL/kg/d = 25 L/d
  - Replacement fluid administration: 10 to 20 mL/kg/h
    - 500 kg × 10 to 20 mL/kg/h = 5 to 10 L/h until deficit volume is replaced
    - Maintenance rate after deficit replacement = 2 to 4 mL/kg/h
      - 500 kg × 2 to 4 mL/kg/h = 1 to 2 L/h
- Pain management
  - Xylazine: 0.3 to 0.5 mg/kg IV
  - Detomidine: 0.006 to 0.02 mg/kg IV
  - Butorphanol: 0.01 to 0.04 mg/kg IV (use in combination with xylazine or detomidine)
  - Nonsteroidal antiinflammatory drugs: Flunixin meglumine (1.1 mg/kg IV)
- Preoperative antibiotics
- Exploratory celiotomy
  - The goal of surgery is to release the strangulation and assess intestinal viability.
  - Palpation of the mesentery aids in determining the direction of the volvulus.

- Reduction can be complicated because of an inability to visualize the strangulation.
- Assessment of intestinal viability to determine the need for resection and anastomosis
- If volvulus is at the root of the mesentery causing ischemia and necrosis of greater than 50% of the length of the small intestine, the potential for postoperative complications increases, and the prognosis worsens.
- Horses surviving after resection of up to 60% to 70% of the small intestine with minimal complications have been reported. The true limit of small intestinal resection in horses is unknown.
- Potential complications caused by short bowel syndrome include malabsorption problems leading to diarrhea, weight loss, and liver damage.

CHRONIC TREATMENT

Provided the horse recovers through the immediate postoperative period, long-term treatment is not needed.

POSSIBLE COMPLICATIONS

- Ileus
- Abdominal pain
- Incisional complications
- Complications at the anastomosis site
- Intraabdominal adhesions
- Complications more common among horses requiring resection and anastomosis

RECOMMENDED MONITORING

Postoperative period
- Cardiovascular status
- Nasogastric reflux
- Recurring signs of colic
- Incisional complications
- Slow return to oral intake

PROGNOSIS AND OUTCOME

- The prognosis depends on the duration and severity of the disease.
- Prognosis is good for horses not requiring resection of small intestine.
- Prognosis for horses requiring resection and anastomosis is fair provided postoperative complications (eg, ileus, endotoxemia) are minimal. In the face of prolonged complications, the prognosis decreases.
- Prognosis worsens slightly with ileocecostomies and jejunocecostomies.
- Short-term survival for horses with small intestinal strangulating disease is 75% to 86%. Long-term survival is reported to be about 75%.

PEARLS & CONSIDERATIONS

- Surgical emergency
- Small intestinal volvulus is a common cause of small intestinal strangulating lesions in foals between 2 and 7 months of age.
- May be seen as a primary or secondary lesion caused by preexisting abnormalities
- Prognosis is significantly improved if surgical intervention occurs within the first 8 hours and before signs of endotoxemia appear.

SUGGESTED READING

Freeman DE: Small intestine. In Auer JA, Stick JA, editors: *Equine surgery*, ed 3, St Louis, 2006, Saunders Elsevier, pp 412–413.

Freeman DE: Diseases of the small intestine. In White NA, Moore JN, Mair TS, editors: *The equine acute abdomen*, ed 2, Jackson, WY, 2008, Teton NewMedia, pp 594–616.

Mueller POE, Moore JN: Gastrointestinal emergencies and other causes of colic. In Orsini JA, Divers TJ, editors: *Equine emergencies treatment and procedures*, St Louis, 2008, Saunders Elsevier, pp 124–125.

Seahorn JL, Seahorn TL: Fluid therapy in horses with gastrointestinal disease. *Vet Clin North Am Equine Pract* 19(3):665–679, 2003.

Stephen JO, Corley KT, Johnston JK, Pfeiffer D: Factors associated with mortality and morbidity in small intestinal volvulus in horses. *Vet Surg* 33:340–348, 2004.

Stephen JO, Corley KT, Johnston JK, Pfeiffer D: Small intestinal volvulus in 115 horses: 1988–2000. *Vet Surg* 33:333–339, 2004.

White NA: Equine colic, VI. Prognosis and prevention. *Proc Am Assoc Equine Pract* 52:169–173, 2006.

AUTHOR: **RANDY EGGLESTON**

EDITORS: **TIM MAIR** and **CERI SHERLOCK**

Smoke Inhalation

BASIC INFORMATION

DEFINITION

Injury caused by exposure to a fire with a great deal of smoke, especially a fire in a confined area such as a barn or arena. Horses are at risk for carbon monoxide poisoning, chemical insult, and direct thermal injury to the respiratory system. The most severe consequence is pulmonary edema and death caused by asphyxia.

SYNONYM(S)

- Carbon monoxide poisoning
- Lung thermal injury
- Lung chemical injury

EPIDEMIOLOGY

SPECIES, AGE, SEX

- Barn fires are one of the most common causes of burns and smoke inhalation in horses of any age.
- Horses housed in at-risk barns (no fire detection or protection systems) are at increased risk for smoke inhalation if a fire occurs.

CLINICAL PRESENTATION

DISEASE FORMS/SUBTYPES Inhalation injury is a common sequela of closed-space fires and develops through three mechanisms

- Direct thermal injury
- Carbon monoxide poisoning
- Chemical insult

HISTORY, CHIEF COMPLAINT

- History of smoke inhalation related to a barn fire
- Commonly an associated burn injury to the skin of various depth and extent (see "Burns" in this section)

PHYSICAL EXAM FINDINGS

- Tachypnea
- Tachycardia
- Pale, blue, or toxic mucous membranes; cool extremities; poor peripheral pulses

ETIOLOGY AND PATHOPHYSIOLOGY

- Direct thermal injury causes edema and obstruction of the upper airway.
- Carbon monoxide interferes with oxygen delivery in several ways because its affinity for hemoglobin is approximately 230 times the affinity between oxygen and hemoglobin (shifts the oxygen-hemoglobin curve to the left).
  - The resultant carboxyhemoglobin is incapable of oxygen transport.
  - Carbon monoxide also binds to myoglobin, impairing oxygen transport to muscles.
  - Carbon monoxide is excreted by the lungs at a rate relative to ambient oxygen tensions. In room air, carbon monoxide has a half-life of more than 3 hours.
  - An increase in oxygen tension promotes the dissociation of carbon monoxide and hemoglobin; thus, 100% oxygen therapy reduces the half-life to 30 to 40 minutes. Hyperbaric oxygen therapy at 2.5 atm further decreases the half-life to 22 minutes.
- Chemical insult depends on the material that was burned.
  - Combustion products such as hydrogen cyanide, hydrochloric acid, phosgene, sulfuric acid, and aldehydes may induce severe tracheobronchitis when combined with the moisture in the airways.
  - Initially, only erythema may be present, but chemical injury continues as long as chemical-covered carbon particles remain attached to the airway mucosa. Particle size

determines where damage will occur within the respiratory tree.
  - Combustion products cause increased pulmonary artery pressure, peribronchial edema, mucosal sloughing, bronchoconstriction, decreased mucociliary transport and bacterial clearance, and altered surfactant action. Subsequent pulmonary ventilation/perfusion mismatches may develop.
- Pulmonary infection is a potential complication in every smoke inhalation patient. Alveolar macrophages, as the primary cellular defense in the lung, are increased in number after the injury but have decreased phagocytic and bactericidal functions.
- Susceptibility to pulmonary infection, pulmonary edema, and lung dysfunction increases greatly in patients that also have cutaneous thermal injury.
  - The interrelationship between inhalation and surface burns is unclear but appears to be additive.
  - Major cutaneous burns alone have been reported to cause pulmonary dysfunction in as many as 25% of patients (see "Burns" in this section).
  - Inhalation injury increases morbidity and mortality rates for a given cutaneous thermal injury.

DIAGNOSIS

DIFFERENTIAL DIAGNOSIS

- Direct thermal injury
- Carbon monoxide poisoning
- Chemical lung injury
- Pulmonary infection

INITIAL DATABASE

- Complete blood count
- Serum chemistry panel

- Serial arterial blood gas analyses
- Upper airway endoscopy

ADVANCED OR CONFIRMATORY TESTING

- Thoracic radiographs
- Tracheal washes for cytology and culture

TREATMENT

THERAPEUTIC GOAL(S)

- Maintenance of airway patency
- Adequate oxygenation and ventilation
- Stabilization of hemodynamic status

ACUTE GENERAL TREATMENT

- Early intervention and respiratory support
  - Essential even before the diagnosis of respiratory injury is confirmed
  - Nasal or tracheal insufflation with humidified 100% oxygen counteracts the effects of carbon monoxide and facilitates clearance by decreasing carbon monoxide half-life in the blood.
  - Oxygen insufflation rates of 15 to 20 L/min can be achieved through a tracheotomy and should be continued until the patient is able to maintain normal oxygenation.
  - Humidification can relieve excessive airway drying or mucous plugging.
  - Nebulizing with *N*-acetylcysteine and heparin and the use of humidified air reduce the formation of pseudomembranous casts and aid in the clearance of airway secretions.
  - Nebulized dimethylsulfoxide helps decrease lung fluid formation.
  - The β-adrenergic agonist albuterol can be aerosolized to reduce bronchospasm.

- Maintenance of optimal fluid status is essential. Patients with concurrent surface burns and inhalation injury require 2 mL/kg more fluid for each percentage of surface area burned than those with cutaneous burns alone to support adequate cardiac and urine output.
- Although pulmonary edema is a concern, especially for smaller patients, adequate circulating volume is the primary goal. Lung function should be monitored during fluid therapy by measuring hemoglobin saturation and arterial blood gasses.
- Systemic antimicrobials are indicated only for proven infections, the incidence of which increases 2 to 3 days after smoke inhalation. Intramuscular penicillin (Procaine penicillin G 22,000 IU/kg IM q12h) is effective against oral contaminants colonizing the airway.

CHRONIC TREATMENT

Therapy should be adjusted based on the clinical response and the results of serial blood gas analyses, complete blood counts, chest radiographs, airway endoscopy, and cultures.

DRUG INTERACTIONS

Antibiotics and corticosteroids do not influence survival rates and should not be routinely administered to smoke inhalation patients.

POSSIBLE COMPLICATIONS

- Hypoxia
- Tracheitis
- Bronchospasm
- Pulmonary infections
- Pseudomembranous necrotic debris within the upper airway

RECOMMENDED MONITORING

- If signs of respiratory disease worsen, transtracheal aspiration should be submitted for culture and sensitivity testing and the antibiotic regimen adapted accordingly.
- Patients with suspected significant smoke inhalation should be observed closely for several hours and hospitalized in the presence of extensive burns.

PROGNOSIS AND OUTCOME

Successful treatment depends on continuous patient reassessment and early, aggressive patient care.

PEARLS & CONSIDERATIONS

- Weight loss of 10% to 15% during the course of illness is indicative of inadequate nutritional intake.
- Gradually increasing the grain, adding fat in the form of 4 to 8 oz of vegetable oil, and offering free-choice alfalfa hay to increase caloric intake.

SUGGESTED READING

Demling RH, Will JA, Belzer FO: Effect of major thermal injury on the pulmonary microcirculation. *Surgery* 83:746, 1978.

Herndon DN, Barrow RE, Traber DL, et al: Extravascular lung water changes following smoke inhalation and massive burn injury. *Surgery* 102:341, 1987.

Muller MJ, Herndon DN: The challenge of burns. *Lancet* 343:216, 1994.

Nguyen TT, Gilpin DA, Meyer DA: Current treatment of severely burned patients. *Ann Surg* 223:14, 1996.

AUTHOR and EDITOR: R. REID HANSON

Sodium Toxicosis

BASIC INFORMATION

DEFINITION

Sodium ion or salt toxicosis may occur from ingestion of excess sodium in either feed or water or from water deprivation.

SYNONYM(S)

- Hypernatremia
- Sodium chloride toxicosis

EPIDEMIOLOGY

RISK FACTORS Sodium intoxication or water deprivation rarely occurs or is rarely reported in horses. The acute toxic dose of sodium chloride in the equine is about 2.2 g/kg body weight (BW). Sodium chloride is generally added at the rate of 0.5% to 1% of concentrate feeds or is fed free choice. The maximum tolerable concentration of sodium chloride in the diet has been set at 6% of intake by the National Research Council. When adequate potable water is available, animals may tolerate feeds with elevated salt concentrations. Animals not acclimated to higher mineral or salt diets are at risk of overconsumption of sodium. Water deprivation may occur during neglect, overcrowding, mechanical failure of watering systems, and frozen or unpalatable water sources.

GEOGRAPHY AND SEASONALITY Because this toxicosis is often dependent on water intake, cases of hypernatremia may be associated with high ambient temperature and humidity or prolonged exercise without access to water. Average water intake is about 5 L/100 kg BW/d for maintenance in horses, but this amount can be affected by temperature, exercise, and other factors.

CLINICAL PRESENTATION

HISTORY, CHIEF COMPLAINT

- Excessive salt intake may result in gastroenteritis, weakness, and dehydration within 1 to 2 days.
- Clinical signs of sodium intoxication or water deprivation generally develop over 4 to 7 days and involve the central nervous system resulting in the following signs
  - Restlessness
  - Thirst
  - Anorexia
  - Aimless wandering
  - Head pressing
  - Circling
  - Blindness
  - Tremors
  - Seizure-like activity
  - Death

PHYSICAL EXAM FINDINGS

- Restlessness
- Thirst
- Weakness
- Dehydration
- Tucked-up abdomen
- Constipation or diarrhea
- Aimless wandering
- Head pressing
- Depression
- Circling
- Ataxia
- Tremors
- Seizure-like activity
- Sudden death (<24 hours) with excess salt ingestion

ETIOLOGY AND PATHOPHYSIOLOGY

- Excessive salt ingestion may cause irritation of mucosal surfaces, electrolyte imbalances, and severe dehydration. The loss of free body water leads to elevated sodium concentrations in serum and throughout the body.
- Sodium diffuses across the blood-brain barrier into the cerebrospinal fluid (CSF) and neurons in the brain. If hypernatremia develops very quickly, cells in the brain are not able to increase their intracellular osmolarity to prevent excessive water loss to the extracellular fluid. Brain cell shrinkage occurs, leading to brain shrinkage and disruption of the blood supply to the brain, hemorrhages, infarcts, seizure-like activity, and death.
- With increased sodium concentrations in brain cells, glycolysis is inhibited, less energy is available to the cells, and sodium cannot be actively transported out of the brain. If unlimited

water is provided and rehydration occurs too quickly, serum sodium decreases but the brain response is delayed, and the osmotic gradient results in water moving into the brain, causing swelling and cerebral edema.
- Increases in cellular osmolarity over several days results in accumulation of osmotically active organic compounds known as *idiogenic osmoles*. Maximum concentrations of idiogenic osmoles occur within 48 to 72 hours of hypernatremia and require a similar time period to return to normal levels. The idiogenic osmoles account for a large increase in cellular osmolarity.

DIAGNOSIS

DIFFERENTIAL DIAGNOSIS

Although elevated sodium concentrations in the serum, CSF, brain tissue, or ocular fluids are diagnostic, other causes of nervous system signs should be considered.
- Other nontoxic causes of neurologic disorders
- Fumonisins
- Poisonous plants, including *Asclepias* (milkweed), *Cicuta* (water hemlock), *Nicotiana* (tobacco), and *Centaurea* (yellow star thistle)

INITIAL DATABASE

- Measuring serum and CSF sodium concentrations is used to diagnose sodium toxicosis. The normal reference range of serum sodium in adult animals is 135 to 155 mEq/L; serum sodium concentrations greater than 160 mEq/L are diagnostic of hypernatremia. Normal CSF sodium concentrations range from 135 to 150 mEq/L.
- Elevated serum chloride may aid in diagnosis of acute sodium chloride intoxication; normal serum chloride ranges from 90 to 105 mEq/L.

ADVANCED OR CONFIRMATORY TESTING

- Brain sodium concentrations greater than 1800 mg/kg (ppm) on a wet weight basis are considered supportive of a diagnosis of sodium toxicosis. There is a paucity of data for normal equine brain sodium levels at this time, although Oklahoma State University's Animal Disease Diagnostic Laboratory is developing a databank on equine brain sodium concentrations.
- Elevated sodium concentrations in ocular fluid may aid in a diagnosis of sodium intoxication. Check with the veterinary diagnostic laboratory performing the test for their normal values in horses.

TREATMENT

THERAPEUTIC GOAL(S)

- Generally, the water deficit must be replaced slowly over 2 to 3 days to prevent cerebral edema and colic. If serum sodium cannot be monitored, limit water intake to 0.5% of BW at 60 minute intervals until the animal is rehydrated. Highly dehydrated horses given 12 L of water at 30-minute intervals have developed colic.
- In cases of acute hypernatremia, before the development of clinical signs and idiogenic osmole formation, animals can be allowed full access to water and experience a rapid decrease in sodium concentrations without risk of cerebral edema. However, the majority of cases of hypernatremia are found when animals show obvious clinical signs, and the clinical course has progressed beyond acute.

ACUTE GENERAL TREATMENT

- For the individual horse, determine the serum sodium (Na) concentration. Calculate the free water deficit (FWD):

$$FWD\ (L) = 0.6 \times BW\ (kg) \times \\ [(\text{Measured serum Na}/ \\ \text{Normal serum Na}) - 1]$$

- No more than 50% of the FWD should be replaced in the initial 24 hours of treatment, with the remaining deficit replaced over the next 24 to 48 hours. The serum sodium concentration should be lowered at a rate of about 0.5 mEq/L/h.
- Intravenous administration of slightly hypertonic saline solutions rather than isotonic solutions is recommended to prevent iatrogenic cerebral edema. The sodium concentration of both parenteral and oral fluids should approximate the serum sodium level of the animal. To achieve the sodium level in oral fluids, consider use of table salt, which contains 17 mEq/g of sodium.
- If the serum sodium level is not known, start with an initial IV fluid of 170 mEq/L of sodium and decrease the concentration as clinical signs improve.
- If possible, monitor serum sodium levels frequently to adjust the sodium levels in the IV fluids.
- When hypernatremia occurs with hypoglycemia and acidosis, which may occur with severe gastroenteritis and diarrhea, fluids should contain sodium bicarbonate and glucose as needed.
- If during treatment the animal's central nervous system signs worsen and tremors of the facial muscles develop, cerebral edema may be occurring.

Consider using mannitol, dexamethasone, or dimethyl sulfoxide to reduce brain swelling.

RECOMMENDED MONITORING

Monitor serum sodium concentrations during treatment to adjust the sodium level in the IV fluid therapy.

PROGNOSIS AND OUTCOME

Prognosis is guarded to poor in animals showing clinical signs from sodium ion intoxication or water deprivation.

PEARLS & CONSIDERATIONS

COMMENTS

Sodium ion toxicosis is not common in horses.

PREVENTION

- Provide unlimited potable water to horses.
- A safe upper level concentration for sodium in water has not been established for horses. Several recommended guidelines for sodium in livestock drinking water are less than 800 to 1000 mg/L.

SUGGESTED READING

Friend TH: Dehydration, stress, and water consumption of horses during long-distance commercial transport. *J Anim Sci* 78:2568–2580, 2000.

National Research Council for the National Academies: Water and water quality. In *Nutrient requirements of horses*, ed 6, Washington, DC, 2007, National Academy Press, pp 128–140.

Niles G: Sodium. In Plumlee KH, editor: *Clinical veterinary toxicology*, St Louis, 2004, Mosby Elsevier, pp 218–221.

AUTHOR: **MICHELLE S. MOSTROM**

EDITOR: **CYNTHIA L. GASKILL**

Sorghum and Sudan Grass Toxicosis

BASIC INFORMATION

DEFINITION

Sorghum grasses have been selected as drought-tolerant forage or grain crops. Although the grain sorghums ("milo") rarely present a toxicity problem, the forage sorghums can accumulate toxic levels of cyanogenic glycosides and nitrates. These two toxins are primarily a problem to ruminant species and rarely to horses. However, the chronic ingestion of sorghum pastures or hay made from sorghum and its hybrids has been associated with a neuropathy in horses, cattle, and sheep that is not related to the cyanogenic glycoside content responsible for acute cyanide poisoning.

SYNONYM(S)

Common names for varieties of sorghum in the United States include Sudan grass, Sudax, sorgo, kafir, durra, milo, shallu, kaoliang, broomcorn, and Johnson grass.

EPIDEMIOLOGY

RISK FACTORS Continuous consumption of sorghum hay or forage over a period of weeks or months

GEOGRAPHY AND SEASONALITY

- Sorghums are warm-season, coarse, annual grasses ranging in height from 2 to 6 feet. Introduced from Africa, sorghums have become well established in North America, with some being useful grain and forage species (*Sorghum bicolor*); others such as Johnson grass (*Sorghum halapense*) are noxious weeds.
- Sudan grass, formerly *Sorghum sudanense*, is now a species of *S. bicolor* (Figure 1).

- Some sorghum hybrids have been selected for their low cyanogenic glycoside content.

CLINICAL PRESENTATION

DISEASE FORMS/SUBTYPES Sorghum poisoning in horses has a slow onset (1–6 months) and is a chronic disease.

HISTORY, CHIEF COMPLAINT

- Ataxia, dribbling urine, soiled hind legs, tail and perineum, weight loss

- Abortion in some pregnant mares
- Arthrogryposis in some foals

PHYSICAL EXAM FINDINGS

- Weakness and ataxia of the hindquarters. In severe cases, the horse collapses when backed.
- Urinary incontinence may lead to urine scalding of the perineum and hind legs. Hematuria and a thickened, atonic urinary bladder can be palpated rectally.

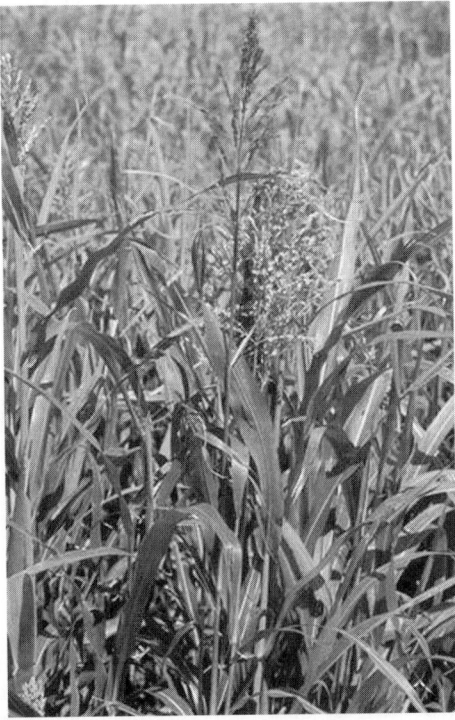

FIGURE 1 Sudan grass hybrid (*Sorghum bicolor*).

- Tail flaccidity, dilatation of the rectum, and abnormal accumulation of feces occur because of an atonic rectum.
- Some foals may be born weak or have arthrogryposis in all legs.

ETIOLOGY AND PATHOPHYSIOLOGY

- The precise etiology is not well defined.
- The condition is not associated with cyanide poisoning.
- The condition is similar to lathyrism in humans associated with the consumption of pea seeds (*Lathyrus* spp.).
- Cyanogenic glycosides or nitriles in sorghums converted to the lathyrogen T-glutamyl-β-cyanoalanine may play a role in pathogenesis.
- Similar signs are reported in cattle and sheep grazing sorghum pastures.
- Not all horses eating sorghum will be affected.

DIAGNOSIS

DIFFERENTIAL DIAGNOSIS

- Equine herpes virus type 1
- West Nile virus
- Polyneuritis
- Spinal cord injury
- Cystitis caused by cystic calculi or neoplasia

INITIAL DATABASE

- Urinalysis: Hematuria, increased leucocytes, bacteria, calcium carbonate crystals
- Hematology: Leukocytosis in chronic cases
- Blood urea nitrogen and creatine: Elevated when pyelonephritis present
- EHV titer: Negative

ADVANCED OR CONFIRMATORY TESTING

- Necropsy: Chronic cystitis with thickening, ulceration, and necrosis of the bladder wall.
- The bladder contains a purulent exudate with large quantities of calcium carbonate adhered to the bladder mucosa.
- Histology: Wallerian degeneration and demyelination of the white matter in the spinal cord.
- Axonal degeneration, demyelination, increased gitter cells throughout spinal cord funiculi.
- Testing for cyanogenic glycosides does not necessarily confirm the potential for sorghum cystitis.

TREATMENT

THERAPEUTIC GOAL(S)

- Very early in the course of the disease, antibiotics may help reduce cystitis and ascending pyelonephritis.
- Remove all sorghum from the horse's diet.
- Supportive treatment with manual removal of rectally impacted feces and expression of the atonic bladder provides symptomatic relief. Vaseline applied to the legs and perineum may help reduce urine scalding.

POSSIBLE COMPLICATIONS

Pyelonephritis and renal failure

PROGNOSIS AND OUTCOME

- Prognosis is poor after the horse becomes incontinent and ataxic.

- Horses with minimal neurologic damage show improvement after prolonged periods.
- Some improvement may occur with the use of antibiotics, but neuropathy is permanent.

PEARLS & CONSIDERATIONS

COMMENTS

- In general, sorghums should not be fed to horses for prolonged periods.
- Selecting sorghum varieties that are low in cyanogenic glycosides may decrease potential toxicity.

PREVENTION

Avoid feeding sorghum species to horses

CLIENT EDUCATION

- If sorghums must be fed to horses, do so for short periods of less than 2 weeks only.
- Grazing or feeding sorghum hay to horses should be avoided whenever possible.

SUGGESTED READING

Adams LG, Dollahite JW, Romane WM, et al: Cystitis and ataxia associated with sorghum ingestion by horses. *J Am Vet Med Assoc* 155:518–524, 1969.

Bradley GA, Metcalf HC, Reggiardo C, et al: Neuroaxonal degeneration in sheep grazing Sorghum pastures. *J Vet Diagn Invest* 7:229–236, 1995.

Morgan SE, Johnson B, Brewer B, Walker J: Sorghum cystitis ataxia syndrome in horses. *Vet Hum Toxicol* 32:582, 1990.

Van Kampen KR: Sudan grass and sorghum poisoning of horses: a possible lathyrogenic disease. *J Am Vet Med Assoc* 156:629–630, 1970.

AUTHOR: **ANTHONY P. KNIGHT**

EDITOR: **CYNTHIA L. GASKILL**

Sperm Abnormalities: Asthenozoospermia

BASIC INFORMATION

DEFINITION

Reduced sperm motility

SYNONYM(S)

Asthenospermia

EPIDEMIOLOGY

SPECIES, AGE, SEX Affects stallions of various ages depending on cause
GEOGRAPHY AND SEASONALITY Sperm cells are very sensitive to environmental factors. Motility may be affected by improper handling, especially in cold climates.
ASSOCIATED CONDITIONS AND DISORDERS Often occurs in combination with teratospermia

CLINICAL PRESENTATION

DISEASE FORMS/SUBTYPES Reduced total motility or reduced progressive motility with adequate total motility
HISTORY, CHIEF COMPLAINT Most stallions present with a reduction in

fertility or complete infertility. Often, these stallions were previously fertile and have either acutely or gradually failed to achieve pregnancies. A complete review of the stallion's breeding records is helpful in determining when the problem or initial insult occurred. Stallions may also present for poor semen motility after cooled transport.
PHYSICAL EXAM FINDINGS A general physical examination is unremarkable unless concurrent systemic disease is present. The reproductive examination

findings may also be within normal limits unless testicular degeneration is present, which may be indicated by smaller, soft testicles. If orchitis is present, the testicles may be slightly enlarged, warm, and painful.

ETIOLOGY AND PATHOPHYSIOLOGY

- Motility of sperm cells is very sensitive to environmental factors. Mishandling of the sample such as exposure to extreme temperatures (hot or cold), temperature fluctuations, toxins (soap residue), or prolonged exposure to light will negatively affect sperm motility.
- Motility and morphology are very closely related; a misshapen sperm will not move correctly. Therefore, causes of teratospermia should be evaluated.

DIAGNOSIS

DIFFERENTIAL DIAGNOSIS

- Inappropriate handling of semen
- Genetics
- Elevated scrotal temperature (pyrexia, elevated ambient temperature, scrotal inflammation, scrotal insulation)
- Malnutrition
- Chemicals, drugs
- Hormonal imbalances
- Testicular degeneration
- Orchitis
- Spermiostasis (plugged ampullae)

INITIAL DATABASE

- A complete semen evaluation should be performed, including morphologic analysis and motility on raw and extended semen. Semen should be allowed to equilibrate after the addition of extender. Some stallions exhibit a decrease in progressive motility (circling) immediately after the addition of semen extender that will resolve after 10 to 15 minutes. Sperm should be extended to a concentration between 30 to 50 million/mL to allow accurate analysis.
  - In practice, motility is often subjectively analyzed using only a single observer and a microscope. Skilled evaluators are able to accurately assess total and progressive motility using this method; however, the evaluator must be trained appropriately.
  - A computer-assisted sperm analysis is available at many universities, specialty clinics, and other large breeding operations. This program will give an accurate, objective analysis of total and progressive motility, including other important sperm characteristics such as velocity and straightness.

- The complete blood count and serum chemistry analysis may be beneficial in assessing the stallion for systemic disease or inflammation that may be affecting the scrotal temperature. If orchitis is present, the stallion may exhibit leukocytosis and hyperfibrinogenemia.
- Ultrasonography of the testicles should be performed to evaluate the parenchyma for abnormalities such as neoplasia and hyperechoic or hypoechoic areas.
- Hormonal assay: Levels of hormones vary considerably in normal and subfertile stallions; therefore, hormonal analysis may be of little value for diagnosis. With severe cases of testicular degeneration, follicle-stimulating hormone and luteinizing hormone levels may be elevated, and the estradiol level may be low. Elevated levels of exogenous androgens lead to a disruption of spermatogenesis. If no other specific causes of teratospermia or asthenozoospermia are found, a hormonal assay should be performed.

ADVANCED OR CONFIRMATORY TESTING

- Sperm chromatin structure assay is an advanced test that evaluates the DNA, or chromatin, of the sperm cells. This test is performed in specific laboratories and may be indicated when other causes of infertility are not identified or an analysis of the sperm chromatin is desired to assess treatment or prognosis.
- Acrosome reaction is an evaluation of the ability of the acrosome to properly undergo the reaction necessary for fertilization. This may be indicated if a large number of abnormal acrosomes or heads are observed. It may also be indicated in cases in which the semen motility is adequate but the stallion is not able to achieve pregnancies.
- Hypoosmotic swelling test is an in-house test that can be performed to assess the membrane integrity of the sperm cell. See Suggested Reading for a description of how to perform this test.

TREATMENT

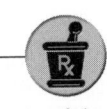

THERAPEUTIC GOAL(S)

To determine the underlying cause of the reduced motility and correct it when possible. If the problem cannot be resolved or improved, more intense breeding management of the stallion may preserve an acceptable seasonal pregnancy rate.

ACUTE GENERAL TREATMENT

- If the reduced motility is caused by teratospermia (diagnosed by a mor-

phologic analysis), see "Sperm Abnormalities: Teratospermia" in this section for treatment options.
- If the morphology of the sperm does not appear to correlate with the reduced motility
  - Assess semen handling technique. Sperm are very sensitive to environmental insult that will cause reduced motility. The entire collection process should be objectively evaluated to identify any problems, including, but not limited to, soap residue on equipment, hot or cold temperature fluctuations, and prolonged exposure to light.
  - Assess raw versus extended semen. Although it is difficult to accurately assess motility on a raw semen sample because of the high concentration of the sperm, comparing the raw with the extended sample may allow the evaluation of the extender on the sperm cells. If motility decreases after the addition of the extender, evaluate different concentrations or extender components.
  - Different sperm or seminal plasma concentration: Some stallions are sensitive to the concentration of seminal plasma, especially after cooled storage. Stallion sperm should be extended to a seminal plasma concentration of at least 5% and no more than 20% (at least a 1:4 dilution) and between 25 and 50 million sperm/mL. If the stallion has low motility at 20% seminal plasma or 50 million sperm/mL, decrease the ratio or concentration and evaluate for improvement.
  - Centrifugation of the sample to decrease the seminal plasma concentration may improve motility in some stallions. The addition of a cushion may further decrease damage to the sperm during centrifugation.

CHRONIC TREATMENT

- If the asthenozoospermia does not improve and the cause does not appear to be heritable, intense management of the stallion may preserve fertility. By breeding very close to ovulation (within 12 hours before or 6 hours after) and using a deep uterine horn insemination technique to place the sperm directly on the oviductal papillae of the mare, many stallions are able to achieve an acceptable seasonal pregnancy rate even with low motility. Increasing the insemination dose to account for the reduced motility may also improve fertility.
- The addition of semen extender may improve motility in stallions that are sensitive to high concentrations of seminal plasma. This may be accom-

plished by either adding extender to the collection bottle before collection or adding the extender immediately after collection.

- Special semen handling techniques are available, but they require some training and practice before applying them to a clinical setting. The ejaculate may be centrifuged through a density gradient such as EquiPure made by Nidacon. This gradient filters out many of the abnormal sperm, leaving a high percentage of normal sperm in the pellet.

DRUG INTERACTIONS

- Exogenous anabolic steroids can negatively affect sperm quality.
- Some herbal supplements can affect sperm quality. All supplements given to the stallion should be assessed individually.

RECOMMENDED MONITORING

- All breeding stallions should have a motility analysis with every collection. This allows the evaluation of trends and observe any underlying environmental factors that may be affecting motility. This also allows the assessment of any treatments on motility.
- If asthenozoospermia occurs with teratospermia, the stallion should be evaluated every 30 to 90 days to assess

improvement. A minimum of 60 days from the resolution of the insult is required for complete recovery (a single spermatogenic cycle).

PROGNOSIS AND OUTCOME

- If the decreased motility is caused by improper handling, the prognosis is excellent provided the problem can be resolved.
- If improvement can be made using different processing techniques, the fertility of the stallion may also be improved.

PEARLS & CONSIDERATIONS

COMMENTS

- Motility analysis should be performed on every semen sample. Total and progressive motility should be recorded to allow the evaluation of trends. Progressive motility is more valuable for predicting potential fertility than total motility.
- Sperm motility alone is not an accurate predictor of fertility. Motility must be assessed with other tests to give a

more reliable prediction of the ability of that stallion to reproduce.

- Because of a wide degree of stallion variability, different techniques such as different extenders, different antibiotics, centrifugation, extending to different concentrations, and so on should be attempted.

PREVENTION

Veterinarians should be well trained in proper semen handling techniques so they are not responsible for iatrogenically reducing sperm motility.

CLIENT EDUCATION

Determining the optimal processing method for each individual stallion may require time and expense. However, if the motility is optimized using a certain technique, fertility will most likely also be optimized.

SUGGESTED READING

Barth AD, Oko RJ: *Abnormal morphology of bovine spermatozoa.* Ames, IA, 1989, Iowa State University.
Turner RM: Testicular abnormalities. In Samper JC, Pycock JF, McKinnon AO, editors: *Current therapy in equine reproduction,* St Louis, 2007, Saunders Elsevier, pp 227–230.

AUTHOR: **AIME K. JOHNSON**

EDITOR: **JUAN C. SAMPER**

Sperm Abnormalities: Azoospermia

BASIC INFORMATION

DEFINITION

A complete absence of spermatozoa in the ejaculate

EPIDEMIOLOGY

SPECIES, AGE, SEX Affects stallions of various ages depending on cause
GEOGRAPHY AND SEASONALITY Spermiostasis usually caused by plugged or blocked ampullae may be more frequently diagnosed at the beginning of the breeding season.
ASSOCIATED CONDITIONS AND DISORDERS Testicular or epididymal hypoplasia, spermiostasis, testicular degeneration, ejaculatory failure

CLINICAL PRESENTATION

DISEASE FORMS/SUBTYPES

- Nonobstructive azoospermia: Occurs when there is a problem with spermatogenesis such as with testicular hypoplasia or degeneration.

- Obstructive oligozoospermia: Occurs when spermatogenesis is normal but sperm cannot be ejaculated because of a physical blockage anywhere between the testicle and the urethra.

HISTORY, CHIEF COMPLAINT

- A complete absence of spermatozoa in the ejaculate, infertility.
- A complete breeding history aids the examiner in narrowing down the differential list. Often, the owners will have records of previous ejaculates, mare records, and seasonal or per cycle pregnancy rate. Stallions may present for acute onset or gradual infertility.
- Typical history for specific causes:
  - Testicular or epididymal hypoplasia: Young stallion; never produced sperm in any ejaculate obtained
  - Plugged ampullae: Oligospermia to azoospermia, low percentage of morphologically normal sperm, high numbers of tailless heads, low percentage of motile sperm, subfertility

  - Testicular degeneration: Recent systemic illness or local injury may cause an acute onset of infertility; aging stallions show a gradual decline in sperm number with gradual infertility
  - Ejaculatory failure: Stallion exhibits a lack of ejaculatory pulses or premature dismount from a phantom or mare

PHYSICAL EXAM FINDINGS

- General physical examination findings unremarkable unless concurrent systemic disease is present. A complete reproductive examination is necessary and can narrow down the differential list.
- Testicular or epididymal hypoplasia: Young or maiden stallion; small, soft testes on external palpation. May be either unilateral or bilateral cryptorchid.
- Plugged ampullae: Distended or enlarged ampullae on transrectal palpation and ultrasonography. Ampullae may contain hyperechoic areas and a prominent lumen, indicating

accumulation of sperm. The tail of the epididymis may be enlarged and turgid.

- Testicular degeneration: Testes may be soft on palpation.
- Ejaculatory failure: Evidence of musculoskeletal or neurologic condition.

ETIOLOGY AND PATHOPHYSIOLOGY

- Testicular hypoplasia: Most often a congenital condition linked to a genetic abnormality or segmental aplasia of the efferent tubules. An intersex condition may be present.
- Plugged ampullae: Physical obstruction in one or both ampullae of unknown cause. This condition may recur after periods of sexual rest in certain stallions.
- Testicular degeneration: Intrinsic factors include defects in the germ cells or supporting cells that may be heritable. Extrinsic factors include temperature changes, endocrine imbalances, vascular insults, toxins, infectious disease, and excessive androgen exposure.
- Ejaculatory failure: Often a result of musculoskeletal pain either before or during ejaculation. Neurologic diseases also cause ejaculatory failure depending on the affected nerve pathway. Behavioral or equipment problems may lead to ejaculatory failure, and these must be evaluated completely in the absence of other clinical signs.

DIAGNOSIS

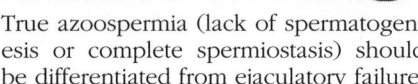

DIFFERENTIAL DIAGNOSIS

True azoospermia (lack of spermatogenesis or complete spermiostasis) should be differentiated from ejaculatory failure.

INITIAL DATABASE

- Testicular hypoplasia: A karyotype may be submitted to check for chromosomal abnormalities leading to some intersex conditions. Testicular hypoplasia should be differentiated from ejaculatory failure by physical examination findings and history. It is common for young stallions to fail to ejaculate during initial collection attempts.
- Plugged ampullae: The ejaculate will range from oligozoospermia to azoospermia. When sperm is obtained, there will be a high percentage of tailless heads and a low percentage of motile sperm. The ampullae may be enlarged and firm on transrectal palpation and ultrasonography. Ampullae may contain areas of dilatation or hyperechogenicity indicating the accumulation of sperm.
- Testicular degeneration: Repeated testicular ultrasonography may show a gradual decline in testicular volume.

Analysis of the ejaculate may show increasing teratospermia or decreasing sperm numbers. Immature (premature) germ cells will also be present in increasing numbers in the ejaculate. The advanced cases will be azoospermic.

- Ejaculatory failure: This condition must be differentiated from other causes of azoospermia. The testes and accessory sex glands should be normal with palpation and ultrasonography.

ADVANCED OR CONFIRMATORY TESTING

- Alkaline phosphatase (ALP): Fluid from the testicles and epididymis has an extremely elevated ALP. The ALP is low (<1000 U/L) when there is no testicular component to the ejaculate. This is the case with ejaculation failure or a blockage in the duct system as with plugged ampullae. With cases of severe testicular degeneration, the ALP is high, indicating fluid contribution from the testicles and epididymis, but there is an absence of sperm cells.
- Testicular biopsy: In practice, a testicular biopsy is rarely indicated, and the risks of the procedure usually outweigh the benefit of the diagnostics. A single sample may not give an accurate representation of the entire testicle, and the risk of hemorrhage or further damage to the already compromised parenchyma must be accounted for. If indicated, histopathology in cases of testicular degeneration will show varying degrees of cytoplasmic vacuolization, increased fibrous tissue, and loss of normal architecture. The number of germ cells will be decreased, and in severe cases, may be absent, leaving only the Sertoli cells and supporting tissues.
- Hormonal assay: Levels of hormones vary considerably in normal and subfertile stallions; therefore, hormonal analysis is of little value for diagnosis. With severe cases of testicular degeneration, follicle-stimulating hormone and luteinizing hormone levels may be elevated, and the estradiol level may be low.

TREATMENT

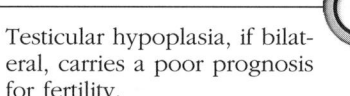

THERAPEUTIC GOAL(S)

- Nonobstructive azoospermia: Treatment is not generally attempted because of a poor prognosis.
- Obstructive azoospermia: Diagnose the underlying condition and resolve the obstruction when possible.

ACUTE GENERAL TREATMENT

Plugged ampullae: Physical transrectal massage of both ampullae for 5 minutes

before each collection to loosen the luminal blockage. Administration of oxytocin (20 IU IV) immediately before collection attempt to stimulate smooth muscle contraction of the ampullae. Increased frequency of ejaculations as often as the stallion can tolerate it, typically several times daily to release the blockage.

CHRONIC TREATMENT

Plugged ampullae: Frequent year-round ejaculations may prevent the accumulation of sperm and subsequent blockage.

POSSIBLE COMPLICATIONS

Plugged ampullae: If a complete blockage is present, administration of oxytocin or aggressive therapy may cause rupture of the ampullae or ductus deferens.

RECOMMENDED MONITORING

The stallion should be examined every 60 days to determine if there is improvement over a single spermatogenic cycle. In cases of plugged ampullae, the stallion's sperm should be collected frequently, as necessary, to prevent recurrence.

PROGNOSIS AND OUTCOME

- Testicular hypoplasia, if bilateral, carries a poor prognosis for fertility.
- Plugged ampullae: Excellent prognosis if the blockage is resolved after treatment. Most affected animals return to their previous levels of fertility.
- Testicular degeneration: May be reversible depending on the cause, but if the problem has progressed to azoospermia, the prognosis for return to function is generally poor. If the degeneration is caused by age-related changes, the problem is most likely permanent.

PEARLS & CONSIDERATIONS

COMMENTS

Causes of oligozoospermia can usually be differentiated based on history and physical examination findings, including a reproductive examination.

CLIENT EDUCATION

In general, horses with complete azoospermia carry a poor prognosis for future fertility; however, treatment should be attempted before castration in valuable animals.

SUGGESTED READING

Love CC, Riera FL, Oristaglio RM, et al: Sperm occluded (plugged) ampullae in the stallion. *Soc Theriogenology Proc* 117–127, 1992.

Turner RM: Testicular abnormalities. In Samper JC, Pycock JF, McKinnon AO, editors: *Current therapy in equine reproduction*, St Louis, 2007, Saunders Elsevier, pp 227–230.

AUTHOR: **AIME K. JOHNSON**

EDITOR: **JUAN C. SAMPER**

Sperm Abnormalities: Oligozoospermia

BASIC INFORMATION

DEFINITION

Deficiency of spermatozoa in the ejaculate

SYNONYM(S)

Oligospermia is defined as low semen volume and should be differentiated from oligozoospermia.

EPIDEMIOLOGY

SPECIES, AGE, SEX Affects stallions of various ages depending on cause
GEOGRAPHY AND SEASONALITY Plugged ampullae may be more frequently diagnosed at the beginning of the breeding season.
ASSOCIATED CONDITIONS AND DISORDERS Orchitis, spermiostasis (plugged ampullae), testicular degeneration, partial ejaculation, overuse

CLINICAL PRESENTATION

DISEASE FORMS/SUBTYPES

- Reduced spermatogenesis: Occurs when there is a problem with spermatogenesis, such as with orchitis or testicular degeneration
- Obstructive oligozoospermia: Occurs when spermatogenesis is normal but sperm cannot be ejaculated because of a physical blockage anywhere between the testicle and the urethra
- Sexual overuse

HISTORY, CHIEF COMPLAINT

- A reduced number of spermatozoa in the ejaculate; subfertility or infertility
- A complete breeding history aids the examiner in narrowing down the differential list. Often, the owners will have records of previous ejaculates, mare records, and seasonal or per cycle pregnancy rate. Stallions may present for acute onset or gradual subfertility.
- Specific causes
  - Testicular or epididymal hypoplasia: Young stallion; reduced total sperm number in the ejaculate
  - Orchitis: Unwilling to ejaculate; urethral discharge; the stallion may have other clinical signs of infection if acute (lethargy, pyrexia)
  - Plugged ampullae: Oligospermia to azoospermia, low percentage

of morphologically normal sperm, high numbers of tailless heads, low percentage of motile sperm, subfertility
  - Testicular degeneration: Systemic illness or recent local injury may cause an acute onset of infertility; aging stallions show a gradual decline in sperm number with gradual infertility.
  - Partial ejaculatory failure: Stallion exhibits a lack of ejaculatory pulses or premature dismount from a phantom or mare.
  - Sexual overuse: Frequent collections or spontaneous ejaculations, decreasing sperm with each subsequent collection

PHYSICAL EXAM FINDINGS

- General physical examination findings unremarkable unless concurrent systemic disease is present. A complete reproductive examination is necessary and can narrow down the differential list.
- Testicular or epididymal hypoplasia: Young or maiden stallion; small, soft testes on external palpation.
- Orchitis: On palpation, the testicles may be enlarged, firm, warm, or painful. Urethral discharge may be present.
- Plugged ampullae: Distended or enlarged ampullae on transrectal palpation and ultrasonography. Ampullae may contain hyperechoic areas and a prominent lumen indicating accumulation of sperm. The tail of the epididymis may be enlarged and turgid.
- Testicular degeneration: Testes may be soft on palpation.
- Partial ejaculatory failure: Evidence of musculoskeletal or neurological condition; may be behavioral.
- Sexual overuse: Normal physical examination results.

ETIOLOGY AND PATHOPHYSIOLOGY

- Testicular hypoplasia: Most often a congenital condition linked to genetic abnormality or segmental aplasia of the efferent tubules. An intersex condition may be present. Oligozoospermia may be caused by reduced spermatogenesis or an obstruction in the efferent duct.

- Orchitis: Infection is generally introduced to the testicle through an ascending infection (from the urethra or the bladder), hematogenous spread, or direct inoculation caused by trauma.
- Plugged ampullae: Physical obstruction in one or both ampullae of unknown cause. This condition may recur after periods of sexual rest in certain stallions.
- Testicular degeneration: Intrinsic factors include defects in the germ cells or supporting cells that may be heritable. Extrinsic factors include temperature changes, endocrine imbalances, vascular insults, toxins, infectious disease, and excessive androgen exposure.
- Partial ejaculatory failure: Often a result of musculoskeletal pain either before or during ejaculation. Neurologic diseases also cause ejaculatory failure depending on the affected nerve pathway. Behavioral or equipment problems may also cause premature dismount and partial ejaculation.

DIAGNOSIS

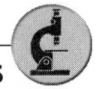

DIFFERENTIAL DIAGNOSIS

True oligozoospermia caused by a testicular or efferent duct problem should be differentiated from partial ejaculatory failure.

INITIAL DATABASE

- Sequential collections should be performed to confirm the diagnosis.
- Testicular hypoplasia: A karyotype may be submitted to check for chromosomal abnormalities leading to some intersex conditions. Testicular hypoplasia should be differentiated from ejaculatory failure by physical examination findings and history.
- Orchitis: A complete blood count may show leukocytosis and hyperfibrinogenemia. Large numbers of neutrophils may be present in the ejaculate. Sperm quality is generally very poor. The affected testicle may be more hypoechoic on ultrasonography compared with the unaffected testicle.
- Plugged ampullae: The ejaculate will range from oligozoospermia to

azoospermia. When sperm is obtained, there will be a high percentage of tailless heads and a low percentage of motile sperm. The ampullae may be enlarged and firm on transrectal palpation and ultrasonography. Ampullae may contain areas of dilation or hyperechogenicity, indicating the accumulation of sperm.

- Testicular degeneration: Repeated testicular ultrasonography may show a gradual decline in testicular volume and sperm number. Analysis of the ejaculate may show increasing teratospermia. Immature (premature) germ cells will also be present in increasing numbers in the ejaculate. The advanced cases will be azoospermic.
- Partial ejaculatory failure: This condition must be differentiated from the other causes of azoospermia. The testes and accessory sex glands should be normal with palpation and ultrasonography.

ADVANCED OR CONFIRMATORY TESTING

- Alkaline phosphatase (ALP): Fluid from the testicles and epididymis has an extremely high concentration of ALP. The ALP is low (<1000 IU/L) when there is no testicular component to the ejaculate. This is the case with a blockage in the duct system as with plugged ampullae. With cases of severe testicular degeneration, ALP is high, indicating fluid from the testicles and epididymis, but there may be a complete absence of sperm cells (see "Sperm Abnormalities: Azoospermia" in this section).
- Bacterial culture of the ejaculate, especially when orchitis is suspected, is helpful to determine the causative organism.
- Testicular biopsy: In practice, a testicular biopsy is rarely indicated, and the risks of the procedure usually outweigh the benefit of the diagnostics. A single sample may not give an accurate representation of the entire testicle, and the risk of hemorrhage or further damage to the already compromised parenchyma must be accounted for. If indicated, histopathology in cases of testicular degeneration will show varying degrees of cytoplasmic vacuolization, increased fibrous tissue, and loss of normal architecture. The number of germ cells will be decreased, and in severe cases, may be absent,

leaving only the Sertoli cells and supporting tissues.
- Hormonal assay: Levels of hormones vary considerably in normal and subfertile stallions; therefore, hormonal analysis is of little value for diagnosis. With severe cases of testicular degeneration, follicle-stimulating hormone and luteinizing hormone levels may be elevated, and the estradiol level may be low.

TREATMENT

THERAPEUTIC GOAL(S)

- Reduced spermatogenesis: Treatment depends on the cause. If caused by inflammation (orchitis), treatment is not generally recommended because of a poor prognosis. If only one testicle is affected, hemicastration is indicated. If oligozoospermia is caused by trauma, treatment to reduce the inflammation initially followed by 60 to 90 days of sexual rest may improve or resolve the condition. If caused by age related testicular degeneration, treatment is not generally attempted because of a poor long-term prognosis.
- Obstructive oligozoospermia: Diagnose the underlying condition and resolve the obstruction when possible.
- Sexual overuse: Determine an appropriate collection schedule for the individual stallion.

ACUTE GENERAL TREATMENT

- Plugged ampullae: Physical transrectal massage of both ampullae for 5 minutes before each collection to loosen the luminal blockage. Administration of oxytocin (20 IU IV) immediately before collection attempt to stimulate smooth muscle contraction of the ampullae. Increased frequency of ejaculations as often as the stallion can tolerate it, typically several times daily to release the blockage.
- Orchitis: Long-term systemic antibiotics based on culture and susceptibility along with antiinflammatory agents and cold water hydrotherapy. If only one testicle is affected, hemicastration may be the best treatment to salvage the remaining unaffected testicle.

CHRONIC TREATMENT

Plugged ampullae: Frequent year-round ejaculations may prevent the accumu-

lation of sperm and subsequent blockage.

POSSIBLE COMPLICATIONS

Plugged ampullae: If a complete blockage is present, administration of oxytocin or aggressive therapy may cause rupture of the ampullae or ductus deferens.

RECOMMENDED MONITORING

The stallion should be examined every 60 days to determine if there is improvement over a single spermatogenic cycle. In cases of plugged ampullae, the stallion's sperm should be collected frequently, as necessary, to prevent recurrence.

PROGNOSIS AND OUTCOME

- Testicular hypoplasia, if bilateral, guarded to grave prognosis for future fertility
- Orchitis: Prognosis for bilateral orchitis is guarded for future fertility. Prognosis improves if the affected testicle is removed, allowing the remaining testicle to return to normal after the inflammatory process is resolved.
- Plugged ampullae: Excellent prognosis if the blockage is resolved after treatment. Most affected animals return to their previous levels of fertility.
- Testicular degeneration: May be reversible depending on the cause. If the degeneration is caused by age-related changes, the problem is most likely permanent.

PEARLS & CONSIDERATIONS

Causes of oligozoospermia can usually be differentiated based on history and physical examination findings, including a reproductive examination.

SUGGESTED READING

Love CC, Riera FL, Oristaglio RM, et al: Sperm occluded (plugged) ampullae in the stallion. *Soc Theriogenology Proc* 117–127, 1992.
Turner RM: Testicular abnormalities. In Samper JC, Pycock JF, McKinnon AO, editors: *Current therapy in equine reproduction*, St Louis, 2007, Saunders Elsevier, pp 227–230.

AUTHOR: **AIME K. JOHNSON**

EDITOR: **JUAN C. SAMPER**

Sperm Abnormalities: Teratospermia

BASIC INFORMATION

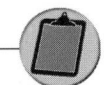

DEFINITION

The presence of sperm with abnormal morphology. As a rule, fertile stallions have greater than 60% morphologically normal sperm, and less than 10% to 15% of any specific defect.

EPIDEMIOLOGY

SPECIES, AGE, SEX Affects stallions at varying ages depending on cause

GENETICS AND BREED PREDISPOSITION Sperm defects have been shown to be hereditary in some species. A detailed history of the stallion's family should be analyzed to determine any heritability.

RISK FACTORS Any disease process, stress, or increase in body or testicular temperature can disrupt spermatogenesis and lead to transient teratospermia. This usually resolves within 60 days (one spermatogenic cycle) once the insult has resolved; if the insult is severe, the damage can be permanent. An increase in the number of abnormal sperm may be seen after periods of sexual rest due to damage caused by increased storage time. In these cases, sperm morphology usually improves with subsequent collections.

GEOGRAPHY AND SEASONALITY
- May be increased after periods of sexual rest, but decreases with subsequent collections
- May be present with higher incidence during very hot summer months, especially in the southern United States

ASSOCIATED CONDITIONS AND DISORDERS Teratospermia tends to occur in combination with asthenozoospermia (low motility).

CLINICAL PRESENTATION

HISTORY, CHIEF COMPLAINT
- Most stallions present with a reduction in fertility or complete infertility. These stallions often were previously fertile and have either acutely or gradually failed to achieve pregnancies. A complete review of the stallion's breeding records is helpful in determining when the problem or initial insult occurred.
- Some stallions have perpetual infertility. These stallions are usually affected by low sperm quality and increased teratospermia that may have begun at puberty.

PHYSICAL EXAM FINDINGS A general physical exam is unremarkable unless concurrent systemic disease is present causing pyrexia or scrotal insulation (edema) that subsequently affects semen quality. The reproductive exam may also be within normal limits. In more advanced cases of testicular degeneration, the testes may be small or soft. If orchitis is present, the testes may be slightly enlarged, warm, and painful to the horse when touched.

ETIOLOGY AND PATHOPHYSIOLOGY
- Genetic factors: The exact genetic factors that lead to teratospermia are not well defined and may overlap with environmental factors.
- Environmental factors: These are the most common causes and result from an insult to the testicle disrupting spermatogenesis. Environmental factors may be any of the following:
  - Elevated scrotal temperature
  - Incomplete testicular descent
  - Malnutrition
  - Chemicals, drugs
  - Hormonal imbalances
- Aging: As stallions age, the efficiency of spermatogenesis may decrease. Older stallions often have a higher number of abnormally shaped sperm.

DIAGNOSIS

DIFFERENTIAL DIAGNOSIS
- Elevated scrotal temperature (pyrexia, elevated ambient temperature, scrotal inflammation, scrotal insulation)
- Incomplete testicular descent (partial cryptorchid, "high flanker")
- Malnutrition
- Chemicals, drugs
- Hormonal imbalances
- Testicular degeneration
- Orchitis
- Spermiostasis (plugged ampullae) (see "Ejaculatory Dysfunction" and "Sperm Abnormalities: Azoospermia" in this section)

INITIAL DATABASE
- CBC and serum chemistry may be beneficial in assessing the stallion for systemic disease or inflammation that may be affecting the scrotal temperature. If orchitis is present, the stallion may exhibit leukocytosis and hyperfibrinogenemia.
- A complete semen evaluation is critical in any case of reduced fertility. A morphologic analysis should be performed every time a fertility problem is diagnosed. The morphology of the sperm is less often affected by artifactual changes (examiner mishandling) than is sperm motility. Morphology should be performed using oil immersion and a good-quality microscope. If using a wet mount, the cells should be examined by phase contrast or differential interference contrast (DIC) microscopy. In practice, most veterinarians will use eosin-nigrosin stain. The stain can also be used to determine the viability of the sperm cells. A normal, viable cell will stain as a white sperm cell on a dark background. If the membrane of the sperm is damaged, the stain will penetrate the cell, causing the spermatozoal head to appear pink.
- All defects—such as abnormal heads, abnormal acrosomes, abnormal midpieces, proximal and distal cytoplasmic droplets, detached or tailless heads, tail defects, and premature germ cells—should be recorded. One hundred cells should be counted and the specific type of defect present recorded. If multiple defects are present on the same sperm cell, they should be counted simultaneously. This gives the examiner a more accurate representation of the frequency of the specific abnormalities present.
- Ultrasound of the testicles should be performed to evaluate the parenchyma for abnormalities such as neoplasia or hyperechoic or hypoechoic areas.
- If defects indicating a problem with transport during ejaculation are present (detached heads, bent tails), palpation and ultrasound of the accessory sex glands should be performed.
- Hormonal assay: Levels of hormones will vary considerably in normal and subfertile stallions; therefore hormonal analysis may be of little value for diagnosis. With severe cases of testicular degeneration, levels of follicle-stimulating hormone and luteinizing hormone may be elevated and estradiol may be low. Elevated levels of exogenous androgens will lead to a disruption of spermatogenesis. If no other specific causes for teratospermia are found, a hormonal assay should be performed.

ADVANCED OR CONFIRMATORY TESTING
- Sperm Chromatin Structure Assay (SCSA) is an advanced test that will evaluate the DNA, or chromatin, of the sperm cells. This test is performed in specific laboratories and may be indicated when other causes of infertility are not identified or an analysis of the sperm chromatin is desired to assess treatment or prognosis.

- Acrosome reaction is an evaluation of the ability of the acrosome to properly undergo the reaction necessary for fertilization. This may be indicated if a large number of abnormal acrosomes or heads are observed. It may also be indicated in cases where the semen analysis is adequate but the stallion is not able to achieve pregnancies.
- Hypoosmotic swelling test (HOS) is an in-house test that can be performed to assess the membrane integrity of the sperm cell. See the references below for a description of how to perform this test.

TREATMENT

THERAPEUTIC GOAL(S)

- Resolve any environmental factors
- Manage stallion to maximize fertility
  - Increase breeding dose of sperm to accommodate for low numbers of normal sperm
  - Cooling trials to determine the best extender and antibiotic combination for each stallion
  - Centrifugation using a density gradient (eg, EquiPure, Molndäl, Sweden) to allow only normal cells in the pellet (see below)
  - Restrict number of mares bred each year to improve pregnancy rates
- Manage mare cycle to maximize fertility
  - Increase palpation frequency to improve prediction of ovulation
  - Use of ovulation induction agents (human chorionic gonadotropin, deslorelin) to time ovulation
  - Breed very close to the time of ovulation (12 hours before or 6 hours after)
  - Inseminate mares every 24 hours until ovulation if longevity of the spermatozoa is reduced
  - Use deep horn insemination techniques to place the sperm as close to the oviductal papillae as possible

ACUTE GENERAL TREATMENT

- If scrotal or testicular insult is identified (edema, inflammation, systemic pyrexia), the inciting cause must be treated, which should resolve the effects on spermatogenesis. If infectious, broad spectrum antibiotics based on culture and sensitivity should be initiated. Antiinflammatories (flunixin meglumine or phenylbutazone) should be administered. Scrotal hydrotherapy and hand walking are indicated in many cases of scrotal or testicular insult.
- If no specific cause of the teratospermia is easily identified, multiple ejaculates should be evaluated to identify

trends. After periods of sexual rest, a larger percentage of teratospermia may initially be present but will tend to resolve with subsequent collections. Complete records of each collection and each specific abnormality will give the veterinarian an accurate assessment of trends. If a specific defect continues to be present in a high percentage, the specific cause should be further identified.

- Specific defects may guide the veterinarian to a specific problem or localization. This is not an all-inclusive list, only the most frequently observed conditions.
  - Detached or tailless heads: Most often indicate spermiostasis. If they are present in more than 10% of the ejaculate, look for blocked or partially blocked ampullae. (See "Sperm Abnormalities: Azoospermia" and "Sperm Abnormalities: Oligozoospermia" in this section for treatment of plugged or blocked ampullae.)
  - Abnormal heads and abnormal midpieces tend to occur together and directly indicate a testicular problem. The specific defect may vary widely from small, large, or misshapen heads to swollen, roughened, or obviously abnormal midpieces.
  - Bent (bowed) midpieces: May occur as a primary testicular problem or as cells lose motility and die, causing circular motility.
  - Bent tails: May be iatrogenic. Exposing sperm to a hypotonic solution will cause a bend in the tail. If these are seen frequently, change the technique for assessing morphology to determine if the bend is iatrogenic or real.
  - Coiled tails and premature germ cells: Indicate sperm that were released prematurely from the testicle. If observed in large numbers (>10%), there has most likely been an insult to the testes. These will also be observed in increasing frequency with testicular degeneration.
  - Proximal cytoplasmic droplets: Caused by a failure of the sperm cell to lose the cytoplasmic droplet during transport through the epididymis. These may be observed in cases of decreased transit time through the epididymis (sexual overuse) or early testicular degeneration. However, the effect of an increased number of proximal droplets on the fertility of stallions is unclear.
  - Distal cytoplasmic droplets: Caused by failure of the droplet to be lost during ejaculation. A high percentage is often observed after cases of

sexual rest, and the frequency will gradually decrease with subsequent collections. The effect of this defect on fertility in the stallion is not clear. Many researchers suspect that stallions with a high percentage of this defect may still remain fertile.

- Abaxial midpieces, where the midpieces and tail are attached to the spermatozoa head laterally to the left or right of midline are considered within normal limits for the stallion.

CHRONIC TREATMENT

- If the teratospermia is permanent and the cause does not appear to be heritable, intense management of the stallion may preserve fertility. By breeding very close to ovulation (within 12 hours before or 6 hours after) and using a deep uterine horn insemination technique to place the sperm directly on the oviductal papillae of the mare, many stallions are able to achieve an acceptable seasonal pregnancy rate even with a low number of morphologically normal sperm (less than 40%). Increasing the insemination dose may also improve fertility.
- Special semen handling techniques are available but require some training and practice before applying them to a clinical setting. The ejaculate may be centrifuged through a density gradient such as EquiPure. This gradient will separate out many of the abnormal sperm, leaving a high percentage of normal sperm in the pellet.

DRUG INTERACTIONS

Misuse of exogenous androgens will cause an increased incidence of teratospermia by disrupting normal spermatogenesis.

RECOMMENDED MONITORING

- All breeding stallions should have a morphologic analysis at the beginning of the breeding season to serve as a reference. Additional analyses may be performed every month in problem stallions or only if a decrease in fertility occurs.
- The stallion should be evaluated every 30 to 90 days to assess improvement. A minimum of 60 days from the resolution of the insult is required for complete recovery (a single spermatogenic cycle).

PROGNOSIS AND OUTCOME

Prognosis depends on the underlying cause and specific defect present.

- Primary testicular abnormalities:
  - Bilateral orchitis: Prognosis for future fertility is poor (see "Sperm Abnormalities: Oligozoospermia" in this section).
  - Age-related testicular degeneration: Intense breeding management may preserve fertility, but the number of mares bred per year may need to be reduced.
  - Systemic illness: If resolved, prognosis for future fertility after a spermatogenic cycle is good.
- Transport abnormalities:
  - Plugged ampullae: Prognosis for future fertility is good with appropriate treatment and management.
  - Cytoplasmic droplets: If due to testicular degeneration, the condition will continue to become progressively worse. The ability of sperm with cytoplasmic droplets to fertilize has not been determined in the stallion. The entire clinical picture should be assessed. This defect has

been observed to be present in a significant percentage (30% or more) in fertile stallions.

PEARLS & CONSIDERATIONS

COMMENTS

- Sperm morphology alone is not an accurate predictor of fertility. Morphology must be assessed with other tests to give a more reliable prediction of the ability of that stallion to reproduce.
- If the veterinarian is not comfortable evaluating sperm morphology, the sample may be preserved in buffered formalin saline and sent to a boarded theriogenologist for analysis.

PREVENTION

All breeding stallions should have a morphologic analysis at the beginning of the breeding season to serve as a reference. Frequent analyses give the veterinarian a

better idea of trends than a single analysis. This also allows the veterinarian to assess response to treatment and predict future fertility.

CLIENT EDUCATION

Although not performed as often as motility assessment, morphologic assessment of the sperm is an important diagnostic tool for analysis of any breeding stallion.

SUGGESTED READING

Turner RM: Testicular abnormalities. In Samper JC, Pycock JF, McKinnon AO, editors: *Current therapy in equine reproduction*, St Louis, 2007, Saunders Elsevier, pp 227–230.

Love CC: Sperm occluded (plugged) ampullae in the stallion. *Soc Theriogenol Proc* 117–127, 1992.

Barth AD, Oko RJ: Abnormal morphology of bovine spermatozoa, Ames, IA, 1989, Iowa State University.

AUTHOR: **AIME K. JOHNSON**

EDITOR: **JUAN C. SAMPER**

Spermatic Cord Rotation and Torsion

BASIC INFORMATION

DEFINITION

- Rotation describes twisting of the spermatic cord along the longitudinal axis, usually 180 degrees or less, and is generally an incidental finding.
- Torsion is an acute clinical condition in which the spermatic cord rotates at least 180 degrees, usually 360 to 720 degrees, compromising blood supply to the testis.

SYNONYM(S)

Testicular torsion

EPIDEMIOLOGY

SPECIES, AGE, SEX Affects stallions of any age

GENETICS AND BREED PREDISPOSITION A genetic basis has not been elucidated; however, Paso Fino horses appear to have a high incidence of spermatic cord rotation, and Standardbreds appear to be overrepresented in cases of spermatic cord torsion.

RISK FACTORS Anatomic variations, including an abnormally long ligament of the tail of the epididymis, proper ligament of the testis, and mesorchium, have been suggested to predispose to spermatic cord torsion.

CLINICAL PRESENTATION

DISEASE FORMS/SUBTYPES Spermatic cord rotation, spermatic cord torsion

HISTORY, CHIEF COMPLAINT

- Spermatic cord rotation, often an incidental finding, may be chronic or intermittent, with the owner relating an abnormal contour to the testis. There is generally no history of pain associated with rotation, but compromise of blood supply by as much as 40% may occur. However, fertility appears to be unaffected.
- In stallions with acute spermatic cord torsion, clinical signs include unilateral scrotal or testicular enlargement (or both), inguinal pain, colic, and a stilted hindlimb gait.
- Occasionally, cases of chronic, recurring spermatic cord torsion are presented with periodic discomfort referable to the inguinal region, abdomen, scrotum, or hindquarters.

PHYSICAL EXAM FINDINGS

- Spermatic cord rotation
  - Tail of the epididymis positioned cranially or nearly so
  - Unilateral testicular or scrotal swelling, distension of the spermatic cord, and pain on scrotal palpation are generally all absent
- Spermatic cord torsion (acute, 360 or 720 degrees)

- Tail of the epididymis positioned at caudal pole of testis but more dorsally than normal
- Unilateral scrotal or testicular enlargement
- Pain on palpation of affected testis
- Spermatic cord distension, firmness, and twisting
- Dorsal displacement or retraction of the spermatic cord and testis
- Hydrocele may be present
- Other clinical signs consistent with colic (eg, tachycardia, tachypnea)
- Spermatic cord torsion (chronic, recurrent)
  - Intermittent unilateral scrotal swelling
  - Mild, transient colic

ETIOLOGY AND PATHOPHYSIOLOGY

- Definitive causes of spermatic cord torsion have not been elucidated. However, several predisposing factors have been suggested as being permissive for rotation of the spermatic cord, including an excessively long ligament of the tail of the epididymis, proper ligament of the testis, and mesorchium.
- Twisting of the spermatic cord around its longitudinal axis and rotation of the testis about its vertical axis result in compromised blood flow to the scrotal contents through the testicular artery and outflow via the pampiniform

plexus. Lymphatic drainage is also interrupted.

- Obstruction of the pampiniform plexus results in hemorrhage and edema within the testicular parenchyma, exerting pressure on the relatively inelastic tunica albuginea and causing pain. Edema and hemorrhage may also develop in the spermatic cord and scrotum.
- Peritoneal fluid may accumulate in the vaginal cavity, resulting in a hydrocele.
- Intra- and extratesticular hemorrhage and edema, inflammation, and hydrocele formation increase the intrascrotal temperature. Scrotal insulation predisposes the affected and contralateral testes to thermally induced degeneration.
- Occlusion of the testicular artery results in ischemia of the affected testis, epididymis, and scrotal skin. Prolonged spermatic cord torsion results in ischemic necrosis and irreversible damage to the testicular parenchyma.

DIAGNOSIS

DIFFERENTIAL DIAGNOSIS

- Inguinal or scrotal hernia
- Scrotal edema secondary to trauma
- Testicular hematoma
- Orchitis or periorchitis
- Testicular neoplasia
- Varicocele
- Spermatic cord vascular thrombosis

INITIAL DATABASE

- Ultrasonography of scrotal contents
  - Useful when marked scrotal edema renders palpation of the testes difficult
  - Alterations in echogenicity of testicular parenchyma: Relatively hypoechoic in acutely presented cases because of vascular stasis; hyperechoic areas consistent with clot formation and fibrin deposition in protracted cases
  - Distension of the central vein of the testis
  - Enlargement of pampiniform plexus distal to torsion (compare with the appearance of the unaffected side)
  - Attendant hydrocele may be present
- Palpation per rectum of the internal inguinal ring
  - Useful in eliminating inguinal herniation as a cause of colic.
  - In cases of spermatic cord torsion, the affected spermatic cord may be enlarged, edematous, and painful to palpation as it enters the inguinal ring.

ADVANCED OR CONFIRMATORY TESTING

Doppler ultrasonography: An absence of blood flow through the central vein and arcuate arteries of the testis as well as the pampiniform plexus confirms vascular occlusion.

TREATMENT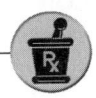

THERAPEUTIC GOAL(S)

- For subclinical spermatic cord rotation, treatment is generally not indicated.
- In cases of spermatic cord torsion:
  - If acute onset, single occurrence, intervene immediately, selecting the course of treatment according to the intended use of the animal.
  - If chronic, recurring case presenting with some discomfort, consider unilateral orchidectomy or orchiopexy, depending on the intended use of the animal.

ACUTE GENERAL TREATMENT

- Provide systemic stabilization and pain management before surgery
- Tetanus prophylaxis
- Prophylactic antimicrobial therapy
- Immediate surgery
  - If use as a breeding animal is unimportant, castrate bilaterally with ligation and transection of affected spermatic cord proximal to the site of torsion.
  - If stallion intended for breeding, perform hemicastration. Consider orchiopexy of the contralateral testis.
  - If the affected testis has been assessed to be viable and preservation is desired, perform orchiopexy by suturing the proper ligament of the testis to the tunica dartos using nonreactive, nonabsorbable suture material followed by routine closure of parietal vaginal tunic and scrotal skin. Alternatively, orchiopexy may be accomplished by fixing the tunica albuginea to the tunica dartos at the cranial and caudal poles of the testis using nonabsorbable suture.

CHRONIC TREATMENT

- Routine postcastration aftercare, including activity restriction for first 24 hours followed by forced exercise to deter formation of scrotal and preputial edema and isolation from mares until surgical site fully healed
- Semen collection and evaluation 2 months after surgery, assuming no complications

POSSIBLE COMPLICATIONS

- Decrease in semen quality from remaining testis caused by testicular degeneration. In most cases, this decrease is transient, and semen quality should improve beginning approximately 2 months after resolution of spermatic cord torsion.
- Experimental evidence in other species suggests possibility of permanent immune-mediated damage to contralateral testis after spermatic cord torsion.

RECOMMENDED MONITORING

- Collect and evaluate semen monthly beginning 2 months after hemiorchidectomy or orchiopexy.
- Monitor the remaining testis for changes in size and consistency as well as orientation, particularly if orchiopexy was not performed because the testis may be prone to rotation or torsion. Expect some change in the shape of the remaining testis because compensatory hypertrophy may render the testis globoid.

PROGNOSIS AND OUTCOME

- With prompt surgical remediation of acute spermatic cord torsion, the prognosis for life is excellent and for future fertility is good.
- In case of hemiorchidectomy, the remaining testis will undergo compensatory hypertrophy, resulting in sperm production greater than 50% of the presurgical total sperm count.

PEARLS & CONSIDERATIONS

- Because most stallions do not service very large books of mares and compensatory hypertrophy of the remaining testis occurs, hemiorchidectomy rather than orchiopexy provides more definitive resolution of spermatic cord torsion while preserving adequate breeding capacity.
- Although the prognosis for return to fertility is generally good after treatment of spermatic cord torsion, owners of breeding stallions should be informed that function of the remaining testis and fertility may be severely compromised if antisperm antibodies have formed during the acute episode.

SUGGESTED READING

Chenier T: Anatomy and physical examination of the stallion. In Samper JC, editor: *Equine breeding management and artificial insemination*, St Louis, 2009, Saunders Elsevier, pp 1–16.

Love CC: Ultrasonographic evaluation of the testis, epididymis, and spermatic cord of the stallion. *Vet Clin North Am Equine Pract* 8(1):167, 1992.

Schumacher J: Testis. In Auer JA, Stick JA, editors: *Equine surgery*, ed 3, St Louis, 2006, Saunders Elsevier, pp 775–810.

Turner RMO: Testicular abnormalities. In Samper JC, Pycock JF, McKinnon AO, editors: *Current therapy in equine reproduction*, St Louis, 2007, Saunders Elsevier, pp 195–204.

Varner DD, Schumacher J, Blanchard TL, et al: Diseases of the spermatic cord. In Pratt PW, editor: *Diseases and management of breeding stallions*, Goleta, CA, 1991, American Veterinary Publications, pp 251–256.

AUTHOR: **DAWNA L. VOELKL**

EDITOR: **JUAN C. SAMPER**

Spinal Injury

BASIC INFORMATION

DEFINITION

Injury to the vertebral column caused by a sudden (mechanical and usually external) force. This section focuses on consequences to the central nervous system (CNS; spinal cord).

SYNONYM(S)

Spinal cord injury (SCI)

EPIDEMIOLOGY

SPECIES, AGE, SEX
- Foals appear more susceptible than adults.
- Young animals are more prone to traumatic (training) accidents.

GENETICS AND BREED PREDISPOSITION
Thoroughbred breeds may be more prone to traumatic accidents because of their temperament and the young age at which (race) training commences.

RISK FACTORS
- Temperament or disposition
- Management: Training and pasture group composition

ASSOCIATED CONDITIONS AND DISORDERS
- Osteomyelitis
- Fractures of vertebral bodies
- Ataxia with a neuroanatomic localization caudal to the foramen magnum

CLINICAL PRESENTATION

DISEASE FORMS/SUBTYPES
- Acute SCI: Such as seen after trauma
- Chronic SCI: Chronic phase of acute SCI or chronic or gradual onset of SCI such as seen in cervical vertebral stenotic myelopathy
- Cervical fractures most common
- Foals: C1-C3 and T15-T18 regions most commonly affected
- Adults: Occipital-atlanto-axial region and C5-T1 and caudal thoracic region

HISTORY, CHIEF COMPLAINT
- Down
- External damage to the body
- Signs of neurologic disease: Unable to get up, ataxic

PHYSICAL EXAM FINDINGS
- Vary depending on severity of insult
- Vary depending on level of lesion
- Range from subtle neurologic deficits to recumbency

ETIOLOGY AND PATHOPHYSIOLOGY
- The severity of SCI is related to the velocity, degree, and duration of impact.
- Cord concussion with transient neurologic deficits is a result of local axonal depolarization and transient dysfunction.
- Permanent paralysis is a result of primary tissue injury followed by spreading of secondary damage.
- Primary damage: Initial mechanical disruption of vasculature and components of the CNS, such as cell bodies (neurons, astrocytes, oligodendrocytes) and axons.
- Secondary damage: A complex cascade of molecular, cellular, and biochemical events that may occur for days to months after the initial insult, resulting in delayed tissue damage and enlargement of the damaged area.
- Systemic alterations such as systemic hypotension further contribute to the tissue damage: Hypoxia, ischemia, infection, breakdown of blood-brain barrier, impaired energy metabolism, altered ionic homeostasis, changes in gene expression, inflammation, and activation or release of autodestructive molecules occur and exacerbate the initial injury.
- Ischemia is exacerbated by spinal cord swelling (hematomas, edema) and cessation of autoregulation of spinal cord blood flow and systemic hypotension.
- *Excitotoxicity* refers to the deleterious cellular effects of excess glutamate and aspartate. When released, these neurotransmitters activate NMDA (*N*-methyl-D-aspartic acid) and AMPA (α-amino-3-hydroxyl-5-methyl-4-isoxazole-propionate) receptors and lead to release of massive amounts of calcium from intracellular stores. Elevation of intracellular calcium concentrations can trigger a multitude of processes that can lethally alter cellular metabolism, generate free radicals, impair mitochondrial function, cause vascular smooth muscle spasm, and bind phosphates.
- Apoptosis, or programmed cell death, is a slowly spreading form of cell death induced by injury. Apoptosis occurs mostly at the lesion margins and at quite remote distances from the point of impact in areas with degenerating axons that were injured at the original lesion site.

DIAGNOSIS

DIFFERENTIAL DIAGNOSIS
- Other causes of recumbency
  - Laminitis
  - Fractures (Figures 1 and 2)
  - Colic
- Other causes of CNS disease with a neuroanatomic localization caudal to foramen magnum
  - Equine herpesvirus-1 myelopathy
  - Equine protozoal myeloencephalitis
  - Equine degenerative myeloencephalopathy
  - Viral encephalitides (Eastern equine encephalomyelitis, Western equine encephalomyelitis, Venezuelan equine encephalomyelitis, rabies, West Nile virus)
  - Meningitis
  - Neoplasia

INITIAL DATABASE
- History
- Complete physical and neurologic examination

ADVANCED OR CONFIRMATORY TESTING
- Imaging of the vertebral column: Radiography, computed tomography, myelography
- Nuclear scintigraphy
- Cerebrospinal fluid (CSF) analysis: Hemorrhage
- Rule out other (infectious) disease through complete blood count, serum titers, and CSF analysis

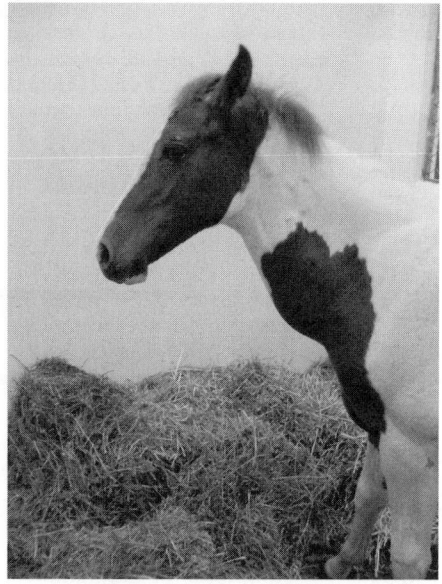

FIGURE 1 Neck fracture.

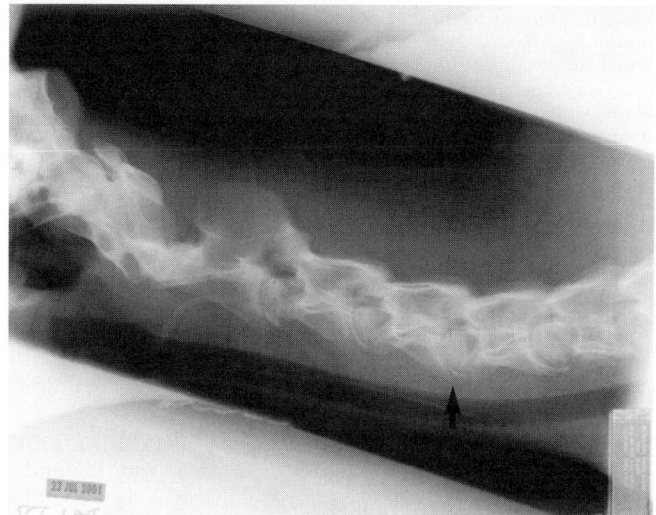

FIGURE 2 Radiograph of neck fracture.

TREATMENT

THERAPEUTIC GOAL(S)

- Prevent further neurologic damage
- Save or salvage undamaged or reversibly damaged components
- Enhance recovery and regeneration

ACUTE GENERAL TREATMENT

- Optimize oxygen delivery
  - Optimize spinal cord blood flow
  - Optimize mean arterial blood pressure and hemoglobin concentration
- Fluid therapy
- Vasopressor or inotropic support (or both)
- Antiinflammatory drugs
  - Corticosteroids: Dexamethasone (0.1–0.25 mg/kg IV q6–24h) or methylprednisolone sodium succinate (0.5–2.5 mg/kg IV q6h); dose and interval depend on severity of clinical signs. Use of corticosteroids for SCI is controversial.
  - Flunixin meglumine: 1.1 mg/kg IV q12–24h
  - Dimethyl sulfoxide (0.5–1.0 g/kg IV q12–24h) must be diluted to a 10% solution or less in an isotonic balanced electrolyte solution.

- Antimicrobial therapy: Not always necessary in the treatment of vertebral or spinal cord trauma; however, indicated in treating open fractures and secondary complications associated with a recumbent horse, such as pneumonia and decubital sores.

CHRONIC TREATMENT

- Sling support in horses that are unable to stand or get up on their own.
- Physiotherapy: Rehabilitation. Exercise has been shown to be beneficial for recovery of function after CNS damage in multiple animal models.

POSSIBLE COMPLICATIONS

- Decubitus ulcers from prolonged recumbency
- Pneumonia from prolonged recumbency

RECOMMENDED MONITORING

- Periodic repeat neurologic examinations to assess response to therapy and recovery of function.
- Monitor appetite and hydration status. Monitor urine and creatinine concentration if treating with possible nephrotoxic drugs.

PROGNOSIS AND OUTCOME

Depends on severity of sustained spinal cord damage

PEARLS & CONSIDERATIONS

PREVENTION

Prevent injuries by increasing safety around the horse and when handling horses.

CLIENT EDUCATION

Clients should be knowledgeable on topics such as (multiple) horse management and safe handling and training.

SUGGESTED READING

Feige K, Fürst A, Kaser-Hotz B, et al: Traumatic injury to the central nervous system in horses: occurrence, diagnosis and outcome. *Equine Vet Educ* 12:220–224, 2000.

Nout YS: Central nervous system trauma. In Reed SM, Furr MO, editors: *Equine neurology*, Ames, IA, 2007, Blackwell Publishing, pp 305–327.

AUTHOR: **YVETTE S. NOUT**

EDITOR: **STEPHEN M. REED**

Splenic Abscess

BASIC INFORMATION

DEFINITION

An encapsulated focus of purulent exudate, usually associated with bacterial infection, in the splenic parenchyma

CLINICAL PRESENTATION

HISTORY, CHIEF COMPLAINT

- Fever
- Colic (variable, usually mild)
- ± Weight loss

PHYSICAL EXAM FINDINGS

- Variable. Fever and poor body condition are usually evident because of chronic infection.
- Rectal examination: No abnormalities are typically noted on palpation of the spleen per rectum, but rarely the abscess may be palpated as an enlarged irregular region of the caudal aspect of the spleen.

ETIOLOGY AND PATHOPHYSIOLOGY

- Hematogenous spread of bacteria from another site of infection rarely may result in formation of a splenic abscess. Organisms most likely to be associated with this are *Streptococcus equi* subsp. *equi* and *Rhodococcus equi* (in foals), although other organisms, such as *Actinobacillus equilli, Streptococcus equi* subsp. *zooepidemicus, Escherichia coli,* or *Corynebacterium pseudotuberculosis,* may be involved.
- Splenic hematomas may (rarely) become infected with any number of bacterial organisms as the spleen functions in its critical role in the reticuloendothelial system.
- Splenic abscess is also a rare but potential complication from splenic biopsy or accidental splenocentesis during attempted abdominocentesis.

DIAGNOSIS

DIFFERENTIAL DIAGNOSIS

- Splenic hematoma
- Splenic neoplasia

INITIAL DATABASE

- Complete blood count and serum chemistry profile: Usually reveal evidence of chronic inflammation with mild anemia, leukocytosis characterized by a mature neutrophilia, hyperfibrinogenemia, or hyperglobulinemia.
- Transabdominal ultrasonography
  - A splenic abscess appears as a focal, irregular, cavitary mixed-echogenic lesion in any part of the splenic parenchyma. Echogenic fluid (pus) may be visible in the cavitary regions of the abscess. The presence of hyperechoic regions that cast anacoustic shadows are consistent with gas (suggesting an anaerobic component) or mineralization in chronic abscesses. The ultrasonographic appearance of a splenic abscess may be very similar to that of a splenic hematoma.
  - Occasionally, multiple splenic abscesses or other intraabdominal abscesses are noted on ultrasonography and can be easily confused with metastatic neoplasia.
  - Percutaneous, ultrasound-guided aspiration of a suspected splenic abscess may be attempted to obtain samples for bacterial culture but carries with it a risk of bacterial contamination of the peritoneal cavity.
- Peritoneal fluid analysis
  - Usually normal because the infection is confined within the splenic capsule, although mildly increased nucleated cell counts (5,000–20,000 cells/µL) or total protein concentration (>2 g/dL) consistent with low-grade peritonitis may be noted.
  - Bacterial culture of peritoneal fluid rarely yields bacterial growth, although *S. equi* and *R. equi* polymerase chain reaction on peritoneal fluid should be submitted.
- Serial blood cultures as well as serology for *S. equi* and *C. pseudotuberculosis* should be submitted if a splenic abscess is suspected.

ADVANCED OR CONFIRMATORY TESTING

Definitive confirmation of splenic abscess requires visualization and sampling via laparoscopy or laparotomy. However, given the difficulty accessing the equine spleen via standard surgical approaches and the typical success of medical management in treatment of splenic abscesses, this is rarely warranted. Thus a presumptive diagnosis is made based on characteristic clinical, clinicopathologic, and ultrasonographic abnormalities and is confirmed via response to antimicrobial therapy.

TREATMENT

THERAPEUTIC GOAL(S)

- Eliminate infection
- Pain management

ACUTE GENERAL TREATMENT

- Antimicrobial therapy
  - Appropriate choices vary with the suspected etiologic agent. Penicillins are the drug of choice for *S. equi,* but many strains are susceptible to cephalosporins or potentiated sulfonamides. *C. pseudotuberculosis* is typically susceptible to most antimicrobials used in horses. In foals, *R. equi* abscesses are best treated with a combination of a macrolide and rifampin.
  - If the specific organism(s) involved is not known, a broad-spectrum antimicrobial with good penetration into tissues is ideal and may include:
    - Chloramphenicol: 35 to 50 mg/kg PO q6–8h.
    - Trimethoprim-sulfamethoxazole (15–30 mg/kg PO q12h) and rifampin (5–10 mg/kg PO q12h).
    - Enrofloxacin: 5 mg/kg IV q24h or 7.5 mg PO q24h.
    - Metronidazole (15–25 mg/kg PO or PR q8h) is indicated if an anaerobic component is suspected.
    - An appropriate duration of antimicrobial therapy is vital. Therapy should be continued until resolution of all clinical, clinicopathologic, and ultrasonographic abnormalities, which may take months with large abscesses.
- Drainage
  - In large abscesses, surgical drainage may be necessary. This occasionally may be accomplished percutaneously if the abscess is adhered to the body wall but is often most safely accomplished via laparotomy or with laparoscopic guidance.
  - Surgical resection of the affected portion of the spleen is not recommended because of difficulty achieving adequate hemostasis.
- Flunixin meglumine (0.5–1.1 mg/kg IV or PO q12h) may be indicated in early therapy for its analgesic and antipyretic effects.

POSSIBLE COMPLICATIONS

Diffuse septic peritonitis secondary to abscess rupture

PROGNOSIS AND OUTCOME

- Fair to good with small or moderately sized abscess and appropriate antimicrobial therapy
- Guarded with large abscesses requiring surgical drainage

AUTHOR: **KELSEY A. HART**

EDITORS: **TIM MAIR** and **CERI SHERLOCK**

PEARLS & CONSIDERATIONS

Splenic abscess, neoplasia, and hematoma may have similar clinical presentations and ultrasonographic appearances.

SUGGESTED READING

Steel CM, Lonsdale RA, Bolton JR: Successful medical treatment of splenic abscesses in a horse. *Aust Vet J* 76(8):541–542, 1998.

Splenic Hematoma

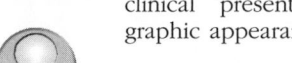

BASIC INFORMATION

DEFINITION
A semisolid mass of blood and blood clots in the splenic parenchyma

SYNONYM(S)
Subcapsular hematoma

EPIDEMIOLOGY
RISK FACTORS
- Abdominal trauma
- Splenic biopsy or accidental splenocentesis during abdominocentesis
- Splenic neoplasia

CLINICAL PRESENTATION
HISTORY, CHIEF COMPLAINT
- Colic (variable)
- ± History of abdominal trauma

PHYSICAL EXAM FINDINGS
- Variable, ranging from within normal limits to signs of hemorrhagic shock, as for hemoperitoneum and splenic rupture (see "Hemoperitoneum" and "Splenic Rupture" in this section).
- Rectal examination: The spleen may be normal, palpably enlarged, irregular, or small and difficult to palpate.

ETIOLOGY AND PATHOPHYSIOLOGY
- External trauma or splenic neoplasia may result in rupture of some splenic vessels and sinusoids, resulting in hemorrhage that remains confined within the splenic capsule.
- A potential complication from splenic biopsy or accidental splenocentesis during attempted abdominocentesis.

DIAGNOSIS

DIFFERENTIAL DIAGNOSIS
- Splenic abscess
- Splenic neoplasia

INITIAL DATABASE
- Packed cell volume (PCV), total solids, complete blood count, and serum biochemistry profile may be within normal limits or consistent with acute hemorrhage (as for hemoperitoneum).

- Coagulation profile should be performed to rule out an underlying coagulopathy.
- Peritoneal fluid analysis
  - Variable. Usually grossly serosanguineous to hemorrhagic, with a PCV ranging from 1% to 2% to levels comparable to peripheral blood if some degree of associated hemoperitoneum is present. Total protein concentrations are also variable but may also be increased from normal levels. May be normal if hemorrhage is entirely confined within the splenic capsule.
  - Fluid obtained via iatrogenic splenocentesis is usually dark red and opaque with a PCV that is substantially higher than peripheral blood (usually 50%–60%).
  - Cytologic evaluation is also variable, ranging from normal to increased numbers of erythrocytes to consistent with frank hemorrhage (if concurrent hemoperitoneum)
- Transabdominal ultrasonography
  - A splenic hematoma appears as a focal, irregular, cavitary mixed echogenic lesion in the splenic parenchyma. Hypoechoic or moderately echogenic fluid may be visible in the cavitary regions of the hematoma.
  - Hematomas may occur in any part of the spleen, but those associated with iatrogenic splenocentesis are found in the cranioventral aspect of the spleen near the location of the attempted abdominocentesis.
  - Splenomegaly, irregular or altered splenic echogenicity, and disruption or irregularity of the splenic contour and capsule are usually apparent with splenic neoplasia. However, the medial side of the spleen usually cannot be adequately visualized, and lesions in this region may be missed. If ultrasonographic findings suggest splenic hematoma is secondary to metastatic or disseminated neoplasia, splenic biopsy can be performed to confirm this.

  - A variable volume of homogeneously echogenic, swirling free peritoneal fluid is usually visible in the ventral abdomen if concurrent hemoperitoneum is present.

TREATMENT

THERAPEUTIC GOAL(S)
- Pain management
- Supportive care and volume replacement (with large hematomas or concurrent hemoperitoneum)

ACUTE GENERAL TREATMENT
- Medical therapy, with IV fluid therapy, whole-blood transfusion, hemostatic support, analgesic therapy, and antimicrobial therapy, as for hemoperitoneum (see "Hemoperitoneum" in this section). Analgesic therapy should be aggressive because significant pain is typically associated with stretching of the splenic capsule.
- If hemorrhage is poorly controlled with medical therapy, splenectomy may be considered.
- Splenectomy is also a potential therapeutic option if splenic hematoma occurs with a focal splenic neoplasia. However, humane euthanasia may be considered with splenic hematoma associated with metastatic neoplasia because of the associated poor long-term prognosis.

POSSIBLE COMPLICATIONS
Splenic rupture

PROGNOSIS AND OUTCOME
- Good with traumatic or iatrogenic splenic hematoma if severe associated hemoperitoneum is absent or quickly resolves
- Guarded to poor with hematoma associated with splenic neoplasia

PEARLS & CONSIDERATIONS

Horses should be monitored closely after accidental splenocentesis for signs associated with splenic hematoma.

SUGGESTED READING

Divers TJ: Hemorrhage into body cavity. In Orsini JA, Divers TJ, editors: *Equine emergencies: treatment and procedures*, ed 3, St Louis, 2008, Saunders Elsevier, pp 253–258.
Ortved K, Witte S, Fleming K, et al: Laparoscopic-assisted splenectomy in a horse with splenomegaly. *Equine Vet Educ* 20(7):357–361, 2008.

AUTHOR: **KELSEY A. HART**

EDITORS: **TIM MAIR** and **CERI SHERLOCK**

Splenic Neoplasia

BASIC INFORMATION

DEFINITION

Neoplasia affecting the spleen

EPIDEMIOLOGY

SPECIES, AGE, SEX

- Uncommon
- More likely in older horses but can occur at any age

CLINICAL PRESENTATION

HISTORY, CHIEF COMPLAINT

- Colic (variable, usually mild, chronic or intermittent)
- Weight loss
- ± Persistent or intermittent pyrexia

PHYSICAL EXAM FINDINGS

- Variable. Poor body condition is usually evident because of systemic effects of neoplasia.
- Rectal examination
  - If the tumor involves the caudal edge of the spleen, it may be palpated as an enlarged irregular region of the caudal aspect of the spleen. If the body or cranial portions of the spleen are involved, the spleen may feel normal on rectal examination.
  - Other tumor masses may be palpable in the case of abdominal metastases (depending on the location of the masses within the abdomen).

ETIOLOGY AND PATHOPHYSIOLOGY

- Splenic neoplasia is usually secondary. Metastatic spread to the spleen from other sites because of the rich vascular supply. Common metastatic neoplasms involving the spleen include Sertoli cell tumor and melanoma.
- Primary splenic tumors are extremely rare. Hemangiosarcoma may occur in the spleen as a primary site.
- Lymphoma (lymphosarcoma) may involve the spleen (usually multicentric but occasionally confined to the spleen initially).
- Amyloid deposition may occur within the spleen secondary to systemic neoplasia (eg, multiple myeloma).

DIAGNOSIS

DIFFERENTIAL DIAGNOSIS

- Splenic hematoma
- Splenic abscess
- Splenomegaly
- Abdominal neoplasia

INITIAL DATABASE

- Complete blood count and serum chemistry profile
  - Usually reveal evidence of chronic inflammation, with mild anemia, leukocytosis characterized by a mature neutrophilia, hyperfibrinogenemia, or hyperglobulinemia
  - In cases of lymphoma, occasionally abnormal (malignant lymphocytes may be present in the peripheral blood)
  - Hypercalcemia of malignancy (pseudohyperparathyroidism) may occur in some cases of neoplasia
- Transabdominal ultrasonography
  - A splenic tumor appears as a focal lesion of abnormal echogenicity (increased or decreased) in any part of the splenic parenchyma. This may be difficult to distinguish from splenic abscess and splenic hematoma.
  - Multiple focal areas of abnormal echogenicity are suggestive of metastatic spread of tumor to the spleen.
  - Percutaneous, ultrasound-guided needle biopsy of a suspected splenic tumor may be attempted to obtain samples for histopathologic examination.
- Peritoneal fluid analysis
  - May be normal, although mildly increased nucleated cell counts (5000–20,000 cells/μL) or total protein concentration (>2 g/dL) consistent with low-grade peritonitis are often noted. Rarely, neoplastic cells may exfoliate into the peritoneal fluid
  - Hemoabdomen may occur with some splenic tumors, especially hemangiosarcoma.

ADVANCED OR CONFIRMATORY TESTING

- Definitive confirmation of splenic neoplasia requires visualization and sampling via laparoscopy or laparotomy.
- Biopsy of a splenic mass may be undertaken at exploratory surgery.
- Evaluation of the rest of the abdomen for metastatic tumor should be undertaken.

TREATMENT

THERAPEUTIC GOAL(S)

- Symptomatic therapy is usually all that is possible.
- Pain management
- Chemotherapy for treatment of lymphoma may be attempted in some cases.
- If the neoplasia is confined to the spleen with no evidence of metastatic or multicentric tumor elsewhere, surgical splenectomy may be curative.

ACUTE GENERAL TREATMENT

Flunixin meglumine (0.5–1.1 mg/kg IV or PO q12h) may be indicated in early therapy for its analgesic and antipyretic effects.

POSSIBLE COMPLICATIONS

Metastatic spread of neoplasm to other sites

PROGNOSIS AND OUTCOME

Poor in most cases

PEARLS & CONSIDERATIONS

Splenic neoplasia, abscess, and hematoma may have similar clinical presentations and ultrasonographic appearances.

SUGGESTED READING

Chaffin, MK, Schmitz DG, Brumbaugh GW, et al: Ultrasonographic characteristics of splenic and hepatic lymphosarcoma in three horses. *J Am Vet Med Assoc* 201:743, 1992.

Kim DY, Taylor HW, Eades SC, Cho DY: Systemic amyloidosis associated with multiple myeloma in a horse. *Vet Pathol* 42:81–84, 2005.

MacGillivary KC, Sweeney RW, Del Piero F: Metastatic melanoma in horses. *J Vet Intern Med* 16:452–456, 2002.

Pratt SM, Stacey BA, Whitcomb MB, et al: Malignant Sertoli cell tumor in the retained abdominal testis of a unilateral cryptorchid horse. *J Am Vet Med Assoc* 222:486, 2003.

Southwood LL, Schott HC 2nd, Henry CJ, et al: Disseminated hemangiosarcoma in the horse: 35 cases. *J Vet Intern Med* 14:105–109, 2000.

AUTHOR: **TIM MAIR**

EDITORS: **TIM MAIR** and **CERI SHERLOCK**

Splenic Rupture

BASIC INFORMATION

DEFINITION

Full-thickness disruption of the splenic parenchyma and capsule

EPIDEMIOLOGY

RISK FACTORS

- Abdominal trauma
- Splenic neoplasia
- Splenomegaly

CLINICAL PRESENTATION

HISTORY, CHIEF COMPLAINT

- Colic (often severe)
- Sweating
- Trembling or muscle fasciculations
- ± Evidence of abdominal trauma

PHYSICAL EXAM FINDINGS

- Clinical signs related to hypovolemia and hemorrhagic shock (as for hemoperitoneum):
  - Tachycardia (often marked)
  - Tachypnea
  - Weak peripheral pulses, cool extremities, and poor jugular refill
  - Pale mucous membranes, prolonged capillary refill time
  - Weakness
  - ± Altered mentation (depression is typical, but violent behavior or severe colic may be seen)
- Rectal examination: The spleen may be normal, palpably enlarged, irregular, or small and difficult to palpate.

ETIOLOGY AND PATHOPHYSIOLOGY

- External trauma, splenomegaly, or splenic neoplasia may result in disruption of the splenic parenchyma and capsule.
- Splenic rupture may also be a complication from an initial splenic hematoma if hemorrhage within the hematoma can not be controlled.

DIAGNOSIS

DIFFERENTIAL DIAGNOSIS

Other causes of hemoperitoneum

INITIAL DATABASE

- Packed cell volume (PCV) and total solids (TS)
  - May be normal in acute stages. A disproportionate decrease in TS concentration is often noted before the PCV decreases significantly.
  - Within 6 to 24 hours of initial hemorrhage, decreased PCV and TS concentration are typically observed.
- Complete blood count
  - Variable hematocrit, as for PCV above.
  - Leukogram is usually normal or consistent with a stress leukogram.
  - Platelet count is usually within reference intervals unless a concurrent coagulopathy (disseminated intravascular coagulation, immune-mediated thrombocytopenia) is present.
- Serum biochemistry profile and blood gas analysis
  - Hypocalcemia is frequently present because of loss of albumin-bound calcium. Ionized calcium may be normal or low.
  - Hypoproteinemia or hypoalbuminemia is usually present.
  - Variable azotemia (prerenal, renal, or both) is often present and is reflective of poor renal perfusion caused by hypovolemia.
  - Hyperlactatemia (>2 mmol/L) or low venous oxygen (PvO_2 <30 mm Hg or SvO_2 <50%) in an anaerobically collected sample indicates significantly decreased oxygen-carrying capacity with associated hemorrhage.
- Coagulation profile should be performed to rule out an underlying coagulopathy.
- Transabdominal ultrasonography
  - A moderate to significant volume of homogeneously echogenic, swirling free peritoneal fluid in the ventral abdomen, as for hemoperitoneum (see "Hemoperitoneum" in this section).
  - With traumatic splenic rupture, the spleen may appear small or seem to be located in an abnormal location within the abdomen, and splenic fragmentation or disruption of the splenic capsule is usually apparent.
  - Splenic hematoma (see "Splenic Hematoma" in this section), splenic neoplasia, or splenomegaly may also be apparent ultrasonographically.
  - Ultrasound-guided splenic biopsy is indicated if splenic neoplasia is suspected.
- Peritoneal fluid analysis
  - Peritoneal fluid is usually grossly hemorrhagic in appearance, with a PCV and TS concentration similar to the peripheral blood.
  - Cytologic evaluation of the peritoneal fluid may reveal platelets in acute or ongoing hemorrhage or hemosiderophages or erythrophagocytosis with previous or chronic hemorrhage (>6–12 hours' duration).

TREATMENT

THERAPEUTIC GOAL(S)

- Pain management
- Supportive care and volume replacement (with large hematomas or concurrent hemoperitoneum)

ACUTE GENERAL TREATMENT

- Medical therapy, with IV fluid therapy, whole-blood transfusion, hemostatic support, analgesic therapy, and antimicrobial therapy, as for hemoperitoneum (see "Hemoperitoneum" in this section).
- If hemorrhage is poorly controlled with medical therapy, splenectomy is a viable although technically challenging therapeutic option.

POSSIBLE COMPLICATIONS

Increased susceptibility to certain infections is reported after splenectomy in other species but has not been described in horses (perhaps because of the rarity of this procedure in horses).

PROGNOSIS AND OUTCOME

Guarded

PEARLS & CONSIDERATIONS

Because of the rarity of splenic rupture, acceptable prognosis of most causes of hemoperitoneum with medical management, and technically challenging nature of the splenectomy procedure in horses, splenic rupture should be confirmed or highly suspected before recommendation of splenectomy.

SUGGESTED READING

Divers TJ: Hemorrhage into body cavity. In Orsini JA, Divers TJ, editors: *Equine emergencies: treatment and procedures*, ed 3, St Louis, 2008, Saunders Elsevier, pp 253–258.

Ortved K, Witte S, Fleming K, et al: Laparoscopic-assisted splenectomy in a horse with splenomegaly. *Equine Vet Educ* 20(7):357–361, 2008.

AUTHOR: **KELSEY A. HART**

EDITORS: **TIM MAIR** and **CERI SHERLOCK**

Splenomegaly

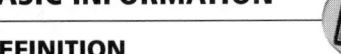

BASIC INFORMATION

DEFINITION

Generalized enlargement of the spleen

CLINICAL PRESENTATION

HISTORY, CHIEF COMPLAINT
- Mild, intermittent colic
- Inappetence
- Lethargy
- ± Weight loss

PHYSICAL EXAM FINDINGS
- Variable
  - Usually no abnormalities if idiopathic splenomegaly.
  - Fever, depression, or poor body condition may be noted if splenomegaly is secondary to splenic neoplasia or other systemic illness.
  - Pale or icteric mucous membranes, tachycardia, tachypnea, and other signs related to anemia may be present if splenomegaly is secondary to immune-mediated hemolytic anemia or equine infectious anemia.
- Rectal examination: The spleen is usually easily palpated in the left caudal abdomen and may appear to extend caudally or medially to an abnormal degree. The splenic contour usually appears rounded, and the surface may be irregular.

ETIOLOGY AND PATHOPHYSIOLOGY
- Splenomegaly may result from
  - Infiltration of the spleen with neoplastic tissue (eg, lymphosarcoma, hemangiosarcoma, melanoma)
  - Acute expansion of the splenic parenchyma with splenic hematoma or edema and inflammation secondary to splenic infarction
  - Splenic congestion and hypertrophy associated with activation of the reticuloendothelial system in infection or immune mediated disease
  - Hypertrophy caused by extramedullary hematopoiesis in chronic anemia
- Rickettsial and viral diseases are commonly associated with splenomegaly in other species, although this is not frequently observed in horses. Diseases that may result in splenomegaly in horses include:
  - Equine infectious anemia (EIA)
  - Babesiosis or theileriosis
  - *Anaplasma phagocytophilia* infection (formerly equine ehrlichiosis)
  - *Borrelia burgdorferi* infection (Lyme disease)
- Idiopathic splenomegaly caused by congestion and hypertrophy has been described as a cause of recurrent colic in two horses.
- Regardless of the cause of splenomegaly, stretching of the splenic capsule is likely the primary cause of the associated abdominal pain.

DIAGNOSIS

INITIAL DATABASE
- Complete blood count and serum biochemistry profile
  - Within reference intervals in idiopathic splenomegaly
  - Variable with splenic neoplasia; may be normal or may have evidence of chronic inflammation
  - Anemia, thrombocytopenia, or alterations in the leukogram may be present with immune-mediated disease or systemic infection
- Transabdominal ultrasonography
  - The spleen is usually visible in the left flank, extending cranially from the paralumbar fossa to approximately the tenth to thirteenth intercostal space and ventrally into the left inguinal region. Extension of the spleen to the right ventral abdomen and rounding of the splenic contour are suggestive of splenomegaly.
  - Multifocal or diffusely increased or decreased splenic echogenicity is usually appreciated in splenic neoplasia.
- Peritoneal fluid analysis: Variable; usually normal but may reveal neoplastic cells

ADVANCED OR CONFIRMATORY TESTING
- Splenic biopsy
  - Should be performed to differentiate idiopathic splenomegaly from splenic neoplasia
  - May be performed percutaneously using ultrasound guidance. Alternatively, larger surgical biopsies or biopsies of specific lesions may be obtained laparoscopically or via laparotomy.
- Serologic testing for EIA, *A. phagocytophilia*, *B. burgdorferi*, and babesiosis should be performed to rule out these possible causes of splenomegaly.
- If immune-mediated anemia or thrombocytopenia is suspected, assessment for antierythrocyte or antiplatelet antibodies should be performed.

TREATMENT

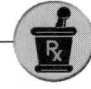

THERAPEUTIC GOAL(S)
- Pain management
- Elimination of primary cause
- Splenectomy for idiopathic splenomegaly

ACUTE GENERAL TREATMENT
- Acute treatment for colic presumed to be associated with splenomegaly should include analgesic therapy with flunixin meglumine (1.1 mg/kg IV

q12h) to alleviate pain associated with stretching of the splenic capsule. If this is ineffective in alleviating pain, more aggressive analgesic therapy with lidocaine infusions (1.3 mg/kg IV slow bolus; then 0.05 mg/kg/min IV constant rate infusion) or opioids may be warranted.

- If splenomegaly is associated with rickettsial disease, appropriate antimicrobial therapy with oxytetracycline (6.6 mg/kg IV diluted q12h) or doxycycline (10 mg/kg PO q12h) may be effective.
- Immunosuppressive therapy with corticosteroids (dexamethasone 0.05–0.1 mg/kg IV or IM q24h or prednisolone 1 mg/kg PO q24h) or azathioprine (2–3 mg/kg PO q24–48h) is indicated in splenomegaly secondary to immune-mediated anemia or thrombocytopenia.
- If lymphosarcoma is confirmed by splenic biopsy, dexamethasone (0.05–0.1 mg/kg IV or IM q24h) or prednisolone (1 mg/kg PO q24h) may also result in transient clinical improvement.
- Splenectomy is reportedly effective in alleviation of colic signs associated with idiopathic splenomegaly. However, the size and depth of the equine abdomen render this a much more challenging procedure than in humans or small animals.

POSSIBLE COMPLICATIONS

- Splenic rupture
- Increased susceptibility to certain infections is reported after splenectomy in other species but has not been described in horses (perhaps because of the rarity of this procedure in horses).

PROGNOSIS AND OUTCOME

Guarded

PEARLS & CONSIDERATIONS

- Splenic size can vary greatly in horses because of stress and hemodynamic related changes, so documentation of persistent splenic enlargement with serial ultrasonography is needed to support a conclusive diagnosis of primary splenomegaly.
- In addition, because of the rarity of this condition, thorough workup to exclude other causes of mild recurrent colic should be performed before making a diagnosis of colic caused by primary splenomegaly.

SUGGESTED READING

Ortved K, Witte S, Fleming K, et al: Laparoscopic-assisted splenectomy in a horse with splenomegaly. *Equine Vet Educ* 20(7):357–361, 2008.

AUTHOR: **KELSEY A. HART**

EDITORS: **TIM MAIR** and **CERI SHERLOCK**

Sporotrichosis

BASIC INFORMATION

DEFINITION
Chronic, slowly invasive subcutaneous mycosis caused by the yeast form *Sporothrix schenckii*. The disease generally manifests as cutaneolymphatic pyogranulomatous inflammation.

EPIDEMIOLOGY
RISK FACTORS
- Wound contaminated with soil and organic debris.
- Immunosuppression (eg, corticosteroids administration) is likely to increase the risk of disease development, progression, and/or recurrence.

CONTAGION AND ZOONOSIS
Although zoonotic potential exists, there are no reports of transmission from an infected horse, presumably because tissues from infected horses have fewer numbers of organisms compared with tissues from infected cats.

ASSOCIATED CONDITIONS AND DISORDERS
- Sporadic infection affecting a number of susceptible hosts, including horses, mules, cattle, dogs, cats, rats, mice, domestic fowl, and humans.
- Similar to horses, the most common form of sporotrichosis in humans is cutaneolymphatic.

- In dogs, the most common forms are cutaneous and cutaneolymphatic; in cats, the disseminated form occurs in addition to the other two.

CLINICAL PRESENTATION
DISEASE FORMS/SUBTYPES
- Cutaneolymphatic form: Most common form in horses
- Cutaneous form: Less common
- Visceral or disseminated form: Extremely rare in horses

HISTORY, CHIEF COMPLAINT
- Insidious onset
- Puncture wound (often lower limb) that may have gone unnoticed
- Development of limb edema associated with nodular and ulcerated cutaneous lesions

PHYSICAL EXAM FINDINGS
- Primary lesions include alopecic nodules and plaques that ulcerate.
- Satellite lesions develop near the primary site.
- The infection spreads via lymphatic vessels, which become thickened, with formation of nodules and punctate ulcers along the lymphatics; pus (resembling rust) often drains from the ulcerated nodules.
- Regional lymph nodes rarely become enlarged or ulcerated.
- The primary cutaneous form, with no lymphatic involvement, is a much less common presentation.

ETIOLOGY AND PATHOPHYSIOLOGY
- *Sporothrix schenckii* is an ubiquitous dimorphic fungi.
  - Mycelial form found naturally in soil, decaying vegetation, sphagnum moss, and tree bark
  - Yeast form in tissues
- Infection is acquired from wound contamination with soil and organic debris from puncture by plant thorns or wood splinters.
- The mycelial form is inoculated into tissues. The fungus changes to the yeast form and slowly proliferates, extending along the lymphatic vessels and causing them to become thick and corded.
- Multiplication of the organism is associated with pyogranulomatous inflammation (although organisms are rarely seen inside neutrophils and macrophages in exudates of horses), leading to the formation of nodules associated with enlargement of lymphatic vessels. Nodules become ulcerated, resulting in a small amount of drainage of thick, red-brown to yellowish exudates or serosanguinous fluid.
- Most lesions develop on distal extremities and rarely affect the upper parts of the body, such as upper forelimb, chest, shoulder, hip, and perineum.
- Infection rarely spreads to regional lymph nodes.

- Dissemination through lymphatics into other organs is extremely rare in horses.

DIAGNOSIS

DIFFERENTIAL DIAGNOSIS

- Ulcerative lymphangitis caused by *Corynebacterium pseudotuberculosis*
- Sporadic bacterial lymphangitis/cellulitis caused by *Streptococcus* spp., *Staphylococcus* spp., *Pseudomonas aeruginosa, Rhodococcus equi*
- Other causes: Foreign body, trauma, insect/arthropod bite
- Cutaneous glanders by *Burkholderia (Pseudomonas) mallei* (exotic to United States; reportable)
- Epizootic lymphangitis by *Histoplasma farciminosum* (exotic to United States; reportable)
- Pythiosis: *Pythium insidiosum* (ulcerated granuloma)
- Cutaneous habronemiasis (ulcerated granuloma)
- Neoplasia: Sarcoid, squamous cell carcinoma (ulcerated granuloma)

INITIAL DATABASE

- No consistent abnormal findings on complete blood count or serum biochemistry are reported.
- Cytologic evaluation of exudates reveals pyogranulomatous inflammation; the organism is unlikely to be seen in exudates from horses.

ADVANCED OR CONFIRMATORY TESTING

Demonstration of the organism by:
- Fungal culture of macerated tissue samples or exudate (best tissue specimens are from biopsy rather than exudate)
- Histopathologic evaluation of biopsy specimen
  - Diffuse to nodular pyogranulomatous dermatitis, multinucleated giant cells are common; fungal elements are nearly impossible to find.
  - Direct fluorescent antibody test aids in the identification of fungal forms.

TREATMENT

THERAPEUTIC GOAL(S)

Clear the fungal infection and ensure regression of lesion(s)

ACUTE AND CHRONIC GENERAL TREATMENT

- Iodides are effective and not too expensive; iodide should be administered daily for at least 1 month after complete regression of lesions.
  - Organic iodides: More efficacious than inorganic iodides

- Ethylene diamine dihydroiodide (EDDI) administered as a feed additive at a dosage of 20 to 40 mg of the powdered form per kilogram of body weight (which corresponds to 1–2 mg of active ingredient per kilogram) q12–24h; this dose may be reduced to half after the first week.
  - Inorganic iodides
    - Sodium iodide:
      □ Dosage of 20 to 44 mg/kg/day as 20% IV solution given slowly for 2 to 10 days, then orally at the same daily dose for the remainder of the treatment
      □ Dosage of 20 to 40 mg/kg/day as 20% IV solution given intravenously slowly for 7 to 10 days
      □ Dosage of 67 mg/kg as 20% IV solution given intravenously slowly twice weekly
    - Potassium iodide: Dose of 20 to 40 mg of the powdered form per kilogram of body weight per day orally (mixed with molasses and given by syringe or given with a small amount of feed or grain)
  - Anecdotal reports of signs of iodism occurring during the first several days as the body adjusts to the medication have prompted some clinicians to initiate therapy with inorganic iodides at a lower dosage for the first few days and then increase to the recommended dosage.
- The affected limb can be cleaned with povidone-iodine and hydrotherapy applied.
- Treatment with itraconazole is an alternative in cases refractory to iodides, pregnancy, or relapse after apparent cure.
  - Treatment should be administered q24h for at least 1 month after complete regression of lesions; overall poor bioavailability (requires acid pH for dissolution; therefore absorption is highly variable).
  - Oral solution licensed for use in humans has a higher and less variable solubility than capsules.
  - Dosage for horses 5 mg/kg PO q24h.

DRUG INTERACTIONS

Itraconazole inhibits P-450 enzymes; thus there are multiple drug-drug interactions.

POSSIBLE COMPLICATIONS

- Premature discontinuation of therapy leading to relapse
- Signs of iodism can develop
  - Lacrimation, salivation, scaling and alopecia, coughing, serous discharge, anorexia, depression, fever,

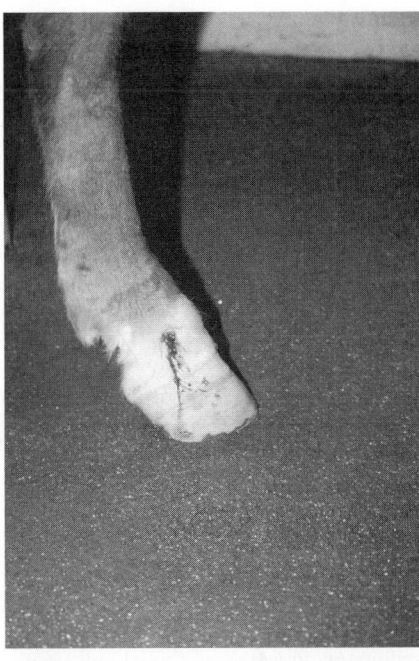

FIGURE 1 Quarter Horse filly with sporotrichosis. Note the limb edema (associated with lymphangitis) and skin nodules, one of which is ulcerated and draining an exudate resembling rust. (Courtesy Dr. M.R. Paradis.)

nervousness, cardiovascular abnormalities, and abortion
- If iodism develops, treatment should be discontinued for 7 days, then reinstituted at a lower dose (eg, three quarters of the dosage at which iodism was noted)

RECOMMENDED MONITORING

- Revaluate every 2 to 3 weeks for clinical signs and side effects associated with treatment.
- If itraconazole is used, monitoring of liver enzymes is recommended (although no adverse effects have been reported in horses).
  - Baseline biochemical profile should be performed to evaluate liver enzymes before administration of itraconazole.

PROGNOSIS AND OUTCOME

Prognosis is fair to good.

PEARLS & CONSIDERATIONS

COMMENTS

- Corticosteroids and other immunosuppressive drugs are contraindicated during and after apparent clinical cure.

○ Corticosteroids can result in relapse of clinical sporotrichosis as long as 4 to 6 months after apparent clinical resolution.
- Considering the zoonotic potential, precautions must be taken when handling horses or samples from horses suspected of sporotrichosis.
  ○ Use gloves, thoroughly clean hands, wrists, and arms with chlorhexidine or povidone-iodide.

CLIENT EDUCATION

Emphasize the zoonotic potential of sporotrichosis and ensure that precautions are taken when handling a horse and suspected samples.

SUGGESTED READING

Scott DW, Miller WH Jr: Fungal skin diseases: subcutaneous mycosis, sporotrichosis. In Scott DW, Miller WH Jr, editors: *Equine dermatology*, St. Louis, 2003, Saunders Elsevier, pp 296–298.

Scott DW, Miller WH Jr: Antifungal therapy. In Scott DW, Miller WH Jr, editors: *Equine dermatology*, St. Louis, 2003, Saunders Elsevier, pp 306–313.

White SD: Diseases of the skin: fungal diseases. In Smith BP, editor: *Large animal internal medicine*, ed 4, St Louis, 2009, Mosby Elsevier, pp 1319–1320.

AUTHOR: **LAIS R. R. COSTA**

Squamous Cell Carcinoma

BASIC INFORMATION

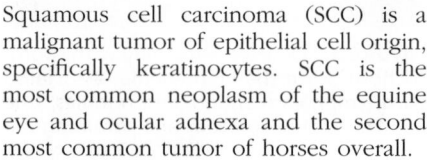

DEFINITION

Squamous cell carcinoma (SCC) is a malignant tumor of epithelial cell origin, specifically keratinocytes. SCC is the most common neoplasm of the equine eye and ocular adnexa and the second most common tumor of horses overall.

EPIDEMIOLOGY

SPECIES, AGE, SEX

- The mean age at diagnosis is approximately 11 years, but a range of 3 to 26 years is reported.
- The gender predisposition of SCC is not well understood. Geldings have been overrepresented in selected studies. However, this finding may simply reflect gender distribution of the general client-owned equine population.

GENETICS/BREED PREDISPOSITION/ RISK FACTORS

- An increased prevalence of SCC is associated with various environmental factors, including geographic influences of increased longitude, decreased latitude, increased altitude, and increased mean annual solar radiation exposure.
- A breed predilection exists for Draft horses, Appaloosas, and Paint horses.

CONTAGION AND ZOONOSIS SCC is not believed to be contagious. There has been one case report of penile SCC identified bovine papillomavirus within SCC tumor nuclei. Current studies are investigating a viral cause in ocular SCC.

GEOGRAPHY AND SEASONALITY Irritation from actinic or ultraviolet (UV) radiation has been thought to promote the development of SCC. Clinically, horses living at higher elevations with increased sunlight exposure have a higher incidence of SCC.

ASSOCIATED CONDITIONS AND DISORDERS Any chronic irritation may promote neoplastic transformation of epithelium into SCC, especially at mucocutaneous junctions (see Etiology and Pathophysiology below).

CLINICAL PRESENTATION

SCC frequently affects the skin, external genitalia (eg, penis; most commonly the glans penis followed by the urethra), nasal and paranasal sinus (especially the caudal maxillary sinus), and eye and periocular areas. Case reports or small case series exist of SCC in many sites such as the hoof wall, thyroid gland, and stomach. Ophthalmic presentations of SCC vary and may involve the corneoconjunctiva, bulbar conjunctiva, third eyelid, and eyelids. The biologic behavior of ocular SCC is reported to differ depending on the location, with the prognosis for eyelid SCC worse compared with other sites of the eye.

HISTORY, CHIEF COMPLAINT

- Suspect SCC with any erosive, erythematous, or raised mass
- Hematospermia for tumors of the glans penis
- Signs referable to paraneoplastic syndromes
  ○ Hypercalcemia of malignancy (often described as pseudohyperparathyroidism)
  ○ Hypertrophic osteopathy (a painful condition of the long bones) has been reported with primary and metastatic pulmonary SCC.
- Signs referable to the location of the tumor
  ○ Tumors of the nasal or paranasal sinuses: Unilateral purulent or mucopurulent nasal discharge with or without epistaxis
  ○ Tumors of external genitalia or bladder: Hematuria, dysuria, urine retention with possible bladder rupture, and reproductive dysfunction
  ○ Tumors of the esophagus or stomach: Weight loss, dysphagia, anorexia, anemia (normochromic and normocytic), neutrophilia, carcinomatosis with peritoneal effusion, high metastatic rate
  ○ Disseminated thoracic SCC: Exercise intolerance, increased respiratory rate and effort at rest, pleural effusion, poor performance, weight loss, inappetence
  ○ Periocular or ocular SCC: Mucopurulent discharge, blepharospasm, tan to reddish raised nodular mass, or erosive plaques

PHYSICAL EXAM FINDINGS Regardless of the location, the most common physical examination finding is a hairless, friable, proliferative mass lesion. Regional lymphadenopathy may be detected in 15% of cases or fewer. Masses often bleed easily with manipulation.

ETIOLOGY AND PATHOPHYSIOLOGY

- SCC has been reported to develop in chronic wounds, at burn sites, and at sites of epithelial scarring (ie, locations consistent with chronic inflammation and prolonged wound healing).
- UV light exposure (with accompanying solar elastosis)
- Overexpression of the tumor suppressor protein p53, possibly mutated because of UV radiation, plays an important role in SCC development in many animals. In two separate studies, 100% of equine ocular SCCs overexpressed p53.
- Cyclooxygenase (COX) enzyme overexpression
  ○ High levels of COX-2 expression have been detected in many human and veterinary neoplasms, including SCC of the head and neck.
  ○ Correlations have been made in humans with head and neck SCC between overexpression of COX-2 in neoplastic tissues and poor prognostic factors.
  ○ A limited number of investigations specifically examining the role of COX in naturally occurring equine ocular and periocular SCC have been conducted to date, and the role of COX expression in the

etiopathogenesis of SCC is as yet undetermined.

DIAGNOSIS

DIFFERENTIAL DIAGNOSIS

- Other tumors (papilloma, melanoma, mastocytoma, basal cell carcinoma, schwannoma, adenoma and adenocarcinoma, hemangioma and hemangiosarcoma, lymphoma and lymphosarcoma), inflammatory lesions (abscesses, granulation tissue, foreign body reaction, solar-induced inflammation, dermatitis, eosinophilic dermatitis, and botryomycosis)
- Affected nasal and paranasal cavities should have other primary tumors (sarcomas), as well as non-neoplastic processes such as maxillary (sinus) cysts, progressive ethmoid hematoma, and inflammatory polyps ruled out.
- Additional differentials to be considered when presented with ocular SCC include other causes of conjunctivitis (lymphoid hyperplasia and follicular conjunctivitis) and parasitic infections (Habronema, onchocerca, Thelazia).

INITIAL DATABASE

- Biopsy of the affected tissue typically confirms a diagnosis and distinguishes SCC from other differential diagnoses. Incisional biopsy should be performed before definitive surgical excision to allow proper surgical planning (wider surgical margins must be attempted with malignant disease as opposed to benign conditions).
- Periocular SCC may be challenging to surgically resect because of the need to maintain near normal eyelid function for globe preservation and the lack of mobile facial equine skin, rendering skin flaps nearly impossible to perform in this species.
- When attempting to diagnose carcinomatosis on cytologic evaluation of peritoneal fluid, sensitivity is low (~50%).
- Thoracic radiographs to detect pulmonary metastasis are typically low yield.

ADVANCED OR CONFIRMATORY TESTING

An assessment of the degree of differentiation and mitotic activity should accompany histology reports because tumors with more mitoses and less differentiation warrant a poorer prognosis.

TREATMENT

THERAPEUTIC GOAL(S)

- Local control via surgery with or without adjuvant therapy such as chemotherapy or radiation therapy in various forms is common. Outcome varies among studies and primary tumor site.
- For SCC of the penis, partial or complete penile amputation and sheath ablation may be required, but the outcome after this procedure is generally good with few long-term complications.

ACUTE GENERAL TREATMENT

- Surgical excision (via sharp dissection or sometimes carbon dioxide laser) is considered the treatment of choice whenever possible.
- Adjunctive therapy is recommended for SCC in locations that are not amenable to complete surgical resection (eg, periocular or cornealconjunctival SCC).
  - Radiation therapy
    - Interstitial brachytherapy (using radioactive implants such as gold-198, iridium-192, iodine-125, or radon-222)
    - Plesiotherapy with strontium-90
    - External-beam radiation therapy (cobalt-60 or linear accelerator) for nasal or paranasal sinus tumors
  - Chemotherapy: Intralesional cisplatin, bleomycin, 5-fluorouracil (5-FU), or topical 5-FU or mitomycin C
- Immunotherapy: Topical imiquimod or intralesional bacillus of Calmette-Guérin
- Radiofrequency hyperthermia
- COX inhibition with piroxicam (80 mg/d PO for an average-sized horse)
- Cryotherapy with nitrous oxide or liquid nitrogen: Local photodynamic therapy
- Depot cisplatin therapy
  - Injected in an oily emulsion
    - 10 mg of cisplatin (lyophilized Platinol) mixed for 1 minute with 1 mL of sterile water and 2 mL of sterile medical-grade sesame oil (creates a viscous, yellow liquid)
    - Target dose of 1 mg/cm^3 every 2 weeks for four treatments
  - Suspended in a mixture of bovine collagen and epinephrine
  - Biodegradable beads
- Topical imiquimod 5% cream used three times weekly for up to 32 weeks as an immune response modifier has been reported to have good efficacy when treating sarcoids (60% complete resolution) and has been anecdotally effective for use with equine SCC.
- SCC arising from the globe or periocular tissue carries a more favorable prognosis when adjunctive therapy is used in conjunction with surgical debulking. Various therapies have been applied (as listed previously).

CHRONIC TREATMENT

- Chronic treatment (beyond an initial surgery or prescribed course of therapy) typically consists either of continued topical 5-FU or imiquimod, or salvage therapy for refractory or relapsed tumors.
- Because there is no single best therapy for SCC, salvage therapy often involves attempting an untried therapy or may necessitate enucleation or exenteration.

DRUG INTERACTIONS

Radioactive gold (gold-198) has been used as an interstitial implant alone and in combination with hyperthermia. There are synergistic effects with this combination because each works best in a different phase of the cell cycle. Radiation affects G2- and M-phase cell cycles, and hyperthermia is most effective in the S phase when cells are radioresistant.

POSSIBLE COMPLICATIONS

Swelling and discharge frequently occur at operated sites. Of importance, if cisplatin treatment has been given, the discharge may contain chemotherapy hazardous to owners and caregivers.

RECOMMENDED MONITORING

Ideally, tumor site(s) should be monitored closely (every 1–3 weeks) to ensure adequate regression, then every month for 3 months, then every 2 to 3 months for the first year, and every 6 months thereafter. Note that exuberant granulation tissue can appear shortly after surgical resection and ancillary therapy, which can appear as tumor regrowth. When in doubt, additional biopsy is recommended.

PROGNOSIS AND OUTCOME

- The long-term outcome for cutaneous tumors can be very good when adequate local control is achieved with 60% to 80% of horses disease-free at time points longer than 2 years. SCC arising in areas difficult to completely excise (eg, larynx, pharynx) carries a more guarded long-term prognosis.
- Surgical excision of penile SCC is generally well tolerated and is effective as a sole treatment option in 55% of cases.
  - Favorable location and smaller size indicate the best surgical candidates.
  - Recurrence is higher (25%) with partial phallectomy, incomplete excision, and in cases with metastasis to regional lymph nodes at the time of surgery. Metastasis is more

common in poorly differentiated tumors.

○ The prognosis for urethral SCC is more guarded than the prognosis for SCC of the glans penis.

- Intralesional cisplatin in oily emulsion
  ○ Perioperative: 92% of horses are disease free at 1 year; the mean relapse-free interval is 3.5 years.
  ○ Perioperative treatment may be superior to postoperative injection, especially in highly proliferative tumors.
  ○ Cisplatin is considered as effective as intratumoral bleomycin and is less expensive.
  ○ Intralesional cisplatin is less effective in cases with measureable disease after surgery, large tumors, and those that had received multiple treatments before cisplatin.
- External-beam radiation therapy (with most reports using cobalt-60 sources) has been used for nasal and paranasal sinus SCC with good results, but the cost and difficulty of repeated general anesthetic episodes and radiation facility availability limit this treatment option.
- Recurrence rates for periocular SCC within 1 year of treatment
  ○ Between 50% to 66.7% with surgery alone, ranging from 25% to 67% with surgery and ancillary irradiation or cryotherapy.
  ○ A 42.4% recurrence rate for ocular SCC with surgical excision, radiofrequency hyperthermia, or both has also been reported.
  ○ In another study, treatments included surgical excision, surgical excision with 90Sr β-irradiation, surgical excision with cryotherapy, surgical excision with radiofrequency, surgical excision with 137Cs interstitial radiotherapy, and/or immunotherapy, and the overall recurrence rate was 30.4%.
  ○ A poorer prognosis is associated with SCC originating at the eyelid

compared with the third eyelid, nasal canthus, or limbus. Larger sized masses, orbital extension, and recurrent SCC are associated with lower survival times.

○ Metastasis of ocular SCC is uncommon and has been reported in isolated case reports or small case series. Metastasis occurs most commonly to the regional (submandibular) lymph nodes, salivary glands, or thorax or extension into the orbit, sinus, and calvarium.

○ Local invasion of the tumor often accompanies ulcerative necrosis and inflammation, resulting in significant ocular discomfort. No single treatment modality has proven to be 100% effective in a large number of cases, and either the SCC itself or treatment complications may threaten both visual outcome and long-term survival.

PEARLS & CONSIDERATIONS

COMMENTS

In general, as is true for most treatment modalities, smaller tumors are treated more successfully and with lower recurrence rates.

PREVENTION

Minimizing sun exposure may abrogate risk. Eyelid tattooing has been proposed as a preventive measure to decrease the risk of eyelid SCC but is not advocated by these authors.

CLIENT EDUCATION

- Both chemotherapy and radiation therapy are effective adjunctive treatments, but both expose the user and equine owner or handler to risk of toxic exposure. Radiation therapy requires specific training, equipment, and licensing.

- Chemotherapy is currently the most cost-effective adjunctive therapy for equine SCC but may expose the user or handler to carcinogenic compounds.
- For these reasons, local photodynamic therapy has shown promise as a useful adjunctive therapy in the treatment of periocular SCC and may prove useful in other primary neoplastic locations. Presently, local photodynamic therapy has not been used for SCC affecting the cornea conjunctiva because of the risk of uveitis or keratomalacia.

SUGGESTED READING

Fortier LA, MacHarg MA: Topical use of 5-fluorouracil for treatment of squamous cell carcinoma of the external genitalia of horses: 11 cases (1988–1992). *J Am Vet Med Assoc* 205:1183–1185, 1994.

Giuliano EA: Equine periocular neoplasia: current concepts in aetiopathogenesis and emerging treatment modalities. *Equine Vet J* 3(suppl), 37:9–18, 2010.

Giuliano EA, Ota J, Tucker SA: Photodynamic therapy: basic principles and potential uses for the veterinary ophthalmologist. *Vet Ophthalmol* 10(6):337–343, 2007.

Hendrix DVH: Equine ocular squamous cell carcinoma. *Clin Tech Equine Pract* 4(1):87–94, 2005.

Hewes CA, Sullins KE: Use of cisplatin-containing biodegradable beads for treatment of cutaneous neoplasia in equidae: 59 cases (2000–2004). *J Am Vet Med Assoc* 229:1617–1622, 2006.

Theon AP, Wilson WD, Magdesian KG, et al: Long-term outcome associated with intratumoral chemotherapy with cisplatin for cutaneous tumors in equidae: 573 cases (1995–2004). *J Am Vet Med Assoc* 230:1506–1513, 2007.

Top JGB, Heer ND, Klein WR, Ensink JM: Penile and preputial squamous cell carcinoma in the horse: a retrospective study of treatment of 77 affected horses. *Equine Vet J* 40:533–537, 2008.

AUTHORS: KIM A. SELTING and ELIZABETH A. GIULIANO

EDITOR: JEFFREY N. BRYAN

Squamous Cell Carcinoma, Periocular

BASIC INFORMATION

DEFINITION

Squamous cell carcinoma (SCC) in tissues around or on the eye

SYNONYM(S)

- Cancer eye
- Skin cancer

EPIDEMIOLOGY

SPECIES, AGE, SEX Mean age of onset is 9 to 12 years.

GENETICS AND BREED PREDISPOSITION Common in Appaloosa, Paint, and Draft horses

RISK FACTORS Horses with light hair and skin have a higher prevalence of periocular SCC.

GEOGRAPHY AND SEASONALITY Increased prevalence of SCC in the United States is associated with an increase in longitude, decreased latitude, increased altitude, and increased mean annual solar radiation.

CLINICAL PRESENTATION

DISEASE FORMS/SUBTYPES The most common location for ocular SCC is the

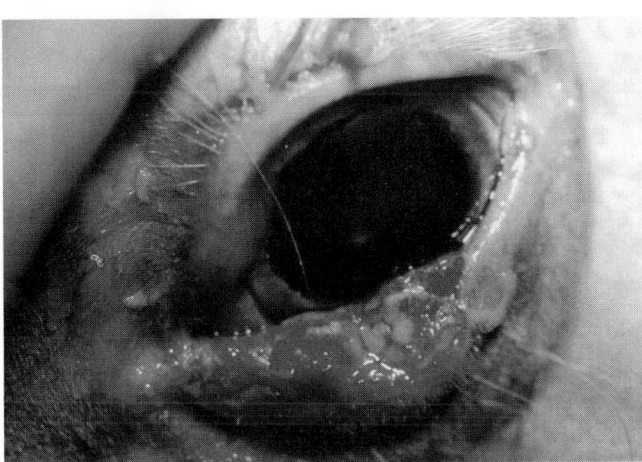

FIGURE 1 Periocular (eyelid) squamous cell carcinoma.

lower eyelid, third eyelid, lateral canthus, and cornea (Figure 1).

HISTORY, CHIEF COMPLAINT Identification of a proliferative pink mass on or near the eye

PHYSICAL EXAM FINDINGS SCC typically starts as a hyperemic area of the eyelid with dark exudates, then progresses to ulceration with hemorrhage to papillomatous masses. The tumors progress to fleshy masses with variable degrees of ulceration, necrosis, and inflammation.

ETIOLOGY AND PATHOPHYSIOLOGY Any chronic irritation may promote neoplastic change of epithelium to SCC, especially at vulnerable locations such as mucocutaneous junctions. Irritation from actinic and/or ultraviolet radiation has been thought to promote the development of SCC. Ultraviolet radiation may promote mutation in the tumor suppressor protein p53, and overexpression plays an important role in the development of most SCCs of animal species studied, including horses.

DIAGNOSIS

DIFFERENTIAL DIAGNOSIS

Tumors (papilloma, melanoma, mastocytoma, basal cell carcinoma, schwannoma, adenoma and adenocarcinomas, heman-gioma and hemangiosarcoma, lymphoma and lymphosarcoma)
- Conjunctivitis (lymphoid hyperplasia and follicular conjunctivitis)
- Inflammatory lesions (abscesses, granulation tissue, foreign body reaction, solar-induced inflammation)
- Parasites (*Habronema, Onchocerca, Thelazia*)

INITIAL DATABASE
- Complete ophthalmic examination
- Biopsy of lesion

ADVANCED OR CONFIRMATORY TESTING

Biopsy of lesion

TREATMENT

THERAPEUTIC GOAL(S)
- Remove neoplasm and prevent recurrence
- Maintain eye and vision

CHRONIC TREATMENT

Medical therapy
- Immunotherapy: Bacillus Calmette-Guérin, 1 mL/cm³ of tumor surface every 2 to 4 weeks
- Chemotherapy: Cisplatin, 1 mg/cm³ every 2 weeks for four treatments

Surgical therapy: Excision with one or more adjunctive therapies
- Cryotherapy: Double or triple freeze-thaw to −25° C
- Hyperthermia: Tissue temperatures between 41° and 45° C
- CO_2 laser ablation
- Gamma irradiation: Brachytherapy
- Mitomycin C
- Photodynamic therapy

POSSIBLE COMPLICATIONS

Local regrowth of the tumor is common after treatment. Subsequent tumor growths are less responsive to therapy.

RECOMMENDED MONITORING

Monitor monthly for 12 months, then annually.

PROGNOSIS AND OUTCOME

Prognosis is poor for nonrecurrence of neoplasm.

PEARLS & CONSIDERATIONS

COMMENTS

Both eyes are at risk and should be monitored.

PREVENTION
- Minimizing ocular sunlight may help prevent the development of periocular SCC.
- Use of a quality fly mask is recommended.

CLIENT EDUCATION

Client communication is essential so that it is understood that treatment is aimed at controlling, not curing, this condition.

SUGGESTED READING

Gilger BC, Stoppini R: Diseases of the eyelids, conjunctiva, and nasolacrimal system. In Gilger BC, editor: *Equine ophthalmology*, St Louis, 2005, Mosby Elsevier, pp 107–156.

AUTHOR: **BRIAN C. GILGER**

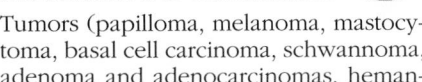

Strangles

BASIC INFORMATION

DEFINITION

Infectious disease caused by the bacterium *Streptococcus equi* subsp. *equi* (often referred to only as *Streptococcus equi*). Affects primarily the upper respiratory tract, although any site may be infected.

SYNONYM(S)

Distemper

EPIDEMIOLOGY

SPECIES, AGE, SEX
- May be more severe in young horses
- Other species rarely affected

RISK FACTORS Commingling with many horses of unknown origin and medical history

CONTAGION AND ZOONOSIS

- Contagious: Spread by direct (horse-to-horse) or indirect (contaminated feed, water, equipment, or handlers) contact
- Source of infection
  - Purulent discharge from horses with active and recovering strangles
  - Nasal secretions of outwardly healthy horses, including horses incubating disease or recovering or subclinical carriers (carrier state develops in up to 10% of affected animals; the guttural pouch is the most common site of prolonged carriage)
  - Prolonged environmental persistence unlikely
- Rare cases identified in humans

GEOGRAPHY AND SEASONALITY Recognized worldwide

ASSOCIATED CONDITIONS AND DISORDERS

- Purpura hemorrhagica: Immune-mediated vasculitis; may occur after exposure to *S. equi* antigens by natural exposure or vaccination
- Immune-mediated myositis or myopathy is similar in pathogenesis to purpura hemorrhagica.

CLINICAL PRESENTATION

DISEASE FORMS/SUBTYPES

- Disease limited to upper respiratory tract and associated lymph nodes (classic strangles)
- Metastatic abscessation

HISTORY, CHIEF COMPLAINT Acute swelling in the submandibular or retropharyngeal area, anorexia, nasal discharge

PHYSICAL EXAM FINDINGS

- Fever
- Anorexia, listlessness
- Nasal discharge: May be initially serous, then mucopurulent
- Lymphadenopathy: Primarily submandibular and retropharyngeal lymph nodes, abscess formation (Figure 1)
- Dysphagia
- Dyspnea, stridor
- Hyperemic nasal and ocular mucosa
- Inconsistent cough
- Other signs depend on specific tissue involvement (eg, chronic weight loss often associated with internal abscessation or abnormal lung sounds associated with pneumonia, colic, neurologic signs, panophthalmitis, other)

ETIOLOGY AND PATHOPHYSIOLOGY

- *S. equi* subsp. *equi*: Gram-positive β-hemolytic coccoid bacterium; several virulence factors, including the surface protein SeM, which is antiphagocytic and immunogenic

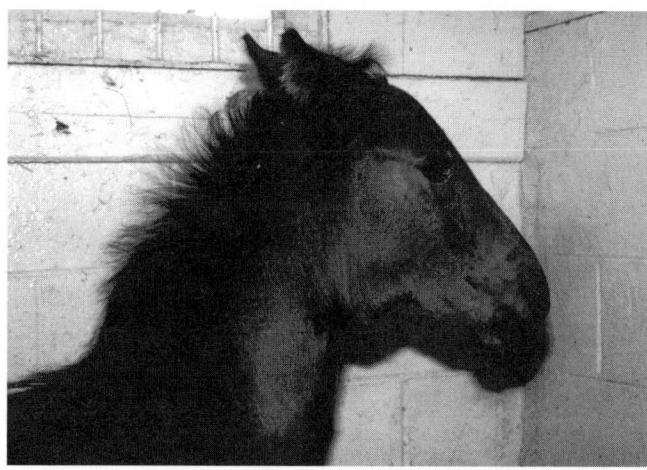

FIGURE 1 Enlarged, abscessed submandibular lymph node in a foal with strangles. (From Sellon DC, Long MT (eds): *Equine infectious diseases*, St Louis, 2007, Saunders Elsevier.)

- Enters via the mouth or nose and attaches to cells in the tonsils; the organism is translocated to the lymph nodes within a few hours.
- Infection results in the production of inflammatory mediators, which attract large numbers of neutrophils, leading to abscess formation.
- First sign of infection is fever, which generally occurs 3 to 14 days after exposure.
- Nasal shedding typically begins 2 to 3 days after onset of fever and generally lasts 2 to 6 weeks after the cessation of clinical signs.
- Disease severity depends on challenge load and duration as well as host factors.
- The majority of exposed horses develop immunity, which lasts for 5 or more years.

DIAGNOSIS

DIFFERENTIAL DIAGNOSIS

- Abscessation caused by other infectious agents
- Foreign body
- Neoplasia
- Salivary gland disease: Duct obstruction resulting in a mucocele and inflammation, sialoadenitis

INITIAL DATABASE

- Complete blood count and fibrinogen: Most often neutrophilic leukocytosis and hyperfibrinogenemia; may see anemia or thrombocytosis, especially in chronic cases
- Serum chemistry: May see hyperglobulinemia; other abnormalities may reflect specific organ involvement such as the liver
- Endoscopic examination: Collapse of the nasopharynx, guttural pouch empyema, and chondroids

- Ultrasonography: May be used to confirm abscessation and identify areas of fluid; useful in evaluation of the thorax and abdomen
- Radiographs: Soft tissue density in the retropharyngeal area, fluid in the guttural pouch, thickening in the roof of the pharynx, distortion of the pharyngeal airway or trachea

ADVANCED OR CONFIRMATORY TESTING

- Identification of *S. equi* from samples
  - Nasal swabs
  - Nasal washes (inject approximately 50 mL of warm saline through a 15-cm soft rubber tube placed into the ventral nasal meatus; collect the saline in a sterile container as it flows from the nostrils)
  - Guttural pouch lavages
  - Aspirated pus
- Guttural pouch lavages and nasal washes appear to be more effective than nasal swabs in detection of small numbers of *S. equi*. Guttural pouch lavages are the most effective but are relatively labor intensive.
- Means of identification of *S. equi*
  - Culture: Colony morphology identical to *S. equi* subsp. *zooepidemicus*; differentiated by inability to ferment lactose and sorbitol
  - Polymerase chain reaction (PCR): Detects DNA sequence of SeM; approximately 3 times more sensitive than culture but does not distinguish dead from live organisms
- Serology: Enzyme-linked immunosorbent assay for measuring SeM-specific antibody (IDEXX Laboratories, West Sacramento, CA)
  - Does not distinguish between vaccine and infection response
  - Considerable individual variation in the immune response to *S. equi*
  - May be useful in confirming recent exposure, determining the need for

vaccination, and diagnosing metastatic abscesses and purpura hemorrhagica

○ Measures antibody concentrations as titers in one of five categories: Negative, weak positive (1:200–1:400), moderate positive (1:800–1:1600), high positive (1:3200–1:6400), and very high positive (>1:12,800)

TREATMENT

THERAPEUTIC GOAL(S)

• Resolution of clinical signs
• Clearance of *S. equi* infection
• Control the spread of *S. equi*

ACUTE GENERAL TREATMENT

• Isolation and hygiene
  ○ Stop movement of horses on and off affected premises.
  ○ Separate horses into affected, exposed, and nonexposed groups. Deal with infectious horses last; monitor rectal temperatures twice daily on all horses to detect infection early.
  ○ Use strict hygiene measures: Dedicated clothing, cleaning, and disinfection of surfaces and equipment, including water troughs. (*S. equi* is susceptible to most disinfectants; follow manufacturers' recommendations.)
  ○ Compost manure and waste feed from infectious horses at an isolated location.
  ○ Contaminated pastures and paddocks should be rested for at least 4 weeks.
  ○ Recovered and exposed horses should be evaluated for shedding of *S. equi* before release from quarantine (culture and PCR of three nasal swabs, nasal washes, or guttural pouch lavages taken at weekly intervals).
• Appropriate treatment of individual horses depends on stage and severity of the disease.
• Antibiotic treatment: Usually not necessary after external lymphadenopathy is present; treatment involves facilitating drainage and supportive care.
• Possible indications for antibiotic treatment
  ○ Cases in the early phase with fever and lethargy but before abscess formation
  ○ Cases with severe systemic illness or dyspnea, especially if a tracheotomy is required
  ○ Metastatic abscessation where drainage is not possible
  ○ Clearance of the carrier state
• Penicillin: Generally considered the antibiotic of choice (procaine penicillin 22,000 IU/kg IM q12h; potassium penicillin G 22,000 IU/kg IV q6h); other antibiotics based on susceptibility testing; generally susceptible to many antibiotics, including cephalosporins and macrolides; trimethoprim sulfa may be effective, although response varies.
• No data confirming an association between the use of antibiotics and the development of metastatic abscessation.
• Nonsteroidal antiinflammatory drugs (NSAIDs) may improve the horse's attitude and decrease swelling; consideration must be given to the potential toxicity of NSAIDs, especially in dehydrated patients.

CHRONIC TREATMENT

• Long-term antibiotic treatment may be required for internal abscesses.
• Treatment of carriers with *S. equi* infection of the guttural pouch
  ○ Guttural pouch lavage followed by topical penicillin therapy (instillation of a penicillin-gelatin solution: dissolve 2 g of gelatin in 40 mL of sterile water; cool to 45° to 50° C and add 10 million U of sodium benzyl penicillin G, which is commercially available through equine pharmacies).
  ○ Systemic antibiotics
  ○ Occasional carriers will have infection at other sites, such as the sinus; local treatment of the sinus is indicated.

POSSIBLE COMPLICATIONS

• Chondroid formation within the guttural pouch
• Metastatic abscessation (bastard strangles): Abscesses at sites other than lymph nodes of the head and neck; seen in approximately 25% to 30% of cases (Figure 2)
• Immune-mediated complications
  ○ Purpura hemorrhagica: Aseptic vasculitis characterized primarily by edema and petechial or ecchymotic hemorrhage
  ○ Myositis: Muscle infarctions or rhabdomyolysis with progressive atrophy
  ○ Glomerulonephritis, myocarditis
• Agalactia
• Neurologic dysfunction associated with lymphadenopathy and guttural pouch infection: Dysphagia, laryngeal hemiplegia, cranial nerve VII or VIII deficits (varying neurologic signs can

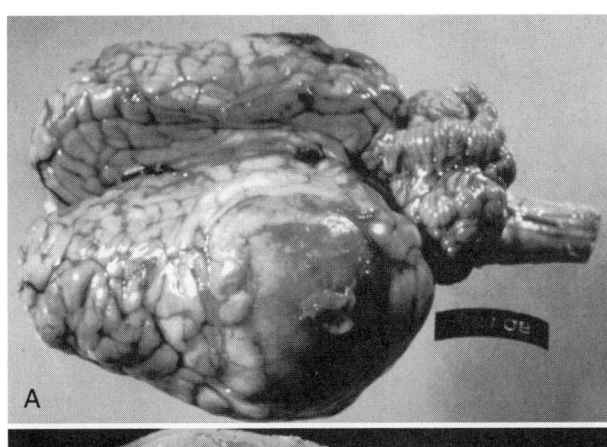
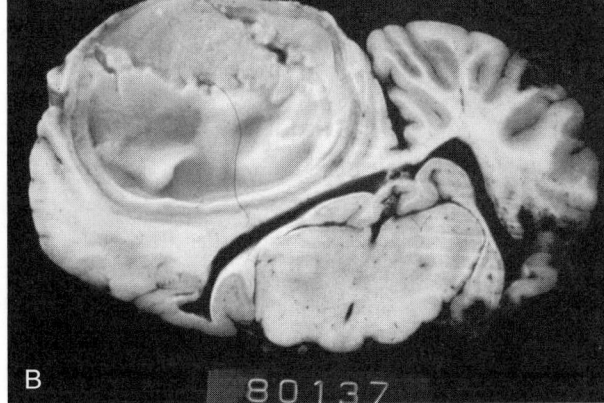

FIGURE 2 **A,** Cerebral abscess of the left hemisphere caused by *Streptococcus equi* infection in a yearling Arabian colt. **B,** Sagittal section through the left hemisphere of the same colt demonstrating the gross extent of the abscess. (From Sellon DC, Long MT (eds): *Equine infectious diseases,* St Louis, 2007, Saunders Elsevier.)

occur with extension of disease to the central nervous system)

RECOMMENDED MONITORING
- Monitor attitude, vital parameters
- Carefully monitor dyspnea; a tracheotomy may be required

PROGNOSIS AND OUTCOME

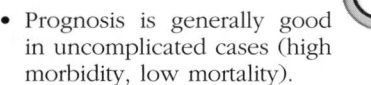

- Prognosis is generally good in uncomplicated cases (high morbidity, low mortality).
- Complications develop in approximately 20% to 30% of cases and significantly increase the case-fatality rate from death or euthanasia, which may approach 40%.

PEARLS & CONSIDERATIONS

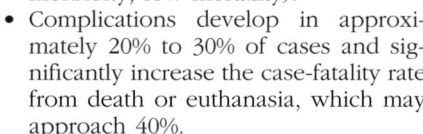

COMMENTS
- First described in 1251 and remains an important equine disease; some aspects are still controversial.
- Eradication strategies have been proposed.

PREVENTION
- Quarantine and bacteriological screening: Ideally, new arrivals should be isolated for 3 weeks and screened for *S. equi* (culture and PCR of three weekly nasal swabs, nasal washes, or guttural pouch lavages).

- Use strict hygiene practices.
- Vaccination: Currently considered a risk-based vaccine according to the American Association of Equine Practitioners Guidelines for Vaccination of Horses (available at http://www.aaep. org/vaccination_guidelines.htm).
  - Vaccination is recommended on premises with persistent endemic strangles and for horses that are at high risk of exposure.
  - Vaccination in the face of an outbreak is controversial and should be carefully considered because the risk of adverse reactions (primarily purpura hemorrhagica) may be increased in exposed horses; management practices are key to outbreak control.
  - Titers can be measured before vaccination; it is recommended that horses with titers greater than 1:1600 not be vaccinated.
  - Vaccines available in the United States have included a killed whole-cell bacterin; extracts of *S. equi* containing SeM; and an attenuated, nonencapsulated live strain of *S. equi* that is administered intranasally; the extract and live vaccines have superseded the use of bacterins.
  - Vaccination attenuates the severity of clinical signs and decreases the incidence of disease but is not completely protective; the attenuated live vaccine stimulated a high level of immunity against experimental challenge.
  - When using the attenuated intranasal vaccine, it is recommended to administer all parenteral vaccinations and other injections first to avoid inadvertent contamination.
  - Vaccination for strangles is an active area of research.

CLIENT EDUCATION
- Clients should be aware of the contagious nature of strangles. Early recognition of clinical signs and good management practices are essential in controlling disease.
- It is also important to understand that given the mobility of Equine populations, exposure risk cannot be completely eliminated at this time.

SUGGESTED READING
Association of Equine Practitioners: http://www.aaep.org/vaccination_guidelines.htm.
Newton JR, Verheyen K, Talbot NC, et al: Control of strangles outbreaks by isolation of guttural pouch carriers identified using PCR and culture of *Streptococcus equi*, *Equine Vet J* 32:515–526, 2000.
Prescott JF, Timoney JF: Could we eradicate strangles in equids? *J Am Vet Med Assoc* 231:377, 2007.
Sweeney CR, Timoney JF, Newton JR, Hines MT: *Streptococcus equi* infections in horses: guidelines for treatment, control, and prevention of strangles, *J Vet Intern Med* 19:123, 2005.
Waller AS, Jolley KA: Getting a grip on strangles: recent progress towards improved diagnostics and vaccines, *Vet J* 173:492, 2007.

AUTHOR: **MELISSA T. HINES**

EDITORS: **MAUREEN T. LONG** and **DEBRA C. SELLON**

Strychnine Toxicosis

BASIC INFORMATION

DEFINITION
Strychnine is a toxic alkaloid from an Indian tree, *Strychnos nux-vomica*, commonly used in gopher, mole, rat, and coyote bait.

SYNONYM(S)
Gopher bait poisoning

EPIDEMIOLOGY
RISK FACTORS
- Usually dyed and coated in milo or in pellets that look like feed to horses
- Often comes in 5-gallon buckets

CLINICAL PRESENTATION
DISEASE FORMS/SUBTYPES
- Low dose
- High dose
HISTORY, CHIEF COMPLAINT
- Muscle stiffness
- Clinical signs within 10 to 120 minutes of ingestion
- Seizures; similar to tetanus but much quicker onset
- Sudden death
PHYSICAL EXAM FINDINGS
- Anxiety
- Muscle stiffness
- Saw-horse stance
- Strained facial expression

- Violent tetanic seizures with opisthotonus and powerful extensor rigidity
- Seizures brought on by external stimuli
ETIOLOGY AND PATHOPHYSIOLOGY
- Readily absorbed
- Metabolized by the liver
- Detected in urine within 2 minutes of exposure
- Blocks the inhibitory effects of glycine
- Skeletal muscles become hyperexcitable
- Potent convulsant with powerful extensor rigidity
- Death by respiratory failure

DIAGNOSIS

DIFFERENTIAL DIAGNOSIS

- Tetanus
- Organophosphates
- Seizures from any central nervous system disease (bacterial, viral, mycotoxin)
- Cardiotoxic plants

INITIAL DATABASE

- Strychnine should be suspected if blue-green milo or blue-green pellets are found in an open bucket, feed trough, or gastric reflux and if slight external stimuli bring on exaggerated stiffness or seizures. Strychnine bait is also available in other colors, such as orange.
- There are no specific serum chemistry or blood abnormalities observed.

ADVANCED OR CONFIRMATORY TESTING

- There are no specific postmortem or histopathologic lesions. The presence of blue-green milo in the stomach contents is almost diagnostic; however, the examiner should be aware that strychnine bait comes in other formulations and colors.
- In a live animal, strychnine can best be detected in gastric reflux and urine. It can also be detected in serum, plasma, liver, and bait with several analytical methods.

TREATMENT

THERAPEUTIC GOAL(S)

- Decrease absorption
- Eliminate the toxin
- Control the seizures

ACUTE GENERAL TREATMENT

- Aggressive treatment with activated charcoal q6–8h
- Pentobarbital (preferred drug) or methocarbamol to control muscular activity without depressing the respiratory center
- Symptomatic and supportive care such as fluids, respiratory assistance, temperature regulation, and traumatic wound treatment from seizures if necessary

CHRONIC TREATMENT

- Muscle relaxation maintained for up to 24 to 48 hours
- Activated charcoal continued q12h on day 2
- Laxative

DRUG INTERACTIONS

- Ketamine is contraindicated (motor stimulatory effects)
- Morphine is contraindicated (respiratory depression)

POSSIBLE COMPLICATIONS

Injury from seizures

RECOMMENDED MONITORING

The horse should be under veterinary care for at least 48 hours if any clinical signs are present.

PROGNOSIS AND OUTCOME

- Guarded, depending on the dose and whether treatment is started immediately after ingestion is observed
- Poor if the horse is having seizures

PEARLS & CONSIDERATIONS

COMMENTS

Strychnine has been used as a malicious poison.

PREVENTION

Do not keep 5-gallon buckets of gopher bait on farms.

CLIENT EDUCATION

Because many rodenticides are in pelleted form or mixed with grain, both of which horses will readily consume, these products should not be used or stored in places accessible by horses.

SUGGESTED READING

Beasley V: Strychnine. In Beasley V, editor: Veterinary toxicology. Available at http://www.ivis.org/advances/Beasley/cpt2b/chapter_frm.asp?LA=1.

Talcott P: Strychnine. In Plumlee KH, editor: *Clinical veterinary toxicology*, St Louis, 2004, Mosby Elsevier, pp 454–456.

AUTHOR: **SANDRA E. MORGAN**

EDITOR: **CYNTHIA L. GASKILL**

Subcutaneous Emphysema

BASIC INFORMATION

DEFINITION

Accumulation of air in the subcutaneous tissues of the skin

RISK FACTORS

- Endoscopic surgery
- Intramuscular injections
- Choke
- Pulmonary disease
- Animal bites
- Axillary or pectoral wounds
- Trauma to the sinuses, trachea, larynx, or thorax

ASSOCIATED CONDITIONS AND DISORDERS

- Pneumothorax
- Pneumomediastinum
- Pneumoretroperitoneum

CLINICAL PRESENTATION

HISTORY, CHIEF COMPLAINT

- History of recent surgery
- History of choke or nasogastric intubation
- History of trauma resulting in wounds on the head, neck, or thorax
- Recent therapy with intramuscular injections
- Suspected or observed snakebite
- Dyspnea
- Abnormal swelling
- Lameness

PHYSICAL EXAM FINDINGS

- Horses may be anxious, dyspneic, tachypneic, or colicky.
- Palpation of subcutaneous swelling may identify crackles.
- Emphysema may be painful to palpation (may be indicative of infectious origin).

ETIOLOGY AND PATHOPHYSIOLOGY

- Infectious causes of emphysema are related to the accumulation of gas produced by anaerobic bacteria (clostridial species most commonly).
- Iatrogenic causes include surgical incisions, transtracheal wash procedures, and escape and accumulation of air related to endoscopic insufflation.
- Respiratory causes of emphysema include disruptions of any portion of

the pulmonary system (sinuses, larynx, trachea, lungs, mediastinum), resulting in a communication to the subcutaneous space.

- Traumatic wounds into the subcutaneous space may result in an accumulation of air because of a valvelike action of the wound opening (axillary wounds, esophageal rupture).

DIAGNOSIS

DIFFERENTIAL DIAGNOSIS

- Infectious
  - Intramuscular injection
  - Esophageal rupture
  - Severe pneumonia, pulmonary bullae rupture
- Iatrogenic
  - Surgery
  - Laryngotomy incisions
  - Transtracheal wash
- Traumatic
  - Tracheal rupture (necrosis) (Figure 1)
  - Skull fractures involving the sinuses
  - Pectoral and axillary wounds
  - Thoracic inlet wounds
  - Esophageal rupture
  - Bite wounds (snake, dog, other horses)
  - Rib fractures penetrating the lung

INITIAL DATABASE

Diagnostics depend on the suspected source of emphysema

- Complete blood count: May show left shift or anemia for infectious causes
- Serum chemistry: Identification of muscle necrosis, renal compromise
- Radiographs: Identify fractures, pneumonia
- Ultrasound: Identify pneumonia, pneumothorax, gas trapped in infected tissues, foreign material
- Endoscopic examination: Identify defects in the upper respiratory tract and trachea
- Arterial blood gas analysis: To identify adequate oxygenation

TREATMENT

THERAPEUTIC GOAL(S)

- Halt accumulation of subcutaneous air
- Remove accumulation of air in thorax
  - Successful for pneumothorax only
  - Air removal from subcutaneous tissues typically nonproductive

ACUTE GENERAL TREATMENT

- If subcutaneous accumulation is severe, oxygen supplementation is warranted because of reduced thoracic expansion.
  - Arterial blood gas will guide therapy.
  - Artifical respiration may be required.
- Pneumothorax and pneumomediastinum
  - Thoracocentesis and indwelling drains remove excess air from the pleural space.
  - Pneumomediastinum has no specific therapy.

- Continuous negative pressure may be applied for tension pneumothorax.
- Pneumonia and pulmonary bullae: Appropriate antibiotic therapy (transtracheal wash may guide choice)
- Esophageal rupture
  - Requires immediate drainage to reduce risk of mediastinitis
  - Esophagus may be sutured primarily (only if rupture is identified early because of contamination).
  - Most ruptures require healing by second intention with an indwelling nasogastric feeding tube.
  - Systemic antibiotics, tetanus prophylaxis, and analgesia are indicated.
    - Include an antibiotic with an anaerobic spectrum.
- Localized infection
  - Bacteria involved may include *Clostridia* spp. and *Bacteroides* spp.
  - May be caused by introduction of bacteria subcutaneously
  - Injection site gangrene is more likely caused by bacterial spores already present in muscle. Irritating substances (eg, procaine penicillin, flunixin meglumine) activate spores (Figure 2).
  - May also be introduced via wounds. Snakebites may be predisposed to clostridial infections.
  - Treatment includes surgical fenestration, debridement, and antibiotics.
    - Metronidazole (20 mg/kg IV q8h): First choice; bacteriocidal and inhibits clostridial α-toxin

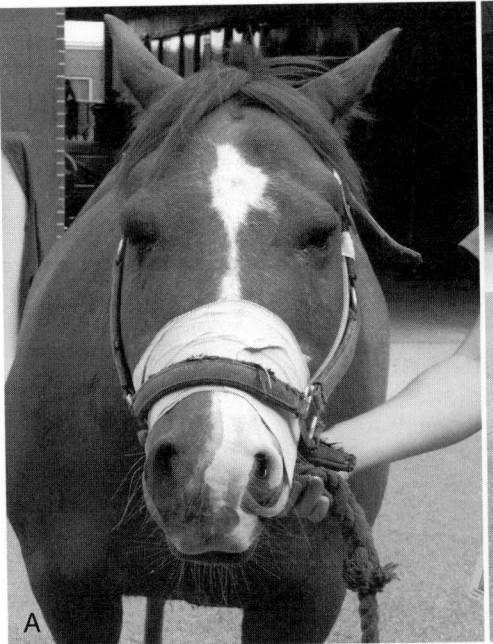
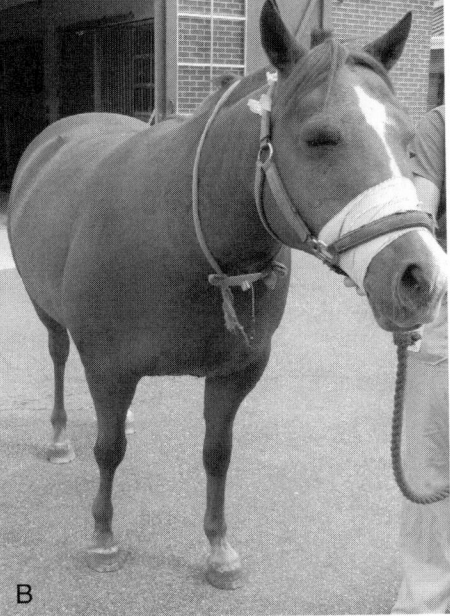

FIGURE 1 **A** and **B,** A mare with subcutaneous emphysema caused by traumatic tracheal rupture. **A,** Note the distended supraorbital fossae and severe swelling of the face, chest, and shoulders. **B,** Off right frontal view to better demonstrate chest and shoulder swelling. (Courtesy Dr. Nelson Pinto.)

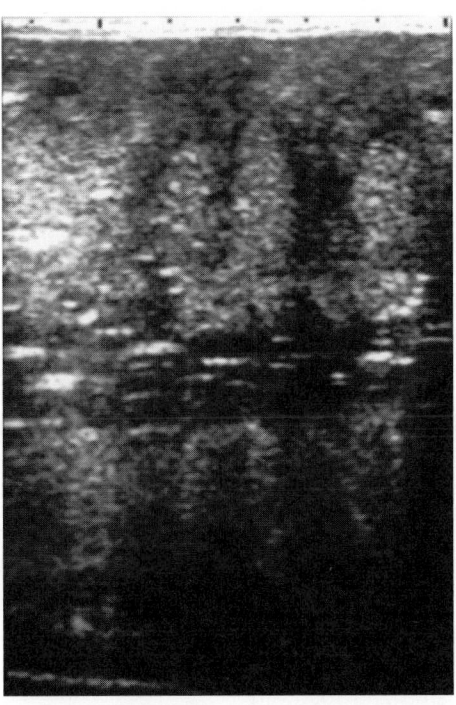

FIGURE 2 Hyperechoic lucencies indicating air in the subcutaneous tissues from a clostridial infection caused by an injection of flunixin meglumine. (Courtesy Dr. Nelson Pinto.)

- Foreign bodies in wounds may result in chronic fistulae.

RECOMMENDED MONITORING

- Arterial blood gas for respiratory compromise
- Complete blood count to monitor response to antibiotics
- Serial hematocrits to diagnose hemolytic anemia

PROGNOSIS AND OUTCOME

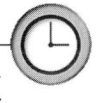

- Most horses with subcutaneous emphysema recover spontaneously in 7 to 21 days.
- Clostridial infections carry a guarded prognosis.

PEARLS & CONSIDERATIONS

COMMENTS

Noninfectious subcutaneous emphysema is not life threatening if addressed early.

CLIENT EDUCATION

Warn owners about the possible infectious sequelae of intramuscular injections.

SUGGESTED READING

Adam EN, Southwood LL: Surgical and traumatic wound infections, cellulitis, and myositis in horses. *Vet Clin North Am Equine Pract* 22(2):335–361, 2006.

Barber SM: Management of neck and head injuries. *Vet Clin North Am Equine Pract* 21(1):191–215, 2005.

Hassel DH: Thoracic trauma in horses. *Vet Clin North Am Equine Pract* 23:67–80, 2007.

Peek SF, Semrad SD, Perkins GA: Clostridial myonecrosis in horses (37 cases 1985–2000), *Equine Vet J* 35(1):86–92, 2003.

Weiss DJ, Moritz A: Equine immune-mediated hemolytic anemia associated with *Clostridium perfringens* infection. *Vet Clin Pathol* 32(1):22–26, 2003.

AUTHOR and EDITOR: **AMELIA MUNSTERMAN**

- Oxytetracycline (6.6 mg/kg, IV q12h) or chloramphenicol (44 mg/kg, PO q6–8h)
- Rifampin may be added for its anti–α-toxin properties (5–10 mg/kg, PO q12h)
  - Secondary immune-mediated anemia may result; responsive to penicillin and steroids.
- Iatrogenic and surgical emphysema
  - Typically resolves without treatment
    - Administer appropriate pain management and analgesics for the primary problem
  - Stall rest horse to limit activity and aspiration of air into incisions
  - Oxygen therapy and ventilation, if required, for severe cases
- Management of traumatic wounds
  - Aseptic exploration, debridement, closure if possible with or without drains
  - Reduce air entry by packing with gauze, occlusion with stent bandages, or plastic occlusive bandages (plastic wrap)
  - Limit movement to reduce further introduction of air through chest or axillary wounds
  - Provide appropriate fixation of skull and rib fractures
  - Trachea rupture may be sutured primarily or left to heal by second intention
  - Systemic antibiotics, tetanus prophylaxis, and analgesia are indicated for all wounds

DRUG INTERACTIONS

Avoid intramuscular injections in areas with emphysema

POSSIBLE COMPLICATIONS

- Esophageal rupture may result in stricture and chronic choke.
- Bacterial infections may result in sepsis, systemic inflammation, pleuritis, and laminitis.

Subsolar Abscess and Penetrating Wound to the Foot

BASIC INFORMATION

DEFINITION

Infection of the subsolar tissues of the foot, primarily including abscessation but also may include penetrating foreign body, septic synovitis of the navicular bursa, distal digital sheath, or tendons and ligaments.

SYNONYM(S)

Sole abscess, gravel, nail, street nail

EPIDEMIOLOGY

RISK FACTORS

- Moist ground conditions that soften the hoof and sole

- Presence of detritus in the stall or pasture that could penetrate the sole (such as nails)

CLINICAL PRESENTATION

DISEASE FORMS/SUBTYPES Slowly progressive sole abscess, acute injury to deeper structures after foreign body penetration that results in acute lameness that subsequently results in deep infection, septic synovitis, tenosynovitis, or osteomyelitis

HISTORY, CHIEF COMPLAINT Acute lameness that becomes more pronounced over several days. Often starts as a mild lameness (grade 2 of 5) that progresses to non–weight-bearing lameness.

PHYSICAL EXAM FINDINGS The horse often points with the affected foot, and that distal limb usually has a pronounced digital pulse. Application of hoof testers to the affected sole usually results in a very painful response directly over the abscess site. Examination of the sole may reveal a tract, site of foreign body penetration, actual foreign body in place, a soft and painful area overlying the abscess, or combination of the above.

ETIOLOGY AND PATHOPHYSIOLOGY

- Softening of hoof, exposure to foreign body penetration, penetration of the sensitive laminae with a high nail at shoeing, poor quality hoof lamellae and white line
- Chronic hoof or sole abscessation frequently occurs with chronic laminitis.

DIAGNOSIS

DIFFERENTIAL DIAGNOSIS

- Sole abscess
- Deep sole bruise
- Laminitis
- Septic arthritis, septic tenosynovitis
- Fracture of the distal phalanges or navicular bone

INITIAL DATABASE

- Lameness evaluation, especially palpation of digital pulses and hoof tester application.
- Radiographs are warranted if a foreign body is in place or to rule out fracture and osteomyelitis.

ADVANCED OR CONFIRMATORY TESTING

- If a tract is present, contrast radiography of the tract or placement of a metal probe in the tract before imaging is indicated.
- If a foreign body appears to penetrate the caudal half of the foot, synovial structure involvement should be ruled out with synoviocentesis of the appropriate structures (distal interphalangeal joint, navicular bursa or digital

sheath) and fluid analysis with bacterial culture as indicated.

TREATMENT

THERAPEUTIC GOAL(S)

- Localize abscess or inflamed or infected tissue
- Provide appropriate drainage and antiseptic or antibacterial access
- Reduce pain and inflammation

ACUTE GENERAL TREATMENT

- The sole of the affected foot should be carefully pared to reveal a clean, uniform sole.
- A combination of hoof tester and finger pressure may be used to localize the likely site of the abscess.
- If the horse is shod, the shoe must often be removed to afford evaluation of the sole margins and the white line, the most common sites for sole abscess.
- Tracts should be pared and followed in the painful region until the abscess is relieved or until further paring of the solar corium develops a slight pink hue (pink color indicates proximity to solar corium). A specialized hoof knife with a tightly curved tip or a bone curette may be useful for following tracts through the sole. Most sole abscesses consist of a grey-colored, malodorous liquid that flows freely when the abscess cavity is breached during paring. Excessive paring may result in hemorrhage from the solar corium. The size of the sole opening used to drain the abscess and permit local treatment is quite small. Excessively large pared sole defects require prolonged healing time and protection of the sole with a pad.
- If the abscess cannot be drained on the initial visit, verify tetanus status and begin poulticing or soaking the foot.
- Poulticing and soaking are done to soften the foot and draw out the abscess. Soaking is done by placing the foot in warm water with diluted povidone–iodine and a handful of Epsom salts (magnesium sulfate) for 10 to 20 minutes once or twice daily. Other agents for poulticing the foot include a combination of sugar and povidone–iodine, ichthammol, and an ointment consisting of magnesium sulphate and menthol (MagnaPaste, Butler Schein Animal Health, Dublin, Ohio). Another method of providing prolonged soaking of the foot is by using a bran mash poultice. Take a strong plastic bag that fits over the foot and add one handful of bran and a small handful of Epsom salts. Add suf-

ficient water to soak the bran and add povidone–iodine (~1 part to 10 parts other constituents). Fit the bag with mixture over the foot and secure with gauze, elastic tape, and duct tape. This poultice should be changed every 24 hours.

- If the abscess was easily drained, apply a gauze soaked in povidone–iodine over the pared defect and protect the sole with an Easyboot (EasyCare Inc., Tucson, AZ) or a bandage. Change the bandage daily for the first few days and then as needed to protect the foot. After the abscess is dry—as soon as 4 to 5 days or as long as 2 weeks—a shoe with a leather pad should be applied to protect the pared area.
- Systemic antibiotics are not administered in uncomplicated sole abscess cases.
- Nonsteroidal antiinflammatory drugs are indicated when lameness is severe.
- If a penetrating foreign body or deep synovial infection is present, surgical debridement of the tract and affected tissue and joint or tendon sheath lavage followed by regional limb perfusion and broad-spectrum parenteral antibacterials are indicated.

CHRONIC TREATMENT

- Deep sole abscesses that cannot be drained through the sole result in prolonged lameness and often break out at the coronary band of the hoof capsule or over the bulbs of the heels.
- If the abscess cannot be accessed from the sole or white line, radiographs may help localize the site. Also, radiographs will determine if the distal phalanx or navicular bone have developed osteomyelitis or osteitis because of the prolonged inflammation and infection. Rarely, persistent sole abscesses must be treated with localized, partial hoof or sole resection or curettage of the distal phalanx.
- After the sole abscess is no longer draining purulent discharge and the soundness has improved, shoeing the horse with a full pad will protect the injured sole and allow a quicker return to complete soundness.

POSSIBLE COMPLICATIONS

Extension of a deep infection within the hoof may result in osteomyelitis, septic tenosynovitis, or septic arthritis.

RECOMMENDED MONITORING

- Repeated evaluation of lameness and degree of discharge and condition of the affected tissues is needed.
- Radiographs should be taken if the abscess and lameness persist for more than 2 weeks.

PROGNOSIS AND OUTCOME

- Most horses with routine sole abscesses have an excellent prognosis for return to soundness in 1 to 3 weeks.
- If bone, synovial structures, or tendons are affected, the prognosis is guarded to fair.

SUGGESTED READING

Celeste CJ, Szoke MO: Management of equine hoof injuries. *Vet Clin North Am Equine Pract* 21:167, 2005.

AUTHOR and EDITOR: **ANDRIS J. KANEPS**

Summer Pasture–Associated Recurrent Airway Obstruction

BASIC INFORMATION

DEFINITION

Seasonal, reversible, inflammatory condition of the lower airways characterized by airway obstruction from bronchoconstriction, mucus hypersecretion, neutrophilic exudation, and pathologic changes of bronchiolitis

SYNONYM(S)

Summer pasture heaves, sumer pasture–associated obstructive pulmonary disease (SPARAO)

EPIDEMIOLOGY

SPECIES, AGE, SEX Affected animals are mature (age 12 ± 6 years)
RISK FACTORS Exposure to pasture environment for extended periods, especially during warm months of the year (airborne particulates inhaled during grazing)
GEOGRAPHY AND SEASONALITY
- Pasture-associated condition first described in southeastern United States; more recently described in England and Scotland; anecdotal reports in various other locations
- During warm months of the year
ASSOCIATED CONDITIONS AND DISORDERS The recurrent, seasonal, clinical exacerbation may progress to a condition of shorter or no clinical remission and irreversible respiratory dysfunction associated with structural changes and chronic obstructive pulmonary disease.

CLINICAL PRESENTATION

DISEASE FORMS/SUBTYPES
- Typically seasonal, reversible condition (signs subside upon removal from triggering environment)
- May be severe and life threatening (similar to status asthmaticus)
- May progress to state of irreversible respiratory dysfunction (no seasonal clinical remission)

HISTORY, CHIEF COMPLAINT
- History of clinical exacerbation occurring during warm months of the year

- Initial signs limited to exercise intolerance and occasional coughing
- Severity and frequency of coughing episodes worsen, often becoming paroxysmal
- Presenting complaints are labored breathing and coughing

PHYSICAL EXAM FINDINGS
- Prominent signs are labored expiratory effort, flared nostrils and coughing.
- Affected horses are alert but anxious because of respiratory difficulty.
- Vital signs are often increased, especially respiratory rate and mildly increased body temperature.
- Affected horses develop a "heave line" (hypertrophy of the external abdominal oblique muscles).
- In mild cases, thoracic auscultation reveals increased bronchovesicular sounds at rest; wheezes and expiratory crackles are evident during forced breathing.
- Thoracic auscultation of severely affected horses at rest reveals wheezes, generally expiratory (sometimes inspiratory), and expiratory crackles. Wheezes may be audible without stethoscope.
- In severe cases, affected horses have a stance with the head and neck extended forward, increased respiratory rate, flared nostrils, and/or end-expiratory effort. These horses are dehydrated and anorexic, undergo weight loss, and may become emaciated.
- Appearance of clinical signs is seasonal and predictable based on time of the year if the animal is kept in the same environment.

ETIOLOGY AND PATHOPHYSIOLOGY
- Exposure to inhaled particulates present in pasture during warm months of the year leads to inflammation and obstruction of lower airways.
- During clinical exacerbation, affected horses develop airway obstruction (from excessive production of viscous mucopurulent secretion, decreased mucociliary clearance, and bronchoconstriction) resulting in expiratory effort and coughing and leading to

ventilation/perfusion inequalities and hypoxemia.

DIAGNOSIS

DIFFERENTIAL DIAGNOSIS
- Lower respiratory tract infections of viral, bacterial, or fungal etiology
- Pharyngeal disease causing chronic coughing and increased respiratory effort
- Verminous pneumonitis
- Anhydrosis
- Cardiac disease with left-sided heart failure

INITIAL DATABASE
- Complete blood count and fibrinogen: Normal or mild leukocytosis, mild mature neutrophilia, mild hyperfibrinogenemia
- Arterial blood gases
  - PaO_2 values often <80 mm Hg and as low as 40 mm Hg in horses with labored breathing
- Thoracic radiographs
  - Increased bronchointerstitial pattern or no abnormalities
  - Flattened diaphragm may be seen

ADVANCED OR CONFIRMATORY TESTING
- Bronchoscopy
  - Copious amount of mucopurulent material
- Tracheal wash/aspirate
  - Mucopurulent material
  - Cytology: Nondegenerate neutrophils (<90%)
  - Presence of fungal elements and bacteria (common and likely reflect impaired mucociliary clearance)
- Bacterial culture of tracheal aspirate may yield bacterial growth (colonization of the lower airways because of impaired mucociliary clearance)
- Bronchoalveolar lavage
  - Preferred diagnostic test because most representative of small airways
  - Cytology: Increased percentage of nondegenerate neutrophils (>20%)

- Pulmonary function testing reveals increased airway resistance
- Histopathologic examination of lung biopsy
  - Mucus metaplasia of small airways
  - Diagnostic value of lung biopsy may be outweighed by the risk of rare, but possibly fatal, bleeding

TREATMENT

THERAPEUTIC GOAL(S)

- Control airway inflammation and decrease airway obstruction.
- Remember that no drug therapy can replace appropriate environmental management.
- Proper control of environmental exposure is best achieved by keeping horses in a dust-free indoor environment and avoiding pasture during warm months of the year.

ACUTE GENERAL TREATMENT

- Severely affected horses must be removed from pasture and kept in a dust-free indoor environment, preferably in a stall with rubber mats and no bedding. They should be fed a complete, forage-based diet. Signs of airway obstruction may subside with simple environmental changes.
- Provide oxygen supplementation to severely distressed/profoundly hypoxemic animals (PaO$_2$ <60 mm Hg)
- Therapy includes a combination of corticosteroids (to control airway inflammation) and bronchodilators (to diminish airway obstruction)
  - Inhaled drugs can be delivered by nebulization, metered-dose inhaler (MDI), or dry-powder inhaler using delivery devices designed for horses (eg, Equine AeroMask, AeroHippus, EquineHaler, EquiPoudre).
- Corticosteroids
  - In severe cases, systemic injectable corticosteroids are recommended:
    - Dexamethasone (0.05 mg/kg IV q24h) until improvement, then taper
    - Isoflupredone acetate (0.02 mg/kg IM q24h) until improvement, then taper
    - Triamcinolone acetonide (0.05 mg/kg IM q24h) single dose = long-lasting and more likely to induce detrimental effects
  - Inhaled corticosteroids are efficacious and have minimal residual effects (response to inhaled corticosteroids takes longer than systemic injectable steroids):
    - Beclomethasone dipropionate (5–7 µg/kg q12h)
    - Fluticasone propionate (4 µg/kg q12h)
- Bronchodilators
  - β$_2$-Adrenergic agonist bronchodilators:
    - Oral β$_2$-adrenergic agonist bronchodilators:
      - Clenbuterol syrup (0.8–3.2 µg/kg q12h) is commonly used
    - Several inhaled β$_2$-adrenergic agonists are effective for horses:
      - Fast-acting and short-lasting: Albuterol MDI (1–2 µg/kg)
      - Slow-acting and long-lasting: Salmeterol MDI (1 µg/kg)
      - Fast-acting and long-lasting: Pirbuterol or fenoterol MDI (1–2 µg/kg)
    - Long-term use of β$_2$-adrenergic agonist may result in tachyphylaxis
  - Parasympatholytic (anticholinergic) bronchodilators
    - Systemically atropine and glycopyrrolate should be avoided because of their adverse effects on the gastrointestinal tract and risk of precipitating colic in horses.
    - Inhaled muscarinic receptor antagonist bronchodilator ipratropium bromide MDI (1–3 µg/kg) is effective in horses and has minimal adverse systemic effects.

CHRONIC TREATMENT

- Disease is manageable with proper control of environmental exposure to triggering factors.
- If medical therapy is necessary, long-term administration of corticosteroids and bronchodilators should be combined with strict environmental control
  - Corticosteroids
    - Oral route
      - Dexamethasone (0.05 mg/kg PO q24h) until improvement, then taper
      - Prednisolone (0.5–2 mg/kg q24h) until improvement, then taper
    - Inhaled
  - Bronchodilators
    - Oral β$_2$-adrenergic agonist bronchodilators
    - Inhaled β$_2$-adrenergic agonist bronchodilators

POSSIBLE COMPLICATIONS

In severe cases, hypoxic vasoconstriction associated with severe hypoxemia can result in pulmonary hypertension and lead to right-sided heart failure.

RECOMMENDED MONITORING

Evaluate respiratory rate and effort daily as well as occurrence of coughing.

PROGNOSIS AND OUTCOME

SPARAO is not a curable disease, but it can be managed by strict management to minimize exposure to environmental triggering factors (pasture during warm months of the year).

PEARLS & CONSIDERATIONS

COMMENTS

- Therapies listed here are based on the author's experience and recommendations for treatment of small airway disease resulting from inhalation of dusty moldy hay and bedding.
- The benefits of other therapies, such as chloride channel blockers (cromones), pentoxifylline, leukotriene inhibitors, and phosphodiesterase inhibitors, in SPARAO is unclear.
- Efficacy of mucolytics, expectorants, and mucokinectic agents (eg, acetylcysteine, dornase, guaifenesin, iodides) in improving signs of SPARAO are limited to anecdotal reports.

PREVENTION

- Because the time of onset of clinical signs is highly predictable for horses kept in the same environmental conditions, removal from pasture exposure before the identified time of the year prevents clinical exacerbation.
- To minimize dietary changes, keep affected horses on the same complete, forage-based diet throughout the year.

CLIENT EDUCATION

- Ideally, affected horses should be maintained away from pasture during the warm months of the year.
- During clinical remission (cooler months of the year), or if the animal is not severely affected during warm months, it may be kept on pasture. The pasture should be cut very short and the horse should be offered a complete, forage-based diet to decrease grazing and inhalation of particulates. However, at early signs of clinical exacerbation, horses must be kept in a dust-free indoor environment.
- Affected horses may have poor pulmonary clearance and should be kept in a low-dust environment when stabled, even during clinical remission.
- Round hay bales should not be offered to affected horses, even during clinical remission.

SUGGESTED READING

Costa LR, et al: Temporal clinical exacerbation of summer pasture-associated recurrent airway obstruction and relationship with climate and aeroallergens in horses. *Am J Vet Res* 67:1635–1642, 2006.

American Association of Equine Practitioners: http://www.aaep.org/health_articles_view.php?id=320

Ainsworth DM: Summer pasture-associated obstructive pulmonary disease. In Smith BP, editor: *Large animal internal medicine*, St Louis, 1999, Mosby, pp 557–558.

AUTHOR: **LAIS R.R. COSTA**

EDITOR: **MELISSA R. MAZAN**

Systemic Inflammatory Response Syndrome

BASIC INFORMATION

DEFINITION

- The pathologic consequences of systemic inflammation in response to septic processes, severe trauma, endotoxemia or burns
- Consensus criteria for the systemic inflammatory response syndrome (SIRS) in equine patients are borrowed from human medicine, in which the systemic inflammatory response is manifested by two or more of the following: (1) hyperthermia; (2) tachycardia; (3) tachypnea or hypocapnia; and (4) leukogram changes, including leukopenia, leukocytosis, or an increased number of band or toxic neutrophils. When SIRS is induced by an infectious process, it is called *sepsis*.

EPIDEMIOLOGY

SPECIES, AGE, SEX

- In foals, SIRS and sepsis may be related to idiopathic bacterial septicemia, clostridial or salmonella enterocolitis, or rotacoccal pneumonia.
- In adults, SIRS and sepsis may be secondary to gastrointestinal disease (anterior enteritis, infectious colitis,

strangulation) or pleuropneumonia, clostridial myositis, endometritis, peritonitis, or severe trauma (Figure 1).
- A pure form of SIRS may develop from the absorption of endotoxins, without an infectious nidus, in cases of surgical colic and colitis.

ASSOCIATED CONDITIONS AND DISORDERS

- Multiple organ dysfunction syndrome (MODS)
- Sepsis

CLINICAL PRESENTATION

HISTORY, CHIEF COMPLAINT History varies because of the numerous inciting causes of SIRS.

PHYSICAL EXAM FINDINGS

- Depression, lethargy
- Injected mucous membranes, increased capillary refill time
- Tachycardia or bradycardia, poor pulse quality, cool extremities
- Tachypnea
- Decreased borborygmi, decreased fecal output, colic
- Fever or hypothermia

ETIOLOGY AND PATHOPHYSIOLOGY

- An insult, whether it is infectious, traumatic, or inflammatory, initiates a proinflammatory and an antiinflammatory

response. If these responses are appropriate and balanced, homeostasis is restored. If inflammation overwhelms the antiinflammatory processes and spills into the systemic system, SIRS develops, which may progress to end-organ dysfunction and MODS.
- Proinflammatory cytokines, including tumor necrosis factor, and interleukin-1, are released from activated macrophages. These cytokines amplify the inflammatory process through additional cytokines and enzymes that produce platelet activating factor, prostaglandin E2, leukotrienes, and nitrous oxide. Neutrophils are activated and marginate, inducing local tissue injury and destruction.
- The coagulation system also becomes dysregulated during SIRS, leading to inappropriate coagulation. The natural anticoagulation mechanisms, including activated protein C, tissue factor pathway inhibitor, and the heparin-antithrombin pathway, are also inhibited. These inhibitors of coagulation are important in preventing elevations in cytokine levels, neutralizing inflammatory mediators and minimizing endothelial cell dysfunction. Fibrinolysis is also impaired through the release of plasminogen activator inhibitor type 1.

DIAGNOSIS

DIFFERENTIAL DIAGNOSIS

Pure SIRS should be differentiated from the systemic inflammatory process caused by sepsis, as well as the severe consequence of SIRS (MODS).

INITIAL DATABASE

- Packed cell volume
- Total protein
- Complete blood count and differential
- Blood lactate
- Blood gas
- Serum chemistry
- Urinalysis
- Coagulation profile
- Arterial blood pressure

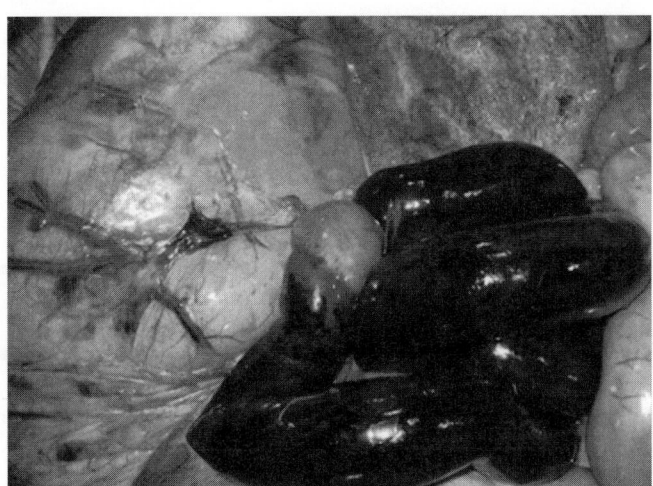

FIGURE 1 Strangulated small intestine that resulted in systemic inflammatory response syndrome.

ADVANCED OR CONFIRMATORY TESTING

Advanced or confirmatory testing depends on the inciting cause of the inflammatory process:

- Cardiovascular system: Cardiac output monitoring, electrocardiography, troponin levels, echocardiography
- Gastrointestinal system: Abdominal ultrasonography, radiography (in foals), nasogastric decompression, transrectal examination, abdominocentesis
- Respiratory system: Thoracic radiography, ultrasonography, arterial blood gas analysis
- Musculoskeletal system: Pedal venography, radiography

TREATMENT

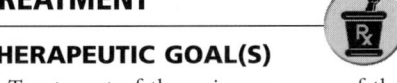

THERAPEUTIC GOAL(S)

- Treatment of the primary cause of the inflammatory process
- Supportive care and optimization of tissue perfusion

ACUTE GENERAL TREATMENT

- Early goal-directed therapy may reduce the risk of tissue hypoxia and shock (see "Early Goal-Directed Therapy" in Section II).
- Fluid therapy
  - Shock-dose fluid administration (see "Shock Dose Fluid Administration" in Section II) when indicated
  - Maintenance fluids to maintain tissue perfusion without causing tissue edema (see "Dehydration" in this section)
- Inotropes and vasopressors for cardiovascular support (see "Shock, Hypovolemic" in this section)
- Oxygen therapy ± mechanical ventilation based on response and blood gas analysis
- Antimicrobial therapy: Broad spectrum initially; narrowed by culture results of the local infectious process
- Antiendotoxin therapy
  - Hyperimmune plasma (against *Salmonella typhimurium* or J5 *Escherichia coli*)

- Antibodies bind and clear endotoxin using the innate immune system.
- Dose: 1.5 mL/kg J5 serum diluted twofold in crystalloid solution.
- Results are conflicting, and therapy may increase the endotoxic effects.
- Drawbacks include high financial cost and the risk of adverse immune reactions.
  - Polymixin B
    - Binds to circulating endotoxin and prevents interaction with its receptors
    - Dosage: 6000 U/kg diluted to 500 mL IV q8–12h
    - Risk of nephrotoxicity in dehydrated horses
  - Nonsteroidal antiinflammatory medications
    - Block the production of eicosanoids and reduces inflammation
    - Flunixin meglumine appears most beneficial in ameliorating clinical signs (1.1 mg/kg IV q12h)
      - The antiendotoxin dose (0.25 mg/kg IV q8h) reduces inflammatory mediators but does not eliminate signs of endotoxemia.
- Closely monitor serum glucose. May reduce mortality and inflammation (noted in human medicine). Insulin may be supplied (0.1–1 IU/kg/h) to maintain normoglycemia.
- Low-dose corticosteroid therapy may be beneficial for patients with corticosteroid insufficiency associated with critical illness.
  - Identified by low serum cortisol and lack of response to exogenous adrenocorticotropin
  - May require low dose prednisolone or hydrocortisone
  - The risk of laminitis with corticosteroid therapy should be considered.
- Treat coagulopathies (see "Disseminated Intravascular Coagulation" in this section)

- Surgically debride septic foci
- Antioxidant therapy
  - Dimethylsulfoxide IV
  - Vitamin E
- Gastrointestinal protectants
  - Glutamine: May provide supportive nutrition to enterocytes to maintain gastrointestinal barrier.
  - Antiulcer medications are commonly prescribed because of the risk of ulcers with anorexia.
  - Omeprazole is preferred, but ranitidine may be effectively used in foals (1.5 mg/kg IV q8h). May increase risk of infection because of the loss of protective gastric acid.

RECOMMENDED MONITORING

- Vital parameters should be monitored closely for change.
- The initial database should be repeated at intervals based on initial findings and new results.

PROGNOSIS AND OUTCOME

The prognosis for SIRS depends on the inciting cause of the inflammatory process and whether SIRS progresses to multiple organ dysfunction.

PEARLS & CONSIDERATIONS

Therapy is most effective if initiated early in the course of SIRS.

SUGGESTED READING

Divers T: Shock and systemic inflammatory response syndrome. In Orsini JA, Divers TJ, editors: *Equine emergencies: treatments and procedures*, St Louis, 2008, Saunders Elsevier, pp 544–552.
Roy MF: Sepsis in adults and foals. *Vet Clin North Am Equine Pract* 20:41–61, 2004.

AUTHOR: **AMELIA MUNSTERMAN**

EDITORS: **R. REID HANSON** and **AMELIA MUNSTERMAN**

Taxus (Yew) Toxicosis

BASIC INFORMATION

DEFINITION

Intoxication as a result of ingesting the yew shrub or tree (Figure 1)

SYNONYM(S)

Taxus, yew

EPIDEMIOLOGY

RISK FACTORS Dried plant material may pose a greater risk because it may

not taste as bitter as fresh material. An approximate lethal dose of plant material in horses is 0.1% to 0.2% of an animal's body weight.

GEOGRAPHY AND SEASONALITY
Yews are commonly encountered orna-

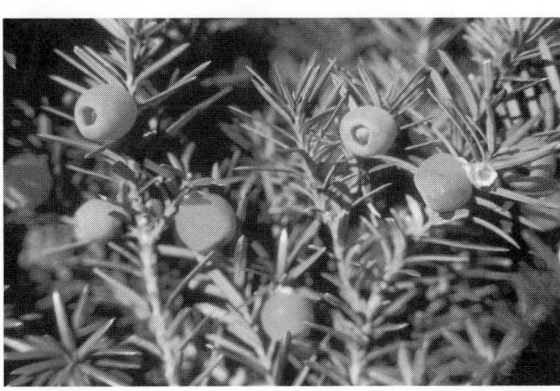

FIGURE 1 Typical yew (*Taxus*) foliage and berries.

mental evergreen shrubs. The Pacific yew is a native tree. These plants are commonly found in landscaped areas, and many animals are exposed to them when shrubs or clippings are removed and discarded in pastures. All parts of the plant are toxic except for the fleshy aril surrounding the seed. The plant is considered toxic either fresh or dried.

CLINICAL PRESENTATION

DISEASE FORMS/SUBTYPES Gastrointestinal (GI) and cardiac problems dominate the disease condition.

HISTORY, CHIEF COMPLAINT The most common complaint is a history of a single or multiple death(s) with few to no premonitory signs. Previously seen clinically normal animals are simply found dead.

PHYSICAL EXAM FINDINGS
- Colic: Not commonly observed
- Dyspnea, respiratory distress
- Weakness
- Muscle tremors
- Collapse
- Death from acute cardiac failure within 15 minutes to 4 hours after exposure

ETIOLOGY AND PATHOPHYSIOLOGY
- Volatile, irritant oils are responsible for the colic observed.
- Taxines interfere with cardiac conduction by inhibiting atrioventricular conduction, thereby slowing atrial and ventricular rates.
- Sodium and calcium channels may be impaired, or hyperkalemia may play a role.

DIAGNOSIS

DIFFERENTIAL DIAGNOSIS

Other cardiotoxic agents, including
- Oleander (*Nerium oleander*)
- Foxglove (*Digitalis* spp.)
- Rhododendron (*Rhododendron* spp.)
- Death camas (*Zigadenus* spp.)
- Ionophores (e.g., monensin, lasalocid, salinomycin, narasin)
- Acute selenium intoxication

INITIAL DATABASE

No specific changes

ADVANCED OR CONFIRMATORY TESTING

- Visual identification of characteristic plant material in GI contents
- Test for taxine in GI contents

TREATMENT

THERAPEUTIC GOAL(S)
- Reduce further GI absorption
- Treat clinical signs

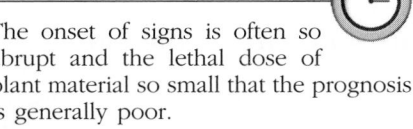

ACUTE GENERAL TREATMENT
- Administer activated charcoal and cathartic in the asymptomatic patient.
- Treat any cardiac arrhythmias observed; atropine or lidocaine may be warranted.

CHRONIC TREATMENT

Repeated use of activated charcoal

RECOMMENDED MONITORING

Monitor possibly exposed but asymptomatic animals for at least 48 hours.

PROGNOSIS AND OUTCOME

The onset of signs is often so abrupt and the lethal dose of plant material so small that the prognosis is generally poor.

PEARLS & CONSIDERATIONS

COMMENTS

This is a very common cause of poisoning and death in horses, mostly because of the popularity of these shrubs as ornamentals.

PREVENTION

Avoid access to the plant material.

CLIENT EDUCATION

Horse owners must be aware of the plants, shrubs, and trees in the area that can pose problems to their animals.

SUGGESTED READING

Burrows GE, Tyrl RJ: Taxus. In Burrows GE, Tyrl RJ, editors: *Toxic plants of North America*, Ames, IA, 2001, Iowa State University, pp 1149–1154.

AUTHOR: **PATRICIA A. TALCOTT**

EDITOR: **CYNTHIA L. GASKILL**

Temporohyoid Osteoarthropathy

BASIC INFORMATION

DEFINITION

Progressive degenerative osteoarthropathy of the articulation between the stylohyoid bone and the styloid process of the petrous temporal bone (temporohyoid articulation) leading to eventual ankylosis of this joint. The condition is generally unilateral, although bilateral involvement or disease can be seen.

EPIDEMIOLOGY

SPECIES, AGE, SEX The disease affects predominantly middle-aged horses of either sex.

RISK FACTORS Hematogenous infection leading to otitis media or interna. The author speculates that cribbing predisposes horses to this condition.

ASSOCIATED CONDITIONS AND DISORDERS
- The enlarging osteoarthropathy of the temporohyoid articulation leads to pain and discomfort and to a compressive

neuropathy with clinical signs dependent on the affected nerve(s). Nerves at risk are VII (facial), VIII (vestibulocochlear), IX (glossopharyngeal), and X (vagus). Finally, ankylosis of the temporohyoid articulation may lead to fracture of the petrous temporal bone, leading to cerebral hemorrhage, which can also cause facial and vestibular nerve damage as well as death.

- Ear polyps are occasionally seen associated with this disorder.

CLINICAL PRESENTATION

DISEASE FORMS/SUBTYPES Temporohyoid osteoarthropathy (THO) presents in one of three forms: Incidental findings, nonneurologic disease, and neurologic disease.

HISTORY, CHIEF COMPLAINT

- In the nonneurologic form, horses present with one or more of the following: Difficulty chewing; head shaking; cessation of cribbing; and behavior problems, especially when being ridden.
- In the neurologic form, horses present with one or more of the following: Ataxia, head tilt, deviation of the nose, falling while eating, and difficulty eating. Depression may also be present.

PHYSICAL EXAM FINDINGS

- In the nonneurologic forms, the following signs are observed: Difficulty chewing; head shaking; and behavior problems, especially when being ridden.
- In the neurologic form, the clinical signs are related to the specific nerve involved.
  - Facial nerve: All branches to the head are affected, causing a deviated muzzle (away from the side of the lesion) and a dropped lower lip, ear, and eyelid on the side of the lesion. Additionally, loss of innervation to the lacrimal gland may lead to keratoconjunctivitis sicca.
  - Vestibulocochlear nerve: Signs vary from mild head tilt and circling to severe horizontal nystagmus (quick phase away from the side of the lesion), recumbency, and seizure-like activity.
  - Glossopharyngeal and vagal nerves: Dysphagia
- In both clinical presentations, pain may be induced by palpation of the base of the ear or by dorsal pressure on the ventral aspect of the basihyoid bone. In addition, ear polyps may be present on the affected side. One may also note abnormalities in both left and right temporohyoid articulations, although signs relating to these lesions occurring in both sides during the same clinical presentation are unlikely.

ETIOLOGY AND PATHOPHYSIOLOGY

- Most commonly a degenerative osteoarthropathy of unknown cause
- Adjacent infection (septic otitis media or interna and temporomandibular joint injection) may by extension lead to this condition.

DIAGNOSIS

DIFFERENTIAL DIAGNOSIS

- Peripheral vestibular disease such as otitis media or interna
- Trauma to the facial nerve
- Skull fractures with other causes

INITIAL DATABASE

- Endoscopy of the guttural pouch to reveal enlargement of the most dorsal aspect of the stylohyoid bone
- Radiographic evidence of enlargement of the affected stylohyoid bone
- Radiographic enlargement and sclerosis of the tympanic bulla

ADVANCED OR CONFIRMATORY TESTING

- Computed tomographic (Figure 1) examination confirms THO by enlargement and degeneration of the temporohyoid articulation. In addition, otitis media or interna may be evidenced by fluid of some tissue density in the tympanic bulla or inner ear.
- Auditory abnormalities occur (brainstem auditory evoked response test).

TREATMENT

THERAPEUTIC GOAL(S)

- Decrease the inflammation
- Provide analgesia and removal of pressure or pain associated with enlarged temporohyoid articulation

- Prevent or control local infection
- Remove the risk of petrous temporal bone fracture

ACUTE GENERAL TREATMENT

- Antiinflammatory and analgesic treatments routinely include phenylbutazone (2 mg/kg q12h IV as needed but generally around 14 days).
- Antiinflammatory treatments also include dimethyl sulfoxide (DMSO). Horses with severe vestibular signs can be treated with a tapering course of corticosteroids (0.04–0.08 mg/kg of dexamethasone).
- Treatment with antimicrobials for either extension of a possible adjacent infection (otitis interna or media, temporomandibular joint) or for prevention of secondary infection in the hemorrhage that follows fracture. Consider ampicillin, trimethoprim-sulfa, enrofloxacin, or chloramphenicol for 2 to 4 weeks.
- If present, treat keratoconjunctivitis sicca associated with facial nerve paralysis with frequent eye lubrication. It is more effective and practical to perform a partial tarsorrhaphy.
- Removal of the pressure on the temporohyoid articulation caused by swallowing is attained by ipsilateral ceratohyoidectomy.
- Elimination of the risk of petrous temporal bone fracture and death is achieved by ipsilateral ceratohyoidectomy.

CHRONIC TREATMENT

Surgery is usually performed in the acute state but can be done in the recovery phase to prevent the likelihood of risk of petrous temporal bone fracture and death.

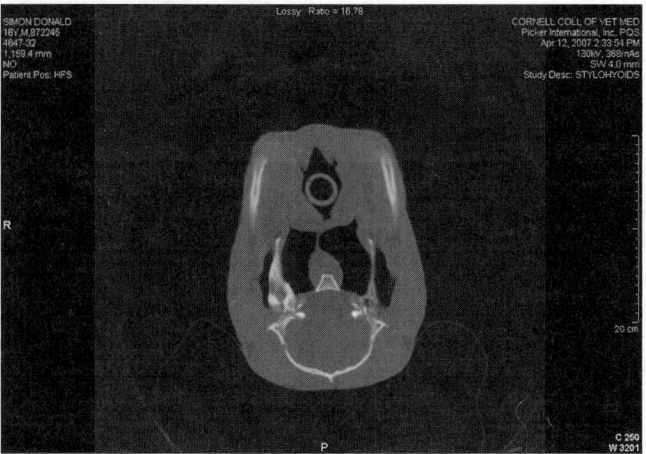

FIGURE 1 Computed tomography examination of a 16-year-old gelding with visible enlargement of the right temporohyoid articulation compared with the normal left side.

POSSIBLE COMPLICATIONS

Petrous temporal bone fracture leading to cerebral hemorrhage and death

RECOMMENDED MONITORING

Reevaluation at 4 months is recommended to assess the improvement in vestibular signs and status of ipsilateral cornea and conjunctiva.

PROGNOSIS AND OUTCOME

The majority of animals respond to treatment, but a significant number (~60%) have some remaining neurologic deficits. However, as illustrated in a recent report, 19 of 20 surviving horses were able to resume their athletic activity despite those deficits.

PEARLS & CONSIDERATIONS

COMMENTS

This is a rare and debilitating disease that is associated with a fair prognosis to return to function. The value of surgery is preventing petrous temporal bone fracture and death and has been neither proven nor dismissed because of the lack of treatment randomization and evidence-based data. Subjectively, the surgery markedly alleviates pain in horses that are dysphagic and thus renders the animal much more comfortable.

CLIENT EDUCATION

Early recognition of neurologic deficit such as head tilt, a deviated nose, and dysphagia are required to initiate aggressive antiinflammatory therapy to preserve nerve function.

SUGGESTED READING

Aleman M, Puchalski SM, Williams DC, et al: Brainstem auditory-evoked responses in horses with temporohyoid osteoarthropathy. *J Vet Intern Med* 5:1196–1202, 2008.

Blythe LL, Watrous BJ: Temporohyoid osteoarthropathy. *Curr Ther Equine Med* 4:323–325, 1997.

Divers TJ, Ducharme NG, de Lahunta A, et al: Temporohyoid osteoarthropathy. *Clin Tech Equine Pract* 5:17–23, 2006.

Pease AP, van Biervliet J, Dykes NL, et al: Complication of partial stylohyoidectomy for treatment of temporohyoid osteoarthropathy and an alternative surgical technique in three cases. *Equine Vet* 36:546–550, 2004.

Walker AM, Sellon DC, Cornelisse CJ, et al: Temporohyoid osteoarthropathy in 33 horses (1993–2000). *J Vet Intern Med* 16:697–703, 2002.

AUTHOR: **NORM G. DUCHARME**

EDITOR: **ERIC J. PARENTE**

Tendinitis and Desmitis

BASIC INFORMATION

DEFINITION

- Tendinitis: Inflammatory conditions of tendons, their muscle or bone attachments, or both encompassing a broad range of injuries from strains to severe fiber pattern disruption
- Desmitis: Inflammatory conditions of the ligaments, their bone attachments, or both encompassing a broad range of injuries from strains to severe fiber pattern disruption

SYNONYM(S)

Sprains, "bowed" tendon (specifically tendinitis of the superficial digital flexor tendon)

EPIDEMIOLOGY

RISK FACTORS

- Tendon and ligament injuries are a leading cause of decreased performance and loss of use in equine athletes. The true incidence is largely unknown but some estimate that as high as 40% of equine athletes develop some degree of tendinitis or desmitis.
- There are significant risk factors for tendon and ligament injuries, particularly in Equine athletes. In addition to those listed below, breed, occupation, age, and level of performance play roles in determining the probability

of injury and which tendon(s) or ligament(s) is involved and the prognosis for return to use. For example, superficial digital flexor tendinitis is a more common and severe injury in racehorses and event horses. Familiarity with the patient's occupation and associated tendon and ligament conditions are invaluable in the diagnosis and treatment of tendon and ligament conditions.

- Training regimen: Poor conditioning or maladaptive remodeling.
- Surface: Deep or inconsistent surfaces are thought to place more stress on tendon and ligaments.
- Contributory lameness: Lameness in the opposite limb or other limb that results in a compensatory tendon or ligament injury because of "overloading."
- Shoeing and trimming (toe length, heel angle and balance): Long toe underrun heels increases the strain on the deep digital flexor tendon; poor medial to lateral balance may increase strain on collateral ligaments and suspensory branches. High heel angles increase stress to the suspensory ligament and superficial digital flexor tendon.
- Conformation: Some conformations may place more stress on tendons and ligaments such as horses that are back at the knee or club footed.

- Poor bandaging technique: May bind or place excessive pressure on tendons. A bandage "bow" is superficial digital flexor tendinitis from poor bandaging.

ASSOCIATED CONDITIONS AND DISORDERS Lameness, poor performance, avulsion fractures, tenosynovitis, sesamoiditis, bursitis, enthesopathy

CLINICAL PRESENTATION

HISTORY, CHIEF COMPLAINT

- The history is variable, from acute swelling with or without significant lameness to insidious lameness with or without significant localizing signs.
- Swelling or heat associated with a tendon or ligament.
- Lameness with or without associated physical signs.

PHYSICAL EXAM FINDINGS

- Visible or palpable swelling with heat and sensitivity. Lameness is variable and may be mild to severe depending on the duration of the injury and the structure involved.
- Lameness without visible or palpable swelling, heat, or sensitivity.
- Visible or palpable distension of synovial structure such as the digital flexor tendon sheath or carpal canal.

ETIOLOGY AND PATHOPHYSIOLOGY

- Single event of supraphysiologic force.
- Maladaptive remodeling: Microdamage accumulates as the tendon or

ligament is unable to adapt to the level of training or exercise placed upon it. This culminates with a strain or fiber pattern disruption but differs from the above in that there is a subclinical phase.
- Trauma: Direct physical force such as an overreaching injury and pressure-induced inflammation as seen in poor bandaging technique.

DIAGNOSIS

DIFFERENTIAL DIAGNOSIS

- Visible or palpable limb swelling
  - Cellulitis
  - Other infection such as swelling secondary to subsolar abscessation or severe dermatitis
  - Bony injury, including fractures and osteomyelitis or osteitis
  - Peritendinous or ligamentous swelling from trauma
  - Synovitis: Generally confined to the limits of the synovial structure
- Without observable or palpable swelling or effusion: Bone, joint, muscle, or neurologic conditions that cause lameness

INITIAL DATABASE

- Physical examination: Emphasis on digital palpation of the tendon and ligaments of the extremities in an effort to isolate regions of heat, swelling, and pain
- Lameness examination: Critical for injuries without obvious localizing signs on physical examination; a complete lameness examination and diagnostic anesthesia may be necessary. Diagnostic anesthesia may be used to support physical findings and diagnosis.
- Ultrasonographic examination: Ultrasonography may be used to localize and document the source of inflammation and determine the severity of fiber pattern compromise if a tendon or ligament is involved. Methodic evaluation and measurement of the cross-sectional area of the structure and the lesion cross-sectional area and evaluation of the fiber pattern are important to document the severity of the injury and serve as a baseline for monitoring rehabilitation. Comparative imaging of the contralateral limb is necessary to establish normal tendon or ligament characteristics for the individual and to rule out bilateral injury, which is common in superficial digital flexor tendinitis and suspensory desmitis.
- Radiographic examination: Radiography is indicated to evaluate the enthesis (bony attachment) in tendon and ligament injuries and to rule out primary bony injuries and potential dystrophic mineralization.

ADVANCED OR CONFIRMATORY TESTING

- Magnetic resonance imaging: Good for soft tissue injuries of the foot and localized lameness in the extremities that appear normal on ultrasonography and radiography.
- Scintigraphy: Especially useful in injuries involving an enthesis. A "soft tissue" phase may show increased radiopharmaceutical uptake in an injured tendon or ligament.

TREATMENT

THERAPEUTIC GOAL(S)

- Reduce inflammation and continued fiber damage
- Prevent further mechanical injury
- Promote healing
- Encourage rapid granulation of areas of fiber pattern loss
- Minimize scarring; encourage early organization of repair tissue

ACUTE GENERAL TREATMENT

- Antiinflammatory drugs
  - Systemic nonsteroidal antiinflammatory drugs (NSAIDs) (phenylbutazone, flunixin meglumine): An optional single systemic dose of corticosteroids, generally triamcinolone (10 mg IM)
  - Local: Icing for 30 to 40 minutes daily for 2 to 4 weeks followed by bandaging with poultice or other antiinflammatory topical treatment
- Rest: Stall rest with handwalking, if sound at the walk, until the injury can be better defined and inflammation is under control.
- Bandaging or compression: For injuries that can be bandaged (generally limited to the extremities) poultice, topical NSAIDs, Furacin, or alcohol can be used with bandaging.
- Intralesional therapies (ie, platelet-rich plasma [PRP] or stem cells): Thought to be most effective in the acute stage of injury before there is significant granulation or scarring of the tendon or ligament.
- Surgical treatments: For select injuries, tendon or ligament decompression (splitting or "desmoplasty") and superior check ligament desmotomy for the treatment of superficial digital flexor tendinitis.

CHRONIC TREATMENT

- Graded controlled exercise program with serial ultrasonographic monitoring.
- Treatment of any contributory conditions such as foot imbalance, long toe, or lameness in other limbs that may result in overloading.
- Extracorporeal shock-wave therapy may provide analgesia and improve healing.
- Intralesional therapies are ideally used in the acute phase but may have benefit for chronic injuries.
- Surgical treatments: Including one or a combination desmoplasty, fasciotomy, and neurectomy.

POSSIBLE COMPLICATIONS

The most common complication is reinjury of the tendon or ligament. Injury of a tendon or ligament in the opposite limb after rehabilitation is also considered a complication.

RECOMMENDED MONITORING

- Daily examination of the injured area to detect inflammation
- Serial ultrasonographic monitoring to evaluate progress by comparing the cross-sectional area, lesion cross-sectional area, and fiber pattern

PROGNOSIS AND OUTCOME

The prognosis for healing and pasture soundness for most tendon and ligament injuries is good. However, the prognosis for a high level of athletic activity for most of the injuries, with the exception of strains, is guarded to poor. Several factors contribute to this prognosis, including the severity of injury, the structure injured, the quality of healing, and the intended future use. The following are generalities.

- Severity of injury: Lesions that involve 0% to 10% of the structure are considered mild, lesions that involve 10% to 25% are considered moderate, and those that involve greater than 25% are considered severe. Reinjuries can almost always be considered severe in terms of prognosis.
- Structure injured: Hindlimb proximal suspensory ligaments, suspensory branches (especially medial), and injuries within the digital sheath are examples of structures that generally carry a more guarded prognosis. Injuries of the accessory ligaments of the deep digital and superficial digital flexor tendons generally have a more favorable prognosis.
- Quality of healing: Much of the therapeutic focus is geared toward improving healing. Injuries that fill in rapidly and develop a near-normal fiber pattern appear to have the best prognosis. Conversely, injuries that maintain significant fiber pattern loss or remain significantly enlarged appear to more consistently reinjure when the

athlete is placed back at a similar level. Surrounding fibrosis and dystrophic mineralization are generally poor prognostic indicators. A good fiber pattern often can be achieved relatively early in the healing process, especially in injuries treated in the acute phase with intralesional therapies. The inclination is to accelerate the rehabilitation process, which can be a mistake because it is difficult to evaluate strength.

- Intended future use: Often horses have an improved prognosis at a lower level or with a less demanding occupation. For example, many racehorses with moderate to severe tendon injuries can have successful careers as lower level sport horses.

PEARLS & CONSIDERATIONS

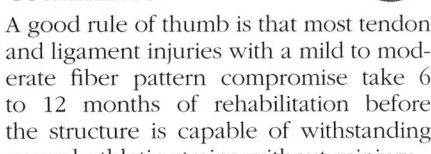

COMMENTS
A good rule of thumb is that most tendon and ligament injuries with a mild to moderate fiber pattern compromise take 6 to 12 months of rehabilitation before the structure is capable of withstanding normal athletic strains without reinjury.

PREVENTION
Attention to the aforementioned contributory factors and client education

CLIENT EDUCATION
The client should be informed of the anatomy of the structure involved and

methods to monitor inflammation. Routine monitoring of the extremities for signs of inflammation should be performed in all equine athletes. Areas showing signs of inflammation should be evaluated by a veterinarian and treated appropriately.

SUGGESTED READING
Gillis C: Ultrasonography for monitoring healing and rehabilitation. *Adv Orthop Clin Tech Equine Pract* 6(3):174–178, 2007.
Ross MW, Dyson SJ: The soft tissues. In Ross MW, Dyson SJ, editors: *Diagnosis and management of lameness in the horse,* St Louis, 2003, Saunders Elsevier, pp 616–723.

AUTHOR: **W. WESLEY SUTTER**

EDITOR: **ANDRIS J. KANEPS**

Tenosynovitis

BASIC INFORMATION

DEFINITION
The digital flexor tendon sheath (DFTS) is the synovial compartment located on the palmar/plantar aspect of the distal extremities surrounding the superficial and deep digital flexor tendons as they pass over the metacarpophalangeal and metatarsophalangeal and proximal interphalangeal joints. The sheath begins approximately at the junction of the middle and distal third of the metacarpus or metatarsus and continues to near the navicular bursa distally.

SYNONYM(S)
Vagina synovialis tendinis, theca tendinis, tendon sheath tendinitis

EPIDEMIOLOGY
RISK FACTORS
- Synovitis with trauma: Athletic activity, overreaching injury, rundown injuries
- Sepsis with trauma: Intrathecal injection, puncture wounds and lacerations, surgery, extension of superficial infection

ASSOCIATED CONDITIONS AND DISORDERS
- Desmitis: Most commonly the proximal annular ligament, but involvement of the digital annular ligaments has been described
- Tendinitis: Deep and superficial digital flexor tendinitis within the sheath as well as injuries to the manica flexoria

CLINICAL PRESENTATION
DISEASE FORMS/SUBTYPES Noninfectious synovitis of the DFTS can be categorized in three stages:
- Stage 1 (effusive): Mild to moderate soft and fluctuant effusion in one or more limbs with no associated lameness and no pain on palpation or significant response to fetlock flexion. This stage generally improves with work.
- Stage 2 (proliferative): Mild to moderate firm distension of the sheath with mild to moderate lameness and a positive response to fetlock flexion and palpation.
- Stage 3 (proliferative with adhesions and synovial masses): Firm and painful on palpation with severe lameness (may be reluctant to place heel down) and significant loss of comfortable range of motion (ROM) in the fetlock.
- Annular ligament syndrome: Often associated with DFTS synovitis. The palmar/plantar annular ligament (PAL) counteracts the forces placed on the proximal sesamoid bones during fetlock extension. This syndrome may be a primary injury or secondary response to chronic inflammation of the DFTS. Fibrosis of the PAL is a contributing factor in lameness associated with the DFTS.
- Infectious synovitis: Generally associated with wounds entering the DFTS but may be iatrogenic with intrathecal injection or surgery. Infection of the axial border of the proximal sesamoid bones may enter the tendon sheath, fetlock joint, or both, depending on

the location and integrity of the intrasesamoidean ligament.
HISTORY, CHIEF COMPLAINT Swelling of the DFTS with or without lameness. This may be an acute or progressive onset.
PHYSICAL EXAM FINDINGS Enlargement of the DFTS sheath, lameness
ETIOLOGY AND PATHOPHYSIOLOGY Traumatic capsulitis or synovitis to the DFTS lining. This may include tearing of the vincula, synovial herniation, or damage to the tendons or manica flexoria and PAL.

DIAGNOSIS

DIFFERENTIAL DIAGNOSIS
- Cellulitis: Swelling and edema around the fetlock as a result of infection not associated with the tendon sheath.
- Fetlock joint synovitis: The swelling is generally confined to the dorsal aspect of the fetlock and the palmar/plantar outpouchings that are dorsal to the suspensory branches.
- Extension of bony injury or infection into the tendon sheath such as osteitis of the axial margin of the proximal sesamoid bones.
- DFTS synovitis: Noninfectious or infectious.

INITIAL DATABASE
- Physical examination: Digital palpation of the tendon sheath noting the character of swelling (fluctuant or firm), pain on palpation, and comfortable ROM.

- Lameness examination: Baseline lameness and response to fetlock flexion.

ADVANCED OR CONFIRMATORY TESTING

- Synovial fluid analysis: Generally used to confirm infectious synovitis.
- Distension of the synovial sheath with saline may be used to confirm communication with a wound.
- Diagnostic anesthesia: Intrathecal injection of an anesthetic agent (generally 8–12 mL of mepivacaine).
- Ultrasonography: This is the primary confirmatory diagnostic tool. Tendon sheath effusion or proliferative synovitis can be confirmed. Tendonitis of the DDFT and superficial digital flexor tendon can often be confirmed by demonstrating areas of tendon enlargement or loss of fiber pattern. The PAL should be evaluated for thickening (>2 mm) or loss of fiber pattern.
- Radiography: Indicated to rule out bony changes associated with DFTS synovitis. The insertions of the PAL and intersesamoidean ligament on the proximal sesamoid bones should be evaluated. Contrast radiography can be used to confirm communication with a wound or evaluate the integrity of the sheath.
- Magnetic resonance imaging: May be beneficial in pinpointing the underlying cause of the DFTS synovitis and evaluating bony involvement.

TREATMENT

THERAPEUTIC GOAL(S)

- Minimize continued inflammation and damage and treat the underlying cause
- If infectious, treat for synovial infection

ACUTE GENERAL TREATMENT

- Noninfectious (DFTS synovitis, PAL syndrome)
  - Systemic antiinflammatory drugs (phenylbutazone or flunixin meglumine) for 5 to 7 days; optional single systemic dose of corticosteroids (dexamethasone phosphate or triamcinolone).
  - Local therapy: Icing 30 minutes twice daily for 5 to 7 days followed by bandaging with antiinflammatory sweat or poultice.
  - Controlled exercise: If sound at the walk, handwalking for 2 to 3 weeks.
  - Intrathecal corticosteroids: 40 to 80 mg of methylprednisolone or 10 mg of triamcinolone; this may be combined with hyaluronic acid. If tendon injury is observed on ultrasonography, intrathecal corticosteroid use is controversial and should not be used to keep the horse in work.
  - Intralesional treatment of concomitant tendon or ligament injuries with platelet-rich plasma (PRP) or stem cells is likely best done in the acute phase.
  - Injuries involving obvious tendon or manica tearing may benefit from tenoscopic debridement in this phase.
- Infectious
  - Culture and antibiotic sensitivity of synovial fluid
  - Systemic broad-spectrum intravenous antibiotics. This generally includes potassium penicillin and gentamicin.
  - Local antibiotic therapy: Including intrathecal antibiotics, regional limb perfusion, or both
  - Lavage ideally with tenoscopy.

CHRONIC TREATMENT

- Noninfectious
  - Graded controlled exercise program.
  - Medical: Intrathecal administration of corticosteroids. The efficacy of intrathecal interleukin-1 receptor antagonist protein, PRP, or stem cells is unknown.
  - Surgical: Diagnostic tenoscopy, debridement of tendon injuries, and generally PAL desmotomy
- Infectious: Same principles as acute treatment but with tenoscopic debridement and open drainage of the tendon sheath

POSSIBLE COMPLICATIONS

Continued inflammation and progressive lameness resulting in loss of use

RECOMMENDED MONITORING

- Noninfectious: Lameness level, synovial distension, loss of comfortable ROM
- Infectious: Lameness level, serial synovial fluid analyses

PROGNOSIS AND OUTCOME

- Noninfectious: Favorable prognosis in acute stages 1 and 2 without significant tendon injury or PAL thickening with medical management. Good prognosis in horses with primary PAL thickening and surgical treatment. Guarded to poor prognosis with stage 3 or horses that have chronic stage 2 or significant tendon injury.
- Infectious: Fair to good prognosis in horses treated rapidly and aggressively with systemic antibiotics, local antibiotics, and lavage. Poor to guarded prognosis in chronic infections.

PEARLS & CONSIDERATIONS

PREVENTION

The early stages of DFTS synovitis may not be preventable. The primary goal is to prevent or slow progression into the more severe stages. This can be achieved by early medical treatment, modification of the exercise program, and continued monitoring.

CLIENT EDUCATION

Monitoring of the DFTS for signs of inflammation or progression from soft fluctuant effusion (stage 1) to more firm and painful effusion.

SUGGESTED READING

Gillis C: Soft tissue injuries to the palmar aspect of the pastern. In White NA, Moore JN, editors: *Current techniques in equine surgery and lameness*, ed 2, Philadelphia, 1998, WB Saunders, pp 334–341.

Schramme MC, Smith RKW: Diseases of the digital synovial sheath, palmar annular ligament and digital annular ligaments. In Ross MW, Dyson SJ, editors: *Diagnosis and management of lameness in the horse*, St Louis, 2003, Saunders Elsevier, pp 674–683.

AUTHOR: W. WESLEY SUTTER

EDITOR: ANDRIS J. KANEPS

Testicular Degeneration

BASIC INFORMATION

DEFINITION

A pathologic process resulting in disruption of the normal histologic architecture of the seminiferous epithelium and of normal sperm production. This is an acquired condition and may have an identifiable cause or may be idiopathic.

SYNONYM(S)

Testicular atrophy

EPIDEMIOLOGY

SPECIES, AGE, SEX The idiopathic form is most commonly diagnosed in middle-aged to older stallions. However, postpubescent stallions of any age may be affected by testicular degeneration, often secondary to a known cause.

CLINICAL PRESENTATION

DISEASE FORMS/SUBTYPES
- Acquired testicular degeneration of known cause (TD)
- Idiopathic testicular degeneration (ITD): Age-related or senile testicular degeneration

HISTORY, CHIEF COMPLAINT
- Intensively managed breeding stallions with TD will be presented for decreased semen quality and pregnancy rates. Changes in testicular size and consistency may have been noted.
- "Acute" onset reduction in fertility: Stallions are often presented with perceived acute onset reduction in fertility in the absence of other overt problems of the reproductive system. Because ITD is an insidious process, changes may go unnoticed until semen quality becomes critically poor.
- Scrotal asymmetry: Stallions not monitored closely may be presented for unilateral testicular enlargement when, in fact, testicular atrophy has occurred contralaterally.
- Included in the history may be external genital trauma, systemic illness including a febrile episode, or administration of anabolic steroids.

PHYSICAL EXAM FINDINGS Palpation of scrotal contents
- ITD: Normally sized testes in early stage, symmetrically small and soft in progressing disease, and symmetrically small and soft with relatively large epididymal tails in advanced cases. In end-stage ITD, testes are symmetrically very small and firm, often with a corrugated tunica albuginea (ribbing).

- TD: In acute cases, no changes in testicular size or consistency may be noted. However, findings referable to the cause of degeneration may be apparent (eg, scrotal edema, hydrocele, hematoma, or puncture wound). In chronic cases, changes in testicular size and consistency, unilateral or bilateral, may be noted. Evidence of prior trauma, including scars, draining tracts, or lack of testicular mobility, may be observed.

ETIOLOGY AND PATHOPHYSIOLOGY
- TD may be unilateral or bilateral, depending on whether the cause is local or systemic. Local insults primarily affect one testis. Degeneration may be induced through direct damage to seminiferous epithelium, increased intrascrotal temperatures ($\geq 2°–3°$ C above normal), or impaired testicular mobility and thermoregulatory efficiency caused by adhesions.
- Trauma
- Orchitis or periorchitis, testicular abscess
- Testicular hematoma
- Circulatory disturbances: Spermatic cord torsion, varicocele
- Testicular neoplasia
- Scrotal edema
- Hematocele
- Hydrocele
- Sperm outflow obstruction
- Incomplete testicular descent: Systemic causes affecting both testes
- Systemic infection with febrile episode
- Administration of exogenous androgens
- Exposure of testes to extreme ambient temperatures, radiation, toxins
- Autoimmune disease resulting in production of antisperm antibodies
- Removal of the cause may result in varying degrees of recovery of testicular function because spermatogonia, Sertoli cells, and Leydig cells are relatively resistant to damage and will reinstitute spermatogenesis.
- Although the pathophysiology of ITD has not been elucidated, preliminary evidence suggests an inherent testicular defect, likely in the Sertoli cell.

DIAGNOSIS

DIFFERENTIAL DIAGNOSIS
- Testicular hypoplasia
- Unilateral testicular enlargement: Upon visual inspection, stallions with asymmetric testes may be incorrectly assessed to have unilateral testicular

atrophy when the smaller testis is normal and the contralateral testis enlarged.

INITIAL DATABASE
- Semen collection and evaluation
  - Libido: Likely normal
  - Ejaculate volume: May be normal
  - Concentration of spermatozoa: Low unless prolonged sexual rest
  - Total sperm count: Low unless prolonged sexual rest
  - Progressive motility of sperm: Low
  - Sperm morphology: Low percentage of morphologically normal sperm; abnormally high percentage of immature spermatogenic or multinucleated giant cells may be present
- Measurement of total scrotal width (TSW) using calipers: Usually significantly smaller than normal; compare TSW with previous measurements and with published data (2- to 3-year-old stallions should have a TSW ≥ 8 cm; older stallions should have a TSW ≥ 9 cm)

ADVANCED OR CONFIRMATORY TESTING
- Ultrasonography of scrotal contents to evaluate for orchitis, testicular abscess, hematoma, neoplasia, and hydrocele are generally unremarkable.
- Measurement of testes using ultrasonography: Obtain the length, width, and height of each testis; calculate the total scrotal volume and total expected sperm output; testicular degeneration or atrophy is confirmed when the actual sperm count is less than the expected sperm count.
- Semen collection and evaluation with the stallion at daily sperm output followed by calculation of sperm production efficiency.
- Reproductive hormone and peptide analysis not routinely applied, although circulating concentrations of estradiol, testosterone, and inhibin tend to be lower and follicle-stimulating hormone higher in subfertile stallions.
- Histopathologic evaluation of testicular biopsy or fine-needle aspirate: Although possible, this is generally not necessary if physical examination and semen evaluation findings support diagnosis. Evaluation of single aspirate or biopsy sample may be nondiagnostic. When the cause has been identified and removed, the risk of the procedure may outweigh the value of the information obtained.

TREATMENT

THERAPEUTIC GOAL(S)

- Treat acute external genital trauma to deter development of prolonged, severe, or irreversible TD.
- Resolve chronic predisposing conditions to halt the progression of ongoing TD.
- In cases of ITD, manage the stallion for breeding to optimize fertility and consider preserving genetics.

ACUTE GENERAL TREATMENT

- Most cases of TD and ITD are presented in the chronic phase, and it is impossible to identify an active cause. Efforts are targeted at managing the stallion to optimize reproductive efficiency.
- In acute cases of mild to moderate external genital trauma, treat with cold hydrotherapy, administer antiinflammatory medications, and provide antimicrobial prophylaxis.
- Prompt hemiorchidectomy of affected testis in cases of spermatic cord torsion, severe trauma, neoplasia, and fulminating orchitis.

CHRONIC TREATMENT

- Reevaluation of semen quality beginning 2 months after resolution of inciting cause or initial evaluation.
- In managing subfertile stallions with testicular degeneration, limit mare book and schedule breedings to maximize sexual rest and allow for accumulation of sperm stores between matings. Add extender to semen to increase sperm longevity and breed mares close to ovulation. Consider sperm cryopreservation and use of assisted reproductive technologies when permitted by breed registry.

RECOMMENDED MONITORING

- Monthly semen evaluations
- Periodic testicular measurements: TSW; testicular volume and sperm production efficiency calculation

PROGNOSIS AND OUTCOME

- When a cause can be identified and removed, variable degrees of recovery of testicular function and semen quality occur. Improvement of semen quality may be partial or complete but requires up to 5 months after resolution of the underlying cause.
- If a cause cannot be identified but ITD is not suspected, semen quality may improve over 2 to 5 months.
- If ITD is suspected, the condition is slowly progressive. With no effective treatment, careful management of the breeding stallion will allow use of subfertile stallions in breeding programs before the animals' becoming azoospermic.

PEARLS & CONSIDERATIONS

COMMENTS

- Testicular degeneration may be present in the absence of decreased testicular size.
- A lag time of approximately 10 days may exist between the inciting cause and the appearance of poor semen quality.
- Because the semen characteristics and histopathologic features of hypoplastic and degenerative testes are similar,

physical examination findings may be helpful in differentiating between these conditions. In a stallion presented with bilaterally symmetrically small testes and limited historical information regarding prior semen quality, the presence of large epididymal tails relative to testes size and easily palpable epididymal bodies may help to differentiate testicular degeneration from testicular hypoplasia, in which the testes and epididymal tails are proportionally small because of concurrent epididymal hypoplasia.

PREVENTION

- There is no known means of preventing ITD.
- Prompt treatment of trauma to the external genitalia and systemic disease may help reduce the duration and severity of resultant TD.
- Routine monitoring of testicular size and consistency along with semen quality in breeding stallions allows for earlier diagnosis and management adjustments.

SUGGESTED READING

Blanchard TL, Johnson L, Roser AJ: Increased germ cell loss rates and poor semen quality in stallions with idiopathic testicular degeneration. *J Equine Vet Sci* 20:263–265, 2004.

Roser JF: Reproductive endocrinology of the stallion. In Samper JC, editor: *Equine breeding management and artificial insemination*, St Louis, 2009, Saunders Elsevier, pp 17–31.

Turner RMO: Pathogenesis, diagnosis, and management of testicular degeneration in stallions. *Clin Tech Equine Pract* 6:278–284, 2007.

AUTHOR: **DAWNA L. VOELKL**

EDITOR: **JUAN C. SAMPER**

Tetanus

BASIC INFORMATION

DEFINITION

Tetanus is an infectious disease of all species that results in persistent hypertonia of the striated muscles with clonic paroxysmal muscular spasms superimposed. The causative agent is *Clostridium tetani* (*C. tetani*).

SYNONYM(S)

Lockjaw

EPIDEMIOLOGY

RISK FACTORS

- Entry of organisms into the animal is usually by inoculation into a deep wound if traumatized or devitalized tissue has become contaminated with spores. The spores can remain dormant until necrosis of the tissue provides the strict anaerobic environment necessary for germination to the vegetative, toxin-producing form.
- Wounds that serve as the initial site of introduction of *C. tetani* may involve unbroken skin or be healed by the

time clinical signs are observed, complicating efforts at diagnosis.
- Other potential sites of entry include surgical sites; the umbilicus of neonatal foals; and the postfoaling reproductive tract, especially if dystocia or a retained placenta occurred.

CONTAGION AND ZOONOSIS The vegetative form of *C. tetani* is susceptible to heat and numerous disinfectants. Production of round terminal spores enables persistence in the environment in the absence of direct sunlight for a prolonged period (years). Spores are resistant to boiling water and many standard disinfection techniques.

GEOGRAPHY AND SEASONALITY *C. tetani* is a common soil inhabitant found throughout the world. It can also be easily isolated from the intestinal tract and feces of a wide range of animals.

CLINICAL PRESENTATION

DISEASE FORMS/SUBTYPES

- Localized tetanus: Muscular rigidity and spasms in the vicinity of the infected wound. This usually progresses to generalized tetanus affecting the entire body. The initial manifestation of tetanus is most often generalized rather than localized.
- Generalized tetanus: Characteristic "sawhorse" stance with an extended rigid tail and stiff gait if the horse remains ambulatory. Extensor muscle rigidity causes difficulty in standing or lying down.

HISTORY, CHIEF COMPLAINT Sudden onset of stiff gait, muscle stiffness, or recumbency

PHYSICAL EXAM FINDINGS

- Fever
- Stiff gait
- Nostril flaring
- Trismus
- Hyperresponsive to tactile and auditory stimuli
- Prolapsed nictitans
- Regurgitation and laryngeal dysfunction
- Elevated tail head
- Signs are exacerbated by external stimuli, however mild. As a result of hyperesthesia, painful reflex muscle spasms may progress to generalized tonic contractions with opisthotonus.
- Disease progression makes voluntary movement impossible because of marked extensor rigidity of all four limbs; this often leads to recumbency.

ETIOLOGY AND PATHOPHYSIOLOGY

- Three toxins are produced of varying effects and importance.
  - Tetanospasmin produces the classical signs of tetanus. Toxin diffuses into adjacent tissues, ascends centripetally along the α motor neurons, and enters the lymphatics and bloodstream. Tetanospasmin blocks the inhibitory synapses of spinal cord motor neurons by preventing neurotransmitter release (glycine and γ-aminobutyric acid [GABA]), thereby inducing a spastic paralysis.
  - Tetanolysin allows the spread of clostridial infection by increasing the amount of local tissue necrosis.
  - Nonspasmogenic toxin
- Death results from respiratory failure, secondary to respiratory muscle spasm, or respiratory arrest caused by medullary intoxication or aspiration

pneumonia secondary to dysphagia or increased airway secretions.
- No characteristic necropsy lesions can be ascribed to the tetanus toxins themselves.

DIAGNOSIS

DIFFERENTIAL DIAGNOSIS

- Seizure activity
- Colic
- Laminitis
- Hepatic encephalopathy
- Meningitis
- Electrolyte derangements: Sodium, calcium
- Intoxication with lead

INITIAL DATABASE

- A presumptive diagnosis of tetanus is based on history, clinical signs, and response to treatment.
- Hematology, serum chemistry, and cerebrospinal fluid analysis are usually unremarkable.
- Neutrophilic leukocytosis with left shift may be observed with wound sepsis or aspiration pneumonia.
- Muscle enzymes may be elevated (creatine kinase and aspartate aminotransferase) because of muscle trauma from sustained contracture and prolonged recumbency.

ADVANCED OR CONFIRMATORY TESTING

- Gram staining of wound aspirates is of limited diagnostic value. Sporulated and vegetative forms of *C. tetani* appear similar to other anaerobic bacteria.
- Isolation of *C. tetani* is difficult because of low concentration of wound-contaminating organisms and the strict anaerobic conditions required for culture.

TREATMENT

THERAPEUTIC GOAL(S)

- Local and parenteral antibiotic therapy to prevent further production of tetanospasmin by eradication of the vegetative form of *C. tetani* at the site of infection
- Neutralizing unbound toxin not yet affecting the central nervous system
- Control of muscular spasms and rigidity with sedatives and muscle relaxants
- Generation of active immunity to tetanus toxins

ACUTE GENERAL TREATMENT

- Penicillin: Drug of choice for eliminating the vegetative form. Recommended to be administered at high dose rates

(50,000 IU/kg) on a schedule appropriate for the formulation. Other antimicrobials that may be effective include the tetracyclines, macrolides (avoid in adults), and metronidazole.
- Tetanus antitoxin (TAT): Sourced from the sera of hyperimmunized horses. After it has been administered to the affected horse, the passively acquired antibodies neutralize unbound toxin both circulating in the blood and present in the wound. Dose rates vary widely, with the efficacy of higher doses debatable. Up to 500 IU/kg is recommended. Intrathecal doses up to 5000 IU are also reported.
- Phenothiazine derivatives: Work at the level of the brainstem depressing descending excitatory input on the lower motor neurons within the spinal cord
- Barbiturates: Depress motor areas of the brain and abolish spontaneous spinal cord activity; potentiated by phenothiazines.
- Benzodiazepines: GABA agonists, indirectly antagonizing tetanospasmin
- Methocarbamol: Centrally acting muscle relaxant.
- Affected horses should be immunized with tetanus toxoid to initiate a protective antibody response. The amount of toxin sufficient to cause clinical disease is inadequate to generate a protective immune response.

CHRONIC TREATMENT

- Supportive care is prolonged, labor intensive, and costly.
- Patients must be maintained in a dark, quiet environment with minimal stimulation and handling.
- If the horse is recumbent, deep, soft bedding and regular turning (every 4 hours) is essential to minimize decubital ulcers and pulmonary congestion.
- If the horse is dysphagic, esophagostomy or gastrostomy tube may be required for feeding.
- Urinary catheterization for bladder emptying, enemas, and manual rectal evacuation of feces are likely required, especially if the horse is recumbent.

DRUG INTERACTIONS

- Phenothiazines are reported to lower seizure threshold, but their effectiveness in management of clinical cases strongly supports their use.
- Subclinical and clinical hepatic disease (Theiler's disease) after TAT administration has been reported.

POSSIBLE COMPLICATIONS

- Decubital ulcers caused by prolonged recumbency
- Regurgitation caused by dysphagia

- Aspiration pneumonia secondary to dysphagia or increased airway secretions in recumbent horses
- Dysuria, cystitis, and ascending urinary tract infection caused by a hypertonic urethral sphincter or catheterization
- Constipation, gaseous distension, and intestinal impaction caused by a hypertonic anal sphincter, lack of exercise, or recumbency
- Death from respiratory failure secondary to the spasm of respiratory muscles or central respiratory arrest from medullary intoxication

PROGNOSIS AND OUTCOME

- The prognosis depends on the incubation period, duration of onset, severity of clinical signs, and presence of any secondary complications. Therefore, a short incubation period, short duration of onset, and rapid progression of signs result in a poor prognosis.
- Binding of tetanospasmin to the α motor neuron is extremely difficult to combat. After the toxin is bound and internalized. it can no longer be neutralized by antitoxin. Therefore the disease will continue to progress after the administration of TAT.
- The recovery period is prolonged, not occurring until new interneuronal synapses have developed to replace those that were inactivated by toxin.
- The ability to swallow is a favorable prognostic sign.
- Dyspnea, dysphagia, and recumbency are significantly more common in nonsurvivors than survivors.

- Younger horses are significantly less likely to survive than older horses.

PEARLS & CONSIDERATIONS

COMMENTS
Recumbency is a grave prognostic indicator.

PREVENTION
- Management of contaminated or necrotic wounds should include thorough debridement, large-volume flushing, and comprehensive cleansing.
- Rational antibiotic therapy should be instituted for all contaminated and at-risk wounds.
- Prophylactic vaccination with tetanus toxoid markedly reduces the occurrence of clinical disease with annual vaccination of all horses recommended.
- Antitoxin: 1500 U of TAT to unvaccinated horses provides immediate passive protection lasting approximately 3 weeks.
- Combined active-passive immunization (tetanus toxoid concurrently with TAT): Rapid and prolonged protection for previously unvaccinated horses with at-risk wounds

CLIENT EDUCATION
- No vaccination or vaccination schedule is absolute. Tetanus toxoid should be administered to horses with susceptible wounds if longer than 6 months has elapsed since the previous vaccination.

- Maternally derived tetanus-specific immunoglobulin G antibodies inhibiting the foal's response to tetanus toxoid are passively transferred via colostrum. Therefore primary immunization of foals born to vaccinated mares should not commence before age 6 months.
- Vaccinal antibody response of younger foals has been shown to be poor, necessitating multiple doses of toxoid. This is especially important for foals born to unvaccinated mares when vaccination programs may be scheduled to begin at a younger age (3 months).
- Recovery from clinical disease does not generate protective immunity; therefore, surviving horses should be vaccinated.
- Owners should be advised of the possible risk of serum-associated hepatitis (Theiler's disease) associated with the administration of tetanus antitoxin, especially to older horses and periparturient mares (see "Theiler's Disease" in this section).

SUGGESTED READING
Furr M: Clostridial neurotoxins: botulism and tetanus. In Furr M, Reed S, editors: *Equine neurology*, Ames, IA, 2008, Blackwell, pp 221–229.
Green SL, Little CB, Baird JD, et al: Tetanus in the horse: a review of 20 cases (1970 to 1990). *J Vet Intern Med* 8:128–132, 1994.
Hatheway CL: Toxigenic clostridia. *Clin Microbiol Rev* 3:66–98, 1990.
Mayhew IG: Toxic diseases. In Mayhew IG, editors: *Large animal neurology*, ed 2, Ames, IA, 2009, Wiley Blackwell, pp 321–359.

AUTHOR: **PETER R. MORRESEY**

EDITOR: **STEPHEN M. REED**

Theiler's Disease

BASIC INFORMATION

DEFINITION
Disease characterized by acute severe hepatic necrosis, most commonly related to recent (within 1–3 months) administration of equine biologic products

SYNONYM(S)
- Serum-associated hepatitis
- Serum sickness
- Idiopathic acute hepatic disease

EPIDEMIOLOGY
SPECIES, AGE, SEX
- Adult horses are overrepresented.
- Females are overrepresented likely because of the practice of administration of tetanus antitoxin in the periparturient period.
RISK FACTORS
- Recent administration of tetanus antitoxin, particularly to a lactating postpartum mare
- Recent plasma or blood transfusion or administration of an equine-originating biologic

CONTAGION AND ZOONOSIS
- Despite reports of outbreaks, no horse-to-horse transmission has been documented.
- Hypothesized similarity to hepatitis B virus in humans, although supportive evidence is lacking
GEOGRAPHY AND SEASONALITY The incidence of disease may be greater in the summer and fall.
ASSOCIATED CONDITIONS AND DISORDERS Clinical signs of Theiler's disease can be indistinguishable from those of acute hepatic failure caused by toxicosis, infectious hepatitis, or immune-mediated hepatitis.

CLINICAL PRESENTATION

DISEASE FORMS/SUBTYPES

- Fulminant acute hepatic failure with signs of hepatic encephalopathy is the most common presentation.
- Rarely, an insidious onset of hepatic failure is reported.

HISTORY, CHIEF COMPLAINT Important historical consideration includes recent (4–10 weeks prior) administration of any biologic product of equine origin (eg, tetanus antitoxin, whole blood, commercial plasma). Owners may observe lethargy, anorexia, stupor, blindness, circling, bruxism, icterus, and fever.

PHYSICAL EXAM FINDINGS Icterus, abnormal mentation, head pressing, circling, blindness, bruxism, fever, ventral edema, photosensitization, colic, and sudden death

ETIOLOGY AND PATHOPHYSIOLOGY

- Exact cause unknown
- Recent (within 1–3 months) administration of equine biologic products
- Suspected type III hypersensitivity reaction to biologic product

DIAGNOSIS

DIFFERENTIAL DIAGNOSIS

- Toxic hepatopathy
- Mycotoxicosis
- Cholangiohepatitis
- Acute biliary obstruction
- Infectious necrotic hepatitis
- Hyperlipemia
- Hemolytic diseases

INITIAL DATABASE

- Packed cell volume: Increased
- Complete blood count: Leukocytosis
- Gamma glutamyltransferase, sorbitol dehydrogenase (SDH): Increased
- Total bilirubin: Increased
- Acidosis
- Blood urea nitrogen: Decreased

- Plasma ammonia concentration: May be increased
- Prothrombin and activated prothrombin times: May be prolonged

ADVANCED OR CONFIRMATORY TESTING

- Gross pathology: Global tissue icterus; the liver may be small or large depending on the course of the disease
- Histopathology: Widespread centrilobular to midzonal hepatocellular necrosis with hemorrhage, moderate to severe centrilobular hepatocyte vacuolar change and granular swelling, hemosiderosis, and bile cast

TREATMENT

THERAPEUTIC GOAL(S)

The goals of therapy include supportive care and prevention of infection; no specific therapy exists.

ACUTE GENERAL TREATMENT

- IV fluids to replace volume, replace electrolytes, and correct acid–base disorders
- IV dextrose to provide energy substrate without requiring hepatic metabolism
- Low–protein, high-carbohydrate diet
- Lactulose and neomycin by nasogastric intubation to reduce plasma ammonia concentrations
- Broad-spectrum antimicrobials to prevent secondary infections
- Nonsteroidal antiinflammatory drugs to reduce inflammation and reduce fever
- See treatment under "Hepatic Encephalopathy" in this section

POSSIBLE COMPLICATIONS

- Persistent polycythemia
- Development of endotoxemia

- Secondary infections
- Hepatic encephalopathy
- Terminal hemolysis

PROGNOSIS AND OUTCOME

- The prognosis is poor, especially if hemorrhage or hemolysis is present.
- Favorable prognostic indicators include waning clinical signs and decreasing serum SDH activity.

PEARLS & CONSIDERATIONS

COMMENTS

May occur without a history of equine biologic administration

PREVENTION

- Vaccinate mares 30 days before parturition with tetanus toxoid.
- Administer tetanus antitoxin only to horses with no history of tetanus vaccination and at high risk for development of tetanus.

SUGGESTED READING

Aleman M, Nieto JE, Carr EA, Carlson GP: Serum hepatitis associated with commercial plasma transfusion in horses. *J Vet Intern Med* 19:120–122, 2005.

Guglick MA, MacAllister CG, Ely RW, Edwards WC: Hepatic disease associated with administration of tetanus antitoxin in eight horses. *J Am Vet Med Assoc* 206:1737–1740, 1995.

Messer NT, Johnson PJ: Idiopathic acute hepatic disease in horses: 12 cases (1982–1992). *J Am Vet Med Assoc* 204:1934–1937, 1994.

AUTHOR: JOHANNA ELFENBEIN

EDITOR: MICHELLE HENRY BARTON

Thrombocytopenia, Immune-Mediated

BASIC INFORMATION

DEFINITION

Excessive bleeding caused by an absence of blood platelets as a result of their destruction by autoantibodies

SYNONYM(S)

Autoimmune thrombocytopenia

EPIDEMIOLOGY

SPECIES, AGE, SEX

- May be primary (idiopathic)
- May be secondary to drug treatment, neoplasia, or other immune-mediated disease

CLINICAL PRESENTATION

HISTORY, CHIEF COMPLAINT

- Multiple sites of small vessel bleeding
- Bleeding possibly confined to a single system such as the respiratory system

with epistaxis or hematomas in the nasal sinus
- May be generalized with widespread petechial hemorrhages on the mucous membranes, epistaxis, and melena
- Mucosal hemorrhage
- Rapidly developing anemia
- Obvious bruising or hematoma formation
- Possible obvious primary disease

ETIOLOGY AND PATHOPHYSIOLOGY

- Antibodies coat the platelet surface and cause their premature removal.
- In primary immune-mediated thrombocytopenia (IMTP), immunoglobulin (Ig) G antibodies produced in the spleen bind to platelet membranes. These antibodies may also bind to megakaryocyte membranes.
- In secondary IMTP, platelets may bind immune complexes formed by antibodies binding to a drug, virus, or neoplastic antigen.
- Removal of the offending antigen may cause rapid remission of secondary IMTP.
- Secondary to equine infectious anemia (see "Anemia, Equine Infectious" in this section), lymphosarcoma, or autoimmune hemolytic anemia

DIAGNOSIS

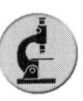

- Clinical diagnosis usually apparent
- Small-vessel hemorrhagic diathesis
- Severe thrombocytopenia with no evidence of disseminated intravascular coagulation (DIC)

DIFFERENTIAL DIAGNOSIS

- DIC
- Warfarin poisoning
- Neonatal isoimmune thrombocytopenia

INITIAL DATABASE

- Complete blood count, including platelet count, hematocrit
- Severe thrombocytopenia (<40,000/μL)
- Prolonged bleeding time
- Abnormal clot retraction
- Anemia accompanied by hypoproteinemia

ADVANCED OR CONFIRMATORY TESTING

Immunoglobulins may be identified on the foal's platelets and megakaryocytes by antiglobulin test or immunofluorescence.

TREATMENT

THERAPEUTIC GOAL(S)

- Prevention of additional blood loss by preventing platelet destruction
- If secondary, removal of the inciting cause

ACUTE GENERAL TREATMENT

- Stop all current medications. Drug-induced IMTP usually resolves within 14 days of drug withdrawal.
- Identify and treat the inciting cause if secondary.
- Provide blood replacement if required.
- Immunosuppressive therapy: Dexamethasone sodium phosphate (0.08 mg/kg IV or PO) given once daily. The platelet counts should increase within 4 to 7 days. When the level reaches >100,000/μL, then the dose of dexamethasone can be gradually reduced by 10% to 20% daily.
- In refractory cases, prednisolone (1 mg/kg IM) should be given q24h.
- Azathioprine (3 mg/kg PO q24h) or (3 mg/kg PO q24h) may be as effective as dexamethasone. After 30 days, half the daily dose should be given for another 30 days.

CHRONIC TREATMENT

Steroid treatment may be discontinued after 10 to 21 days provided the platelet count has been normal for at least 5 days.

POSSIBLE COMPLICATIONS

- Infections secondary to steroid treatment
- Laminitis secondary to steroid treatment

RECOMMENDED MONITORING

- Platelet counts on a weekly basis
- Hematocrit

PROGNOSIS AND OUTCOME

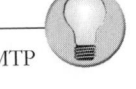

Horses with IMTP have a good prognosis and usually recover by 21 days.

PEARLS & CONSIDERATIONS

- Chronic or recurrent IMTP has been reported.
- Chronic refractory IMTP is probably secondary, and the underlying disease should be identified.

SUGGESTED READING

Clabough DL, Gebhard D, Flaherty MT, et al: Immune-mediated thrombocytopenia in horses infected with equine infectious anemia virus. *J Virol* 65:6242–6251, 1991.

Humber KA, Beech J, Cudd TA, et al: Azathioprine for treatment of immune-mediated thrombocytopenia in two horses. *J Am Vet Med Assoc* 199:591–594, 1991.

McGurrin MK, Arroyo LG, Bienzle D: Flow cytometric detection of platelet-bound antibody in three horses with immune-mediated thrombocytopenia. *J Am Vet Med Assoc* 224:83–87, 2004.

Sellon DC, Levine J, Millikin E, et al: Thrombocytopenia in horses: 35 cases (1989–1994). *J Vet Intern Med* 10:127–132, 1996.

AUTHOR and EDITOR: IAN TIZARD

Thrombocytopenia, Neonatal

BASIC INFORMATION

DEFINITION

Loss of blood platelets in newborn foals as a result of destruction by maternal antibodies

SYNONYM(S)

Alloimmune thrombocytopenia of neonates

EPIDEMIOLOGY

SPECIES, AGE, SEX

- Occurs in foals from multiparous mares
- Usually first seen in third and fourth foals

CLINICAL PRESENTATION

HISTORY, CHIEF COMPLAINT

- Depression
- Failure to suckle
- Multiple sites of small vessel bleeding

- Rapidly developing anemia
- Prolonged excessive bleeding from the umbilical stump
- Obvious bruising or hematoma formation

ETIOLOGY AND PATHOPHYSIOLOGY

- Mares make antibodies against paternal platelet antigens during foaling or pregnancy.
- Multiple foalings boost antibody levels. These antibodies are concentrated in mares' colostrum and ingested by foals.

- Antibodies ingested by foals destroy their lymphocytes, preventing blood coagulation.

DIAGNOSIS

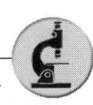

- Clinical diagnosis usually apparent
- Small-vessel hemorrhagic diathesis
- Severe thrombocytopenia with no evidence of disseminated intravascular coagulation (DIC)

DIFFERENTIAL DIAGNOSIS

- Warfarin poisoning
- Neonatal sepsis
- Neonatal isoerythrolysis

INITIAL DATABASE

- Complete blood count, hematocrit
- Severe thrombocytopenia (<40,000/μL)
- Prolonged bleeding time
- Abnormal clot retraction
- Anemia accompanied by hypoproteinemia

ADVANCED OR CONFIRMATORY TESTING

Immunoglobulins may be identified on the foal's platelets, and antibodies to these platelets can be found in the mare's serum.

TREATMENT

THERAPEUTIC GOAL(S)

- Prevention of additional blood loss by preventing platelet destruction
- Replacement of lost blood or fluids

ACUTE GENERAL TREATMENT

- Prevent further antibody absorption by stopping suckling.
- Provide fresh colostrum from known negative mares.
- Mild cases may require only careful nursing.
- Supportive treatment in the form of oxygen therapy, fluid and electrolyte therapy, and maintenance of the acid-base balance. Warmth, adequate hydration, and antimicrobial therapy are also critically important.
- Blood transfusion may be required in acute cases. A red blood cell (RBC) count less than $3 \times 10^6/\mu L$ or a packed cell volume (PCV) of less than 15% warrants a blood transfusion.
  - Transfused equine RBCs have a half-life of only 2 to 4 days, so the transfusion has only a temporary effect.
  - The donor should not only be Aa or Qa negative but should also lack antibodies to these antigens.
  - Washed cells from the mare: About 3 to 4 L of blood is collected in sodium citrate and centrifuged, and the plasma is discarded. The RBCs are washed once in saline and transfused slowly into the foal. The blood is given in divided doses about 6 hours apart.
- If thrombocytopenia is anticipated as a result of the prior birth of a thrombocytopenic foal, stripping off the mare's colostrum and giving the foal colostrum from another mare may prevent its occurrence.

CHRONIC TREATMENT

- The foal should not be allowed to suckle its mare for 24 to 36 hours.
- The mare's colostrum should be stripped out and discarded.
- Identification of stallion/mare combinations that give rise to thrombocytopenia

RECOMMENDED MONITORING

When suckling is permitted, the foal should only be allowed to take small quantities at first and should be observed carefully for adverse side effects. It may be prudent to monitor PCV for several days after suckling resumes.

PROGNOSIS AND OUTCOME

Good if irreversible organ damage has not occurred

PEARLS & CONSIDERATIONS

COMMENTS

- Commonly associated with neonatal isoimmune anemia.
- The prognosis is good if the condition is diagnosed sufficiently early and the appropriate treatment is instituted rapidly.
- Mildly affected foals (PCV of 15%–25% and an RBC count $>4 \times 10^6$) will continue to nurse. Those with a PCV of less than 10% will stop nursing and become recumbent.
- Many subacute cases recover without treatment.

PREVENTION

- Sensitization of a mare sufficient to cause disease in foals requires multiple pregnancies to boost antibody titers to a dangerous level.
- Mares that have previously given birth to affected foals should not be permitted to suckle their foals. They should, however, be milked out and the colostrum discarded. Foals from such mares should be given fresh colostrum from donor mares with colostrum to spare.
- After the colostrum has been replaced by milk, foals may be permitted to suckle from their mothers.

CLIENT EDUCATION

Once identified as originating from specific breeding combinations, the disease can be readily prevented. Steps should be taken to minimize sensitization of mares by repeated breeding to a single sire.

SUGGESTED READING

Bentz AI, Wilkins PA, MacGillivray KC, et al: Severe thrombocytopenia in 2 thoroughbred foals with sepsis and neonatal encephalopathy. *J Vet Intern Med* 16:494–497, 2002.

Perkins GA, Miller WH, Divers TJ, et al: Ulcerative dermatitis, thrombocytopenia, and neutropenia in neonatal foals. *J Vet Intern Med* 19:211–216, 2005.

Ramirez S, Gaunt SD, McClure JJ, Oliver J: Detection and effects on platelet function of anti-platelet antibody in mule foals with experimentally induced neonatal alloimmune thrombocytopenia. *J Vet Intern Med* 13:534–539, 1999.

AUTHOR and EDITOR: IAN TIZARD

Toxic Metritis

BASIC INFORMATION

DEFINITION

Uterine inflammatory condition that extends to the myometrium marked by the presence of septicemia, endotoxemia, or both

SYNONYM(S)

Metritis-septicemia-laminitis complex, septic metritis, postpartum metritis

EPIDEMIOLOGY

SPECIES, AGE, SEX Postpartum intact female horses

RISK FACTORS
- Dystocia, fetotomy, cesarean section
- Retained fetal membranes
- Unhygienic foaling conditions or obstetrical manipulations
- Poor perineal conformation
- Bacterial late-term abortion
- Vaginal or cervical trauma

ASSOCIATED CONDITIONS AND DISORDERS Abortion

CLINICAL PRESENTATION

HISTORY, CHIEF COMPLAINT
- History of recent parturition with or without complications
- Fetid dark-red or dark-brown vulvar discharge
- Fever, depression, inappetence

PHYSICAL EXAM FINDINGS
- Tachycardia
- Tachypnea
- Elevated body temperature
- Hyperemic or toxic mucous membranes
- Increased digital pulses, lameness, increased recumbency, hot hooves, solar sensitivity to a hoof tester if laminitis develops
- Colic
- Decreased intestinal motility

ETIOLOGY AND PATHOPHYSIOLOGY
- Ascending bacterial contamination of the uterus occurs during parturition, dystocia, retained fetal membranes, or obstetric manipulations.
- Accumulated intrauterine fluid, autolytic fetal membranes, necrotic or devitalized tissue, and debris provide favorable conditions for bacterial proliferation and release of endotoxins.
- Septicemia and endotoxemia result from disruption of the uterine mucosal barrier and absorption of bacteria or endotoxins into systemic circulation through the highly vascularized postpartum uterus.
- Endotoxemia may also result from transmural movement of endotoxins into the peritoneal cavity.

DIAGNOSIS

DIFFERENTIAL DIAGNOSIS

- Fever, depression, or colic
  - Postpartum hemorrhage
  - Uterine rupture
  - Necrotic vaginitis
  - Colon torsion
  - Ileus
  - Intestinal or mesenteric rupture or trauma
  - Bladder rupture
- Vulvar discharge: Normal lochia (≤6 days postpartum, dark red-brown, associated with a normally involuting uterus)

INITIAL DATABASE

- Complete blood count (CBC): Leukopenia and neutropenia with toxic changes and left shift, hyperfibrinogenemia, hemoconcentration caused by dehydration
- Serum biochemistry profile: Azotemia caused by dehydration or renal damage by endotoxins ± elevated muscle enzymes caused by increased recumbency
- Transrectal palpation: Enlarged, thin-walled, flaccid uterus
- Transrectal ultrasonography: Large amount of free intrauterine fluid of varying degrees of echogenicity, edematous uterine wall
- Vaginal speculum examination: Dark-red or dark-brown fluid pooled in the cranial vagina and originating from the uterus
- Uterine culture: Growth of a mixed bacterial flora, including gram-positive (*Streptococcus equi* subsp. *zooepidemicus*, β-hemolytic streptococci, *Staphylococcus* spp.), gram-negative (*Escherichia coli*, *Klebsiella pneumoniae*), or anaerobic bacteria (*Bacteroides fragilis*, *Clostridium* spp.); endotoxemia is associated with the presence of gram-negative bacteria
- Endometrial cytology: ± Toxic changes in neutrophils

ADVANCED OR CONFIRMATORY TESTING

Abdominocentesis: ± Increased protein concentration and white blood cell count

TREATMENT

THERAPEUTIC GOAL(S)

- Control bacterial growth
- Evacuate uterine contents
- Prevent complications

ACUTE GENERAL TREATMENT

- Control of bacterial growth
  - Potassium penicillin for gram-positive and some anaerobic bacteria: 22,000 IU/kg IV q6h.
  - Gentamicin for gram-negative bacteria: 6.6 mg/kg IV or IM q24h.
  - Metronidazole for anaerobic bacteria: 15 to 25 mg/kg PO q6h–12h.
  - Antibiotics should be adjusted based on the results of the culture and sensitivity test.
- Evacuation of uterine contents
  - Oxytocin: 10 to 40 IU IM or IV q2–6h.
  - Uterine lavage: 2 to 6 L of warm saline solution (sterile or water with 9 g of table salt/L) repeatedly infused and siphoned off via a sterile nasogastric tube until the effluent is clear. Performed daily or twice daily based on clinical and ultrasonographic findings.
- Treatment of dehydration and endotoxemia
  - Polyionic solutions at a volume and rate determined by the degree of dehydration
  - Calcium gluconate solution (125 mL of 23% solution) can be added to a 5-L bag of crystalloid fluid
  - Flunixin meglumine: 0.25 mg/kg IV or PO q8h (antiendotoxic) or 0.55 to 1.1 mg/kg IV or PO q12h (anti-inflammatory and antipyretic)
  - Phenylbutazone: 2 to 4 mg/kg IV or PO q12h
  - Polymyxin B: 6000 U/kg IV q12h in 1L of saline over 30 to 60 minutes for 1 or 2 days
  - Antiendotoxin serum: 1.5 mL/kg diluted at least twofold in balanced IV fluids
  - Hyperimmune plasma: 2 to 10 mL/kg IV
  - Pentoxifylline: 7.5 mg/kg PO q12h
- Treatment of laminitis
  - Flunixin meglumine or phenylbutazone as above
  - Acetylpromazine maleate: 0.02 to 0.04 mg/kg IM or IV q4–6h
  - Provide extra bedding and pads for frog support
- Lactation failure: Domperidone (1.1 mg/kg PO q12–24h)

DRUG INTERACTIONS

- Aminoglycosides and polymyxin B can be nephrotoxic. Ensure good hydration before and during treatment.
- Aminoglycosides are ineffective in anaerobic environments. Enrofloxacin can be used as an alternative if extensive tissue damage and necrosis are present.
- Nonsteroidal antiinflammatory drugs can cause gastrointestinal (GI) ulceration and potentiate nephrotoxicity of aminoglycosides and polymyxin B.
- Penicillin can cause disruption of the intestinal flora and diarrhea, as well as anaphylactic reactions.

POSSIBLE COMPLICATIONS

- Septicemia
- Endotoxemia
- Laminitis
- Death
- Delayed uterine involution
- Lactation failure

RECOMMENDED MONITORING

- Monitor the CBC frequently to determine the response to treatment.
- Monitor the digital pulses and gait for signs of laminitis. Radiographs may be needed to determine rotation or sinking of the third phalanx.

- Monitor for signs of colic or ileus that may result from release of inflammatory mediators that alter GI activity or intestinal blood flow. Monitor fecal output and consistency and administer mineral oil (0.5–1.0 gallon) or bran mash if necessary.
- Monitor uterine involution via transrectal palpation and ultrasonography. An absence of free intrauterine fluid and the presence of good uterine tone indicate response to treatment and adequate uterine involution.

PROGNOSIS AND OUTCOME

- The prognosis depends on severity, duration, and complications of metritis.
- The reported survival rate is 77%.
- The prognosis is guarded if laminitis develops.

PEARLS & CONSIDERATIONS

COMMENTS

Early aggressive treatment is key to prevent complications associated with metritis.

PREVENTION

- Promptly treat mares with retained fetal membranes.
- Maintain good hygienic conditions during foaling and obstetric manipulations.

CLIENT EDUCATION

- Toxic metritis can be life threatening, and laminitis can arise as a complication of endotoxemia.
- The veterinarian must be contacted immediately if a postpartum mare develops inappetence, depression, fever, colic, or lameness.

SUGGESTED READING

Blanchard TL, MacPherson ML: Postparturient abnormalities. In Samper JC, Pycock JF, McKinnon, editors: *Current therapy in equine reproduction*, St Louis, 2007, Saunders Elsevier, pp 465–475.

Card C, Lopate C: Infectious diseases of the puerperal period. In Youngquist RS, Threlfall WR, editors: *Current therapy in large animal theriogenology*, ed 2, St Louis, 2007, Saunders Elsevier, pp 138–143.

AUTHOR: **MARIA S. FERRER**

EDITOR: **JUAN C. SAMPER**

Tracheal Collapse

BASIC INFORMATION

DEFINITION

- Tracheal collapse is a condition characterized by dorsoventral narrowing of the tracheal lumen associated with flaccidity of the dorsal membrane and loss of the circular contour of the tracheal rings.

EPIDEMIOLOGY

SPECIES, AGE, SEX

- Age distribution may be bimodal, with approximately one third of cases reported in foals and two thirds of cases reported in horses, donkeys, and mules older than 10 years.

GENETICS AND BREED PREDISPOSITION

- Most reported cases have been in ponies and Miniature Horses, suggesting a breed predisposition. Cases have also been reported in donkeys and mules.

GEOGRAPHY AND SEASONALITY

- Animals may be more affected during hot, humid months of the year.

CLINICAL PRESENTATION

HISTORY, CHIEF COMPLAINT

- Clinical signs noted by the owner may include exercise intolerance, respiratory noise, dyspnea, and paroxysmal coughing (classic honking).

PHYSICAL EXAM FINDINGS

- Auscultation of the thorax and trachea can be used to determine the point of maximal intensity of the respiratory noise. In addition, the phase of respiration during which stridor is apparent may help determine the location of collapse (expiration = intrathoracic; inspiration = extrathoracic). Palpation of the trachea may induce a cough. The trachea may have prominent lateral borders on palpation.

ETIOLOGY AND PATHOPHYSIOLOGY

- Etiology is currently unknown. However, congenital and degenerative defects in the tracheal cartilage have been proposed as well as neuromuscular disorders associated with weakening of the trachealis muscle and changes in respiratory tract pressures associated with lung disease.

- In most cases, the decrease in dorsoventral distance is related to flattening of the circular shape of the tracheal cartilages and collapse of the trachealis muscle. Separation of the trachealis muscle from the tracheal cartilages dorsally without a change in the cartilage shape has also been seen.

DIAGNOSIS

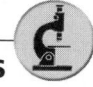

DIFFERENTIAL DIAGNOSIS

- Tracheal stenosis
- Other upper respiratory disease associated with stridor: obstruction in the nasal passages, pharynx and larynx
- If dyspnea without stridor is present, lower airway disease should be a differential

INITIAL DATABASE

- Endoscopy provides rapid and accurate diagnosis
- Radiographs of the extrathoracic and intrathoracic trachea during both phases of respiration

ADVANCED OR CONFIRMATORY TESTING

- Fluoroscopy can be used to further evaluate the dynamic nature of the disease and the extent of trachea involved.
- Computed tomography, magnetic resonance imaging, and ultrasound can be used to determine the diameter of the trachea, which would be necessary for any surgical planning.

TREATMENT

THERAPEUTIC GOAL

- Restore adequate airway to prevent dyspnea and/or respiratory distress

ACUTE GENERAL TREATMENT

- Tracheal collapse worsens as the animal becomes more distressed due to increased respiratory pressures. Treatment includes intranasal oxygen, cooling, and sedation with acepromazine.
- Inflammation will further narrow the airway. Treat with nonsteroidal antiinflammatory drugs or corticosteroids (inhaled or systemic), a low-allergen environment, and antitussives (butorphanol) to decrease turbulent airflow.
- Maximize lower airway diameter. Treat with bronchodilators (systemic or inhaled).

- If severe collapse is present, an endotracheal tube may be required to maintain an airway. If collapse is present in the distal and/or intrathoracic trachea, placement of the endotracheal tube may require tracheotomy.

CHRONIC TREATMENT

- Medical: If tracheal collapse is not severe (<50% decrease in luminal diameter is used in dogs), continuation of medical management initiated during acute treatment may be adequate to maintain respiratory function.
- Surgical: If tracheal collapse is severe and/or medical management has failed, surgical treatment can be attempted. Described surgical treatments include extraluminal and intraluminal stent placement.

PROGNOSIS AND OUTCOME

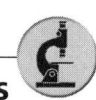

- Due to the limited number of cases reported in the literature, it is difficult to determine an accurate prognosis.
- Although medical management may be successful when cases are diagnosed early and symptoms are mild, it is likely, due to the assumed nature of the disease, that collapse will progress over time.

- In two cases, intraluminal stents provided temporary (1.5- to 2-year) successful treatment, which was eventually limited by continual production of granulation tissue.
- Extraluminal stents have been used with some success as well (author experience and personal communication).

PEARLS & CONSIDERATIONS

COMMENTS

- Tracheal collapse is an uncommon disease in horses. However, it should be considered in Miniature Horses and ponies with appropriate clinical signs.

SUGGESTED READING

Dixon PM, Schumacher J, Collins N: Tracheal disorders. In McGorum BC, Dixon PM, Robinson NE, et al, editors: *Equine respiratory medicine and surgery*, New York, 2007, Saunders Elsevier, pp 543–561.

Epstein K. *Tracheal collapse in horses*. 2007 ACVS Veterinary Symposium Proceedings. Chicago, 2007.

Wong DM, Sponseller BA, Riedesel EA, et al: The use of intraluminal stents for tracheal collapse in two horses: case management and long-term treatment. *Equine Vet Educ* 20(2):80–90, 2008.

AUTHOR: **KIRA L. EPSTEIN**

EDITOR: **ERIC J. PARENTE**

Tracheal Perforation

BASIC INFORMATION

DEFINITION

Disruption of the tracheal lumen

SYNONYM(S)

Tracheal wounds, tracheal trauma

CLINICAL PRESENTATION

HISTORY, CHIEF COMPLAINT Tracheal perforation is associated with trauma to the trachea. The trauma can result in an open wound or swelling associated with soft tissue trauma and air leaking into the subcutaneous space.

PHYSICAL EXAM FINDINGS

- Crepitus associated with subcutaneous emphysema is an important physical examination finding.
- The emphysema may travel down fascial planes into the mediastinum, resulting in pneumomediastinum and, if severe, pneumothorax. If pneumothorax is present, auscultation of the

lungs will reveal no lung sounds in the dorsal lung fields.
- If infection (cellulitis) is present, heat and pain may be associated with the swelling, and the infection can travel down the fascial planes, leading to septic mediastinitis and pleuritis.

ETIOLOGY AND PATHOPHYSIOLOGY

Trauma

DIAGNOSIS

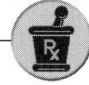

DIFFERENTIAL DIAGNOSIS

Esophageal perforation or trauma

INITIAL DATABASE

- Endoscopy of the trachea and esophagus to rule out esophageal perforation
- Radiography of the chest to evaluate for pneumomediastinum and pneumothorax
- Complete blood count and fibrinogen to evaluate for evidence of infection

TREATMENT

THERAPEUTIC GOAL(S)

- Restore the integrity of the tracheal lumen
- If present, manage pneumothorax, open wound, and infection

ACUTE GENERAL TREATMENT

- Small tears generally respond to medical management with pressure bandages, antiinflammatory drugs, and antimicrobials.
- If the tear is large, surgical treatment may be required. Wounds can be debrided and closed primarily. Tracheal resection and anastomosis may be required if the wound is very extensive or complete tracheal rupture has occurred.
- If pneumothorax is associated with clinical signs of dyspnea or respiratory distress, thoracocentesis can be performed.

- If there is an open wound, debridement, bandaging, and healing by second intention are generally successful and preferred by some authors over primary closure.

POSSIBLE COMPLICATIONS

Tracheal stenosis can occur after large tracheal perforation (>50% of the circumference) or after resection and anastomosis.

RECOMMENDED MONITORING

Patients should be closely monitored for signs of pneumothorax and infection.

PROGNOSIS AND OUTCOME

- The prognosis for small wounds treated with medical management is very good.
- The prognosis decreases as size of defect in trachea increases.

PEARLS & CONSIDERATIONS

Tracheal perforation should be considered whenever subcutaneous emphysema is present in the neck.

SUGGESTED READING

Dixon PM, Schumacher J, Collins N: Tracheal disorders. In McGorum BC, Dixon PM, Robinson NE, Schumacher J, editors: *Equine respiratory medicine and surgery*, New York, 2007, Saunders Elsevier, pp 543–561.

Stick JA: Trachea. In Auer JA, Stick JA, editors: *Equine surgery*, ed 3, St Louis, 2006, Saunders Elsevier, pp 608–615.

AUTHOR: **KIRA L. EPSTEIN**

EDITOR: **ERIC J. PARENTE**

Tracheal Stenosis

BASIC INFORMATION

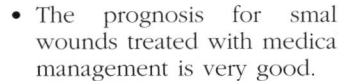

DEFINITION

A fixed narrowing or stricture of the trachea

EPIDEMIOLOGY

SPECIES, AGE, SEX Specific causes of stenosis may be more common in certain ages (eg, neoplasia in older horses, abscessation of lymph nodes in younger horses, congenital stenosis in younger horses)

CLINICAL PRESENTATION

HISTORY, CHIEF COMPLAINT
- Clinical signs noted by the owner may include exercise intolerance, respiratory noise, and dyspnea.
- Horses with acquired strictures may have a history of an injury to the neck or previous tracheotomy.
- Horses with external compression may have a history of *Streptococcus equi* infection.

PHYSICAL EXAM FINDINGS
- Auscultation should be performed to determine the point of maximal intensity for stridor.
- Examination of the neck may reveal scars from previous injury or tracheotomy, enlarged lymph nodes, or masses.
- Palpation of the trachea may reveal an abnormal contour of the tracheal rings.

ETIOLOGY AND PATHOPHYSIOLOGY
- The decrease in diameter of the trachea may be caused by intraluminal obstruction, abnormalities in the architecture of the trachea, or extraluminal compression.
- Intraluminal lesions have been associated with granulation tissue secondary to tracheotomy, transtracheal wash, and intratracheal antibiotic administration.
- Abnormalities in the architecture of the trachea may be congenital or acquired and may affect the cartilage or soft tissue of the trachea. Congenital abnormalities are rare. Acquired abnormalities in the cartilage may occur after tracheotomy or potentially with prolonged traumatic intubation.
- Extraluminal compression is most common secondary to lymph node abscess formation with *S. equi*. Other sources of compression include neoplasia and other abscesses.

DIAGNOSIS

DIFFERENTIAL DIAGNOSIS

- Tracheal collapse
- Other upper respiratory disease associated with stridor: obstruction in the nasal passages, pharynx, and larynx
- If dyspnea without stridor is present, lower airway disease should be included in the differential diagnoses.

INITIAL DATABASE

- Endoscopy to evaluate the lumen of the trachea
- Imaging of the area surrounding the trachea with radiographs and ultrasonography to evaluate for external compression
- Complete blood count and fibrinogen to evaluate for evidence of infection

ADVANCED OR CONFIRMATORY TESTING

Advanced imaging with computed tomography or magnetic resonance imaging can be used to further evaluate the nature and extent of the region of stenosis and surrounding structures.

TREATMENT

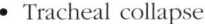

THERAPEUTIC GOAL(S)

- Relieve respiratory distress or difficulty
- Restore normal tracheal diameter

ACUTE GENERAL TREATMENT

- If obstruction is severe, establishment of a secure airway is required rapidly.
- If the obstruction is in the cervical region, perform tracheotomy.
- If the obstruction is too low in the cervical region or within the thorax, place an endotracheal tube to establish a more rigid airway against compression by an extraluminal mass.
- Adjunctive treatment to decrease inflammation contributing to the decrease in diameter (see "Tracheal Collapse" in this section).

CHRONIC TREATMENT

- Intraluminal granulation tissue has been treated with endoscopic laser debridement.
- Horses with abnormalities in the architecture of the trachea may be treated with resection and anastomosis (up to five rings), stent placement, or chondrotomy with or without stent placement.
- Horses with extraluminal abscesses may be treated with drainage, antimicrobial agents, or both. Other masses may require resection. If tracheal compression has been chronic, stenting with or without chondrotomy may be required.

POSSIBLE COMPLICATIONS

If resection and anastomosis is used for treatment, stricture at the anastomosis site is possible.

RECOMMENDED MONITORING

Reassessment with physical examination and endoscopy should be performed with any change in respiratory effort or noise noted by the owner.

PROGNOSIS AND OUTCOME

- Successful treatment of intraluminal granulation tissue and extraluminal compression in the cervical region has been reported.

- Horses with mediastinal neoplasia have a poor prognosis.
- The prognosis for abnormalities in the architecture of the trachea depends on the severity of the decrease in diameter and the expectations of the owner. It is difficult to establish a normal diameter with surgical intervention.

PEARLS & CONSIDERATIONS

COMMENTS

Tracheal stenosis is an uncommon disease in horses. The prognosis varies depending on the cause of the obstruction.

PREVENTION

Care should be taken when performing tracheotomy to avoid transection of more than 180 degrees of the annular ligament or the cartilage rings.

SUGGESTED READING

Dixon PM, Schumacher JA, Collins N: Tracheal disorders. In McGorum BC, Dixon PM, Robinson NE, Schumacher J, editors: *Equine respiratory medicine and surgery*, New York, 2007, Saunders Elsevier, pp 543–561.

Mair TS, Lane JG: Disease of the equine trachea. *Equine Vet Educ* 17(3):146–149, 2005.

AUTHOR: **KIRA L. EPSTEIN**

EDITOR: **ERIC J. PARENTE**

Transitional Cell Carcinoma

BASIC INFORMATION

DEFINITION

Neoplasia of the transitional cells in the mucosa of the urinary system

EPIDEMIOLOGY

SPECIES, AGE, SEX More common in adult and elderly horses

RISK FACTORS In cattle and sheep, ingestion of bracken fern has been associated with occurrence of urinary bladder neoplasia, but this has not been documented in horses.

ASSOCIATED CONDITIONS AND DISORDERS

- Pyelonephritis
- Anemia
- Hydronephrosis

CLINICAL PRESENTATION

HISTORY, CHIEF COMPLAINT

- Hematuria
- Stranguria
- Pollakiuria
- Weight loss
- Fever
- Colic
- Depressed or obtunded

PHYSICAL EXAM FINDINGS

- Hematuria
- Palpation of the bladder per rectum may reveal a thickened bladder wall or a firm mass. A palpably enlarged or abnormal kidney is possible with renal involvement.

ETIOLOGY AND PATHOPHYSIOLOGY

- Normal equine bladder mucosa contains scattered islands of squamous epithelium

- Some squamous cell carcinomas of the bladder may arise from squamous metaplasia in transitional cell tumors.

DIAGNOSIS

DIFFERENTIAL DIAGNOSIS

- Urolithiasis
- Pyelonephritis

INITIAL DATABASE

- Complete blood count often indicates anemia caused by severe hematuria.
- Endoscopic examination of the urinary bladder and urethra
- Transrectal ultrasonographic examination of the bladder wall may demonstrate bladder masses.
- Urinalysis usually confirms hematuria, proteinuria, and possibly pyuria.

ADVANCED OR CONFIRMATORY TESTING

- Biopsy and histopathologic examination of the mass may confirm transitional cell carcinoma.
- Cytologic examination of urine sediment may reveal neoplastic transitional epithelial cells.
- Abdominocentesis and cytologic examination of abdominal fluid may sometimes recover neoplastic cells.

TREATMENT

THERAPEUTIC GOAL(S)

Surgical debridement or removal and local injection of antineoplastic drugs if

discovered early in the course of the disease

ACUTE GENERAL TREATMENT

Primarily palliative

CHRONIC TREATMENT

Intracystic infusion of 5-fluorouracil (100 mg in 50 mL of isotonic saline q24h for four treatments; then q48h for four treatments) markedly reduced hematuria in one case; however, treatment was ultimately unsuccessful, and the horse was euthanized.

PROGNOSIS AND OUTCOME

Poor

PEARLS & CONSIDERATIONS

- Squamous cell carcinoma is the most commonly reported bladder neoplasia in horses, but transitional cell carcinoma is frequently reported.
- Transitional cell carcinomas are most often found in the bladder but can also affect the kidney.
- Most cases have extensive metastasis at necropsy.

SUGGESTED READING

Fischer AT, Spier S, Carlson GP, Hackett RP: Neoplasia of the equine urinary bladder as

a cause of hematuria. *J Am Vet Med Assoc* 186:1294–1296, 1985.
Traub-Dargatz JL: Urinary tract neoplasia. *Vet Clin Pract Equine North Am* 14:495–504, 1998.

AUTHOR: **JENNIFER TAINTOR**

EDITOR: **BRYAN M. WALDRIDGE**

Trypanosomiasis

BASIC INFORMATION

DEFINITION

A disease caused by a bloodborne parasite of subtropical and tropical climates consisting of several species or subspecies of trypanosomes that are differentiated by clinical disease, morphology, and country of origin

SYNONYM(S)

Surra, dourine, African animal trypanosomiasis, mal de caderas, naga, sleeping sickness

EPIDEMIOLOGY

SPECIES, AGE, SEX

- Affects horses, mules, and donkeys.
- Anecdotally, females appear less likely to die from infection than are males.

GENETICS AND BREED PREDISPOSITION
Light breeds may experience more severe disease than draft breeds; indigenous breeds may also demonstrate higher survival.

RISK FACTORS
Trypanosomiasis is transmitted both biologically and mechanically by insects, and the risk of disease is related to exposure to these various insects. For Surra, the transmitting vectors include mechanical transmission by biting flies (*Tabanus* and *Stomoxys* spp.) and by the bite of vampire bats. Tsetse flies (*Glossina* spp.) transmit African animal trypanosomiasis, and cattle are the likely reservoir. Direct sexual contact occurs with animals infected with causative agent of dourine, *Trypanosoma equiperdum*. Donkeys have chronic infection and are the likely reservoir.

GEOGRAPHY AND SEASONALITY

- The actual trypanosome and syndrome are geographically related. Surra is a syndrome of South and Central America, Northern Africa, the Middle East, Asia, Indonesia, and Philippines.
- African animal trypanosomiasis occurs in Central and Southern Africa starting mainly along the southern edge of the Sahara, Angola, Zimbabwe, and Mozambique.

CLINICAL PRESENTATION

DISEASE FORMS/SUBTYPES

- Surra
- African animal trypanosomiasis
- Dourine

HISTORY, CHIEF COMPLAINT This is an insidious disease with animals exhibiting cyclical episodes of hemolymphatic disease characterized by pale mucous membranes, icterus, and lymphadenopathy. Horses usually have edema, hyperemia, and petechiation of conjunctiva and mucous membranes.

PHYSICAL EXAM FINDINGS

- Surra can be an inapparent infection, yet these animals are capable of transmitting the disease to vectors. With clinical disease, the onset is variable with insidious signs composed of fever, progressive anemia, and weight loss with a normal appetite. Edema is common on the ventral abdomen and distal limbs. There are frequently petechial hemorrhages on the mucous membranes. Horses commonly have neurologic signs such as weakness and ataxia.
- African animal trypanosomiasis usually starts with an initial infection of skin that is called a chancre. The animal progresses to systemic signs of intermittent fever with accompanying anemia, edema, and weight loss. *Trypanosoma brucei* infection may be associated with neurologic signs similar to surra. Abortion and infertility may occur.
- Dourine is mainly a sexually transmitted disease with transmission from male to female most commonly occurring. After incubation (short or prolonged), animals can become asymptomatic carriers. Clinical disease is characterized by paraphimosis and cutaneous plaques with accompanying neurologic signs in males. Females have swollen vulvar and vaginal tissues and mucopurulent discharge. Mares are frequently uncomfortable and polyuric. The genital symptoms usually are cyclical. The development of characteristic cutaneous lesions follows. These lesions are circular, elevated plaques of thickened skin ranging from 1 to 10 cm in diameter that are observed mostly on the neck, hip, and ventral abdomen.
- With neurologic signs in these diseases, horses become restless and exhibit leg shifting, progressive weakness, and incoordination, and they eventually progress to recumbency. Cranial nerve paralysis, usually cranial nerve VII, may occur.

ETIOLOGY AND PATHOPHYSIOLOGY

- The following *Trypanosoma* spp. infect horses: *T. evansi, T. congolense, T. vivax,* and *T. brucei* subsp. *brucei*
- Surra and mal de caderas: *T. evansi, T. equinum*
- African animal trypanosomiasis, nagana, sleeping sickness: *T. congolense, T. vivax, T. brucei* subsp. *brucei*
- Dourine: *T. equiperdum*

DIAGNOSIS

DIFFERENTIAL DIAGNOSIS

- Anemia, vasculitis, edema
  - Equine infectious anemia virus
  - Equine viral arteritis
  - African horse sickness
  - *Babesia caballi, Babesia equi*
  - *Anaplasma phagocytophilum*
  - Systemic *Clostridium* spp. infections
  - Immune-mediated hemolytic anemia
  - Heinz body anemia
  - *Corynebacterium pseudotuberculosis*
  - Purpura hemorrhagica
- Central nervous system disease
  - Flavivirus encephalitis: West Nile virus, Japanese encephalitis virus, Kunjin virus
  - Alphavirus encephalitis: Eastern, Western, and Venezuelan equine encephalitis virus
  - Ross River virus
  - Getah virus
- Reproductive disease
  - Contagious equine metritis (*Taylorella equigenitalis*)
  - Vesicular exanthema
  - Equine herpesvirus-3

INITIAL DATABASE

- Complete blood count
  - Erythron: Decreased packed cell volume, decreased red blood cell count, decreased hemoglobin
  - Leukon: Leukopenia, lymphocytosis, monocytosis, thrombocytopenia
- Serum biochemical analysis
  - Metabolic acidosis
  - Hyperglobulinemia
  - Azotemia

ADVANCED OR CONFIRMATORY TESTING

- Thick or thin smears, scrapings, and reproductive fluids stained with Giemsa or Leish protocol
  - Blood smear
  - Lymph node aspirate
  - Hematocrit centrifuge buffy coat stain
- Mouse inoculation with detection of parasitemia in 48 to 72 hours and the presence of organism in tissues
- Antigen- and antibody-based tests: enzyme-linked immunosorbent assay, card agglutination, immunofluorescent assay, complement fixation
  - Sensitivity and specificity of these tests are problematic
  - CF test cannot differentiate *T. equiperdum* from *T. evansi, T. ambience,* or *T. brucei.*

TREATMENT

THERAPEUTIC GOAL(S)

- Discouraged because of concerns of induction of persistence and then spread beyond endemic countries and to naïve animals (especially cases of dourine).
- Supportive care.
- Clearance if no chronic exposure.
- The goal is to identify the organism as accurately as possible because some strains are resistant because of widespread use of these treatments in other species and horses.

ACUTE GENERAL TREATMENT

- Suramin (Germanin): As early single treatment only, 10% solution, 7 to 10 mg/kg IV every 7 days for three doses. Will enhance quinapyramine sulphate and diminazene.
  - Recommended for *T. brucei, T. evansi,* and *T. equiperdum*
- Quinapyramine sulphate: 5% solution, 3 to 5 mg/kg q6h by injection IM or SC
  - Recommended for *T. congolense, T. vivax, T. evansi,* and *T. equiperdum*
  - Resistance to *T. brucei*
- Isometamidium chloride: Multiple treatment regimens depending on the organism
  - *T. vivax:* 0.5 mg/kg IM divided in three doses given q6h
  - *T. brucei* and *T. congolense:* 0.5 to 1.0 mg/kg IM divided in doses given q6h
- Diminazene (Berenil): 11 mg/kg IM q24h for 2 days
  - *T. brucei*

POSSIBLE COMPLICATIONS

- Quinapyramine sulphate and isometamidium chloride can cause severe sloughing of tissues; doses should be split into two or three smaller injections.
- Quinapyramine prosalt causes extremely severe local reactions.

RECOMMENDED MONITORING

Quinapyramine sulphate has been extensively used, and some strains are resistant. Retesting over a 3- to 6-month period is necessary to fully confirm clearance.

PROGNOSIS AND OUTCOME

- Guarded for full cure even in early stages of disease
- Poor after clinical signs become extensive
- Reinfection is highly likely unless the animal has been moved from its endemic location.

PEARLS & CONSIDERATIONS

COMMENTS

- These are considered foreign animal diseases for United States, and testing and importation are regulated by the United States Department of Agriculture.
- Contact Area Veterinarians in Charge (AVIC): http://www.aphis.usda.gov/vs/area_offices.htm

PREVENTION

- Reinfection common: Prevention with continuous therapy
- Quinapyramine prosalt: 0.25 mL/kg SC q3mo in stallions and 18 days before breeding in mares. Suramin enhances efficacy.
- Isometamidium chloride: 0.5 to 11 mg/kg IM in several sites once q2–4mo
- Combination Suramin and quinapyramine: 10 mg/kg SC q6mo
- Segregation, quarantine, vector control

SUGGESTED READING

Fenger CK: Antiprotozoal drugs. In Bertone JJ, Horspool LJ, editors: *Equine clinical pharmacology,* St Louis, 2004, Saunders Elsevier, pp 49–62.

Katz JB: Dourine. In Biological Standards Commission of the Organisation Mondial de la Sante Animale, editor: *Manual of diagnostic tests and vaccines for terrestrial animals.* Available at http://http://www.oie.int/fr/normes/mmanual/A_00080.htm.

Luckins AG: Surra. In Biological Standards Commission of the Organisation Mondial de la Sante Animale, editor: *Manual of diagnostic tests and vaccines for terrestrial animals.* Available at http://www.oie.int/fr/normes/mmanual/A_00093.htm.

Schalter J, Van Den Bossche P: Trypanosomiasis (*Tsetse*-transmitted). In Biological Standards Commission of the Organisation Mondial de la Sante Animale, editor: *Manual of diagnostic tests and vaccines for terrestrial animals.* Available at http://www.oie.int/fr/normes/mmanual/A_00066.htm.

AUTHOR: **MAUREEN T. LONG**

EDITORS: **DEBRA C. SELLON** and **MAUREEN T. LONG**

Typhlitis

BASIC INFORMATION

DEFINITION

Inflammation of the cecum

EPIDEMIOLOGY

RISK FACTORS

- Stress: Shipping, routine changes, illness, hospitalization
- Recent diet changes
- Recent antimicrobial administration
- Nonsteroidal antiinflammatory drug therapy

CLINICAL PRESENTATION

HISTORY, CHIEF COMPLAINT
- Usually depression, fever, inappetence, and mild colic signs
- Diarrhea is uncommon.

PHYSICAL EXAM FINDINGS
- Depression
- Variable signs of abdominal pain, usually mild to moderate.
- Pyrexia
- Variable tachycardia and tachypnea.
- Mucous membranes are often injected and hyperemic with a "toxic line."
- Capillary refill time may range from brisk (<1 sec) in the early stages to prolonged (2–4 sec) as dehydration progresses.
- Hypermotile, "fluidy" gastrointestinal borborygmi in the right abdominal quadrants
- Severe diarrhea is typically not observed unless concurrent colitis is present, although the feces may be soft in horses with primary typhlitis.
- Rectal examination: The ventral cecal band is often taut, and the cecum may be pulled cranially and ventrally. Occasionally, fluid contents are palpable within the cecum, although this is not consistently observed.

ETIOLOGY AND PATHOPHYSIOLOGY
- *Salmonella, Clostridium difficile* and *Clostridium perfringens,* and larval cyathastominosis are the most likely causes of typhlitis, either on its own or in conjunction with colitis.
- Idiopathic typhlitis, in which a specific cause cannot be determined, is also fairly common.
- The cecal mucosal barrier is damaged via the same mechanisms as the colonic mucosal barrier in acute colitis (see "Colitis/Diarrhea, Acute, in Adult Horses" in this section), resulting in loss of fluid and electrolytes into the cecal lumen and systemic exposure to bacterial toxins.

DIAGNOSIS

DIFFERENTIAL DIAGNOSIS
- Salmonellosis
- *C. difficile* or *C. perfringens* infection
- Cyathostominosis
- Cecal motility disorder
- Other causes of colitis

INITIAL DATABASE
- Complete blood count
  - Leukopenia characterized by a neutropenia with increased band neutrophils and toxic changes in neutrophils is typically seen.
  - The hematocrit varies with hydration status, but is often increased (40%–50%).
- Serum biochemistry profile
  - Variable electrolyte derangements may be seen, with hypokalemia, hyponatremia, hypochloremia, and hypocalcemia most common.
  - Hypoproteinemia is less common than with acute colitis but may occur.
  - Variable azotemia is common and may be caused by prerenal or renal causes (or both).
  - Metabolic acidosis and hyperlactatemia (>2 mmol/L) suggests impaired peripheral perfusion and tissue oxygenation caused by hypovolemia.
- Transabdominal ultrasonography
  - Increased cecal mural thickness (>5 mm) and fluid contents in the cecum are usually appreciated.
  - Colonic mural thickness is normal in primary typhlitis but may be increased (>5 mm) focally or diffusely with concurrent colitis.
- Peritoneal fluid analysis: Usually normal or with a mildly increased nucleated cell count and total protein concentration (>2 g/dL).

ADVANCED OR CONFIRMATORY TESTING
- Diagnostic testing for specific etiologies of typhlitis in adult horses should include the following:
  - Fecal flotation for intestinal parasites
  - Fecal polymerase chain reaction (PCR) or culture for *Salmonella* spp.
  - Fecal Gram stain and fecal toxin assays for *C. perfringens* and *C.difficile* toxins
- If diarrhea or concurrent colitis is present, the following are also indicated:
  - Serology or whole blood PCR for Potomac horse fever
  - Fecal sedimentation and abdominal radiography for sand accumulation
  - ± Urine analysis for cantharidin
- See "Cyathostominosis," "Salmonellosis," "Diarrhea, Clostridial," "Potomac Horse Fever," "Sand Enteropathy," and "Blister Beetle Toxicosis" in this section for more details.

TREATMENT

THERAPEUTIC GOAL(S)
Supportive care

ACUTE GENERAL TREATMENT
- As for acute colitis (see "Colitis/Diarrhea, Acute, in Adult Horses" in this section)
- Larvicidal deworming with fenbendazole (10 mg/kg PO q24h for 5 days) should be performed in all horses with primary typhlitis because of the predilection of the encysted cyathostomes for the cecum.
- As for clostridial diarrhea, metronidazole therapy (15–25 mg/kg PO or PR q8h), di-tri-octahedral smectite (BioSponge) and *Saccharomyces boulardii* may be beneficial for patients with primary typhlitis if a clostridial cause is suspected (see "Diarrhea, Clostridial" in this section).

POSSIBLE COMPLICATIONS
- Laminitis
- Thrombophlebitis
- Peritonitis
- Cecal infarction (rare)
- Secondary cecal dysmotility and cecal impaction

PROGNOSIS AND OUTCOME
- Fair to good with adequate supportive care in patients that maintain a good appetite
- May be more guarded in patients with severe typhlocolitis

PEARLS & CONSIDERATIONS

In general, horses with primary typhlitis seem to be less systemically compromised than horses with colitis, although this is not always the case.

SUGGESTED READING

David JB: Diarrheal diseases. In Orsini JA, Divers TJ, editors: *Equine emergencies: treatment and procedures,* St Louis, 2008, Saunders Elsevier, pp 159–165.

Jones SJ: Medical disorders of the large intestine: acute diarrhea. In Smith BP, editor: *Large animal internal medicine,* St Louis, 2009, Mosby Elsevier, pp 743–744.

AUTHOR: **KELSEY A. HART**

EDITOR: **TIM MAIR**

Tyzzer's Disease

BASIC INFORMATION

DEFINITION

Tyzzer's disease is caused by infection with *Clostridium piliforme* (formerly known as *Bacillus piliformis*), a motile, spore-forming, obligate intracytoplasmic bacterium causing acute necrotizing hepatitis and rapidly progressing hepatic failure.

EPIDEMIOLOGY

SPECIES, AGE, SEX Foals ages 6 to 45 days are most susceptible.

CONTAGION AND ZOONOSIS
- Disease incidence is sporadic and rare and thus not believed to be contagious.
- The mode of transmission is unknown, although it is speculated that foals ingest feces containing spores of the organism from carrier horses with resulting colonization of the intestinal tract and liver.
- Other species affected include rodents, birds, cats, dogs, cattle, primates, and humans.

GEOGRAPHY AND SEASONALITY The disease has been reported in the United States, Canada, South Africa, England, and Australia.

ASSOCIATED CONDITIONS AND DISORDERS Clinical signs can be indistinguishable from other diseases causing lethargy, recumbency, and seizures in foals.

CLINICAL PRESENTATION

HISTORY, CHIEF COMPLAINT Foals are normal at birth and thrive appropriately. Peracute onset of loss of suckle, lethargy, recumbency, seizures, coma, and sudden death.

PHYSICAL EXAM FINDINGS Tachycardia, tachypnea, fever, icterus, seizures, lethargy, recumbency, shock, and coma

ETIOLOGY AND PATHOPHYSIOLOGY
- *C. piliforme* is excreted in the feces of healthy horses and can survive in the soil
- Ingestion of *C. piliforme* spores from contaminated soil.
- Colonization of intestinal tract and liver

- Acute hepatic centrilobular necrosis with peripheral hepatic degeneration and inflammation

DIAGNOSIS

DIFFERENTIAL DIAGNOSIS
- Sepsis
- Meningitis
- Iron hepatotoxicity
- Perinatal equine herpesvirus-1 infection
- Atresia of the bile duct
- Portosystemic shunt

INITIAL DATABASE
- Packed cell volume: Increased
- White blood cell count: Decreased
- Fibrinogen: Increased
- pH: Decreased
- Bicarbonate: Decreased
- Glucose: Decreased
- γ-Glutamyl transferase, sorbitol dehydrogenase: Increased
- Bilirubin: increased

ADVANCED OR CONFIRMATORY TESTING
- Abdominal ultrasonography: Hepatomegaly with increased hepatic echogenicity
- Polymerase chain reaction test on liver sample: Only way to make definitive diagnosis antemortem
- Gross pathology: Hepatomegaly; multifocal discoloration of liver, visceral, and subcutaneous icterus
- Histopathology: Definitive diagnosis by demonstration of intracellular filamentous bacteria at the periphery of lesions within the liver. Warthin-Starry silver stain used to identify the organism. Other findings include multifocal hepatic necrosis and inflammation, lymphofollicular necrosis, necrotic splenic follicles, and myocarditis.

TREATMENT

THERAPEUTIC GOAL(S)
- There have been rare reported cases of successful treatment.

- The goal of therapy is to replace glucose, correct metabolic acidosis, maintain hydration, and eradicate the organism.

ACUTE GENERAL TREATMENT
- IV fluids to replace volume, correct electrolyte disorders, and correct metabolic acidosis
- IV dextrose to replace glucose in hypoglycemic animals and provide energy substrate without requiring liver metabolism
- IV antimicrobial therapy: *C. piliforme* is reportedly sensitive to penicillin, tetracycline, and erythromycin.
- Parenteral nutrition with close attention paid to blood urea nitrogen and ammonia concentrations because impaired liver metabolism of amino acids may occur.

RECOMMENDED MONITORING
- Frequent assessment of glucose, electrolyte, and acid-base status
- Liver specific enzymes

PROGNOSIS AND OUTCOME

- Grave prognosis with intensive care
- Successful treatment rarely reported

PEARLS & CONSIDERATIONS

Foals of multiparous mares and foals born on premises where mares have been housed for years seem to be less likely to develop disease, suggesting a role of colostral antibodies in the prevention of disease.

SUGGESTED READING

Borchers A, Magdesian KG, Halland S, et al: Successful treatment and polymerase chain reaction (PCR) confirmation of Tyzzer's disease in a foal and clinical and pathologic characteristics of 6 additional foals (1986–2005). *J Vet Intern Med* 20:1212–1218, 2006.

AUTHOR: **JOHANNA ELFENBEIN**

EDITOR: **MICHELLE HENRY BARTON**

Ulcerative Duodenitis

BASIC INFORMATION

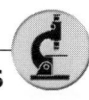

DEFINITION

Focal or diffuse duodenal ulceration of unknown origin

SYNONYM(S)

Gastroduodenal ulcer disease (GDUD)

EPIDEMIOLOGY

SPECIES, AGE, SEX Seen predominantly in foals and occasionally in young horses (<2 years)

CLINICAL PRESENTATION

HISTORY, CHIEF COMPLAINT

- Colic (usually mild and recurrent, but may be acute)
- Inappetence, fever, diarrhea, and weight loss (most frequently described)
- ± Spontaneous nasal reflux of gastric contents
- ± Signs associated with concurrent gastroesophageal ulceration (bruxism, hypersalivation, colic associated with eating; see "Gastric Ulceration in Foals" in this section)

PHYSICAL EXAM FINDINGS

- No significant abnormalities may be identified or poor body condition, dehydration, or variable tachycardia (caused by pain associated with gastric distension) may be present.
- If duodenal stricture and pyloric outflow obstruction have occurred, large-volume gastric reflux is usually obtained on passage of a nasogastric tube, although this may not be present if a concurrent gastric impaction is present.

ETIOLOGY AND PATHOPHYSIOLOGY

- The specific cause of ulcerative duodenitis is unknown.
- Damage to the duodenal mucosa as a result of exposure to excess gastric acid and pepsin, as in gastric ulceration (see "Gastric Ulcers in Foals" and "Gastric Ulcers in Adult Horses" in this section), has been theorized to play a role in the development of ulcerative duodenitis.
- However, reports of possible outbreaks of ulcerative duodenitis in several foals on a single farm suggest an infectious cause may be involved in some cases, although a specific pathogen has not been identified to date.
- Clinical signs of abdominal pain and fever are associated with duodenal inflammation in the early stages of the disease.

- In the later stages, fibrosis occurs as a result of chronic inflammation and may lead to duodenal stricture and gastric outflow obstruction (see "Pyloric Stenosis" in this section).

DIAGNOSIS

DIFFERENTIAL DIAGNOSIS

- Gastric ulcers
- *Rhodococcus equi* enterocolitis in foals
- In later stages, with duodenal stricture
  - Mechanical gastric outflow obstruction secondary to proximal small intestinal obstruction or pyloric stenosis from other causes
  - Proximal enteritis

INITIAL DATABASE

- Complete blood count: Evidence of chronic inflammation, with leukocytosis, hyperfibrinogenemia
- Serum biochemistry profile
  - Variable, may be within normal limits
  - Serum liver enzymes (sorbitol dehydrogenase and γ-glutamyl transpeptidase) activity and serum bile acid concentration may be increased because of secondary ascending cholangiohepatitis.
  - A hypochloremic metabolic alkalosis may be present with concurrent stricture and gastric outflow obstruction.
- Transabdominal ultrasonography
  - The duodenum may be dilated or hypomotile or have increased wall thickness (>5 mm), although this is not consistently seen.
  - Caudal displacement of the gastric contour beyond the left fifteenth intercostal space consistent with gastric distension may be noted if gastric outflow obstruction is present. However, the sonographic location of the gastric contour may vary dramatically and occasionally extends to this location in the absence of gastric distension.

ADVANCED OR CONFIRMATORY TESTING

- Gastroduodenoscopy
  - This is the best method for confirming a diagnosis of ulcerative duodenitis, although in foals with more distal lesions this may be inconclusive.
  - A 2- to 3-mm endoscope is necessary to reach the duodenum in most foals. Focal or diffuse mucosal

ulceration is usually apparent in the region of the pylorus and duodenal ampulla.
  - The presence of enterogastric reflux through the pylorus suggests duodenal disease and may be helpful if a more distal lesion (one that cannot be visualized endoscopically) is present.
  - Concurrent severe gastric ulceration (in the squamous and glandular regions) is often present. The persistence of gastric ulceration despite appropriate treatment should warrant consideration of ulcerative duodenitis.
- Contrast radiography: Serial abdominal radiographs, immediately after administration of barium (30%, 5 mL/kg via a nasogastric tube) and then q20–30 min for 2 to 6 hours can reveal delayed gastric emptying and may be helpful in locating a duodenal stricture.
- Exploratory celiotomy: May be indicated to rule out another type of duodenal or small intestinal abnormality if duodenoscopy is inconclusive.

TREATMENT

THERAPEUTIC GOAL(S)

- Support mucosal healing and prevent further ulceration and scarring
- Promote gastric emptying

ACUTE GENERAL TREATMENT

- Acid suppression:
  - Proton pump inhibitors (PPIs)
    - Omeprazole: 4 mg/kg PO q24h
      - May require 24 to 72 hours to persistently increase gastric pH
      - The parenteral form (Losec 0.5 mg/kg IV q24h) is useful in foals in which gastric reflux prevents PO administration (not available in the United States).
    - Pantoprazole: 1.5 mg/kg IV q24h
      - Has been shown to effectively raise gastric pH in foals
      - Available in the United States
  - Histamine H2-receptor antagonists
    - Cimetidine (16–25 mg/kg PO or 6.6 mg/kg IV q6–8h): Inhibits hepatic cytochrome P450 oxidase and thus alters metabolism of other drugs; use with caution in patients taking concurrent medications.

- Ranitidine: 6.6 mg/kg PO or 1.5 mg/kg IV q8h.
- Famotidine: 2.8 to 4.0 mg/kg PO or 0.23 to 0.5 mg/kg IV q8–12h.
- Because of the need for more frequent administration, these agents are most useful to rapidly decrease gastric pH during the initial 24 to 72 hours of PPI therapy but are also effective when used alone.
- Mucosal protectants
  - Sucralfate: 20 mg/kg PO q6–8h
    - Adheres to ulcerated mucosa, providing protection from gastric acid, and stimulates local production of protective prostaglandins and cytokines to promote mucosal healing
    - Appears to effectively improve comfort in foals with severe lesions
    - Should be used in conjunction with acid suppression as above
  - Misoprostol: 2.5 to 5.0 μg/kg PO q12–24h
    - A PGE2 analogue that inhibits acid secretion, promotes mucosal blood flow, and enhances bicarbonate and mucus production.
    - Useful in nonsteroidal antiinflammatory drug (NSAID)–induced gastric ulceration and duodenal ulceration in humans.
    - Side effects may include abdominal pain and diarrhea.
    - *Should not be handled by women who are or may become pregnant*

- Promotility agents: Bethanechol (0.02–0.04 mg/kg SC q8h or 0.22–0.45 mg/kg PO q8h). May result in significant abdominal discomfort in some horses, especially in those with duodenal stricture
- Antiinflammatory and analgesic therapy
  - NSAIDs and steroids should be avoided because of their potential to exacerbate duodenal ulceration.
  - Opioids and lidocaine (1.3 mg/kg IV slow bolus then 0.05 mg/kg/min IV continuous-rate infusion should be considered in foals with persistent abdominal pain.
- Diet modifications
  - Feed should be restricted for 1 to 3 days during initial therapy, especially if gastric reflux or colic is present. Parenteral nutrition during this period is vital in young foals and should also be considered in older foals.
  - Eliminate hay and maintain on a low complete pelleted feed.
  - Some horses can tolerate pasture if the grass is kept clipped short.

CHRONIC TREATMENT

- If the above medical therapy is unsuccessful, surgical therapy is indicated. Gastrojejunostomy is indicated with severe duodenal fibrosis and stricture.
- The surgical procedure is technically challenging because of limited surgical access to the pylorus in horses.
- In addition, the patient requires intensive postoperative care, because

normal, coordinated gastroenteric motility patterns take weeks to be established at the anastomosis site.
- Thus, this is most often a last resort and carries a guarded to poor prognosis for successful long-term outcome. Medical therapy as above should be continued in the perioperative period to promote motility and prevent further mucosal ulceration.

PROGNOSIS AND OUTCOME

- Guarded to fair with early and aggressive treatment
- Guarded to poor with duodenal stricture and need for surgical bypass

PEARLS & CONSIDERATIONS

Ulcerative duodenitis is not common but should be considered as a differential diagnosis in foals and young horses with recurrent colic, fever, diarrhea, and weight loss.

SUGGESTED READING
Davis JL: Medical disorders of the small intestine: ulcerative duodenitis. In Smith BP, editors: *Large animal internal medicine*, St Louis, 2009, Mosby Elsevier, pp 723–725.

AUTHOR: **KELSEY A. HART**

EDITORS: **TIM MAIR** and **CERI SHERLOCK**

Ulcers, Buccal and Lingual

BASIC INFORMATION

DEFINITION

Ulcers found on the buccal aspect of the cheeks and lateral aspect of the tongue, typically associated with sharp enamel points of the cheek teeth

SYNONYM(S)

Cheek and tongue ulcers

EPIDEMIOLOGY

ASSOCIATED CONDITIONS AND DISORDERS Sharp enamel points of the cheek teeth

CLINICAL PRESENTATION

HISTORY, CHIEF COMPLAINT
- Bit avoidance
- Headshaking
- Quidding
- Dysphagia

PHYSICAL EXAM FINDINGS
- Areas of partial or full-thickness mucosal ulceration adjacent to the lateral edges of the upper cheek teeth and lingual edges of the lower cheek teeth that are painful to the touch (in some cases).
- Healed ulcers may present as slightly depressed, irregularly shaped areas in the cheek that are subjectively thickened on palpation.

ETIOLOGY AND PATHOPHYSIOLOGY
Ulcers are invariably associated with sharp enamel points (or edges) of the adjacent cheek teeth.

DIAGNOSIS

DIFFERENTIAL DIAGNOSIS

- Trauma
- Systemic disease
- Poisoning

INITIAL DATABASE

Complete oral examination

TREATMENT

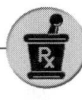

THERAPEUTIC GOAL(S)

Restitution of the oral mucosa

ACUTE GENERAL TREATMENT

Occlusal equilibration and removal of sharp lateral edges of the upper cheek teeth and medial (lingual) edges of the lower cheek teeth

RECOMMENDED MONITORING

Recheck in 6 months

PROGNOSIS AND OUTCOME

Excellent

PEARLS & CONSIDERATIONS

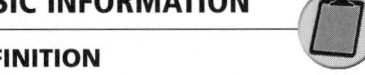

COMMENTS

Buccal ulceration is extremely common and relatively easy to treat.

PREVENTION

Routine oral examination and dental equilibration

SUGGESTED READING

Baker GJ: Abnormalities of wear and periodontal disease. In Baker GJ, Easley J, editors: *Equine dentistry*, ed 2, New York, 2005, Saunders Elsevier, pp 111–119.

AUTHOR and EDITOR: **JAMES. L. CARMALT**

Umbilical Infection in the Neonate

BASIC INFORMATION

DEFINITION

Umbilical infection encompasses infection of the umbilical arteries and veins, urachus, and umbilical stump.

SYNONYM(S)

Navel ill

EPIDEMIOLOGY

SPECIES, AGE, SEX Most infections of the umbilical structures are apparent in the first 2 weeks of life, although infections occasionally become apparent later.
RISK FACTORS Poor sanitation, failure of passive transfer, inappropriate care of the umbilicus
ASSOCIATED CONDITIONS AND DISORDERS Septicemia

CLINICAL PRESENTATION

DISEASE FORMS/SUBTYPES Infection of any single structure or combination of structures may occur. Most common is inflammation or infection of the umbilical stump followed by the urachus, the umbilical vein, and the umbilical arteries.
HISTORY, CHIEF COMPLAINT Usually the owner notices some size change to the umbilicus or fluid discharge (blood, urine, serum, pus). If umbilical infection is a part of septicemia, recumbency, anorexia and lethargy can also be seen. Pyrexia is also common.
PHYSICAL EXAM FINDINGS Umbilical structures can be swollen, hot, or painful to pressure. If septicemia is associated with umbilical infection, foals can be depressed, have diarrhea, or exhibit joint swellings associated with infection of the joint or growth plate.
ETIOLOGY AND PATHOPHYSIOLOGY Most umbilical infections are presumed to be ascending as a result of contamination of the stump of the umbilicus.

However, deep arterial infections have been seen not associated with external infection, suggesting that hematogenous infection is possible.

DIAGNOSIS

DIFFERENTIAL DIAGNOSIS

- Blood clots in the umbilicus or vessels
- Urine accumulation in the urachus

INITIAL DATABASE

- All neonates with suspected infection of their umbilicus should have a complete blood count (CBC) performed and a serum immunoglobulin G concentration determined.
- Transabdominal ultrasonography of umbilical structures (5–10 MHz) strongly support the diagnosis of infection if abnormalities of the size, shape, and echogenicity of the umbilical structures are detected. Blood clots give an enlarged appearance to the vessels, but the echogenicity is homogeneous compared with the heterogeneity commonly seen in infections. The vessel wall is also usually thickened if infected. Urine accumulation may be seen around the urachus but is hypoechoic.

ADVANCED OR CONFIRMATORY TESTING

Culture of discharge can be performed but may be misleading because of the presence of contaminants. Positive blood culture results are more likely to represent causative organisms.

TREATMENT

THERAPEUTIC GOAL(S)

Resolve the local infection and prevent septicemia

ACUTE GENERAL TREATMENT

- Any external necrotic tissue, purulent discharge, or ligatures placed around the umbilicus should be removed. Systemic antimicrobial therapy should be administered based on likely local pathogens. Initial IV therapy with bactericidal drugs is best and can be replaced with oral therapy if necessary. Nonsteroidal antiinflammatory drugs can be used if local inflammation is severe but are usually not necessary long term.
- Other local therapy should be limited to gentle cleaning only as necessary and stump dipping with a nonirritating antiseptic such as chlorhexidine. Cauterizing with silver nitrate or other products leads to excessive inflammation and does not work.

CHRONIC TREATMENT

- Serial ultrasonography is the best method to determine the effectiveness of medical therapy. A good response is exhibited when the size of enlarged structures is decreasing, which should occur within 1 week of treatment initiation. Enlarging structures suggests that therapy is ineffective.
- Foals with urachal infection or inflammation usually have a patent urachus and a thickened urachal wall and usually respond well to oral trimethoprim-sulfa antibiotics.
- Some infections (usually in foals older than neonates) will not resolve with medical therapy, and surgical therapy is indicated. Large or expanding abscesses may require surgery. The decision to remove an umbilical remnant abscess is best made after a few days of IV therapy to allow local inflammation to subside. Complications of surgery can include peritonitis, adhesions, and incisional infections. Surgical therapy of extensive umbilical

vein abscesses that appear to enter the liver (more common in draft horse foals) should be avoided if possible. Marsupialization of remaining infection (as is recommended for calves) may lead to complications such as herniation and adhesions in foals.

POSSIBLE COMPLICATIONS

Rarely, peritonitis or abdominal adhesions may result from a severe infection that results in necrosis of an abscess or severe local inflammation.

RECOMMENDED MONITORING

Serial ultrasonography is best to determine the local progress, and serial CBCs help define systemic and other remote septic processes.

PROGNOSIS AND OUTCOME

The prognosis for horses with uncomplicated infections is very good. Umbilical hernias may occur after therapy but are not as common as in calves.

PEARLS & CONSIDERATIONS

COMMENTS

- Local and medical therapies are often effective.
- Ultrasonography is an invaluable diagnostic aid.

PREVENTION

Appropriate umbilical care immediately after birth, clean foaling areas, and assurance of transfer of passive immunity decrease all septic conditions of the neonate, including those of the umbilicus.

CLIENT EDUCATION

- The umbilical stump should be dipped in a mild astringent two to three times the first day of life. Use of strong antiseptics or overdipping should be avoided.
- The location for foaling should be clean and dry whether a stall or paddock.

SUGGESTED READING

Reef VB: Equine pediatric ultrasonography. *Compend Contin Educ Pract Vet* 13:1277–1285, 1991.

AUTHOR: **ELIZABETH M. SANTSCHI**

EDITORS: **PHOEBE A. SMITH** and **ELIZABETH M. SANTSCHI**

Urachal Diverticulum

BASIC INFORMATION

DEFINITION

A diverticulum from the cranial bladder to the umbilicus that is closed at the umbilicus and open at the bladder

EPIDEMIOLOGY

RISK FACTORS Neonatal umbilical infections or abscesses
ASSOCIATED CONDITIONS AND DISORDERS Urachal abscess or infection

CLINICAL PRESENTATION

HISTORY, CHIEF COMPLAINT
- Dysuria
- Pollakiuria
- Apparent urinary incontinence
PHYSICAL EXAM FINDINGS
- Urine scalding of the hindlimbs
- Possible urovagina in females
ETIOLOGY AND PATHOPHYSIOLOGY
- Urachal diverticula are speculated to result from incomplete closure of the proximal urachus or neonatal umbilical infections and abscesses.
- Affected horses cannot completely empty the bladder as a result of bladder adhesion to the umbilicus.

DIAGNOSIS

DIFFERENTIAL DIAGNOSIS

- Cystic calculi
- Cystitis

- Urinary bladder neoplasia
- Neurologic bladder incontinence
- Partial urethral obstruction
- Ectopic ureter

INITIAL DATABASE

- Neurologic examination
- Complete blood count and fibrinogen concentration
- Serum chemistries
- Urinalysis

ADVANCED OR CONFIRMATORY TESTING

- Cystoscopy
- Ultrasound examination (probably more reliable in foals)
- Contrast cystograms (practical only in foals)
- Rectal examination in mature horses may reveal an abnormality of the cranial bladder

TREATMENT

THERAPEUTIC GOAL(S)

Resolve dysuria and restore normal bladder anatomy

ACUTE GENERAL TREATMENT

Surgical removal of the urachal remnant as is performed in foals to remove umbilical remnants has been curative in one reported case.

PROGNOSIS AND OUTCOME

Apparently good with surgical removal of the urachal remnant

PEARLS & CONSIDERATIONS

COMMENTS

- Urachal diverticulum is a rare cause of dysuria.
- Cystoscopy is the most useful diagnostic procedure to confirm urachal diverticulum.

PREVENTION

- Routine neonatal umbilical antiseptic therapy
- Antibiotic therapy or surgical removal of infected umbilical remnants (or both)

SUGGESTED READING

Dean PW, Robertson JT: Urachal remnant as a cause of pollakiuria and dysuria in a filly. *J Am Vet Med Assoc* 192:375–376, 1988.

AUTHOR and EDITOR: **BRYAN M. WALDRIDGE**

Urinary Bladder and Urethral Rupture

BASIC INFORMATION

DEFINITION

Rupture of the urinary bladder or urethra caused by increased intraabdominal pressure, occlusion, or localized infection

SYNONYM(S)

- Uroabdomen
- Uroperitoneum

EPIDEMIOLOGY

SPECIES, AGE, SEX Urinary bladder rupture is reportedly more common in colts during the first few days of life. Urethral rupture is more common in male horses.

RISK FACTORS

- Urinary bladder rupture may be a postfoaling sequela in mares.
- Meconium impaction may induce bladder rupture caused by straining and increased intra-abdominal pressure (IAP).
- Omphalophlebitis or sepsis in foals can seed areas of the bladder that may become necrotic and perforate.

ASSOCIATED CONDITIONS AND DISORDERS

- Urolithiasis
- Recent foaling

CLINICAL PRESENTATION

HISTORY, CHIEF COMPLAINT

- Colic
- Stranguria
- Pollakiuria
- Swollen prepuce
- Abdominal distension
- Depression or obtundation

PHYSICAL EXAM FINDINGS

- Possible abdominal distension
- Swollen prepuce, ventral midline, or both
- Balanoposthitis
- Depression or obtundation
- Tachypnea or increased respiratory effort

ETIOLOGY AND PATHOPHYSIOLOGY

- In foals, the urinary bladder usually ruptures dorsally where it is thinnest. The long, narrow urethra in colts may predispose them to bladder rupture because of high IAP with the mare's contractions during foaling. In some cases, sepsis may create an area of bladder necrosis that eventually perforates.
- Mares may spontaneously rupture the bladder during foaling.
- Urethral occlusion, usually with urolithiasis, can lead to urethral or bladder rupture in adult male horses.

DIAGNOSIS

DIFFERENTIAL DIAGNOSIS

- Acute abdominal pain (colic)
- Urinary tract obstruction
- Peritonitis
- Gastrointestinal tract rupture
- Urachal (foals) or ureteral rupture

INITIAL DATABASE

- Complete blood count and fibrinogen concentration.
- Serum chemistries
- Serum electrolyte abnormalities classically include hyperkalemia, hyponatremia, and hypochloremia. It is possible that acutely recognized cases may not have had sufficient time for equilibration of electrolytes and water across the peritoneum.
- Abdominocentesis
- Peritoneal fluid/serum creatine concentration ratio of 2:1 or above confirms uroperitoneum, although occasionally some affected foals have a lower ratio.

ADVANCED OR CONFIRMATORY TESTING

- Ultrasonography of the abdomen will reveal much free fluid within the abdominal cavity if the bladder has ruptured. The bladder can appear very small and collapsed. Sometimes the defect can be directly observed (Figure 1).
- Retrograde infusion of agitated sterile saline into the bladder during ultrasound examination may reveal gas bubbles leaking from the defect into the peritoneal cavity.
- If urinary bladder rupture cannot be diagnosed by other methods, then retrograde infusion of sterile dye (methylene blue or fluorescein) and ensuing abdominocentesis may confirm the diagnosis.
- Urethroscopy, cystoscopy, or both

TREATMENT

THERAPEUTIC GOAL(S)

- Surgically repair the defect of the urinary bladder or urethra
- Correct hyperkalemia and other electrolyte abnormalities

ACUTE GENERAL TREATMENT

- IV fluids to replace any fluid deficit. Potassium-containing fluids should be avoided, which necessitates use of 5% dextrose or 0.9% saline. Dextrose solutions have the advantage of promoting intracellular movement of potassium.
- Broad-spectrum prophylactic antibiotics, especially those that are eliminated in the urine (aminoglycosides, penicillins, and cephalosporins)
- Calcium gluconate (4 mg/kg IV slowly) can offset the arrhythmogenic effects of hyperkalemia.
- Horses with severe electrolyte abnormalities usually benefit from having urine drained from the abdominal cavity while attempting to correct electrolyte imbalances. The abdomen can be drained using peritoneal drains or large-gauge IV catheters.

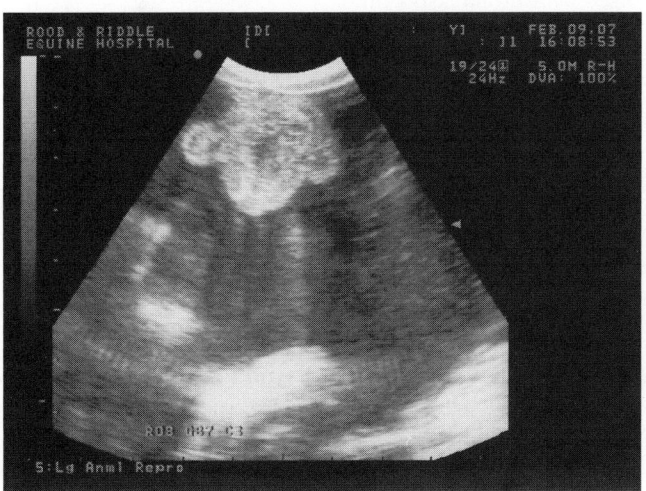

FIGURE 1 Uroperitoneum in a neonatal foal. Note the small and collapsed bladder and urachus with the paired umbilical arteries at *top*.

- Surgical correction of the urethral or bladder defect and removal of any possible occlusion. Unilateral nephrectomy is often necessary for ureteral rupture.

CHRONIC TREATMENT

Small tears in the bladder can sometimes be managed with indwelling catheters in the peritoneal cavity and urinary bladder, mainly in adult horses.

DRUG INTERACTIONS

Potassium-containing balanced electrolyte solutions should not be administered to avoid complicating hyperkalemia. Isotonic saline should be administered to best correct electrolyte abnormalities.

RECOMMENDED MONITORING

- Serial electrolyte concentrations before and during anesthesia
- Electrocardiographic abnormalities may be present in some horses with significant hyperkalemia (bradycardia, elevated T waves, flattened P waves, and prolonged P-R interval)
- Blood urea nitrogen, creatinine, and electrolyte concentrations for several days postoperatively

PROGNOSIS AND OUTCOME

Good with timely diagnosis and surgical correction of urinary tract rupture

PEARLS & CONSIDERATIONS

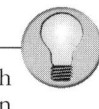

- Most horses and foals with ruptured urinary bladders can still urinate normally.
- The diagnosis of uroperitoneum is usually straightforward using ultrasonography and measurement of the ratio of peritoneal fluid to serum creatinine.

SUGGESTED READING

Conwell R: Uroperitoneum. *Curr Ther Equine Med* 5:857–858, 2003.

AUTHOR and EDITOR: **BRYAN M. WALDRIDGE**

Urolithiasis/Cystic Calculi

BASIC INFORMATION

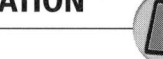

DEFINITION

Cystic calculi are usually singular, round or egg-shaped stones found in the bladder.

SYNONYM(S)

- Cystic urolith
- Bladder stone

EPIDEMIOLOGY

SPECIES, AGE, SEX Cystic calculi are more frequently found in male horses.
RISK FACTORS Horses previously treated for bladder stones or pyelonephritis are at increased risk of developing cystic calculi.
ASSOCIATED CONDITIONS AND DISORDERS Horses with urolithiasis of the lower urinary tract should be examined for disease of the upper urinary tract because pyelonephritis can be a predisposing cause of cystic calculi.

CLINICAL PRESENTATION

DISEASE FORMS/SUBTYPES
- Type I urolith: Most common urolith, yellow to green and spiculated; composed primarily of calcium carbonate. Type I uroliths are often imbedded in mucosa and tend to be larger and more friable than type II uroliths.
- Type II urolith: Smooth, firm, and white; composed of calcium carbonate, phosphate, and magnesium

HISTORY, CHIEF COMPLAINT Hematuria observed after exercise is the most common clinical sign and is virtually

pathognomonic for a cystic calculus. Other clinical signs of cystic or urethral calculi include pollakiuria, dribbling of urine, dysuria, and prolonged periods of penile protrusion. The hindlimbs are often stained with urine or blood. A cystic calculus may cause a stilted hindlimb gait.

PHYSICAL EXAM FINDINGS The presence of a cystic calculus can usually be confirmed by palpation of the bladder per rectum. The pelvic portion of the urethra should be palpated, as well as the bladder, so that a calculus in this location is not overlooked. A cystic calculus is more likely to be detected if only the hand and wrist are inserted into the rectum to palpate the bladder.

ETIOLOGY AND PATHOPHYSIOLOGY Horses excrete a large amount of calcium carbonate crystals in their urine. Mineralization of these crystals around a nidus is thought to be the initiating event. In other species, the nidus is often desquamated epithelial cells. Exfoliated epithelial cells may also act as a nidus for formation of cystic calculi because some horses with urinary calculi are found to have infection of the upper urinary tract.

DIAGNOSIS

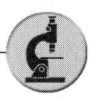

DIFFERENTIAL DIAGNOSIS

- Urethral rents in male horses
- Bacterial cystitis
- A granuloma involving the urethral process, caused by larvae of *Draschia* and *Habronema* spp.

- Renal infection with *Halicephalobus gingivalis* or *Strongylus vulgaris*
- Renal or vesicular neoplasia
- Blister beetle toxicosis (Equine cantharidiasis; see "Blister Beetle Toxicosis" in this section)

INITIAL DATABASE

- Unless the bladder wall is thickened, the diagnosis can often be made or ruled out by palpation of the bladder per rectum.
- Ultrasound examination of the bladder should reveal the cystolith, which should have an acoustic shadow distal to the stone (Figure 1).

ADVANCED OR CONFIRMATORY TESTING

- Endoscopic examination of the urethra and bladder (Figure 2).
- Because pyelonephritis has been found to occur concomitantly in some horses with cystic calculi, renal ultrasonography and bacterial culture of urine may be warranted.
- Evaluation of serum concentrations of urea nitrogen, creatinine, and electrolytes may help to determine if the horse has concomitant renal disease.

TREATMENT

THERAPEUTIC GOAL(S)

Surgical removal of the calculus without leaving behind fragments that can act as a nidus for recurrent stone formation

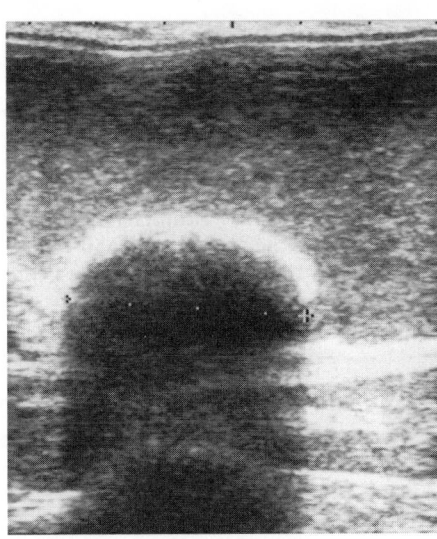

FIGURE 1 Ultrasound image of a cystolith. Note the acoustic shadowing ventral to the stone.

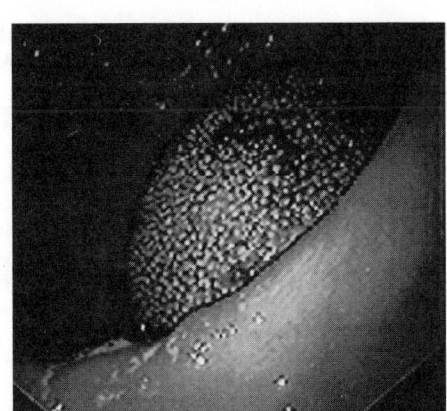

FIGURE 2 Type I urolith in the bladder as observed using endoscopy.

ACUTE GENERAL TREATMENT

A calculus can be removed by laparocystotomy, standing perineal urethrotomy, and standing pararectal cystotomy. During the standing perineal urethrotomy, a calculus can be fragmented with crushing forceps, laser lithotripsy, or extracorporeal shock waves.

RECOMMENDED MONITORING

- Because of the possibility of recurrence, horses with uroliths should be observed for reappearance of clinical signs.
- Occasional recheck ultrasonography or rectal examination may be useful to check for formation of new cystoliths.

PROGNOSIS AND OUTCOME

Most equine surgical texts describe a favorable prognosis for horses with cystic uroliths, but several retrospective studies cite a high rate of recurrence.

PEARLS & CONSIDERATIONS

COMMENTS

- A retrospective study of urolithiasis in horses reported uroliths in the bladder in 69% of affected horses. Approximately 9% of horses had urolithiasis at more than one location.
- Reports of laser lithotripsy in horses are limited, and it appears that certain lasers cannot be assumed to be uniformly successful against all types of uroliths.
- One case report describes use of a radial extracorporeal shockwave therapy device to fragment a urethrolith in a draft horse gelding.

PREVENTION

- A low-calcium diet is recommended to prevent recurrence. The diet should meet, but not exceed, the horse's calcium requirements. This can be accomplished by feeding mature grass pasture or hay or a cereal-grain hay and grain with no added calcium. Early growth grass and legume forages should be avoided.

- Urinary acidification with ammonium chloride, ammonium sulfate, or ascorbic acid is often prescribed to prevent recurrence of urinary tract calculi. However, these are unpalatable to most horses, and there are no studies that compare the likelihood of recurrence of calculi among horses that have received urinary acidifiers and horses that have not received urinary acidifiers. The urinary pH at which formation of calcium carbonate calculi is inhibited in horses is unknown.

SUGGESTED READING

Duesterdieck-Zellmer KF: Equine urolithiasis. *Vet Clin Pract Equine North Am* 23:613, 2007.
Laverty S, Pascoe JR, Ling GV, et al: Urolithiasis in 68 horses. *Vet Surg* 21:56–62, 1992.
Schott HC: Recurrent urolithiasis associated with unilateral pyelonephritis in 5 equids. In *Proceedings Am Assoc Equine Pract* 48:136–137, 2002.

AUTHOR: **JOHN SCHUMACHER**

EDITOR: **BRYAN M. WALDRIDGE**

Uroperitoneum

BASIC INFORMATION

DEFINITION

Free urine within the peritoneal cavity. Although commonly the result of urinary bladder or urachal rupture, various congenital, septic, or traumatic defects of the proximal urinary tract are reported.

SYNONYM(S)

Uroabdomen

EPIDEMIOLOGY

GENETICS AND BREED PREDISPOSITION Foals within the first 2 weeks of life are affected. The majority of the patients are colts; however, fillies may also be affected.

RISK FACTORS Rupture of a foal's bladder usually occurs because of compressive forces associated with parturition. Congenital defects and necrosis caused by infection slightly later in life are also possible.

GEOGRAPHY AND SEASONALITY Uroperitoneum is frequently observed during the foaling season because of its prevalence in neonates.

ASSOCIATED CONDITIONS AND DISORDERS In a medically unstable foal, the clinical signs of uroperitoneum can mimic those of severe dehydration and electrolyte abnormalities, metabolic acidosis, and overall ill thrift.

CLINICAL PRESENTATION

HISTORY, CHIEF COMPLAINT

- Foals are initially normal in clinical appearance, but by 1 to 3 days of age, they may begin to show signs of depression, lethargy, anorexia, mild to moderate colic, and abdominal distension. If the abdominal distension becomes severe, foals may appear dyspneic.
- Other historical findings consist of increased frequency and reduced volume of urine flow. When the defect is the result of necrosis, clinical signs may not be seen until 10 to 14 days of age.

PHYSICAL EXAM FINDINGS Depression, lethargy, anorexia, colic, dyspnea, abdominal distension, pollakiuria, and oliguria

DIAGNOSIS

DIFFERENTIAL DIAGNOSIS

- Ruptured bladder
- Ruptured urachus
- Ruptured ureter

INITIAL DATABASE

- Electrolyte abnormalities
  - Hyperkalemia
  - Hyponatremia
  - Hypochloremia
  - Dehydration
  - Metabolic acidemia
- Abdominocentesis:
  - Clear, yellow, odorless fluid
  - Low specific gravity (<1.008)
  - Increased creatinine and urea nitrogen value
- Serum peritoneal creatinine ratio: Diagnostic when ratio is greater than 1:2

ADVANCED OR CONFIRMATORY TESTING

- Abdominal ultrasonography
  - Increased amounts of free abdominal fluid.
  - Identification of a rent in the urinary bladder.
  - "Bubblegram": Sterile saline shaken and instilled into the bladder can identify rupture after ultrasonographic evaluation of air bubbles exiting a rent and entering the peritoneal cavity.
- Abdominal radiographs: Lateral views can be valuable after retrograde injection of contrast medium. After the contrast reaches the bladder, the presence and location of a rupture may be identified.

TREATMENT

THERAPEUTIC GOAL(S)

- Medical stabilization is a priority and essential before anesthetic induction. Recognition of concurrent disease is also necessary before surgery for correction of a bladder rupture.
- After the foal has been stabilized, elimination of the constant urine leakage into the peritoneum is necessary.

ACUTE GENERAL TREATMENT

- Immediate treatment should include correction of dehydration and electrolyte abnormalities. Because of the frequency of hyperkalemia with uroperitoneum, dehydration should be managed with administration of sterile saline (0.9%).
- IV sodium bicarbonate can also be used to correct the metabolic acidosis.
- Urine should be drained from the abdomen before surgery to facilitate ventilation and improve cardiovascular status. Abdominal lavage with warmed sodium chloride can be effective to further reduce serum potassium concentrations.
- Hyponatremia potentiates cardiotoxic effects of hyperkalemia, so serum sodium concentrations should be maintained within the normal range.

CHRONIC TREATMENT

- After the horse has been stabilized, surgical management for large tears in the bladder can be achieved via a ventral midline celiotomy and cystorrhaphy.
- Smaller tears can be managed conservatively with medical support and

drainage of the bladder via a Foley catheter placed via perineal urethrostomy.
- However, after surgery, urinary catheters are not recommended.

POSSIBLE COMPLICATIONS

Possible complications after a ventral midline celiotomy include abdominal adhesion formation, ventral midline hernia formation, and peritonitis. These are uncommon after repair of a ruptured bladder.

RECOMMENDED MONITORING

Monitor for signs of continued pollakiuria, oliguria, depression, anorexia, or signs of colic.

PROGNOSIS AND OUTCOME

- Very good after medical stabilization and correction of bladder rupture.
- Severely debilitated and sick foals are at risk for death if immediate correction of electrolyte abnormalities and dehydration is not achieved.

PEARLS & CONSIDERATIONS

COMMENTS

Uroperitoneum can be successfully treated after early recognition and correction of electrolyte abnormalities and dehydration.

CLIENT EDUCATION

Signs of anorexia, depression, frequent urination, decreased volume of urine per event, colic, or abdominal distension should necessitate contacting the regular veterinarian, especially during the first week of life.

SUGGESTED READING

Hackett RP: Rupture of the urinary bladder in neonatal foals. *Comp Cont Educ Pract Vet* 6:S488–S491, S494, 1984.

Richardson DW: Urogenital problems in the neonatal foal. *Vet Clin North Am Equine Pract* 1:179, 1985.

Richardson DW, Kohn CW. Uroperitoneum in the foal. *J Am Vet Med Assoc* 182(3):267–271, 1983.

AUTHOR: JARRED WILLIAMS

EDITOR: ELIZABETH M. SANTSCHI and **PHOEBE A. SMITH**

Urospermia

BASIC INFORMATION

DEFINITION

The presence of urine in the ejaculate, which, by changing the pH and osmolarity of the semen, causes infertility

EPIDEMIOLOGY

SPECIES, AGE, SEX Occurs in stallions; may be sporadic in the same stallion

RISK FACTORS
- Neurologic diseases
- Uroliths
- Bladder surgery

ASSOCIATED CONDITIONS AND DISORDERS
- Neurologic diseases
- Painful conditions

CLINICAL PRESENTATION

HISTORY, CHIEF COMPLAINT
- Abnormally large volume of ejaculate
- Semen with the characteristic color and odor of urine
- Decreased to no spermatozoa motility
- Decreased pregnancy rates in bred mares

PHYSICAL EXAM FINDINGS
- Presence of urine in collected semen
- Stallions usually clinically healthy with no systemic signs of illness

ETIOLOGY AND PATHOPHYSIOLOGY
- Asynchrony of the emission or ejaculation and bladder neck closure
- Unknown but appears to be an all-or-none response. Proposed functional abnormality in neuronal control of both ejaculation and urination (α-adrenergic innervation). Occurs by a different mechanism than that which results in retrograde ejaculation (ejaculation into the bladder).

DIAGNOSIS

DIFFERENTIAL DIAGNOSIS

- For neurologic diseases:
  - Cauda equina neuritis
  - Equine herpesvirus type 1
  - Sorghum or Sudan grass toxicity
- For urospermia in healthy stallions with no systemic disease: Pain during breeding; sequelae of neurologic disorders

INITIAL DATABASE

- Examination of collected semen
  - Color (yellow)
  - Volume (can be quite large depending on the amount of urine that was in the bladder at that time)
  - Odor
  - Decreased to absent spermatozoa motility
- Examination of the stallion
  - Rule out systemic diseases: Complete neurologic examination
  - Demonstration of normal libido and sexual performance
  - Videotape stallion during mounting and ejaculation
  - Semen collection using an open-ended artificial vagina

ADVANCED OR CONFIRMATORY TESTING

- Semen pH may be elevated
- Test for the presence of urine
  - Creatinine levels: >2 mg/dL
  - Urea nitrogen level in semen: >30 mg/dL
  - Use of semiquantitative tests for detection of urea nitrogen (Azostix)
    - Rinse after 10-second exposure to semen
    - Color change from yellow to green is significant
  - Use of semiquantitative tests for detection of nitrite (Multistix)
    - Expose to sample for 3.5 minutes
    - Color change from yellow to orange
  - Microscopic examination for urine crystals
- Advanced neurologic examination in all stallions with urospermia

TREATMENT

THERAPEUTIC GOAL(S)

Elimination of urine in the ejaculate to restore or improve fertility

ACUTE GENERAL TREATMENT

- Because the cause of urospermia is often unknown, treatment options include management practices and pharmacologic treatment to prevent urination during collection or breeding.
- Encourage the stallion to urinate before collection or breeding.
  - Exposure to mares in estrus
  - Exposure to fecal piles of other stallions

- Place in a freshly bedded stall
- Placement of a urinary catheter
- Pharmacologic treatment to prevent urination during ejaculation
  - Not shown to be very effective
  - Furosemide, bethanechol, flavoxate, oxytocin not shown to be effective
  - Imipramine: 500 to 800 mg PO before breeding
- Collection of semen by fractions
  - Use an open-ended artificial vagina
  - Can diagnose timing of urination during ejaculation
- Collection of semen into extender
  - "Wash" semen after collection
  - If live cover, can infuse extender directly into the mare's uterus

POSSIBLE COMPLICATIONS

From urinary catheter placement: Urethritis, cystitis, trauma (could lead to stricture or urethral defects)

PROGNOSIS AND OUTCOME

- Generally poor for idiopathic urospermia.
- The unknown cause of urospermia means it is challenging to treat.
- Many stallions have been managed successfully by implementing changes in management and collection. Pharmacologic treatments are rarely reported to be effective.

SUGGESTED READING

Griggers S, Paccamonti DL, Thompson RA, et al: The effects of pH, osmolality and urine contamination on equine spermatozoal motility. *Theriogenology* 56:613–622, 2001.

Lowe JN: Diagnosis and management of urospermia in a commercial Thoroughbred stallion. *Equine Vet Educ* 13:4–7, 2001.

Sepulveda MLH, Rocha GFQ, Brumbaugh GW, et al: Lack of beneficial effects of bethanechol, imipramine, or furosemide on seminal plasma of three stallions with urospermia. *Reprod Domestic Anim* 34: 489–493, 1999.

Turner RM: Urospermia and hemospermia. In Samper JC, Pycock JF, McKinnon AO, editors: *Current therapy in equine reproduction*, St Louis, 2007, Saunders Elsevier, pp 258–265.

AUTHORS: **LISA K. PEARSON, JACOBO S. RODRIGUEZ,** and **AHMED TIBARY**

EDITOR: **JUAN C. SAMPER**

Urovagina

BASIC INFORMATION

DEFINITION
Accumulation of incompletely voided urine in the vaginal fornix

SYNONYM(S)
- Urine pooling
- Vesicovaginal reflux

EPIDEMIOLOGY
SPECIES, AGE, SEX Urovagina can be most often identified in older or multiparous mares.
RISK FACTORS
- Abnormal perineal conformation
- Low body condition score
- In some cases, the mare may only pool urine during estrus when the reproductive tract is under the influence of increased estradiol concentrations.
- Transient urine pooling may occur peripartum because of urethral bruising or from shifting of the urethral angle caused by a heavy uterus.

ASSOCIATED CONDITIONS AND DISORDERS
- Urometra
- Pneumovagina

CLINICAL PRESENTATION
HISTORY, CHIEF COMPLAINT
- Urine dripping from the vulva during exercise or at rest
- Urine scalding on the caudal medial thighs
- History of infertility or reduced fertility
PHYSICAL EXAM FINDING Vaginal speculum examination shows a pool of urine in the ventral aspect of the vaginal fornix and a cranioventral slope of the vaginal vault with inflammation of the cranial vagina and cervix.
ETIOLOGY AND PATHOPHYSIOLOGY
In normal young mares, the reproductive tract slopes craniodorsally, and the vestibule and vagina are mostly contained within the pelvic cavity. The vagina may slope cranioventrally and fall below the level of the pelvic floor because of increased age. After multiple pregnancies, stretching and relaxation of the reproductive tract occurring during vaginal delivery may also lead to urine pooling. This often worsens with each foaling. Because of these physical changes, urine may collect in the cranial vagina, where it provides a spermicidal environment and irritates the vaginal mucosa, predisposing to vaginitis, cervicitis, and endometritis. Affected mares often have some degree of abnormal perineal conformation such as a sunken anus or dorsally sloped vulva. Poor perineal conformation may be caused by loss of pelvic fat.

DIAGNOSIS

DIFFERENTIAL DIAGNOSIS
- Uterine infection with an accumulation of exudate in the vagina
- Postbreeding endometritis
- Vaginitis (acute or chronic)
- Chronic accumulation of urine sediment in the vagina and uterus from chronic urine pooling may resemble a foreign body or even air in the uterus during ultrasound evaluation.

INITIAL DATABASE
- Examination of the mare on several occasions and finding urine accumulated in the cranial vagina confirms the diagnosis.
- Diagnosis is easiest during estrus when the vaginal tissue is more relaxed, allowing for urine accumulation.

ADVANCED OR CONFIRMATORY TESTING
- Uterine lavages can be diagnostic in some cases because of the character of the effluent from the lavage (eg, presence of urine crystals, urine odor).
- In chronic cases, endometrial biopsies may be indicated to assess reproductive capacity.

TREATMENT

THERAPEUTIC GOAL(S)
- Evacuate fluid accumulated in the vagina
- Prevent further inflammation to the vaginal mucosa
- Prevent urometra
- Prevent urine backflow into the vagina
- Allow for future fertile breedings

ACUTE GENERAL TREATMENT
- Manual evacuation of urine from the cranial aspect of the vagina before breeding may improve conception rates, but this does not provide any permanent improvement of the condition.
- Mares that accumulate significant amounts of uterine fluid may be treated with daily uterine lavage with saline and frequent doses of oxytocin (20 IU q4–6h IM).
- Treatment for urine scalding of the skin includes regular washing to remove urine residue and application of protective ointments (eg, zinc oxide).
- Removal or evacuation of accumulated and possibly adhered urine sediment from the vagina and uterus.

CHRONIC TREATMENT
- Surgical procedures to prevent the cranial flow of urine include
  - Vaginoplasty
  - Urethral extension
- Definitive surgical treatment for urine pooling involves modification of the external urethral orifice.
  - The urethral extension is a conduit to channel urine caudally so that it does not accumulate in the vagina.
  - A variety of surgical techniques are commonly used to perform urethral extensions.
- When poor body condition predisposes to urine pooling, weight gain is often beneficial.

RECOMMENDED MONITORING
Reproductive soundness examination before breeding season

PROGNOSIS AND OUTCOME

- This condition decreases the chances of the mare's conceiving and carrying a pregnancy to term.
- The prognosis varies depending on the degree and chronicity of endometritis and surgical success. Early diagnosis and successful surgical treatment often carry a good future reproductive prognosis.
- In some cases, endometrial biopsies may be needed to assess the patient's reproductive future.
- If the condition is left untreated or is not corrected, there is an increased risk and predisposition for cervical irritation and fibrosis, leading to an ascending placentitis or infertility.

PEARLS & CONSIDERATIONS

- When diagnosis is made in a postpartum mare, the decision of surgical intervention should be delayed until after foal heat.

- Mares with postpartum urovagina can pool very large volumes of fluid in the uterus that can delay uterine involution.
- Often, these animals have had a Caslick's procedure performed to correct conditions such as pneumovagina.

SUGGESTED READING

Easley J: Correction of vesicovaginal reflux. In McKinnon A, Voss J, editors: *Equine reproduction*, Philadelphia, 1992, Lea & Febiger, pp 428–436.

McCue P: The problem mare: management philosophy, diagnostic procedures, and therapeutic options. *J Equine Vet Sci* 28(11):619–626, 2008.

Pycock J, Ricketts S: Perineal and cervical abnormalities. *Proceedings of the 10th International Congress of World Equine Veterinary Association*, Russia; 2008, pp 257–265.

Troedsson MHT, Christensen BW: Disease of the reproductive system. In Smith BP, editor: *Large animal internal medicine*, ed 4, St Louis, 2009, Mosby Elsevier, pp 1419–1483.

Trotter G, McKinnon A: Surgery for abnormal vulvar and perineal conformation in the mare. *Vet Clin North Am Equine Pract* 4:389–405, 1988.

AUTHOR: **HERNÁN J. MONTILLA**

EDITOR: **JUAN C. SAMPER**

Urticaria

BASIC INFORMATION

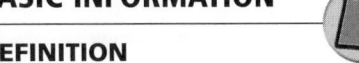

DEFINITION

An acute or chronic edematous skin disorder that may be caused by immunologic or nonimmunologic mechanisms. This is a reaction pattern in the skin of horses with numerous underlying causes.

SYNONYM(S)

Hives

EPIDEMIOLOGY

GENETICS AND BREED PREDISPOSITION There is a genetic predisposition to atopic dermatitis, one of many causes of urticaria.

GEOGRAPHY AND SEASONALITY May be seasonal or nonseasonal depending on causative factors

ASSOCIATED CONDITIONS AND DISORDERS Angioedema, atopic dermatitis, insect hypersensitivity

CLINICAL PRESENTATION

DISEASE FORMS/SUBTYPES
- Conventional urticaria involves wheals ranging in size from 2 mm to 5 cm in diameter. Small wheals (3–6 mm) are called *papular urticaria*, and large wheals (≤40 cm) are termed *giant urticaria*.
- Linear urticaria is characterized by linear bands of urticaria vertically along the trunk.
- Chronic urticaria is defined as urticaria lasting longer than 8 weeks.

HISTORY, CHIEF COMPLAINT Acute or chronic, persistent or recurrent wheals typically occurring on the trunk, neck, or legs

PHYSICAL EXAM FINDINGS The wheals should pit on digital pressure and typically do not remain in the same location for more than 48 hours. They are generally nonpainful and variably pruritic. In severe cases, they may ooze serum and have overlying serous crusts.

ETIOLOGY AND PATHOPHYSIOLOGY
Urticaria results from mast cell basophil degranulation. This may be immunologic and caused by atopic dermatitis, adverse reactions to foods, insect hypersensitivity, drug or vaccine reactions, or contact dermatitis. Nonimmunologic factors include cold, heat, pressure (dermatographism), exercise, or stress. Idiopathic factors are common.

DIAGNOSIS

DIFFERENTIAL DIAGNOSIS

Erythema multiforme, vasculitis, lymphoma, sterile or infectious granulomas, amyloidosis

INITIAL DATABASE

Diagnosis of urticaria is made by history, clinical findings, response to therapy (urticaria is steroid responsive), and ruling out other differential diagnoses. The cause of the urticaria requires further workup.

ADVANCED OR CONFIRMATORY TESTING

- Histopathology can be confirmative and rule out other differentials. Mild to moderate perivascular to interstitial dermatitis with eosinophils and variable dermal edema. In some cases, the edema is diminished during processing of the slide.
- After urticaria is diagnosed, a methodical workup or history evaluation is necessary to determine the underlying cause. If seasonal, there is concern for atopy, insects, seasonal plants or food items, cold, or heat. Assess if there is an association with the administration of drugs, vaccines, topical medications, supplements, or food items or if the lesions occur only in certain locations, with certain tack, or upon exercise.
- If atopy is suspected, intradermal allergy testing can help to identify specific allergens involved.
- Adverse reactions to foods can be assessed with a 4-week novel protein diet trial.
- Cold or heat urticaria can be induced by applying ice or hot packs to the skin.
- Exercise-induced urticaria can be diagnosed if lesions occur after vigorous exercise.
- Pressure urticaria (dermatographism) may be induced by applying digital pressure to the skin.

TREATMENT

THERAPEUTIC GOAL(S)

Control the active disease and prevent recurrence

ACUTE GENERAL TREATMENT

- Avoidance of the offending item or activity that elicits the reaction
- Epinephrine in severe cases
- Corticosteroids
  - Prednisone or prednisolone: 1 to 2 mg/kg PO q24h; then tapered to the lowest possible alternate-day dose
  - Dexamethasone: 0.1 to 0.2 mg/kg PO q24h; then tapered to the lowest possible q72h dose
- Antihistamines: Most effective as preventatives
  - Hydroxyzine: 1 to 2 mg/kg PO q8–12h (antihistamine of choice)
  - Doxepin: 1 mg/kg PO q12h
  - Amitriptyline: 1 mg/kg PO q12h
  - Chlorpheniramine: 0.25 to 0.5 mg/kg PO q12h
  - Diphenhydramine: 1 to 2 mg/kg PO q8–12h

CHRONIC TREATMENT

- Atopic patients: Allergen-specific immunotherapy (ideally based on intradermal testing) is the most specific treatment. The success rates range from 80% to 90% and is indicated only in chronic cases.
- Symptomatic therapy with antihistamines or low alternate-day dosing of prednisolone.

POSSIBLE COMPLICATIONS

Angioedema is a severe form of urticaria that can be life threatening if it obstructs the upper airways. It is most often associated with drug reactions.

PROGNOSIS AND OUTCOME

Good

PEARLS & CONSIDERATIONS

COMMENTS

Immunotherapy for chronic urticaria secondary to atopic dermatitis is a highly effective, safe, and relatively inexpensive mode of therapy.

PREVENTION

Atopic animals should not be considered for breeding.

SUGGESTED READING

Rees CA: Response to immunotherapy in six related horses with urticaria secondary to atopy. *J Am Vet Med Assoc* 218:753–755, 2001.

Scott D, Miller WH: Skin immune system and allergic skin disease. In *Equine dermatology*, St Louis, 2003, Saunders Elsevier, pp 395–449.

AUTHOR: DAVID SENTER

EDITOR: DAVID A. WILSON

Uterine Torsion

BASIC INFORMATION

DEFINITION

Rotation or displacement of a uterine horn more than 45 degrees around the long axis of the uterus

EPIDEMIOLOGY

SPECIES, AGE, SEX

- Pregnant mares
- Rare in ponies and miniature horses
- Comprises 5% to 10% of all obstetrical problems
- Mares having fewer than four previous foals have a higher risk, according to one report

RISK FACTORS Mid to late gestation to term. Most are seen in 7 months to term.

CLINICAL PRESENTATION

HISTORY, CHIEF COMPLAINT

- Mares may be presented with mild to intermittent colic or extreme pain depending on the severity of torsion.
- Severe torsion presents with
  - Discomfort
  - Sweating
  - Anorexia
  - Frequent urination
  - Looking at the flank
  - Kicking at the abdomen and rolling

PHYSICAL EXAM FINDING

- Normal or increased pulse, respiration, and temperature
- Normal or decreased gastrointestinal (GI) sounds
- Chronic uterine torsion, anemia, and pyrexia associated with uterine rupture, fever, tachycardia, and hypovolemia

ETIOLOGY AND PATHOPHYSIOLOGY

Not well understood. Hypotheses include:

- A combination of fetal activity and sudden recumbency and rolling of the mare
- Increased elasticity of the broad ligament along with malposition of the fetus

DIAGNOSIS

DIFFERENTIAL DIAGNOSIS

GI disorders such as impactions, volvulus, intussusceptions

INITIAL DATABASE

- Complete blood count and serum chemistry to assess the degree of dehydration and vascular compromise
- Transabdominal and transrectal imaging to assess the health of the fetus, uterus, and placenta

ADVANCED OR CONFIRMATORY TESTING

- Transrectal palpation of the broad ligaments: Palpation of the taut broad ligament will be extremely painful. The broad ligament on the side of the torsion tends to be more caudal and is palpable as a tight vertical band that disappears under the uterus.
- In counter-clockwise 180-degree uterine torsion, the right broad ligament will be stretched over the uterus, and the left broad ligament will be shorter and run under the uterus.
- In clockwise 180-degree uterine torsion the left broad ligament will be horizontally stretched over the uterus, and the right ligament will be shorter and tucked under the uterus.
- Uterine torsions greater than 360 degrees are rare.

- Equine uterine torsion rarely involves the cervix, and vaginal examination may often not be helpful.
- Ultrasound examination of the mare is important for determining if the uterine wall is compromised (uterine edema) and to assess fetal viability and well being. In some cases, a tortuous middle branch of the uterine artery may be detected by Doppler ultrasound examination.

TREATMENT

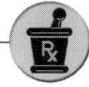

THERAPEUTIC GOAL(S)

- Correction of the torsion
- Supportive therapy to improve fetal viability
- Supportive therapy if the mare is compromised

ACUTE GENERAL TREATMENT

- The method of correction of torsion depends on many factors such as the size of the mare, uterine wall compromise, and compromise of fetal viability.
- Nonsurgical: Rolling the mare under general anesthesia
  - Preferred method in the field
  - Not recommended in draft mares because of complications because of size
  - Drop the mare in lateral recumbency on the side to which the torsion is directed
- Surgical: Standing flank laparotomy
  - One or two sides
  - Highly recommend in younger gestations and in draft mares
- Surgically, ventral abdominal midline: Recommended if the mare has GI involvement, uterine rupture, uterine

tear, death of the foal, or edema in the broad ligament.
- It is important to perform a transrectal palpation and ultrasonography examination after the uterine torsion has been corrected.

CHRONIC TREATMENT

- Depends of ease of correction, results of fetal and placental evaluation, and mare status
- Tocolytic agents
  - Clenbuterol: 0.06 µg/kg orally two to four times daily for the first 4 to 6 days after uterine torsion
  - Altrenogest: 0.088 mg/kg PO once daily for 2 to 3 weeks
- Flunixin meglumine: 0.5 mg/kg IV q6h for 3 to 5 days
- Pentoxifylline
- Antimicrobial therapy if correction was surgical

POSSIBLE COMPLICATIONS

- Uterine rupture
- Uterine tears

- Uterine artery rupture with signs of hypovolemic shock
- Peritonitis

RECOMMENDED MONITORING

- Monitor mare for any further signs of colic, vaginal discharge, or premature lactation
- Abortion
- Premature birth
- Premature placental separation

PROGNOSIS AND OUTCOME

According to one study, both the mare and foal have improved chances of survival if the uterine torsion occurred before 320 days of gestation (97% and 72%, respectively) than if torsion occurred after 320 days of gestation (65% and 32%, respectively).

PEARLS & CONSIDERATIONS

COMMENTS

Surgical or nonsurgical correction of the torsion does not affect the mare for future pregnancy unless cesarean section is performed.

CLIENT EDUCATION

Monitor all pregnant mares for signs of discomfort and mild colic.

SUGGESTED READING

Chaney KP, Holcombe SJ, LeBlanc MM, et al: The effect of uterine torsion on mare and foal survival: a retrospective study, 1985–2005. *Equine Vet J* 39:33–36, 2007.
LeBlanc M: Common peripartum problems in the mare. *J Equine Vet Sci* 28(11):709–715, 2008.

AUTHORS: **JACOBO S. RODRIGUEZ, LISA K. PEARSON**, and **AHMED TIBARY**

EDITOR: **JUAN C. SAMPER**

Uveitis, Equine Recurrent

BASIC INFORMATION

DEFINITION

Recurrent and often progressive inflammation of any to all parts of the uveal tract. Immune-mediated panuveitis has an approximately 2% to 25% prevalence rate in horses in the United States.

SYNONYM(S)

Moon blindness, iridocyclitis, periodic ophthalmia

EPIDEMIOLOGY

GENETICS AND BREED PREDISPOSITION

- Common in Appaloosa, Paint, and Draft Horses
- Appaloosa horses may have a genetic predisposition for equine recurrent uveitis (ERU)

CLINICAL PRESENTATION

DISEASE FORMS/SUBTYPES Three main clinical syndromes are observed in ERU: classic, insidious, and posterior.
- Classic type: Most common and is characterized by active inflammatory episodes in the eye followed by periods of minimal ocular inflammation. The acute, active phase of ERU predominantly involves inflammation of the iris, ciliary body, and choroid, with concurrent involvement of the

cornea, anterior chamber, lens, retina, and vitreous. After treatment with nonspecific antiinflammatory medications such as corticosteroids, the signs of active, acute uveitis can recede, and the disease enters a quiescent or chronic phase. After variable periods of time, the quiescent phase is generally followed by further and increasingly severe episodes of uveitis. The recurrent, progressive nature of the disease is responsible for development

of cataracts, intraocular adhesions, and phthisis bulbi (scarred eye) (Figure 1).
- Insidious type: The inflammation never completely resolves, and a low-grade inflammatory response continues that leads to chronic clinical signs of ERU. Frequently, these horses do not demonstrate overt ocular discomfort, and owners of these horses may not recognize the presence of disease until a cataract forms or the eye becomes blind. This type of uveitis is

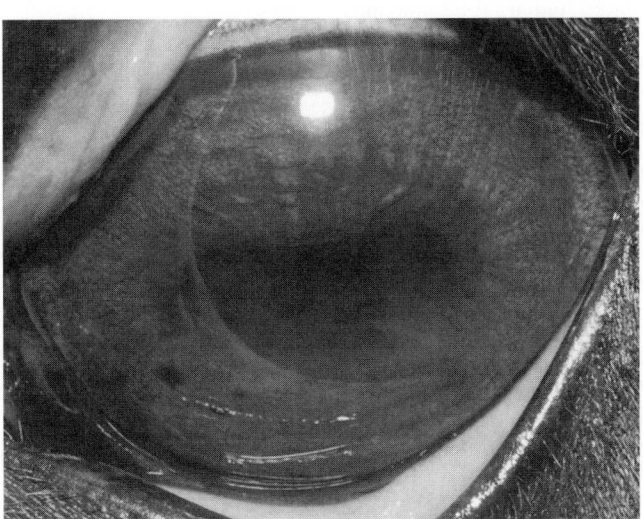

FIGURE 1 Acute uveitis in a horse with ERU.

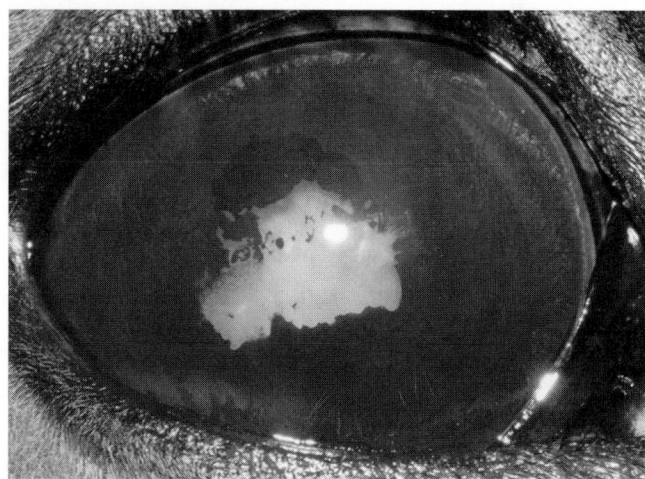

FIGURE 2 Chronic changes in an eye after multiple bouts of ERU.

most commonly seen in Appaloosa and Draft Horses.

- Posterior type: Has clinical signs existing entirely in the vitreous and retina, with little or no anterior signs of uveitis. In this syndrome, there are vitreal opacities and retinal inflammation and degeneration.

HISTORY, CHIEF COMPLAINT Persistent or recurrent blepharospasm, epiphora, ocular cloudiness, and blindness

PHYSICAL EXAM FINDINGS

- Typical clinical signs of active RU are similar to signs of uveitis in other species: Photophobia, blepharospasm, corneal edema, aqueous flare, hypopyon, miosis, vitreous haze, and chorioretinitis.
- Clinical signs of chronic RU include corneal edema, iris fibrosis and hyperpigmentation, posterior synechia, corpora nigra degeneration (smooth edges), miosis, cataract formation, vitreous degeneration and discoloration, and peripapillary retinal degeneration (Figure 2).
- The classic and insidious types of RU can have either predominantly anterior (cornea, iris, lens, and ciliary body inflammation) or posterior (ciliary body, vitreous, and chorioretinal inflammation) segment involvement. Ultimately, even with aggressive treatment, many horses develop a chronically painful eye and blindness as a result of secondary cataract, synechia (intraocular adhesions), scarring, glaucoma, and development of phthisis bulbi.

ETIOLOGY AND PATHOPHYSIOLOGY

- ERU is a nonspecific immune-mediated condition that results in recurrent or persistent inflammatory episodes in the eye. To diagnose the syndrome of ERU, it must be differentiated from non-ERU uveitis. There is a long list of infectious and noninfectious agents responsible for causing acute uveitis in

horses. Although any of these causes may allow horses to develop ERU, not all of these acute uveitis cases will develop into ERU.

- The recurrent episodes typical of ERU are thought to develop because of one of these pathogeneses:
  - Incorporation of an infectious agent or antigen into the uveal tract after the initial uveitis episode. These inciting antigens become established in the ocular tissues, and their continued presence causes periodic episodes of inflammation. Recent studies have suggested that *Leptospira* organisms may be one of the sequestered antigens.
  - Persistence of an immune competent sensitized T lymphocyte in the uveal tract that reactivates when given a signal. The original antigen ("molecular mimicry"), an altered self-antigen, or a decreased immunologic feedback downregulation of the T cell may be the inciting signal for reactivation of the T cell and inflammation.

DIAGNOSIS

Clinical diagnosis of ERU is based on a history of documented recurrent or persistent episodes of uveitis and the presence of characteristic clinical signs (corneal edema, aqueous flare, posterior synechia, corpora nigra atrophy, cataract formation, vitreous degeneration, retinal edema or degeneration with or without signs of associated ocular discomfort such as epiphora, periocular swelling, and blepharospasm).

DIFFERENTIAL DIAGNOSIS

Differentiate from non-ERU uveitis and other causes of recurrent or persistent

ocular inflammation, such as herpesvirus keratitis or immune-mediated keratitis.

INITIAL DATABASE

Complete ophthalmic examination

ADVANCED OR CONFIRMATORY TESTING

Leptospiral serology of aqueous humor and serum

TREATMENT

THERAPEUTIC GOAL(S)

- The main goals of therapy for ERU are to preserve vision and reduce and control ocular inflammation in an attempt to limit permanent damage to the eye.
- When a definite inciting cause has been identified, treatment is directed at eliminating the primary problem, and initial tests to isolate an inciting agent are performed. These tests may consist of a complete blood count, biochemistry profile, conjunctival biopsy, and serology for bacterial and viral agents.
- More often, however, one particular cause cannot be isolated. In these instances, therapy is directed at alleviating symptoms and reducing ocular inflammation.

ACUTE GENERAL TREATMENT

- In acute cases, treatment in the form of systemic and local therapy consisting of antibiotics, corticosteroids, and antiinflammatory drugs is used, many times simultaneously. Initial therapy is instituted for at least 2 weeks and should be tapered off over an additional 2 weeks after the resolution of clinical signs.
- In severe cases, local subconjunctival injections of corticosteroids may be indicated as an adjunct to therapy. In most instances, a subpalpebral lavage catheter is placed to facilitate delivery of topical medications.

CHRONIC TREATMENT

- Many horses respond well to intermittent topical or systemic therapy of their active episodes of ERU. Other horses, however, do not respond to traditional therapy and may experience frequent recurrences of uveitis.
- Traditional treatments used for ERU (corticosteroids and nonsteroidal antiinflammatory drugs) are aimed at reducing inflammation and minimizing permanent ocular damage at each active episode. They are not effective in preventing recurrence of disease. Other medications used to prevent or decrease the severity of recurrent

episodes, such as aspirin, phenylbutazone, and various herbal treatments, have limited efficacy and potential detrimental effects on the gastrointestinal and hematologic systems when used chronically in horses.

- Suprachoroidal cyclosporine sustained-release devices: The goal of cyclosporine therapy is to prevent further inflammatory episodes and thereby prevent additional chronic damage to eyes. Implants are placed surgically and have been demonstrated to control uveitis for up to 3 years.

POSSIBLE COMPLICATIONS

- Secondary glaucoma is possible after chronic uveitis.
- Secondary corneal infectious keratitis is common after long-term topical corticosteroid therapy.

RECOMMENDED MONITORING

Examine weekly until uveitis is controlled, then every 3 months

PROGNOSIS AND OUTCOME

Prognosis is poor for nonrecurrence of uveitis.

PEARLS & CONSIDERATIONS

COMMENTS

Both eyes are at risk and should be monitored.

PREVENTION

- Practices that decrease ocular injury or minimize the inflammatory stimuli may decrease or eliminate the development of recurrent episodes of uveitis in ERU. It may be possible to eliminate environmental triggers (eg, allergens, antigens) of the recurrent episodes of uveitis by changing the horses' pasture, pasture mates, or stable; increasing insect and rodent control; decreasing sun exposure; or changing bedding type.

- Trauma to the eye(s) can also be decreased by eliminating sharp edges, nails, and hooks in the stable; removing low tree branches in the pasture; lightening training and show schedule; minimizing trailering; and constant use of a quality fly mask. Finally, ensuring that horses have proper hoof care, optimal vaccination and anthelmintic schedules, and proper diet may also minimize uveitis episodes.

CLIENT EDUCATION

Client communication is essential so it is understood that treatment is aimed at controlling, not curing, this condition.

SUGGESTED READING

Dwyer A, Gilger BC: Equine recurrent uveitis. In Gilger BC, editor: *Equine ophthalmology*, St Louis, 2005, Elsevier, pp 285–322.

Gilger BC, Salmon JH, Wilkie DA, et al: A novel bioerodible deep scleral lamellar cyclosporine implant for uveitis. *Invest Ophthalmol Vis Sci* 47:2596–2605, 2006.

AUTHOR and EDITOR: **BRIAN C. GILGER**

Vaginal Hemorrhage

BASIC INFORMATION

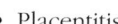

DEFINITION

Bloody vaginal discharge seen during pregnancy, most often caused by ulceration of vaginal varicose veins

SYNONYM(S)

Blood spotting

EPIDEMIOLOGY

SPECIES, AGE, SEX

- Incidence is higher in old multiparous mares
- Occurs in the last trimester of gestation

RISK FACTORS Large varicose vestibulovaginal veins

CLINICAL PRESENTATION

HISTORY, CHIEF COMPLAINT

- Large blood clots are usually present in the stall when the mare lies down or after micturition.
- Dried blood is seen on the perineum, tail hairs, and hindlimbs.

PHYSICAL EXAM FINDINGS

- Presence of blood in the vestibule and vulvar lips or under the tail
- Blood spotting when mare lies down
- Some mares may show severe anemia with pale mucous membranes.

ETIOLOGY AND PATHOPHYSIOLOGY

- Increasing abdominal size leads to retrograde venous pressure distending vaginal veins with subsequent diapedesis and rupture.
- Prolonged progesterone influence may increase dryness of the vagina and ulceration of the veins.

DIAGNOSIS

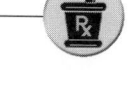

DIFFERENTIAL DIAGNOSIS

- Placentitis
- Premature placental separation
- Impending abortion
- Urinary tract disease (cystitis, urolithiasis, neoplasia)
- Remnants of the hymen at the level of the vestibular sphincter
- Vulvar or vaginal trauma

INITIAL DATABASE

- Vaginal examination using a Polansky speculum: Varicose veins are commonly found laterally and dorsally in the vaginal wall. They are more obvious at the level of the vestibulovaginal sphincter.
- Pale and closed cervix rules out the compromise of the fetoplacental unit.

- In some cases, it is necessary to do an endoscopic vaginal examination for definitive diagnosis.

TREATMENT

ACUTE GENERAL TREATMENT

- Local treatment with astringents: Phenylephrine (hemorrhoid cream) or swab moistened in 10% formalin.
- Ligation of the vessel is necessary in severe persistent hemorrhage.
- Cauterization

RECOMMENDED MONITORING

After foaling, it is important to differentiate if the blood comes from these vaginal varicose veins or from the uterus or cervix.

PROGNOSIS AND OUTCOME

Treatment is generally successful, and no recurrence has been reported during pregnancy.

SUGGESTED READING

Bresciani C, Parmigiani E, Ianni F, et al: A clinical case of bleeding vaginal varicose veins causing severe anaemia in a late-term pregnant mare. *Reprod Domest Anim* 43(suppl 3):157, 2008.

AUTHORS: **JACOBO S. RODRIGUEZ, LISA K. PEARSON**, and **AHMED TIBARY**

EDITOR: **JUAN C. SAMPER**

Vaginitis, Necrotic

BASIC INFORMATION

DEFINITION

Localized necrosis of vaginal mucosa

EPIDEMIOLOGY

SPECIES, AGE, SEX
- Observed mostly in miniature horses and donkeys
- Mares with difficult foaling are at very high risk

GENETICS AND BREED PREDISPOSITION Fetal maternal disproportion and dystocia

ASSOCIATED CONDITIONS AND DISORDERS Vaginal manipulations to relieve dystocias, fetotomy

CLINICAL PRESENTATION

HISTORY, CHIEF COMPLAINT
- Clinical signs may not be apparent for the first 3 to 5 days postpartum
- Systemic signs (eg, depression, inappetence)
- Tenesmus
- Reluctance to defecate or urinate
- Pelvic pain

PHYSICAL EXAM FINDINGS
- Elevated tail
- Swollen vulva
- Walking with an arched back
- Pyrexia not normally present unless the horse has additional periparturient problems (eg, endometritis, retained fetal membranes)
- Fetid discharge or foul vaginal smell

ETIOLOGY AND PATHOPHYSIOLOGY
- Necrotic vaginitis is commonly a sequela of dystocia caused by fetal-pelvic disproportion and the foal remaining in the vagina for a prolonged period.
- Pressure on the walls of the vagina by the fetus or obstetrician causes bruising of vaginal mucosa, leading to localized necrosis, which in turn becomes infected by secondary bacterial contamination. This process may be precipitated by a lack of cleanliness and excessive force by operators during correction of dystocia.
- Severe trauma (other than dystocia) and infection of the vagina may also be followed by necrotic vaginitis.
- Rapid formation of adhesions follows this condition.

DIAGNOSIS

DIFFERENTIAL DIAGNOSIS

- Metritis
- Retained fetal membranes
- Uterine trauma
- Vaginitis (nonnecrotic)
- Peritonitis
- Rectal trauma (prolapse)
- Retroperitoneal abscess
- Lacerations

INITIAL DATABASE

- Diagnose by visual vaginal examination.
  - Development of dark gray to green plaques on the surface of the mucosa (which become gangrenous) are often visualized within the vulvar lips and may extend forward along the vaginal wall.
  - Vaginal speculum or endoscopic examination may show evidence of purulent discharge from the uterus if the horse has concurrent metritis. The speculum should be very well lubricated.
- The rectal examination should be carefully performed to assess the size, state of involution, and consistency of the uterus to rule out the presence of a concurrent uterine infection.
- Aerobic and anaerobic cultures and antibiotic susceptibility.

ADVANCED OR CONFIRMATORY TESTING

- Blood chemistry to assess for potential systemic involvement
- Complete blood count to assess for white blood cell left shift
- Vaginal endoscopy

TREATMENT

THERAPEUTIC GOAL(S)

- Prevent secondary infections
- Promote a patent vaginal canal and prevent vaginal adhesions

ACUTE GENERAL TREATMENT

- Urethral catheterization should be performed if necrosis on the vaginal floor is near the urethral opening or if the transverse fold is involved.
- Analgesics (eg, systemic, epidural, constant rate infusion)
- Antiinflammatory agents (eg, nonsteroidal antiinflammatory drugs)
- Gentle manual removal of necrotic tissue (unless removal results in bleeding)
- Twice-daily application of a soft emollient cream (eg, udder balm), topical antibiotics, or steroid-impregnated ointments can help prevent mural adhesions.
- A well-lubricated partially inflated beach ball may be useful to keep the vaginal lumen patent.
- Systemic antibiotics (include sensitivity for aerobic and anaerobic agents)
- Fecal softeners
- Fly repellent around the perineum may be beneficial if the possibility of fly strike is present.
- Tetanus toxoid and antitoxin
- The inciting cause (if still present) should be treated.

POSSIBLE COMPLICATIONS

- Severe, necrotic vaginitis is a life-threatening condition.
- Transvaginal intrauterine manipulations, even gentle manipulations, should be avoided because necrotic tissue and bacteria may be carried into the uterus, resulting in metritis.

RECOMMENDED MONITORING

Reproductive soundness examination before breeding season

PROGNOSIS AND OUTCOME

- The prognosis for horses with severe necrotic vaginitis is guarded.
- Vaginal stenosis and adhesions may follow this condition.

PEARLS & CONSIDERATIONS

COMMENTS

The vaginal mucosa is initially very inflamed, hard, and painful. Manual vaginal examination may be extremely painful and should be avoided.

PREVENTION

Necrotic vaginitis may be prevented by avoiding or reducing trauma to the vagina when relieving the dystocia by choosing the most appropriate methods and using minimal extractive force.

SUGGESTED READING

Jackson PGG: Postparturient problems in large animals. In Jackson PGG, editor: *Handbook of veterinary obstetrics*, ed 2, St Louis, 2004, Saunders Elsevier, pp 209–231.

Leblanc M: Reproductive emergencies session III. *Proceedings of the Ninth AAEP Resort Symposium*. Mexico, 2007.

AUTHOR: **HERNÁN J. MONTILLA**

EDITOR: **JUAN C. SAMPER**

Venereal Diseases in Stallions: Bacterial

BASIC INFORMATION

DEFINITION

- Bacterial venereal disease (BVD)
- Contagious equine metritis (CEM) caused by the bacterium *Taylorella equigenitalis*. This is the major BVD in the stallions and the family Equidae.
- *Pseudomonas aeruginosa, Klebsiella pneumoniae* (capsule types K1, K2, and K5, potentially types K7 and K39), *Escherichia coli*, and *Streptococcus equi* subsp. *zooepidemicus* are other BVDs in horses.

EPIDEMIOLOGY

RISK FACTORS

- Venereal transmission of *P. aeruginosa, K. pneumoniae, E. coli*, and *S. equi* subsp. *zooepidemicus* can be associated with local overgrowth of these opportunistic pathogenic bacteria on the stallion's penis or associated with normal breeding practices involving susceptible mares.
- Although all factors associated with the colonization of the penis by these organisms have not been fully elucidated, intact penile skin with natural epithelial desquamation and normal commensal microorganisms suppress overproliferation of pathogenic bacteria.
- Improper environmental hygiene of stallion stables and runs may impact the number and type of organisms harbored on the external genitalia.
- Local overgrowth has been associated with improper washing practices.
  - Use of harsh washing solutions, such as povidone-iodine, chlorhexidine, and others, disrupt the normal commensal microflora, allowing opportunistic overgrowth.
  - Excessive washing even with mild soaps may disrupt normal microflora and allow opportunistic overgrowth.
- These organisms can also be acquired from an infected mare at the time of coitus, from an improperly cleaned artificial vagina, or from contaminated equipment such as a phantom.

CONTAGION AND ZOONOSIS

- In most situations, opportunistic bacterial pathogens are asymptomatic residents on the genital epithelium; however, they may be found throughout the stallion's reproductive tract, and accessory sex glands may harbor the organisms. Stallions with an opportunistic bacterial overgrowth can shed and transmit large numbers at breeding or at semen collection via an artificial vagina. This bacterially contaminated semen can cause endometritis with a subsequent reduction in fertility in susceptible mares.
- Although it is rare, there is zoonotic potential with *P. aeruginosa, K. pneumoniae*, and *E. coli*; however transmission to nonimmunocompromised individuals is considered to be rare. The other organisms addressed above are generally considered specific to Equidae.

GEOGRAPHY AND SEASONALITY The geographical distribution of *P. aeruginosa, K. pneumoniae, E. coli*, and *S. equi* subsp. *zooepidemicus* is worldwide and associated with cutaneous microflora of Equidae.

ASSOCIATED CONDITIONS AND DISORDERS All of the bacterial infections listed above, including CEM, *P. aeruginosa, K. pneumoniae, E. coli*, and *S. equi* subsp. *zooepidemicus*, have similar presentations in mares. Stallions, with few exceptions, are asymptomatic. Uncommonly, cutaneous infections can become apparent after abrasions or lacerations that allow subcutaneous tissue penetration and colonization, leading to purulent accumulations on the penis.

CLINICAL PRESENTATION

DISEASE FORMS/SUBTYPES Obvious clinical signs of bacterial infection of the external or internal genitalia are often not apparent in stallions, with the exception of orchitis. Infection becomes suspected based on decreased fertility in inseminated mares or when routine cultures are obtained from the reproductive tract and semen. Although some bacterial overgrowths are short lived, others become persistent and must be treated to restore balance to the commensal microflora.

HISTORY, CHIEF COMPLAINT

- Mares may exhibit overt signs of endometritis after coitus with an affected stallion. The major exception is CEM in mares, which typically produces a significant volume of odorless, grayish-white, mucopurulent vulvar discharge.
- Stallions: Generally, there are no abnormal findings; the primary complaint is decreased fertility in mares being bred. As with CEM in stallions, most other bacteria behave as commensal organisms, causing no clinical signs of infection or inflammation.

PHYSICAL EXAM FINDINGS With few exceptions, there are no abnormal findings on physical examination of stallions affected by an opportunistic pathogenic bacteria overgrowth.

ETIOLOGY AND PATHOPHYSIOLOGY *P. aeruginosa, K. pneumoniae* (capsule types K1, K2, and K5, potentially types K7 and K39) are the pathogenic bacteria primarily associated with venereal transmission in Equidae through coitus and artificial insemination. *S. equi* subsp. *zooepidemicus, E. coli, P. aeruginosa*, and *K. pneumoniae* are most commonly isolated from mares with endometritis. They are also often cultured as commensal, not associated with posthitis.

DIAGNOSIS

DIFFERENTIAL DIAGNOSIS

- Because affected stallions are generally asymptomatic, all causes of infertility must be considered in the differential diagnosis list. These range from infertility with its many facets in mares to all forms of infertility in stallions.
- A differential list of infectious causes of infertility includes all of the bacteria and protozoa listed above and a possibility of a myriad of others, as well as venereally transmitted viruses, such as equine arteritis virus and coital exanthema (equine herpesvirus-3).

INITIAL DATABASE

- Collection of cutaneous swabs for bacterial isolation from the stallion include
  - Unwashed or minimally washed prepuce (vigorously rubbed)
  - Fossa glandis, including the diverticulum
  - Urethral sinus
  - Distal urethra (before and after ejaculation)
  - May include swabs taken from raw semen
  - Culture swabs should be transported refrigerated in Amie's medium with charcoal and plated within 48 hours to increase the likelihood of culturing bacteria of concern.
- External and internal genitalia examination, including accessory sex gland palpation per rectum with ultrasonographic evaluation

ADVANCED OR CONFIRMATORY TESTING

A definitive diagnosis of opportunistic bacterial overgrowth is made by isolating a pure culture of the suspected microorganism.

- This can be supported by the isolation of the same microorganism with a similar sensitivity pattern from the recently bred mares.
- Although a majority of the discussion has been on colonization of the external genitalia, occasionally bacteria can infect the accessory sex glands. In those cases, ultrasonography, urethroscopy, and cystoscopy may aid in localizing infection of the accessory sex glands in stallions.

TREATMENT

THERAPEUTIC GOAL(S)

The primary goal of treatment is the restoration of the normal epithelial microflora.

ACUTE GENERAL TREATMENT

- Treatment of opportunistic bacterial overgrowth on the penis depends on the bacteria isolated and their sensitivity pattern.
- Use of systemic antibiotics or antibiotic ointments is unrewarding and is usually contraindicated; however, extending the semen with semen extenders containing the appropriate antibiotic is useful in breeds allowing artificial insemination.
- Thoroughly washing the stallion's penis with copious amounts of water and removing loose squamous cells and smegma as much as possible along with thoroughly drying decreases bacterial counts.

- Replacing the artificial vagina if collection takes more than one intromission also facilitates reduced bacterial counts.
- Performing postbreeding uterine lavage 4 to 6 hours after breeding followed by an appropriate antibiotic infusion can be a control measure for infected stallions.
- In breeds requiring natural cover, the penis should likewise be washed and scrubbed thoroughly.
- Prebreeding infusion of semen extender containing the appropriate antibiotic, coupled with a postbreeding uterine lavage and antibiotic infusion, as mentioned above, may be effective.
- Stallions with penile colonization by *Klebsiella* or *Pseudomonas* spp. may require penile washes with a weak solution of HCl (0.2%) or sodium hypochlorite (bleach 5.25%), respectively.
- Daily rinsing with sodium hypochlorite (40 mL of bleach per gallon of water) after smegma is removed with copious amounts of water for 2 weeks may be effective.
- Additionally, anecdotal observations of thorough washing followed by packing with either plain yogurt or probiotic paste or with inoculation of the prepuce with smegma from a "normal" stallion have been suggested as beneficial in reestablishing normal commensal microflora.

POSSIBLE COMPLICATIONS

Treatment of some stallions infected with seemingly stubborn strains of *Klebsiella* or *Pseudomonas* spp. may have to be repeated one or more times before the pathogens are replaced by normal flora.

RECOMMENDED MONITORING

Careful monitoring of mares for postbreeding fluid accumulation suggestive of endometritis and monitoring of breeding records are required.

PROGNOSIS AND OUTCOME

- With appropriate treatment, most affected stallions can return to normal without complications.
- Elimination of opportunistic bacterial overgrowth can be successfully achieved with one or more courses of treatment.

PEARLS & CONSIDERATIONS

COMMENTS

- The solution to pollution is dilution. Copious amounts of warm water with

careful desquamation of loose epithelial cells and smegma is the major aim of washing a stallion's penis.
- There is virtually no need to use soaps or detergents in washing a stallion's penis.
- If more than two jumps are required to collect semen from a stallion, you may wish to consider changing out the artificial vagina.

PREVENTION

- For detection of reportable diseases such as CEM, more widespread screening of stallion and mare populations and tighter quality controls over laboratories providing diagnostics would increase detection of carrier animals.
- For bacterial overgrowth prevention, wash appropriately, avoiding excess use of even mild soaps.
- Do not use harsh detergents, disinfectants, or soaps in washing.
- Use disposable liners, phantom covers, and sterilized equipment and supplies in breeding barns and collection centers.

CLIENT EDUCATION

- Avoid using harsh soaps, detergents, or disinfectants for routine washing of the stallion penis.
- Use disposable liners, phantom covers, and sterilized equipment and supplies in breeding barns and collection centers.
- Regulatory veterinarians are our partners in protecting animal health.

SUGGESTED READING

Conboy HS: Significance of bacteria affecting the stallion's reproductive system. In Samper JC, Pycock JF, McKinnon AO, editors: *Current therapy in equine reproduction*, St Louis, 2007, Saunders Elsevier, pp 121–125.

Hughes JP, Loy RG: The relation of infection to infertility in the mare and stallion. *Equine Vet J* 7(3):155–159, 1975.

Ley WB, Slusher SH: Infertility and diseases of the reproductive tract of stallions. In Youngquist RS, Threlfall WR, editors: *Current therapy in large animal theriogenology*, St Louis, 2007, Saunders Elsevier, pp 15–23.

Samper JC, Tibary A: Disease transmission in horses. *Theriogenology* 66:551–559, 2006.

Varner DD: External and internal genital infections of stallions. In *Proceedings of the Stallion Reproduction Symposium*. Society for Theriogenology, Baltimore, 1998, pp 84–94.

Wood JLN, Cardwell JM, Castillo-Olivares J, Irwin V: Transmission of diseases through semen. In Samper JC, Pycock JF, McKinnon AO, editors: *Current therapy in equine reproduction*, St Louis, 2007, Saunders Elsevier, pp 266–274.

AUTHOR: GILBERT REED HOLYOAK

EDITOR: JUAN C. SAMPER

Venereal Diseases in Stallions: Protozoal

BASIC INFORMATION

DEFINITION

- Dourine, caused by *Trypanosoma equiperdum*, is a tissue-borne protozoa that mainly infects horses, donkeys, and mules.
- Piroplasmosis (caused by *Babesia caballi* or *Theileria equi*) is most often spread by ticks, but mechanical transmission has also been documented, and possible venereal transmission is a possible concern if blood from an infected horse contaminates the semen. However, this mode (ie, venereal) has not been demonstrated.

SYNONYMS

Protozoal venereal disease (PVD)

EPIDEMIOLOGY

GENETICS AND BREED PREDISPOSITION Dourine mainly affects horses, donkeys, and mules. These species appear to be the only natural reservoirs for *T. equiperdum*. Zebras have tested positive by serology, but there is no conclusive evidence of infection. Within affected species, there is no reported predisposition difference among breeds.

RISK FACTORS

- Transmission of *T. equiperdum* is unusual in that it is a tissue rather than a blood parasite and is present in associated seminal fluid and mucous exudates of the penis and prepuce as well as in vaginal mucus.
- Artificial insemination would, therefore, be as effective at transmitting dourine as natural breeding.
- Noninfectious periods, more common late in the disease, may last for weeks to months.
- Male donkeys can be asymptomatic carriers.

CONTAGION AND ZOONOSIS Dourine is the only known trypanosome not transmitted by insect vectors. Transmission of *T. equiperdum* is almost exclusively at coitus between mares and stallions and is more readily spread from stallions to mares than vice versa. There are also reports of mares' milk being infectious.

GEOGRAPHY AND SEASONALITY Although the geographical distribution of *T. equiperdum* was once widespread through equine movement during World War I, it has since been eradicated from many countries. The disease is currently endemic in parts of Africa and parts of Asia, including Russia and Mongolia. Occurrences occasionally have been reported in other areas, including the Middle East and Europe, and may exist in some areas where routine testing is not performed. Dourine primarily occurs during the breeding season.

ASSOCIATED CONDITIONS AND DISORDERS

- Coital exanthema
- Surra
- Anthrax
- Equine infectious anemia
- Equine viral arteritis
- Causes of purulent bacterial endometritis

CLINICAL PRESENTATION

DISEASE FORMS/SUBTYPES Dourine is characterized mainly by swelling of the genitalia, cutaneous plaques, and neurologic signs. The symptoms vary with the virulence of the strain, the nutritional status of the horse, and stress factors. The clinical signs often develop over weeks or months. Clinical signs frequently wax and wane, and relapses may be precipitated by stress. Recrudescence of clinical signs can occur several times before the animal either dies or experiences an apparent recovery.

HISTORY, CHIEF COMPLAINT

- Edema of the reproductive organs, including the prepuce and glans penis, and a mucopurulent urethral discharge are often the first signs. Edematous enlargement of the glans may lead to paraphimosis. The swelling may spread to the scrotum, perineum, ventral abdomen, and thorax.
- Neurologic signs can present soon after reproductive tract edema develops or lag weeks to months behind.
- Conjunctivitis and keratitis are common and may be some of the first clinical findings.

PHYSICAL EXAM FINDINGS

- The initial physical presentation is usually marked swelling of the external genitalia.
- Neurologic signs may include restlessness and weight shifting, weakness, incoordination, and eventually paralysis, depending on the duration and rate of disease progression. Facial paralysis, usually unilateral, may be seen in some animals.
- Conjunctivitis and keratitis are common findings.
- Anemia and intermittent fever may also be found.
- Additionally, vesicular ulcerations may erupt on the genitalia, leaving permanent white scars referred to as leukodermic patches.

ETIOLOGY AND PATHOPHYSIOLOGY

- *T. equiperdum* belongs to the subgenus *Trypanozoon* and *Salivarian* section of the genus *Trypanosoma*.
- Strains of *T. equiperdum* vary in their pathogenicity.
- The course of the disease varies with the strain. Some strains cause chronic, relatively mild disease that persists for years. Other strains cause a fairly acute form of disease that lasts only 1 to 2 months, and in rare cases, can progress to the end stage in as little as 1 week.
- The incubation period ranges from a few weeks to several years.
- A waxing and waning of genital edema and swelling may occur in both stallions and mares. With the resolution of the local swelling, a progression occurs of permanently thickened plaques noted on the prepuce and penile shaft.
- Neurologic signs may develop soon after the genital edema or weeks to months after the acute phase of infection.
- Although most cases are fatal, some recoveries have been described. Debate persists as to whether reported patients fully recovered from this disease or merely remained latent at the time of reporting.

DIAGNOSIS

DIFFERENTIAL DIAGNOSIS

For dourine, the differential diagnosis includes coital exanthema, surra, anthrax, equine infectious anemia, and equine viral arteritis.

INITIAL DATABASE

Dourine is best confirmed by

- Serology with diagnostic clinical signs using the complement fixation test
- Detection of *T. equiperdum* in samples is difficult; very small numbers of organisms are usually present.
- Organisms may sometimes be found in vaginal or preputial washings or scrapings taken 4 to 5 days after infection.

ADVANCED OR CONFIRMATORY TESTING

- Although polymerase chain reaction has not been fully validated, it has been reported to markedly improve detection of *T. equiperdum*.
- The most widely used test for dourine and probably the most reliable is complement fixation.

- Other serologic tests include enzyme-linked immunosorbent assays, radioimmunoassay, card agglutination, agar gel immunodiffusion, and counter immunoelectrophoresis.

TREATMENT

THERAPEUTIC GOAL(S)

- Dourine is a reportable disease that is controlled through eradication.
- Quarantines and cessation of breeding prevent transmission.
- Serologic-positive animals are identified and euthanized.
- *T. equiperdum* does not survive outside of its host and will die shortly after euthanasia of its host.

ACUTE GENERAL TREATMENT

- There is no confirmed treatment for dourine.
- *T. equiperdum* can be destroyed by a variety of disinfectants such as sodium hypochlorite (1%) and glutaraldehyde (2%). It is also sensitive to heat at above 50° C.
- The use of trypanocidal drugs has been reported but has not been tested thoroughly.

RECOMMENDED MONITORING

Careful monitoring for development of disease postbreeding, such as swelling of the genitalia progressing to neurologic deficits

PROGNOSIS AND OUTCOME

- Dourine is a reportable disease that is best controlled through eradication.
- The prognosis is grave.

PEARLS & CONSIDERATIONS

PREVENTION

- Dourine must be reported to state or federal authorities.
- New animals should be tested and quarantined in endemic and surrounding areas and with horses coming from those areas.
- If infection is suspected, all breeding activity should be stopped.
- All infected animals should be euthanized.

CLIENT EDUCATION

Regulatory veterinarians are our partners in protecting animal health.

SUGGESTED READING

Conboy HS: Significance of bacteria affecting the stallion's reproductive system. In Samper JC, Pycock JF, McKinnon AO, editors: *Current therapy in equine reproduction*, St Louis, 2007, Saunders Elsevier, pp 121–125.

Hughes JP, Loy RG: The relation of infection to infertility in the mare and stallion. *Equine Vet J* 7(3):155–159, 1975.

Ley WB, Slusher SH: Infertility and diseases of the reproductive tract of stallions. In Youngquist RS, Threlfall WR, editors: *Current therapy in large animal theriogenology*, St Louis, 2007, Saunders Elsevier, pp 15–23.

Samper JC, Tibary A: Disease transmission in horses. *Theriogenology* 66:551–559, 2006.

Varner DD: External and internal genital infections of stallions. In *Proceedings from the Stallion Reproduction Symposium.* Society for Theriogenology, Baltimore, 1998, pp 84–94.

Wood JLN, Cardwell JM, Castillo-Olivares J, Irwin V: Transmission of diseases through semen. In Samper JC, Pycock JF, McKinnon AO, editors: *Current therapy in equine reproduction*, St Louis, 2007, Saunders Elsevier, pp 266–274.

AUTHOR: **GILBERT REED HOLYOAK**

EDITOR: **JUAN C. SAMPER**

Venereal Diseases in Stallions: Viral

BASIC INFORMATION

DEFINITION

- The major viral venereal diseases in the stallion and the family Equidae are equine viral arteritis (EVA) and coital exanthema caused by equine herpesvirus-3 (EHV-3) (see "Arteritis, Equine Viral" in this section).
- EHV-3 is a self-limiting venereal disease usually transmitted via direct contact during the acute phase of infection through ruptured vesicle fluid or ulcer exudates. It is characterized by the formation of small vesiculopustular lesions on the penis and prepuce or on the vaginal or vestibular mucosa and external genitalia and occasionally on the perineum of mares.

EPIDEMIOLOGY

GENETICS AND BREED PREDISPOSITION Appears to be exclusive to Equines.

RISK FACTORS

- Transmission of EHV-3 is primarily through coitus-associated direct transfer of infectious pustular exudates. Additionally, there is evidence of spread through infected fomites such as artificial insemination equipment or gynecologic examination instruments.
- The source of infection during EHV-3 outbreaks within closed breeding herds is most likely from reactivation of an asymptomatic carrier.

CONTAGION AND ZOONOSIS

- The contagious material associated with vesicles, pustules, ulcers, and scabs of the acute infection are contagious.
- EHV-3 infection is generally mild to subclinical, with lesions often unseen on the vaginal or vestibular mucosa in mares and on the prepuce in stallions.
- However, experimentally induced recrudescence has shown latent infection exists, adding weight to circumstantial evidence from field outbreaks of latency and reactivation.

- EHV-3 has been isolated from a lesion on the nostril of a 2-month-old foal after venereal transmission from an infected stallion to the foal's dam, demonstrating nonvenereal horse-to-horse transmission.
- EHV-3 is not zoonotic.

GEOGRAPHY AND SEASONALITY Reported to have a worldwide geographical distribution and has been isolated from Equids in many countries, including the United States, Australia, Canada, Denmark, England, India, Japan, and Norway. Transmission is primarily associated with the breeding season.

ASSOCIATED CONDITIONS AND DISORDERS Pustule formation and occasionally vulvar edema may be seen. Secondary bacterial infections may occur locally and exacerbate the severity of clinical disease.

CLINICAL PRESENTATION

DISEASE FORMS/SUBTYPES Papules, pustules, ulcers, and scabs that when healed leave areas of cutaneous depigmentation. Occasionally, a low-grade fever and mild depression may be detected, but systemic illness is not usually seen with EHV-3 infection.

HISTORY, CHIEF COMPLAINT The chief complaint is the pustules and ulcers during the active phase of infection. These lesions usually resolve completely within 3 to 4 weeks. During the active phase of infection, some stallions may be reluctant to breed because of pain associated with lesions on the penile shaft.

PHYSICAL EXAM FINDINGS The initial physical presentation ranges from early herpesvirus infection lesions of small, raised, fluid-filled vesicles to a range of vesicles, papules, and pustules to healing ulcers with well-defined margins. Occasionally, stallions are more severely affected than mares, becoming mildly lethargic and febrile.

ETIOLOGY AND PATHOPHYSIOLOGY

- EHV-3 is an α-herpesvirus separate from EHV-1 and EHV-4.
- Although not confirmed with EHV-3, it is assumed that viral entry into the cells of the genital epithelium is via cell-dependant caveolar endocytosis, similar to EHV-1. Intracellular viral replication in its lytic infection phase leads to the development of vesicopustular lesions on the penis and prepuce and sometimes the scrotum of stallions and on the vestibulovaginal mucosa and vulva and sometimes the perineum of mares. These vesiculopustular lesions progress to well-demarcated ulcers, which heal with visible scabs, leaving an area of cutaneous depigmentation.
- During occurrences of EHV-3 infection, conception is not prevented, and abortions do not occur in mares with active lesions of coital exanthema. Normal pregnancy rates occur in mares bred to stallions with active infection.

DIAGNOSIS

DIFFERENTIAL DIAGNOSIS

- EHV-1
- Dourine
- EVA
- Bacterial posthitis or balanoposthitis
- Any other inflammatory process that may present with roughly similar lesions
- Vesicular stomatitis may rarely affect the genitalia.

INITIAL DATABASE

- Characteristic lesions and clinical symptoms
- Isolation of EHV-3
- Demonstration of neutralizing antibodies in the sera of recovered mares and stallions

ADVANCED OR CONFIRMATORY TESTING

Although polymerase chain reaction (PCR) has not been fully validated, an EHV-3 specific PCR assay targeted to the highly conserved gC gene has been developed.

TREATMENT

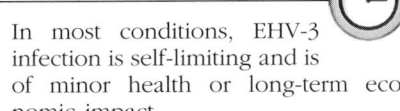

THERAPEUTIC GOAL(S)

Recovery from acute infection and avoidance of virus spread

ACUTE GENERAL TREATMENT

- Sexual rest until a full clinical recovery has been achieved.
- Debridement and cleansing of ulcers and topical antibiotics to avoid secondary bacterial infections may be beneficial.

CHRONIC TREATMENT

There is no chronic treatment for EHV-3.

POSSIBLE COMPLICATIONS

- Secondary bacterial infections may develop within the cutaneous ulcers.
- Latent infections may develop.

RECOMMENDED MONITORING

Careful monitoring of all horses coming into and from breeding facilities for clinical signs of disease

PROGNOSIS AND OUTCOME

- In most conditions, EHV-3 infection is self-limiting and is of minor health or long-term economic impact.
- With appropriate treatment, most affected stallions can return to normal without complications.
- Other than cutaneous depigmentation of previously infected areas and the potential of latency, there is no other apparent long-lasting effect of EHV-3 infection.

- Recrudescence of EHV-3 has been experimentally induced, demonstrating that the virus exhibits a latency-reactivation behavior similar to that of other α-herpesviruses.

PEARLS & CONSIDERATIONS

COMMENTS

Reactivation of latent EHV-3 may have a role in clinical occurrences of coital exanthema within a breeding population without actual evidence of virus transmission.

PREVENTION

- There is no vaccine available for EHV-3.
- Prevention centers on the cessation of breeding of animals with active lesions.
- Breeding and semen collection should not be continued where clinical or epidemiologic evidence indicates an active infection.
- Proper breeding barn hygiene and proper disinfection and sterilization of equipment should be used to prevent fomite transmission.

CLIENT EDUCATION

- At the first sign of EHV-3 infection, all breeding activity should cease.
- Institute appropriate biosecurity measures.

SUGGESTED READING

Barrandeguy M, Vissani A, Olguin C, et al: Experimental reactivation of equine herpesvirus-3 following corticosteroid treatment. *Equine Vet J* 40:593–595, 2008.

Ley WB, Slusher SH: Infertility and diseases of the reproductive tract of stallions. In Youngquist RS, Threlfall WR, editors: *Current therapy in large animal theriogenology*, St Louis, 2007, Saunders Elsevier, pp 15–23.

Samper JC, Tibary A: Disease transmission in horses. *Theriogenology* 66:551–559, 2006.

Varner DD: External and internal genital infections of stallions. In *Proceedings of the Stallion Reproduction Symposium*. Society for Theriogenology, Baltimore, 1998, pp 84–94.

Wood JLN, Cardwell JM, Castillo-Olivares J, Irwin V: Transmission of diseases through semen. In Samper JC, Pycock JF, McKinnon AO, editors: *Current therapy in equine reproduction*, St Louis, 2007, Saunders Elsevier, pp 266–274.

AUTHOR: **GILBERT REED HOLYOAK**

EDITOR: **JUAN C. SAMPER**

Venomous Snakebite

BASIC INFORMATION

DEFINITION

Most venomous snakes in the United States belong to the pit viper family and are either of the *Crotalus* or *Sistrurus* genus (rattlesnakes) or *Agkistrodon* genus (cottonmouths and copperheads). The only poisonous snake endemic to the United States that is not a pit viper is the coral snake. Being familiar with the snakes endemic to your area and having an understanding of the toxic components of their venom will allow you to most appropriately treat the patient.

EPIDEMIOLOGY

RISK FACTORS Residing in an area endemic to poisonous snakes
GEOGRAPHY AND SEASONALITY
- There are many detailed resources that will help locate the poisonous snakes endemic to your area. It is recommended to have this information available in your practice for quick reference.
- Most bites occur during the warm months but can occur on unseasonably warm winter days when snakes briefly come out of hibernation, seeking the warmth of the sun.

ASSOCIATED CONDITIONS AND DISORDERS
- Horses should be carefully examined every 3 to 4 months for 1 year after being bitten to detect any cardiac abnormalities that may have occurred secondary to the bite. Careful cardiac auscultation is important, and an electrocardiogram (ECG) may be necessary.
- Changes in behavior have also been noted after rattlesnake bites.

CLINICAL PRESENTATION

HISTORY, CHIEF COMPLAINT Mild to very severe focal swelling of a distal limb or the muzzle; the patient may or may not be in respiratory distress
PHYSICAL EXAM FINDINGS
- The area surrounding the bite wound will be mildly to markedly swollen depending on the amount of venom injected, the duration of time that has passed since the bite occurred, and the species of snake.
- If the horse is bitten on the muzzle, the swelling can cause occlusion of the nasal passages, resulting in respiratory distress.
- If the horse is bitten on a distal limb, marked lameness may be present.

- The bite wound may or may not be visible. If it is visible it is common to see serum or blood leaking from the wound. Hemorrhage at the site of the wound may persist for hours to days.

ETIOLOGY AND PATHOPHYSIOLOGY
- Snake venoms are complicated mixtures of toxins that have various effects on the body.
- Major effects of immediate clinical concern
  - Effects on hemostasis
  - Tissue necrosis
  - Cardiac toxicity
  - Neurotoxicity (only certain species; commonly Mojave and Timber rattlesnakes; others may exist in your area)
- Hemostasis
  - Affects coagulation cascade in multiple locations
  - Dysfunction or destruction of platelets
  - Persistent bleeding from bite site, mucosal petechiation, potential spontaneous hemorrhage
- Tissue swelling and necrosis
  - Multiple toxins resulting in diffuse tissue swelling and necrosis (eg, myotoxin A causes increased intracellular calcium and cell destruction)
  - Necrosis can be quite severe depending on species of snake and amount of venom injected. This is most detrimental in bites involving the distal limb.
- Cardiac toxicity has been noted with rattlesnake bites.
  - May have persistent tachycardia or other arrhythmias
  - The mechanism is unknown.
  - Cardiac damage may be permanent in some cases.
- Neurotoxicity: Toxins primarily affect the peripheral nervous system, causing respiratory paralysis, general weakness, or flaccid paralysis.

DIAGNOSIS

DIFFERENTIAL DIAGNOSIS

Puncture wound, clostridial myositis, anaphylactic or allergic reaction

INITIAL DATABASE
- Baseline complete blood count and serum chemistry profiles can be useful for assessing hydration and monitoring platelet count.
- A blood smear should be examined for echinocytosis, which may occur with rattlesnake envenomation.

ADVANCED OR CONFIRMATORY TESTING
- If signs of bleeding are present, a coagulation panel can be performed.
- If tachycardia is persistent or an arrhythmia is ausculted, an ECG is indicated.
- Cardiac troponin I can be measured to determine if cardiac damage has occurred. An elevation in this enzyme may be delayed, so repeated samples may be necessary if cardiac abnormalities persist.

TREATMENT

THERAPEUTIC GOAL(S)
- Reduce swelling
- Alleviate pain
- Reduce adverse effects of the venom

ACUTE GENERAL TREATMENT
- Establish an airway in horses bitten on the muzzle. This can be done by inserting a pliable rubber tube into the nostril (eg, garden hose, nasogastric tubing) and securing it in place. The tube should be as long as the distance from the medial canthus of the eye to the muzzle.
- Antiinflammatory drugs should be administered to decrease inflammation. If swelling is severe, corticosteroids should be used initially. If swelling is mild to moderate, nonsteroidal antiinflammatory drugs (NSAIDs) should be used in place of corticosteroids. Antiinflammatory drugs may need to be administered for up to 1 week. Caution is warranted when using NSAIDs in cases with severe thrombocytopenia and coagulopathy because NSAID effects on platelet function may potentially worsen coagulopathy.
- Horses bitten on the muzzle may be unable to prehend food and drink water. Closely monitor hydration status and administer IV fluids as necessary to maintain adequate hydration, especially when administering NSAIDs.
- Horses with distal leg wounds with extensive amounts of tissue necrosis should be treated with broad-spectrum antibiotics such as penicillin or gentamicin.
- Other analgesics such as opioids are indicated with severe pain that is unresponsive to NSAIDs.
- Administer antivenin (most critical in cases with hemostatic dysfunction or neurotoxicity).

CHRONIC TREATMENT

If cardiac inflammation is detected, long-term corticosteroids may be indicated to decrease cardiac muscle fibrosis.

POSSIBLE COMPLICATIONS

Mortality with snake envenomation is most commonly caused by asphyxiation followed by hemorrhage and neurotoxicity. Serum sickness may occur secondary to administration of equine-origin antivenin products.

RECOMMENDED MONITORING

Monitor heart rate and rhythm for signs of cardiac toxicity. Examinations should occur every 3 to 4 months for 1 year after a bite.

PROGNOSIS AND OUTCOME

The overall prognosis for life is good with many venomous snake bites; however, if horses experience cardiac effects, the prognosis for full return to function may be guarded to poor.

PEARLS & CONSIDERATIONS

COMMENTS

- It is very important to remember when giving antivenin that even a low dose can be helpful. Do not discount using the product because you think a "horse dose" is too expensive. Any amount that you give should reduce circulating venom and therefore reduce the overall toxic effects. Dosing of antivenin is based on the suspected dose of venom injected by the snake, not the size of the animal that received the bite.
- The newer ovine Fab product Crofab is still extremely expensive; therefore the polyvalent equine-origin product is still the more commonly used antivenin.

PREVENTION

A vaccine against rattlesnake venom has been developed for dogs and is being developed for horses. This vaccine has reduced the effects of rattlesnake envenomation in dogs.

CLIENT EDUCATION

Clients should understand that treatment is not only for tissue wounds and swelling. The venom affects many parts of the body that cannot be seen, and the damage may be long term.

SUGGESTED READING

Dickinson CE, Traub-Dargatz JL, Dargatz DA, et al: Rattlesnake poisoning in horses: 32 cases (1973–1993). *J Am Vet Med Assoc* 208(11):1866–1877, 1996.
Lawler JB, Frye MA, Bera MM, et al: Third degree atrioventricular block in a horse secondary to rattlesnake envenomation. *J Vet Intern Med* 22(2):486–490, 2008.
Parrish M: *Poisonous snakebites in the United States*, New York, 1980, Vantage Press.
Tu AT: *Rattlesnake venoms: their actions and treatment*, New York, 1982, Marcel Dekker.

AUTHOR: **LYNDI L. GILLIAM**

EDITOR: **CYNTHIA L. GASKILL**

Venous Air Embolus

BASIC INFORMATION

DEFINITION

Imbibement of air, typically through a jugular catheter, into the venous system

EPIDEMIOLOGY

SPECIES, AGE, SEX Horses are at increased risk because of their large veins, the use of large-gauge catheters, and the fact that their heads are elevated above their hearts.

RISK FACTORS
- Downward placed jugular catheters
- Distal end of the catheter is toward the heart
- Large-gauge jugular venous catheters

CLINICAL PRESENTATION

PHYSICAL EXAM FINDINGS
- Ataxia
- Agitation
- Head pressing
- Hypermetric gait
- Cerebral signs: Delayed onset of central blindness
- Pruritus
- Tachypnea, abnormal pulmonary auscultation

- Tachycardia, arrhythmias, hear murmurs ("mill wheel" character)

ETIOLOGY AND PATHOPHYSIOLOGY
- Negative pressure created in the thorax on inspiration pulls air through the catheter when the head is above the heart.
- Cardiovascular issues result from the physical obstruction of blood flow from the right ventricle (an "air lock" is formed).
- Pulmonary edema may result from air in the microvaculature, causing inflammation and increased vascular permeability, resulting in surfactant inactivation and atelectasis.
- Air may enter the systemic vasculature through cardiac shunts (patent foramen ovale) or by pulmonary arteriovenous physiologic shunts, resulting in systemic and cerebral issues.
- Cerebral disorders may be attributed to local ischemia and necrosis directly caused by air occlusion of the vessel, cerebral edema caused by irritation of the vascular wall and loss of the blood-brain barrier, and transient hypoxia caused by hyperventilation reducing cerebral perfusion.

DIAGNOSIS

DIFFERENTIAL DIAGNOSIS

- Neurologic disease or pathology (toxic, metabolic, infectious, traumatic)
- Anesthetic complications
- Allergic reaction
- Respiratory disease

INITIAL DATABASE

- Physical examination
- Arterial blood gas
- Blood pressure
- Pulse oximetry
- End-tidal CO_2 (if anesthetized)

ADVANCED OR CONFIRMATORY TESTING

- Echocardiography may identify air in the right heart.
- Computed tomography or magnetic resonance imaging to identify cerebral emboli

TREATMENT

THERAPEUTIC GOAL(S)

- Reduce further air imbibement
- Remove air embolus

- Provide immediate resuscitation
- Reduce pulmonary inflammation and edema
- Reduce cerebral inflammation and edema

ACUTE GENERAL TREATMENT

- Stop further entry of air through the catheter
  - Occlude the catheter
  - Fluid therapy to increase blood pressure will reduce air aspiration
  - Place the head at a level below the heart (if anesthetized) to reduce aspiration
  - Positive-pressure ventilation increases thoracic pressure and reduces air aspiration
- Remove air emboli in the heart (feasible in foals only); air in the right ventricle may be vacuumed from the heart using a central venous line
- Provide emergency cardiopulmonary resuscitation
  - Mechanical ventilation if indicated by dyspnea or apnea. General anesthesia may reduce the short-term effects of air embolus.
  - Oxygen therapy to treat hypoxia and reduce the size of the embolus by diffusion
  - Fluid therapy to maintain blood pressure and cerebral perfusion
- Treat sequelae of air embolus
  - Pulmonary inflammation and edema
    - Nasal oxygen therapy (5–15 L/min)
    - Furosemide (1–2 mg/kg IV initially then 0.25–1.0 mg/kg IV q12–24h maintenance) for edema
    - Nonsteroidal antiinflammatory drugs (NSAIDs; flunixin meglumine: 1.1 mg/kg IV q12h)
  - Cerebral infarction
    - Maintain blood pressure within normal range with fluid therapy
    - Nonsteroidal antiinflammtory drugs

- Dimethylsulfoxide (1 g/kg, 10% solution, IV q12h) for free radical scavenging and edema
- Alleviate seizures
  - Diazepam (adults: 0.05–0.44 mg/kg IV; foals: 0.1–0.2 mg/kg IV)
  - Phenobarbital (5–15 mg/kg IV slowly)
- Reduce edema
  - Hypertonic saline (2–4 mL/kg IV)
  - Mannitol (0.2–2.0 g/kg, 20% solution, IV over 30–45 min)
  - Hyperbaric oxygen therapy (if available)
    - Physically reduces size of air bubbles
    - Increases tissue oxygenation
    - Reduces cerebral edema

CHRONIC TREATMENT

- Supportive care should be provided if the horse is unable to function in a normal manner.
  - Provide hydration and nutrition.
  - Nursing care and positional adjustments for down horses
- Further therapy will depend on the clinical signs.

POSSIBLE COMPLICATIONS

Bronchodilators are indicated for pulmonary edema but cause pulmonary vascular relaxation that may increase the release of air emboli to the systemic circulation.

RECOMMENDED MONITORING

Serial arterial blood gas, pulse oximetry, and blood pressure can monitor the response to therapy.

PROGNOSIS AND OUTCOME

Signs of encephalopathy may indicate a poor prognosis.

PEARLS & CONSIDERATIONS

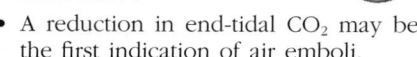

COMMENTS

- A reduction in end-tidal CO_2 may be the first indication of air emboli.
- Up to 0.25 mL/kg of air may safely be aspirated into a vessel.
  - The toxic dose may have individual variation based on the rate of embolization or position of the head relative to the heart.

PREVENTION

- Monitor all IV catheters and any extensions of fluid lines to ensure proper connection and prevent air entry.
- Catheters may be placed with the distal end cranial in the jugular (away from the heart).
  - Reduces risk of aspiration
  - Increases the risk of thrombophlebitis
- Smaller catheters may reduce the risk of air imbibement

SUGGESTED READING
Bradbury LA, Archer DC, Dugdale AH, et al: Suspected venous air embolism in a horse. *Vet Rec* 156(4):109–111, 2005.
Heckmann JG, Lang CJ, Kindler K, et al: Neurologic manifestations of cerebral air embolism as a complication of central venous catheterization. *Crit Care Med* 28(5):1621–1625, 2000.
Holbrook TC, Dechant JE, Crowson CL, et al: Suspected air embolism associated with post-anesthetic pulmonary edema and neurologic sequelae in a horse. *Vet Anaesth Analg* 34(3):217–222, 2007.
van Hulst RA, Klein J, Lachmann B, et al: Gas embolism: pathophysiology and treatment. *Clin Physiol Funct Imaging* 23(5):237–246, 2003.

AUTHOR: **AMELIA MUNSTERMAN**

EDITORS: **R. REID HANSON** and **AMELIA MUNSTERMAN**

Ventricular Fibrillation

BASIC INFORMATION

DEFINITION
Fatal ventricular tachyarrhythmia attributable to reentry, causing ventricular activation to be so rapid and uncoordinated that contractile function is lost. Cardiac output is essentially zero.

EPIDEMIOLOGY
RISK FACTORS
- Any cause of severe electrolyte imbalance (eg, ruptured bladder)
- Severe cardiac disease
- Hypoxia
- Severe systemic disease

CLINICAL PRESENTATION
HISTORY, CHIEF COMPLAINT
- Weakness, collapse
- Signs of cardiac failure
- Suspicion of intoxication (cardiac glycosides)
- Electrical cardioversion
- Sudden death

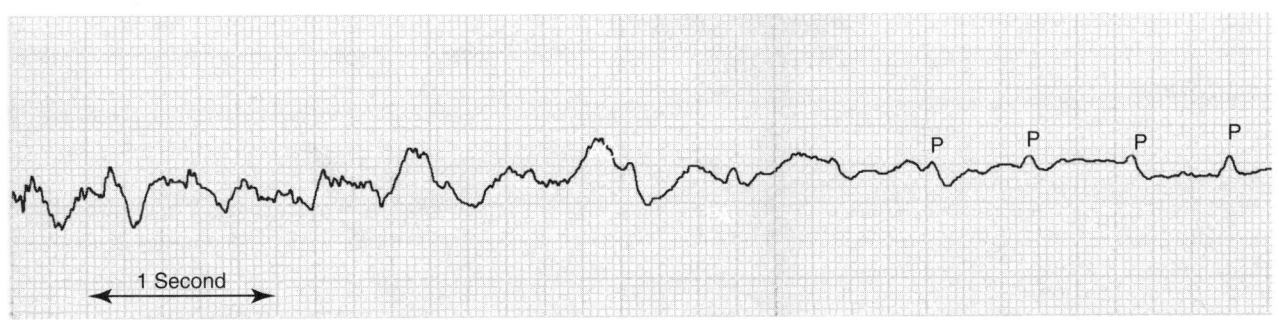

FIGURE 1 Ventricular fibrillation in a horse with oleander intoxication. P waves can still be identified immediately after the onset of fibrillation.

PHYSICAL EXAM FINDINGS

- Physical examination findings immediately before the onset of ventricular fibrillation (VF)
  - Signs of ventricular ectopy: Ventricular premature complexes (VPCs) or ventricular tachycardia (VT)
  - Signs of severe cardiac disease
  - Signs of severe systemic disease
  - Signs of bladder rupture
- Physical examination findings when VF occurs (Figure 1)
  - Instantaneous collapse with no palpable pulse. A weak pulsation may occasionally be observed in the jugular vein caused by atrial contractions.
  - Death within seconds to minutes; always fatal.

ETIOLOGY AND PATHOPHYSIOLOGY

- Ventricular ectopy (VPCs or VT) usually precedes VF and is caused by enhanced automaticity or triggered activity because of cardiac disease, electrolyte imbalances, systemic disease, drugs, or toxicity.
- Ventricular ectopy during the vulnerable period of the ventricular myocardium (ie, during the T wave) may suddenly initiate reentry, which results in VF. This reentry phenomenon can be initiated by:
  - A single VPC during the vulnerable period
  - Deterioration of ventricular tachycardia or ventricular flutter into VF
  - Deterioration of torsades de pointes
  - Electrical cardioversion
    - Caused by spontaneous occurrence of ventricular ectopy after shock delivery.
    - Caused by inappropriate shock delivery on the T wave (eg, during transvenous electrical cardioversion of atrial fibrillation). Whenever electrical cardioversion is applied for tachyarrhythmias other than VF, it is mandatory to deliver the shock in "synchronous mode." In synchronous mode, the defibrillator will automatically deliver the shock synchronous with the R wave on the surface electrocardiogram (ECG). However, when the defibrillator incorrectly detects T waves as R waves, shock delivery may occur on the T wave, which carries a very high risk of fatal VF induction. Therefore, electrodes must always be repositioned until correct R wave (without T wave) detection is obtained. VF (or cardiac arrest) is the only tachyarrhythmia in which shock delivery is instantaneous, not synchronized with the R wave because there are no R waves.
- After reentry is initiated, VF will never terminate spontaneously because this self-sustaining arrhythmia is very stable in the large ventricular myocardium in horses.
- During VF, ventricular activation is so rapid and chaotic that the myocardium only trembles without any coordinated contraction. As a result, cardiac output is absent, and death occurs.
- Antiarrhythmic drug administration (eg, quinidine) or intoxication (eg, cardiac glycosides) may be associated with VF because of ventricular ectopy or changes in ventricular electrophysiology that promote reentry.

DIAGNOSIS

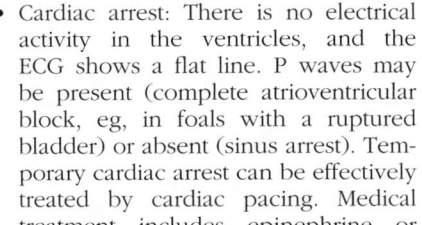

DIFFERENTIAL DIAGNOSIS

- Cardiac arrest: There is no electrical activity in the ventricles, and the ECG shows a flat line. P waves may be present (complete atrioventricular block, eg, in foals with a ruptured bladder) or absent (sinus arrest). Temporary cardiac arrest can be effectively treated by cardiac pacing. Medical treatment includes epinephrine or vasopressin and atropine.
- Ventricular tachycardia (high rate): Rapid (often regular) QRS complexes and T waves; R-on-T might be present.
- Torsades de pointes: Wide QRS tachycardia in which the QRS and T twist around the baseline with changing amplitude; this arrhythmia may rapidly deteriorate into VF.
- Artifacts: Always double check the position of electrodes, connection of the cables, and condition of wires (for damage) to obtain a good-quality recording.

INITIAL DATABASE

- Electrocardiography: The ECG shows irregular and bizarre waves, and QRS complexes and T waves can no longer be identified. VF may be coarse (large oscillations) or fine (small oscillations). During fine VF, it is possible that P waves can still be identified because the atria may continue at their own rate for a short period (Figure 1). The arrhythmia is always fatal within seconds or minutes. Attempts at treatment must start immediately.
- Electrolyte status
- Blood gas, acid-base status

ADVANCED OR CONFIRMATORY TESTING

In case the horse (most likely a foal) survives, diagnostic procedures for ventricular ectopy must be performed (see "Ventricular Premature Complex/Ventricular Tachycardia" in this section).

TREATMENT

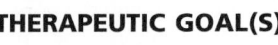

THERAPEUTIC GOAL(S)

- Terminate VF
- Restore sinus rhythm

ACUTE GENERAL TREATMENT

- Establish an airway and ventilation
- Establish cardiac compression
- Provide immediate electrical defibrillation
  - Biphasic shocks are more effective than monophasic shocks.
  - Shocks are delivered as soon as possible and are not synchronized (there is no R wave).
  - Use contact gel and place the paddle on each side of the thorax slightly ventral to the apex beat area.

○ Deliver 2 J/kg (foals).
○ If unsuccessful, administer epinephrine or lidocaine and repeat defibrillation at 4 J/kg. Repeat shock delivery with 50% increasing energy if unsuccessful. Between cardioversion attempts, 1 to 2 minutes of chest compression need to be performed (foals).
○ The success of electrical defibrillation strongly depends on ventricular size and thus the size of the animal. It can be effective in foals, has a low efficacy in animals that weigh more than 200 to 300 kg, and is very unlikely to be effective in mature horses.
• Fluid administration

RECOMMENDED MONITORING
Monitor ECG until normalization.

PROGNOSIS AND OUTCOME

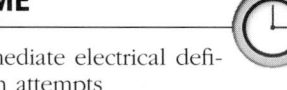

• For immediate electrical defibrillation attempts
  ○ In foals or ponies that weigh less than 200 kg: Guarded to grave prognosis
  ○ In larger animals: Usually fatal
• For medical treatment alone: Usually fatal

SUGGESTED READING
Corley KTT, Axon JE: Resuscitation and emergency management for neonatal foals. *Vet Clin North Am Equine Pract* 21:431–455, 2005.
Geddes LA, Tacker WA, Rosborough JP, et al: Electrical dose for ventricular defibrillation of large and small animals using precordial electrodes. *J Clin Invest* 53:310–319, 1974.
Geddes LA, Tacker WA, Rosborough J, et al: The electrical dose for ventricular defibrillation with electrodes applied directly to the heart. *J Thorac Cardiovasc Surg* 68:593–602, 1974.
Palmer JE: Neonatal foal resuscitation. *Vet Clin North Am Equine Pract* 23:159–182, 2007.
van Loon G, De Clercq D, Tavernier R, et al: Transient complete atrioventricular block following transvenous electrical cardioversion of atrial fibrillation in a horse. *Vet J* 170:124–127, 2005.
Witzel DA, Geddes LA, Hoff HE, McFarlane J: Electrical defibrillation of the equine heart. *Am J Vet Res* 29:1279–1285, 1968.

AUTHOR: GUNTHER VAN LOON

EDITOR: MARY M. DURANDO

Ventricular Premature Complex and Ventricular Tachycardia

BASIC INFORMATION

DEFINITION
• Ventricular premature complex (VPC): A spontaneous premature ventricular depolarization that originates from the ventricles, resulting in a QRS' complex and T' wave on the surface electrocardiogram (ECG) that have a different morphology (and duration) (Figure 1).
• Ventricular tachycardia (VT): More than three consecutive VPCs, resulting in an increased heart rate.
• Idioventricular rhythm: An independent pacemaker in the ventricles discharging at a relatively slow rate, dominating the cardiac rhythm, resulting in a normal or almost normal heart rate.
• Fusion beat: A VPC that originates almost simultaneously with the normal ventricular depolarization. The morphology of this fusion beat is a mixture between the normal QRS and the VPC morphology.

SYNONYM(S)
• Ventricular premature contraction
• Ventricular premature beat
• Ventricular premature depolarization
• Ventricular extrasystole
• Ventricular tachyarrhythmia
• Ventricular ectopy (used for both VPC and VT)

EPIDEMIOLOGY
RISK FACTORS
• Ventricular myocardial disease
• Aortic regurgitation
• Aortocardiac fistula
• Ventricular dilatation
• Maximal exercise
• Electrolyte and metabolic disturbances
• Hypoxia, anemia
• Fever, toxemia
• High sympathetic tone
• Drugs (eg, epinephrine)
• Toxicity (eg, cardiac glycosides, monensin)

ASSOCIATED CONDITIONS AND DISORDERS Association with respiratory disease has been suspected in some cases but rarely confirmed.

CLINICAL PRESENTATION
DISEASE FORMS/SUBTYPES
• Depending on the number of VPCs
  ○ Isolated ventricular premature contractions versus VT
• Depending on the morphology of the QRS' complex (Figure 2)
  ○ Monomorphic (originating from the same focus; unifocal, uniform) VPCs or VT versus polymorphic (originating from different foci; multifocal, multimorphic, multiform) VPCs or VT
• Depending on the duration of VT
  ○ Paroxysmal (short, self-terminating bout) versus sustained (continuous) VT

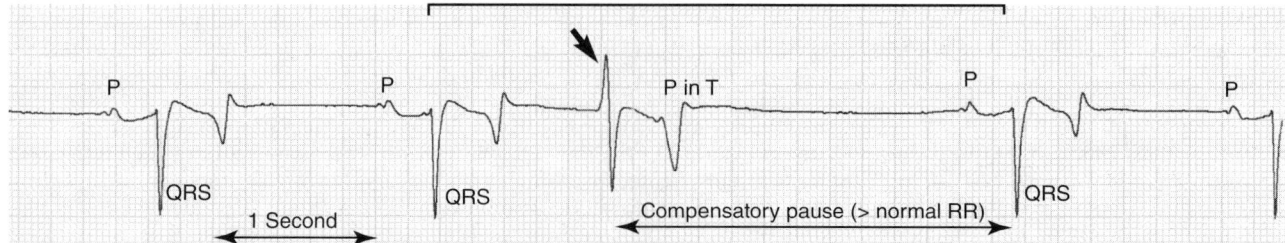

Normal-VPC-Normal = 2 × normal RR interval

P   P   P in T   P   P

QRS   QRS   Compensatory pause (> normal RR)   QRS

1 Second

FIGURE 1 A VPC occurs earlier than expected, has no preceding P wave, and shows an abnormal morphology and duration. The ectopic beat is followed by a compensatory pause to "fall back" into the underlying sinus rhythm. The duration of the interval normal–abnormal–normal equals twice the normal RR interval.

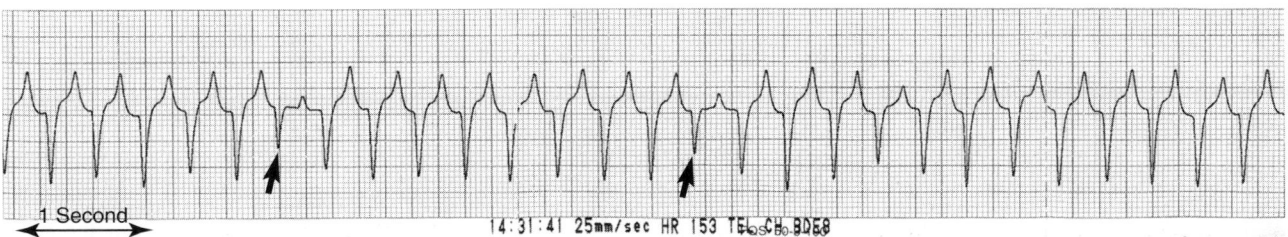

FIGURE 2 Paroxysms of monomorphic VT are interrupted by a normal QRS complex (*arrows*). Compared with the normal QRS complexes, the ectopic beats have a different morphology and longer duration.

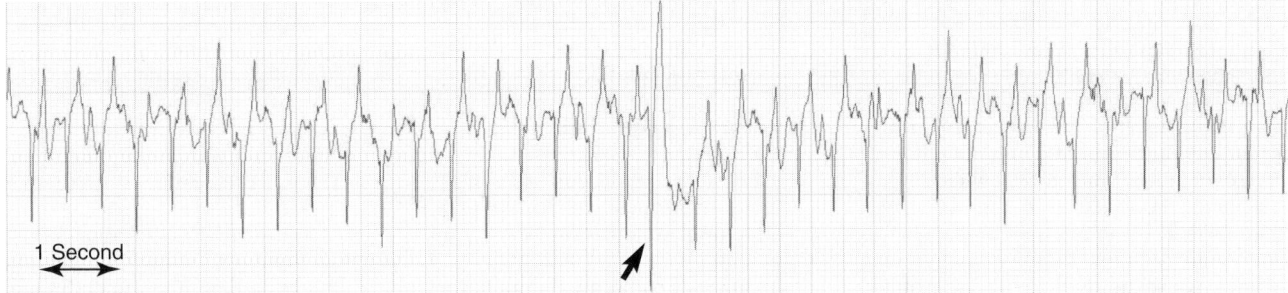

FIGURE 3 This horse shows one VPC (*arrow*) during recovery from fast work. The ectopic beat is easily recognizable by its prematurity, abnormal morphology, and the compensatory pause. Because no other abnormalities were found in this horse, the ectopic beat was considered to be normal.

HISTORY, CHIEF COMPLAINT

- Incidental finding
- Exercise intolerance
- Anorexia, weakness
- (Pre)syncope
- Underlying systemic disease (fever, toxemia, colic, renal disease, neoplasia)
- Intoxication
- Drug administration

PHYSICAL EXAM FINDINGS

- VPCs
  - Irregular rhythm on auscultation. The VPC may have an increased intensity of the first heart sound and is usually followed by a compensatory pause.
  - Depending on the prematurity, a pulse deficit may be palpated.
- VT
  - An increased heart rate: Generally more than 50 beats/min; sustained monomorphic VT usually results in a heart rate above 100 to 120 beats/min.
  - The rhythm is regular (monomorphic) or irregular (monomorphic or polymorphic).
  - A weak pulse or pulse deficit
  - At excessively high rates, not every QRS' is associated with semilunar valve opening and heart sounds. Therefore, calculation of heart rate by auscultation may underestimate the actual heart rate.
  - Horses with sustained VT develop jugular pulsation, ventral edema, hydrothorax, or even pulmonary edema, hydropericardium and ascites.

- Signs of underlying cardiac disease such as congestive heart failure, diastolic murmur, weakness, or (pre) syncope
- Signs of underlying disease resulting in fever, toxemia, hypoxia, and electrolyte imbalance

ETIOLOGY AND PATHOPHYSIOLOGY

- Spontaneous impulse formation (by increased automaticity, triggered activity or reentry) occurs in the ventricles usually because of primary cardiac disease.
  - Myocardial inflammation, degeneration, or necrosis caused by infection (bacterial, viral, parasitic), intoxication (cardiac glycosides, monensin), or neoplasia
  - Aortic regurgitation
  - Aortocardiac fistula
- Underlying systemic disorders may cause or enhance ventricular ectopy
  - Electrolyte imbalances (especially potassium, calcium, magnesium)
  - Hypoxia
  - High sympathetic tone
  - Fever, toxemia
- Other causes
  - Drug administration or intoxication (cardiac glycosides, antiarrhythmic drugs, anesthesia)
  - Maximal exercise: An occasional ectopic beat (usually during recovery) should be considered as normal in maximally exercising horses (Figure 3)
  - Iatrogenic: During cardiac catheterization or transvenous electrical cardioversion of atrial fibrillation (AF)

- The ectopic impulse depolarizes both ventricles but follows a different route through the myocardium, resulting in a QRS' complex with a different morphology and a longer duration.
- Depending on the site of origin, the QRS' complex may be completely abnormal or may be difficult to distinguish from the normal complexes (when it originates high in the ventricle near the His-Purkinje system).
- Isolated ectopic beats have limited hemodynamic consequences and may not result in obvious clinical signs.
- VT has an important impact on hemodynamics. Sustained VT at high rates leads to cardiac failure within days.
- VT of less than about 140 beats/min, especially if polymorphic, is usually caused by increased automaticity. Monomorphic VT of more than about 140 beats/min is usually caused by a rapidly firing focus, triggered activity, or reentry.
- Any ventricular ectopic rhythm carries a risk for sudden initiation of high rate VT or flutter (signs of weakness, ataxia, and [pre]syncope) or even ventricular fibrillation (VF; sudden death).

DIAGNOSIS

DIFFERENTIAL DIAGNOSIS

- Supraventricular tachycardia (sinus tachycardia or atrial tachycardia): QRS complexes of normal morphology and duration are preceded by P waves

(P waves may be buried in the preceding T waves).

- VF: The ECG shows a bizarre wavy line, and QRS complexes can no longer be identified. VF warrants immediate therapy because it is always fatal within seconds to minutes.
- Aberrant conduction in horses with AF: In AF, sympathetic stimulation or exercise may result in extremely high ventricular rates (up to >400 beats/min). Occasionally, QRS broadening and an R-on-T phenomenon may be found. Although AF and VPC/VT may occur concurrently, these extremely high rates are probably supraventricular in origin (sudden conduction of atrial impulses through the atrioventricular (AV) node because of the change in autonomic tone) whereby an aberrant conduction to the ventricles results in broader QRS complexes and R-on-T.
- Ventricular escape rhythm: Because of the absence of a normal ventricular depolarization, an ectopic beat is generated in the ventricles, resulting in a QRS' complex that occurs later than normal and has an abnormal morphology and duration.
- Artifacts, especially during muscle twitching, body movement, and exercise. Important criteria for differentiation include
  - The normal QRS complex is the fastest depolarization of the ventricles. Sharp deflections of shorter duration are artifacts (eg, muscle twitching).
  - Artifacts do not have T waves.
  - During the artifacts, normal sinus rhythm persists.
  - During exercise, large irregular deflections of the baseline caused by muscle activity may distort the normal QRS complexes. Verify whether the RR interval is irregular. Do not interpret the ECG if quality is insufficient.
  - Look at the other leads when doubt exists about an artifact.
  - Record all events during ECG recording. It is unlikely that an occasional VPC exactly coincides with a sudden body motion.

INITIAL DATABASE
- Ambulatory ECG
  - "Typical" criteria for a VPC
    - QRS' occurs earlier than normal (shortened RR' interval).
    - There is no preceding P wave.
    - QRS' morphology is abnormal.
    - QRS' duration is increased (>140 msec).
    - A compensatory pause usually follows the VPC. The reason for this pause is that the P wave occurring just before, during, or just after the VPC is not conducted toward the ventricles because the AV node is still refractory after being depolarized by the VPC. As the atria continue at their own rate, the next normal QRS complex only occurs after the next P wave. As such, the interval from VPC to the following normal QRS is longer than the normal RR interval and is called the *compensatory pause*. The interval normal QRS–VPC–normal QRS is equal to (or slightly greater than) twice the normal RR interval.
  - It is very important to realize that all of these criteria are not always present.
    - The VPC may occur at (almost) the same time as the normal QRS, resulting in a "fusion beat" from which the morphology is a mixture of the normal and abnormal QRS. In this case, the RR' interval can be almost normal.
    - A normal P wave may, by coincidence, precede the VPC (or fusion beat) but not be the trigger for the ventricular depolarization.
    - When the VPC originates near the His bundle or Purkinje system, the "route" of depolarization through the ventricles may be almost identical to normal and therefore the QRS' morphology and duration may only slightly change. As such, the QRS' duration may be within normal limits (<140 msec). It is possible that abnormal QRS' morphology is easily overlooked in one lead while obvious in another lead. Recording of more than one lead significantly contributes to the diagnosis of these VPCs.
    - In horses, the heart rate at rest is slow. Instead of the compensatory pause, the VPC may be interlaced or interpolated, which means that the VPC occurs without disrupting the underlying rhythm. In this situation, the VPC occurs between two normal beats, and the AV node and ventricular myocardium have already regained their excitability when the second P wave occurs. This results in normal conduction of this P wave to the ventricle.
  - More than three consecutive VPCs are called VT.
  - Regarding QRS' morphology
    - Ectopy from a single source: Monomorphic or uniform VPCs or VT
    - Ectopy from multiple sources: Polymorphic or multiform VPCs or VT
  - Regarding VT duration
    - Paroxysmal VT: One or more short bouts of VT that terminate spontaneously
    - Persistent (or sustained) VT: VT is continuously present and does not terminate spontaneously.
  - R-on-T phenomenon: The QRS complex occurs simultaneous with the preceding T wave, which carries a high risk for development of VF and death.
  - Torsades de pointes: Wide QRS tachycardia in which the QRS and T twist around the baseline; may rapidly deteriorate into VF and death.
- Exercise ECG is needed (unless the condition of the horse precludes it) to examine the response of the VPC or VT.
  - Occasionally, occurring VPCs may be overridden by the normal sinus tachycardia. These VPCs are less likely to affect performance. However, additional examinations should be performed to find the cause.
  - VPCs or VT may worsen during exercise. These horses should be rested and treated before continuing work (along with determination of the underlying cause).
  - VPCs or VT may be absent at rest and only occur during exercise.
    - Occasional VPCs at the end of maximal exercise and particularly during the recovery phase may be considered normal. Trains of VPCs or VT are an abnormal finding and warrant further examination.
    - VPCs or VT occurring at lower levels of exercise are abnormal.
- Echocardiography to identify myocardial dysfunction (eg, cardiomyopathy caused by ionophore toxicity), myocardial lesions (eg, aortocardiac fistula), or predisposing cardiac disease (eg, aortic regurgitation)
- Electrolyte status (serum, fractional urinary excretion)
- Complete blood cell count and biochemistry to look for underlying disease
- Myocardial markers (cardiac troponin I, creatine kinase–MB fraction)
- Digoxin and digitoxin plasma levels in case of suspected cardiac glycoside intoxication (foxglove, oleander, and adonis)

ADVANCED OR CONFIRMATORY TESTING
- Arterial blood gas analysis
- Vitamin E and selenium levels
- Long-term ECG recording (24-hour Holter monitor) allows analysis of the frequency of the arrhythmia, diagnosis

of intermittent arrhythmias, and monitoring of the effect of treatment. Generally, fewer than 30 isolated, unifocal VPCs in a 24-hour period are considered normal.

- Repeated monitoring of the electrolyte status to look for a correlation with the arrhythmia
- Analyses for possible intoxication (eg, ionophores)
- Right ventricular endomyocardial biopsies may be taken, especially when generalized myocardial disease is suspected.

TREATMENT

THERAPEUTIC GOAL(S)

- Rest
- Reduce inflammatory reaction
- Antiarrhythmic therapy: Only if VPCs are frequent (resulting in clinical signs) or when rapid or polymorphic VT or the R-on-T phenomenon is present. Patients with intermittent VPCs generally do not need antiarrhythmic therapy because they usually do not result in a clinical problem, and treatment may be associated with undesirable side effects.
- Treat the underlying, predisposing disease.
- Terminate drug administration, if possible, association with arrhythmia.

ACUTE GENERAL TREATMENT

- First confirm that the arrhythmia is ventricular in origin! Remember that all antiarrhythmic drugs may have adverse effects and can be proarrhythmic.
- For intermittent VPCs (<~10/min)
  - Rest (1–2 months)
  - Treat the underlying condition.
  - Corticosteroid therapy (dexamethasone, prednisolone) can sometimes be useful to reduce the number of VPCs (when there is no indication of an infectious process).
  - In addition, oral phenytoin can be administered (20 mg/kg q12h for 2 days followed by 10–15 mg/kg q12h; reduce the dose when signs of sedation, lip and facial twitching, or gait deficits occur; monitor plasma levels; keep dose at lowest for effective suppression of the arrhythmia) to suppress ectopy.
- For VT resulting in clinical signs at rest attributable to the arrhythmia or for VT with an excessively high rate (>120 beats/min), an R-on-T phenomenon, or that is polymorphic
  - Intranasal oxygen and fluid therapy
  - Control anxiety by administering diazepam, if needed.

- Lidocaine IV (without epinephrine [adrenaline]) is often the first choice because of its availability, safety, and cost.
  - 0.25 to 0.5 mg/kg slow bolus q5min for a maximum dose of 2 to 4 mg/kg
  - Ataxia, excitability, or seizure may occur: Administer 0.05 mg/kg of diazepam IV
  - Therapeutic plasma level is 1.5 to 5 µg/mL
- Quinidine gluconate at 1.0 to 2.2 mg/kg IV q10min to effect or a maximum total dose of 12 mg/kg
- Procainamide at 1 mg/kg/min IV up to 20 mg/kg total dose
- Amiodarone
  - 5 mg/kg/h IV for 1 hour followed by 0.83 mg/kg/h for q24–48h.
  - Potential adverse effects include weight shifting and diarrhea.
- Phenytoin
  - 5 to 10 mg/kg IV followed by 1 to 5 mg/kg IM q12h or 10 to 15 mg/kg PO q12h.
  - 20 mg/kg PO BID for 2 days followed by 10 to 15 mg/kg q12h.
  - Reduce the dose when signs of sedation, lip and facial twitching, or gait deficits occur.
  - Monitor plasma levels.
  - Phenytoin is the treatment of choice for treatment of cardiac glycoside intoxication.
- Magnesium sulphate at 2 to 6 mg/kg/min IV to effect up to a 55 mg/kg total dose.
- Propafenone IV at 1 mg/kg in 5% dextrose over 5 to 8 minutes.
- Propranolol IV at 0.03 mg/kg q12h.
- Bretylium tosylate IV at 3 to 5 mg/kg slow bolus up to a 10 mg/kg total dose.
- Intracardiac electrical cardioversion may be attempted in unresponsive VT.
  - Similar procedure as for transvenous electrical cardioversion of AF but with a cardioversion catheter in the right and left ventricle.
  - Concurrent antiarrhythmic therapy might increase the success rate.
  - Under general anesthesia, biphasic synchronized shocks at 150 to 360 J are delivered.
  - Important risks include VF and risks associated with anesthesia of a cardiovascularly compromised horse.
- After successful cardioversion, the horse should be further rested for at least 2 months and further examinations should be performed to identify the cause.
- Treat electrolyte imbalance.
- Treat the predisposing underlying disorders.

- After the rest period and before returning to training, ECG recordings at rest and during exercise should confirm normalization of the condition.

CHRONIC TREATMENT

- Ongoing management of the underlying cause
- Rest period of 1 to 2 months
- Corticosteroid (tapering regimen) treatment may be given during the rest period for 2 to 4 weeks.
- Oral phenytoin treatment may be given to suppress ventricular ectopy.
- After the rest period, the horse should be reassessed using ECG at rest and during exercise before returning to training.

DRUG INTERACTIONS

- Serum digoxin levels increase with concurrent administration of quinidine.
- Should not give digoxin if suspected digitalis intoxication as a cause for VT

POSSIBLE COMPLICATIONS

VF may suddenly occur and is virtually always fatal in horses.

RECOMMENDED MONITORING

- Continuous ECG monitoring during treatment, especially in an unstable animal with VT
- Periodic ECG monitoring until normalization of the condition
- Periodic echocardiographic reexaminations (every 6 months to 1 year) if structural cardiac disease (eg, aorto-cardiac fistula or aortic regurgitation) is associated with ventricular arrhythmias

PROGNOSIS AND OUTCOME

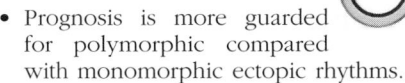

- Prognosis is more guarded for polymorphic compared with monomorphic ectopic rhythms.
- Sustained VT carries a more guarded prognosis than isolated VPCs or paroxysmal VT.
- The prognosis depends on the management of underlying systemic disease.
- The prognosis is guarded when the arrhythmia develops as a result of cardiac disease.
- The prognosis is good when the arrhythmia is caused by an electrolyte disorder or by drug administration.
- The prognosis is grave for patients with sustained high-rate VT unresponsive to treatment because cardiac failure will rapidly develop.
- Successfully treated VT may recur within 6 months to 1 year.

PEARLS & CONSIDERATIONS

COMMENTS

- Both VPCs and ventricular ectopic beats occurring in an escape rhythm look similar on an ECG. However, an escape rhythm occurs because the heart rate is too slow and is therefore lifesaving, so it should never be treated with antiarrhythmic drugs.
- Recording multiple leads is very useful to detect ventricular ectopic beats because some VPCs may be difficult to detect on a single lead.
- Double check the ECG or make additional recordings when there is any doubt about artifacts or ventricular ectopy.

- Avoid overinterpretation of a bad recording, especially during exercise.

PREVENTION

Manage underlying disease, if possible

CLIENT EDUCATION

- When ventricular arrhythmias with a normal or only slightly elevated heart rate are present, clinical signs may not be very obvious to the owner. However, the owner should be informed that VF and death may suddenly occur without warning.
- Successfully treated horses that return to training should be monitored (clinical signs, periodic auscultation) for recurrence of the arrhythmia during the first months (for approximately 1 year).

SUGGESTED READING

Baggot JD: The pharmacological basis of cardiac drug selection for use in horses. *Equine Vet J Suppl* 19:97–100, 1995.

Hughes KJ, Hoffmann KL, Hodgson DR, et al: Long-term assessment of horses and ponies post exposure to monensin sodium in commercial feed. *Equine Vet J* 41:47–52, 2009.

Kiryu K, Machida N, Kashida Y, et al: Pathologic and electrocardiographic findings in sudden cardiac death in racehorses. *J Vet Med Sci* 61:921–928, 1999.

Marr CM, Reef VB, Brazil TJ, et al: Aortocardiac fistulas in seven horses. *Vet Radiol Ultrasound* 39, 22-31, 1998.

McGuirk SM, Muir WW: Diagnosis and treatment of cardiac arrhythmias. *Vet Clin North Am Equine Pract* 1, 353-370, 1985.

Reimer JM, Reef VB, Sweeney RW: Ventricular arrhythmias in horses: 21 cases (1984–1989). *J Am Vet Med Assoc* 201:1237–1243, 1992.

AUTHOR: **GUNTHER VAN LOON**

EDITOR: **MARY M. DURANDO**

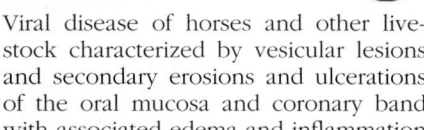

Vesicular Stomatitis

BASIC INFORMATION

DEFINITION

Viral disease of horses and other livestock characterized by vesicular lesions and secondary erosions and ulcerations of the oral mucosa and coronary band with associated edema and inflammation

EPIDEMIOLOGY

SPECIES, AGE, SEX No age or sex predilection is known, but the disease has not been reported in foals.

GENETICS AND BREED PREDISPOSITION Horses, cattle, swine, and rarely llamas

RISK FACTORS
- Access to pasture
- High insect populations
- Source of water close to animal housing

CONTAGION AND ZOONOSIS
- Primarily transmitted by insects, especially sandflies and blackflies.
- No evidence of direct transmission between horses.
- Potential for vertebrate reservoirs for the virus
- Outbreaks after transport of infected horses have occurred.
- The disease is zoonotic, and humans that handle affected animals or tissues are most commonly affected.
- Although affected humans may be asymptomatic, clinical signs may include fever, malaise, nausea, and muscle soreness and present much like the flu.

GEOGRAPHY AND SEASONALITY
- Only identified in the Western hemisphere.
- Disease outbreaks have occurred across the United States, primarily in the Southwestern states.
- Seasonality is related to vector exposure, so it is most likely to occur in the late spring to early fall.

CLINICAL PRESENTATION

DISEASE FORMS/SUBTYPES
- Stomatitis, gingivitis, or lesions of the feet and coronary band
- Subclinical cases (seroconversion without clinical signs) common during outbreaks

HISTORY, CHIEF COMPLAINT
- Fever, lethargy, inappetence
- Ptyalism
- Swelling and edema of the lower limbs

PHYSICAL EXAM FINDINGS
- Raised ulcerations of the oral mucosa, most commonly on the tongue but can also occur at the mucocutaneous junctions, palate, and gingival surfaces.
- Vesicles present in the acute stages, but after rupture, only ulcers remain.
- The muzzle, ventrum, prepuce, and udder may exhibit crusts and scabs.
- Edema and coronitis of the lower limbs may also occur.

ETIOLOGY AND PATHOPHYSIOLOGY
- Viruses are single-stranded RNA viruses of the Rhabdoviridae family.
- Virus penetrates the epithelium, and as with most viral infections, invasion

results in further production of virus and cell death.
- This causes edema and necrosis of the epithelium, influx of inflammatory cells, and subsequent formation of vesicles as the mucosa separates from the underlying tissue.
- Lesions occur 48 hours after experimental infection.

DIAGNOSIS

DIFFERENTIAL DIAGNOSIS

- Trauma
- Causes of oral ulcerative lesions
- Cantharidin (blister beetle) toxicosis
- Corrosive or irritating oral medication such as enrofloxacin or nonsteroidal antiinflammatory drugs
- Squamous cell carcinoma
- Exposure to wood shavings containing quassin or neoquassin
- Equine herpesvirus (rare)
- Equine arteritis virus (rare)
- Horses do not contract foot and mouth disease, but this disease should be considered in cattle and swine.
- Differentials for crusty skin lesions
- Sunburn
- Pemphigus foliaceus
- Exfoliative eosinophilic dermatitis

INITIAL DATABASE

Routine laboratory testing is generally unremarkable.

ADVANCED OR CONFIRMATORY TESTING

- Contact your state veterinarian if a case is suspected to assess risk in your area as well as diagnostic options.
- Quarantine is recommended during disease investigation.
- Diagnostic testing includes antibody detection via virus neutralization, enzyme-linked immunosorbent assay (ELISA) or complement fixation test (CFT), virus isolation from vesicle swabs or fluid, or polymerase chain reaction on tissue samples or swabs.
- The World Animal Health Organization (OIE) recognizes the CFT as the test required for international trade. The competitive ELISA is the test of choice during an outbreak.
- Positive test results are confirmed by virus neutralization or CFT.

TREATMENT

THERAPEUTIC GOAL(S)

Because the disease is self-limiting and short lived, therapy is directed at cleansing of the ulcerations and supportive care.

ACUTE GENERAL TREATMENT

- Rinsing of the mouth with mild antiseptic solutions may decrease the incidence of secondary bacterial infections.
- Provide a soft, palatable diet.
- More advanced supportive care is rarely required.

POSSIBLE COMPLICATIONS

Secondary bacterial infection of ulcerative lesions

RECOMMENDED MONITORING

- Monitoring of the lesions for bacterial infection or worsening is recommended.
- Feed and water intake should also be monitored because of oral pain.

PROGNOSIS AND OUTCOME

Prognosis for recovery is good.

PEARLS & CONSIDERATIONS

COMMENTS

- Biosecurity is mandatory.
- Quarantines will be implemented by state and federal veterinarians if a diagnosis is confirmed.

PREVENTION

No vaccine is currently available.

CLIENT EDUCATION

In the event of a suspected case, strict biosecurity measures should be followed. All personnel should limit contact with the infected horse given its zoonotic potential.

SUGGESTED READING

McCluskey BJ: Vesicular stomatitis. In Sellon DC, Long MT, editors: *Equine infectious diseases*, St Louis, 2007, Saunders Elsevier, pp 219–225.
McCluskey BJ, Mumford EL: Vesicular stomatitis and other vesicular, erosive, and ulcerative diseases of horses. *Vet Clin North Am Equine Pract* 16:3, 2000.

AUTHOR: **L. NICKI WISE**

EDITORS: **DEBRA A. SELLON** and **MAUREEN T. LONG**

Water Hemlock Toxicosis

BASIC INFORMATION

DEFINITION

Water hemlocks are native plants of North America that are highly poisonous to horses, livestock, and humans. There are four recognized species: Western water hemlock (*Cicuta douglasii*), spotted water hemlock (*Cicuta maculata*, which is the most widely distributed), bulblet-bearing water hemlock (*Cicuta bulbifera*), and Mackenzie's water hemlock (*Cicuta virosa*).

SYNONYM(S)

Cow bane, beaver poison, poison parsnip, spotted parsley, spotted water hemlock, musquash root

EPIDEMIOLOGY

RISK FACTORS Early growth and the roots pose the greatest risk, but all parts of the plant should be considered toxic.

GEOGRAPHY AND SEASONALITY

- Water hemlock species are found throughout North America, preferring wet, marshy habitats along rivers, irrigation ditches, swamps, and ponds. Early spring and late summer when other forages are scarce make water hemlock more accessible to animals.
- Typically, water hemlock are erect plants 0.5 to 2 meters tall with smooth, branching stems, swollen at the base, rarely purple-striped or mottled (especially *C. maculata*), hollow except for partitions at the junction of the root and stem, with thick tuberous roots. Leaves are alternate, compound, and pinnate with serrated margins (Figure 1). Leaf veins extend to the leaf notches. Many small white flowers are produced in umbrella-shaped terminal clusters.

CLINICAL PRESENTATION

HISTORY, CHIEF COMPLAINT

- Animals are often found dead with no previous clinical signs noted.
- Horses placed in new pasture that has suitable habitat for water hemlock are at risk.

PHYSICAL EXAM FINDINGS Excessive salivation, frothing at the mouth, nervousness, and incoordination rapidly followed by tremors, muscular weakness, violent seizures, and respiratory failure. Death occurs within hours of ingesting water hemlock.

ETIOLOGY AND PATHOPHYSIOLOGY

- All parts of the plant, but especially the tuberous roots, contain cicutoxin and cicutol.
- Cicutoxin is a yellow-colored, unsaturated acetylenic alcohol that is rapidly absorbed through the mucous membranes.
- Cicutoxin acts primarily on the brain and skeletal muscles.
- Cicutoxin blocks Na^+ and K^+ channels and inhibits γ-aminobutyric acid pathways.
- Violent convulsions are common.
- Death results from respiratory failure.
- Death can occur within 15 minutes of ingesting the cicutoxin.
- Lethal dosage is 0.5% body weight or less.
- The tuberous roots are the most toxic part of the plant, with 3 to 5 oz being potentially fatal to an adult horse.

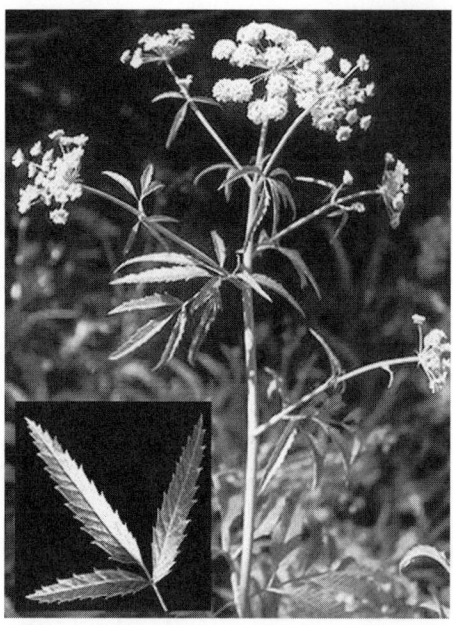

FIGURE 1 Spotted water hemlock (*Cicuta maculata*). *Inset,* Typical leaf.

DIAGNOSIS

DIFFERENTIAL DIAGNOSIS

- Ionophore toxicity
- Oleander poisoning
- Yew poisoning
- Organophosphate toxicity
- Organochlorine toxicity

INITIAL DATABASE

Death occurs rapidly, but marked elevations of muscle enzymes may be present.

ADVANCED OR CONFIRMATORY TESTING

- Stomach contents can be analyzed for cicutoxin by gas chromatography/mass spectrometry.
- Diffuse acute myopathy histologically

TREATMENT

THERAPEUTIC GOAL(S)

- Early recognition and heavy sedation or anesthesia helps prevent severe myopathy and violent convulsions.

- Experimentally, sheep given lethal doses of cicutoxin survive if anesthetized before convulsions develop.

ACUTE GENERAL TREATMENT

- Sedation and anesthesia to help prevent myopathy and seizures
- Other therapy may include activated charcoal and supportive care, including IV fluids.

RECOMMENDED MONITORING

Muscle and hepatic enzymes

PROGNOSIS AND OUTCOME

- Animals showing convulsions have a poor prognosis.
- Cicutoxin is rapidly excreted within 4 to 6 hours, and animals still alive after this time period may survive.

PEARLS & CONSIDERATIONS

COMMENTS

- Water hemlock should be routinely removed from animal pastures.
- Water hemlock poisoning should be considered in all sudden death cases of pastured horses because it is clinically indistinguishable from other acute toxicities such as yew and oleander poisoning.

PREVENTION

Correct identification of the plant is essential. Water hemlock should be pulled or dug up and destroyed. Spot spraying with an approved herbicide is also effective for controlling water hemlock.

CLIENT EDUCATION

- Recognition of all growth stages of water hemlock will help prevent exposing animals to the plants.
- A number of plants, including poison hemlock (*Conium maculatum*), Queen Anne's lace or wild carrot (*Daucus carrota*), and water parsnip (*Sium suave*), are similar in appearance and should be identified by a botanist.

SUGGESTED READING

James LF, Ralphs MH: Water hemlock. *Utah Sci* 47:67–69, 1986.
Panter KE, Keeler RF, Baker DC: Toxicoses in livestock from the hemlocks (*Conium maculatum* and *Cicuta* spp.). *J Anim Sci* 66:2407–2413, 1988.
Panter KE, Baker DC, Kachele PO: Water hemlock (*Cicuta douglasii*) toxicosis in sheep: pathologic description and prevention of lesions and death. *J Vet Diag Invest* 8:474–480, 1996.
Smith RA, Lewis D: Cicuta toxicosis in cattle: a case history and simplified analytical method. *Vet Hum Toxol* 29: 240–241, 1987.

AUTHOR: **ANTHONY P. KNIGHT**

EDITOR: **CYNTHIA L. GASKILL**

West Nile Encephalitis

BASIC INFORMATION

DEFINITION

A single-stranded RNA virus of the genus *Flavivirus* that causes a diffuse or multifocal polioencephalomyelitis

EPIDEMIOLOGY
RISK FACTORS

- Residence in an endemic area
- Turnout during dawn and dusk
- Vaccination status
- Lack of mosquito control programs

CONTAGION AND ZOONOSIS

- Vector: Mosquitoes, especially *Culex* spp.
- Reservoir: Birds
- Aberrant dead-end hosts: Domestic animals, especially horses, and humans

GEOGRAPHY AND SEASONALITY

- Peak transmission in the Western hemisphere from July through October
- Year-round infections in subtropical and tropical regions
- Increased incidence in areas with increased temperature and moisture

CLINICAL PRESENTATION

HISTORY, CHIEF COMPLAINT

- Initially depression and anorexia with or without a fever during initial viremia
- Ataxia
- Weakness, especially in the pelvic limbs
- Asymmetric neurologic signs

PHYSICAL EXAM FINDINGS

- Depression
- Fever
- Tremors or muscle fasciculations
- Muscle rigidity
- Recumbent or difficulty rising
- Weakness, ataxia, and dysmetria (affecting one to multiple limbs)
- Droopy lip
- Change in mentation: Hyperexcitable, aggressive, somnolence, or hyperesthesia
- Lameness
- Abdominal pain or colic
- Sudden sleeplike activity revealing narcolepsy

ETIOLOGY AND PATHOPHYSIOLOGY

- Viremia occurs 3 to 5 days after inoculation of the virus into the host by a mosquito.
- Translocation into the central nervous system (CNS) occurs in approximately 10% of horses.
- Clinical signs occur 7 to 10 days after inoculation.

DIAGNOSIS

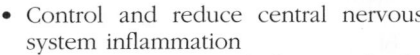

DIFFERENTIAL DIAGNOSIS

- Rabies
- Botulism
- Equine protozoan myeloencephalitis
- Cervical vertebral myelopathy
- Equine herpes virus myelopathy
- Equine degenerative myelopathy
- Western equine encephalitis, eastern equine encephalitis, Venezuelan equine encephalitis

INITIAL DATABASE

- Complete blood count: Mild lymphopenia
- Serum chemistry

- Cerebrospinal fluid (CSF) analysis: Plasmacytic or lymphocytic pleocytosis with elevated total protein
- Neurologic examination

ADVANCED OR CONFIRMATORY TESTING

- Preferred test: West Nile virus (WNV) immunoglobulin M capture enzyme-linked immunosorbent assay using CSF or serum
- Plaque reduction neutralization or complement fixation using serum
- Virus isolation from whole blood, serum, CSF, and brain or spinal cord tissues: Not recommended because of zoonotic potential
- Postmortem: Reverse transcriptase polymerase chain reaction of the CNS tissues; immunohistochemistry or histopathology

TREATMENT

THERAPEUTIC GOAL(S)

- Control and reduce central nervous system inflammation
- Supportive care, including IV fluids, vitamin E, dimethyl sulfoxide (DMSO), and mannitol

ACUTE GENERAL TREATMENT

- Nonsteroidal antiinflammatory drugs: Flunixin meglumine (1.1 mg/kg q12h IV)
- Mannitol and DMSO to decrease cerebral edema and spinal cord swelling
- IV fluids
- Antibiotics for secondary infections caused by recumbency
- WNV-specific IV immunoglobulin
- Interferon-α

CHRONIC TREATMENT

- Sling support for recumbent horses
- Dexamethasone sodium: 0.5 to 0.1 mg/kg q24h IV (controversial)
- Mannitol (0.25–2.0 g/kg q24h IV) to decrease cerebral edema
- Detomidine to provide prolonged tranquilization
- Equine protozoal myeloencephalitis treatment until *Sarcocystis neurona* is ruled out or WNV is confirmed (see "Equine Protozoal Myeloencephalitis" in this section)

POSSIBLE COMPLICATIONS

Sudden death caused by overwhelming encephalomyelitis

RECOMMENDED MONITORING

- Periodic repeat neurologic examinations to assess response to therapy
- Continual monitoring of hydration status and renal function with possible nephrotoxic drugs

PROGNOSIS AND OUTCOME

- Suggested mortality rates of 30% to 40%.
- About 30% of horses progress to complete paralysis of one or more limbs.
- Many horses improve in 3 to 7 days from the onset of clinical signs. If initial improvements are made, approximately 90% of horses are expected to recover fully.

PEARLS & CONSIDERATIONS

PREVENTION

- Reduce mosquito breeding sites through the use of larvicides and adulticides.
- Stable horses in an insect-proof facility during dusk and dawn in mosquito seasons and avoid lights when inside.
- Eliminate areas of standing water.
- Vaccination once to twice per year depending on geographical location. Vaccinate before the onset of mosquito season.

CLIENT EDUCATION

- Environmental control is an important control measure. Remove standing water and other larval breeding sites.
- Change water tanks at least once a week to break the mosquito life cycle.
- Human application of a DEET-based product is recommended in areas with endemic disease.

SUGGESTED READING

Castillo-Olivares J, Wood J: West Nile virus infection of horses. *Vet Res* 35:467, 2004.

Goehring L: Viral diseases of the nervous system. In Furr M, Reed S, editors: *Equine neurology*, Ames, IA, 2008, Blackwell, pp 178–180.

Long M: Flavivirus infections. In Sellon D, Long M, editors: *Equine infectious diseases*, St Louis, 2007, Saunders Elsevier, pp 198–206.

AUTHOR: CAMERON M. CHILDERS

EDITOR: STEPHEN M. REED

White Snakeroot and Rayless Goldenrod Toxicosis

BASIC INFORMATION

DEFINITION

White snakeroot (*Ageratina altissima*), and rayless goldenrod (*Isocoma pluriflora*), members of Asteraceae, contain similar toxins collectively referred to as *tremetol*.

SYNONYM(S)

- White snakeroot: Richweed, snakeroot, *Eupatorium rugosum*
- Rayless goldenrod: Southern goldenbush, jimmyweed, burroweed, *Haplopappus heterophyllus, Isocoma wrightii*

EPIDEMIOLOGY

SPECIES, AGE, SEX

- All animals that graze on white snakeroot or rayless goldenrod are susceptible to the toxic effects of the plants.
- Lactating animals eating the plants secrete the toxin through their milk, thereby exposing their nursing young to the toxin.
- Humans drinking this milk will be similarly affected, developing "milk sickness."

RISK FACTORS

- Poisoning by white snakeroot and rayless goldenrod is historically sporadic because of the considerable variation in the quantity of the tremetol present in the plants in different locations and growing conditions. Toxicity is highest in the green plant, but dried plants remain toxic. There are at least 26 species of *Ageratina* (*Eupatorium*) worldwide, and many are considered toxic. In the genus *Isocoma*, with 16 species, only three are reported to be toxic; *I. pluriflora, I. tenuisectus, I. coronopifolia*. However, all species should be considered toxic until proven otherwise.
- Animals eating 1% to 10% of their body weight of green white snakeroot can be fatally poisoned. Rayless goldenrod in the amount of 1% to 2% of body weight over a period of weeks can be lethal to horses.

GEOGRAPHY AND SEASONALITY

- White snakeroot is a woodland plant of eastern North America extending as far west as North Dakota and south to Texas. It is an erect, branching, perennial plant growing 3 to 4 feet tall, with opposite, oval, pointed leaves with toothed edges. The flowers are small and white and are produced in flat-topped clusters at the ends of the branches (Figure 1).
- Rayless goldenrod, a common plant of the southwestern United States and northern Mexico, is a drought-tolerant perennial, growing 3 to 4 feet tall, with numerous, erect woody stems, and alternate, hairy, lanceolate, often resinous leaves. Yellow flowers are compact heads produced terminally. Seeds have a pappus of coarse whitish-brown bristles (Figure 2).

CLINICAL PRESENTATION

HISTORY, CHIEF COMPLAINT Muscle tremors ("trembles"), generalized weakness, and "acetone breath"

PHYSICAL EXAM FINDINGS

- Horses may be found down, and death may occur in 1 to 2 days in severely poisoned animals. Typically, horses develop severe depression, muscle tremors, and weakness to the extent that they have difficulty holding up their heads. Ataxia, especially of the hindquarters, with leg crossing is common. Impaired swallowing caused by myopathy may cause difficulty in swallowing and choking. Severe sweating, rapid respirations, cardiac dysrhythmias, and sudden death may occur.
- Foals suckling mares that are eating white snakeroot or rayless goldenrod can show similar signs even if the mare appears normal.

ETIOLOGY AND PATHOPHYSIOLOGY

- Trematol, a mixture of complex sterols and methyl ketone benzofuran derivatives, is present in both white snake root and rayless goldenrod.
- Trematol has a cumulative effect, causing poisoning when eaten in small amounts over time.
- Trematol acts to inhibit citrate synthase in the tricarboxylic acid (TCA) cycle, thereby causing hypoglycemia and ketoacidosis as a result of impairment of the TCA cycle.
- Cardiac and skeletal muscle degeneration and liver and kidney injury are typical.
- Renal tubular nephrosis is more pronounced in rayless goldenrod poisoning.

DIAGNOSIS

DIFFERENTIAL DIAGNOSIS

- Monensin, oleander, and milkweed toxicity; rabies; selenium and vitamin E deficiency

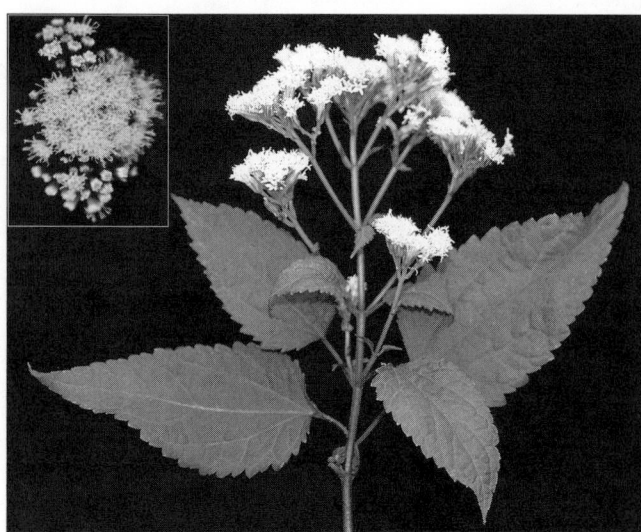

FIGURE 1 White snakeroot.

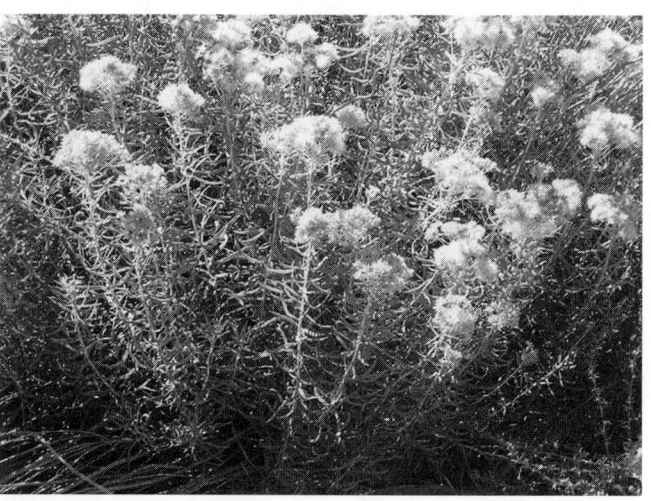

FIGURE 2 Rayless golden rod (*Isocoma pluriflora*). (Courtesy Samantha R. Uhrig, DVM, Carlsbad, NM.)

- Seasonal pasture myopathy in horses and atypical myopathy reported in Europe produce very similar clinical signs and histopathologic findings.

INITIAL DATABASE

- Serum enzymes: Lactate dehydrogenase, aspartate aminotransferase, Creatine phosphokinase, and alkaline phosphatase elevated
- Urine analysis: Myoglobinuria, myoglobin casts, ketonuria

ADVANCED OR CONFIRMATORY TESTING

- Pathologic lesions: Degenerative myopathy in cardiac and skeletal muscle
- Liver and kidney tissue can be analyzed for tremetol

TREATMENT

THERAPEUTIC GOAL(S)

There is no specific treatment for trematol intoxication.

ACUTE GENERAL TREATMENT

- IV fluids to correct the metabolic acidosis and hypoglycemia and to maintain renal function

- Provide symptomatic and supportive care as needed.
- Activated charcoal may be administered orally (3 g/kg body weight) for acute exposures.

POSSIBLE COMPLICATIONS

Rhabdomyolysis from prolonged recumbency

PROGNOSIS AND OUTCOME

- Early recognition of signs and removal of the animals from the plant source dictate a good prognosis.
- Recumbency from severe myopathy and cardiac irregularities warrants a poor prognosis.

PEARLS & CONSIDERATIONS

- Prevent access to green white snakeroot and rayless goldenrod and to hay contaminated with these plants.

- The plant can be controlled by pulling and burning the plant or through the use of herbicides.

SUGGESTED READING

Beier RC, Norman JO: The toxic factor in white snakeroot: identity, analysis and prevention. *Vet Hum Toxicol* 32(suppl):81–88, 1990.

Finno CJ, Valberg SJ, Wünschmann A, Murphy MJ: Seasonal pasture myopathy in horses in the midwestern United States: 14 cases (1998–2005). *J Am Vet Med Assoc* 229:1134–1141, 2006.

Lee ST, Davis TZ, Gardner DR, et al: Quantitative method for the measurement of three benzofuran ketones in rayless goldenrod (*Isocoma pluriflora*) and white snakeroot (*Ageratina altissima*) by high-performance liquid chromatography (HPLC). *J Agric Food Chem* 57:5639–5643, 2009.

Sharma OP, Dawra RK, Kurade NP, Sharma P: A review of the toxicosis and biological properties of the genus *Eupatorium*. *Nat Toxins* 6:1–14, 1998.

Smetzer DL, Coppock RW, Ely RW: Cardiac effects of white snakeroot intoxication in horses. *Equine Pract* 5:26–32, 1983.

AUTHOR: **ANTHONY P. KNIGHT**

EDITOR: **CYNTHIA L. GASKILL**

Wound Infection

BASIC INFORMATION

- Infection is a major factor contributing to:
  - Delayed wound healing
  - Reduced gain in tissue tensile strength
  - Dehiscence after wound closure
- Infection rates in veterinary medicine
  - Infection occurs in approximately 10% of equine orthopedic surgical patients overall and 8% of orthopedic patients undergoing clean surgical procedures.
  - Contaminated wounds with lesser concentrations of microorganisms can become infected when
    - Foreign bodies are present
    - Excessive necrotic tissue is left in the wound
    - Development of hematoma
    - Impaired local tissue defense (burn or immunosuppressed patients)
    - Altered vascular supply

- Dirty wounds have a 25-fold greater infection rate than do clean wounds.
  - Wounds contaminated with dirt have a higher risk of infection because of specific infection-potentiating fractions, which
    - Decrease the effect of white blood cells
    - Decrease humoral factors
    - Neutralize antibodies
  - Wounds contaminated with feces are highly susceptible to infection; feces contain up to 10^{11} microorganisms per gram.
- Hemoglobin liberated from hemorrhage suppresses local wound defenses.
- Hematoma formation is considered a leading factor in decreased local wound resistance to infection.
- Mechanism of injury
  - Lacerations caused by sharp objects are generally more resistant to infection.
  - Shear wounds from barbed wire, sticks, nails, and bites are more susceptible to infection because of the degree of soft tissue damage.

  - Soft tissue trauma from entanglement or entrapment or impact with a solid object or a kick are more susceptible to infection because of the degree of soft tissue injury and resultant reduction in blood supply.
  - Susceptibility to infection increases in multiple trauma patients even though the injury(ies) occurs at a site other than the surgical site; reduced tissue perfusion is believed to be the cause.

SUGGESTED READING

Wilson DA: Principles of early wound management. *Vet Clin North Am Equine Pract* 21:45–62, 2005.

AUTHORS: **CHRISTINE THÉORÊT** and **TED S. STASHAK**

EDITOR: **DAVID A. WILSON**

This entry is adapted from Orsini JA, Divers TJ, editors: *Equine emergencies: treatment and procedures*, ed 3, St Louis, 2008, Saunders Elsevier.

Wry Nose

BASIC INFORMATION

DEFINITION
Congenital lateral deviation of the nasal bones, the maxilla or premaxilla (incisive bones), and the nasal septum with associated unilateral shortening of the affected bones or cartilage

SYNONYM(S)
Campylorrhinus lateralis, rhinocampylus lateralis

EPIDEMIOLOGY
SPECIES, AGE, SEX Equine: Congenital; no known sex predisposition
GENETICS AND BREED PREDISPOSITION May occur in all breeds; the incidence seems to be higher in Arabians, which has led to so far unproven speculation that there may be a genetic component to this malformation in this breed. No cases of inherited campylorrhinus lateralis have been reported in the literature.
RISK FACTORS Primiparous mares
ASSOCIATED CONDITIONS AND DISORDERS
- Palatoschisis (cleft palate)
- Torticollis

CLINICAL PRESENTATION
HISTORY, CHIEF COMPLAINT
- Lateral nasal deviation (≤90 degrees) with associated incisor occlusion deficiency and possibly protrusion of the tongue. The deformity may cause problems nursing or grazing.
- Depending on the degree of nasal septum deviation, the respiratory symptoms may vary from exercise intolerance to respiratory stridor at rest.
PHYSICAL EXAM FINDINGS
- Lateral nasal deviation
- Incisor malocclusion
- Reduced airflow from one or both nostrils
- Malodorous breath because of food retention at the concave angle of the premaxilla or maxilla
- Respiratory stridor
- Exercise intolerance
- Frequently with associated abnormal concavity of the nasal bones and hard palate rostral to the cheek teeth
ETIOLOGY AND PATHOPHYSIOLOGY
- Fetal malpositioning in utero
- Caudal or transverse presentation of fetus
- Bicornuate gestation

DIAGNOSIS

INITIAL DATABASE
- Oral examination
- Lateromedial radiograph to determine the location of the deviation in the premaxilla or maxilla
- Dorsoventral radiograph to assess the degree of nasal septum deviation
- Endoscopy to confirm the patency and size of the remaining airway

TREATMENT

THERAPEUTIC GOAL(S)
- Improve airflow
- Improve incisor occlusion
- Cosmesis

ACUTE GENERAL TREATMENT
Ensure adequate airflow and caloric intake until the foal reaches an age older than 6 months. (In foals younger than 6 months, the nasal septum seems to provide support for the developing nasal bones, and nostrils and nasal septum resection before that age can lead to nasal bone collapse.)

CHRONIC TREATMENT
Two different treatment options
- Osteotomy of the premaxillae or maxillae and nasal bones at the site of maximum curvature is performed, a section of rib equivalent in length to the length difference between the convex and the concave premaxilla is harvested to be grafted at the concave side of the osteotomy, the bones are aligned, the rib section is inserted, and the bones are stabilized using internal fixation (Steinman pins inserted into the medullary cavity of the premaxillae and ipsilateral maxillae or using 2.7-mm reconstruction plates). The nasal bones are transected at the point of their maximum curvature and straightened using a wedge ostectomy or insertion of a rib graft. The nasal bones are then stabilized using 2.7-mm reconstruction plates. The nasal septum is removed using the three-wire method or a modification thereof. The nasal passages are packed with rolled gauze, the nostrils are sutured closed, and a tracheotomy tube is inserted.
- Distraction osteogenesis: Partial osteotomy of the premaxillae or maxillae at the site of maximum curvature is performed bilaterally, and the bones are then stabilized by application of a monolateral distraction external skeletal fixator (two pins are inserted caudally to the osteotomy site and two pins are inserted rostrally). Seven days after surgery, linear distraction is started on the concave side at a rate of 1 mm every 24 hours. After the desired alignment is achieved, an external skeletal fixator without distraction has to be kept in place for 6 weeks to allow healing of the osteotomy.

POSSIBLE COMPLICATIONS
- Hemorrhage
- Nasal bone collapse
- Collapse of the alar fold, the ventral aspect of the nasal diverticula, or the nostrils
- Formation of excessive granulation tissue of the caudal stump of the resected nasal septum
- Adhesions of the stump of the resected nasal septum to the conchae after subtotal resection.
- Breakdown of the fixation
- Implant infection

RECOMMENDED MONITORING
- Packed cell volume and total proteins during surgery
- Airflow before removal of the tracheotomy tube

PROGNOSIS AND OUTCOME

- The prognosis for athletic performance is guarded to poor depending on the degree of athleticism expected. (One horse was reported to race after facial reconstruction for wry nose.)
- The prognosis for life and breeding is good.

SUGGESTED READING
Baker GJ: Abnormalities of development and eruption. In Baker GJ, Easley J, editors: *Equine dentistry*, ed 2, Philadelphia, 2005, Saunders Elsevier, pp 69–77.

Doyle A, Freeman DE: Extensive nasal septum resection in horses using a 3-wire method. *Vet Surg* 34:167–173, 2005.

McKellar GM, Collins AP: The surgical correction of deviated anterior maxilla in a horse. *Aust Vet J* 70:112–114, 1993.

Puchol JL, Herrán R, Durall I, et al: Use of distraction osteogenesis for the correction of deviated nasal septum and premaxilla in a horse. *J Am Vet Med Assoc* 224:1147–1150, 2004.

Schumacher J, Brink P, Easley J, Pollock P: Surgical correction of wry nose in 4 horses. *Vet Surg* 27:142–148, 2008.

AUTHOR: **FLORIEN JENNER**

EDITOR: **ERIC J. PARENTE**

Yeast Dermatitis

BASIC INFORMATION

DEFINITION

Yeast dermatitis is a rare disorder in horses that may be caused by different species of *Candida* spp. or *Malassezia* spp. It can be either a primary dermatitis or secondary to underlying disease. This type of dermatitis can occasionally look like other skin conditions such as food allergies or atopy.

EPIDEMIOLOGY

CONTAGION AND ZOONOSIS Malassezia can potentially affect immune-compromised humans.

CLINICAL PRESENTATION

HISTORY, CHIEF COMPLAINT The main complaint is presence of rubbed areas on the tail, perineum, and ventral midline caused by variable pruritus.
PHYSICAL EXAM FINDINGS The affected skin is dry, has evidence of crusts that are greasy to the touch, and has evidence of exudate. Pruritus is variable, and areas of the tail, perineum, and ventrum are rubbed. In some cases, mares can have intense pruritus in between their mammary glands.
ETIOLOGY AND PATHOPHYSIOLOGY
- The exact species of *Malassezia* affecting horses is still under investigation.
- Among the multiple species that have been identified are *Malassezia pachydermatis*, *M. furfur*, *M. slooffiae*, *M. obtusa*, *M. globosa*, and *M. restricta*.
- The most common species isolated for horses is *M. pachydermatis*, which can be found in both healthy and affected horses.
- A species tentatively named *M. equi* has been recently identified in healthy horses.
- Isolation of *Malassezia* spp. can be an incidental finding and may not be causing any clinical signs.

DIAGNOSIS

DIFFERENTIAL DIAGNOSIS

- Dermatophytosis
- Pemphigus foliaceus
- Culicoides or insect hypersensitivity
- Mange
- Chronic skin rubs

INITIAL DATABASE

- Cytology will identify multiple organisms on the skin.
- Biopsy and histopathologic information in affected animals has not been specified, but in other species, findings include epidermal acanthosis and hyperkeratosis with parakeratotic crusts.
- *M. pachydermatis* is easily cultured in Sabouraud agar gel, but other species will not grow in the agar.
- *Candida* spp. is part of the normal microflora, so diagnosis needs to be confirmed by culturing the organism in Sabouraud agar gel and by performing cytology and histopathology.
- Histopathology of *Candida*-affected areas reveals blastoconidia and pseudohyphae with evidence of nodular to diffuse dermatitis, perivascular dermatitis, or folliculitis furunculosis.

TREATMENT

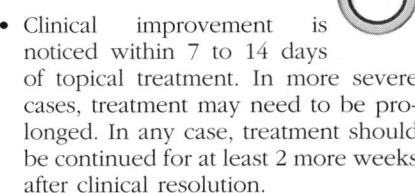

THERAPEUTIC GOAL(S)

- Rapid response to therapy by elimination of lesions and pruritus if present.
- Treatment is individualized depending on the severity of lesions.

ACUTE GENERAL TREATMENT

- *Malassezia* infection
  - Antifungal ointments or sprays containing miconazole work well for small focal areas.
  - In severe cases, use of shampoos and rinses containing miconazole and chlorhexidine may need to be used.
  - If skin is extremely waxy, scaly, and greasy, use of keratolytic degreasing shampoos may be required before use of other products.
- *Candida* infection
  - Correction of any underlying diseases to prevent yeast from affecting the patient.
  - Avoid excessive moisture and wetting of affected areas.
  - Use of antifungals such as nystatin, miconazole, or clotrimazole for mild cases.
  - In severe cases, systemic treatment with antifungals may be required.

PROGNOSIS AND OUTCOME

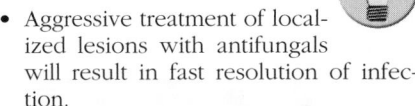

- Clinical improvement is noticed within 7 to 14 days of topical treatment. In more severe cases, treatment may need to be prolonged. In any case, treatment should be continued for at least 2 more weeks after clinical resolution.
- The prognosis for complete recovery from *Malassezia* infection and mild cases of *Candida* is good.
- In cases of severe candidiasis infections, prognosis can be poor because of systemic involvement and a compromised immune system that prevents the patient from being able to fight the infection. These patients may be treated with systemic nystatin, ketoconazole, or amphotericin B.

PEARLS & CONSIDERATIONS

- Aggressive treatment of localized lesions with antifungals will result in fast resolution of infection.
- It is important to continue treatment for a minimum of 2 weeks despite clinical resolution to prevent recurrence of the problem shortly after therapy has been discontinued.

SUGGESTED READING

Nell A, James SA, Bond CJ, et al: Identification and distribution of a novel *Malassezia* species yeast on normal equine skin. *Vet Rec* 150(13):395–398, 2002.
White SD: Equine bacterial and fungal diseases: a diagnostic and therapeutic update. *Clin Tech Equine Pract* 4:302–310, 2005.

AUTHOR: **ALFREDO SANCHEZ LONDOÑO**

EDITOR: **DAVID A. WILSON**

Yellow Star Thistle and Russian Knapweed Toxicosis

BASIC INFORMATION

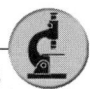

DEFINITION

Yellow star thistle and Russian knapweed cause a unique syndrome in horses characterized by the inability to prehend and chew food because of hypertonicity of the facial muscles. Prolonged continuous consumption of either plant is necessary to produce this irreversible and ultimately fatal poisoning.

SYNONYM(S)

- Yellow star thistle, St. Barnaby's thistle (*Centaurea solstitialis*)
- Russian knapweed (*Acroptilon repens*)
- Nigropallidal encephalomalacia
- Chewing disease

EPIDEMIOLOGY

GEOGRAPHY AND SEASONALITY Both plants were unintentionally introduced to North America and have become highly invasive noxious weeds in much of the western United States. Yellow star thistle is a very common annual or biennial in the west coastal states and is sporadic in most other states (Figure 1). Russian knapweed is a particularly problematic perennial in the intermountain states but is present in all states (Figure 2).

CLINICAL PRESENTATION

HISTORY, CHIEF COMPLAINT The sudden onset of involuntary facial movements and hypertonicity of the facial muscles inhibits the ability of the horse to bite off and chew its food. Affected horses often have continuous chewing movements because they are unable to move food to the oropharyngeal area for swallowing.

PHYSICAL EXAM FINDINGS

- Hypertonicity of the facial muscles may give a stiff, wooden appearance to the face.
- The lips and tongue are hypertonic, and the jaw may be held open or tightly closed.
- Chewing and prehension of food are impaired. Food may be held in the mouth. Dehydration, severe weight loss, and depression develop rapidly.
- The swallowing reflex is unimpaired. Some horses may learn to drink by submerging their head into a deep bucket or trough of water.

ETIOLOGY AND PATHOPHYSIOLOGY

- A specific toxin has not been identified in the plants, but repin, the most abundant sesquiterpene lactone found in both plants, is the probable toxin. The neurotoxin causes selective necrosis of the globus pallidus and the substantia nigra.
- The neurotoxin affects the dopaminergic pathways of cranial nerves V, VII, and IX.
- Horses must continuously eat large quantities of the plants to become affected (60% to 71% and 86% to 200% of their body weight of Russian knapweed and yellow star thistle, respectively). Ruminants fed large quantities of the plants are not affected.
- Interrupted consumption of the plants does not produce poisoning.
- Both the green and dried plants are potentially toxic.
- Neurologic signs are irreversible.

DIAGNOSIS

DIFFERENTIAL DIAGNOSIS

- Choke
- Teeth problems
- Mouth ulcers: Vesicular stomatitis virus
- Rabies

INITIAL DATABASE

Hematocrit, serum protein: Elevated because of dehydration

ADVANCED OR CONFIRMATORY TESTING

- Pathologic lesions: Bilateral, symmetrical yellowish-brown discoloration of the globus pallidus and substantia nigra.
- In chronic cases, cavitation of the affected necrotic areas may be present.
- Histologically, nigropallidal encephalomalacia is diagnostic.
- Magnetic resonance imaging: Focal necrosis in the globus pallidus and substantia nigra.

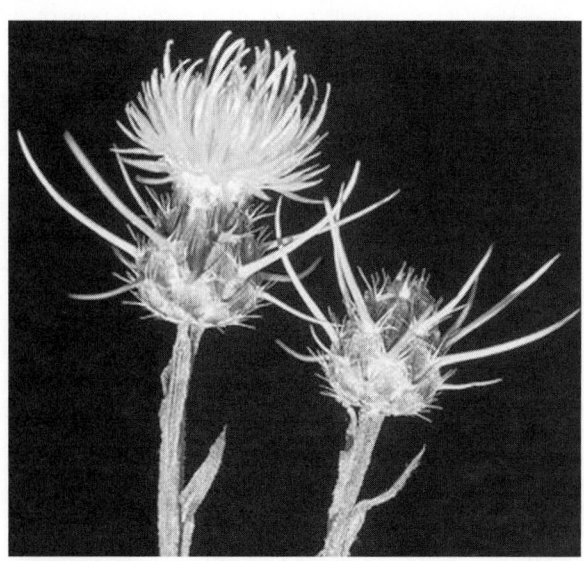

FIGURE 1 Yellow star thistle (*Centaurea solstitialis*).

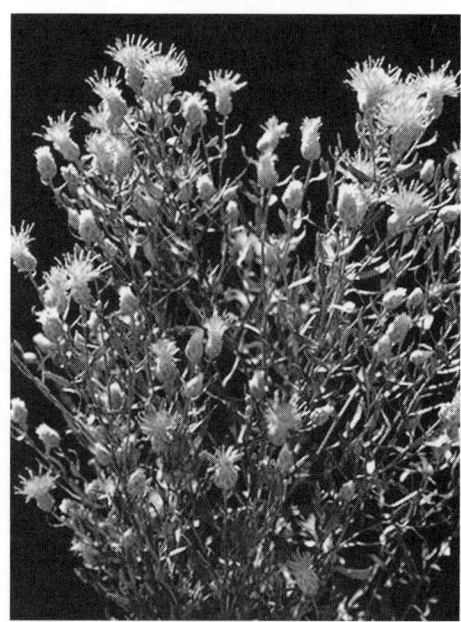

FIGURE 2 Russian knapweed (*Acroptilon repens*).

TREATMENT

THERAPEUTIC GOAL(S)

After clinical signs are evident, there is no specific treatment.

ACUTE GENERAL TREATMENT

Affected horses should be given supportive fluid and electrolyte therapy.

CHRONIC TREATMENT

- Provide supportive nutrition.
- Glutamine synthetase plus a bovine brain ganglioside extract has shown beneficial effect.

POSSIBLE COMPLICATIONS

Inhalation pneumonia

PROGNOSIS AND OUTCOME

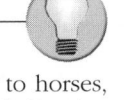

After clinical signs are present, the disease is typically fatal as a result of starvation; therefore euthanasia is recommended.

PEARLS & CONSIDERATIONS

COMMENTS

Aside from their neurotoxicity to horses, both yellow star thistle and Russian knapweed are noxious weeds that will displace useful forages in a pasture, decreasing the value of the property.

PREVENTION

- Identification of these plants will facilitate appropriate management.
- Interrupted grazing of the plants prevents a threshold of toxicity developing because the toxin is not cumulative.
- Herbicides to control these invasive species is recommended.
- Biological control: Specific insects and heavy grazing by sheep and goats.

CLIENT EDUCATION

Recognition of the plants will prevent their continuous consumption.

SUGGESTED READING

Knight AP: Guide to poisonous plants. Colorado State University. Available at http://southcampus.colostate.edu/poisonous_plants.

Roy DN, Peyton DH, Spencer PS: Isolation and identification of two potent neurotoxins, aspartic acid and glutamic acid, from yellow star thistle (*Centaurea solstitialis*). *Nat Toxins* 3:174–180, 1995.

Robles M, Wang N, Kim R: Cytotoxic effects of Repin, a principle sesquiterpene lactone of Russian knapweed. *J Neuro Science* 47:90–97, 1997.

Sanders SG: A putative neurotoxin in nigropallidal encephalomalacia and other Parkinson-like diseases. *Proceedings ACVIM 20th Forum*, 2002.

Sanders SG, Tucker RL, Bagley RS, Gavin PR: Magnetic resonance imaging features of equine nigropallidal encephalomalacia. *Vet Radiol Ultrasound* 42:291–296, 2001.

AUTHOR: **ANTHONY P. KNIGHT**

EDITOR: **CYNTHIA L. GASKILL**

Zearalenone Toxicosis

BASIC INFORMATION

DEFINITION

Zearalenone is a nonsteroidal estrogenic mycotoxin produced by numerous Fusarium molds—including *Fusarium graminearum* (*Gibberella zeae*), *Fusarium culmorum, Fusarium verticilliodes, Fusarium avenaceum, Fusarium tricinctum, Fusarium oxysporum,* and *Fusarium nivale*—that can contaminate corn and grains and occasionally hays, straws, and silages.

SYNONYM(S)

- RAL (resorcylic acid lactone)
- F-2
- Pink ear rot

EPIDEMIOLOGY

SPECIES, AGE, SEX The most adverse effects have been observed in females. Horses are not considered a sensitive species to zearalenone; however, young horses are generally more sensitive than older animals, and cycling animals are more sensitive than pregnant animals.

RISK FACTORS

- Low toxicity except for reproductive effects. Adverse effects are proportional to the zearalenone concentration in the diet. Zearalenone is a stable compound in the environment and not readily altered.
- Cycling mares dosed orally with purified zearalenone, which approximated 1 mg/kg (ppm) in feed, for 8 to 10 days had no changes in luteal or follicular activity.
- One report of enlarged uteri and vulvas and vaginal prolapses in mares and flaccid genitalia in stallions fed barley straw and corn screenings for 30 days; approximately 2.7 mg/kg zearalenone was detected in feed by thin-layer chromatography.

GEOGRAPHY AND SEASONALITY

- Occurs worldwide, especially in northern temperate climates and in high moisture grains and hays containing greater than 22% moisture.
- Zearalenone production is favored by alternating warm days (20°–25° C) and cool nights (7° C) during corn maturation and harvesting and in the fall haying during wet, cold conditions. Zearalenone can be found particularly in stored ear corn and in maturing corn after hail storms.

CLINICAL PRESENTATION

DISEASE FORMS/SUBTYPES Hyperestrogenism includes clinical signs of prolonged estrus, anestrus, infertility, delayed return to estrus, increased mammary or udder development and abnormal lactation, swollen external genitalia, and atrophy of ovaries or testicles.

HISTORY, CHIEF COMPLAINT Estrogenic clinical signs

PHYSICAL EXAM FINDINGS

- Enlarged or swollen genitalia
- Edematous uterus and vulva and prolapsed vulva
- Abnormal mammary gland enlargement
- Testicular and ovarian atrophy

ETIOLOGY AND PATHOPHYSIOLOGY

- Zearalenone and metabolites bind to cytosolic receptors for 17β-estradiol and stimulate specific RNA synthesis and signs of estrogenism. Increased estrogenic feedback on the pituitary gland reduces follicle-stimulating hormone concentrations and ovarian follicle maturation and ovulation.
- Zearalenone is absorbed from the gastrointestinal tract and metabolized by the liver to α- and β-zearalenol (which can exhibit higher estrogenic activity than zearalenone) and may be subsequently reduced to α- and β-zearalanol. Zearalenone and metabolites are conjugated and excreted in the urine and feces. Enterohepatic cycling can extend the half-life of zearalenone and prolong adverse effects.

DIAGNOSIS

DIFFERENTIAL DIAGNOSIS

Phytoestrogens such as coumestrol and high concentrations of isoflavones in alfalfa and clover (legume) forages can cause estrogenic signs.

INITIAL DATABASE

Diagnosis is based on clinical observations and the detection of zearalenone in feed sources. The possibility of chronic zearalenone exposure elevating serum progesterone concentrations in horses is unknown.

ADVANCED OR CONFIRMATORY TESTING

- Confirm exposure through chemical analysis of feedstuffs for zearalenone. Testing using liquid or gas chromatography and mass spectrometry can confirm concentrations in feed.
- Analysis of zearalenone and metabolites in serum, urine, and tissues may be of diagnostic value, but few laboratories offer these analyses.

TREATMENT

THERAPEUTIC GOAL(S)

- Remove animals from the contaminated feed. Clinical signs in affected animals generally improve in 2 to 8 weeks.
- No Food and Drug Administration–approved mycotoxin binders are available.

ACUTE GENERAL TREATMENT

Treatment of secondary complications may be required. Generally, animals will return to normal productivity without treatment.

PROGNOSIS AND OUTCOME

No permanent effects are expected from exposure, and animals generally return to normal state of productivity if secondary complications (eg, prolapsed rectums) are treated.

PEARLS & CONSIDERATIONS

COMMENTS

Few credible reports have been published on zearalenone toxicosis in horses suggesting that equine species are not very sensitive to the effects of zearalenone.

PREVENTION

Preventing mold growth on crops in the field or during harvesting and storage by using good management practices is the best approach to prevent zearalenone contamination of feed.

CLIENT EDUCATION

Avoid feeding moldy grain or forages to horses. Analyze suspect feed for the presence of mycotoxins.

SUGGESTED READING

Juhasz J, Nagy P, Kulcsár M, et al: Effect of low-dose zearalenone exposure on luteal function, follicular activity and uterine oedema in cycling mares. *Acta Vet Hung* 49:211–222, 2001.

Meerdink GL: Zearalenone. In Plumlee KH, editor: *Clinical veterinary toxicology*, St Louis, 2004, Mosby Elsevier, pp 273–275.

AUTHOR: **MICHELLE S. MOSTROM**

EDITOR: **CYNTHIA L. GASKILL**

Zinc Phosphide Toxicosis

BASIC INFORMATION

DEFINITION

Zinc phosphide is a rodenticide used to kill gophers, ground squirrels, and other burrowing animals as well as mice and rats. Zinc phosphide and related compounds occasionally cause poisoning in horses, creating a diagnostic challenge. Zinc phosphide has no direct effect on coagulation, unlike the more commonly used anticoagulant rodenticides. Zinc phosphide baits typically are grain based, often containing oats, and may resemble horse feed.

SYNONYM(S)

Magnesium phosphide and aluminum phosphide may have similar activity to zinc phosphide. Aluminum phosphide is used as a grain fumigant.

EPIDEMIOLOGY

RISK FACTORS

- Horses with access to rodenticides used on farms have a higher risk of poisoning
- Rodenticide bait mixed with oats

CONTAGION AND ZOONOSIS Zinc phosphide—related compounds produce phosphine gas, which is toxic to humans as well as horses. A veterinarian may be poisoned after passing a stomach tube or performing a necropsy on a horse that has ingested one of these compounds.

GEOGRAPHY AND SEASONALITY Rodenticides are used over most of the world.

CLINICAL PRESENTATION

HISTORY, CHIEF COMPLAINT

- Zinc phosphide bait used around farms
- Aluminum phosphide used to fumigate grain

- Rapid onset of clinical signs (within 4 hours of exposure) or occasionally delayed
- Colic
- Muscle tremors
- Sweating
- Dyspnea
- Depression
- Recumbency, thrashing
- Often rapidly lethal

PHYSICAL EXAM FINDINGS Cardiac arrhythmias

ETIOLOGY AND PATHOPHYSIOLOGY

- Zinc phosphide releases phosphine gas in the presence of acid (stomach acid).
- Aluminum and magnesium phosphides release phosphine gas in the presence of water.
- The mechanism of action of phosphine is not entirely understood, but it may inhibit oxidative phosphorylation in mitochondria, resulting in cell death.

DIAGNOSIS

DIFFERENTIAL DIAGNOSIS

Other rapidly acting toxins, such as cholinesterase inhibitors

INITIAL DATABASE

Clinical pathology findings are nonspecific.

ADVANCED OR CONFIRMATORY TESTING

- Testing for phosphine is available at some laboratories. Stomach contents or suspect material should be packed in an air-tight container and frozen immediately for transport to the diagnostic laboratory.
- Pathologic lesions are nonspecific and may include evidence of gastrointestinal irritation and pulmonary congestion and edema. Renal tubular degeneration and necrosis have also been reported.

TREATMENT

THERAPEUTIC GOAL(S)

- Stabilization
- Detoxification
- Symptomatic and supportive
- No specific antidote exists for zinc phosphide

ACUTE GENERAL TREATMENT

- Stabilization with symptomatic and supportive care
  - Correction of acidosis
  - Respiratory support
  - Seizure control
- Attempts to detoxify with activated charcoal or mineral oil have not been successful in horses.
- Use of antacids to prevent phosphine gas release has not been successful in horses.
- Stomach tube may release the phosphine gas.
  - Only do this in a well-ventilated area.
  - If you can smell the gas (garlic or rotten fish odor), you are in danger.

RECOMMENDED MONITORING

- Respiration
- Acid/base status
- Liver enzymes
- Renal function
- Seizure activity possible

PROGNOSIS AND OUTCOME

Guarded to poor in symptomatic animals; rapidly fatal

PEARLS & CONSIDERATIONS

COMMENTS

The LD_{50} dose has not been determined for horses but is approximately 40 mg/kg for most other domestic species.

PREVENTION/CLIENT EDUCATION

- Avoid rodenticide use around horses
- Do not store rodenticides near feeds
- Maintain sheds and other storage facilities to prevent animals from accessing stored pesticides

SUGGESTED READING

Albretsen JC: Zinc phosphide. In Plumlee KH, editor: *Clinical veterinary toxicology*, St Louis, 2003, Mosby Elsevier, pp 456–458.
Gupta RC: Non-anticoagulant rodenticides. In Gupta RC, editor: *Veterinary toxicology basic and clinical principles*, New York, 2007, Academic Press, pp 548–560.
Plumlee KH: Pesticide toxicosis in the horse. *Vet Clin North Am Equine Pract* 17:491–500, 2000.

AUTHOR: **KARYN BISCHOFF**

EDITOR: **CYNTHIA L. GASKILL**

Zygomycosis

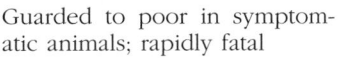

BASIC INFORMATION

DEFINITION

Deep, progressive, and rapidly invasive subcutaneous mycosis caused by fungi belonging to the class Zygomycetes (includes Entomophthorales and Mucorales)

SYNONYM(S)

Phycomycosis, entomophthoromycosis, conodiobolosis, rhinophycomycosis, basidiobolosis, mucormycosis

EPIDEMIOLOGY

GEOGRAPHY AND SEASONALITY

- Zygomycosis occurs mostly in tropical and subtropical areas (Americas, Australia, Asia, and Africa).
- In the United States, zygomycosis is most common in states along the Gulf of Mexico.

ASSOCIATED CONDITIONS AND DISORDERS

Relatively rare opportunistic fungal infection in humans manifested with gastrointestinal, pulmonary, cutaneous, renal, or meningeal involvement. It generally affects only immunocompromised individuals.

CLINICAL PRESENTATION

DISEASE FORMS/SUBTYPES

- Entomophthoromycosis
  - Conodiobolosis: Ulcerative granulomas on mucosa
  - Basidiobolosis: Ulcerative cutaneous granulomas
- Mucormycosis: Ulcerated cutaneous granulomas

HISTORY, CHIEF COMPLAINT

- Insidious onset of cutaneous granulomas, potentially fast-growing lesions.
- Nasal granulomas can go unnoticed, and the only clinical signs might be red-tinged nasal discharge and dyspnea.

PHYSICAL EXAM FINDINGS

- Basidiobolus infects the lateral aspects of the head, neck, trunk, and body (Figures 1 and 2).
  - Lesions are usually single and large, nodular eroded to ulcerative granulomas associated with moderate to severe pruritus and oozing of serosanguineous discharge.
  - Moderate to severe pruritus
  - If excised, tissue has a thickened fibrotic dermis (pink) and might contain small, scattered areas of red surrounding a white to yellow central core ("leeches") smaller than those seen with pythiosis.
- Conidiobolus affects almost exclusively the mucosa of the nares, nasal passages, and possibly the mouth and nasopharynx.
  - Serosanguinous nasal discharge
  - Single or multiple ulcerative pyogranulomas may lead to mechanical blockage of the airway, resulting in dyspnea.
    - If on the external nares: Lesions appear similar to basidiobolus infection.

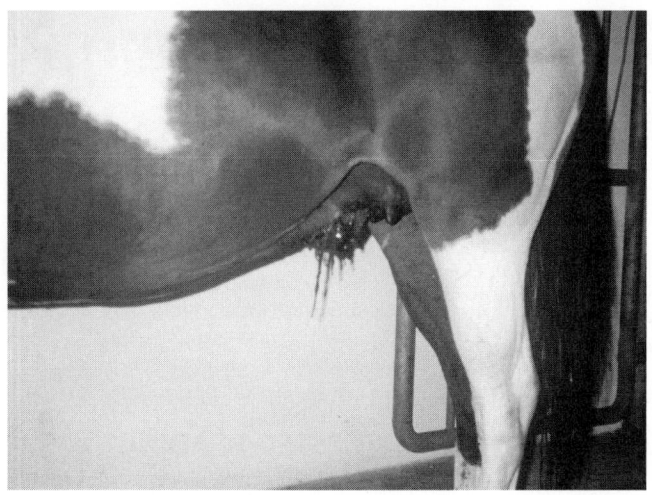

FIGURE 1 Basidiobolus infection.

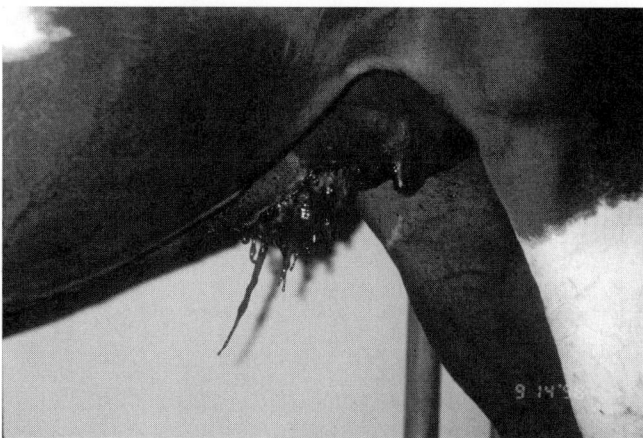

FIGURE 2 Example of zygomycosis.

- If in nasal passages and nasopharynx: Firm nodules covered by edematous, focally ulcerated mucosa.
- Mucormycosis: Single or multiple ulcerated cutaneous granulomas of the limbs, muzzle, and lips

ETIOLOGY AND PATHOPHYSIOLOGY

- Zygomycetes are ubiquitous saprophytic fungi in soil and decaying vegetation and may be present as part of the normal flora of skin and haircoat of horses.
- Infection may be caused by several related fungal species belonging to two orders under the class Zygomycetes, phylum Zygomycota:
  - Entomophthorales (includes genera *Conidiobolus* and *Basidiobolus*)
  - Mucorales (includes genera *Rhizopus, Mucor, Absidia,* and *Mortierella*)
- Infections are thought to develop secondary to wound inoculations.
- After inoculation, the fungi develop in the dermis, resulting in a pyogranulomatous inflammation.

DIAGNOSIS

DIFFERENTIAL DIAGNOSIS

- Exuberant granulation tissue
- Cutaneous habronemiasis
- Foreign body granuloma
- Pythiosis
- Bacterial pseudomycetoma or botryomycosis (limb, lips, head, mammary area, scrotum)
- Cutaneous actinomycosis (generally head and neck)
- Cutaneous nocardiosis (generally distal limb)
- Phaeohyphomycoses and eumycotic mycetomas
- Ulcerated neoplasia such as squamous cell carcinoma

- Neoplasia such as sarcoid, squamous cell carcinoma (ulcerated granulomas), and possibly cutaneous lymphoma, melanoma (generally not ulcerated)

INITIAL DATABASE

Abnormalities in the complete blood count and biochemistry profile are not reported.

ADVANCED OR CONFIRMATORY TESTING

- Cytologic evaluation of aspirate or direct smear: Pyogranulomatous to granulomatous inflammation with numerous eosinophils.
- Definitive diagnosis requires demonstration of the organism by histopathology evaluation or fungal culture of biopsy specimen.
  - Thickened fibrotic dermis with diffuse to nodular, pyogranulomatous to granulomatous inflammation containing numerous eosinophils.
  - Scattered areas with a central core of necrotic tissue, which often contains hyphal forms (poorly or occasionally septated) surrounded by eosinophilic infiltrate of the Splendore-Hoeppli phenomenon; hyphae are often poorly stained and may appear as clear spaces.
  - Tissue sections stained with Giemsa reveal large, branching occasionally septate, 4- to 20-μm, hyphae.
  - Immunohistochemistry of histologic sections allows identification of the organism.
  - Biopsy specimen for culture (in Sabouraud dextrose agar) should not be macerated.
- A serum agar gel immunoprecipition test is useful for the diagnosis of conidiobolomycosis.

TREATMENT

THERAPEUTIC GOAL(S)

- Attempt to reduce fungal burden via both medical and surgical management.
- Treatment should be instituted as soon as possible.

ACUTE AND CHRONIC GENERAL TREATMENT

- Surgical excision should be performed if possible. Surgical excision should be followed by chemotherapy.
- Drug therapy depends on the causative agent.
- Entomophthoromycosis
  - Iodides are effective and not too expensive; iodide should be administered daily for at least 1 month after complete regression of lesions
    - Organic iodides: More efficacious than inorganic iodides. Ethylene diamine dihydroiodide (EDDI) administered as a feed additive at a dosage of 1 to 2 mg/kg q12–24h for 7 days; then reduce to 0.5 to 1.0 mg/kg q24h for the remainder of the treatment
    - Inorganic iodides
      - Sodium iodide: Dose of 10 to 40 mg/kg/d as a 20% solution given IV slowly; the length of treatment varies: 2 to 5 days and then orally for the remainder of the treatment.
      - Potassium iodide: Dose of 20 to 40 mg/kg/d PO mixed with molasses and given by syringe or given with a small amount of feed or grain.
      - Anecdotal reports of signs of iodism occurring during the first several days as the body adjusts to the medication have prompted some clinicians to

initiate therapy with inorganic iodides at lower doses for the first few days and then increase to the recommended dose.

- Azoles can be attempted in cases refractory to iodides, pregnancy, or relapse after apparent cure; treatment should be administered daily for at least 1 month after complete regression of lesions.
  - Itraconazole: Overall poor bio-availability (requires acid pH for dissolution; therefore, absorption is highly variable).
    - Oral solution licensed for use in humans has higher and less variable solubility than capsules.
    - Dosage for horses: 5 mg/kg q24h.
  - Fluconazole: Successfully used to treat zygomycosis in pregnant mares. Recommended dosage: Loading dose of 14 mg/kg PO followed by 5 mg/kg q24h.
- Mucormycosis
  - Iodides are not effective against Mucorales (Rhizopus, Mucor, Absidia).
  - Amphotericin B given systemically after surgical excision must be dissolved in 5% dextrose and water.
    - The initial dose should be low and gradually increased. The initial daily dose is 0.3 mg/kg, and every third day, the dose is increased by 0.1 mg/kg until a maximum dose of 0.8 to 0.9 mg/kg/d is reached.
    - Treatment is continued daily or every other day for a total of 30 days.

DRUG INTERACTIONS

Azoles inhibit P450 enzymes; therefore there are multiple drug-drug interactions (greater with itraconazole than fluconazole).

POSSIBLE COMPLICATIONS

- Premature discontinuation of therapy may lead to relapse.
- Iodides have unpleasant taste and might cause nausea (requiring molasses to mask it). For oral inorganic iodides, potassium iodide is often preferred.
- Tolerance to iodides is variable, and some horses show signs of iodism.
  - Signs of iodism include lacrimation, salivation, scaling and alopecia, coughing, serous discharge, anorexia, depression, fever, nervousness, cardiovascular abnormalities, and abortion.
  - If signs of iodism develop, treatment should be discontinued for 7 days and then reinstituted at a lower dose (eg, 75% of the dose responsible for the toxic signs).
- Sodium iodide is very hydroscopic.
- Amphotericin B is nephrotoxic (poses greater risk in dehydrated animals and if concurrent nephrotoxic therapy is administered).

RECOMMENDED MONITORING

- Revaluate every 2 to 3 weeks for clinical signs and side effects associated with treatment.
- If azoles are used, monitoring of liver enzymes is recommended (although no adverse effects have been reported in horses). Baseline biochemical profile should be performed to evaluate liver enzymes before administration of azoles.
- If amphotericin B is used, there is a high risk nephrotoxicity. Water intake, urine output, and blood urea nitrogen and creatinine concentrations must be closely monitored.

PROGNOSIS AND OUTCOME

Horses with chronic lesions have a poorer prognosis.

PEARLS & CONSIDERATIONS

COMMENTS

- Identification of the causative agent is critical for effective chemotherapy.
- Treatment, including surgical excision and chemotherapy, should be instituted as soon as possible (horses undergoing early treatment have a much more favorable prognosis).

CLIENT EDUCATION

- All subcutaneous dermatomycoses carry a fair to guarded prognosis (worse prognosis if complete surgical excision cannot be achieved).
- Treatment duration is at least 1 month but often much longer.
- Treatment can be expensive if itraconazole or amphotericin B is used.

SUGGESTED READING

Scott DW, Miller WH Jr: Fungal skin diseases—subcutaneous mycosis—zygomycosis. In *Equine dermatology*, St Louis, 2003, Elsevier, pp 293–295.

Scott DW, Miller WH Jr: Antifungal therapy. In *Equine dermatology*, St Louis, 2003, Elsevier, pp 306–313.

White SD: Diseases of the skin—fungal diseases. In Smith BP, editor: *Large animal internal medicine*, ed 4, St Louis, 2009, Mosby Elsevier, p 1320.

AUTHOR: **LAIS R.R. COSTA**

EDITOR: **DAVID A. WILSON**

Procedures and Techniques

Abdominocentesis

BASIC INFORMATION

SYNONYM(S)

Belly tap
Abdominal tap
Paracentesis
Abdominal paracentesis

OVERVIEW AND GOAL(S)

Obtain a representative sample of peritoneal fluid in a safe, aseptic manner.

INDICATIONS

- Colic
- Increased peritoneal effusion
- Post–exploratory laparotomy complications (fever, colic)
- Weight loss
- Chronic diarrhea
- Fever of unknown origin

CONTRAINDICATIONS

- Distended viscus on ventral midline
- Overtly painful horse unwilling to stand without proper restraint available

EQUIPMENT, ANESTHESIA

- Sedation (xylazine)
- Experienced horse handler with a properly applied nose twitch may be necessary for young, excited, or fractious patients
- Stocks, if available, are preferred for improved restraint and protection of operator
- Clippers
- Surgical scrub solution-impregnated gauze and alcohol gauze for aseptic prepping of skin
- 3 mL of lidocaine with 25-gauge needle for local anesthesia
- Teat cannula, bitch catheter, 3-inch 18-gauge spinal needle, or 1.5-inch 18-gauge needle
- Sterile gloves
- Sterile gauze
- No. 15 blade
- Evacuated glass tube and several evacuated tubes containing EDTA
- Syringe (3 or 6 mL)
- Ultrasound for identification of appropriate tap site

ANTICIPATED TIME

Approximately 10 to 15 minutes

PREPARATION: IMPORTANT CHECKPOINTS

- Ultrasound the most dependent portion of abdomen to determine the best location for abdominocentesis. It is usually on right side of midline caudal to the xiphoid.
- Locate an area where there is free peritoneal fluid if possible, and avoid the spleen and large distended viscera.

POSSIBLE COMPLICATIONS AND COMMON ERRORS TO BE AVOIDED

- Enterocentesis: Ingesta (green, foul smelling, with particulate matter) will flow from cannula or needle. Remove cannula or needle from abdomen immediately and administer systemic antibiotics.
- Splenic laceration: Most commonly occurs when a needle is used to perform abdominocentesis but may also happen with a teat cannula, resulting in hemorrhage into the peritoneal cavity.

PROCEDURE

- Locate tap site with ultrasound, if available.
- Shave adequate (approx. 10 cm square) area over site with clippers.
- Aseptically prep shaved area.
- Use a 25-gauge needle and place a local block with 3 mL of 2% Lidocaine at the desired tap site.
- Apply a subsequent aseptic prep.
- Put on sterile gloves.
- If using a needle:
  - Acquire an 18-gauge 1.5-inch or 18-gauge 3-inch needle sterilely.
- If the tap is performed on midline—or, in a small pony, to the right of midline, a 1.5-inch needle should be adequate. However, if the spleen or a large viscus is over midline and one must go to the right of midline in a fat adult horse, a 3-inch needle will be needed to reach the peritoneal space.
- Grasp the needle firmly approximately 1 cm down the shaft and insert it slowly through the skin bleb.
- Insert the needle slowly a few millimeters at a time, stopping to check for fluid every few millimeters. At each point, rotate the needle hub to ensure the needle stays free of material that may prevent fluid from flowing through it.
- If a 1.5-inch needle is not long enough to reach the peritoneal space, replace with 3-inch needle.
- If using a teat cannula:
  - Make a small hole in one sterile 4 × 4 sponge with the No. 15 blade and place the teat cannula through this hole.
  - Use a sterile No. 15 blade to make a stab incision through the lidocaine bleb. Hold the blade firmly at the base of the blade portion with the blade facing caudally. Insert the blade through the skin, then continue inserting it until your fingers are firmly pressed against the body wall. This will ensure the external rectus sheath has been penetrated. Rotate the blade 90 degrees (vertical axis) laterally or 45 degrees (horizontal axis) caudally then remove.
  - Insert the teat cannula in the skin incision and allow the gauze to catch any blood that may be dripping from the skin.
  - Patiently locate the incision in the external fascia with the tip of the teat cannula.
  - Grasp the teat cannula firmly approximately 1 cm down from the skin and gently insert the cannula. Aim perpendicular to the body wall at all times to avoid dissecting through the tissue plains of the muscle.
  - The cannula should glide smoothly through the muscle then one pop should be felt (the internal rectus sheath).
  - Continue advancing the cannula a few millimeters at a time in a controlled conscious manner, always firmly holding the cannula a few millimeters from the skin surface.
    - A second pop should be felt; this will be the peritoneum. At this point the peritoneal cavity has been entered.
- TROUBLESHOOT: If fluid is not obtained immediately:
  - Rotate the cannula.
  - Gently insert it further.
  - Slowly remove the cannula.
  - Gently redirect the cannula.
  - Try a bitch catheter and insert it further.
  - If these measures fail to acquire fluid, a second tap site can be tried with either a cannula or a needle.
- TROUBLESHOOT: If you doubt you are in the peritoneal space:
  - If you are in doubt that the end of the cannula or needle is in the peritoneal space or still in the muscle, use a 3-mL syringe to inject air into the needle or cannula. If a squeaking noise or rush of air is heard when the syringe is removed, the needle or cannula it is most likely not in the peritoneal space.
  - Catch fluid in one evacuated glass tube (red top tube) for culture and sensitivity and several EDTA tubes (purple top tubes) for cytologic

evaluation, protein concentration, and nucleated cell count. If the fluid is originally red-tinged but then clears, it may be blood-contaminated and the clearest sample should be submitted for analysis.

- TROUBLESHOOT: If only a small amount of fluid is available:
  - Shake the excess EDTA out of the tube prior to collection so as not to dilute the small volume of sample.

This can falsely increase the protein concentration.

POSTPROCEDURE

Wipe tap site with alcohol gauze.

AUTHOR: **CHRISTINE WIMER**

Adrenocorticotropic Hormone (ACTH) Stimulation Test: Adults

BASIC INFORMATION

- Take pre-ACTH administration blood sample in heparinized or plain tubes.
- Administer ACTH gel (1 IU/kg IM) between 8 and 10 AM.
- Take post-ACTH blood samples 2 and 4 hours after ACTH administration.

- Horses with a functional adrenal cortex should have more than twofold increases in cortisol concentrations.
- In the cosyntropin stimulation test, 0.5 to 1 mg of synthetic ACTH (cosyntropin; Cortrosyn) is administered IV between 8 AM and noon.
- Take pre-ACTH blood sample, administer cosyntropin, and take post-ACTH blood sample 2 hours later.

- Interpret as for the ACTH stimulation test.
- Cortisol should be twice baseline 2 hours later.
- A lack of cortisol response suggests adrenal insufficiency.

AUTHOR: **RAMIRO TORIBIO**

Adrenocorticotropic Hormone (ACTH) Stimulation Test: Foals

BASIC INFORMATION

- Take pre-ACTH administration blood sample in heparinized or plain tubes.
- Administer 10 or 100 μg of synthetic ACTH (cosyntropin; Cortrosyn).

- Collect blood sample at 30 minutes for the 10 μg dose.
- Collect blood sample at 90 minutes for the 100 μg dose.
- Cortisol concentrations should be more than twice the baseline values in

30 minutes (10 μg) or 90 minutes (100 μg).
- A lack of response to cosyntropin is highly indicative of adrenal insufficiency.

AUTHOR: **RAMIRO TORIBIO**

Arthrocentesis

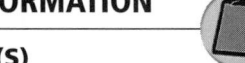

BASIC INFORMATION

SYNONYM(S)

Joint tap

OVERVIEW AND GOAL(S)

Aseptic technique and anatomic landmarks are used to access a joint, bursa, or synovial sheath and sample synovial fluid and/or inject appropriate medications.

INDICATIONS

Sampling the synovial space is necessary to rule in or rule out sepsis. Treatment of a joint or synovial space may be necessary to treat sepsis, osteoarthritis, or traumatic synovitis.

CONTRAINDICATIONS

The needle should not be placed through an area of cellulitis or infection.

EQUIPMENT, ANESTHESIA

- The horse is sedated with medications that also provide analgesia such as a combination of detomidine and butorphanol.
- A standard aseptic surgical preparation of the injection site will be required.
- Sterile gloves, sterile 18- to 20-g, 1- to 1.5-inch needles, several 6-mL sterile syringes, sampling tubes (usually EDTA, heparin, and plain Vacutainer tubes, and culture transport media) and any appropriate joint medications.

ANTICIPATED TIME

20 minutes

PREPARATION: IMPORTANT CHECKPOINTS

- Identify the anatomic landmarks of the sampling site (see "Lameness Examination: Diagnostic Local Anesthesia" in this section). The site does not need to be clipped or shaved, but this may be helpful to specifically identify the site.
- Sedation/analgesia should be administered so that the maximal effect is present at the time of arthrocentesis (for example, administer detomidine and butorphanol 10 minutes before injection).

- Standard aseptic preparation should be made using povidone-iodine or chlorhexidene gluconate scrub for 10 minutes of contact time. Alcohol should be applied as the final preparation.

POSSIBLE COMPLICATIONS AND COMMON ERRORS TO BE AVOIDED

Fluid may not be obtained if the joint is "dry" or the needle is improperly positioned. In some locations, such as the palmar/plantar pouch of the fetlock joint, synovial fronds may obstruct the needle or iatrogenic hemorrhage may result.

PROCEDURE

- After the final preparation of alcohol is applied, smartly and quickly introduce the needle into the synovial space.
- Have an assistant prepared to catch any fluid that drips from the needle hub with a small EDTA tube.
- Attach the syringe and gently aspirate until 3 to 5 mL of synovial fluid is obtained.

- If medication is being injected in a joint with effusion, remove the approximate volume to be injected from the joint before administering the medications(s).

POSTPROCEDURE

- Transfer the remaining sample to the appropriate sampling containers.
- Wipe the arthrocentesis site with an alcohol gauze.
- On distal limb sites a protective clean bandage may be applied and left in place for 12 to 24 hours.

AUTHOR: **ANDRIS J. KANEPS**

Artificial Insemination: Deep Horn Pipette

BASIC INFORMATION

SYNONYM(S)

Deep artificial insemination (AI), low-dose AI

OVERVIEW AND GOAL

- Deposit a low dose of semen (3 to 50 × 10^6 progressively motile sperm) at the tip of the uterine horn ipsilateral to the preovulatory follicle-bearing ovary
- Requires one assistant

INDICATIONS

- Increasing number of doses for large booked stallions or when limited doses are available after death of a stallion
- Subfertile stallions
- Use of sex-sorted and epididymal semen

EQUIPMENT, ANESTHESIA

- Cleaning material: Chlorhexidine/povidone-iodine, soap, and water
- Special flexible insemination pipette for deep horn AI, sterile palpation glove, sterile lubricant

ANTICIPATED TIME

Insemination timing: Same as AI in the uterine body

PREPARATION: IMPORANT CHECKPOINTS

- Mare preparation:
  - Sedation may be required depending on the mare's behavior.

  - Place the mare in stocks with its tail wrapped and tied. Empty the rectum, perform three alternate scrubs/rinses of the perineal area, and dry the area.
- Semen preparation:
  - With fresh semen coming from fertile stallions, centrifugation is required to reduce the final volume of the insemination dose. Cushioned and layered centrifugation may be performed in subfertile stallions. In both cases, final concentration is obtained by mixing the semen pellet with an extender and seminal plasma (10% of the final volume) to obtain a final concentration of 25 to 100 × 10^6 sperm/mL.

POSSIBLE COMPLICATIONS AND COMMON ERRORS TO BE AVOIDED

- Pipette insufficiently advanced in the horn
- Endometrial trauma

PROCEDURE

- Draw the semen into the inner catheter of a prewarmed flexible pipette (65 cm long insemination pipette; Minitube, Tieffenback, Germany); with a 5 mL syringe, aspirate 2 mL air + semen + 1 mL air. Seal the inner catheter in the pipette.
- The assistant holds the syringe and the external extremity of the pipette during its placement.
- Direct the tip of the pipette to the desired horn by bending it slightly.

- Use transrectal palpation to identify the pipette within the horn and guide it toward the tip of the horn.
- Deposit the semen into the tip of the horn.
- Insufflate 3 mL of air in the inner catheter before removing it. Absence of semen in the inner catheter should be monitored when removed.
- Remove the pipette and keep the horn elevated for 3 minutes. (Alternatively, the ovary may be pushed down.)

POSTPROCEDURE

Same as AI in the uterine body

ALTERNATIVES AND THEIR RELATIVE MERITS

Deep horn AI under hysteroscopy: Visualization of the papilla of the uterotubal junction

SUGGESTED READINGS

Brinsko SP: Insemination doses: how low can we go? *Theriogenology* 66:543–550, 2006.

Brinsko SP, Rigby SL, Lindsey AC, et al: Pregnancy rates in mares following hysteroscopic or transrectally guided insemination with low sperm numbers at the utero-tubal papilla, *Theriogenology* 59:1001–1009, 2003.

Lyle SK: Low dose insemination: why, when and how, *Theriogenology* 64:572–579, 2005.

Morris L: Advanced insemination techniques in mares, *Vet Clin North Am Equine Pract* 22:693–703, 2006.

Samper JC: Rectally guided or hysteroscopic insemination: is there a difference? *J Equine Vet Sci* 28:640–644, 2008.

AUTHORS: **FRANÇOIS-XAVIER GRAND** and **REJEAN CLÉOPHAS LEFEBVRE**

Artificial Insemination: Deep Hysteroscopy

BASIC INFORMATION

SYNONYM(S)

Hysteroscopic insemination

OVERVIEW AND GOAL(S)

- The semen is deposited onto the oviductal papilla of the ipsilateral horn on the side of the preovulatory follicle using an endoscope.
- This technique allows the visualization of the oviductal papilla.
- Although it may give better results when the insemination dose is close to the oviductal sperm reservoir capacity, it requires two assistants and it is more time-consuming.

INDICATIONS

- Breeding with a very low dose ($<5.0 \times 10^6$ progressively motile sperm) and very small volume (<20–$500\ \mu L$) of semen from a subfertile, booked, or old stallion, or using sex-sorted semen
- When the insemination dose is close to the oviductal sperm reservoir capacity

EQUIPMENT

- Sedation: Combination of detomidine-butorphanol
- Sterilized and prewarmed ($37°$ C) endoscope (at least 1.2 m long) with inner insemination catheter

ANTICIPATED TIME

Insemination timing: See "Artificial Insemination: Uterine Body" in this section.

PREPARATION: IMPORANT CHECKPOINTS

- Mare preparation: See "Artificial Insemination: Uterine Body" in this section.
- Endoscope preparation:
  - Draw the semen into the inner catheter with a 5 mL syringe: 2 mL air + Semen + 1 mL air.
  - Pass the insemination catheter in the endoscope channel.

POSSIBLE COMPLICATIONS AND COMMON ERRORS TO BE AVOIDED

- Failure to recognize the utero tubal junction (UTJ).
- Excess of air insufflation in the uterus prevents the semen from sticking to the UTJ.

PROCEDURE

- Place the sterile endoscope into the uterine body through the cervix.
- Remove the gloved hand from the vagina.
- Bring the endoscope to the tip of the horn under rectal guidance.
- Close the horn around the scope at two-thirds of its length and insufflate a moderate amount air only in the distal third of the horn (endometrial folds should still be visualized).
- Bring the endoscope in close contact with the papilla of the UTJ.
- Inject the semen onto the oviductal papilla.
- Remove the air from the uterus by endoscope suction or transrectal massage.
- As an alternative to step 2, the inseminator's hand may stay in the vagina:
  - Close the cervix around the endoscope.
  - Insufflate a moderate amount of air in the uterus.
  - Advance the endoscope to the tip of the horn ipsilateral to the ovary where ovulation has occurred (or where the preovulatory follicle is): Closely monitor the orientation of the scope to go in the designated horn.

POSTPROCEDURE

See "Artificial Insemination: Uterine Body" in this section.

SUGGESTED READING

Sanchez R, Gomez I, Samper JC: Artificial insemination with frozen semen. In Samper JC, editor: *Equine breeding management and artificial insemination*, ed 2, St Louis, 2009, Elsevier, pp 175–184.

AUTHORS: **FRANÇOIS-XAVIER GRAND** and **REJEAN CLÉOPHAS LEFEBVRE**

Artificial Insemination: Uterine Body

BASIC INFORMATION

SYNONYM(S)

Conventional artificial insemination (AI)

OVERVIEW AND GOAL(S)

- Essential tool for reproductive management in the horse industry (Box 1).
- Approximately 50% of mares bred by AI are bred with fresh semen; 40% receive cooled transported semen, and 10% receive frozen semen.
- Estrus, follicular development, and ovulation should be accurately monitored to optimize AI efficiency.
- Success mainly depends on two factors: Mare management (before and after insemination) and semen quality.

BOX 1   Physiologic Events Involved in the Fertilization Process by Insemination

- Cellular membrane changes occurring during the freezing process reduce the longevity of frozen/thawed sperm.
- After the placement of semen in the uterine body, the interaction between the endometrium and semen results in a physiologic inflammatory reaction. Seminal plasma modulates this inflammatory reaction.
- Migration of sperm from the uterine body to the oviduct occurs within 4 hours, and a retrograde sperm loss of approximately 43% is observed.

- The oviduct serves as a reservoir for sperm by attaching and selecting the most viable, motile, and morphologically normal sperm. These subpopulations of sperm are eventually delivered to the fertilization site.
- Sperm capacitation (4 hours) and hyperactivation are necessary for fertilization.
- Oocyte competence for fertilization lasts only 6 to 8 hours after ovulation. Oocyte quality decreases in aged and exercised mares.

TABLE 1 Expected Sperm Survival Time in the Mare Reproductive Tract

Type of Semen	Expected Mean Time of Sperm Viability in the Female Genital Tract	Conventionally Required Number of Sperm
Fresh extended	48 h (few hours to 6 days)	500×10^6 PMS
Cooled	48 h	1×10^9 PMS precooling
Frozen/thawed	12 h (few minutes to 18 h)	200×10^6 PMS postthawing

PMS, Progressively motile sperm

INDICATIONS

- To improve semen availability (time, location, quantity)
- To control venereal diseases
- To reduce risks of injuries in mares and stallions
- To increase the genetic pool
- Breeding with a conventional dose of semen from a fertile stallion (Table 1)

CONTRAINDICATIONS

Not allowed in Thoroughbreds

EQUIPMENT

- Cleaning material: Chlorhexidine/povidone iodine, soap, and water
- Insemination pipette, sterile palpation glove, sterile lubricant
- Thawing equipment if frozen semen is used: Thermometer, 37° C water, chronometer

MARE SELECTION

- Avoid transitional heats.
- General body condition: 4/9 to 6/9 and no concomitant disease.
- Normal perineal conformation.
- Absence of urine pooling and vaginal tears on vaginal examination.
- Normal reproductive tract and normal cyclicity on transrectal examination.
- Normal cytologic and bacteriologic endometrium.
- Endometrial biopsy suggested in repeatedly bred mares and in mares with a history of early embryonic death or abortion. Mares with uterine biopsy results of Kenney and Doig grade IIB and III have a lower probability of carrying a pregnancy to term.

ANTICIPATED TIME

- AI timing with cooled semen: Inseminate within 48 hours before ovulation with a single dose.
- Order the semen when the following signs are observed: 33 to 35 mm follicle concomitant with endometrial edema and a relaxed cervix. It is suggested to induce ovulation at the same time as the insemination (not earlier because of possible delayed semen arrival).
- Ideally, the semen dose is inseminated within 24 hours of cooling.

- If two doses are shipped together, both doses should be inseminated upon receipt if ovulation is imminent and total insemination volume is less than 120 mL.
- Mares sensitive to persistent mating-induced endometritis are preferably bred only once and closer to ovulation.
- A dual-shipment strategy can be chosen for mares with a history of ovulating small follicles. The first AI may be performed when the dominant follicle is at preovulatory size (33 to 35 mm in diameter). If the mare has not ovulated after 48 hours, a second AI is performed when the dominant follicle will respond to ovulation induction.
- AI timing with frozen semen: Inseminate within 6 hours of ovulation.
- Single-dose postovulation insemination protocol: Ultrasonographic monitoring of ovulation every 6 hours starting 12 to 24 hours after inducement. Insemination is performed as soon as ovulation is noted.
- Multiple-dose insemination protocol: Ultrasonographic monitoring daily until the preovulatory follicle reaches 35 mm in diameter. Ovulation is then induced and the mare is inseminated twice, at 24 and 42 hours after human chorionic gonadotropin administration. A third insemination is performed if the mare has not ovulated 52 hours after human chorionic gonadotropin administration. This method is not recommended in older mares and those that are susceptible to developing post-mating–induced endometritis.
- Both protocols show similar pregnancy rates.

PREPARATION: IMPORANT CHECKPOINTS

Mare preparation:
- Sedation may be needed in a few mares.
- The mare is placed in a stock with its tail wrapped and tied. The rectum is emptied, three alternate scrubs/rinses of the perineal area are performed, and the area is dried.

Semen preparation:
- Cooled semen should not be warmed before insemination.
- For frozen semen, the veterinarian should strictly follow the thawing instructions provided by the laboratory that processed the semen. If no specific thawing protocol is recommended, 30 seconds in a 37° C water bath should be adequate for 0.5 mL straws. Straws must be dried carefully before their seals are removed.

POSSIBLE COMPLICATIONS

Post-mating–induced endometritis

PROCEDURE

The tip of the insemination pipette is cupped within the gloved hand and sterile gel is deposited on the dorsal part of the inseminator's hand. The hand cupping the pipette is introduced into the vagina and the cervix is identified with the index finger. Once the cervix lumen is identified, the pipette is guided with the index finger and advanced 6 to 8 cm into the uterine body. With the pipette placed at the opening of the uterine body, the cervix is closed around the pipette and the semen is delivered into the uterine body. After AI, a drop of semen may be recovered from the straw for semen quality assessment.

POSTPROCEDURE

Monitor uterine fluid accumulation to detect exacerbated post-mating–induced endometritis.

EXPECTED PREGNANCY RATES PER CYCLE

- Fresh semen: 65% to 70% per cycle
- Cooled semen: 50% to 60% per cycle
- Frozen semen: 40% to 50% per cycle

ALTERNATIVES AND THEIR RELATIVE MERITS

Deep horn AI: Optimal results with subfertile stallions (see "Aritificial Insemination: Deep Horn Pipette" in this section).

SUGGESTED READING

Bedford-Guaus SJ: Transported stallion semen and breeding mares with cooled or frozen-thawed semen, *Clin Tech Equine Pract* 6:239–248, 2007.

Miller CD: Optimizing the use of frozen-thawed equine semen, *Theriogenology* 70:463–468, 2008.

Samper JC: Artificial insemination with fresh and cooled semen. In Samper JC, editor: *Equine breeding management and artificial insemination,* ed 2, St Louis, 2009, Elsevier, pp 165–174.

Samper JC, Estrada AJ, McKinnon AO: Insemination with frozen semen. In Samper JC, Pycock JF, McKinnon AO, editors: *Current therapy in equine reproduction,* St Louis, 2007, Elsevier, pp 285–288.

AUTHORS: **FRANÇOIS-XAVIER GRAND** and **REJEAN CLÉOPHAS LEFEBVRE**

Aspiration Cytology Culture: Draining Tract from Jaw

BASIC INFORMATION

OVERVIEW AND GOAL(S)

Percutaneous sampling technique for the determination of etiologic organisms in maxillary and mandibular draining wounds.

INDICATIONS

Swellings on the mandible or maxilla, from which there is drainage of serous, mucoid, mucopurulent, or purulent debris.

CONTRAINDICATIONS

Little is to be gained by "swabbing" this region after prolonged antimicrobial therapy.

EQUIPMENT, ANESTHESIA

- Sedation: Local anesthesia or perineural analgesia (if required)
- Antiseptic scrub and isopropyl alcohol
- Sterile gloves
- Sterile transport swabs (aerobic and anaerobic)
- Blood culture medium
- 3-mL syringes and 20-gauge 1-inch needles

ANTICIPATED TIME

10 minutes

PREPARATION: IMPORTANT CHECKPOINTS

- Complete physical examination
- Complete oral examination
- Radiographic examination of affected region

POSSIBLE COMPLICATIONS AND COMMON ERRORS TO BE AVOIDED

Care must be taken to sample the internal surface of the fistula tract only to avoid extraneous contamination.

PROCEDURE

- Sedate horse.
- Clip the hair and prepare skin aseptically.
- Using sterile gloves, insert the sterile transport swab as deep into the draining tract as possible.
- Repeat using an anaerobic swab.
- Seal, label, and submit to the laboratory.
- If there is no draining tract, however, a subcutaneous pocket has been detected during the physical examination stage of the evaluation, the skin can be aseptically prepared and the pocket of fluid can be sampled using a percutaneous aspiration technique.
  - A 3-mL syringe with a 20-gauge or 18-gauge 1-inch needle will suffice.
  - If material is easy to obtain, then either transport this to a local (in-house) laboratory or transfer to standard transport swabs.
  - If sample is not easy to obtain, standard techniques of aspiration should be followed; that is, repeated withdrawal of the syringe plunger and subsequent expulsion of material onto a clean slide for cytologic and Gram stain evaluation.

AUTHOR: **JAMES L. CARMALT**

Aspiration Cytology Culture: Nasomaxillary Sinus

BASIC INFORMATION

SYNONYM(S)

Sinus culture

OVERVIEW AND GOAL(S)

To obtain a diagnostic sample of nasomaxillary sinus secretions for the determination of infectious etiology or to rule out the presence of neoplasia or paranasal sinus cyst

INDICATIONS

Unilateral purulent nasal discharge, facial distortion

EQUIPMENT, ANESTHESIA

- Sedation
- Local analgesia
- Jacobs chuck and Steinmann pin (4 mm)
- Extension set for intravenous catheter
- Bacterial transport swabs
- Needles and syringes

ANTICIPATED TIME

15 minutes

PREPARATION: IMPORTANT CHECKPOINTS

Complete physical, radiologic, and endoscopic examination

POSSIBLE COMPLICATIONS AND COMMON ERRORS TO BE AVOIDED

Attempting to sample the incorrect sinus: Inadequate prior workup or incorrect external landmarks

PROCEDURE

- Restrain the horse (either using a handler or placing within stocks).
- Select appropriate site for sinocentesis:
  - Frontal sinus: Midway between the supraorbital foramen and the midline
  - Caudal maxillary sinus: 2 cm rostral and 1 cm ventral to the medial canthus of the eye
  - Rostral maxillary sinus: One-half-way along and 4 cm ventral to a line connecting the medial canthus of the eye to the nasoincisive notch (the path of the bony portion of the nasolacrimal duct)
- Insert bleb of local anesthetic under skin and into the periosteum.
- A small stab incision is made through the skin to the level of the periosteum and the skin edges separated using a hemostat.
- To access the sinus, use a Jacob's chuck and appropriately sized Steinmann pin.
- In some cases, sinus material is immediately apparent. In other cases, a needle may have to be inserted into the sinusotomy site and the material aspirated using a syringe in standard fashion.
  - Infectious sinusitis material may be liquid or cheese-like in consistency.
  - Fluid from a paranasal sinus cyst is usually straw-colored and nonviscous containing refractive crystals.

○ Neoplastic masses may require a core biopsy to obtain sufficient material for a definitive diagnosis.

ALTERNATIVES AND THEIR RELATIVE MERITS

Flap sinusotomy under general anesthesia. Greater exposure and good ability to clear infected tissue; however, it is an invasive procedure.

AUTHOR: **JAMES L. CARMALT**

Biopsy: Bone/Soft Tissue

BASIC INFORMATION

OVERVIEW AND GOAL(S)

Percutaneous sampling technique for investigation of bone or soft tissue pathology to determine etiology

INDICATIONS

Investigation of bone lesions (primary and secondary) as well as soft tissue lesions suspected of being neoplastic or infectious in origin.

EQUIPMENT, ANESTHESIA

- Local anesthesia or perineural analgesia (if required). In some cases, especially lesions in the oropharynx, general anesthesia may be necessary.
- Antiseptic scrub and isopropyl alcohol
- Scalpel blade
- Sterile gloves
- 10% formalin or specific fixation medium
- Skin biopsy instrument or Jamshidi needle. In some cases a Michelle or Galt trephine is indicated.

ANTICIPATED TIME

20 minutes

PREPARATION: IMPORTANT CHECKPOINTS

- Complete physical examination
- Complete oral examination
- Radiographic examination of affected region

POSSIBLE COMPLICATIONS AND COMMON ERRORS TO BE AVOIDED

- Iatrogenic nerve and vessel damage: Good knowledge of anatomy essential
- Diagnostically useless sample

PROCEDURE

- Sedate horse and perform appropriate additional analgesic procedures.
- Clip the hair and prepare skin aseptically.
- Using sterile gloves:
  ○ Soft tissue biopsy: Tissue in question is sampled by elevating the tissue with Adson forceps and resected with a pair of scissors. Alternatively, skin punch biopsy punches (4–6 mm in diameter) can be used to collect tissue. Samples should include normal tissue, the margin of normal and grossly abnormal tissue. Each sample is clearly identified and submitted for histologic examination. If possible, the examiner in question should be a dermatohistopathologist for best results.
  ○ Bone biopsy: Skin sectioned sufficiently to allow introduction of biopsy instrument. Bone is sampled as above, with sections of normal and grossly abnormal bone as well as marginal regions.

POSTPROCEDURE

- Soft tissue biopsy: None
- Bone biopsy: Skin may be closed with a single suture or skin staple; however, in most cases the incision is left to close by second intention.

AUTHOR: **JAMES L. CARMALT**

Biopsy: Liver

BASIC INFORMATION

SYNONYM(S)

Percutaneous liver biopsy, ultrasound-assisted or ultrasound-guided liver biopsy

OVERVIEW AND GOAL(S)

A liver biopsy can provide both diagnostic and prognostic value in horses with liver disease. Because many hepatic diseases in horses result in diffuse pathology, a representative sample is usually easily obtained using either a "blind" or an ultrasound-assisted technique. In animals with focal sonographic abnormalities, an ultrasound-guided technique can aid in obtaining diagnostic biopsy samples.

INDICATIONS

- To provide diagnostic and prognostic information in horses with liver disease
- To obtain a representative liver sample for bacterial culture
- In horses with clinical and ultrasonographic findings consistent with metastatic neoplasia (focal or multifocal masses), a liver biopsy sample may be more easily obtained than a sample at the primary tumor site and thus may aid in diagnosis and characterization of neoplastic disease if hepatic metastases are present.

CONTRAINDICATIONS

- A liver biopsy should be performed with caution in horses with documented coagulopathies; hemorrhage is a potential complication even when clotting function is normal.
- Percutaneous liver biopsy is also discouraged in horses in which the liver cannot be visualized ultrasonographically; the risk of penetration of other structures (right kidney, pancreas, large colon, diaphragm, spleen) is increased in these cases.

EQUIPMENT, ANESTHESIA

- Appropriate sedation and/or a twitch
- Clippers with a No. 40 blade
- Disinfectant scrub material and sterile gauze for sterile preparation of the skin
- Sterile gloves
- 2% lidocaine or another local-acting anesthetic
- One 5 to 10 mL syringe and several 22 or 25 gauge needles
- No. 15 scalpel blade, sterile

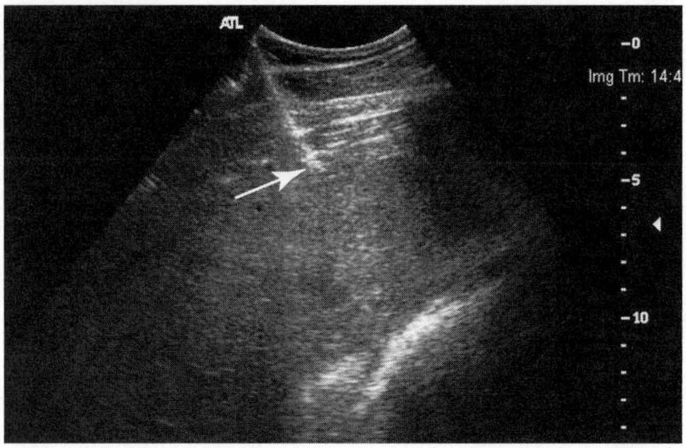

FIGURE 1 Ultrasound-guided liver biopsy. The *arrow* indicates the tip of the echogenic biopsy needle as it is about to enter the liver. This image was obtained at the right twelfth intercostal space, using a 3 to 5 MHz transducer, displayed to a depth of 15 cm.

- Sterile gauze pads (3 × 3 or 4 × 4 inches)
- A 14 gauge, 15 to 16 cm biopsy instrument, such as one of the following:
  - Tru-Cut (Baxter-Travenol, St. Louis, MO) biopsy instrument
  - Franklin-modified Vim-Silverman (Mueller & Co, Chicago, IL) biopsy instrument
  - A semiautomatic or automatic biopsy "gun" (such as EZ-Core, Products Group International, Lyons, CO; or ProMag 2.2 Biopsy System, Mannan Medical Products, Northbrook, IL)
- If using ultrasound assistance or guidance:
  - Ultrasound machine with a 2.5 to 5.0 MHz transducer
  - Sterile ultrasound probe covers or extra sterile gloves
  - Sterile ultrasound contact gel
- Nonabsorbable suture material and needle drivers
- 10% formalin to preserve samples for histopathologic evaluation
  - Foam-filled tissue cages are useful for maintaining the integrity of small biopsy samples
- Transport media for aerobic and anaerobic bacterial culture of biopsy samples

ANTICIPATED TIME

30 to 45 minutes

PREPARATION: IMPORANT CHECKPOINTS

- A complete blood count and coagulation profile should be completed before a liver biopsy is performed. In general, if platelet counts are decreased or clotting times are prolonged, appropriate procoagulant therapy (eg, fresh or fresh-frozen plasma) should be administered before biopsy to support hemostasis.

- Ensure that the patient is appropriately restrained. For most horses, this is best accomplished with chemical sedation and restraint in stocks. A twitch may provide adequate restraint in very compliant or very ill horses.
- If possible, use percutaneous ultrasonography before the sterile preparation to identify the liver and determine the desired biopsy site.
- If an ultrasound-guided biopsy of a small focal lesion is desired, it is helpful to have an extra person with sterile gloves on so that one person can guide and operate the biopsy instrument while the other person maintains the appropriate ultrasound image (Figure 1).

POSSIBLE COMPLICATIONS AND COMMON ERRORS TO BE AVOIDED

- The most common complications include:
  - Hemorrhage (even in the absence of a coagulopathy)
  - Penetration of other viscera, including the diaphragm, colon, pancreas, right kidney, spleen (if biopsying on the left), lung, or heart (rarely)
  - Peritonitis secondary to penetration of a hepatic abscess or if severe bacterial cholangiohepatitis is present
  - Hepatic rupture (rare, seen with biopsy of markedly enlarged livers due to hepatic lipidosis)
  - Bile peritonitis (rare)
- These complications can be minimized by evaluation of hemostasis and treatment of impaired coagulation before biopsy and accurate visualization of the liver, hepatic vasculature, and associated viscera with ultrasonography before and during liver biopsy. If penetration of a hepatic abscess or severe bacterial cholangiohepatitis

is suspected, prophylactic broad-spectrum antimicrobial therapy is warranted. Liver biopsy should be avoided in hyperlipemic patients with dramatic hepatic enlargement and hyperechoic hepatic parenchyma because of the risk of biopsy-related liver rupture.

- It is important to note that even if histopathologic evaluation of a liver biopsy is consistent with severe hepatic pathology, it may not be possible to determine the specific cause of the liver disease from a liver biopsy sample. In addition, if the hepatic pathology is localized or multifocal rather than diffuse, it may be difficult to obtain a representative sample of the affected area to provide diagnostic and prognostic information.

PROCEDURE

- Determine the specific biopsy site
  - For a "blind" liver biopsy, the skin incision is made in the right thirteenth or fourteenth intercostal spaces on a line drawn from the tuber coxae to just below the point of the shoulder.
  - For an ultrasound-localized or ultrasound-guided biopsy, the specific site may deviate somewhat from this line or may even be on the left side of the abdomen if the liver is more easily visualized there. If ultrasound assistance is used, determine the depth (in centimeters) the biopsy instrument will need to penetrate to reach the desired site in the liver.
- Clip and aseptically prepare the skin at the biopsy site, and infiltrate 3 to 6 mL of local anesthetic subcutaneously at the site for the skin incision.
- Open sterile gloves, scalpel blade, sterile gauze, and biopsy instrument using aseptic technique.
- Put on sterile gloves and ensure that the biopsy instrument is functional and you are comfortable operating it.
- Make an approximately $\frac{1}{4}$-inch stab incision through the skin with the No. 15 blade. Sterile gauze may be used to blot skin bleeding as needed.
- Insert the biopsy instrument through the skin incision and advance it cranially and ventrally to the desired depth. To avoid the intercostal vessels, the instrument should be inserted at the rostral edge of the ribs. If an alteration in angle is necessary, the biopsy instrument should be withdrawn to the skin and the position changed rather than redirect the instrument once it has penetrated the body wall or liver.
- Stabilize the biopsy instrument at the desired depth and fire the biopsy instrument as directed by the manu-

facturer. Withdraw the instrument without changing its angle.

- Remove samples from the biopsy instrument carefully over your sterile field or over the formalin jar. A sterile 18 or 20 gauge needle may be used to ease samples out of the instrument if needed.
- Additional samples may be obtained by using the same biopsy instrument providing aseptic technique is maintained. It is ideal to obtain separate samples for histopathologic analysis and bacterial culture. Samples may be obtained from distinct locations (via additional skin incisions) if desired by using ultrasound guidance or may be obtained via the same incision if the biopsy instrument is advanced at a slightly different angle on repeat attempts.
- When desired biopsy samples have been obtained, close the skin incision with a single interrupted or cruciate suture.

- Submit formalin-fixed samples to a veterinary pathologist for interpretation and additional samples for aerobic and anaerobic bacterial culture.

POSTPROCEDURE

- Monitor the patient closely for the following 24 to 36 hours for any signs associated with significant hemorrhage (eg, tachycardia, tachypnea, pallor, anemia, hypoproteinemia).
- Development of pyrexia after liver biopsy may indicate development of peritonitis. Abdominocentesis with cytologic analysis of peritoneal fluid and broad-spectrum antimicrobial therapy may be indicated in these cases.
- A small amount of subcutaneous emphysema occasionally develops at the site of the skin incision if the lung was penetrated. This is usually not a problem, though development of signs of respiratory distress should warrant evaluation for a biopsy-related pneumothorax or hemothorax.

ALTERNATIVES AND THEIR RELATIVE MERITS

Surgical liver biopsy samples may be obtained laparoscopically or via laparotomy.

- These procedures are more invasive and expensive than percutaneous biopsy but can be helpful in cases with focal lesions that are difficult or dangerous to sample via a percutaneous approach, in patients in which the liver is difficult to visualize with transabdominal ultrasonography, or in patients in which a larger sample of liver is desired due to previous nondiagnostic biopsy samples obtained percutaneously.
- In addition, if obstructive cholelithiasis is strongly suspected based on clinical or sonographic findings, laparotomy also provides a means for surgical intervention and resolution of a biliary obstruction.

AUTHOR: **KELSEY A. HART**

Biopsy: Rectal

BASIC INFORMATION

OVERVIEW AND GOAL(S)

- The rectal biopsy procedure is used as a minimally invasive technique for assessment of the gastrointestinal tract.
- Common disease states in which rectal biopsies may assist in diagnosis include:
  - Chronic weight loss
  - Chronic diarrhea
  - Chronic hypoproteinemia
  - Suspected equine grass sickness

CONTRAINDICATIONS

- Enteropathies are often not generalized and often do not extend to the rectum; therefore biopsies may be of low diagnostic yield.
- Approximately 33% of rectal biopsies are diagnostically useful in horses with chronic enteropathies.

EQUIPMENT, ANESTHESIA

- Sedation (xylazine/romifidine/detomidine ± butorphanol)

- Rectal sleeve
- Rectal lubricant
  - Biopsy instrument: A variety of instruments have been used such as human rectal biopsy instruments, human cervical biopsy instruments, or equine uterine biopsy instruments. An ideal feature for this instrument is a folding upper jaw that cuts against a rigid lower jaw.
- 10% buffered formalin (10:1 formalin to tissue ratio)

ANTICIPATED TIME

15 to 20 minutes

PROCEDURE

- Sedate and adequately restrain the horse (preferably in stocks) as for a rectal examination.
- Manually empty the rectum of feces using a rectal sleeve and rectal lubrication.
- Insert the uterine biopsy instrument guarded by the hand so the wrist is just inside the rectal sphincter (20–25 cm into the rectum).

- At the 11 o'clock position, pinch the rectal mucosa between the thumb and index finger and feed this into the biopsy instrument. Close the jaws tightly.
- Remove the biopsy (mucosa and submucosa) and place it in formalin for histopathologic assessment. Ensure that biopsy specimens are <1 cm × <1 cm to allow fixation of the tissues.
- Repeat the procedure at the 1 o'clock position if necessary. Either place in formalin again or if needed for bacteriologic culture, place in a sterile glass tube containing sterile saline.
- Using the 11 o'clock and 1 o'clock positions minimizes the risks of injury to the dorsal vasculature of the rectum. Some mild rectal bleeding is normal after this procedure; however, as biopsies are only partial wall thickness, adverse consequences are extremely uncommon and this is considered a safe, easy procedure.

AUTHOR: **CERI SHERLOCK**

Biopsy: Skin

BASIC INFORMATION

SYNONYM(S)

- Cutaneous biopsy, punch biopsy
- Excisional biopsies: Removal of the whole lesion
- Wedge biopsies: Full-thickness skin lesion is excised with a scalpel blade through the abnormal tissue to include a small rim of normal skin.
- Both excisional and wedge biopsies may provide more tissue to more accurately diagnose the underlying skin disease.
- Skin biopsies may also be used to obtain tissue for a macerated tissue culture.

OVERVIEW AND GOAL(S)

It is important to take multiple samples of skin lesions that reflect the spectrum of the skin disease present (old and new, severe and milder, centre of lesion versus periphery) and preserve for further processing at the laboratory.

INDICATIONS

Skin biopsies submitted for histopathologic examination can assist in making a diagnosis, confirming a clinical diagnosis or, at a minimum, ruling out certain diseases.

EQUIPMENT, ANESTHESIA

Disposable 6 and 8 mm diameter punch biopsies, No. 10 scalpel blade and handle, Brown-Adson thumb forceps, straight or curved iris scissors, suture material, container with 10% buffered formaldehyde, local anaesthesia (2% lidocaine, may add small amount of sodium bicarbonate to reduce the stinging of the lidocaine), possible sedation. General anaesthesia is usually not required.

ANTICIPATED TIME

10 to 30 minutes

PREPARATION: IMPORANT CHECKPOINTS

- Gently clip hairs without disturbing the surface of the skin.
- **Do not prep the surface.** Crusts can have very important clues for the diagnosis that could be easily lost if scrubbed before the biopsy sample is taken (eg, pemphigus foliaceous: acantholytic cells may be in the surface crust of a pustule). Use clean technique (wash hands and use sterile instruments) but sterile prep techniques with scrubbing of the surface are usually not advised.
- 1 mL of 2% lidocaine (more for excisional or wedge biopsies) in subcutaneous tissue under each lesion with or without nerve block; sedation is rarely needed with an α_2-agonist (eg, xylazine, detomidine).

POSSIBLE COMPLICATIONS AND COMMON ERRORS TO BE AVOIDED

- Do not scrub the surface crusts off; they may provide important clues to the diagnosis.
- In rare cases, biopsy sites (larger excisional biopsies) may form a seroma.
- Like all wounds, the biopsy site may form a small but visible scar.

PROCEDURE

- Use sterile, sharp 6 to 8 mm punch biopsies (bigger is better when it comes to skin biopsies).
- Center the punch over lesion. It is usually not necessary to include normal tissue, although sometimes it is helpful to include the transition from normal to abnormal tissue.
- Slowly twist the punch with gentle pressure.

- Push the metal part all the way in; horse dermis is thick and often has important information in the deeper parts.
- Slowly twist the punch with gentle pressure.
- Avoid repeated lifting of the punch, which can create artificial clefts.
- Remove the tissue by gently grasping subcutaneous tissue with thumb forceps, lifting it up, and cutting close to the body with iris scissors.
- Remove any excess blood by gently blotting.
- Place subcutaneous tissue down on cardboard or tongue depressor in 100% neutral buffered formalin.
- Close biopsy site with one to three sutures.
- Submit biopsy sample to dermatopathologist or pathologist experienced in equine dermatopathology. (General pathologists may miss less common diagnoses of dermatologic diseases, for which biopsies are needed the most.)
- Include patient's signalment, description of lesion, differential diagnoses, response to previous treatment and, if possible, photos of the lesions.

POSTPROCEDURE

The biopsy sites should be kept clean and dry. It is also important to keep flies from getting in the wound by applying fly repellents or a light bandage.

ALTERNATIVES AND THEIR RELATIVE MERITS

Alternatives include direct impression cytology of the surface of the lesion or, if the lesion is deeper, fine needle aspiration. Neither procedure typically provides an adequate amount of tissue for a diagnosis.

AUTHOR: **ANNETTE PETERSEN**

Blood Transfusion: Adults

BASIC INFORMATION

SYNONYM(S)

Transfusion
Blood transfusion
Bloodgiving

OVERVIEW AND GOAL(S)

- Overview: a transfusion is the administration of blood and/or partial blood constituents from one horse (donor) to another (recipient) in which the recipient has a clinical disease that necessitates these components as therapy to prolong life.

- There is usually a history of prior disease or trauma that results in a reduction in the functional circulating erythrocyte mass.
- Reduced numbers of red cells occurs from loss (hemorrhage), destruction (hemolysis), or failure

to replace red blood cells (erythropoietic failure).

- Clinical signs are dependent on the cause of the anemia, the rapidity in which the anemia developed, and the type of anemia.
- The underlying type of the anemia should be determined as hypovolemic (eg, hemorrhagic) or euvolemic (hemolytic or erythropoietic failure).
- For hemorrhagic anemia, the cause should be determined as either internal or external hemorrhage.
- In the case of hemolysis, the anemia should be classified as extravascular or intravascular.
- Goal of therapy: to increase the delivery of oxygen (DO_2) to the tissues to treat/prevent global and local tissue hypoxia.
  - Global and local tissue hypoxia causes ineffective cellular metabolism, cell dysfunction, and cell death (apoptosis and necrosis).
  - Certain organs are more sensitive to low oxygen tension, which can lead to significant organ dysfunction (ie, brain, heart, kidney, and gut).
  - Increased oxygen delivery is achieved by reducing the loss of the red cell mass (ie, stopping hemorrhage and/or hemolysis) and exogenously increasing the red cell mass of the animal through compatible transfusion and oxygen therapy.

INDICATIONS

- There are no age or sex predispositions for the need for blood transfusions in adult horses.
  - This is in contrast to neonatal isoerythrolysis (see "Neonatal Isoerythrolysis" in Section I), where only foals with the ability to ingest and absorb colostral anti-erythrocyte antibodies from their mare may develop hemolysis requiring blood component therapy.
- Risk factors for the need of whole blood transfusion include surgical procedures, notably procedures that involve the paranasal sinuses.
- Disease conditions such as guttural pouch mycosis (where fatal hemorrhage from the internal carotid artery can occur) may also increase the likelihood for transfusion.
- Traumatic events such as limb lacerations, long bone fractures (notably femoral), and penetrating chest wounds are also high-risk conditions that may require transfusion.
- Pregnancy, parturition, and dystocia can result in urogenital trauma and hemorrhage.
  - Middle uterine artery bleeding into the broad ligament is a condition that may require transfusion.

- Congenital and acquired coagulopathic disorders including disorders of platelets and/or coagulation factors may result in hemorrhage and necessitate transfusion.
- Ingestion of hemolytic toxins including red maple leaf and onion weed may require packed erythrocyte transfusion.
- Endogenous production of hemolytic antibodies (immune mediated hemolytic anemia) in certain diseases (ie, clostridial and streptococcal diseases) may necessitate packed erythrocyte transfusion.
- Bone marrow disorders resulting in significant erythroid hypoplasia/aplasia may necessitate packed erythrocyte transfusion.
  - In the case of bone marrow disorders, the primary disease is often incurable (eg, leukemia, lymphoma) and transfusion therapy is considered palliative, unless a reversible underlying disease is found (ie, iron deficiency).

CONTRAINDICATIONS

- Interspecies transfusion is contraindicated and will result in severe transfusion reaction leading to death.
  - Horse recipients should only receive horse blood or blood products.
  - Donkey recipients should only receive donkey blood or blood product.
- Interbreed transfusions may be compatible, but specific compatibility testing is recommended before administration to a recipient.

EQUIPMENT, ANESTHESIA

- Clippers, prep, nonsterile and sterile gloves
- 3 to 5 mL of lidocaine to block the skin of each horse at the site of catheter insertion
- 14-gauge catheter (one for donor and one for recipient)
- Suture or superglue for temporary catheter placement
- Collection bag (plastic preferred to preserve platelets)
- Anticoagulant (use one-third of recommended amount for autotransfusion)
  - If administered immediately
    - Acid-citrate-dextrose (1:9 ratio of citrate to donor blood)
    - Heparin (3 U/mL donor blood)
  - For blood storage
    - Citrate-phosphate-dextrose-adenine (1:9 ratio of citrate to donor blood)
    - Blood administration set
    - Crystalloid fluids for the donor if large volume harvested

ANTICIPATED TIME

Time depends on the amount of blood to be transfused

PREPARATION: IMPORTANT CHECKPOINTS

- Initial database: Packed cell volume (PCV) and total protein (TP)
  - Acute hemorrhagic anemia: PCV is often normal; TP is often decreased.
  - Chronic hemorrhagic anemia: PCV and TP are usually decreased.
  - Acute and chronic intravascular hemolytic anemia: PCV is low; TP is normal or increased; serum free hemoglobin concentration may be increased.
  - Acute and chronic extravascular hemolytic anemia: PCV is low; TP is often normal or increased.
  - Erythropoietic failure: PCV is low; TP is often normal; blastic cells may be present in circulation from primary marrow disease; azotemia with isosthenuria may indicate primary renal failure.
- Compatibility testing: Compatibility between donor and recipient blood is important to minimize transfusion reactions (this step may be skipped in an emergency if this is the first transfusion for the horse, with the understanding that a reaction may occur).
- Cross matching:
  - This test assesses agglutination or hemolysis (incompatibility) when donor red cells are mixed with recipient serum (major cross-match) and when donor serum is mixed with recipient red cells (minor cross-match).
  - Agglutination or hemolysis is considered incompatible findings.
- Blood typing:
  - This test accurately reports the specific blood type of a horse.
  - An ideal donor for a recipient would be one in which the blood type is exactly the same.
  - Some blood types have a higher rate of incompatibility through production of anti-erythrocyte antibodies that either agglutinate or hemolyze recipient red cells.
- Blood types Aa and Qa are notable for this.
- Donkey and donkey-crosses have a specific erythrocyte surface antigen termed "donkey-factor" that results in a greater risk of incompatibility.
  - Donkey recipients should be cross-matched with blood from a donkey donor.

POSSIBLE COMPLICATIONS AND COMMON ERRORS TO BE AVOIDED

- Transfusion reactions are the most common and serious complication of transfusion therapy (up to 16% of transfusions may result in some type of reaction)

○ Acute reactions (time of onset within 1–30 min):
- Often immediate hypersensitivity reaction characterized by hyperthermia, tachycardia, tachypnea, urticaria, sweating, piloerection, and cardiovascular collapse (anaphylactic) in the extreme
- Immediately stop transfusion
- If only mild signs are noted, monitor closely for progressive deterioration
- If severe signs develop, administer epinephrine (0.005 to 0.02 mg/kg of 1:1000 IV)

○ Immune-mediated reactions (any time):
- Acute immune-mediated reactions include the development or worsening of hemolysis (notably intravascular) and subsequent production of anti-donor erythrocyte antibodies, or increased sensitization to additional transfusions.
- Mares receiving transfusion may be at a higher risk of producing a foal that could be affected by neonatal isoerythrolysis (NI) if the foal inherits a similar blood type as that from the donor horse used to provide previous transfusion.

- Transmission of zoonotic disease:
  ○ Equine infectious anemia virus and piroplasmosis (*Babesia/Theileria* spp.) can be transmitted by transfusion.
  ○ Similarly, donors should be equine viral arteritis negative, be free of rickettsial disease (eg, *Anaplasma phagocytophilia*) and not be anemic themselves.

PROCEDURE

- Assess patient for clinical signs of poor perfusion requiring transfusion.
  ○ Tachycardia (>60 beats/min)
  ○ Tachypnea (>32 beats/min)
  ○ Pale mucous membranes
  ○ Colic, sweating, trembling
  ○ Uncontrollable bleeding
  ○ Cool extremities, weak pulses
  ○ Systolic blood pressure <80 mm Hg or persistent hypotension after fluid resuscitation

○ Estimated blood loss >33% estimated blood volume
○ Packed cell volume <12%, hemoglobin <7 g/dL, total protein <4 g/dL

- May not reflect acute losses
  ○ Venous L-lactate >4 mmol/L
  ○ PvO_2 <25 mm Hg

- Perform compatibility testing (skip to collection in emergency).
  ○ Crossmatching (major and minor)
  ○ Blood typing (if known)

- Calculate deficit.
  ○ If signs of hypovolemic hemorrhagic shock are present, estimate at least 25% of blood volume lost.
  ○ If losses are external, they may be directly measured.
  ○ Liters of blood lost can also be estimated by the following (if not acute hemorrhage):
    - (normal PCV − patient PCV)/ normal PCV × (0.08) × (patient weight in kg)
  ○ Goal of transfusion is to supply 40% of losses to allow bone marrow stimulation to still occur in the recipient.

- Roughly 2.2 mL of whole blood per kilogram body weight will increase the PCV by 1%.

- Blood collection
  ○ If compatibility unknown, choose a healthy, large, adult gelding of the same breed, with no history of being a previous transfusion recipient.
  ○ Draw blood sterilely with a large gauge catheter into a plastic collection bag primed and filled with anticoagulant.
  ○ Donor may require sedation and crystalloid fluid administration if a large volume is removed.

- Up to 20% of the donor's blood volume may be harvested.

- Begin administration.
  ○ Use blood administration set with filter.
  ○ Change administration set every 3 to 4 L.
  ○ Start administration at 0.1 mL/kg for 10 to 15 minutes to monitor for reaction.
  ○ The remainder of blood may be bolused (20–30 mL/kg/h).
  ○ Stop transfusion if any reaction occurs.

POSTPROCEDURE

- Monitoring:
  ○ Transfused erythrocytes have a half life of <4 days; therefore, additional transfusions may be needed for continued anemia or hemolysis.
  ○ PCV, TP, and hemoglobin concentrations are insensitive indicators of global DO_2.
  ○ Venous L-lactate, venous oxygen saturation (SvO_2), and venous oxygen tension (PvO_2) are more sensitive markers of oxygen delivery.

- Decreased PvO_2 and SvO_2 with increases in L-lactate indicate hypoxia
  ○ Serum ionized calcium should be monitored after large-volume transfusions with citrated anticoagulants, which may chelate this ion.

- Prognosis:
  ○ The prognosis for survival is largely determined by the severity of anemia, how fast the anemia developed, the underlying cause for anemia, and response to therapy.
  ○ In one retrospective, the overall short-term survival rate for adult horses receiving blood transfusion therapy was 54%, where horses treated for hemorrhagic anemia had the greatest survival rate (66%) followed by erythropoietic failure (40%) and hemolytic anemia (37.5%).

- In mares with postparturient hemorrhage, the prognosis for survival is better (86%).

ALTERNATIVES AND THEIR RELATIVE MERITS

Bovine hemoglobin products may provide a more compatible, and more expensive, short-term alternative to whole blood.

SUGGESTED READING

Arnold CE, et al: Periparturient hemorrhage in mares: 73 cases (1988–2005), *J Am Vet Med Assoc* 232:1345, 2008.

Hurcombe SD, et al: Clinical and clinicopathologic variables in adult horses receiving blood transfusions: 31 cases (1999–2005), *J Am Vet Med Assoc* 231:267, 2007.

Magdesian KG: Acute blood loss, *Compendium Equine* 3(2):80–90, 2008.

AUTHOR: SAMUEL D. A. HURCOMBE

Body Conditioning Score

BASIC INFORMATION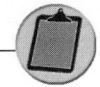

OVERVIEW AND GOAL(S)

- Developed at Texas A&M University over 25 years ago as an applicable method to compare horses based on their stored body fat.
- Fat deposition
  - In most mammals, fat deposition occurs in a very dependable pattern.
  - Initial body fat deposition occurs in the areas of the vital organs, the ribs, and spine, providing both protection and a local source of maintenance energy.
  - Fat then begins to accumulate in those areas of greatest need, the major muscle groups.
  - In the horse, fat is deposited across the rump and along the shoulders. If additional excess energy continues to be consumed, fat is deposited along the neck and thighs.
  - Internal fat deposition differs from species to species. The horse is unique in that the vast majority of stored body fat lies on the outside of the musculature. Horses have relatively little internal body fat under normal conditions. Therefore using these areas to estimate body fat content in the horse is very accurate.

POSSIBLE COMPLICATIONS AND COMMON ERRORS TO BE AVOIDED

- Problems with the body condition scoring system:
  - The first problem lies in the accuracy of the system. This system is designed to estimate body condition by estimating stored body fat. It is a subjective score based on objective measurements. Accuracy of scoring by the same individual is quite high. However, accuracy between evaluators will vary. Competent evaluators should be within one body condition score of each other on the same animal.
  - Another problem is the tendency of evaluators to overestimate horses on the high end of the system. From the original research, a number 9 horse will have approximately 30% body fat. With the exception of horses with endocrine problems, encountering a true number 9 is very rare.
  - Finally, there is often a misconception between fatness and fitness.

Examination of mammals that depend on athleticism for survival (speed, strength, quickness) indicates that the individual animal strives to maintain fat reserves that produce the most efficient bioenergetics for muscle utilization. Their body tends to regulate energy intake with energy need. Some horses perform best as a number 7 while others are best as a 4. Ideal body condition of an equine athlete should depend on the performance of the individual, not on the preconceived ideas of the owner. Exercise does a much better job of regulating energy intake and fat deposition than does restricting feed intake and produces far fewer digestive problems.

PROCEDURE

- Determining the body condition score for a horse:
  - The system should be based on evaluation of the total horse.
  - Conformation differences between horses may make some areas less accurate in some horses.
  - Horses that are not heavy muscled over the loin may never develop a crease.
  - Lighter muscled horses in the rump may appear to carry less fat in that area. In these cases, those areas influenced by conformation should be discounted, but not ignored, in making the final determination of the condition score.
- The body condition scoring system:
  - Most accurate when the horse is manually evaluated.
  - The evaluator must distinguish between feeling muscle or fat.
  - The physical condition of the horse does not influence its score.
  - Knowing a horse's fitness level should also not influence the evaluator.
  - The score depends on the evaluator's unbiased feel of the horse.
  - Other factors to consider: Conformation, pregnancy status, and gaining or losing weight.
- Evaluating the horse's ribs:
  - Best done halfway between the shoulder and last rib and one-third to one-half-way down from the spine.
  - Measuring above this point may get into the muscling covering the upper rib, producing an artificially high estimate.

- Measuring too low on the rib often results in a low estimate, especially in aged brood mares.
- Evaluating the spine:
  - Estimate the fat cover over the lumbar vertebrae. Pressing down on the vertebrae will allow the evaluator to determine the amount of fat cover.
  - At very low condition scores the vertebrae feel sharp.
  - As body condition increases, the vertebrae feel smoother, then rounder, then the area between them starts filling in with fat.
  - At high scores, the individual vertebrae become hard to differentiate.
  - In heavily muscled animals, a crease may appear.
- Evaluating the rump:
  - Best estimated close to the tail head.
  - Fat will begin to feel spongy as it builds up in this area.
  - As a horse loses weight, most often the rump is the first area that declines, even before the neck and thighs.
- Evaluating the withers:
  - Similar to feeling the loin.
  - The vertebrae initially feel sharp, then smooth, then rounded, and then hard to differentiate.
  - Finally fat begins to accumulate along the sides.
  - The wither area is an area that can be significantly influenced by conformation. Horses with prominent withers often feel thinner in this area than they actually are overall. Therefore adjustments may be needed in determining the final score.
- Evaluating the neck and thighs:
  - Usually the last areas to be utilized for fat storage.
  - At high condition scores, fat becomes deposited along the sides of the neck. The neck thickens and a crest may form in some breeds. At the same time, fat is deposited along the inside and outside of the thighs. The striated musculature of the thigh becomes hard to distinguish. Fat will continue to accumulate as a smooth covering.
  - At extremely high body condition, fat deposits along the neck and thighs may appear patchy. Raised areas of fat may appear dimpled and/or lumpy.
- Body condition score of 9:
  - The true body condition score 9 is rare.

Horse Body Condition Scorecard

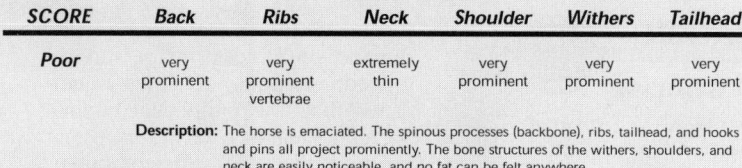

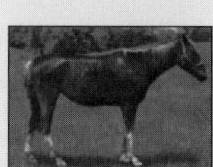

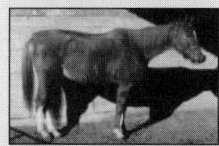

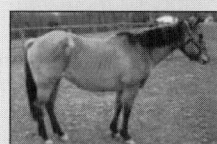

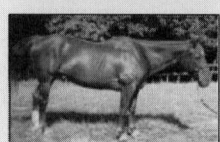

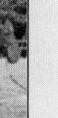

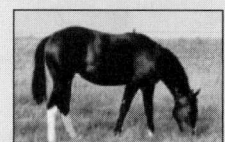

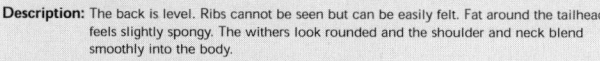

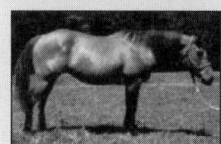

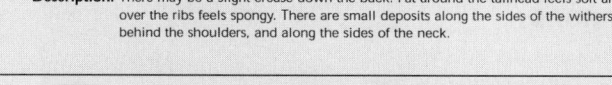

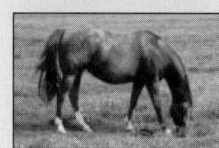

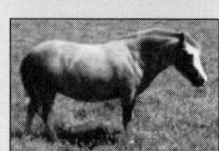

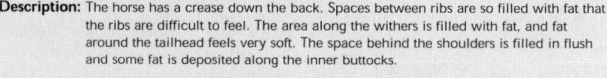

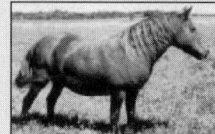

SCORE	Back	Ribs	Neck	Shoulder	Withers	Tailhead
Poor	very prominent	very prominent vertebrae	extremely thin	very prominent	very prominent	very prominent

Description: The horse is emaciated. The spinous processes (backbone), ribs, tailhead, and hooks and pins all project prominently. The bone structures of the withers, shoulders, and neck are easily noticeable, and no fat can be felt anywhere.

Very Thin	prominent vertebrae	prominent	very thin	very thin	very thin	very thin

Description: The spinous processes are prominent. The ribs, tailhead, and pelvic bones stand out, and bone structures of the withers, neck, and shoulders are faintly discernable.

Thin	vertebrae fat ½ way up	see easily	thin	thin	thin	prominent

Description: The spinous processes stand out, but fat covers them to midpoint. Very slight fat cover can be felt over the ribs, but the spinous processes and ribs are easily discern-able. The tailhead is prominent, but individual vertebrae cannot be seen. Hook bones are visible but appear rounded. Pin bones cannot be seen. The withers, shoulders, and neck are accentuated.

Moderately Thin	negative crease	can see outline of ribs	moderately thin	moderately thin	moderately thin	some fat

Description: The horse has a negative crease along its back and the outline of the ribs can just be seen. Fat can be felt around the tailhead. The hook bones cannot be seen and the withers, neck, and shoulders do not look obviously thin.

Moderate	level (no crease)	cannot see, easily feel	blend into shoulder	blend smoothly into body	rounded	moderate fat

Description: The back is level. Ribs cannot be seen but can be easily felt. Fat around the tailhead feels slightly spongy. The withers look rounded and the shoulder and neck blend smoothly into the body.

Moderately Fleshy	slight crease	cannot see, can feel	little fat	little fat	little fat	moderate fat

Description: There may be a slight crease down the back. Fat around the tailhead feels soft and fat over the ribs feels spongy. There are small deposits along the sides of the withers, behind the shoulders, and along the sides of the neck.

Fleshy	crease	barely feel	average fat	average fat	average fat	fleshy fat

Description: There may be a crease down the back. Individual ribs can be felt, but there is notice-able fat between the ribs. Fat around the tailhead is soft. Fat is noticeable in the with-ers, the neck, and behind the shoulders.

Fat	obvious crease	difficult to feel	fat	flush behind	fat filled	very soft fat

Description: The horse has a crease down the back. Spaces between ribs are so filled with fat that the ribs are difficult to feel. The area along the withers is filled with fat, and fat around the tailhead feels very soft. The space behind the shoulders is filled in flush and some fat is deposited along the inner buttocks.

Extremely Fat	very obvious crease	cannot feel (patchy fat)	bulging fat	bulging fat	bulging fat	bulging fat

Description: The crease down the back is very obvious. Fat appears in patches over the ribs and there is bulging fat around the tailhead, withers, shoulders, and neck. Fat along the inner buttocks may cause buttocks to rub together, and the flank is filled in flush.

BCS adapted from Henneke, 1983. Description source: Texas A&M University.

For custom feeding suggestions to help you maintain or change your horse's body condition score, call the FORAGE FIRST™ EQUINE NUTRITION HELPLINE at 1-800-680-8254.

○ Given adequate exercise, most horses will not become this obese. Most often horses with patchy neck and thigh fat have endocrine disorders that interfere with natural metabolism.

AUTHOR: **DON HENNEKE**

EDITOR: **DANIEL J. BURKE**

Breeding with Frozen Semen

BASIC INFORMATION

SYNONYM(S)

- Fresh cooled semen may also be referred to as *cooled shipped* or *fresh chilled semen*. Semen is collected from a stallion with an artificial vagina, filtered to remove debris and gel and extended with a commercial milk-based semen extender. Cooled semen is inseminated into a mare within 24 to 72 hours after collection.
- Frozen semen is collected from a stallion with an artificial vagina, filtered, and centrifuged, and a special freezing extender is added. Semen is then generally placed into 0.5 mL straws for freezing. The dose (typically 1 to 8 straws) depends on the post-thaw motility achieved. There is significant variability with regard to semen quality and fertility when breeding with frozen semen.
- Live cover, natural cover, or natural service refers to a stallion directly mating with a mare.

OVERVIEW AND GOAL(S)

- To place semen into the mare prior to or just after ovulation.
- With cooled semen, insemination may occur 24 to 48 hours before ovulation, with good results for most stallions.
- With frozen semen, insemination should occur within 6 to 8 hours of ovulation.
- If ovulation has occurred, best fertility rates are obtained within 6 to 8 hours, with decreasing success up to 12 to 18 hours postovulation.

INDICATIONS

- Fresh cooled semen is preferred to frozen semen for breeding, when available, because most sperm have decreased longevity when the semen is frozen. In addition, some mares may have more of an inflammatory uterine reaction to frozen semen (post–mating-induced endometritis). Fresh cooled semen is commonly used when mares are not located within convenient driving distance to a stallion for natural cover or the stallion is not available for live cover.
- Frozen semen may be used when the stallion is not available due to a busy show schedule, being overseas, or being deceased.

CONTRAINDICATIONS

- Frozen semen may have a decreased success rate in older mares prone to post–mating-induced endometritis. However, with proper mare selection, good technique, and quality semen, similar pregnancy rates may be achieved between fresh chilled and frozen semen.
- Human chorionic gonadotropin (hCG) may be less effective in inducing ovulation in older broodmares who have received hCG multiple times.
- Stallions with poor sperm longevity ("poor shipper") may not be candidates for either fresh cooled or frozen semen. A longevity test, looking at spermatozoal motility over time, can differentiate a poor shipper. Stallions may have decreased longevity with either fresh cooled and/or frozen semen. Occasionally, a stallion may not perform well with one method but may be better with the alternative method.
- An alternative breeding method in the case where both fresh cooled and frozen semen longevity are poor would be natural cover.

EQUIPMENT, ANESTHESIA

- Breeding pipettes, sterile sleeve, sterile lubricant, microscope, slides, cover slips, incubator (warming plate or warm water bottle to lay slides on).
  ○ Breeding pipettes that use an internal metal stylet (multiple-use insemination gun) allow direct insemination of 0.5 mL frozen semen straws and should be used with frozen semen to maximize deposition of the entire dose into the uterus.
  ○ Frozen semen should not be directly aspirated or poured into a syringe because too much loss will occur from wetting of plastic surfaces (syringe and pipette), thus decreasing the breeding dose.
  ○ Aspirating semen into the breeding pipette, rather than directly into the syringe, for delivery is an intermediate method that results in less wetting of surfaces but is not as good as direct placement of the straws such as occurs with the metal stylet method.
- Sterile lubricant that is osmotically and pH-balanced should be used to avoid negative effects on spermatozoal quality.

ANTICIPATED TIME

- 20 to 30 minutes to tail wrap, wash the mare, and breed her.
- An extra 10 minutes should be allocated to thaw frozen semen.
- An extra 10 to 15 minutes should be added to ultrasound the mare per rectum.
- Total time may vary from 30 to 60 minutes depending on breeding method.

PREPARATION: IMPORTANT CHECKPOINTS

- Place a tail wrap on the mare and tie the tail to side.
- Wash the perineum in concentric circles outward from vulva.
- Repeat two to three times until clean.
- Pass a fairly dry wipe from the dorsal commissure of the vulva to the ventral commissure of the vulva just inside the lips of vulva to remove any fecal material that may have wicked into the vestibule.
- Dry the perineum.
- With frozen semen, prepare a water bath long enough for the entire straw to be submerged. Typically, most 0.5 mL frozen semen straws are thawed at 37° C for 30 to 35 seconds. Frozen semen may also come in other sized straws, ampoules, or packets.
- Semen should be evaluated for total and progressive motility before insemination.

POSSIBLE COMPLICATIONS AND COMMON ERRORS TO BE AVOIDED

Semen evaluation:

- A warm slide and cover slip should be used to examine spermatozoal motility; this provides a better estimation of what motility would be like in the mare's reproductive tract.

- When warming semen to examine for motility, do not place cold semen on a warm slide or place warm semen on a cold slide; this may give an erroneous interpretation of motility by negatively affecting sperm physiology.
- With cooled semen, place a single drop of semen on a room-temperature slide and then warm.
- With frozen semen, after warming, place a single drop of semen on a warm slide and examine.
- The drop of semen is typical for a disposable pipette and should not cause the cover slip to float on the slide. Too little and the motility may appear depressed; too much and liquid movement (flow) will make it difficult to evaluate motility.
- With frozen semen, if there is only one 0.5 mL straw for breeding, it may be prudent to make a slide without a cover slip and limit the volume to a very small drop to maximize the inseminated volume.
- Make sure the slide stays warm or the semen is examined quickly after warming the slide; motility will decrease significantly as the slide cools.

With postpartum mares, their cervix may be difficult to discern and their uterine body may be ventrally located. It is important that semen be placed into the uterine body and not into the cervical canal.

PROCEDURE

- Drugs to induce ovulation (typically only one is given):
  - hCG, 1500 to 2500 IU, IM, or IV: Ovulation occurs within 48 (28–96) hours after administration in most cases.
  - Deslorelin, 1.5 mg IM: Ovulation occurs in about 40 (36–42) hours after administration in most cases.
  - Deslorelin, 2.1 mg subcutaneous implant: Ovulation occurs in about 40 (36–42) hours after administration in most cases. The implant is removed after ovulation to avoid downregulation of gonadotropin axis. Typically, implant is placed in the vulvar mucosa for ease of removal.
  - Equine luteinizing hormone, 750 µg IV: Ovulation occurs within 48

hours of administration in most cases.

- Ovulatory drugs should be administered to mares in estrus when at least a 35 mm follicle and evidence of uterine edema on ultrasound are evident. This timing may vary depending on breed of horse and previous follicular ovulation size.
- Fresh chilled semen:
  - Open the shipping container and use the paperwork to confirm the stallion's identity and shipping conditions.
  - Spermatozoa will have settled out in the container, so remix the semen.
  - If already packaged in a syringe, the semen may be then directly deposited into the uterus.
  - If in a bag or centrifuge tube, the semen should be aspirated into a syringe (ideally one without lubricant or rubber plunger).
  - Using a sterile glove, lubricant, and pipette, deposit the semen into the uterine body after passing the pipette through the cervix.
  - After insemination, withdraw the pipette and gently hold the external cervical os closed for approximatey 15 seconds to encourage retention of semen.
  - If two doses of fresh chilled semen are provided, one may be inseminated immediately and one the next day if adequate total motile spermatozoa are present and the mare is not in the process of ovulating. If the mare can handle the fluid volume within her uterus, the mare is close to ovulation, and/or the spermatozoa numbers are low, both doses may be placed intrauterine.
- Frozen semen:
  - Semen is transported in the mail in a vapor shipper.
    - The vapor shipper will hold a liquid nitrogen charge for a predefined time depending on the size of the vapor shipper (typically 5 to 7 days).
    - The vapor shipper may be weighed to determine the remaining amount of nitrogen charge per shipper instructions.
    - Semen should be used or transferred to a permanent liquid nitrogen tank before depletion of the vapor shipper's charge.

- Paperwork should detail the stallion, number of straws per dose, and expected post-thaw motility.
- Semen should be thawed according to instructions.
- Semen is placed either into the uterine body, or a pipette may be passed into the uterine horn ipsilateral to the ovary with the dominant follicle (see "Artificial Insemination: Deep Horn" in this section).
  - If two doses of frozen semen are provided, semen may be placed at 24 and 40 hours after administration of the ovulatory drug. Alternatively, one dose may be placed and the second held for placement after ovulation. If one dose is provided, the mare should be examined frequently for ovulation (q6–8h) and bred after ovulation.

POSTPROCEDURE

- Mares should be examined for ovulation and for the presence of excessive uterine fluid or increase of uterine edema after breeding.
- Excessive uterine edema after ovulation may signify uterine inflammation.
- Mares with uterine fluid may require the use of ecbolics (oxytocin or prostaglandins) and/or uterine lavage (with lactated Ringer's solution). Examination/treatment for uterine fluid may be performed as early as 4 hours after breeding for treatment as spermatozoa have already colonized the oviduct and uterine therapy will not decrease conception rates.

ALTERNATIVES AND THEIR RELATIVE MERITS

- Mares may be live covered (natural cover) if cooled or frozen semen quality is poor. Cooled shipped semen may be sent via airplane for same-day insemination if longevity is poor (counter-to-counter shipment).
- Semen may be collected and directly inseminated into a mare without cooling (fresh semen). This is performed when the mare will not allow the stallion to mate safely or to decrease contamination during breeding.

AUTHORS: JOHN J. DASCANIO and **LEEAH R. CHEW**

Bronchoalveolar Lavage

BASIC INFORMATION

SYNONYM(S)

Lung wash

OVERVIEW AND GOAL(S)

It is commonly agreed that tracheal wash cytology, endoscopy, and radiography are not sufficient diagnostic techniques for the diagnosis of inflammatory airway disease (IAD) in horses; bronchoalveolar lavage (BAL) provides the "gold standard" diagnosis. The goal of the BAL is to obtain a representative sample of lower airway respiratory secretions to diagnose diseases that diffusely affect the lower airways, such as IAD and exercise-induced pulmonary hemorrhage (EIPH).

INDICATIONS

- Indications for BAL include
  - Diffuse lung disease such as IAD
  - Alveolar hemorrhage such as EIPH
  - Nonresolving pneumonia
  - Diffuse lung infiltrates
  - Alveolitis
  - Nonresolving bronchitis
  - Silicosis, other dust exposure
  - Research

CONTRAINDICATIONS

- BAL is relatively contraindicated in patients with borderline oxygenation.
- Care should be used in animals with tachypnea, tachycardia, or dysrhythmias.
- Should not be performed within 24 hours of anticipated exercise.

EQUIPMENT, ANESTHESIA

- Bronchodilator (360 μg of albuterol or 84 μg of ipratropium bromide) using an aerosol delivery device (AeroHippusR, Trudell Medical International, London, Ontario, Canada) 15 minutes before BAL
- Sedation (xylazine hydrochloride 0.5–0.75 mg/kg IV or detomidine 0.005–0.01 mg/kg IV). The addition of butorphanol tartrate (0.02–0.04 mg/kg IV) to the sedation will decrease coughing
- Twitch
- Bivona tube (VBAL30) with outside diameter 11 mm, 244 cm length, Smith Medical or a long (2–3 m) endoscope
- 30 mL of warmed lidocaine to inject on the glottis and additional 30 mL for anesthesia of the trachea
- 2 × 250 mL bolus of warmed sterile saline in bottle or large syringes that can be prefilled

- Administration set with pressure bulb and three-way stopcock
- Ice for chilling sample
- Tubes with EDTA or other fixative only if sample cannot be refrigerated
- Table top centrifuge or cytocentrifuge
- Transfer pipette
- Slides
- Fan for drying slides
- Diff-Quik or similar stain if staining in-house
- Toluidine blue if staining in-house

ANTICIPATED TIME

With practice, the procedure itself should take no more than 10 minutes, with an additional 10 minutes for making slides

PREPARATION: IMPORTANT CHECKPOINTS

- It is important to warn the owner that the horse will likely cough and gag during the procedure.
- It is important to sedate the horse adequately for the procedure. A plane of sedation similar to that before standing surgery is appropriate.
- Make sure to check the cuff of the Bivona BAL tube before inserting it into the horse's respiratory tract.

POSSIBLE COMPLICATIONS AND COMMON ERRORS TO BE AVOIDED

This is a low-risk procedure, but in teaching students, the author has witnessed the Bivona tube be inserted in one nostril and come out the contralateral nostril: This can be remedied with more sedation, lubrication, and gentle traction. The author has also witnessed the Bivona tube emerge in the oropharynx and be chewed by the horse. Exacerbation of emphysema has been seen in humans. Horses may have a transient elevation in rectal temperature in the 24 hours following the procedure.

PROCEDURE

- Give the horse albuterol or ipratropium via metered dose inhaler 10 to 15 minutes before the procedure.
- Sedate the horse as suggested above.
- Apply a twitch: This will help to steady the head (Figure 1).
- Warn the owner that the horse will cough.
- Pass the tube in a fashion similar to a nasogastric tube, but stretch the head and neck out as far horizontally as possible.
- When a swallow is felt, administer 30 mL lidocaine to anesthetize the glottis.
- Continue to pass the tube down the trachea. You should feel a lack of resistance and an inability to palpate the tube in the esophagus, and there should be no negative pressure on aspiration of air from the tube.
- Once the trachea is reached, the head may be held in a more relaxed

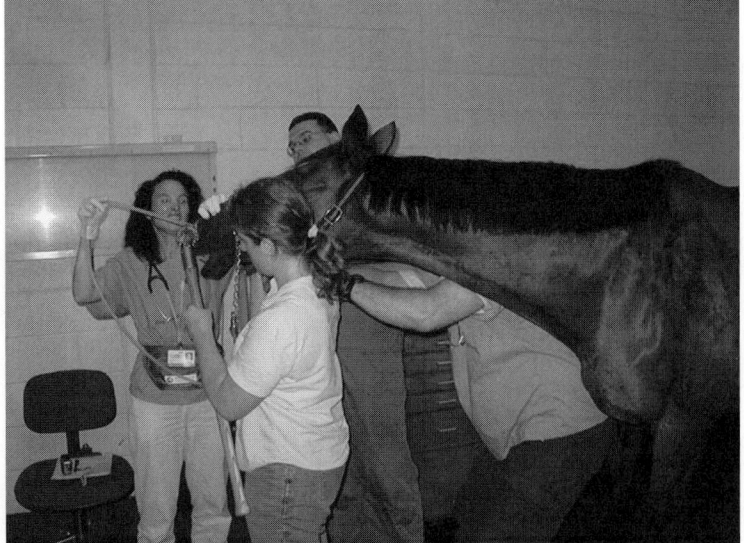

FIGURE 1 The horse must be well sedated before beginning the BAL. A twitch helps to stabilize the head. The neck and head should be extended as far as possible to facilitate the passage of the BAL tube into the airway.

position. You may administer additional lidocaine if the horse coughs while the tube is being passed further. Continue to pass the tube until it wedges in a fourth or fifth subsegment: If you are doing this blindly it will usually be in the caudal lobe.

- Seal the cuff with 10 mL of air. At this point the horse usually settles and relaxes.
- Rapidly instill 250 mL of prewarmed saline; rapidly withdraw the fluid.
- Examine the fluid for foam. If it is not foamy, it is likely that you have not wedged in a distal subsegment of the bronchi.
- Instill and withdraw an additional 250 mL of sterile saline, then pool your samples.
- Place the fluid in red top tubes on ice until the sample can be processed.
- Centrifuge using a table top centrifuge or a cytocentrifuge, keeping the *g* low.
- If using a table top centrifuge, pour off the supernatant, then mix the pellet with the small amount of remaining fluid. Use approximately 0.25 mL of the resultant fluid to make a smear.
- Avoid using pressure when making the smear, to avoid crushing the cells.
- Dry the slides rapidly with a fan or at least wave the slides vigorously to avoid drying artifacts.
- Stain with Diff-Quik or a similar stain. Prepare one slide with toluidine blue to look for mast cells. In our laboratory, we fix the slide, and then incubate it in toluidine blue at room temperature for 30 minutes before rinsing.
- Count at least 400 cells using a brightfield microscope at 630 to 1000× magnification.
- Macrophages should constitute 50% to 70% of cells, lymphocytes 30% to 50%, neutrophils <5%, mast cells <2%, and eosinophils <0.01%. Epithelial cells are rare (Figures 2 to 5).

POSTPROCEDURE

Horses should not be exercised for at least 24 hours after the BAL.

ALTERNATIVES AND THEIR RELATIVE MERITS

The tracheal wash and endoscopy are sometimes substituted for the diagnosis of IAD. Both modalities are less sensitive and less specific than the BAL. BAL has been shown to relate better than tracheal wash cytology to the clinical signs and pathophysiologic consequences of IAD.

AUTHOR: **ANDREW M. HOFFMANN**

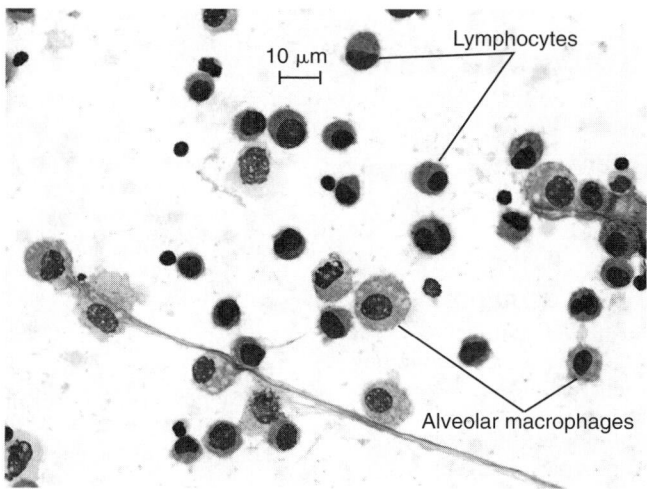

FIGURE 2 The normal BAL is composed primarily of alveolar macrophages with lesser amounts of lymphocytes. There is scant mucus. Stained with Diff-Quik, 200× magnification.

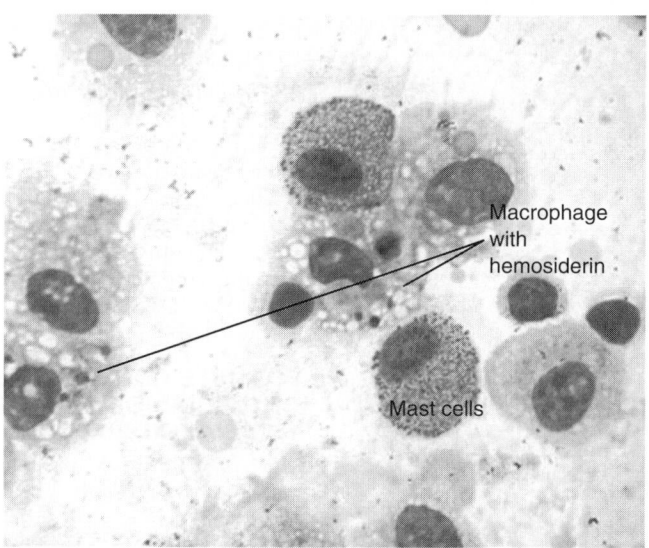

FIGURE 3 A toluidine blue stain is frequently necessary to demonstrate the presence of mast cells. Hemosiderin particles within macrophages (hemosiderophages) are easily visualized using Diff-Quik. 600× magnification.

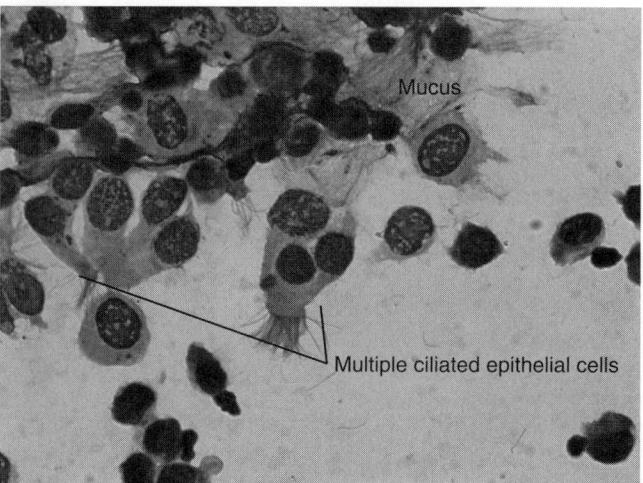

FIGURE 4 Ciliated epithelial cells may be present with viral disease or due to excessive coughing in IAD or heaves. Stained with Diff-Quik, 400× magnification.

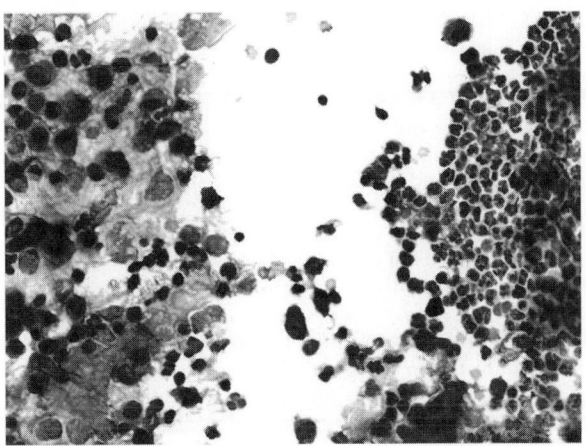

FIGURE 5 The BAL in a horse with heaves will show plentiful mucus and is markedly neutrophilic: In some cases 90% neutrophils or more. Stained with Diff-Quik, 200× magnification.

Cardiac Auscultation

BASIC INFORMATION

OVERVIEW AND GOAL(S)

- Cardiac auscultation is the systematic examination of the heart using a stethoscope.
- Auscultation is both expedient and relatively sensitive for detection of serious heart disease when performed by a knowledgeable and experienced examiner.
- This examination is most useful for measurement of heart rate, recognition of persistent arrhythmias, and detection of congenital heart malformations and acquired valvular diseases.
- Pericardial diseases also may be recognized by auscultation.
- This procedure is conducted in the context of a medical history and general physical examination, which includes assessment of the precordium and pulses, auscultation of the thorax, and inspection for edema and abnormal ventilatory patterns.

INDICATIONS

Auscultation is indicated as part of every clinical examination. It is particularly important in horses with signs of potential heart disease, including exercise intolerance, reduced performance, falling, tachypnea, abnormal jugular pulses, ventral edema, and weight loss. Auscultation also is important before sedation or anesthesia.

EQUIPMENT, ANESTHESIA

- A good-quality stethoscope is required, but the specific instrument used is a matter of personal preference.

- The diaphragm should be applied firmly and used for most of the examination.
- The bell should be applied lightly, creating an air seal against the skin, and is most useful for detecting low-frequency sounds (third sound) and soft diastolic murmurs.
- Combination chest pieces use a "tunable diaphragm" in which mild pressure accentuates lower pitched sounds (bell function) and progressively firmer pressure optimizes higher frequency sounds.

ANTICIPATED TIME

Precordial palpation and cardiac auscultation should take approximately 2 minutes on the left thorax and 1 minute or less on the right. Palpation or inspection of the pulses should add no more than an additional 1 to 2 minutes.

PREPARATION: IMPORANT CHECKPOINTS

- The horse should be restrained by an assistant whenever possible.
- The examination should be conducted in a quiet area.
- The examiner must be knowledgeable of the procedure, with an understanding of both normal and abnormal heart sounds.
  - Normal equine heart sounds include the fourth, first, second, and third sounds, designated by their historical discovery. The general cadence of these sounds is "ba-lub ... dup-ah" (4-1...2-3).
  - The fourth, or atrial, sound is presystolic and follows the P wave of the electrocardiogram and vibra-

tions of the atrial contraction. It is isolated following a blocked P wave of atrioventricular block and is absent in atrial fibrillation. When closely timed to the following first sound, a "pseudo-split" sound is detected. The P-R interval determines the proximity of the atrial to the first heart sound.
  - The long and lower pitched first sound follows the QRS complex and indicates the onset of ventricular systole. The higher frequency second sound heralds the onset of ventricular diastole. These sounds can be closely split in healthy animals.
  - The third sound occurs near the termination of rapid ventricular filling and is the softest, lowest pitched, and most variable of the normal sounds.
- The heart sounds should be correlated to the cardiac impulse and the arterial and venous pulses.
  - The left apical (cardiac) impulse occurs near the fifth intercostal space and represents the area just ventral to the mitral valve. The first sound, and often the third, are loudest at this point. The external impulse develops during early systole and forms a useful timing clue for the cardiac cycle.
  - The arterial pulse can be identified in the facial artery, carotid artery, and forelimbs. This event is timed approximately to mid-systole. Arrhythmias can cause rapid, slow, irregular, or variable pulses. Significant aortic regurgitation or the rare aortocardiac fistula can create a

hyperkinetic or bounding pulse. Heart failure, pericardial effusion, and volume depletion cause hypokinetic pulses and often resting sinus tachycardia in the 60 to 70 beats/min range. Marked respiratory variation in pulse pressure can be observed with pericardial effusion (pulsus paradoxicus).

○ Pulsations and diameter of the jugular veins are reflective of right atrial pressures that vary from positive to subatmospheric during the cardiac cycle. When the head is elevated, the jugular vein should not be distended and pulsations should be limited to the lower third of the neck. The finding of jugular venous distension suggests right heart failure, cardiac tamponade, or a cranial mediastinal mass. Jugular pulsations are usually physiologic and relate to atrial contraction. Pathologic retrograde venous pulses can be caused by congestive heart failure, tricuspid regurgitation, and some heart rhythm disturbances.

POSSIBLE COMPLICATIONS AND COMMON ERRORS TO BE AVOIDED

Cardiac auscultation is noninvasive and unlikely to lead to complications. However, a number of examination or interpretation pitfalls can be identified.

- Subtle abnormalities may be missed in a noisy environment, if the approach is not systematic, or if the examiner is not sufficiently attentive to the task at hand.
- Failure to listen over the right thorax may lead to a missed murmur of tricuspid regurgitation or a ventricular septal defect.
- Inability to time systole and diastole can foster erroneous conclusions. The left apical impulse and arterial pulse are both systolic events. However, even with these clues, some heart murmurs can be confusing, such as with the late systolic, crescendo murmur of mitral valve prolapse and the variable presystolic murmur related to atrial contraction.
- The functional ejection murmur and the murmur of mitral regurgitation (MR) are the primary murmurs to distinguish on the left side; distinction is made based on timing and point of maximal intensity (see below).
- The functional protodiastolic (filling) murmur and the murmur of aortic regurgitation (AR) are usually distinguished by age (older horses acquire AR) and timing (AR is generally holodiastolic). However, early or very mild AR can also be protodiastolic in timing.
- Prominent jugular pulsations can be misinterpreted in otherwise normal

horses in relation to head position (too low), misinterpretation of normal collapse and refill as a pathologic pulse, and not appreciating that the carotid artery pulse can be transmitted across the jugular vein.

PROCEDURE

Auscultation should be preceded by (1) inspection of the jugular pulses and pressure, (2) palpation of the facial artery or digital artery pulse, and (3) palpation of the thorax over the heart (the precordium) for vibrations (a precordial thrill).

The heart rate and rhythm should be assessed from the pulse and while listening between the left apex and left base (ie, between the mitral and aortic valve areas).

- If the rhythm is irregular, the most common possibilities are sinus arrhythmia, sinus pause or arrest, second-degree atrioventricular block, conduction or nonconduction atrial premature complexes, atrial flutter or fibrillation, and ventricular premature complexes.
- Healthy mature horses can demonstrate markedly irregular heart rhythms. Blood pressure is regulated by altering vagal tone, which leads to variation in sinus node discharge rate and physiologic (second-degree) atrioventricular block. Auscultation of a regular rhythm immediately after sympathetic stimulation induced by startle or exercise can be useful for recognizing vagally induced arrhythmias. Rapid resumption of vagal arrhythmia is common.
- Persistently elevated heart rates with regular rhythms may indicate a sustained sinus, atrial, junctional, or ventricular tachycardia. Ectopic rhythms should be strongly considered if the rate consistently exceeds 90 to 100 beats/min. Tachycardias with variable intensity sounds are more likely to be ventricular in origin.
- Irregularly irregular rhythms without a consistent atrial sound are suggestive of atrial flutter or fibrillation.
- Sudden pauses in an otherwise regular rhythm are typical of atrial and ventricular premature complexes. Careful auscultation may reveal premature first (± second) sounds, which are more likely to be split or muddled if ventricular in origin. The pauses follow the premature beats.

In addition to heart rate and rhythm, the individual heart sounds should be scrutinized and the presence or absence of cardiac murmurs noted. A systematic approach is needed to localize the valve areas and the related heart sounds and murmurs. One method involves identifying the left apical impulse by palpation followed by localization of the aortic

valve area by auscultation. The typical sounds and murmurs identified over these areas can be summarized as follows:

- The **mitral valve area** is located over and immediately dorsal to the palpable left apical impulse near the fifth intercostal space.
  - The first heart sound is loudest over the mitral area. Accentuation of the first heart sound is common in thin animals or associated with sympathetic activity. Conversely, the first (and second) sound in barrel-chested or overweight horses may be soft. Marked muffling of sounds is typical of pericardial effusion; conversely, with pleuropneumonia and pulmonary consolidation the heart sounds may transmit over a wider area of the thorax.
  - The third (ventricular) sound is often loudest at or adjacent to the left apex. Accentuation of the third sound is sometimes heard during tachycardia in healthy, trained horses and in horses with severe mitral regurgitation (MR) or with congestive heart failure.
  - The murmur of MR is typically holosystolic (plateau shaped) but also can be crescendo, starting after the first sound and peaking in late systole to obscure the second sound. Murmurs of MR often radiate dorsally and to the right. Causes of MR include valvular degeneration (perhaps accentuated by heavy training), ruptured or stretched chordae tendineae, cardiomyopathy or myocarditis leading to ventricular dilation or papillary muscle dysfunction, infective endocarditis, malformation (rare), and possibly fibrosis or infarction of a papillary muscle. Transient MR may be heard during ventricular ectopy.
  - The physiologic protodiastolic murmur of rapid left ventricular filling may be evident over the left ventricular inlet. Occasionally this murmur is musical or squeaky or sounds like a "rusty gate" in young horses.
  - A brief presystolic murmur following left atrial contraction may be evident here or cranial to this valve area.
- The **aortic valve area** is one intercostal space craniodorsal to the mitral area and is the location where the second sound is most prominent. The aorta projects craniodorsally from this valve.
  - The fourth heart sound (atrial sound) is often loudest near or adjacent to this location, though it also may be heard well at the apex and over the right thorax.

- The diastolic murmur of AR is loudest over this area and often radiates to the tricuspid area on the right. Murmurs of AR can be soft or loud, and the character has been described as blowing, vibratory, cooing, buzzing, or "dive bombing." This murmur is most often caused by valvular degeneration and prolapse in older horses, but it also can be due to infective endocarditis, aortic root abscess, ventricular septal defect, truncus arteriosus, and congenital fenestrations.
  - Prolonged and loud ejection murmurs over the aortic and pulmonary areas are sometimes evident in foals with severe cardiac malformations such as persistent truncus arteriosus or pulmonary atresia.
- The **pulmonic valve area** is one intercostal space cranioventral to the aortic area. The pulmonary artery extends immediately dorsally and crosses the ascending aorta.
  - The second sound may be physiologically or pathologically split at this location in a variable fashion.
  - A tympanic second heart sound over the pulmonary area is suggestive of pulmonary hypertension and may be evident with left-sided congestive heart failure or severe pulmonary disease.
  - Functional ejection murmurs ("innocent" or "athletic" murmurs) are heard best over the pulmonic and aortic valves and their respective great vessels. These murmurs typically peak in early to mid-systole and are silent at end systole, allowing the second sound to be readily detected.
  - Particularly loud systolic murmurs over this region may indicate relatively rare defects such as subarterial ventricular septal defect or valvular pulmonic stenosis.

- A loud diastolic murmur loudest over the pulmonic valve can be caused by pulmonary regurgitation associated with moderate to severe pulmonary hypertension or florid insufficiency caused by infective endocarditis.
- The **tricuspid valve area** is located at the third to fourth intercostal space on the right, opposite the aortic valve.
  - Heart sounds are generally softer over the right thorax.
  - Murmurs of tricuspid regurgitation are loudest at this area and can be decrescendo, holosystolic, or crescendo in configuration. This murmur tends to radiate dorsally on the right and sometimes projects to the left-cranioventral thorax. Tricuspid regurgitation is common in highly trained equine athletes and also can develop from infective endocarditis, ruptured chordae tendineae, pulmonary hypertension, causes of right ventricular dilatation, and malformation (rarely).
  - The physiologic protodiastolic murmur of rapid right ventricular filling or a brief presystolic murmur following right atrial contraction may be evident at this valve area.

Cardiac murmurs should be characterized by general timing in the cardiac cycle, configuration or "shape," point of maximal murmur intensity, radiation, and quality and pitch. These points are detailed in "Heart Murmur" in Section I.
- The systolic murmur of paramembranous ventricular septal defect is usually most intense along the cranioventral right thorax and radiates to the left cranial base. A precordial thrill is common.
- Diastolic or continuous murmurs may be heard in horses with one or more ruptures of an aortic sinus of Valsalva into the right atrium, right ventricle, or pulmonary artery.

- Pericardial friction rubs are uncommon in horses but can be confused with heart murmurs. These are typically multiphasic, occurring in systole, early diastole, and sometimes late diastole. Friction rubs may be evident over multiple valve areas.
- An algorithmic approach to cardiac murmurs is presented in the algorithm "Cardiac Auscultation in the Horse" in Section V.

ALTERNATIVES AND THEIR RELATIVE MERITS

- Electrocardiography is the procedure of choice to document heart rhythm disturbances or to confirm, if necessary, the presence of a vagally induced arrhythmia such as sinus arrhythmia or second-degree atrioventricular block.
- Echocardiography with Doppler studies is considered the noninvasive gold standard for recognition of congenital heart disease, valvular disease, pericardial effusion, and cardiomyopathies. However, results of echocardiography are best interpreted in conjunction with the auscultatory findings because Doppler techniques are highly sensitive; even normal valves can show evidence of "backflow" or mild regurgitation. In short, the Doppler findings should be congruous with those of auscultation.

SUGGESTED READING

Kriz NG, Hodgson DR, Rose RJ: Prevalence and clinical importance of heart murmurs in racehorses. *J Am Vet Med Assoc* 216(9):1441–1445, 2000.

Young LE, Rogers K, Wood JLN: Heart murmurs and valvular regurgitation in thoroughbred racehorses: epidemiology and associations with athletic performance. *J Vet Intern Med* 22:418–426, 2008.

AUTHOR: **JOHN D. BONAGURA**

Cardiac Output Monitoring

BASIC INFORMATION

OVERVIEW AND GOAL(S)

- Cardiac output is used to assess overall cardiovascular function and is useful to determine the contribution of cardiac dysfunction to hemodynamic derangements. It allows direct interpretation of the heart's ability to deliver oxygen globally and allows calculations of other important hemodynamic parameters that may help to improve patient management.
- Cardiac output can be measured by several methods; however, only the lithium dilution cardiac output (LiDCO) method is described here, as it is relatively noninvasive, is accurate, is simple to use, and has been validated in the horse.
- LiDCO is an indicator dilution method, relying on the principle that volume A × concentration A = volume B × concentration B. Therefore when a known mass of a substance is injected into an unknown volume, and the final concentration of the substance measured, the volume it is diluted in (cardiac output) can be calculated.
- LiDCO was developed to avoid the need for a pulmonary artery catheter, as required by other indicator dilution methods. It also avoids the need for a pulmonary artery catheter and measurement of oxygen consumption/CO_2

production as required by the Fick method.

INDICATIONS

- Aid in the management of critically ill neonates.
- Aid in the management of horses with cardiac disease.
- Aid in the management of horses under general anesthesia.
- Aid in the management of horses with circulatory compromise or abnormal hemodynamic status.

CONTRAINDICATIONS

- For lithium dilution cardiac output measurement:
  - Those of jugular venous catheter placement
  - Those of peripheral arterial catheter placement
  - Horses with significant blood loss/anemia, particularly if small neonates such as miniature horses

EQUIPMENT, ANESTHESIA

- LiDCO:
  - LiDCOplus or LiDCO computer (LiDCO Ltd., Sawston, Cambridge, UK)
  - Peristaltic pump
  - Blood collection bag (waste)
  - Extension tubing
  - Lithium sensor (disposable)
  - Arterial catheter
  - Narrow bore extension tubing
  - Three-way stopcocks
  - Jugular venous catheter
  - T-port or short extension set
  - Lithium chloride solution
  - 500-mL bag heparinized saline (10 units heparin/mL)
  - 20- to 30-mL syringes
  - 3-mL syringes
  - Sodium concentration analyzer (serum/plasma)
  - Hemoglobin concentration analyzer (blood)

ANTICIPATED TIME

Approximately 15 minutes if venous and arterial catheters are already in place.

PREPARATION: IMPORTANT CHECKPOINTS

- Arterial and jugular catheters should be placed prior to set-up.
- Weight of horse should be determined: Appropriate dose of lithium chloride calculated and precisely drawn up.
- Sensor should equilibrate to room temperature and be flushed with saline to remove air bubbles and saturate.
- Horse's sodium and hemoglobin concentrations should be predetermined.
- For horses under general anesthesia, arterial pressure cannot be monitored

while the LiDCO measurement is occurring (over a few minutes) (unless a second arterial catheter is placed); this should be taken into consideration when timing the measurement of cardiac output (CO) in unstable horses.

POSSIBLE COMPLICATIONS AND COMMON ERRORS TO BE AVOIDED

- Potential for excessive blood to be withdrawn from patient if multiple readings are performed and the amount of blood withdrawn for each reading is not monitored. This is more likely to occur if the patient is very small and/or anemic.
- If repeated injections of high concentrations of lithium are performed, excessive background lithium can build up, interfering with accurate calculation of CO and resulting in significant overestimation of CO. However, with the standard doses used in standing adult horses or in neonates, this is unlikely to occur.
- If the injection of lithium is made before the baseline has stabilized, erroneous results may be obtained.
- The sensor and extension tubing must be free of air bubbles and clots; either will interfere with the sensor's determination of lithium concentrations and the calculated CO.
- Dilution methods are not accurate in the presence of intracardiac shunts; therefore if a ventricular septal defect (VSD) or other cardiac shunts are present, the measurements will not be reliable.

PROCEDURE

- Arterial blood sample for measurement of sodium and hemoglobin

concentrations. This is used by the computer algorithm to calculate CO from the lithium concentration measured by the sensor.

- Mass of lithium to be injected (in mmol) and arterial sodium and hemoglobin concentrations are entered into the computer at the prompts. The height and weight can be ignored (any number entered) as the computer calculates a body surface area using a human algorithm, which has not been validated in horses, and is not used.
- A narrow bore extension set should be attached to the arterial catheter with a three-way stopcock at the end. The input of the lithium sensor is connected to the stopcock (as per manufacturer's instructions), and the output attached to a second three-way stopcock, extension tubing, and a peristaltic pump leading to the blood collection bag (Figure 1). The sensor should be allowed to come to room temperature and be free of air bubbles before connecting.
- After everything is connected but before making measurements, the line between the arterial catheter and the sensor should be open, the pump should be turned on, and blood allowed to flow from the arterial line through the sensor (this allows it to equilibrate and obtain a stable baseline). Pump speed is typically 4 to 8 mL/min during injection of lithium and calculation of CO.
- Once a stable baseline is present, the lithium solution can be injected. Before actually injecting, the "inject" button on the computer must be depressed (screen or foot pedal); the time between pressing the button and injecting depends upon the expected

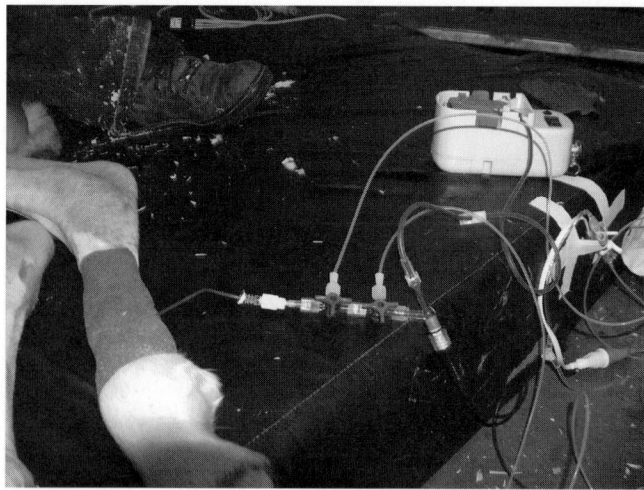

FIGURE 1 Foal instrumented with an arterial catheter in the metatarsal artery connecting to the input of the lithium sensor via two three-way stopcocks. The output of the sensor is then connected to a peristaltic pump and waste blood collection bag. (Courtesy Kevin Corley.)

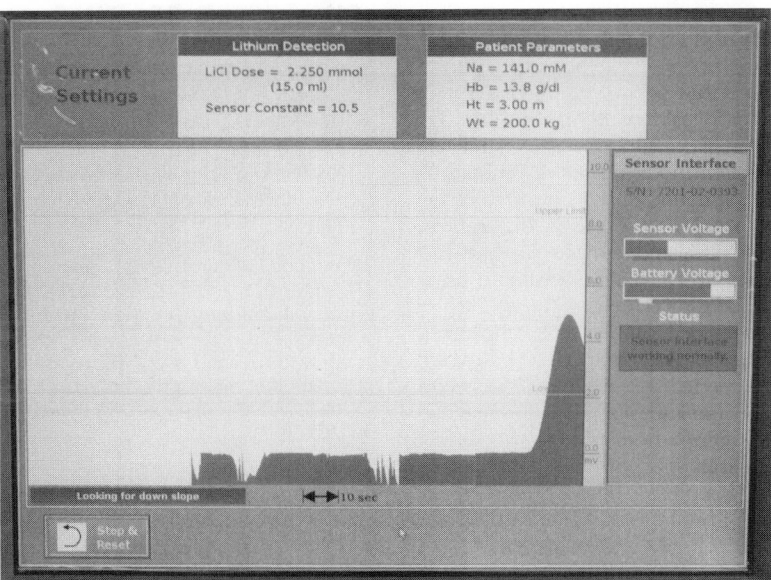

FIGURE 2 Example of lithium dilution converted to voltage, displaying a stable baseline and lithium injection. (Courtesy Kevin Corley.)

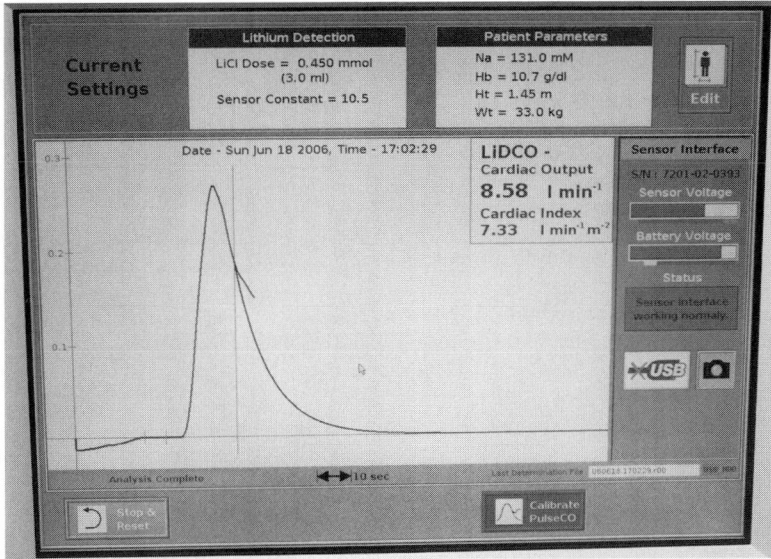

FIGURE 3 Example of a typical lithium dilution curve, with the area under the curve calculated by the computer program and cardiac output displayed in L/min. (Courtesy Kevin Corley.)

CO of the horse (the larger the CO, the longer the lead time). Typical masses injected are 20 mL of 150 mmoL/L or 10 mL of 300 mmoL/L lithium chloride for a standing adult horse and 5 mL of 150 mM lithium chloride for a neonate.

- Injections should be performed as rapidly as possible, using as precisely measured lithium chloride solution as possible. For this reason, it is easiest to use a T-port, rather than an extension set connected to the jugular venous catheter. The T-port and catheter should be primed with the lithium solution.

- The lithium sensor detects the lithium concentration in the blood over time and draws a curve from this information (Figure 2). CO is generated by calculating the area under the curve, and is given in L/min (Figure 3). This should be divided by the body weight in kilograms and multiplied by 1000 to give cardiac index in mL/kg/min. The computer-derived cardiac index should not be used.

- Once the computer has calculated a value, the pump should be turned off so that blood is no longer flowing from the arterial line through the sensor and the arterial catheter and

sensor flushed thoroughly with heparinized saline to prevent blood clots. Care should be taken to prevent the sensor from drying out between readings.

- The sensor has a relatively limited lifespan and may not be usable over multiple patients or more than 1 day.

- If it is desired to monitor trends in CO, or when significant changes may occur, PulseCO can be used in combination with LiDCOplus. This allows a continuous display of hemodynamic parameters, including CO, using the arterial blood pressure monitor. Pulse contour analysis of the arterial waveform is used to assess changes in cardiovascular status.

- This is based on the principle that each individual has a unique arterial waveform based partially on the elastic recoil of the artery. The waveform generated from the arterial catheter is calibrated to the LiDCOplus.

- This requires the arterial catheter to be connected to a pressure monitor (usually via an extension set from the three-way stopcock).

- After the LiDCO curve is obtained by the computer, the arterial catheter and the pressure monitor are reconnected and the PulseCO software calibrates to the LiDCO. Two measurements of CO should be obtained for calibration. This allows a continuous reading of CO, heart rate (HR), stroke volume (SV), mean arterial pressure (MAP), and systemic vascular resistance (SVR). The pulse contour should be recalibrated periodically, especially if large swings in hemodynamic status occur.

POSTPROCEDURE

- The pump should be turned off, the arterial catheter should be flushed with heparinized saline, and the three-way stopcock turned off to the horse.

- The sensor should be flushed thoroughly to avoid blood clots if it is to be used later or on a different patient. However, it is not likely to be usable over more than 1 day or on multiple patients.

- If no additional measurements are to be made and the arterial catheter removed, pressure should be applied over the artery for several minutes to avoid hematoma formation.

ALTERNATIVES AND THEIR RELATIVE MERITS

- Physical exam parameters (HR/intensity of heart sounds, peripheral pulse quality, venous filling, mucous membrane color, capillary refill time, temperature of extremities, urine output): These parameters are essential to monitor in all patients; however, they only give an indirect assessment

of cardiac function, global oxygen delivery, and hemodynamic status.
- Arterial blood pressure (direct and indirect): Critical in the determination of adequate tissue perfusion; however, does not distinguish between abnormalities in SVR and CO.
- Central venous pressure: Although this gives some indication of cardiac function, it is highly dependent on preload. It is influenced by circulating blood volume and vascular tone, as well as cardiac function. In addition, it does not give systemic hemodynamic variables such as arterial blood pressure and SVR.

- Lactate concentration: A good indicator of anaerobic metabolism; however, if it is abnormal, it does not discriminate among hypovolemia, inadequate blood oxygen content, cardiac dysfunction, local/global changes in tissue perfusion, or increases in metabolic rate.
- Arteriovenous O_2 or CO_2 differences/central or mixed venous O_2 and CO_2 tensions: These values estimate tissue oxygen delivery and balance, which is influenced by CO; however, other factors can influence the overall balance (regional tissue perfusion, hemoglobin content, cellular metabolism, pulmonary function).

SUGGESTED READING

Corley KTT, Donaldson LL, Furr MO: Comparison of lithium dilution and thermodilution cardiac output measurements in anesthetized neonatal foals. *Eqine Vet J* 34:598–601, 2002.

Corley KTT, Donaldson LL, Durando MM, et al: Cardiac output technologies with special reference to the horse. *J Vet Int Med* 17:262–272, 2003.

Durando MM: Cardiac output measurement. In Corley K, Stephen J, editors: *The Equine Hospital Manual*, London, 2008, Blackwell, pp 55–58.

Linton RA, Band DM, Haire KM: A new method of measuring cardiac output in man using lithium dilution. *Br J Anaesth* 71:262–266, 1993.

AUTHOR: **MARY M. DURANDO**

Cardiopulmonary Cerebral Resuscitation in Neonatal Foals

BASIC INFORMATION

SYNONYM(S)

CPCR
CPR
Cardiopulmonary resuscitation

OVERVIEW AND GOAL(S)

- Cardiopulmonary cerebral resuscitation is instituted to return the foal to spontaneous and effective circulation and ventilation, with minimal hypoxic organ damage.
- Resuscitation attempts performed after respiratory arrest alone are more successful (50% survive) than those performed after cardiac arrest (10% survive).
- Prognosis for any CPCR event due to primary cardiac failure or severe disease is guarded to grave.

INDICATIONS

- Impending signs of cardiopulmonary arrest in hospitalized foals include tachycardia or bradycardia, depression, oliguria, weak to absent pulses, poor capillary refill time, hypothermia, sporadic respirations, and an abdominal component to respiration.
- Causes of cardiopulmonary arrest fall in two categories: Primary cardiac failure and secondary cardiac arrest
  - Primary cardiac failure
    - Rare in foals
    - Etiology includes hypoxic-ischemic injury, sepsis-induced cardiac damage, or congenital defects.
    - CPCR is initiated immediately for a lack of heart beat or nonperfusing rhythm.

  - Arrhythmias noted range from ventricular tachycardia/fibrillation, asystole, to pulseless electrical activity (PEA).
  - Note that certain arrhythmias are common and normal in foals for the first 15 minutes of life, and require no resuscitative effort.
    - Atrial fibrillation
    - Premature atrial or ventricular contractions
  - Secondary cardiopulmonary arrest
    - Systemic disease leads to pulmonary or cardiac failure, causing metabolic acidosis due to hypoxia.
    - Hypoxia leads to respiratory arrest, followed by bradycardia, PEA, and asystole.
    - Causes include dystocia, hypoxic-ischemic encephalopathy, sepsis, hypovolemic shock, electrolyte abnormalities, hypoglycemia, and hypothermia.
  - Respiratory issues are noted in first 20 seconds after birth.
    - Failure to sit upright, heart rate <50 bpm, lack of spontaneous breaths or irregular gasping.
    - Supply nasal oxygen until assessment is finished, and stimulate respirations with towel drying.
    - Initiate ventilatory support within 30 seconds of birth if irregular breathing or dyspnea continues.
    - CPCR is initiated for a lack of perfusing rhythm, heart rate <40 bpm, or asystole.

CONTRAINDICATIONS

- CPCR should not be attempted if the underlying cause cannot be addressed and treated with success after resuscitation.
  - CPCR is discouraged in foals with severe systemic illness or congenital defects.
  - CPCR is recommended for normal foals with a hypoxic event during or after birth or under anesthesia.

EQUIPMENT, ANESTHESIA

- Recommended:
  - Towels
  - Bulb syringe
  - Cuffed endotracheal tubes (7–12 cm diameter, 55-cm long)
- 5 mL syringe for cuff inflation
  - Ambu bag (Ambu Inc., Glen Burnie, MD) or C.D. Foal resuscitator (McCulloch Medical, Auckland, NZ)
  - Flashlight
  - Medications (epinephrine, vasopressin, atropine, lidocaine, magnesium)
  - 2-mL syringes and 20-gauge needles
  - Two to four 1-L bags of crystalloid fluids (Normosol-R, Plasmalyte 148, lactated Ringer's)
  - 50% dextrose solution
  - IV catheters (16 and 14 gauge)
  - Fluid administration set
- Optional:
  - Sterile gloves
  - 14-gauge needles (for intraosseous access)
  - 6F red rubber catheter (for intratracheal drug administration)
  - Oxygen

- ○ Electrocardiogram (ECG)
- ○ Capnography
- ○ Suction unit
- ○ Point of care meter for blood gas, lactate, glucose, and electrolytes
- ○ Mechanical ventilator

ANTICIPATED TIME

- The majority of CPCR events last less than 15 minutes.
- Success rates decline rapidly after 10 minutes due to lack of adequate cerebral oxygenation.

PREPARATION: IMPORTANT CHECKPOINTS

- CPCR will not be successful without organized equipment, personnel, and a CPCR plan including chain of command.
- A CPCR code should be practiced on a regular basis to ensure everyone knows their roles and expectations.
- Resuscitation status should be determined for all foals admitted and clear communication of the expectations of all involved should be established if an unplanned code occurs (see "Neonatal Resuscitation Assessment" in Seccion V).
- Equipment should be checked on a regular basis, and medications assessed to ensure they have not reached their expiration dates.
- Data sheets should be readily available to record the event.
- A postresuscitation assessment should be performed for every CPCR event to identify areas of improvement.

POSSIBLE COMPLICATIONS AND COMMON ERRORS TO BE AVOIDED

- Inaccurate dosages can be avoided by composing a chart of doses for average foal weights in 5-kg increments (remember miniature foals) using the concentrations of medications available in your hospital.
- Hyperventilation of the foal is common due to the stress of the situation, and an end-tidal CO_2 monitor may reduce the risk by providing feedback.
- Excessive fluid administration may occur in normovolemic newborns and result in pulmonary edema; therefore fluid boluses should be carefully administered based on hydration status.
- ECG results, pulse assessment during CPCR, and pulse oximetry cannot be relied on for assessing perfusion; only pupil size and the end-tidal CO_2 monitoring are accurate.
- Long breaks in cardiac compressions (>10 seconds) significantly reduce the success of CPCR.

PROCEDURE

Based on the cause of the arrest, either compressions or ventilation are started first (see "Cardiopulmonary Cerebral Resuscitation" in Seccion V).

- Primary cardiac arrest
  - ○ Initiate compressions immediately.
  - ○ Ventilation is secondary.
- Primary ventilatory arrest, with a minimally perfusing rhythm
  - ○ Ventilation is the primary concern.
  - ○ Compressions are initiated when perfusion halts (pulse <40 beats/min).

The following events may occur nearly simultaneously depending on the number of personnel:

ESTABLISH AN AIRWAY AND PROVIDE VENTILATION

- Place foal in lateral recumbency on firm surface; broken ribs, if any, down.
  - ○ If ribs are broken bilaterally, place side with more cranial fractures down.
- If a newborn, remove airway secretions/amniotic fluid with bulb syringe.
  - ○ Suction units can evacuate lungs and damage alveoli: Use cautiously and briefly.
  - ○ Continuous suction may also stimulate vagal responses and cause bradycardia.
- Ventilation can be provided three ways.
  - ○ Mouth to nose ventilation
    - ▪ Occlude down nostril and extend the head to open airway.
    - ▪ Occlude esophagus if possible with opposite hand to reduce aerophagia.
  - ○ Mask ventilation
  - ○ Endotracheal intubation through nose or mouth
    - ▪ Place tube blindly without elevating head (position preserves cerebral blood flow).
    - ▪ Palpate placement in trachea.
    - ▪ Inflate cuff.
- Provide adequate respirations.
  - ○ Rate should be minimal with primary cardiac arrest.
    - ▪ 8 to 10 breaths/minute, with a 1-second inspiratory time to maximize time in diastole.
    - ▪ Positive intrathoracic pressures reduce the time in diastole and therefore cardiac output.
      - □ Cardiac filling and coronary perfusion occurs in diastole.
    - ▪ Perfusion is only a third of normal in CPCR; therefore less air is required for complete oxygenation.
  - ○ Rate should be faster, but still less than normal, with primary respiratory arrest prior to asystole.
    - ▪ 10 to 20 breaths/min, with a short inspiratory time.

- ▪ Perfusion is better than with full CPCR; therefore more air is required for diffusion than during cardiac arrest.
- ○ Breaths and compressions do not have to coincide to be effective.
- ○ Room air is adequate for CPCR, but 100% oxygen may maximize diffusion with ventilation-perfusion mismatching that is occurring in CPCR.
- ○ Look for adequate chest rise.
  - ▪ Avoid pressures above 30 cm H_2O to prevent barotrauma.

SUPPORT PERFUSION WITH CARDIAC COMPRESSIONS

- Start immediately if primary cardiac arrest.
- Begin after 30-second evaluation notes a decline in heart rate in respiratory arrest.
- Goal is 100 compressions/minute.
  - ○ Use heel of fist with opposite hand wrapped over it to compress the thorax either over heart or at highest point of chest.
  - ○ Bend at waist and keep elbows locked for quick hard strokes.
  - ○ The key to perfusion is a short compression phase and long recoil time.
    - ▪ Recoil of thorax is how blood moves forward.
    - ▪ Cardiac or venous valves prevent backward flow.
  - ○ Compressions should never stop for more than 10-second intervals to increase success.

PROVIDE MEDICATIONS AND VASCULAR ACCESS

- Medications may be administered IV, intraosseous (IO), or intratracheal (IT).
  - ○ IO medications are administered at the same dose as IV, and IV drugs can be given IO.
  - ○ IT medications are injected down the endotracheal tube with a long catheter or with a needle transtracheally.
    - ▪ Epinephrine, atropine, lidocaine, and naloxone are absorbed in the lung.
    - ▪ Chase IT medications with air (2–3 breaths) to deliver to lung.
    - ▪ Tracheal doses must be doubled.
      - □ Drugs are poorly absorbed.
      - □ Deposits in lungs may provide a drug reservoir that may be absorbed later.
- Medications commonly administered in CPCR (Table 1)
- Fluid therapy
  - ○ For hypovolemic or septic shock use the shock dose of crystalloids (10–20 mL/kg).
    - ▪ Normasol-R, Plasmalyte 148, lactated Ringer's
  - ○ For respiratory arrest in normovolemic foals use 5 to 10 mL/kg crystalloid solution to avoid pulmonary edema.

TABLE 1 Drugs Commonly Used In CPCR

Drug	Class	MOA	Use	Negatives	Dose	Comments
Epinephrine 1:1000, 1 mg/mL	Catecholamine	α- and β-adrenergic receptor agonist	Increase coronary perfusion through increased diastolic aortic pressure (heart is perfused in diastole during CPCR) Small inotropic effect	May increase myocardial oxygen use May decrease coronary perfusion at high doses	0.01–0.02 mg/kg IV or IO q3min; 0.05–0.1 mg/kg IT	Incompatible with bicarbonate High-dose epinephrine (0.1–0.2 mg/kg) may negatively effect neurologic outcomes
Vasopressin	Vasoconstrictor	Antidiuretic hormone receptor agonist	As a vasopressor for cardiac arrest, especially asystole May be more effective than epinephrine in asystole	May reduce splanchnic perfusion after circulation is restored	0.6 U/kg IV or IO q10–20min	Vasopressor effect in normal individuals is blunted by bradycardia
Atropine	Antimuscarinic	Counters excess vagal tone	For PEA, decreased HR, SVR, and BP only after CPCR and epinephrine are deemed unsuccessful Do not use in newborns	May increase heart rate/ oxygen demand in the face of hypoxia	0.02 mg/kg IV or IO q5min (double dose IT) Only give 2 doses	Vagal tone is rarely a cause of PEA; bradycardia is usually due to hypoxia. Ventilate first to reduce vagal stimulation by hypoxia/hypercapnia. Incompatible with bicarbonate
Lidocaine	Class 1B antidysrhythmic	Suppresses ventricular arrhythmias through decreased automaticity and deceased conduction	For ventricular fibrillation or pulseless ventricular tachycardia		1 mg/kg IV or IO followed by CRI 20–50 μg/kg/min (double dose IT), max. 3 mg/kg	Neurologic toxicity: depression, paraesthesia, seizures Cardiovascular depression
Magnesium	Electrolyte		For torsades des pointes in ventricular fibrillation	Ineffective for other forms of ventricular fibrillation	25–50 mg/kg diluted in 5% dextrose to 10 mL Give over 5–20 min (over 60 min if patient has pulse)	Rapid dosing may cause hypotension Incompatible with bicarbonate
Calcium	Electrolyte		For hyperkalemia, hypermagnesemia, or hypocalcemia	No benefit in CPCR	20 mg/kg of 23% Ca gluconate (0.9 mL/kg)	May speed cell death Incompatible with bicarbonate

IV, Intravenous; *IO,* intraosseous; *IT,* intrathoracic; *PEA,* pulseless electrical activity; *HR,* heart rate; *SVR,* systemic vascular resistance; *BP,* blood pressure; *CRI,* continuous-rate infusion.

- ○ Dextrose is administered only if hypoglycemic (hyperglycemia may decrease prognosis).
- • Apply external monitoring equipment last, if available.
  - ○ ECG, capnography
    - ▪ Assess rhythm to determine need for additional therapy.
- • Defibrillation
- • Antiarrhythmic medications
  - ○ Monitor electrolytes, blood gas, packed cell volume, and lactate intermittently.
- • Defibrillation:
  - ○ Indicated for ventricular fibrillation or tachycardia.
  - ○ Converts a large group of cardiac myocytes back to organized depolarization.
  - ○ Requires shaved skin and electrode gel.

- ○ Begin at 2 J/kg, and increase to 4 J/kg for each shock thereafter.
- ○ Start as soon as a ventricular arrhythmia is noted for best effect.
- ○ Defibrillate 30 to 60 seconds after epinephrine dose is administered.
- ○ Resume cardiac compressions immediately.
- ○ Perform 2 minutes of compressions between each shock.
- • Assess overall success of CPCR every 2 to 3 minutes during a code.
  - ○ Stop compressions for <10 seconds, and assess rhythm and pulse.
    - ▪ Pulses measured during CPCR are not effective at measuring success.
  - ○ Monitor end-tidal CO_2 during CPCR.
    - ▪ 12 to 18 mm Hg ideal (indicative of perfusion and pulmonary gas exchange)

- ○ Monitor pupil size.
  - ▪ Neutral size indicates cerebral perfusion.
- • Stop resuscitation when:
  - ○ Regular heart rate (>60 beats/min) is present immediately after compressions stop.
  - ○ Respirations are spontaneous.
    - ▪ Assess respirations if a perfusing rhythm is present by disconnecting bag for 30 seconds.
    - ▪ Rate should be >15 breaths/min and regular to stop ventilation.

POSTPROCEDURE

- • Treat underlying cause or the foal will rearrest.
- • Monitor vitals continuously, or every 30 minutes for the first 4 hours.
  - ○ Assess perfusion.
    - ▪ Heart rate and rhythm
    - ▪ Mucous membranes

- Peripheral temperature
- Peripheral pulses
- Urine output
- Mentation
- Blood pressure
- Lactate
- Central venous pressure
  - Assess ventilation.
    - Respiratory rate and effort
    - Blood gas
    - Capnography
    - Lactate
- Additional supportive measures that are recommended:
  - Nursing care: Positioning, hygiene, eye lubrication, physical therapy
  - Oxygen therapy
  - Active warming
  - Fluid therapy

- Parenteral nutrition
- Cerebral protectants
  - Osmotic agents: Mannitol
  - Antioxidants: dimethyl sulfoxide, vitamin C, vitamin E, magnesium sulfate
- Inotropic medications and vasopressors
- Mechanical ventilation
- Most foals will requires transfer to a facility that can provide 24-hour intensive care and monitoring.

ALTERNATIVES AND THEIR RELATIVE MERITS

CPCR for neonatal foals is extrapolated from neonatal human CPCR and new information is available weekly regarding success and failure of CPCR methods in humans. There is currently a paucity of literature available that provides direct evidence for the procedures and medications currently recommended in veterinary CPCR. The reader is encouraged to prepare their resuscitation team by assessing the most recent available literature and the validity of their claims to extrapolate a CPCR protocol for their hospital.

SUGGESTED READING

Corley KT, et al: Resuscitation and emergency management for neonatal foals. *Vet Clin North Am Equine Pract.* 21:431–455, 2005.
Palmer JE: Neonatal foal resuscitation. *Vet Clin North Am Equine Pract.* 23:159–182, 2007.

AUTHOR: **AMELIA MUNSTERMAN**

Cecal Trocarization

BASIC INFORMATION

SYNONYM(S)

Percutaneous cecal decompression

OVERVIEW AND GOAL(S)

Reduce abdominal distention and thoracic compression by alleviating the gas distention of the cecum and colon.

INDICATIONS

- Severe abdominal distention with well-defined audible ping in the right paralumbar fossa.
  - This may be helpful to ease ventilation in cases in which horses are dyspneic due to abdominal distention (compartment disease) prior to induction of general anesthesia.
  - Used to reduce gas distention of cecum and large colon in cases with suspected large colon displacement and no surgical option. The reduction in size of the cecum and large colon may allow the latter to "slip" back into place.

CONTRAINDICATIONS

- Ill-defined or no ping in the right paralumbar fossa
- Repeated trocarization: With repeated trocarization there is greater risk for peritoneal contamination and subsequent peritonitis.

EQUIPMENT, ANESTHESIA

- Sedation (ie, xylazine, detomidine, and/or butorphanol may be necessary depending on how painful/fractious the patient is)

- Experienced horse handler with a properly applied nose twitch may be necessary for young, excited, painful, or fractious patients
- Stocks if available are preferred for improved restraint and protection of operator but are inappropriate if the horse may become recumbent due to pain
- Stethoscope
- Clippers
- Surgical scrub solution soaked gauze and alcohol gauze for aseptic preparation of skin
- 12 mL Lidocaine with 21-gauge 1.5-inch needle
- 14-gauge over the needle IV catheter
- Extension set
- Nonsterile cup with water
- Sterile gloves
- 6 to 12 mL procaine penicillin in syringe

ANTICIPATED TIME

Approximately 10 to 15 minutes

PREPARATION: IMPORTANT CHECKPOINTS

- Locate the area where the ping is of maximal intensity in the right paralumbar fossa (dorsally between the last rib and the tuber coxae). This should be approximately one-third to one-half of the distance from the last rib to the tuber coxae. Do not trocarize at the caudal edge of the last rib as laceration of the vessels or nerve caudal to the last rib is possible. If the ping is cranial to this point, the trocarization can be performed between the last two ribs just cranial to the last rib.

- The center of the ping is the optimal location to trocarize the cecum. If the top of the ping is entered as the gas is evacuated from the base of the cecum, it may collapse down and pull away from the catheter. Conversely, by entering the bottom of the ping the catheter may fill with cecal fluid and be clogged by ingesta also increasing the risks of peritonitis.

POSSIBLE COMPLICATIONS AND COMMON ERRORS TO BE AVOIDED

- Peritonitis
- Bowel laceration

PROCEDURE

- Locate the area where the ping is of maximal intensity dorsally in the right paralumbar fossa.
- Clip an adequate area round this location (approximately 15 cm square).
- Aseptically prepare the area.
- Place a block in the skin and muscle with a 20-gauge needle and 12 mL of 2% lidocaine.
- Perform a subsequent aseptic preparation of the site.
- Put on sterile gloves.
- Acquire a 14-gauge 5-inch over the needle intravenous catheter sterilely.
- Insert the catheter through the bleb perpendicular to the body wall at a very slight cranial and ventral directed angle.
- Continue to insert the catheter slowly until the resistance decreases or gas is heard or smelled coming from the catheter. At this point, the base of the cecum has been entered.

- TROUBLESHOOT:
  - If gas is not obtained and the catheter has been inserted in the desired site, remove the catheter, listen for the ping, and redefine your location; then start over.
- At this point the catheter stylet may be removed.
  - Removal of the stylet may decrease the chance of bowel laceration if the cecum base deflates away from the catheter. However, the musculature of the body wall may crush and occlude the lumen of the catheter once the stylet has been removed.
  - If the stylet is left in, take care to not move the catheter excessively.
- Attach the sterile extension tubing to the catheter at this time and hand the end to a nonsterile helper. This end may then be submerged in the cup of water. Bubbles in the cup indicate that the gas is flowing readily from the catheter.
- When gas ceases to drain from the catheter do not attempt to redirect the catheter as the relative location of the bowel and the catheter are unknown. Movement of the catheter at this stage increases the likelihood of bowel laceration and peritoneal contamination.
- Remove the catheter slowly while injecting procaine penicillin G to decrease the chance of infection in the catheter tract.

POSTPROCEDURE

- Wipe the area with an alcohol gauze.
- Listen to the ping again; if the ping is still prominent and adequate decompression was not acquired, the procedure can be repeated in a different location if desired.

AUTHOR: **CHRISTINE WIMER**

Central Venous Pressure Monitoring

BASIC INFORMATION

OVERVIEW AND GOAL(S)

Central venous pressure (CVP) is very useful to assess venous return to the heart (preload) and to monitor fluid therapy. CVP gives an indication of the patient's fluid requirements and the ability of the cardiovascular system to handle the administered fluid load. It is a reflection of cardiac function, circulating blood volume, and vascular tone.

INDICATIONS

- Management of horses on fluid therapy with an increased risk of overhydration, such as those in renal failure with decreased urine production, those with significant cardiac disease, or those that are very young and/or very small.
- Assessment of whether the administered fluid therapy is sufficient to meet the needs of the patient. This is particularly useful in horses with gastrointestinal diseases.

CONTRAINDICATIONS

Only those of jugular venous catheter placement

EQUIPMENT, ANESTHESIA

- Jugular venous catheter (10- to 14-gauge)
- Sterile polyethylene (PE) tubing, at least 100 cm in length, outer diameter small enough to fit through 10- to 14-gauge catheter (eg, PE 190, PE 210, or PE 240)
- Blunt needle
- Alternatively, a specialized CVP catheter can be used, providing it is long

enough to reach just cranial to the right atrium
- Three-way stopcock
- Narrow-bore extension tubing
- 500 mL bag of sterile saline or heparinized saline (10 units heparin/mL saline)
- IV drip set
- Manometer measurement
  - Manometer: Alternatively, fluid extension tubing taped to a vertically held ruler can be used
- Electronic measurement
  - Pressure transducer
  - Patient monitor with capability of measuring blood pressure and electrocardiogram (ECG)

ANTICIPATED TIME

If a jugular venous catheter is in place, 15 to 20 minutes to place CVP catheter and record measurements

PREPARATION: IMPORTANT CHECKPOINTS

- An IV catheter in the jugular vein is needed. If sterile PE tubing is used, premeasure to distal cranial vena cava to determine appropriate length to pass.
- If a commercial CVP catheter is used, it should be premeasured to ensure that it will reach to a level just cranial to the right atrium and to determine how far distally in the jugular vein it must be placed.

POSSIBLE COMPLICATIONS AND COMMON ERRORS TO BE AVOIDED

- Primarily risks associated with IV catheter placement, such as introduction of infection or thrombosis.

- If catheter is passed into the right atrium, supraventricular dysrhythmias may be induced.
- The lines must be free of obstructions to accurately measure CVP.
  - They should be flushed periodically with heparinized saline and fluid be allowed to flow through frequently to prevent blood clots.
  - Care must be taken to ensure that air bubbles are not within the lines.
- The manometer must be placed at a constant height with respect to the horse (by convention, the heart base), especially if multiple measurements are to be made over time.
- If there is significant right-sided cardiac disease present, this will greatly affect CVP, regardless of intravascular blood volume.
- CVP is a reflection of intravascular blood volume; therefore if significant interstitial edema is present, the animal could have a decreased CVP in the face of fluid overload.

PROCEDURE

Because of the size of adult horses, it is often necessary to measure CVP by passing sterile PE tubing through a 10- to 14-gauge jugular venous catheter.
- The appropriate length of the PE tubing should be premeasured from the jugular catheter to just cranial to the heart base (approximately the second to third intercostal space) and the distance marked.
- The end of the PE tubing should have a blunt needle of appropriate gauge carefully placed into it to create a Luer connection and a three-way stopcock attached to the needle.
- A 500-mL fluid bag with IV drip set is also connected to the stopcock.

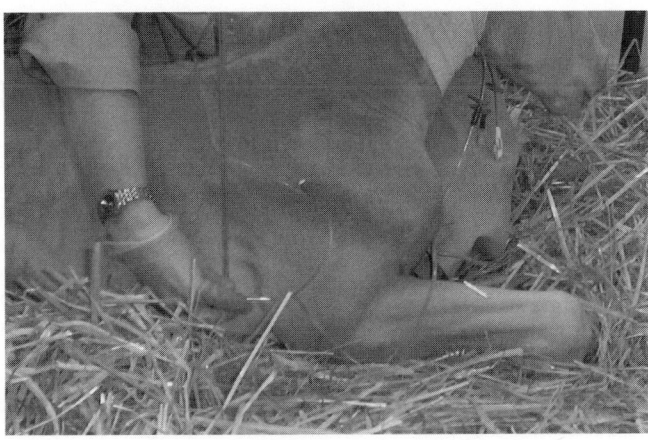

FIGURE 1 CVP measurement in a foal, with the zero point of the manometer at the heart base. An extension set connects the catheter to the manometer. (Photo courtesy Gary Magdesian.)

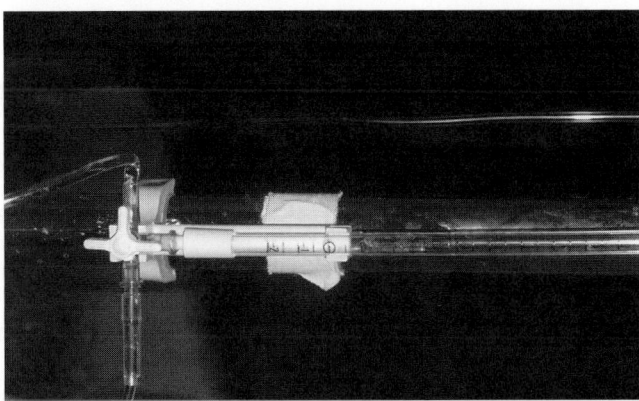

FIGURE 2 Manometer with stopcock open between the horse and the manometer and the zero point on a level with the right atrium (point of shoulder).

- After priming the PE tubing with sterile saline from the fluid bag and turning the stopcock off to the PE tubing (so fluid remains within the line), it is passed through the injection cap on the IV catheter to the distal aspect of the cranial vena cava.
- The PE tubing is connected to a manometer or electronic pressure transducer via the third port of the stopcock and narrow-bore extension tubing.
- The manometer or pressure transducer is placed at the level of the heart base (point of shoulder) as a standardized way to zero the instrument and record pressures (Figure 1).
- With the stopcock open to the extension tubing and manometer (off to the PE tubing and horse), saline from the fluid bag is allowed to fill the line and the manometer, to within a few centimeters of the extremity (top), and all air bubbles removed.
- If a pressure transducer is used, saline should flow through the transducer to remove air bubbles.
- The stopcock is then turned to open the lines between the PE tubing within the jugular catheter and the manometer or pressure transducer (off to the fluid bag) (Figure 2).
- A catheter of sufficient length designed for central venous monitoring may be used in place of the PE tubing and jugular catheter. Once placed, it is connected to a three-way stopcock, which is connected to a manometer as above.
- NOTE: If serial measurements from a patient are to be recorded, the manometer or pressure transducer should be attached to a fluid stand at a fixed height, to ensure that the zero point remains the same.
- Reading the CVP from a manometer
  - Once the PE tubing and manometer are connected and the PE tubing is

in its proper place, the fluid column within the manometer should rise and fall with respiration, reflecting intrathoracic pressure changes. The CVP is read as the height of the fluid column in centimeters.
  - Normal CVP in adult horses is approximately 7 to 12 cm H_2O if referenced to the point of the shoulder.
- Reading the CVP from an electronic transducer
  - If an electronic pressure transducer is used, the extension set is connected to the transducer rather than a manometer, and secured to a fluid stand at a level of the heart base. It is then primed with saline as above.
  - The transducer is connected to a pressure-monitoring device that also records simultaneous ECGs and is zeroed prior to readings.
  - To decrease the effects of respiration on the CVP value (particularly those under general anesthesia and mechanically ventilated), the CVP is read as the a-wave at end-expiration. The a-wave occurs during the PR interval on the ECG; inspiration is seen as a decrease in pressure, and expiration as an increase in pressure in spontaneously breathing animals, this is reversed in mechanically ventilated animals.
- NOTE: It is very important to ensure all air has been removed from the lines and that fluid flows freely without blood clots present, as this will interfere with accurate pressure measurements.

POSTPROCEDURE

- The stopcock should be turned off to the horse, and the fluid lines and manometer or transducer should be disconnected.

- After the PE tubing is removed, the catheter should be flushed with heparinized saline.

ALTERNATIVES AND THEIR RELATIVE MERITS

- Other indices of relative hydration status such as packed cell volume/total solids (PCV/TS) or urine specific gravity (USG) may be used.
- PCV/TS can indicate hydration status (increased PCV/TS hemoconcentration, decreased PCV/TS hemodilution) but is also commonly confounded in horses with protein-losing situations such as colitis, by a decrease in TS in the face of inadequate intravascular fluid volume.
- A decrease in USG can indicate successful fluid therapy; however, horses on IV fluids may have decreased urine specific gravity regardless of their circulatory status. In addition, USG is very dependent on normal kidney function.
- Blood pressure monitoring is another way to monitor cardiovascular status and will reflect circulatory status; however, it is influenced by cardiac function and vascular tone, as well as circulating blood volume.

SUGGESTED READING

Daily EK, Schroeder JS: Central venous and right atrial pressure monitoring. In Daily EK, Schroeder JS, editors: *Techniques in Bedside Hemodynamic Monitoring*, St Louis, 1994, Mosby, pp 79–98.

Durando MM: Central venous pressure measurement. In Corley K, Stephen J, editors: *The Equine Hospital Manual*, London, 2008, Blackwell, pp 47–49.

Hall LW, Nigam JM: Measurement of central venous pressure in horses, *Vet Rec* 97:66–69, 1975.

AUTHOR: **MARY M. DURANDO**

Cerebrospinal Fluid Analysis

BASIC INFORMATION

- Cerebrospinal fluid (CSF) is a clear, colorless fluid produced as an ultrafiltrate of plasma and is actively secreted by ependymal cells and the choroid plexus.
- CSF is absorbed by microvilli located in the venous sinuses, collections of which are called *arachnoid granulations*.
- CSF is produced at a constant rate in humans and other species; however, the rate of CSF production in horses has not been determined.
- Because the production rate is constant and independent of intracranial pressure, the rate of absorption is the primary regulator of intracranial pressure.
- CSF fills the brain ventricular system, central canal of the spinal cord, and the subarachnoid space.

OVERVIEW AND GOAL(S)

Function:
- Suspends and helps nourish the brain and spinal cord as well as give them a degree of physical protection from trauma
- Helps maintain the appropriate ionic and pH environment for the central nervous system (CNS).
- Aids in the regulation of intracranial pressures.
- Serves as a medium to transport neurotransmitters.

Evaluation:
- May help with the diagnosis of problems affecting the CNS of horses.

- Can be performed after collection from either the atlanto-occipital or lumbosacral space.
- Most useful in the diagnosis of neurologic diseases when the problem is the result of either an inflammatory or infectious cause.

Analysis:
- Spinal fluid can be analyzed for protein content, red and white blood cell numbers, creatine kinase, glucose, and antibodies against infectious agents such as *Sarcocystis neurona* or *Neospora hughesi*.
- Normal CSF should be crystal clear and should not clot.
- CSF that is slightly pinkish may be a result of iatrogenic damage to a blood vessel and will often clear within a few seconds of flow.

Normal values:
- Protein: 0 to 100 mg/dL
- Immunoglobulin G (IgG): 3 to 8 mg/dL
- Red blood cells: Less than 50/mL
- White blood cells: 0 to 5/mL
- Creatine kinase: 0 to 7 IU/L
- Glucose: 30% to 70% of plasma values

Abnormal findings:
- Samples containing blood may indicate a spinal cord injury.
- Xanthochromia may indicate elevated protein levels, a recent hemorrhage, or equine herpesvirus-1 myeloencephalopathy.
- Cloudy CSF may be due to high protein concentration, increased red blood cells, bacterial or fungal infection, epidural fat, or high white blood cell numbers in the fluid. Cytologic examination should help determine the cause of the turbidity.

- In equine protozoal myelitis (EPM):
  - Often shows no increase in either protein concentration or cell count.
  - In some cases, may be negative for antibodies against the causative organism on Western blot, immunofluorescent assay, or enzyme-linked immunoassay.
  - If clinical signs persist, testing should be repeated in 1 to 2 weeks to allow the antibodies to increase to a detectable level.
  - A positive test result for EPM increases the probability that a horse showing clinical signs likely has the disease.
  - Identification of an increase in the IgG index and albumin quotient provides further evidence that the organism has entered the CNS.

Normal findings and neurologic disease:
- A finding of normal CSF does not preclude the possibility of neurologic disease. The findings should be used along with the history and clinical signs demonstrated by the horse.
- Even in the face of obvious neurologic disease in a horse, the CSF may appear normal.
- Reasons for normal CSF in the face of neurologic disease may include:
  - Collection of the sample either too soon or too late after the onset of a disease.
  - Collection from a site too distant from the pathology in the CNS.
  - The signs may be a result of an extradural lesion such as vertebral stenosis, an extradural tumor, or a synovial cyst.

AUTHOR: **STEPHEN M. REED**

Cerebrospinal Fluid Collection

BASIC INFORMATION

SYNONYM(S)

- CSF tap
- Lumbar puncture

OVERVIEW AND GOAL(S)

Cerebrospinal fluid (CSF) is collected most often from the lumbosacral space in the horse because it can be done on an awake, standing animal with minimal risk to the patient.

INDICATIONS

The procedure is indicated when horses show signs of neurologic disease and the cause is not known. CSF analysis can also be useful when diagnostic procedures such as myelography are needed.

CONTRAINDICATIONS

The biggest contraindication is when the horse is too ataxic to tolerate standing while the procedure is performed or when the horse is too fractious to safely perform the procedure.

EQUIPMENT, ANESTHESIA

The standing lumbosacral procedure requires a safe, quiet location such as a stall or procedure room, tranquilization, local anesthetic, and a 6-inch, 18-gauge spinal needle with a stylet. Stocks may be used but are not preferred by the author.

ANTICIPATED TIME

The procedure normally requires about 10 minutes of preparation time and 10 minutes to complete the procedure.

PREPARATION: IMPORTANT CHECKPOINTS

The most important checkpoint is to know the anatomic landmarks and be deliberate but persistent in performing the procedure.

POSSIBLE COMPLICATIONS AND COMMON ERRORS TO BE AVOIDED

One of the most common problems identified with this procedure is to overtranquilize or to tranquilize too early. If the horse has its head in very ventral posture, it may be difficult to maintain adequate CSF pressure for the fluid to readily flow from the spinal needle.

PROCEDURE

The horse should stand squarely with weight bearing on all four limbs.
- Identify the lumbosacral space that is never further forward than the caudal limits of the tuber coxae.

- Palpate along the dorsal midline until the depression of the lumbosacral space is identified. Ultrasound guidance may help identify the space.
- The depression represents the caudal edge of the dorsal spine of the last lumbar vertebrae and the cranial edge of the sacrum as well as the medial sides of the left and right tuber sacrale.
- Block the skin and subcutaneous area with local anesthetic and perform a sterile scrub of the area.
- Tranquilize the horse and perform the procedure using an 6-inch, 18-gauge needle directed along the median plane.
- The subarachnoid space is identified at an approximate 5-inch depth.
- A slight popping will be noted when penetrating the lumbosacral interarcuate ligament due to a loss of resistance. If this is not felt, the needle can be slowly advanced until it hits the

floor of the canal and can then be slightly withdrawn.
- As the needle is advanced, the clinician's hands should rest comfortably on the animal's back to help steady and slowly advance the needle.
- To determine the correct location, remove the stylet and use a 5 to 6 mL syringe to apply gentle pressure.
- If CSF does not readily flow into the syringe, replace the stilette before advancing the needle.
- As soon as the dura is penetrated, stop and collect CSF in 5 to 6 mL syringes.

POSTPROCEDURE

Remove the needle and wipe the area with alcohol and rinse with warm water. Return the horse to its stall when the horse is alert enough walk.

AUTHOR: **STEPHEN M. REED**

Cervical Damage Repair

BASIC INFORMATION

SYNONYM(S)
- Cervical laceration repair
- Cervical muscle defect repair
- Cervical adhesion repair

OVERVIEW AND GOAL(S)
Repair cervical muscle defect in the mare to improve fertility.

INDICATIONS
Presence of cervical muscle defect or adhesion

CONTRAINDICATIONS
Fibrotic or malformed cervix

EQUIPMENT, ANESTHESIA
EQUIPMENT
- Equine stocks for restraint
- Modified Finochietto-type retractor with 28 cm detachable blades
- Long-handled instruments (Metzenbaum scissors, scalpel handle, needle drivers, suture scissors, Allison tissue forceps)
- Suture (no. 2 polyglactin 910, no. 0 polyglactin 910)
- Sterile 4 × 4 gauze

ANESTHESIA
- Sedation: Combination of detomidine (0.01–0.04 mg/kg) and xylazine (0.5–1.1 mg/kg) IM and IV
- Epidural: Xylazine (85 mg) and 2% lidocaine (20 mg) diluted to a total

volume of 6 mL with 0.9% sodium chloride administered into the epidural space

ANTICIPATED TIME
2 hours

PREPARATION: IMPORANT CHECKPOINTS
- Epidural in place
- Evacuate rectum of feces
- Sterile perineal preparation
- Open previous closed vulvoplasty (Caslick's) if present
- Procaine penicillin G (22,000 IU/kg IM)
- Gentamicin sulphate (6 mg/kg IV)
- Flunixin meglumine (1.1 mg/kg IV or PO)
- Tetanus toxoid (1 mL IM)

POSSIBLE COMPLICATIONS AND COMMON ERRORS TO BE AVOIDED
- Avoid removing excess cervical mucosa or muscle.
- Attempt repair when mare is in diestrus (under the influence of progesterone).

PROCEDURE
Surgical technique: Cervical muscle defect
- Place the modified Finochietto-type retractor with 28 cm detachable blades

in the vaginal vault and anchor to the base of the tail.
- Place 2 to 3 stay sutures of no. 2 polyglactin 910 on either side and across from the defect in the cervix to retract the cervix caudally.
- Long-handled instruments are necessary to perform the procedure in the vagina.
- Freshen the edges of the defect by incising or cutting along the edges of the defect from the external os of the cervix to beyond the cranial aspect of the lesion with a no. 10 scalpel blade or sharp, long-handle Metzenbaum scissors.
- A three-layer closure technique is used with no. 0 polyglactin 910.
  - Cervical lumen mucosa: Continuous horizontal mattress pattern
  - Cervical muscle: Simple continuous pattern
  - Vaginal mucosa layers: Simple continuous pattern

Surgical technique: Cervical adhesions
- The mare and perineal area are prepared as previously described.
- The cervical adhesion(s) are located by palpation per vagina and reduced by sharp or blunt dissection.
- Excess scar tissue may be trimmed as needed.

POSTPROCEDURE
- Flunixin meglumine (1.1 mg/kg IV or PO) q24h for 3 days.

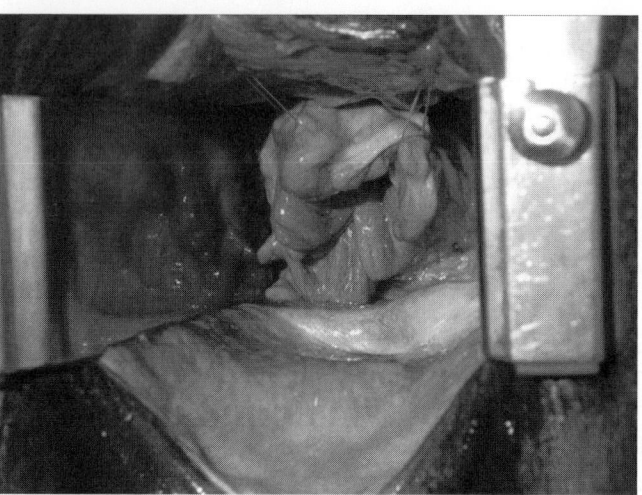

FIGURE 1 Cervix with stay sutures in place.

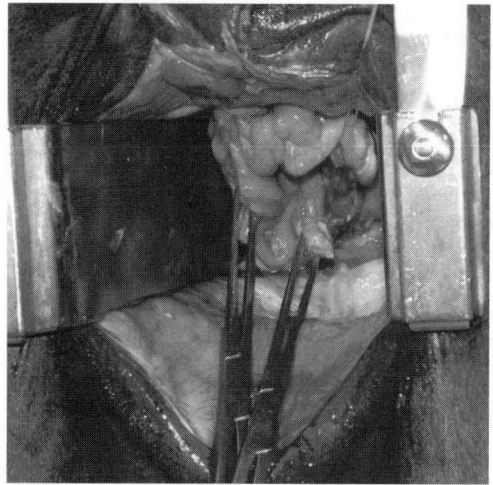

FIGURE 2 Freshening edges of the cervical muscle defect.

- Mares are returned to normal exercise and diet.
- Mares with cervical muscle defect repair are to have nothing per vagina for 3 weeks postoperatively.

- Mares treated for cervical adhesions are treated topically with nystatin/thiostrepton/neomycin sulphate/triamcinolone acetonide ointment once daily for 7 days or Seprafilm Adhesion

Barrier on days 4 and 8 postoperatively.

AUTHOR: **CHELSEA MAKOLSKI**

Clinical Pharmacokinetics and Pharmacodynamics

BASIC INFORMATION

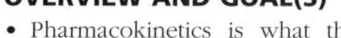

OVERVIEW AND GOAL(S)
- Pharmacokinetics is what the body does to the drug.
- Pharmacodynamics is what the drug does to the body, cell, or pathogen.

PROCEDURE
PHARMACOKINETICS
- ADME: Mathematical evaluation of the rates of drug absorption (A), distribution throughout the body (D), along with metabolism (M), and ultimate excretion from the body (E).
- Absorption
  ○ Indicates the process whereby drug is transferred from the site of administration to the systemic circulation.
  ○ An intravenously administered drug is 100% absorbed.
  ○ Bioavailability (F) is the fraction of the dose administered extravascular that reaches intact the systemic circulation.
    ■ Determined by comparing the area under the plasma drug concentration curve versus time (AUC) after extravascular (EV) administration to the AUC after intravenous (IV) administration.

$$F = (AUC_{ev}/AUC_{iv}) \times 100 = \% \text{ bioavailable}$$

  ■ If the EV AUC is significantly less than the IV AUC, then the drug dose must be adjusted for the EV route.

Adjusted dose = $dose_{iv}/F$

  ○ Reasons for low bioavailability of drugs in horses:
    ■ Extensive "first pass effect"
    ■ Poor dissolution of drug in gastrointestinal fluids
    ■ Drug instability in gastric juices
    ■ Transporter interactions (eg, ABCB1/MDR1/P-glycoprotein in intestine)
    ■ Drug interactions leading to poor solubility, enzyme induction
    ■ For IM or SC injections: Poor circulation at injection site, improper injection technique, insoluble complex formation
    ■ If a drug has a narrow therapeutic margin and the F is low, with substantial variation between horses, then there may be no ideal dose for that formulation.
    ■ The oral F for enrofloxacin in horses is approximately 50%, so suggested oral doses are twice the IV doses.
    ■ The oral F for ciprofloxacin is approximately 6%, so it is not feasible to use oral ciprofloxacin in horses.

- Drug distribution
  ○ Determined by the drug's ability to cross biologic membranes and reach tissues outside the systemic circulation.
  ○ Volume of distribution (Vd) (L/kg): The apparent volume of the body in which a drug is dissolved, but it does not correspond to any specific physiologic compartment.
  ○ Vd is used to calculate the dose of drug given to produce a desired plasma drug concentration, (eg, a loading dose).
  ○ Vd is determined by transporter function and the physical characteristics of the drug, including:
    ■ Protein binding
    ■ Ionization
    ■ Lipid solubility
    ■ Molecular size
  ○ Although Vd describes the extent of distribution of a drug, it does not confirm penetration of a drug to specific tissues.
    ■ When penetration into specific tissues is unknown, a large Vd drug (Vd > plasma volume) is more likely to distribute there than a low Vd drug.
  ○ Vd can change with specific physiologic or pathologic conditions.
    ■ Any condition that changes extracellular fluid volume affects the

plasma concentrations of drugs with low Vd values (eg, competition with endogenous substances for protein binding sites).

- Aminoglycosides and nonsteroidal antiinflammatory drugs (NSAIDs) have low Vd values and plasma concentrations and risks of toxicity are increased in dehydrated horses.
- Drugs with high Vds are not significantly affected by changes in body water status but may be affected by changes in body fat.
- Moxidectin distributes into fat, therefore higher plasma concentrations and a greater risk of toxicity are seen in foals or debilitated adult horses.

- Protein binding
  - Many drugs in circulation are bound to plasma proteins.
    - Albumin
    - Lipoprotein
    - Glycoprotein
  - If the protein binding is reversible, then a chemical equilibrium will exist between the bound and unbound states:

Protein + drug $\rightleftharpoons$ Protein-drug complex

  - Bound drug is too large to pass through biologic membranes, so only free drug is available for delivery to the tissues and to produce the desired pharmacologic action.
  - With few exceptions, only free drug is available for metabolism and excretion.
  - Bound drug may act as a drug reservoir or depot, from which the drug is slowly released as the unbound form.
    - Responsible for the long dosing interval for ceftiofur compared to other cephalosporins.
    - Drug-drug interactions from protein displacement are rarely clinically significant and typically do not require dosage adjustment.
    - Increased anticoagulant effects seen with concurrent administration of phenylbutazone and warfarin are due to inhibition of hepatic metabolism of warfarin from phenylbutazone and not from displacement from protein binding sites.
- Lipid solubility and drug ionization (the pH-partition hypothesis)
  - The degree of lipid solubility determines how readily a drug will cross biologic membranes.
  - Most drugs are weak acids or weak bases.
  - Ionized drug is hydrophilic and poorly lipid-soluble.

- Nonionized drug is lipophilic and can cross biologic membranes.
- The degree of ionization for a weak acid or weak base depends on the pKa of the drug and the pH of the surrounding fluid.
- It is calculated from the Henderson-Hasselbach equation:
  - For a weak acid: pH = pKa + log (ionized drug/nonionized drug)
  - For a weak base: pH = pKa + log (nonionized drug/ionized drug)
  - When the pH is equal to the pKa of the drug, then the drug is 50% ionized and 50% nonionized (log 1 = 0).
- Basic drugs can be "ion trapped" when they move from the plasma to sites where fluids are more acidic than plasma such as cerebrospinal fluid, milk, and infected tissues.

- Flip-flop kinetics
  - Oral and injectable "long-acting "drug formulations are often slowly absorbed into the systemic circulation.
  - This causes the drug elimination rate to be limited by the drug absorption rate.
  - Flip-flop kinetics is identified by comparing the plasma concentration versus time curve for the extravascular route of administration to the curve after the drug is given intravenously. If the slopes of the elimination phases are not parallel, then absorption is limiting elimination (Figure 1).
- Drug elimination
  - The irreversible removal of drug from the body by all routes of elimination.
  - Excretion is the removal of the intact drug.
  - Most drugs are excreted by the kidney into the urine.

- Drug can also be excreted into bile, sweat, saliva, or milk.
- Biotransformation or drug metabolism converts the drug in the body to a metabolite that is more readily excreted.
- Enzymes involved in biotransformation are mainly located in the liver.
- Other tissues such as the kidney, lung, small intestine, and skin also contain biotransformation enzymes.

- Clearance (Cl)
  - Measure of drug elimination from the body without reference to the mechanism of elimination.
  - Cl is the sum of all tissue clearances, where renal clearance (Cl_R) and hepatic clearance (Cl_H) are the major routes of elimination.
  - The body is considered a compartment of fluid with a definite volume (Vd) in which a drug is dissolved.
  - Cl is the volume of fluid containing drug that is cleared of drug per unit of time (ml/kg/min), calculated by:

$$Cl = Dose/AUC$$

- Renal clearance (Cl_R)
  - Includes glomerular filtration, active tubular secretion, and tubular reabsorption:

$$Cl_R = Cl_F + Cl_S - FR$$

  - Cl_F = clearance attributed to glomerular filtration
  - Cl_S = clearance attributed to active tubular secretion
  - FR = fraction reabsorbed from the tubule back to circulation
- Hepatic clearance (Cl_H)
  - Nonrenal drug elimination is due primarily to biotransformation (hepatic metabolism) and biliary excretion.
  - Hepatic clearance is determined by hepatic blood flow and the intrinsic ability of the liver to extract the drug.

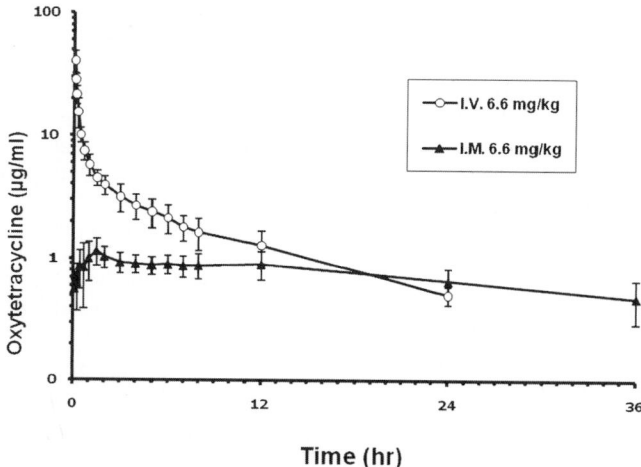

FIGURE 1 Flip-flop kinetics.

- First-pass effect: orally administered drugs may undergo presystemic metabolism in intestine, liver, and portal blood before being distributed to the rest of the body.
- Because of first-pass effects, lidocaine and diazepam cannot be administered orally.
- Hepatic metabolism
  - Necessary for removal of lipophilic drugs from the body. Depends on:
    - Activity of major drug metabolism enzymes
    - Hepatic volume (perfusion rate)
    - Drug accessibility to and extraction by hepatic metabolic enzyme sites
    - Physicochemical properties of the drug
  - Biotransformation of a parent drug results in metabolites that may be active or inactive themselves.
  - A prodrug is a drug administered in an inactive form, which must be biotransformed to its active form.
    - Prednisone is a prodrug for the active form prednisolone.
    - Enalapril is a prodrug for the active form enalaprilat.
  - Drug metabolic pathways are divided into phase I and phase II reactions.
    - Phase I reactions add or expose functional groups to/on the drug molecule necessary for phase II reactions.
    - Phase II reactions include conjugation reactions, which increase the water solubility of drugs, facilitating their excretion by the kidney.
    - Species differences in drug metabolic rates are the primary sources of variation in drug activity and toxicity.
- Induction and inhibition of metabolism
  - Metabolism can be affected by enzyme induction or inhibition by other drugs or chemicals.
  - A drug may alter its own metabolic fate by induction or inhibition.
  - Hepatic enzyme inducers can increase the rate of metabolism and hepatic clearance of concurrently administered drugs, typically resulting in a decreased pharmacologic effect.
    - Phenobarbital induces its own metabolism.
    - Rifampin induces the metabolism of azole antifungal drugs.
  - Hepatic induction is important in the pathogenesis of hepatotoxicity and therapeutic failure of many drugs.
  - Induction occurs slowly, requiring several weeks to reach maximum effect.

- Hepatic enzyme inhibition typically results in decreased hepatic clearance of concurrently administered drugs.
- Inhibition increases the potential for toxicity or for an exaggerated pharmacologic response.
  - Erythromycin and fluoroquinolones decrease the metabolism of theophylline, leading to neurotoxicity.
  - In contrast to induction, inhibition occurs rapidly (within 3–5 days).
- Elimination half-life
  - The elimination rate constant, k, is the sum of the drug eliminated by excretion and metabolism:

$$k = k_m + k_e$$

  - Elimination half-life ($t_{1/2}$) is the time required for drug concentration to decrease by one half in the matrix where it is measured:

$$t_{1/2} = 0.693/k$$

  - $t_{1/2}$ determines
    - Drug dosage interval
    - How long a toxic or pharmacologic effect will persist
    - Drug withdrawal times for performance horses
  - It is not the time for half of the administered dose to be eliminated.
  - Plasma half-life is influenced by the extent of drug distribution and clearance.
  - It takes 10 half-lives to eliminate 99.9% of drug from the plasma.
    - 0.1% may still be easily detected by medication control laboratories.
- Accumulation
  - To predict plasma drug concentrations, it is necessary to decide whether or not successive doses of a drug will have any effect on the previous dose.
  - As equal doses are given at a constant dosage interval, the plasma concentration-time curve plateaus and a "steady-state" is reached.
  - At steady-state, plasma drug concentrations fluctuate between a C_{max} (peak) and C_{min} (trough).
  - C_{max} and C_{min} are constant and remain unchanged from dose to dose.
  - Time to steady-state depends solely on the elimination half-life.
    - It takes approximately 6 half-lives to reach 99% steady-state levels.
- Dose and dosage frequency influence the values of C_{max} and C_{min} at steady-state.

- Dosage frequency and elimination half-life influences the fluctuation between C_{max} and C_{min}.
- Clinical consequences of dosage interval $<t_{1/2}$:
  - C_{max} at steady-state is greater than C_{max} after a single dose.
  - There is minimal fluctuation between C_{max} and C_{min}.
  - Missing a dose will not affect plasma concentrations greatly.
  - There is a lag time to reach the desired plasma concentration, and there will be a lag time for plasma concentration to change in response to a dose change.
- Clinical consequences of dosage interval $>t_{1/2}$:
  - C_{max} is less than when the dosage interval was $<t_{1/2}$.
    - As the dosage interval increases, C_{max} becomes closer in value to the C_{max} of a single dose.
    - If the dosage interval is >10 half-lives drug accumulation does not occur.
  - There is marked fluctuation between C_{max} and C_{min}.
  - Missing a dose will affect plasma concentrations greatly.
  - There is minimal lag time to achieve the desired plasma concentration.

PHARMACODYNAMICS
- Dose-effect relationships
  - For most drugs, action is crucially dependent on chemical structure as the drug "fits" into a specific cellular or subcellular receptor.
    - Very small structural changes have significant effects on drug activity.
    - The combination of a drug with its receptors starts a cascade of time-dependent biologic reactions.
  - Agonists interact with receptors to initiate the response.
  - Antagonists occupy the receptors without initiating the response while blocking the agonists from interaction with the receptors.
- Drug receptor interactions are categorized by:
  - Affinity: Attraction between a drug and a receptor
  - Efficacy: Quantifies the ability of agonists to induce a response
    - Full agonists: $e = 1$; cause maximal responses
    - Partial agonists: $0 < e < 1$
    - Pure antagonists: $e = 0$
  - Potency: The required drug concentration to cause a response
  - Sensitivity: The steepness of the concentration/dose-response curve
- Pharmacodynamic indices for antimicrobial drugs
  - Minimum inhibitory concentration (MIC): The lowest drug concentra-

tion that inhibits bacterial growth in vitro.
- Minimum bactericidal concentration (MBC): The lowest drug concentration that kills 99.9% of bacteria in vitro.
- Pharmacodynamic indices for other drugs
  - A wide range of endpoints can be used for evaluating drug effect, such as:
    - Physical responses: heart rate, respiratory rate, degree of swelling, lameness, stride length
    - Physiologic responses: depth of anesthesia, analgesia; changes in cell counts; changes in inflammatory exudate concentrations.

DOSAGE REGIMEN DESIGN
- Drug action depends on the concentration-time profile at the site of action.
- Although not identical to the plasma-concentration profile, typically there is a proportional relationship.
- PK/PD relationships for antimicrobials
  - PK parameters used are the area under the plasma concentration versus time curve (AUC) from 0 to 24 hours, the maximum plasma concentration (C_{max}), and the time (T) the antimicrobial concentration exceeds a defined PD threshold.
  - The most commonly used PD parameter is the bacterial MIC.
  - For concentration-dependent antimicrobials, high plasma concentrations relative to the MIC of the pathogen (C_{max}:MIC) and the area under the plasma concentration-time curve that is above the bacterial MIC during the dosage interval (area under the inhibitory curve, $AUC_{0\text{-}24\,hr}$:MIC) are the major predictors of clinical efficacy.
    - These PK/PD relationships are not independent, because as C_{max} increases, so does AUC.
    - For fluoroquinolones, clinical efficacy is associated with achieving either an $AUC_{0\text{-}24\,hr}$:MIC > 125 or a C_{max}:MIC > 10.
    - For aminoglycosides, achieving a C_{max}:MIC > 10 is considered optimal for efficacy.
    - Other antimicrobials that appear to have concentration-dependent activity include metronidazole and azithromycin.
  - For time-dependent antimicrobials, the time during which the antimicrobial concentration exceeds the MIC of the pathogen determines clinical efficacy (T > MIC).
    - Penicillins, cephalosporins, macrolides, tetracycline, chloramphenicol, and potentiated sulfonamides are time-dependent.

- How much above the MIC and for what percentage of the dosing interval concentrations should be above the MIC is specific to individual bacteria-drug combinations.
  - Exceeding the MIC by 1 to 5 multiples for between 40% to 100% of the dosage interval is appropriate for most time-dependent killers.
  - T>MIC should be closer to 100% for bacteriostatic drugs and for patients that are immunosuppressed.
- PK/PD relationships for NSAIDs
  - Plasma concentrations of NSAIDs and their actions at the molecular level are not in phase, with action lagging behind concentration.
  - The delay is primarily due to the time between cyclo-oxygenase (COX) inhibition and reduction in the concentration of the marker eicosanoids.
  - A wide range of PD parameters are assessed and used in dosage determination.
- Efficacy: Change in lameness, stride length, swelling, heat, inhibition of inflammatory mediators
- Potency: Relationship of dose to effect
  - COX-1:COX-2 inhibition ratios
  - Sensitivity: Slope of the concentration-response curve

THERAPEUTIC DRUG MONITORING (TDM)
- The drugs for which TDM is commonly used are characterized by:
  - Serious toxicity (eg, digoxin, phenobarbital)
  - A steep dose-response curve, where a small increase in dose can cause a marked increase or decrease in response (eg, theophylline)
  - Marked PK variability between individual patients so that dose is poorly predictive of plasma drug concentration (eg, phenobarbital)
  - Easily saturated elimination mechanisms that lead to nonlinear kinetics
  - Cost of therapy justifies confirming a desired plasma drug concentration
- Performing therapeutic drug monitoring
  - Submit samples when plasma drug concentrations have reached steady-state in the patient (approximately 6 half-lives).
  - When steady-state concentrations must be reached immediately, a loading dose ($Dose_l$) can be administered:

$$Dose_l = Dose_m / (1 - e^{-k\tau})$$

- $Dose_m$ is the maintenance dose
- κ is the elimination rate constant (or $0.693/t_{1/2}$)
- τ is the dosage interval in the same units as $t_{1/2}$
- The risk of adverse drug reactions is obviously increased with a loading dose, so TDM can be used to proactively determine the proper maintenance dose.
- When administering a loading dose, TDM should be done after the loading dose to establish a baseline.
- The second time should be at one drug administration interval later to ensure that the maintenance dose is able to maintain the concentrations achieved by the loading dose.
- If the drug concentrations at the second sample do not match the first sample, the maintenance dose can be adjusted at this time rather than waiting the usual recommended time period, with the risk of therapeutic failure or toxicity.
- For the aminoglycosides, TDM is performed on C_{max} and C_{min} samples to determine the appropriate dosing regimen.
- The C_{max} is correlated with antimicrobial efficacy and the C_{min} is correlated with nephrotoxicity.
- To allow for the distribution phase, blood sampling for the peak concentration is done at 0.5 to 1 hour after administration and the trough sample is usually taken prior to the next dose.
- The peak and trough concentrations can then be used to estimate the terminal half-life for the individual patient.
- An increase in the elimination half-life during therapy is a very sensitive indicator of early tubular insult.
- If using a once-daily dosage regimen, a blood sample just prior to the next dose will be well below the recommended trough concentrations and may even be below the limit of detection of the assay. For these patients, an 8-hour postdose sample will provide a more accurate estimate of the terminal half-life.
- Serum concentrations should be 0.5 to 2 µg/mL before the next dose for gentamicin or less than 6 µg/mL for amikacin.

SUGGESTED READING

Lees P, Cunningham FM, Elliot J: Principles of pharmacodynamics and their applications in veterinary pharmacology. *J Vet Pharmacol Ther* 27:397–414, 2004.

Lees P, Giraudel J, Landoni MF, et al: PK-PD integration and PK-PD modeling of nonsteroidal anti-inflammatory drugs: principles and applications in veterinary pharmacology. *J Vet Pharmacol Ther* 27:491–502, 2004.

Lees P, Landoni MF, Giraudel J, et al: Pharmacodynamics and pharmacokinetics of non-steroidal anti-inflammatory drugs in species of veterinary interest. *J Vet Pharmacol Ther* 27:479–490, 2004.

McKellar QA, Sanchez Bruni SF, Jones DG: Pharmacokinetic/pharmacodynamic relationships of antimicrobial drugs used in veterinary medicine. *J Vet Pharmacol Ther* 27:503–514, 2004.

Toutain PL, Lees P: Integration and modeling of pharmacokinetic and pharmacodynamic data to optimize dosage regimens in veterinary medicine. *J Vet Pharmacol Ther* 27:467–477, 2004.

AUTHORS: **PATRICIA M. DOWLING** and **FRANCESCA SAMPIERI**

EDITOR: **PATRICIA M. DOWLING**

Colostrum Banking

BASIC INFORMATION

OVERVIEW AND GOAL(S)

Colostrum is essential to the neonatal foal as a source of immunoglobulins. Foals that fail to obtain the necessary colostrum from their own dams can be successfully supplemented with the colostrum of another mare, provided this occurs within the immediate neonatal period, when the foal is still capable of immunoglobulin (Ig) G absorption. It is therefore useful to store a supply of good quality colostrum in advance because mares producing colostrum are not always immediately available.

INDICATIONS

Colostrum can be collected and stored from any foaling mare, provided it is of good or excellent quality.

CONTRAINDICATIONS

- Mares producing deficient colostrum. This occurs most often in maiden mares or those that begin lactation prematurely, but can occur in any mare.
- Mares known to have produced foals affected with neonatal isoerythrolysis, or mares that have tested positive for red cell alloantibodies.
- Mares nursing weak foals that may require more colostrum to thrive.

MARE SELECTION AND PREPARATION

Foaling mares selected for colostrum harvesting should be of second parity or greater and should have received booster vaccinations at 30 days before foaling.

POSSIBLE COMPLICATIONS AND COMMON ERRORS TO BE AVOIDED

- The dam's own foal must be allowed to nurse sufficiently before colostrum removal.
- Colostrum must be collected within 3 hours of parturition because IgG levels decline with time.
- Colostrum must be tested before banking to ensure adequate IgG levels. When measured by a direct assay,

only colostrum with greater than 1000 mg IgG/dL should be saved for use. A colostrometer or Brix refractometer can also be used to measure IgG levels indirectly. Alternatively, a bioassay may be used in which colostrum is only saved if the foal's serum IgG levels reach at least 800 mg/dL.

- Colostrum should be tested for the presence of hemolytic antibodies and should be discarded if results are positive.

PROCEDURE

- Milk approximately 500 to 600 mL of colostrum from one side of the mare's udder. The remaining side should be reserved for the nursing foal; if the foal was lost during parturition, the entire quantity of colostrum can be harvested.
- Filter the collected colostrum through a cheesecloth, milk filter, or gauze to remove debris.
- Store the colostrum in a durable, plastic container with a lid. Label the container with the date of collection, name of mare, and quality of colostrum (mg IgG/dL).
- The colostrum can be frozen at −17° C and stored for up to 2 years; for short-term use it can be stored in the refrigerator for several hours.

USE OF BANKED COLOSTRUM

- Colostrum should be thawed in a water bath at approximately 37.5° C. Excessively high temperatures will cause denaturation of immunoglobulin proteins.
- Colostrum should be administered to the foal within 16 to 18 hours of birth and is most effective when administered before 12 hours. Nasogastric intubation is recommended over bottle feeding due to the risk of aspiration pneumonia, particularly in foals with poor or low suckling reflex.
- The amount of colostrum needed depends on both the quality of colostrum and the degree of failure of passive transfer in the foal. An average 50 kg foal with complete failure of passive transfer will require

96,000 mg IgG to reach plasma levels of 400 mg IgG/dL.

- Colostrum should be administered several times if needed at intervals of 40 to 60 minutes. A 50 kg foal will tolerate approximately 400 to 500 mL at a time.
- Plasma IgG of the foal should be tested 8 to 12 hours after colostrum administration.

ALTERNATIVES AND THEIR RELATIVE MERITS

- Plasma transfusion can be used to provide the IgG requirements for a foal affected with failure of passive transfer, and is especially useful in those greater than 16 to 18 hours of age that can no longer absorb IgG through the gut. Supplemental colostrum in foals less than 16 hours of age is recommended over plasma transfusion because it provides additional IgM and IgA antibodies.
- Bovine colostrum has been used as an alternative to equine colostrum. Bovine IgM and IgG are both readily absorbed by the foal; however, they have a shortened half-life in circulation compared with equine immunoglobulins. In addition, bovine colostrum is unlikely to protect the foal against some equine pathogens.
- Equine colostrum supplements consisting of concentrated serum or IgG are commercially available. Preliminary investigations of these products have shown that they are ineffective in raising serum IgG levels above 800 mg/dL in normal foals nursing from mares with suboptimal colostrum. Their use is not recommended as a replacement for colostrum.

SUGGESTED READING

Perryman L: Diseases of the immune system. In Colahan P, Mayhew IG, Merritt A, et al (eds). Equine medicine and surgery, vol II, ed 5, St Louis, 1999, Mosby, pp 2034–2040.

Vivrette SL, Young K, Manning S, et al: Efficacy of Seramune in the treatment of failure of passive transfer in foals. *Proc Am Assoc Equine Pract* 44:136–137, 1999.

AUTHOR: **ALANA KING**

Computed Tomography: Dental Disease

BASIC INFORMATION

SYNONYM(S)

CT
Computed axial tomography
CAT scan

OVERVIEW AND GOAL(S)

- Computed tomography (CT) is a cross sectional x-ray imaging modality.
  - Cross-sectional images eliminate the problems encountered in radiograph interpretation that are caused by superimposition of the complex anatomy of the skull.
  - Uses x-ray technology so the gray shades within the images represent variations in tissue density making it an excellent modality for the evaluation of osseous and dental tissues.
  - Provides information to complement or enhance the clinical and radiographic examinations.

INDICATIONS

- CT is indicated anytime information is needed to augment the clinical, oral, and radiographic examinations.
  - Most commonly used when dental abnormalities are complicated by secondary disease such as osteomyelitis or sinusitis, granuloma or cementoma formation, or osseous deformation.
  - Used to identify abnormalities that are sufficiently subtle to be unidentifiable by more routinely available techniques such as radiography.
  - Exceedingly useful when further characterization of the disease is

necessary for planning treatments such as surgery of the supporting structures (sinus flap) or dental-related procedures (extraction, endodontic therapies).

CONTRAINDICATIONS

- There are no reported contraindications for CT.
- Contraindications are limited to contraindications for general anesthesia and/or heavy sedation (where standing CT is available).

EQUIPMENT, ANESTHESIA

- CT scanner: helical scanning is preferable for dental disease.
- Equine CT table: A table linked to the CT scanner capable of supporting a horse is necessary.
- Trained technical or veterinary staff: To position the horse and prescribe the CT scan acquisitions.
- Viewing station: A workstation equipped with high-quality monitors and appropriate software.
- General anesthesia: Routine methods of induction, maintenance, and recovery are needed. Anesthetic agents should be suitable for maintaining the horse for a 20- to 60-minute procedure.
- CT scanners capable of imaging the standing sedated horse are infrequently available. These scanners require that the horse be sedated.

ANTICIPATED TIME

10 to 60 minutes. The scan time is dependent on the speed of the CT scanner. The

actual time to acquire images with a modern helical scanner is approximately 60 to 120 seconds for the entire skull. The remaining time allotted is for positioning and acquisition planning.

PREPARATION: IMPORTANT CHECKPOINTS

- Calibration and warm up of the CT scanner.
- Check function of the scanner and table.
- General anesthesia.
- Positioning: dorsal recumbency, the skull must be positioned so that midline is parallel to the central axis of the CT scanner (Figure 1).

POSSIBLE COMPLICATIONS AND COMMON ERRORS TO BE AVOIDED

Improper positioning causes artefacts that confound CT image interpretation.

PROCEDURE

- Acquire scout or pilot images (Figure 2).
- Use the scout images to plan the CT scan.
- Obtain images through the entire arcade of interest. For some scanners this may require obtaining images 5- to 10-mm thick.
- Obtain additional 1- to 2-mm images through the abnormal regions.
- Consider repeating the scan after the administration of systemic contrast media.

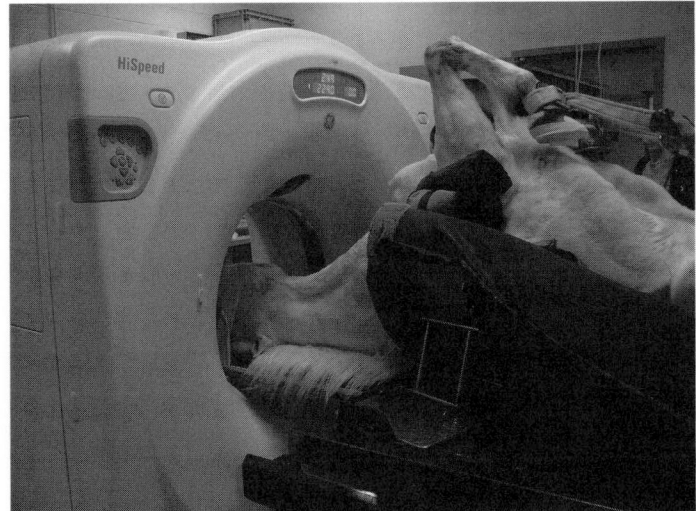

FIGURE 1 A horse is positioned in dorsal recumbency within the gantry of the CT scanner.

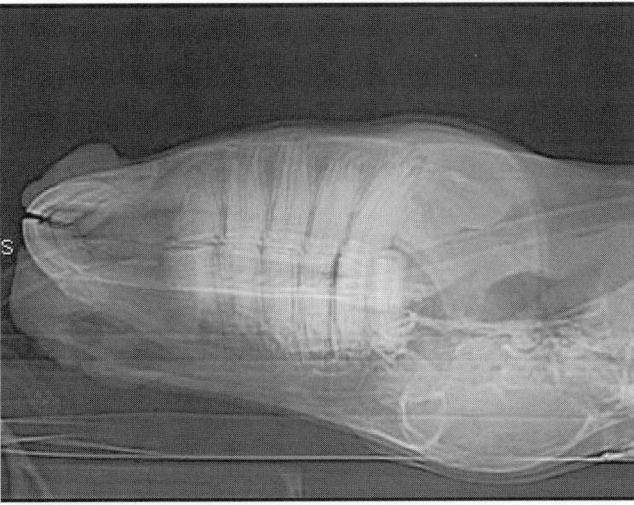

FIGURE 2 A scout image is acquired to plan the remainder of the CT scan.

POSTPROCEDURE

Routine postanesthetic monitoring should be observed.

ALTERNATIVES AND THEIR RELATIVE MERITS

- Magnetic resonance imaging (MRI) is an alternative cross-sectional imaging modality.
  - Yields excellent soft tissue contrast resolution, which allows for the evaluation of associated soft tissue inflammatory or infectious pathology.
  - Hard tissues (bone and dental) yield a signal void (black signal) on MRI images and variations in bone density or dental tissue density cannot be identified. Information about these tissues must be inferred from changes in bone fluid signal as in osteomyelitis or shape change of bone or dental structures.
- Nuclear medicine has been used successfully for the identification and characterization of some equine dental diseases.
  - Uses a phosphate analogue (methylene diphosphonate) attached to a radioactive substance (technetium 99m) and a gamma camera to produce images.
  - The radiopharmaceutical accumulates in areas of increased bone metabolism and these areas are mapped by the gamma camera.
  - Very sensitive for detecting osseous abnormalities of the skeletal structures supporting the dentition, but it is not specific.
  - Infectious or inflammatory bone pathology cannot be distinguished from traumatic pathology such as fracture.
  - Dental tissues (cementum, enamel, or dentin) do not incorporate the radiopharmaceutical and so the teeth are not imaged within the practical limits associated with the radioactive material. The dental abnormalities must be inferred by the changes in the surrounding structures.

AUTHOR: **SARAH M. PUCHALSKI**

Computed Tomography: Musculoskeletal

BASIC INFORMATION

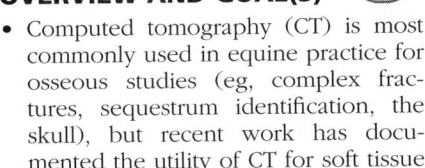

OVERVIEW AND GOAL(S)

- Computed tomography (CT) is most commonly used in equine practice for osseous studies (eg, complex fractures, sequestrum identification, the skull), but recent work has documented the utility of CT for soft tissue evaluation.
- The relatively small size of the CT opening (gantry or bore) limits usefulness to the extremities, from the carpus and tarsus distally, the skull, and proximal to mid-cervical spine, in most adult horses. In addition, special tables are required for adult horses because the limit for most CT scanners is around 400 lb.
- CT uses a rotating x-ray tube to produce axial (transverse or cross-sectional) tomographic images of the patient as the CT table advances in predetermined small distances after each slice of data acquisition. These axial images are organized into spatially consecutive, parallel image sections (tomographic slices).
- Reconstruction of axial CT images into sagittal or dorsal image planes is possible. Reconstructions into any plane necessary for image analysis are also possible, including three-dimensional images. This is unlike magnetic resonance imaging (MRI), in which each image plane must be acquired separately, increasing the time of MRI studies relative to CT.
- In CT, a computer stores x-ray attenuation data and generates a matrix of picture elements termed *pixels*. The x-ray attenuation data of each pixel are represented as a shade of gray.
- Each shade of gray is assigned a CT number in Hounsfield units (HU). In this scale, water is equal to 0 HU, pure air is equal to −1000 HU, and cortical bone is 1000 HU or greater. The density level of almost all soft tissue organs is between 10 and 90 HUs.
- The viewed CT image is thus composed of a series of pixels forming the matrix; the matrix is a square series of pixels forming the field of view (FOV). Typical matrix size for CT scanners is 512 × 512 pixels, or more than 260,000 pixels comprising the image.
- Because CT acquires tomographic slices, each pixel actually represents a small volume of tissue, a *voxel*. For example, a 1 × 1 mm pixel may represent a 1 × 1 × 10 mm volume of tissue if the tomographic slice is 10 mm thick. It is important to remember that matrix size and slice thickness are responsible in large part for image resolution; each pixel (and therefore voxel) can only represent one particular HU value (only one shade of gray).
- There are two types of image resolution that are important: spatial resolution and contrast resolution. Spatial resolution is the ability to differentiate small anatomic structures from one another. CT excels in spatial resolution. Conversely, MRI has much better tissue contrast resolution than CT. This is why MRI has become the standard for orthopedic injuries and neurologic disease in human and veterinary medicine.
- CT is capable of differentiating 3000 to 4000 levels of HUs. The viewing monitor can display a maximum of 256 gray tones at one time, whereas the human eye is able to discriminate only about 20.
- CT displays of various tissues and regional anatomy are therefore selected and enhanced by operator-adjustable viewing parameters, termed *window level* and *window width*. Adjusting the gray scale is a feature of CT that allows viewing a large range of tissues from a single acquisition series. This is unlike MRI, in which multiple sequences must be obtained to view various tissues and tissue characteristics. This is one reason why CT studies typically require much less time to acquire than MRI studies.
- The window level (L) is the center point of HU value display. Window level should be set close to the mean density level of the tissue to be critically examined. The window width (W) is a range of HU values displayed and influences the contrast of the image.
- Commonly used terminology includes "bone window" when window and level are set to maximize bone detail and "soft tissue" window when parameters are set to maximize soft tissue differentiation (Figure 1).

EQUIPMENT, ANESTHESIA

Positioning:

- The patient is typically positioned in lateral recumbency, usually with the limb of interest dependent to minimize respiratory motion.
- Initial pilot images ("scout films") are made to center the limb and position

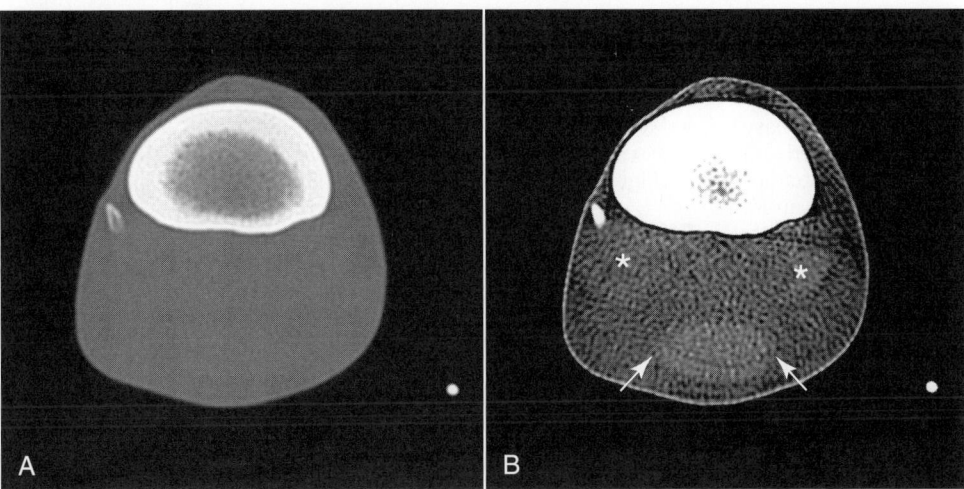

FIGURE 1 Effects of window width and window level settings when viewing CT images. Axial image of the distal third metacarpus. **A,** Bone window width (3000 HU) and level (450 HU). Note the exquisite detail of the cortical and trabecular bone. The palmar soft tissues cannot be differentiated from one another. **B,** Same image as **A** but viewed in a soft tissue window width (300 HU) and level (150 HU). The superficial digital and deep digital flexor tendons can be seen (*arrows*); the branches of the proximal suspensory ligament (*asterisk*) are poorly demarcated. Note that third metacarpal bone is now viewed as nearly solid bone; the trabecular medullary tissue is not differentiated from cortical bone.

it perpendicular to the plane of gantry/ table translation.

Equipment:

- In conventional CT, a series of equally spaced images (tomographic slices) is acquired sequentially through a specific region. The x-ray attenuation data are obtained on a slice-by-slice basis, with the CT table advancing by predetermined set distances after each slice data acquisition.
  - Table translation: Requires a specialized table that can support and translate a patient weighing more than 1000 lb through the gantry since equine CT uses equipment designed for human patients. Several vendors have developed such tables.
  - Gantry translation: This type of CT scanner does not require a specialized table to move the patient. Rather, the gantry (containing the x-ray tube) translates along the long axis of the imaged region. These scanners (eg, Philips Tomoscan) were commonly used for equine applications because any equine transport table could be used to obtain CT images. The downside to the Tomoscan CT is that it uses relatively low mA (10 to 30 mA), resulting in images that have lower signal to noise ratio and thus more "noise."
- Types of CT scanners:
  - Axial (single slice) versus helical (spiral) systems:
    - Axial: Obtain one slice of acquisition before translation. Nonhelical scanners are typically slower in acquisition.
    - Helical: Perform a continuous (spiral) acquisition. Helical

systems have faster acquisition times and typically produce a smoother volume reconstruction.
  - Single-row versus multiple-row detectors:
    - Single-row detector CT scanners acquire a single axial slice per gantry revolution. These may be helical or nonhelical in design.
    - Multiple-row detectors acquire multiple axial slices in a single gantry rotation. This allows very rapid image acquisition.
    - Multiple-row detector CT units provide the ultimate in resolution of multiple plane and volume reconstructions, essentially equal to native axial image resolution.
    - Depending on the manufacturer, design, and generation, multiple-row CT scanners are capable of 4 to 64 or even more slices per each gantry revolution. This allows CT images of large anatomic areas to be acquired in as little as several seconds in some instances.

PREPARATION: IMPORTANT CHECKPOINTS

- General anesthesia is required for the CT examination.
- Metal (eg, shoes) needs to be removed from the area to be examined. Anatomic areas of interest that contain metallic implants will be poorly visualized due to x-ray beam hardening artifact.
- Dirt and debris should be removed from the haircoat and hoof wall.
- Any iodine-based cleaners or medications should be avoided due to their highly attenuating properties.

PROCEDURE

- Slice thickness (termed *collimation*) will vary depending on anatomic region and may range from as thin as 1 mm to as thick as 10 cm.
- Thinner slices allow greater spatial resolution, but the tradeoff is longer scan times.
- A minimum slice thickness is required to maintain a reasonable signal to noise ratio. This minimum value is machine dependent but usually 1 to 2 mm.
- Thicker slices yield faster scan times but offer less resolution because of slice thickness averaging.
- Axial images can be obtained in a continuous (contiguous slices) or overlapped fashion (nonhelical systems). Overlap of the acquisition improves the smoothness of reconstruction.
- The amount of overlap in helical systems is defined by *pitch*. It has been determined that a pitch of 1.4 is optimal for reconstruction while maintaining the speed of acquisition.
- Higher kVp and mAs yield the best CT images. Typical high-quality scan parameters would be 120–150 kVp at 100 mAs or higher.
- Regional limb perfusion with iodinated contrast material has been used in recent research to view and characterize soft tissue abnormalities of the equine limb. This typically requires specialized injectors.

POSTPROCEDURE

- Evaluation of CT images is somewhat intuitive because of familiarity with evaluation of radiographs; radiographs and CT images are both created by x-ray interaction with the patient so it is easy to evaluate air, fat, soft tissues, and bony structures.

- The cross-sectional nature of CT makes interpretation relatively easy since there are no interfering overlying structures as when viewing a radiograph. CT typically shows a more extensive nature of radiographically identified lesions or identifies pathology not seen on radiographs.
- However, unfamiliarity with cross-sectional anatomy may be challenging, and anatomic references become a commonly used resource.
- CT images are routinely viewed one slice at a time, but often in fairly rapid succession, like a slow-moving movie. Scrolling back and forth is very helpful in gaining a three-dimensional understanding of the pathology.
- Evaluation of CT images with bone and soft tissue must be performed at different window settings for each tissue type, as explained above (see Figure 1).

- Evaluation of complex fractures is greatly simplified compared with radiography, given the nature of the modality.
- Multiplanar reformatting is valuable in assessment of tomographic images (Figures 2 and 3).

SUGGESTED READING

Collins JN, Galuppo LD, Thomas HL, et al: Use of computed tomography angiography to evaluate the vascular anatomy of the distal portion of the forelimb of horses. *Am J Vet Res* 65:1409–1420, 2004.

Hanson JA, Seeherman HJ, Kirker-Head CA, et al: The role of computed tomography in evaluation of subchondral osseous lesions in seven horses with chronic synovitis. *Equine Vet J* 28(6):480–488, 1996.

Puchalski SM: Computed tomography in equine practice. *Equine Vet Educ* 19(4):207–209, 2007.

Puchalski SM, Snyder JR, Hornof WJ, et al: Contrast enhanced computed tomography of the equine distal extremity. *Proc Am Assoc Equine Pract* 51:389–394, 2005.

Rose PL, Seeherman H, O'Callaghan M: Computed tomographic evaluation of comminuted middle phalangeal fractures in the horse. *Vet Radiol Ultrasound* 38(6):424–429, 1997.

Thrall D: *Textbook of veterinary diagnostic radiology*, ed 5, St Louis, 2007, Saunders Elsevier.

Tomlinson JE, Redding WR, Berry C, et al: Computed tomographic anatomy of the equine tarsus. *Vet Radiol Ultrasound* 44(2):174–178, 2003.

Tucker RL, Sande RD: Computed tomography and magnetic resonance imaging of the equine musculoskeletal conditions. *Vet Clin North Am Equine Pract* 17(1):145–157, 2001.

Whitton RC, Buckley C, Donovan T, et al: The diagnosis of lameness associated with distal limb pathology in a horse: a comparison of radiography, computed tomography and magnetic resonance imaging. *Vet J* 155(3):223–229, 1998.

AUTHORS: **JOHN S. MATTOON, JASON W. BRUMITT, JONATHAN HAYLES, DANA A. NEELIS, GREGORY D. ROBERTS,** and **TOM WILKINSON**

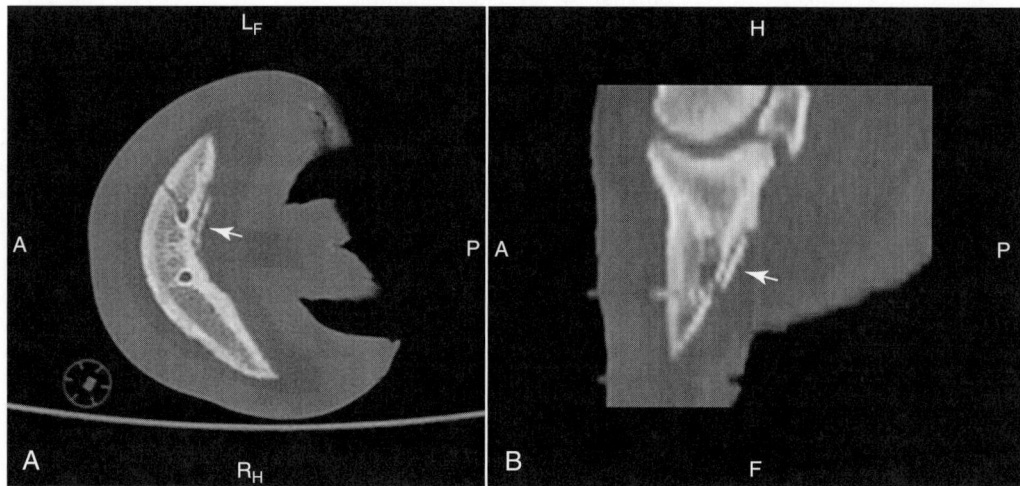

FIGURE 2 Axial and sagittal reconstruction CT images of a sequestrum of the third phalynx. **A,** Axial CT image of the foot showing the small sliver of sequestered bone (*arrow*). The sequestrum could not be seen on radiographs. **B,** Reconstruction from the axial image data shows the sequestrum in sagittal plane (*arrow*). Note the sagittal reconstruction has less detail than the axial image, with slight blurriness and a "notchiness" not seen in the original axial image. This is a fundamental problem with reconstructions from single-slice CT data acquisition (both axial and helical). Reconstruction images made from multidetector CT units do not show image degradation. Images are shown with a window width of 2500 HU and window level of 450 HU.

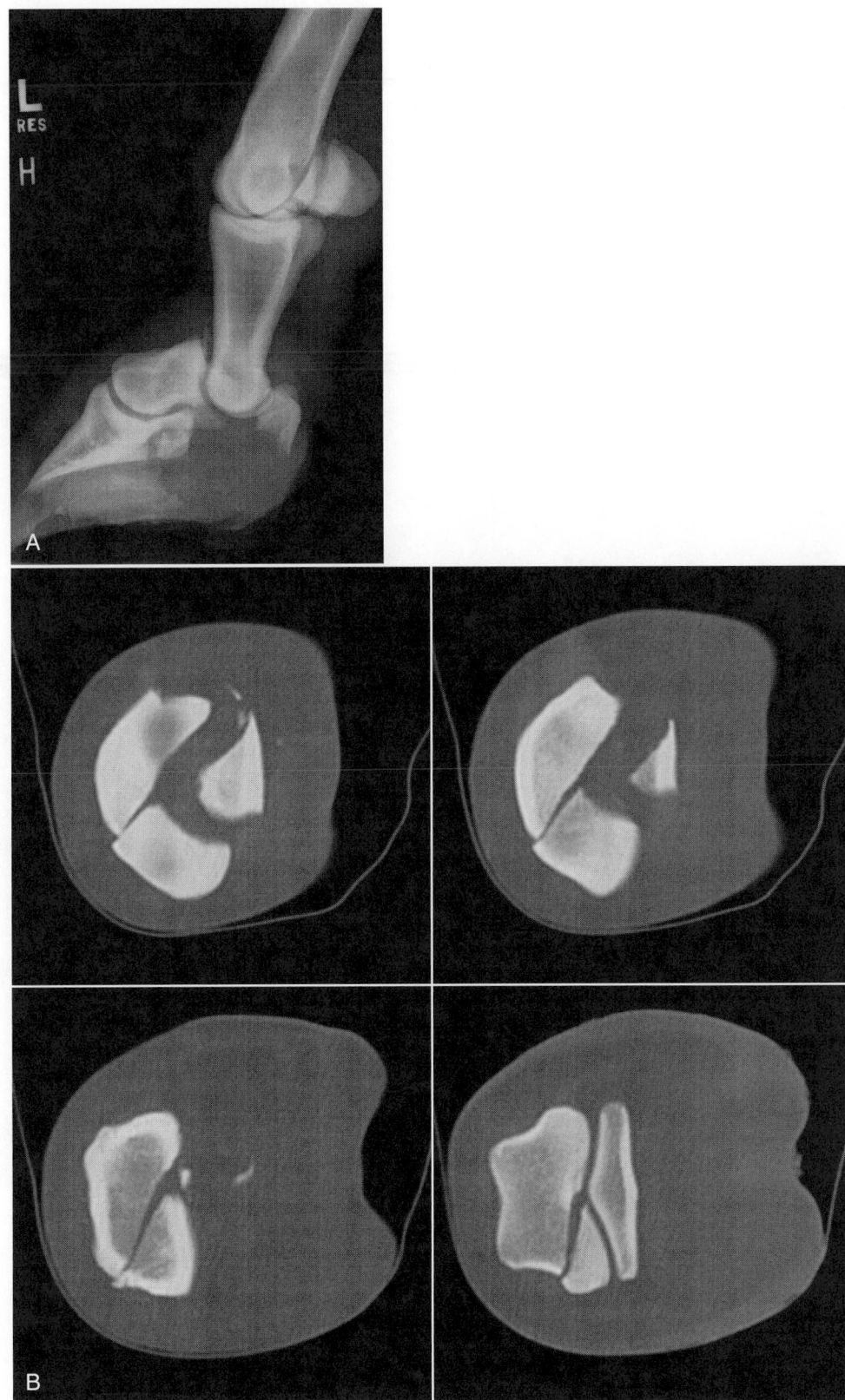

FIGURE 3 Complex second phalynx fracture. **A,** Lateral radiograph of second phalynx fracture of the left hindlimb. **B, 1** to **4,** Selected axial CT images of second phalynx fracture from proximal to distal.

Continued

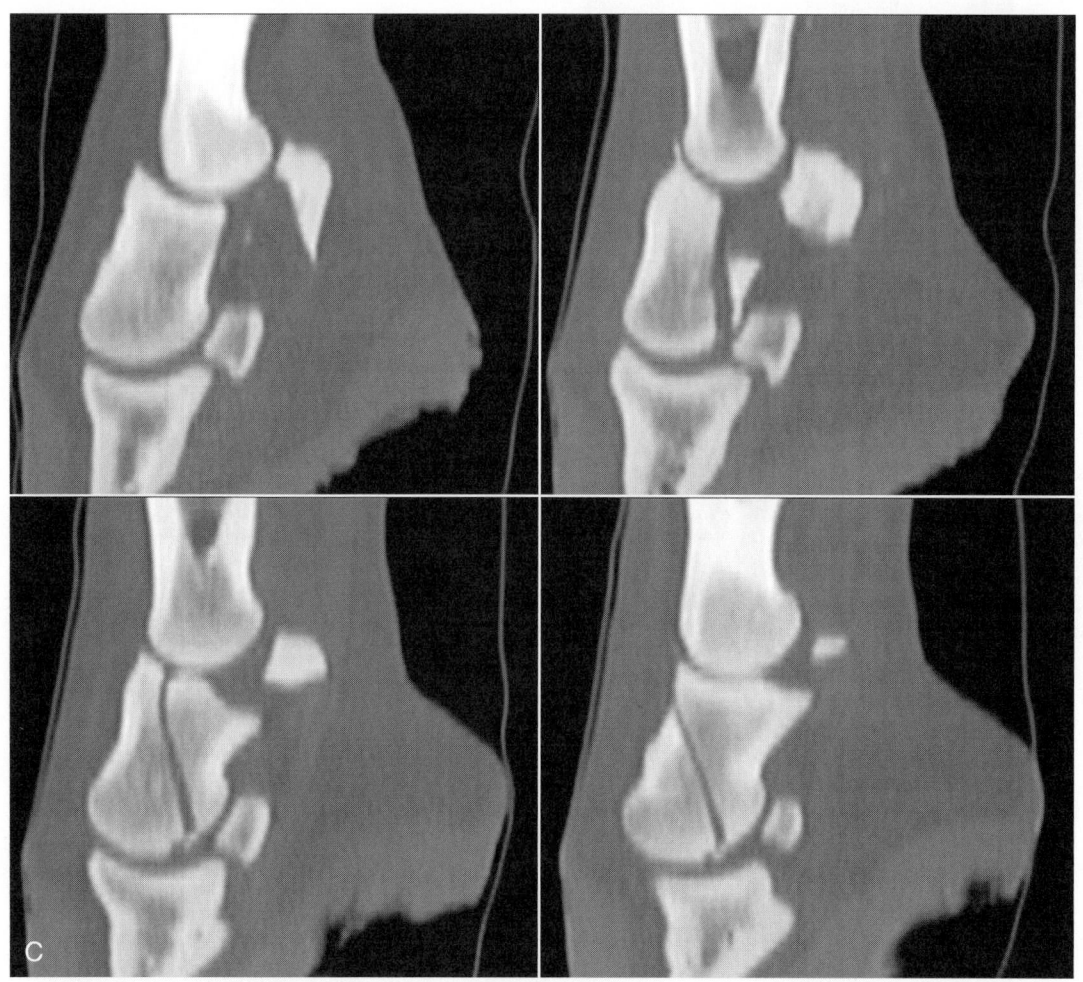

FIGURE 3, cont'd C, 1 to 4, Selected sagittal reconstruction CT images of second phalynx fracture.

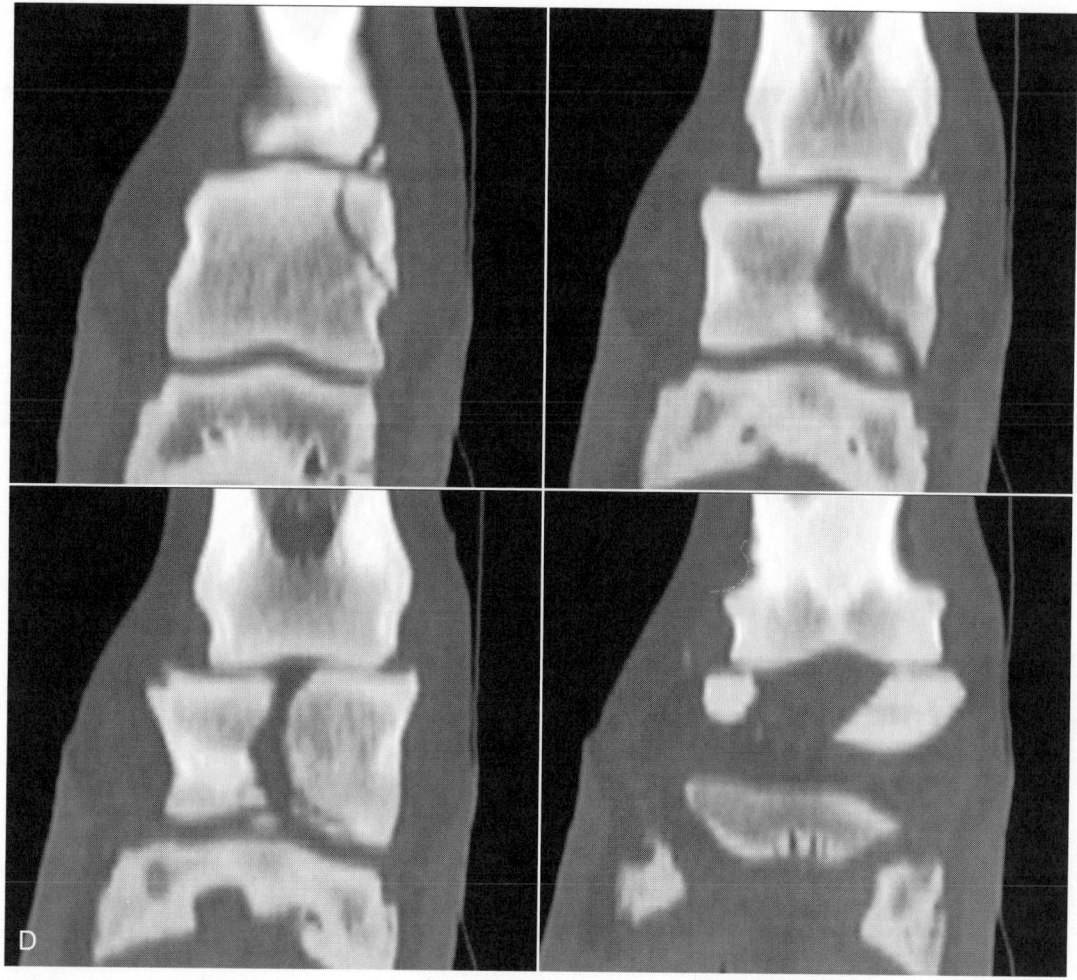

FIGURE 3, cont'd D, 1 to 4, Selected dorsal reconstruction images of second phalynx fracture from dorsal to plantar. The axial images were made using 3 mm slices with 1 mm overlap. The 1 mm overlap allows a smoother and more representative reconstruction than contiguous slices. Note that the sagittal reconstructions are smoother than the sagittal reconstruction shown in Figure 2, *B*. Not all slices are shown. Images are shown with a window width of 3000 HU and a window level of 600 HU.

Dental Nerve Blocks

BASIC INFORMATION

SYNONYM(S)

Perineural analgesia

OVERVIEW AND GOAL(S)

To provide analgesia to the relevant branches of the fifth cranial nerve (trigeminal nerve) for invasive dental and surgical techniques

INDICATIONS

For use in exodontia, sinus surgery, periodontal treatments, and fracture repair

CONTRAINDICATIONS

None

EQUIPMENT, ANESTHESIA

- 20-gauge 1.5-inch needles, 20-gauge 3.5-inch needles, and 20-gauge 9-inch spinal needles
- 3, 5, and 12 mL syringes
- Anesthetic agent: Lidocaine 2%, mepivacaine 2%, or bupivacaine 0.75%

ANTICIPATED TIME

5 minutes

PREPARATION: IMPORANT CHECKPOINTS

The maxillary nerve block is the only perineural injection that the author treats as a joint injection. The site is aseptically prepared, sterile gloves are worn, and sterile technique is rigidly followed.

POSSIBLE COMPLICATIONS AND COMMON ERRORS TO BE AVOIDED

Anatomically, nerve tissues parallel vascular tissue, and the maxillary and mandibular nerves are no different. Therefore hemorrhage may occur due to inadvertent puncture of these large vessels. Because of the position of these structures, it is unlikely that significant external blood loss will be appreciated; however, in the case of the maxillary nerve, hemorrhage may lead to exophthalmos and possibly a retrobulbar abscess. Therefore clients should be forewarned of the risk and aseptic technique should be adhered to during the procedure.

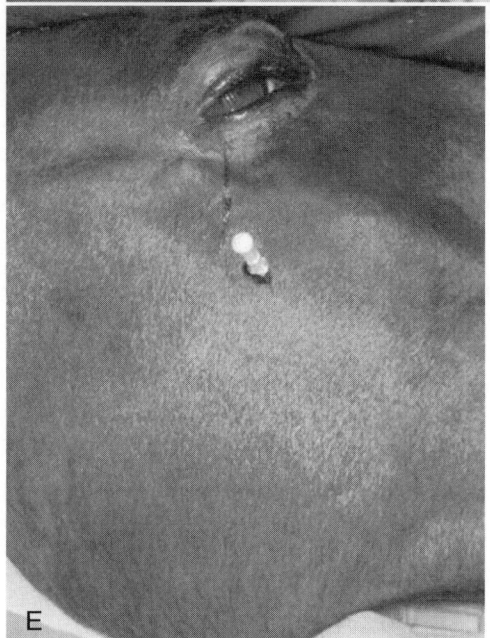

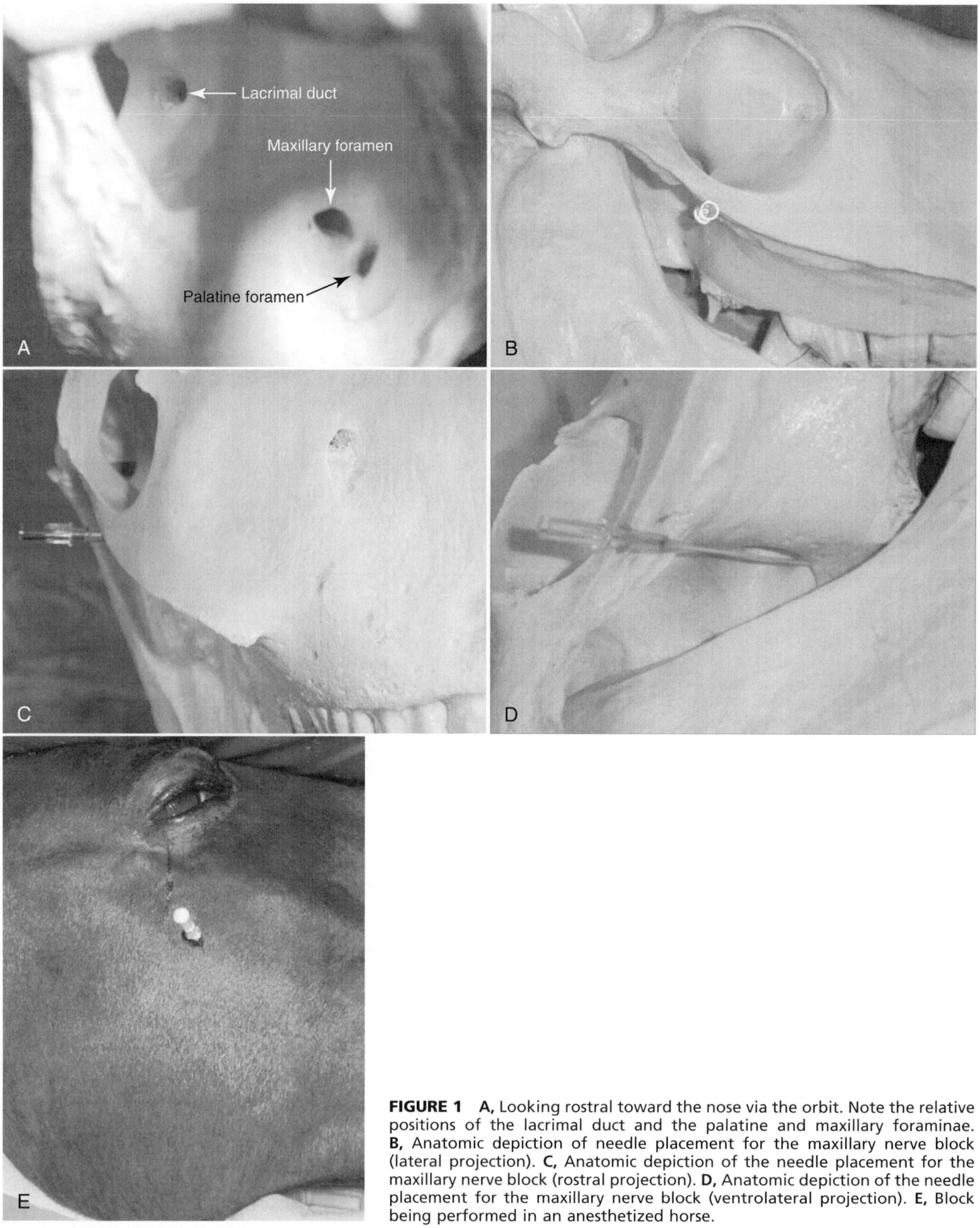

FIGURE 1 **A,** Looking rostral toward the nose via the orbit. Note the relative positions of the lacrimal duct and the palatine and maxillary foraminae. **B,** Anatomic depiction of needle placement for the maxillary nerve block (lateral projection). **C,** Anatomic depiction of the needle placement for the maxillary nerve block (rostral projection). **D,** Anatomic depiction of the needle placement for the maxillary nerve block (ventrolateral projection). **E,** Block being performed in an anesthetized horse.

PROCEDURE

- Block: Maxillary nerve (Figure 1)
  - Desensitized region: All sensation to maxillary teeth (including incisors), sinuses, and skin of muzzle
  - Anatomic landmarks: Rostral limit of the caudal third of the palpebral fissure, under the zygomatic arch, angle slightly up
  - Needle size and length: 20-gauge, 3.5 inch
  - Note: The needle depth should be at least 3 inches, and the sharp end of the needle should be against bone for correct positioning. If the end of the needle is not on bone, the needle position is incorrect.

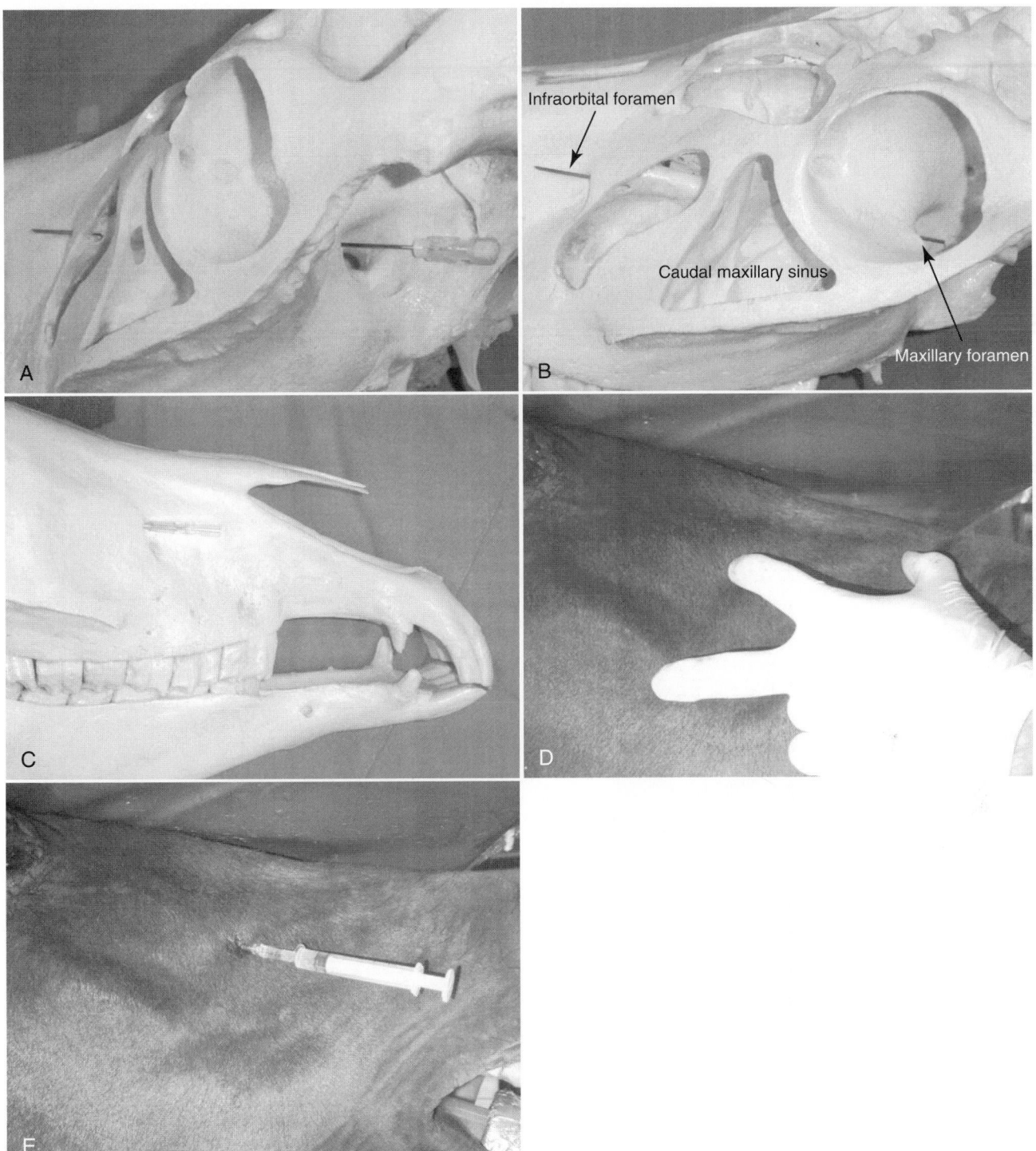

FIGURE 2 **A,** Path of the infraorbital nerve via the infraorbital canal, which traverses the paranasal sinuses innervating the cheek teeth (ventrolateral view). **B,** Path of the infraorbital nerve via the infraorbital canal, which traverses the paranasal sinuses innervating the cheek teeth (dorsolateral view). **C,** Modification of the perineural analgesic technique (lateral view). **D,** Location of the infraorbital foramen. **E,** Block being performed in an anesthetized horse.

- Block: Infraorbital nerve (Figure 2)
  - Desensitized region: Skin to muzzle, canines and upper incisors
  - Modification (thumb occlusion of the infraorbital canal): Block sensation to teeth as far caudal as the last cheek tooth (M3 or 1/211).
  - Anatomic landmarks: Nasoincisive notch (thumb), facial crest (middle finger); lift levator nasolabialis a few millimeters with the index finger and palpate the infraorbital foramen.
  - Needle size and length: 20-gauge, 1-inch.
  - Note: Horses do not tolerate this block well. Administer adequate sedation.

- Block: Mandibular nerve (Figure 3)
  - Desensitized region: Bone of mandible, all lower cheek teeth, and lower lip.
  - Anatomic landmarks: At the intersection of a line from joining the point of greatest curvature of the mandible to the lateral canthus of the eye and a line parallel to the

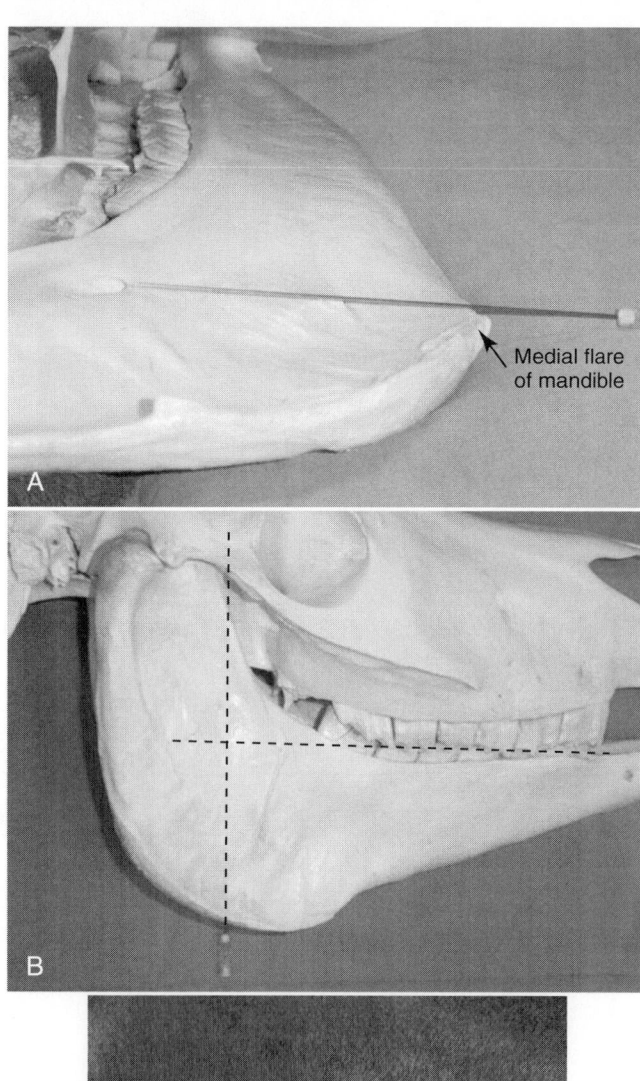

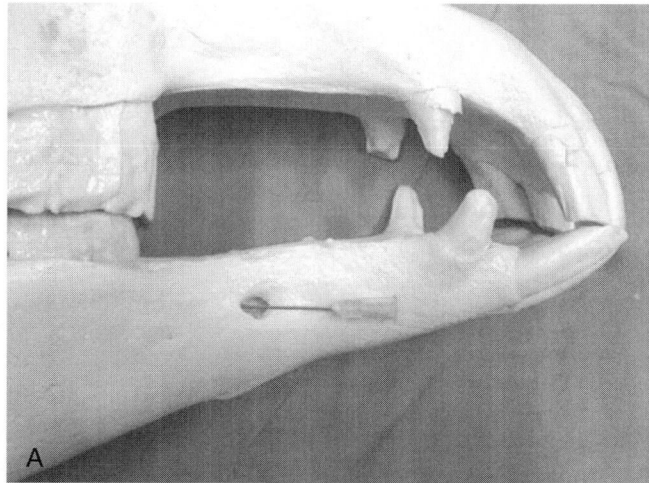

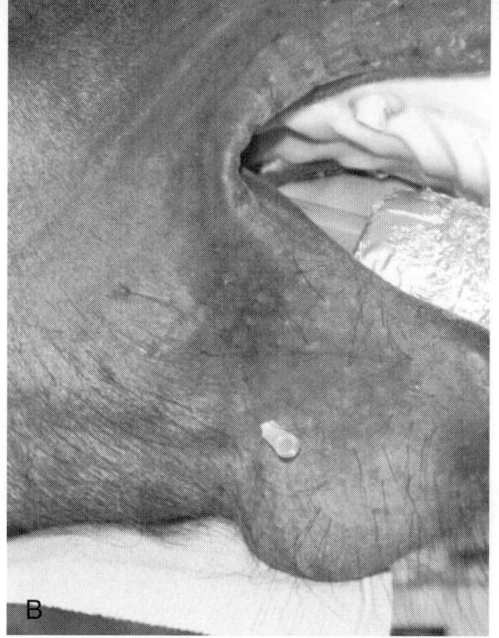

FIGURE 4 A, Location of the mental foramen with needle in position. **B,** Block being performed in an anesthetized horse.

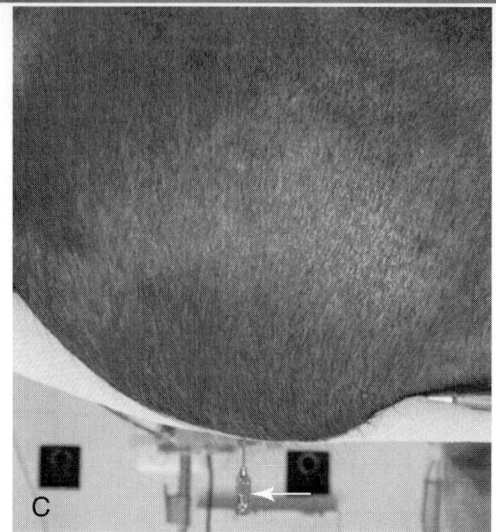

FIGURE 3 A, Location of the mandibular foramen on the inside of the vertical ramus of the mandible. Needle in position. **B,** External position of the foramen can be determined using the intersecting line technique (*dotted lines*). **C,** Block being performed in an anesthetized horse.

occlusal surface of the upper cheek teeth (as palpated externally).
- Needle size and length: 20-gauge, 5- to 9-inch
- Note: Horses tolerate this block incredibly well. Minimal sedation is

necessary. Take care to angle the needle abaxially (to the outside) once you are through the skin. The presence of the medial flare will cause the needle tip to be approximately 1 inch too medial if this is not performed.

- Block: Mental nerve (Figure 4)
  - Desensitized region: Canine tooth, ipsilateral incisors, and lip.
  - Anatomic landmarks: At the chin crease, palpate the rostral limit of the mental foramen and associated nerve.
  - Note: Place a 45-degree bend on the needle before placing it at the entrance to the mental foramen. This will enable the hub of the syringe to be connected without interference from the strong, mobile fibrous tissue of the equine lower lip.

AUTHOR: **JAMES L. CARMALT**

Dentistry: Occlusal Equilibration

BASIC INFORMATION

SYNONYM(S)

Floating
Balancing
Performance floating

OVERVIEW AND GOAL(S)

- Eliminating or reducing factors contributing to abnormal occlusal wear and/or restrictions in normal masticatory biomechanics to eliminate pain, restore dental health, optimize masticatory function, and prolong the useful life of the dentition.
- A thorough knowledge of normal equine masticatory biomechanics is critical to successfully equilibrate equine dentition. These fundamentals are outside the scope of this text and are detailed elsewhere.
- Consider referral for any cases outside the operator's expertise.

INDICATIONS

Every horse over the age of 18 months will benefit from occlusal equilibration at least once yearly.

CONTRAINDICATION

Any disease condition that prohibits the safe use of standing sedation

EQUIPMENT, ANESTHESIA

- Equipment:
  - Full-mouth speculum
  - Patient head support
  - Bright light source
  - Oral cavity flush
  - Abrasive dental tools (hand tools, rotary grinders, reciprocating grinders, disc grinders, according to operator preference and expertise)
  - Dental mirrors
  - Cheek retractor
  - Cooling irrigation if necessary to avoid thermal injury to dentition
  - Disinfectant for tools
  - Safety equipment such as operator eye protection, hearing protection if necessary, and exam gloves
- Anesthesia:
  - Standing sedation
  - Variable, but typically α_2 agonists alone or in combination with another α_2 agonist or a narcotic such as butorphanol
  - Choice of sedation protocol: Depends on operator preference and anticipated duration of procedure

ANTICIPATED TIME

30 to 60 minutes depending on operator expertise

PREPARATION: IMPORTANT CHECKPOINTS

- A thorough dental and health history should be obtained before treatment.
- A thorough oral examination should be performed prior to or in conjunction with the equilibration procedure.
- Allow adequate time for onset of full sedation effect before attempting treatment, usually at least 5 minutes.

POSSIBLE COMPLICATIONS AND COMMON ERRORS TO BE AVOIDED

- Overly aggressive correction techniques can result in injury to sensitive dental tissue or excessive loss of occlusal surface either of which can manifest in prolonged dysphagia or other signs of dental pain or dysfunction, such as hypersalivation, quidding, or inappetence.
- Unprotected grinding equipment can injure soft tissues, which may result in dysphagia. Lingual lacerations are particularly painful to the horse.
- Soft tissue disruption through direct abrasive injury or less demonstrable mechanical forces can seed oral bacteria to local lymph nodes or distant organ systems. Caution should be exercised in patients with periodontal disease and in patients with compromised immune function. Judicious prophylactic antimicrobial use may be indicated in selected cases.

PROCEDURE

- Following administration of the selected standing sedation protocol, manually move the mandible through its masticatory range of motion to assess preprocedure occlusion via both sound and palpable sensations.
- Raise the sedated patient's head to an ergonomic position for the horse, which is also compatible with visual observation by the operator. Using a cheek retractor and strong light source, visually evaluate the quality of occlusion along the entire length of both arcade pairs through the lateral excursion.
- Place the full-mouth speculum and open wide enough to allow digital access and visual evaluation but not so much as to place nonphysiologic strain on the patient's joints and soft tissues. Adequate sedation is critical.

- Assuming a thorough oral exam has been previously performed, quickly begin a systematic occlusal equilibration protocol, which will result in improved biomechanical function, elimination of oral pain, and increase in functional life of the teeth.
  - Judiciously reduce tall crowns or portions thereof to eliminate abnormal wear on opposing teeth and allow more normal masticatory movement. Normal equine masticatory biomechanical function has been described elsewhere, a thorough knowledge of which should guide a safe and effective equilibration plan.
  - Current research suggests that crown reductions greater than about 3 mm can damage sensitive tissues. Similarly, mechanical abrasive tools generate varying amounts of heat. Thermal injury due to excessive grinding must be avoided.
  - Sufficient occlusal contact must be maintained or restored to allow the patient to continue grinding roughage while the dentition is adapting to any changes made. Do not make changes greater than the patient can easily tolerate.
  - During the equilibration procedure, make sure that all sharp enamel points, mainly those on the buccal aspect of maxillary cheek teeth and lingual aspect of the mandibular cheek teeth, are smoothed to prevent laceration or ulceration of the soft tissues. It is not necessary to disturb the occlusal surfaces to accomplish this smoothing. A thorough knowledge of equine dentition, anatomy, and eruption mechanisms dictates proper technique. Pay particular attention to those cheek teeth that can be impacted by a bit or other tack. Make sure all cheek teeth are addressed. Special tools are necessary to reach the caudal molars.
- Upon completion of equilibration procedures for the cheek teeth, remove the full-mouth speculum and again visually assess the quality and quantity of occlusion along the entire length of both arcade pairs by observing the occlusal planes as the mandible moves through its lateral excursion. If insufficient occlusion remains for normal function, or inadequate corrections were achieved, carefully make additional changes to allow successful mastication and reduce the severity of

malocclusions. It is best to adopt a conservative approach to equilibration because it is always possible to remove a bit more crown if necessary, but it is not possible to replace it once removed.

- Finally, evaluate the incisor arcades for malocclusions such as ventral or dorsal curvatures, diagonal incisor malocclusions, missing or stepped teeth, and so forth.
  - Equilibration of the incisor arcades involves reducing tall crowns to restore normal masticatory biomechanics. No portion of the incisor arcade should interfere with optimal cheek teeth function.
    - Current research suggests that reduction of greater than approximately 3 mm of any single incisor crown should be avoided so as not to damage sensitive tissues.
    - Again, a thorough understanding of normal masticatory biomechanics is required to safely and effectively equilibrate equine incisor arcades. Uninformed reduction of incisor crown can result in significantly decreased interocclusal space at the premolar/molar arcades, a situation that can carry severe consequences for the patient. Consider referral for any case outside the operator's expertise.
- Once the horse's head is down off the head support, again assess the excursion and occlusal contact with the head in this more physiologic position because the mandible changes position as head position is changed. Compare parameters to preprocedure findings.

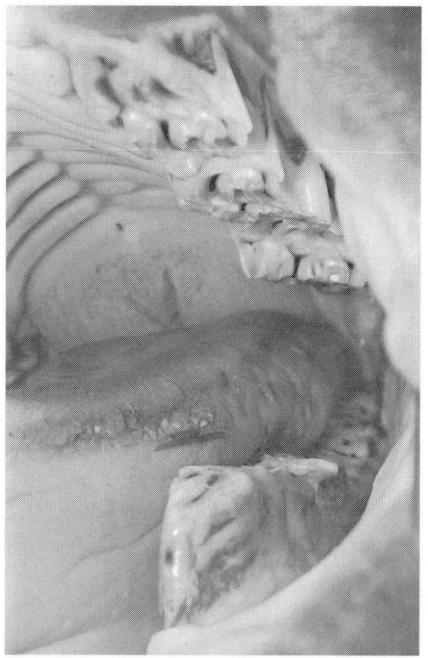

FIGURE 1 Severe "step mouth" before initial equilibration procedure.

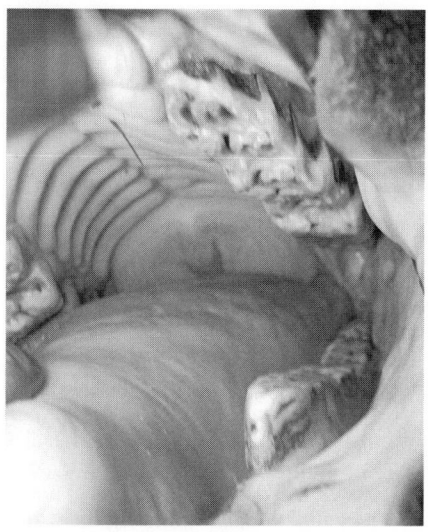

FIGURE 2 Same mouth as Figure 1 following initial equilibration procedure. Note that only a partial correction is performed due to severity of malocclusions. More complete corrections may have resulted in removal of unsafe amounts of crown. Further corrective procedures are recommended in approximately 4 to 6 months.

POSTPROCEDURE

- Patients should be held off feed for 1 to 3 hours following sedation and dental equilibration to prevent choke or ileus-induced gas colic.
- Consider partial reversal of α_2 agonists when profound sedation is needed.
  - Tolazoline is Food and Drug Administration (FDA) approved in horses.
  - Yohimbine use is off-label.

ALTERNATIVES AND THEIR RELATIVE MERITS

Limited scope procedures to remove sharp enamel points are useful to prevent most soft tissue lacerations/ulceration but will not correct malocclusions and therefore will not prevent premature wear and expiration of the dentition.

AUTHOR: **MARY S. DeLOREY**

Dexamethasone Suppression Test

BASIC INFORMATION

- Draw a baseline blood sample (use plasma or serum) and administer dexamethasone (40 μg/kg IM; ~20 mg/500 kg horse) at 5 PM (4–6 PM).
- Blood samples can be collected in ethylenediamine tetraacetic acid or plain blood collection tubes.

- Take blood samples at 15 and 19 hours (8 AM and noon the next day).
- Expect plasma cortisol concentrations to be less than 1 μg/dL in horses with normal hypothalamus-pituitary-adrenal function. Horses with cortisol concentrations higher than 1 μg/dL are considered positive for pituitary pars intermedia dysfunction (equine Cushing's disease).

- It is important to avoid putting the horse in a stressful position when performing this test.
- Avoid glucocorticoid administration 1 week before performing this test.

AUTHOR: **RAMIRO E. TORIBIO**

Dexamethasone/Thyrotropin-Releasing Hormone Test (DST/TRH), Combined

BASIC INFORMATION

- Collect baseline blood sample (first sample).
- Administer dexamethasone (40 μg/kg IV) between 8 and 10 AM and collect a blood sample 3 hours later (second sample).
- Administer 1 mg IV thyrotropin-releasing hormone (TRH) and collect an additional blood sample 30 minutes

latter (third sample, 3.5 hours from dexamethasone administration).
- Collect last blood sample 24 hours after dexamethasone administration (fourth sample).
- The test is considered positive if cortisol concentration is less than 1 μg/dL at 24 hours or cortisol concentration increases by more than 66% 30 minutes after TRH administration.
- This test has a sensitivity of 88% and a specificity of 76%.

- Advanges: This method has increased sensitivity and specificity compared with the dexamethasone suppression test (DST) and TRH test administered separately.
- Disadvantages: Additional expenses and collection of multiple samples.
- Blood samples can be collected in ethylenediamine tetraacetic acid (EDTA) or plain blood collection tubes.

AUTHOR: **RAMIRO E. TORIBIO**

Early Goal-Directed Therapy

BASIC INFORMATION

OVERVIEW AND GOAL(S)

- Early goal-directed therapy is hemodynamic optimization through the use of resuscitation endpoints to guide therapy and improve tissue oxygenation in an effort to reduce mortality.
- Involves a three part strategy:
  - Maintain preload: The circulating fluid volume
  - Maintain afterload: The systemic peripheral resistance
  - Maintain cardiac contractility

INDICATIONS

- Severe injury, trauma, or septic disease where tissue oxygen delivery is reduced or variable, cell oxygen uptake is dysfunctional, or myocardial depression is present
- Parameters monitored to identify patients at risk, their prognosis and ideal therapy required are:
  - Central venous pressure (CVP)
  - Mean arterial pressure (MAP)
  - Lactate and pH
  - Central or mixed venous oxygen saturation

CONTRAINDICATIONS

- Each factor alone cannot be used to predict prognosis.
- Lactate, especially, can be affected by cellular dysfunction as well as perfusion, and serial measurements should be taken into consideration for all predictions.

- Excessive resuscitation (to hyperphysiologic levels) is likely not beneficial.
- Monitor heart rate and rhythm if vasoactive agents are used.

EQUIPMENT, ANESTHESIA

- Central venous catheter
- Sphygmomanometer or direct electronic transducer
- Lactate meter
- Blood gas analysis meter
- Crystalloid fluids
- Vasopressor agents (dobutamine, dopamine, norepinephrine)
- Electrocardiogram (ECG)

ANTICIPATED TIME

Horse should optimally reach goals of therapy in 6 hours.

POSSIBLE COMPLICATIONS AND COMMON ERRORS TO BE AVOIDED

- Delay in resuscitation results in cellular dysfunction and tissue inflammation/necrosis that reduces the likelihood of successful resuscitation.
- No single resuscitation parameter should be used to assess therapy.

PROCEDURE

- Administer fluid therapy to increase volume, venous return, and cardiac output (CO).
  - Shock-dose fluids may be required (see "Shock-Dose Fluid Administration" in this section).
  - Colloids may supplement vascular fluid volume.

- Hypertonic saline may increase circulating volume in adults.
- Lack of positive response to adequate fluid therapy indicates need for vasopressors and inotropism.
  - Dobutamine: 1 to 15 μg/kg/min (dilute to 100 μg/mL in 0.9 % saline)
  - Dopamine: 1 to 20 μg/kg/min
  - Norepinephrine: 0.05 to 1 μg/kg/min
- Monitor response q1–2h to determine if goals have been met:
  - Central venous pressure (CVP) of 8 to 12 mm Hg
  - MAP of 65 mm Hg or greater
  - Urine output of 0.5 mL/kg/h or greater
  - Venous oxygen saturation of 70% or greater
  - pH >7.32
  - Lactate <1.5 mmol/L

POSTPROCEDURE

Address primary cause of sepsis and shock.

ALTERNATIVES AND THEIR RELATIVE MERITS

Traditional endpoints of resuscitation (mentation, heart rate, capillary refill time, pulse quality, temperature) may normalize with compensated shock, preventing identification of occult oxygen debt without goal-directed endpoints.

SUGGESTED READING

Bedenice D: Evidence-based medicine in equine critical care. *Vet Clin North Am Equine Pract* 23:293–316, 2007.

Prittie J: Optimal endpoints of resuscitation and early goal-directed therapy. *J Vet Em Crit Care* 16(4):329–339, 2006.

AUTHOR: **AMELIA MUNSTERMAN**

Echocardiography

BASIC INFORMATION

SYNONYM(S)
- Echo
- Cardiac ultrasound
- Transthoracic echocardiography

OVERVIEW AND GOAL
Echocardiography has tremendously increased the equine clinician's ability to recognize and diagnose cardiac diseases. The purposes of a complete echocardiographic exam are to:
- Recognize congenital or acquired disorders/structural abnormalities
- Evaluate valvular function
- Evaluate ventricular function
- Evaluate the effect of any observed hemodynamic abnormalities on cardiac chamber size
- Evaluate the pericardium and pericardial effusion

INDICATIONS
Any suspected acquired or congenital cardiac diseases (eg, loud or new murmur, unexplained elevated heart rate, abnormal heart rhythm, muffled heart sounds, clinical signs consistent with right- or left-sided cardiac disease, unexplained poor performance or exercise intolerance, collapse, unexplained pleural effusion, unexplained or complicated respiratory distress, suspected pulmonary hypertension).

CONTRAINDICATIONS
- Horse should be stable enough to handle restraint.
- Life-threatening problems should be addressed before prolonged echocardiography is performed.

EQUIPMENT, ANESTHESIA
- Clippers with no. 40 blade
- Ultrasonic coupling gel
- Isopropyl alcohol
Ultrasound machine:
- Two-dimensional (2D), motion-mode (M-mode), and Doppler (color-coded, pulsed-wave, continuous-wave) capabilities.
- Simultaneous electrocardiogram (ECG) to allow accurate timing of cardiac measurements and proper interpretation of Doppler signals.

- Cine loop capabilities, allowing review of a number of previous cardiac cycles after freezing the image.
- Displayed image depth of at least 30 cm for adult horses; less depth is needed for ponies and foals. If the depth is less than 30 cm, the entire heart of an adult horse will not fit on the screen and the exam must be performed from both the right and left sides.
Ultrasound probes:
- Phased array or sector scanning transducer.
- For adult horses, a low-frequency (2.5 MHz or lower) transducer.
- For yearlings, foals, and ponies, a higher frequency transducer (3.5–5.0 MHz) can be used.
- Anesthesia is not used in horses for transthoracic cardiac ultrasound.

Sedation is not desirable because it will affect cardiac function; it should be used only in uncooperative patients.

ANTICIPATED TIME
Variable, depending on complexity of problem, patient cooperation, and examiner experience

PREPARATION: IMPORANT CHECKPOINTS
- Image quality is aided by clipping the hair over the right third and fourth intercostal spaces (ICS) between the olecranon and the point of the shoulder (ie, over the caudal aspect of, and just caudal to, the triceps muscle) and in a comparable location over the left third, fourth, and fifth ICS. Clipping may not be necessary in horses with a fine summer haircoat, particularly in smaller, thinner horses. In this case, more liberal use of alcohol and ultrasound gel will be helpful.
- Isopropyl alcohol to clean the area and ultrasound coupling gel are applied after clipping.

POSSIBLE COMPLICATIONS AND COMMON ERRORS TO BE AVOIDED
Common errors or pitfalls to be avoided:
- Inability to find the heart: Transducer is located too far caudal; relocate one ICS cranial.

- Beware of excessive gain, particularly in the near field.
- Reverberation artifacts are common and cardiac masses are rare; do not overinterpret.
- It is advisable to try to reproduce any visible abnormalities in another image plane to avoid misinterpretation or overinterpretation.
- The muscle of the outermost portion of the posterior free wall of the left ventricle appears hypoechoic compared with the inner portion. Do not confuse with pericardial effusion.
- Hyperechoic areas within the myocardium are common and may not be associated with dysrhythmias or other clinical signs.
- Measurements made from left parasternal images cannot be directly compared with measurements made from a right parasternal approach because they are made across a different axis. Normal values or serial comparisons must be obtained from the same side.

PROCEDURE
- The horse should be standing quietly; stocks are often used but are not necessary if unavailable or the horse is unable or unwilling to stand in stocks.
- The electrocardiogram (ECG) electrodes should be placed according to the ultrasound manufacturer's instructions. These are usually placed in a base-to-apex configuration. Clipping is not necessary, but sufficient alcohol or water to saturate the area is needed to have a trace with adequate electrode contact and without artifact.
- A systematic approach using standard views is critical to avoid overlooking important information, reduce variability, and be able to convey important findings to others.
- Right parasternal images:
  - The examination is initially performed from the right side and is facilitated by placing the horse's right leg forward (Figure 1).
  - Six standard 2D views (three long-axis and three short-axis) are obtained from the right parasternal window, although permutations of these views may be used to more thoroughly explore an abnormality.
  - Right parasternal long-axis views:

- The transducer is held in the left hand and oriented vertically, with the reference marker under the examiner's left thumb (this indicates the edge of the imaging sector on the screen, which is customarily displayed on the right side of the screen).
- Transducer is placed in the fourth ICS (in most horses, just caudal to the triceps musculature if the right leg is placed forward), between the olecranon and the point of the shoulder (see Figure 1).
- Right ventricular outflow tract: With the reference marker in the 11 to 12 o'clock position, the transducer is angled slightly cranial and dorsal, angling toward the opposite side (left) point of the shoulder. The right atrium, tricuspid valve, right ventricle, pulmonary artery, aorta, and coronary artery can be seen (Figure 2).

- Left ventricular outflow tract and aorta: The transducer is angled slightly caudal from the first view to look straight across the chest and rotated slightly clockwise (to approximately the 1 o'clock position) (Figure 2, *B*). The aorta and left ventricle are seen horizontally crossing the center of the image, and the right atrium, tricuspid valve, and right ventricle are seen closer to the skin surface. The pulmonary artery can be seen deep to the aorta as a circular structure.
- Four-chamber view: The transducer is angled slightly caudally and rotated slightly counterclockwise back to the 12 o'clock position (no rotation) (Figure 2, *C*). This allows visualization of the left and right atria and ventricles, with the interventricular septum oriented horizontally across the image. This view can be the most difficult one to obtain in heavily muscled horses because the triceps can interfere with proper placement of the transducer. Therefore it is emphasized that placing the horse's right front leg forward is very helpful.
  - Right parasternal short-axis views are obtained by rotating the probe in a clockwise direction, so the

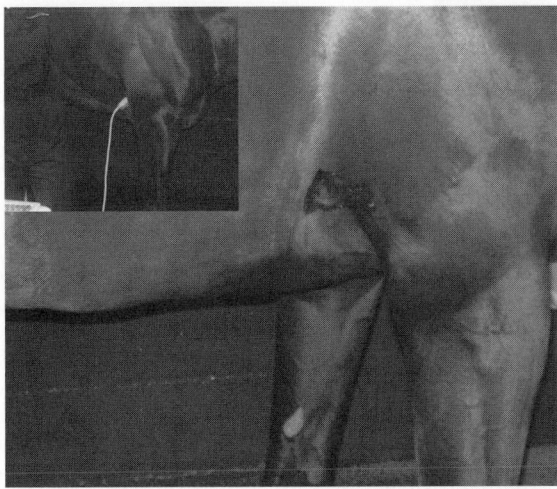

FIGURE 1 Horse in position for an echocardiogram.

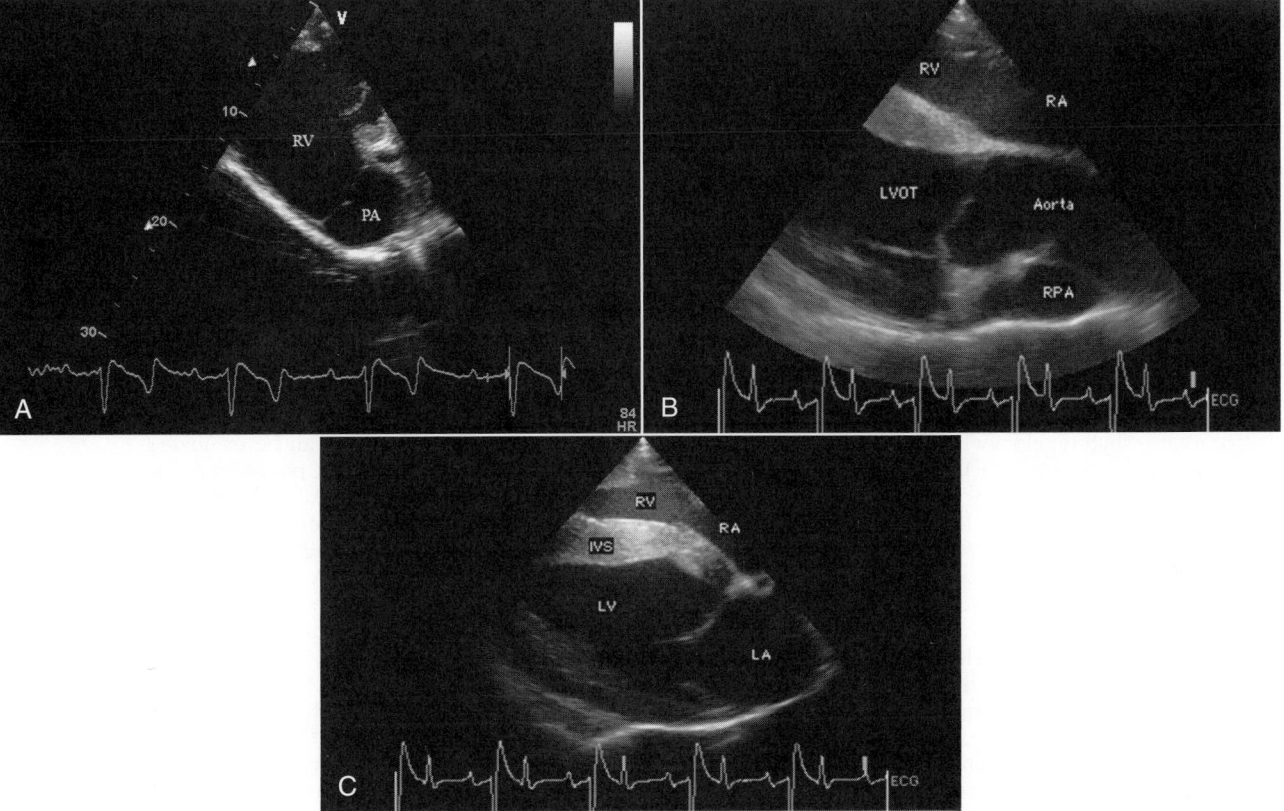

FIGURE 2 Right parasternal long-axis views. **A,** Right ventricular outflow tract. **B,** Left ventricular outflow tract. **C,** Four-chamber view.

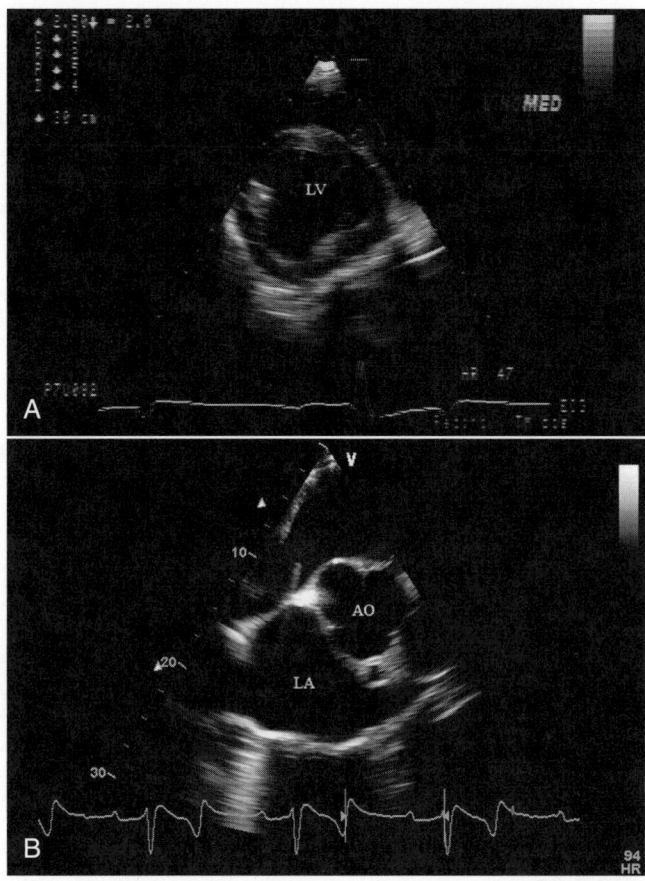

FIGURE 3 Right parasternal short-axis views. **A,** Left ventricle at chordal level. **B,** Aorta.

marker is at 4 o'clock, while maintaining the same location on the thorax.

- With ventral angulation, the cross-section of the left ventricle at the level of the papillary muscles and ventricular apex is obtained. As the probe is angled slightly dorsally, the left ventricle at the chordal level is visualized (Figure 3).
- Continuing dorsally, the mitral valve will come into view.
- By slight dorsal and cranial angulation from this position, the aorta in cross-section can be seen (Figure 3, *B*). It is often necessary to rotate slightly clockwise, to approximately the 5 o'clock position, to see the three cusps of the valve clearly. In this view the left atrium is seen, allowing comparison of the relative sizes of the left atrium and aorta to assess left atrial enlargement.

Note: For all views, only subtle changes in rotation or angulation are needed because small changes result in large differences at this depth.

- M-mode images: One-dimensional views of the heart displayed over time. By combining M-mode with the simultaneously recorded ECG, specific times within the cardiac cycle can be selected, which allows accurate comparisons of intracardiac dimensions between exams or patients.
- The continuously displayed 2D image allows it to be used to guide proper placement of the M-mode cursor.
- End-diastolic measurements are taken at the onset of the QRS complex, and systolic measurements are taken at the maximum excursion of the ventricular septum, with measurements made using the "leading edge" method, as recommended by the American Society of Echocardiography.
- From the right hemithorax, three M-mode images are recorded from the three short-axis views. It is very important to have precise cursor placement in standard views that are obtained correctly because small inconsistencies will yield inaccurate and unreliable measurements.
  - To obtain an M-mode of the left ventricle, the short-axis view at the chordal level is obtained, and the cursor placed perpendicular to the septum and left ventricular free wall to evenly bisect the left ventricle (Figure 4). The following structures are measured: Left ven-

tricular internal diameter in systole (LVIDs) and diastole (LVIDd), interventricular septum in systole (IVSs) and diastole (IVSd), left ventricular free wall in systole (LVFWs) and diastole (LVFWd), and right ventricular internal diameter in systole (RVIDs) and diastole (RVIDd).

- From these measurements, the percentage of fractional shortening (FS) of the left ventricle can be calculated, giving an assessment of the contractility. The formula is:

$$\%FS = \frac{LVIDd - LVIDs}{LVIDd} \times 100$$

Note: If the maximal depth of the ultrasound image is 24 cm or less, the ventricular free wall of adult horses will not be on the 2D image, and measurement of the LVID and the LVFW cannot be made from the M-mode. In this situation, the left ventricle can be measured from M-modes of the left parasternal short-axis views.

- To obtain an M-mode at the level of the mitral valve, the 2D image of the mitral valve is obtained, and the cursor is positioned perpendicular to the IVS and ventricular free wall, bisecting the ventricle and mitral valve (Figure 4, *B*). This allows assessment of the movement of the mitral valve as well as information on left ventricular dilation by measuring the distance between the maximal opening of the mitral valve in early diastole (E point) and the interventricular septum.
- The final M-mode image recorded from the right hemithorax is of the aorta. A short-axis view of the aorta at the level of the aortic valve is obtained, and the cursor is positioned to bisect it (Figure 4, *C*). In this image, one cusp of the valve should clearly be seen during systole and diastole. The diameter of the aortic root is measured from leading edge to leading edge, and the movement and timing of opening and closing of the valve can be evaluated.
- Left parasternal images:
  - Allow better visualization of the left atrium and mitral and pulmonic valves.
  - Are useful if the entire heart does not fit on the screen from the right parasternal approach.
  - May allow better alignment with blood flow for Doppler studies of the mitral and aortic valves.
  - It is helpful to have the horse's left leg forward when on the left side, as for scanning from the right side.

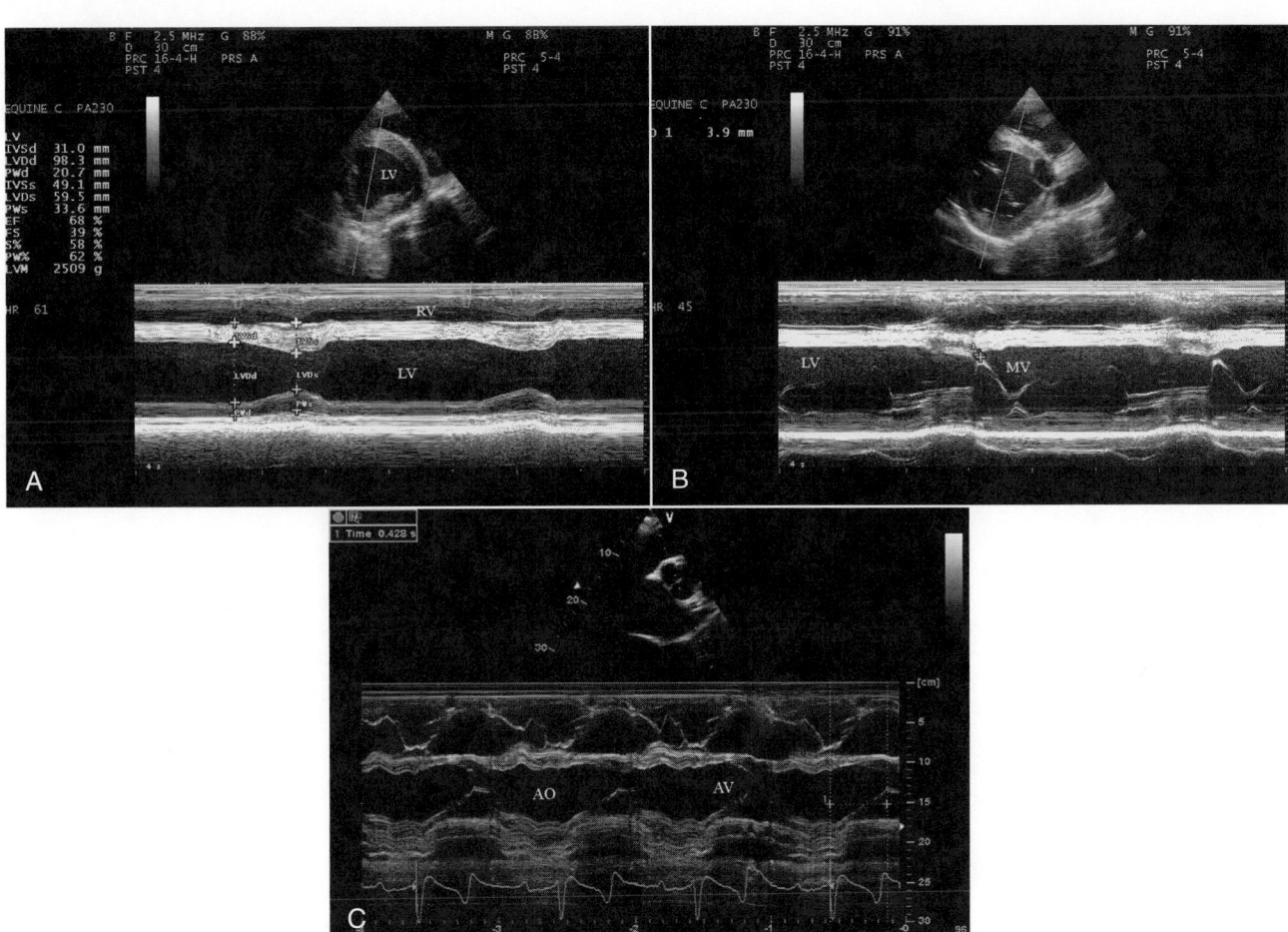

FIGURE 4 M-mode images. **A,** At the level of the left ventricle. **B,** At the level of the mitral valve. **C,** At the level of the aorta.

○ The transducer should be held in the right hand, with the reference marker oriented vertically (12 o'clock position).

■ The left parasternal two-chamber view is obtained by holding the transducer perpendicular to the body wall in the fifth ICS (just caudal to the triceps musculature). The transducer is placed caudal to and above the olecranon process, dorsal to the apical impulse. In this view, the left atrium and mitral valve are optimized and often allow superior Doppler evaluation of abnormal blood flow across the mitral valve (Figure 5). Measurements of the left atrium are more sensitive for detecting left atrial enlargement than those made from the right side. It may be necessary to angle the transducer slightly cranially or slide it ventrally and angle dorsally if the lungs obscure the left atrium.

■ Placing the transducer one space cranially (fourth ICS) in the same orientation allows visualization of the aorta and left ventricular outflow tract in long axis (Figure 5, *B*). With some horses, it may be helpful to rotate the probe slightly counterclockwise.

■ The final long-axis view is obtained by placing the probe in the third ICS and angling it slightly caudally. This enables visualization of the pulmonary artery and pulmonic valve, right ventricle, and aorta (Figure 5, *C*). Many horses object to this image, which can be difficult to obtain in heavily muscled horses; therefore it is very helpful to ensure the horse's left leg is placed forward.

• The short-axis views are obtained by rotating the probe, as for the right-sided views, and are needed if the depth is inadequate for examination of the entire heart from the right hemithorax.

• M-mode images can be obtained from these short-axis views, as with the right side. However, if the entire heart can be seen from the right, the left parasternal short-axis views and M-modes are often not done.

Note: Measurements made from left parasternal images are usually larger than the corresponding views from the right hemithorax.

POSTPROCEDURE

Remove ECG electrodes and wipe off ultrasound gel.

ALTERNATIVES AND THEIR RELATIVE MERITS

• For large animals, there are currently no other practical diagnostic alternatives allowing a detailed examination of heart size, structure, and function.

• Although ECGs are critical for evaluation of cardiac rhythm, they do not give reliable information on cardiac size in horses.

• Radiography is a very insensitive means of assessing the cardiac silhouette. In addition, radiographs do not distinguish between cardiac enlargement and pericardial effusion.

• Transesophogeal echocardiography allows detailed images and excellent alignment with blood flow for Doppler studies; however, the equipment is not routinely available for horses, and the procedure requires general anesthesia.

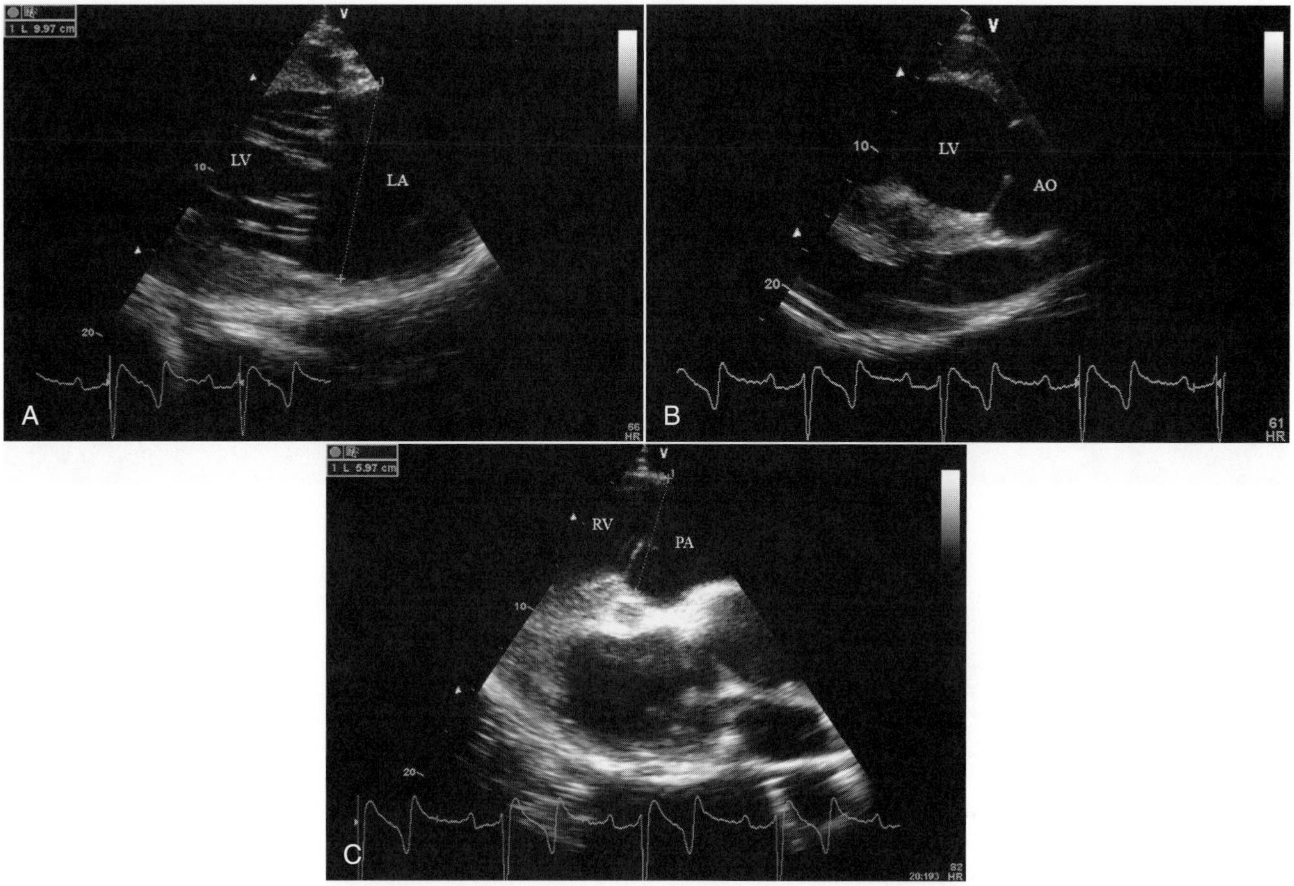

FIGURE 5 Left parasternal long-axis views. **A,** Two-chamber view. **B,** Aorta. **C,** Pulmonary artery.

SUGGESTED READING

Bonagura JD, Blissit KJ: Echocardiography. *Equine Vet J Suppl* 19:5–17, 1995.

Long KJ, Bonagura JD, Darke PG: Standardized imaging technique for guided M-mode and Doppler echocardiography in the horse. *Equine Vet J* 24:226–35, 1992.

Reef VB: Echocardiographic examination in the horse: the basics. *Compend Contin Educ Pract Vet* 12:1312, 1990.

Reef VB: Heart murmurs in horses: determining their significance with echocardiography. *Equine Vet J Suppl* 19:71, 1995.

AUTHORS: **MARY M. DURANDO, LESLEY E. YOUNG,** and **KAREN BLISSITT**

Electrocardiography

BASIC INFORMATION

SYNONYM(S)

ECG
EKG

OVERVIEW AND GOAL(S)

- An electrocardiogram records the depolarization and repolarization process in atria and ventricles during the cardiac cycle.
- Electrocardiography is used to evaluate cardiac rate and rhythm. It allows the diagnosis of the nature of a dysrhythmia (eg, origin of ectopy, type of conduction disturbance).

INDICATIONS

- Monitoring:
  - Routine monitoring during general anesthesia and intensive care
  - Monitoring during treatment procedure (eg, antiarrhythmic drug administration such as quinidine)
  - Monitoring a patient at risk for developing arrhythmias (eg, due to electrolyte imbalance)
- Diagnosis of the presence and origin (ectopy, conduction disturbance) of an arrhythmia:
  - An arrhythmia detected on auscultation
  - Exercise intolerance
  - Clinical signs suggestive of syncope
  - Underlying cardiac or systemic disorders that might predispose to arrhythmias

EQUIPMENT, ANESTHESIA

- Electrocardiograph (ECG machine) to make the recording. This can be a large or small (handheld) recorder, or a recorder that transmits data wirelessly to a computer with appropriate software (Figures 1 and 2).
- Cable to connect the machine to the electrodes on the patient.
- Electrodes: Best results are obtained with self-adhesive (equine) electrodes. These are well tolerated, easy to use, and produce few artifacts. Crocodile clamps are more painful and produce more movement artifacts, although they are also often used.

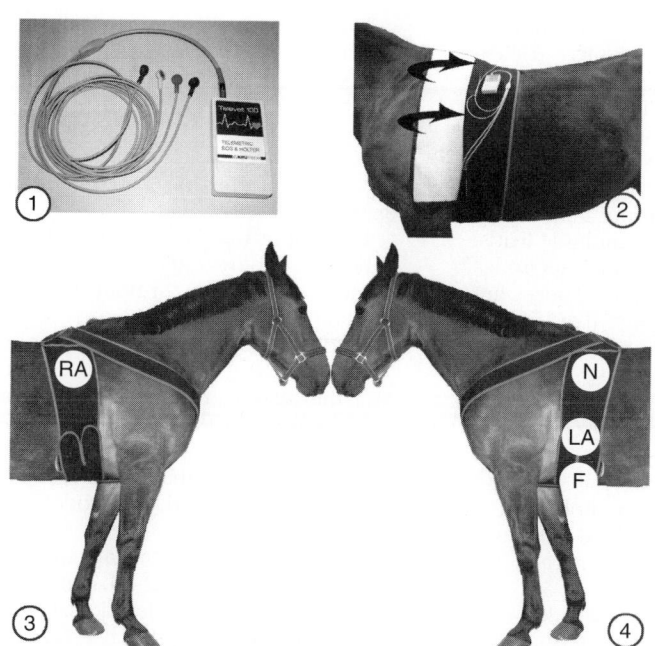

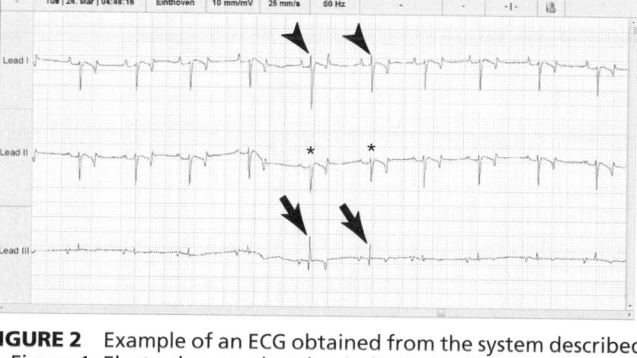

FIGURE 1 Example of recording an ECG using one type of ECG (wireless) equipment. **1,** A battery powered recorder (Televet100) records the ECG digitally and transmits it wireless to a computer. **2,** Using an elastic girth (OrthoHorse) with Velcro, the recorder and wires are fixed within the girth by closing the tissue flap (*arrows*). **3** and **4,** Proper placement of self-adhesive electrodes under the girth (so that they do not fall off during recording) results in good quality recordings from leads I, II, and III.

FIGURE 2 Example of an ECG obtained from the system described in Figure 1. Electrodes are placed as indicated in figure 1 to record three leads in this horse. Leads I and II produce the largest deflections. However, ventricular premature complexes are hard to differentiate from the normal complexes on lead II (*). The difference is more obvious on lead I (*arrowheads*) but most easily seen on lead III (*arrows*), which shows the smallest deflections.

PROCEDURES AND TECHNIQUES

- The ECG trace can be displayed on a screen, recorded on paper, or digitally recorded (digital media, computer).
- A single lead recording is satisfactory in most cases. However, multiple lead recordings may be helpful in some situations.

ANTICIPATED TIME

- Ambulatory ECG: 5 minutes
- Any duration for long-term ECG recordings

PREPARATION: IMPORTANT CHECKPOINTS

- Check recording unit for paper supply, batteries (ink: rarely used).
- Take measures to protect equipment with animals at risk for collapse.
- Take measures to protect equipment when horses are free in a box or paddock during long-term recording (eg, to prevent damage during recumbency or rolling).

POSSIBLE COMPLICATIONS AND COMMON ERRORS TO BE AVOIDED

- It is very important to realize that in horses an ECG can only be used for evaluation of rate and rhythm. Vector electrocardiography cannot be applied to horses because of a different Purkinje network. Therefore myocardial lesions or the place of origin of ven-

tricular ectopy cannot be accurately diagnosed from the surface ECG.
- Although cardiomegaly often results in small P and QRS changes, the ECG should not be applied to diagnose cardiac chamber enlargement. Echocardiography is used to diagnose structural changes.
- In horses, the T wave is very variable. It can be positive, negative, or biphasic without clinical importance. When heart rate increases (exercise, stress) the T wave will be opposite to the QRS complex. This means that in the same, normal horse, the T wave might show large changes between rest and exercise.
- Artifacts should be minimized.
  ○ Use self-adhesive electrodes instead of crocodile clamps. These electrodes contain a small amount of gel, which is sufficient for a good contact. Unless the hair coat is very long (ponies) clipping is not necessary and even undesirable as the electrodes generally stick better on the hair than on the skin.
  ○ For an ambulatory ECG, reduce motion artifacts by keeping the horse calm and standing still. Motion artifact will always be present during an exercise test.
  ○ Recording multiple leads is very useful to diagnose certain arrhythmias (eg, atrial premature contrac-

tions, ventricular premature contractions) and is also useful to differentiate between ectopy and an artifact.
  ○ Watch the horse during the procedure and record body movements so these can be related to the artifacts (eg, sudden defensive reaction, synchronous diaphragmatic flutter).

PROCEDURE

- The horse can be placed in stocks, held by hand, or if portable/wireless equipment is used, given free access to a box or paddock.
- Specific color codes are used for the different electrodes and these are different between Europe and the United States.
- Specific bipolar leads are recorded between the different electrodes:
  ○ Lead I: Between RA (−) and LA (+)
  ○ Lead II: Between RA (−) and F (or LL) (+)
  ○ Lead III: Between LA (−) and F (or LL) (+)
- General principles for placement of the electrodes:
  ○ To obtain a good quality recording with large deflections, electrodes should be placed along the major direction of depolarization of atria and ventricles. This means that one electrode (positive) is placed

ventrally, near the left ventricular apex (ie, on the left thorax, near the elbow). The second electrode (negative) is placed more dorsally and if possible slightly more cranially and/or to the right. Exact location of the electrode is not that important because vector electrocardiography is not applied in horses.

- Standard electrode positions have been described in horses (see later), but the electrode position can be adapted according to suitability for the clinician (eg, position of the horse in recumbency or anesthesia), suitability during an exercise test (to fix the electrodes to the horse and minimize movement artifact), or suitability for the rider during an exercise test.
- Recording of additional leads can be very helpful:
  - To differentiate between artifact and arrhythmia
  - To detect ectopic beats with a morphology similar to normal complexes
  - To continue recording when one lead falls off (eg, exercise test)
- Ambulatory ECG recording at rest: The base-apex recording is most commonly used:
  - Left arm electrode (L or LA, +) is placed near the left ventricular apex (left thorax, near the elbow)
  - Right arm electrode (R or RA, −) is placed in the lower third of the right jugular furrow or over the right shoulder (spina scapulae)
  - The ground electrode (N or RL) is placed anywhere remote from the heart (eg, left shoulder, right dorsal neck area)

- Lead I is recorded. In normal horses, the P wave will be positive (bifid), the QRS complex predominantly negative, and the T wave positive, negative, or biphasic.
- 24-hour ECG: Electrode position is slightly changed to reduce movement artifacts, to allow proper fixation to the horse and to record multiple leads. A girth is used to keep the electrodes and recorder in place. There are several different systems that can be used, with varying numbers of leads and cable configurations, and thus ways to position the leads on the horse. See "Holter Monitor/Telemetry Recording" in this section for more information and detail on 24-hour ECG recordings. One example of lead placement with a four-lead system is as follows (other combinations are possible):
  - All self-adhesive electrodes are placed under an elastic girth.
  - Foot or left leg electrode (LL) is placed near the left ventricular apex (left thorax, about 5 cm below the elbow).
  - Left arm electrode (L or LA) is placed 10 to 15 cm dorsal to the LL electrode.
  - Right arm electrode (R or RA) is placed on the flat portion of the dorsal right thorax (about 20 cm below the withers).
  - The ground electrode is placed on any other location, for example, on the flat portion of the dorsal left thorax (about 20 cm below the withers).
  - The slight separation of the two ventrally positioned electrodes allows making an additional record-

ing between these electrodes so that lead I, II, and III (and aV_L, aV_R, aV_F) will produce a useful recording.
- Exercise ECG: See "Holter Monitor/Telemetry Recording" in this section for more information and detail on exercising ECG:
  - Lunging or treadmill exercise: Identical procedure and electrode placement as for the 24-hour ECG, if using a four-lead system
  - Ridden exercise, if using four leads:
    - Similar to the 24-hour ECG with the elastic girth cranial to or underneath the front part of the saddle. The advantage of the elastic girth is that motion artifact is reduced and electrode dislodgement is less likely.
    - The electrodes (RA and ground) can also be attached cranial to the saddle, in the left dorsal neck region, and the other two (LL and LA) caudal to the saddle girth (LL most ventral and LA 10 cm more dorsal) with the recorder attached to the saddle. The advantage of placing the electrodes in a visible area is that it is easy to check whether they fall off during the exercise test.
  - Trotters:
    - Similar as for the 24-hour ECG with the elastic girth just caudal to the harness.

POSTPROCEDURE

Remove electrodes after recording.

AUTHOR: **GUNTHER VAN LOON**

Embryo Cryopreservation

BASIC INFORMATION

SYNONYM(S)

Embryo vitrification

OVERVIEW AND GOAL(S)

- Cryopreservation by vitrification is preferred to conventional slow freezing for equine embryos. The vitrification technique is simple and can be performed on a farm with commercially available media.
- Vitrification involves exposing the embryo to high concentrations of cryoprotectants, which triggers a glass-like state, to avoid ice crystal formation.

INDICATIONS

- 6- to 6.5-day-old embryo (morula stage) <300 μm in diameter
- Good-quality embryo (grade 1)

EQUIPMENT, ANESTHESIA

- A user-friendly vitrification kit is available (Bioniche, Belleville, ON, Canada)
- 0.25 mL nonirradiated polyvinyl chloride straw

PREPARATION

- After embryo recovery, the embryo is washed as described previously.
- The embryo should not stay in the washing media for more than 20 minutes.

POSSIBLE COMPLICATIONS AND COMMON ERRORS TO BE AVOIDED

Leaving the embryo too long in the last vitrification solution

PROCEDURE

- The embryo is transferred sequentially into three different vitrification solutions (VS) containing increasing concentrations of cryoprotectants at room temperature.
- Transfer embryo from the holding medium to VS1 (with only a very small volume of holding medium). Leave embryo in VS1 for 5 minutes.

- Transfer embryo to VS2. Leave the embryo in VS2 for 5 minutes.
- Transfer the embryo into a 30 μL drop of VS3 and leave the embryo for less than 1 minute.
- Load the embryo into a 0.25 mL straw: Draw up 90 μL of dilution solution (DS) media followed by (1) an air bubble of 5 μL, (2) 30 μL of the VS3 media containing the embryo, (3) an additional 5 μL of air, and (4) 90 μL of DS media.
- Expose the straw to nitrogen vapor for 1 minute (in a plastic goblet) before submerging it in liquid nitrogen.

POSTPROCEDURE

- Thaw the straw.
- Remove the straw from liquid nitrogen tank.

- Hold the straw in the air at room temperature for 10 seconds.
- Plunge into a 20° to 22° C water bath for 10 seconds.
- Dry the straw and place it horizontally on a table for 4 to 5 minutes.
- Evaluate the embryo under stereoscope while it is in the horizontal straw.
- Transfer the embryo using the technique described for a fresh embryo.

EXPECTED PREGNANCY RATES

Pregnancy rates of up to 70% have been reported for small frozen embryo transfer (<300 μm in diameter) even if embryos are cooled for transport before being vitrified. For larger embryos, pregnancy rates decrease to 10% to 20%. These success rates require careful selection of

embryos. Lower pregnancy rates may be expected with less than fresh embryos.

SUGGESTED READING

Carnevale EM: Vitrification of equine embryos. *Vet Clin North Am Equine Pract* 22:831–841, 2006.

Carnevale EM, Elderidge-Panuska WD, Caracciolo di Brienza V: How to collect and vitrify equine embryo for direct transfer. *Proc Am Assoc Equine Pract* 50:402–405, 2004.

McKinnon AO, Squires EL: Embryo transfer and related technologies. In Samper JC, Pycock JF, McKinnon AO, editors: *Current therapy in equine reproduction*, St Louis, 2007, Elsevier, pp 319–334.

AUTHORS: **FRANÇOIS-XAVIER GRAND** and **LEFEBVRE REJEAN CLÉOPHAS**

PROCEDURES AND TECHNIQUES

Embryo Transfer to Recipient

BASIC INFORMATION

SYNONYM(S)

Embryo transplantation

OVERVIEW AND GOAL(S)

See "Embryo Transfer: Embryo Collection" in this section.

INDICATIONS

Establishment of a pregnancy in a surrogate dam after transfer of embryo collected from a valuable donor

EQUIPMENT, ANESTHESIA

- Mare cleaning supplies
- Embryo transfer gun and sanitary sheath

ANTICIPATED TIME

- Mare's synchronization:
  - The day of donor's ovulation is designated as day 0.
  - Availability of pool of recipient mares that can be matched with donors is ideal.
  - Need at least two, and preferably three, recipients per donor if synchronization of ovulation is used.
- Option 1: Prostaglandin F2α (PGF2α) and human chorionic gonadotropin or deslorelin (less effective)
  - Cyclic recipients are examined by palpation and ultrasonography at regular intervals and daily during estrus. With similar follicular development, luteolysis is induced 2 days later in recipients. Once in estrus, all mares (recipients and donors) are monitored daily and ovulations

are induced 1 day later in recipient mares than in the donor. With different follicular development, estrus induction is performed earlier in mares with the smaller follicle, and ovulation is induced later in mares with a larger preovulatory follicle.

- Option 2: Progesterone and estradiol (most commonly used technique)
  - Give combined progesterone (150 mg) and 17β-estradiol (10 mg, P&E) daily for 10 days to the recipients and donor. Administer PGF2α or analogue on tenth day
  - Monitor follicular development, induce ovulation, and breed donor accordingly to artificial insemination guidelines and induce ovulation in recipients 1 day after the donor.
- Option 3: Use of ovariectomized hormone treated mares
  - Progestins (altrenogest, Regu-Mate, 0.088 mg/kg) are administered for 6 days before the embryo transfer. Some have recommended estradiol prior to the administration of progestins, but others have found it not to be necessary. After the transfer, the recipient mare is maintained on long-acting progesterone or progestins for the first 120 days of pregnancy.
- Embryo transfer timing:
  - Ideal recipient should have ovulated on the same day or up to 2 days after donor.
  - Recipients that have ovulated a day before and up to 3 days after donor may be used.

PREPARATION: IMPORANT CHECKPOINTS

- Recipient selection:
  - Should be in good body condition and health
  - Age 5 to 10 years with a prior normal pregnancy, delivery, and lactation
  - Good temperament
  - Current on vaccinations
  - No history of infertility or genital disorders and biopsy grade I
  - Have a good cervical tone at the time of transfer
- Mare preparation: See "Artificial Insemination: Uterine Body" in this section.
- Embryo loading in embryo transfer gun (use side delivery embryo transfer gun).
- Transfer gun in sanitary sheath.
- The double-sleeve technique and rinsing of the inner face of the vulva are recommended to minimize the risk of uterine contamination.
- Rapidity of execution of the technique is important.

POSSIBLE COMPLICATIONS AND COMMON ERRORS TO BE AVOIDED

- Incomplete emptying of the straw triggering to embryo stocked in the transfer gun
- Monitor transfer gun sheath after transfer under stereomicroscope

PROCEDURE

- Place transfer gun into a sanitary sheath (Chemisette), then place into the vagina.

- Gently dilate cervix with the index finger and insert the tip of the embryo transfer gun.
- Rip the sanitary sheath and advance the gun gently through the cervix.
- The gun can be advanced gently until it reaches the wall of the uterus, then pull it back 1 to 2 cm.
- The embryo is then delivered by advancing the stylet.

POSTPROCEDURE

- Pregnancy diagnosis at day 10 or 11 after ovulation
- Pregnancy rate for fresh embryos: 65% to 75%

ALTERNATIVES AND THEIR RELATIVE MERITS

- Some practitioners verify placement of the embryo transfer gun by transrectal palpation, but this procedure is not necessary.
- Many practitioners administer flunixin meglumine before transfer.
- Some prefer to have all recipients on altrenogest or long-acting progesterone until pregnancy is diagnosed.

SUGGESTED READING

Daels P: Equine embryo transfer. In *Proceedings of the North American Veterinary Conference*, Orlando, FL, 2007.

Hurtgen JP: Management of embryo donor mares with chronic infertility. *Proc Am Assoc Equine Pract* 54:414–417, 2008.

McKinnon AO, Squires EL: Embryo transfer and related technologies. In Samper JC, Pycock JF, McKinnon AO, editors: *Current therapy in equine reproduction*, St Louis, 2007, Elsevier, pp 319–334.

Riera FL: Equine embryo transfer. In Samper JC, editor: *Equine Breeding management and artificial insemination*, ed 2, St Louis, 2009, Elsevier, pp 185–200.

AUTHORS: FRANÇOIS-XAVIER GRAND and LEFEBVRE REJEAN CLÉOPHAS

Embryo Transfer: Collection

BASIC INFORMATION

SYNONYM(S)

Embryo transplantation

OVERVIEW AND GOAL(S)

- Embryo transfer (ET) consists of transferring an embryo collected from a donor mare to a recipient mare (Box 1).
- Commercial ET programs include multiple steps leading to the transfer of the embryo: Donor and recipient selection and synchronization, donor insemination, recovery, and transfer of the embryo.
- The major limiting factor in most equine embryo transfer programs is recipient management. Veterinary practitioners may provide a donor management and embryo collection service and ship cooled embryos to an embryo recipient facility (within 24 hours).

INDICATIONS

- Multiple foals from individual genetically superior mares are desired in a short period of time
- Mares in competition
- Subfertile mares (unable to maintain a pregnancy to term)

CONTRAINDICATIONS

- Infertile donor or recipient mares in which cervix, uterine, oviductal, or ovarian disorders have been identified.
- Some breeds do not register foals born from ET (eg, Thoroughbreds).
- Most breeds limit the number of foals registered per year per mare.

EQUIPMENT, ANESTHESIA

- Sedation: Acepromazine is preferred because there is less occurrence of pneumovagina complicating uterine manipulations.
- Collection equipment and supplies:
  - Several types of Foley catheters are available; choice is generally based on individual experience and preference.
  - Different sizes of bores and balloons are available; choice is dictated by breed and size of the mare.
  - Two types of catheters may be used: two-way or three-way. Most practitioners use a two-way catheter with a Y-junction.
  - Prewarmed collection media: Ready-made commercial embryo flushing media are available. Some are complete and ready for use; others may need addition of fetal calf serum (at least 3 L). Alternatively, Ringer's lactate may be used.
  - Embryo filter: Several 0.75 μm filters are available.
- Embryo search material:
  - Stereoscope
  - Petri dishes
  - Washing plates
  - Washing and holding media
  - 0.25 mL straw and tuberculin syringe

ANTICIPATED TIME

Collection days:

- Day 6 to 6.5: Smaller embryos are suitable for cryopreservation (< 300 μm)
- Day 7 to 8: Optimal time under normal circumstances
- Day 8 to 8.5: Older mares or when frozen semen is used

In case of double asynchronous ovulation (1-day interval), it may be preferable to plan the embryo recovery 8 days after the first ovulation.

PREPARATION: IMPORANT CHECKPOINTS

- Mare preparation: Same as AI in the uterine body
- Embryo recovery material: Connect the three-way tubes to the filter, the uterine catheter, and the fluid. Fill the entire system with fluid.

BOX 1 Characteristics of Equine Embryos

The embryo travels from the oviduct to the uterus about 6.0 to 6.5 days after ovulation. At day 6 (morula stage), the embryo is about 200 μm (range, 130–750 μm) in diameter. At day 7 (young blastocyst stage), the mean diameter is approximately 400 μm (range, 130–1400 μm), and at day 8 (blastocyst stage), the embryo is about 1100 μm (120–3900 μm) in diameter. For embryos that are 300 to 2000 μm in diameter, the pregnancy rate reaches 50% to 60%, with an expected 10% embryonic loss. Embryo loss rises to 20% for embryos smaller than 300 μm or larger than 2000 μm in diameter. Embryos bigger than 2000 μm are also more fragile and require adequate handling to obtain comparable pregnancy rates. The recovered embryos can be transferred fresh, cooled, or cryopreserved. Embryos larger than 300 μm in diameter do not tolerate cryopreservation well, but survive better in cooled storage.

POSSIBLE COMPLICATIONS AND COMMON ERRORS TO BE AVOIDED

- Misplaced catheter: Too deep in the uterus (single horn flushed)
- Overinflated balloon
- Overdilation of the cervix (loss of fluid in the vagina)
- Contamination of the uterus
  Note: Fluid should be allowed to rest in the uterus for 2 minutes before recuperation.

PROCEDURE

Embryo recovery:
- Dilate the cervix with one finger.
- Introduce the catheter through the cervix until the caudal edge of the balloon is at the tip of the finger.
- Inflate the catheter balloon with 40 to 90 mL of air or medium and pull back the catheter until the balloon is snug against the internal cervical os.
- Fill the uterus with 300 to 500 mL of flushing media. Then allow the fluid to flow back by gravity into the filter.
- The manipulation may be repeated several times with the hand in the vagina or by transrectal massage.
- Monitor return; should recuperate 98% of the fluid placed in the uterus.
- Repeat procedure three to six times. In general, 3 to 4 L of media are used per collection.
- Oxytocin may be given after the last filling, and the fluid may be allowed to stay 3 minutes in the uterus before recovery.

Embryo search:
- Some prefer direct searching in the embryo filter if it is designed for this purpose.
- Filter should be rinsed and fluid recovered into a Petri dish.
- Start a methodic search for the embryo with a stereoscope at about ×15 magnification.
- Once identified, wash the embryo several times (International Embryo Transfer Society recommends 10 times) in enriched media.
- Examine the embryo at higher magnification (×100) to grade the morphologic features (McKinnon grading scale).
- Load the embryo into a sterile 0.25 mL straw by aspiration with a tuberculin syringe attached to the cotton end of the straw in the following manner. Draw up 90 μL of media followed by (1) an air bubble of 10 μL, (2) 30 μL of media containing the embryo, (3) an additional 10 μL of air, and (4) 90 μL of media until full. The first column of fluid must come in contact with the cotton plug in the straw to prevent fluid leakage.
- Once the embryo is in the straw, it can be transferred immediately into the appropriate recipient mare or cooled. Equine embryos are quite resistant to temperature variations (25° to 37° C). However, efforts should be made to prevent extreme temperature changes.

POSTPROCEDURE

- The embryo may be transferred or preserved (cooled or cryopreserved) for delayed transfer.
- If an embryo is not recovered after the first collection (3 L of media), the mare's uterus may be flushed again immediately or the following day with an additional 2 L.
- Embryos that are 6 to 6.5 days old may not be recovered because of a greater specific gravity.
- Several other reasons may also account for the absence of an embryo (ovulation and fertilization problem, sperm and embryo transport problem, or embryo survival within the uterus).
- If an embryo is not recovered after three collections performed at three different estrous cycles, the mare should be removed from the ET program and causes of infertility investigated.

- Luteolysis may be induced in the donor on the recovery day.
- Storage options for transport:
  - Embryos tolerate cooling well. Therefore overnight shipment in a zwiterrionic buffer media is possible before transfer in a synchronized recipient mare.
  - A 5 mL sterile tube (do not use blood sampling tubes, which have a silicone coating) can be filled with transport media (EmCare, ICP, Auckland, NZ; or Vigro Holding Solution Plus, A-B Technology, Pullman, WA) and placed in a 50 mL tube filled with room temperature water for packaging in an Equitainer-type shipment box. Another easy option is to introduce the loaded embryo straw in a bacteriologic sampling tube instead of the swab.
  - Pregnancy rates with properly cooled and transported embryos are similar to those obtained using fresh embryos.

ALTERNATIVES AND THEIR RELATIVE MERITS

An open system using fluid bottle is commonly used in Europe.

SUGGESTED READING

Daels P: Equine Embryo transfer. In *Proceedings of the North American Veterinary Conference*, Orlando, FL, 2007.

Hurtgen JP: Management of embryo donor mares with chronic infertility. *Proc Am Assoc Equine Pract* 54:414–417, 2008.

McKinnon AO, Squires EL: Embryo transfer and related technologies. In Samper JC, Pycock JF, McKinnon AO, editors: *Current therapy in equine reproduction*, St Louis, 2007, Elsevier, pp 319–334.

Riera FL: Equine embryo transfer. In Samper JC, editor: *Equine breeding management and artificial insemination*, ed 2, St Louis, 2009, Elsevier, pp 185–200.

AUTHORS: **FRANÇOIS-XAVIER GRAND** and **LEFEBVRE REJEAN CLÉOPHAS**

PROCEDURES AND TECHNIQUES

Endodontics

BASIC INFORMATION

OVERVIEW AND GOAL(S)

Preservation of the structure and function of the nonvital, endodontically infected tooth or the vital tooth with iatrogenic or traumatic pulp exposure.

DEFINITIONS

- Vital pulp therapy: Treatment of the damaged clinical crown that has resulted in exposure of vital pulp tissue with the goal of maintaining a vital tooth.
- Root canal therapy: Treatment of a tooth that involves removal of all pulp tissues, sterilization and obturation of the root canal, and restoration to obtain a hermitically sealed tooth.

INDICATIONS

- Vital pulp therapy
  - The indication for vital pulp therapy is recent traumatic crown fracture with pulp exposure.

- May be iatrogenic, as in overreduction of the incisors, canines, or first cheek teeth during occlusal equilibration.
- More commonly, this occurs with traumatic injury to the crown (idiopathic tooth fracture).
- Root canal therapy
  - The indication for root canal therapy is irreversible pulpitis of a permanent tooth.
  - Presents as a draining tract from ventral mandible, a facial fistula, or unilateral nasal discharge, depending on the cheek tooth involved.
  - Apical infection of cheek teeth may be hematogenous (anachoretic), via coronally exposed pulp horns (endodontic), or as an extension of periodontal disease (combined endodontic-periodontal lesion).

CONTRAINDICATIONS

Advanced periodontal disease is a contraindication for traditional root canal therapy. There are no published studies assessing the prognosis of vital pulp therapy as a function of time from pulp exposure. In brachyodont species, the prognosis for vital pulpotomy and direct pulp capping is good when the procedure is performed within 48 hours of pulp exposure. The equine tooth is probably more forgiving, and the author would attempt vital pulp therapy within 1 week of traumatic/iatrogenic pulp exposure.

EQUIPMENT, ANESTHESIA

- Dental radiography is required; both intraoral and extraoral dental radiographs are often needed to assess the subgingival status of the affected tooth and to guide the practitioner through the endodontic treatment.
- Root canal therapy requires a wide array of endodontic instrumentation. Because of the large size of the equine root canal, some instruments are not commercially available and must be fabricated by the practitioner. For most practitioners, the infrequent indication for root canal therapy will not justify the large investment in equipment and advanced training.
- Vital pulp therapy requires a high-speed dental handpiece (with water irrigation) and burs for pulpotomy, sterile paper points, and calcium hydroxide or mineral trioxide aggregate as a pulp dressing.
  - The restoration of the tooth is generally performed with a layer of glass ionomer followed by a composite resin filling material.
  - Restoration of the endodontically treated tooth is a highly technique-sensitive procedure and requires an array of restorative materials, including a curing light for the light-activated restorative materials and a dental unit with high and low speed handpieces and an air-water spray.
- Vital pulp therapy and root canal therapy of incisors can be performed on the sedated standing horse under local anesthesia. Root canal therapy of the cheek teeth requires general anesthesia.

ANTICIPATED TIME

- Vital pulp therapy (vital pulpotomy and direct pulp capping): 30 to 60 minutes
- Root canal therapy of incisors: 1 to 2 hours
- Surgical root canal therapy of cheek teeth: 2 to 4 hours

PREPARATION: IMPORANT CHECKPOINTS

Vital pulp therapy success depends on the elapsed time from pulp exposure; quick referral to a specialist is recommended. Diagnosis of apically infected cheek teeth and incisors requires high-quality dental radiography, which may also necessitate referral.

POSSIBLE COMPLICATIONS AND COMMON ERRORS TO BE AVOIDED

Failure of root canal therapy requires either repeating the treatment or extracting the tooth. If vital pulp therapy fails, the likely outcome is a nonvital, apically infected tooth that requires either root canal therapy or extraction.

PROCEDURE

- Vital pulpotomy is performed with a carbide or diamond bur on a high-

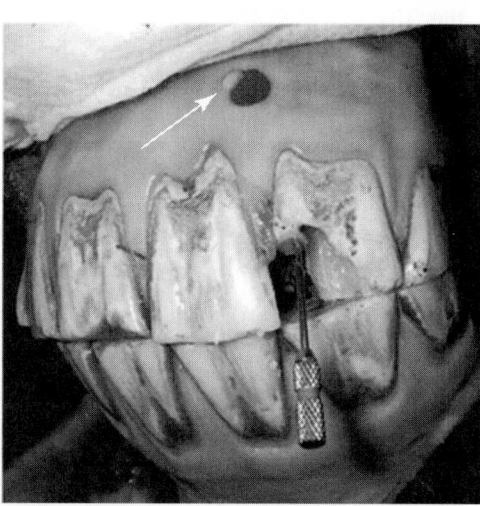

FIGURE 1 Left maxillary second incisor (202) fractured about 2 weeks previously in a 5-year-old Morgan stallion. An endodontic file placed into the exposed pulp chamber resulted in purulent drainage from the fistula near the mucogingival line (*arrow*).

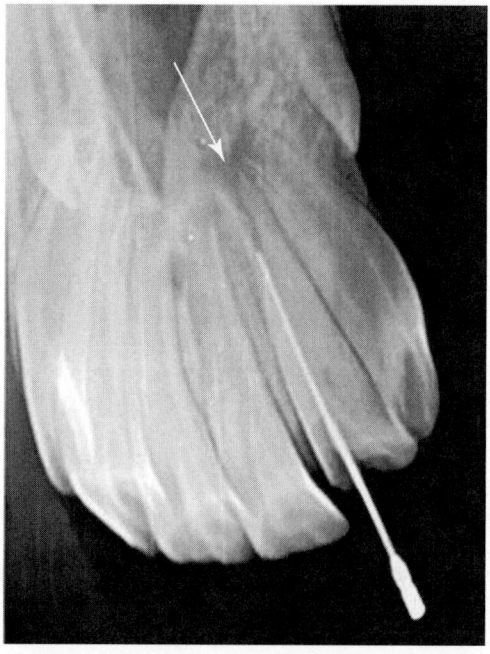

FIGURE 2 Intraoral radiograph of maxillary incisors with an endodontic file in the root canal of the fractured second incisor (202) with a necrotic pulp in a 5-year-old Morgan stallion. This incisor has an open apex (*arrow*).

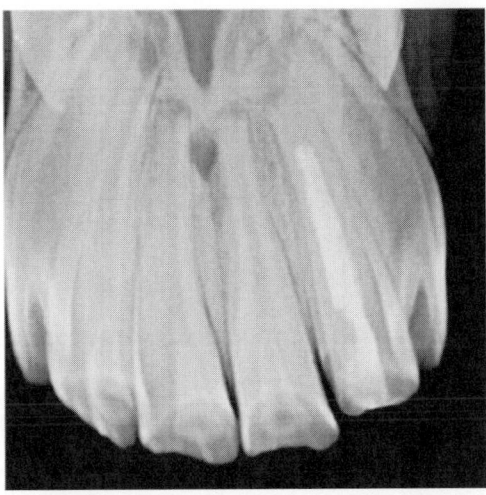

FIGURE 3 Intraoral radiograph taken after completed endodontic therapy of a fractured left maxillary incisor (202) in a 5-year-old Morgan stallion. The fractured incisor had a necrotic pulp and an open root apex at the time of presentation. Endodontic therapy consisted of induction of hard tissue closure of the apex (apexification) by endodontic placement of calcium hydroxide, followed 12 months later by obturation with an endodontic sealer, compacted gutta percha, and a composite restoration.

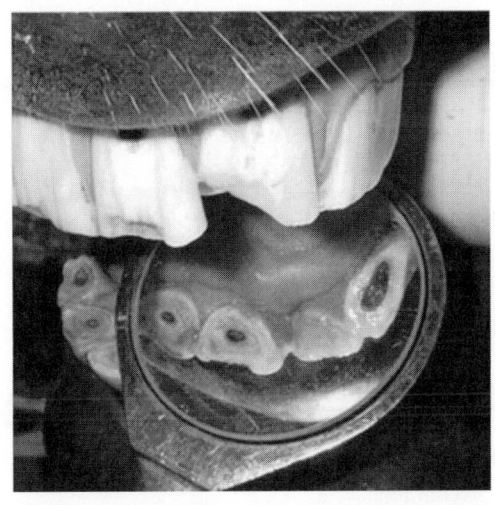

FIGURE 4 Oral photograph of the completed root canal therapy of the second incisor (202) shown in Figures 1 through 3.

speed dental handpiece with water irrigation.

o Approximately 10 mm of pulp is removed; hemorrhage is controlled by application of saline-moistened paper points.

o A 2- to 3-mm layer of mineral trioxide aggregate is layered directly on the pulp and gently tamped down with the blunt paper point.

o A 2- to 3-mm layer of glass ionomer (dual cure or light cure) is then placed over the mineral trioxide aggregate.

o The walls of the canal are cleaned with endodontic spoon curettes, acid etched (37% phosphoric acid) for 30 seconds, rinsed with water, and dried with an air stream.

o A bonding agent is applied to the conditioned canal walls according to the manufacturer's recommendations and then light cured.

o Light-cured composite material(s) are then used to incrementally fill the coronal aspect of the canal.

• Root canal therapy of the incisors uses techniques adapted from those in widespread use in humans and small animals.

o Obturation and restorative materials have not been specifically developed for or critically evaluated in the hypsodont dentition of the horse. Root canal therapy of the cheek teeth requires a surgical approach to the tooth apex as well as retrograde instrumentation and obturation, and is considered investigational or experimental at this time.

POSTPROCEDURE

Radiographic follow-up at 3 and 6 months, then annually, is recommended for endodontically treated teeth.

ALTERNATIVES AND THEIR RELATIVE MERITS

The horse appears to be able to respond to idiopathic tooth fracture resulting in pulp exposure in the majority of cases.

• The pulpal response is retraction of the pulp and formation of a dentinal bridge. Therefore the clinical finding of an exposed pulp does not carry the same prognosis as in other species.

• Radiographic assessment of a dentinal bridge warrants conservative therapy (occlusal equilibration and follow-up radiographs).

• Exodontia is the alternative to endodontic treatment in apically infected teeth.

SUGGESTED READING

Baker GJ, Easley J: *Equine dentistry*, ed 2, Edinburgh, 2005, Saunders Elsevier.

Baratt RM: Equine incisor endodontics. In *Proceedings of the 22nd Annual Veterinary Dental Forum*, Jacksonville, 2008, FL, pp 113–123.

Cohen S, Burns RC: *Pathways of the pulp*, ed 8, St Louis, 2002, Mosby.

Dacre I, Kempson S, Dixon PM: Equine idiopathic cheek teeth fractures. Part 1: pathological studies on 35 fractured cheek teeth, *Equine Vet J* 39(4):310–318, 2007.

Wiggs RB, Loprise HB: Veterinary dentistry: principles and practice, Philadelphia, 1997, Lippincott-Raven.

AUTHOR: **ROBERT M. BARATT**

Endoscopy: Oral

BASIC INFORMATION

OVERVIEW AND GOAL
To obtain a better visual appreciation of oral pathology

INDICATIONS
Determination of size of diastemata, position and extent of occlusal crown fractures, and periodontal disease

CONTRAINDICATIONS
A nonsedated animal

EQUIPMENT, ANESTHESIA
- Intravenous sedation
- Full-mouth speculum (eg, Hausmann/McPherson or Stubbs)
- Fiberoptic/videoendoscope and associated electrical equipment or LED dental stick

ANTICIPATED TIME
10 minutes

PREPARATION: IMPORANT CHECKPOINTS
- Complete oral examination under sedation
- Oral flush with water to remove feed material

POSSIBLE COMPLICATIONS AND COMMON ERRORS TO BE AVOIDED
If the horse is able to extract its incisors from the biteplate of the full mouth speculum, there is a significant risk of irreversible damage to the imaging equipment (LED dental stick) unless it is sheathed appropriately.

PROCEDURE
- Sedate horse
- Oral flush with water
- Place full-mouth speculum
- Insert endoscopic instrument and continue with oral examination

ALTERNATIVES AND THEIR RELATIVE MERITS
Oral examination with a mirror and light source

AUTHOR: **JAMES L. CARMALT**

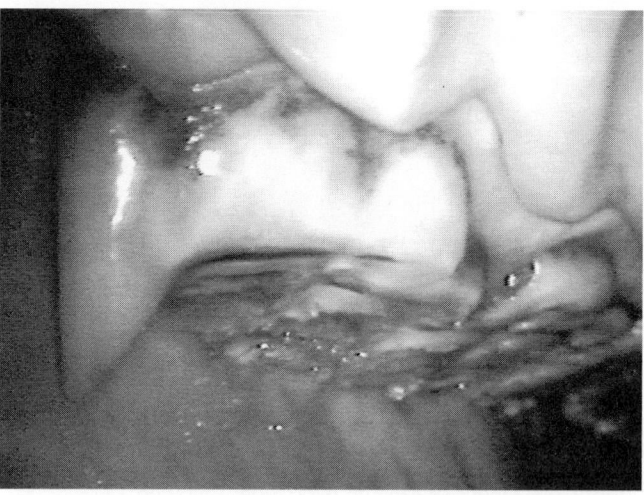

FIGURE 1   Large hook on rostral aspect of tooth 106.

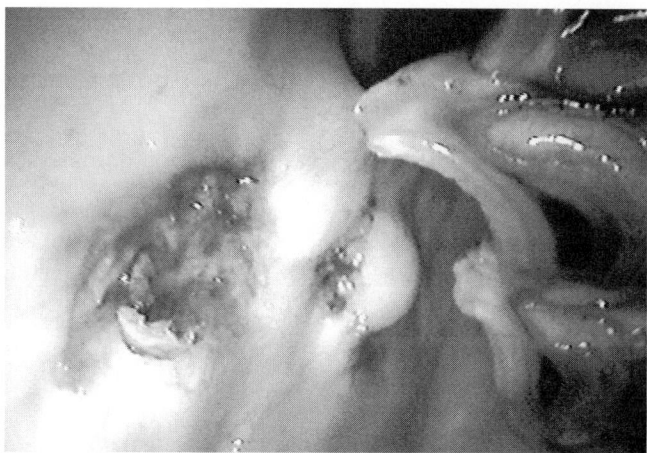

FIGURE 2   Cheek ulcers associated with sharp lateral cingulae on upper cheek teeth.

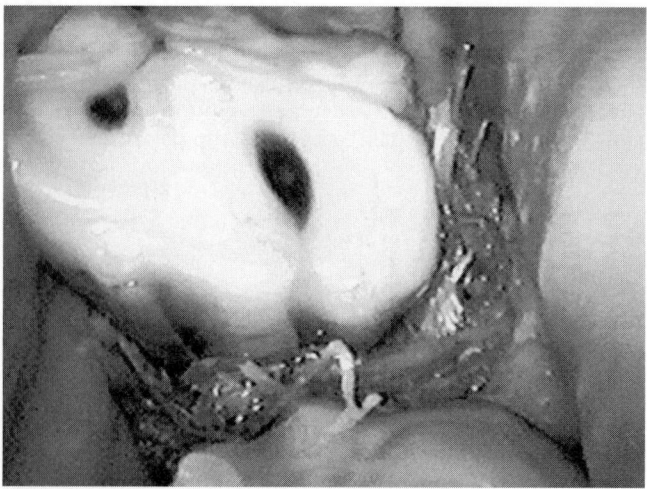

FIGURE 3   A diastema with associated feed packed between teeth.

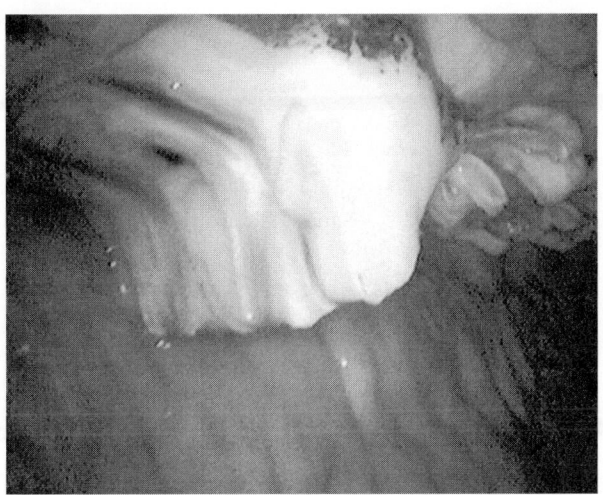

FIGURE 4 Hook on caudal half of tooth 110 associated with a missing or as yet unerupted 410.

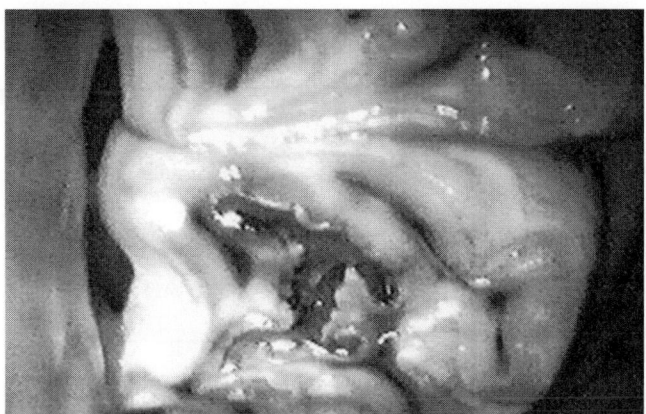

FIGURE 5 Infundibular necrosis.

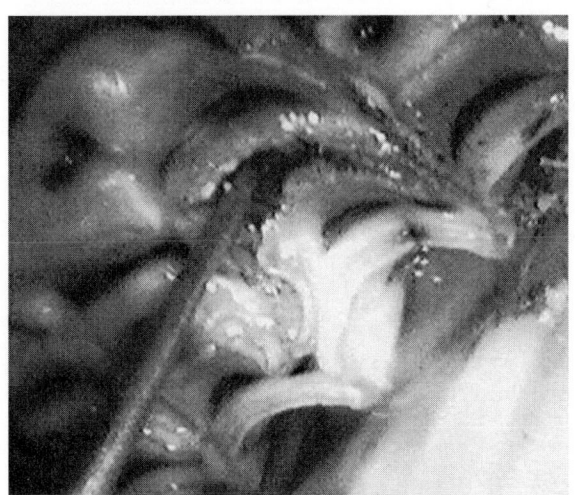

FIGURE 6 Probe within an infundibulum displaying necrosis.

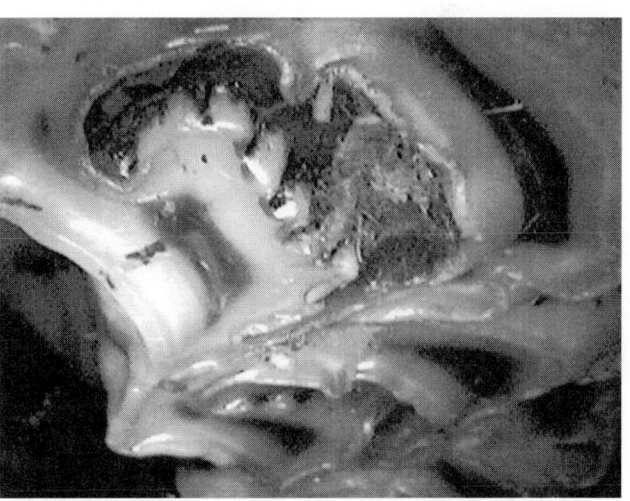

FIGURE 7 Advanced infundibular necrosis.

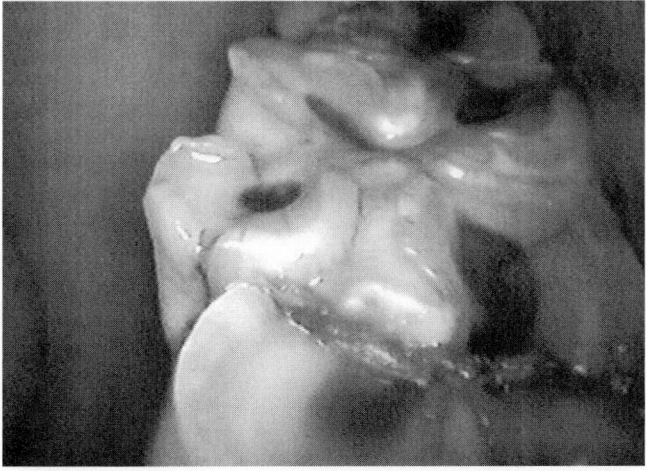

FIGURE 8 Diastema (valve/closed) with feed packed in the interdental space. This tooth is also slightly medially displaced.

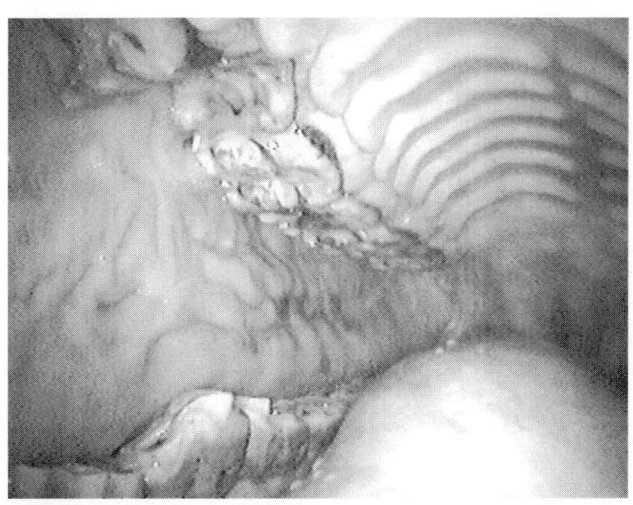

FIGURE 9 Rostral displacement of tooth 106 and abnormal wear of 107 with an associated stepped 407/8.

Endoscopy: Urinary Tract

BASIC INFORMATION

SYNONYM(S)

Transurethral cystoscopy
Urethrocystoscopy
Uroendoscopy

OVERVIEW AND GOAL(S)

Urethrocystoscopy involves the use of a flexible endoscope for examination of the urethra, accessory sex glands, urinary bladder, ureteral orifices, and occasionally the ureters. Endoscopy of the urinary tract is useful to diagnose suspected unilateral renal hematuria, urethral rents, urolithiasis, and neoplasia.

INDICATIONS

- Urethrocystoscopy is performed to evaluate the source of hematuria or pyuria; cause of stranguria, pollakiuria, incontinence; and rarely for the investigation of weight loss, fever of unknown origin, or chronic colic.
- Urethrocystoscopy is useful for the evaluation of the urethra and bladder for calculi, inflammation, masses, assessment of bladder atony, and sabulous urolithiasis.
- Biopsy and lavage of the urethra and urinary bladder can be performed under endoscopic guidance.
- Visualization of the ureteral orifices can reveal the source of hematuria or pyuria of renal origin, the location of ectopic ureters, or other congenital defects.
- Ureterocystoscopy can be performed with a narrow diameter endoscope in a nondilated ureter, but ureteral diseases frequently result in hydroureter and dilation of the ureter allowing passage of a standard endoscope.

EQUIPMENT, ANESTHESIA

- A 1-m long and <12 mm external diameter flexible endoscope is usually used to assess the urethra and bladder in adult female horses and small male horses. A >1.5-m long endoscope may be required in larger male horses. The large urethral orifice of the mare will accommodate any size endoscope.
- Light source and light cables
- Accessory implements including sterile biopsy forceps, cytology brushes, stone retrieval baskets
- Sterile endoscopic catheters for passage into the ureters if unilateral ureteral or renal disease is suspected
- Ability to perform cold sterilization of the endoscope

- Documentation equipment (digital imaging [prints or video]), videotapes, printer
- Sedation

ANTICIPATED TIME

10 to 20 minutes for visualization but longer for biopsy, stone retrieval, or lavage procedures

PREPARATION: IMPORTANT CHECKPOINTS

- The use of sterilized equipment and attention to hygiene is of the utmost importance when assessing possible perforation of the bladder or urethra.
- Knowledge of normal appearance of anatomical features of the lower urinary tract.
- Cold sterilization should be performed by soaking the flexible endoscope for 30 minutes and then rinsing the outer surface, water channel, and biopsy port with sterile saline in an aseptic manner. The sterilized instrument can be temporarily stored in a sterile rectal sleeve prior to the procedure.
- Tranquilization is recommended, especially in male horses where exteriorization of the penis is necessary. The use of acepromazine for penile relaxation should be reserved for geldings, while larger dosages of alpha$_2$ agonists such as detomidine are required for stallions.
- Thorough cleansing of the distal end of penis or vulva and the use of sterile gloves to pass the endoscope is recommended.
- Aseptic collection of a urine sample for possible culture is best performed using a Foley catheter in a mare or a stallion catheter in a male horse rather than obtaining the urine sample via the endoscope. The bladder can be evacuated of urine using the catheter prior to endoscopy.

POSSIBLE COMPLICATIONS AND COMMON ERRORS TO BE AVOIDED

- Mistaking the urethral fossa for the urethral orifice in male horses.
- Overinterpretation of catheter or endoscope-induced minor trauma (often resulting in mural hyperemia and rarely irritation and hemorrhage), which is often mistaken for urethritis.
- It is not uncommon for multidrug resistant *Pseudomonas* to be cultured from samples collected via an endoscope, even if cold sterilization has been performed. Urine samples should

be collected via passage of a sterile catheter and a quantitative urine culture and urine sediment examination should always be performed prior to a diagnosis of cystitis.
- Iatrogenic urinary tract infections from inadequate hygiene or compromised innate defense mechanisms, especially detrusor muscle atony and inability to completely evacuate the urinary bladder.
- Rupture of the urethra or urinary bladder due to inappropriate technique or severe pre-existing disease.
- Operator reliance on visual impressions rather than histopathologic or cytologic evaluation.
- Insufflation is usually performed using room air without incident. However, there are occasional anecdotal reports of sudden death associated with air emboli during cystoscopic procedures and ideally insufflation should be performed using CO_2. Insufflation of the bladder should not be performed until the bladder is fairly empty of urine. Urinary mucus is very viscous and excessive bubbling of urine will greatly diminish ability to visualize and examine the entire bladder.

PROCEDURE

- After cleaning the distal end of the penis or vulva, the sterilized endoscope should be passed into the urethra using aseptic technique by an operator wearing sterile gloves.
  - Some contamination from the animal's vulva or prepuce is inevitable, but passage of the endoscope should be as clean as possible.
  - A small amount of sterile lubricant aids in smooth passage of the endoscope.
- In female horses, the endoscope is passed into the urethral opening, which is located approximately one hand's length in the vulva on the ventral floor of the vestibule.
- Air inflation makes passage up the urethra easier.
  - With dilation, the pale pink mucosa may appear redder than normal and may show a prominent linear vascular pattern.
  - Longitudinal mucosal folds will flatten with air insufflation.
- If the bladder has not previously been emptied via catheterization, then suction can be used to empty the bladder of urine via the biopsy channel of the endoscope. Care should be taken not to apply suction to the

bladder wall to avoid iatrogenic ery-thematous lesions.

- Rinsing the bladder with sterile saline can be performed to remove residual mucous and crystals.
- Insufflation of the bladder with air or sterile saline allows complete examination of the bladder mucosa. External indentation of the bladder by bowel is not uncommon.
- The subtle ureteral orifices are located in the caudodorsal aspect of the bladder at approximately 10 and 2 o'clock positions (Figure 1). These are best visualized in an empty bladder, just cranial to the trigone. Pulsatile flow of urine is intermittently observed from each ureteral orifice approximately once every minute.
- The bladder is examined in a methodical manner including visualization of each urethral orifice and inserting sufficient length of the endoscope to retroflex and look caudally at the trigone region. The bladder should be examined for the presence of calculi, sabulous material (Figure 2), inflammatory foci, or masses.
- Production of abnormal urine (hematuria or pyuria) from one urethral orifice or evidence of unilateral renal disease suspected by renal ultrasound should prompt ureteral catheterization to obtain a urine sample for cytology and culture.
- It is easier to examine the male urethra as the endoscope is removed at the end of the procedure. Mild erythema or irritation of the urethra is a normal finding.
- Biopsies of mural lesions can be collected for histopathologic examination and culture.
- Urethral rents in male horses are found in the region of the ischial arch where the urethra widens into the ampullar portion. The colliculus seminalis is seen in the roof of the pelvic urethra, distal to urethral sphincter.

Ureteral Catheterization:

- Ureteral endoscopy is performed to evaluate unilateral disorders of the upper urinary tract, to localize pyelonephritis, renal hemorrhage, and neoplasia. Dilation of the ureter and secondary hydroureter can allow passage of the fiberscope in some cases.
- Sterile polyethylene tubing can be passed up the biopsy channel of the fiberscope and through the ureteral orifice into each ureter to obtain individual urine samples (Figure 3).
- In mares, ureteral catheterization can also be performed without an endoscope using a No. 8- to 10-Fr sterile polypropylene catheter. After all urine is removed from the bladder via catheterization, the urethra is manually

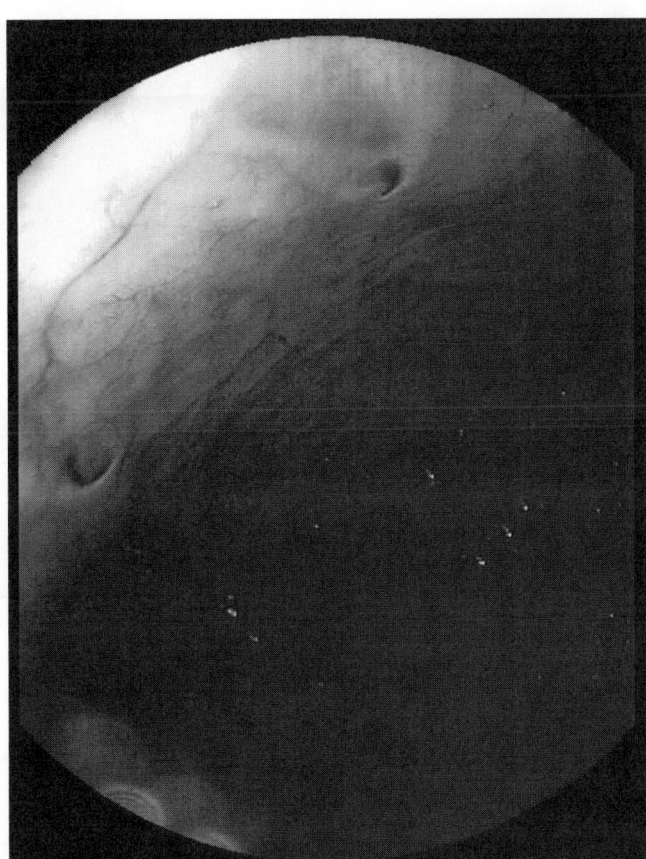

FIGURE 1 The U-shaped ureteral orifices are located in the caudodorsal bladder wall just cranial to the trigone.

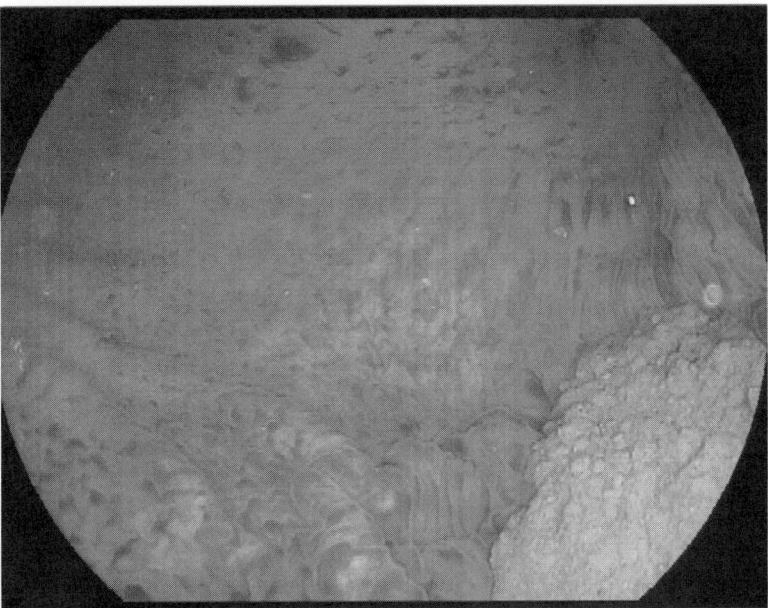

FIGURE 2 Sabulous urolithiasis (*bottom right corner*) with moderate bladder mucosal irritation in an atonic bladder.

dilated until two fingers can pass into bladder. The ureteral orifices are palpable dorsally and the catheter can be guided into the ureter between the two fingertips, which are positioned at the ureteral orifice. The catheter is advanced 5 to 10 cm, and negative pressure is applied via an attached syringe to collect a urine sample from one individual ureter, while the ureteral orifice is sealed with the two finger tips.

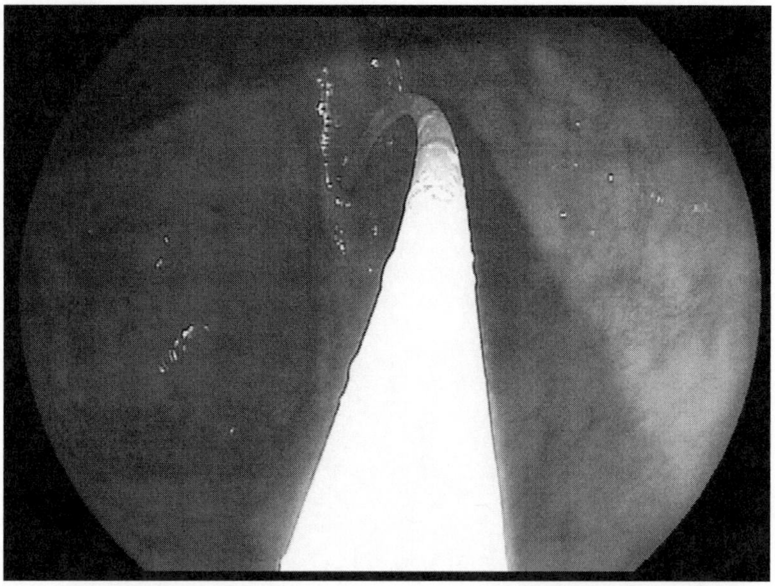

FIGURE 3 Polyethylene tubing inserted into a ureter under endoscopic guidance to obtain a urine sample.

POSTPROCEDURE

- Analgesic therapy is not usually required unless indicated by the diagnosis of the underlying entity.
- Routine antibiotic therapy is not usually required unless indicated by the underlying disease process or breaches in aseptic technique.

ALTERNATIVES AND THEIR RELATIVE MERITS

Perineal urethrotomy may be required in male horses if urethral obstruction prevents passage of an endoscope from the distal urethra.

AUTHOR: **ALLISON J. STEWART**

Enema, Barium

BASIC INFORMATION

SYNONYM(S)

Contrast enema

OVERVIEW AND GOAL(S)

Provides information on the gross structure of the rectum and colon and identifies intraluminal obstructions when present

INDICATIONS

- Suspected meconium impactions without palpable meconium in rectum
- Suspected colonic aganglionosis (lethal white foal syndrome)
- Suspected cases of atresia coli

CONTRAINDICATIONS

Suspected bowel perforation

EQUIPMENT, ANESTHESIA

- Sedation: Diazepam (0.1–0.2 mg/kg IV), butorphanol (0.05 mg/kg IV)
- Equipment: Radiographic equipment, barium sulphate suspension, 30 cm Foley catheter with 30 cc balloon, 60 mL catheter tip syringe, hemostat

ANTICIPATED TIME

10 minutes

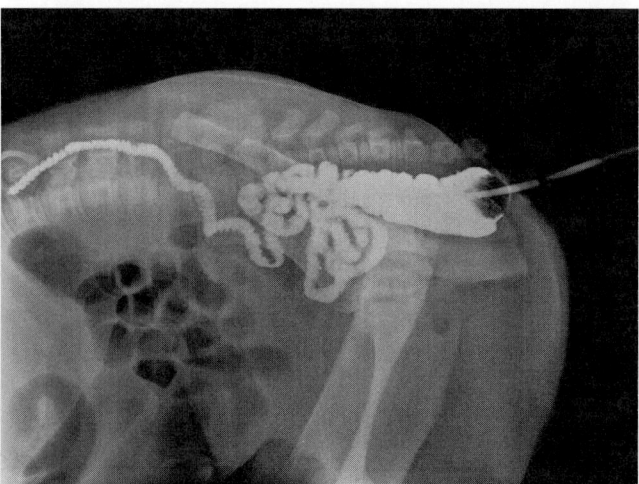

FIGURE 1 Barium enema in a colicky 1-day-old Paint colt illustrating the small diameter of the distal colon, supporting a diagnosis of lethal white foal syndrome. Intraluminal obstruction (meconium) was not evident.

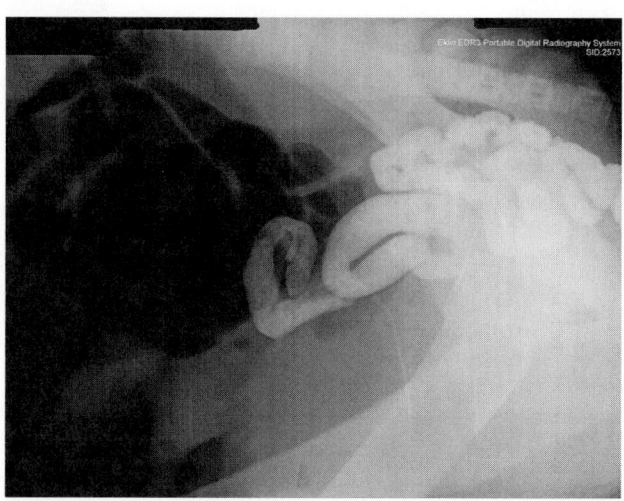

FIGURE 2 Barium enema in a colicky 1-day-old Thoroughbred colt illustrating a blind-ended colon. Intraluminal obstruction (meconium) was not evident.

PREPARATION: IMPORANT CHECKPOINTS

- Prepare 200 mL barium sulphate suspension
- Ensure adequate sedation of the foal to minimize straining and movement during radiographs

POSSIBLE COMPLICATIONS AND COMMON ERRORS TO BE AVOIDED

- Inadequate volume of barium administered. Expect to use 150–200 mL barium suspension for a 45 kg foal.
- Rapid administration of barium may result in rectal tearing.

- Inadequate sedation will result in foal straining and nondiagnostic images.

PROCEDURE

- Place sedated foal in lateral recumbancy on the radiograph plate.
- Obtain preliminary radiographs of abdomen to set radiographic technique.
- Insert well-lubricated Foley catheter 2 to 4 cm into the rectum and slowly inflate the balloon with saline or water until the rectum is occluded.
- Attach a 60 mL catheter tip syringe case to the free end of the Foley catheter; pour in barium suspension, using gravity for filling.

- Clamp the Foley with a hemostat once gravity flow is impeded or 200 mL has been administered.
- Obtain radiographic views of cranial and caudal abdomen/

POSTPROCEDURE

Deflate balloon and remove Foley catheter.

ALTERNATIVES AND THEIR RELATIVE MERITS

Abdominal ultrasound and plain film radiographs do not allow visualization of the diameter of the colon.

AUTHOR: **PHOEBE A. SMITH**

Enema, Retention/High

BASIC INFORMATION

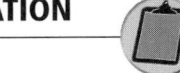

SYNONYM(S)

High enema, acetylcysteine enema

OVERVIEW AND GOAL(S)

Meconium impactions are the most common cause of colic in the neonatal foal. Routine enemas often resolve simple meconium impactions, whereas more aggressive therapy is warranted for cases that do not readily resolve with simple routine enemas.

INDICATIONS

Meconium impactions that have not resolved with routine enema administration

CONTRAINDICATIONS

Cases of suspected bowel perforation

EQUIPMENT, ANESTHESIA

- Sedation: Diazepam (0.1–0.4 mg/kg IV), butorphanol (0.05 mg/kg IV), and/or xylazine (0.3–0.5 mg/kg IV)
- Equipment: 30 cm Foley catheter with 30 cc balloon, lubricant, hemostats, 60 mL catheter tip syringe, acetylcysteine, sodium bicarbonate

ANTICIPATED TIME

45 minutes

PREPARATION: IMPORANT CHECKPOINTS

- Administration of glucose-containing intravenous fluids during the procedure is recommended (eg, lactated Ringer's solution + 2.5% dextrose at 5 mL/kg/h)

- An appropriate location for a recumbent foal should be prepared. Ambient temperature should be considered as well as temperature of enema fluid to be used.
- Preparation of a 4% acetylcysteine solution by combining 40 mL of the 20% solution with 160 mL of sterile water or by combining 100 g of powdered N-acetylcysteine with 200 mL sterile water. The final solution (prepared either way) can be mixed with 20 g of sodium bicarbonate (4 tsp baking soda) to improve the efficacy of the acetylcysteine solution.

POSSIBLE COMPLICATIONS AND COMMON ERRORS TO BE AVOIDED

- Rapid administration of the enema fluid can result in rectal tears; therefore administration should be by gravity flow only.
- Rapid filling of the Foley catheter balloon may also result in rectal mucosal trauma.
- Administration of adequate sedation is recommended; many foals react to the distension of the rectum and small colon.
- Filling the Foley catheter balloon with saline or water results in superior occlusion of the rectum than does the use of air in the balloon.

PROCEDURE

- Sedate the foal adequately for lateral recumbancy.
- A well-lubricated 30 cm Foley catheter is inserted 2.5 to 5 cm into the rectum.

The balloon is slowly distended with warm saline or water until the rectum is occluded.
- Attach a 60 mL catheter tip syringe case to the free end of the Foley and pour in 200 mL of 4% acetylcysteine solution (with sodium bicarbonate already added); allow the solution to flow by gravity.
- Clamp the Foley with the hemostat; leave in place for 30 to 45 minutes.
- Fluids may be administered during this time to ensure normal hydration and glucose availability.
- A single dose of an antiinflammatory may also be administered to reduce postprocedural straining (flunixin meglumine 1.1 mg/kg IV).
- After 30 to 45 minutes of retention time, remove the hemostats, deflate the Foley balloon, and remove the Foley catheter.

POSTPROCEDURE

Monitor meconium production and postprocedural signs of straining to defecate and colic signs. The retention enema may be repeated in 12 hours if needed.

ALTERNATIVES AND THEIR RELATIVE MERITS

Routine enemas may not be sufficient to resolve difficult meconium impactions. Surgical correction of meconium impactions is rarely required, and the need for surgical intervention has been shown to be decreased with the advent of retention enema use.

AUTHOR: **PHOEBE A. SMITH**

Esophagram, Barium

BASIC INFORMATION

SYNONYM(S)

Contrast esophagram

OVERVIEW AND GOAL(S)

A contrast agent allows evaluation of the esophageal diameter and the course of the esophagus from its proximal end to the stomach.

INDICATIONS

- Cases of dysphagia not isolated to the head or pharynx (swallowing is normal)
- Evidence of esophageal obstruction (esophageal foreign body, esophageal stricture)

CONTRAINDICATIONS

- Evidence or risk of esophageal perforation.
- If esophageal perforation is suspected, nonionic iodinated contrast agents may be used (iohexol).

EQUIPMENT, ANESTHESIA

- Sedation: If needed for restraint and placement of a nasogastric tube (diazepam 0.1–0.2 mg/kg IV)
- Radiographic equipment, small nasogastric tube, barium sulphate suspension or iodinated contrast agent, 60 mL catheter tip syringe

ANTICIPATED TIME

20 minutes

PREPARATION: IMPORANT CHECKPOINTS

- Obtain survey films of cervical and thoracic esophagus.
- Place nasogastric tube (stallion catheter works well) in the most proximal esophagus.
- Handler, injector of contrast agent, and radiographer should be in position before the contrast agent is administered.

POSSIBLE COMPLICATIONS AND COMMON ERRORS TO BE AVOIDED

- Aspiration of contrast agent if nasogastric tube is not appropriately placed and maintained.
- Insufficient volume of contrast used, resulting in misdiagnosis.
- Delayed radiographs yields spurious results because the contrast agent is moved aborally through the esophagus.

PROCEDURE

- Sedation: If needed (diazepam 0.1–0.2 mg/kg IV)
- Foal should be standing or maintained in sternal recumbancy.
- Administer the contrast agent by gravity flow via the indwelling nasogastric tube.
- Take radiographs immediately after contrast administration, imaging the cervical esophagus first, then the thoracic esophagus and stomach.
- Repeat contrast administration if needed to evaluate suspicious areas.

POSTPROCEDURE

Ensure there is no contrast in the nasogastric tube before removing it by administering a small amount of water or air through the tube.

ALTERNATIVES AND THEIR RELATIVE MERITS

Esophageal images obtained by plain film radiographs do not reliably delineate strictures or foreign bodies. Ultrasound of the esophagus is limited to the cervical region.

AUTHOR: **PHOEBE A. SMITH**

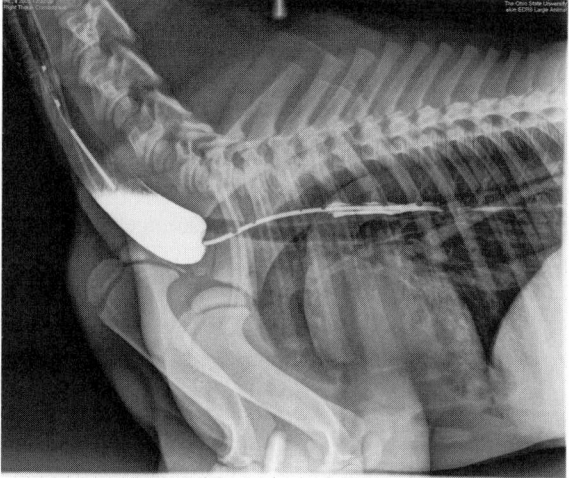

FIGURE 1 Barium esophagram in a 2-day-old Quarter Horse filly with milk regurgitation; dilation, barium pooling proximal to the thoracic inlet, and marked narrowing of the esophagus at the thoracic inlet are visible.

Estrus Suppression

BASIC INFORMATION

OVERVIEW AND GOAL(S)

- Estrus behavior is a problem in performance mares.
- Many have temperament changes and become more difficult to handle during the estrus period.
- Some mares show aggression, pain, and reduced performance while in heat.
- An accurate diagnosis is necessary to avoid confusion with other health issues that can cause refractory or chronic pain (gastric ulcers, lameness, back soreness, muscle soreness, etc.)

INDICATIONS

- The abnormal behavior creates a problem, especially in mares used for performance careers.
- Many mares fail to perform at their best due to strong sexual behavior and may become more difficult to manage or even appear lame when in heat.

- This behavior usually corresponds to the follicular phase of the estrous cycle.
- There may also be behavioral and physical effects of the estrogens, such as increased joint laxity, that can adversely affect performance.
- This behavior may also be related to pain associated with growing follicles that stretch the ovarian tunic, or from rupture of the follicle at ovulation. Many mares exhibit pain during ovarian palpation immediately after ovulation.

TREATMENTS
NON PHARMACOLOGIC
- Ovariectomy or surgical removal of both ovaries will eliminate the cyclicity of mares.
  - Advantage: Long-term or definitive treatment.
  - Disadvantages: This procedure eliminates any future reproductive potential; low effectiveness on estrus inhibition. As many as 30% of mares may exhibit behavioral signs of estrus even after ovariectomy.
  - If the unwanted behavior is not related to the estrous cycle it will not be modified by the surgery.
- Intrauterine marble: The use of a 35-mm intrauterine glass ball induces a state of false pregnancy and prolongs the luteal phase.
  - Advantage: Nonpharmacologic treatment to suppress estrus behavior.
  - Disadvantage: Effective in only 40% of the mares in a report by Nie et al in 2001. As a foreign body, the marble may become a nidus for uterine infection.
- Induced pseudopregnancy by disruption of the conceptus development in pregnant mares after maternal recognition of pregnancy (between days 16–22), can prolong the diestral phase in some mares for almost 3 months. To maximize effectiveness, the pregnancy may be terminated after the formation of the endometrial cups (after day 45), which should prevent estrus behavior for 120–150 days.
  - Advantage: Nonpharmacologic alternative to suppress estrus behavior.
  - Disadvantage: Ethical issues as it involves aborting a viable pregnancy. If the pregnancy is not aborted appropriately, the mare may carry the pregnancy to term and deliver a foal. Any fetal membranes or tissue that are retained may be a source for infection or lead to generalized sepsis.

HORMONAL TREATMENTS
- Natural progesterone: Suppresses estrus behavior, simulates diestrus.

Estrus behavior occurs when the mare's progesterone plasma concentration is less than 1 to 2 ng/mL.
  - Dose: Progesterone in oil 100 to 150 mg IM q24h; May take 2 to 3 days for mare to go out of behavioral estrus.
  - Advantage: Very effective
  - Disadvantage: Daily intramuscular injection is impractical and may be associated with local tissue reactions. Also, daily injections may lead to injection aversion in some mares.
- Long-acting progesterone: Compounded long-acting injectable formulation.
  - Dose: 10 mL/animal (150 mg/mL) dose once weekly can achieve serum concentrations sufficient to block behavioral estrus for up to 45 days.
  - Advantage: Effective treatment. Daily injections are not necessary.
  - Disadvantage: May induce injection site reactions.
- Synthetic progesterone compounds: Most studies about synthetic progesterone products in the mare have shown them to be ineffective (norgestomet, medroxyprogesterone acetate, megestrol acetate). The most widely used synthetic progesterone and the only one with proven effectiveness is altrenogest (Regumate). Altrenogest claims to be effective in reducing behavioral estrus in 95% of mares (dose: 0.044 mg/kg/day PO). Altrenogest suppresses behavioral estrus in mares within 2 to 3 days of the start of administration.
  - Advantage: Effective in estrus behavior suppression. Oral.
  - Disadvantages: Necessity of daily treatment, which can make mares reluctant to be handled around the mouth. Costly and impractical for long-term use. Continued daily exposure of horse owners may affect human health such as "disruption of the menstrual cycle, uterine or abdominal cramping, uterine bleeding, prolongation of pregnancy, and headaches." (Regumate, package insert).
- Immunization against GnRH: Neutralization of GnRH is achieved by inducing an immune response and production of specific antibodies after vaccination with a GnRH carrier protein and an adjuvant (Equity, Pfizer Animal Health P/L, West Ryde, NSW, Australia).
  - Advantage: Long-term treatment.
  - Disadvantages: Contradictory reports on effectiveness of suppressing estrus behavior. Not available in the United States at this time.

- GnRH antagonist: inhibit the action of GnRH, thereby suppressing ovarian activity (Antarelix, Europeptides. Argenteuil, France)
  - Disadvantages: Requires frequent administration. The behavioral estrus signs are inconsistent because of suppressed ovarian activity.
- GnRH agonist: Treatment with deslorelin acetate (Ovuplant, Fort Dodge Animal Health, IA) inhibits the action of GnRH, by overstimulation that causes a down regulation of pituitary gonadotropin secretion thereby suppressing ovarian activity.
  - Disadvantages: Inconsistent results
- Oxytocin Injection: Vanderwall et al (2007) showed that administration of oxytocin (60 IU IM q12h for 7 days) was an efficacious method to extend luteal function in mares.
  - Advantages: Induce estrus suppression for 30 to 40 days.
  - Disadvantages: Just one study was performed and used a low number of mares; also, behavioral estrus was not monitored in this study. Multiple injections of a relatively high dose of oxytocin may cause excessive discomfort, cramping, and pain.

SUMMARY
- Expression of behavioral estrus in mares can have a profound negative effect on training and performance.
- Clinical signs attributed to performance problems include attitude changes, tail swishing, difficulty in training, squealing, excessive urination, kicking, and colic-like discomfort associated with ovulation.
- The only effective treatments to suppress estrus behavior in mares are the use of natural progesterone or Altrenogest. At this time, however, there is no single long-term treatment available to suppress estrus signs in mares that is also safe, effective, and convenient.

PEARLS & CONSIDERATIONS

COMMENT
- It should be noted that the manifestation of estrus behavior in anovulatory mares is a phenomenon that has been described after any treatment that inhibits ovarian function including vaccination against GnRH, treatment with GnRH antagonists, and ovariectomy due to low circulating progesterone.
- Different treatments may work differently in each mare. Treatment options should be discussed with owners and the best treatment for that mare and owner should be attempted.

CLIENT EDUCATION

Always wear gloves to manipulate Regumate® (altrenogest) as it can be absorbed through intact skin, affecting manipulator's health.

SUGGESTED READING

Elhay M, Newbold A, Britton A, et al: Suppression of behavioral and physiological oestrus in the mare by vaccination against GnRH. *Aust Vet J* 85(1&2):39–45, 2007.

Gee EK, DeLuca C, Stylski JL, et al: Efficacy of medroxiprogesterone acetate in suppression of estrus in cycling mares. *J Equine Vet Sci* 29(3):140–145, 2009.

Imboden I, Janett F, Burger D, et al: Influence of immunization against GnRH on reproductive cyclicity and estrous behavior in the mare. *Theriogenology* 66:1866–1975, 2006.

Lefranc AC, Allen WR: Non pharmacological suppression of oestrus in the mare. *Equine Vet J* 36(2):183–185: 2004.

Nie GJ, Johnson KE, Wenzel JGW: Use of glass ball to suppress behavioral estrus in mares. *Proc Am Assoc Equine Pract* 47:246–248, 2001.

Pryor P, Tibary A: Management of estrus in the performance mare. *Clinical Techniques in Equine Practice* 4(3):197–209, 2005.

Vanderwall DK, Rasmussen DM, Woods GL: Effect of repeated administration of oxytocin during diestrus on duration of function of corpora lutea in mares. *J Am Vet Med Assoc* 231(12):1864–1867, 2007.

Watson ED, Pedersen HG, Thomson SRM, Fraser HM: Control of follicular development and luteal function in the mare: effect of a GnRH antagonist. *Theriogenology* 54:599–609, 2000.

AUTHOR: **GHISLAINE DUJOVNE**

EDITOR: **JUAN C. SAMPER**

Exodontia (Oral Extraction)

BASIC INFORMATION

SYNONYM(S)

Pulling a tooth

OVERVIEW AND GOAL(S)

To remove the affected tooth in its entirely via the oral cavity, creating as little collateral damage as possible.

INDICATIONS

Severe periapical infection, periodontal disease, or teeth fractured beyond salvagability.

EQUIPMENT, ANESTHESIA

- Perineural nerve blocks (dental blocks)
- Adequate sedation
- Molar spreaders (in various degrees of angulation)
- Molar extraction forceps
- Variety of fulcrums
- Anesthetic agent: Lidocaine 2%, mepivacaine 2%, or bupivacaine 0.75%

ANTICIPATED TIME

20 minutes to several days

PREPARATION: IMPORANT CHECKPOINTS

Quality radiographs, oral examination, and advanced imaging (computed tomography) if necessary. Ensure that exodontia remains the only means of controlling the problem and improving the quality of life.

POSSIBLE COMPLICATIONS AND COMMON ERRORS TO BE AVOIDED

- Inadvertent removal of the incorrect tooth
- Fracturing the tooth such that intraoral extraction becomes impossible
- Inadvertently leaving dental fragments within the alveolus, which could subsequently sequester

PROCEDURE

- Sedate sufficiently to allow perineural analgesia.
- Additional sedation may be necessary.
- Place the full-mouth speculum and light source such that the tooth to be removed can be adequately visualized.
- Apply the molar spreaders to the interdental space caudal to the affected tooth. Slowly apply force to drive the wedges together. NOTE: This takes time and should not be rushed. The handles of the instrument can be taped together to reduce operator fatigue. This stage can take up to 20 minutes or longer (Figure 1).
- Apply the molar spreaders to the interdental space rostral to the affected tooth. Use the same technique as above.
- Elevate the gingiva on all sides of the tooth (Figure 2).
- DO NOT APPLY MOLAR FORCEPS UNTIL THE TOOTH IS DEMONSTRABLY LOOSE. At this stage, the alveolus will be bleeding readily and "squishing" sounds can be heard when the tooth is manually grasped and rocked.
- Apply molar extraction forceps (Figure 3). Insert fulcrum to allow the handles of the instrument to be moved toward the occlusal surface of the tooth. DO NOT ROCK THE INSTRUMENT IN A DORSOVENTRAL DIRECTION. If molar forceps application has occurred at the correct time, pressure against the fulcrum will result in elevation of the tooth from the alveolus as a single, intact unit. (Figure 4).
- Remove from the mouth and check that the specimen is intact.
- Check the alveolus manually and radiographically for retained fragments.
- Pack alveolus if necessary. A variety of products are available, such as iodine-soaked gauze and plaster of Paris. The author currently recommends a Silastic pack (Splash Putty Pak, regular putty, firm setting (European distributor: EMDAR BV, El Arnhem, The Netherlands; North American distributor: Discus Dental Inc., Culver City, CA).

POSTPROCEDURE

Ensure that pack is still in position or replace it if necessary (depending on pack design).

AUTHOR: **JAMES L. CARMALT**

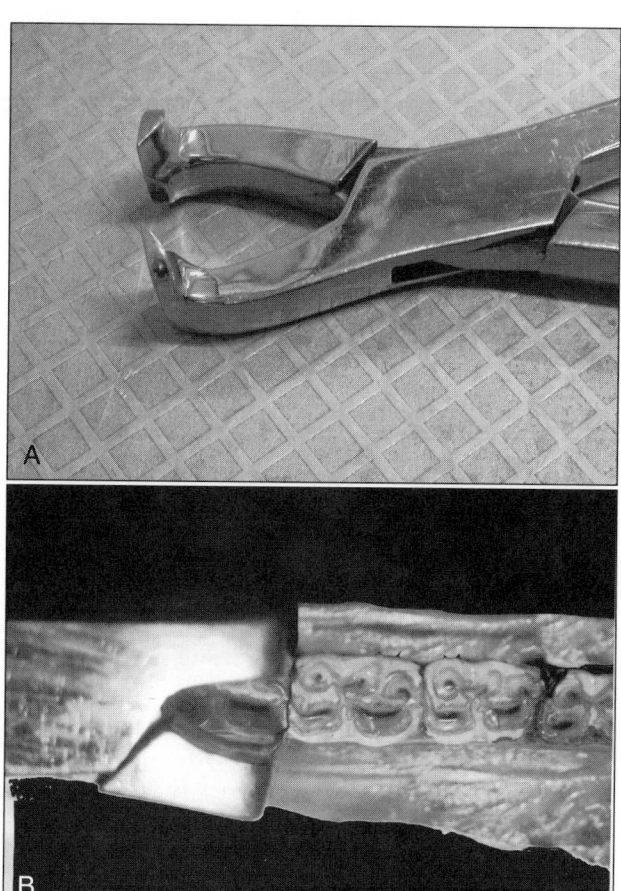

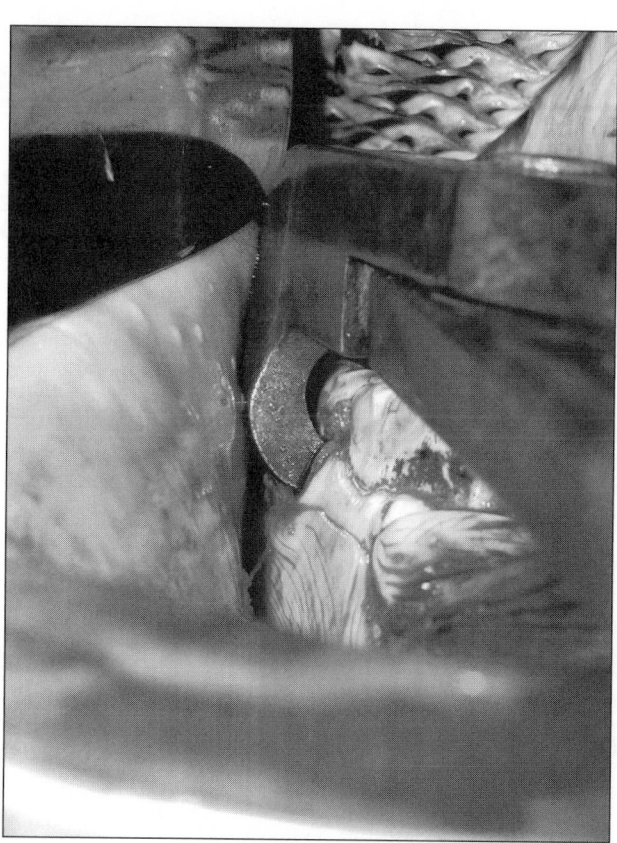

FIGURE 3 The molar extractors are placed on the tooth to be extracted in an attempt to gain maximal contact between forceps and tooth. (From Baker GJ, Easley J [eds]: *Equine dentistry*, ed 2. New York, 2005, Saunders Elsevier, pp 267–294.)

FIGURE 1 **A**, Molar separators with varied head designs achieve different degrees of separation. **B**, The molar separators (**A**) are placed in the interdentium rostral and caudal to the affected tooth and cautiously closed to stretch the mesial and distal periodontal attachments (**B**). (From Baker GJ, Easley J [eds]: *Equine dentistry*, ed 2. New York, 2005, Saunders Elsevier, pp 267–294.)

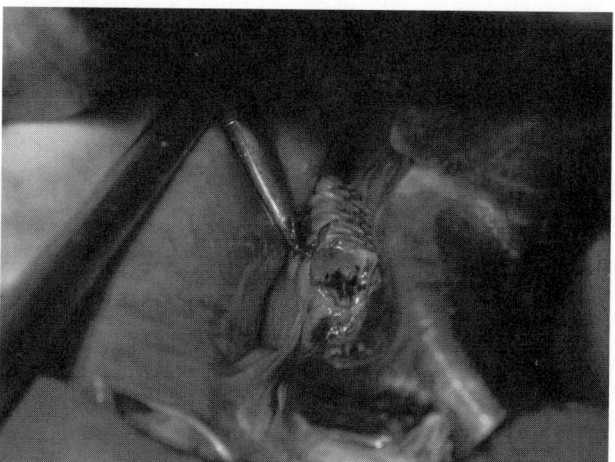

FIGURE 2 Flat-bladed periodontal elevators are used to gently elevate the gingival and periodontal attachments from the buccal and lingual aspects of the tooth. (From Baker GJ, Easley J [eds]: *Equine dentistry*, ed 2. New York, 2005, Saunders Elsevier, pp 267–294.)

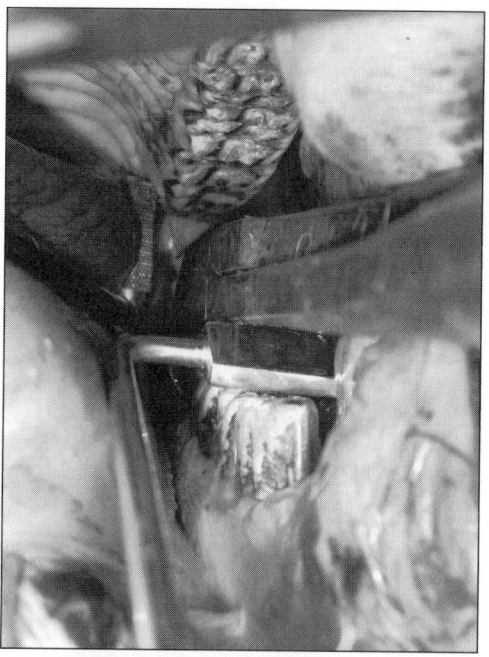

FIGURE 4 Once the fulcrum is positioned carefully, extraction can be performed by exerting a firm force on the handles of the extractors to elevate the tooth from the alveolus. (From Baker GJ, Easley J [eds]: *Equine dentistry*, ed 2. New York, 2005, Saunders Elsevier, pp 267–294.)

Exodontia: Lateral Buccotomy Extraction

BASIC INFORMATION

SYNONYM(S)

Punching a tooth
Repulsing a tooth

OVERVIEW AND GOAL(S)

To remove the affected tooth, the whole tooth, and nothing but the affected tooth by resection of the lateral alveolar plate and either extracting the entire tooth laterally or using this method to repulse the tooth into the oral cavity

INDICATIONS

Severe periapical infection, periodontal disease, and teeth fractured beyond repair that cannot be removed via the oral approach and have no chance of survival if left in place

EQUIPMENT, ANESTHESIA

- Perineural nerve blocks (dental blocks)
- General anesthesia
- Molar spreaders (various degrees of angulation)
- Radiographic guidance
- Anesthetic agent: Lidocaine 2%, Mepivacaine 2%, or Bupivacaine 0.75%

ANTICIPATED TIME

90 minutes

PREPARATION: IMPORTANT CHECKPOINTS

- Quality radiographs, oral examination, and advanced imaging computed tomography (CT) if necessary
- Ensure that exodontia remains the only means of controlling the problem and improving the quality of life.

POSSIBLE COMPLICATIONS AND COMMON ERRORS TO BE AVOIDED

- Inadvertent removal of the incorrect tooth.
- Inadvertently leaving dental fragments within the alveolus that could subsequently sequester.

PROCEDURE

- Place horse under general anesthesia.
- Perform perineural analgesia.
- Place full-mouth speculum and light source such that the tooth to be removed can be adequately visualized.
- Apply the molar spreaders to the interdental space caudal to the affected tooth.
  - Slowly apply force to drive the wedges together. NOTE: This takes time and should not be rushed.
  - The handles of the instrument can be taped together to reduce operator fatigue.
  - This stage can take up to 20 minutes or longer.
- Apply the molar spreaders to the interdental space rostral to the affected tooth. Technique as above.
- Elevate gingiva on all sides of the tooth.
- Clip hair from lateral aspect of head in region of surgical field.
- Surgically prepare the skin.
  - Using radiographic guidance, place 18-gauge needles through the cheek at the level of the gingiva such that one needle is rostral and one is caudal to the tooth in question.
- Elevate a semicircle of skin with periosteum between these needles.
- Using an oscillating saw, sterile cast cutter, or osteotome and mallet, remove the lateral alveolar plate of bone over the affected tooth.
- Remove entire tooth from this incision.
- Close the periosteum, subcutaneous tissue, and skin in three separate layers.
- Pack alveolus if necessary.
  - A variety of products are available such as iodine-soaked gauze, plaster of Paris. The author currently recommends a silastic pack (Splash Putty Pak, Regular Putty, firm setting [EU Distributor: EMDAR BV, Ijsselburcht 3, Pob 5486, 6802 El Arnhem, The Netherlands, 31 263-653-375], [North American Distributor: Discus Dental Inc., Culver City, CA 90232 1-800-422-9448]).
- Recover the horse.

POSTPROCEDURE

- Ensure that pack is still in position or replace if necessary (depending on pack design).
- Judicious nonsteroidal antiinflammatory medication. The author typically uses 2 g phenylbutazone by mouth once daily for 3 days, followed by 1 g by mouth once daily for a further 2 days.
- Antimicrobial therapy is generally not necessary.

ALTERNATIVES AND THEIR RELATIVE MERITS

Exodontia: oral approach. This is the preferred method, with a published success rate of 87% first-time resolution of clinical problems.

AUTHOR: **JAMES L. CARMALT**

Exodontia: Retrograde Repulsion

BASIC INFORMATION

SYNONYM(S)

Punching a tooth
Repulsing a tooth

OVERVIEW AND GOAL(S)

To remove the affected tooth, the whole tooth, and nothing but the affected tooth by repulsing it and any associated fragments into the oral cavity

INDICATIONS

Severe periapical infection, periodontal disease, and teeth fractured beyond treatment that cannot be removed via the oral approach

EQUIPMENT, ANESTHESIA

- Perineural nerve blocks (dental blocks)
- Adequate sedation or general anesthesia
- Molar spreaders (various degrees of angulation)
- Variety of blunted Steinmann pin or dental punches
- Radiographic guidance
- Anesthetic agent: Lidocaine 2%, mepivacaine 2% or bupivacaine 0.75%

ANTICIPATED TIME

20 minutes to several hours

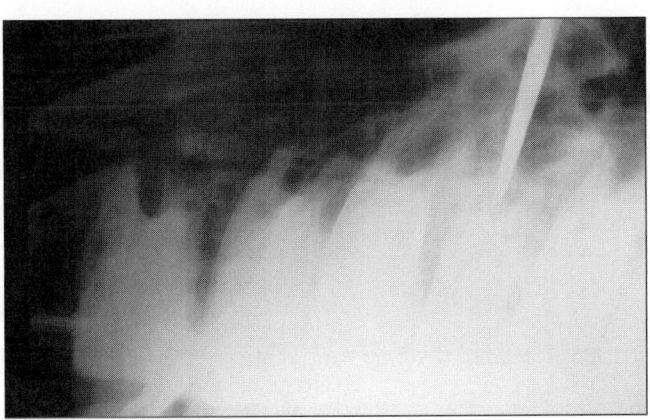

FIGURE 1 Oblique intraoperative radiograph showing a metallic marker used to check the line of repulsion for the extraction of 209. (From Tremaine WH, Lane JG: Exodontia. In Baker GJ, Easley J, editors: *Equine dentistry*, ed 2, New York, 2005, Saunders Elsevier, pp 267–294.)

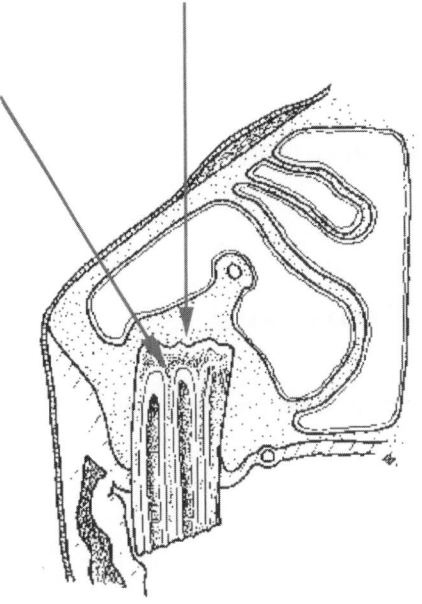

FIGURE 2 Diagram to illustrate the correct positioning of the trephine hole directly over the apex of the tooth to be extracted. (From Tremaine WH, Lane JG: Exodontia. In Baker GJ, Easley J, editors: *Equine dentistry*, ed 2, New York, 2005, Saunders Elsevier, pp 267–294.)

PREPARATION: IMPORTANT CHECKPOINTS

- Quality radiographs, oral examination, and advanced imaging such as computed tomography (CT) if necessary
- Ensure that exodontia remains the only means of controlling the problem and improving the quality of life.

POSSIBLE COMPLICATIONS AND COMMON ERRORS TO BE AVOIDED

- Inadvertent removal of the incorrect tooth.
- Inadvertently leaving dental fragments within the alveolus that could subsequently sequester.

PROCEDURE

- Sedate sufficiently to allow perineural analgesia.
- Additional sedation may be necessary.
- Place full-mouth speculum and light source such that the tooth to be removed can be adequately visualized.
- Apply the molar spreaders to the interdental space caudal to the affected tooth.

- ○ Slowly apply force to drive the wedges together. NOTE: This takes time and should not be rushed.
- ○ The handles of the instrument can be taped together to reduce operator fatigue.
- ○ This stage can take up to 20 minutes or longer.
- Apply the molar spreaders to the interdental space rostral to the affected tooth. Technique as above.
- Elevate gingiva on all sides of the tooth.
- Using radiographic and manual guidance, remove a circle of bone using a Michelle or Galt trephine over the tooth root in question (Figure 1).
- Place blunt Steinmann pin or dental punch above the tooth roots and using firm, repeated tapping motions with the mallet, drive the pin/punch onto the tooth until it is well seated.
- Ensure that the correct tooth is being removed (digital palpation per os) will allow the operator to feel the vibration of the tooth immediately underneath the punch (Figure 2).
- Drive the tooth into the mouth and extract manually.

- Remove from mouth and check that the specimen is intact. If not, repeat the motion to remove all palpable dental fragments and confirm radiographically.
- Pack alveolus if necessary. Variety of products are available such as iodine-soaked gauze, plaster of Paris. The author currently recommends a silastic pack (Splash Putty Pak, Regular Putty, firm setting [EU Distributor: EMDAR BV, Ijsselburcht 3, Pob 5486, 6802 El Arnhem, The Netherlands, 31 263-653-375], [North American Distributor: Discus Dental Inc., Culver City, CA 90232 1-800-422-9448]).

POSTPROCEDURE

Ensure that pack is still in position or replace if necessary (depending on pack design).

ALTERNATIVES AND THEIR RELATIVE MERITS

Exodontia: oral approach. This is the preferred method, with a published success rate of 87% first-time resolution of clinical problems.

AUTHOR: **JAMES L. CARMALT**

Gait Analysis

BASIC INFORMATION

SYNONYM(S)
Kinematic lameness evaluation, evaluation of lameness

OVERVIEW AND GOAL(S)
Evaluation of lameness while observing the horse moving is current standard of care. However, agreement for evaluation of mild to moderate lameness is poor. Gait analysis has determined the movement parameters most sensitive for detection of lameness in horses. Although altered limb movement may be helpful in select cases, asymmetry of vertical movement of the torso is more sensitive and specific.

INDICATIONS
Mild or multiple limb lameness, evaluating lameness after blocking, prepurchase evaluations, evaluating recovery after treatment

EQUIPMENT
Two accelerometers and one gyroscopic sensor (for right forelimb), tablet computer, USB Bluetooth receiver, head bumper, pastern pouch, tape

ANTICIPATED TIME
15 minutes

PREPARATION: IMPORTANT CHECKPOINTS (Figure 1)
- Attach the head sensor to the head bumper.

- Attach the pelvis sensor to a strip of 3M Dual Lock tape on the dorsal midline and tape in place.
- Place the gyroscopic sensor in the right forelimb pastern pouch on the dorsal aspect of the limb.
- Place sensor labels face up (head and pelvis sensors) or out (right forelimb sensor).
- Face the light-emitting diodes of sensors forward (head and pelvis sensors) or up (right forelimb sensor). Collect at least 25 strides.

POSSIBLE COMPLICATIONS AND COMMON ERRORS TO BE AVOIDED
- Placing gyroscopic sensor on a limb other than right forelimb
- Placing gyroscopic sensor upside down or backwards
- Switching head and pelvic accelerometer

PROCEDURE

FORELIMB LAMENESS (Figure 2)
- *Pain in first half of stance:*
  - Neck muscles reduce weight bearing by restricting fall of the head and neck.
  - Measure the difference in minimum head position (HEADDIFFMIN) between left and right limb stances.
    - By convention, HEADDIFFMIN is positive when the head falls less during right forelimb stance and negative when the head falls less during left forelimb stance.

- The horse may also push off the opposite, sound limb harder.
- Measure the difference in maximum head position (HEADDIFFMAX) between left and right limb stances.
  - By convention, HEADDIFMAX is positive when the head rises more after left forelimb push-off and negative when the head rises more after right forelimb push-off.
- Lameness closer to beginning of stance will cause greater asymmetry in HEADIFFMAX than in HEADDIFFMIN.
- Lameness closer to midstance will cause greater asymmetry in HEADDIFFMIN than in HEADDIFFMAX.
- Horses with positive HEADDIFFMIN and HEADDIFFMAX have lameness in the first half of right forelimb stance.
- Horses with negative HEADDIFFMIN and HEADDIFFMAX have lameness in the first half of left forelimb stance.
- *Pain in second half of stance:*
  - Neck muscle activity reduces force on limb by raising the head and neck.
  - Measure the difference in maximum head position (HEADDIFFMAX) after push-off between right and left limbs.
    - By convention, HEADDIFFMAX is negative when the head rises more after push-off of the right forelimb and negative when the

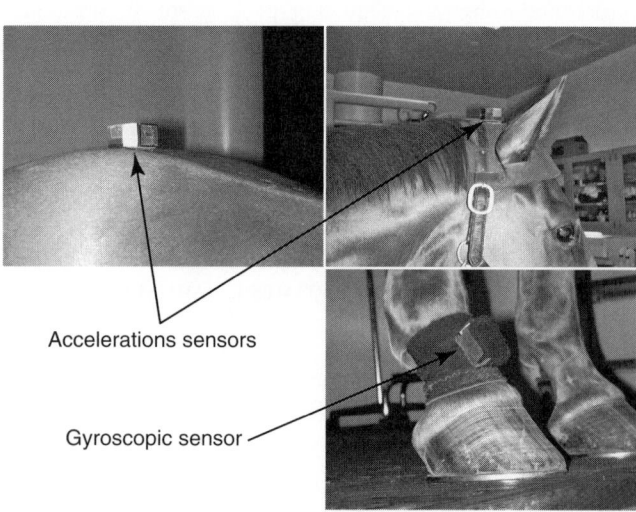

FIGURE 1 Lameness Locator (Equinosis) body-mounted sensors.

Accelerations sensors

Gyroscopic sensor

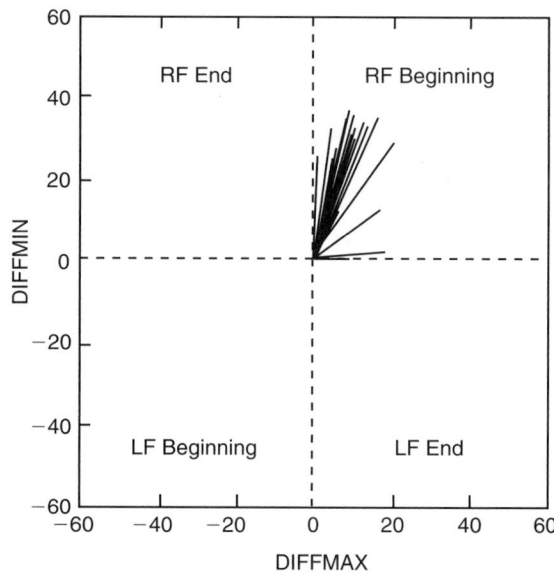

FIGURE 2 Right forelimb beginning of stance lameness, positive HEADDIFFMAX and positive HEADDIFFMIN.

head rises more after push-off of the left forelimb.

- Lameness closer to breakover will cause greater asymmetry in HEAD-DIFFMAX than in HEADDIFFMIN.
- Horses with negative HEADDIFF-MAX and positive HEADDIFFMIN have lameness in the second half of the right forelimb stance.
- Horses with positive HEADDIFF-MAX and negative HEADDIFFMIN have lameness in the second half of the left forelimb stance.

- Forelimb lameness is displayed as a ray diagram (see Figure 2). The *x*-axis is HEADDIFFMAX and the *y*-axis is HEADDIFFMIN.
  - Each blue ray is one stride.
  - Length of ray indicates amplitudes of HEADDIFFMIN and HEADDIFF-MAX and represents severity of lameness of stride.
  - Mean HEADDIFFMIN and HEAD-DIFFMAX are calculated over all strides.
  - Ray orientation indicates limb involved (left/right) and timing (beginning/end of stance) of lameness.
    - Rays in quadrant 1 indicate right forelimb beginning of stance lameness
    - Rays in quadrant 2 indicate right forelimb end of stance lameness
    - Rays in quadrant 3 indicate left forelimb beginning of stance lameness
    - Rays in quadrant 4 indicate left forelimb end of stance lameness
  - Thresholds for HEADDIFFMIN and HEADDIFFMAX between normal and lameness are estimated (±6 mm).

HINDLIMB LAMENESS (Figure 3)

- *Pain in first half of stance:*
  - Extensor muscles reduce pelvic falling.
  - Measure the difference of minimum pelvic height (PELVISDIFFMIN) between right and left hindlimb stance phase.
    - By convention, PELVISDIFFMIN is positive when the pelvis falls less during stance phase of the right hindlimb and negative when pelvis falls less during stance phase of the left hindlimb.
  - Positive PELVICDIFFMIN indicates lameness in the first half of right hindlimb stance.
  - Negative PELVICDIFFMIN indicates lameness in the first half of left hindlimb stance.
- *Pain in second half of hindlimb stance:*
  - Reduced rate of pelvic upward thrust.
  - Measure the difference in maximum pelvic height (PELVISDIFFMAX)

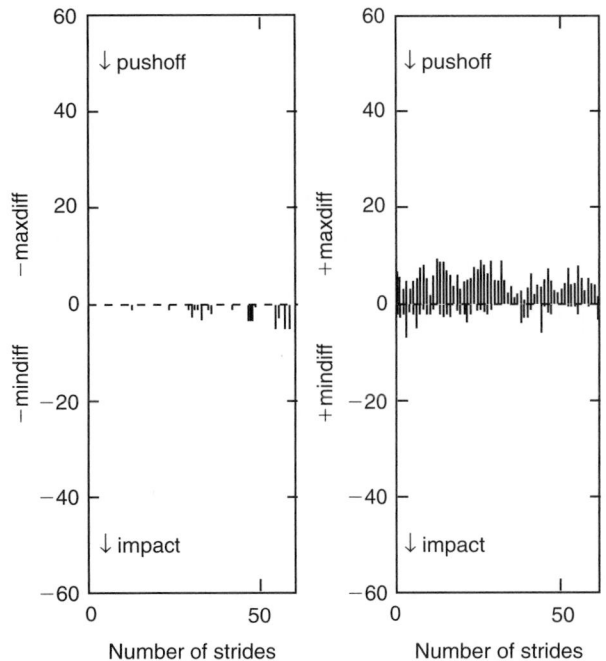

FIGURE 3 Right hindlimb push-off lameness, positive PELVICDIFFMAX.

between right and left hindlimb push-off.
- By convention, PELVISDIFFMAX is positive when the pelvis rises less after push-off of the right hindlimb and negative when the pelvis rises less after push-off of the left hindlimb.
  - Positive PELVICDIFFMAX indicates right hindlimb push-off lameness.
  - Negative PELVICDIFFMAX indicates left hindlimb push-off lameness.
- Most horses with hindlimb lameness display components of both impact and push-off lameness.
  - Hindlimb lameness displayed as "deficiencies" in impact and/or push-off (see Figure 3).
  - Left plot indicates left and right plot right hindlimb deficiencies.
  - For each limb, "deficiency" of impact/push-off is indicated with the first stride on the extreme left and last on the extreme right of each plot.
  - The amplitude of each red, upwardly directed line above the horizontal (PELVICDIFFMAX) is an indicator of the "deficiency" of that hindlimb's push-off for that stride.
  - The amplitude of each green, downwardly directed line below horizontal (PELVICDIFFMIN) is an indicator of "deficiency" of that hindlimb's impact for that stride.
  - Mean PELVICDIFFMAX and PEL-VICDIFFMIN are calculated over all strides.
    - More and longer red rays pointing upward on the left indicate left hindlimb push-off lameness.

- More and longer red rays pointing upward on the right indicate right hindlimb push-off lameness.
- More and longer green rays pointing downward on the left indicate left hindlimb impact lameness.
- More and longer green rays pointing downward on the right indicate right hindlimb impact lameness.
  - Thresholds for PELVICDIFFMIN and PELVICDIFFMAX between normal and lameness are estimated (±3 mm).

COMPENSATORY LAMENESS

- *Compensatory forelimb lameness:*
  - During the trot, a horse with primary hindlimb lameness may shift its center of gravity forward during weight bearing of the lame hindlimb by moving its head forward and downward.
  - The head moves down farther during contralateral forelimb stance, giving the appearance of ipsilateral forelimb lameness.
  - Sometimes primary hindlimb lameness is very mild and apparent, but false compensatory head movement is quite dramatic.
  - Increased sensitivity of inertial sensors for measuring pelvic movement asymmetry protects against concentrating on false compensatory forelimb lameness (Figure 4).
- *Compensatory hindlimb lameness:*
  - During the trot, a horse with primary forelimb lameness may shift its

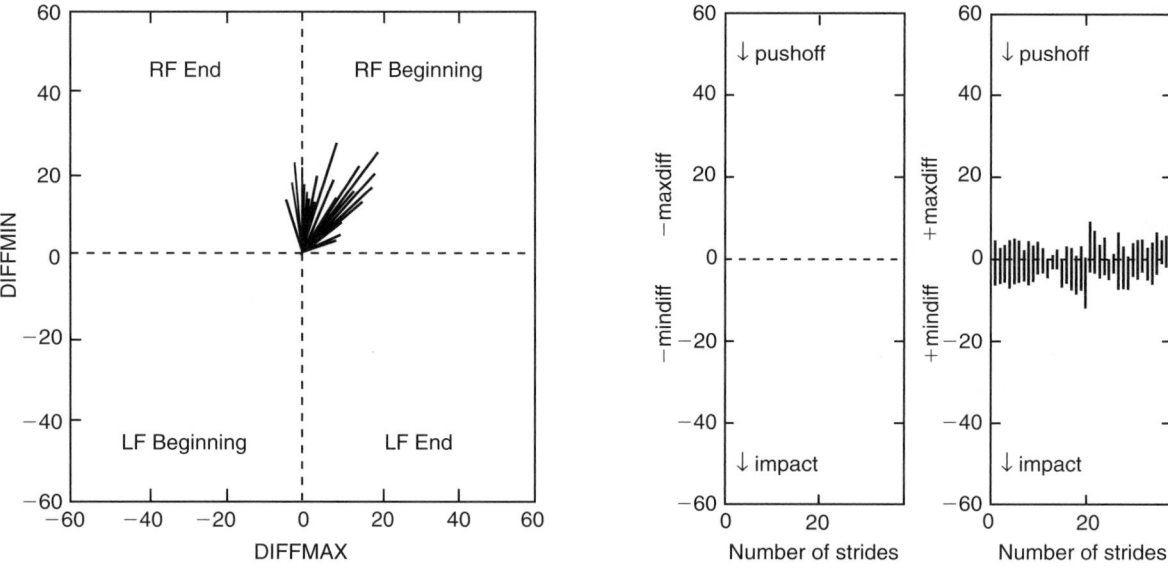

FIGURE 4 Primary right hindlimb lameness with compensatory right forelimb.

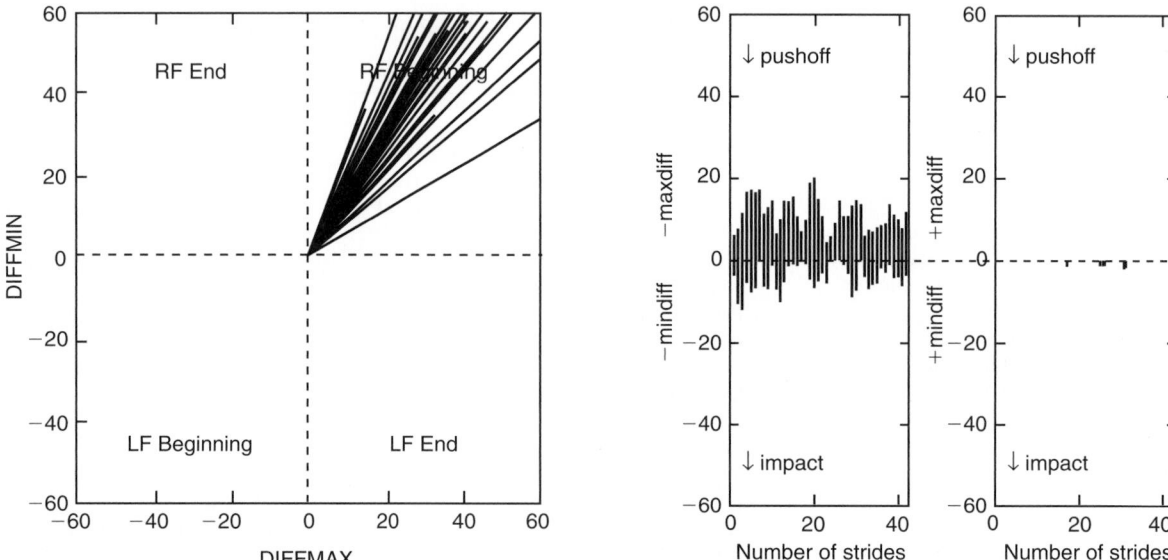

FIGURE 5 Primary right forelimb lameness with compensatory contralateral left hindlimb push-off lameness.

center of gravity backward during weight bearing of the lame limb by moving its head backward and upward.

○ Shifting weight backward causes the pelvis to fall more during contralateral hindlimb stance, giving the appearance of ipsilateral hindlimb impact lameness.

○ During the succeeding stance phase in opposite diagonal, the horse will normally push off harder, giving the appearance of contralateral hindlimb push-off lameness.

○ Compensatory contralateral hindlimb push-off deficiency usually is more prominent than compensatory ipsilateral hindlimb impact deficiency.

○ Compensatory hindlimb deficiency is usually only seen when primary forelimb lameness is severe.

○ Compensatory deficiencies in pelvic movement with primary forelimb lameness can be easily seen with an inertial sensor system and can be used to assist in the evaluation of forelimb lameness (Figure 5).

LUNGING

• Lunging horses may have asymmetric head and torso movement because the torso is tilted toward the center of the circle. This may cause subjective appearance of lameness.

• In normal horses, asymmetric lunging in one direction will be equal in amplitude but opposite in direction to lunging in the other direction.

• Lunging on soft surface:
  ○ Head movement asymmetry may mimic outside forelimb push-off lameness.
  ○ Pelvic movement asymmetry may mimic inside hindlimb impact lameness and outside hindlimb push-off lameness (Figure 6).

• Lunging on hard surface:
  ○ Head movement asymmetry may mimic an inside forelimb impact lameness.
  ○ Pelvic movement asymmetry may mimic an inside hindlimb impact lameness.

• Deviations from expected asymmetry may indicate lameness (Figure 7).

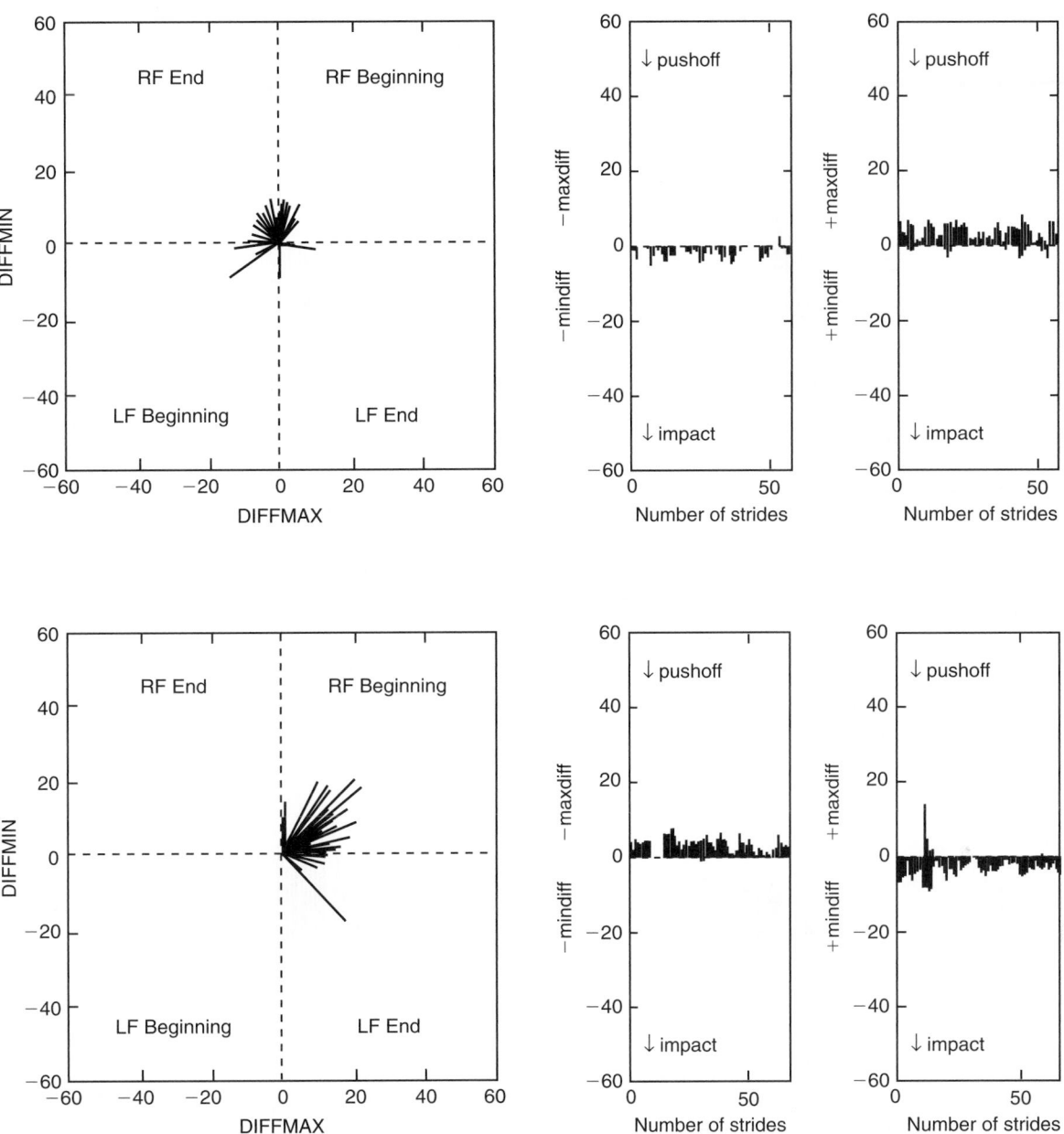

FIGURE 6 Equal but opposite pelvic movement asymmetry when horse is lunging to the left and then to the right. Lunging to the left has apparent left hindlimb (inside hindlimb) impact lameness and right hindlimb (outside limb) push-off lameness. Lunging to the right has apparent right hindlimb impact lameness and left hindlimb push-off lameness. This horse has mild right forelimb lameness when lunging to the right but no hindlimb lameness.

ALTERNATIVES AND THEIR RELATIVE MERITS

Three inertial sensor systems are available (Equusense by Equusys [www.equusys.com], Lameness Locator by Equinosis [www.equinosis.com], and Equimetrix by Centaure-Metrix [www.centaure-metrix.com]) to evaluate lameness in horses. The primary advantage of inertial sensor systems is the ability to collect multiple, contiguous strides in an over-ground setting in a single trial. Camera-based kinematic analysis systems can collect multiple, noncontiguous strides over ground by collecting many trials.

AUTHOR: **KEVIN KEEGAN**

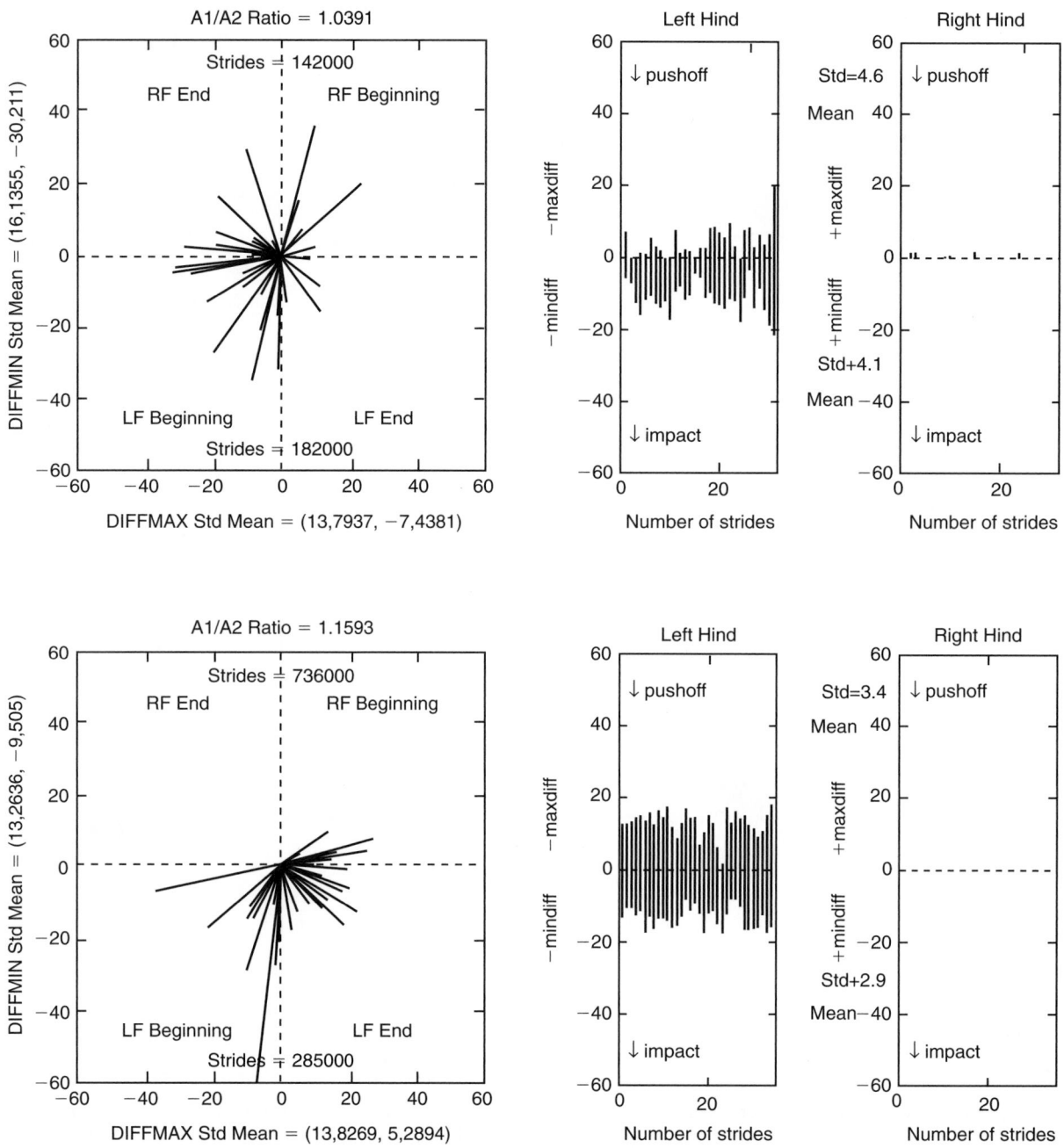

FIGURE 7 Horse with left hindlimb lameness lunging to the left and then lunging to the right. While lunging to left, there is mild left hindlimb push-off lameness. The left hindlimb impact deficiency is expected while lunging to the left. While lunging to the right, the horse displays significant left hindlimb impact lameness. The left hindlimb push-off deficiency is expected while lunging to the right. The horse also displays a mild and erratic left forelimb lameness while lunging to the left and right (all rays pointing downward), which is probably compensatory to the primary left hindlimb lameness.

Glucose Tolerance Test (GTT)

BASIC INFORMATION

- Easy to perform.
- Place the intravenous catheter the day before testing to reduce stress.
- Administer glucose (0.2–0.5 g/kg IV in 50% dextrose solution).

- Collect blood samples every 30 minutes for 3 hours.
- Insulin is released immediately after glucose administration.
- Serum glucose concentrations should return to baseline by 3 hours.

- A delayed return in glucose concentrations to baseline (>3 hours) suggests insulin resistance (equine metabolic syndrome).

AUTHOR: **RAMIRO E. TORIBIO**

Glucose/Insulin Test (CGIT), Combined

BASIC INFORMATION

- The test is easy to perform.
- Place the IV catheter the day before testing.
- Administer glucose (150 mg/kg IV) and immediately after administer regular insulin (0.1 IU/kg IV).
- Collect blood samples at 0, 1, 5, 15, 25, 35, 45, 60, 75, 90, 105, 120, 135, and 150 minutes.

- The test can be limited to 90 minutes.
- Glucose concentrations do not decrease below baseline before 90 minutes in horses with insulin resistance (IR) and equine metabolic syndrome (EMS).
- Glucose concentrations above baseline at 45 minutes are consistent with IR and EMS.
- Avoid α_2 adrenergic receptor agonists (xylazine, detomidine) because they interfere with the glucose tolerance

test and CGIT in healthy horses, with glucose remaining elevated for more than 75 minutes (false-positive result).
- Avoid stressful conditions and the use of glucocorticoids.
- Withhold grain and grass for 24 hours; water and grass hay do not affect the results.
- For additional information see "Insulin Resistance" in Section I.

AUTHOR: **RAMIRO E. TORIBIO**

Heel Extension

BASIC INFORMATION

OVERVIEW AND GOAL(S)

Heel extensions are placed on the weight-bearing surface of the digit of neonatal foals to prevent hyperextension of the joints of the digit.

INDICATIONS

- Hyperextension of the joints of the digit
- Also supports weak flexor tendons in foals with hypoplastic tarsal bones, reducing compression dorsally

CONTRAINDICATIONS

Should not be used in foals unless stall confined.

EQUIPMENT, ANESTHESIA

- Extensions can be made of many lightweight but strong materials including aluminium and fiberglass. The author prefers 4-inch triangular door hinges cut in half with the points bent up to form a 50-degree angle. The toe of the foot is glued in the angle.
- The extensions are applied to the hooves with polymethylmethacrylate or hoof adhesive products such as Equi-thane Adhere (Vettec Hoof care products).
- There are commercial shoes available for this purpose including Babi-cuff (Ibex, Farrier Supplies, West Midland, UK) shoes and Dalric cuffs (Nanric Inc., Lawrenceburg, KY).

ANTICIPATED TIME

Application to two hooves requires 20 to 30 minutes.

PREPARATION: IMPORTANT CHECKPOINTS

The hoof should be clean and dry.

POSSIBLE COMPLICATIONS AND COMMON ERRORS TO BE AVOIDED

- The major complication is loss of the heel extension, which occurs at about 1 week. The extensions can be easily reapplied.
- The most common error is insufficient foot preparation. The adhesives must

be applied to dry horn, and the foot must be clean. Lightly rasping the horn to provide a rough surface for adhesion may provide some benefit.

PROCEDURE

- The foot is cleaned and trimmed to provide a flat bearing surface and a slightly squared toe (Figure 1).
- The hoof wall can be lightly roughened with a rasp.
- The shoe, either commercial or purpose-made should fit the foot and

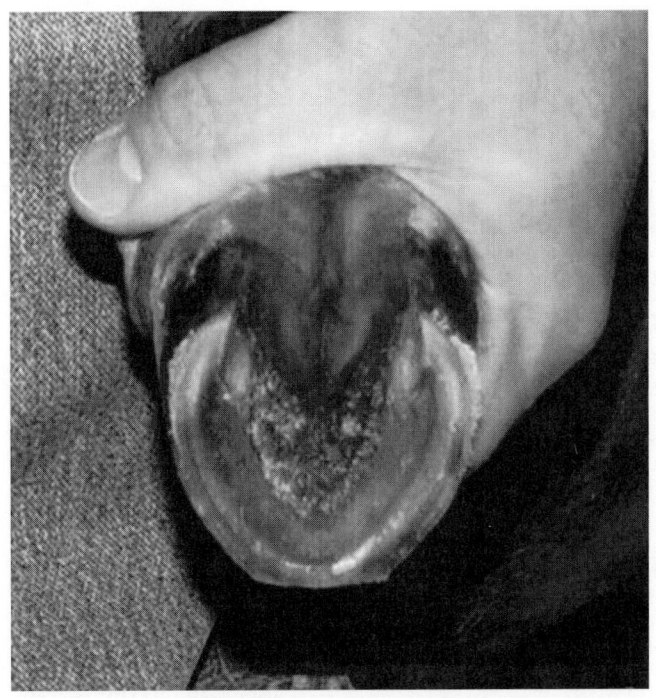

FIGURE 1 Well-trimmed foal foot. Note flat bearing surface and squared off toe.

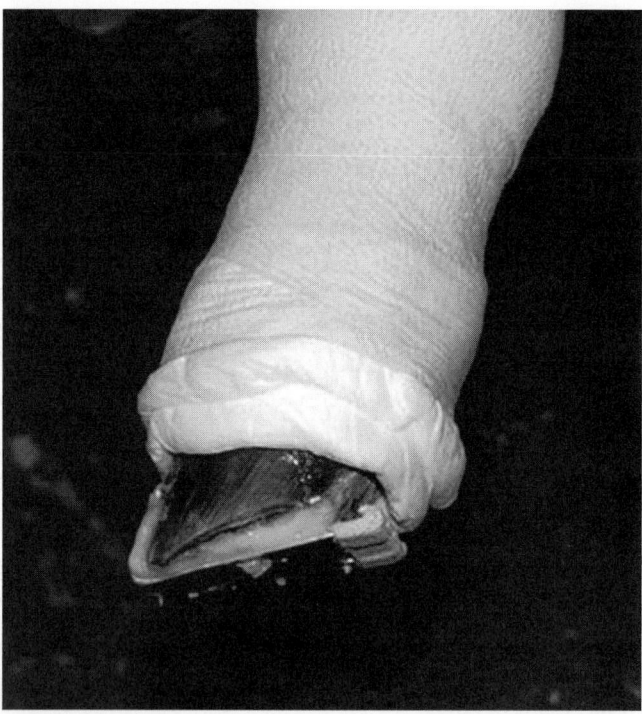

FIGURE 2 Recumbent foal with heel extension made from door hinge. Note bent up apex, and adhesive attaching hinge to foot. The caudal aspect of the hinge is taped to avoid self-trauma.

allow room for adhesive to grip the shoe (Figure 2).

- Holes drilled through the shoe allow adhesive to flow through and form "buttons" to help attach the shoe to the foot.
- Shoes should be held in place until the adhesive is set, which usually requires sedation of the foal.
- Fast-setting adhesives are preferred, and substances that set with a strong exothermic reaction are not preferred due to the possibility of heat damage to the laminae.

POSTPROCEDURE

Large stall confinement to allow some exercise to promote musculoskeletal maturation but also protect immature structures.

ALTERNATIVES AND THEIR RELATIVE MERITS

Trimming the foot flat can help foals with mild flexor laxity and requires no additional effort.

AUTHOR: **ELIZABETH M. SANTSCHI**

Holter Monitor/Telemetry Recording

BASIC INFORMATION

SYNONYM(S)

Ambulatory electrocardiographic (ECG) monitoring, telemetric ECG, cardiac telemetry, telemetry

OVERVIEW AND GOAL(S)

To provide continuous monitoring of heart rhythm over a prolonged period (eg, 24–48 hours). It allows observation while the horse is in its natural environment so that heart rate and rhythm are not influenced by the procedure.

INDICATIONS

- To monitor for suspected intermittent or paroxysmal dysrhythmias (Holter or telemetry)
- To assess number of dysrhythmias over time (Holter)
- To monitor horses with episodes of syncope or collapse (Holter or telemetry)
- To monitor rhythm during exercise in horses with suspected exercise-induced dysrhythmias or unexplained poor performance (Holter or telemetry)

- To monitor effects of antidysrhythmic drugs during conversion of dysrhythmias (telemetry)

EQUIPMENT, ANESTHESIA

- Clippers (no. 40 blade)
- Isopropyl alcohol
- Ultrasound coupling gel
- Sponges
- Surcingle and padding
- Disposable cardiac electrode adhesive patches
- Holter monitor (either digital recording device or magnetic tape for recording) or transmitter (for telemetry), with leads attached
- New batteries
- Receiver (for telemetry) with or without a printer
- Computer and system to read and interpret Holter recordings with or without a printer
- White adhesive surgical tape

ANTICIPATED TIME

- 10 to 20 minutes to apply leads and monitor
- Recording periods are typically up to 24 to 48 hours, although some monitors can record for 7 days (with enough battery life)

PREPARATION: IMPORTANT CHECKPOINTS

- Determine whether monitoring is required (through a combination of history, physical examination, cardiac examination, and routine bloodwork).
- Ensure monitor is functioning properly.
- Ensure battery life is sufficient for the recording period.
- If equipment allows, ensure that the trace is of acceptable quality before starting recording (Holter).
- If the Holter monitor is to be sent out for placement and maintenance at home, equipment care must be discussed with the owner (keeping it clean and dry, preventing horse from rolling on it or rubbing or biting the leads).

POSSIBLE COMPLICATIONS AND COMMON ERRORS TO BE AVOIDED

- Horses should not get wet while wearing the monitor, and care should be taken to keep the monitor and leads out of reach of damage.
- Electrode/lead placement must be periodically checked. If an electrode

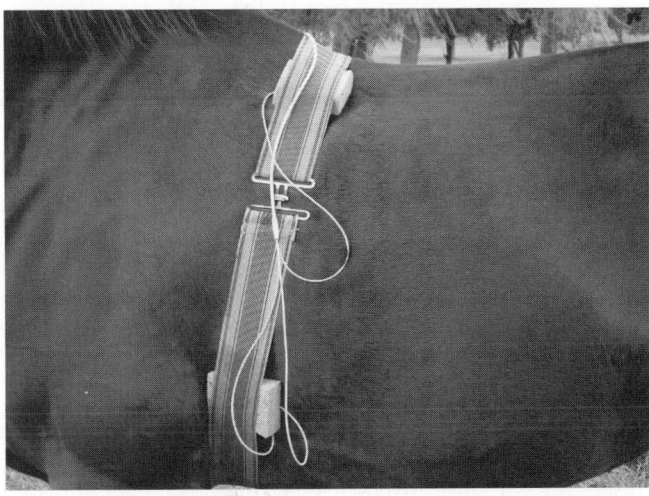

FIGURE 1 Example of a horse with a Holter monitor in place in a base-apex configuration. The surcingle holds the electrodes, leads, and sponges in place. It has not yet been secured with tape or had leads tucked in.

becomes dislodged, replace it; if a lead unsnaps from an electrode, snap it in place; if a lead becomes unattached from the monitor, reattach it.

- Electrodes should be periodically checked to ensure they are damp and contact is good. They can be moistened directly or the sponges can be resaturated with water or alcohol. This is more critical in winter or dry climates.
- Make sure batteries are new, with enough life for the recording period.
- Make sure the horse stays within range of the receiver (for telemetry).

PROCEDURE

- Placement of electrode patches should be predetermined and may vary depending on the system and number of cables used.
- If the haircoat is long (eg, in winter) or the contact is poor, the areas of electrode placement should be clipped.
- If the hair is not clipped, the area will need to be saturated with alcohol.
- In general, electrodes are either placed in a base-apex configuration or over the heart on both the right and left sides of the horse for many Holter systems. Refer to the manufacturer's instructions.
- In many telemetry systems, the electrodes are often placed in a simple or modified base-apex arrangement.
  - The negative (RA) lead is placed on the left side, behind the dorsal portion of the scapula.

  - The positive (LA) lead is placed on the left side in the axillary region or on the sternum, and the ground lead (if present) placed remotely.
  - In this configuration, the ECG is recorded on lead 1 and the QRS should be negative.
  - These areas should be cleaned with alcohol to remove skin oils.
- The electrode patches are applied after saturating the contact area (center) with ultrasound coupling gel.
- The leads are snapped into the electrode patches according to the appropriate color scheme.
- Once the leads are snapped into place, an elastic surcingle is cinched snugly around the electrodes and leads to secure them and keep them protected (Figure 1). The wires should be tucked under the surcingle so they are not protruding or visible and taped into place. It is important to tighten the surcingle to apply enough pressure for good contact (without causing the horse discomfort).
- Soaking sponges with water and placing them between the electrodes and the surcingle help maintain moisture and prolong contact time (see Figure 1). These should be taped in place once electrodes, leads, and sponges are in position. Sponges can be periodically moistened during the recording period to keep the electrodes damp and ensure better contact and a cleaner recording.
- It is often necessary to put padding between the horse's withers and the

surcingle to prevent rub sores from developing on the horse and to allow the surcingle better stabilization and contact with the sides of the horse's thorax, particularly if the surcingle is stiff or will be in place for a prolonged period.

- Once the electrode patches, leads, and surcingle are in place, a new battery should be inserted into the Holter monitor or transmitter (for telemetry) and the monitor attached to the leads.
- Telemetry recording:
  - The receiver should be turned on and the recording tested to confirm it is of adequate quality.
  - Confirm that the horse remains within the monitoring perimeter of the receiver. Some equipment allows additional antennas to boost the signal and enlarge the recording area.
- Holter recording:
  - The monitor should be configured according to the manufacturer's instructions. This includes patient information and recording start time.
  - If possible, a test ECG should be run to determine recording quality.
  - Recording should be started, with actual time synchronized with the monitor clock time (zero) in the medical record if the actual start time cannot be entered in the monitor.
- It is very helpful for the owner to keep a diary to correlate time and observed activity with any rhythm abnormalities.
- Once the telemetry or Holter equipment has been started, the monitor should be securely taped to the surcingle near the horse's withers.

POSTPROCEDURE

- Telemetry: Turn off receiver, unhook transmitter, remove battery from device, and remove surcingle and leads.
- Holter: Remove cassette or memory card for downloading, unhook monitor, remove battery from device, and remove surcingle and leads.

ALTERNATIVES AND THEIR RELATIVE MERITS

ECG: Better recordings, with fewer motion or contact artifacts are possible; however, the recording time is very limited, and the setting is in an artificial environment, which may influence results.

AUTHOR: **MARY M. DURANDO**

Induction of Estrus

BASIC INFORMATION

OVERVIEW AND GOAL

Induce accurate and predictable onset of estrus

INDICATION

- Timed artificial insemination or mating
- Limited availability of a stallion
- Breeding with cooled or frozen semen
- Induction of estrus in mares that fail to demonstrate outward signs of estrus (silent estrus)
- Treatment of prolonged diestrus
- Induction of estrus behavior for use as teaser mares for semen collection

CONTRAINDICATIONS

Pregnancy

ANTICIPATED TIME

Variable with protocol selected and objectives. Time to estrus and ovulation depends on the degree of follicular development at the time of treatment with prostaglandins. 17β-estradiol induces estrous behavior within 3 to 6 hours of administration. If estradiol cipionate is used, estrous signs are expected within 2 to 3 days.

PREPARATION: IMPORANT CHECKPOINTS

Teasing, transrectal palpation, and ultrasonography at time of treatment to identify the phase of the estrous cycle and the follicular population.

POSSIBLE COMPLICATIONS AND COMMON ERRORS TO BE AVOIDED

Treatment with prostaglandin F2α (PGF2α) or its analogues can produce undesirable side effects, including sweating, trembling, increased heart rate, and even signs of colic. These signs present within 15 minutes of administration and resolve within 1 hour.

PROCEDURE

- Termination of the luteal phase of the estrous cycle with PGF2α
  - Dinoprost
    - 5 to 10 mg IM
    - Two injections of 0.5 mg IM, 24 hours apart, have been shown to be effective with fewer side effects
  - Cloprostenol
    - Not labeled for horses
    - 100 to 250 μg IM
    - Has been shown to have fewer side effects than Dinoprost
- Induction of estrous behavior in mares that fail to demonstrate outward signs of estrus
  - 17β-estradiol 0.5 to 10 mg IM 6 hours before breeding.
  - Estradiol cipionate 10 mg IM 2 to 3 days before breeding.
  - Cipionate is available through compounding pharmacies in the United States.
  - Estradiol can be used in anestrus or ovariectomized mares for use as teasers.

POSTPROCEDURE

- Estrous behavior is expected in 3 to 5 days and ovulation in 7 to 9 days after PGF2α injection.

- Ovulation could occur within 72 hours without signs of estrus if a large growing follicle is present at the time of PGF2α administration.
- Ovulation could occur as late as 14 days after PGF2α administration if a large regressing follicle is present at the time of treatment.
- Complete luteolysis may not occur if PGF2α is administered fewer than 5 days after ovulation. Repeat the injection if signs of estrus are not present when expected.
- 17β-estradiol induces estrous behavior within 3 to 6 hours after injection that will last for 24 hours.
- Estradiol cipionate induces estrous behavior within 2 to 3 days that persists for 3 to 4 days.

ALTERNATIVES AND THEIR RELATIVE MERIT

Intrauterine infusions of 100 mL saline or lavage with 1 to 3 L saline solution. The mechanism behind it is production of inflammation and prostaglandin release from the endometrium that will produce luteolysis. There is a potential risk of introduction of bacteria into the uterus and development of a uterine infection.

SUGGESTED READING

Pinto CRF, Meyers PJ: Control and synchronization of the estrous cycle and ovulation. In Younquist RD, Threlfall WR, editors: *Current therapy in large animal theriogenology*, St Louis, 2007, Saunders Elsevier, pp 91–98.

AUTHOR: MARIA CLARA SARDOY

Induction of Lactation

BASIC INFORMATION

OVERVIEW AND GOAL(S)

Lactation induction can be used to produce nurse mares without requiring the production of a foal. Hormones are administered to mimic the physiologic events of pregnancy and parturition, with the goal of inducing sufficient milk production to foster an adopted foal.

INDICATIONS

- Production of a nurse mare when there is loss of the maternal mare in the peripartum period, poor milk production in the maternal mare, or lack of acceptance of the foal by the maternal mare
- Failure of the commercial nurse mare to become pregnant and foal, resulting in loss of use

CONTRAINDICATIONS

- Mares that have shown inadequate or aggressive behavior toward their own foals
- Mares affected with mastitis or mammary neoplasia

PREPARATION: MARE SELECTION

Nonpregnant mares that have successfully foaled and nursed at least once are potential candidates for lactation induction; mares that have shown good maternal behavior on previous foalings are preferred. Mammary glands should be inspected for mastitis or other abnormalities before selection. Mares can be cycling or anestrus at the time of induction.

POSSIBLE COMPLICATIONS AND ERRORS TO BE AVOIDED

Induction of colostrum production is largely unsuccessful, with only a small percentage of mares yielding colostrum before an induced lactation. Thus this procedure should not be used to replace colostrum banking on the farm or colostrum or plasma administration to orphan foals (see "Colostrum Banking" in this section).

PROCEDURE

- 5 mg estradiol benzoate IM once on day 1
- 22 mg altrenogest PO, once daily for 7 days, beginning on day 1
- 1 mg/kg sulpiride IM q12h *or* 2.2 mg/kg domperidone PO q24h beginning on day 1. Either galactogogue can be used for several days after foal adoption occurs for a maximum of 20 days.
- Milking should begin when the mammary gland has greatly enlarged or has milk drops at the teats. This should be done five to seven times daily, either by hand, with a goat milking machine, or with an aggressively suckling foal if the mare will

allow it (the foal should be supplemented with formula until the milk production is sufficient). Five units of oxytocin can be administered IM 1 to 2 minutes before milking to facilitate letdown.

POSTPROCEDURE

The mare is usually ready for foal adoption after 3 to 5 days of milking. Foal introduction should be assumed under supervision, with measures taken to ensure handler safety.

- A bar is placed across the length of the stall at the level of the hip of the mare, with just enough room behind the bar for the mare to stand comfortably.
- The foal is held at the mare's head while the mare receives vaginal-cervical stimulation. Vigorous stimulation of the external os of the cervix and attempts to dilate the cervix are applied twice for 2 minutes, with a 10-minute interval. The mare is allowed to have contact with the foal during this time.
- Most mares will accept the foal within 24 to 48 hours with this technique. Interaction between mare and foal should be closely supervised at all times until adoption is complete.

SUCCESS RATES

Success of this procedure is generally good, with most mares producing suffi-

cient milk and accepting foal adoption. It should be noted, however, that some mares will not produce milk; it may be advisable to prepare more than one mare if a nurse mare is needed immediately.

ALTERNATIVES AND THEIR RELATIVE MERITS

- Mares that have lost their foals in the peripartum period as well as commercially available nurse mares are useful alternatives to this procedure. These mares will reliably produce colostrum for the first 48 hours, which can be advantageous to the orphan foal if it is grafted to the mare within 24 to 48 hours of birth and before the end of the colostrum production period. These mares will also produce milk without labor-intensive treatment.
- Orphan foals can be bucket fed with milk replacement formula. This is a simple solution, but it often results in a horse with inappropriate social behavior.

SUGGESTED READING

Daels P: Induction of lactation and adoption of the orphan foal. In *8th AAEP Annual Resort Symposium,* 2006.

Steiner J: How to induce lactation in pregnant mares. *Proc Am Assoc Equine Pract* 52:259–260, 2006.

AUTHOR: **ALANA KING**

Induction of Parturition

BASIC INFORMATION

SYNONYM(S)

Foaling Induction

OVERVIEW AND GOAL(S)

Induction of parturition permits observation and professional assistance at the time of delivery. With proper preparation and assessment of fetal maturity, the goal of a smooth induction that mimics the mare's natural process can be accomplished.

INDICATIONS

Mares requiring close supervision/assistance during foaling
- Ruptured prepubic tendon
- Pelvic fracture
- History of dystocia
- Premature placental separation
- Suspected or diagnosed twin pregnancy

- Neonatal isoerythrolysis
- Rupture/weakening of abdominal wall
- Prolonged gestation
- Near-term colic
- Uterine inertia
- Convenience/research or teaching purposes

CONTRAINDICATIONS

Convenience for mare owner

EQUIPMENT, ANESTHESIA

Obstetric equipment: Lubricant, clean bucket, towels, obstetric chains and handles, gloves, oxygen and administration set, enema bucket, foal nasogastric tube, foal nasal catheter, tail wrap, nonirritating soap (eg, Ivory).

ANTICIPATED TIME

From 40 to 90 minutes
- Rupture of the chorioallantoic membrane will occur approximately 30

minutes after administration of oxytocin.
- Delivery of the foal will commence approximately 30 to 60 minutes after administration of oxytocin and will take roughly 20 to 30 minutes.
- Fetal membranes should be passed within 2 hours.

PREPARATION: IMPORANT CHECKPOINTS

Criteria before induction:
- Minimum 330 days' gestation.
- Colostrum in the udder.
- Relaxation of the pelvic ligaments and cervix.
- Mammary secretions of >400 ppm (10 mmol) calcium and inversion of the Na:K ratio; K+ should be greater than Na+ in mammary secretions.
- Normal presentation of fetus.

POSSIBLE COMPLICATIONS AND COMMON ERRORS TO BE AVOIDED

- Administration of high-dose oxytocin causes more rapid and violent delivery and may cause injuries to the foal (fractured ribs) or mare (cervical tears).
- Inaccurate assessment of fetal maturity results in delivery of a premature foal with a poor chance of survival.
- Induction is often indicated in high-risk pregnancies; therefore dystocia should be anticipated and precautions taken.

PROCEDURE

- Place intravenous catheter (optional).
- Wash perineal area and apply tail wrap.
- Administer low-dose oxytocin 5 to 10 IU intravenous bolus or 5 IU intramuscular and 5 IU intravenous bolus. An alternative is to administer 10 IU in 200 mL physiologic saline over 15 minutes.
- Provide the mare with a quiet area in which to foal.
- Periodically perform vaginal examinations to asses fetal position and pro-

gression after administration of oxytocin (15–20 minutes).
- Monitor for rupture of the chorioallantoic membrane; manual rupture may be necessary.
- Oxytocin rarely needs to be repeated as long as induction criteria are met.

POSTPROCEDURE

- Allow mare and foal time to acclimate after foaling.
- Ensure that the foal is able to stand and nurse.
- Postpartum examination of mare, including examination of placenta.
- Physical examination of foal and neonatal care, including application of navel dip and administration of enema, if required.
- Determine the foal's immunoglobulin G blood levels at 8 to 12 hours of age.

ALTERNATIVES AND THEIR RELATIVE MERITS

- Prostaglandin $F_{2\alpha}$ ($PGF_{2\alpha}$) administration alone for induction is unreliable and is associated with increased incidence of premature placental separation and dystocia due to the rapidly developing events. In addition, $PGF_{2\alpha}$ can be associated with fractured ribs in foals and damage to the cervix.

- Fluprostenol can be used to induce mares with a closed cervix (2.2 µg/kg). The time to delivery is about 4 hours, and it causes less myometrial stimulation then $PGF_{2\alpha}$. The explosive nature of the birth can cause cervical damage or foals with broken ribs.
- Dexamethasone, 100 mg at 24-hour intervals until parturition occurs, can be used but is less reliable than oxytocin, with an average induction time of 4 ± 1.6 days. Colostrum quality is questionable, and foals need to be supplemented. It is a viable solution when mares are over 315 days' gestation and with severe physical impediments.

SUGGESTED READING

Camillo F, Marmorini P, Romagnoli S, et al: Clinical studies on daily low dose oxytocin in mares at term. *Equine Vet J* 32:307, 2000.

Macpherson ML, Chaffin MK, Carroll G, et al: 3 Methods of oxytocin-induced parturition and their effects on foals. *J Am Vet Med Assoc* 210:799, 1997.

Ousey JC, Kolling M, Allen WR: The effects of maternal dexamethasone treatment on gestation length and foal maturation in Thoroughbred mares. *Anim Reprod Sci* 94:436, 2006.

AUTHORS: **TRACY PLOUGH** and **JUAN C. SAMPER**

Intracytoplasmic Sperm Injection

BASIC INFORMATION

OVERVIEW AND GOAL(S)

- A micromanipulator is used to mechanically insert a spermatozoon into an in vivo or in vitro matured oocyte.
- Fresh or frozen spermatozoa may be used.
- Injected oocytes may be transferred directly to the oviduct or cultured in vitro and transferred to the uterus or frozen.

INDICATIONS

- Postmortem salvage of oocytes
  - Mare death or euthanasia
- Reproduce mares with severe reproductive problems preventing ovulation, fertilization, or early embryo development
  - Chronic persistent mate-induced endometritis
  - Oviduct function failure (eg, salpingitis, oviductal blockage)
  - Ovulation failure (eg, repeated anovulatory hemorrhagic follicle)

  - Repeatedly unsuccessful embryo collection
  - Cervical compromise
  - Pyometra
- Avoid in vivo insemination complications (timing, persistent mate-induced endometritis, etc.)
- Severely subfertile stallions

EQUIPMENT

This is a specialized technique requiring:
- Oocyte collection (in vivo or in vitro)
- Cell culture facilities
- Special micromanipulator with a Piezo drill

POSSIBLE COMPLICATIONS AND COMMON ERRORS TO BE AVOIDED

Because of a low success rate, several oocytes are usually transferred to a single recipient. This can lead to multiple pregnancies and associated complications.

PROCEDURE

Fresh or frozen semen can be used for ICSI. This technique requires a very small

amount of semen, but the highest quality should be used. A single spermatozoon is required per oocyte. Only the oocytes capable of developing are transferred, maximizing the efficiency of the transfer. ICSI may be performed on the oocytes of euthanized mares.

EXPECTED PREGNANCY RATES

- Blastocyst development rates range from 25% to 35%.
- Pregnancy rate is approximately 50%.
- With a pregnancy loss greater than 50%, overall success rate is approximately 20%.

ALTERNATIVES AND THEIR RELATIVE MERITS

In vitro fertilization in horses is not successful.

SUGGESTED READING

Alvarenga MA, Da Cruz Landim-Alvarenga F: New assisted reproductive techniques applied for the horse industry. In Samper JC, editor: *Equine breeding management and artificial insemination*, ed 2, St Louis, 2009, Elsevier, pp 209–221.

Hinrichs K: Update on equine ICSI and cloning. *Theriogenology* 64:535–541, 2005.
McKinnon AO, Trounson AO, Silber SJ: Intracytoplasmic sperm injection. In *Proceedings* of the 11th annual resort symposium of the American Association of Equine Practitioners, 2009, pp 58–80.

AUTHORS: **FRANÇOIS-XAVIER GRAND** and **LEFEBVRE REJEAN CLÉOPHAS**

Joint Flush in the Neonate

BASIC INFORMATION

SYNONYM(S)

Joint lavage

OVERVIEW AND GOAL(S)

- Septic arthritis is a common sequelae of neonatal septicemia and is also a common cause of euthanasia due to the potential to cause life-long athletic limitations.
- The goal of joint lavage is to remove the debris and inflammatory products resulting from synovial infection.

INDICATIONS

- Any joint with effusion and lameness in a neonate should have an arthrocentesis performed to determine if infection is present.
- If there are elevations in white blood cell count (especially if the polymorphonuclear cells are elevated) and total protein, the joint should be flushed and cultured.
- Joints should be flushed every other day until the lameness resolves.

CONTRAINDICATIONS

- If properly performed, the only contraindication could be introduction of bacteria into the joint if inflamed tissue must be punctured to enter the joint.
- Although attempts should be made to avoid swollen tissues when performing arthrocentesis, this fear is thought to be overstated and delaying therapy is a greater risk.

EQUIPMENT, ANESTHESIA

- Short-term injectable anesthesia such as a combination of xylazine, duazeoan (Valium), and ketamine is recommended for joint flushes in foals. Sedation alone can result in inadvertent movement.
- Equipment required includes:
  - Clippers
  - Surgical preparation materials
  - Sterile isotonic fluid for flushing
  - Needles
  - Sterile gloves
- Some clinicians favor additives to the flush fluids, but these must be carefully selected to avoid inciting further inflammation, and the author does not use them.
- A pressurized bag to squeeze the fluid bag can be used to hasten fluid flow.
- Light bandages are often applied after the flush is finished.

ANTICIPATED TIME

The time for the procedure is dependent on the volume of flush and the size of egress needle, but 30 minutes is usually sufficient.

PREPARATION: IMPORTANT CHECKPOINTS

- Due to the short length of anesthesia, the following should be available at the time of induction:
  - Clippers
  - Surgical preparation
  - Flush fluids
  - Needles
  - Sterile gloves

POSSIBLE COMPLICATIONS AND COMMON ERRORS TO BE AVOIDED

- Hemarthrosis and extravasation of flushing fluids into soft tissues are common complications and are self-limiting.
- A compression bandage after the flush can be applied to assist in subcutaneous fluid elimination.

PROCEDURE

- A through and through lavage is preferred over a single needle injection and aspiration, and large volumes (at least a liter for most joints) of sterile fluid are recommended for each joint lavage.
- The needles used for lavage should be at least 18-gauge, and larger should be used for egress if possible to remove larger fibrin clumps.
- If there is significant fibrin accumulation, or if infection is recalcitrant, small (1 cm) arthrotomies can be performed to promote drainage.
- A sterile bandage is required after an arthrotomy.
- It is very common to inject a water-soluble antimicrobial such as Amikacin into the joint after flushing.

POSTPROCEDURE

For a routine joint lavage, bandages are left in place for at least 1 day and the limb re-evaluated for swelling and lameness.

AUTHOR: **ELIZABETH M. SANTSCHI**

Lameness Examination

BASIC INFORMATION

OVERVIEW AND GOAL(S)

- A normal horse moves in a balanced manner with all limb movements in equilibrium.
- If lameness is present, movement is unbalanced or asymmetrical.

- The examiner's task:
  - Identify the gait abnormality
  - Locate the source of the lameness
  - Identify the likely cause(s)
  - Recommend appropriate treatment
- Evaluation of lameness requires:
  - An ability to visualize gait abnormalities

  - Skill in applying techniques that localize the abnormality to a specific site
  - Obtaining and interpreting appropriate images of the site(s). These findings must be consolidated to determine a diagnosis.

INDICATIONS

Gait abnormality

EQUIPMENT, ANESTHESIA

- Hoof tools
  - Hoof testers
  - Local anesthesia
  - Lunge line
  - Access to even, flat surfaces preferably both firm and soft
- Site to have horse ridden during the examination is helpful for low-level lameness

ANTICIPATED TIME

30 minutes to 2+ hours

PROCEDURE

- History
  - Reasons for a complete anamnesis of a horse presented for lameness
    - Helps to narrow the list of differential diagnoses
    - Determines the effect of previous treatment or shoeing protocols
    - May help to narrow the focus of the examination
  - The signalment of the horse (age, sex, breed, and use of the horse) should be clearly elucidated.
  - Specific questions to ask during the history:
    - Date and circumstances of lameness onset
    - When is the lameness most obvious?
    - Have you noticed any swelling or thickenings?
    - Has the horse undergone any treatment for this condition?
    - When was your horse last shod?
    - Is this a new condition or a continuation of a previous injury?
- Visual examination at rest
  - Before observing the horse in motion
    - Carefully evaluate the horse's conformation, stance, and limbs.
    - Evaluate the horse from a distance to view its stance, general conformation, areas of swelling or atrophy, and attitude.
    - Evaluate wear patterns of the hoof or shoes.
  - Closer inspection should involve:
    - Palpation of each limb in its entirety.
    - Subtle effusion of the carpal joints and medial femorotibial joints may only be noticed with palpation.
    - Swollen regions should be palpated to evaluate tissue temperature and the degree of sensitivity to deep palpation. A swelling that is sensitive to touch and is warmer than surrounding areas is likely undergoing active inflammation. A cold, insensitive swelling may be a lesion that has healed and is no longer actively inflamed.
    - Digital pulses should always be palpated.
    - Elevated pulses are associated with injury or inflammation in the distal limb and may help localize the lesion to medial or lateral aspects of the limb.
    - Tendons and ligaments should be palpated with the limb in both weight bearing and flexed positions. Tendon sheath effusions are best evaluated with the limb bearing weight. When the limb is flexed the tendons and ligaments on the palmar or plantar surface are more easily defined and separated. Deep palpation of the mid to proximal suspensory ligament often elicits some discomfort in the normal horse. Compare contralateral limbs if there is a concern regarding palpation sensitivity.
- In-motion examination
  - Examination of the lame horse in motion is necessary to characterize the nature and intensity of the gait abnormality.
  - The lameness should be graded using a consistent scale.
  - The AAEP scale is most commonly used:
    - Grade 0 = no lameness
    - Grade 1 = intermittent lameness evident under special circumstance such as lungeing or following manipulations
    - Grade 2 = consistent lameness evident under special circumstances
    - Grade 3 = consistent lameness readily evident without special circumstances
    - Grade 4 = severe, consistent lameness
    - Grade 5 = non–weight bearing lameness
  - The in-motion lameness exam should be conducted in controlled surroundings to add consistency to the findings.
  - The ideal location to examine a horse for lameness
    - A flat, firm surface.
    - At least 30 to 40 m without obstructions or distractions.
    - An asphalt surface has the advantage of allowing the examiner to both visualize and listen to the horse's footfalls. The sound of the lame limb impacting the surface will be diminished when compared to the unaffected contralateral limb. A common finding with subtle gait abnormalities may be the unaffected limb of a pair impacting the surface louder than the affected limb.
    - There should be a safe place to work the horse in a circle, preferably on a lunge line. The surface should be firm, but safe enough to permit circles from 10 to 20 m in diameter without risk of the horse slipping.
    - Horses with subtle gait abnormalities may need to be observed while being worked in normal tack or under saddle. In select circumstances an examiner with sufficient experience may find it useful to work or ride the horse. This is particularly useful in harness race horses that only demonstrate their gait abnormalities at speed.
  - Watch the horse initially at a walk.
    - Evaluate footfall patterns to familiarize the horse with the environment in which the examination will take place.
    - Each foot should normally land heel first, then toe with the lateral and medial aspects of the hoof landing nearly equally in time. Deviations from normal footfall may indicate dynamic imbalance of the limb that could be due to abnormalities of conformation, hoof shape, shoeing, or pain.
    - The swinging phase of the limb in a correctly conformed horse should be a straight track without any predilection to swinging-in or swinging-out.
    - Toe-in or toe-out conformations predispose the horse to swinging-out ("paddling") or swinging-in ("winging-in"), respectively.
  - Evaluate the horse at a trot.
    - The most useful gait to evaluate lameness
    - It is a symmetrical, two-beat gait.
    - Diagonal limb pairs are simultaneously in the stance phase. The horse should be trotted at a comfortable, unhurried speed with the head allowed to move freely up and down.
    - The horse should be trotted directly away and returned directly toward the examiner. Subtle imbalances in gait may easily be missed if the examiner is not directly aligned with the center of the long axis of the horse (the vertebral column).
    - The examiner should also observe the horse from the side as it trots by for characteristics of stride length and to determine if there is any toe dragging. Viewing the horse from the side at the trot may provide better evaluation of some hindlimb lameness.

- Lameness is evident to the observer as an asymmetry of the gait (see "Gait Analysis" in this section).
  - Forelimb lameness is usually evident as a head bob:
    - The head rises immediately prior to and during weight bearing of the lame limb.
    - The head drops as the sound limb contacts the ground and bears weight.
- Stride length may also be altered by gait abnormalities.
  - A shortened anterior phase to the stride (shuffling gait) may be associated with:
    - Heel pain as the horse is reluctant to extend the affected limb and bear full weight on the heel.
    - Pain during the swing phase of the gait, such as may be encountered with bicipital bursitis/tendonitis of the forelimb.
    - Subtle forelimb lameness may only be evident as an unequal shift in weight with the unaffected limb bearing more weight than the lame limb. Such subtle weight shifts are best observed with the horse trotting directly toward the examiner.
- Hindlimb gait abnormalities may be evident as elevation of the hip (hip hike, gluteal rise), dropping of the hip (hip drop, gluteal drop), toe dragging, and decreased stride length.
  - These responses to hindlimb lameness are mechanisms the horse uses to avoid discomfort during various portions of the stride and are due to the nature of the abnormality.
  - Elevation of the hip occurs when the horse shifts weight away from the lame limb during the weight bearing phase of the stride.
  - Dropping of the hip occurs if pain is most acute during the posterior phase of the weight bearing portion of the stride. Often this movement is associated with abnormalities of the caudal/plantar aspect of the hindlimb such as suspensory desmitis, flexor tendinitis, desmitis of the distal suspensory apparatus, and injury to the semimembranosus/semitendinosus muscle group.
  - Dragging of the toe is associated with reluctance to raise the limb during the swing phase of the stride and is usually associated with upper hindlimb joint lameness such as bone spavin and

abnormalities of the stifle or coxofemoral joints.
  - When hindlimb lameness is observed at the trot from the rear of the horse, the tuber coxae of the lame limb usually has greater amplitude (up-and-down motion) compared with the tuber coxae of the sound limb. Severe hindlimb lameness (>grade 3) is often associated with a head bob. At the trot the hindlimb and the contralateral forelimb are simultaneously in the same stride phase (working as a diagonal pair).
  - If lameness of the hindlimb is severe enough, as the affected limb contacts the ground the horse will shift weight forward (off of the lame hindlimb) using the neck resulting in an observable head drop as the contralateral forelimb enters the weight bearing phase of the stride. Kinematic analysis has found a measurable head bob with even mild hindlimb lameness. The examiner needs to be aware of this process as moderate to severe hindlimb lameness may be confused with a lameness of the ipsilateral forelimb.
- When the examiner encounters difficulty in determining which limb is lame, it may be easier to determine "which limb is sound." At times it is simpler to visualize and/or hear which limb is bearing more weight (the sound limb).
  - Manipulative tests should be used when lameness is subtle.
- Manipulative tests
  - Lunge line
    - Most sport horses may be safely worked in a circle on a lunge line.
    - Working the horse in a 10- to 20-m diameter circle will put additional weight and stress on the innermost limbs and the medial aspect of the outermost limbs. The additional stress on the limbs helps the examiner identify subtle lamenesses and in some cases will help localize the region of soreness to a portion of the limb. A round pen of appropriate size may be similarly used.
  - Evaluation of the foot
    - Evaluate for balance, general condition of the hoof and sole, and the degree of wear of shoes and hoof walls. Abnormalities such as: dished hoof, long toe, low heels, sheared heels, contracted heels, hoof cracks, thrush, flaky sole, hard sole, sole bruis-

ing, and white line disease should be noted.
  - Percuss the hoof wall with the hoof tester or a hammer. Hollow-sounding areas may correspond to a deep abscess or hoof wall separation. Areas of pain on concussion may be indicative of a tightly clinched nail or a nail that has penetrated the sensitive laminae and is causing a local abscess.
- Use of hoof testers
  - Hoof testers are squeezed on the sole and hoof capsule to determine if there are any sensitive areas present.
  - Hoof tester pressure on normal hoof or sole does not result in a significant withdrawal response.
  - If a sensitive area is found the hoof tester pressure should be repeated to verify the finding, then pressure should be maintained for 20 to 30 seconds and the horse should be trotted off to determine if pressure on the sensitive area causes an exacerbation of the lameness.
  - Significant sensitive areas should be closely evaluated by paring out the foot.
- Flexion tests
  - Flexion tests are used to apply stress or pressure on an anatomical region of the limb for a set period of time (Table 1).
  - Following the flexion period the horse is trotted off and observed for the effects of the test on gait. Recalling the baseline level of lameness during both trotting on the lead rope and on the lunge line (if appropriate) is crucial to objectively evaluate the results of both flexion tests and diagnostic local anesthesia.
  - The amount and duration of pressure applied may affect the outcome of flexion tests.
  - Consistency of application is also a key to correct interpretation of flexion tests.
  - The flexion test, particularly of the distal limb, should not be over interpreted.
  - Each flexion test should be completed in anatomical pairs (eg, distal flexions of both fore limbs) with the sound limb flexed first.
  - Tests should progress from the distal to proximal aspect of the limbs.
  - Moderate and equal pressure should be applied for each flexion test.
  - Consistency is improved by having the same individual

TABLE 1 Flexion Tests

Sequence of Flexion Tests	Technique	Duration of Test
Forelimb		
Distal limb	Stand to the front or side of the horse with the carpus relaxed. Grasp the toe with one hand using the other hand placed on the palmar aspect of the distal metacarpus as a fulcrum. Alternatively, stand in front of the horse and grasp the toe with both hands placing the dorsal aspect of the fetlock on your knees and flex the distal joints. Distal limb flexion stresses the metacarpophalangeal, proximal and distal interphalangeal joints, and the navicular region.	30 seconds
Carpus	Stand to the side of the horse; grasp the distal dorsal aspect of the metacarpus with one hand. Flex the carpus maximally. A full range of motion is evident when the palmar metacarpus contacts the caudal aspect of the antebrachium. The metacarpus may be adducted and abducted during flexion to provide more stress to the medial and lateral aspects of the joints.	30 seconds
Metacarpus	Direct pressure on the flexor tendons or suspensory ligament	30 seconds
Proximal forelimb	The shoulder and elbow are difficult to isolate. The bicipital bursa of the shoulder may be evaluated by applying direct pressure over the bicipital tendon at the point of the shoulder or by retracting the upper fore limb caudally to its full extent. The upper limb should be abducted and adducted to stress the medial and lateral support structures of the joints.	30–60 seconds
Hindlimb		
Distal hindlimb	Techniques are similar to that used in the forelimb. Flexion is performed with the tarsus and stifle relaxed.	30 seconds
Full hindlimb	Also referred to as the "spavin test." This flexion test stresses all of the hindlimb joints to some degree because of their connection via the reciprocal apparatus; however, the tarsus and stifle joints are stressed more than others. The hindlimb is grasped with both hands around the distal metatarsus and the full limb is flexed maximally.	45–90 seconds
Stifle	This joint is stressed during application of the full limb flexion. The cruciate ligaments may be stressed by abruptly forcing the tibial crest caudally using a hand on the tibial crest while the horse is fully weight-bearing on the limb. The medial collateral ligament of the stifle may be stressed by picking up the limb, grasping the mid-metatarsus and using placing the examiner's shoulder over the lateral aspect of the stifle. Abruptly abduct the distal limb using the examiner's shoulder as the fulcrum.	15–30 seconds
Coxofemoral joint	With the limb not bearing weight and nearly extended "stir" the limb in an arc. An alternative method is to adduct the limb. For example: To stress the right coxofemoral joint stand on the horse's left, pick up the right hindlimb while maintaining limb extension and pulling the distal limb to the horse's left side.	30 seconds

perform all of the tests during an examination.
- Results of flexion tests may be recorded as:
  □ Negative: No change in lameness
  □ Slight positive or 1+: Slight exacerbation of lameness fol-

lowing flexion that is noticed during only a portion of the trotting course
  □ Moderate positive or 2+: Lameness is exacerbated while the horse is trotting away from the examiner, but not on the return

  □ Severe positive or 3+: Marked exacerbation of lameness during the outbound and return portions of the trotting course

AUTHOR: **ANDRIS J. KANEPS**

Lameness Examination: Diagnostic Local Anesthesia

BASIC INFORMATION

SYNONYM(S)
Nerve block
Joint block

OVERVIEW AND GOAL(S)
- Diagnostic local anesthesia is often performed to localize lameness. Important considerations are:

  ○ Understanding the anatomy to provide accurate placement of the anesthetic
  ○ Being aware of different options for administering anesthetic to a site as clinical situations may dictate one approach over another
  ○ Maintaining strict asepsis when penetrating synovial spaces
  ○ Always using a fresh bottle of local anesthetic

- Technique
  ○ The most painful portion of the injection is needle penetration of the skin and joint capsule.
  ○ Confident, quick insertion of the needle in the correct anatomical site minimizes discomfort for the horse.
  ○ A skin bleb of local anesthetic may be helpful in making the joint injection less uncomfortable, particularly when a larger-gauge needle must be used.

- The sequence of diagnostic local anesthesia:
  - Begins with the most distal nerves being injected first and gradually working proximally until the lameness has been localized.
  - Regional anesthesia usually results in less effective analgesia of intra-articular soreness than direct intra-articular anesthesia.
  - If the lameness has been improved noticeably, but not completely, following regional nerve anesthesia, intra-articular anesthesia of the suspect joint should be conducted.

INDICATIONS

Localization of lameness

CONTRAINDICATIONS

Do not inject through a potentially contaminated site such as a wound or a region of cellulitis.

EQUIPMENT, ANESTHESIA

- Mepivacaine HCl 2% (Carbocaine-V, Winthrop Laboratories) is the preferred local anesthetic for regional and joint anesthesia in horses.
  - It is less irritating to tissues and has a comparable onset yet a longer duration of action than does lidocaine.
- Local anesthetics cause blockade of sodium channels that results in inhibition of nerve conduction. The effectiveness of local anesthesia depends on local tissue pH (local anesthetics are much less effective in acid pH), accuracy of deposition, and the size of nerves being blocked (small, unmyelinated fibers are more sensitive than large, myelinated fibers).
- The toxic dose of local anesthetic is approximately 13 mg/kg (~6 mg/lb) and may result in heart block, bradycardia, and convulsions. Toxicity is usually only a concern in smaller animals.
- Onset of action for regional nerve blocks is 10 to 25 minutes with smaller diameter nerves desensitized earlier than larger nerves.
- Onset of intra-articular analgesia is 5 to 10 minutes with a gradual increase in analgesia over that time.
- Check the effects of the local anesthetic in most joints at 20 minutes and in complex joints such as the stifle in 30 minutes. Mepivacaine inhibits nerve sensation for 90 to 180 minutes.

PREPARATION: IMPORTANT CHECKPOINTS

- The site for local peripheral nerve anesthesia does not need to be clipped and is prepared by wiping with 70% isopropyl alcohol until clean.

- The site for intra-articular anesthesia may be clipped, but clipping the site has not been found to improve results of skin surface bacteriologic cultures.
  - A 7- to 10-minute scrub with povidone-iodine or chlorhexidine should be made with the injection site being carefully wiped with 70% isopropyl alcohol immediately prior to injection.
  - The operator should wear sterile surgical gloves.
  - Adequate assistance should be available for restraining the horse.

POSSIBLE COMPLICATIONS AND COMMON ERRORS TO BE AVOIDED

- Local swelling at the injection site resolves following bandaging.
- Joint sepsis is unlikely but may occur due to a break in aseptic technique.

PROCEDURE

REGIONAL DIAGNOSTIC ANESTHESIA

- See Tables 1 and 2 for forelimb and hindlimb nerve blocks.

INTRA-ARTICULAR ANESTHESIA

Navicular bursa

- Strict asepsis must be adhered to particularly at this site.
- A subcutaneous bleb of local anesthetic should be placed on the palmar aspect of the distal pastern in the mid-sagittal cleft immediately proximal to the heel bulbs.
- An 18-gauge, 3-inch (1.2 × 90 mm) spinal needle is advanced until it contacts the flexor surface of the navicular bone.
- The needle should be aimed at a point 1 cm distal to the coronary band and midway between its most dorsal and palmar extent.
- Correct placement of the needle should be confirmed with radiography or ultrasonography.
- 3 to 5 mL of local anesthetic is injected.
  - Comparing the results of navicular bursa, distal interphalangeal joint and palmar digital nerve local anesthesia may aid localization of distal limb lameness. However, mepivacaine has been found to diffuse widely following injection in the distal equine limb.

Distal interphalangeal (DIP) joint

- The DIP joint has a large dorsal pouch that is easily entered with a needle.
- Anesthetic injected in the DIP joint will desensitize other nearby structures.
- Dorsal approach: This injection is best made with the horse fully weight-bearing using a 20- to 18-gauge, 1.5-inch (0.9–1.2 × 40 mm) needle.
  - The needle is inserted 1.5 to 2 cm proximal to the coronary band and

a like distance lateral or medial to the extensor process of the distal phalanx and directed toward the extensor process.
  - A skin bleb may be made at this site to facilitate needle placement.
  - Alternatively, the needle may be directed perpendicular to the dorsal cortex of the second phalanx and walked distally until the joint is entered.
  - The needle usually penetrates the skin approximately 1 inch (25 mm) before entering the joint.
  - 4 to 6 mL of anesthetic is injected.
  - Hemorrhage often occurs from the coronary corium when the needle is withdrawn. Counter pressure and a light bandage will control any bleeding and help protect the region from contamination until the needle puncture seals.
- Lateral approaches: Two dorsolateral approaches have been described with the needle inserted either cranial or proximal to the collateral cartilage.
  - The most cranial extent of the collateral cartilage is palpated and the needle is inserted at that point approximately 1 to 2 cm proximal to the coronary band with the horse fully weight bearing. The needle is first inserted parallel to the ground then immediately angled 30 degrees distally.
  - Needle placement proximal to the collateral cartilage may be performed with the horse non–weight bearing. The needle is inserted just proximal to the collateral cartilage midway between the dorsal and palmar aspect of the second phalanx and is directed along the palmar surface of the second phalanx by aiming at the center of the frog.

Proximal interphalangeal (PIP) joint

- A dorsolateral or palmar approach may be used to enter the PIP joint.
- Dorsal approach: The horse should be weight bearing for this approach. A 20-gauge, 1.5-inch (0.9 × 40 mm) needle is directed through the skin approximately 1 to 2 cm distal to the distal eminence of the first phalanx and under the extensor tendon. Orient the needle parallel with the dorsal joint surface. Inject 4 to 5 mL of local anesthetic.
- Palmar approach: The limb should be picked up and held with the distal joints in moderate flexion.
  - The palmar pouch of the PIP joint is bounded by the palmar first phalanx, the palmarodistal eminence of the first phalanx, and the insertion of the lateral branch of the superficial digital flexor tendon. When the pastern is moderately

TABLE 1 Peripheral Nerve Blocks: Forelimb

Sequence of Diagnostic Local Anesthesia	Anatomic Site of Injection	Region Desensitized	Needle Size and Anesthetic Volume	Onset of Action
Palmar digital nerves (PDN)	Palmar aspect of pastern, immediately proximal to the collateral cartilages	Palmar heel, entire sole	25–22 g × 1 inch 0.5–0.7 × 16 mm 1.5–2 mL/nerve	10–15 minutes
Dorsal branch of PDN	Same as above, redirect needle dorsally approximately 1 inch (25 mm)	All structures within the hoof	As above	As above
Abaxial sesamoid (palmar nerves)	Abaxial aspect of proximal sesamoid bones	All structures within the hoof and most of structures from mid-pastern distal	25–22 g × 1 inch 0.5–0.7 × 16 mm 2–2.5 mL/nerve	As above
Low four-point (palmar nerves and palmar metacarpal nerves)	At the level of the distal aspect of MCII and MCIV (splint bones). Palmar nerves are injected subcutaneously between the suspensory branch and the deep digital flexor tendon immediately proximal to the digital sheath. Palmar metacarpal nerves are injected subcutaneously immediately dorsal and distal to the splint buttons.	Fetlock joint and all distal structures	22 g × 1 inch 0.7 × 25 mm 4–5 mL per palmar nerve, 3 mL per palmar metacarpal nerve	15 minutes
High four-point (palmar nerves and palmar metacarpal nerves)	At the most proximal aspect of the metacarpus that a palpable groove between the deep digital flexor tendon and suspensory ligament is palpable. The palmar nerves are injected in this groove. The palmar metacarpal nerves are injected by redirecting the needle to the axial surface of MCII and MCIV.	All structures distal to the point of injection. Inadvertent injection within the carpal canal or carpometacarpal joint may occur.	22 g × 1 inch 0.7 × 25 mm 4–5 mL per palmar nerve, 3 mL per palmar metacarpal nerve	15 minutes
Base of the accessory carpal bone	The lateral and medial palmar metacarpal and lateral palmar nerves lie together at a site between the flexor retinaculum and the carpal sheath at a point midway between the head of MCIV and the base of the accessory carpal bone and immediately distal to the accessoriometacarpal ligament. The medial palmar nerve is injected as previously described at the axial aspect of proximal MCII. An alternate method may be used by to block the lateral palmar nerve and deep branch on the axial aspect of the accessory carpal bone. The needle is placed in the distal two thirds of a longitudinal groove in the fascia on the medial aspect of the accessory carpal bone directed from medial to lateral. When the needle contacts bone, inject 1.5 to 2 mL of anesthetic.	All structures distal to the point of injection including The origin of the suspensory ligament. Inadvertent injection within the carpal canal or carpometacarpal joint may occur.	22 g × 1 inch 0.7 × 25 mm 3–4 mL at base of accessory carpal bone, 3 mL at medial palmar metacarpal nerve Alternate technique 1.5–2 mL on medial aspect of accessory carpal bone	15 minutes
Suspensory ligament origin	The needle is inserted directly into the origin of the suspensory ligament. A large needle is used to reduce the chance of breakage. (High four-point, base of accessory carpal, and suspensory origin blocks may be interchanged depending on operator preference.)	The entire suspensory ligament and structures distal to the injection point. Inadvertent injection within the carpal canal or carpometacarpal joint may occur.	18 g × 1–1.5 inch 1.2 × 25–40 mm 4–6 mL	First check in 10 minutes, then again after 20 minutes
Median/ulnar/ musculocutaneous	The median nerve is injected on the caudomedial aspect of the radius immediately distal to the pectoral muscle mass. The needle is partially removed and redirected subcutaneously to a point just cranial to the cephalic vein for the musculocutaneous nerve. The ulnar nerve is injected 25 mm deep to the skin at a point 6 to 8 cm proximal to the accessory carpal bone between the flexor carpi ulnaris and ulnaris lateralis muscles.	The entire limb distal to points of injection including the carpus, suspensory origin.	22–20 g × 1.5 inch 0.7–0.9 × 40 mm 6–8 mL at median nerve, 4–6 mL at musculocutaneous nerve, 4–6 mL at the ulnar nerve	20–30 minutes

TABLE 2 Peripheral Nerve Blocks: Hindlimb

Sequence of Diagnostic Local Anesthesia	Anatomic Site of Injection	Region Desensitized	Needle Size and Anesthetic Volume	Onset of Action
Plantar digital nerves (PDN)	See forelimb			
Dorsal branch of PDN				
Abaxial sesamoid (plantar nerves)				
Low six-point (plantar, plantar metatarsal, and dorsal metatarsal nerves)	At the level of the distal aspect of MTII and MTIV (splint bones). Plantar nerves are injected subcutaneously between the suspensory branch and the deep digital flexor tendon immediately proximal to the digital sheath. Planar metatarsal nerves are injected subcutaneously immediately dorsal and distal to the splint buttons. Dorsal metatarsal nerves are injected immediately lateral and medial to the long digital extensor tendon.	Fetlock joint and all distal structures	22 g × 1 inch (0.7 × 25 mm) 4–5 mL per plantar nerve, 3 mL per plantar metatarsal nerve, 3 mL per dorsal metatarsal nerve	15 minutes
High six-point (plantar, plantar metatarsal, and dorsal metatarsal nerves)	At the most proximal aspect of the metatarsus, a groove is palpable between the deep digital flexor tendon and suspensory ligament. The plantar nerves are injected in this groove. The plantar metatarsal nerves are injected by redirecting the needle to the axial surface of MTII and MTIV. Dorsal metatarsal nerves are injected immediately lateral and medial to the long digital extensor tendon.	All structures distal to the point of injection. Inadvertent injection within the tarsometatarsal joint may occur.	22 g × 1 inch (0.7 × 25 mm) 4–5 mL per plantar nerve, 3 mL per plantar metatarsal nerve, 3 mL per dorsal metatarsal nerve	15 minutes
Suspensory ligament origin	The needle is inserted directly into the origin of the suspensory ligament. A large needle is used to reduce the chance of breakage. (High six-point and suspensory origin blocks may be interchanged depending on operator preference.)	The entire suspensory ligament and structures distal to the injection point. Inadvertent injection within the tarsometatarsal joint may occur.	18 g × 1–1.5 inch (1.2 × 25–40 mm) 4–6 mL	First check in 10 minutes, then again after 20 minutes
Tibial/peroneal	The tibial nerve is injected subcutaneously on the medial aspect of the limb approximately 6 to 8 cm proximal to the tuber calcis and immediately deep to the calcaneal tendon. The peroneal nerves are injected on the lateral aspect of the tibia with the needle inserted between the muscle bellies of the lateral and long digital extensor muscles. Injections are made 25 mm deep to the skin (deep peroneal n.) and subcutaneously (superficial peroneal n.).	The entire limb distal to points of injection including the tarsus, suspensory origin.	20 g × 1.5 inch (0.9 × 40 mm) 6–8 mL at tibial nerve, 4 mL at each peroneal nerve	20–30 minutes

flexed these structures form a "V" on the palmar first phalanx.

○ Avoid the palmar digital neurovascular bundle that lies directly over the needle insertion site. The bundle may be retracted palmar with the thumb of the operator. The needle is placed through the skin dorsal to the neurovascular bundle within the region of the distal 25% of the first phalanx and directed distally and toward midline. Joint fluid is commonly aspirated.

Metacarpophalangeal/ metatarsophalangeal joint

- The fetlock joint is commonly injected for diagnostic and therapeutic reasons.
- Three approaches may be used: dorsal, palmar/plantar pouch, and palmar/plantar approach through the collateral sesamoidean ligament.
- The collateral sesamoidean ligament approach is best used if arthrocentesis

is an objective because synovial fluid free of blood contamination is more readily obtained.

- For administration of local anesthesia the palmar/plantar pouch approach is preferred.
- Palmar/plantar pouch:
  ○ The approach is made with the horse weight bearing.
  ○ The palmar/plantar pouch is bounded by the third metacarpus/ metatarsus dorsally, distally by the apex of the sesamoid bone, and palmar/plantar by the suspensory ligament.
  ○ A 20-gauge, 1.5-inch (0.9 × 40 mm) needle is inserted through the skin in the center of this site and directed distally and toward midline. Synovial fluid commonly will drip from the needle if effusion is present, but aspiration with a syringe often

results in plugging of the needle with synovial tissue.
  ○ 4 to 6 mL of local anesthetic is injected.
- Dorsal approach:
  ○ This approach should only be used if effusion is present because of the possibility of abrading joint cartilage with the needle.
  ○ The horse should be weight-bearing.
  ○ The needle is placed from the lateral side into the proximal aspect of the dorsal joint capsule and directed toward midline and under the extensor tendon.
  ○ Care should be taken to not abrade the sagittal ridge.
- Collateral ligament approach:
  ○ The limb should be held up with the fetlock joint flexed.
  ○ This procedure is facilitated by an assistant holding the limb.

- The lateral palmar/plantar aspect of the distal metacarpal/metatarsal condyle and the dorsal surface of the proximal sesamoid bone are palpated.
- The collateral sesamoidean ligament may be rarely palpated.
- The neurovascular bundle over the abaxial surface of the sesamoid bone does not interfere with this approach because it is displaced palmar when the joint is flexed.
- The needle is inserted in the palpable space between the third metacarpus/metatarsus and the proximal sesamoid bone.
- Entry into the joint is easily determined because the needle may be inserted easily up to its hub.

Carpal joints

- The radiocarpal joint is always separate from the middle carpal and carpometacarpal joints, which are always considered to communicate.
- Complete intra-articular anesthesia of the carpus requires injecting local anesthetic into the radiocarpal and middle carpal joints.
- The joints are traditionally injected with the limb flexed but may also be injected with the horse weight-bearing on the limb.
- Dorsal approach:
  - The limb is flexed and the joint spaces of the middle and radial carpal joints are easily palpated medial or lateral to the extensor carpi radialis tendon.
  - A 20-gauge, 1- to 1.5-inch (0.9 × 25–40 mm) needle is most often inserted medial to the extensor carpi radialis tendon.
  - If inserted lateral to the extensor carpi radialis tendon, care must be taken to avoid the common digital extensor tendon.
  - The most common difficulty encountered when inserting the needle is penetrating into articular cartilage. To avoid this, visualize the plane of the carpal articular surfaces distal to the intended needle insertion site.
  - Direct the needle parallel to the joint surfaces on insertion.
  - Inject 10 mL of local anesthetic per joint.
- Caudolateral approach:
  - The carpal joints may also be injected with the horse standing on the limb.
  - The joint spaces may be identified by palpation of the lateral aspect of the carpus by inducing slight carpal flexion.
  - The radiocarpal joint is immediately cranial to the accessory carpal bone at roughly 50% of its proximal-distal length.

- The middle carpal joint is immediately cranial to the distal aspect of the accessory carpal bone.

Cubital (elbow) joint

- This joint is injected from the lateral aspect of the limb just cranial to the lateral collateral ligament.
- The joint space may be palpated in most horses by identifying the humeral condyle and tracing it with your finger.
- The procedure may be done with the horse standing or by having an assistant elevate the forelimb slightly to open the joint space dorsally.
- An 18- to 20-gauge, 1.5-inch (0.9–1.2 × 40 mm) needle is inserted perpendicular to the limb and 15 to 20 mL of local anesthetic is injected.
- An alternate approach may be used by inserting the needle on the cranial aspect of the olecranon at a point approximately 3 cm distal to its most proximal extent. The needle is directed distally and axially.

Scapulohumeral (shoulder) joint

- Craniolateral approach:
  - This is the most common approach used to inject the scapulohumeral joint.
  - Identify the cranial and caudal parts of the greater tubercle on the craniolateral aspect (point) of the shoulder.
  - An intradermal bleb of anesthetic will facilitate insertion of the spinal needle.
  - An 18-gauge, 3.5-inch (1.2 × 90 mm) spinal needle with a stylet is inserted in the notch between the cranial and caudal parts of the greater tubercle and directed slightly distally and toward the opposite tarsus (roughly a 30–40-degree angle to the long axis of the horse). The needle is inserted 2 to 3 inches (50–75 mm) to reach the joint.
  - Synovial fluid is rarely aspirated to confirm the needle is within the joint.
  - Injection of 20 to 30 mL of anesthetic with minimal resistance initially, followed by increased resistance as the joint fills, confirms that the needle is correctly positioned.
  - Diffusion of local anesthetic into the surrounding tissues may cause temporary anesthesia of the suprascapular nerve. While this nerve is desensitized, the horse will not have use of the infraspinatus and supraspinatus muscles, which results in abaxial displacement of the shoulder during weight bearing. This may be avoided by injecting the minimum volume of anesthetic that will affect joint desensitization

and by minimizing multiple needle punctures of the joint capsule.
- Lateral approach:
  - A skin bleb of anesthetic may be placed immediately caudal to the infraspinatus tendon at the level of the proximal humerus.
  - Insert the needle immediately caudal to the infraspinatus tendon, roughly perpendicular to the long axis of the horse and directed slightly distally.
  - The needle is inserted 1.5 to 2 inches (40–50 mm) to enter the joint.
  - Synovial fluid is more commonly obtained with this approach.

Bicipital bursa

- The bicipital bursa lies between the bicipital tendon and the dorsoproximal aspect of the humerus.
- The bursa is injected using an 18-gauge, 1.5-inch (1.2 × 40 mm) needle entering perpendicular to the skin at a point proximal to the deltoid tuberosity and distal to the proximal humeral tuberosity.
- 10 to 15 mL of local anesthetic is injected.

Tarsal joints

- The tarsocrural (tibiotarsal) and proximal intertarsal (PIT) joints are thought to always communicate.
- Communication between the distal intertarsal (DIT) and tarsometatarsal (TMT) joints is reported to occur 8% to 38% of the time.
- For accurate diagnosis or complete treatment of the distal tarsal joints, separate injections must be made in the DIT and TMT joints.
- Use of 22-gauge (0.7 mm) needles with metal hubs facilitates injections of the distal tarsal joints, particularly when medications are being administered. The small needle size makes placement within the joint easier and the syringe is more securely seated in a metal than a plastic hub needle. The more secure syringe attachment decreases the inadvertent leakage of costly medications.

Tarsocrural (tibiotarsal) and proximal intertarsal joints

- These joints are approached on the dorsomedial aspect of the proximal tarsus.
- An 18- to 20-gauge, 1.5-inch (0.9–1.2 × 40 mm) needle is inserted either lateral or medial to the medial saphenous vein at a point 1 to 3 cm distal to the medial malleolus.
- 8 to 10 mL of local anesthetic is injected.
- If joint effusion is present, the needle may be inserted in the plantarolateral pouch of the tarsocrural joint.

Tarsometatarsal joint

- The TMT joint may be injected from a plantarolateral or medial approach.
- Plantarolateral approach:
  - The plantarolateral approach is the easiest method because the landmarks are easily palpated and the needle can usually be inserted securely into the joint.
  - The site for plantarolateral injection is directly proximal to the head of the lateral splint bone (metatarsal IV).
  - The plantar edge of the splint and the indentation at its proximal aspect is identified.
  - A 22- to 20-gauge, 1-inch (0.7–0.9 × 25 mm) needle is directed toward the opposite forelimb and distally at approximately 10 to 15 degrees.
  - When correctly placed, the needle is inserted nearly to its hub and 3 to 4 mL of local anesthetic is injected.
- Medial approach:
  - No landmarks are palpable when injecting the TMT from the medial approach.
  - The needle is inserted perpendicular to the medial surface of the tarsus approximately 1 cm distal to the DIT joint (see later).
  - A 22-gauge (0.7 mm) needle should be used and the joint is found by probing with the needle until it enters the joint.

Distal intertarsal joint

- The DIT joint is injected by placing a 22-gauge, 1-inch (0.7 × 25 mm) needle in a small space between the fused first and second tarsal bones, and the third and central tarsal bones.
- The space is immediately distal to the cunean tendon on the medial aspect of the tarsus.
- Firm digital pressure is necessary to identify the space.
- The needle is inserted perpendicular to the medial tarsal surface and some probing is often necessary to fall into the joint space.
- If the needle does not enter the joint easily, inject 1 to 2 mL of local anesthetic subcutaneously. This will make repeated needle insertions more comfortable for the horse.
- Probing for the joint space often causes a burr to form on the needle

tip. Formation of a burr will be made obvious by the increased friction and rough feel of the needle during continued probing. If this is noticed, change to a fresh needle.
- Inject 3 to 4 mL of local anesthetic.

Stifle joints

- The stifle includes three large volume joints: the femoropatellar, lateral femorotibial, and medial femorotibial.
- The femoropatellar and medial femorotibial joints communicate in 60% to 80% of horses.
- The lateral and medial femorotibial joints do not communicate under normal circumstances.
- Each joint should be separately injected to ensure complete analgesia of the stifle.

Femoropatellar joint

- Insert an 18-gauge, 3.5-inch (1.2 × 90 mm) spinal needle at the cranial aspect of the stifle between the middle and medial or middle and lateral patellar ligaments at a point approximately 2 cm proximal to the tibial crest with the limb fully weight bearing.
- Direct the needle slightly proximad to a depth of approximately 2 to 3 inches (50–75 mm).
- Synovial fluid is rarely aspirated using this approach, but entry into the joint is assumed when there is minimal resistance during injection of 30 to 50 mL of local anesthetic.
- An alternative approach may be used to enter the lateral proximal pouch of the femoropatellar joint.
  - An 18-gauge, 1.5-inch (1.2 × 40 mm) needle is placed immediately caudal to the proximal aspect of the lateral trochlear ridge and the lateral patellar ligament and directed lateral to medial and somewhat distally.
  - The insertion point is approximately 5 cm proximal to the lateral tibial condyle.
  - This approach avoids abrasion of articular cartilage and results in greater quantity of synovial fluid aspiration than the cranial approach.

Lateral femorotibial joint

- Have the limb fully weight-bearing and identify the space between the proximal tibia and the distal lateral trochlear ridge of the femur between the lateral patellar ligament and the lateral collateral ligament.

- The space is a small triangle of soft tissue that you may indent with digital palpation.
- An 18- to 20-gauge, 1.5-inch (0.9–1.2 × 40 mm) needle is inserted perpendicular to the skin and may be placed nearly to its hub.
- Inject 15 to 20 mL of local anesthetic.
- The approach is similar for the medial femorotibial joint with the needle being placed between the medial patellar and medial collateral ligaments.

Coxofemoral joint

- Accurately injecting local anesthetic into the coxofemoral joint is not easily accomplished.
- The landmarks may be difficult to palpate in heavily muscled horses and the joint is very distant to the insertion point of the needle.
- This procedure may be facilitated with ultrasonographic guidance of the needle.
- The horse should be standing squarely in stocks and a bleb of local anesthetic in the skin should be placed at the needle insertion point.
- The paired eminences of the major trochanter of the femur lie on a line approximately two-thirds of the distance from the tuber coxa to the tuber ischium.
- The proximal aspect of the cranial part of the greater trochanter lies approximately 5 cm distal to the proximal extent of the caudal part.
- An 18-gauge, ⅝-inch (1.2 mm × 15–20 cm) needle is inserted immediately proximal to the cranial part of the greater trochanter.
- The needle is directed in nearly a horizontal plane, slightly cranial and distal, toward the coxofemoral joint.
- The joint capsule is thick and may require vigorous pressure on the needle to penetrate.
- A volume of 20 to 40 mL of local anesthetic is injected.

SUGGESTED READING

Kaneps AJ: Diagnosis of lameness. In Hinchcliff KW, Kaneps AJ, Geor RJ, editors: *Equine sports medicine and surgery,* Philadelphia, 2004, Saunders Elsevier, pp 250–258.

AUTHOR: **ANDRIS J. KANEPS**

Liver: Diagnostic Imaging

BASIC INFORMATION

SYNONYM(S)

Trans-abdominal ultrasonography
Radionucleotide imaging (hepatic or biliary scintigraphy)
Mesenteric contrast portography

OVERVIEW AND GOAL(S)

- Trans-abdominal ultrasonography is the most commonly used imaging modality to evaluate the equine liver. It allows determination of hepatic size and contour, as well as detection of alterations in the hepatic parenchyma (abscesses, neoplastic masses, diffuse hepatitis, hepatic lipidosis) or evidence of obstruction of the biliary tree (dilated bile ducts, choleliths).
- Radionucleotide imaging of the liver and mesenteric contrast portography are occasionally used to provide additional information regarding aspects of hepatic function and blood flow but require specialized equipment and technical expertise. Ultrasonographic evaluation of the liver is discussed in detail in the following sections. As the use of radionucleotide imaging and contrast portography is typically confined to referral institutions, these modalities are covered briefly in the "Alternatives and Their Relative Merits" section in this chapter.

INDICATIONS

- To evaluate hepatic size, contour, and parenchyma in horses and foals with clinical or clinicopathologic evidence of liver disease
- To evaluate the liver for metastases from distant neoplasms
- To aid in obtaining a percutaneous liver biopsy sample

CONTRAINDICATIONS

None, although personnel safety should be considered when attempting to image patients with severe hepatic encephalopathy

EQUIPMENT, ANESTHESIA

- Clippers, with a No. 40 blade
- Alcohol
- Ultrasound contact gel
- 2.5 to 5.0 MHz (adult horses) or 5 to 7.5 MHz (foals) sector scanner or linear-array transducer
- Good quality ultrasound image viewing and recording equipment
- ± supplies for a percutaneous liver biopsy (see "Biopsy: Liver" in this section)

ANTICIPATED TIME

20 to 40 minutes

PREPARATION: IMPORTANT CHECKPOINTS

- Ultrasonographic evaluation of the liver may be performed in a standing, unsedated adult horse and in a standing or recumbent foal.
- The patient may be sedated as necessary to ensure patient compliance for a comprehensive examination or if an ultrasound-guided liver biopsy is anticipated.
- The right and left flanks should be clipped as follows:
  ○ Right: From the sixth to sixteenth intercostal spaces, ventral to a line extending from the right olecranon to the right tuber coxae
  ○ Left: From the fifth to sixth to ninth intercostal space, ventral to a line extending from the left olecranon to the left tuber coxae
- After clipping, the skin should be wiped with alcohol and coated with a thin layer of ultrasound contact gel.

POSSIBLE COMPLICATIONS AND COMMON ERRORS TO BE AVOIDED

- No specific complications are associated with the ultrasound procedure itself.
- It is important to note that the entire liver is not visible with trans-abdominal ultrasound in the adult horse and in most foals, due to the position of the liver relative to the lung fields, diaphragm, stomach, and large colon. In addition, some atrophy of the right liver lobe is common in older horses and can limit visualization of the liver in these cases. Thus difficulty imaging the liver does not always imply hepatic pathology or diminished hepatic mass.
- Ultrasonography provides no information regarding hepatic function, and ultrasonographic abnormalities are not always found even with severe hepatic disease or hepatic failure. Thus a normal hepatic ultrasonographic appearance does not exclude the possibility of hepatic disease.

PROCEDURE

- Begin scanning on the right side of the abdomen, just cranial to the right kidney at approximately the right sixteenth intercostal space.
- Scan from dorsal to ventral in each intercostal space, moving from caudal to cranial, until the liver is visualized ventral to the lung margin.
- The normal hepatic parenchyma is homogeneous and of moderate echogenicity (Figure 1). In general, the hepatic echogenicity should be in between the echogenicity of the kidney and the spleen.
- The branching hepatic vasculature is easily visualized (Figure 2) and aids in recognition of the liver. The portal vein walls are more echogenic than the hepatic vein walls, due to increased amounts of connective tissue in the portal vasculature.
- Four to 10 cm of liver are typically visible in an adult (not aged) horse from the right side of the abdomen,

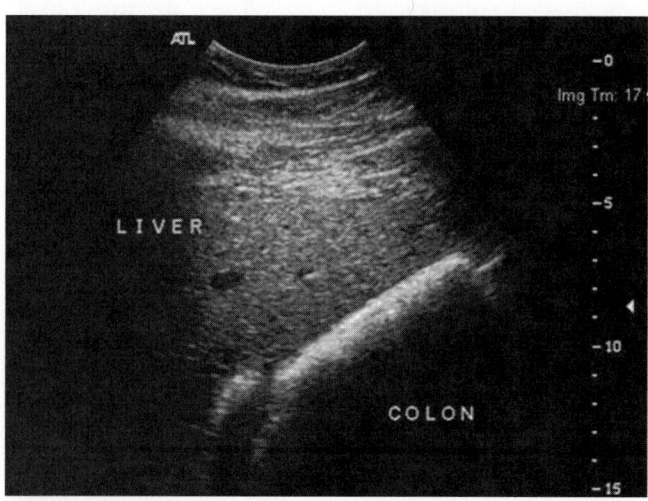

FIGURE 1 Normal echogenicity of the hepatic parenchyma. This image was obtained at the eleventh right intercostal space using a 3- to 5-MHz transducer, displayed to a depth of 15 cm.

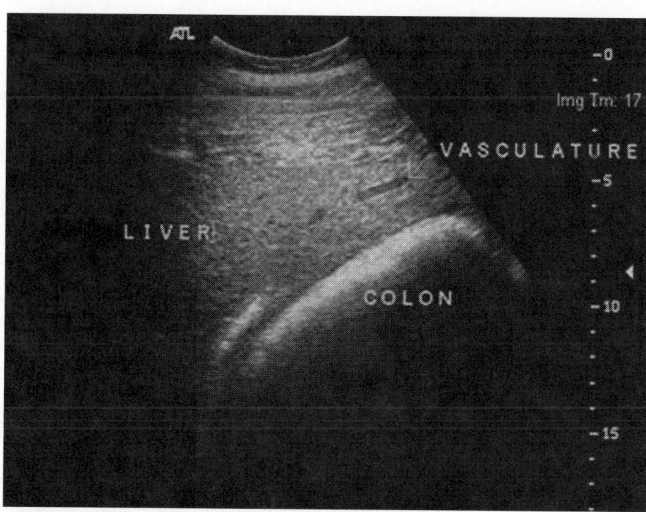

FIGURE 2 Portal vasculature is distinguished by the presence of echogenic walls. This image was obtained at the eleventh right intercostal space using a 3- to 5-MHz transducer, displayed to a depth of 18 cm.

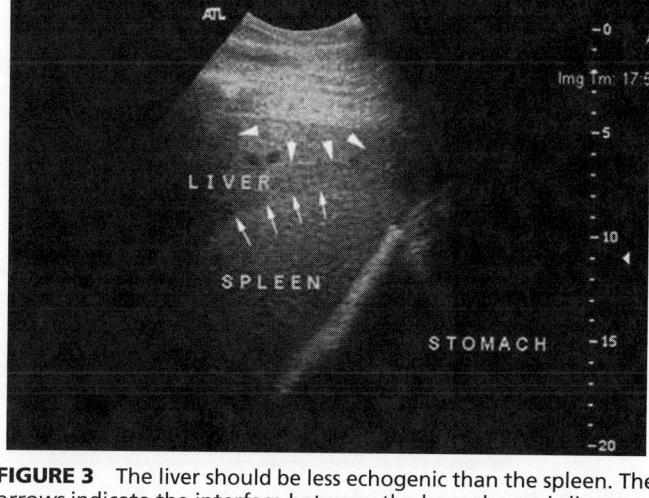

FIGURE 3 The liver should be less echogenic than the spleen. The *arrows* indicate the interface between the less echogenic liver and the spleen. The *arrowheads* within the liver mark a focal area of increased echogenicity within the liver. This image was obtained at the left ninth intercostal space.

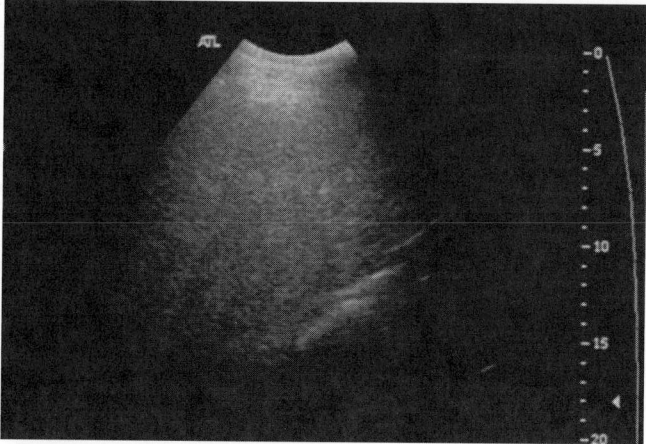

FIGURE 4 An abnormal generalized increase in hepatic echogenicity (compare to Figure 1). This horse had hepatic lipidosis. This image was obtained at the twelfth right intercostal space using a 3- to 5-MHz transducer, displayed to a depth of 20 cm.

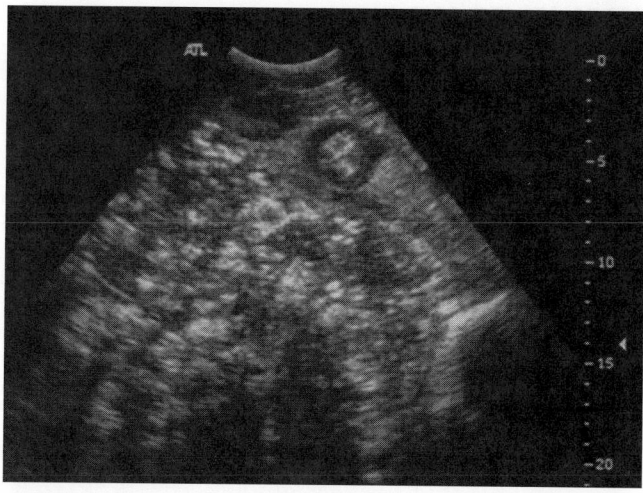

FIGURE 5 Abnormal hepatic parenchyma of mixed echogenicity (compare to Figure 1). This patient had metastatic hepatic lymphoma. This image was obtained at the twelfth right intercostal space using a 3- to 5-MHz transducer, displayed to a depth of 21 cm.

although this amount can vary greatly depending on the relative position of the lungs and large colon in relation to the liver.

- The caudal vena cava and common bile duct are not visible ultrasonographically in an adult horse. The bile ducts and biliary tree are not normally visible.

- Continue scanning from dorsal to ventral in each intercostal space, moving from caudal to cranial, noting the relative size of the liver, the echogenicity of the parenchyma, and the contour of the hepatic margins (which should be smooth and sharp).

- When the entirety of the liver has been imaged on the right side of the abdomen, the left lobe of the liver should be evaluated in the left cranioventral abdomen.

- Begin scanning the left side in the ninth intercostal space, at approximately the level of the point of the shoulder, and scan from dorsal to ventral in each intercostal space, again moving from a caudal location to cranial.

- The liver is found cranial to the stomach and medial or lateral to the spleen in this location. It is typical to visualize approximately 3 to 7 cm of liver from the left side, although again this can vary greatly.

- The liver is less echogenic than the spleen and is also differentiated from the spleen by the easily visible hepatic vasculature as described above (Figure 3).

- The entirety of the liver on both sides of the abdomen should be scanned in both dorsal and transverse planes to ensure a comprehensive evaluation.

- Alterations in hepatic parenchymal echogenicity (increased or decreased, focal or diffuse), rounded hepatic borders, dilated or difficult to visualize hepatic vasculature, dilated or thickened bile ducts (which are not normally seen), or a rounded hepatic contour may indicate clinically significant liver disease (see Figures 3, 4, 5, and 6). However, histopathologic evaluation of biopsy samples of areas of concern on ultrasonographic evaluation is necessary for definitive diagnosis.

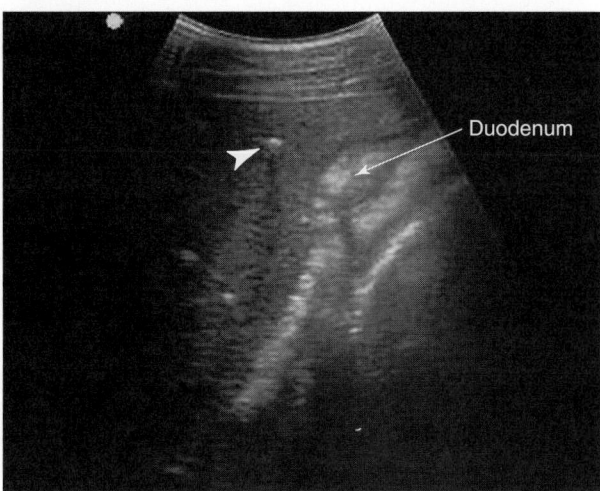

Duodenum

FIGURE 6 Hyperechoic foci with an anacoustic shadow (*arrowhead*) are consistent with a cholelith. This image was obtained at the eleventh right intercostal space using a 3- to 5-MHz transducer, displayed to a depth of 20 cm.

ALTERNATIVES AND THEIR RELATIVE MERITS

RADIONUCLEOTIDE IMAGING

- Two types of scans may be performed.
  - Hepatic scan with technetium-99m-labelled sulfur colloid
    - A two-dimensional representation of relative radioactivity in the hepatic parenchyma is obtained after hepatic macrophages phagocytose the radiolabeled sulfur colloid.
    - This is most commonly performed to provide information regarding hepatic blood flow when a portosystemic shunt is suspected, in which decreased radionucleotide uptake is seen in the liver.
    - In addition, large alterations in structure such as abscesses or masses may be detectable.
  - Biliary scan with technetium-99m-labelled iminodiacetic acid
    - Hepatocytes extract, conjugate, and excrete the radiolabeled iminodiacetic acid in the bile, and a two-dimensional representation of the radioactivity within the biliary tree is generated.

- This test is performed to provide more information regarding bile production and flow when biliary system dysfunction or obstruction is suspected.
  - Although these procedures provide more information regarding hepatic function, blood flow, and biliary flow than hepatic ultrasound can, they are expensive and require specialized equipment to perform, and thus their use is limited to referral institutions and cases in which hepatic ultrasound and biopsy are inconclusive.

MESENTERIC CONTRAST PORTOGRAPHY

- In this procedure, radiopaque contrast material is injected into a mesenteric vein, and rapid serial abdominal survey radiographs are obtained, providing information regarding portal blood flow.
- This test is indicated when a portosystemic shunt is suspected based on clinical or radionucleotide imaging findings and allows determination of the specific location of the portosystemic shunt (intrahepatic vs. extrahepatic).
- This procedure requires surgical access to the mesenteric vasculature via a laparotomy and the capacity to obtain intraoperative abdominal radiographs. Thus its use is limited to specialty practices and referral institutions, and primarily to foals with suspected portosystemic shunting.

AUTHOR: **KELSEY A. HART**

Magnetic Resonance Imaging: Dental

BASIC INFORMATION

SYNONYM(S)

MRI

OVERVIEW AND GOAL(S)

- Magnetic resonance imaging (MRI) generates images based on the response of tissue to radiofrequency (RF) pulses while present within a strong magnetic field.
  - The images depict the tissues based on a number of different factors that include but are not limited to the composition of and the environment in and around the tissue of interest.
  - Factors such as degree of proton movement (fluid vs. collagen) and

local magnetic fields (the ferrous portions of degrading blood products respond to the external magnetic field) influence the imaging characteristics in the area of interest.
  - MRI is particularly useful for the evaluation of soft tissues and fluid as expected in chronic inflammatory conditions and sinusitis.
  - Tissues containing a high percentage of collagen or hydroxyapatite, a main component of bone and dental tissue, produce no or very low signal when exposed to an external magnetic field and RF pulses. For this reason, dental and osseous structures appear black.
  - MRI can be useful to infer disease of the hard tissues by pathology

detected in the surrounding structure and shape and margination change of the hard tissues themselves.
  - Excess fluid content in bone as found in osteomyelitis can be detected using MRI.

INDICATIONS

- MRI is uncommonly used to evaluate dental and dental-related disease.
  - Similar to computed tomography, MRI is indicated when the oral examination and radiographic examination do not provide sufficient information to plan therapeutic strategies, when dental disease is complicated by secondary problems such as osteomyelitis and sinusitis.

CONTRAINDICATIONS

Contraindications for MRI are limited to contraindications for general anesthesia.

EQUIPMENT, ANESTHESIA

- MRI scanner: RF coils appropriate for skull scanning
- Equine MRI table
- Trained technical or veterinary staff: To position the horse and prescribe the MRI scan acquisitions
- Viewing station: A workstation equipped with high-quality monitors and appropriate software
- General anesthesia: routine methods of induction, maintenance and recovery are needed. Anesthetic agents should be suitable for maintaining the horse for a 60- to 120-minute procedure.

ANTICIPATED TIME

45 to 90 minutes of scanning time. Additional time is needed for positioning and planning of the MRI scan.

PREPARATION: IMPORTANT CHECKPOINTS

MRI scanners are limited in availability. Prior to scanning, quality assurance tests should be run on the MRI scanner. The equine table function should be checked and the horse should be prepared for a moderately lengthy general anesthesia. Most facilities using MRI will be well versed in preparation for an MRI scan.

POSSIBLE COMPLICATIONS AND COMMON ERRORS TO BE AVOIDED

MRI is a less appropriate technique than computed tomography for the evaluation of sinonasal and dental disease. A discussion with a veterinarian versed in all imaging modalities (radiologist) should be undertaken prior to subjecting a horse to a lengthy and potentially suboptimal or inappropriate imaging study.

PROCEDURE

- The horse will be positioned within the MRI scanner in either dorsal or lateral recumbency.
- Pilot images are obtained in several planes that allow the MRI operator to plan the subsequent diagnostic series.
- The imaging study will include several different imaging sequences (spin echo, gradient echo, and/or inversion recovery sequences) in transverse, dorsal, and parasagittal planes.
- After a sufficient number of images are acquired to obtain a diagnostic study, the study is terminated and the horse recovered from general anesthesia.
- Higher field strength magnets will obtain images more rapidly and with higher resolution than low field strength MRI systems.

POSTPROCEDURE

Routine postanesthetic monitoring should be observed.

ALTERNATIVES AND THEIR RELATIVE MERITS

Computed tomography uses x-ray technology to produce images based on tissue x-ray density. Similar to MRI, CT produces cross-sectional images that provide high detail and eliminate the problems caused by superimposition on routine radiographs. CT is considerably more rapid than MRI, limiting the total general anesthesia time.

AUTHOR: **SARAH M. PUCHALSKI**

Magnetic Resonance Imaging: Musculoskeletal

BASIC INFORMATION

OVERVIEW AND GOAL(S)

- Magnetic resonance imaging (MRI) produces images based on the magnetic properties of the hydrogen protons within the body.
- MRI provides exquisite detail of the soft tissues. Osseous structures are also well visualized, particularly bone marrow and subchondral bone. However, due to the minimal resonance produced by normal cortical bone, periarticular proliferation and small osseous bodies can be easily overlooked compared with computed tomography (CT).
- MRI differs from CT in that multiple scan planes are acquired rather than being reconstructed from a single axial plane. This leads to much longer scanning times.
- The patient is placed within a relatively strong magnetic field (see "Equipment" below), aligning the hydrogen protons of the body.
- A pulse sequence is applied to the anatomic area of interest, and the response of the protons to that pulse

sequence produces an image. Within the pulse sequence, a radiofrequency (RF) pulse is introduced into the patient from a transmit coil, energizing the tissue. As the tissue reverts to its original state, RF energy is emitted from the patient and recorded by a receiving coil.

- The differences in the magnetic properties of tissues are demonstrated by using multiple types of pulse sequence. By altering these parameters, the contrast of various tissues is altered, allowing differentiation of anatomic structures.
- Spin-echo sequences use multiple introductions of RF signal that include a 180-degree rephasing pulse. This rephasing pulse corrects for magnetic susceptibility.
- The most commonly used scanning sequences are:
  - ○ T1 spin-echo: T1 recovery is a measure of the exchange of energy with the surrounding environment. T1 sequences have high signal-to-noise ratio and are more subject to small changes in the local magnetic field, making them ideal for contrast studies.
  - ○ T2 spin-echo: T2 relaxation is a measure of transfer of magnetization between adjacent protons. T2 sequences have high contrast but a decreased signal-to-noise ratio compared with T1 and proton density sequences.
  - ○ Proton density (PD): The signal intensity is based on the number of protons in a voxel. PD sequences have a high signal-to-noise ratio, similar to T1 and better than T2.
  - ○ Gradient echo (GRE): GRE sequences can be T1 or T2 weighted. They are not a true spin-echo sequence and are prone to magnetic susceptibility artifact. Volume acquisitions can be obtained, allowing for thinner slices. Because these are not spin-echo sequences, they are also rapidly acquired.
  - ○ Short tau inversion recovery (STIR): Sequences that null the signal from fat. This allows for identification for abnormalities within the medullary cavity of bone. Image detail is reduced compared with T1, T2, and PD pulse sequences, but the STIR sequence is very sensitive in the

TABLE 1 Comparison of MRI Units

	Standing	Low-Field	High-Field	Comments
Initial cost	$	$	$ to $$$	Cost of high-field MR units are highly variable, especially when used equipment is considered.
Operating and maintenance costs	$	$	$ to $$$	The largest proportion of costs with high-field MR involve helium replenishment. Newer designs minimize replenishment requirements.
Image Quality	+	+	++ to +++	Standing magnet image quality can be hampered by patient motion. Higher field magnet image quality can vary depending on field strength and gradient strength.
Scan Time	↑↑ to ↑↑↑	↑↑	↑	Patient motion can greatly increase scan time with standing patients. In general, with higher field strength signal-to-noise ratio is increased and scan time is decreased.

detection of abnormal fluid signal in bone.

- Fat saturation sequences are similar in end result to STIR sequences (decreased signal from fat). These sequences can have various names depending on the manufacturer.
  ○ Cartilage imaging: Manufacturer-specific sequences have been created to better visualize articular cartilage (eg, spoiled gradient echo).

INDICATIONS

- Generally reserved for patients with a localized source of lameness.
- Other imaging modalities have failed to identify a lesion believed to cause lameness or the severity or duration evident clinically.
- Lameness localized to areas that are not amenable to accurate ultrasound evaluation of the soft tissues, such as the foot or proximal suspensory ligaments.

EQUIPMENT, ANESTHESIA

Positioning:

- It is imperative that patient positioning be accurately entered into the initial patient setup to avoid mislocalization of lesions. Additional markers, commonly vitamin E capsules (used because of the bright fat signal produced), can be used to delineate right and left sides.
- Sand bags or foam wedges are commonly used to stabilize the limb and minimize respiratory motion. This is especially important with the nondependent limb because it is more prone to motion.

Equipment:

- Types of magnets:
  ○ Low field (<1 T): The majority of low-field magnets used in equine imaging are permanent magnets that do not require cooling.
  ○ The Hallmarq magnet is a permanent low-field magnet designed for image acquisition in the standing, sedated horse.

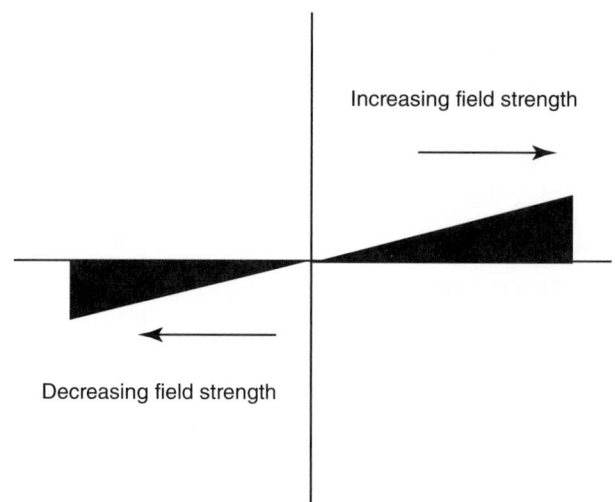

FIGURE 1 Gradient coil.

(figure labels: Increasing field strength; Decreasing field strength)

  ○ High field (≥1 T): These units require supercooling with helium. As the field strength of a magnet increases, the signal to noise ratio increases (in general) and better quality images are obtained (Table 1).
- Coils: The coils used with MRI function like an antenna, receiving or transmitting (or both) RF signals. Multiple coils are in use during image acquisition performing different tasks, and multiple coil types are available to receive the signal from the patient that produces the image information.
  ○ Gradient coils: This coil system coordinates the anatomy being scanned into a matrix by producing a gradient of magnetic strengths along each axis. As the strength of the gradient increases, the spatial resolution increases (measured in mT/m) (Figure 1).
  ○ Receive coils: Dedicated wire that detects signal from the patient for image formation.
  ○ Transmit/receive coils: Perform both send and receive functions of RF pulses.
    - Surface coils: Receive coils that detect signal from the patient.

These coils have good signal to noise ratio, with the signal degrading as distance from the coil increases.
    - Quadrature coils: Typically a transmit/receive coil. Provides a more homogenous signal of a volume of interest compared with surface coils.
    - Array coils: Multiple small coils that can be combined to surround anatomy. Allows better anatomic coverage than a single surface coil.
- Shielding: Proper RF shielding must be installed surrounding the MR suite to avoid interference from outside RF signals because the RF pulse used to generate the signal during the examination is similar to the RF pulses used for radio transmission. Outside RF interference can have deleterious effects on image quality. Access to the suite during the examination should be limited, and doors should remain closed to avoid artifact.
- Shielding is also required for high field strength magnets to avoid interference with electronic equipment *outside* the MR suite; most magnets are internally shielded.

- Manufacturers and specialized construction companies are available to assist in the design of an MR suite.

Safety

- The magnetic field strength associated with MRI machines is much stronger than the Earth's magnetic field; therefore any metallic object placed near the magnet has the potential to become a projectile (eg, anesthetic machines, oxygen tanks, mops, buckets, vacuums, instruments). These are not only a danger to the patient and operators, but small magnetic items that have gone undetected in the bore of the magnet will cause artifacts and/or damage to the apparatus.
- Patients or operators with metallic implants, including pacemakers, vascular clips, cochlear devices or orthopedic implants, should not go near the magnet. Pacemakers in particular can malfunction when in the proximity of the magnet.
- Anyone entering the MRI suite should remove all objects from their pockets, including credit cards, identification badges, cell phones, watches, keys, and pagers because these objects can malfunction or become projectiles. Information encoded in the magnetic strip of credit cards or identification cards will be erased in the presence of the magnetic field.

PREPARATION: IMPORTANT CHECKPOINTS

- All metal, including nails and shoes, must be removed to prevent signal voids created by magnetic susceptibility artifact. To ensure all metal has been removed, radiographs should be taken before MRI examination.
- Do not use blue modeling compound (ie, Play-Doh) to pack the feet for radiographs before an MRI examination because this material causes magnetic susceptibility artifact.
- Except for Hallmarq standing MRI equipment, general anesthesia is required.

PROCEDURE

- Common sequences used in equine imaging:
  - T1 spin-echo: The high signal-to-noise ratio shows pathology well with contrast and good anatomic detail.
  - T2 spin-echo: Provides good contrast with high signal from fluid and adipose tissue. Signal-to-noise ratio is lower than PD or T1.
  - PD: High signal-to-noise ratio with better contrast than T1.
  - GRE: Typically volume acquisitions; allows for thinner slices and better spatial resolution. Highly sensitive to magnetic susceptibility. A good sequence for the detection of hemorrhage.
  - STIR: Nulls signal from normal adipose tissue and is therefore very useful in detection of abnormal fluid signal within bone (edema). With T1, PD, and T2 images, medullary bone (adipose tissue) is high in signal (hyperintense, bright). A hyperintense fluid signal is difficult to differentiate from fat with PD and T2 but is highly contrasted from the nulled signal from fat with STIR imaging.
  - Fat saturation: Same principle as STIR, but with saturation of fat rather than nulling; signal-to-noise ratio is improved.
- Common imaging planes: Multiple imaging planes are required. Abnormalities should be confirmed in multiple planes to differentiate from artifact and allow more definitive localization.
  - Axial: Slices are obtained perpendicular to the long axis of the limb.
  - Sagittal: Imaging parallel to the long axis of the limb.
  - Coronal: Parallel to the long axis but in the frontal or dorsal plane.
- Scanning of both limbs over the area of interest is extremely valuable for comparison and highly recommended.

POSTPROCEDURE

- Knowledge of normal anatomy is imperative to interpretation of the MRI examination.
- Comparison between limbs is essential for identifying individual variations of normal.
- Normal tendons and ligaments for the most part lack signal and are therefore black. This is because of the relative lack of free hydrogen protons within these tissues.
- Hyperintensity within tendons and ligaments often represents pathologic alteration in structure.
  - Some of these injuries will maintain high signal chronically, making determination of active versus chronic lesions difficult.
- STIR sequences are extremely valuable in the assessment of medullary bone.
  - Hyperintensity within the medullary bone is often termed *bone marrow edema* in the literature. Based on histologic study, this high signal has been attributed not only to edema but also various cellular alterations of the medullary cavity. Therefore the term "bone edema" has recently fallen out of favor. In an acutely lame patient, bone contusion is a likely cause of subchondral bone hyperintensity on STIR sequence (Table 2; Figures 2 and 3).

Artifacts:

- Motion and blood flow artifact
  - Patient motion causes marginal blurring, typically in nonconsecutive slices (slice image information is usually obtained in an "every other slice" order.
    - Positional devices are used to minimize this artifact.
  - Standing systems use motion correction software to attempt to minimize motion artifact.
  - Motion from moving blood in vessels will produce repeating artifacts vertically or horizontally along the entire image (depending

TABLE 2 MRI Sequence Comparison

	T1 weighted	T2 weighted	PD	STIR	GRE
Fluid	Hypointense	Hyperintense	Intermediate intensity (low)	Hyperintense	Variable depending on weighting
Fat/intramedullary bone	Hyperintense	Hyperintense	Hyperintense	Hypointense	Variable
Tendon/ligament	Hypointense	Hypointense	Hypointense	Hypointense	Hypointense
Muscle	Intermediate intensity (low)	Intermediate intensity (high)	Intermediate intensity (low)	Intermediate intensity (high)	Intermediate intensity (high)
Cortical bone	Hypointense	Hypointense	Hypointense	Hypointense	Hypointense
Hemorrhage	Variable depending on time	Variable depending on time	Variable depending on time	Variable depending on time	Hypointense

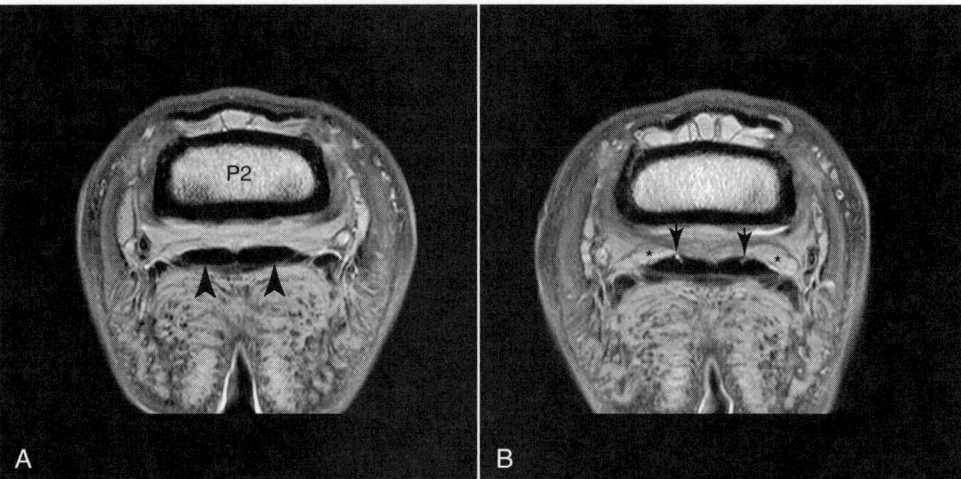

FIGURE 2 Normal deep digital flexor (DDF) tendon (**A**) and DDF tendonitis (**B**) in the forelimbs of a horse. These are axial PD images made at the level of the mid second phalanx (P2). **A,** The normal medial and lateral portions of the DDF tendon are in the center of the image, seen in cross-section as black, thin elliptical structures (*arrowheads*). The second phalanx (P2) is seen as hyperintense (white) central bone marrow surrounded by a thick black rim of cortical bone. The thin black common digital extensor tendon can be seen dorsal to P2. **B,** In the contralateral forelimb, a short hyperintense linear tear is present within the medial and lateral portions of the DDF tendon (*arrows*). The *asterisks* denote abnormal fluid within the navicular bursa.

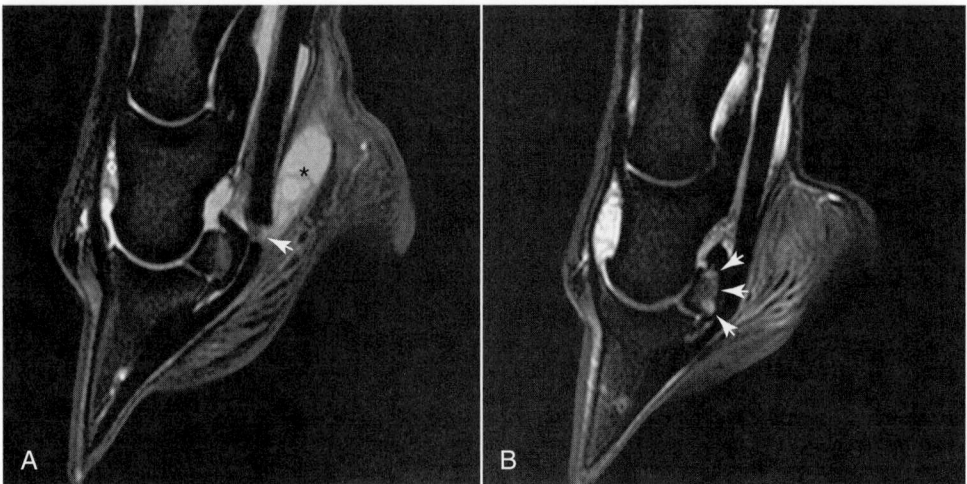

FIGURE 3 STIR sagittal images of the distal extremity of two horses demonstrating soft tissue and osseous abnormalities. **A,** Disruption of the deep digital flexor (DDF) tendon just proximal to the navicular bone (*arrow*), with a large hyperintense focus of fluid accumulation palmar to this region (*asterisk*). There is also an abnormal hyperintense signal within the medullary cavity of the navicular bone. The diagnosis was a penetrating wound to the bulb of the heel and laceration of the DDF tendon. **B,** Uneven hyperintensity within the medullary cavity of the navicular bone is present (*arrows*). This is due to bone contusion, bone marrow edema, or osseous inflammation. This is a common MRI finding in horses with navicular degeneration.

on the phase encoding direction) (Figure 4)
- Similar axial scans with different weighting will often use different phase encoding direction to "flip" the artifact in the opposite direction between scans.
- Magic angle artifact
  - Tendinous/ligamentous structures that should be hypointense are artificially increased in signal intensity due to their angle relative to the main magnetic field. This is evident when the structure of interest is

coursing at an angle of 55 ± 10 degrees relative to the main magnetic field. This artifact is not present with sequences that have a long TE (echo time), such as T2-weighted sequences (Figure 5).
- Magnetic susceptibility artifact
  - This artifact is created by ferrous metals within the magnetic field. The effects may be minimal (Figure 6) or quite severe, rendering the MRI study useless (Figure 7).
  - Removal of all metallic debris possible is essential to minimize this artifact.

- Gradient echo sequences are inherently more sensitive to this artifact given their lack of an 180-degree rephasing pulse.

SUGGESTED READING

Denoix J: *The equine distal limb: an atlas of clinical anatomy and comparative imaging,* London, 2000, Manson Publishing Ltd.

Westbrook C: MRI at a glance, Ames, IA, 2002, Blackwell Science.

AUTHORS: **JOHN S. MATTOON, JASON W. BRUMITT, JONATHAN HAYLES, DANA A. NEELIS, GREGORY D. ROBERTS,** and **TOM WILKINSON**

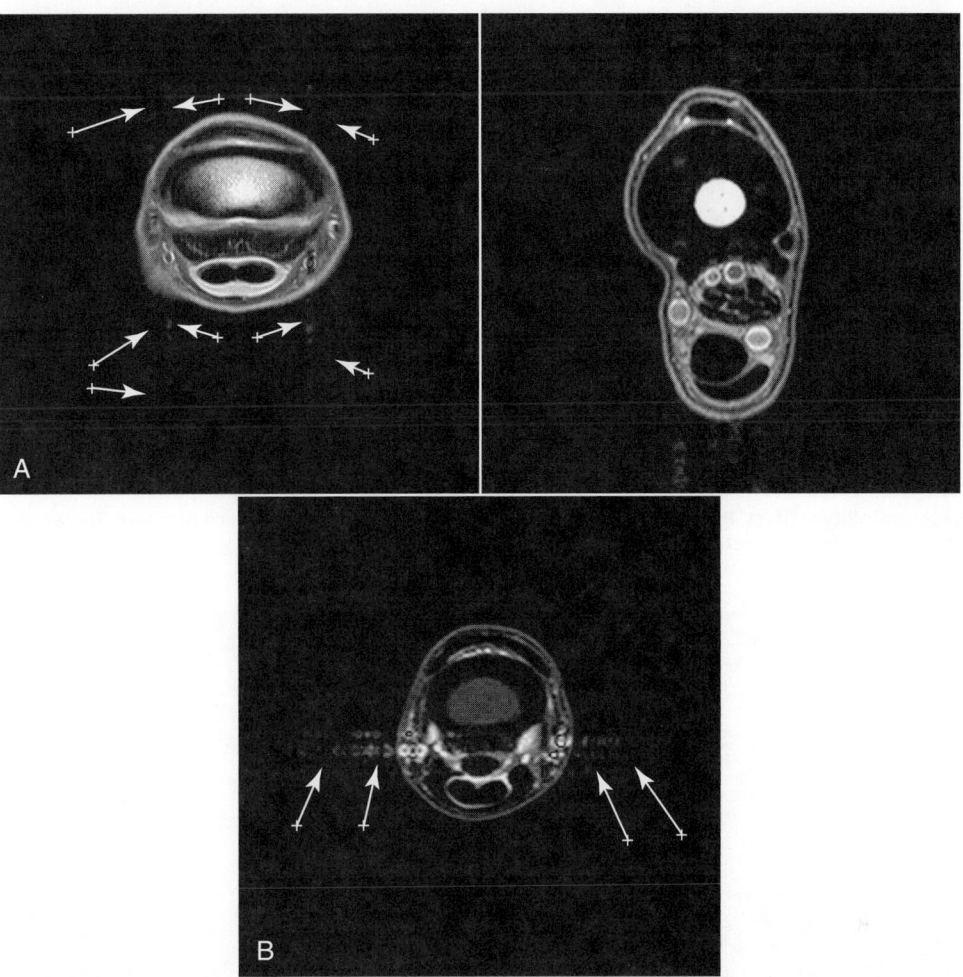

FIGURE 4 Blood flow artifact. **A,** The flow artifact is repeating dorsally and plantarly on this PD axial image at the level of the metatarsus. The four vertical whitish streaks can be seen to be composed of intermittently continuous white circular images, representing blood flow within of the cross-section of the four plantar blood vessels. When these artifacts overlay tendons or ligaments, they can be mistaken for hyperintense lesions. In this image, hyperintense foci can be seen over the dark cortical bone and the extensor and flexor tendons. **B,** The flow artifact is now repeating laterally and medially (horizontally) on this axial STIR image at the same level of the metatarsus as in **A**. Note the artifactual focal hyperintensities now positioned over the suspensory ligament and the DDF. The phase and frequency encoding directions have been reversed between sequences (a user-defined field).

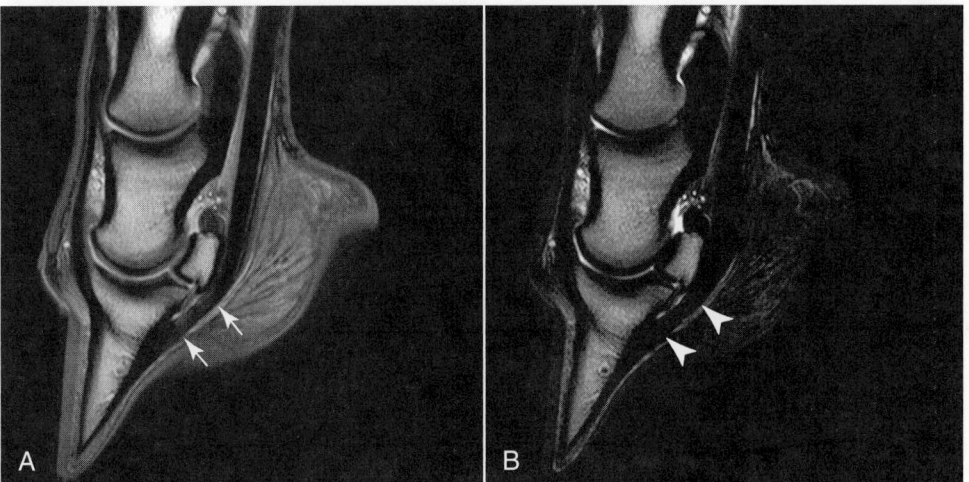

FIGURE 5 Magic angle artifact. **A,** Artifactual hyperintensity of the deep digital flexor (DDF) tendon distal to the navicular bone on PD sequences is seen (*arrows*). **B,** On the T2 weighted image the DDF tendon is now black, without the presence of the hyperintensity artifact.

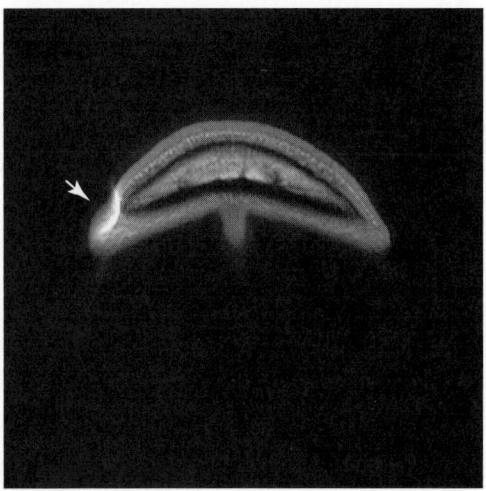

FIGURE 6 Magnetic susceptibility artifact. PD axial image through the distal portion of the third phalanx. The *arrow* indicates a magnetic susceptibility artifact created by ferrous metal within the hoof wall (shoe nail remnant).

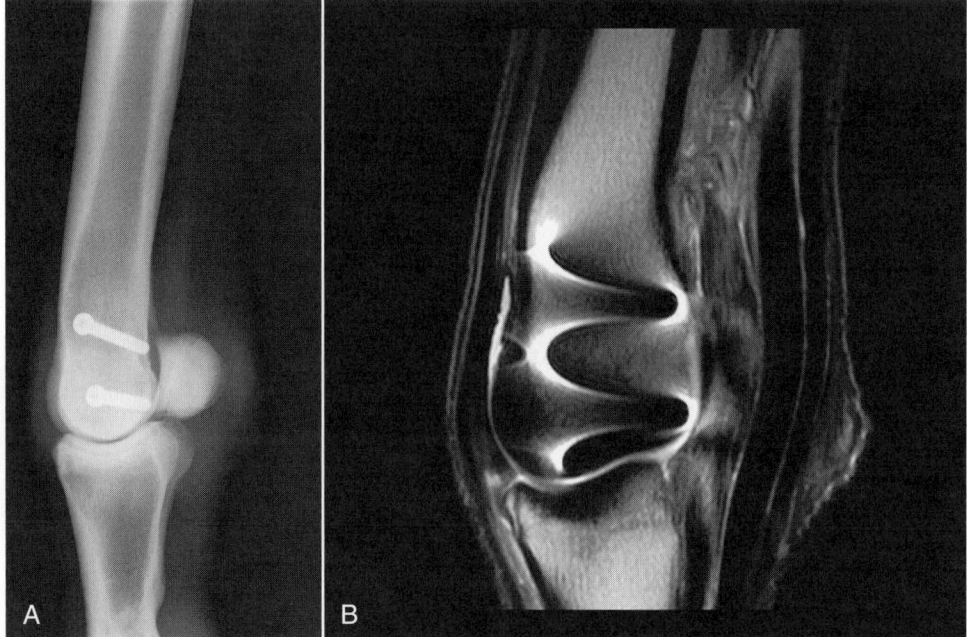

FIGURE 7 Magnetic susceptibility artifact. **A,** Lateral radiographic image of the third metatarsus after fracture repair using bone screws. **B,** PD sagittal MRI image of the third metatarsus fracture repair showing severe distortion created by the bone screws.

Metered-Dose Inhalation Therapy

BASIC INFORMATION

SYNONYM(S)

Nebulization

OVERVIEW AND GOAL(S)

- The purpose of inhaled therapy is to deliver an amount of medication that ensures therapeutic concentrations in the lower respiratory tract. Inhalation therapy is an alternative to parenteral dosing, allowing treatment with small doses of drug to minimize toxicity and side effects.
- Different types of inhalation devices are available including:
  - Nebulizers (jet and ultrasonic)
  - Metered-dose inhalers (MDI)
  - Dry powder inhalers (DPI)

INDICATIONS

- Inhalation therapy is recommended for treatment of many respiratory disorders that occur with broncho-constriction, inflammation, and/or infection of the lower respiratory tract.
- The most common conditions in which inhaled therapy is used in horses include:
  - Recurrent airway obstruction
  - Small airway disease
  - Pneumonia (bacterial, parasitic, fungal, or viral)
  - Exercise-induced pulmonary hemo-rrhage

- The most common medications and doses used in inhalation therapy are listed in Table 1.

CONTRAINDICATIONS

- Sensitivity to the medication
- Corticosteroid therapy is only recommended if infection has been ruled out.
  - Negative culture of transtracheal wash (TTW) fluid can identify infection.

EQUIPMENT, ANESTHESIA

- Inhalation therapy has been achieved with diverse devices such as nebulizers (jet and ultrasonic), MDIs, and DPIs.
  - The most commonly used are MDIs, which do not require expensive and fragile equipment (ultrasonic nebu-

lizer), or other devices that can produce loud noise (jet nebulizer).
- Several devices have been used to maximize the efficiency of the MDI, including:
  - AeroMask (Figure 1)
  - Equine Haler (Figure 2)
  - Era Mask (Figure 3)
  - Equine Inhaler
  - AeroHippus (Figure 4)
- The adequate delivery of medication with MDIs requires an airtight junction (minimizing drug leakage and subdosing), which has particular importance when devices such as the Equine Haler or the AeroHippus are used.

ANTICIPATED TIME

- In general, adults and foals tolerate inhalation therapy without behavior problems.

- If the horse is conditioned to the device the time to prepare the patient for treatment is minimal.
  - Horses usually become accustomed to the device after several uses.
- Depending on the dose and the amount of puffs, the session lasts for 3 to 5 minutes for each dose.
- Duration of the treatment depends on the condition.
  - In the case of small airway disease or recurrent airway obstruction, it can be as long as 10 weeks.

PREPARATION: IMPORTANT CHECKPOINTS

- Proper maintenance (cleaning) of the delivering device before each treatment is required.
- Some degree of training in use of an MDI is required.

TABLE 1 Dosage of Common Medications Available in MDIs

Class	Substance	Dose	Frequency	Comments
Bronchodilator (anticholinergic)	Ipratropium bromide	360 µg–1 mg	q6–8 h	
Bronchodilator (β₂ agonist)	Albuterol	720 µg	q3–6 h	Effective in 5 min Lasts 30 min
	Fenoterol	0.9–2 mg		Effects in <5 min
	Pirbutenol	1.2–2.4 µg/kg	q3 h	Effective in 5 min Lasts 7 h Do not exceed 6 µg/kg
	Salmeterol	63–210 µg	q8 h	Effective in 5 min Lasts 6-8 h
Mast cell stabilizer	Sodium cromoglycolate	8–12 mg	q12 h	
	Nedocromil sodium	16–24 mg	q12 h	
Corticosteroid	Fluticasone	1–2 mg	q12 h	High potency
	Beclometasone	1500–3750 µg	q12 h	Medium potency

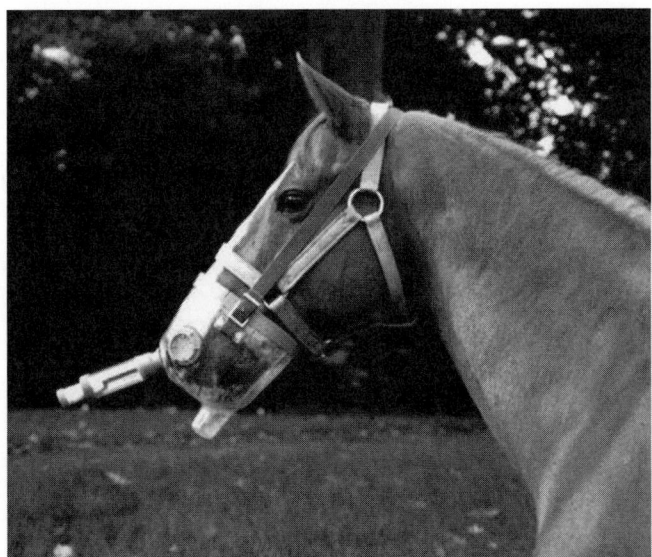

FIGURE 1 AeroMask (Trudell Medical International, London, Canada).

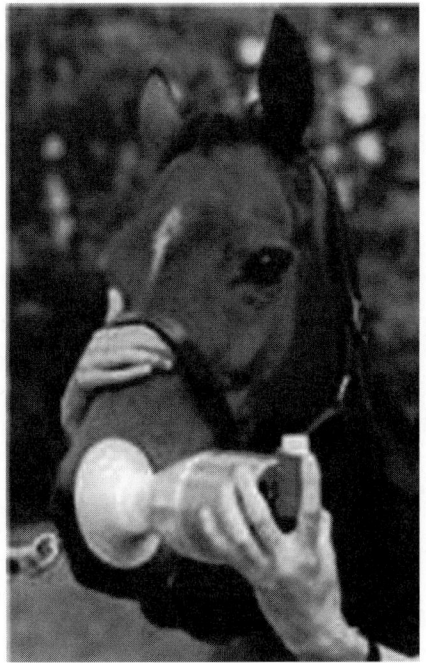

FIGURE 2 Equine Haler (APS, Equine Healthcare, Hillerod, Denmark).

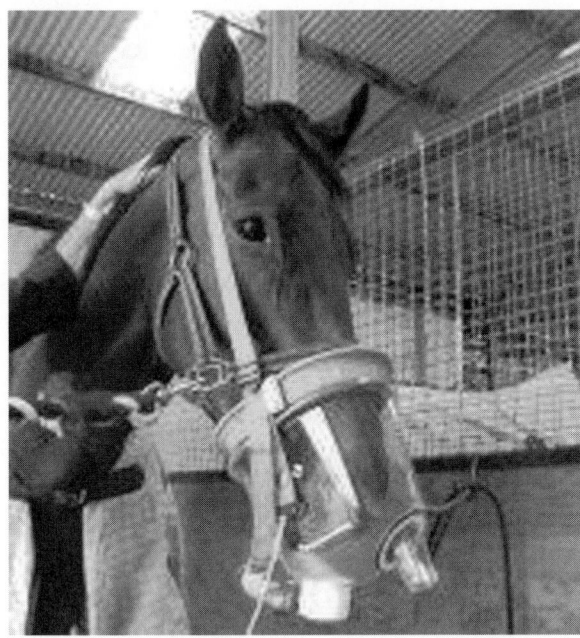

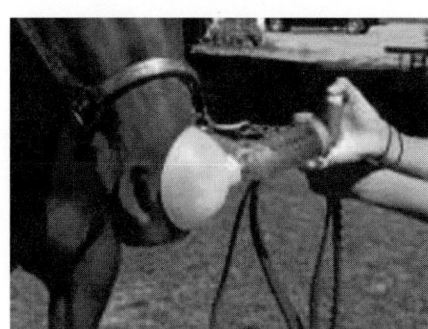

FIGURE 4 AeroHippus (Trudell Medical International, London, Canada).

FIGURE 3 Era Mask (Biomedtech Australia PTY LTD).

- Initially, in the case of mask type devices, easy release is recommended to avoid accidents.

POSSIBLE COMPLICATIONS AND COMMON ERRORS TO BE AVOIDED

- Fungal infection of the larynx associated with use of MDIs has been reported in humans but not in horses.
- Treatment with inhaled corticosteroids without a negative culture of the TTW can increase the risk of exacerbating bacterial pneumonia.
- Corticosteroids (inhaled and parenteral) are contraindicated in cases of fungal pneumonia.

PROCEDURE

- Clean the horse's face.
- Place the mask or inhaler device, ensuring that no air leak is present.

- Let the horse breathe several times, release one puff, then allow the horse to breath for 20 to 30 seconds and then release another puff.
- For some devices it is very important to synchronize with the inspiration.
- Repeat this step until the proper dose is administered.
- After the last puff wait for a few seconds before removing the device.

POSTPROCEDURE

Clean the device and the horse's nose.

ALTERNATIVES AND THEIR RELATIVE MERITS

- Pneumatic and ultrasonic nebulizers can be used but are relatively expensive.
  - They allow the possibility to use different medications that are not available in MDI.

- Some devices (AeroMask and Era Mask) are easily attached to the nebulizer.
- Nebulizers require thorough cleaning after each use, which can be time-consuming.

SUGGESTED READING

Rush BR: *Aerosolized Drugs.* Proceedings North American Veterinary Conference 2006. Available at www.ivis.org.

Bayly WB: *Inhalation Therapy and Respiratory Disease.* Proceedings of the annual meeting of the Italian Association of Equine Veterinarians 2005. Available at www.ivis.org.

Rush BR: Treatment of inflammatory airway disease: aerosol delivery devices and medications. *Proc Am Assoc Equine Pract* 48:218–227, 2002.

AUTHOR: **NELSON I. PINTO**

Nasogastric Intubation

BASIC INFORMATION

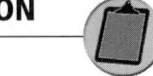

SYNONYM(S)

Tube
Gastric decompression
Reflux

OVERVIEW AND GOAL(S)

- To decompress the stomach to relieve pain and decrease risk of gastric rupture

- Instill fluids or medication into the stomach

INDICATIONS

- Colic
- Tachycardia of unknown origin
- Abdominal distension
- Administration of medication, fluids, or nutrition

CONTRAINDICATIONS

- Respiratory distress
- Decreased upper airway patency
- Pharyngeal obstruction

EQUIPMENT, ANESTHESIA

- Nasogastric tube of appropriate size for horse and a second smaller one available
- Pump

- Bucket with clean water and empty bucket
- Fluids, medication, or nutritional supplementation if desired
- Lidocaine (10–20 mL)
- Lube (optional)
- Twitch (optional)
- Sedation (optional)
- Towel
- Horse handler
- If tube is to be indwelling:
  ○ Tape
  ○ 6-mL syringe plunger with rubber stopper removed or glove finger with small hole in the end
  ○ Muzzle

ANTICIPATED TIME

10 minutes

PREPARATION: IMPORTANT CHECKPOINTS

- Sedation if appropriate (xylazine should provide adequate sedation for passing of the tube)
- A skilled horse handler should hold the horse with a twitch properly applied. Not all horses need to be twitched but it is helpful in most patients and creates a safer situation in most cases. One should not attempt to struggle with a horse that is throwing its head as this increases the danger of getting the tube in the wrong place (ethmoids, trachea).
- The buckets and pump should be at the ready with a helper to operate or hold the buckets.
- Alternatively the buckets can be placed on a shelf or cart or hung at nose level.

POSSIBLE COMPLICATIONS AND COMMON ERRORS TO BE AVOIDED

- Epistaxis from mucosal trauma or ethmoturbinate damage
- Pneumonia or death due to water or other liquids being inadvertently instilled into the lungs due to improper passing of the tube
- Pharyngeal or laryngeal trauma

PROCEDURE

- Stand on the same side of the horse as the nostril you wish to pass the tube in (ie, stand on the left to pass it through the left nostril).
- Mark the depth of the pharynx on the tube by placing the tube alongside the horse's head and approximating the length from the nostril to the pharynx on the tube.
- Place the tube once behind your neck, and place the pump end in your mouth.
- With your hand closest to the horse, gently grasp the nostril with your thumb and forefinger. Take care not

to occlude the opposite nostril with your other fingers.
- With your opposite hand, direct the rounded smooth end of the tube ventrally and medially in the nostril into the ventral meatus.
- Keep pressing the tube ventromedially with your thumb of the hand closest to the horse as you slowly advance the tube with the opposite hand.
- Once you have entered the pharynx, rotate the tube 90 degrees and have the horse handler flex the neck at the poll. This directs the tube more dorsally toward the opening of the esophagus rather than towards the trachea. However, this may cause the tube to become lodged in the dorsal pharyngeal recess causing pharyngeal trauma. One must be careful not to be excessively forceful when advancing the tube for this reason.
- Gently tap the dorsal portion of the arytenoids while blowing into the tube, until the horse swallows.
- When the horse swallows, pass the tube into the esophagus. This portion of the procedure requires patience and should not be rushed, due to the risk for pharyngeal or laryngeal trauma.
- TROUBLESHOOT: If one encounters difficulty getting the horse to swallow:
  ○ Try inserting a finger into the horse's mouth to stimulate swallowing.
  ○ After several attempts try passing from the other nostril.
  ○ The tube selected may simply be too large; try passing one size smaller tube.
  ○ One may also try pumping a very small amount of water in the tube to stimulate swallowing. CAUTION: Use a very small amount of water and withdraw the tube slightly prior to pumping in the water to decrease the likelihood of water entering the trachea.
- Once in the esophagus, insert the tube several more inches. There should be some drag, but not moderate or severe resistance. At this point suck back on the tube; if you are in the esophagus, you should feel negative pressure as the mucosa occludes the end of the tube. If you are in the trachea, you will be able to readily suck air back, because the ridged structure of the trachea dose not occlude the tube.
- Ensure you are in the esophagus, not the trachea.
  ○ Negative pressure when one sucks back on the tube suggest that you are in the esophagus.
  ○ One should be able to palpate both the trachea and the nasogastric tube within the esophagus (the two-tube effect) rather than just the trachea if the tube were within the trachea.

CAUTION: In very athletic horses, the thick strap muscles may feel like a tube in the esophagus. Do not rely on this method in these horses.
  ○ One should be able to palpate or see the tube passing through the esophagus as it enters the pelvic inlet on the left side.
  ○ Grasp the trachea and shake it back and forth: If the tube is in the trachea you may appreciate a rattling sound/feeling.
  ○ Give a short, sharp blow into the tube: If it is situated in the esophagus you should see the bolus of air distend the esophagus on the left side of the neck.
- If the tube is inadvertently passed into the trachea, withdraw the tube several centimeters back into the nasopharynx and try to repass it as described above.
- Once the tube is in the esophagus, slowly advance it while blowing into the tube to inflate the esophagus.
- Once you have entered the stomach, you should be able to smell gastric content. If air is blown into the tube one should hear gurgling as gas exits the tube.
- TROUBLESHOOT: If one encounters resistance prior to entering the stomach:
  ○ The tube may be stuck at the cardia. The cardia can be very tight in cases where the stomach is distended. Do not assume just because you cannot get in the stomach there is no reflux.
  ○ If repeated attempts to enter the stomach fail, 10 to 20 mL of 2% lidocaine can be put in the tube and blown down to the cardia. Allow this to sit for a minute or two and try to advance the tube again.
  ○ Alternatively pump a small amount of water into the tube in attempt to stimulate the cardia to open.
  ○ The tube may also turn back on itself at the cardia and curl up in the esophagus. The tube will usually kink when this happens and air will no longer flow through it. If this happens, withdraw the tube partially and try to advance it again.
  ○ The tube may also fold double in the pharynx. This will feel like the tube springs or pushes back slightly when pressure on the tube is released and the horse will most often respond poorly when pressure is applied. If this happens, withdraw the tube several centimeters, rotate the tube 90 degrees, and try again.
- If the stomach is severely distended with fluid, it will spontaneously reflux from the tube. If this happens hold the end of the tube low in the reflux collection bucket and allow the reflux to flow out.

- If fluid does not spontaneously flow from the tube, one should check for reflux by creating a siphon. This should be done even if the only goal is to distill fluid or medication into the stomach.
- Water should always be the first thing you pass down the tube. CAUTION: If the horse coughs when water is pumped into the tube, check the placement of the tube as it may in fact be in the lungs.
- Pump water into the tube to create a siphon. Then disconnect the pump and immediately occlude the end of the tube with thumb.
- Hold end of tube low in the reflux collection bucket and remove thumb. Allow fluid to flow from tube into bucket.
- TROUBLESHOOT: If reflux stops flowing:
  - If the reflux stops flowing abruptly then starts again for a moment then stops abruptly over and over again, it is likely that stomach mucosa is becoming drawn in the end of the tube. Pull the tube a short distance out of the nose to move it away form the mucosa.
  - If air starts to move up the tube or the reflux slows down, pull the tube several inches out of the nose in a steady motion to reestablish the siphon.
  - The siphon can also be reestablished in either situation by small abrupt tugs on the end of the tube out of the nose. This may work, but it will likely cause more mucosal irritation and more resentment from

the horse especially in horses that have indwelling tubes for a significant period of time.
  - Refrain from sucking reflux from the tube. Reflux can contain *Salmonella* or *Clostridium* spp. both of which cause significant disease in humans.
  - This process can be repeated several times until no net reflux is obtained. The net refluxed fluid is the amount of water pumped in subtracted from the amount of reflux received.
- If you wish to instill medication or fluid:
  - Check for reflux as described above.
  - If there is any question that you are in the correct location, obtain gastric content via reflux prior to pumping anything but water down the tube.
  - If no reflux is obtained, pump desired fluid into the stomach followed by several pumps of water.
- If you wish to remove the tube, blow the tube clear, and while blowing kink the tube. Then smoothly pull the tube forward and down out of the nose.
- TROUBLESHOOT:
  - An excessive amount of blowing is not necessary; this will only distend the stomach with air. One only needs to blow until they feel the tube clear indicated by decreased resistance to air flow.
  - Kinking of the tube is very important to prevent fluid from entering the trachea.
  - Have the handler steady the head while pulling the tube. If the horse moves its head violently during extubation, the end of the tube may

flip up and hit the ethmoids causing epistaxis.
  - It may be best to hold the hand closest to the horse on the nose to steady the tube and pull down and out on the tube with the opposite hand.
- If you wish to leave the tube in situ for ease of frequent refluxing:
  - Position the tube such that it will not need to be inserted further to reflux the horse in future sessions.
  - Affix the tube to the noseband and D rings of the halter with tape. Thread the remaining portion of the tube through the side of the halter in a comfortable position.
  - Place the plunger of a 6-mL syringe, with the stopper removed, in the end of the tube to stop air from building up in the stomach. Alternatively tape a glove finger over the end of the tube with a hole in the end. The glove finger acts as a one-way valve, allowing gas and fluid to flow out but not in.
  - Place a muzzle on the horse so it is not able to remove the tube by rubbing it.
- If horses are to be left with a tube in, they should be kept NPO. The presence of an indwelling tube may cause pharyngeal dysfunction and lead to aspiration.

POSTPROCEDURE
- Monitor closely if tube is left in place.
- Monitor closely for colic signs if fluid or medication was instilled in the stomach.

AUTHOR: **CHRISTINE L. WIMER**

Neurologic Examination: Evaluation of Cranial Nerve Function

OVERVIEW AND GOAL(S)
Evaluation of cranial nerve (CN) function can provide information on:
- Sight
- Hearing
- Swallow reflex
- Breathing
- Facial symmetry and expression
- Sensation
- Jaw tone
- Larynx and pharynx

Evaluation of the CNs and cervicofacial reflexes:
- Head and neck posture are influenced by the cerebellar and vestibular systems.
- Horses with cerebellar disease often show fine resting tremors of the head

that become exaggerated by intentional movements.
- The level of consciousness can be evaluated as alert, depressed, stuporous, semicomatose, or comatose.
- The response of an animal to its environment is controlled by the cerebrum and brainstem. The normal horse should appear alert and responsive to external stimuli.
- Lesions of the cerebral hemispheres can result in comatose or semicomatose animals, whereas severe systemic illnesses can produce depression.
- Horses with cerebral disease may demonstrate inappropriate behavior, head pressing, or compulsive walking and circling.

- Recumbent horses with spinal cord disease often appear bright and alert, at least during the early stages of the problem.
- Horses with vestibular disease often have a head tilt in which the poll is deviated toward the side of the lesion. There will be weakness on this side as well, with increased tone on the opposite side that often results in circling toward the side of the lesion.
- CN examination can help localize a problem in horses with neurologic disease along the brainstem.

CN I: THE OLFACTORY NERVE
- Deficits of the olfactory nerve are rarely observed in the horse.

CN II: THE OPTIC NERVE

- Courses from the eye to the optic chiasm, where a significant number of the fibers cross over to the contralateral side (about 80%).
- From the optic chiasm, the fibers travel to the pretectal nucleus in the midbrain and from there to the Edinger-Westphal nucleus in the brainstem, which provides input to the oculomotor nerve (CN III) and ciliary ganglia.
- Evaluation of visual perception:
  - Requires input from the retina along the optic nerve to the optic chiasm, where it crosses over and continues along the optic tract to the lateral geniculate nucleus in the midbrain.
  - From this point, information follows the optic radiation along the brainstem to the occipital cortex. The fibers seem to course from the brainstem through tracts in the cerebellum to the occipital cortex of the brain.
  - Horses with cerebellar abiotrophy fail to blink to bright light and do not have a menace response.
  - The menace response can be used to evaluate visual perception by making a menacing gesture toward the eye and observing for a blink as well as the horse moving the head away from the examiner. It is important to avoid touching the eye or generating excessive air currents while performing this test. The blink response relies on both cranial nerves II and VII for a normal response.
  - Evaluation of vision can also be done by placing the horse in a maze or strange environment and observing its activity.
  - Other helpful tests to evaluate vision:
    - Examination of pupil size and position
    - Evaluation of the pupillary light response (PLR)

CN III: THE OCULOMOTOR NERVE

- The PLR provides information about cranial nerves II and III.
  - The pupil is under the control of CN III.
  - Parasympathetic fibers in this nerve are responsible for pupil *constriction*; pupillary *dilation* is under the influence of the sympathetic nervous system.
  - Examine the pupils for size and symmetry.
  - If unequal in size (anisocoria), determine which one is abnormal.
    - If one pupil fails to dilate when the animal is placed in dark light, it is an indication of damage to the sympathetic system.
    - If one pupil fails to constrict when the animal is placed in bright light, it is an indication of damage to the oculomotor nerve.
  - Use a bright light to evaluate PLR.
  - Dazzle response: A normal animal will blink when a bright light is initially shined into a normal eye.
  - Direct PLR: Constriction of the ipsilateral eye when bright light is directed into the eye.
    - In the direct PLR, light is directed into one eye and travels along the optic nerve to the optic chiasm, where crossing occurs. From here, the impulse follows the optic tract to the pretectal nucleus in the midbrain and then to the oculomotor nucleus. The signal is sent along the oculomotor nerve to the ciliary ganglion and pupil, where constriction then occurs. The indirect PLR is a result of crossing of the fibers between the eye to the optic cortex. In most large animal species, approximately 90% of the fibers cross over. Thus lesions of the eye or optic nerve often result in an abnormal PLR, whereas lesions along the optic tract present as blindness in both eyes.
  - Consensual PLR: Constriction of the contralateral pupil is also observed in normal horses.
  - Swinging light test: Used when observing the consensual response is difficult.

CNS II, IV, AND VI: VESTIBULAR NERVES

- A normal response provides information about the extraocular muscles as well as the connections along the medial longitudinal fasciculus in the brainstem.
- Clinical features that result from damage to the oculomotor (III), trochlear (IV), or abducens (VI) nerves:
  - Strabismus, an abnormal positioning of the eye within the orbit
  - Enophthalmos

CN V: TRIGEMINAL NERVE

- Contains both motor and sensory fibers.
- Clinical features associated with damage or abnormalities of this nerve include:
  - Decreased sensation to the skin and mucous membranes of the head
    - Sensory function can be evaluated by palpation of the ears, eyelids, and local response along the face as well as inside the nares. Most normal horses respond with a flick of the ear, blink, or dilation of the nostril along with a cerebral response.
  - Atrophy of the masseter muscle
  - Loss of innervation to the masseter muscles will cause a dropping of the jaw and drooling of saliva.

CN VII (FACIAL NERVE) AND CN VIII (VESTIBULOCOCHLEAR NERVE)

- Damage to CNs VII and VIII are two of the most commonly recognized abnormalities of the CNs seen in horses.
- CN VII contains branches to the ears, the eyelids, and the muzzle.
  - Unilateral damage to CN VII will result in deviation of the muzzle to the unaffected side as well as an inability to blink the eyelid and deviation of the ear.
  - CN VII contains parasympathetic fibers that control part of the tear production; injury to this nerve results in the inability to blink along with a loss of normal tear production in the affected eye.
- Cranial nerve VIII controls hearing and balance.
  - Unilateral damage to CN VIII will present with a head tilt toward the affected side along with atypical positioning of the limbs and nystagmus, with the fast phase directed away from the side of the lesion.
- Central damage to the vestibular nucleus will cause the nystagmus to be irregular and depend on the positioning of the head. With central vestibular disease, the horses will often have gait deficits of ipsilateral weakness and contralateral hyperextension.

CN IX (GLOSSOPHARYNGEAL NERVE), CN X (VAGUS NERVE), AND CN XI (SPINAL ACCESSORY NERVE)

- Laryngeal and pharyngeal paralysis can be due to lesions located in CNs IX to XI, which originate in the medulla.
- These nerves contain both motor and sensory fibers for the pharynx, larynx, and esophagus.
- Horses with laryngeal paralysis will present with upper respiratory noise.
- Horses with pharyngeal paralysis will present with difficulty swallowing food and water.

CN XII: HYPOGLOSSAL NERVE

- Damage to CN XII results in loss of motor function to the tongue.
- Horner syndrome: May present with a raised temperature of the face, asymmetric facial sweating, congestion of the nasal and conjunctival membranes, a prolapsing third eyelid, and irregularly responding pupils.

SUGGESTED READING

Reed SM, Andrews FM: Disorders of the neurologic system. In Reed SM, Bayly WM, Sellon DC, *Equine internal medicine*, ed 3, St Louis, 2010, Saunders, pp 545–681.

AUTHOR: **STEPHEN M. REED**

Neurologic Examination: General and Peripheral

BASIC INFORMATION

Disorders of the nervous system are serious and sometimes debilitating problems affecting horses. Many diseases, disorders, and toxins can affect the nervous system of the horse. The goal of the neurologic examination is to identify the neuroanatomic location of the lesion(s).

OVERVIEW AND GOAL

Ancillary diagnostic aids:
- Radiography
- Ultrasonography
- Electroencephalography
- Electromyography
- Myelography
- Computed tomography
- Magnetic resonance imaging
- Evaluation of cerebrospinal fluid
- Specialized techniques
  - Auditory, somatosensory, or visual evoked response testing
  - Nerve conduction velocity measurement

Many gait deficits caused by neurologic diseases are difficult to distinguish from a musculoskeletal problem; therefore, a lameness examination should be a part of the neurologic assessment.

INDICATIONS

Signalment and history:
- Obtain whenever possible.
- An accurate history can sometimes help narrow the list of differential diagnoses, especially when trauma, certain infectious diseases, or exposure to a specific toxin has occurred.
- The signalment may aid the examiner because certain diseases or developmental problems typically affect certain breeds, genders, or ages.

An incorrect diagnosis may delay the initiation of appropriate therapy and lead to a worse prognosis or result in the potential use of an expensive but unnecessary medication.

PROCEDURE

- Generally divided into five parts:
  - Head and neck
  - Trunk
  - Tail and anus (perineum)
  - Gait
  - Posture
- Begin with observation of the horse
  - Behavior
  - Mental awareness
  - Head posture
  - Coordination
  - Limb position

- Symmetry of the muscles of the head, neck, and body
- Lesion localization in the head (see "Neurologic Examination: Evaluation of Cranial Nerve Function" in this section)
- Lesion localization beyond the head
  - Several reflexes may be helpful to localize a lesion, including the local cervical and cervicofacial responses
    - Pressure applied with a sharp object along the side of the neck down to the approximate level of the third cervical vertebrae will normally result in a response in which a smile is initiated in the corner of the mouth on the affected side.
    - Caudal to the third cervical vertebrae there is a local response of the skin and muscles along the side of the neck.
    - Abnormalities of these reflexes have been noted in horses with cervical spinal cord disease.
  - Cutaneous trunci reflex
    - Pressure applied to the skin on the side of the body locally sends an afferent impulse to the spinal cord where it ascends in tracts to the brainstem and the efferent or motor response (contracture of the cutaneous trunci muscles) occurs along the entire side of the body.
- Evaluation of the tail and anus
  - Stimulation of the anus should cause the anal sphincter to contract and the tail to clamp down. Damage to the sacrococcygeal spinal cord segments can result in loss of the normal response of tail and anal tone as well as loss of sensation in the region of the perineum.
  - Evaluation of gait: Both lameness and neurologic examinations
    - Differentiating between a mild thoracic or pelvic limb lameness and subtle ataxia is often difficult.
    - Gait deficits identified on the neurologic examination are scored to describe severity. The scale, previously described by Mayhew, ranges from Grade 0 to 4:
      - Grade 0 = Normal
      - 1 = Very subtle gait deficits that become slightly more obvious when the head is elevated
      - 2 = Moderate abnormalities that are readily noted at a walk even by the most casual observers

- 3 = Easily recognizable and become noticeably more severe when the animal is negotiating obstacles, walked on a slope, or walked with its head elevated
- 4 = Falls or nearly falls at normal gaits and activities
- 5 = Recumbent
- Clinical signs used to describe neurologic gait deficits:
  - Ataxia: A proprioceptive abnormality expressed in the horse as truncal sway, weaving, pivoting on an inside limb while turning, outward deviation of a pelvic limb while circling, or pacing when walking.
  - Paresis: Arises from a lack of muscular power while walking.
  - Weakness: Horses often knuckle, stumble, drag their limbs, drop their trunk when bearing weight and have a lower arc of flight in one or more limbs while walking. Can be a result of damage to the upper motor neuron or lower motor neuron or primary muscle disease.
    - Damage to the upper motor neuron or its axons in the cerebral cortex, subcortical white matter, brainstem, or spinal cord can result in weakness or paresis. Weakness as a result of damage to the lower motor neurons is often accompanied by muscle atrophy and in some cases sensory deficits.
  - Dysmetria: A gait deficit in which the limb is either hypometric or hypermetric
    - A hypometric limb often has a low arc of flight, and the limb may appear stiff or spastic.
    - A hypermetric gait often appears to have exaggerated joint flexion and movements.
  - Spasticity: A stiff, short stride and a lack of joint flexion; likely a result of damage to the upper motor neurons with a sudden release after achieving a maximum tension
- Gait evaluation
  - Observe the horse at a walk and trot.
  - Evaluate subtle deficits with additional obstacles and tests such as walking the horse up and down an incline or over a curb, walking the horse with its head elevated, and backing and circling may be necessary.
  - Gait deficits can be most readily detected when circling if the circle

is started in slow, wide (about 15 feet diameter) position with the horse moving forward and gradually tightening the circle until the horse is pivoting around the handler.

- Tests to evaluate strength and stability
  - Sway test: Performed with the animal at rest. A normal horse will respond to pressure applied to the shoulder or pelvic region by pushing back against the pressure and maintain its balance; as the pressure persists the horse will eventually step away with its opposite limb.
  - Tail pull: Performed while the animal is in motion. The examiner

should walk alongside the horse and pull its tail at various times during the horse's stride to evaluate both strength as well as the horse's ability to catch itself and prevent falling.

POSTPROCEDURE

After conclusion of the neurologic examination and grading of the gait deficits, the examiner needs to determine whether a lesion is present and, if so, where the lesion is located.

- If the horse exhibits no signs of brain, brainstem, or cranial nerve abnormalities the lesion must be caudal to the foramen magnum.

- If the horse exhibits signs of proprioceptive and gait abnormalities in all four limbs, the lesion is most likely located within the cervical spinal cord.
- Gait deficits involving only the pelvic limbs indicate the lesion is caudal to the second thoracic vertebra.
- Weakness or focal muscle atrophy along with areas of sensory loss indicates either focal peripheral nerve damage, generalized lower motor neuron disease, or polyneuritis equi.

SUGGESTED READING

Reed SM, Andrews FM: Disorders of the neurologic system. In Reed SM, Bayly WM, Sellon DC, *Equine internal medicine*, ed 3, St Louis, 2010, Saunders, pp 545–681.

AUTHOR: **STEPHEN M. REED**

Nuclear Scintigraphy

BASIC INFORMATION

OVERVIEW AND GOAL(S)

- Medical nuclear medicine is the science of using radioactive substances (termed *radionuclides* or *radioactive isotopes*) to evaluate specific metabolism and physiology. As a radionuclide decomposes (to a more stable state) it releases energy in the form of radioactivity, termed *radioactive decay*. This emitted energy can be captured and quantified in assessment of various disease processes.
- The most commonly performed nuclear medicine study in equine practice is a bone scan. Bone scans are useful for identifying occult or nonlocalizable causes of lameness referable to the musculoskeletal system.
- Bone scans are performed by injecting bone-seeking radiopharmaceuticals that allow detection of abnormal bone metabolism and/or altered blood flow. The most commonly used radiopharmaceutical is technetium-99m (^{99m}Tc, commonly referred to as "tech"). During the decay process, 140keV gamma rays are emitted, easily detected for diagnostic imaging purposes using a gamma camera. Gamma rays are identical to x-rays, differing only in origin (nuclear vs. x-ray machine, respectively).
- *Radiopharmaceuticals* are drugs (compounds or materials) labeled ("tagged" or linked) to a radionuclide. In many cases, radiopharmaceuticals function much like materials found in the body and do not produce special pharmacologic effects.

- For bone scans, ^{99m}Tc is labeled to an inorganic phosphate that is essential for bone metabolism. The most commonly used radiopharmaceutical for bone scans is ^{99m}Tc methylene diphosphonate (^{99m}Tc-MDP); ^{99m}Tc hydroxymethylene diphosphonate (^{99m}Tc-HMDP) is less commonly used.
- There are three phases of a musculoskeletal nuclear medicine scan, classified by the temporal sequence of the scan: vascular, soft tissue, and bone phases.
  - In the vascular phase, the region of interest is scanned immediately after injection of the radiopharmaceutical. As the name implies, this phase assesses arterial and venous blood flow. It lasts 1 to 2 minutes and is rapidly replaced by the soft tissue phase. The vascular phase is not commonly performed.
  - The soft tissue phase represents distribution of the radiopharmaceutical throughout the tissues of the body before incorporation into the bone matrix. This phase is performed minutes after injection and is useful for conditions such a myositis or abscesses.
  - The bone phase is performed 2 to 4 hours after injection, allowing time for the radiopharmaceutical to be incorporated into the inorganic bone matrix.
    - Incorporation of radiopharmaceutical occurs in all areas of living bone, but more so in bone that is actively remodeling. As the radiopharmaceutical decays, more gamma ray emission is detected in areas of increased

bone turnover, thereby allowing localization of active remodeling. This is termed a *hot spot* (Figure 1). Occasionally pathologic decreased or absent bone metabolism is present, termed a *cold spot* (eg, a bone infarction).

- Nuclear imaging studies can yield valuable information regarding the site of abnormal blood flow and altered physiology, but the images have relatively poor anatomic detail.
- Rarely can a *specific* diagnosis be made based on abnormal radiopharmaceutical uptake identified on a bone scan; however, these studies can direct the clinician to one or a few limited anatomic regions for further imaging and clinical evaluation.

EQUIPMENT, ANESTHESIA

Positioning:

- The patient should be standing squarely for the examination.
- Sedation is necessary to avoid motion artifact.
- The distance between the patient and the gamma camera surface is important and should be minimized at all times.
  - Increased patient distance from the gamma camera leads to a decrease in detectable radiopharmaceutical uptake, degrading image quality.
  - When imaging bilateral structures simultaneously (Figure 2; also see Figure 1, *A*) it is important that the structures are equidistant from the gamma camera to avoid differences in apparent radiopharmaceutical uptake.

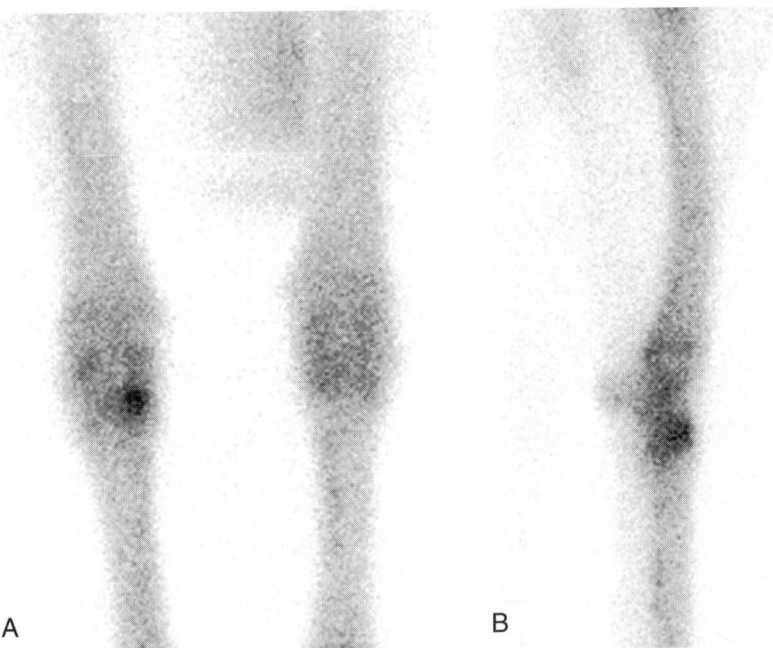

A   B

FIGURE 1 Increased radiopharmaceutical uptake in the right third carpal bone (hot spot). **A,** Dorsal image of the right and left carpi. The right carpus (on the *left*) shows a highly focal area of increased radiopharmaceutical uptake in the medial aspect of the distal row of carpal bones. Note that both radii, carpi, and metacarpi are similar in size and detail, indicating proper, equidistant placement of the limbs to the gamma camera. **B,** Lateral image centered at the right carpus shows the abnormal increased activity of the dorsal portion of the distal row of carpal bones. The left limb cannot be seen (it is shielded from the gamma camera). The final diagnosis was a slab fracture of the third carpal bone.

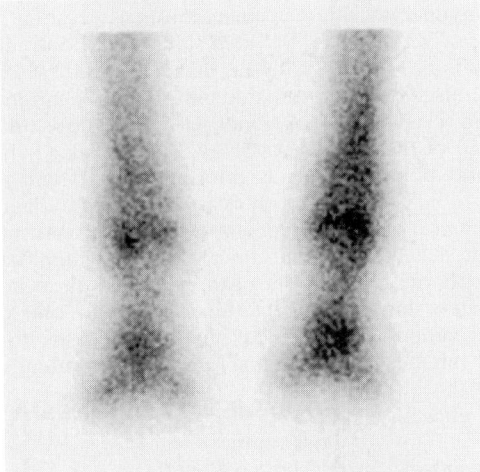

FIGURE 2 Artifactual asymmetry of radiopharmaceutical uptake in forelimb distal extremities caused by nonequidistant limb positioning to the gamma camera. The forelimb on the right is closer to the gamma camera than the forelimb on the left. Therefore the limb on the right appears to have more uptake than the contralateral limb and could be falsely interpreted as diseased.

- A lead shield should be used to block gamma radiation from reaching the gamma camera from nonimaged contralateral limbs. For example, a lead blocker should be used along the medial aspect of the left front leg when obtaining a lateral image of the right front leg (see Figure 1, *B*).

Equipment:
- A gamma camera is used to detect the gamma radiation produced from radionuclide decay. Several different cameras and detector assemblies are available.
- Lead blockers are necessary to block gamma emissions from adjacent structures that could reduce image quality. They come in various sizes and shapes, including semicylinders and flat panels. These can be purchased commercially or constructed using PVC pipe or plastic paneling lined with lead shielding material.

- The technician or handler should wear a laboratory coat, disposable booties, and gloves to avoid contact with the radiopharmaceutical.
- A bucket should be available to catch urine and avoid contaminating the floor and distal extremities.
- For distal extremity imaging, the gamma camera must be placed distal to the solar margin of the foot. This can be accomplished by elevating the patient with wooden blocks or ramps. Alternatively, a pit can be constructed to allow the camera to be positioned below the level of the floor.
- A radiation detection device is necessary to assess radiation levels.

Safety:
- Nuclear medicine and radiation safety practices are tightly regulated by state and federal regulations. Veterinarians interested in using nuclear scintigraphy in their practice are required to undergo proper training and certification by their state.
- The majority of the ^{99m}Tc-MDP is excreted by the kidneys. Radioactive urine is the primary source of potential radioactive contamination in personnel and can create image artifacts by soiling the patient.
- All animals that have been injected with radioactive materials must be confined in an area properly identified as a "radioactive" area, with limited human contact. The stall should not be cleaned until contaminated bedding

reaches background levels of radiation. This usually occurs within 10 half-lives of the radiopharmaceutical being used (for ^{99m}Tc, approximately 60 hours).

PREPARATION: IMPORTANT CHECKPOINTS

- The horse should be in some level of work prior to a scintigraphy study to ensure that any areas of inflammation or increased metabolism are active.
- A jugular catheter should be placed before administration of the radionuclide.
- Temperature plays a large role in the vascular distribution of radiopharmaceutical to the tissues. This can be facilitated by leg wraps, housing in a heated stall, or brisk exercise before the injection.
- Removable wraps can be placed on the feet before scanning. If the patient urinates before the scan, the wraps help protect the feet from urine contamination and potential misdiagnoses. The wraps are removed immediately before scanning.
- Patient weight should be obtained for accurate dosage of the radiopharmaceutical.

PROCEDURE

Techniques:
- Suggested technetium dose: 7 to 11 MBq/ kg (0.2–0.3 mCi/kg) by intravenous injection. In practice, injected doses are not very specific. Typical doses are roughly 125 to 200 mCi per horse.
  - The curie (Ci) is the unit commonly used in the United States to measure radiation. One curie is equivalent to 3.7×10^{-10} disintegrations per second.
  - Becquerels (Bq) are the SI unit (international system) of radioactivity. One becquerel is equivalent to one disintegration per second (dps).
  - The conversion factor is 37MBq = 1 mCi.
- Radiopharmaceuticals should be ordered from a commercial radiopharmacy.

- Doses are injected intravenously as a single bolus via a jugular catheter.
- Timing of the studies after injection:
  - Vascular studies are obtained in the first **30 seconds** after injection.
  - Soft tissue studies should be performed within the first **5 minutes** after injection.
  - Sufficient bone uptake of radiopharmaceutical (bone phase) is generally achieved **2 to 4 hours** after injection.

Standard views:
- The images acquired should be governed by the clinical presentation of the patient.
- Routine views (bone phase):
  - Forelimb: Lateral and cranial/dorsal views of the radius, carpus, fetlock, and distal limb
  - Hindlimb: Lateral and caudal/plantar views of the stifle, tarsus, fetlock, and distal limb
  - Pelvis: Dorsal and dorsal oblique projections of the pelvis
  - Spine: Dorsal and lateral projections of the spine

Additional views:
- In racehorses, specific long bone projections are warranted (eg, humerus, tibia, scapula).
- With a foot lameness, soft tissue phase images of the feet can be obtained as well as bone phase images of the solar margin of the distal phalanx (solar views made with the foot on the gamma camera).

POSTPROCEDURE

- Nuclear medicine images can be viewed in a variety of displays. Black dots on white background are preferred by many. However, white dots on black background and many different color maps are available (Figure 3).
- Normal patterns of radiopharmaceutical uptake differ based on exercise regimen and age of the patient. These patterns are variable and beyond the scope of this text.
- Symmetry is evaluated with lateral and dorsal/plantar projections and between contralateral limbs.

- Asymmetry in radiopharmaceutical uptake and artifactual differences in uptake can be caused by:
  - Poor positioning (see Figure 2)
  - True asymmetry in bone uptake
    - Any lesion that causes increased bone turnover will cause increased uptake, such as sclerosis, fracture, osteomyelitis, osteophytosis (see Figure 1).
  - Asymmetric vascular distribution (eg, cold extremities)
  - Persistent soft tissue uptake (eg, rhabdomyolysis)
  - Asymmetry of overlying soft tissues leading to differences in gamma radiation attenuation (eg, muscle atrophy)
  - Radioactive contamination (eg, urine)
- Artifacts:
  - Motion:
    - Newer software packages can be used to correct for motion artifact (Figure 4).
  - Radioactive urine (within the urinary bladder and external contamination)
  - Edge packing:
    - A misrepresentation of the edge of the gamma camera based on the counts from the photomultiplier tube, which creates a higher count in the periphery of the field. Modern gamma cameras correct for this artifact.
    - To correct for this artifact, anatomic areas of high radiopharmaceutical uptake on the edge of the field of view should be repositioned in the center of the field.

SUGGESTED READING

Daniel GB, Berry CR, editors: *Textbook of veterinary nuclear medicine*, ed 2, Harrisburg, PA, 2006, American College of Veterinary Radiology.

Ross MW, Stacy VS: Nuclear medicine. In Ross MW, Dyson SJ, editors: *Diagnosis and management of lameness in horses*, St Louis, 2003, Saunders Elsevier.

Dyson SJ, Martinelli MJ, Pilsworth R, et al: *Equine scintigraphy* Newmarket, UK, 2003, Equine Veterinary Journal Ltd.

AUTHORS: **JOHN S. MATTOON, JASON W. BRUMITT, JONATHAN HAYLES, DANA A. NEELIS, GREGORY D. ROBERTS,** and **TOM WILKINSON**

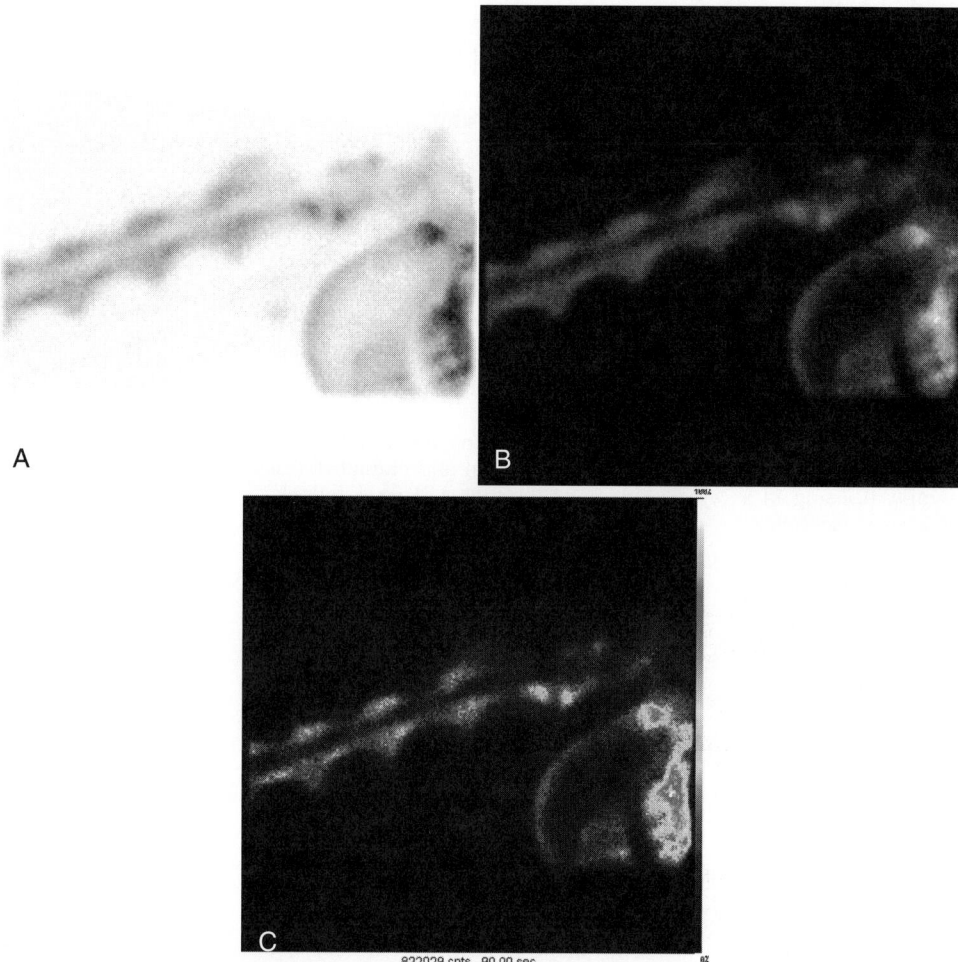

FIGURE 3 Various image displays of the right side of a cervical spine and portion of the skull. **A,** Black on white. The more dark dots present, the more radioactivity. **B,** White on black. The more white dots present, the more radioactivity. **C,** Color display. This color map displays the highest radioactivity levels as white, with decreasing levels seen as shades of red, orange, yellow, green, blue, and purple. The color scale bar can be seen along the right vertical margin of the image.

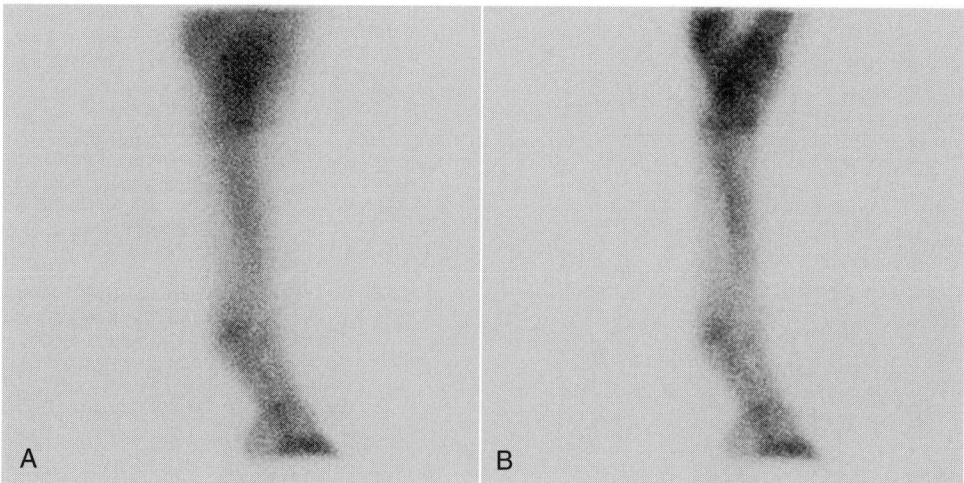

FIGURE 4 Degradation of image quality due to patient motion and motion correction. **A,** Right lateral image of the hindlimb. Patient motion (swaying) causes the image to be slightly blurry. **B,** Same image as in **A** but with motion correction software applied, yielding a much sharper image.

Nutrition: Amino Acids

BASIC INFORMATION

INDICATIONS

PROTEIN

- Essential for the development and maintenance of tissues in the body
- Required for the synthesis of enzymes, hormones, and antibodies
- Made of amino acids; therefore the ultimate need is for amino acids, not protein

AMINO ACIDS

- There are approximately 20 amino acids categorized as either essential or nonessential.
- Essential amino acids: Considered to be of greater concern when formulating diets because they cannot be manufactured in the horse's body at an adequate rate or amount to satisfy the horse's needs.
- There are 10 essential amino acids: Arginine, histidine, methionine, isoleucine, leucine, lysine, phenylalanine, threonine, tryptophan, and valine.
- Lysine is the first limiting amino acid (most likely amino acid to be in short supply compared to demand).
- Threonine is speculated to be the second limiting amino acid.
- Recent interest in developing "ideal" amino acid profile for the horse.

PROTEIN DIGESTIBILITY

- Protein digested in the foregut via enzymes yields amino acids for absorption into the bloodstream.
- Protein fermented in the hindgut yields ammonia.
- Therefore the goal is to have the majority of protein digested in the foregut in order for the horse to enhance the amino acid pool for use in the body.
- Concentrates tend to have higher foregut digestibility compared to forages and would therefore be a better source of amino acids. It is possible to provide a horse with a high protein diet from a forage like alfalfa yet not provide enough lysine or other amino acids due to the amino acid profile of the protein source and the digestibility of the protein source. Consideration should also be made for horses with a lowered ability to digest feeds such as aged horses.
- Digestibility of the protein source will affect the supply of amino acids in the body.
- Concentrates tend to provide higher quantities of amino acids and are generally more digestible especially in the foregut.

- At least 60% of the total protein in the diet should be provided by the concentrate portion of the diet for growing horses and lactating mares.
- Older horses may require additional dietary protein and amino acids due to decreased digestibility with age.

LYSINE

- The first limiting amino acid for growing horses
- Increasing the lysine content of the diet has resulted in an improvement in average daily gain (ADG) for growing horses of all ages (foals, weanlings, yearlings).
- Diet content of lysine for the lactating mare becomes of utmost importance not only to ensure an adequate supply in milk for the foal but help the mare maintain her own body tissues without resorting to using reserves in muscle mass to support milk production.
- In exercising horses, supplemental lysine has resulted in improved muscle mass compared to those that did not receive supplementation.
- Management guidelines:
  - Be sure to provide adequate lysine, especially for growing horses and lactating mares.
  - Use only high-quality sources of protein to ensure a good amino acid profile to the protein source (milk-based protein for young; soybean meal for all functions)
  - Synthetic forms of lysine are available to improve the quality of the protein in the diet should the source of protein be of poor quality.

THREONINE

- The second limiting amino acid for horses based on improved average daily gain observed in yearling horses
- Improvement in muscle mass for exercising horses was also observed for horses receiving both supplemental lysine and threonine.
- Management guidelines:
  - Be sure to provide a good quality source of protein to ensure a good amino acid profile to the protein source (milk-based protein for young; soybean meal for all functions).
  - Synthetic forms of threonine are available to improve the quality of the protein in the diet should the source of protein be poor quality.

OTHER AMINO ACIDS

- The branch chain amino acids (BCAAs; leucine, isoleucine, and valine)
  - BCAAs are unique in that they are metabolized by muscle to yield energy.

- Particularly important for the exercising horse. However, research into the potential benefits of BCAA supplementation is inconclusive and limited.
- BCAAs are utilized in muscle during exercise for energy; however, supplementation has not been proven to be beneficial.
- Caution should be taken when evaluating the need for BCAA supplements for the exercising horse.

PROTEIN DEFICIENCY

- Will result in a lack of adequate supply of amino acids
- Initial symptoms include a decreased appetite and poor coat.
- Without adequate amino acids (particularly the limiting amino acids), a decrease in production will result. Examples of this would include slower or retarded growth in growing horses, decreased milk production in lactating mares, and potentially smaller foals or fetal loss in pregnant mares (although this has not been specifically studied).
- Management guidelines:
  - Be sure to provide minimum amounts of crude protein to prevent deficiency symptoms.
  - Utilize highly digestible feeds and higher protein concentrations in the diets of growing horses and lactating mares.

PROTEIN EXCESS

- Protein provided in excess of needs is processed by the liver resulting in urea production and excretion. Therefore increased urea excretion (measured in blood or urine) can be an indicator of excessive consumption of protein.
- Excess urea excretion results in management issues such as dirty stabling conditions (wet bedding), respiratory issues (ammonia fumes), and even changes in water consumption to compensate for increased urination.
- Excretion of urea (ultimately nitrogen) also contributes to contamination of the environment.
- Kidney damage following excessive protein consumption has not been documented in the horse.
- Management guidelines:
  - Minimize excessive consumption of protein to reduce urea excretion (good for stall cleanliness and the environment).
  - More protein in the diet is not necessarily better for the horse.
  - Kidney damage has not been documented in horses due to excess protein intake.

IDEAL PROTEIN

- The concept was developed in swine and poultry.
- Based on the premise that the dietary supply of amino acids should closely mimic the end product produced by the body with the amino acids, which is mainly muscle mass
- Nitrogen balance studies along with total muscle amino acid profiles have been used to develop ideal protein for swine and poultry in various states of production.
- Ideal protein has not been developed yet in horses.
- Improvement in the amino acid profile of the diet:
  - Improves production but will decrease waste and nitrogen excretion, which is an environmental concern
  - Results in improved production (ADG primarily) and a decrease in blood urea nitrogen levels
  - Different sources of protein have different amino acid supplies and would therefore have different abilities to provide amino acids to the horse.

- Meta-analysis of nitrogen balance studies has found different amounts of crude protein on a body weight basis required to maintain nitrogen balance and this is presumably due to the difference in supply of amino acids.

MANAGEMENT GUIDELINES

- Be aware of protein source and amino acid profile.
- Formulate diet to match protein source amino acid profile with end-product amino acid profile.
- A protein source with a better amino acid profile will be required at a smaller quantity than one with a poor amino acid profile.

PROCEDURE

- Provide the horse with a high-quality source of protein to ensure a good supply of amino acids.
- Provide horses with a minimum amount of crude protein (CP) per day as outlined in the table. If a high-quality protein is used, these amounts should ensure an adequate supply of the limiting amino acids especially lysine.

Function	CP, g/kg BW/d (minimum)
Maintenance	1.3
Exercise	1.4–2.0*
Pregnant	1.6
Lactation	3.0
Growth	2.8–3.0†

*Depending on intensity (light to heavy).
†Depending on stage (weanling, yearling).

- Lysine concentrations in the diet should equate to 4.3% of the crude protein (CP) to utilize formulating a diet for crude protein and still meet amino acid needs for all functions but lactation.
- Lactating mares should receive lysine at a rate of 5.4% of the CP.
- There is not enough information at this time to make specific threonine recommendations.

SUGGESTED READING

National Research Council: Proteins and amino acids. In *Nutrient requirements for horses*, ed 6, Washington, DC, 2007, National Academy Press, pp 54–68.

AUTHOR: **PATTY GRAHAM-THIERS**

EDITOR: **DANIEL J. BURKE**

Nutrition: Breeding Farm, Management

BASIC INFORMATION

INDICATIONS

- Inadequate or excessive calorie intake
- Unbalanced diets
- Failure to group horses appropriately when individual feeding is not practiced
- Consumption of endophyte-infected tall fescue pasture or hay in late gestation (relative to mares experiencing long gestations and weak/dead foals)
- Appropriate nutritional management on the breeding farm is necessary for reproductive efficiency and for promoting normal skeletal development in growing horses. Common problems resulting from inappropriate nutritional management include reduced conception and live foal rates, increased services per conception, and developmental orthopedic disease.
- The most common presentation of inappropriate nutrition
  - Broodmares: Suboptimal body condition. See chapter on Body Condition Scores. Condition scores below 5 are associated with more services per conception, lower conception

rates, and a delay in the first normal ovulation in the spring. Foals that are born weak may indicate a nutritional or feed related problem. Selenium deficiency may result in weak foals. Consumption of endophyte-infected tall fescue by late-gestation mares may cause prolonged gestation, thickened placentas, dystocia, and weak/dead foals.
  - Stallions: Excess body condition. Stallions should be maintained in a body condition score of about 5. Body condition has not been shown to affect semen quality but could potentially affect the ability of the stallion to mount mares without difficulty or fatigue.
  - Growing horses: Poor growth, very fast growth, or an increased incidence of developmental orthopedic issues.

OVERVIEW AND GOAL(S)

- Brood mares:
  - Maintain a body condition score of at least 5 throughout the year.
  - Feed a nutrient adequate diet.
  - Avoid endophyte-infected tall fescue pasture and hay.

- Stallions:
  - Maintain a body condition score of about 5 throughout the year
  - Feed a nutrient adequate diet
- Growing horses:
  - Moderate, even growth
  - At 4 months of age most horses will have achieved about 34% of their expected mature weight; at 8 months of age they will have achieved about 50% of their expected mature weight.
  - Feed a nutrient-adequate diet.

PREPARATION: IMPORTANT CHECKPOINTS

- Amounts of feed offered should be weighed.
- Samples of all feeds, especially hay and pasture, should be analyzed for nutrient content.

PROCEDURE

- Dietary assessment
- The amount of nutrients consumed = nutrients in concentrate + nutrients in forage + nutrients in supplements.
- Nutrients provided = weight of feed × composition of feed.

TABLE 1 Approximate Nutrient Composition of Typical Feeds Used on a Breeding Farm

	DE (Mcal/lb)	% Crude Protein	%Ca	%P	Cu (mg/lb)	Zn (mg/lb)	Se (mg/lb)
Grass/legume forage*	0.8–1.1	12–16	0.4–0.8	0.2–0.4	3–4	10–15	0.01–0.03
Concentrate	1.3–1.4	13–16	0.6–1.0	0.6–0.8	12–25	35–60	0.15–0.3
Balancer pellet	1.2–1.3	25–30	3–4	1–2	60–80	200–300	0.6–1.0

*Mineral content will reflect soil characteristics. *Ca*, Calcium; *CP*, crude protein; *Cu*, copper; *DE*, digestible energy; *P*, phosphorus; *Se*, selenium.

- A small hanging scale can be purchased to weigh feed. Different feeds will have different densities; therefore it is not accurate to assume that a 2-pound scoop will contain 2 pounds.
- The dietary assessment of lactating mares should also consider feed consumption by the foal. After 2 months of age most foals will be eating some of their dam's feed unless the foal is fed separately. By 4 months of age some foals may be eating 1 to 4 pounds of concentrate from the dam's feed.
- Concentrates/grains
  - The nutrient composition on the feed tag or bag may not include information about all nutrients. Some feed manufacturers will provide the needed information if asked, otherwise it may be necessary to submit a sample to a laboratory.
  - Accurate information about nutrient composition will only be obtained if the lab receives a representative sample of the feed. Therefore feed should be obtained from several bags, mixed, and then a subsample submitted.
- Forages (hay and grain)
  - The amount of hay offered can be weighed, but it is also important to assess the amount of hay wasted to calculate the amount consumed.
  - A representative sample of hay must be obtained for analysis by sampling several bales. The best method is to use a hay-coring device. Some county extension offices will have these devices.
  - It is difficult to quantify pasture intake. When pasture is abundant, most horses will consume at least 2% of body weight in dry matter in pasture per day (24-hour turn-out). Lactating mares and weanlings/yearlings may be able to consume more than 2% of body weight. As pasture quantity declines, dry matter intake will also decline.
  - Pasture quantity and quality can be assessed by walking a zigzag pattern in the pasture and evaluating amount available every 50 steps. Samples of pasture can also be obtained using grass shears at each

location. The composite sample can then be mixed and subsampled for analysis.
- Supplements
  - The nutrient content of the diet should be calculated initially without supplements to determine whether the forage and concentrate are sufficient and if any additional supplements are necessary.
  - Many diets will be low in sodium and chloride and a salt block will be necessary.
- Endophyte-infected tall fescue
  - Unless a horse owner knows that endophyte-free tall fescue was planted in a pasture, any tall fescue should be considered suspect for endophyte contamination
  - Pasture samples can be tested for the presence of the endophyte as well as the amount of ergovaline present.
    - The endophyte is not uniformly active during the entire year and pastures that have low ergovaline concentrations at one point in time may have high levels at another time.

SPECIFIC NUTRIENTS TO BE ADDRESSED

- Energy (calorie) intake will determine body condition in mature horses and will influence rate of gain in growing horses. Therefore energy intake should be evaluated first.
- Protein quantity and quality (amino acid intake) will influence growth and also maintenance of lean tissue in mature horses.
- Broodmares and growing horses must have adequate calcium and phosphorus. Imbalanced calcium:phosphorus ratios (more P than Ca) can result in skeletal issues. Mares may mobilize bone mineral to meet the needs of gestation and lactation unless the diet provides adequate calcium and phosphorus.
- Trace minerals and vitamins are important for normal reproduction and development. Deficiencies increase the incidence of developmental issues, but excess supplementation does not provide additional benefits.

RECOMMENDED DIETS

- There are three basic feeds that can be combined to meet the needs of most horses on a breeding farm.
  - A good-quality grass legume forage (pasture or hay)
  - A commercially manufactured concentrate formulated for broodmares and growing horses
  - A commercially manufactured balancer pellet
- The approximate compositions of these feeds are shown in Table 1. These values are suggested as a guide for selecting feeds and not all essential nutrients are shown.
- Good quality pasture and/or hay may provide enough energy to maintain a body condition score (BCS) above 5 without much concentrate supplementation. However, forage alone may not meet the mineral requirements of gestating mares. The National Research Council suggests that the nutrient requirements of pregnant mares start to increase above maintenance in the fifth month of gestation. This is a new recommendation; previously it was suggested that nutrient needs did not increase until the ninth month of gestation. If pregnant mares are not receiving any concentrate, a supplement should be given at least once a day. A convenient supplement source is a "balancer pellet" that is sold by many feed companies. Feeding 1 to 2 pounds of a typical balancer pellet during early and mid-gestation should ensure adequate daily mineral intakes of mares that are grazing pasture.
- Pregnant mares should be maintained at a BCS of at least 5. A slightly higher BCS will ensure that the mares have a buffer of body stores at foaling and in early lactation. When forage quality or quantity is not enough to maintain body condition, concentrate should be added to the diet. As mares approach the end of gestation, appetite may decline, so concentrate intake may have to be increased. A typical diet for a Quarter Horse–type mare in the 10th or 11th month of gestation might be 20 pounds of good quality hay and 3 to 6 pounds of a concentrate. Thoroughbred-type mares may require larger amounts of concentrate. If

mares live outside during the winter, additional feed will often be necessary. To ensure adequate nutrient intakes, pregnant mares in late gestation should be fed a concentrate that is formulated for broodmares. If mares are maintaining adequate body condition without concentrate, 1 to 2 pounds of balancer pellet should be given to meet mineral needs. The balancer pellet is not needed if the mare receives at least 3 to 4 pounds of concentrate per day.

- Lactating mares may consume 25 to 30 pounds (or more) of hay (or equivalent pasture) per day. The use of very good-quality forage reduces the need for concentrate in the diet. Broodmares should be fed a concentrate that is formulated for the needs of mares and foals. Concentrate intakes will usually range from 5 to 10 pounds per day in early lactation and then decrease as the mare approaches weaning. To maximize rebreeding efficiency, mares should foal with a BCS of at least 5 and then maintain that condition score. Loss of body condition during lactation indicates that nutrient intake is not sufficient and that the diet should be changed.
- As foals approach 2 months of age they will be eating some forage and concentrate. By 4 months of age they will be obtaining about 40% to 60% of their required nutrients from forage and concentrate, and the rest from milk. Typical concentrate intakes for 4- to 8-month-old foals with an expected mature weight of 1,250 pounds will range from about 0.5 to 1.5 pounds per month of age per day. Less concentrate will be needed when forage quantity and forage quality are high and more will be needed as forage quantity and quality decline.
- Growing horses will consume large amounts of forage. Hay allowances should be approximately 2% of body weight per day, but more hay may be consumed by many growing horses.
- In most cases, weaning involves an abrupt change in diet for foals. In the immediate postweaning period, foal growth may slow. The period of slow growth may be followed by a period of rapid growth. To minimize this period of erratic growth, foals should be adapted to eating concentrate and forage prior to weaning and weaning methods that minimize stress should be used.
- Developmental orthopedic diseases cannot be entirely prevented by nutritional management. However, poor dietary management may increase the incidence or severity of problems. The following strategies are suggested to minimize the incidence of developmental orthopedic disease in horses:
  - Moderate, even growth
  - Diets that contain adequate amounts of all nutrients should be fed throughout gestation and lactation as well as during growth.
  - Limit stall confinement to brief periods.

POSTPROCEDURE

- All horses should be body condition-scored on a monthly basis and dietary changes imposed to achieve the desired condition score.
- Young horses should be weighed if possible on a monthly basis to ensure an even, moderate growth rate. Monitoring is especially important after weaning when weight gains can be erratic. Foals that are growing too rapidly can be fed less concentrate to reduce energy intake. However, diets should be examined to ensure that other nutrients are adequate. Foals growing too slowly can be fed more concentrate. All changes should be made gradually.
- Horses that are fed in groups should be observed at feeding to ensure that all horses receive the appropriate amount of feed.
- Mares that foal at a condition score below 5 will have a difficult time increasing condition during early lactation. Changes in body condition are easiest to accomplish when mares are not lactating or in late gestation.
- If mares have been exposed to endophyte-infected tall fescue during late gestation, the feasibility of medical intervention with domperidone should be considered.

ALTERNATIVES AND THEIR RELATIVE MERITS

- When horses are maintained and fed in groups, it may be desirable to sort them by nutrient needs. It is common to sort broodmares by breeding or foaling dates, but it may be more desirable to sort them by condition score or temperament to make certain that timid mares have the same access to feed as aggressive mares.
- If it is not possible to sort mares, access to food can be manipulated by individually feeding the mares in stalls or by using nose bags on mares kept in paddocks.
- Foals that aggressively consume their dam's feed may become fat. Access to the mare's feed can be restricted by using a nose bag on the mare or by hanging her feed tub high enough to limit the foal's access.
- After foaling a mare's feed intake may increase rapidly. This increase in feed intake should be managed gradually, the same as any other change in diet.

COMMENTS

- Good-quality forage is the basis of nutrition on breeding farms. The better the forage, the less supplementation will be necessary with concentrates or other feeds. In addition, horses will waste less when fed good-quality forage than when fed low-quality forage.
- Hay should be supplied when pasture quantity declines. Because growing conditions affect pasture availability, there are no hard and fast dates to start or end hay feeding to pastured horses. The best way to determine whether hay is needed is to offer good-quality hay in the pasture and observe the behavior of the horses. If hay is readily consumed, then supplemental hay is probably warranted.
- Horses should be fed an amount of hay that they will clean up readily.
- Excessive tail chewing among weanlings and yearlings may suggest that the amount of forage provided is not sufficient.

SUGGESTED READING

National Research Council: *Nutrient requirements of horses*, Washington, DC, 2007, National Academy Press.

AUTHOR: **LAURIE M. LAWRENCE**

EDITOR: **DANIEL J. BURKE**

Nutrition: Carbohydrates

BASIC INFORMATION

OVERVIEW AND GOAL(S)

- The horse is anatomically designed as a grazing, hind-gut fermenting herbivore, with a range of carbohydrates—hydrolyzable to fermentable—as its primary energy source.
  - Pastures and hay contain fermentable carbohydrates that provide constant energy and maintain the integrity of the microbial population in the equine hindgut.
  - Grain concentrates contain hydrolyzable carbohydrates that provide efficient fuel for performance.

CARBOHYDRATE DIGESTION AND END PRODUCTS

- Carbohydrates may be hydrolyzed or fermented in horses, depending on the chemical linkage of their molecules.
  - Hydrolyzable carbohydrates include simple sugars (eg, glucose, fructose), disaccharides (eg, sucrose, maltose, lactose), and starch. Starch consists of long chains of glucose.
  - Small intestinal enzymes hydrolyze starch and disaccharides into simple sugars.
  - Absorbed simple sugars fuel equine performance, especially prolonged or high-intensity exercise, through efficient production of ATP in the Krebs cycle, and replenishment of muscle glycogen.
- Fermentable carbohydrates resistant to digestion by mammalian enzymes include the following:
  - Soluble fibers (eg, gums, mucilages, pectins)
  - Fructans and galactans (medium-chain sugars containing fructose or galactose)
  - Starches resistant to enzymatic hydrolysis (encased in a seed coat or due to chemical structure)
  - Insoluble fibers, hemicellulose, cellulose, and lignocellulose
- Horses rely on microbial fermentation in the hindgut to break down structural carbohydrates. Fermentation produces mainly volatile fatty acids (acetate, propionate, butyrate, and, to a lesser extent, lactate), gas, heat, and B-complex vitamins. Absorption of volatile fatty acids is integral to maintaining colon pH above 6, as required for optimal populations of microbes.
- Proportions of volatile fatty acids produced are dependent on substrates. Slow fermentation is desired:

- Forage diets high in fiber favor slow fermentation and production of acetate and butyrate.
- Increasing grain over forage favors rapid fermentation, decreases efficiency of fiber utilization, and alters the microbial ecosystem.
- "Grain overload" or "starch overload" occurs when excessive starch intake overloads the capacity of small intestinal hydrolysis and passes into the hindgut. When starch exceeds 4 g per 100 kg body weight per meal (approximately 5 lb of a traditional grain concentrate), it is rapidly fermented in the hindgut.
- Fructans pass through the small intestine and are rapidly fermented in the hindgut.
- Rapid fermentation favors proliferation of *Lactobacilli* spp. and production of lactate, which is poorly absorbed and may cause osmotic diarrhea, colic, and increased risk of laminitis and founder.

CARBOHYDRATES IN HORSE FORAGES AND FEEDS

- Forages: During photosynthesis, green plants produce simple sugars. When sugar production exceeds the energy requirements of the plant, sugars are converted to storage carbohydrates, either starch or fructans.
  - Cool season pasture grasses accumulate fructans. Legumes and warm season grasses accumulate starch.
  - Fructan and starch concentrations in pastures fluctuate with season and diurnally from night to day or shade to sunlight.
  - Fructan and starch concentrations generally rise during the morning, peak in the afternoon, and decline to a low overnight.
  - Seasonal and circadian patterns in glucose and insulin in grazing horses correspond to changes in pasture starch and fructan.
  - High pasture starch and fructan may increase risk of laminitis or "grass founder" by exacerbating insulin resistance (see "Insulin Resistance" in Section I).
  - After frost, the palatability of fructan-rich cool season grasses increases dramatically, and high intakes increase risk of overload, laminitis, and founder.
- Grains
- Horse owners supplement grain concentrates to meet energy demands of performance and provide a carrier for

micronutrients that are marginal or deficient in forages.
  - Oat starch appears to be the most digestible of the cereal starches fed to horses.
  - Digestion is hindered when starch is contained within whole grain or waxy seed coats, such as corn, or entrapped within rigid cell walls, as in soybeans. Processing increases digestibility.
  - Barley is relatively resistant to hydrolysis and may be fermented rapidly in the hindgut.
  - Grain concentrates formulated with balanced nutrients are recommended over oats, corn, or other plain grains.
- "Super fibers" are feeds containing highly digestible fiber available for microbial fermentation.
  - Common super fibers include beet pulp, soybean hulls, and almond hulls, and to a lesser extent, oat hulls, rice bran, and citrus pulp.
  - Super fibers are purported to contain calories similar to oats and barley while not producing symptoms of grain overload.
  - Some super fibers contain starch in amounts that are significant in horses with carbohydrate-associated disorders.
  - Wheat bran contains less fiber than whole oats. Bran mashes for horses are not recommended. They contain enough starch to disturb the balance of intestinal microflora and may affect calcium and phosphorus balance.

CARBOHYDRATES AND GLYCEMIC INDEX

- The glycemic index is a reflection of glucose and insulin responses to a meal, an in vivo estimate, not a chemical analysis. Glycemic indices are used in human nutrition to formulate therapeutic diets for diabetics.
  - The glycemic index of a horse feed provides information about the feed and is not meant to provide information about a specific horse.
  - Multiple factors affect glycemic response, including meal size, starch, sugar, fiber and fat content, processing, intake time, chewing behavior, gastric emptying, digestibility, and rate of absorption.
  - Glycemic indices for horses are reported using oats as a standardized reference, with the calculated response for oats set to a value of 100. Glycemic indices of common feeds follow:

- Beet pulp, 1; alfalfa hay, 26; timothy hay, 32; carrots, 51
- Oats, 100; barley, 101; corn, 117
- Glycemic indices may aid formulation of diets for horses with carbohydrate-associated disorders.

INDICATIONS

CARBOHYDRATES AND PERFORMANCE

- Exercising horses require dietary starch to efficiently fuel performance.
  - Horses have an opportunity for small intestinal metabolism of starch and sugars to glucose, which is more metabolically efficient than hindgut fermentation of fibers to volatile fatty acids.
  - Compared to fat, glucose (and its stored form, glycogen) is aerobically metabolized twice as fast to generate ATP for muscle contraction.
  - As speed and exertion increase, glycogen metabolism is favored.
  - Depletion of glycogen causes fatigue.
  - Feeds with high glycemic index may aid glycogen repletion in performance horses after strenuous exercise.

CARBOHYDRATE-ASSOCIATED DISORDERS

- Grain concentrates have been associated with several digestive and metabolic disorders, including colic, laminitis, gastric ulcers, developmental orthopedic disease, insulin resistance, equine metabolic syndrome, and polysaccharide storage myopathy.
  - The abundant starch in grain concentrates has been implicated as the culprit, leading to marketing of "low starch" concentrates for horses.
  - Although low-starch grain concentrates provide an energy source critical for horses with carbohydrate-associated disorders, they are

not a "one fits all" solution (see carbohydrates and Performance, Above).

PROCEDURE

- Carbohydrate components are analyzed in the laboratory as follows:
  - Nonstructural carbohydrate (NSC) is a measure of hydrolyzable carbohydrate, mainly sugar and starch. In some laboratories, fructan is included in NSC.
  - Neutral detergent fiber (NDF) includes insoluble fibers, hemicellulose, cellulose, lignocellulose, and lignin. NDF reflects total bulk of the feedstuff and is an indicator of intake potential.
  - Acid detergent fiber (ADF) is a subset of NDF, including cellulose, lignocellulose, and lignin. ADF is the least digestible portion of the feedstuff, so higher ADF equals lower calories. Feedstuffs with high ADF may be poorly accepted.
  - Nonfiber carbohydrate (NFC) is calculated, not directly analyzed. NFC includes NSC, fructans, galactans, soluble fibers, and resistant starch, calculated as follows:

$$\% \text{ NFC} = 100 - \% \text{ water} - \% \text{ crude protein} - \% \text{ crude fat} - \% \text{ NDF} - \% \text{ ash}$$

  - Lignin is a component of woody plant tissue and included in standard carbohydrate analysis. Lignin is indigestible.

SUMMARY AND OVERALL RECOMMENDATIONS

- Fermentable carbohydrates provide constant energy and maintain the integrity of the microbial population in the equine hindgut.
- Excess grain or lush pasture rich in starch or fructan may cause rapid fer-

mentation and excess lactic acid in the hindgut, causing osmotic diarrhea, colic, and perhaps laminitis and founder.

- To avoid starch overload, limit intake to 5 pounds or less of grain per meal (4 g starch per 100 kg body weight per meal).
- Starch and fructan content of pasture fluctuates with season, night to day, and shade to sunlight. Glucose and insulin concentrations in grazing horses reflect these changes. Horses with carbohydrate-associated disorders should have restricted or night-only grazing.
- The glycemic index of a feed provides information about the feed and is not meant to provide information about a specific horse, as multiple factors affect glycemic response.
- Hydrolyzable carbohydrates efficiently fuel equine performance, especially prolonged or high-intensity exercise, and replenish muscle glycogen.

SUGGESTED READING

Hoffman RM: Carbohydrate metabolism in horses. In Ralston SL, Hintz HF, editors: *Recent Advances in Equine Nutrition*, 2003. International Veterinary Information Service. http://www.ivis.org/advances/Ralston/hoffman/chapter_frm.asp?LA=1

Hoffman RM, et al: Hydrolyzable carbohydrates in pasture, hay, and horse feeds: direct assay and seasonal variation. *J Anim Sci* 79:500–506, 2001.

Potter GD, et al: Digestion of starch in the small or large intestine of the equine. *Pferdeheilkunde* 1:107–111, 1992.

Rodiek A: Glycemic index of practical horse feeds. *Agricultural Research Institute Publication*, #00-2-034-1B, Fresno, 2006, California Agricultural Technology Institute, California State University.

AUTHOR: RHONDA M. HOFFMAN

EDITOR: DANIEL J. BURKE

Nutrition: Fats

BASIC INFORMATION

OVERVIEW AND GOAL(S)

- A high-fat diet is a disaster if you are planning your own diet, but potentially beneficial for many types of horses.
- Research has established many benefits of feeding fat.
- Benefits of a high-fat diet include:
  - Increasing energy content of the diet

  - Enhanced body condition in thin horses
  - Diminished excitability, and increased oxidative capacity in performance horses
  - As a carrier for the fat-soluble vitamins
- What is fat?
  - Fats (lipids) fed to horses are triglycerides.
  - Triglycerides consist of three fatty acids and a glycerol molecule.

  - Chemical structure of the fatty acids determines if the fat is saturated or unsaturated.
  - Saturated fats (tallow/lard) are solids at room temperature.
  - Unsaturated fats (vegetable oil) are liquids at room temperature.
  - Examples: corn oil, soybean oil, canola oil
  - The location of double bonds within the fatty acid is used to identify omega-6 and omega-3 fatty acids.

- Omega-3 and omega-6 fatty acids have different fates within the body.
  - Research is ongoing to determine the proper amount and ratio of omega-3 and omega-6 fatty acids need to be in the diet.
- Sources of fat
  - Saturated animal fat is not typically fed to horses.
  - Unsaturated fat (vegetable oil) is primarily supplemented in horse diets.
  - Common vegetable oil sources include:
    - Corn oil, soybean oil, rice oil, and canola oil
  - Vegetable oil is 100% fat.
  - Other common fat sources fed to horses include:
    - Spray dried vegetable fat (99% fat)
    - Stabilized rice bran (20% fat)
    - Horse feed supplemented with fat (6%–12% fat)
  - Each fat source is palatable given the horse has been slowly adapted to the fat source.
  - Fish oil is high in omega-3 fatty acids but is less palatable.
    - Fish oils can be more palatable with a slow adaptation period.
- Is fat digestible?
  - Unsaturated vegetable oil is highly digestible, in excess of 95% digestible by horses.
  - Vegetable oil is digested in the small intestine.
  - Horses can digest large amounts of vegetable oil, up to 20% of the diet.
- How many calories are in fat ?
  - Vegetable oil contains approximately 2.5 times as much digestible energy as an equal weight of oats.
    - 2.3 times as much digestible energy as an equal weight of cracked corn
  - Vegetable oil is the most calorie-dense ingredient used in horse diets.
- Is fat safe to feed?
  - Fat should be gradually introduced into a horse's diet over a 14-day adaptation period.
  - Too much fat added to the diet will result in feed refusal.
    - If too much fat is consumed in a single meal, a transient diarrhea may result.
    - Unlike grain, oversupplementation with fat will not result in colic or laminitis.
  - Coronary heart disease has not been demonstrated in horses supplemented with fat.
  - A horse on a "high-fat" diet may get 20% of its calories from fat.
    - Our typical diet provides 40% to 70% of calories from fat.

- By comparison to a human diet, a high-fat diet for a horse is really a misnomer.
- How much fat can be fed?
  - Horses are capable of digesting large amounts of fat.
  - In controlled experiments, horses have been fed as much as 230 g of oil/kg of diet.
    - This equates to approximately 11 cups of oil/day.
  - Practically, the maximum amount of oil top-dressed to feed would not exceed 2 cups/day for a 1000-pound horse.
    - In special circumstances horses can be fed more vegetable oil.
    - In all feeding situations, gradually introduce vegetable oil into the diet to avoid feed refusal and diarrhea.

INDICATIONS

- Safe calorie source for weight gain
  - Vegetable oil contains approximately 2.5 times more energy than any single ingredient in the horse's diet.
  - Feeding fat is a safe, effective method to put extra calories in the horse's diet.
  - Calories from fat boost body condition in thin horses.
  - Calories from fat assist performance horses in meeting their high energy requirements.
  - Adding fat to the diet decreases the amount of grain that must be fed, thereby potentially decreasing the risk of digestive upset or colic.
- Tying-up syndrome
  - High-grain diets are a potential problem for horses with two chronic forms of exertional rhabdomyolysis.
  - Unfit horses with polysaccharide storage myopathy (PSSM) benefit from daily exercise, removal of grain, and the addition of fat to provide necessary calories.
  - Fit horses with recurrent exertional rhabdomyolysis (RER) can maintain high calorie intake if the amount of grain in the diet is reduced and the amount of fat in the diet is significantly increased.
  - In both of these forms of tying-up, dietary fat helps to minimize symptoms.
- Exercise performance
  - Performance horses require large amounts of energy.
  - Feeding large amounts of grain risks digestive upset, colic, and laminitis.
  - Fat is a safe means to add calories to the diet.
  - Horses that are adapted to fat in the diet have:
    - Increased oxidative capacity

- Spare muscle and liver glycogen during exercise
  - Fat is a major energy source when exercise is below 75% of maximum aerobic capacity (VO$_2$Max).
  - Many types of performance horses can use large amounts of fat during exercise.
- Broodmares
  - Energy balance and body fat are major factors in reproductive performance of mares.
  - Dietary fat can assist mares in maintenance of energy balance and body fat reserves.
    - Primarily when feed intake capacity is reduced in late pregnancy
  - Dietary fat helps lactating mares meet the high energy needs associated with milk production.
- Sales preparation and show horses
  - A sleek, shiny hair coat is desirable for both show and sale horses.
  - A quality hair coat is partially dependent on providing horses with essential fatty acids.
  - Supplementing with vegetable oil is both a reliable and common practice to deliver essential fatty acids to improve hair and skin.

SUMMARY

- Fat (lipid) in the form of triglycerides is added to equine diets.
- Saturated fat is solid at room temperature. Examples of saturated fats include tallow and lard. These fats are not typically fed to horses.
- Unsaturated fat (vegetable oil) is liquid at room temperature. Examples of unsaturated fats are corn, soybean, and canola oil.
- Unsaturated vegetable oil is highly digestible, greater than 95% digestible in horses.
- Fat is extremely energy dense, containing approximately 2.5 times the digestible energy as an equal weight of corn or oats.
- Fat is very safe to feed. Feeding too much fat will result in feed refusal or diarrhea but will not cause colic or laminitis.
- Large amounts of fat can be fed provided the horses are properly adapted to fat. Normally a maximum of 2 cups/day can be top-dressed to feed for a 1000-pound horse.
- Fat is recognized as a safe energy source for weight gain.
- Fat can help alleviate symptoms of tying-up in certain horses.
- Fat has a positive influence on exercise performance provided the horses are adapted to having fat in the diet. These horses will spare muscle glycogen and have an increased oxidative capacity.

- Fat is useful in broodmare diets to assist in maintenance of energy balance and body fat reserves.
- Fat provides essential fatty acids that are necessary for healthy hair and

skin. Show horses and sales horses benefit from the addition of fat to the diet.

AUTHOR: **STEPHEN DUREN**

EDITOR: **DANIEL J. BURKE**

Nutrition: Feeding for Seniors

BASIC INFORMATION

OVERVIEW AND GOAL(S)

No exact chronological threshold for old age in horses has been identified. Although 20 years of age has been suggested as a threshold for old age in horses; the age at which horses show physical signs of aging (eg, body condition score chronically below 5, loss of muscle mass over the top-line yielding a swayback appearance, hollowing out of the grooves above the eyes, graying of the coat and dental disease) varies considerably between horses. Therefore the combination of chronological age and physical signs of aging may be the most effective means of establishing the old-age threshold for individual horses.

NUTRITION REQUIREMENTS

- Currently there are no published nutrient requirements specific to senior horses. Requirements for adult horses are used with modifications discussed below.
- For specific nutrient requirements of horses the reader is referred to NRC Nutrient Requirements of Horses, 6th edition. The NRC Model program can be accessed free online at http://nrc88.nas.edu/nrh/ and used to generate requirements for specific feeding classes of horses.

REQUIREMENTS POTENTIALLY AFFECTED BY OLD AGE:

- Calories:
  - The actual metabolic requirement for calories probably does not increase with age and may actually decrease due to loss of lean body mass. However the ability to digest fibrous feeds (eg, forage and other roughage) that typically provide a large proportion of calories for adult horses may decrease with age due to age-related changes in dentition. Therefore, high quality forage (ie, low level of plant maturity; relatively high leaf:stem) should be used in feeding older horses to help counter the effect of potential reduction in fiber digestibility. Additionally, routine dental care should be maintained.

- Low body-condition score (ie, body condition score <5) and subsequent lack of insulation from fat covering may increase heat loss from old horses in cold climates. Increased heat loss increases metabolic and dietary requirements for energy. Therefore, appropriate shelter should be available for old horses with low body-condition score during the late fall and winter months.
  - The sixth edition of the NRC Nutrient Requirements of Horses provides three different estimates for maintenance digestible energy requirements: low, average, and high. Using the "high" estimate may be prudent for senior horses having difficulty maintaining a body condition score of 5 (ie, ribs cannot be seen, but are easily felt). The high maintenance digestible energy (DE) requirement is 36.3 kcal DE/kg of BW or 18.2 Mcal DE / 500 kg BW.
- Protein and Amino Acid Requirements:
  - The effect of aging on protein and amino acid requirements in horses is unknown.
  - Some evidence suggests that older horses may have reduced apparent crude protein digestibility; however, more recent observations found no difference when older horses were compared to younger adult horses. Fortunately, forage-based rations generally contain much more crude protein than is required. Therefore, even if digestibility is slightly reduced, the total amount absorbed for metabolism is likely to be more than adequate.
  - Supplemental lysine (0.25% of DM or 20 g/day) and threonine (0.2% of DM or 15 g/day) have been suggested to maintain muscle mass in old horses.
- Micronutrient requirements:
  - The effect of aging on micronutrient requirements of horses is unknown.
  - Phosphorus apparent digestibility was decreased in senior horses (26 ± 5 years of age) versus younger horses (2.3 ± 0.5 years of age).

However, additional reports have found no difference between senior and younger adult horses.
- An initial study reported lower vitamin C status in senior versus younger adult horses. However, more recent evidence does not support this finding.
- Senior horses can have reduced immune function relative to younger horses. Several micronutrients (eg, Cu, Zn, Mn, Se, vitamin A, and vitamin E) play roles in immune function. Although the effect of micronutrient status on immune function in senior horses is not well studied, it seems prudent to ensure that adequate amounts of these nutrients are present in the ration. The reader is referred to the NRC Nutrient Requirements of Horses for specific mineral and vitamin requirements.

PROCEDURE

- Feeding Senior Horses:
  - Senior horses free from disease, having adequate dentition, and having no difficulty in maintaining body condition may thrive on rations similar to those fed to younger mature horses.
  - Senior horses that cannot maintain body weight or condition when fed rations that are effective for younger mature horses should follow the protocol outlined below:
    - Total amount of feed offered per day should be 2.25% to 2.75% of body weight on an as-fed basis (eg, 11.25 to 13.75 kg per day for a 500-kg horse). This total daily amount should be divided into at least two feedings per day. Amounts of feed should be obtained by use of a scale. If the horse gains body weight and condition beyond that desired (eg, body condition score of 5 to 6) then the total amount of feed can be reduced to 2% of body weight on an as-fed basis.
    - Begin by feeding high-quality forage (immature alfalfa or alfalfa-grass mix; or well-

managed pasture) at the above rate in addition to a vitamin-mineral supplement complementary to the forage. See the Suggested Readings for an example of a suitable mineral-vitamin supplement. High-quality hay should be introduced slowly by replacing 25% of the previously fed hay every 3 or 4 days until the complete switch has been made.

- If the forage + mineral-vitamin supplement ration above fails to maintain body weight and condition after 30 to 40 days of feeding, then replace 20% of forage with a fortified (ie, contains supplemental minerals and vitamins) grain-mix-concentrate formulated for growing horses or lactating

mares, and remove the mineral-vitamin supplement used above, as the grain-mix-concentrate will provide adequate mineral-vitamin nutrition. In addition, up to 2 cups of vegetable oil can be top-dressed on the grain-mix-concentrate.

- Alternatively, a commercially formulated feed designed specifically for senior horses can be used as the sole ration. Some long-stem forage should be provided to alleviate boredom.
- A source of clean water and free choice white salt (iodinized) should also be provided.
- House and feed horses in a manner that prevents competition for feed with other horses.

- Body weight and condition score should be monitored monthly on senior horses to ensure that the ration fed is effective.
- Maintain routine (every 6 months to 1 year) dental care and an effective parasite prevention program.

SUGGESTED READING

National Research Council: *Nutrient requirements of horses*, revised ed 6, Washington, DC, 2007, National Academy Press.
Siciliano, PD: Nutrition and feeding of the geriatric horse. *Vet Clin North Am Equine Pract* 18:491–508, 2002.

AUTHOR: PAUL D. SICILIANO

EDITOR: DANIEL J. BURKE

Nutrition: Herbs and Other Supplements

BASIC INFORMATION

OVERVIEW AND GOAL(S)

- Forage is the main component of any horse's diet, but intensely exercising horses require supplementation to meet increased nutrient demands.
- Supplementation
  - The basic principle is to give a horse one or more dietary ingredients above what are normally required to meet nutrient requirements.
  - Given with the goal of improving performance, preventing a problem from occurring, and combating or managing a problem after it arises.
  - Many commercial supplement products contain ingredients that provide one or more vitamins, minerals, amino acids (protein), fuel sources (carbohydrates and fats), herbs, and direct-fed microbials (bacteria and yeast).
  - This chapter focuses on specific supplements that are commonly used in the horse industry.
  - Published literature is scarce concerning supplements, so research in human and other species is included to better illustrate their benefits.

INDICATIONS

Specific Supplements
Oral Chondroprotectants
- Possible ingredients: Glucosamine, chondroitin sulfate, hyaluronic acid, and methyl-sulfonyl-methane (MSM)

  - Low absorption rates (2.5% for glucosamine and 32% for chondroitin sulfate)
  - Should see an effect in 1 month's time, if no improvement is seen after 2 months, it is assumed that the individual is a nonresponder.
- Glucosamine has antiinflammatory properties, ultimately preventing cartilage degradation and preserving the integrity of the joint.
- Chondroitin sulfate initiates glycosaminoglycan (GAG) synthesis, enhancement of synovial fluid viscosity and antiinflammatory processes.
- Hyaluronic acid theoretically helps restore viscoelasticity and provides joint lubrication while exhibiting antiinflammatory and antioxidant properties.
- Low incidence of toxicity in laboratory animals and humans; nothing found in horses.

ANTIOXIDANTS

- Ingredients include vitamins (eg, vitamins E, C and A), minerals (eg, selenium), enzymes (eg, superoxide dismutase, glutathione peroxidase, catalase) and nutrient derivatives (eg, glutathione, lipoic acid).
  - Decrease negative effects of reactive oxygen species (ROS) or free radicals.
  - Oxidative stress occurs when the antioxidant defense system in the body is overwhelmed with ROS.
    - Increase in ROS may occur due to:
      - Increased exposure to oxidants from the environment

      - Increased production within the body from an increase in oxygen metabolism during exercise
      - An imbalance in antioxidants
- Antioxidants are most effective when used in combination with each other as they can recycle antioxidant radicals that are formed during the scavenging of ROS.

ERGOGENIC AIDS

- Ergogenic aids are compounds that enhance exercise performance.
- Increasing speed, power, muscle mass, or endurance capacity are some of the claims provided by advertisements.
  - Not proven effective in horses as well as humans and other animals.
  - β-hydroxy β-methylbutyrate (HMB), carnitine, creatine, coenzyme Q10, and γ-oryzanol are a few of the many products theorized to increase anaerobic or aerobic capacity.

PROBIOTICS

- Probiotics or direct-fed microbials are used to help increase the population of beneficial microorganisms in the gastrointestinal (GI) tract.
- No evidence to prove that providing probiotics to animals with healthy GI flora would have any effect.
  - Bacterial populations including the *Lactobacillus* species might effectively treat some conditions, like diarrhea.
  - Yeast, including *Saccharomyces cerevisiae*, has been found to increase feed digestibility and milk production in mares and increased growth rate in foals.

HERBAL SUPPLEMENTS

- Herbal supplements that affect the immune system can be classified as adaptogens, immunostimulants, or both.
  - Adaptogens increase resistance to stressors: physical, chemical, or biologic.
  - Immunostimulants activate the nonspecific or innate defense mechanisms against viral, bacterial, or cellular infections.
- Most of the studies to date in laboratory animals, humans, and other species have determined that the immunologic effect of herbal supplements does not enhance normal immune response but may help if the immune system is compromised.
- Devil's claw (*Harpagophytum procumbens*):
  - Known properties: Antiinflammatory
  - Uses: Painkilling and antiinflammatory properties
  - Active ingredients: Iridoid glycosides, acetylated phenolic glycosides, and terpenoids
  - Human studies: >50 mg of harpagoside (a glycoside) per day are helpful in alleviating lower back pain in humans.
  - Laboratory animal studies: Topical application decreases the expression of cyclooxygenase (COX)-2.
  - Horse studies: A polyherbal composite containing devil's claw on osteoarthritis reduced PGE_2 in synovial fluid.
  - Side effects: Potential to cause gastrointestinal upset linked to gastric ulcers.
- Echinacea (*Echinacea* spp.):
  - Known properties: Immunostimulant, or "cold fighter," antiinflammatory and antioxidant
  - Uses: Immune booster
  - Active ingredients: Polysaccharides, glycoproteins, alkamides, and cichoric acid
  - Horse studies: Supplemented for 42 days at a level equivalent to 1000-mg standardized extract were immune stimulated, found increased lymphocyte count, decreased neutrophil count, increased red blood cell count and hemoglobin.
- Garlic (*Allium sativum*):
  - Known properties: Antibacterial, antiviral, antifungal, and antiparasitic, antioxidant
  - Active ingredients: Organosulphur compounds, phytochemicals, cysteine sulfoxides, and γ-glutamylcysteines
  - Uses: Expectorant and fly control
  - Horse studies: A polyherbal composite with garlic decreased respiratory rate in horses with symptomatic chronic obstructive pulmonary disease (COPD) and freeze-dried garlic fed at >0.4 g/kg per day resulted in symptoms indicative of Heinz body anemia
  - Dog studies: 5 g/kg of fresh garlic increased oxidation of hemoglobin within red blood cells and decreased total hemoglobin
  - Side effects: Gastric irritation, decreased sperm production, Heinz body anemia, and occupational asthma
- Ginger (*Zingiber officinale*):
  - Known properties: Antithrombotic, antioxidant, antiinflammatory, and antibacterial
  - Active ingredients: Paradol, gingerol, and myoga
  - Horse studies: A single dose of ginger in intensely exercised horses reduced recovery time; however, also a tendency to increase proinflammatory cytokines tumor necrosis factor (TNF)-α and interferon (IFN)-γ
  - Side effects: Gastric ulcers
- Ginseng (*Panax* spp.):
  - Known properties: Immunostimulating and antioxidant
  - Active ingredients: Glycosidal saponins called ginsenosides, essential oils, phytosterols, amino acids, peptides, vitamins, and minerals
  - Studies: Found to inhibit IL-1β and IL-6 gene expression, decrease TNF-α production by macrophages, decrease COX-2 expression, and suppress histamine and leukotriene release.
- Valerian (*Valeriana* spp.):
  - Known properties: Tranquilizing, sedative, and antispasmodic
  - Active ingredients: Valerenic acids, such as monoterpenes and sesquiterpenes, and iridoid glycosides
  - Studies: Effects neuromediators such as γ-aminobutyric acid (GABA), decreases central nervous system (CNS) activity in mice equal to that of phenobarbital.
  - Human studies: Treating insomnia and other sleep disorders in humans
  - Warnings: Banned substance in certain show organizations, such as the International Federation for Equestrian Sports (FEI)
- Yucca (*Yucca schidigera*):
  - Known properties: Antiinflammatory, antioxidant, antispasmodic, and antiplatelet
  - Active ingredients: Steroid-like saponins (yucca stem contains 10%), resveratrol, and yuccaols A-E (found in yucca bark)
  - Uses: Joint pain relief, decrease respiratory problems
  - Studies: Reduced the level of ROS in blood platelets, change production of superoxide radicals, inhibit free radicals activated by thrombin, and decrease lipid peroxidation.
- Spices:
  - Fenugreek (*Trigonella foenum*):
    - Uses: Increase weight gain, quite palatable to horses
    - Known properties: Antidiabetic and antioxidant effect
    - Active ingredients: Omega-3 fatty acids, flavonoids, and polyphenols vitamins B_1, B_2, niacin, folic acid, vitamin C, and the minerals sodium, phosphorous, potassium, calcium, iron, magnesium, and zinc (3.7 g of seeds contains 12 kcal)
  - Cinnamon (*Cinnamomum zeylanicum*):
    - Uses: Decrease fasting blood glucose, maintain a healthy digestive tract
  - Turmeric (*Curcuma domestica*),
    - Uses: Antioxidant and antiinflammatory, hypoglycemic effects
    - Active ingredients: Curcumin and sesquiterpenoids

OTHER NUTRACEUTICALS

- Flaxseed (*Linum usitatissimum*):
  - Active ingredients: Omega-3 fatty acids, α-linolenic acid, phytoestrogens, flavonoids, various amino acids, and minerals
  - Uses: Enhance coat, skin, and hoof quality of horses, laxative in humans
  - Horse studies: As a treatment for Culicoides or "sweet itch" found a significant improvement in a skin test response
  - Side effects: Some concern for cyanide poisoning in horses; however, the stomach acid inactivates enzymes within the seeds.
- Bee pollen and propolis:
  - Known properties: Antioxidant, antimicrobial, antifungal, antiinflammatory, and immunoregulatory actions
  - Active ingredients: Polyphenols, flavonoids, beta-carotene, caffeic acid, kaempferol, and phenethyl caffeate, p-hydroxyacetophenone, benzyl hydroxybenzoate, coumaric and cinnamic acid
  - Uses: Oxygen utilization, lower heart rates, and firmer muscle tone
  - Horse studies: a 55% bee pollen supplement for 42 days did not alter physical fitness or immunologic variables, did increase feed intake and nutrient retention.

POSSIBLE COMPLICATIONS AND COMMON ERRORS TO BE AVOIDED

HERB-DRUG INTERACTIONS Herbs can have a druglike action that can interact with other components in the horse's diet. Some herbs contain prohibited substances like salicylates, digitalis, heroin, cocaine, and marijuana. Drug-herb interactions can create various side effects ranging from mild to severe; thus caution needs to be taken when determining which "natural product" to use. A few are listed below:

- *Valerian*: Prolong the action of barbiturates, interact with alcohol, inhibit cytochrome P450.
- *Echinacea*: Hepatotoxic effects, should not be taken with other hepatotoxic drugs like steroids.
- *Garlic*: Heinz body anemia, gastrointestinal upset, allergic reactions and dermatitis in humans, decreased systolic and diastolic blood pressure.
- *Ginger*: Inhibit thromboxane synthetase and increase bleeding time.

- *Ginseng*: Hypertension, insomnia, vomiting, headache, nervousness, sleeplessness, and epistaxis in humans, also discontinue use of warfarin, heparin, aspirin, and other nonsteroidal antiinflammatory drugs (NSAIDs).

SUMMARY

Various supplements, including herbs and nutraceuticals, are being used in the equine industry. Despite many anecdotal reports of efficacy, most of the supplements have never been proven safe and effective in horses; therefore caution must be taken when selecting a supplement. Herb–drug interactions are also a potential problem and if a horse is at risk of developing a potential toxicity or drug interaction, a veterinarian or nutritionist should be contacted.

SUGGESTED READING

Burk AO, Williams CA: Feeding management practices and supplement use in top level event horses. *Comp Exerc Physiol* 5:85–93, 2008.

Geor RJ: The role of nutritional supplements and feeding strategies in equine athletic performance. *Equine Comp Exerc Physiol* 3:109–119, 2006.

Goodrich LR, Nixon AJ: Medical treatment of osteoarthritis in the horse—a review. *Vet J* 168:204–209, 2004.

Harris PA, Harris R: Ergogenic potential of nutritional strategies and substances in the horse. *Livestock Prod Sci* 92:147–165, 2005.

Poppenga RH: Risks associated with the use of herbs and other dietary supplements. *Vet Clin North Am Equine Practice* 17:455–477, 2001.

AUTHOR: **CAREY A. WILLIAMS**

EDITOR: **DANIEL J. BURKE**

Nutrition: Managing Starvation and Neglect Cases

BASIC INFORMATION

OVERVIEW AND GOAL(S)

- The role of the veterinarian is to provide medical services to the neglected horse(s) and to maintain a lead role in the educational needs, report cases to regulatory authorities, and provide expertise in the legal proceedings.
- Starvation of horse(s) may be due to a variety of factors including economic hardship, ignorance, apathy, illness or injury, and possibly other crimes such as domestic violence.
- Prolonged severe weather conditions (eg, drought, floods, heavy snow) may precipitate conditions of starvation and neglect.
- Seasonal changes in pasture and/or overgrazing may limit the nutritional capacity.
- Pathologic conditions such as cancer, insulin resistance, infections, or diseases of the liver, kidney, pancreas, or heart can elicit symptoms associated with emaciation.
- Salmonellosis and other bacterial infections may occur due to the compromised immune system and starvation.
- Conditions such as lactation, pregnancy, or old age may increase dietary requirements.

DEFINITIONS

- **Neglect** is the failure to provide proper feed, water and shelter; may include failure to provide veterinary care to a horse that is ill or injured.

- **Starvation** is the severe or lack of nutrient intake over a prolonged period of time.
- **Malnutrition** is the lack or unbalanced intake of nutrient(s) (eg, protein, vitamins) or the compromised utilization of available nutrients.
- **Emaciation** refers to loss of body condition, becoming extremely thin in appearance.
- **Abuse and cruelty** includes the intentional act, omission, or neglect whereby unnecessary or unjustifiable physical pain or suffering is caused or permitted. Examples include poking with a sharp stick or excessively beating, intentionally scaring, or poisoning a horse.

INDICATIONS

Animal control officers, public reports, or owners may observe the following:
- Loss of weight
- Lack of feed, water, or shelter
- General lethargy and weakness
- Lack of veterinary care to ill or injured horses
- Health of each horse should be evaluated using these guidelines:
  ○ Physical examination of each horse should be performed. The symptoms of the starved horse over time include:
    ▪ Behavioral changes with a depressed reactivity to external stimuli occurs usually 3 to 4 days to a week after the severe restriction of feed (Kronfeld, 1993).

  ▪ Immune compromise occurs 3 to 4 days after total feed deprivation, with a decrease in circulating lymphocyte count and a compromise in phagocytic response (Naylor and Kenyon, 1981).
  ▪ Body weight loss becomes noticeable after 1 to 2 weeks of feed deprivation. Assign and document body condition score.
  ○ Injuries should be documented along with their location and severity.
  ○ Evaluate existing parasite control program.
  ○ Examine dental condition of horses.
  ○ Evaluate hoof condition. Photograph overgrown hooves with a ruler to provide a reference for the length of hoof.
- Causes of starvation: Multifactorial including (Kronfeld, 1993):
  ○ Lack of quantity and quality of feed, especially the nutrient content and balance of energy and protein. Deficiencies or excesses of certain minerals and vitamins over the long-term can contribute to malnutrition and/or emaciation.
  ○ Seasonal declines in the primary feed source such as pasture.
  ○ Malabsorption of nutrients associated with diarrhea or poor dental function.
  ○ Parasites can be either a primary or secondary contributor to starvation/emaciation.

- Evaluating animal condition:
  - History of the horse in the preceding weeks or months should be initiated through discussion with the owner. However, the owner may provide misleading or false information. Contacting their veterinarian and/or feed supplier may assist an objective assessment. Others involved in the investigation may provide information on the timeline of events.
  - Identification of specific horses should include a written record and/or photographs using the following as a guide:
    - General characteristics, including gender, breed, age, coat color, markings, and hot or freeze brands
    - Specific identifying marks, such as scars, swirls on forehead, blindness, or other unique conformation characteristics (ie, frostbitten ear, sway back, or "Roman-nose")
    - Photographs of side, rear, and front stances are helpful in identifying horses, especially with seasonal changes in coat color and fluctuations in body condition.
  - Body condition or weight should be assessed on the initial visit and at weekly intervals during rehabilitation.
    - Scoring method is based on visual appraisal and palpable fat in six body areas with scores ranging 1 to 9:
      - Score of 1 is designated as "extremely emaciated" with no fatty tissue felt.
      - Score of 9 is considered obese or extremely fat and described as having patchy, bulging fat depots.
      - Scores of 5 and 6 are desirable in most healthy horses.
    - Heart girth tapes measure the circumference of the heart girth size, which will decrease with losses in body condition.
    - Scales provide the most accurate body weight measurement.
  - Document the amount and condition of feed accessible to the horses and stored on premises; note consumption or refusal of offered feed.
    - Identify any poisonous weeds in feed or pasture.
    - Consider sampling pasture or feed for nutrient content by chemical analysis at an approved laboratory.
    - Document the water source and the cleanliness, and consider submitting water for analysis of any toxins or pathogens.

PREPARATION: IMPORTANT CHECKPOINTS

- Reporting: Start and maintain a logbook recording all communication and visits. Include the date and time with each entry. Record both positive and negative observations.
  - Record the property address and names of the contact people, owners, and witnesses.
  - Write summaries of all phone calls, meetings, and in-person discussions.
  - Record, in detail, all oral and written recommendations and instructions.
  - Samples submitted to commercial laboratories should be recorded and the proper chain of custody procedures should be followed.
  - Document presence and condition of any other animals on premises.
  - Record information on the environment such as facility design, feed storage, barn/stall design and maintenance, flooring, bedding, feeders, and water supply, and outside pen conditions (ie, appropriate fencing, presence of mud, and hazardous objects or materials).
  - Record information on sanitation, including manure management, water cleanliness, presence of pests, or other conditions that impact horse health.

POSSIBLE COMPLICATIONS AND COMMON ERRORS TO BE AVOIDED

Minimize stress associated with transport, novel handling or housing, disrupting social bonds (eg, mare and foal), or environmental impacts such as very cold temperatures, wind, or rain.

PROCEDURE

- Recommendations for immediate care or treatment of horses should be discussed and presented in written form to the owner and any authorities. Less urgent recommendations can be written as an educational document to the owner or report to enforcement authorities.
- Initiate supportive nutritional programs. In severely starved horses, consider feeding small meals of alfalfa and withholding any soluble carbohydrates such as grain or concentrates to minimize "refeeding syndrome." (See "Nutrition: Refeeding the Starved Horse" in this section.)
- Provide medical treatment for severe injuries and disease conditions. Initiate appropriate nutritional programs. Minimize stressful conditions and handling.
- Perform or submit dead animals for necropsy with consideration to the following (Kronfeld, 1993):
  - Atrophy of fat depots occurs first with the coronary and perirenal adipose tissues, followed by the subcutaneous tissues, and then the abdominal fat depots. Muscle wasting occurs with prolonged starvation.
  - Parasites should be identified.
  - Tissues for histology should be submitted for liver and kidney, and when appropriate, thymus, pancreas, intestinal wall, or lymph nodes.
  - Other conditions, such as cancer (lymphoma) or adenoma, can be identified with necropsy.

POSTPROCEDURE

- Provide health programs, housing, and nutritional regimens appropriate to the needs of individual horses.
- Provide safe environment for horses.
- Initiate preventative health programs and any necessary state or federal disease monitoring and surveillance programs.
- Once a horse loses more than 50% of its body weight, the prognosis for survival is extremely poor. Horses that are recumbent for long periods of time are also poor candidates for nutritional rehabilitation.
- Some weight gain can be achieved in 1 month, but usually 3 to 6 months are needed to achieve normal body condition.

COMMENTS

- Safety: Safety is a concern for the veterinarian. Proceed with caution because the cause of neglect is unknown and the suspected perpetrator may be psychologically unstable. Do not trespass to help a horse, as this act may result in criminal charges, jeopardize your credibility, and damage any existing legal proceedings against the owner.
- Reporting neglect, abuse, or cruelty may be mandatory under some governmental authorities. If reporting is not compulsory, "good faith" reporting is warranted for the veterinary professional.
  - There is a strong connection between animal cruelty and human violence including child or spousal abuse. Reporting human abuse is mandatory under some governmental authorities. If not, veterinarians aware of suspicious circumstances should consider reporting to the proper agency. Social services may assist with an animal neglect case if there is suspected human violence or other human safety or health needs.

SUGGESTED READING

Kronfeld DS: Starvation and malnutrition of horses: recognition and treatment. *J Equine Vet Sci* 13(5):298–304, 1993.

Naylor JM, Kenyon SJ: Effect of total calorific deprivation on host defence in the horse. *Research Vet Sci* 31:369–372, 1981.

National Research Council (NRC): *Nutrient Requirements of Horses*, ed 6, Washington, DC, 2007, National Academy Press.

Solomon SM, Kirby DF: The re-feeding syndrome: a review. *J Parenteral Enteral Nutr* 14:90–97, 1990.

Witham CL, Stull CL: Metabolic responses of chronically starved horses to refeeding with three isoenergetic diets. *J Am Vet Med Assoc* 212(5):691–696, 1998.

Veterinary Medicine Extension Animal Welfare: http://www.vetmed.ucdavis.edu/vetext/animalwelfare/

AUTHOR: CAROLYN L. STULL

EDITOR: DANIEL J. BURKE

Nutrition: Parenteral

PROCEDURES AND TECHNIQUES

BASIC INFORMATION

SYNONYM(S)

PN
Partial parenteral nutrition (PPN)
Total parenteral nutrition (TPN)

OVERVIEW AND GOAL(S)

- Parenteral nutrition (PN) is nutritional support administered intravenously.
- The goal of PN is to supply a portion (PPN) or the horse's complete nutritional needs (TPN) to maintain hypermetabolic patients (ie, sepsis, burns) or caloric deficient patients (ie, gastrointestinal disease).
- The objective of PN is to reduce catabolism and the deleterious effects of malnutrition on immunity, wound healing, and survival rates

INDICATIONS

- Intravenous nutrition is indicated in diseases or disorders that prevent adequate intake or absorption of enteral feeds.
  - Gastrointestinal ileus (anterior enteritis, postoperative ileus)
  - Infectious or inflammatory bowel disease (necrotizing enterocolitis, salmonellosis)
  - Dysphagia (encephalopathy, botulism)
  - Hyperlipemia/insulin resistance (miniature horses, ponies, donkeys)
  - Concurrent pregnancy/lactation with systemic illness
  - Severe trauma/burns

CONTRAINDICATIONS

- If an animal is able to take in feed enterally, or will be fed within the next 5 days in adults (or next 2 days in foals), enteral feeding is preferred to PN to maintain enterocyte health.
- Thromboembolic disease or coagulation disorders may increase the risk of venous thrombosis.

EQUIPMENT, ANESTHESIA

- Catheter
  - Catheter material should be silicone or polyurethane to reduce risk of thrombosis.
  - A large vessel is required (typically the jugular vein) due to the hypertonicity of these solutions.
  - Multilumen catheters are preferred to allow the solution to enter through a dedicated catheter and line to reduce contamination and drug interactions without increasing the number of veins catheterized.
    - If a single jugular catheter is used, flush with 100 mL of fluid before and after medications.
  - All catheters should be placed under sterile conditions.
- Parenteral nutrient mixture
  - Amino acid mixture (3%–10% concentration) to supply a protein base
    - Hypertonic and basic (will irritate endothelium)
  - Carbohydrate source (dextrose 10%–50% solution) for a nonprotein energy source
    - Hyperosmolar: Dilute to <10% solution or infuse concurrently with crystalloids
    - May separate lipid emulsions due to an acidic pH
  - Lipid emulsion (10%–20%) provides additional (optional) calories, especially for insulin resistance.
    - Optional
    - Should be avoided in hyperlipemic states (triglycerides >300 g/dL)
  - Electrolytes may be supplied with the amino acids or provided separately in the fluids administered.
  - Fat-soluble vitamin and mineral parenteral admixtures may be added but typically are not needed if therapy will be administered for less than 2 weeks in duration.
- Fluid administration pumps are recommended for accurate delivery and to provide a constant infusion.
- Continuous monitoring by nurses is required to ensure catheter patency and PN delivery.

- Serum chemistry analysis to monitor electrolytes is indicated as needed by response to therapy (typically q6h until administration stabilized).
  - Electrolytes may require monitoring q6h initially.
  - Additional intermittent serum glucose (q2h initially) is recommended until administration rate stabilizes.
  - White blood cell counts are recommended every other day to monitor for infection.
  - Triglycerides should be assessed once a day initially, and then as needed.

ANTICIPATED TIME

PN is typically administered for 3 to 14 days.

PREPARATION: IMPORTANT CHECKPOINTS

- Due to the costs and complications of PN, PN solutions should be used only:
  - In adult horses that are anticipated to be anorexic >5 days
  - In foals held off oral feeding >48 hours
  - Those patients with severe catabolic issues in addition to their primary illness (pregnancy, lactation)

POSSIBLE COMPLICATIONS AND COMMON ERRORS TO BE AVOIDED

- Overfeeding is common due to hypometabolic state of most patients: Hyperglycemia, hyperlipemia, hypercapnia, and immune suppression may result.
  - For hyperglycemia: Reduce PN rate or supplement with insulin.
  - For hyperlipemia: Reduce or eliminate lipid emulsion.
- Fluid overload may result if intravenous fluids are not calculated to include the contribution from PN.
  - Adjustments must be made for each alteration in PN infusion rate.
  - Various electrolyte abnormalities may result and should be corrected by supplementing the crystalloids to

allow for rapid changes and reduce the risk of contamination.

- Catheter-related complications are common due to the hyperosmolality of PN.
  - Any suspect catheter (heat, swelling, discharge) should be replaced and the catheter tip cultured.

PROCEDURE

- Calculate the resting energy requirement (RER) for the horse.
  - Increased by surgery, trauma, sepsis, pregnancy, lactation
  - Decreased by hypometabolism, stall rest
    - Estimated at approximately 30 kcal/kg/day for adults.
    - >50 kcal/kg/day for a recumbent foal (increases to 75 kcal/kg/day or more for growth).
- Determine the proportion of protein in the PN.
  - Ideal is 4 to 6 g protein per 100 kcal digestible energy (calculated from RER).
  - Amino acids provide 4 kcal/g.
    - Divide protein calories desired by 4 kcal/g = grams amino acid required.
    - Divide the grams amino acid required by the concentration of the amino acid solution (g/mL solution) = volume (mL) amino acid solution required.
  - Additional cross-check: determine the percent nitrogen contribution to determine if protein content is adequate but not excessive.
    - Divide the sum of the dextrose and lipid calories by the grams of protein, divided by 6.35.
    - 6.35 g of protein provides 1 g of nitrogen.
      - Low ratio (100–150) indicates high protein (indicated for severe sepsis, trauma, burns).

- Moderate ratio (150) is moderate protein (indicated for growth, sepsis, catabolic states).
- High ratio (>200) indicates low protein (for liver disease, renal failure).
- Determine the proportion of carbohydrate in the PN.
  - Carbohydrates can comprise up to 60% of PN solution.
  - 50% dextrose provides 1.7 kcal/mL.
- Determine the proportion of lipids in the PN.
  - Lipids can comprise up to 70% of PN.
  - 20% lipids emulsions provide 2 kcal/mL.
- Determine if additional vitamins, minerals, or electrolytes will be added.
- Mix PN solution (sterile conditions if possible).
  - Mix amino aids and glucose first, then add lipids to prevent emulsion disruption.
- Determine the infusion rate by dividing by 24 hours.
  - Infusion rates generally start at a quarter to third of the total dose and gradually adjust to full rate over 12 to 24 hours.
  - For foals, the rate is typically started at RER of 50 kcal/kg/day and adjusted over 3 days to 75 kcal/kg/day, if possible.

POSTPROCEDURE

- PN solution may need modifications for disease.
  - Hypermetabolic disease states are often insulin resistant and protein deficient.
  - Cardiovascular disease may have reduced renal function and less tolerance to protein.
  - In hepatic dysfunction, fatty acids may increase free bilirubin, increas-

ing risk of kernicterus (bilirubin toxicity).
- Amino acid and glucose metabolism is altered.
- Renal disease may reduce the ability to clear amino acids.
- Solution should be changed every 24 hours if left at room temperature, and all administration lines should be replaced every 48 to 72 hours.
  - All lines should be handled with gloves and kept sterile (no injections into the PN line).
  - Solution should be mixed twice daily to prevent settling.
  - Protect from light to prevent amino acid and vitamin degradation and lipid peroxidation.
  - PN solutions may be stored at 4° C for 2 days.
- PN should be discontinued slowly, reduced by 25% at a time over 1 to 3 days, depending on duration of therapy,

ALTERNATIVES AND THEIR RELATIVE MERITS

Enteral feeding should be used, if possible, due to its beneficial nutritional effects on enterocytes, as well as its cost effectiveness.

SUGGESTED READING

Bercier DL: How to use parenteral nutrition in practice. *Proc Am Assoc Equine Pract* 49:268–273, 2003.

Beuchner-Maxwell VA: Nutritional support for neonatal foals. *Vet Clin North Am Equine Pract* 21:487–510, 2005.

Cruz AM, Cot N, McDonnell WN, et al: Postoperative effects of anesthesia and surgery on resting energy expenditure in horses as measured by indirect calorimetry. *Can J Vet Res* 70:257–262, 2006.

Hardy J: Nutritional support and nursing care of the adult horse in intensive care. *Clin Tech Eq Pract* 2(2):193–198, 2003.

AUTHOR: AMELIA MUNSTERMAN

Nutrition: Refeeding the Starved Horse

BASIC INFORMATION

SYNONYM(S)

Refeeding syndrome
Nutritional rehabilitation

OVERVIEW AND GOAL

- Starvation of horse(s) may be due to a variety of factors including lack of feed availability, illness or injury, or owner factors such as economic hardship, ignorance, apathy, illness or

injury, and possibly other crimes such as domestic violence.
- Causes of starvation: Multifactorial including (Kronfeld, 1993):
  - Lack of quantity and quality of feed, especially the nutrient content and balance of energy and protein. Deficiencies or excesses of certain minerals and vitamins over the long-term can contribute to malnutrition and/or emaciation.
  - Seasonal declines in the primary feed source such as pasture.

- Malabsorption of nutrients associated with diarrhea, poor dental function, or geriatric condition.
- Parasites can be either a primary or secondary contributor to starvation/emaciation.

INDICATIONS

- Conditions such as lactation, pregnancy, or old age may increase dietary requirements.
- Pathologic conditions such as cancer, insulin resistance, infections, or

diseases of the liver, kidney, pancreas, or heart can elicit symptoms associated with emaciation.

- Salmonellosis and other bacterial infections may occur due to the compromised immune system and starvation.
- Loss of body weight, with body condition scores less than 2.5 on a 9-point scale

PREPARATION: IMPORTANT CHECKPOINTS

- Physical examination should be performed; symptoms of the starved horse over time include:
  - Behavioral changes with a depressed reactivity to external stimuli occurs usually 3 to 4 days to a week after the severe restriction of feed (Kronfeld, 1993).
  - Immune compromise occurs 3 to 4 days after total feed deprivation, with a decrease in circulating lymphocyte count and a compromise in phagocytic response.
  - Body weight loss becomes noticeable after 1 to 2 weeks of feed deprivation. Assign and document body condition score.
    - Injuries should be documented along with their location and severity.
    - Evaluate existing parasite control program and dental condition.
    - History of the horse in the preceding weeks or months should be acquired through discussion with the owner/caregiver.
    - Body condition or weight should be assessed on the initial visit and at weekly intervals during rehabilitation (see "Body Condition Score" in this section).
      - Heart girth tapes measure the circumference of the heart girth size, which will decrease with losses in body condition.
      - Scales provide the most accurate body weight measurement.
- Document the availability of water and the amount and condition of feed accessible to the horses and stored on premises; note consumption or refusal of offered feed.
- No single or group of laboratory tests have been identified to confirm starvation. Elevated free fatty acids in plasma, compromised serum electrolyte concentrations, and depressed red blood cell indices are supportive of a long-term starved state, but not exclusively.
  - Perform or submit dead animals for necropsy with consideration to the following (Kronfeld, 1993):
    - Atrophy of fat depots occurs first with the coronary and perirenal adipose tissues, followed by the subcutaneous tissues, and then the abdominal fat depots. Muscle wasting occurs with prolonged starvation.
    - Parasite identification; pathologic conditions, such as cancer (lymphoma) or adenoma.

POSSIBLE COMPLICATIONS AND COMMON ERRORS TO BE AVOIDED

Mild hypophosphatemia may develop during the first 10 days of refeeding of alfalfa diets but will be more severe with greater carbohydrate intake. Severe hypophosphatemia limits cell metabolism in red blood cells and leads to impaired oxygen delivery to tissues. Cardiac and respiratory failure may result in death usually in the first 10 days of refeeding.

PROCEDURE

- Minimize stress associated with transport, novel handling or housing, disrupting social bonds (eg, mare and foal), or environmental impacts such as very cold temperatures, wind, or rain.
- Initiate preventative health programs and any necessary state or federal disease monitoring and surveillance programs.
- A physical exam prior to an exercise/riding program is advisable to ascertain any organ (eg, heart) damage.

NUTRITIONAL MANAGEMENT

THERAPEUTIC GOAL(S)

Abrupt refeeding of starved horses may cause death in 3 days due to severe hypophosphatemia, hypomagnesemia, and/or hypokalemia. Initiate supportive nutritional programs in severely starved horses by frequent small meals of high-quality forage diet and withholding any soluble carbohydrates such as grain or concentrates to minimize the postprandial insulin and glucose effects that contribute to the "refeeding syndrome."

DIETARY ASSESSMENT

- Select palatable, high-quality forage such as alfalfa. Alfalfa hay is more supportive than oat hay in refeeding starved horses because of the greater content of phosphorous and magnesium (Witham and Stull, 1998).
- Limit or eliminate all concentrates or other high carbohydrate feeds, which may stimulate the release of insulin. Release of insulin causes influx into cells of glucose, phosphorous, potassium, and other electrolytes. Hypophosphatemia results because there is a depletion of total body phosphorous during starvation along with the intracellular shift of phosphorous during refeeding.

- Supplementing corn oil with forage diets does not prevent or minimize hypophosphatemia or hypomagnesemia during the initial 10 days of refeeding starved horses (Stull et al, 2003).

SPECIFIC NUTRIENTS TO BE ADDRESSED

- High-quality leafy forage (eg, alfalfa) that is low in starch (3%), high in crude protein (20%), and high in phosphorous and magnesium content is supportive of a refeeding program.
- High-fiber forage such as oat hay (crude fiber 28%) is bulky and may cause diarrhea. Also, oat hay is low in magnesium and phosphorous content, thus not supportive of successful rehabilitation.

RECOMMENDED DIETS

- Provide clean, fresh water ad libitum.
- Small frequent meals are offered initially because gastric volume and emptying time and absorptive capability may be compromised.
- The following table is based on a horse with a projected normal weight of 1000 pounds and alfalfa hay (digestible energy 2.28 Mcal/kg):

Day	Number of Meals/Day	Feed (lb)/Meal	% DE/Day
Days 1–3	6 (every 4 hours)	1.0–1.25 lb alfalfa	50
Days 4–5	6 (every 4 hours)	1.75–2.0 lb	75
Days 6–10	3 (every 8 hours)	Increase to 5 lb	100

DE, Digestible energy.

- Do not add concentrates (grain) for several months or until the horse has achieved a body condition score of 3.5 to 4 (out of a possible 9) or more.

POSTPROCEDURE

- The nutritional program of starved horses should be carefully monitored for 10 days since most serious complications from refeeding syndrome develop within the first 5 days of refeeding.
- Monitoring serum electrolytes, especially phosphorous and magnesium, during the initial refeeding period may assist in evaluating rehabilitation progress and detecting deficiencies.
- Once a horse loses more than 50% of its body weight, the prognosis for survival is extremely poor. Horses that are recumbent for long periods of time, are also poor candidates for nutritional rehabilitation.
- Some weight gain can be achieved in 1 month, but usually 3 to 6 months are needed to achieve normal body condition.

- Deworming and correcting dental problems will enhance prognosis.

SUGGESTED READING

Kronfeld DS: Starvation and malnutrition of horses: recognition and treatment. *J Equine Vet Sci* 13(5):298–304, 1993.
National Research Council: Nutrient requirements of horses, rev ed 6, Washington, DC, 2007, National Academy Press.

Solomon SM, Kirby DF: The re-feeding syndrome: a review. *J Parenteral Enteral Nut* 14:90–97, 1990.
Stull CL, Hullinger PJ, Rodiek AV: Fat supplementation to alfalfa diets for refeeding the starved horse. *Prof Anim Scientist* 19(1):47–54, 2003.
Witham CL, Stull CL: Metabolic responses of chronically starved horses to refeeding with three isoenergetic diets. *J Am Vet Med Assoc* 212(5):691–696, 1998.
Veterinary Medicine Extension Animal Welfare: http://www.vetmed.ucdavis.edu/vetext/animalwelfare/

AUTHOR: **CAROLYN L. STULL**

EDITOR: **DANIEL J. BURKE**

Nutrition: Supplements

BASIC INFORMATION

SYNONYM(S)

Animal dietary supplements
Nutraceuticals
Food supplement
Nutritional supplement
Functional foods

OVERVIEW AND GOAL(S)

- As defined by National Research Council (NRC, 2009), an animal dietary supplement is a substance for oral consumption by horses, whether in or on feed offered separately, intended for specific benefit to the animal by means other than provision of nutrients recognized as essential, or for provision of essential nutrients for intended effect on the animal beyond normal nutritional needs, but not including legally defined drugs.
- Ingredients in animal dietary supplements include but are not limited to:
  ○ Herbs and other botanicals
  ○ Extracts and concentrates
  ○ Enzymes and metabolites
  ○ Organ glandular tissues
  ○ Vitamins, minerals, and amino acids (provided above known nutrient requirements)

REGULATION OF DIETARY SUPPLEMENTS IN THE UNITED STATES

- There are currently no laws and regulations that address animal dietary supplements as a specific group or entity.
- Animal dietary supplements are typically regulated as "food" under the Federal Food, Drug, and Cosmetic Act; however, there are plans to regulate some animal dietary supplements as drugs.
- The 1994 Dietary Supplement Health and Education Act applies to the regulation of dietary supplements for use by humans but not for use by animals.
- At the state level, the Association of American Feed Control Officials (AAFCO) is charged with the regulation of animal feeds.
- All ingredients in animal feeds must be codified as GRAS (generally recognized as safe), approved food additives, or otherwise sanctioned for use in animal feed.
- Many animal dietary supplements contain ingredients that do not meet the legal requirements to be marketed as foods or drugs.
- Animal dietary supplements cannot claim that they can be used to diagnose, prevent, mitigate, treat, or cure disease; products that make such claims are considered to be illegal drugs by the Food and Drug Administration (FDA).

SAFETY OF DIETARY SUPPLEMENTS

- Very few of the ingredients commonly included in animal dietary supplements have undergone adequate testing to determine their safety for use in horses.
- Proof of reasonable assurances of safety are required for food additives, new food ingredients, and drugs, but proof of safety is not currently enforced for animal dietary supplements.
- GRAS designation of an ingredient signifies safety only under specified conditions of use (eg, amount fed, intended use in food, species fed).
- Although an ingredient may be "all natural" or have GRAS status, it can still be toxic.
- At present, there are no federal- or state-enforced good manufacturing practices applicable to animal dietary supplements; thus they may be contaminated, adulterated, or mislabeled.
- The National Animal Supplement Council (NASC) is a private, nonprofit, self-regulated organization representing paid members who manufacture animal health supplements.
- NASC has set standards for manufacturing, labeling, and adverse event reporting for their membership in an effort to improve supplement quality.
- Membership in or registration of an animal dietary supplement with NASC does not guarantee the safety of that product when administered to horses.

REDUCING THE RISK OF ADVERSE EVENTS FROM ANIMAL DIETARY SUPPLEMENTS

- Evaluate the risks and benefits of including animal dietary supplements in treatment protocols.
- Recommend the use of dietary supplements only when deemed necessary.
- Select from animal dietary supplements manufactured by reputable companies who have conducted safety analyses on their products in horses.
- Encourage clients to fully disclose all supplements and medications administered to their horses to more accurately evaluate propensity for negative interactions.
- Educate clients on the proper administration of all animal dietary supplements, as well as monitor clinical signs that may indicate negative reactions to the supplement.
- Report any adverse events—no matter how minor—to the dietary supplement manufacturer and/or the Poison Control Center of the American Humane Society.
- Do not use an ineffective animal dietary supplement in lieu of using an approved drug that could reasonably be expected to lead to a cure or amelioration of a disease.

SUGGESTED READING

National Research Council (NRC): *Safety of dietary supplements for horses, dogs, and cats*, Washington, DC, 2009, National Academy Press.

AUTHOR: **LORI K. WARREN**

EDITOR: **DANIEL J. BURKE**

Nutrition: Total Diet Assessment

BASIC INFORMATION

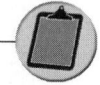

OVERVIEW AND GOAL(S)

- It is important to realize that forages (hay and pasture) provide a significant portion of the horse's daily nutrient requirements. Proper nutritional principles require that we recognize the contribution of forages and adjust the concentrate (grain) portion of the diet accordingly to meet the horse's requirements. Recommending a feed and/or supplement without assessing the total diet may adversely affect the horse's health and performance.
- Thus selection of the concentrate and/or supplement should be based on the forage being fed and supply the portion of the horse's requirements not met by that forage. Furthermore, adding supplements to the horse's diet is more a rule than an exception in today's horse industry. So understanding how to assess the total diet is the responsible path to follow.

KEY POINTS

- All feedstuffs offered to horses have some level of most nutrients.
- Horses typically consume more forage than concentrate (grains). Consider the contribution of forage to meeting the horse's requirements.
- Certain nutrient requirements may be met by the forage alone.
- One must understand what the forage is providing before designing or selecting the appropriate concentrate.
- The nutrient requirements of the horse are determined by the National Research Council (NRC) Committee on Horse Nutrition (2007).

PROCEDURE

DETERMINING TOTAL INTAKE

- Total intake is determined by calculating the amount of each nutrient that is supplied by all feeds offered to the horse—hay, pasture, grain, and supplements.
- Commercial software programs are available to perform these calculations and compare the results to NRC 2007 requirements without the tedious calculations outlined later.
- NOTE: Calculations for nutrients whose requirements are not addressed by NRC 2007 will be the same as described here, but the relevance is more subjective. Nutrients such as starch, sugar (nonstructural carbohydrates [NSC] = sugar + starch), acid detergent fiber (ADF), neutral deter-

gent fiber (NDF), lignin, and ash may have value, but no established requirements exist.

- Values for certain vitamins, minerals, and amino acids are often listed on feed tags, but assessing the relevance is purely speculation when no requirement has been established.
- Nutrient concentration values for forages can be obtained most accurately by laboratory analysis, but NRC and other database values can be used in lieu of laboratory analyses.
- Most laboratories have information on proper sampling techniques for hay, pasture, and concentrates. Valid results are only obtained when proper sampling techniques are followed.
- Nutrient concentration values for grains, concentrates, and supplements will be found on the product labeling but can also be submitted for laboratory analysis. Take care to note possible differences in label concentrations with respect to feeding recommendations, especially with supplements. Supplement concentrations are often listed as "per pound," but feeding recommendations are in ounces or grams.

In general, how is the amount of nutrient supplied by a feed calculated?

$$\text{Amount of feed being fed (pounds or kilograms)}$$

$$\times$$

$$\text{Concentration of that nutrient in the feed (ie, \% or mg/kg)}$$

Charts 1 to 4 demonstrate the contribution of grass or legume hay to meeting the NRC 2007 nutrient requirements of either an idle, mature horse or a lactating mare. As you can see, the gap between the NRC requirement (depicted as the "100%" line) and what is supplied by the forages varies with the type of animal and the forage source.

SPECIFIC CALCULATIONS

- Assessing digestible energy (DE) supplied
  - DE concentration of a feed is expressed in a forage analysis or on a feed tag as Mcal/lb or Mcal/kg with daily requirement expressed as Mcal.
  - The amount of DE in Mcal supplied by a feed is:

$$\text{Mcal/lb} \times \text{lb of feed} = \text{Mcal}$$

or

$$\text{Mcal/kg} \times \text{kg of feed} = \text{Mcal}$$

- Example: A client is feeding 15 pounds (6.8 kg) of a grass hay with a digestible energy (DE) of 0.8 Mcal/lb (1.76 Mcal/kg.).
  - The amount of DE in Mcal supplied by a feed is:

$$0.8 \text{ Mcal/lb} \times 15 \text{ lb of hay} = 12 \text{ Mcal}$$

or

$$1.76 \text{ Mcal/kg} \times 6.8 \text{ kg of feed} = 12 \text{ Mcal}$$

- Assessing crude protein, lysine, calcium, phosphorous, magnesium, potassium, sodium, chlorine, or sulfur supplied
  - The concentration of these nutrients in a feed is expressed in a forage analysis or on a feed tag as a percent with daily requirement expressed as grams.
  - The amount of these nutrients in grams supplied by a feed is:

$$\% \text{ nutrient (as decimal)} \times \text{lb of feed} \times 454 \text{ g/lb} = \text{grams}$$

or

$$\% \text{ nutrient (as decimal)} \times \text{kg of feed} \times 1000 \text{ g/kg} = \text{grams}$$

- Example: A client is feeding 5 pounds (2.3 kg) of a grain mix that is 1.2% calcium. The amount of calcium in grams supplied by this feed is:

$$0.012 \text{ (decimal for 1.2\% Ca)} \times 5 \text{ lb of feed} \times 454 \text{ g/lb} = 27 \text{ g}$$

or

$$0.012 \text{ (decimal for 1.2\% Ca)} \times 2.3 \text{ kg of feed} \times 1000 \text{ g/kg} = 27 \text{ g}$$

- Assessing cobalt, copper, iodine, iron, manganese, selenium, zinc, thiamine, or riboflavin supplied
  - The concentration of these nutrients in a feed is expressed in a forage analysis or on a feed tag as parts per million (ppm) or mg/kg with daily requirement expressed as mg.
  - The amount of these nutrients in mg supplied by a feed is:

$$\text{mg/kg (or ppm)} \times (\text{lb feed}/2.2 \text{ lb/kg}) = \text{mg}$$

or

$$\text{mg/kg (or ppm)} \times \text{kg of feed} = \text{mg}$$

- Example: A client is feeding 2 lb (0.91 kg) of a supplement with a copper concentration of 200 mg/kg. The amount of copper in mg supplied by this feed is:

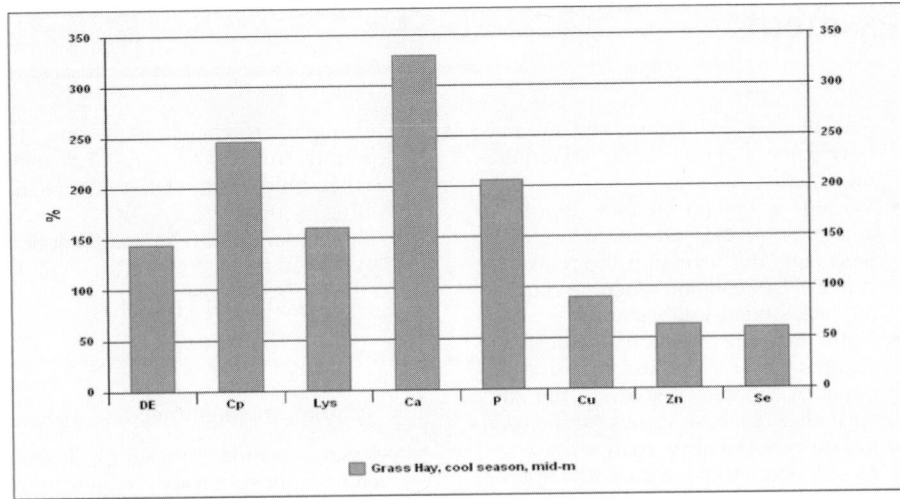

Nutrients Supplied by Ingredient as Percent of Daily Requirements

Grass Hay, cool season, mid-m

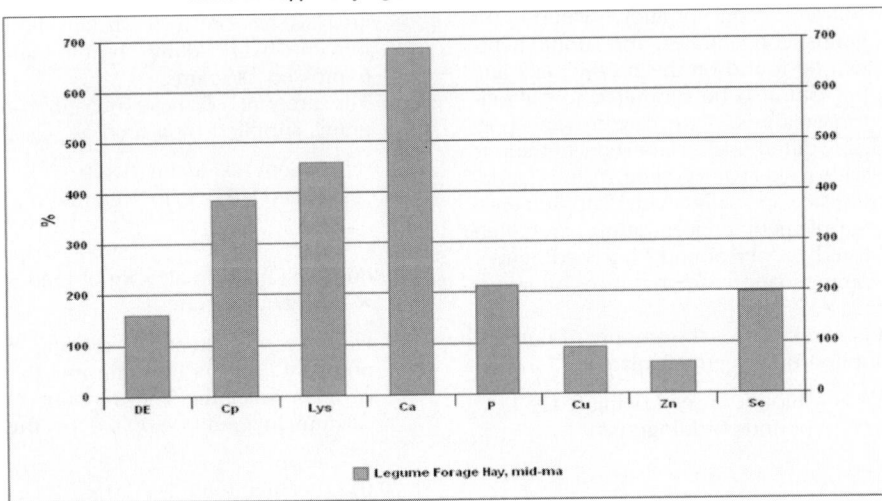

Nutrients Supplied by Ingredient as Percent of Daily Requirements

Legume Forage Hay, mid-ma

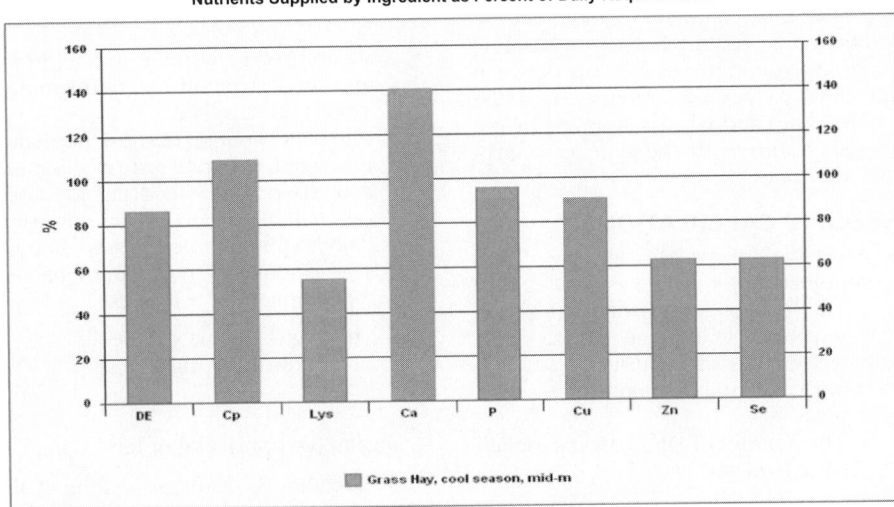

Nutrients Supplied by Ingredient as Percent of Daily Requirements

Grass Hay, cool season, mid-m

200 mg/kg (or ppm) × (2 lb feed/2.2 lb/kg) = 182 mg

or

200 mg/kg (or ppm) × 0.91 kg of feed = 182 mg

- Assessing vitamin A, D, or E supplied
  - The concentration of vitamins D and E in a feed is expressed in a forage analysis (very seldom are vitamins included in forage analysis due to the expense) or on a feed tag as International Units (IU)/lb with daily requirement expressed as IU. Vitamin A requirement is listed as kIU (IU × 1000).
  - The amount of vitamin A, D, or E in IU supplied by a feed is:

    IU/lb × lb feed = IU

    or

    IU/lb × (kg of feed × 2.2 lb/kg) = IU

  - Example: A client is feeding 5 pounds of a concentrate with a Vitamin A concentration of 4,000 IU (4 kIU)/lb.
  - The amount of vitamin A in IU supplied by this feed is:

    4,000 IU/lb × 5 lb feed = 20,000 IU (20 kIU)

    or

    4,000 IU/lb × (2.3 kg of feed × 2.2 lb/kg) = 20,000 IU (20 kIU)

- Using the above calculations or a software program, include assessment for all nutrients of interest for the forage, concentrate/grain, as well as any supplements provided to the horse. Total the amounts for each feed and compare to the horse's requirement in NRC 2007.
- For specific nutrient requirements of horses see *NRC Nutrient Requirements of Horses,* 6th edition. The NRC model program is available online at http://nrc88.nas.edu/nrh/ and can be used to generate requirements for specific classes of horses.
- Many horse owners only concern themselves with the concentration of a nutrient, especially protein and starch, without regard to the amount of the feed offered to the horse.
- As one can appreciate, the concentration of a nutrient is only one step in the analysis: By varying concentration and amount, the horse's requirement can be met by feeds with higher nutrient concentrations by feeding less feed or vice versa.

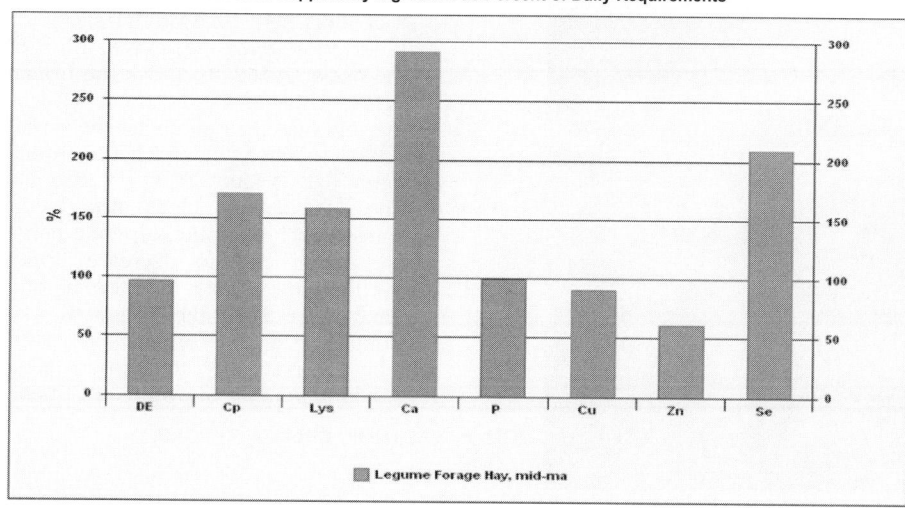

Nutrients Supplied by Ingredient as Percent of Daily Requirements

Legume Forage Hay, mid-ma

SUMMARY

- Proper nutritional guidance can only be offered when the total diet of the horse is considered.

- Include assessment of all sources of nutrients offered to the horse, including forages, concentrates, and supplements.

- Overfeeding most nutrients is, at a minimum, wasteful, but it can also affect the health and general well-being of the horse.
- Commercial ration evaluation software:
  - Creative Formulations Concepts, LLC. Horse Ration Formulation — 2007, 1831 Forest Drive, Suite H, Annapolis, MD 21401, http://www.agri-data.com/.
  - Equi Balance Software, Performance Horse Nutrition, 967 Haas Road, Weiser, ID 83672, http://www.performancehorsenutrition.com/.

SUGGESTED READING

National Research Council: Nutrient Requirements of horses, rev ed 6, Washington, DC, 2007, National Academy Press.

AUTHOR AND EDITOR: **DANIEL J. BURKE**

Ocular Nerve Blocks: Standard

BASIC INFORMATION

SYNONYM(S)

Palpebral nerve blocks
Frontal nerve blocks

OVERVIEW AND GOAL(S)

Because of the strength of the horse's periocular muscles, palpebral and/or frontal nerve denervation (nerve block) with lidocaine or mepivacaine (or equivalent) is required to enable the veterinarian to thoroughly examine the eyes.

INDICATIONS

Complete examination of the eye of the horse

CONTRAINDICATIONS

Known sensitivity to lidocaine or mepivacaine (or similar medication)

EQUIPMENT, ANESTHESIA

- Lidocaine HCL (2.0%) or mepivacaine HCL (2.0%) (or similar medication)
- 25-gauge needles
- 3-mL syringes

ANTICIPATED TIME

Approximately 5 minutes

PREPARATION: IMPORTANT CHECKPOINTS

The best tranquilizer for ophthalmic procedures in the horse is detomidine HCL

(0.01–0.02 mg/kg IV). This medication has a rapid onset and is effective for 30 to 45 minutes. The major advantage of this drug is that during its effect the horse's head remains still and does not tremor.

POSSIBLE COMPLICATIONS AND COMMON ERRORS TO BE AVOIDED

Complications include:
- Hypersensitivity reactions to medications

- Infections due to needlesticks
- Possible ocular or eyelid trauma due to poorly restrained or tranquilized horses

PROCEDURE

- The palpebral nerve is a branch of the facial nerve that controls the motor activity of the upper orbicularis oculi muscle, which controls upper eyelid function. To adequately block the palpebral nerve, 2 mL of 2% lidocaine HCL is injected subcutaneously along the dorsal zygomatic arch (Figure 1).

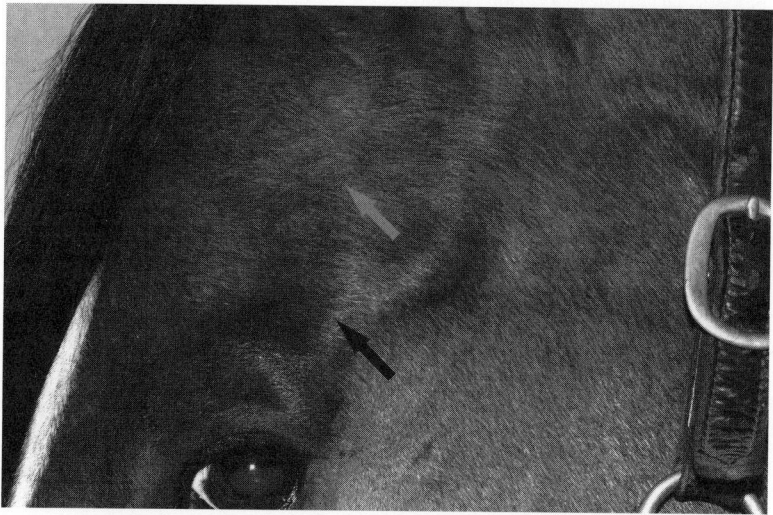

FIGURE 1 Location of the palpebral nerve injection site.

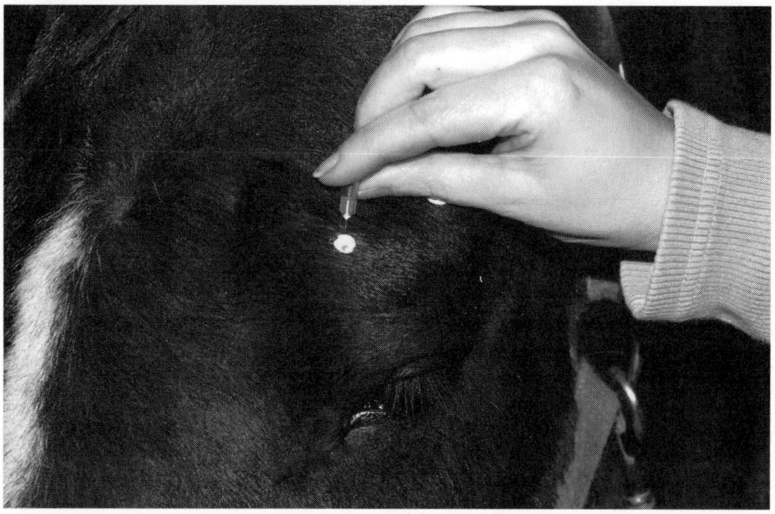

FIGURE 2 Location of the frontal nerve (supraorbital foramen) injection site.

- The frontal nerve is the branch of the trigeminal nerve that provides sensory innervation to the medial two-thirds of the upper eyelid. To block the frontal nerve, 1 mL of 2% lidocaine HCL is injected over the opening to the supra-orbital foramen, in which the frontal nerve exits (Figure 2).
- The frontal nerve block also denervates branches of the palpebral nerve and thus helps to decrease upper eyelid motor activity; therefore a combination of both the palpebral and frontal nerve block provides an excellent denervation to the upper eyelid resulting in minimal eyelid movement.

AUTHOR: **BRIAN C. GILGER**

Ocular Surgery: Standing

BASIC INFORMATION

SYNONYM(S)

Ocular surgery without general anesthesia in the horse

OVERVIEW AND GOAL(S)

- There are many advantages to performing standing surgical procedures and avoiding general anesthesia in horses.
  - Horses with orthopedic or other medical problems may be at higher risk to develop anesthesia-related complications and should not undergo routine general anesthesia.
  - Even healthy horses can injure themselves on recovery from general anesthesia and are predisposed to develop colic, cecal impactions, and myositis in the postanesthetic period.
  - Standing surgical procedures can also decrease the time needed for hospitalization compared to horses receiving general anesthesia. This is advantageous because hospitalized horses, in general, are predisposed to developing pneumonia, laminitis, salmonellosis or other forms of colitis, and laminitis.
  - Therefore learning the correct and latest methods for performing standing ocular surgery will increase a veterinarian's ability to provide excellent service without a major outlay of infrastructure expense.

- Because the cornea and conjunctiva of the horse's eye are thin and delicate, ophthalmic surgery must be precise to avoid damage.
  - The use of small instruments, needles, and suture is generally required.
  - In most instances, the surgeon will benefit from the use of magnification, which allows precise cutting of tissues and suture placement but exaggerates patient movement when the horse is not anesthetized.
  - To perform ocular microsurgery, the eye must be immobile. In general, the use of microsurgical technique and magnification during equine ocular surgery requires general anesthesia. However, with appropriate tranquilization, ocular nerve blocks (especially the retrobulbar nerve block) and restraint, many ocular surgeries can be performed adequately in standing horses.
  - The purpose of this chapter is to describe the equipment needed and technique for performing ocular surgical procedures in the standing horse.

INDICATIONS

Surgical procedures that can be done with the horse standing include those involving the eyelids, conjunctiva, and cornea (tumor removal, keratectomy, eyelid laceration, third eyelid removal) that take less than 30 minutes to perform). Also, minimally invasive intraocular pro-

cedures such as iris cyst laser disruption, laser cyclophotocoagulation, or anterior chamber centesis can be performed adequately with the horse standing.

CONTRAINDICATIONS

Surgeries for perforating lesions of the cornea (or lesions pending perforation, such as corneal descemetoceles or infected deep corneal ulcers) or intraocular surgical procedures such as cataract surgery

EQUIPMENT, ANESTHESIA

- Lidocaine HCL (2.0%) or mepivacaine HCL (2.0%) (or similar medication)
- 25-gauge needles
- 3-mL syringes
- 22-gauge 2.5-inch spinal needle
- 1% Proparacaine HCL

ANTICIPATED TIME

Approximately 30 minutes

PREPARATION: IMPORTANT CHECKPOINTS

- The best tranquilizer for ophthalmic procedures in the horse is detomidine HCL (0.01–0.02 mg/kg IV). This medication has a rapid onset and is effective for 30 to 45 minutes. The major advantage of this drug is that during its effect the horse's head remains still and does not tremor.
- Use of xylazine and/or butorphanol should be avoided because each causes head movement and exaggerated response to stimuli.

POSSIBLE COMPLICATIONS AND COMMON ERRORS TO BE AVOIDED

Complications include:

- Hypersensitivity reactions to medications
- Infections due to needlesticks
- Possible ocular or eyelid trauma due to poorly restrained or tranquilized horses

PROCEDURE

Palpebral and frontal nerve blocks should be performed as previously described.

- Retrobulbar nerve block:
  - The orbital fossa above the dorsal orbital rim and zygomatic arch is first clipped and aseptically prepped with Povidone-iodine scrub and alcohol. Care must be taken to avoid getting surgical scrub or alcohol on the ocular surface because severe irritation and corneal ulceration may develop.
  - Once prepped, a 22-gauge, 2.5-inch spinal needle is placed through the skin perpendicular to the skull, in the orbital fossa, just posterior to the posterior aspect of the boney dorsal orbital rim.
  - The needle is advanced posterior to the globe until it reaches the retrobulbar orbital cone. When the needle advances to this location, the eye will have a slight dorsal movement as the needle passes through the fascia of the dorsal retrobulbar cone into the retrobulbar space (Figure 1).
  - Once positioned, 10 to 12 mL of 2% lidocaine HCL is injected into the retrobulbar space. During the injection, the globe is pushed externally (ie, slight exophthalmos) indicating an accurate placement of lidocaine. The lidocaine will take effect and anesthetize the eye in 5 to 10 minutes. The duration of effect is approximately 1 to 2 hours.
- Application of topical medications:
  - Once the retrobulbar block has been given, cultures of the ocular surface should be done, if needed, prior to surgical preparation of the globe (if indicated).
  - Topical anesthetic (0.2 mL of 0.5% proparacaine HCL) and 2.5% phenylephrine are applied to enhance ocular surface anesthesia and to constrict blood vessels in the cornea and conjunctiva to enhance hemostasis and visibility during surgery.
  - The topical medications can be repeated every 15 to 20 minutes as needed to maintain effect.
- Surgical procedures:
  - After following the above steps, the eye is now prepared for surgery. A list of possible ocular surgical procedures that can be done in a standing horse is listed in Table 1.
  - Use of a twitch or other manual restraint is rarely required because the eye is anesthetized; however, certain horses do require additional restraint methods, such as use of a twitch, or additional intravenous tranquilizer, especially when the preparation and procedure lasts longer than 30 to 40 minutes.
- When the appropriate nerve blocks and procedures are done as described in the methods, the eye will be immobile during the surgery.
  - The retractor oculi muscles will be paralyzed so that the eye cannot be retracted and therefore the third eyelid will not move anteriorly.
  - Visual and tactile stimuli will be reduced because the optic nerve and ophthalmic branch of the trigeminal nerve are anesthetized. This reduces stimuli to the horse and decreases induced head and body movements.
  - This lack of movement of the eye allows the surgeon to adequately perform short ocular microsurgical procedures.

POSTPROCEDURE

- Because the eye is anesthetized after the nerve blocks, sensation, blink reflex, and vision will also be compromised. Therefore stall rest and protection of the eye with lubricants is recommended for 2 to 4 hours after anesthesia.
- If the horse must be transported soon after the procedure or will not be monitored closely, a single temporary tarsorrhaphy suture can be placed laterally to protect the eye for the first 24 hours after surgery.
- Other medications, such as topical ophthalmic antibiotics, topical atropine, and oral nonsteroidal antiinflammatory medications are prescribed frequently after ocular surgery. The frequency and duration depends on the severity and type of the ocular condition.

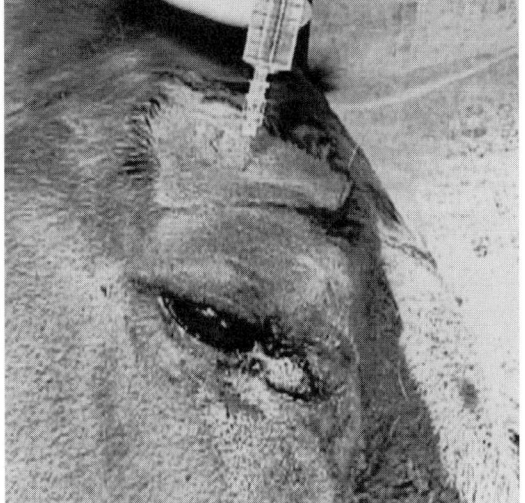

FIGURE 1 Location for the retrobulbar nerve block.

TABLE 1 Ocular Surgical Procedures That May Be Done in a Standing Horse

Adnexal	Corneal	Intraocular
Small eyelid mass removal	Corneal scraping for cytology	Aqueocentesis
Eyelid mass biopsy	Ulcer debridement	Intraocular injection (ie, TPA)
Eyelid lacerations—small	Grid keratotomy	Iris cyst laser ablation
Conjunctival biopsy	Superficial keratectomy—small	Laser cyclophotocoagulation for glaucoma
Third eyelid laceration repair	Suture of non-perforating corneal laceration	Intraocular mass laser ablation
Third eyelid mass removal or biopsy	Removal of superficial corneal foreign body	

AUTHOR: **BRIAN C. GILGER**

Oocyte Transfer

BASIC INFORMATION

OVERVIEW AND GOAL

- Transfer of mature oocytes from a donor into the oviduct of a recipient for their in vivo fertilization and development until the uterine stage (compact morulae or early blastocysts).
- Blastocysts are collected and transferred to other recipients to establish pregnancy or are collected (morula and early blastocyst) for cryopreservation.

INDICATIONS

- Postmortem salvage of oocytes
  - Mare death or euthanasia
- Mares with severe reproductive problems preventing ovulation, fertilization, or early embryo development
  - Persistent mate-induced endometritis
  - Oviduct function failure (salpingitis, oviductal blockage)
  - Ovulation failure (eg, repeated anovulatory hemorrhagic follicle)
  - Repeatedly unsuccessful embryo collection.
  - Cervical compromise
  - Pyometra

EQUIPMENT, ANESTHESIA

- Sedation: Detomidine
- Aspirating cannula or transvaginal aspirating 12-gauge needle (with sector ultrasound probe and needle guide)
- Follicular lavage system

PREPARATION: IMPORANT CHECKPOINTS

Mare preparation: See "Artificial Insemination: Uterine Body" in this section.

POSSIBLE COMPLICATIONS AND COMMON ERRORS TO BE AVOIDED

- Less than 0.1% risk of rectal tears, peritonitis, hemorrhage, ovarian abscess, oviductal damage, and mild colic. Ovarian fibrosis occurs, but ovarian function remains normal.
- Higher risk of postbreeding endometritis in oocyte recipients.
- Some preovulatory follicles located on the medial aspect of the ovary may be difficult to aspirate by flank transcutaneous aspiration.

PROCEDURE

- Oocyte aspiration:
  - Transvaginal ultrasound-guided aspiration under standing sedation is the preferred technique. Transabdominal percutaneous oocyte aspiration is also possible.
  - Large and palpable preovulatory follicles can be collected through a cannula (flank aspiration) or a transvaginal ultrasound-guided aspiration needle with follicular lavage media.
  - Oocyte collection success rates range from 65% to 75%.
  - Oocytes are very fragile and sensitive to temperature variations. They must be handled and transported with maximum care to maintain viability under field collection conditions.
  - The best pregnancy rates are achieved with preovulatory follicles. Depending on the laboratory, oocytes are collected 20 to 36 hours after human chorionic gonadotropin administration. Fertile stallions with high-quality semen are recommended for oocyte transfer to optimize success rates.
- Oocyte transfer:
  - Similar pregnancy rates are achieved with cyclic and acyclic recipient mares.
  - Recipients are ideally inseminated 12 to 16 hours before oocyte transfer.
  - As the recipient mare is inseminated, her own oocyte must be removed.
  - Oocyte transfer is performed through a standing flank laparotomy approach. The ovary is exposed through the incision, the oviduct localized, and the oocytes transferred into the oviduct using a pipette.

POSTPROCEDURE

- A pregnancy rate greater than 35% is achievable with oocyte transfer in young mares; overall success rate is 25%.
- A pregnancy rate of 30% has been reported for oocyte aspirations performed on euthanized mares.
- Oocytes may be cryopreserved for subsequent fertilization. However, success rates are still too low to offer this technique on a commercial basis.
- Monitor postbreeding endometritis in oocyte recipients.

SUGGESTED READING

Alvarenga MA, Da Cruz Landim-Alvarenga F: New assisted reproductive techniques applied for the horse industry. In Samper JC, editor: *Equine breeding management and artificial insemination*, ed 2, St Louis, 2009, Elsevier, pp 209–221.

Carnevale EM: Clinical considerations regarding assisted reproductive procedures in horses. *J Equine Vet Sci* 28:686–690, 2008.

Carnevale EM, Maclellan LJ: Collection, evaluation, and use of oocytes in equine assisted reproduction. *Vet Clin North Am Equine Pract* 22:843–856, 2006.

Colleoni S, Barbacini S, Necchi D, et al: Application of ovum pick-up, intracytoplasmic sperm injection and embryo culture in equine practice. *Proc Am Assoc Equine Pract* 53:554–559, 2007.

AUTHORS: **FRANÇOIS-XAVIER GRAND** and **REJEAN CLÉOPHAS LEFEBVRE**

Ophthalmic Examination

BASIC INFORMATION

SYNONYM(S)

Eye examination of the horse

OVERVIEW AND GOAL(S)

Appropriate diagnostic methods to examine equine eyes are reviewed and described.

INDICATIONS

- Complete examination of the eye of the horse
- Routine physical examination
- Examination of ocular disease
- Prepurchase examination

CONTRAINDICATIONS

- Known sensitivity to lidocaine or mepivacaine (or similar medication)
- Tropicamide HCL, proparacaine HCL, or any contraindications for ocular mydriasis (ie, presence of glaucoma, lens luxation)

EQUIPMENT, ANESTHESIA

- Medications:
  - Lidocaine HCL (2.0%) or mepivacaine HCL (2.0%) (or similar medication)
  - Tropicamide HCL (1.0%)
  - Proparacaine HCL (0.5%)
- Equipment:
  - 25-gauge needles
  - 3-mL syringes
  - Bright, focal light source: A Finnoff transilluminator is ideal
  - Direct, panoptic, or indirect ophthalmoscope
  - Graefe fixation forceps
  - Open-ended Tomcat urinary catheter for nasolacrimal catheterization
  - Sterile fluorescein strips
  - Sterile culture swabs
  - Kimura spatula for obtaining cytology
  - Tonometer (Tono-Pen or TonoVet)
  - Glass slides
  - Sterile eyewash

ANTICIPATED TIME

Approximately 20 to 30 minutes

PREPARATION: IMPORTANT CHECKPOINTS

- Initial examination of the horse eye should take place in adequate illumination, prior to tranquilization.
  - Facial, orbital, and eyelid symmetry, the presence of ocular discharge and/or blepharospasm, and cranial nerve evaluation are all performed. Specifically, cranial nerves II, III, IV, V, VI, and VII are evaluated. These are assessed through pupillary light and menace response (CN II, III, and VII evaluation), maze testing, globe position and mobility (CN III, IV, VI), sensation of ocular and adnexal structures (CN V), and eyelid position and function (CN VII). To accurately evaluate direct and consensual pupillary light responses, a bright, focal light source and a darkened examination area are often required.
- Vision should also be evaluated by performing a menace response and possible maze testing in bright and dim light.
- Complete ocular examination usually requires tranquilization, regional nerve blocks, and topical anesthesia. These are described in other chapters (see "Ocular Nerve Blocks: Standard" in this section.

POSSIBLE COMPLICATIONS AND COMMON ERRORS TO BE AVOIDED

- Complications include:
  - Hypersensitivity reactions to medications
  - Infections due to needle sticks
  - Possible ocular or eyelid trauma due to poorly restrained or nontranquilized horses

PROCEDURE

- Ophthalmic examination can be performed in a darkened stall or the horse can be placed in stocks depending on the temperament of the horse and availability of equipment.
- The area of examination should be quiet and away from the distraction of other horses, dogs, and so forth.

- The examiner should position himself or herself at the side of the head, not in front of the horse.
  - If the horse has been sedated, an assistant may be required to elevate the head to the same level as the examiners' eyes.
  - If an auriculopalpebral nerve block has not been used, avoid attempting to elevate the superior eyelid, instead examine the eye with minimal handling of the adnexal tissues.
- Direct and consensual pupillary light reflexes should be assessed by shining a bright light source (Finnoff transilluminator) into the eye (direct pupillary light reflex) while having an assistant assess the pupillary constriction of the opposite eye (consensual pupillary light reflex).
  - Similarly, also assess the horse's dazzle reflex by shining a bright light source into the eye and observing blinking or avoidance by the horse, which suggests a positive reflex. Positive pupillary light and dazzle reflexes indicate a least minimal functioning retina.
- Culture of the ocular surface followed by ocular cytology should be performed prior to application of any substance into the eye.
  - A sterile swab is used to collect the culture at the periphery of the lesion.
  - Cytology is collected next, preferably with a Kimura spatula or the sterile handle end of a Bard-Parker surgical blade. Topical anesthetic may need to be applied prior to collection of the cytologic sample (Figure 1).
- Fluorescein staining of the cornea is best performed by placing a sterile

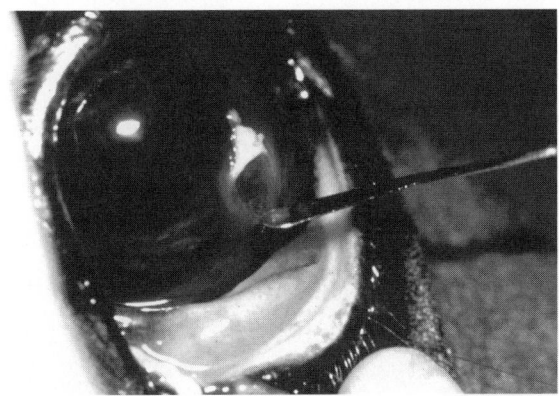

FIGURE 1 Cytology collection using a Kimura spatula.

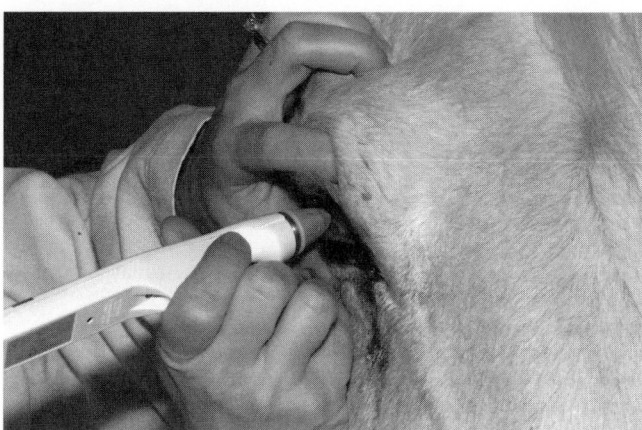

FIGURE 2 Measurement of the intraocular pressure using a Tono-Pen tonometer.

fluorescein strip in a 3-mL syringe, filling the syringe with sterile eyewash, and placing the solution of fluorescein directly on the cornea.

- Fluorescein staining is followed by topical anesthesia with proparacaine 0.5%, examination for a foreign body, and examination of the nasolacrimal system, third eyelid, conjunctiva, and anterior and posterior segments.
- The superior and inferior fornix and anterior and posterior surfaces of the third eyelid are evaluated.
- The anterior surface of the third eyelid is examined by retropulsion of the globe resulting in passive prolapse of the third eyelid.

- To evaluate the posterior surface, the third eyelid is gently grasped with Graefe fixation forceps or manipulated using a strabismus hook. Foreign bodies or debris are commonly found in the conjunctival cul de sacs and behind the third eyelids.
- Following examination of the ocular adnexa, the intraocular pressure should be measured. This is done using a digital tonometer (Tono-Pen; Tonovet; Figure 2). The normal intraocular pressure for the horse is between 12 and 30 mm Hg.
  - If the intraocular pressure is normal, then the pupil should be dilated to allow complete examination of intraocular structures. Use of 1.0% tropicamide topically is preferred

for mydriasis because it dilates the pupil in 15 to 20 minutes and keeps the pupil dilated for only 4 to 6 hours in most horses.
- The ocular media (cornea, aqueous humor, lens, and vitreous) are evaluated for clarity and transparency using a transilluminator and direct ophthalmoscope.
  - Position and size of the lens, shape and mobility of the pupil, and appearance of the corpora nigra, optic nerve, retinal blood vessels, and tapetal and nontapetal fundus are all evaluated.
  - The ocular fundus is best visualized in the horse with indirect ophthalmoscopy and a 20-diopter hand lens. Alternatives to use of an indirect ophthalmoscope are the direct ophthalmoscope or the panoptic ophthalmoscope. Both the direct and panoptic ophthalmoscopes allow the examiner to visualize the ocular fundus, but only a small area of the ocular fundus is visible at one time.

POSTPROCEDURE

Complete eyelid function should return prior to trailering the horse (generally 1 hour after nerve blocks). Also, if the pupil is dilated, the horse should not be worked. Short-acting mydriatics generally allow the pupil to return to normal size within 6 hours after administration.

AUTHOR: **BRIAN C. GILGER**

Pericardiocentesis

BASIC INFORMATION

SYNONYM(S)

Pericardial tap

OVERVIEW AND GOAL(S)

To obtain access to the pericardial space for therapeutic and/or diagnostic purposes.

INDICATIONS

- Pericarditis
- Pericardial effusion
- Cardiac tamponade

CONTRAINDICATIONS

Inadequate pericardial fluid to perform the procedure safely

EQUIPMENT, ANESTHESIA

- Sedation will likely be required.
- Pericardiocentesis site preparation: Clippers, scrub material, local anesthetic (eg, 2% lidocaine), needle and syringe for infiltration of the site with local anesthetic, scalpel blade for skin and intercostal muscle incision.
- Large-bore trocar catheter (eg, 16–28 Fr thoracic catheter) or a 10- to 14-gauge over-the-needle catheter if the fluid accumulation is small enough to make large-bore trocar catheter placement dangerous.
- Hemostats
- Suture material
- One-way Heimlich valve or condom for the end of the pericardial tube if left indwelling.

ANTICIPATED TIME

20 to 30 minutes to perform procedure if a site has already been chosen

PREPARATION: IMPORTANT CHECKPOINTS

- An echocardiogram is necessary to determine the optimal location for pericardiocentesis.
- The procedure is usually performed in the left fifth intercostal space approximately 6 cm ventral to the point of the shoulder and dorsal to the lateral thoracic vein.
- The depth of the pericardial fluid (between parietal pericardium and epicardium) should be at least 5 cm to proceed safely with a trocar catheter without risk to the myocardium.
- Continual monitoring by electrocardiography should be performed throughout the procedure.

- An intravenous catheter should be in place before the procedure.
- The size of the pericardial catheter should be as large as can be accomodated by the animal.

POSSIBLE COMPLICATIONS AND COMMON ERRORS TO BE AVOIDED

- Arrhythmias, particularly if the epicardium is inadvertently touched with the trocar or catheter.
- Myocardial perforation resulting in hemopericardium and/or fatal hemorrhage.
- Hypotension from fluid shifts if large volumes of fluids are drained quickly without intravenous fluid support.
- Pneumopericardium, pneumothorax, septic pericardium, or septic thorax can be introduced during the procedure.
- Fibrinous effusions can clog the catheter, resulting in the impression that drainage is complete despite a significant volume of fluid remaining.

PROCEDURE

- Initial physical exam and clinicopathologic workup (complete blood count, serum chemistry panel).
- Cardiac exam (including a complete echocardiogram and electrocardiogram) before pericardiocentesis:
  - To determine the volume and character of pericardial fluid and select the optimal site for catheter placement.
  - To examine the pericardial space (fluid allows enhanced visualization).
  - If necessary, the exam can be abbreviated and completed after centesis.
- The site for pericardiocentesis should be clipped and scrubbed using aseptic technique.
- Local anesthetic should be injected subcutaneously and as deeply as possible along the path of the trocar catheter, then allowed to sit for at least 5 minutes before starting the procedure.
- An incision should be made through the skin and intercostal muscles with a No. 10 scalpel blade.
- A large-bore trocar catheter should be advanced through the skin incision and pushed through the intercostal muscles toward the pericardium.
  - A "pop" may be felt as the catheter is advanced through the parietal pericardium into the pericardial space.
  - To check if the catheter is within the pericardial space, the trocar can be slightly withdrawn; fluid should fill the catheter readily.
- Once the pericardial space has been entered, the catheter is advanced over

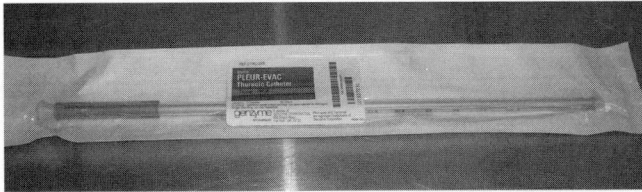

FIGURE 1 An example of a trocar catheter that can be used for pericardiocentesis (Pleur-Evac Thoracic Catheter, Genzyme Corporation, Fall River, MA).

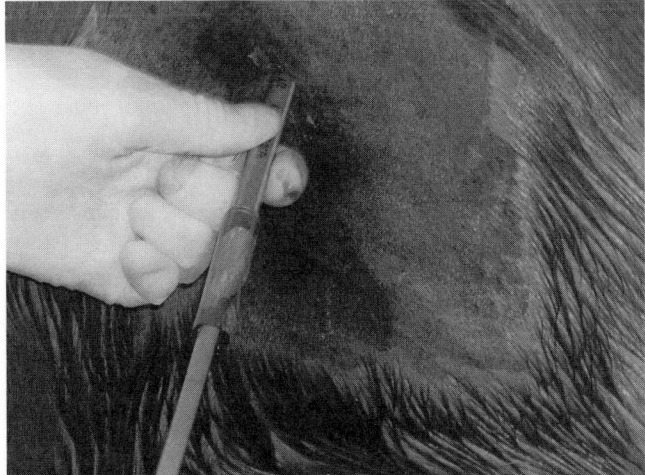

FIGURE 2 The trocar catheter has been inserted in the left fifth intercostal space by ultrasound guidance. The catheter is filling with pericardial fluid as the stylet is being withdrawn.

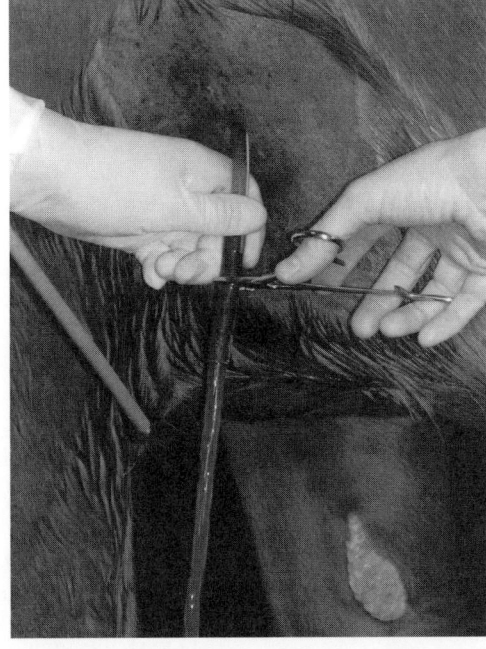

FIGURE 3 The stylet has been removed from the trocar catheter and pericardial fluid is flowing freely. A hemostat is in place for clamping the catheter as flow stops.

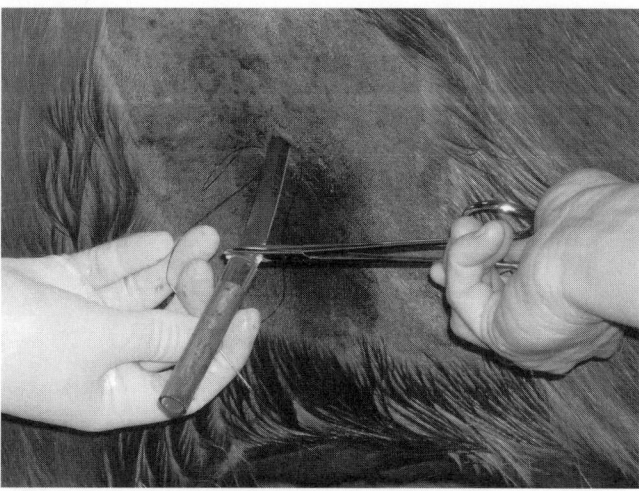

FIGURE 4 A purse string suture is being placed around the trocar catheter so that it can be left indwelling. The catheter will be further secured with a Chinese finger tie.

the trocar until only 5 to 10 cm remain external to the body wall or the heart can be felt beating against the tip of the catheter (if this occurs, the catheter should be withdrawn a few centimeters or until movement can no longer be felt).

- The catheter is then secured in place by a purse string suture and Chinese finger tie.
- Drainage of the pericardial fluid is then performed.
  - Some clinicians prefer that this be done slowly to avoid large hemodynamic fluctuations and the potential for hypotension.
- As drainage slows, a hemostat can be used to clamp the catheter closed until

a one-way Heimlich valve or a condom is placed on the end of the catheter to prevent air from entering.

- Pericardial lavage with 5 L warm isotonic fluids and subsequent redrainage can be performed every 12 hours.
  - Allows flushing and dilution of inflammatory cells and mediators, fibrin, infectious organisms, and immune complexes.
  - Should be continued until minimal fluid is recovered from the initial drainage.
  - Local medications can be instilled in 1 L of fluids after redrainage of lavage fluid to remain until the next drainage and lavage.

POSTPROCEDURE

- Intravenous fluids should be given during or just after pericardial drainage so that blood volume is adequate as cardiac output increases.
- Indwelling pericardial tubes must be closely monitored to avoid pneumopericardium or septic pericarditis and to ensure that they remain patent and positioned appropriately.
- The site should be monitored for subcutaneous swelling, heat, pain, or discharge around the catheter. Petroleum jelly or other soothing creams or ointments should be spread around the ventral aspect of the site so that local discharge does not result in skin scalding.
- Once the effusion is less than 1 L per day, the catheter can be removed and the skin closed.
- Ideally, this should be confirmed with echocardiography first because fibrin clots in the catheter or repositioning of the catheter may prevent fluid drainage, even if significant fluid remains.

ALTERNATIVES AND THEIR RELATIVE MERITS

- There are no good alternatives to pericardiocentesis. When cardiac tamponade is present, the procedure must be performed as quickly as possible. The size of the catheter used and the decision of whether to leave it indwelling will vary from case to case.
- Pericardial surgery (exploration, pericardectomy, pericardial stripping) is very risky and should only be considered as a last resort (usually in cases of constrictive pericarditis).

AUTHOR: **SOPHY A. JESTY**

Periodontics

BASIC INFORMATION

SYNONYM(S)

Periodontal disease, periodontal pockets, diastema with periodontium attachment loss, periodontal ligament attachment loss, periodontitis

OVERVIEW AND GOAL

- *Periodontium* is composed of the gingiva, periodontal ligament, cementum, and alveolar bone.
- *Periodontitis* is active inflammation of the periodontium.
- *Diastema* is a space between teeth within the same arcade.

  - In the equine dentition, this would be abnormal except for the spaces between the third incisor and canine and the canine and first premolar (or second premolar).
  - An abnormal diastema tends to collect feed material. Periodontal disease may or may not be present. The presence of a diastema does not mean that periodontal disease is present.
- A *periodontal pocket* is a defect in the attachment apparatus (periodontium) that typically allows food to collect below the gingiva. There are two types of periodontal pockets: suprabony and infrabony. A suprabony

pocket refers to attachment loss in which the bottom of the pocket is coronal to the alveolar bone. An infrabony pocket refers to attachment and bone loss in which the bottom of the pocket is apical to the normal level of alveolar bone.

- *Periodontal disease* is a collective term referring to all stages of periodontal inflammation (Box 1). The stages are determined by the amount of attachment and bone loss. The bone loss can be estimated by radiology. When evaluating alveolar bone with radiology, one must be cognizant of the three-dimensional aspect of bone loss:

BOX 1   Stages of Periodontal Disease

Stage 1: Gingivitis, no attachment loss, <5 mm
Stage 2: Early; <25% attachment or bone loss (typically 5–12 mm)
Stage 3: Moderate; <50% attachment or bone loss (typically 12–18 mm)
Stage 4: Severe; >50% attachment or bone loss (typically 18–25 mm)

○ A cyclic process with periods of periodontitis that creates stages of progressive attachment loss.
○ Reported to be as high as 60% in horses older than 15 years.
○ Progression appears to be related to food stasis. In the brachyodont dentition (dog, cat, human), the build-up of plaque and calculus is correlated with the progression of periodontal disease.
○ Periodontal disease is staged according to the amount of periodontium attachment loss.
○ Treatment goals for periodontitis are to prevent further bone and attachment loss and to allow for periodontium healing with reattachment.
○ The ultimate goal is to prevent premature tooth loss.

INDICATIONS

• Periodontal disease is classified based on the veterinary periodontal disease index, which evaluates the amount of periodontium attachment loss.
• The amount of loss should be assessed by oral and radiographic examination.
• If the percentage of attachment loss is less than 50% (stages 0 to 3), periodontal treatment is indicated.

CONTRAINDICATIONS

If the attachment loss is greater than 50% (stage 4: severe periodontal disease), tooth loss is eminent and extraction is the most logical treatment.

EQUIPMENT, ANESTHESIA

• Dental speculum, dental mirror, and periodontal probe are necessary for a complete oral examination.
• Intraoral and extraoral radiographs are used in conjunction with the oral exam to evaluate and stage the degree of periodontal disease. A complete radiologic exam includes intraoral and extraoral cassettes.
• Standard dental floating equipment (hand or power instruments) is sufficient for occlusal adjustment treatment.
• Periodontal curettes and a NaHCO₃/air abrasion unit are limited in their ability to debride a periodontal pocket.
• A tapered diamond burr with a high-speed handpiece will debride decayed cementum; however, one must be careful to not damage healthy cementum, enamel, or dentin.
• A piezoelectric ultrasonic scaler does a moderate to good job of debridement of the periodontal pocket and surrounding decayed cementum. It is also noninvasive to healthy periodontal and dental tissues.
• Multiple barrier materials (CaCO₃, CaSO₄ hemihydrate, vinyl polysiloxane, etc.) and antibiotics (doxycycline, metronidazole) have been used.

ANTICIPATED TIME

• Oral examination and radiographic evaluation: 60 to 90 minutes
• Occlusal adjustment: 20 to 30 minutes
• Local debridement: 30 to 45 minutes
• Barrier and local antibiotic placement: 15 to 20 minutes

PREPARATION: IMPORTANT CHECKPOINTS

• Document the depth and diameter (cross-section) of the periodontal pocket(s).
• With follow-up examinations, these measurements can be compared as periodontal healing is monitored.
• Periodontal pockets less than 7 mm in depth usually respond well to occlusal adjustment.
• If periodontal pockets are deeper than 7 mm, local debridement should be considered.
• Periodontal pockets of 10 mm or more should be considered for barrier placement and local antibiotic placement.

POSSIBLE COMPLICATIONS AND COMMON ERRORS TO BE AVOIDED

• Avoid placing vinyl polysiloxane deep into the pocket; this could potentially inhibit healing.
• When using a piezoelectric ultrasonic scaler, the short handle makes it difficult to access pockets further back in the mouth (PM 4, M1-3). Currently there is no commercially available unit designed specifically for the equine mouth.

PROCEDURE

• Treatment of equine periodontal disease is centered on three basic concepts:
  1. Occlusal adjustment to help prevent food stasis

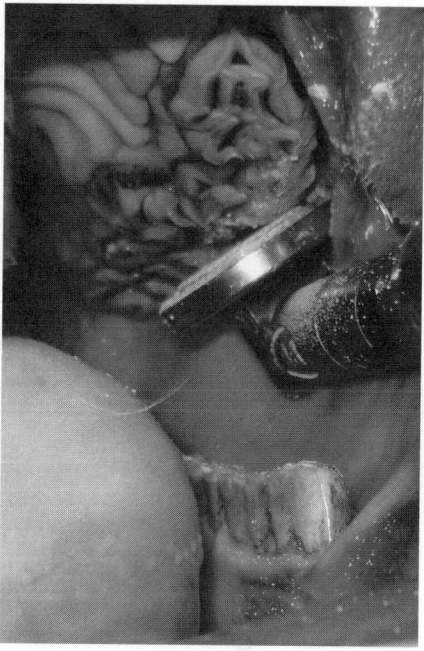

FIGURE 1 Occlusal adjustment: removal of sharp enamel points along the buccal aspect of the maxillary cheek teeth and the lingual aspect of the mandibular cheek teeth.

  2. Local debridement of the periodontal pocket and decayed cementum
  3. Local placement of a barrier and/or antibiotic to allow healing and reattachment of the periodontium
• Occlusal adjustment involves removing sharp enamel points and correcting arcade abnormalities (hooks, ramps, waves, steps, etc).
  ○ Be careful not to make extreme adjustments at one time.
  ○ It is better to make minor corrections and repeat 3 to 4 months later. This will give the pulp time to "retreat" as tertiary dentin/secondary reparative dentin is formed to repair the exposed dentinal tubules (Figure 1).
• Local debridement of the periodontal pocket entails removal of food and debris from the periodontal pocket.
  ○ Decayed cementum should also be locally debrided.
  ○ Both techniques should be performed with the goal of conserving healthy tissues to allow periodontium reattachment.
  ○ These procedures may need to be repeated at 1- to 3-month intervals (Figure 2).
• Placement of barriers and local antibiotic:
  ○ Accomplished by crushing an antibiotic into a powder (or removing the gelatin coating of a capsule) and blending with a barrier in the powder form (CaSO₄/CaCO₃ hemihydrate). Plaster of Paris is a

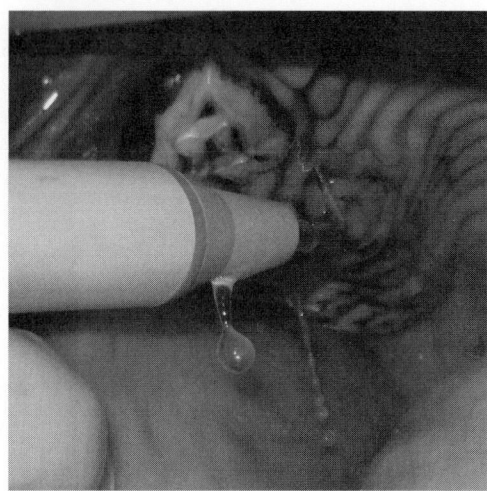

FIGURE 2 Local debridement of the periodontal pocket and decayed cementum using a piezoelectric ultrasonic scaler.

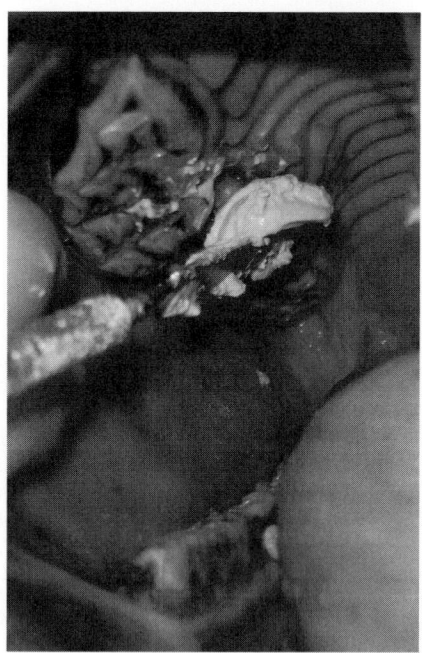

FIGURE 3 Barrier placement using a mixture of an antibiotic with CaSO$_4$/CaCO$_3$ hemihydrate.

common and economical source of CaSO$_4$ and CaCO$_3$ hemihydrate.

○ Once mixed, a slight amount of water is added to make the mixture into a "dry" paste that aids placement into the periodontal pocket. The dried mixture typically will last 1 to 2 weeks.

○ A thin layer of vinyl polysiloxane placed over the barrier/antibiotic may help maintain closure of the pocket for an additional 1 to 2 weeks (total of 3 to 4 weeks) (Figure 3).

• All these treatments have a common goal of preventing food stasis.

• By implementing these techniques, the periodontium tends to heal very well.

• As a general rule, occlusal adjustment is the first line of defense and treatment of periodontal disease.

• Early stages of periodontal disease (stage 1 and 2) may show complete healing with this treatment alone.

• Stage 3 periodontal disease will show some improvement with occlusal adjustment; however, local debridement and barrier/local antibiotic placement are typically indicated.

POSTPROCEDURE

• After treatment of periodontal disease, regular and complete follow-up examinations are necessary.

• Follow-up examination should include radiography to monitor bone and attachment healing.

• Pocket debridement, barrier placement, and local antibiotic treatment may need to be repeated for complete healing.

SUGGESTED READING

Baker GJ: Abnormalities of wear and periodontal disease. In Baker GJ, Easley J, editors: *Equine dentistry*, ed 2, St Louis, 2005, Saunders Elsevier, pp 116–200.

Earley ET: How to manage maleruptions of upper fourth premolars in the miniature horse. *Proc Am Assoc Equine Pract* 53:487–497, 2007.

Epstein S, Valen M: An alternative treatment for the periodontal infrabony defect. *Dent Today* 25(2):92–97, 2006.

Klugh DO: Equine periodontal disease. *Clin Tech Equine Pract* 4:135–147, 2005.

Klugh DO: A review of equine periodontal disease. *Proc Am Assoc Equine Pract* 52:551–558, 2006.

Newman MG, Takei HH, Klokkevold PP, et al: *Carranza's clinical periodontology*, ed 10, St Louis, 2006, Saunders Elsevier, pp 434–451.

Wiggs RW, Lobprise HB: Veterinary dentistry, principles and practice, Ames, IA, 1997, Wiley Blackwell, pp 202–212.

AUTHOR: **EDWARD T. EARLEY**

Peritoneal Drains

BASIC INFORMATION

OVERVIEW AND GOAL(S)

A drain is a tube that is placed in a cavity to promote fluid egress from a space or cavity. Peritoneal drains are placed to remove fluid from the peritoneal cavity.

INDICATIONS

• Drains are used to remove fluid (including urine), inflammatory materials, and cellular debris.

• Drains can be egress only, or used for both ingress and egress.

• Drains are placed either for only the length of a sedated procedure, or as indwelling drains for use over several days.

CONTRAINDICATIONS

Drains are difficult to place safely when there is distended bowel or very little abdominal fluid.

EQUIPMENT, ANESTHESIA

- In neonates, short-term abdominal drains can be placed under sedation and local anesthesia.
- Indwelling abdominal drains are best placed under general anesthesia, often at a celiotomy.
- Teat cannulas are usually used for short-term drains, although other softer materials such as plastic and Teflon are suitable.
- Long-term drains are usually made of plastic.

ANTICIPATED TIME

- Placement of a short-term drain takes 10 minutes.
- Placement of an indwelling drain takes between 15 and 30 minutes and depends on how the abdomen is approached.

PREPARATION: IMPORTANT CHECKPOINTS

- Appropriate foal control is essential.
- Sedation is sufficient for short-term drains and some long-term drains.
- If a foal is very active, anesthesia will be necessary for the placement of indwelling drains.
- Percutaneous ultrasound can help choose the best location for a drain to place it in the abdominal cavity.
- If peritoneal lavage is to be used, fluids should be warmed before the procedure.

POSSIBLE COMPLICATIONS AND COMMON ERRORS TO BE AVOIDED

- The worst complication is bowel damage by the drain and should be avoided by careful placement and pre-procedure ultrasound.
- The biggest problem with short-term drains is occlusion by the omentum. Often, two teat cannulas are placed, one to trap the omentum and another to drain the fluid.

PROCEDURE

- Placement of a short-term drain like a teat cannula is often done to drain urine preoperatively in cases of uroperitoneum.
  - The foal is placed in right lateral recumbency to avoid puncturing the cecum.

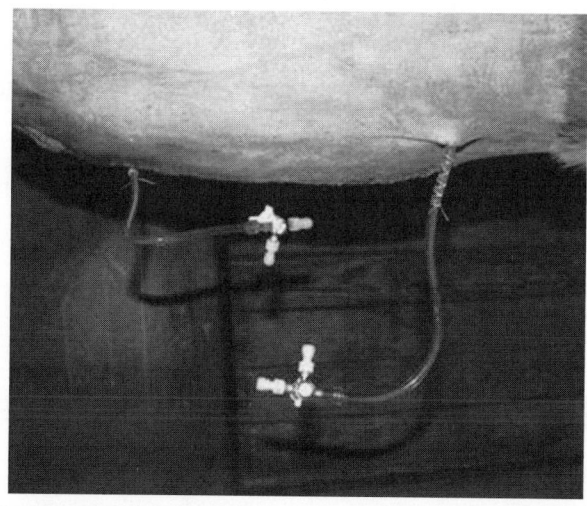

FIGURE 1 Center fenestrated abdominal drain placed in a foal at celiotomy for abdominal pain.

- The ventral aspect of the foal's abdomen is placed at the edge of the surface it is lying upon.
- The sites for drainage are surgically prepared and local anesthetic is placed in the skin, subcutaneous tissues, and muscle if appropriate.
- A No. 15 blade is used to cut a 5- to 7-mm hole in the skin and linea or external sheath of the rectus (depending on the location of the drain insertion).
- The teat cannula is inserted into the incision and pushed into the abdomen using controlled pressure.
- A distinct pop will usually be felt upon entering the peritoneum, and the foal will often react as this area is rarely adequately blocked.
- The author usually places two teat cannulas on the ventral aspect of the abdomen, and often a third in the left flank to instill warmed sodium chloride for peritoneal lavage.
- Long-term drains can be placed during celiotomy by puncturing the abdominal wall away from the incision and leaving a fenestrated drain in the abdomen (Figure 1).
  - The author prefers to use a 0.25-inch center fenestrated drain that exits the abdomen with both ends of the nonfenestrated portion of the drain. This allows two portals for egress and ingress.
  - The ends of the drain are sutured to the skin at the two ends of the incision.
  - Long-term drains placed without a celiotomy are placed similar to short-term drains, except that only one end of the drain tube is inserted and the external portion is sutured to the skin.
  - All fenestrations should be in the peritoneum.

POSTPROCEDURE

- Systemic antibiotics should be administered while the drain is in place.
- Instillation of fluid for flushing the peritoneal cavity can be performed readily, although occasionally drainage is hindered, usually by omental interference.
- Drains are pulled when deemed unnecessary (usually 2–3 days in peritonitis) and the openings left to heal by second intention.

ALTERNATIVES AND THEIR RELATIVE MERITS

Open peritoneal drainage can be performed but has a high complication rate.

AUTHOR: **ELIZABETH M. SANTSCHI**

Poisoning: Basic Treatment

BASIC INFORMATION

OVERVIEW AND GOAL(S)

Six general steps should be considered when treating poisoned horses.

1. **Stabilize the patient if necessary.** Goal: keep the animal alive long enough to make a diagnosis and begin more specific treatment. This step should be addressed first if needed. All other steps can be performed concurrently once the patient is stable.

2. **Evaluate the patient.** Goal: to determine what is wrong with the patient, the severity of the condition, treatment required, and how aggressive treatment should be. The clinical evaluation is based on a combination of:
   - Physical examination
   - History
   - Basic diagnostic tests (complete blood count, serum chemistry profile, other tests as needed). Note: very few rapid tests for specific toxins exist, so in most cases treatment must be initiated without benefit of specific confirmatory toxicologic testing.
   - Dosage calculation if the amount of toxin the animal was exposed to is known
   - On occasion, environmental investigation will also be necessary.

3. **Decontaminate the patient if appropriate.** Goal: to decrease the amount of toxin absorbed into the body. This step is unique to the treatment of poison cases and must be done soon after exposure. Decontamination methods depend on the route of exposure:
   - Ocular
   - Dermal
   - Gastrointestinal (GI). Decontamination methods include:
     - Gastric lavage to remove toxin still remaining in the stomach.
     - Administration of activated charcoal to bind toxin remaining in the GI tract.
     - Administration of a cathartic to hasten movement of activated charcoal-bound toxin out of the GI tract. Efficacy and safety of cathartic use in poisoned horses is unclear.
     - Note: emesis should NOT be induced in horses.

4. **Enhance elimination of absorbed toxin.** Goal: to hasten the removal of toxin that has been absorbed systemically to diminish the severity and duration of toxic effects. Methods:
   - Diuresis. Goal: to increase urine flow and excretion rate of renally excreted toxins.
   - Repeated doses of activated charcoal. Goal: to decreased enterohepatic recycling of toxins excreted via the biliary system.
   - Ion trapping. Goal: to alter urine pH to inhibit resorption of acidic or basic toxins from urine.
   - Chelation. Goal: to alter the diffusion gradient for metal or metalloid toxins.
   - Other methods such as dialysis are impractical in most settings and are not discussed in this entry.

5. **Administer an antidote if available and appropriate.** Goal: to inactivate or otherwise prevent the toxin from causing adverse effects. Very few poisons have specific antidotes, which is why other treatment steps are so important for most cases.

6. **Provide symptomatic and supportive care.** Goal: to restore or preserve homeostasis for all organ systems. This step is often the only treatment possible because many cases present too late for decontamination and no specific antidote exists.

INDICATIONS

- **Stabilization:** Indicated for patients with immediately life-threatening conditions such as severe airway, breathing and circulation abnormalities, or seizures, shock, severe hypothermia or hyperthermia, or life-threatening electrolyte abnormalities.
- **Clinical evaluation:** Indicated in all cases.
- **Decontamination:** Indicated only if unabsorbed toxin is still present on the body or in the GI tract. Guidelines:
  - **Gastric lavage:** Indicated only if some of the toxin might still be in the stomach, if the toxin is of a size and consistency that can be removed via nasogastric tube, and if the amount and type of toxin might pose a serious risk to the patient. Liquid toxins can quickly pass through the stomach; forages, grains and other solid substances can remain in the stomach for many hours but may be too large to pass through a stomach tube. As a general rule, lavage may be indicated if:
    - Ingestion of the toxin has been within approximately 3 to 5 hours of lavage.
    - The toxic substance can pass through a nasogastric tube.
    - The toxin ingested and estimated dosage are dangerous enough to outweigh risks of lavage.
    - None of the contraindications for lavage exist (see Contraindications).
  - **Activated charcoal:** Indicated if some amount of toxin might still remain in the GI tract.
    - The sooner after toxin exposure that activated charcoal is administered the better, but it is never too late as long as any toxin remains in the GI tract.
    - Activated charcoal can be administered after lavage or can be given alone without lavage.
    - Activated charcoal does not adsorb to all toxins and is not necessarily useful in all poison cases. The following toxins are reportedly NOT well bound by activated charcoal: acids and alkalis, cyanide, detergents, ethanol and other alcohols, ethylene glycol, iron, fluoride, nitrate, petroleum distillates, sodium, and other salts and metals. However, lack of efficacy is generally NOT a contraindication for the use of activated charcoal, with a few exceptions (see Contraindications).
  - **Cathartics:** may be indicated if activated charcoal has been given and either the risk of constipation is high or the risk from the toxin is high enough to outweigh risks from the cathartic. However, due to the risk of colic and other complications, cathartics should be used with caution in poisoned horses.
- **Enhanced elimination of absorbed toxin:** Indicated if systemically absorbed toxin still remains in the body.
  - Diuresis is indicated if the toxin is excreted renally, is in high concentration in the plasma, and is not highly protein bound. Diuresis can be considered even if the toxin is unknown.
  - Multiple doses of activated charcoal are indicated to decreased enterohepatic recirculation for toxins excreted primarily via the biliary system. This can be used for toxins that enter the body via any route as

long as the toxin is excreted via the biliary system. Repeat doses of activated charcoal can be considered even if the toxin is unknown.

○ Ion trapping can be considered if the toxin is known to be acidic or basic and is renally excreted, not highly protein bound, not conjugated, and not highly lipid soluble.

○ Chelators are often considered antidotes (see Antidotes).

- **Antidotes:** Indicated if an antidote for the particular toxin exists, its use in horses is appropriate, and the risks from the toxin outweigh risks from the antidote.

- **Symptomatic and supportive care:** Indicated in any patient that has clinical signs resulting from toxin exposure. Treatments should address abnormalities with all systems, including cardiovascular, respiratory, renal, digestive, musculoskeletal, cutaneous, and central nervous systems. Also address thermoregulation, electrolyte imbalances, patient comfort, hydration, and nutrition status.

CONTRAINDICATIONS

- There are no specific contraindications for stabilization, clinical evaluation, and symptomatic care.
- **Decontamination:**
  ○ **Gastric lavage** is generally contraindicated if the ingested toxin is:
    ■ Caustic or corrosive (eg, acid or alkali)
    ■ A volatile petroleum hydrocarbon (with a few exceptions)
    ■ If an increased risk of gastric perforation exists
  ○ **Activated charcoal** is contraindicated in cases with:
    ■ Perforated GI tract
    ■ Severe dehydration or electrolyte imbalances (correct these first)
    ■ Caustic or corrosive agents
  ○ **Cathartics** are contraindicated if the patient:
    ■ Already has diarrhea or is likely to develop diarrhea from the toxin
    ■ Is likely to develop colic from the toxin
    ■ Has a GI obstruction or blockage
    ■ Is dehydrated or has electrolyte imbalances (correct these first)
    ■ If the toxin is osmotically active (eg, salt)
    ■ Do not use magnesium-containing cathartics if the patient has central nervous system depression, ileus, renal disease, or has been previously treated with docusate
- Enhanced elimination:
  ○ Diuresis: contraindicated in cases of oliguria and anuria

○ Multiple doses of activated charcoal: contraindicated in cases with severe constipation

○ Ion trapping: contraindicated in patients with preexisting acidosis or alkalosis for acidifying urine or alkalinizing urine, respectively

- **Antidotes:** All antidotes have the potential to cause toxicity. Use of an antidote is contraindicated if risks from the antidote outweigh risks from the toxin itself.

EQUIPMENT, ANESTHESIA

Standard medical instrumentation and equipment are used for stabilization, clinical evaluation, toxin elimination procedures, and symptomatic/supportive care.

- Decontamination:
  ○ Gastric lavage:
    ■ Anesthesia is not required for gastric lavage in horses, although the procedure can be performed in an anesthetized patient if the airway is protected with a cuffed endotracheal tube.
    ■ Equipment: the largest nasogastric tube that can safely fit through the nasal passages.
  ○ Activated charcoal:
    ■ Anesthesia is not required for administration of activated charcoal.
    ■ Equipment: activated charcoal is best administered via nasogastric intubation in horses.
- **Antidotes:** See Procedure.

POSSIBLE COMPLICATIONS AND COMMON ERRORS TO BE AVOIDED

- **Clinical evaluation**
  ○ Physical examination: Be sure to evaluate the entire patient, not just the most obvious abnormalities.
  ○ History: Be sure to obtain a complete history to avoid missing vital information. Have the owner bring any packaging from known toxin exposures so dosages can be calculated and ingredients can be confirmed.
- **Decontamination.** Possible complications:
  ○ Gastric lavage
    ■ Aspiration
    ■ Trauma to the nasal passages, esophagus or stomach from intubation
    ■ Inappropriate placement of nasogastric tube into the lungs
  ○ Activated charcoal:
    ■ Osmolarity changes and possibly hypernatremia (uncommon)
    ■ Constipation (uncommon)
    ■ Aspiration

○ Cathartics
    ■ Colic, excessive diarrhea
    ■ Dehydration
    ■ Electrolyte imbalances
    ■ Magnesium intoxication with magnesium-containing cathartics

- Enhanced elimination of the absorbed toxin. Possible complications:
  ○ Diuresis: pulmonary edema, cerebral edema, acid-base and electrolyte abnormalities
  ○ Multiple doses of activated charcoal: electrolyte imbalances, constipation, aspiration
  ○ Ion trapping: Acidifying urine—metabolic acidosis, central nervous system depression. Alkalinizing urine—metabolic alkalosis, electrolyte imbalances

- **Antidotes.** All antidotes have the potential to cause adverse side effects. Be sure to use proper dosages and understand all potential adverse effects before using any antidote.

PROCEDURE

The procedures for stabilization, clinical evaluation, and symptomatic and supportive care are basic medicine and not specific for poison cases; hence these procedures will not be discussed.

- Decontamination:
  ○ Ocular: Copious lavage with a dilute saline solution or water.
  ○ Dermal: Bathing, clipping. For bathing, use a mild dish soap or shampoo and copious water.
  ○ Gastrointestinal:
    ■ Gastric lavage:
      □ Place the largest nasogastric tube that will reasonably fit in the standing horse. Light sedation may be needed in some cases, but general anesthesia is not required. The procedure can be performed in a comatose patient or a patient anesthetized for other purposes if the airway is protected with a cuffed endotracheal tube.
      □ Use gravity flow to instill water into the stomach. The amount of water to use depends on the size of the horse. As a general rule, a gallon of water per cycle can be used for the average 1000 lb adult horse, and more or less for larger or smaller horses.
      □ Lower the end of the tube and drain as much fluid from the stomach as possible by gravity flow or suction with a dosing syringe. Suction from a dosing syringe may be needed to dislodge chunks of material that block the tube. Note: lavage fluid may not return until additional fluid is instilled. Always

remember the small size of the equine stomach and be careful not to overfill the stomach.

□ Repeat the cycle multiple times (10–20 cycles) until the return lavage fluid is clear.

□ The first lavage recovery fluid can be saved for chemical analysis if necessary.

□ After the last lavage cycle, instill activated charcoal before removing the stomach tube.

■ Administration of activated charcoal:

□ Standard dosage range is 1 to 4 g activated charcoal per kilogram of body weight per os.

□ Target is 10 parts activated charcoal to every 1 part of toxin, but the amount of toxin ingested is often not known.

□ Formulations of activated charcoal include:

• *Powder formulation.* Mix calculated dosage of activated charcoal with just enough water to achieve moderately thick consistency. If the solution is too thick, it will not pass through the tube. If too thin, the volume needed will be too large for the stomach size. Pros: cheap. Cons: messy and difficult to get into solution. Note: 1 Tbsp of activated charcoal powder weighs approximately 5 g.

• *Premixed solutions.* Pros: easy to administer. Cons: expensive and impractical for adult horses; may contain other ingredients such as cathartics that might not be appropriate. More practical to use premixed solutions for foals than for adult horses.

• *Granular formulations.* Pros: easy to mix into solution, not very messy, not cost prohibitive. Cons: none.

• *Tablets and capsules*: not appropriate for poison cases because they take too long to be dissolved, hence delaying the adsorptive effects.

□ Place the nasogastric tube into the stomach and slowly administer activated charcoal solution by gravity flow or dosing syringe.

■ Administration of a cathartic:

□ The efficacy and safety of cathartic use in poisoned horses are not well docu-

mented, and cathartic dosages are not well established. Many practitioners do not routinely use cathartics in poisoned horses. However, if a cathartic is deemed necessary, guidelines include:

□ Use cathartics only in conjunction with activated charcoal.

□ Use only osmotic cathartics. Examples:

• Sorbitol: Can purchase as a powder or a solution; also comes premixed with activated charcoal in some solutions.

• Magnesium salts: Magnesium sulfate (Epsom salts), magnesium hydroxide (Milk of Magnesia), magnesium citrate (Citro-Mag).

• Refer to drug formularies for dosage recommendations.

□ Mix cathartic with activated charcoal dose and administer via nasogastric tube.

□ Do not repeat cathartics.

□ Do not use stimulant cathartics (castor oil, bisacodyl) or emollient laxatives (psyllium, bran).

□ Mineral oil is generally not recommended for poison cases because it will interfere with activated charcoal.

• Enhance elimination of the absorbed toxin:

○ Diuresis for renally excreted toxins: Administer fluids at a diuresis rate to increase urinary flow rate. Diuretics such as furosemide and dextrose can also be used in conjunction with the fluids.

○ Multiple doses of activated charcoal for toxins excreted via the biliary system: After the first dose of activated charcoal is given, repeat doses can be given every 6-8 hours until the toxin is eliminated from the body. Repeat doses are usually half of the original dose. Examples of toxins excreted via the biliary system include ivermectin and barbiturates.

○ Ion trapping: Information available for individual specific toxins will indicate if the toxin in acidic or basic and if ion trapping should be considered. See drug formularies for dosing information.

■ For weak basic toxins, acidify urine by administering ammonium chloride.

■ For weak acidic toxins, alkalinize the urine by administering sodium bicarbonate.

■ Monitor urine pH to be sure the dosages are correct and the targeted pH is achieved.

■ Monitor serum electrolytes and acid-base status.

■ Ion trapping should be used with caution. Risks may outweigh benefits, and efficacy is often not well established.

• **Administration of an antidote:** Very few antidotes exist. Refer to monographs on individual toxins for specific antidote indications and refer to current veterinary formularies such as *Plumb's Veterinary Drug Handbook* for dosing information and adverse effects for various antidotes. Additional resources include the Web site of the American Board of Veterinary Toxicology (www.abvt.org). Antidote cost and availability can sometimes be problematic. A number of antidotes that are not available from veterinary suppliers can be obtained from veterinary compounding pharmacies or human hospitals. Contact a veterinary clinical toxicologist for more information on dosage recommendation, availability, and sources for various antidotes.

ALTERNATIVES AND THEIR RELATIVE MERITS

Notes on adsorbents:

• Adsorbents other than activated charcoal can be used but in general are not superior to activated charcoal. Other adsorbents include kaolin, pectin, bismuth, and ion exchange resins.

• Bio-Sponge (di-tri-octahedral smectite) is a product marketed for adsorbing bacterial toxins in the GI. The product is not marketed for use against other types of toxins, and very few studies have been done evaluating its efficacy against other toxins. The few studies that have been performed have shown that Bio-Sponge is significantly less effective than activated charcoal at adsorbing the toxin. Therefore, use of Bio-Sponge as a general adsorptive agent in place of activated charcoal for treatment of intoxication is not recommended at this time.

• Mineral oil should not be used in place of activated charcoal as it does not adsorb to toxins, but it can be used if activated charcoal is not available

• Mineral oil and activated charcoal should not be administered together because mineral oil can decrease the efficacy of activated charcoal.

• A "universal antidote" product that contains activated charcoal and other ingredients is available, but dosing information may be inadequate and the product is unlikely to be superior to activated charcoal.

AUTHOR: **CYNTHIA L. GASKILL**

Postpartum Breeding

BASIC INFORMATION

DEFINITIONS

- Foal heat is the first postpartum estrus. Behavioral estrus and ovulation typically accompany foal heat. Expression of behavioral signs of estrus, however, can be absent or subtly demonstrated in individual mares, especially those nursing their first foal.
- *Second natural estrus* refers to the second postpartum estrus period when no manipulation occurs to hasten the beginning of this estrus (ie, a normal intraestrus period occurs).
- *Short cycling after foal heat ovulation* is the hastening of the second estrus period by inducing luteolysis. To achieve the shortest parturition-to-conception interval, if the mare is not bred on foal heat, the corpus luteum is typically lysed at 5 to 6 days postovulation with prostaglandin $F_{2\alpha}$ ($PGF_{2\alpha}$) or one its analogues.
- *Delaying foal heat* is a breeding strategy in which the foal heat ovulation is delayed by exogenous steroid hormone administration.

SYNONYM(S)

- First postpartum estrus is also known as *foal heat* or *9-day heat*.
- Second natural postpartum estrus is also known as *30-day heat*.

GOALS

- January 1 is the universal birthday for many breed associations in the Northern Hemisphere. Foals born earlier in the calendar year command superior sales prices to yearlings and 2-year-olds. Thus the goal is to produce healthy foals early in the year.
- Because horses have an average gestation length of 333 to 345 days (range, 320 to 360 days), postpartum mares must become pregnant within 1 month of foaling to maintain a 12-month foaling interval.

OVERVIEW

Foal heat:
- Begins, on average, 5 to 12 days after parturition.
- Foal heat ovulation occurs, on average, 10 to 16 days after parturition.
- Parturition to foal heat ovulation intervals tends to decrease with increasing day length. According to Loy (1980), 33.3% of mares in January and February, 55.3% in March, 64.8% in April, and 82.9% in May had intervals less than 10 days.

Second natural estrus:
- Should begin approximately 15 to 16 days after foal heat ovulation, with this ovulation occurring 19 to 22 days after the foal heat ovulation.
- First cycle interovulatory intervals less than 14 to 16 days are considered abnormal. Diagnostics to determine causes of early luteolysis should be considered. Potential diagnostics include transrectal palpation and ultrasonography, vaginal examination, endometrial culture, endometrial cytology, and endometrial biopsy.

Seasonal anestrus:
- Short photoperiods are the primary cause of the higher anestrous periods earlier in the year.
  - A 5-year retrospective study of a breeding farm composed of 120 to 150 broodmares in southeast Texas had the following anestrous incidence rates: 26.6% (December and January), 23.3% (February), 14.0% (March), 2.6% (April), and 0% (May).
- See Adjunct Therapies below for prevention of seasonal anestrus.

Influences of nutrition, body condition, and lactation:
- Mares fed low nutritive rations for the last 3 months of pregnancy and the first month postpartum have lower pregnancy rates and higher embryonic loss rates than mares fed high nutritive rations.
- Mares with thin body condition have longer intervals from parturition to reproductive cyclicity than do mares with good to obese body condition.
- Lactational anestrus in mares is controversial. Season (photoperiod), nutrition, and body condition should be examined when lactational anestrus is suspected.

Involution:
- Normal foaling mares:
  - Histologic uterine involution is complete by postpartum day 14.
  - Gross uterine involution is complete, on average, by postpartum day 23 (range, 13 to 29 days).
  - Lochia is commonly expelled from the uterus between postpartum days 3 and 6. Normal lochia should not be malodorous. It is initially blood-tinged, but it becomes brown-tinged, then dark mucoid, and finally transparent mucoid as the cellularity of the fluid decreases.
  - Intrauterine luminal fluid decreases in quantity and quality (ie, ultrasonographic changes from mildly echogenic to anechoic) between postpartum days 3 and 15. No fluid is typically detected ultrasonographically by day 15.
  - Pregravid secretory function of the endometrium appears to return by postpartum day 16.
  - Bacterial presence within the lumen of the postpartum uterus is generally transient:
    - *Escherichia coli* is the most common microorganism isolated early postpartum. It can be slowly replaced by β-hemolytic *Streptococcus* spp. during advancing involution.

Rationale for foal heat breeding:
- Pros:
  1. Potential to achieve the shortest parturition-to-conception interval
  2. Reduces the odds of postpartum mares entering anestrus after the foal-heat ovulation.
     - This phenomenon is rare but tends to occur at a higher frequency earlier in the year during shorter photoperiods.
  3. Seasonal pregnancy rates for mares bred on foal heat can be comparable to those of mares first bred on subsequent estrous cycles. The similarities in seasonal pregnancy rates can be explained by the following:
     - Pregnancy rates for estrous cycles after foal heat are similar between mares bred and mares not bred on foal heat.
     - Mares bred on foal heat that do not conceive are typically bred on subsequent estrous cycles.
- Cons:
  1. Foal heat breedings may result in potentially 20% lower pregnancy rates than breedings during later postpartum estrus periods.
     - Effect of time of ovulation: Pregnancy rates are higher when mares ovulate more than 10 days postpartum.
     - Uterine fluid: The presence of fluid during the first postpartum ovulatory period results in significantly lower pregnancy rates (33%) than when no fluid is detected (84%).
     - Age of mares: Older mares have significantly lower foal heat pregnancy rates.
     - Method of breeding: Foal heat pregnancy rates are higher with artificial insemination than natural cover.
  2. Foal heat pregnancies may have a greater potential for loss than later postpartum estrous periods.

- Pattern of embryonic fixation relative to previous gravid horn:
  - Approximately 60% to 86% of embryonic fixation in postpartum mares occurs in the previous nongravid horn (PNGH).
  - The frequency of embryonic fixation in the previous gravid horn (PGH) increases in older mares.
  - PGH pregnancies have an embryonic loss rate approximately 8% to 12% higher than that of PNGH pregnancies.
- Intrauterine fluid: Pregnancies obtained on foal heat breedings are lost more frequently when treatment (oxytocin and/or uterine lavage) is required during the foal heat.

PROCEDURE

Determination of the most suitable postpartum breeding strategy for the individual mare:
- The mare should be examined 5 to 8 days postpartum. The examination should include:
  - History of the most recent pregnancy, delivery, and postpartum interval
  - Assessment of body condition score
  - Visual inspection of the perineum
  - Transrectal palpation and ultrasonography of the reproductive tract and caudal abdomen
  - Vaginal speculum examination (palpable if needed)
  - Examination findings that would preclude foal heat breeding:
    - Uterine discharge, especially if voluminous or malodorous
    - Evidence of trauma to the reproductive tract
    - Urine pooling
    - Pneumovagina
    - Excessive intrauterine luminal fluid
    - History of dystocia
    - History of retained placenta
  - Because pregnancy rates tend to be lower, mares that ovulate 10 or fewer days postpartum may be considered questionable foal heat breeders. This decision is based on the above examinations as well as the overall management of the mare (eg, full pasture turnout versus stall confinement, adequate nutritional plane).

Foal heat breeding:
1. Beginning 5 to 8 days postpartum, examine mare every few days until a 30 to 35 mm follicle is observed.
2. Monitor the mare daily to determine proper timing of breeding. Breeding

mares with intrauterine fluid should be avoided because of decreased pregnancy rates and increased embryonic loss rates.
3. Proper administration of an ovulatory induction agent (human choriogonadotropin [hCG] or deslorelin) is recommended to reduce the breeding to ovulation interval.
4. Monitor daily for ovulation and to determine the need for postbreeding treatment with ecbolics and/or uterine lavage.

Short cycle after foal heat ovulation:
1. This strategy allows mares not bred on foal heat more time for uterine involution and resolution of problems identified at the 5- to 8-day postpartum examination. Parturition-to-conception interval is increased by approximately 9 days compared with foal heat breeding.
2. Monitor the mare as needed after the 5- to 8-day postpartum examination to institute any necessary therapy and determine the day of ovulation.
3. Examine and administer PGF$_{2\alpha}$ or an analogue 5 to 6 days after ovulation to cause luteolysis.
4. Following steps 1 to 4 of foal heat breeding above except for step 2. Modification of step 2: Intrauterine luminal fluid should be evaluated and properly treated. Depending on the amount and character of the fluid, diagnostics (culture, cytology, ± endometrial biopsy) and treatment (ecbolics, uterine lavage, and antibiotics if a positive culture is obtained) should be considered. The decision to breed on this estrus should also be reevaluated.

Second natural estrus breeding:
1. This strategy allows mares time for potentially complete uterine involution and resolution of problems identified at the 5- to 8-day postpartum examination. Parturition-to-conception interval is increased to more than 18 to 21 days compared with successful foal heat breeding.
2. Monitor the mare as needed after the 5- to 8-day postpartum examination to institute any necessary therapy and determine the day of ovulation.
3. Examine the mare 14 to 16 days after ovulation to evaluate reproductive health and follicular status.
4. Follow step 4 of the short cycle after foal heat ovulation.

ALTERNATIVE PROCEDURE

Delaying the foal heat:
1. The goal of this strategy is to delay the first postpartum ovulation past 10 days postpartum.

2. Starting within the first 24 hours postpartum, mares are administered 150 mg of progesterone and 10 mg of estradiol-16β for 3 or 4 days. Some veterinarians advise that the first injection be administered within the first 6 hours postpartum to maximum efficacy.
3. Examine the mare at 5 to 8 days postpartum as previously described to reevaluate qualifications of foal heat breeding.
4. Follow steps 1 to 4 of foal heat breeding, as described above.

ADJUNCT THERAPIES

- Sixteen-hour artificial photoperiod to decrease the incidence of postpartum anestrous early in the breeding season.
  - Start 60 or more days before foaling and continue through confirmation of pregnancy or until natural day length is adequate to maintain cycling.
- Ecbolics such as oxytocin and PGF$_{2\alpha}$ or an analogue (eg, dinoprost tromethamine and cloprostenol) can be used alone or in combination with uterine lavage with physiologic saline or lactated Ringer's solution to remove uterine fluid and debris.
- Exercise encourages gross uterine involution and expulsion of intrauterine luminal fluid.
- A Caslick's vulvoplasty is recommended as soon as reasonably possible (ie, at foal heat check or at the 5- to 8-day postpartum examination) for mares with pneumovagina or poor perineal conformation.

SUGGESTED READING

Blanchard TL, Thompson JA, Brinsko SP, et al: Mating mares on foal heat: a five-year retrospective study. *Proc Am Assoc Equine Pract* 50:525–530, 2004.

Ginther OJ: *Reproductive biology of the mare: basic and applied aspects*, ed 2, Cross Plains, WI, 1992, Equiservices, pp 466–486, 504–506.

Loy RG: Characteristics of post-partum fertility in the mare. *Vet Clin North Am Large Anim Pract* 2:345–359, 1980.

MacPherson ML, Blanchard TL: Breeding mares on foal heat. *Eq Vet Educ* 16:44–52, 2005.

McKinnon AO, Squires EL, Harrison LA, et al: Ultrasonographic studies on the reproductive tract of mares after parturition: effect of involution and uterine fluid on pregnancy rates in mares with normal and delayed first postpartum ovulatory cycles. *J Am Vet Med Assoc* 192:350–353, 1988.

AUTHOR: SHELBY HAYDEN

Pregnancy Diagnosis up to 60 Days

BASIC INFORMATION

SYNONYM(S)

Pregnancy check, early pregnancy monitoring

OVERVIEW AND GOAL(S)

- Accurate early diagnosis and evaluation of pregnancy and nonpregnancy are essential for optimal reproductive efficiency.
- Determination of pregnancy is critical for the establishment of effective veterinary management of broodmares. Not only does early detection of pregnancy provide information on whether the mare is pregnant and for arranging rebreeding of nonpregnant mares, it also helps establish a medical approach for abnormal pregnancy (eg, twinning) in the most advantageous manner.
- Several methods of pregnancy detection (behavior, transrectal palpation, ultrasonography, hormonal tests) are available. The choice of technique ultimately depends on the stage of pregnancy.

INDICATIONS

All mares included in a breeding program

CONTRAINDICATIONS

- Mare with a disease that could compromise the integrity of the rectal mucosa
- Mare with an explosive temperament

EQUIPMENT, ANESTHESIA

- The mare must be adequately restrained. Depending on the mare's temperament, stocks, lip chain, twitch, or sedation should be used before the reproductive tract is examined. In general, mares tolerate the procedure without major restraint.
- The veterinarian can, while wearing a glove, palpate the internal genital organs of the mare per rectum.
- A B-mode real-time ultrasound system consisting of a monitor and a linear array 5 to 7 MHz transducer is adequate for most needs encountered in equine reproduction.

ANTICIPATED TIME

- **Days 12 to 25 of pregnancy:** Objective is to confirm the pregnancy status
  - *Monitoring sexual behavior* by daily teasing with a stallion can be performed. Failure to return to estrus between days 16 and 20 suggests the mare is pregnant. Estrous behav-

ior occasionally may be displayed in pregnant mares around days 14 to 18 after ovulation. Furthermore, absence of estrous behavior may occur in nonpregnant mares: those with a persistent corpus luteum, early embryonic death, or a diestrus ovulation (1% to 2% of mares). Young or dominant mares may also not show estrous behavior as well as mares with a foal at foot.
  - *Transrectal palpation* is the most common means of early pregnancy testing. Since pregnancy in the mare is associated with a tonic and tubular uterus and a tight, firm, and elongated cervix, transrectal palpation of both structures between days 17 and 20 can indirectly determine pregnancy status. The embryonic vesicle is usually not detectable by transrectal palpation between days 16 and 20 (15–24 mm in diameter). Because of possible false-negative results, reexamination is always necessary to confirm pregnancy.
  - *Transrectal ultrasonography* is the most sensitive and specific pregnancy test. The ultrasound machine allows visualization of the embryonic vesicle as early as day 9.5 (3 mm in diameter), with an accuracy rate reaching 99% by days 14 to 15 after ovulation with a vesicle of 17 to 22 mm in diameter. Ultrasonography also allows assessment of the growth of the embryonic vesicle and early detection of multiple pregnancies (twins). In ultrasonographic images from a cross-section of a uterine horn, the vesicle appears as a spherical, anechoic (dark) structure surrounded by a lighter area of uterine tissue. Between days 10 and 15, the embryonic vesicle progresses from 6 to 22 mm in diameter (~3.0 mm/day). At day 17 to 18, the vesicle has a triangular shape like a guitar pick. The embryo itself can first be seen in the ventral portion of the yolk sac at day 21. Presence of a corpus luteum with an elevated progesterone concentration in the blood of the mare beyond day 15 of the estrous cycle is associated with pregnancy. Blood progesterone levels cannot be used as the sole diagnostic method of pregnancy. Nonetheless, a progesterone concentration less than 1 ng/mL of serum between 18 and 21 days after

ovulation points to nonpregnant status.
- **Days 25 to 35 of pregnancy:** Objective is to confirm normal progression of the pregnancy and viability of the embryo. By days 25 to 30, the embryonic vesicle has expanded to 30 to 60 mm in diameter.
  - The *transrectal examination* is meticulously performed on the whole uterine horn because the spherical or ovoid bulge (size of a golf ball) of early pregnancy is often noted on the anteroventral aspect at the base of one horn near the junction of the uterine body and feels like a fluid-filled structure. The cervix and uterine tone have similar characteristics as the previous stage.
  - By day 25, the *transrectal ultrasonography* allows an accurate determination of the embryonic heartbeat, confirming its viability. The absence of a heartbeat after 25 days of gestation is a reliable sign of embryonic death. An increase in fluid echogenicity, inadequate size and shape of the embryonic vesicle, and an irregular outline of the embryo are signs of embryonic death. At day 26, the allantois occupies approximately 25% of the embryonic vesicle. By day 30 of gestation, the dorsal regressing yolk sac is about equal in size to the developing allantois. The major advantage of transrectal ultrasonography for early pregnancy diagnosis is the potential detection of twin embryos so that one can be removed as well as detection of embryonic death, leading to a rapid return to rebreeding.
- **Days 35 to 45 of pregnancy:** Objective is to confirm viability of the embryo and provide measurements of its growth rate. During this period, the embryonic vesicle grows from 60 (lemon size) to 100 mm (orange size) in diameter.
  - On *transrectal palpation*, the vesicle shows resilience and is oblong, approximately the size of a baseball at the base of one uterine horn.
  - On *ultrasonography* between 32 and 33 days of pregnancy, the allantois occupies approximately 75% of the embryonic vesicle, and at day 40 the embryo is located at the dorsal pole of the vesicle, hanging by its umbilical cord. The allantoic cavity occupies the entire vesicle surrounding the amniotic vesicle.

After day 40, the umbilical cord elongates and the fetus moves down in the embryonic vesicle and reaches the ventral wall of the gravid horn by day 48 (when it is grapefruit size). After day 26, the conceptus grows at approximately 1.8 mm per day until day 50.

○ *An endocrinological test* is available for diagnosing pregnancy. Between days 36 and 40 of pregnancy, endometrial cups are present and persist until day 120 of pregnancy, secreting equine chorionic gonadotropin (eCG). Concentrations of serum eCG peak between days 55 and 65 and decrease to baseline between days 120 and 150. The eCG assays are valuable methods when breeding date and ovulation time are known and more particularly in miniature or touchy mares that do not tolerate transrectal palpation and ultrasonography. A false-positive test result can occur when pregnancy is lost after day 36 of gestation.

- **Days 45 to 65 of pregnancy:** Objective is to monitor fetal well-being and sexing. Although the physical characteristics of the cervix do not change as pregnancy advances, the uterus becomes less tonic and progressively fills and expands into the uterine body.
  ○ On *transrectal palpation*, the uterine bulge loses resiliency and the uterus begins to descend into the abdominal cavity, having the size and shape of a small football.

○ On *transrectal ultrasonography*, several elements of the conceptus can be measured to assess fetal well-being, such as size of the fetus, heartbeat, echogenicity of the allantoic fluid, appearance of the umbilical cord, and fetal membranes. However, very little information is available in the literature on early pregnancy in mares.

○ Measurement of eCG serum levels is a useful endocrinological test for the diagnosis of pregnancy. Evaluation of serum, urine, and fecal estrogen levels is another endocrinological test that can be performed in mares. Equilin and equilenin are estrogens unique to the mare. A statistically different increase in the serum concentration of estrogen is only detectable at day 60 of the pregnancy. It peaks at day 180 to 240 of gestation before progressively declining toward parturition. The Cuboni test can measure levels of estrogens in the urine with 90% accuracy after 100 days of gestation.

POSSIBLE COMPLICATIONS AND COMMON ERRORS TO BE AVOIDED

- Possible complication: Rectal irritation or injuries
- Differential diagnosis:
  ○ Multiple pregnancies
  ○ Pyometra
  ○ Mucometra
  ○ Endometrial cyst

○ Anembryonic vesicle
○ Dying embryo
○ Pneumouterus
○ Small amount of uterine fluid with or without embryonic loss
○ Gestation in the uterine body

PROCEDURE

Steps for transrectal palpation and ultrasonography of the reproductive organs to precisely evaluate pregnancy status:

- Wrap the tail and move it to the side.
- Lubricate the plastic sleeve well.
- Remove all fecal matter from the rectum.
- Systematically palpate the cervix and the uterus in their entirety by transrectal palpation.
- Advance a well-lubricated hand with or without the transducer over the cervix, the body of the uterus until the bifurcation of the uterus, and the tip of one horn. At the tip of the horn, move the hand/transducer toward the ipsilateral horn until the tip is reached. The genital tract needs to be examined in its entirety twice by keeping the cross-section view of the tract in the center of the monitor screen and by slightly rotating the transducer around the horn.

POSTPROCEDURE

Clean the perineal area.

AUTHORS: **GABRIEL BORGES COUTO, REJEAN CLÉOPHAS LEFEBVRE, FRANÇOIS-XAVIER GRAND,** and **IGNACIO RAGGIO**

Pulse Oximetry

BASIC INFORMATION

SYNONYM(S)

Hemoglobin saturation

OVERVIEW AND GOAL

Pulse oximetry is used as an estimate of hemoglobin saturation with oxygen in the capillary beds. Saturation is estimated by the absorption of light as it passes through (transmission) or is reflected from (reflectance) the tissues. Oxygenated hemoglobin absorbs less light at 660 nm than reduced hemoglobin, and vice versa at 940 nm. The difference is used to determine hemoglobin saturation.

INDICATIONS

Serial pulse oximetry is indicated to monitor hemoglobin desaturation.

CONTRAINDICATIONS

- Hypovolemic shock
  ○ Vasoconstriction may provide false readings.

EQUIPMENT, ANESTHESIA

Pulse oximeter

ANTICIPATED TIME

15 seconds to a reading

POSSIBLE COMPLICATIONS AND COMMON ERRORS TO BE AVOIDED

- At low saturation, transmission pulse oximetry underestimates saturation, whereas reflectance pulse oximetry overestimates saturation.
- Pulse oximetry is most accurate when saturation is >80% and underestimates saturation if it is less than 80%.

- Carboxyhemoglobin and methemoglobin can interfere with absorption (pulse oximetry cannot differentiate them from oxyhemoglobin).
- Pulse oximetry cannot determine saturations over 100%.
- Calculated hemoglobin saturation by a machine uses the human oxyhemoglobin desaturation curve, which may not be accurate for horses.
- Pigmented tissues interfere with pulse oximetry results.

PROCEDURE

- Apply the pulse oximeter to the tongue or ear 4 cm from the tip.
  ○ Tissues must be nonpigmented.
  ○ The coccygeal artery is useful in foals but underestimates saturation.
  ○ Rectal probes may also be used in foals.

- Obtain reading.
  - Reposition probe ever 45 minutes to prevent falsely low readings.
  - Saturation <95% correlates with hypoxemia.

POSTPROCEDURE

Pulse oximetry is best used as a repeated measured to determine trends in hemoglobin desaturation.

ALTERNATIVES AND THEIR RELATIVE MERITS

Packed cell volume and arterial blood gas values are required to accurately determine the oxygen content of the blood.

SUGGESTED READING

Magdesian KG: Monitoring the critically ill equine patient, *Vet Clin North Am Equine Pract* 20:11–39, 2004.

AUTHOR: **AMELIA MUNSTERMAN**

Radiation Therapy

BASIC INFORMATION

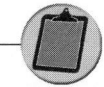

SYNONYM(S)

External beam radiation, brachytherapy, interstitial therapy

OVERVIEW AND GOAL

- Used to treat tumors that cannot be adequately treated with surgery.
- Primary effect on cancer cells is to damage the DNA and cause cell death when the cells try to divide.
- Radiation can treat visible tumor mass as well as surrounding areas affected microscopically by tumor so that areas a surgeon may not be able to remove may also be treated.
- Does not selectively seek cancer cells, but damage to normal tissue is reduced by fractionating the dose of radiation into many small doses or spreading the dose out over time through slow, constant delivery of dose. This allows normal tissues time to repair, repopulate, and survive the radiation insult.
- The total dose of radiation used is the dose needed to kill the tumor. This also determines the severity of the early effects that occur after irradiation. These early effects occur in rapidly dividing tissues, including epithelial surfaces of skin and mucosa.
- The fraction size is chosen based on the normal tissues being treated; some tissues will not tolerate large doses of radiation administered rapidly. These late-responding tissues, such as bone, muscle, and nervous tissue, divide slowly. They are intolerant of large doses per fraction. Adverse effects in these tissues can take years to appear.
- The period over which the radiation is delivered ideally is chosen based on the speed at which the tumor is growing.
- Total dose, fraction size, and total time in treatment must also take into account the increased difficulty to anesthetize and position horses. Therefore the number of fractions is often limited compared with smaller animal patients.
- Damage in normal tissues that do not contain tumor is also limited by delivering the dose of radiation as precisely as possible into the tumor. This requires treatment volumes that are as small as possible and shaped to match the tumor and its potential margins. This is termed *treatment planning*.

INDICATIONS

- In equine patients, external tumors and those of the extremities or head are easiest to position under the therapy beam or locally implant with radioactive seeds.
- Tumors need to have low metastatic potential to be good candidates for radiation therapy.
- Sarcoids and squamous cell carcinomas have been most commonly treated in the past.
- Localized low-grade lymphoma, sinonasal tumors, and malignant melanomas can also be treated.

CONTRAINDICATIONS

- Metastatic tumors
- Tumors involving areas greater than 25 cm in diameter.
- Tumors deep-seated in the chest or abdomen.

EQUIPMENT, ANESTHESIA

- Special training and equipment are required for radiation therapy. For these treatments, the animal must be referred to a radiation treatment facility with the ability to treat horses.
- The source of radiation used can vary:
  - **Plesiotherapy,** or very close range radiation, uses a very small strontium-90 source that emits beta-radiation into the tissues and travels only 2 to 3 mm deep. The most common indications for plesiotherapy are ocular and periocular lesions that are small or have been surgically debulked to minimal disease.
  - **Brachytherapy**, or short-distance radiation, uses implantation of radioactive seeds of a variety of sources directly into the tumor.
  - **Teletherapy,** or external beam radiation, involves equipment that houses a radioactive source or a linear accelerator that generates radiation. Linear accelerators have an advantage because they often have the ability to generate two forms of radiation with different energies and abilities to penetrate tissues. The differing energy beams and their differing levels of penetration are important to treatment planning.
- Anesthesia is required for each treatment with a linear accelerator or strontium probe because the horse must remain motionless while undergoing therapy.
- Placement of interstitial implants can be done under sedation, but anesthesia is often used so the implantation can be done quickly and efficiently, thereby limiting human exposure to the radioactive sources.

ANTICIPATED TIME

- Horses treated with plesiotherapy generally receive a single treatment, often accompanying surgery.
- Interstitial implants are left in place for a period determined by how active the implanted sources are and their rate of decay. In general, this is approximately 3 to 7 days.
- External beam radiation requires fractionation of the dose, with overall treatment time generally 4 weeks or longer and the horse being treated at least three times per week.

PREPARATION: IMPORANT CHECKPOINTS

- It is important to have a definitive tumor diagnosis and to make as good a judgment as possible that the tumor has not metastasized.

- In equine patients, thorough cancer screening can be nearly impossible, but the local lymph nodes should be examined and the tumor itself may need to be imaged by advanced means to ensure the entire tumor is treated.

POSSIBLE COMPLICATIONS AND COMMON ERRORS TO BE AVOIDED

- If tumors are allowed to grow several times after inadequate surgical removal, they will usually become more difficult to irradiate. Radiation needs to be considered early in the treatment of tumors and not as a last attempt at salvage.
- Radiation therapy itself is fraught with potential complications if not done properly and requires the services of a specialist.

PROCEDURE

- Brachytherapy: Radioactive seeds are passed into catheters that have been surgically placed in the tumor. The horse is left in a stall as isolated from people as possible. The seeds are generally removed after adequate radiation dose has been delivered.
- External beam radiation: The horse is anesthetized and moved into the radiation therapy vault for treatment. The horse is then positioned as precisely as possible so that the dose of radiation can be accurately delivered to the tumor (Figure 1). Once the fraction has been delivered, the horse is removed from the treatment vault and taken to a recovery stall. This procedure is repeated for each fraction delivered, which can be as few as three fractions given 1 week apart or

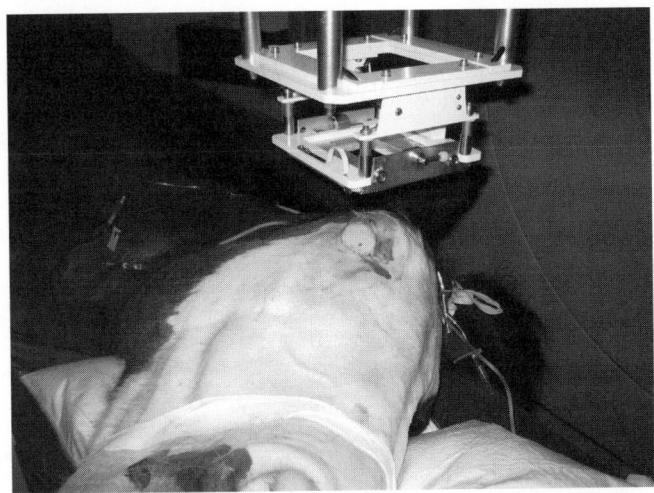

FIGURE 1 A horse positioned for therapy of a squamous cell carcinoma of the medial canthus. The eye is shielded with a piece of wax, which approximates the density of tissue and blocks the radiation from reaching the cornea. The linear accelerator is being used to generate an electron beam (for superficial treatments), and the field is shaped with an electron cone and block so that only a confined area is treated.

as many as 18 fractions given once daily.

POSTPROCEDURE

- Early effects of radiation include hair loss, erythema, moist desquamation in the skin of the treatment field, mucositis, and conjunctivitis.
- Late effects can include keratitis sicca cataracts if the eye is treated and skin fibrosis or bone necrosis if large fraction sizes are used.

ALTERNATIVES AND THEIR RELATIVE MERITS

- Surgery if the tumor can be removed.
- Incomplete surgical removal should be treated with radiation shortly after surgery, and the tumor should not be

allowed to regrow before using radiation.

SUGGESTED READING

Mosunic CB, Moore PA, Carmicheal KP, et al: Effects of treatment with and without adjuvant radiation therapy on recurrence of ocular and adnexal squamous cell carcinoma in horses: 157 cases (1985-2002). *J Am Vet Med Assoc* 225:1733–1738, 2004.

Theon AP: Radiation therapy in the horse. *Vet Clin North Am Equine Pract* 14:673–688, 1998.

Walker MA, Schumacher J, Schmitz DG, et al: Cobalt 60 radiotherapy for treatment of squamous cell carcinoma of the nasal cavity and paranasal sinuses in three horses. *J Am Vet Med Assoc* 212:848–851, 1998.

AUTHOR: **JANEAN L. FIDEL**

Radiography: Dental

BASIC INFORMATION

SYNONYM(S)

Radiographs
x-Rays

OVERVIEW AND GOAL(S)

- Radiography is an ancillary technique for the evaluation of pathology of the dentition and its supporting structures including the paranasal sinuses.
- Production and interpretation of dental radiographs require an understanding of the regional anatomy, radiographic anatomy, and dental pathology as well as the anticipated effect of dental

pathology on the surrounding structures.
- Radiographs must be interpreted in light of changes associated with continuous eruption of equine (hypsodont) teeth, which makes their radiographic appearance variable with advancing age.

INDICATIONS

- The oral examination is limited to the erupted portions of teeth and the surrounding oral tissues. Frequently, primary dental disease results in secondary infectious or inflammatory lesions of the unerupted portions of

teeth, the periodontal tissues, skeletal structures, and paranasal sinuses.
- Dental radiography is indicated for any dental condition suspected to extend beyond the oral cavity, or when the clinical signs relate to the secondary effects of dental disease.
  - Secondary signs can include but are not limited to nasal discharge, osseous swelling, maxillofacial deformity, draining tracts, ozena (malodorous breath), pain on mastication or prehension, or even performance problems related to bitting.

○ Radiography is also indicated for evaluation of the temporomandibular joint disease.

CONTRAINDICATIONS

- Few contraindications to radiography exist per se.
- Radiography uses ionizing radiation.
- Care should be taken to keep the radiation dose to the staff and patient as low as reasonably achievable (ALARA).
- Children and pregnant women should not be permitted to be in the presence of a radiographic examination.
- The use of sedation and restraint for acquisition of radiographs should be considered in light of the patient's clinical status.

EQUIPMENT, ANESTHESIA

- X-Ray generator: The generator should be capable of 80 to 100 kVp and 1.0 to 2.0 mAs. Specific recommendations for kVp and mAs settings depend upon the radiography equipment being used.
- Cassettes: Large size cassettes (14 × 17 inch) are preferable. Small-sized cassettes and many digital detectors require two projections to complete the evaluation of the entire arcade.
- Safety equipment:
  ○ Cassette holders reduce personnel exposure.
  ○ Lead aprons must be worn by all persons involved in the study and within range of both primary beam and scatter radiation.
  ○ Lead gloves must be worn by the person holding the cassette even if they are using a cassette holder.
  ○ Radiation dosimeters must be worn by personnel with occupational radiation exposure.
- Markers: Lead markers to indicate left and right should be placed on the cassette. A lead marker such as a BB

should be considered to mark the external site of soft tissue swelling or draining tract.
- Personnel: Two persons, one to hold the cassette/detector and one to operate the generator
- Rope halter
- Wooden block: 2 × 4 inch or other radiolucent block to place between incisor teeth to produce open-mouth oblique projections

ANTICIPATED TIME

The production of a complete radiographic study is dependent on patient compliance (level of sedation) and the number of views necessary to completely evaluate the problem or anatomic region. Generally 20 to 40 minutes.

PREPARATION: IMPORTANT CHECKPOINTS

- Sedation: The goal for sedation is to keep the head low and immobile. This must be done in the face of equipment moving around and above the horse's head. Most commonly an α_2 agonist ± an opioid (butorphanol) is used.
- The radiographer must check five features to produce each radiographic projection.
  ○ Obliquity: Varies with anatomic region of interest
  ○ Beam center
  ○ Beam angle
  ○ Film focal distance
  ○ kVp and mAs

POSSIBLE COMPLICATIONS AND COMMON ERRORS TO BE AVOIDED

Inadequate sedation or poor patient compliance will result in motion artefact or poor positioning.

PROCEDURE

- A complete radiographic examination should include a minimum of four

views. The views should be chosen based on the clinical and oral examinations. The lateral and oblique projections can be made with a block between the incisor teeth to obtain open-mouth views. The open mouth views improve visualization of the occlusal and interdental regions.
- Dorsoventral (DV) projection (Figure 1): The cassette is placed ventral to and against the mandible. The generator is positioned so that the beam passes from dorsal and approximately 5 degrees caudal to a line perpendicular to the dorsal surface of the frontal bone to ventral. Care should be taken to shoot the radiographic beam straight through the skull in a direction that is parallel to the nasal septum, thereby positioning the dental arcades equidistant from midline (Figure 2).
- Maxillary laterolateral projection (Figure 3): The long axis of the cassette should be parallel and dorsal to the dorsal surface of the horse's frontal bone. The beam center is dependent on cassette size but should be approximately at the level of the rostral facial crest (large cassette). The beam should pass through the maxillary arcade and sinuses parallel to the dorsal surface of the face (Figure 4).
- Mandibular laterolateral projection: The long axis of the cassette should be parallel to the ventral surface of the mandible. The beam center should be at the middle of the mandibular arcade. The beam is parallel to a line crossing the ventral borders of the mandibular bodies.
- Sinus oblique (dorsal 55 degrees lateral to ventrolateral oblique: Figure 5): The x-ray generator is positioned 55 degrees lateral, measuring from a point directly dorsal to the dorsal surface of the frontal bone. The beam center should be near the rostral aspect of the facial crest but care

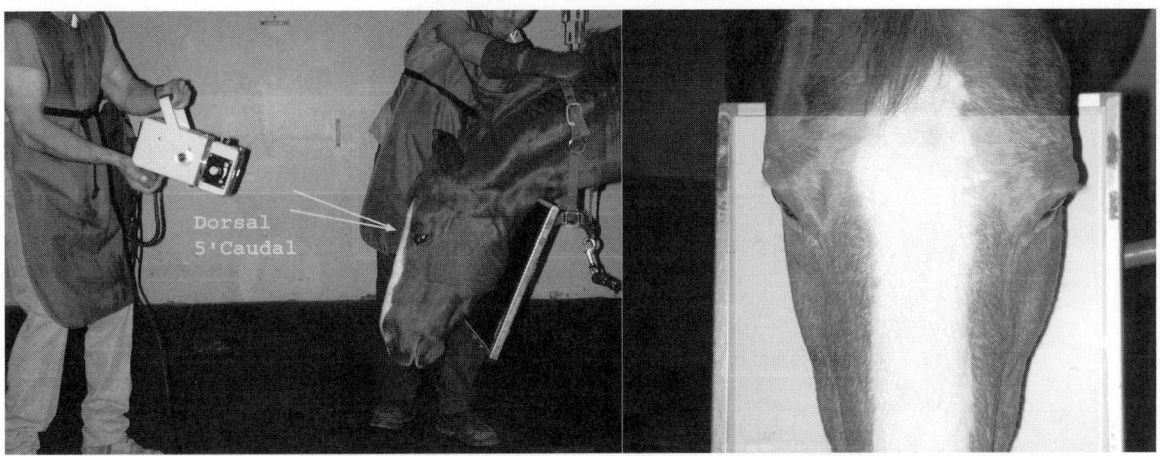

FIGURE 1 Production of a dorsoventral radiograph.

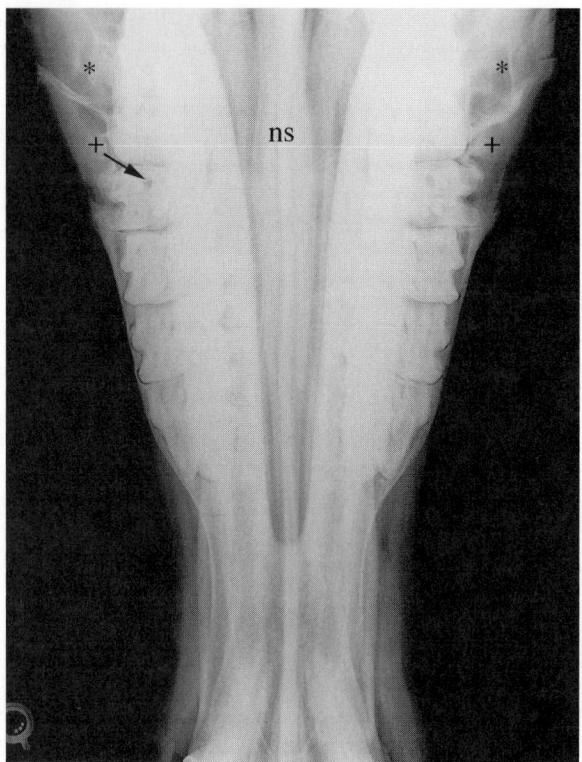

FIGURE 2 A well-positioned dorsoventral radiograph. *ns,* Nasal septum; *, caudal maxillary sinus; +, rostral maxillary sinus. The black arrow shows an irregular lucent lesion present on both maxillary 09s that represents infundibular caries.

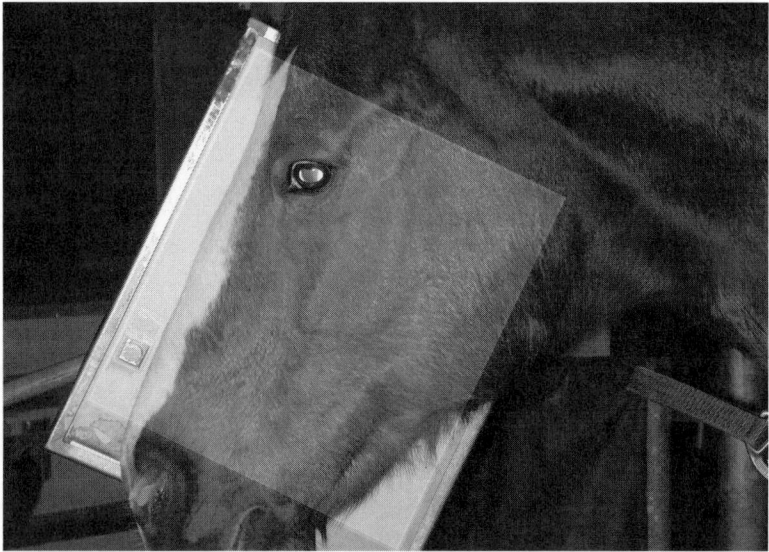

FIGURE 3 Production of a maxillary lateral radiograph.

should be taken to incorporate the most caudal portions of the arcade and caudal maxillary sinus. This can be achieved by including the contralateral zygomatic arch within the collimator shadow on the cassette. NOTE: Always include the opposite oblique view for comparison. Annotate left and right accurately. A dorsal 55 degrees left to ventral right oblique should have a right marker at the top of the cassette and a left marker at the bottom.

- Mandibular body oblique (dorsal 45 degrees lateral to ventrolateral oblique): The cassette should be placed parallel and ventral to the mandible. The degree of obliquity is slightly less in order to visualize separation between the mandibular bodies.
- Mandibular ramus oblique or temporomandibular oblique (lateral 30 degrees caudal 5–10 degrees ventral to lateral cranial dorsal oblique): The beam center should be at the level of the guttural pouches and passing slightly ventral to dorsal. The collimator light should extend to the base of the ear. The cassette should be placed opposite the point of entry and perpendicular to the x-ray beam.

POSTPROCEDURE

No specific postprocedure steps are recommended.

ALTERNATIVES AND THEIR RELATIVE MERITS

- Intraoral radiographs provide improved evaluation of the individual teeth and their relationship with the supporting structures.
- Specialized or modified equipment is required to examine the cheek teeth.
- Readily available radiographic equipment is appropriate and adequate to provide intraoral evaluation of the incisor teeth.
- In both cases, chewing motions should be minimized by either performing the examination at peak sedation or by using a higher level of sedation.
- The cassette (detector) is placed within the oral cavity.
- Beam angle is dependent on the tissue of interest.

AUTHOR: **SARAH M. PUCHALSKI**

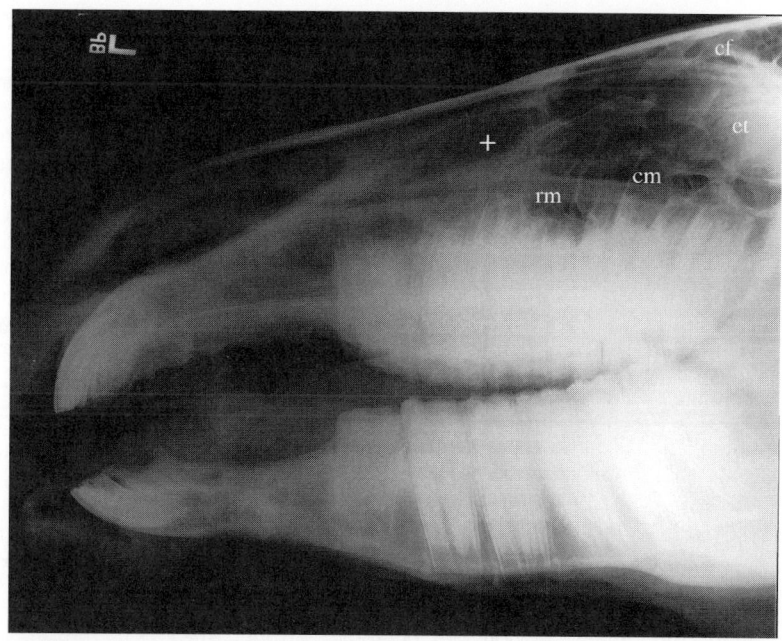

FIGURE 4 Open mouth lateral radiograph. *cf,* Conchofrontal or frontal sinus; *et,* ethmoturbinates; *cm,* caudal maxillary sinus; *rm,* rostral maxillary sinus; +, dorsal conchal sinus.

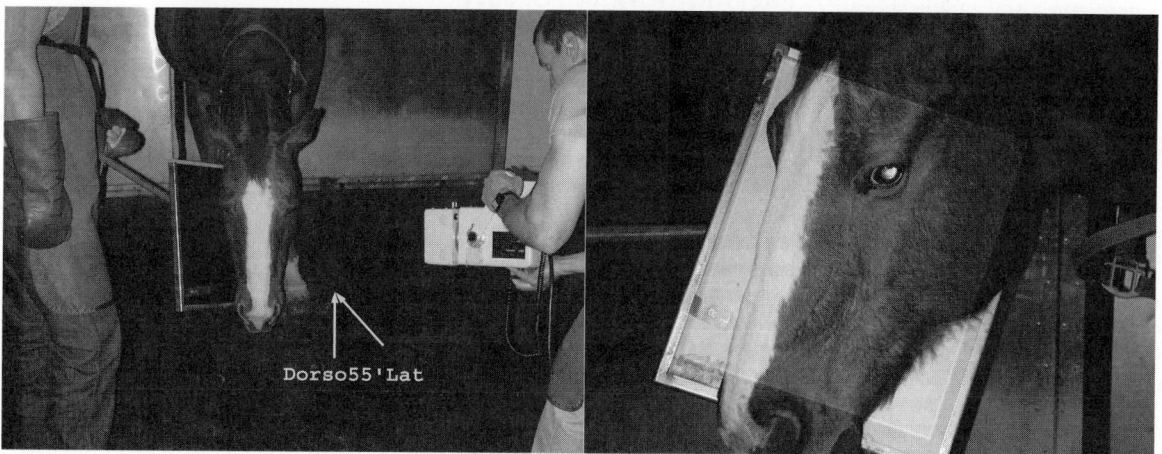

FIGURE 5 Production of a maxillary arcade oblique projection.

Radiography: Musculoskeletal

BASIC INFORMATION

EQUIPMENT, ANESTHESIA

Types of radiographic systems:
- Film/screen radiography (ie, conventional radiography) consists of a cassette with radiographic film. The wavelength of light emitted by the intensifying screens within the cassette must match the film sensitivity for best results (eg, blue light–emitting screens must be paired with blue-sensitive film).

- Digital radiography (DR) is now commonplace in equine practice due to its ease of use and obvious advantages over analog film. There are two basic types of digital radiography available: computed radiography (CR) and flat panel detectors. One advantage of digital radiography is the ability to obtain quality radiographic images within a larger range of techniques. This reduces the number of retake examinations caused by improper exposure factors. Postprocessing algorithms can be applied to alter contrast and latitude. Storage and transfer of digital images is a major advantage over conventional film radiography.

- CR is similar to conventional radiography in that it uses an imaging cassette, in which is placed a reusable imaging plate coated with phosphostimulable phosphor (PSP) that stores the latent radiographic image for later processing. Once the radiographic exposure is made, the imaging plate is processed with a dedicated computer (digital processor, reader unit) yielding a digital radiographic image to be viewed at a radiographic work station. CR is portable and replacement of a damaged cassette is relatively inexpensive.

- Flat panel detectors (often referred to incorrectly as DR) have the advantage of immediate capture and transfer of a digital image to a computer without the need for the reader unit. A current limitation of flat panel detectors is that the detector plate and computer are directly connected via an electrical cord, somewhat limiting maneuverability. Another is that damage to the panel is expensive to repair or replace (tens of thousands of dollars).

- Depending on facilities and workload, x-ray machines can range from less than 10 lb handheld units to large ceiling-mounted gantries. The majority of equine practitioners use portable units. The largest factor when purchasing a portable unit is the power output. The larger the tube, the more the power output (kilovoltage potential [kVp] and milliamperage [mA]) and the greater the ability to radiograph thicker anatomic structures (eg, adult shoulder, adult thorax, skull). Most portable x-ray units can generate between 40 and 100 kVp using high-frequency generator technology, ranging from 10 to 40 mA.

- Positioning items include a cassette tunnel, slotted wooden block, cassette holder, and a tripod x-ray machine stand.

Safety

- Safety is of utmost importance when working with radiation. Radiation is known to cause deleterious effects ranging from cataracts to cancer. However, with proper safety precautions, radiographic exposure to personnel can be minimized.

- The fundamentals of limiting personnel radiation exposure are:
  - Time: Limit the amount of time spent in the radiographic suite during radiographic procedures. Minimize the number of retake exposures.
  - Distance: When holding a cassette or patient, the handler should be as far from the primary x-ray beam as possible. The distance from the primary beam can be increased by the use of radiographic cassette holders. Remember that doubling the distance decreases the amount of x-ray exposure four-fold (the inverse square law).
  - Shielding: Lead aprons, lead thyroid protectors, and lead gloves should be worn by all personnel when radiographs are being obtained. Lead shielding effectively eliminates

human exposure to scatter radiation. Lead protection does not protect from primary x-ray beam exposure; no human body parts should be exposed to the primary x-ray beam. Lead shielding should be periodically inspected for damage or wear (cracks, tears). Rolling your lead apron for transport is preferred over folding, which increases the likelihood of cracking the lead.
  - Collimating the x-ray beam to the smallest field of view over the area of interest is critical. "Tight" collimation decreases scatter radiation exposure to personnel and considerably increases image detail and contrast.

- Clinics are responsible for monitoring personnel dosimetry.
  - Rules and regulations for radiation exposure vary by state; more information can be found through the State Veterinarian or Department of Health.

PREPARATION: IMPORANT CHECKPOINTS

- Patient preparation is very important to minimize artifacts and misdiagnoses, in particular the foot and hair coat.

- A small amount of sedation is generally sufficient to minimize patient motion; excessive sedation may lead to patient instability and motion artifact.

- Dry dirt and debris within the hair coat should be removed with a firm brush.

- Boots/wraps, bandages, blankets, and halters with metallic clasps should be removed from the area to be radiographed when possible. Rope halters work well (vs. nylon). Temporary halters can be made of rolled gauze for evaluation of the head in cooperative horses.

POSSIBLE COMPLICATIONS AND COMMON ERRORS TO BE AVOIDED

- A radiographic technique chart is specific for body part, equipment, and film-screen combination. A technique chart specifies kVp, mAs, and focal film distance (FFD), the distance from the x-ray tube to the cassette. A properly set up and used technique chart should minimize the number of retakes due to inappropriate exposures.

- Technique charts should be developed and procedures for designing a technique chart can be found in a highly recommended textbook, *Equine Radiography* (see "Suggested Readings" below).

PROCEDURE

Techniques:

- In addition to kVp and mAs, FFD will greatly alter the exposure. Inconsistent FFD is the most common cause of fluctuating film exposure. Consistent FFD is determined by using a tape measure (often incorporated into the x-ray machine), a yardstick, or focused laser pointers.

- All radiographs should be labeled with the following information: Name of owner and patient, name and address of clinic, patient's age, sex and breed, and date of the films. Lead markers should be placed on the cassette to identify the leg and should be positioned on the lateral or dorsal aspect of the radiograph.

- If the radiographic image is overexposed (too dark), reducing the kVp by 10% to 15% will noticeably lighten the image. Conversely, a film that is underexposed can be corrected by increasing kVp by 10% to 15%.

- Overexposure or underexposure can also be effectively corrected by altering mAs.

- Doubling or halving mAs proportionally doubles or halves radiographic film density. Appropriate film density (film background blackness) is sufficient when you cannot see your hand behind the film while viewing.

- Altering the kVp also inversely alters image contrast. Higher kVp produces a radiographic image that has less contrast (more shades of gray; higher latitude or long-scale contrast); lower kVp produces a more black and white image (fewer shades of gray, higher contrast, short-scale contrast). While tempting to produce equine extremity radiographs with the highest contrast to maximize bony detail, doing so reduces or eliminates visualization of the surrounding soft tissues. Assessment of tendons, ligaments, and joint effusion becomes difficult or impossible. Altering mAs does not have a significant effect on film contrast.

- Probably the most common technical error when using digital radiography is gross overexposure. This results in "burned out" peripheral anatomic structures, in turn mimicking osteolysis (Figure 1).

- Grids can be used to increase radiographic detail by decreasing the amount of scatter radiation reaching the cassette. Grids are sometimes used to increase detail of the third phalanx and navicular bone. Grids are more commonly used with high radiation exposure techniques for thick body parts such as the spine, shoulder, elbow, and skull. The grid is placed adjacent to the cassette or imaging plate.

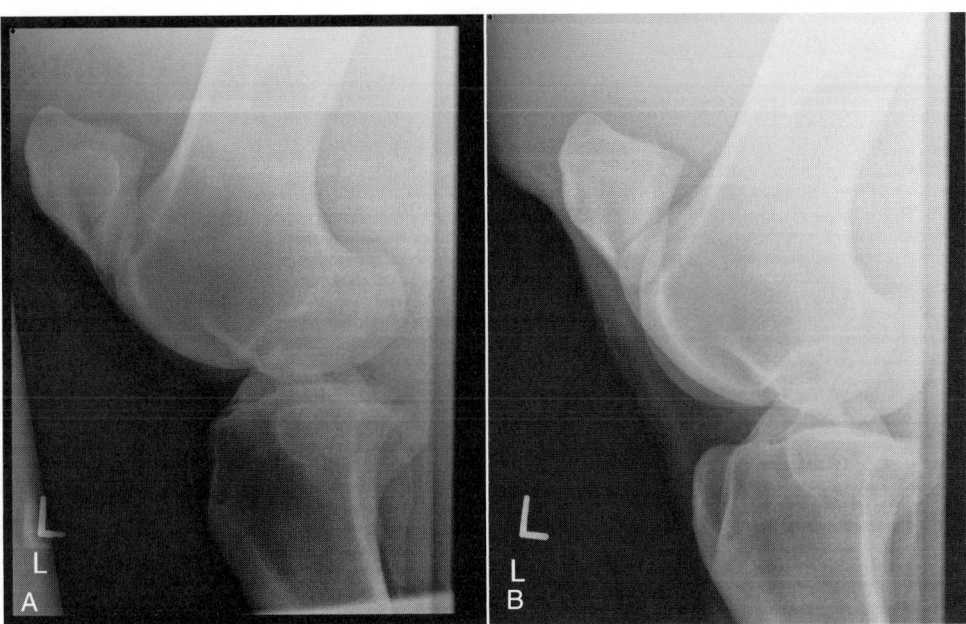

FIGURE 1 An example of digital overexposure (**A**) and a correct exposure (**B**). In **A**, portions of the lateral trochlear ridge of the femur and the cranial proximal tibia cannot be seen due to overexposure. This can easily be misinterpreted as lytic bone pathology. Note the black overexposure band cranial to the stifle. In the properly exposed digital image (**B**), the normal lateral trochlear ridge and the cranial proximal tibia are clearly visualized. *L,* Left stifle.

- The grid is a thin plate composed of parallel lead strips alternating with radiolucent material. Grids are classified by grid ratio and line pairs/inch. The higher the grid ratio (12 : 1 vs. 6 : 1) and greater the number of line pairs (eg, 104 pairs per inch), the more effective the grid is at decreasing scatter, yielding higher radiographic detail and image contrast. The downside is that twofold to fourfold increases in mAs must be used to make a proper exposure when a grid is used. The grid must also be aligned perfectly with the primary x-ray beam, or grid "cut off" occurs. Grids are focused and must be used within a specified FFD. For these reasons, grids are rarely used in the field. Remember, tight x-ray beam collimation is the best way to maximize image detail.

Radiographic views:

Standard radiographic projection nomenclature is determined by the direction of the x-ray beam to the cassette. Degree values (e.g., 60 degrees) indicate positioning of the x-ray machine and direction of the x-ray beam from its initial starting point. This may be from proximal to distal or from midline to medial/lateral or combinations of both. As an example, a D60°L-PaMO view of the carpus refers to the x-ray machine beginning dorsal (D) to the limb on midline and then moved 60 degrees laterally (L), directing the x-ray beam to the palmar (Pa) and medially (M) located cassette.

These descriptions can become cumbersome, and most practitioners use some form of abbreviation or slang ter-minology. Unfortunately, abbreviated terminology is not standardized. To some, a "medial oblique" refers to a DLPMO; to others, it describes the exact opposite view, the DMPLO. For many, a "DL" view would refer to moving the x-ray machine laterally from dorsal (a DLPMO view); a "DM" would refer to a DMPLO view.

Foot preparation:

- Careful foot preparation is essential. Evaluation of foot radiographs is challenging enough without the added contribution of confusing artifacts. Time spent preparing the foot properly absolutely pays dividends with more confident evaluation and diagnoses.

- If possible, shoes should be removed. Even with proper removal, metal fragments or rust may remain in the nail tracts. These are generally inconsequential unless advanced imaging such as MRI or CT is to be performed.

- Use a wire brush to remove loose debris from the hoof wall. A hoof pick can be used to remove dirt from the sole. Pare away redundant sole.

- The crevices of the foot should be filled in with a modeling compound (eg, Play-Doh) to minimize artifacts (Figure 2). Careful packing of the foot must be performed to limit trapping of air or excessive opacity from overpacking. The packing material should be level with the surrounding soft tissues of the sole and not extend beyond the apex of the frog to minimize artifacts of the solar margin of P3. When working in the field, stand-ing the horse on a canvas tarp can help reduce debris accumulation on the prepared sole of the foot.

- Some forms of modeling clay are too opaque to be used as foot packing material. Also, blue Play-Doh is more opaque than other colors and should be avoided.

- If necessary, a metal opaque marker can be used to delineate the dorsal hoof wall (eg, flexible wire or barium paste) or coronary band (eg, BB pellet) in laminitis cases. A better alternative is to take a second slightly underexposed lateral radiograph (eg, reduce kVp by 10) to ensure evaluation of the soft tissues.

Technique:

- The distal extremity examination (DEE) assesses the navicular bone, the third (P3), the second (P2), and most of the first (P1) phalanges, and the distal (coffin) and proximal (pastern) interphalangeal joints. In most cases, the DEE includes evaluation of the pastern, especially if special views are considered. The fetlock joint is examined in a different, dedicated radiographic study described later.

- The foot is positioned on a block or cassette tunnel for all of the views.

- There are five recommended radiographic projections to fully evaluate the equine foot. These include the lateral view, three variations of the dorsopalmar (DP) view, and a skyline (flexor) view of the navicular bone. If specific pathology is seen or if radiographic abnormalities are not present on the standard views, supplemental

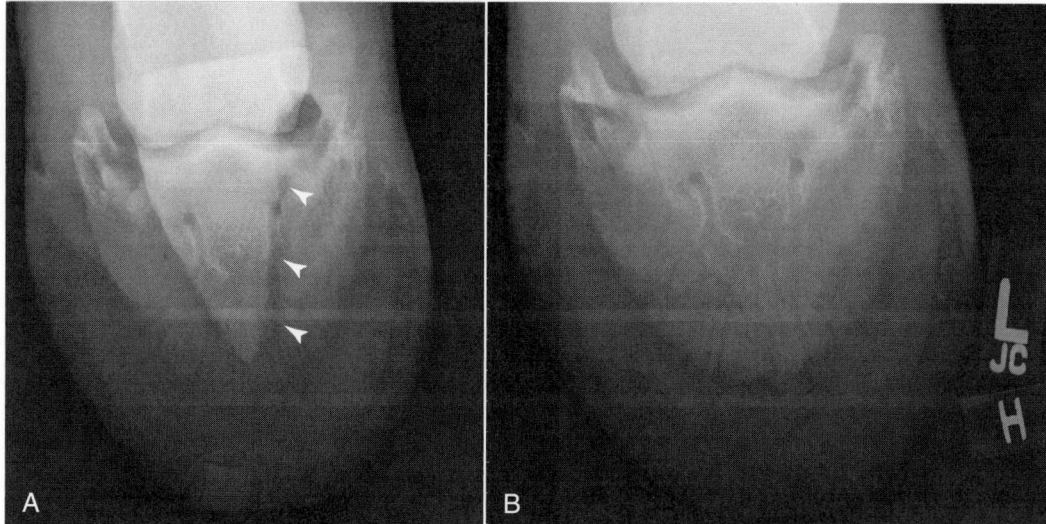

FIGURE 2 An example of a nonprepared foot for the DEE examination (**A**) and the same foot properly prepared (**B**) by packing the sulcus with Play-Doh. **A,** Note the V-shaped soft tissue opacity of the frog, bordered by areas of radiolucency overlying the third phalanx and distal interphalangeal joint. This artifact is created by gas within the unpacked deep sulcus of the foot. In this case, the gas within the medial sulcus was suspicious for a fracture of P3 (*arrowheads*). **B,** The sulcus of the foot has been properly packed with elimination of the confusing gas radiolucencies, though faint linear gas lucencies persist within the medial sulcus. Note that on both views the exposure latitude allows assessment of the distal interphalangeal joint and the soft tissues of the foot. These examples are DP views of P3 (D65°Pr-PDiO of P3, or 65°DP-P3), left hind (*LH*) foot, marker placed laterally.

views may be indicated (noted at the end of this section).

- The lateromedial view (lateral view) is made by placing the foot on a wood block, raising it enough off the ground to be able to radiograph the sole. The x-ray beam is aligned with the bulbs of the heel and is horizontal to the ground and perpendicular to the cassette (this assumes that the limb is positioned truly vertically; if the horse is leaning, the x-ray beam and cassette must be positioned accordingly).
- With the foot still on the block, the 45-degree DP view is obtained by placing the cassette parallel to the angle of the distal phalanges (either on the ground or within a slot in the block), with the x-ray beam perpendicular to the angle of the cassette. This view allows assessment of all three joints of the distal extremity and provides the least distorted view of the proximal margin of the navicular bone.
- Some practitioners prefer a 0-degree, horizontal beam DP view of distal extremity (D0°Pr-PDi [*Pr,* proximal; *Di,* distal], or P3 extensor process view). This view is made with the cassette positioned vertically palmar/plantar to the limb, with the x-ray beam parallel to the ground and perpendicular to the cassette. This view allows a more thorough evaluation of the extensor process and medial and lateral margins of P3 and the sole of the foot. Both of these DP views are valuable for evaluating lateromedial foot balance and in some cases both

may be necessary for complete evaluation of the foot.

- With the foot placed on a cassette tunnel, three of the five views of the distal extremity are obtained. These include DP views of P3 (D65°Pr-PDiO of P3, or 65°DP-P3; see Figure 2) and the navicular bone (D65°Pr-PDiO [*O,* oblique] of the navicular bone (65°DP-conedown navicular), and the navicular skyline view (P50°Pr-PDiO, skyline navicular or flexor view).
- The 65°DP of P3 and the navicular bone are made with the foot positioned exactly the same; the only difference is the navicular view must use a twofold or threefold increase in mAs to adequately evaluate the navicular bone (the solar margins of P3 will be overexposed on this view, whereas the navicular bone will be underexposed on the P3 view). The x-ray beam is centered on the coronary band. Using digital radiography, it is sometimes possible to make a single exposure that is satisfactory for evaluation of the solar margins of P3 and the navicular bone using different brightness and contrast settings at the viewing station. Tight collimation over the navicular bone (or "cone-down") will noticeably increase detail. A grid may be used to further increase detail.
- The P50°Pr-PDiO (skyline navicular or flexor view) is made with the limb in an extended palmar/plantar direction ("opening up" the bulbs of the heel) with the foot on the cassette tunnel. Directing from proximal to distal along

the palmar or plantar aspect of the distal extremity, the x-ray beam is centered on the bulbs of the heel. This view is often obtained while handholding the x-ray machine, and the FFD is often less than 26 to 30 inches due to interference by the ventral body wall of the horse.

- Commonly used supplemental views of the foot include horizontal and angled DP oblique projections, both with the foot on a cassette tunnel and on a block.
- Examples include evaluation of the solar and articular margins of P3 and the navicular bone with a D65°Pr45°L(or M)-PDiO view (*L,* lateral; *M,* medial); the x-ray beam is directed away from midline 45 degrees medial or lateral and aimed at the coronary band, with the foot on a cassette tunnel. This is commonly referred to as an *oblique heel view.*
- Evaluation of the palmar/plantar medial and lateral aspects of P3, navicular bone, P2, and the interphalangeal joints can also be made using horizontal beam or 45-degree DP oblique views with the foot on a block and the cassette placed either vertical to the ground or parallel to the distal limb axis.

The fetlock:

- There are five standard views of the fetlock including lateral (lateromedial), flexed lateral (flexed lateromedial), DP (D30°Pr-PDiO), and both oblique projections (D30°Pr60°L-PDiMO and D30°Pr60°M-PDiLO).

- True lateral and flexed lateral views are identified by perfectly superimposed metacarpal/tarsal condyles, proximal sesamoid bones, and "open" joint spaces.
- The flexed lateral view is needed for assessment of the sagittal ridge of distal MC/MT3 for osteochondral lesions.
- For DP (D30°Pr-PDiO) and oblique views, the cassette is positioned along the palmar surface of the limb approximating the angle of the distal limb axis, resting on the floor. The x-ray beam is directed perpendicular to the cassette.
- The 60-degree oblique views (D30°Pr60°L-PDiMO and D30°Pr60°M-PDiLO) are best for evaluation of the dorsomedial and dorsolateral eminences of proximal P1, where chip fractures and osteophytes commonly occur close to midline.
- For evaluation of the proximal sesamoid bones oblique views of 45 degrees (closer to dorsal) are best (D30°Pr45°L-PDiMO and D30°Pr45°M-PDiLO), allowing more of one sesamoid bone to be highlighted palmarly/plantarly, including periarticular margins, subchondral bone, and abaxial surfaces.
- A palmaroproximal-palmarodistal sesamoid skyline view can be used to identify occult or difficult to visualize sesamoid bone fractures. The x-ray beam can also be moved laterally or medially to produce yet another variation of a sesamoid skyline oblique view.
- Special DP radiographs of varying proximal to distal angulation are sometimes necessary to evaluate otherwise difficult incomplete P1 fractures or lesions of the palmar/plantar condylar surface of distal MC/MT3. For the latter, an extended D0°Pr-PDiO view can be obtained with the foot on a block and forward extension of the leg. This view projects the proximal sesamoid bones distally, so they are bisected by the fetlock joint. For assessment of the palmar condyle of the distal metacarpus, a flexed DPa (non-weight-bearing with the foot off the ground) or D15°Di-PaPr view is recommended. For either of these views the angle between the x-ray beam and the dorsal surface of MC/MT 3 is 125 degrees to ensure visualization of the palmar aspect of the condyle.
- D30°Pr70°L-PaDiMO and D30°Pr 70°M-PaDiLO to identify palmar proximal phalanx fragments.
- M45°PrLDiO to view the abaxial surface of the lateral proximal sesamoid bone (and vice versa for the medial proximal sesamoid bone). The

cassette should be perpendicular to the floor.
- Although rarely necessary, the dorsal surface of the sagittal ridge of distal MC/MT3 can be evaluated by a dorsodistal skyline view. In this case, the fetlock is flexed with the cassette placed adjacent to the dorsal surface of the distal limb, parallel to the ground; the x-ray beam is directed from dorsoproximal to dorsodistal, highlighting the projecting sagittal ridge.
- For the hind limb non-weight-bearing flexed DP view, the dorsum of the foot is in contact with the ground.

Metacarpus/metatarsus:
- The use of long cassettes (17 inches) is often necessary to image the entire metacarpus/metatarsus.
- Four standard views of the metacarpus/metatarsus include lateral (lateromedial), DP, and both oblique projections (D45°L-PMO and D45°M-PLO). This degree of obliquity highlights the lateral and medial splint bones separate from MC/MT3 palmarly/plantarly.
- Oblique views positioned more toward lateral (eg, D65°L-PMO and D65°M-PLO) may be necessary when evaluating dorsal cortical stress fractures.

Carpus:
- Standing lateromedial, flexed lateromedial, DP, and both obliques (D60°L-PMO, D60°M-PLO) are considered standard views by some.
- In addition, three skyline views of the dorsal carpus are routinely preformed. These include skyline views of the distal radius and the proximal and distal rows of carpal bones.
- Since much of carpal pathology occurs dorsally (chip and corner fractures), it is sometimes necessary to perform oblique views that are closer to lateral than described above (eg, D75°M-PLO, D75°L-PMO). Indeed, a common error is making oblique radiographs of the carpus that are closer to dorsal than lateral, which highlights the more medial and lateral surfaces rather than the more commonly affected dorsolateral and dorsomedial aspects of the carpus.
- The skyline view of the dorsodistal radius is used to assess chip fractures and bony change associated with the gliding surface of the extensor tendons. It is made by flexing the carpus at 90 degrees with the radius vertically positioned and the distal extremity parallel to the ground. The cassette is placed along the metacarpus parallel to the ground and the x-ray beam is angled from dorsoproximal to dorsodistal such that the distal dorsal surface of the radius is silhouetted by the collimator light onto the cassette. The view is correctly described as a flexed

D65°Pr-DDiO projection of the carpus. Correct positioning can be recognized by the familiar contour of the distal radius with the projecting intertendinous eminence located centrally, separating the shallow concavities of the extensor carpi radialis and common digital extensor tendons.
- The skyline view of the proximal row of carpal bones is positioned differently from above. For this view, the carpus is maximally flexed and pushed cranially. The cassette is positioned along the metacarpus and the x-ray beam is directed from dorsoproximal to dorsodistal such that the dorsal surface of the proximal row of carpal bones is projected as a shadow by the collimator light onto the cassette. The angle of the x-ray beam is not as steep as for the distal radius skyline view. The view is properly termed the flexed-D45°Pr-DDiO projection and can be recognized by the symmetrical dorsally projected radial and intermediate carpal bone; the distal radius may be visible deep within the image.
- The most common skyline view of the carpus is that of the distal row of carpal bones, in particular the third carpal bone. Most practitioners consider this part of a routine examination. The limb and cassette are positioned as for the proximal row of carpal bones, but the x-ray beam is much closer to horizontal. The view is named the flexed-D30°Pr-DDiO projection. Because of the extreme angle of the x-ray beam relative to the cassette, there is a large degree of geometric distortion elongating the third and fourth carpal bones. Nevertheless, this is an extremely important view for assessment of the third carpal bone for fractures and facet sclerosis. This view is recognized by the large third carpal bone projected dorsally with the smaller fourth carpal bone seen laterally.
- Circumferential oblique views taken at small degree intervals are helpful when evaluating for occult slab fractures of the cuboidal bones.
- It should be noted that sometimes "creative" views are needed to fully assess pathology. These may include flexed oblique views, variation of skyline views, etc.
- When evaluating angular limb deformity centered at the carpus (or tarsus), the use of long cassettes (17 inch) to include as much of the long bones proximal and distal to the joint is desired.

Elbow:
- Lateral and craniocaudal views of the elbow can be obtained in most instances in the field. The lateral view

is sometimes all that is necessary when evaluating olecranon fractures.

- The "lateral" view is often easiest to obtain as a mediolateral projection with the limb extended.
- The craniocaudal view is obtained by pulling the limb cranially and placing the cassette caudal to the elbow. The x-ray beam is angled to be perpendicular to the long axis of the radius, aiming at the elbow joint. The degree of angulation needed varies. Due to the thickness of the distal brachium only the distal-most portion of the humerus can usually be seen.
- Sometimes a CrM-CdLO view is useful to better evaluate the joint.

Shoulder:

- The lateral view can be made for smaller horses in the field. In some horses this view is best performed under anesthesia, where use of a grid significantly enhances bony detail.
- The "lateral" view is obtained as a mediolateral projection by having an assistant pull the leg as far cranially as possible.
- A skyline view (CrPr-CrDiO) of the humeral head and tubercles can be obtained in the field.
- Oblique views (eg, CdL-CrMO) can be made when evaluating for fractures.

Tarsus:

- Standard views should include the lateral, DP (D0°Pr-PDiO, or D10°Pr-PDiO), D45°L-PMO, and D5°Pr60°M-PDiLO (obtaining the view from underneath the horse), or P5°Di60°L-DPrMO (view from behind the horse). The x-ray beam is centered at the level of the central tarsal bone.
- For the lateromedial view of the tarsus, a very slight downward angulation of the x-ray beam (approximately 3 degrees) will "open" the intertarsal and tarsometatarsal joint spaces better than a horizontal x-ray beam. Caution: if you angle too much the joints will be artifactually narrowed.
- A flexed lateral view is valuable for evaluation of the caudal distal tibial physis and epiphysis in foals as well as the tarsocrural joint.
- For DP radiographs, when the x-ray beam is parallel to the floor (0 degrees or horizontal DP) the medial side of the distal intertarsal joint will appear normal in width ("open") while the lateral side will artifactually appear narrow. With 10 degrees of proximal to distal angulation of the x-ray beam (10 degree DP), the lateral aspect of the distal intertarsal joint will appear normal width while the medial aspect will appear narrow.
- The approximate angle of the x-ray beam on DP radiographs of the tarsus can be determined by noting the position of the heads of MT4/2 in relation

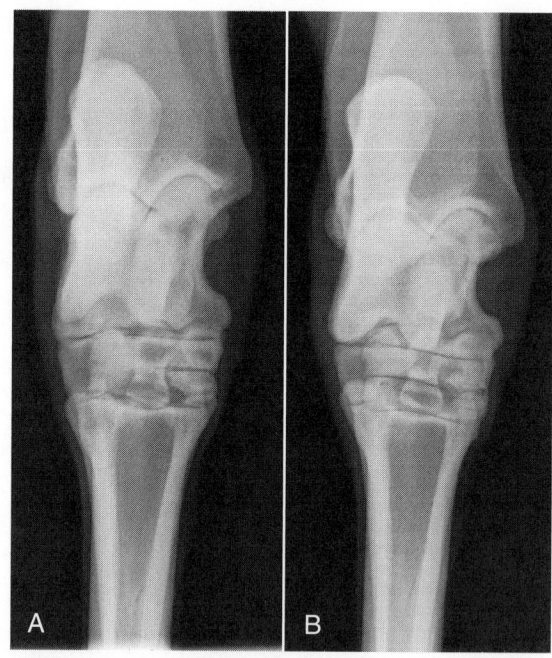

FIGURE 3 DP tarsal views illustrating the effect of x-ray beam orientation on the appearance of the distal intertarsal joint. **A,** Horizontal beam DP view (D0°Pr-PDiO). The x-ray beam is horizontal to the ground (perpendicular to the tarsus). This view "opens up" the medial portion of the distal intertarsal joint and to a lesser extent the proximal intertarsal and tarsometatarsal joints. The lateral portion of the distal intertarsal joint is radiographically "closed". This view is identified radiographically by the position of proximal MT2/4 (heads of the splint bones) at the level of the tarsometatarsal joint. **B,** Angled DP view (D10°Pr-PDiO). The x-ray beam is angled approximately 10° downward. This view "opens up" the lateral portion of the distal intertarsal joint while "closing" the medial distal intertarsal joint, and to a lesser extent the proximal intertarsal and tarsometatarsal joints. This view is identified by the position of proximal MT2/4 (heads of the splint bones) at the level of the distal intertarsal joint.

to the tarsometatarsal joint. When the heads are even with the tarsometatarsal joint, a horizontal beam was used and when projected proximal (above) the tarsometatarsal joint, the x-ray beam was angled (Figure 3).

- A commonly used supplemental view is the D10°L-PMO for better visualization of the medial malleolus of osteochondral lesions (OCD). Many practitioners replace the true DP view with this view in horses younger than 3 years.
- Circumferential oblique views taken at small-degree intervals are helpful when evaluating for occult slab fractures of the central and third tarsal bones.
- The calcaneal skyline view is invaluable when assessing injury to the calcaneus, including the tuber and the sustentaculum tali. The tarsus is flexed, the cassette is placed along the plantar surface of the calcaneus and metatarsus and the x-ray beam is directed in a plantaroproximal to plantarodistal direction. The shadow of the calcaneus on the cassette produced by the collimator light indicates proper positioning. This view is properly termed the Flexed-P75°Pr-PDiO.

Stifle:

- Lateromedial and caudocranial views are standard and can be routinely obtained in the field.
- The key to an adequate lateromedial view is to push the cassette as far proximal as possible. This can be difficult in some patients; failure to do so results in cutting off portions of the patella and distal femur.
- For the caudocranial view, the x-ray beam is centered at the level of the indentation of the stifle; the x-ray beam is directed perpendicular to the long axis of the tibia (usually horizontal to angled downward slightly). A radiographic image with artifactual "collapse" of the stifle joint (due to overlap of the distal femur and proximal tibia) can often be corrected by angling the x-ray beam downward.
- Oblique views (Cd60°L-CrMO or Cd45°L-CrMO) are often included in a standard study to separate the femoral condyles and trochlear ridges for osteochondrosis assessment.
- A flexed lateromedial view is sometimes helpful in further assessing the patella, femoral trochlea, or proximal tibia.
- A skyline view of the patella is invaluable in assessment of potential sagittal

patellar fractures and patellar osteo-chondrosis. The stifle is flexed and the cassette is placed nearly horizontal to the ground along the cranial tibia. The x-ray machine is above the rump of the horse cranial to the stifle, the x-ray beam angled caudodistally, projecting the cranial margin of the patella on the cassette. The stifle can be rotated outward to separate the patella away from the body wall.

Cervical spine:

- Lateral views (usually three to four radiographs are needed to include the base of the skull to C7-T1 vertebrae).
- Field radiography in the standing horse may not be possible due to the high radiographic exposure required and patient motion; anesthesia is often necessary.
- Obtaining true lateral radiographs is a key element in making diagnostic quality cervical radiographs for assessment of cervical stenotic myelopathy and other cervical spinal diseases. This is actually easier in a standing horse, provided the horse is not too unsteady. Under anesthesia, sponges must be placed to compensate for "bowing" of the cervical spine while the patient is in lateral recumbency. True lateral radiographs are recognized by perfect overlap of the transverse processes.

POSTPROCEDURE

Interpretation:

- Just as equine radiography is an art, so is radiographic interpretation. Veterinarians must be keenly aware of anatomy, not only the bony structures, but the complex relationship of the associated soft tissues such as the various ligaments, tendons and joint capsules. Anatomy, radiology and equine reference textbooks ease interpretation and increase confidence of diagnosis.
- Radiographs of the contralateral limb can be performed as an appropriate comparison when specific questions arise regarding the normalcy or potential pathology of a specific area.
- There are numerous artifacts that can hinder interpretation. Some are associated with patient preparation. Geometric distortion of anatomic structures caused by the intricate relationship of the x-ray beam, position of the patient, and the cassette, and those caused by over and underexposure and processing are all present on nearly every radiographic examination and must be recognized.
- When interpreting any radiographic study, a systematic approach should be used. Many variations exist and

each of us develops our own methodology. Consistency yields thoroughness and is the most important aspect in not overlooking pathologic change.

- An appropriate environment for evaluation of radiographs is very important. The following should be considered when evaluating conventional radiographic film or digital images on the computer:
  - Ambient light: Room light should not be too bright or too dark. When viewing digital images, ambient light should minimize glare on the computer screens.
  - Bright light boxes ("hot lights") should be available for evaluation of darker areas of the film.
  - Noise: The room should be quiet to minimize distractions.
- Finally, when a radiographic diagnosis is made, the question should be "Are these radiographic findings compatible with the clinical presentation?" If not, further imaging may need to be performed. Radiographic abnormalities may exist but are not necessarily clinically relevant.

AUTHORS: **JOHN S. MATTOON, JASON W. BRUMITT, JONATHAN HAYLES, DANA A. NEELIS, GREGORY D. ROBERTS,** and **TOM WILKINSON**

Regional Limb Perfusion

BASIC INFORMATION

SYNONYM(S)

Intravenous regional perfusion
Intraosseous regional perfusion
Regional perfusion

OVERVIEW AND GOAL(S)

Regional limb perfusion is a technique adapted from human medicine by which a selected part of an extremity's vascular supply can be isolated by the use of a tourniquet, and in this manner treated independently to the rest of the body. It is used to provide high levels of a pharmaceutical, commonly antibiotics, in the selected and isolated region of the lower extremity.

INDICATIONS

- Septic arthritis
- Osteomyelitis
- Recalcitrant infections

EQUIPMENT, ANESTHESIA

- The intravenous variant of this technique requires:

  - Tourniquet (12-inch rubber tubing or pneumatic tourniquet applied to a pressure above systolic)
  - 20- or 22-gauge catheter or butterfly needle
  - Extension set
- The intraosseous variant of this technique requires:
  - Tourniquet (12-inch rubber tubing or pneumatic)
  - Cannulated screw (commercially available or custom-made of 4.5 mm diameter) (Figure 1)

  - 3.2-mm drill bit and 4.5-mm tap
  - 3.2-mm drill guide/tissue protector
  - Air or electric drill
  - Extension set
- Both procedures (intravenous or intraosseous) can be performed in the standing horse under heavy sedation. The intraosseous variant requires local anesthetic in the region and a small incision to place the drill bit against the bone, commonly the third metacarpal or metatarsal, where a unicortical hole is drilled into the medullary cavity (Figures 2 and 3).

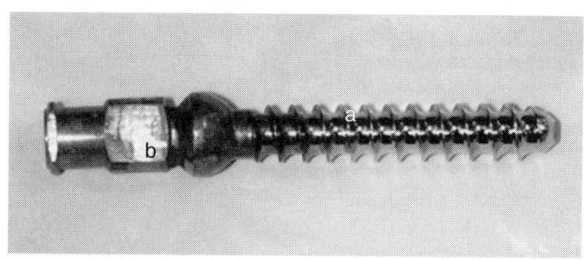

FIGURE 1   Cannulated screw. Image of a custom-made cannulated 4.5-mm cortical screw with a welded luer connector.

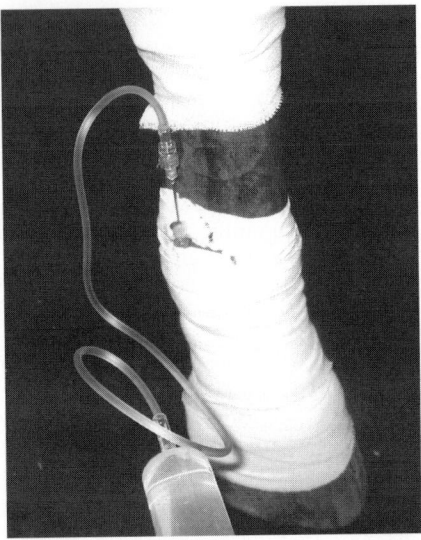

FIGURE 2 Regional intravenous perfusion. Image of regional intraosseous perfusion being performed. An intravenous set is connected to the luer connector of the screw, which protrudes through the skin.

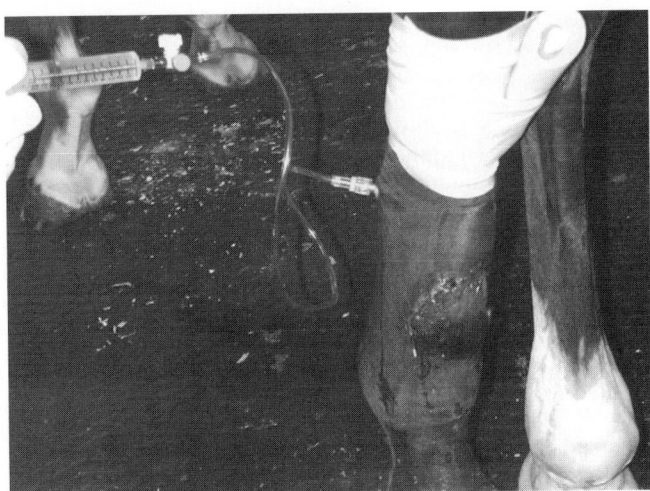

FIGURE 3 Cannulated screw placed in the third metacarpal bone for intraosseous perfusion. Note the tourniquet applied proximal to the cannulated screw.

ANTICIPATED TIME

- The tourniquet should be in place for 30 minutes postinjection.
- The total time for the entire intravenous procedure is approximately 45 minutes.
- The placement of a cannulated screw under sterile conditions will take approximately 30 minutes or less.

PREPARATION: IMPORTANT CHECKPOINTS

- Horse must be adequately sedated and restrained.
- Thrombosis of the vessels used may occur, so it is important to adhere to meticulous technique.
- The cannulated screw may break at the attachment to a luer lock.
- A 3- to 10-mL volume of lidocaine may be infused in the intraosseous technique prior to injection of the agent to minimize pain associated with increased intraosseous pressure.

POSSIBLE COMPLICATIONS AND COMMON ERRORS TO BE AVOIDED

- Inadequate catheterization of the vessel may lead to extravascular injection and potential thrombosis.
- The screw must be well positioned and protected to avoid breakage.
- The volume to be injected is commonly 60 mL and antibiotics commonly used are Amikacin (500 mg) or Ceftiofur (500 mg).

- The operator must resist the urge to inject the 60 mL quickly as this may provoke vascular damage. It is important to inject the agent over a period of 3 to 5 minutes.
- Horses may resent the increased intraosseous pressure associated with intraosseous infusion. To avoid this, 3 to 10 mL of local anesthetic could be infused into the medullary cavity prior to injection.

PROCEDURE

- Place the horse in stocks or cross-tie.
- Administer an effective dose of an alpha-2 sedative and 15 mg of butorphanol tartrate or similar.
- Place tourniquet above region to be infused (above hock or carpus).
- Identify saphenous (hindlimb) or cephalic (forelimb).
- The area to approach the vessel can be prepared now or prior to tourniquet placement.
- If a cannulated screw is going to be used, incise the skin with a No. 15 blade enough to place a 3.2-mm drill bit.
- Make a unicortical hole, tap the hole with a 4.5-mm tap, and place the screw making sure that the end of the screw will be in the medullary cavity.
- For intravenous administration, catheterize the vessel with the indicated materials.
- Connect the end of the screw or catheter to an injection extension set.

- Inject slowly.
- Maintain the tourniquet for 30 minutes after infusion.
- After infusion you may remove the vessel catheter or needle, apply a gauze pad, and firmly bandage over the injection site to reduce vessel leakage.

POSTPROCEDURE

For the intraosseous procedure, ensure that the luer lock connection to the screw is protected by a heavy bandage.

ALTERNATIVES AND THEIR RELATIVE MERITS

- Intravenous or intraosseous variants have been described. The intraosseous variant is slowly being abandoned in favor of the more user-friendly intravenous variant. However, in situations where cellulitis prevents the identification of a vessel, the intraosseous route is preferred.
- Studies performed following intravenous and intraosseous variants reveal different results, although from a clinical perspective, both variants seem to accomplish antimicrobial concentrations in bone and synovial fluid, severalfold of the minimum inhibitory concentration for most bacteria.

AUTHOR: **ANTONIO M. CRUZ**

Shock-Dose Fluid Administration

BASIC INFORMATION

SYNONYM(S)

Fluid resuscitation

OVERVIEW AND GOAL(S)

Shock doses of fluids are indicated to support the cardiovascular system and provide adequate tissue perfusion and oxygenation to compromised patients with hypovolemia shock (ie, patients with low blood pressure, high heart rates, endoxemia, and poor peripheral perfusion).

INDICATIONS

- Maintain adequate hydration for normal metabolic processes.
- Restore fluid losses due to dehydration or relative losses from fluid shifts due to endotoxemia.
- Replenish ongoing fluid losses due to diarrhea, nasogastric reflux, or excessive sweating.
- Preload the cardiovascular system to prevent cardiovascular collapse due to an acute loss of third-space fluid through a drain (peritonitis, pleuritis).

CONTRAINDICATIONS

- Oral fluids: Contraindicated with concurrent nasogastric reflux, suspected small intestinal obstruction or severe dehydration (>8%).
- Large volume resuscitation: Contraindicated with cardiac disease, pulmonary or cerebral edema or anuria.
- Coagulation disorders: IV catheters may result in thrombophlebitis.
- Hypertonic saline cannot be administered to foals.

EQUIPMENT, ANESTHESIA

- Local anesthesia (2–5 mL anesthetic, 25-gauge needle)
- Catheter (large bore, short length to speed fluid delivery)
- Extension set
- Fluid administration set
- Fluids (balanced electrolyte crystalloids, hypertonic saline, colloids)

ANTICIPATED TIME

- Initial dose should be administered as a bolus.
- Reassessment should occur hourly to identify the need for additional doses (up to three total).

PREPARATION: IMPORTANT CHECKPOINTS

- Physical examination and hematocrit provide an estimate of the level of dehydration (<5% is undetectable).
  - Heart rate 40 to 60 bpm, capillary refill time (CRT) <2, packed cell volume (PCV) = 40%, total protein (TP) = 7.0 g/dL is 6% dehydration.
  - Heart rate 61 to 80 bpm, CRT <3, PCV = 45%, TP = 7.5 g/dL is 8% dehydration.
  - Heart rate 81 to 100 bpm, CRT <4, PCV = 50%, TP = 8.0 g/dL is 10% dehydration.
  - Heart rate >100 beats/min, CRT >4, PCV >50%, TP >8.0 g/dL is >10% dehydration.
- Any concurrent losses (nasogastric reflux, hemorrhage) must be considered.

POSSIBLE COMPLICATIONS AND COMMON ERRORS TO BE AVOIDED

- Excessive initial fluid resuscitation results in widespread tissue edema, including pulmonary edema, because only one-third of crystalloids administered remain intravascular after 1 hour.
- Extremely dehydrated horses are at risk of air embolus during catheter placement: Hold off vein until extension is firmly attached.
- Colloids, notably hydroxyethyl starch, may increase clotting times at doses >20 mL/kg.
- Certain medications may react with electrolytes in crystalloid solutions (ie, bicarbonate and calcium).
- Avoid lactate buffers in horses with severe liver dysfunction that may inhibit conversion of lactate to bicarbonate.

PROCEDURE

- Example resuscitation plan for a 500-kg horse:
  - The shock-dose calculation for initial crystalloid administration is 60 to 90 mL/kg
  - 90 mL/kg × 500 kg = 45 L needed (Normasol-R, lactated Ringer's, Plasma-Lyte 148).
  - Administer one-fourth to one-third of shock dose = 11 to 15 L.
  - Does not correct for dehydration or ongoing losses.

- Administer 20 mL/kg in patients who cannot handle high fluid volumes (cardiac disease, head trauma).
- Low-sodium fluids (half-strength lactated Ringer's, Plasma-Lyte 56) may be preferred in foals.

POSTPROCEDURE

Reassess patient's physical parameters hourly, and determine if additional bolus therapy is required or if a maintenance fluid rate (calculated from dehydration, losses, and maintenance needs) is adequate.

ALTERNATIVES AND THEIR RELATIVE MERITS

- To resuscitate faster than with crystalloid fluid boluses, hypertonic saline or colloids can be used to maintain fluid in the vascular space but require concurrent crystalloid administration to maintain effects and replenish interstitial fluid losses:
  - Hypertonic saline (7.5% sodium chloride): 4 mL/kg bolus, duration of effect 45 minutes
    - Induces intravascular hypertonicity to pull fluid from the interstitium and intracellular spaces
    - May also increase tissue perfusion by selective vasodilation and vasoconstriction at the capillary level
    - Contraindicated with severe dehydration or hypernatremia
  - Colloids: hydroxyethyl starch (6%): 10 to 20 mL/kg, duration of effect 1 to 3 days
    - Hyperoncotic substituted sugar
    - Expands intracellular fluid volume to a level equal to the volume infused
    - May provide additional volume support by occluding pathologic gaps in the endothelium
    - Hydroxyethyl starch is preferred over dextrans in shock; due to its higher molecular weight, less likely to leak from damaged endothelium

SUGGESTED READING

Dreissen B, Brainard B: Fluid therapy for the traumatized patient. *J Vet Em Crit Care* 16(4):276–299, 2006.

AUTHOR: AMELIA MUNSTERMAN

Splinting

BASIC INFORMATION

SYNONYM(S)
Temporary external coaptation

OVERVIEW AND GOAL(S)
A splint is an external rigid support applied to provide temporary external fixation of a limb.

INDICATIONS
- Indications for splinting in adults include temporary support of fractures and adjunct therapy for internal fixation of fractures, tendon lacerations, and wound management.
- Splints are also used in foals as treatment for incomplete ossification of the carpal or tarsal bones to prevent further cartilage damage, or as a definitive therapy for tendon contracture.

CONTRAINDICATIONS
Any horse that will not tolerate immobilization without further injuring itself

EQUIPMENT, ANESTHESIA
- A bandage should be applied to the leg prior to splint application.
  - The bandage should be thick enough to prevent rubs but not too thick to allow the bones to move beneath the bandage.
  - Materials needed for the bandage beneath the splint include cotton combine or roll cotton, brown gauze, Vet-wrap, and elastic tape.
- The splint can be made of PVC pipe (schedule 40 or 80), wood, metal, or cast material.
  - Wood is a difficult material to use because small pieces do not provide enough strength while large pieces do not conform to the leg well.
  - PVC also does not conform to the leg well but may be bent to improve fit.
  - Cast material conforms well to the leg but does not provide as much support as a true cast when placed over a bandage.
  - Premade stainless steel splints are very convenient for immobilization of distal limb injuries but alone provide little lateral to medial support.
- Extra cotton and nonelastic tape (duct tape, white tape) should be available to pad the top of splints.

ANTICIPATED TIME
A typical splint takes 15 to 20 minutes to apply.

PREPARATION: IMPORTANT CHECKPOINTS
- All wounds should be addressed and bandaged prior to applying a splint over them.
- The horse may be sedated to allow splint application, but sedation should be kept light to prevent excessive weight bearing on the injured limb.

POSSIBLE COMPLICATIONS AND COMMON ERRORS TO BE AVOIDED
The splint should be steadied by a second person to prevent rotation when applying the nonelastic tape.

PROCEDURE
Splinting is divided into four anatomical levels based on the type of splint required (Figure 1):

LEVEL 1
- Fractures of distal metacarpus/metatarsus, first and second phalangeal bones, and proximal sesamoid bones
- Luxation of the pastern or fetlock joints
- Flexor tendon laceration at the pastern or the metacarpus/metatarsus
- Goal: Align the dorsal cortices of the bones
- Procedure:
  - Apply a light Robert Jones bandage from the carpus, distal.
  - Have handler hold leg by radius or tibia to suspend the leg in the air.
  - Place a dorsal splint on the forelimb or a plantar splint on the hindlimb from the ground to the proximal edge of the third metacarpal/metatarsal bone.
  - Secure splint in place with nonelastic tape in two to three layers.
  - Alternative: Kimzey Leg Saver (Kimzey Welding Works, Inc., Woodland, CA) commercial metal splint may be used (Figure 2).

LEVEL 2
- Fractures of the mid- to proximal third metacarpal bone and carpal bones
- Fractures of the mid- to proximal third metatarsal bone and tarsal bones
- Goal: Align bones and prevent abduction of the limb
- Procedure:
  - Apply a Robert Jones bandage from the olecranon to the ground with the forelimbs or from the top of the calcaneus to the ground on the hindlimbs.
  - For the hindlimb: align the solar hoof surface with the flexor tendons.
  - Use 2 to 3 layers of cotton to provide 2 to 3 times the limb circumference.
  - Apply brown gauze or Vet-wrap to each layer of cotton used to ensure compression of injured limb.
  - Apply the caudal or plantar splint first and tape over the splint with 2 to 3 layers of nonelastic tape from the ground to the top of the olecranon or calcaneus (Figure 3).
  - Apply a lateral splint second and tape over splint with 2 to 3 layers of nonelastic tape from the ground to the top of the olecranon or calcaneus.

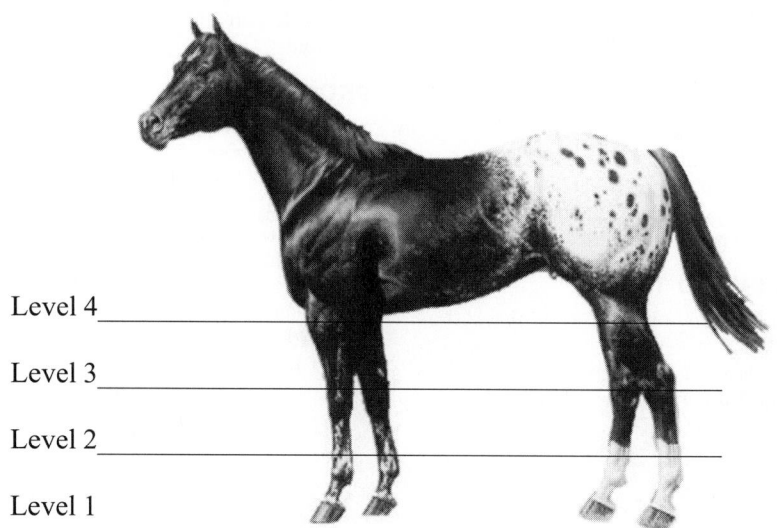

Level 4 _____

Level 3 _____

Level 2 _____

Level 1

FIGURE 1 Splinting chart.

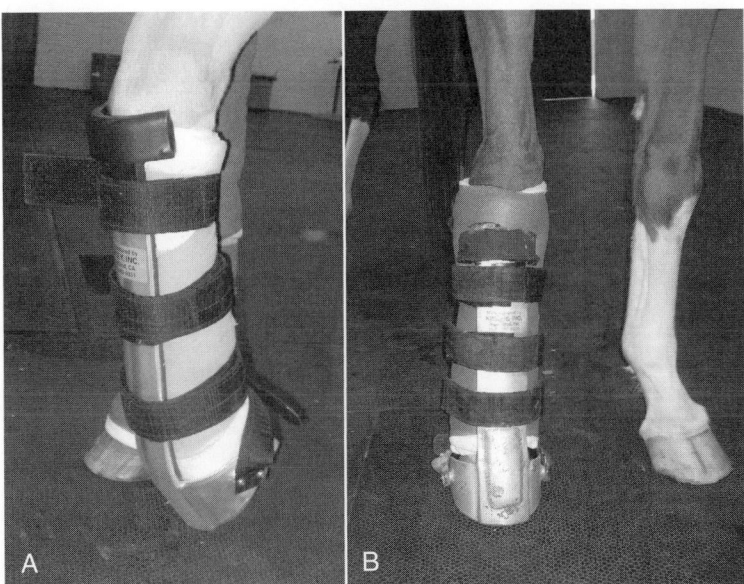

FIGURE 2 Lateral (**A**) and dorsal (**B**) view of level 1 stabilization with a Kimzey splint.

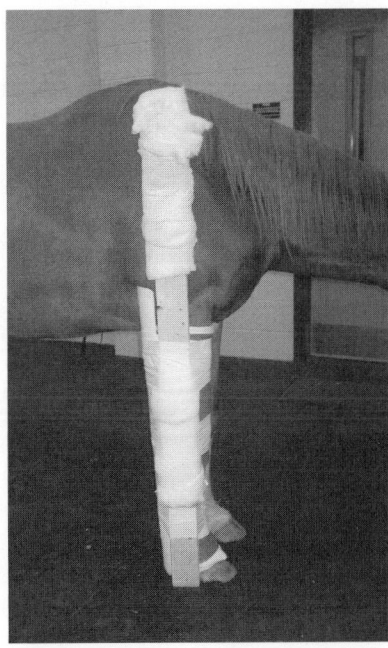

FIGURE 4 Lateral view of level 3 forelimb stabilization with palmar PVC splint and lateral board splint extending to the top of the scapula. Two to three layers of nonelastic tape should be applied over the splints from the ground to the olecranon.

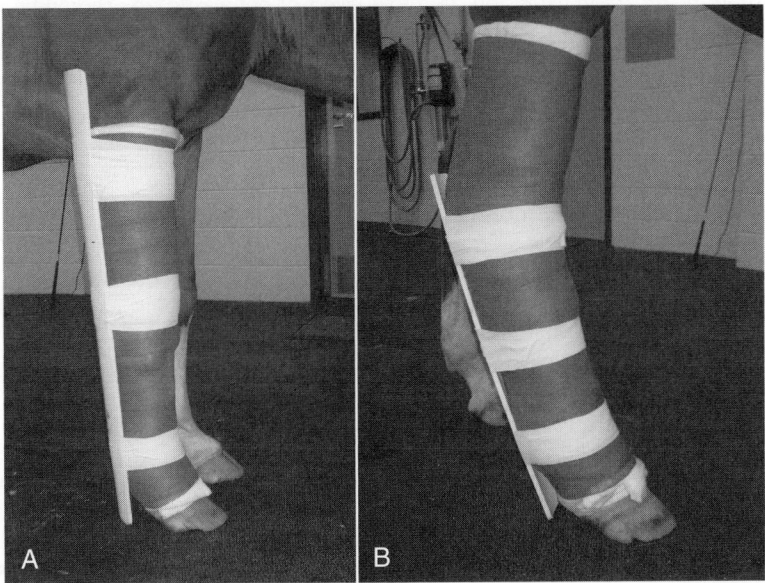

FIGURE 3 **A**, Lateral view of level 2 forelimb stabilization with palmar PVC splint. **B**, Lateral view of level 2 hindlimb stabilization with plantar PVC splint. A second PVC splint can also be applied on the lateral aspect of either limb for greater stabilization. Two to 3 layers of nonelastic tape should be applied over the splints from the ground to the olecranon or calcaneus.

LEVEL 3: FORELIMB
- Fractures of the radius
- Goal: Prevent abduction and flexion of the limb
- Procedure:
  - Apply a Robert Jones bandage from the top of the olecranon to the ground.
  - Use 2 to 3 layers of cotton to provide 2 to 3 times the limb circumference.
  - Apply brown gauze or Vet-wrap to each layer of cotton used to ensure compression of injured limb.

  - Apply the caudal splint first and tape over the splint with 2 to 3 layers of nonelastic tape from the ground to the top of the olecranon to fix the carpus.
  - Second, apply a lateral splint extending to the top of the scapula and tape over the splint with 2 to 3 layers of nonelastic tape from the ground to the top of the olecranon (Figure 4).
  - A figure of eight can be performed with Elastikon or white tape around the proximal portion of the lateral

splint to secure the splint to the thorax.

LEVEL 3: HINDLIMB
- Fractures of the hock or tibia
- Goal: Prevent abduction of the limb
- Procedure:
  - Apply a Robert Jones bandage from the stifle to the ground.
  - Use 2 to 3 layers of cotton for 2 to 3 times the limb circumference.
  - Apply brown gauze or Vet-wrap to each layer of cotton used to ensure compression of injured limb.
  - Apply a lateral splint with angulation at the hock, if possible, from the tuber coxae to the ground (Figure 5).
  - Tape the splint onto the limb with 2 to 3 layers of nonelastic tape.
  - A figure of eight can be performed with Elastikon or tape around the proximal portion of the splint to secure the splint to the rump.

LEVEL 4: FORELIMB
- Fractures of the humerus, scapula, or olecranon
- Goal: Provide rigid fixation of the carpus
- Procedure:
  - Apply a Robert Jones bandage from the top of the olecranon to the ground.
  - Use 2 to 3 layers of cotton for 2 to 3 times the limb circumference.

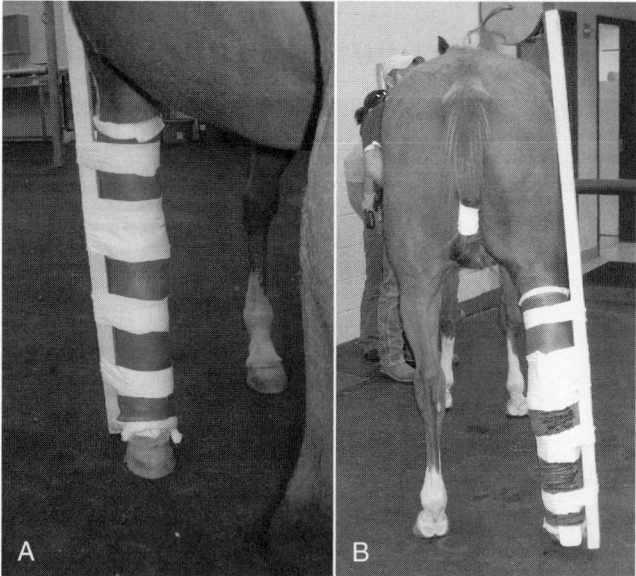

FIGURE 5 Cranial (A) and caudal (B) views of level 3 hindlimb stabilization with plantar splint to the level of the calcaneus and lateral board splint to the level of the tuber coxae. Two to 3 layers of nonelastic tape should be applied over the splints from the ground to the calcaneus.

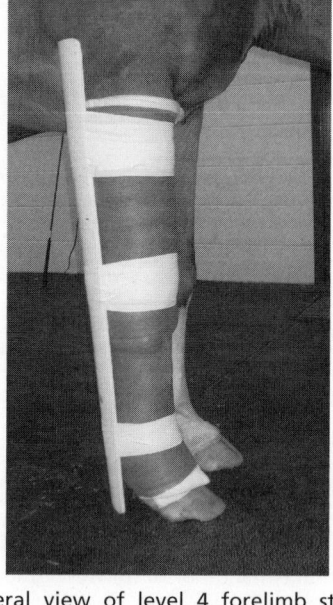

FIGURE 6 Lateral view of level 4 forelimb stabilization with palmar splint to the level of the olecranon applied to fix the carpus in extension. Two to 3 layers of nonelastic tape should be applied over the splints from the ground to the olecranon.

○ Apply brown gauze or Vet-wrap to each layer of cotton used to ensure compression of injured limb.
○ Apply the caudal splint with 2 to 3 layers of nonelastic tape from the ground to the top of the olecranon to fix the carpus (Figure 6).

LEVEL 4: HINDLIMB
• Fractures of the femur, pelvis, or stifle joint

• Procedure:
  ○ No splint is possible that will reduce fracture displacement.
  ○ A splint plantar or distal to the calcaneus increases distraction on the fracture.

POSTPROCEDURE

Definitive therapy for the injury is required.

ALTERNATIVES AND THEIR RELATIVE MERITS

In foals, a thick Robert Jones bandage may be sufficient depending on the stability of the fracture.

SUGGESTED READING

Smith JJ: Emergency fracture stabilization. *Clin Tech Equine Pract* 5:154–160, 2006.

AUTHOR: CHRISTINA HEWES

Superovulation

BASIC INFORMATION

OVERVIEW AND GOAL(S)
• Superovulation consists of a hormonal treatment to promote recruitment and development of several follicles to the preovulation stage.
• The goal is to eliminate any dominant follicle and improve the number of ovulations in a cycle.
• Superovulation is achieved by eliminating the inhibitory mechanism of the dominant follicle (immunization against inhibin) or by promoting development of a subordinate follicle using follicle-stimulating gonadotropins.
• The most effective commercially available treatment is based on the use of purified equine pituitary extract (eFSH, Bioniche Animal Health, Belleville, ON, Canada).

INDICATIONS
Increasing the number of embryos or oocytes recovered per cycle in young mares with no history of infertility that are inseminated with fresh semen.

CONTRAINDICATIONS
Anestrus mares

EQUIPMENT, ANESTHESIA
eFSH

HORMONAL PROTOCOL
• Monitor mare by ultrasound starting 5 days after ovulation.

• Start treatment with eFSH when the ovaries present several follicles of 22 to 25 mm diameter.
• Administer eFSH at 12.5 mg IM q12h.
• Administer prostaglandin $F_{2\alpha}$ on day 2 of eFSH treatment.
• Continue eFSH at the same dose and interval until most follicles are between 32 to 35 mm in diameter.
• Induce ovulation 30 to 36 hours after the last eFSH dose with either human chorionic gonadotropin (2500 IU or IV) or deslorelin (1.5 mg IM).
• Inseminate or collect oocytes as per standard procedure.

EXPECTED RESULTS
Under commercial breeding conditions, 3.1 ovulations are observed and 1.5 embryos are recovered per mare per cycle.

LIMITATIONS

- Inconsistency in the response to superovulation
- Expensive
- Requires intensive monitoring
- Drug treatment not always available

SUGGESTED READING

McCue PM, Patten M, Denniston D, et al: Strategies for using eFSH for superovulating mares. *J Equine Vet Sci* 28:91–96, 2008.

McCue PM, LeBlanc MM, Squires EL: eFSH in clinical equine practice. *Theriogenology* 68:429–433, 2007.

AUTHORS: **FRANÇOIS-XAVIER GRAND** and **REJEAN CLÉOPHAS LEFEBVRE**

Thyroid-Stimulating Hormone (TSH) Test

BASIC INFORMATION

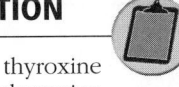

- Determine baseline thyroxine (T4) and triiodothyronine (T3) concentrations.
- Administer thyroid-stimulating hormone (TSH) 5 IU or thyrotropin-releasing hormone (TRH) 0.5 to 1.0 mg IV.
- Collect blood sample at 2 and 4 hours.
- Animals with normal thyroid function should have a twofold increase in T3 at 2 hours and T4 at 4 hours after TSH administration.
- Blood samples can be collected in ethylenediamine tetraacetic acid (EDTA) or plain blood collection tubes.

AUTHOR: **RAMIRO E. TORIBIO**

Thyrotropin-Releasing Hormone (TRH) Test

BASIC INFORMATION

- Administer thyrotropin-releasing hormone (TRH) 0.5 to 1 mg IV.
- Collect blood before TRH administration and every 15 minutes for 2 hours.
- Horses with pituitary pars intermedia dysfunction (equine Cushing's disease) will have an increase in cortisol concentrations within 15 minutes of TRH administration; these concentrations remain elevated for 90 minutes.
- Horses with normal thyroid function should have a twofold increase in triiodothyronine (T3) at 2 hours and thyroxine (T4) at 4 hours after TRH administration.
- Blood samples can be collected in ethylenediamine tetraacetic acid (EDTA) or plain blood collection tubes.

AUTHOR: **RAMIRO E. TORIBIO**

Tube Cast of the Forelimb in the Neonate

BASIC INFORMATION

SYNONYM(S)

Sleeve cast

OVERVIEW AND GOAL(S)

- Tube casts are placed on the forelimbs of foals to protect the carpal joints (bone, ligament, and cartilage) from asymmetric load if malaligned and to reduce load if incompletely ossified.
- Tube casts are used in the forelimbs and span the limb from the axilla to the distal metacarpus.
- Tube casts are rarely applied to hindlimbs as they are very difficult to manage and make it difficult for foals to get up.

INDICATIONS

- Carpal ligamentous laxity
- Carpal hypoplasia

CONTRAINDICATIONS

- Casts should not be used in foals unless they are stall confined.
- Casts impede access to portions of the limb if required.

EQUIPMENT, ANESTHESIA

- Fiberglass casting material in 2- and 3-inch widths
- 3M custom support foam
- 2-inch stockinet
- Cast felt
- Water bucket
- Casting gloves
- General anesthesia rather than sedation is recommended for this procedure because it is important that the foal not move during placement of the casts.
  - Injectable anesthesia such as the combination of xylazine, Valium, and ketamine is quite adequate.

ANTICIPATED TIME

Once the foal is anesthetized, placement of two forelimb tube casts should require 30 to 45 minutes.

PREPARATION: IMPORTANT CHECKPOINTS

All materials should be assembled before casting begins. Once the cast material is exposed to air, it begins to set rapidly and is useless if not quickly applied.

POSSIBLE COMPLICATIONS AND COMMON ERRORS TO BE AVOIDED

- The greatest complication is cast sores.
  - This complication is somewhat lessened for tube casts as compared to casts that incorporate the digit.
  - However, the skin of the foal is very thin and cannot tolerate abrasion or point pressure.

○ The operator must keep this in mind when applying padding under the cast.

   ▪ Appropriate padding is important; however, too much padding can compress and shift over time and be counterproductive.

   ▪ Although open to individual preference, the author prefers to use two layers of stockinet, which has circumferential strips of cast felt at the proximal and distal aspects of the cast.

○ The top of the cast should fit comfortably in the foal's axilla.

○ The bottom of the cast should end just proximal to the fetlock at approximately the level of the physeal scar.

○ The bottom of the cast should not contact the dorsal aspect of P1 when the fetlock is extended.

   ▪ This can be difficult to accurately determine in the recumbent foal, so make certain that the bottom cast padding strip is wide enough (3 cm is sufficient) to still be present if some of the distal cast material and felt must be trimmed from the distal dorsal aspect of the cast to allow full fetlock extension.

○ After placement of the stockinet and felt, small (2–3 cm) squares of felt are taped over areas where cast sores commonly occur.

   ▪ In the forelimb these areas include the caudal aspect of the accessory carpal bone and the medial distal radius.

   ▪ Tube casts are very difficult to execute successfully in the hindlimb, but if used, squares of padding should be placed over the point of the hock and medial malleolus of the tibia.

○ After placement of the stockinet and any felt squares, the cast padding is applied.

PROCEDURE

• After placement of the underlayer composed of stockinet, cast felt, and

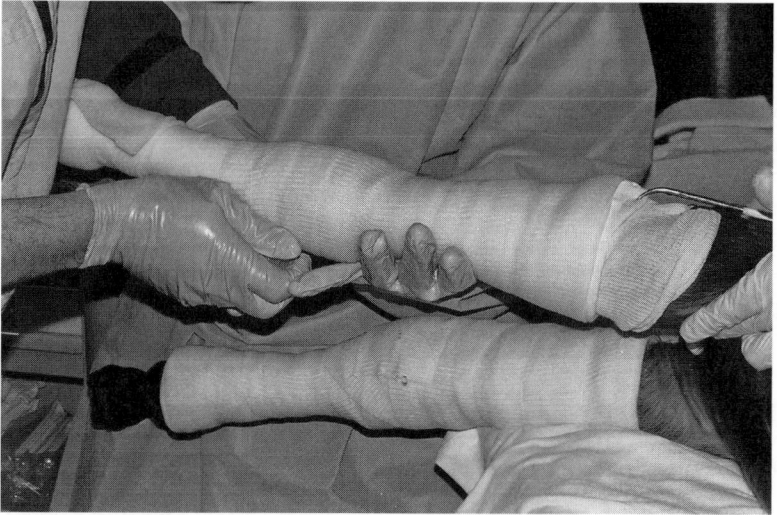

FIGURE 1 Application of bilateral forelimb tube casts in a neonatal foal.

cast padding, the casting tape is applied.

○ Casting tape of 2-inch width is used for the first layer (usually two rolls) as the thinner material conforms better to the limb and wrinkles less.

○ Cast tape is overlapped by 50% of width and applied rapidly and smoothly with very light tension.

○ After the 2-inch tape is applied, two rolls of 3-inch tape are applied. Care is taken at the ends of the casts to keep felt at the ends of the casts, as cast material is rigid and abrasive and should not directly contact the foal's skin.

○ After the casting tape is applied, the stockinet is folded over the cast felt and cast and taped to the cast. This can also be done right before the last layer of the casting tape is applied but should not be done before to avoid cast lamination (Figure 1).

POSTPROCEDURE

• Casts should be checked for fit, cracking, heat, and drainage at least twice daily.

• Foals should be monitored for lameness.

• In neonates, 14 days is the maximum duration a cast can be applied as growth inside a rigid cast can cause real damage to the limbs.

ALTERNATIVES AND THEIR RELATIVE MERITS

• Splints can also be used effectively but are not as effective at keeping the limb rigidly aligned.

   ○ They need to be frequently (usually daily) reset and in the author's experience are more likely to cause pressure-induced skin lesions than a properly applied cast.

   ○ An exception is coaptation of the hindlimbs for tarsal hypoplasia. Foals must flex the hocks to rise, so casts are not useful.

   ○ An articulated splint such as hinged splints for anterior cruciate ligament injuries in humans (small) have been used successfully (DonJoy Playmaker splint). A soft padded bandage is often needed underneath the splint for small foals.

AUTHOR: **ELIZABETH M. SANTSCHI**

Ultrasound: Abdominal, in Neonatal Foals

BASIC INFORMATION

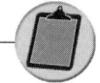

SYNONYM(S)

Abdominal scan

OVERVIEW AND GOAL(S)

Abdominal ultrasound provides a means of evaluating abdominal organs and peritoneal space for diagnostic purposes.

INDICATIONS

• Sepsis: Investigate for possibility of localized infection

• Colic: Evaluation of gastrointestinal tract, peritoneal space

• Lethargy: Investigate possible uroabdomen, hemoabdomen

EQUIPMENT, ANESTHESIA

Ultrasound machine, 3.5–7.5 MHz sector, linear, or convex array probe can be used

ANTICIPATED TIME

5 to 10 minutes

PREPARATION—IMPORTANT CHECKPOINTS

- Clipping of hair on ventral abdomen may be necessary for long or coarse haircoats.
- Contact is improved with application of alcohol or ultrasound gel.

POSSIBLE COMPLICATIONS AND COMMON ERRORS TO BE AVOIDED

Experience reading the ultrasound image is imperative for accurate interpretation.

PROCEDURE

Foals can be scanned standing or recumbent. If scanning a recumbent foal, be certain to image the down side of the abdomen. Familiarity with normal is essential for recognition of abnormalities. The entirety of the abdomen should be imaged readily in the neonate. Voluminous, anechoic free fluid is consistent with ascites or uroperitoneum. Echoic fluid may indicate peritonitis or hemoabdomen. Small intestinal wall thickness is normally <3 mm and the lumen should

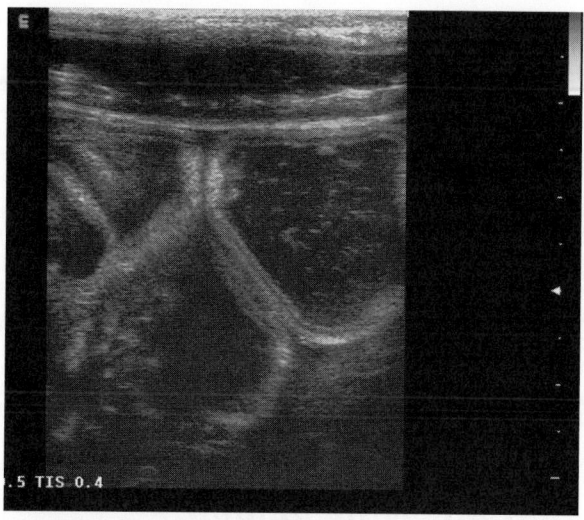

FIGURE 1　Multiple loops of distended small intestine visualized in the ventral abdomen of a colicky 7-day-old Thoroughbred filly.

be imaged only as segments contract. Meconium images as echogenic masses within the large and/or small colon.

POSTPROCEDURE

Clean alcohol or gel from skin.

ALTERNATIVES AND THEIR RELATIVE MERITS

Contrast radiography is useful in identifying meconium impactions, congenital atresia, colonic aganglionosis and bladder rupture or urachal leakage, but is less sensitive than ultrasound for localizing infection, characterizing fluid, and identifying thickened bowel and ileus.

AUTHOR: **PHOEBE A. SMITH**

EDITORS: **PHOEBE A. SMITH** and **ELIZABETH SANTSCHI**

Ultrasound: for Dental Disease

BASIC INFORMATION

SYNONYM(S)

Ultrasound (US)

OVERVIEW AND GOAL(S)

Ultrasound is a readily available, inexpensive cross-sectional imaging modality that can provide an excellent evaluation of the soft tissues and bone surfaces of the jaw and sublingual region. High-frequency (7.5–12 MHz) linear, or curvilinear probes can be exceedingly useful for the characterization of swellings, draining tracts, and masses. Ultrasound should be used to identify the underlying cause of clinical disorders and to obtain diagnostic samples for culture and/or cytology. Ultrasound is also very useful for characterization of temporomandibular joint disease.

INDICATIONS

- Swellings, draining tracts, or masses of the mandibular, maxillary, or sublingual regions; temporomandibular joint pain or swelling
- Trauma to the mandible or maxilla for identification of fractures

CONTRAINDICATIONS

There are no known contraindications for ultrasound. Its use should be considered in light of the patient's clinical status, as sedation is often necessary to obtain diagnostic ultrasound images.

EQUIPMENT, ANESTHESIA

- High-frequency (7.5–12 MHz) linear or curvilinear probes
- Ultrasound machine

ANTICIPATED TIME

Highly variable with operator experience and size of imaging area

PREPARATION: IMPORTANT CHECKPOINTS

- Clip hair.
- Wash the skin surface to remove debris, matted hair, and scurf. This is particularly important in horses with chronic draining tracts where dried exudate and scabs can impede the ultrasound beam.
- Plan your examination:
  - Review the regional anatomy.
  - Review the expected normal ultrasonographic findings (muscle, bone surface).
  - Prepare to compare to the contralateral jaw.
- Sedate as needed.

POSSIBLE COMPLICATIONS AND COMMON ERRORS TO BE AVOIDED

Insufficient preparation, inadequate equipment, and poor scanning technique will compromise the quality of the examination and therefore the interpretation of the imaging findings.

PROCEDURE

Soft tissue swellings and masses should be methodically evaluated. The region should be evaluated in a minimum of two planes. Follow draining tracts from their point of exit to the point of origin in a slow and methodical fashion. Compare to the contralateral side when scanning unfamiliar anatomy. Document and label images that represent important normal and abnormal findings.

ALTERNATIVES AND THEIR RELATIVE MERITS

- Fistulography is a technique in which positive contrast media or a metallic probe is introduced into a draining tract and radiographs are made. The contrast media is expected to fill the tract from its point of exit to its point of origin thereby making the draining tract evident on radiographs. This technique can be used as an alternative to ultrasound. Often this technique will make the source of the

draining tract more obvious when the source is an abnormal tooth as compared to ultrasound for the same purpose.
- Computed tomography and magnetic resonance imaging both provide cross-sectional images of soft and hard tissues. The lack of availability and need for general anesthesia with these techniques make them much less practical and much more expensive than ultrasound.

AUTHOR: **SARAH M. PUCHALSKI**

Ultrasound: Musculoskeletal

BASIC INFORMATION

OVERVIEW

Ultrasound involves sending high-frequency sound waves into the patient and "listening" to the waves as they reflect off tissue. Depending on the amount of reflection, scatter, and absorption, the returning echoes produce varying degrees of bright dots, forming a two-dimensional real-time image along the axis of the handheld transducer.

PREPARATION: IMPORTANT CHECKPOINTS

- Patient preparation is very important to minimize artifacts and misdiagnoses.
- Sedation is often necessary to allow proper positioning and expedite the exam. A small amount of sedation is generally sufficient to minimize patient motion; excessive sedation may lead to patient instability.
- Dry dirt and debris within the hair coat can be removed with a firm brush. A mild detergent or scrub can be used to further clean a clipped area.
- The hair coat must be clipped for an optimal image to be acquired. This is because hair and the air trapped between the hair shafts act as an acoustic barrier to the insonating ultrasound beam and the returning echoes.
- Applying 70% alcohol to the clipped area helps reduce small air bubbles remaining in the undercoat.
- Applying an acoustic coupling gel allows optimal transfer of sound waves from the transducer into and out of the patient.

EQUIPMENT

- Many different machines are available. These include handheld ultraportable units designed specifically for minor

applications to large units mounted on four-wheeled carts designed for stationary use. The majority of equine ultrasound is performed on laptop or portable units.
- The most important aspects of transducer choice are frequency and configuration. Transducers come in several configurations, each having a preferred application.
- Newer transducers are electronic, consisting of multiple (several hundred) small piezoelectric elements, or arrays. The configuration of the piezoelectric crystals is what defines the size, shape, and application of the transducer. Electronic transducers include linear, curvilinear, microconvex, and phased arrays.
- Linear array transducers are the only suitable choice for equine tendon and ligament examination because of excellent near-field width and high resolution (Figure 1).

- Curvilinear, microconvex, and phased array transducers all produce a form of a sector image (pie shaped).
- Curvilinear transducers have a large radius, a large patient contact area (footprint), and a relatively large near-field view. They are used for deeper areas such as abdominal imaging.
- Microconvex transducers have a very small "tip," allowing a small area of contact with the patient and producing a sector image with very little usable information in the near field.
- Phased array transducers also produce a sector image and generally have the highest penetration (depth) of any of the transducers. Phased array transducers are the choice for cardiac imaging because high achievable frame rates provide the best visualization of cardiac motion.
- All the sector transducers can be used for evaluating deeper anatomy; musculoskeletal applications include eval-

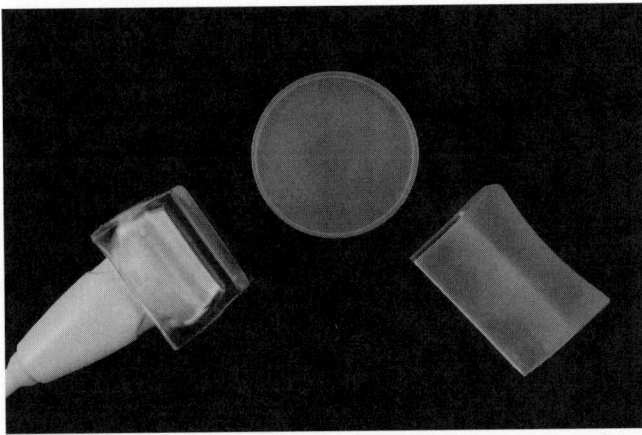

FIGURE 1 *Left,* A linear array transducer with a fitted standoff pad attached designed specifically for this transducer. *Center,* A universal application standoff pad in the shape of a disc. On the *left* is a universal semifitted standoff pad for use with linear array transducers.

uation for deep-seated abscesses and assessing continuity of deeper bony surfaces for fractures.

- Electronic transducer design has many advantages over older mechanical transducer technology, including wide band width (eg, 4–13 MHz) and focusing.
- Wide bandwidth allows the user to preferentially select the frequency range that is most appropriate for the depth of penetration necessary and resolution of image detail. As an example, a linear array transducer capable of operating between 4 and 13 MHz allows visualization of deeper structures at a lower frequency range while very near-field structures can be studied at higher resolution (image detail) using the highest frequency.
- Focusing is a method to increase lateral (side-to-side) resolution with electronic transducers. The focal point (or multiple focal points) provides the best resolution at the selected depth(s). Use of multiple focal points results in a reduction in frame rate (how many times per second the image is updated) which can be bothersome while scanning.
- Older transducers are of the mechanical type, in which a single piezoelectric crystal was oscillated to produce a sector (pie-shaped image), or in some designs consisted of three crystals of different frequencies that rotated to form a sector image. These transducers have a fixed single focus and their frequency cannot be adjusted, except for the annular array design. Mechanical transducers are not available in linear array configuration. These transducers are still operational for imaging deeper areas of the patient such as the heart and abdomen but have little utility today for most extremity tendon and ligament examinations.
- *Use the highest frequency transducer available that allows imaging the anatomic area of interest.* The higher the frequency of the ultrasound transducer, the better the axial resolution, the trade-off being less penetration of the ultrasound beam. Lower frequency transducers trade less resolution for greater depth of penetration. This is why the broad-bandwidth electronic transducers are so user friendly; one transducer can image a wide range of depth by just varying the available frequency range.
- Most equine musculoskeletal examinations are performed with a high frequency linear transducer, typically from 7.5 to 13 MHz or even 18 MHz. These frequencies allow a usable scanning depth of up to 4 or 5 cm, making them ideal for most tendon and ligament work. A linear probe is

used because of its large flat footprint and excellent near-field resolution. The linear configuration emits the ultrasound beam perpendicular to tendon/ligament fibers when properly aimed, in turn yielding the best overall image.

- A standoff pad is made of a flexible, sonolucent material. The purpose of the standoff is to allow better visualization of very superficial structures. Standoff pads may be form-fitted to the transducer or be of a universal application and disposable (see Figure 1). A few newer, dedicated near-field transducers have build-in permanent standoffs. The key to using a standoff pad properly is to ensure adequate acoustic coupling by liberal use of acoustic gel between the transducer and the standoff and the standoff and the patient.

BASIC MACHINE SETTINGS FOR OBTAINING A QUALITY IMAGE

- *Gain* controls the brightness of the ultrasound image by *uniformly* amplifying the returning echoes. The overall gain needed is variable depending on patient preparation, size, skin thickness, etc. The ultrasound image should be bright enough to easily see all structures in the field of view. An entire image that is too dark despite a maximum gain setting is usually due to poor acoustic coupling (hair not clipped, scaly or uneven skin surface, lack of acoustic coupling gel). This emphasizes the importance of achieving the best acoustic coupling of the transducer to the patient as possible. Figure 2 illustrates improper gain settings.
- Increasing the power output of the ultrasound machine can be useful in making an image brighter. The power

output is really the volume of the ultrasound being transmitted into the patient. Ultrasound machines are limited in their output by the Food and Drug Administration. The power control may be labeled as P (power) or MI (mechanical index).

- Another common cause of images that are too dark is the presence of high levels of ambient light or reflected light on the monitor. A darkened room is essential. Positioning the patient so that the ultrasound machine is in a shadow may be your only hope to obtain an adequate image in a field setting.
- Time gain compensation (TGC): This is a depth-dependent gain adjustment controlled by a series of sliders or knobs. These controls are set such that the level of image brightness is even from the near field to the far field. In most applications, the near-field gain must be reduced (since near-field echoes are inherently louder because they are not attenuated to the same degree as echoes originating from deeper areas), whereas the far field gain must be boosted. Figure 3 illustrates incorrect TGC settings, rendering the images nondiagnostic. Figure 4 illustrates properly adjusted, diagnostic-quality images.
- When the far field remains too dark despite a maximum overall gain, power setting, and far-field TGC boost, use a lower frequency to obtain adequate penetration.
- The *focal zone* is the narrowest portion of the ultrasound beam and therefore is the depth of the image that has the best resolution. The focus should be placed at the level of the structure of interest to obtain optimal resolution (see Figure 4). The use of multiple

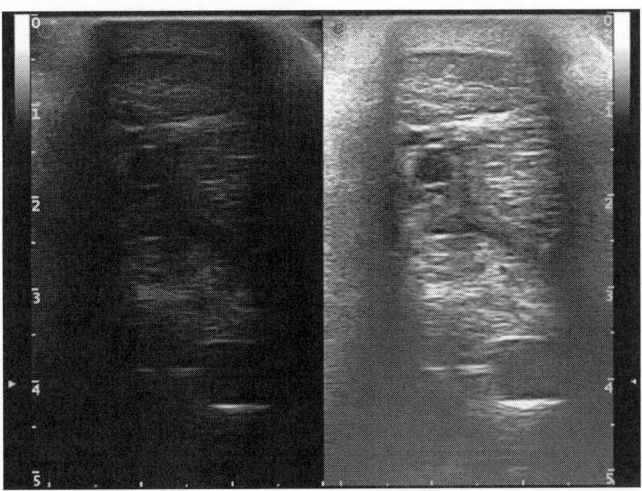

FIGURE 2 Improper overall gain settings. *Left,* This image has the gain set too low; as a result, the image is uniformly too dark. *Right,* This image has the overall gain control set too high and is much too bright. Neither of these images is diagnostic nor acceptable.

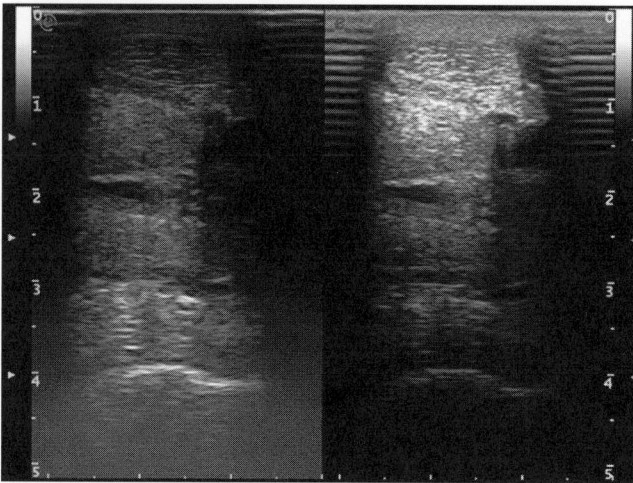

FIGURE 3 Improper TGC settings. *Left,* This image has the near-field gain reduced inappropriately, whereas the far-field gain is boosted too high. The result is an image that is dark in the near field and too bright in the far field. *Right* This image has the TGC controls inappropriately set in the opposite direction. The near field has too much gain and is therefore too bright; the far field is too dark because the gain at this depth was reduced. TGC should be adjusted so that the image brightness is the same for the entire depth of field. Uniform increase or decrease in image brightness is controlled by the overall gain setting.

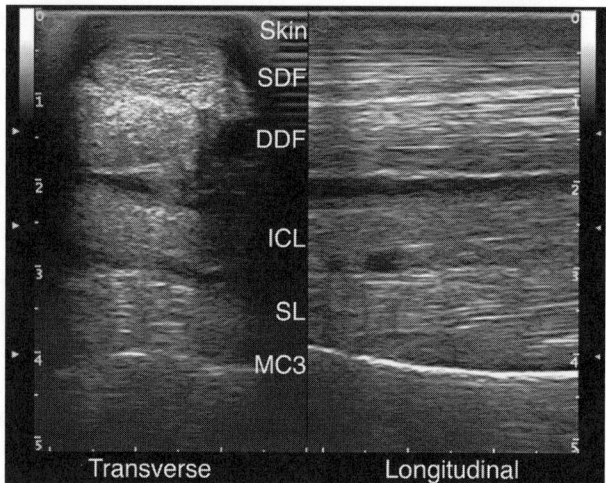

FIGURE 4 Properly adjusted images of normal proximal metacarpal tendons and ligaments in transverse and long-axis image planes, displayed in split-screen mode. In the long axis, these structures have a notable hyperechoic, linear, striated fiber pattern. The dorsal and palmar edges are well delineated by bright, linear margins due to the ultrasound beam interacting with the surfaces at right angles, creating maximum reflectivity. In the transverse section, the tendons and ligaments are hyperechoic with an even, mottled echotexture, created by the fibers in cross-section. The dorsal and palmar margins are clearly defined as noted for the long axis image; however, note that laterally and medially there is very poor margin identification. This is normal and is a result of severe off-incident interaction of the ultrasound beam, striking the edges of these structures tangentially. To view these margins, transducer orientation must be changed. Lack of margin visualization hinders precise mensuration in many cases. The overall gain and TGC are set correctly to achieve balanced image brightness from near field to far field. A standoff pad was not used. *SDF,* Superficial digital flexor tendon; *DDF,* deep digital flexor tendon; *ICL,* inferior check ligament; *SL,* suspensory ligament; *MC3,* surface of the third metacarpal bone.

focal zones yields the best image, but the tradeoff is a reduced frame rate, seen as "flicker" when the transducer is moved along its path too quickly.
- There are numerous additional user-defined settings available to adjust the appearance of the ultrasound image.

These can be considered fine tuning. An explanation of some of these settings is provided in Figure 4.

PROCEDURE

- Before starting the examination, select a probe that will provide the most

detail and penetration to evaluate the anatomic structures of interest. The higher the frequency, the better the resolution but with less penetration. For example, a lower frequency would be required for the suspensory ligament than for the superficial flexor tendon.
- Tendons and ligaments should be scanned in transverse and longitudinal planes for thorough evaluation (see Figure 4).
- Tendons and ligaments are normally highly reflective tissues due to their parallel fiber composition. When the ultrasound beam strikes the fibers at 90 degrees, maximum reflection (echoes) occurs, yielding a bright (very echogenic) image (see Figure 4).
- Conversely, slight proximal to distal rocking of the transducer puts the incident ultrasound beam at non-90-degree angles and creates a very common hypoechoic artifact that must be recognized and differentiated from pathology. This occurs more easily in the transverse plane (also possible, but to a lesser extent, in the longitudinal plane). For optimal imaging, the ultrasound beam or probe must be *perpendicular* to the fibers. In some cases, however, slight off-incidence scanning will reveal a true lesion not seen with perpendicular to the main fiber axis (Figure 5).
- Ultrasound artifacts are many and are very easy to produce in musculoskeletal ultrasound. You will notice artifacts on every scan that you perform. Familiarity and recognition of artifacts is imperative to avoid misinterpretation and misdiagnoses.

INTERPRETATION GUIDELINES

- Knowledge of anatomy is crucial for performing and interpreting an ultrasound examination. Comparison of the diseased limb with the contralateral limb is very helpful in many cases. The Suggested Readings below are excellent sources of information.
- The ease of use and safety of ultrasound make it ideal for serial recheck examinations. Information from recheck exams is maximized when detailed anatomic and quantitative information has been recorded or documented.
- The examination should be recorded, using anatomical landmarks or zones, either with hard or soft copy images. Lesions should be referenced to a fixed palpable landmark, such as the accessory carpal bone or point of the hock, for more accurate follow-up (see Figure 5). A cloth tape measure secured at its proximal end by a wrap of hook-and-loop tape is handy. Alternatively, ultrasonographic zones have

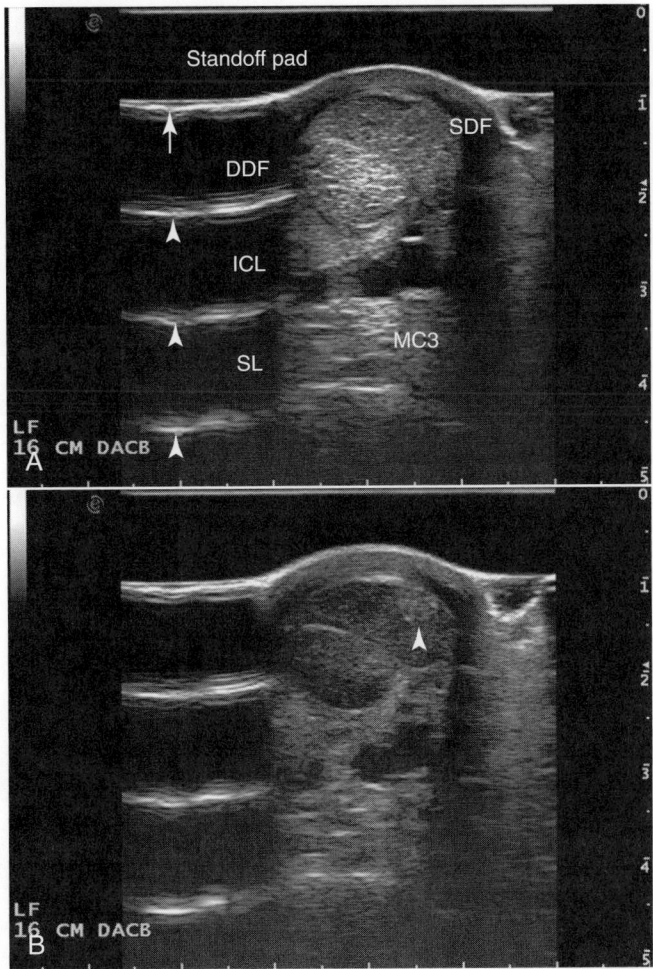

FIGURE 5 Transverse ultrasound images of the palmar metacarpal soft tissues showing the effect of off-incidence scanning of tendons. The overall gain and the TGC controls are properly set to give an image that is of the same brightness from the near to far field. The small *arrowhead* adjacent to the centimeter scale on the right of the images signifies the location of the focus, maximizing image detail at a depth of approximately 2 cm. The images of the left forelimb (LF) were made at a measured distance of 16 cm distal to the accessory carpal bone (DACB) **A,** The superficial digital flexor tendon (SDF), deep digital flexor tendon (DDF), distal check ligament (ICL), the distal portion of the body of the suspensory ligament (SL), and the echogenic surface of metacarpal 3 (MC3) are seen. A standoff pad is seen as anechoic near field space. Strong echo at the standoff-air interface (*arrow*) creates a series of repeating reverberation artifact (*arrowheads*). The SDF tendon is enlarged and slightly less bright (hypoechoic) than the underlying DDF tendon. **B,** This image is made at the same location as Figure 2, *A,* but the incident ultrasound beam is not perpendicular to the tendons and ligaments, made by slight angulation of the transducer up or down. Note how the SDF and DDF tendons are now much less echogenic (bright). This is artifact caused by off-incident ultrasound beam interaction with the tendon fibers. In some cases, this can create artifacts that mimic hypoechoic tendon or ligament lesions. Also note that the ICL is now more echogenic than the SDF and DDF. This is due to mild convergence of the ICL as it joins the DDF. The ICL does not course parallel to these tendons and therefore it is difficult in most cases to critically review all three of these structures with a single transducer angle and image plane. The off-incidence evaluation revealed a focal hyperechoic healed lesion within the SDF tendon (*arrowhead*).

been described in an attempt to standardize lesion localization (eg, Figures 1 through 3 from proximal to distal metacarpus). Regardless of method, the examiner should be consistent for repeatability, recheck evaluations, and of course accuracy.

- Basic evaluation parameters should be followed. These include the *size* of tendons and ligaments evaluated, their *shape,* alterations in *echogenicity,* disruption of the normal echogenic *fiber pattern,* and the presence or absence of focal lesions within the structure.

- The cross-sectional area and/or thickness of the tendon or ligament can be measured with electronic measurement applications on the ultrasound machine. The size of the lesion or area of damaged fibers should also be mea-

sured. The percent of the cross-sectional area affected can be calculated and has been used in determining prognosis (Figure 6).

NORMAL TENDONS AND LIGAMENTS

- In a transverse section, normal tendons and ligaments have a finely speckled appearance due to the cross-sectional nature of the fibers. This has been compared to looking at the cut end of a rope end-on. Borders should be echogenic, thin, and smoothly marginated (see Figure 4).

- In the longitudinal axis, tendons and ligaments have a very structured appearance of echogenic parallel fibers (see Figure 4).

TENDON AND LIGAMENT INJURY

- In nearly all cases, tendons and ligaments increase in size and lose their normal echogenic fiber pattern when injured. They lose their normal highly echogenic appearance and become hypoechoic to anechoic. This is due to disruption of the fibers and ensuing edema, hemorrhage, and inflammation (see Figure 6).

- Healing takes a minimum of several months, and in ideal circumstances is seen as "filling in" of the previously detected hypoechoic areas with echogenic, realigning fibers.

- In some cases, healed tendons and ligaments become hyperechoic compared with normal, but often the ultrasound healing is never complete, with residual hypoechoic areas persisting for months to years (see Figure 5, *B*).

MUSCLE

- Muscle is a relatively hypoechoic tissue compared with tendons and ligaments. It also has a coarse echotexture, created by highly echogenic fibrous fascial planes sparsely interspersed between hypoechoic muscle.

- Muscle bellies can be followed to their transition to tendons for musculotendonous junction injury.

- Intuitively, muscle injury appears as disruption of the normal echotexture and echogenicity. Fibrous lesions such as fibrotic myopathy will render the muscle tissue more echogenic than normal.

- Abscesses within muscle have a central area of anechoic to very echogenic fluid, which may be surrounded by a capsule (Figure 7). The echogenic fluid can usually be diagnosed by movement of the echoes with transducer pressure, but there are some abscesses that are so echogenic and viscous that they resemble tissue. The capsule can be more or less echogenic than surrounding muscle tissue, and with chronicity may even be lamellar.

- Ultrasound can be used to safely guide needles into abscess pockets for sample collection and drainage.

PROCEDURES AND TECHNIQUES

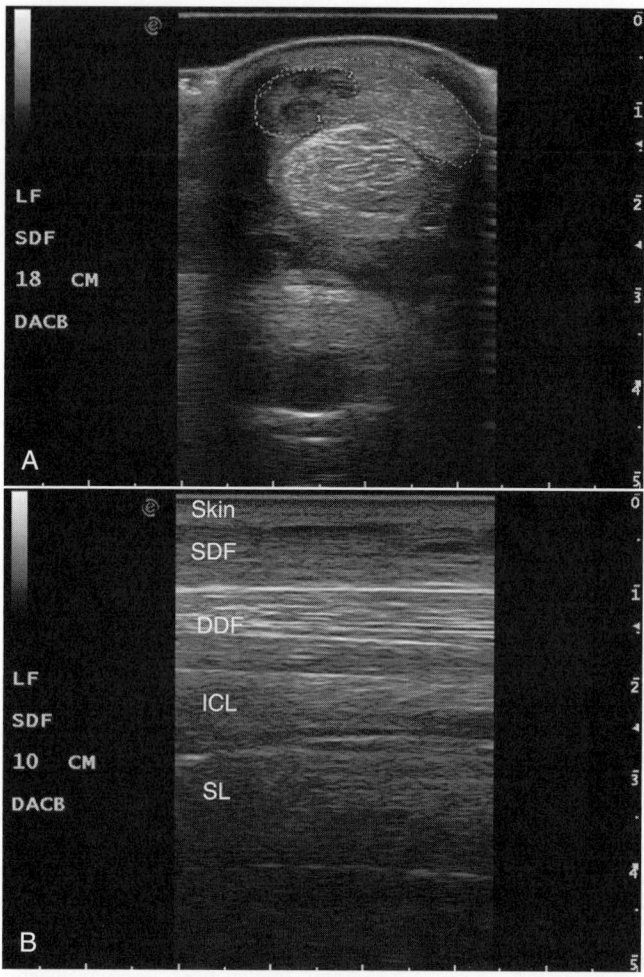

FIGURE 6 Superficial digital flexor tendonitis. **A,** Transverse image. The superficial digital flexor tendon has a well-marginated, mottled, hypoechoic lesion in its lateral aspect. The lesional area is 1.66 cm² (defined by electronic boundary 2) at 18 cm distal to the accessory carpal bone (18 cm DACB). The overall size of the superficial digital flexor tendon in the region of the lesion is enlarged with a cross-sectional area of 3.35 cm² (electronic boundary 1). There are four measurements given: A1 is the areas of the lesion, P1 is the circumference (periphery), A2 is the area of the superficial digital flexor (SDF) tendon, P2 is the circumference. **B,** Longitudinal image. The near field SDF tendon is hypoechoic and has lost the majority of its fiber pattern. This image was made 10 cm distal to the accessory carpal bone (10 cm DACB). This SDF lesion began approximately 7 cm distal to the accessory carpal bone and continued to 27 cm distal (the entirety of the lesion is not shown. *DDF,* Deep digital flexor tendon; *ICL,* inferior check ligament; *SL,* suspensory ligament.

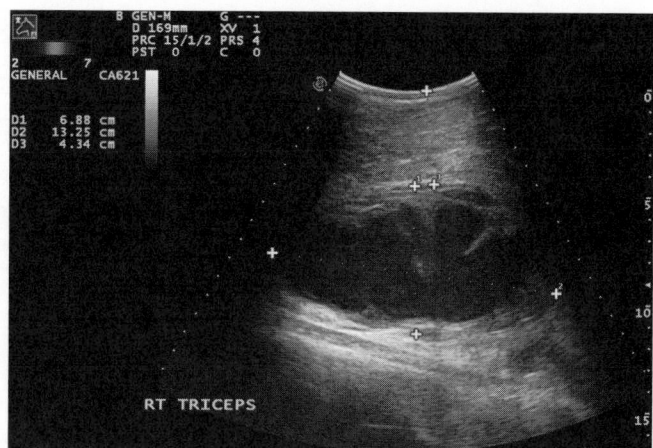

FIGURE 7 Abscess. A large (approximately 13 cm in length and 7 cm in depth) abscess is present within the right triceps muscle. The abscess contains a pocket of hypoechoic fluid and several hyperechoic septa. A poorly defined hyperechoic capsule surrounds the abscess. When measured from the lateral skin surface, the abscess was more than 4 cm deep.

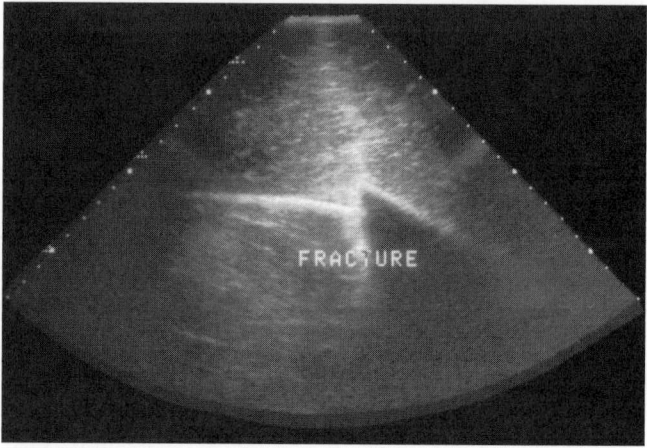

FIGURE 8 Fracture of the ilium. The bony surface of the ilium is seen as the highly echogenic linear structure coursing across the central part of the image. Note the discontinuity of the bony surface and abrupt angle of the displaced fracture. This image was made using an older phased array sector transducer. Note the comparatively reduced image quality.

BONE

- The bony surface is highly effective at attenuating (absorbing) the ultrasound beam. This creates a very echogenic (bright), linear interface.
- Ultrasound cannot penetrate bone; any image displayed deep to the bone interface is artifact. This artifact is termed *acoustic shadow.*
- A bone surface can be evaluated with ultrasound and has been used to diagnose fractures in areas where radiography may be limited or impossible, such as the ilium or femur.

- A fracture can be recognized as an interruption of the normal linear contour of bone surface (Figures 8 and 9).

ARTICULAR CARTILAGE

- Articular cartilage of the fetlock, tarsus, and stifle is often evaluated by ultrasound.
- Normal articular cartilage is visualized with high-frequency transducers and is seen as a thin band of hypoechoic to anechoic tissue paralleling the subchondral bone (Figure 10).

METAL AND GAS

Metal and gas are both highly reflective and thus can be detected quite readily with ultrasound. The ultrasound beam reflects vigorously off of gas and metal, seen as a very echogenic focus. Since ultrasound does not penetrate any further, an acoustic shadow artifact is encountered, seen as a trail of hypoechoic to anechoic area directly deep to the gas or metal. Another form of artifact seen is a reverberation artifact (comet tail), in which multiple, repeating echoes continue deep into the tissues.

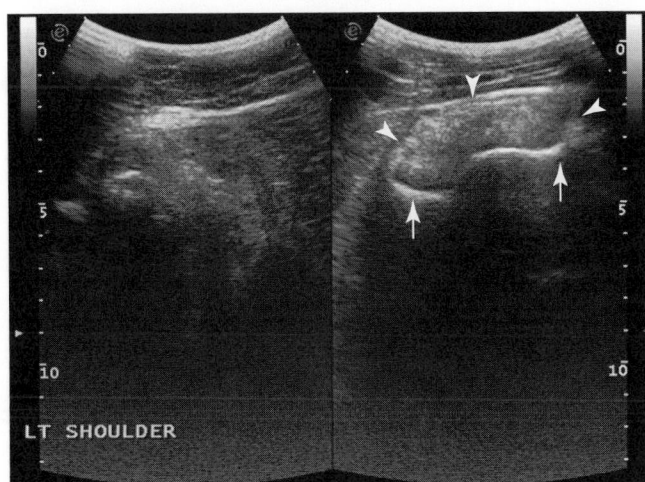

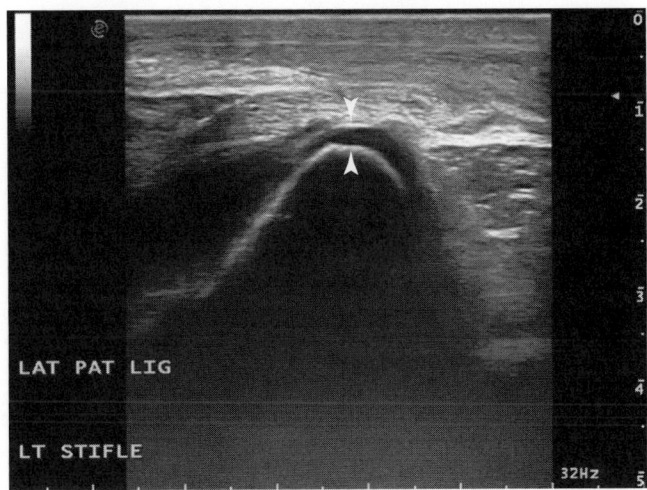

FIGURE 9 Proximal left humeral fracture with normal right humerus for comparison, displayed in split screen mode. The right normal biceps tendon (*arrowheads*) can be seen within the inter-tuberal (bicipital) groove (*arrows*), defined by the echogenic bone surface of the proximal humerus. Comparison with the fractured proximal humerus on the left, distortion of the biceps tendon and loss of normal bony contour of the proximal humerus can be easily and confidently appreciated.

A lower frequency (2–7 MHz) curvilinear transducer was used to examine the humerus because of the depth required to visualize the thick shoulder tissues. In these images it was operating within its mid-band range (approximately 5 MHz; note the central location of the frequency graph in the upper left corner, and the B GEN-M designation in the header). Note the large curved near-field contact area with the patient. The true diverging extent of the sector image cannot be appreciated due to the two images overlapping on this split-screen function. The focus is seen at 9 cm. Repositioning it to the level of the fracture (approximately 5 cm) would have optimized the image at the depth of the pathology.

FIGURE 10 A transverse image of a normal lateral trochlear ridge of the femur, showing articular cartilage as a hypoechoic to anechoic layer of tissue (between *arrowheads*) adjacent to the underlying echogenic subchondral bone surface.

SUGGESTED READINGS

Denoix J: *The equine distal limb: an atlas of clinical anatomy and comparative imaging*, London, 2000, Manson Publishing Ltd.

McKinnon AO: *Equine diagnostic ultrasonography*, Philadelphia, 1998, Lippincott Williams & Wilkins.

Reef VB: *Equine diagnostic ultrasound*, Philadelphia, 1998, WB Saunders.

Reimer J: *Atlas of equine ultrasonography*, St Louis, 1998, Mosby–Year Book.

Ross MW, Dyson SJ: *Diagnosis and management of lameness in the horse*, St Louis, 2003, Saunders Elsevier.

AUTHORS: **JOHN S. MATTOON, JASON W. BRUMITT, JONATHAN HAYLES, DANA A. NEELIS, GREGORY D. ROBERTS**, and **TOM WILKINSON**

Ultrasound: Umbilicus

BASIC INFORMATION

SYNONYM(S)

Umbilical scan

OVERVIEW AND GOAL(S)

Ultrasound of the internal remnants of the umbilicus allows the practitioner to obtain images to establish a baseline in hospitalized neonates and to identify localized infection.

INDICATIONS

- Foals admitted to neonatal intensive care units
- Foals with fever of unknown origin, septic arthritis, pneumonia, bacteremia/sepsis, or leukocytosis
- Foals with enlargement or moisture of the external umbilical stump

EQUIPMENT, ANESTHESIA

An ultrasound machine with a 5.0 MHz linear transducer is best.

ANTICIPATED TIME

5 to 10 minutes

PREPARATION: IMPORANT CHECKPOINTS

- Clipping the hair of the ventral midline from xiphoid to inguinal region may be necessary in foals with coarse or long haircoats.
- Contact is improved by use of alcohol or ultrasound gel.

POSSIBLE COMPLICATIONS AND COMMON ERRORS TO BE AVOIDED

Experience reading the ultrasound image is imperative for accurate interpretation.

Familiarity with normal image findings is essential to accurate assessment of ultrasound images.

PROCEDURE

- The umbilical structures may be scanned with foals in a standing or laterally recumbent position.
- Sedation with diazepam (0.1–0.2 mg/kg IV) or butorphanol (0.05 mg/kg IV) may be required.
- The umbilical structures should be scanned in both transverse and longitudinal planes.
- To image the umbilical vein in transverse section, orient the probe perpendicular to the spinal column on the cranial border of the umbilical stump. The umbilical vein is a thin-walled, ovoid structure 0.5 to 1.0 cm in diameter visible 1 to 2 cm deep to the skin

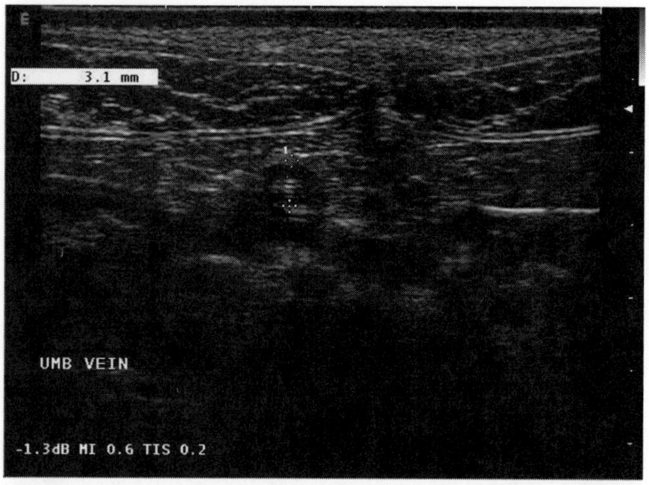

FIGURE 1 Normal umbilical vein in the short axis imaged 2 cm cranial to the external umbilical stump in a 12-day-old Standardbred colt with pneumonia.

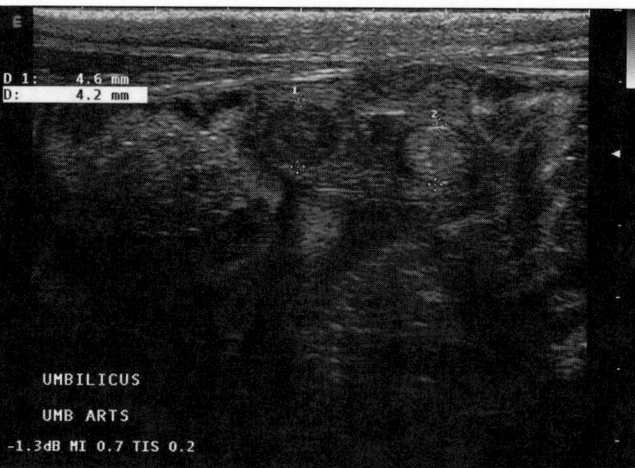

FIGURE 2 Umbilical arteries in the short axis imaged in the caudal abdomen of a 10-day-old Arabian colt with a fever. Arteries appear normal in size and echogenicity.

surface (Figure 1). Follow the umbilical vein cranially as it courses toward the liver. The umbilical vein is generally largest just cranial to the external stump.

- The umbilical arteries are imaged caudal to the external stump, also 1 to 2 cm deep to the skin surface (Figure 2). Both right and left umbilical arteries appear as thick-walled vessels and may be asymmetrical in size in normal foals. Normal diameter averages 1.2 cm. Just cranial to the apex of the bladder, the arteries are imaged together along with the urachus. Collectively, these structures at this location should measure 2.5 cm or less. The arteries diverge along either side

of the bladder and disappear at the caudal aspect of the bladder.
- The urachus extends caudally from the umbilical stump to the apex of the bladder but is often collapsed and difficult to image. When fluid filled, it is easily recognized as abnormal. A valuable view of the urachus is made in longitudinal section at its attachment to the apex of the bladder. A patent urachus is imaged as communication between the bladder and urachus.
- The external umbilical stump is imaged by holding onto the tip and scanning along its length in both longitudinal and transverse axis planes. Small fluid pockets that are unrecognizable grossly are imaged this way. Standard

sizes have not been established for the umbilical stump diameter, and considerable variation exists among foals of different sizes.

POSTPROCEDURE

Clean gel from foal's abdomen and external umbilical stump.

ALTERNATIVES AND THEIR RELATIVE MERITS

Imaging the internal umbilical structures can only be achieved with ultrasound. Inspection and palpation of the external stump do not provide information about the internal structures.

AUTHOR: **PHOEBE A. SMITH**

Ultrasound: Urinary Tract

BASIC INFORMATION

OVERVIEW AND GOAL(S)

The left and right kidneys can be imaged transabdominally in horses. Umbilical structures and the urinary bladder can be imaged transabdominally in foals. The urinary bladder and caudal pole of the left kidney can be imaged transrectally in adult horses.

INDICATIONS

- Stranguria
- Dysuria
- Hematuria
- Weight loss
- Abdominal pain
- Colic

CONTRAINDICATIONS

Transrectal imaging in an animal that has had a previous rectal tear

EQUIPMENT, ANESTHESIA

- Transrectal imaging of the urinary bladder and caudal pole of the left kidney is best performed using a 5-MHz linear-array rectal transducer.
- The urethra in male horses can be imaged, depending on the location, either transcutaneously using 7.5- to 10.0-MHz transducer or transrectally using a 5.0- to 7.5-MHz linear-array transducer.
- The right kidney is imaged transabdominally using a 2.5- to 5.0-MHz sector-scanner transducer and the left

kidney and urinary bladder using a 2.5- to 3.5-MHz transducer.

ANTICIPATED TIME

10 minutes

PREPARATION: IMPORTANT CHECKPOINTS

- Clipping hair over the paralumbar fossa region and cranially to the sixteenth to seventeenth intercostal space on the left and between the fourteenth to seventeenth intercostal spaces on the right is desirable prior to ultrasound evaluation of the kidneys.
- Sedation and restraint in stocks is ideal for transrectal imaging.

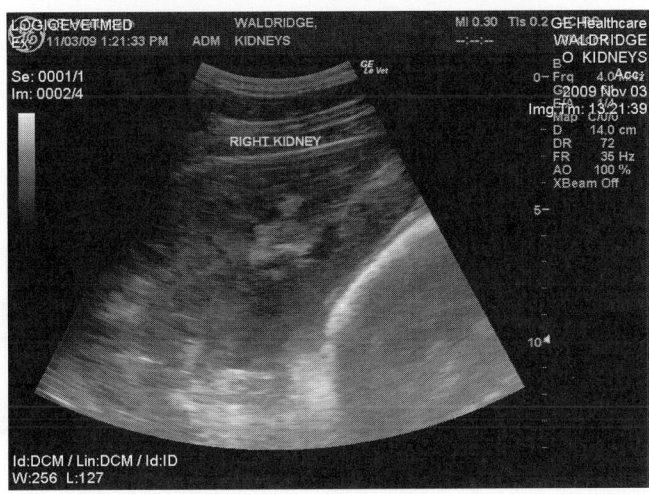

FIGURE 1 A normal right kidney.

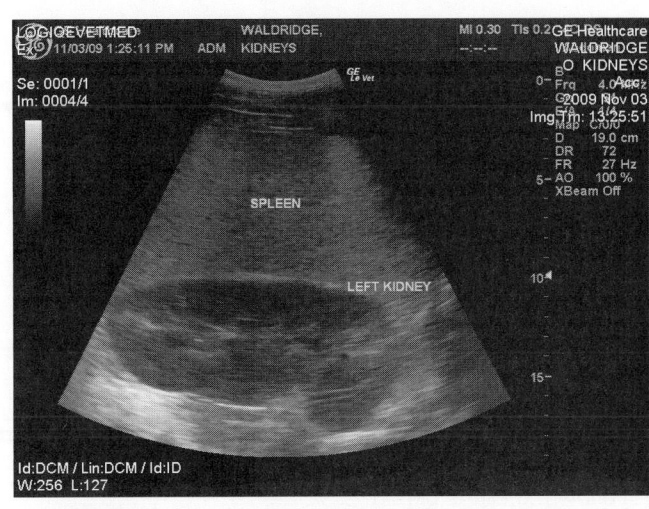

FIGURE 2 A normal left kidney, deep to the spleen.

- Application of ultrasound gel or iso-propyl alcohol will improve image quality.

POSSIBLE COMPLICATIONS AND COMMON ERRORS TO BE AVOIDED

- Rectal tears are a potential risk of transrectal imaging. Sedation and/or manual restraint are suggested for fractious horses.
- The ureters are not normally observed using ultrasonography.
- The high mucus content of equine urine produces many acoustic artifacts.

PROCEDURE

BLADDER

- The urinary bladder may be imaged on the floor of the ventral abdomen just cranial to the pelvic brim.
- The bladder can be examined either transrectally (5.0-MHz linear array transducer) or transabdominally (2.5–5.0 MHz sector-scanner transducer) if the urinary bladder is distended with urine.
- The urinary bladder is best imaged when full of urine.
- The thickness of the wall of the bladder varies with distension but is normally between 3 to 6 mm.
- Equine urine appears as a heterogeneous mixed echogenic fluid due to the presence of mucus and crystals. Crystals can accumulate as sediment in the ventral aspect of the bladder. The sediment can be made to swirl if the bladder is balloted.
- Cystic calculi have an echogenic appearance and produce an acoustic shadow.
- Intramural masses can be imaged in the wall of the urinary bladder.
- Normal ureters and ureteral openings into the urinary bladder can occasion-

ally be imaged transrectally using a high-frequency transducer but become obvious with hydroureter.

URETHRA

- The entire urethra of male horses can be examined ultrasonographically.
  - The pelvic urethra is imaged rectally and the perineal and penile portions of the urethra are examined transcutaneously.
- Due to the urethra's superficial location, higher frequency transducers should be used for optimal image quality.

KIDNEYS

- The right kidney is triangular to horse-shoe shaped and is imaged transabdominally via the last three intercostal spaces, ventral to the tuber coxae (Figure 1).
  - The right kidney measures approximately 15 to 18 cm wide, 13 to 15 cm long, and 5 cm thick.
- The left kidney is imaged via the last two intercostal spaces or in the paralumbar fossa at the level of the tuber coxae.
  - The left kidney is bean-shaped and lies deep to the spleen (Figure 2).
  - The left kidney is 15 to 18 cm long, 11 to 15 cm wide, and 5 to 6 cm thick.
  - A very good image of the caudal pole of the left kidney can be obtained by transrectal imaging.
- Assessment of the size, shape, architecture, and echogenicity of both kidneys should be performed in dorsal, sagittal, transverse, and oblique views.
- The renal cortex is approximately 1- to 2-cm thick and is hypoechoic compared with surrounding tissues.
- The medulla is less echogenic than the cortex.
- The renal pelvis is the most echogenic due to its fat and fibrous tissue.

  - In the transverse plane, the renal pelvis appears as two echogenic diverging lines leading toward the crescent-shaped renal crest.
- The terminal recesses are visible in the cranial and caudal extremities of each kidney and appear as moderately echogenic lines measuring 1 to 3 mm within the medulla.
- The proximal right ureter is strongly echogenic, while the proximal left ureter is difficult to differentiate.
- The renal vessels can be imaged at the kidney hilus, with the renal artery and/or branches located cranial to the renal vein.
- Enlargement of the kidneys can be seen in acute renal failure. Look for perirenal edema, widening of renal cortex, and loss of a distinct cortico-medullary junction.
- In chronic renal failure, kidney size may be decreased and kidneys may appear more echogenic.
- Cystic or mineralized areas indicate chronic renal disease, congenital abnormalities, or calculi in the renal pelvis.
  - Small mineralized areas within the kidney are often an incidental finding, especially in horses frequently treated with nonsteroidal antiinflammatory drugs.
  - Calculi will produce a characteristic acoustic shadow.
  - Hydronephrosis and hydroureter may be due to congenital renal dysplasia or secondary to obstructive calculi.

ALTERNATIVES AND THEIR RELATIVE MERITS

- Radiography is useful only in foals and miniature horses.
- Excretory urography is performed under general anesthesia and is used

to identify ectopic ureters or nonfunctional or hypoplastic kidneys.
- Retrograde contrast ultrasonographic studies may detect ectopic ureters,

ruptured bladder, strictures, or masses in the urethra or bladder or evaluate ureters in mares. Saline or agitated saline with air bubbles may improve visualization of some structures.

- Contrast ultrasound examinations can be difficult to interpret, even with extensive diagnostic ultrasound experience.

AUTHOR: **ALLISON J. STEWART**

Ultrasound: Uterine Edema

BASIC INFORMATION

INDICATIONS
- Follow the estrus period
- Determine normalcy of the endometrium
- Determine time of insemination

EQUIPMENT, ANESTHESIA
Ultrasound equipment with a 5 to 7.5 mHz probe

ANTICIPATED TIME
With experience, 1 to 2 minutes

PREPARATION: IMPORTANT CHECKPOINTS
- The mare should be well restrained.
- Some mares might need light sedation.
- Evacuate rectum as per transrectal palpation.

POSSIBLE COMPLICATIONS AND COMMON ERRORS TO BE AVOIDED
The most common complication is a rectal tear. With experience, good glove lubrication, and proper restraint, the risk is minimal.

PROCEDURE
Endometrial edema in mares with a normal healthy uterus should increase progressively and, after reaching its maximal point, start to dissipate as the mare approaches ovulation. No uterine edema should be present during diestrus. A subjective scoring system ranging from 0 (no edema) to 5 is used to determine the degree of endometrial edema of the mare during the estrus cycle. All endometrial edema scores are determined by evaluating a cross-section of the uterine horn ipsilateral to the ovary that has the dominant follicle.
- **Grade 0** (UE0): A uterus with no edema is characterized by a homogenous echotexture and the presence of an active corpus luteum (Figure 1).
- **Grade 1** (UE1): A mare that is just starting to come in heat is characterized by a moderately soft cervix at palpation and the presence of a 25 to 35 mm follicle depending on breed

and size of the mare. However, UE1 can also be present on a mare that is very close to ovulation. The presence of a large softening follicle with uterine folds of a uterus with UE1 can be difficult to identify; unless there is a record of a previous examination, it could be undetectable. However, the difference in echotexture with UE0 is noticeable but no individual folds are identifiable (Figure 2).
- **Grade 2** (UE2): As shown in Figure 3, *A,* this demarcates the first real sign of uterine edema in the mare and most often is detected at the cervix and visualized ultrasonographically as a fish-bone appearance (Figure 3, *B*). Follicles can be 35 mm or longer, and often you can easily identify some of the endometrial folds on ultrasonography. UE2 can also be present as the mare approaches ovulation with a follicle greater than 40 mm in diameter and a very soft cervix.
- **Grade 3** (UE3): Grade 3 edema is easily identifiable and a "cartwheel" pattern is observable (Figure 4). The echotexture of the uterus is completely heterogenous. The folds are identifiable individually and are slightly thicker at the base compared with the image of the grade 2 folds. Follicles are 38 to 40 mm or longer, and the endometrial folds can easily be observed throughout the uterus. Mares with UE3 are good candidates for treatment with ovulation-inducing agents, with ovulation occurring between 36 and 48 hours after treatment.

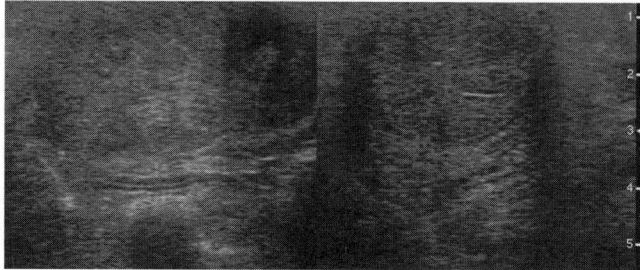

FIGURE 1   Grade 0 uterine edema.

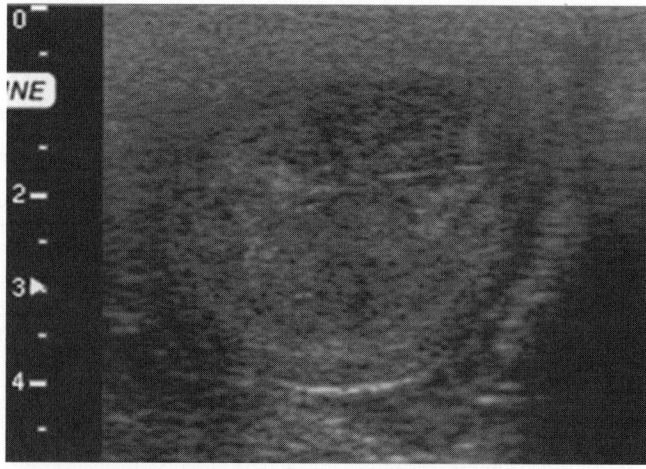

FIGURE 2   Grade 1 uterine edema.

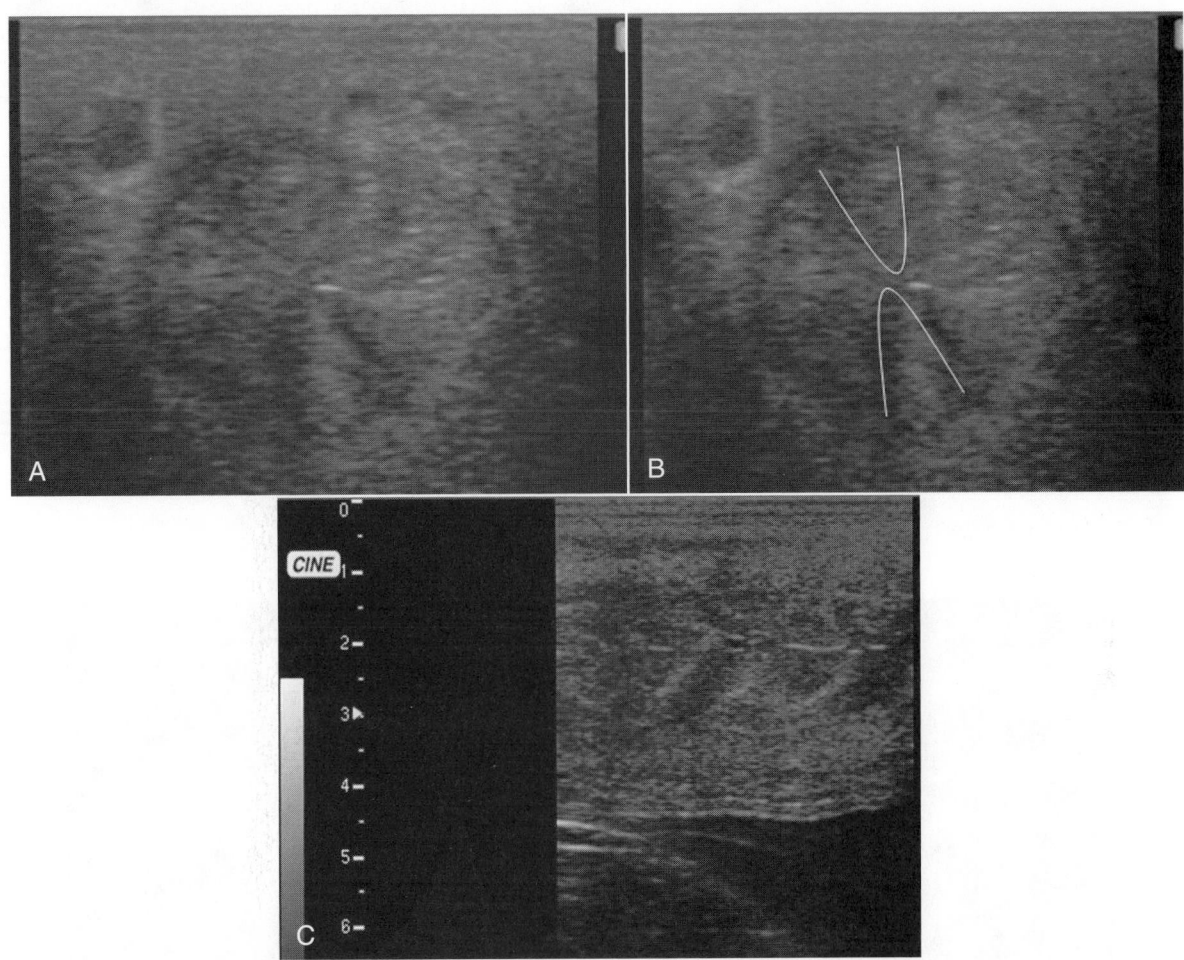

FIGURE 3 Grade 2 uterine edema.

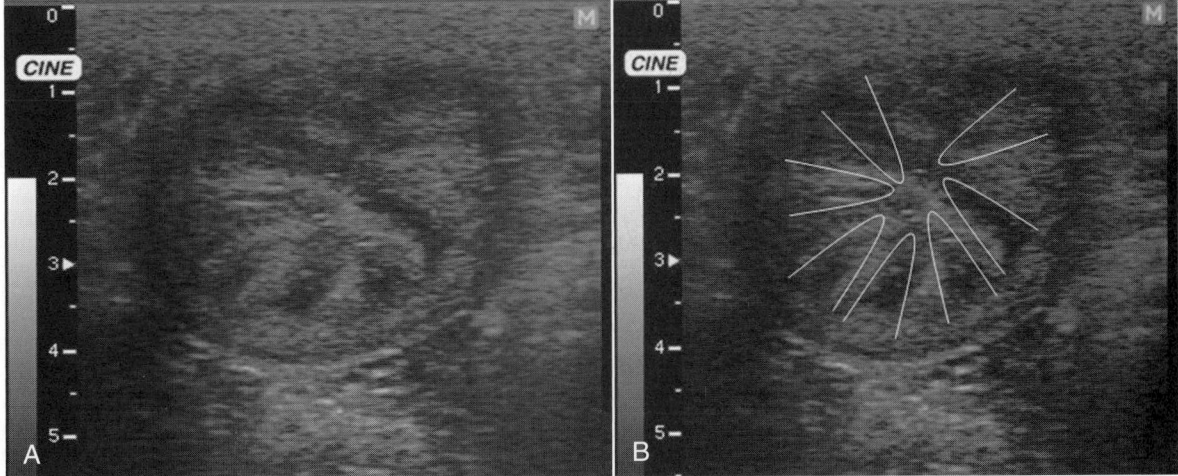

FIGURE 4 Grade 3 uterine edema.

- **Grade 4** (UE4): This is the maximal grade of edema considered normal with the presence of a hard 40 mm or longer dominant follicle. The folds are thickened and possibly hyperplastic, resulting in a typical increase of the width of the endometrial folds. Ultrasonographically, the folds have hyperechoic borders and a hypoechoic center. However, the ultrasonographic uterine architecture of the cartwheel is still maintained (Figure 5).

- **Grade 5** (UE-5): As shown in Figure 6, this type of edema has several characteristics:
  - Abnormally thick endometrial folds, making the uterus lose the normal architecture of the cartwheel pattern—hence the term *hyperedema*.
  - Folds are very thick with bright borders and mottled centers.
  - Often there is the presence of detectable amount of uterine fluid in the body or in the cervical lumen. However, due to the increase in surface area of the uterus, fluid can

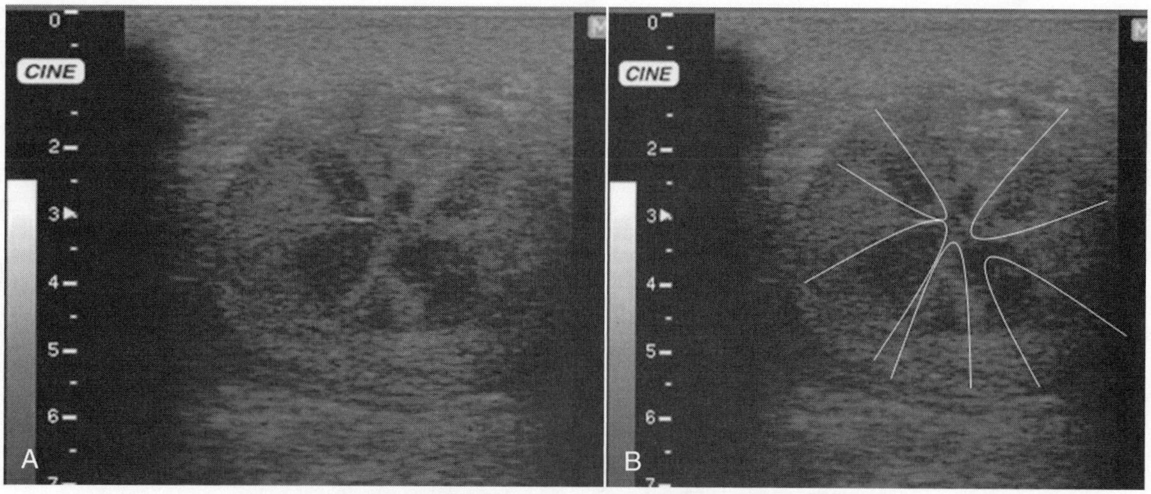

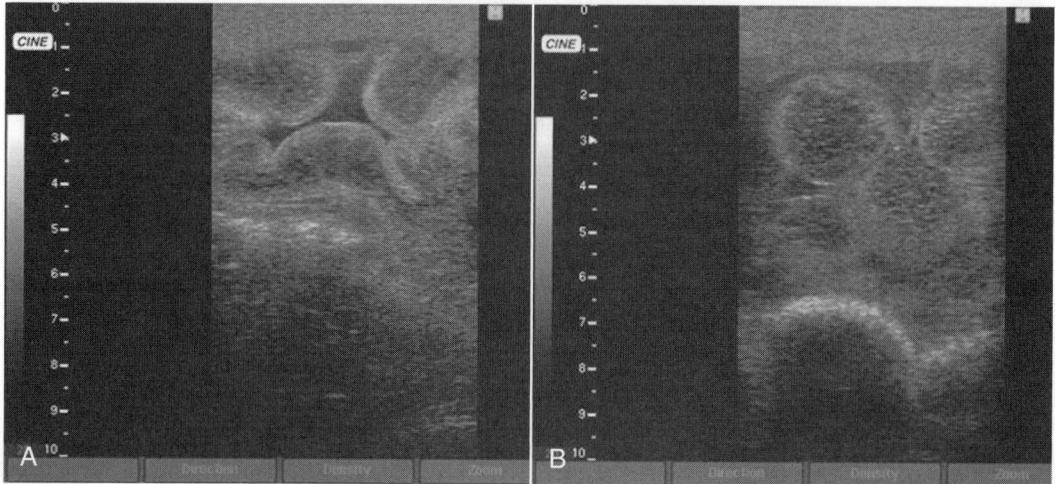

FIGURE 5 Grade 4 uterine edema.

FIGURE 6 Grade 5 uterine edema.

often be dissipated between the folds and not be detected. Treatment with dexamethasone helps reduce the degree of endometrial edema.

POSTPROCEDURE

Pregnancy rates per cycle are 14% higher for mares that have uterine edema grades of 1, 2, or 3 at 6 to 48 hours after breeding compared with mares that have edema scores of 4 or 5. The presence of uterine fluid at the time of ovulation is significantly lower for mares with edema grades 1 and 2 at 6 to 48 hours after breeding compared with mares ovulating with edema grades of 3, 4, or 5. Most mares with hyperedema have a positive culture and/or cytology, and their seasonal and per-cycle pregnancy rates are lower.

ALTERNATIVES AND THEIR RELATIVE MERITS

Interpretation of endometrial edema requires a good-quality ultrasound and evaluation of the mare on a regular basis during late diestrus and estrus until ovulation is detected. If used critically and consistently, the pattern of uterine edema can aid the practitioner in determining uterine health and guide the veterinarian for possible diagnostic or therapeutic procedures that may help increase the fertility of mares. Following the pattern of endometrial edema is a key tool to help veterinarians manage mares reproductively and can help detect pregnancy in a given breeding cycle. Endometrial edema cannot be assessed accurately by rectal palpation.

AUTHOR: **JUAN C. SAMPER**

Urinalysis

BASIC INFORMATION

OVERVIEW AND GOAL(S)

Urinalysis usually involves examination of urinary sediment and determination of urine contents with a commercially available dipstick.

INDICATIONS

Suspected urinary tract disease

EQUIPMENT, ANESTHESIA

- Urine dipstick
- Centrifuge tube
- Centrifuge
- Microscope
- Slides

ANTICIPATED TIME

30 minutes

PREPARATION: IMPORANT CHECKPOINTS

Urinalysis should be performed as soon as possible because the normally alkaline urine of horses may dissolve some casts.

POSSIBLE COMPLICATIONS AND COMMON ERRORS TO BE AVOIDED

- Dipstick analysis in horses is only accurate for pH, glucose, protein (except in alkaline urine), pigment, and bilirubin. Dipsticks should not be used to assess specific gravity or presence of white blood cells. Ketones are rarely detected in equine urine.
- pH: Equine urine is normally alkaline (7.0–9.0). Vigorous exercise or bacteriuria can lead to acidic urine. Bacteria can break down urea with urease and produce ammonia, which has a characteristic odor. Feeding concentrates decreases urine pH toward neutral. Foals with dilute urine have a neutral pH that is free of crystals. Aciduria is typically attributed to metabolic acidosis. Dehydrated or anorectic horses may have aciduria. Patients with hypochloremic metabolic alkalosis may have paradoxic aciduria due to an underlying hypokalemia or whole-body potassium deficit.
- Proteinuria: Urine reagent strips can give false-positive results for protein when testing alkaline urine. Proteinuria is assessed more accurately by a chemistry analyzer (<100 mg/dL

protein is normal). Measurement of urine protein/creatinine ratio (UP/UCr) is recommended to remove the effects of urine concentration. A ratio greater than 2:1 suggests proteinuria, which may be due to exercise, glomerular disease, bacteriuria, or pyuria. Protein-losing glomerulopathies lead to a loss of albumin rather than globulins. Severe chronic renal disease can result in hypoproteinemia and hypoalbuminemia, but this is very rare in horses compared with other species. Hyperglobulinemia consistent with chronic inflammatory response is more common in inflammatory or infectious renal disease.

- The renal threshold for glucose is approximately 160 to 180 mg/dL. Hyperglycemia (150–175 mg/dL) occurs secondary to stress, sepsis, exercise, pituitary adenoma, or diabetes mellitus and can result in glucosuria. Glucosuria can occur after administration of α_2 agonists, exogenous corticosteroid therapy, or glucose-containing fluids and parenteral nutrition. If glucosuria exists without hyperglycemia, suspect primary tubule dysfunction (Fanconi syndrome).
- Pigmenturia or blood on reagent strips reflects hemoglobin, myoglobin, or erythrocytes. To differentiate, assess plasma for hemolysis, muscle enzyme activity to distinguish myoglobinuria from hematuria or hemoglobinuria, and urine sediment for the presence of erythrocytes. Fewer than five erythrocytes should be seen per high power field (hpf). Hematuria can be due to inflammation, infection, neoplasia, toxemia, or intense exercise.
- Bilirubinuria is associated with intravascular hemolysis, hepatic necrosis, and obstructive hepatopathies. Hemolysis and hepatic disease are detected by abnormally elevated serum bilirubin concentrations, and increased hepatic enzyme activity is present with liver disease.
- Casts consist of sloughed tubular cells and Tamm-Horsfall glycoprotein. Presence of casts indicates tubular damage, inflammation, or infection.
- More than 10 leukocytes/hpf is associated with infectious or inflammatory disease. Normal equine urine has few to no bacteria, but the absence of bacteria does not rule out infection.

- Equine urine is normally rich in crystals; the majority are calcium carbonate. Calcium phosphate and occasionally calcium oxalate crystals are also found.
- Urine specific gravity measures urine concentration but is determined more accurately by urine osmolality because large molecules such as glucose and protein lead to overestimation of urine concentration using specific gravity.
  - Normal horses have urine specific gravity of 1.025 to 1.050 and urine osmolality of 900 to 1200 mOsm/kg (three to four times more than serum).
  - Hyposthenuria: Urine is more dilute than serum; specific gravity is less than 1.008 and osmolality is less than 260 mOsm/kg.
  - Isosthenuria: Urine and serum are of similar osmolality; specific gravity is 1.008 to 1.014 and osmolality is 260 to 300 mOsm/kg.
  - Hypersthenuria: Urine is more concentrated than serum; specific gravity is greater than 1.014 and osmolality is greater than 300 mOsm/kg.
  - Foals usually have hyposthenuric urine as a consequence of the large volume of water in their milk diet. With dehydration, foals can have a concentration of 1.030.
  - Chronic renal failure typically manifests with isosthenuria and inability to concentrate (specific gravity >1.025) or dilute (specific gravity <1.008) urine.

PROCEDURE

DIPSTICK URINALYSIS

- Pipette urine onto reagent strips and read results as directed by the manufacturer's label.

SEDIMENT EXAMINATION

- Centrifuge 10 mL of urine at 1000 rpm for 3 to 5 minutes, discard the supernatant, resuspend the pellet in a few drops of urine, and then transfer onto a glass slide.
- Urine sediment should be evaluated within 30 to 60 minutes of collection.
- Evaluate sediment for casts, erythrocytes, leukocytes, epithelial cells, and bacteria.

AUTHOR: **ALLISON J. STEWART**

Urinary Catheterization

BASIC INFORMATION

OVERVIEW AND GOAL(S)

Urinary catheters can be placed to collect a sterile urine sample or to drain or lavage the bladder.

INDICATIONS

- Whenever a sterile sample of urine is needed
- Bladder paralysis
- To reduce bladder pressure postoperatively and allow healing of bladder incisions
- To allow urine flow and collection in recumbent or debilitated patients

EQUIPMENT, ANESTHESIA

- Sterile stallion catheter (males), mare catheter, or large-diameter Foley catheter (females)
- Sterile lube
- Sterile gloves
- Scrub for aseptic preparation of the penis or vulva
- Sedation (often unnecessary for females)

ANTICIPATED TIME

15 minutes

PREPARATION: IMPORTANT CHECKPOINTS

Sedation with α_2 agonist drugs (xylazine, detomidine) will decrease urine specific gravity; therefore urine should be collected as soon as possible after sedation for urinalysis.

POSSIBLE COMPLICATIONS AND COMMON ERRORS TO BE AVOIDED

- Breaks in aseptic technique or improper sterilization of equipment may cause iatrogenic urinary tract infections.
- Closed urine collection systems are difficult to maintain in nonrecumbent patients.

PROCEDURE

- Males
  - The penis, internal preputial laminae, and urethral fossa are cleaned of debris and aseptically scrubbed. The use of antiseptic soaps should be avoided on stallions to prevent disruption of the normal preputial flora.
  - Sterile gloves and sterile lube should be used when passing the urinary catheter into the urethral orifice.
  - When the urinary catheter passes the ischial arch, the male horse will raise its tail (flags).
  - Air can usually be heard entering the bladder when the catheter enters, due to negative pressure.
  - Urine can be suctioned using a catheter-tipped syringe if it does not flow freely.
- Females
  - The tail is wrapped and tied off of the perineum.
  - The vulva and perineum are cleaned of debris and aseptically scrubbed.
  - Sterile gloves and sterile lube should be used when passing the urinary catheter through the vulva and into the urethral orifice.
  - The urethral orifice is located as a definite protrusion, ventrally on the floor of the vagina about 10 cm cranial to the vulva.
  - A finger is introduced into the urethral orifice and the urinary catheter is then inserted alongside the finger. The urethral orifice in mares is large and can easily dilate.
  - Otherwise, similar as described for male horses.
- Indwelling urinary catheters
  - Urinary catheters are passed as described above.
  - The balloon should be filled with sterile saline, which will add weight to the end of the catheter, help maintain its position in the bladder, and better prevent catheter dislodgement.
  - A tape butterfly can be placed distally and sutured into place to prevent catheter displacement.
  - If desired, many commonly used tubing and attachments can be fitted to make a closed urine collection system that drains into recycled intravenous fluid bags (Figure 1). This allows for accurate measurement of urine production and prevents urine scald in recumbent patients.
- Be certain that all scrub has been rinsed from the external urinary tract, perineum, or vulva to avoid local irritation.
- Observe for any signs of urinary tract infection for several days.
- Antibiotics are rarely necessary, except for indwelling urinary catheters or if urinary tract infection was suspected before catheterization.

ALTERNATIVES AND THEIR RELATIVE MERITS

Although cystocentesis is possible in foals, it is very rarely attempted due to the risk of enterocentesis.

AUTHOR: **BRYAN M. WALDRIDGE**

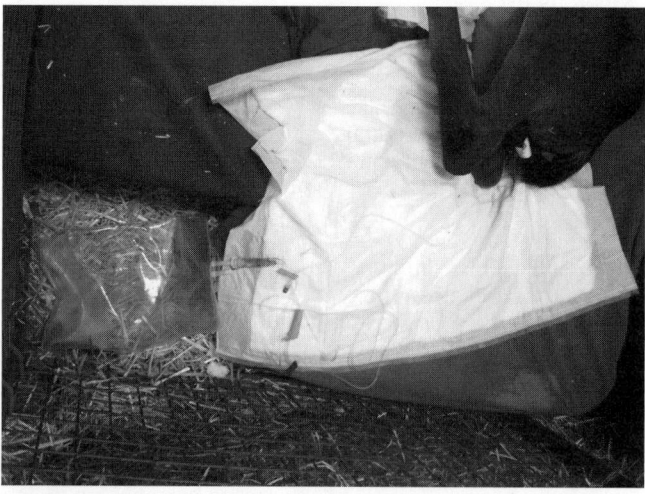

FIGURE 1 An indwelling urinary catheter and closed urine collection system made of a drip set and empty intravenous fluid bag in a recumbent foal.

Urinary Fractional Excretion of Electrolytes

BASIC INFORMATION

SYNONYM(S)

Fractional excretion, fractional clearance

OVERVIEW AND GOAL(S)

- Electrolyte losses, which reflect tubular function, can be expressed as excretion rates (amount of electrolytes excreted during a given period [mEq/min]) and require timed urine collections (typically a 24-hour collection).
- Fractional excretion (FE) can be used to determine electrolyte loss in urine by using simultaneously collected samples of urine and serum. By expressing the clearance of an electrolyte as a fraction of creatinine clearance, timed urine collections are not required.
- Equine kidneys conserve more than 99% of filtered sodium and chloride ions, whereas potassium is only conserved when whole-body depletion (anorexia, prolonged exercise) is present.
- FE of sodium helps differentiate prerenal azotemia and intrinsic renal failure. Tubular capacity to reabsorb sodium is decreased in renal failure, resulting in urinary sodium wasting:

    Urine/serum creatinine ratio >50:1

      and FE Na <1%

      = Prerenal azotemia

    Urine/serum creatinine ratio <37:1

      and FE Na >0.8%

      = Primary renal disease

INDICATIONS

- Excessive dietary phosphorus intake increases the FE of phosphorus, and inadequate calcium intake decreases the FE of calcium. Increased FE of phosphorus and decreased FE of calcium can indicate nutritional imbalances that lead to developmental orthopedic diseases or nutritional secondary hyperparathyroidism. For accurate assessment of urine calcium concentration, acetic acid should be added to urine to dissolve calcium carbonate crystals prior to measurement of calcium.
- Decreased FE of potassium indicates potassium deficiency and is more indicative of whole-body potassium status than are serum potassium concentrations.
- Hyponatremia and hypochloremia are common in renal disease due to impaired tubular resorption of sodium and chloride. Increased FE of sodium and phosphorus can be signs of early renal tubular damage.
- Abnormal FE of electrolytes with renal disease usually indicates impaired tubular secretion or resorption of electrolytes and decreased renal ability to maintain homeostasis.
- Low FE shows the need for electrolyte supplementation in athletes.

EQUIPMENT, ANESTHESIA

Serum chemistry machine

ANTICIPATED TIME

30 to 60 minutes

PREPARATION: IMPORANT CHECKPOINTS

Serum and urine should be collected at approximately the same time and electrolyte and creatinine concentrations are measured in both the serum and urine samples.

POSSIBLE COMPLICATIONS AND COMMON ERRORS TO BE AVOIDED

- Increases of FE of sodium and chloride can occur as a response to excess dietary salt or psychogenic salt consumption.
- Determine FE prior to fluid therapy because FE can be artifactually increased in horses receiving intravenous fluids.
- Medications (furosemide) and light exercise increase urine flow and FE of sodium and chloride.

PROCEDURE

- FE of electrolyte A is compared with clearance of creatinine using the following formula:

$$Cl_A/Cl_{Cr} = (Serum_{Cr}/Urine_{Cr} \times Urine_A/Serum_A) \times 100$$

- Reference ranges for fractional clearance:
  - Sodium: <1%
  - Potassium: 15% to 65%
  - Chloride: 0.04% to 1.6%
  - Phosphorus: <0.5%

AUTHOR: **ALLISON J. STEWART**

Urinary Tract Disease: Clinical Pathology

BASIC INFORMATION

OVERVIEW AND GOAL

An inflammatory or infectious disease process may result in an elevated leukocyte count, neutrophilia, hyperglobulinemia, hyperfibrinogenemia, low serum iron concentration, and mild anemia secondary to inflammation or decreased erythropoietin.

INDICATIONS

- Suspected renal failure or infectious disease of the urinary tract

- To monitor for renal compromise in patients at risk for dehydration and/or receiving potentially nephrotoxic drugs

EQUIPMENT, ANESTHESIA

- Needles, syringes, appropriate blood tubes
- Serum chemistry analyzer
- Hematology analyzer

ANTICIPATED TIME

15 to 60 minutes

POSSIBLE COMPLICATIONS AND COMMON ERRORS TO BE AVOIDED

- Mild anemia can occur in chronic renal failure secondary to decreased erythropoietin and shortened erythrocyte lifespan.
- Blood urea nitrogen (BUN) and serum creatinine (Cr) are used as indexes for renal function, especially as estimators of glomerular filtration rate (GFR). However, BUN and Cr increase only when approximately 75% of the nephrons are nonfunctional. BUN and Cr are insensitive indicators of minor

changes of GFR, but once elevated they provide sensitive indicators of further deterioration. Azotemia is increased BUN and/or Cr concentrations in the serum.
- Prerenal: Decreased renal perfusion (hypovolemia, dehydration); BUN and Cr elevations generally mild to moderate.
- Renal: Primary renal disease with moderate elevations in BUN and/or Cr concentrations.
- Postrenal: Obstructive urinary disease or disruption of the urinary tract (ruptured bladder, urolithiasis). Marked elevations in BUN and Cr concentrations can occur.
- BUN/Cr ratio: Higher for prerenal azotemia (increased reabsorption of urea with low renal tubule flow rates) and postrenal azotemia (diffusion of urea across peritoneal membranes). The BUN/Cr ratio is lower with intrinsic renal failure. However, there is a large overlap between animals with prerenal and renal azotemia; therefore this ratio can only be used as a guide.

- The BUN/Cr ratio is more useful to distinguish acute from chronic renal failure:
  - Acute: BUN/Cr ratio usually <10:1
  - Chronic: BUN/Cr ratio usually >10:1
- Prerenal failure is often accompanied by altered glomerular and tubular function resulting in proteinuria and cast formation, impaired concentrating ability, and changes in electrolyte excretion due to a combination of renal and prerenal azotemia. Renal damage is usually reversible, but permanent damage of nephrons is possible.
- Urine specific gravity and osmolality: Elevations in BUN and Cr concentrations should prompt assessment of urine concentrating ability. Determination of urine specific gravity by refractometer is easily performed, but measurement of urine osmolality is more accurate. Measurements are only valid if made before fluid therapy and treatments that can affect urine outflow and concentration (α_2 agonists,

furosemide). With prerenal azotemia, urinary concentrating ability is maintained, urine specific gravity is greater than 1.020, and urine osmolality is greater than 500 mOsm/kg. With intrinsic renal failure, urinary concentrating ability is lost in the face of dehydration, urine specific gravity is less than 1.020, and urine osmolality is less tan 500 mOsm/kg.
- Electrolytes: Hyponatremia and hypochloremia are common in renal disease due to impaired tubular reabsorption of sodium and chloride. Serum potassium concentrations can be normal to elevated in acute or chronic renal failure. Hyperkalemia frequently occurs with urinary tract disruption or uroperitoneum. Serum calcium and phosphorus concentrations vary in renal disease. Hypercalcemia and hypophosphatemia are common in chronic renal disease, especially when horses are fed alfalfa hay. Hypocalcemia and hyperphosphatemia are more common in acute renal disease.

AUTHOR: **ALLISON J. STEWART**

Urine Culture

BASIC INFORMATION

OVERVIEW AND GOAL

Quantitative culture of urine confirms urinary tract infection and allows selection of effective antibiotic therapy.

INDICATIONS

Suspected urinary tract infection

EQUIPMENT, ANESTHESIA

- Sterile urine specimen cup
- Microbiology laboratory

ANTICIPATED TIME

2 to 3 days for full culture and sensitivity results

PREPARATION: IMPORANT CHECKPOINTS

Ensure aseptic technique and preparation of the external urinary tract to reduce the possibility of bacterial contamination.

POSSIBLE COMPLICATIONS AND COMMON ERRORS TO BE AVOIDED

- Collection of urine via an endoscope often yields multiple resistant *Pseudomonas* spp., which are common contaminants.
- Contamination of urine samples is common with free-catch or catheterization techniques, and a definitive diagnosis of infection requires a quantitative culture with growth of more than 10,000 colony-forming units

(CFUs) per milliliter and concurrent evidence of pyuria based on a urine sediment examination.
- Foals receiving antibiotics may occasionally develop fungal (*Candida albicans*) urinary tract infections.

PROCEDURE

- Collect urine with a sterile Foley catheter in mares or a stallion catheter in male horses. Cystocentesis can be performed in neonates. Although less than ideal, a free-catch midstream urine sample can be used.
- Submit urine samples for urinalysis (including sediment examination) and bacterial and/or fungal culture.

AUTHOR: **ALLISON J. STEWART**

Venous Catheterization: Alternate Sites

BASIC INFORMATION

SYNONYM(S)

Lateral thoracic vein catheterization
Cephalic vein catheterization
Saphenous vein catheterization

OVERVIEW AND GOAL(S)

Placement of a catheter in alternate vessels including the saphenous, cephalic, and lateral thoracic veins

INDICATIONS

For administration of intravenous fluids and medications when jugular catheterization is not possible

CONTRAINDICATIONS

- Cellulitis in surrounding tissues
- Phlebitis of the vein to be catheterized
- Saphenous veins are not safely accessible in most adults

EQUIPMENT, ANESTHESIA

- Clippers
- Sterile prep
- Exam gloves for scrub preparation
- Sterile gloves
- 2- to 3-mL lidocaine with a 25-gauge needle attached
- Catheter/extension set/catheter injection cap
- Heparinized saline
- Suture (2-0, polypropylene)
- White tape
- Scissors
- Bandage material depending on placement

ANTICIPATED TIME

Approximately 15 minutes, including scrub

PREPARATION: IMPORTANT CHECKPOINTS

- If catheterizing the lateral thoracic vein, ultrasound-guided identification of the cranial and caudal direction the vein is coursing under the skin assists in catheterization.
- Landmarks can be marked with a permanent marker on the skin outside the prepped area.

POSSIBLE COMPLICATIONS AND COMMON ERRORS TO BE AVOIDED

Avoid large volumes of subcutaneous block, which can compress the vein or shift it deeper.

PROCEDURE

- Restrain the horse with sedation, or a twitch.
  - For foals, restrain with light sedation in lateral recumbency.
- Clip, sterile prep and block the catheter site, and apply a final prep.
  - For adult horses, perform a stab incision at the site of entry by pulling the skin away from the vein, so that the vein is not disrupted.
- Catheter placement with a Seldinger (guidewire) technique:
  - Insert the trocar or stylet from the same size catheter into the vein.
  - Pass the guidewire through the stylet until the majority lies in the vein.
  - Hold the end of the wire and withdraw the stylet, leaving the wire in the vein.
  - Do not let go of the wire at any time.
  - Thread the catheter over the wire until the wire exits the injection port.
  - Grasp the wire and seat the catheter hub flush with the skin.
  - Remove guidewire, flush catheter with heparinized saline, and suture the catheter in place.
  - Bandage the limb if a cephalic or saphenous vein was used.

POSTPROCEDURE

- Monitor catheter closely for phlebitis (heat, swelling, or discharge at the insertion site).
- Flush four to six times daily with heparinized saline.

ALTERNATIVES AND THEIR RELATIVE MERITS

- Lateral thoracic catheterization:
  - Advantages:
    - Less morbidity than jugular vein catheters
    - Less prone to kinking and dislodgement
  - Disadvantages:
    - Placement is more difficult than in a jugular vein (caudal to cranial)
  - Guidelines:
    - A guidewire is recommended to aid in placement and for long-term catheterization.
    - A 14- or 16-gauge, 5- to 8-inch silicone or polyurethane catheter is recommended.
    - The typical lifespan of catheters in this vessel can be longer than 14 days.
- Cephalic vein catheterization:
  - Advantages:
    - Few
  - Disadvantages:
    - Catheters are easy to dislodge, therefore bandaging is recommended.
    - Horses may chew at these catheters or their bandage.
  - Guidelines:
    - The vessel is highly mobile and difficult to catheterize.
    - A 16-gauge, 3-inch catheter is recommended.
    - The typical lifespan of catheters in this vessel is 5 to 7 days.
- Saphenous vein catheterization:
  - Advantages:
    - Few
  - Disadvantages:
    - Catheters are easy to dislodge.
    - Recommended only in foals.
  - Guidelines:
    - This vessel is highly mobile.
    - A 16-gauge, 3-inch catheter is recommended.
    - The typical lifespan of catheters in this vessel is 5 to 7 days.

AUTHOR: **AMELIA MUNSTERMAN**

Wound Closure and Healing

BASIC INFORMATION

INDICATIONS

- **Primary closure** performed within several hours of injury is appropriate for fresh, minimally contaminated wounds, with a good blood supply, not involving vital structures; wounds of the head region; flap wounds with a good blood supply; and wounds of the upper body when a good cosmetic outcome is desired.
- **Delayed primary closure** performed before granulation tissue formation is appropriate for severely contaminated, contused, or swollen wounds and those that involve a synovial structure.
- **Secondary closure** performed after granulation tissue formation is used for chronic wounds with a compromised blood supply. The wound is sutured after a healthy bed of granulation tissue develops.
- **Second intention healing** allows a wound to close by wound contraction and epithelialization and relied upon for large wounds with a tissue deficit involving the body and for highly mobile areas such as the pectoral and gluteal regions.
- **Skin grafting** is used when tissue deficits exceed the capability of wound contraction and epithelialization.
- **Reconstructive surgery** is used to improve the cosmetic and functional outcome of a wound.

PROCEDURE

- Local anesthetics
  - Effects
    - Intralesional injection of 2% concentrations inhibits collagen synthesis and formation of granulation tissue. Epinephrine exacerbates this effect via vasoconstriction.
    - Lidocaine reduces the effects of oxygen radicals, leukocyte migration, and inflammation.
    - Intralesional injection of 0.5% lidocaine has no significant effect on wound healing.
  - What to do:
    - Regional is best.
    - Intralesional; <2% solutions are acceptable.
    - Avoid epinephrine.
- Suturing techniques and suture material

This monograph is adapted from Orsini JA, Divers TJ, editors: Equine emergencies: treatment and procedures, ed 3, St Louis, 2008, Saunders Elsevier.

- Suturing technique and material influence wound healing.
  - Synthetic monofilament sutures are superior; less reactive, stronger and if absorbable, degrade at a constant rate.
- Simple interrupted (SI) when compared to simple continuous sutured skin wounds exhibit:
  - Less edema
  - Increased microcirculation
  - 30% to 50% greater tensile strength after 10 days
  - In horses, SI sutured linea alba compared to continuous sutured linea alba show:
    - No difference in bursting strength at 0 and 21 days
    - Greater bursting strength at 5 to 10 days
  - SI sutures cause less inflammation than vertical mattress and far-near-near-far patterns.
  - What to do: Use interrupted sutures where impaired healing is anticipated and excessive tension is present.
- Suturing technique:
  - Loosely approximated wounds are stronger at 7, 10, and 21 days postoperatively than wounds tightly closed with sutures.
  - What to do:
    - Appose wound edges anatomically. Avoid overreduction of tissues.
    - Use the least number of sutures. Increased number of sutures results in increased infection rates.
    - Deep suture only fascial planes, tendons, and ligaments
- Tension sutures
  - Used to reduce tension on the primary suture line.
  - Widely placed vertical mattress sutures with or without supports, using buttons, gauze, or rubber tubing, are effective in reducing tension on the primary suture line.
  - Sutures with supports are used in areas that cannot be effectively bandaged (eg, upper body and neck regions).
  - Sutures without supports are used in areas that are bandaged or to which a cast is applied.
  - Tension sutures are removed in 4 to 10 days, depending on the appearance of the wound; staggered removal is preferred.
- Hematoma and seroma
  - Hematoma formation is considered a leading factor in decreasing local wound resistance to infection.

- Mechanical separation of wound edges, thereby delaying healing
  - Fluid pressure can alter blood supply.
  - Excellent media for bacterial growth
  - Hemoglobin inhibits local tissue defenses; iron necessary for bacterial replication and virulence.
- Drains
  - Used when a large dead space remains after suture closure.
  - Must be maintained in a sterile environment.
    - Use sterile bandage for extremities.
    - Use sterile stent bandage for upper body.
  - Should be buried and sutured dorsally/proximally and:
    - Traverse a wound that is parallel to the limb's long axis, adjacent to but not directly underlying the sutured skin edges and exit adjacent to the distal extremity of the wound or
    - Cross underneath sutured transverse wound edges and exit either ventrally or distally or
    - Be placed underneath a skin flap
  - Should exit from a separate incision adjacent to the wound edge and be sutured. This reduces the risk of retrograde infection directly involving the suture line.
  - Usually left in place for 24 to 48 hours but may remain longer if drainage persists.
  - NOTE: Drains are a two-way street and meticulous postoperative care of the drain exit site is essential to decrease the risk of infection.
  - Although the use of drains is somewhat controversial because they represent a foreign body within the wound, if drainage of a hematoma from "dead space" is needed, the consequences of not using a drain are considerably more serious than the potential complications that may arise from the drain.

SUGGESTED READING

Céleste C, Stashak TS: Selection of suture materials, suture patterns and drains for wound closure. In Stashak TS, Theoret CL, editors: *Equine Wound Management*, ed 2, Ames, IA, 2008, Wiley-Blackwell Publishing, pp 193–224.

Rodeheaver GT: Wound cleaning, wound irrigation, wound disinfection. In Krasner D, Rodeheaver G, Sibbald G, editors: *Chronic Wound Care*, ed 3, Wayne, PA, 2001, HMP Communications, pp 389–393.

Stashak TS: Selection of approaches to wound closure. In Stashak TS, Theoret CL, editors:

Equine Wound Management, ed 2, Ames, IA, 2008, Wiley-Blackwell Publishing, pp 177–192.

Theoret CL: Physiology of wound healing. In Stashak TS, Theoret CL, editors: *Equine*

Wound Management, ed 2, Ames, IA, 2008, Wiley-Blackwell Publishing, pp 5–28.

Wilson DA: New and innovative approaches to wound closure. In Stashak TS, Theoret CL, editors: *Equine Wound Management*,

ed 2, Ames, IA, 2008, Wiley-Blackwell Publishing, pp 225–238.

AUTHORS: **CHRISTINE THÉORÊT** and **TED STASHAK**

EDITOR: **DAVID A. WILSON**

Wound Dressing

BASIC INFORMATION

OVERVIEW AND GOAL(S)

- Wound dressings
- >300 wound dressings available, ranging from passive adherent/nonadherent to interactive and bioactive products that contribute to healing
- Most newer dressings are designed to favor "moist wound healing," which allows wound fluids and mediators to remain in contact with the wound therefore promoting "autolytic debridement" and subsequently accelerating wound healing.
- No single material can produce the optimal microenvironment for all wounds or for all the stages of the healing process.
- Wound dressings are broadly classified as either adherent or nonadherent and as absorbent or nonabsorbent.
  - Adherent dressings are frequently made from gauze, and are mostly passive. Gauze dressings are highly absorbent and are used for heavily contaminated, exudative wounds.
  - Nonadherent dressings have variable absorbency and are subdivided into occlusive, semiocclusive, and biologic types.

This monograph is adapted from Orini JA, Divers TJ, editors: Equine emergencies: treatment and procedures, ed 3, St Louis, 2008, Saunders Elsevier.

INDICATIONS

- Protection of wounds from further contamination
- Reduction of edema via exerted pressure
- Absorption of exudate
- Increased temperature and reduced CO_2 loss from the wound surface, thus reducing pH
- Immobilization and prevention of additional trauma (eg, wound at dorsal surface of hock)
- Bandaged distal extremity wounds heal 30% faster than do nonbandaged wounds.

POSSIBLE COMPLICATIONS AND COMMON ERRORS TO BE AVOIDED

Exuberant granulation tissue may develop in bandaged wounds of the distal extremities.

PROCEDURE

- Selection of a wound dressing for the treatment of wounds destined to heal by second intention or to be treated by delayed closure is important to the outcome.
- Clean acute wounds are best dressed with an occlusive dressing until a healthy bed of granulation tissue develops.
- During the transition from acute inflammation to fibroplasia, alginate dressings are recommended. These

dressings can also be used to kick-start healing of chronic wounds.
- Once granulation tissue develops, a semiocclusive dressing is recommended.
- Heavily contaminated or infected wounds are best treated with adherent dressings, particulate dextranomers, or antimicrobial dressings until a healthy bed of granulation tissue develops, after which a semiocclusive dressing is selected for the repair phase.
- Although reports on biologic, bioactive dressings are limited and in some cases conflicting, these dressings represent an important category that will undoubtedly generate more use in the future.

SUGGESTED READING

Gomez JH, Hanson RR: Use of dressings and bandages in equine wound management. *Vet Clin North Am Equine Pract* 21:91–104, 2005.

Gomez J, Stashak TS: Bandaging and casting techniques for wound management. In Stashak TS, Theoret CL, editors: *Equine Wound Management*, ed 2, Ames, IA, 2008, Wiley-Blackwell Publishing, pp 623–658.

Stashak TS, Farstvedt E: Update on wound dressings: Indications and best use. In Stashak TS, Theoret CL, editors: *Equine Wound Management*, ed 2, Ames, IA, 2008, Wiley-Blackwell Publishing, pp 109–136.

AUTHORS: **CHRISTINE THÉORÊT** and **TED STASHAK**

EDITOR: **DAVID A. WILSON**

Wound Dressing: Absorbent Dressings

BASIC INFORMATION

PROCEDURE

ABSORBENT/ADHERENT AND NONADHERENT DRESSING (ADs)

- ADs are used during the inflammatory phase of healing to assist with debride-

This monograph is adapted from Orsini JA, Divers TJ, editors: Equine emergencies: treatment and procedures, ed 3, St Louis, 2008, Saunders Elsevier.

ment. Wide mesh gauze usually promotes better adherence and wound debridement. AD may be applied dry or wet.
  - Dry dressings are used if wound fluids have low viscosity.
  - Wet dressings are used when wound fluids have high viscosity or a scab has developed. Sterile saline is often used as the wetting agent with or without the addition of

soluble antiseptics, antibiotics, or enzymes.
  - Can be used for packing deep wounds.
  - Discontinued when a healthy bed of granulation tissue develops.
- Kerlix AMD (Tyco Healthcare Kendall, Mansfield, MA) is effective:
  - For debriding wounds
  - For reducing bacterial numbers on the wound surface. The antimicrobial dressing is impregnated with

0.2% polyhexamethylene biguanide, which has a broad antimicrobial spectrum and is effective against *Pseudomonas aeruginosa.*
- Large roll is ideal for packing deep wounds; packing is changed daily with progressively less gauze used to pack the wound.
- Curasalt (Tyco Healthcare Kendall, Mansfield, MA), a hypertonic 20% saline dressing, appears to provide effective osmotic nonselective wound debridement. Recommended for

infected, necrotic, heavily exuding wounds only. Applied once and removed the following day.
- Animalintex (3M Animal Care Products, St. Paul, MN) is discussed elsewhere under antimicrobial dressings.
- Gamgee (3M Animal Care Products, St. Paul, MN):
  - Used as a wound dressing while providing protection, support and insulation.
  - Highly absorbent, its proposed best use is for highly exudative limb

wounds during the inflammatory phase of healing.

SUGGESTED READING
Stashak TS, Farstvedt E: Update on wound dressings: indications and best use. In Stashak TS, Theoret CL, editors: *Equine Wound Management*, ed 2, Ames, IA, 2008, Wiley-Blackwell Publishing, pp 109–136.

AUTHORS: **CHRISTINE THÉORÊT** and **TED STASHAK**

Wound Dressing: Antimicrobial Dressings

BASIC INFORMATION

INDICATIONS

Bacterial colonization and infection remain predominant factors contributing to delayed wound healing. Because the widespread use of systemic and topical antibiotics has resulted in increasing numbers of resistant bacterial strains (methicillin-resistant *Staphylococcus aureus* and vancomycin-resistant *Enterococcus faecalis* and *Pseudomonas aeruginosa*), the judicious use of antimicrobial dressings (eg, Tyco Healthcare Kendall, Mansfield, MA), notably those containing certain antiseptics, can be important in infection control and in promoting healing.

PROCEDURE

- Iodine containing dressing
  - Iodosord (Smith & Nephew, Hull, UK) is manufactured from cross-linked polymerized dextran that contains iodine. As the dressing hydrates in the moist wound environment, elemental iodine is released to exert an antibacterial effect and to interact with macrophages to produce proinflammatory mediators that can indirectly influence wound healing.
    - Best use would be for contaminated wounds early in the inflammatory phase of repair.
  - Iodoflex (Smith & Nephew, Hull, UK), a slow-release iodine dressing, designed to maintain adequate local levels of active iodine for at least 48 hours. The slow release of povidone iodine (PI) in this product does not slow wound healing.

  - PI powder dressing (PRN Wound Dressing, PRN Pharmacal, Pensacola, FL) has 1% available iodine, a broad antimicrobial spectrum, and is also fungicidal.
  - Biozide Gel—Hydrogel containing 1% available PI complex in a polyglycol base (Performance Products Inc. [www.mwivet.com]). A theoretical advantage of this product is that even though it is an occlusive dressing it can be safely applied to a heavily contaminated or infected wound because of the antiseptic PI incorporated in the product.
  - No objective studies attesting to the effect of any of these products on wound healing in horses are presently available. One study documented that there was no delay in wound healing in horses treated with 10% PI ointment compared to another antimicrobial dressing.
- Antimicrobial gauze dressing (AMD) (Kerlix Antimicrobial Dressing, Tyco Healthcare Kendall, Mansfield, MA) (see "Wound Dressing: Absorbent Dressing" in this section).
- Poultice pad
  - Animalintex Poultice and Hoof pad (3M Animal Care Products, St. Paul, MN)
  - Made of nonwoven cotton with a plastic backing.
  - Contains boric acid (mild antiseptic) and Tragacanth, a natural poultice agent.
  - Pad is shaped to fit sole; can be applied hot, cold, or dry.
  - Proposed best use
    - Apply hot for infected hoof wounds (eg, abscesses, dirty wounds); can be used as a poultice for other regions of the body.
    - Apply cold for sprains and strains.
- Silver chloride-coated nylon dressing: (Ag-WD)
  - Silverlon Argentum, Lakemont, GA; Acticoat Antimicrobial Barrier,

dressing, Westaim Biomedical Corp, Ft. Saskatchewan, AB, Canada; Actisorb Silver 220, Johnson & Johnson Products Inc, New Brunswick, NJ, are available. The silver released from the dressing is bactericidal.
  - Silverlon shown effective in killing five common equine pathogens (in vitro); also antifungal. The dressing should be moistened before application and it should be changed every 3 to 4 days.
  - Best use is during the inflammatory to repair phase of wound healing.
- Activated charcoal dressing
  - Activate (3M Animal Care Products, St. Paul, MN, and Actisorb, Johnson & Johnson Products Inc, New Brunswick, NJ). One of the dressings, Activate, is packaged as a multilayered nonwoven nonadherent material.
  - Proposed advantages:
    - Provides a moist wound healing environment for autolytic debridement.
    - Effectively absorbs bacteria.
    - Prevents the formation of exuberant granulation tissue in horses.
    - Reduces wound odor.
  - Best use is for the heavily infected wound during the inflammatory phase to the repair phase. Good healing is anecdotally reported in a limited number of cases through the repair phase of wound healing.

SUGGESTED READING
Stashak TS, Farstvedt E: Update on wound dressings: indications and best use. In Stashak TS, Theoret CL, editors: *Equine Wound Management*, ed 2, Ames, IA, 2008, Wiley-Blackwell Publishing, pp 109–136.

AUTHORS: **CHRISTINE THÉORÊT** and **TED STASHAK**

EDITOR: **DAVID A. WILSON**

This monograph is adapted from Orsini JA, Divers TJ, editors: Equine emergencies: treatment and procedures, ed 3, St Louis, 2008, Saunders Elsevier.

Wound Dressing: Biologic Dressings

BASIC INFORMATION

PROCEDURE

- Equine amnion (EA): EA is believed to have most of the qualities of an ideal dressing. Despite its occlusive properties in the horse it did not encourage the formation of exuberant granulation tissue, but did result in more rapid wound healing when compared to a synthetic semiocclusive control dressing. Best used to suppress the formation of exuberant granulation tissue and to accelerate epithelialization.
- Equine peritoneum and split-thickness allogeneic skin: A study done in horses found that wounds dressed with equine peritoneum or split-thickness allogeneic skin did not heal faster than similar wounds dressed with a control synthetic dressing
- Collagen dressing (CDs): CDs made into gels (Collasate, PRN Pharmacal, Pensacola, FL), porous and nonporous membranes, particles (Collamend, Veterinary Products Laboratory, Phoenix, AZ), and sponges reportedly enhance wound healing in humans and laboratory animals. Studies evaluating bovine porous and nonporous collagen membranes or gel dressings in horses found no benefit for this dressing over semiocclusive control dressings.

This monograph is adapted from Orsini JA, Divers TJ, editors: Equine emergencies: treatment and procedures, ed 3, St Louis, 2008, Saunders Elsevier.

- Extracellular matrix scaffolds (ECMs)
  - ECMs are available as porcine urinary bladder lamina propria (ACell Vet Scaffold, ACell, Inc, Jessup, MD) and as a scaffold made of chemically cross-linked glycosaminoglycans (EquitrX, Sentrx Animal Care, Salt Lake City, UT).
  - ECMs have the capability of recruiting the body's stem cells to migrate into the acellular scaffold resulting in "constructive remodeling" of the severely damaged or missing tissue. The healed remodeled tissue has differentiated cell and tissue types. Minimal scar tissue formation is found in the healed wounds. Preliminary findings in horses show that distal limb wounds treated with multiple applications of the EquitrX film heal with superior cosmesis.
- Solcoseryl (S): S is a protein-free, standardized dialysate/ultrafiltrate derived from calf blood (Solcoseryl, Solco Basle Ltd, Birsfelden, Switzerland). In an equine study, S provoked a greater inflammatory response with faster formation and contraction of granulation tissue. Subsequently S inhibited repair by causing protracted inflammation and delayed epithelialization. Perceived best use is for deep wounds during the early inflammatory phase; treatment should be discontinued at the first signs of epithelialization.
- Platelet-rich plasma (PRP): PRP is a volume of plasma with a platelet concentration well above baseline. Where the normal platelet counts in whole

blood average $200,000/\mu L$, the platelet counts in PRP should average $1,000,000/\mu L$. Lesser concentrations of platelets cannot be relied upon to enhance wound healing while greater concentrations have not yet been shown to further enhance wound healing. Upon activation, platelets release 70% of their stored growth factors and close to 100% within the first hour. Because of this, clotting of the PRP (via addition of thrombin or $CaCl_2$) should be induced just before delivery to the surface of the wound.
- Lacerum (L): L, a natural equine-specific wound healant (Lacerum, PRP Technologies, Roanoke, IN) containing a homologous source of activated platelets and their released growth factors, was shown in a preliminary study to induce repair of an avulsion injury involving bone and tendons.
- Activated macrophage supernatant (AMS): In vitro studies suggest AMS may improve wound healing in horses and ponies by inhibition of dermal fibroblast proliferation. No significant in vivo effects were found. The supernatant is not commercially available.

SUGGESTED READING

Stashak TS, Farstvedt E: Update on wound dressings: Indications and best use. In Stashak TS, Theoret CL, editors: *Equine Wound Management*, ed 2, Ames, IA, 2008, Wiley-Blackwell Publishing, pp 109–136.

AUTHORS: **CHRISTINE THÉORÊT** and **TED STASHAK**

EDITOR: **DAVID A. WILSON**

Wound Dressing: Occlusive Dressings

BASIC INFORMATION

PROCEDURE

- Hydrogels (Polyethylene oxide occlusive dressings)
  - 3D network of hydrophilic polymers with 90% to 95% water content
  - Available as sheets or gels
    - Sheet hydrogels believed to possess most of the properties of an ideal wound dressing (eg,

This monograph is adapted from Orini JA, Divers TJ, editors: Equine emergencies: treatment and procedures, ed 3, St Louis, 2008, Saunders Elsevier.

BioDres, DVM Pharmaceuticals, Inc. Miami, FL; Tegagel dressing, 3M Center St. Paul, MN; Nu-gel, Johnson & Johnson Products Inc, New Brunswick, NJ). When applied to dry wound they effectively hydrate it, creating an environment for moist wound healing.
- Amorphous hydrogels also possess a "moisture donor" effect for necrotic wounds that require autolytic debriding.
- Hydrogels containing acemannan (CarraVet, Veterinary Products Laboratories, Phoenix, AZ; Carrasorb,

Carrington Laboratories, Irving, TX) stimulate healing over exposed bone.
- Some hydrogels contain hyaluronic acid and chondroitin sulfate within a chemically crosslinked glycosaminoglycan (GAG) hydro-film (Tegaderm, 3M Center, St. Paul, MN), which reportedly increases epithelialization and fibroplasia compared to Tegaderm alone.
- Other products contain gauze impregnated with a hydrogel (eg, FasCure, Ken Vet, Greeley, CO; Curafil, Tyco Healthcare Kendall, Mansfield, MA) and another

contains 25% propylene glycol (Solugel, Johnson & Johnson Medical, North Ryde, Australia).
- A study evaluating the effects of Solugel on second intention healing in horses found no beneficial effects when compared to the control saline-soaked gauze dressing.
- In another study on equine limb wounds, the hydrogel sheet dressing (BioDres, DVM Pharmaceuticals, Inc.) was associated with excess exudate and prolonged wound healing (2× compared to controls) along with an increased need to trim exuberant granulation tissue, believed to result from continued application of the BioDres during the repair phase.
- What to do:
  - Apply dressing within 6 hours of wounding and maintain for at least 48 hours before changing.
  - Dressing should be discontinued at the earliest evidence of granulation tissue.
  - Prior to application of a sheet hydrogel dressing, skin around the wound should be cleaned and dried and the wound surface gently rinsed with a dilute antiseptic solution.
  - Dressing should be cut to appropriate size for the wound and the thin sheet on one side peeled off. Dressing is then covered with a secondary and tertiary bandage layer. Dressing should be left in place for 2 days. If skin surrounding the wound begins to appear

macerated because of excess moisture, dressing should be replaced with a nonadherent semiocclusive dressing.
  - Best used on clean acute wounds during the inflammatory phase of wound healing.
- Ketanserin gel (Vulketan gel, Janssen Animal Health, Beerse, Belgium) was recently evaluated in a large multicenter randomized controlled field study. This dressing was found to be more effective than other standard treatments in preventing exuberant granulation tissue and infection.
- Hydrocolloid
  - Consists of an inner, often adhesive layer, a thick absorbing hydrocolloid "mass" and an outer, thin, water-resistant and bacteria-impervious polyurethane film.
  - Available as (Duoderm, ER Squibb Inc. Princeton, NJ; Dermaheal, Solvay Animal Health, Mendota Heights, MN) or carboxymethylcellulose particles embedded in an elastotic mesh (Comfeel, Coloplast, Marietta, GA).
  - Duoderm is oxygen impermeable, supposed to promote the rate of epithelialization and collagen synthesis and to decrease the pH of the wound exudate, thus reducing bacterial count.
    - Acceleration of epithelialization has not been documented in all studies.
    - A study on horses showed Dermaheal or Duoderm dressings

promote the formation of granulation tissue directly from the surface of denuded bone and on the surface of frayed tendons and ligaments. Also showed that wound infection can develop under dressing; when it does, application should be discontinued until the wound is healthy.
  - Best use in horses appears to be during the early inflammatory phase until granulation tissue fills the wound. Dressing should be applied to a clean wound, free of infection, and discontinued before the development of exuberant granulation tissue.
- Silicone dressing (SD): SD (CicaCare Smith & Nephew, Hull, UK) was recently investigated in experimental distal limb wounds in horses. The study showed that the silicone dressing surpassed a conventional nonadherent absorbent dressing in preventing the formation of exuberant granulation tissue. Contraction and epithelialization progressed faster in the first 2 weeks of repair. Furthermore, tissue quality exceeded that of wounds treated conventionally.

SUGGESTED READING

Stashak TS, Farstvedt E: Update on wound dressings: indications and best use. In Stashak TS, Theoret CL, editors: *Equine Wound Management*, ed 2, Ames, IA, 2008, Wiley-Blackwell Publishing, pp 109–136.

AUTHORS: **CHRISTINE THÉORÊT** and **TED STASHAK**

EDITOR: **DAVID A. WILSON**

Wound Dressing: Particulate Dextranomers

BASIC INFORMATION

PROCEDURE

- Particulate dextranomers
  - Beads (eg, Debrisan, Johnson & Johnson Products Inc, New Brunswick, NJ), flakes (eg, Avalon, Summit Hill Laboratories, Avalon, NJ), and powders (eg, Intrasite, Smith & Nephew, Hull, UK; Intracell, Macleod Pharmaceuticals, Inc., Fort Collins, CO)
    - Absorb the aqueous component, including prostaglandins, from wound exudate.

- Remove microorganisms from the wound bed, primarily by capillary action.
- Activate chemotactic factors that attract polymorphonuclear and mononuclear cells to the wound bed.
- Best use appears to be for debridement of sloughing, exuding wounds. Should be discontinued when a healthy bed of granulation tissue develops. Contraindicated in dry wounds.
- NOTE: Because particulate dextranomers are not biodegradable they should be rinsed from the wound with saline before the wound dries to avoid residue build-up and the subsequent development of a granuloma.

- Maltodextrin
  - Intracell (Macleod Pharmaceuticals, Inc., Fort Collins, CO) is commercially available as a powder or gel.
  - Hydrophilic soluble powder "pulls" fluids up through wound tissues, bathing the wound from inside, encouraging moist wound healing.
  - Yields glucose from hydrolysis of polysaccharide, providing energy for cell metabolism to promote healing.
  - Powder and gel cause chemotaxis of macrophages, polymorphonuclear cells, and lymphocytes into the wound, enhancing debridement.
  - The powder should be applied over the wound to a thickness of approximately 1 cm. A primary nonadherent semiocclusive dressing should

This monograph is adapted from Orsini JA, Divers TJ, editors: Equine emergencies: treatment and procedures, ed 3, St Louis, 2008, Saunders Elsevier.

be applied over the powder, followed by an absorbent wrap and tertiary bandage.
- Bandages are changed daily, the wound lavaged, after which more powder is applied.
- Proposed best use is for debridement to cleanse and promote healing in contaminated and infected wounds.
- The powder is best used on exudative wounds and the gel is best used for drier wounds.
- Calcium alginate (CA)
  - Classified as a fibrous dextranomer; made from salts of alginic acid obtained from *algae phaeophyceae* found in seaweed.
  - Available from a variety of sources (Curasorb, Ken Vet, Greeley, CO; C-Stat, R. S. Jackson Inc., Alexandria, VA; Nu-Derm, Johnson & Johnson Products Inc, New Brunswick, NJ; Kalginate, DeRoyal, Powell, TN).

- Hydrophilic; dressing absorbs 20 to 30 times its weight in wound fluid.
- Promotes moist environment conducive to wound healing.
- Manufacturer reports accelerated epithelialization and granulation tissue formation; this was not found in one study done in horses.
- Improves clotting.
- Activates macrophages within a chronic wound bed, promoting granulation tissue formation.
- Some alginates have the ability to "kick start" the healing cascade by causing lysis of mast cells resulting in release of histamine and 5-hydroxytryptamine.
- Because of these attributes, calcium alginate dressings are considered bioactive.
- Proposed best use:
  - Moderately to heavily exuding wound during transition from the acute inflammatory to repair phase of healing

- Wounds with substantial tissue loss, such as degloving injuries
- Kick starts the healing in a chronic wound bed.
- Dressing should be premoistened before application to a chronic dry wound requiring stimulation of fibroplasia. A semiocclusive nonadherent pad should be placed over the calcium alginate dressing, followed by secondary and tertiary bandage layers.

SUGGESTED READING

Stashak TS, Farstvedt E: Update on wound dressings: Indications and best use. In Stashak TS, Theoret CL, editors: *Equine Wound Management*, ed 2, Ames, IA, 2008, Wiley-Blackwell Publishing, pp 109–136.

AUTHORS: CHRISTINE THÉORÊT and TED STASHAK

EDITOR: DAVID A. WILSON

PROCEDURES AND TECHNIQUES

Wound Dressing: Semiocclusive Dressings

BASIC INFORMATION

- Commercially available as:
  - Petrolatum-impregnated gauze (NU Gauze sponges, Johnson & Johnson Products Inc, New Brunswick, NJ; Vaseline Petrolatum Gauze, Tyco Healthcare Kendall, Mansfield, MA; Xerofoam, Tyco Healthcare Kendall, Mansfield, MA; Jelonet, Smith and Nephew, Hull, UK)
  - Petrolatum emulsion dressing (Adaptic, Johnson & Johnson Products Inc, New Brunswick, NJ), oil emulsion knitted fabric (Curity, Tyco Healthcare Kendall, Mansfield, MA), rayon/polyethylene fabric (Release, Johnson & Johnson Products Inc, New Brunswick, NJ), petrolatum impregnated gauze with 3% bismuth tribromophenate (Adaptic + Xerofoam, Johnson & Johnson Products Inc, New Brunswick, NJ)
  - Absorbent adhesive film (Mitraflex, Polymedica Industries Inc., Wheat Ridge, CO)
  - Perforated polyester film filled with compressed cotton (Telfa, Tyco Healthcare Kendall, Mansfield, MA)
  - Study evaluating the effects of two semiocclusive dressings (Telfa

and Mitraflex), a biologic dressing (equine amnion) and an occlusive dressing (Biodres) on the healing of surgically created full-thickness distal limb wounds in horses, showed wounds dressed with Biodres developed more exuberant granulation tissue, excess exudate, and suffered delayed healing (2× compared to Telfa). Wounds dressed with amnion required minimal trimming of granulation tissue; those dressed with Telfa healed the fastest.

- Polyurethane semiocclusive dressings
  - Available as film (eg, Op-Site, Smith & Nephew, Hull, UK; Tegaderm, 3M Center, St. Paul, MN; Bioocclusive, Johnson & Johnson Products Inc., New Brunswick, NJ) or foam (eg, Hydrosorb, Ken Vet, Greeley, CO; Hydrosorb, Wound Care Products, Avitar Inc., Canton, MA; Sof-Foam, Johnson & Johnson Products Inc., New Brunswick, NJ)
  - Film is transparent, waterproof, semipermeable to vapor, oxygen-permeable, adhesive to dry skin while nonadhesive to the wound and has an analgesic effect.
    - Although considered nonadherent, one product (Op-Site) has a tendency to strip away newly formed epidermis from the surface of a healing wound.

- Although the proposed best use for the sheet dressings in horses is during the repair phase, their unique characteristics allow them to be used during the entire healing period of a clean wound.
- Foam sponges come as sheet dressings, in situ formed foams, and adhesive foams (eg, Tielle hydropolymer adhesive, Johnson & Johnson Products Inc, New Brunswick, NJ).
- Highly conforming, vapor-permeable, absorptive, easy to apply, and provides an effective barrier against bacterial penetration. Moisture is absorbed into the dressing, reducing tissue maceration while providing a moist healing environment.
- Proposed best use for the sponge is during early inflammatory phase of healing, when there is considerable exudate in the wound. Under these circumstances bandage should be changed daily or as indicated according to the amount of fluid produced by the wound. Because of their semiocclusive nature they are also indicated during the repair phase of wound healing. An alternate use of the sponge is to deliver liquid medication or wetting agents to the wound by

This monograph is adapted from Orsini JA, Divers TJ, editors: Equine emergencies: treatment and procedures, ed 3, St Louis, 2008, Saunders Elsevier.

saturating the sponge before placing it on the wound. The same sponge, however, cannot be used for both absorption and medication delivery.

SUGGESTED READING

Stashak TS, Farstvedt E: Update on wound dressings: indications and best use. In Stashak TS, Theoret CL, editors: *Equine Wound Management*, ed 2, Ames, IA, 2008, Wiley-Blackwell Publishing, pp 109–136.

AUTHORS: **CHRISTINE THÉORÊT** and **TED STASHAK**

EDITOR: **DAVID A. WILSON**

Wound Infection: Techniques to Reduce Infection in a Surgical Wound

BASIC INFORMATION

PROCEDURE

- Anesthesia
  - Reduce depth. Excessive depth of anesthesia causes reduced tissue perfusion resulting in reduced oxygen tension, acidosis, and impaired resistance to infection.
  - Reduce length. Prolonged anesthesia impairs alveolar macrophage function, depresses neutrophil function/migration, chemotaxis of white blood cells (WBCs), and phagocytic capabilities. Wound infection rates increase by 5% per minute after 60 minutes of anesthesia. Wound infection rates double after 90 minutes of surgery and triple when surgery exceeds 120 minutes.

This monograph is adapted from Orsini JA, Divers TJ, editors: Equine emergencies: treatment and procedures, ed 3, St Louis, 2008, Saunders Elsevier.

- Avoid propofol. Propofol has been shown to increase infection rates 3.8 times in clean wounds.
- Clipping: Clipping hair >4 hours before induction of anesthesia increases likelihood of surgical infection by three times. Recommendation: Clip and shave hair after induction of anesthesia. When clipping hair, protect the wound with sterile moist gauze sponges, clip a wide area of hair around the wound. Dampen hair with water or coat lightly with K-Y water-soluble jelly to prevent hair from falling into the wound. Sponges used to pack the wound are discarded and replaced by new ones.
- Surgical technique
  - Limit use of electrocautery.
  - Decrease surgery time.
  - Use aseptic technique:
    - Provide meticulous hemostasis.
    - Eliminate dead space and use a suction or passive drain if necessary.

- Use nonreactive sutures, proper suturing techniques.
- Antibiotics
  - Generally not needed for patients in good health with adequate immunity, if surgery is <60 minutes and performed in clean environment.
  - Generally needed in cases with tissue ischemia, if an enterotomy is performed, and if surgery time exceeds 60 minutes.
  - Perioperative antibiotics, when used, should be administered within 2 hours preceding surgery and for 24 hours following surgery.

SUGGESTED READING

MacDonald DG, Morley PS, Bailey JV, Barber SM, Fretz PB: An examination of the occurrence of surgical wound infection following equine orthopaedic surgery (1981–1990). *Equine Vet J* 26:323–326, 1994.

AUTHORS: **CHRISTINE THÉORÊT** and **TED STASHAK**

EDITOR: **DAVID A. WILSON**

Wound Infection: Techniques to Reduce Infection in a Traumatic Wound

BASIC INFORMATION

PROCEDURE

- Principles are the same as for elective surgery.
- Patient sedation and wound analgesia:
  - Avoid using phenothiazine tranquilizers in hypovolemic patients.
  - Perineural anesthesia is useful for wounds of distal extremities, while regional infiltration of local anesthetic is used elsewhere.

This monograph is adapted from Orini JA, Divers TJ, editors: Equine emergencies: treatment and procedures, ed 3, St Louis, 2008, Saunders Elsevier.

- Direct infiltration of the wound is acceptable only after wound has been cleaned.
- Wound cleansing:
  - One of the most important components of effective wound management
  - In acute wounds <3 hours duration, water or saline may be all that is needed for adequate wound cleansing. For field use, saline solution is made by adding 10-mL salt to 1-L boiling water (8 teaspoons to a gallon).
  - Commercial wound cleansers are recommended when enhanced wound cleansing is needed. Constant-Clens (Tyco Healthcare

Kendall, Mansfield, MA) appears to be the least toxic of wound cleansers. Antiseptics should not be added to wound cleanser as they increase the cytotoxic effects.
  - Vetericyn (Oculus Innovative Sciences, Inc., Petaluma, CA) has many of the attributes of an ideal wound cleanser. It is a super-oxidized solution with a neutral pH, has broad antimicrobial spectrum against bacteria, fungi, viruses, and spores, and reportedly has 15 seconds of bactericidal effect. It also has a shelf life >12 months.
  - Use smooth sponges to scrub the wound.

- ○ Scrubbing the wound with antiseptic soaps is not recommended because of cytotoxicity. Additionally, Povidone-iodine surgical scrub was shown to be ineffective in reducing bacterial levels in wounds.
- Wound lavage/irrigation
  - ○ In acute wounds <3 hours duration lavage effectively reduces the number of bacteria residing on the wound surface.
  - ○ Lavage solutions are most effective when delivered by a jet of at least 7 psi at an oblique angle to the wound. Pressures of 10 to 15 psi have been shown to be 80% effective in removing infection potentiating factors and adherent bacteria from a wound. This pulsatile pressure can be achieved by forcefully expressing lavage solutions from a 35- or 60-mL syringe through an 18-gauge needle, using a spray bottle, a "Water Pik," or a Stryker inter-pulse irrigation system (Stryker InterPulse irrigation system, Med-Vet Innovations, Inc., Penrose, CO). Wounds should not be irrigated with fluids delivered at pressures >15 psi, which would force contaminants into tissue.
  - ○ Sterile isotonic saline or lactated Ringer's solutions are commonly used. Tap water delivered from a hose can be used for large wounds, initially. Solutions are often combined with antiseptics/antimicrobials.
  - ○ Volume of fluid for lavage/irrigation depends on size of wound and degree of contamination. Minimally, gross contaminants should be removed. Discontinue before tissue becomes water-logged.
- Antiseptics used for wound lavage/ irrigation
  - ○ Povidone-iodine solution [PI] (10%)
    - ▪ Commonly used because of its broad antimicrobial spectrum against gram-positive and gram-negative bacteria, fungi, and *Candida* organisms. Bactericidal effect is 15 seconds. Bacterial resistance has not been identified.
    - ▪ Diluting the solution uncouples the bond, making more free iodine available for antimicrobial activity. 0.1 and 0.2% (10–20 mL/L) concentrations are recommended.
    - ▪ Disadvantages include:
      - □ Inactivated by organic material and blood
      - □ <0.1 % concentrations are inactivated by large number of neutrophils
      - □ Concentrations >1% are required to kill *Staphylococcus aureus*

- ○ Chlorhexidine diacetate solution [CHD] (2%)
  - ▪ Broad antimicrobial spectrum. NOTE: Ineffective against fungi and *Candida* organisms, while *Proteus* and *Pseudomonas* organisms have developed or have an inherent resistance to CHD.
  - ▪ When applied to intact skin, antimicrobial effect is immediate and has a lasting residual effect caused by binding to protein in the stratum corneum.
  - ▪ Currently, 0.05% CHD (1 : 40 dilution [25–975 mL] of the 2% concentrate) solution is recommended for wound lavage. Greater concentrations can be harmful to wound healing.
  - ▪ Dilution in a sterile electrolyte solution results in precipitation within 4 hours. This does not affect the antibacterial effects of CHD.
  - ▪ 0.05% CHD has more bactericidal activity than PI.
  - ▪ Continued activity in the presence of blood and pus.
  - ▪ Disadvantages include:
    - □ Ocular toxicity
    - □ Full-strength CHD delays wound healing to a greater extent than does alcohol.
    - □ >0.5% solutions inhibit epithelialization and formation of granulation tissue.
    - □ <0.05% concentration results in significant survival of *S. aureus*.
    - □ Narrow margin of dilution safety
- ○ Hydrogen peroxide (3%)
  - ▪ Narrow antimicrobial spectrum
  - ▪ Damaging to tissues, cytotoxic to fibroblasts, and causes thrombosis in the microvasculature.
  - ▪ Not recommended for wound care/lavage
- ○ Sodium hypochlorite solution (0.5%) (Dakin's solution)
  - ▪ Release of chlorine and oxygen kills bacteria
  - ▪ More effective than PI and CHD in killing *S. aureus*
  - ▪ Cytotoxic to fibroblasts and retards epithelialization
  - ▪ Decreases blood flow in microvessels
  - ▪ Chemically debrides the wound
  - ▪ Recommend one-quarter strength (0.125%) for wound treatment
  - ▪ NOTE: In a pinch, dilute 5% sodium hypochlorite with tap water to achieve a 0.025% solution.
- ○ Conclusions, Antiseptics:
  - ▪ Kill surface bacteria only.
  - ▪ Most effective in reducing bacterial numbers in acute contami-

nated wounds and not in chronic wounds or wounds with established infection.
  - ▪ Wounds with established infection should be treated by debridement as well as systemic and topical antibiotics.
- NOTE: Surgeons should never select a wound irrigation solution they are unwilling to put in their own conjunctival sac!
- Wound exploration
  - ○ Once wound is cleaned and free of devitalized tissue/debris, it is explored digitally using sterile gloves.
  - ○ A sterile probe is useful in identifying wound depth, if a foreign body is present, or if bone is contacted, and can be used in conjunction with radiography.
  - ○ Synovial fluid is identified by stringing it between the thumb and forefinger; a sample should be submitted for cytologic examination and culture/sensitivity.
  - ○ If synovial cavity penetration is suspected, a needle is placed in the synovial cavity at a site remote to the wound (Figure 1). If synovial fluid can be retrieved, it is submitted for cytology and culture/ sensitivity. Following fluid retrieval, sterile saline solution is injected into the synovial structure; if the joint capsule has been violated, fluid is seen at the wound. If a synovial structure is involved, it is lavaged with 3 to 5 L of sterile saline or crystalloid solution. Intrasynovial instillation of antibiotics is also recommended.
  - ○ Radiographic examination
    - ▪ Standard
    - ▪ Contrast/fistulography
  - ○ Ultrasound examination can document injury to tendons, ligaments, and joint capsules. It can identify foreign bodies not apparent on radiographs, gas accumulation, and muscle separation (Figure 2).
  - ○ Arthroscopy can be helpful in identifying radiographically occult lesions, particularly those involving cartilage, and in identifying foreign bodies within the joint (eg, hair, dirt, or other foreign bodies) (Figure 3).
- Wound debridement
  - ○ Debridement reduces the number of bacteria and removes contaminants (dead tissue, foreign bodies) that alter local defense mechanisms.
  - ○ The standard approach is sharp debridement, converting a contaminated wound to a clean one. The types of debridement include:
    - ▪ Excisional (layered) (Figure 4)
    - ▪ En bloc

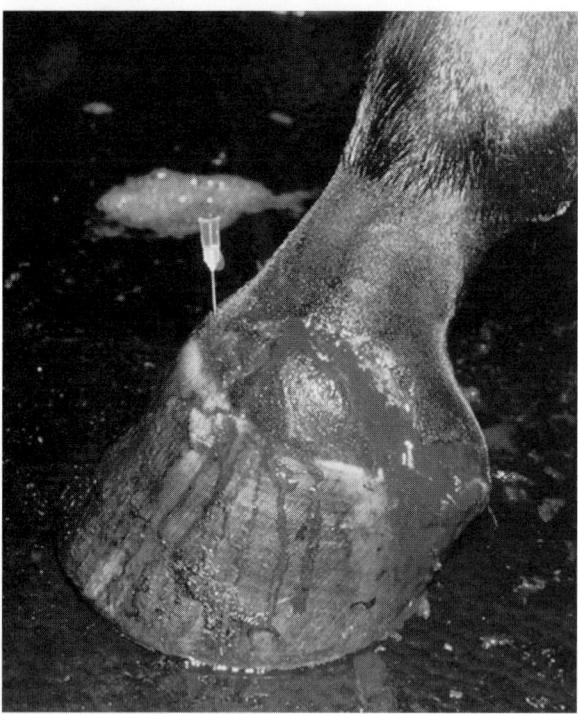

FIGURE 1 An example of a needle placed in the distal interphalangeal (coffin) joint at a site remote to the wound. (From Stashak TS: *Proc Am Assoc Equine Pract* 52:270–280, 2006. In Orsini JA, Divers TJ, editors. *Equine Emergencies: Treatment and Procedures,* ed 3. St Louis, 2008, Saunders.)

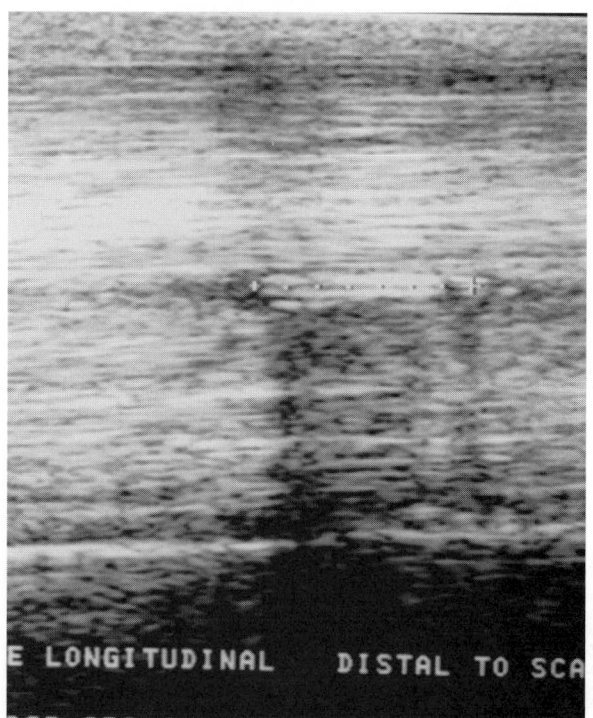

FIGURE 2 A longitudinal ultrasound examination identifying a piece of wood (*cursors*) located at the distal extent of the carpal canal at the attachment of the carpal check ligament to the deep digital flexor tendon. (From Stashak TS: *Proc Am Assoc Equine Pract* 52:270–280, 2006. In Orsini JA, Divers TJ, editors. *Equine Emergencies: Treatment and Procedures,* ed 3. St Louis, 2008, Saunders.)

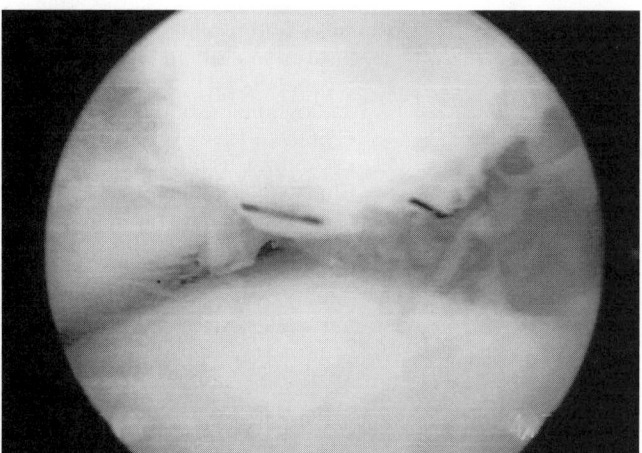

FIGURE 3 Arthroscopic view of the distal interphalangeal (coffin) joint. Note the hair (*dark particles*) in the joint. This horse had sustained a puncture wound to the cornet band region 1 week earlier. (From Stashak TS: *Proc Am Assoc Equine Pract* 52:270–280, 2006. In Orsini JA, Divers TJ, editors. *Equine Emergencies: Treatment and Procedures,* ed 3. St Louis, 2008, Saunders.)

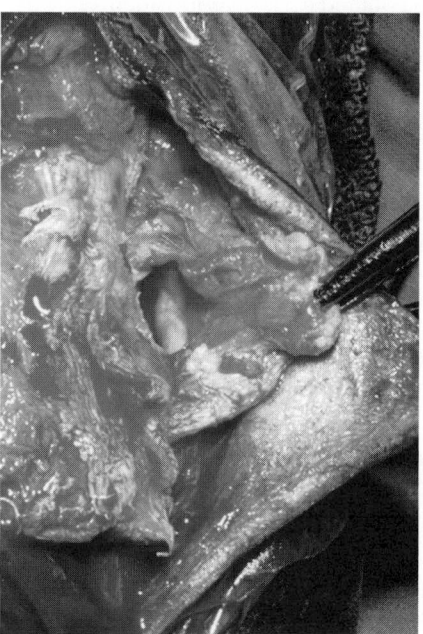

FIGURE 4 An example of extensive layered debridement of a wound of a 6-hour duration entrapment injury involving the dorsolateral fetlock region. Note that the damaged joint capsule was also debrided, exposing the joint. (From Stashak TS, Theoret CL: Wound healing, management, and reconstruction. In Orsini JA, Divers TJ, editors. *Equine Emergencies: Treatment and Procedures,* ed 3. St Louis, 2008, Saunders.)

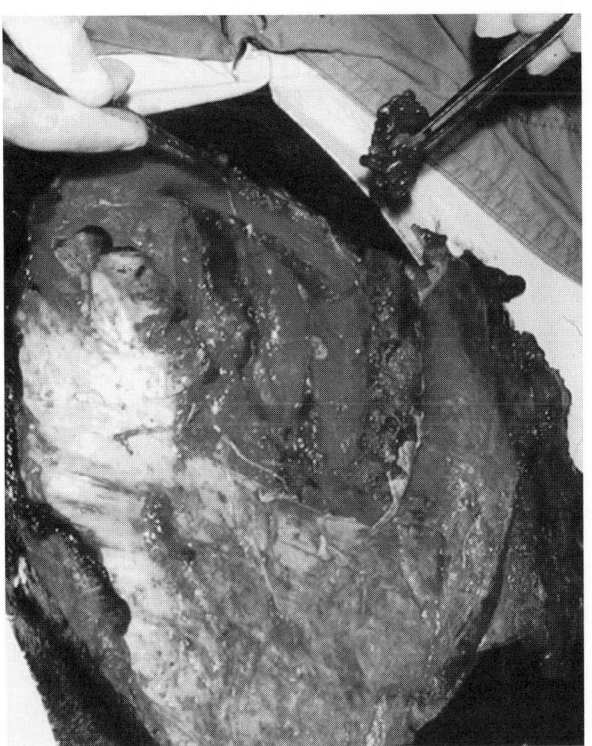

FIGURE 5 A large wound involving the lateral thoracic region is a good example of where piecemeal debridement can be used. (From Stashak TS: *Proc Am Assoc Equine Pract* 52:270–280, 2006. In Orsini JA, Divers TJ, editors. *Equine Emergencies: Treatment and Procedures,* ed 3. St Louis, 2008, Saunders.)

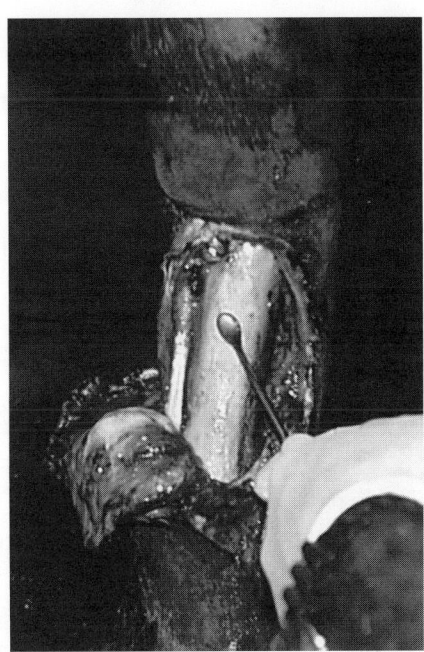

FIGURE 6 A large avulsion injury of the dorsal metatarsal region with exposed ischemic bone (chalky appearance). The bone is being partially decorticated (debrided) with a hip arthroplasty rasp. (From Stashak TS, Theoret CL: Wound healing, management, and reconstruction. In Orsini JA, Divers TJ, editors. *Equine Emergencies: Treatment and Procedures,* ed 3. St Louis, 2008, Saunders.)

- Simple or piecemeal (used for very large wounds of the body) (Figure 5)
- Staged (used over a number of days). This approach prevents the inadvertent removal of viable tissue. Governing criteria are color and attachment. White, tan, black, or green tissue that is poorly attached is debrided. Pink to dark purple tissue that is well attached is left.
- NOTE: Exposed ischemic, contaminated cortical bone should be debrided (partial decortication) sufficiently to reach bleeding/serum-oozing bone. Partial decortication can be accomplished with a pneumatic-driven burr or a bone rasp. (Figure 6)
- Enzymatic
  - Wound surface coagulum and bacterial biofilm encompass contaminants and bacteria, thus preventing access by topical antibiotics/antiseptics and systemic antibiotics.
  - Proteolytic enzymes degrade the coagulum and biofilm.
  - Indications: When surgical debridement could result in damage to or removal of valuable tissue needed for reconstruction of a wound and when a wound approximates nerves and vessels
  - Products include:
    - Pancreatic trypsin (Granulex, Dertek Pharmaceuticals, Research Triangle Park, NC)
    - Streptodornase or Streptokinase (Varidase, Lederle Lab, Wayne, NJ)
    - Collagenases, proteinases, fibrinolysin, and deoxyribonuclease (Elase, Fujisawa Health Care, Deerfield, IL)
  - Debridement dressings include:
    - Adherent open mesh gauze (eg, 4 × 4 gauze sponges)
    - Wet to dry using 4 × 4 mesh gauze or sheet cotton
    - Kerlix AMD (Tyco Healthcare Kendall, Mansfield, MA) excellent choice because it contains broad-spectrum antiseptic and shown to kill bacteria on the wound surface and prevent "strike through" (penetration through the dressing)

SUGGESTED READING

Orsini JA, Elce YA, Kraus B: Management of severely infected wounds. In Stashak TS, Theoret CL, editors: *Equine Wound Management,* ed 2, Ames, IA, 2008, Wiley-Blackwell Publishing, pp 543–567.

Stashak TS: Selected factors that negatively impact healing. In Stashak TS, Theoret CL, editors: *Equine Wound Management,* ed 2, Ames, IA, 2008, Wiley-Blackwell Publishing, pp 71–84.

Stashak TS: Management practices that influence wound infection and healing. In Stashak TS, Theoret CL, editors: *Equine Wound Management,* ed 2, Ames, IA, 2008, Wiley-Blackwell Publishing, pp 85–106.

Stashak TS, Theoret CL: Wound healing, management and reconstruction. In Orsini JA, Divers TJ, editors: *Equine Emergencies—Treatment and Procedures,* ed 3, St. Louis, MO, 2008, Elsevier-Saunders, pp 189–236.

Theoret CL, Wilmink JM: Treatment of exuberant granulation tissue. In Stashak TS, Theoret CL, editors: *Equine Wound Management,* ed 2, Ames, IA, 2008, Wiley-Blackwell Publishing, pp 445–462.

AUTHORS: **CHRISTINE THÉORÊT** and **TED STASHAK**

EDITOR: **DAVID A. WILSON**

Wound Therapy: Antibiotic Therapy for Traumatic Wounds

BASIC INFORMATION

PROCEDURE

- Antibiotics used in wound lavage/irrigation.
  - Addition of antibiotics to the lavage solution markedly reduces the number of bacteria in a wound.
  - 1% neomycin solution is effective in preventing infection in wounds experimentally contaminated with feces.
  - In a double-blind study done on 260 sutured lacerations, penicillin sprayed on the wound before closure reduced infection by 75%.
- Antibiotics systemic: General comments
  - Decision is easy: Selection depends on type and location of wound.
  - Systemic: (±broad spectrum)
  - Pulse dosing improves antibiotic penetration.
  - Parenteral recommended initially. IV is preferred because its effects are predictable. IM absorption is often prolonged and variable and depends on the site selection and amount of exercise.
  - Oral is used after adequate blood levels have been achieved.
- Antimicrobial choices
  - Superficial wounds: Generally not needed in clean wounds <3 hours duration that are sutured or left to heal by second intention. Generally needed for heavily contaminated wounds >3 hours duration. Antibiotics used include penicillin (22,000–44,000 IU/kg IV q6 or IM q12h) alone or in combination with TMS (15 mg/kg PO q12h).
  - Deeper wounds involving synovial cavities: Penicillin, ampicillin (6.6–11 mg/kg IM or IV q8–12h), or cefazolin (11 mg/kg IV or IM q6–8h) in combination with an aminoglycoside
    - Gentamicin (6.6 mg/kg IV or IM q24h) or amikacin (15–25 mg/kg IV or IM q24h). Combination is synergistic.
    - Ceftiofur (adult = 2.2–4.4 mg/kg IM or IV q12h; foals 4–6 mg/kg IV or IM q12h) or enrofloxacin (5 mg/kg IV q12–24h or 7.5 mg/kg PO q24h [not recommended for foals]) reserved for bacteria

resistant to all previously mentioned antibiotics.
  - Deep fascial cellulitis/septic myositis due to *Clostridia*
    - High doses of penicillin, ampicillin, or cephazolin and metronidazole (15 mg/kg PO q6–8h) or rifampin (5–10 mg/kg PO q12–24h) or ceftiofur.
  - Pyonecrotic processes
    - Metronidazole and penicillin
- Duration of antimicrobial therapy
  - Minimum course: 3 to 5 days
  - Established soft tissue infection: 7 to 10 days
  - Established synovial infection: 10 to 21 days
  - Established bone infection: 3 to 6 months
  - NOTE: Wounds contaminated with 10^9 microorganisms/g of tissue will develop infection despite antibiotic treatment.
- Topical antibiotics (TAs)
  - Can retard wound healing, especially some ointments or creams (eg, nitrofurazone [Furacin] and Gentamicin cream).
  - Solutions most effective when applied to wounds before closure or as lavage/irrigation solutions.
  - Creams and ointments remain in contact with the wound longer, prevent desiccation of the wound surface, and are best used under bandages and on exposed wounds.
  - Most effective when applied within 3 hours of wounding. However if a wound >3 hours or a chronically infected wound is debrided, a "new" wound is created, making TA use appropriate. In the latter, systemic antibiotics are also recommended.
  - Triple antibiotic ointment (TAO) (bacitracin/polymyxin B/neomycin) has wide antimicrobial spectrum but is ineffective against *P. aeruginosa*. The zinc component of bacitracin stimulates epithelialization (25% increase) but can retard wound contraction. TAO is poorly absorbed, therefore toxicity is rare.
  - Silver sulfadiazine (SS) has wide antimicrobial spectrum, including against *Pseudomonas* organisms and fungi. SS has been shown to accelerate epithelialization by 28% in some studies, but in others it slows epithelialization.
  - Nitrofurazone ointment (NO) has good antimicrobial spectrum against gram-positive and gram-negative

organisms but has little effect against *Pseudomonas* organisms. Shown to decrease epithelialization and wound contraction in horses.
  - Gentamicin sulfate (GS) has narrow antimicrobial spectrum but may be applied to wounds infected with gram-negative bacteria, particularly *P. aeruginosa*. Treatment with 0.1% oil-in-water cream base slows wound contraction and epithelialization.
  - Cefazolin is effective against gram-positive and some gram-negative organisms. When applied at 20 mg/kg, cefazolin yields a high wound fluid concentration (above minimal inhibitory concentration [MIC]) for longer periods than does systemically administered cefazolin at same dose. Powder form provides more sustained tissue concentration than does solution. Because of this property, cefazolin may be effective in the management of established infections.
  - NOTE: Antibiotic-resistant bacterial strains are a major health concern; therefore, new emphasis is placed on the development and use of alternative wound care products, particularly those with no known induction of bacterial resistance.
- Management of synovial penetration
  - Synovial lavage, irrigation, and drainage
    - Lavage with sterile salt solution (1–3 L) + 10% DMSO (1 L)
    - Arthroscopy/tenoscopy ± synovectomy
    - Arthrotomy can be used for nonresponsive, chronic infections.
    - Closed suction drainage
    - Ingress/egress system
  - Intrasynovial injection of antimicrobials
    - Less than one systemic dose q24h. Bactericidal effects of aminoglycosides are concentration dependent. High peak concentration is also associated with longer postantibiotic effect.
    - Amikacin (250 mg q24h). Amikacin has good activity against most equine orthopedic pathogens and resistance to amikacin is less likely than to gentamicin.
    - Gentamicin (150–250 mg q24h). Gentamicin is effective against 85% of the bacterial isolates obtained from musculoskeletal infections in the horse. It is also shown to be active in equine

This monograph is adapted from Orsini JA, Divers TJ, editors: Equine emergencies: treatment and procedures, ed 3, St Louis, 2008, Saunders Elsevier.

infected synovial fluid. Intra-articular administration of 150 mg of gentamicin results in peak concentrations, which remain significantly higher than the MIC for *E. coli* for more than 24 hours.
- Penicillin 5×10^6 IU q24h
- Ceftiofur (150 mg). Intrasynovial treatment with 150 mg of ceftiofur results in synovial fluid concentrations significantly higher than those achieved after IV administration (2.2 mg/kg). Synovial fluid concentration following IA administration remains above MIC for 24 hours; following IV administration, concentration remains above MIC for only 8 hours.
- Local antimicrobial therapy (see "Regional Limb Perfusion" in this section)
  - Antimicrobial-impregnated beads
    - Beads are made from either polymethylmethacrylate or hydroxyapatite cement.
    - Increase local concentrations of the antimicrobial 200 times that achieved by systemic administration.
    - MIC persist for 80 days after implantation.
    - Serum levels do not reach toxic levels.
    - Gentamicin and amikacin most often used.

  - Ceftiofur-impregnated beads are unlikely to provide long-term bactericidal concentrations.
  - Biodegradable drug delivery systems
    - Poly (DL) lactide ± co-glycolide flat discs + 500 mg of gentamicin (Boehringer Ingelheim)
    - Gentamicin-impregnated collagen sponge + 130 mg of gentamicin (Collatamp G; Schering Plough, Kenilworth, NJ)
    - Used commonly in humans for soft tissue surgery and injury.
    - Reportedly higher concentrations of antibiotic are reached for 3 days (first day 15 times, third day 2 times) in wound exudate than achieved with PMMA beads.
    - Collagen sponge absorbed within 12 to 49 days depending on the vascular supply to the region.
    - Seven of eight horses with moderate to severe traumatic septic synovial cavities (arthritis and tenosynovitis) responded favorably to this treatment. Collagen sponges are implanted in the synovial cavity through the arthroscope cannula.
    - A study done in horses, using purified bovine type 1 colla-

gen sponge impregnated with 130 mg of gentamicin placed in the tarsocrural joint, showed a rapid rise in peak concentration of gentamicin >20 times MIC within 3 hours. Rapid decline occurred by 48 hours; no substantial joint inflammation was seen.
  - Continuous intrasynovial infusion
    - Catheter + balloon infuser placed in the tarsocrural joint
    - 17 of 24 remained functional
    - Gentamicin dosage 0.02 to 0.17 mg/kg/h resulted in concentrations 100 times the MIC for common equine pathogens.

SUGGESTED READING

Baxter GM: Diagnosis and management of wounds involving synovial structures. In Stashak TS, Theoret CL, editors: *Equine Wound Management*, ed 2, Ames, IA, 2008, Wiley-Blackwell Publishing, pp 463–488.

Brumbaugh GW: Use of antimicrobials in wound management. *Vet Clin North Am Equine Pract* 21:63–72, 2005.

Farstvedt E, Stashak TS, Othic A: Update on topical wound medications. *Clin Tech Equine Pract* 3:164–172, 2004.

Farstvedt E, Stashak TS: Topical wound treatments and wound care products. In Stashak TS, Theoret CL, editors: *Equine Wound Management*, ed 2, Ames, IA, 2008, Wiley-Blackwell Publishing, pp 137–160.

AUTHORS: **CHRISTINE THÉORÊT** and **TED STASHAK**

EDITOR: **DAVID A. WILSON**

Wound Therapy: Topical Agents

BASIC INFORMATION

PROCEDURE

- Live yeast cell derivative (LYCD): Water-soluble yeast extract reported to stimulate angiogenesis, epithelialization and collagen formation. Associated with improved wound healing in dogs. In horses, it prolonged wound healing and resulted in excessive granulation tissue formation.
- Aloe vera (AV)
  - Reported to have both anti-thromboxane and anti-prostaglandin properties that favor vascular patency and prevent dermal ischemia.

- AV extract gel with allantoin is reported to stimulate epithelialization.
- AV extract gel with acemannan shown experimentally to encourage epithelialization and wound healing in open pad wounds in dogs at 7 days.
- Therapeutic efficacy in horses not yet investigated and at least one study showed that AV delayed wound healing in this species.
- Honey (H)
  - Beneficial in the treatment of chronic infected wounds
  - Proposed advantages include wound debridement, antibacterial effect, and promotion of wound healing. Honey-treated wounds show little neutrophilic infiltration but marked proliferation of angioblasts and fibroblasts.

- Sugar (S)
  - Bacteriostatic, reduces edema, attracts macrophages, debrides the wound, provides energy, and creates moist wound healing.
  - Sugar should be placed on the wound 1 cm thick then covered with an absorbent dressing.
  - Best used in necrotic, infected wounds.
- Miscellaneous topical agents
  - Vitamin E: One study found that 90% of treated wounds had a poorer cosmetic outcome and 33% developed a contact dermatitis.
  - Gentian violet shown to be carcinogenic.
  - Scarlet oil contains 30% isopropyl or benzyl alcohol, which delays wound healing. Scarlet red, the wound dressing used in burn patients, has no alcohol and has been shown to promote epithelialization.

This monograph is adapted from Orsini JA, Divers TJ, editors: Equine emergencies: treatment and procedures, ed 3, St Louis, 2008, Saunders Elsevier.

- ○ Red Kote, a germicidal, nondrying, softening wound dressing and healing aid. Indications: Treatment of surface wounds, cuts, lacerations, and abrasions. No studies available.
- ○ Vetericyn, a super-oxidized salt solution with a neutral pH and a broad antimicrobial spectrum against bacteria, fungi, viruses, and spores. Reportedly has 15-second cidal effect with a shelf life >12 months. Intended for use in moistening, irrigation, debridement, and bacterial load reduction of acute and chronic wounds, ulcers, cuts, abrasions, and burns.
- ○ Amino Plex, a solution made up of amino acids, trace minerals, peptides, electrolytes, and nucleosides. Reported properties: Reverses cell damage, increases glucose and oxygen uptake, enhances collagen synthesis, and accelerates epithelialization in humans. No controlled studies in the horse.
- ○ Addison lab-Zn7 Derm, a patented solution with a neutral pH. Reportedly enhances wound healing, promotes hair regrowth, and is antimicrobial. No controlled studies in the horse.
- ○ Kinetic, Proud flesh formula, contains polyethylene glycol, nitrofurazone, dexamethasone, and scarlet oil. Recommended use: Apply to granulating wounds to suppress exuberant granulation tissue and treat superficial dermatitis. No studies in horses.
- • Recombinant growth factors
  - ○ Transforming growth factor (TGF)–β_1 shown to exert no beneficial effects on experimental wound healing in ponies and horses at the doses used.
  - ○ Platelet-derived growth factor shown to be effective in the treatment of chronic nonhealing diabetic ulcers in humans. No studies in the horse. Commercially available as Regranex, Ethicon Products, Somerville, NJ).
  - ○ NOTE: It appears that a "combination" of growth factors is required to have an effect.

SUGGESTED READING

Dart AJ, Dowling BA, Smith CL: Topical treatments in equine wound management. *Vet Clin North Am Equine Pract* 21:77–90, 2005.

Farstvedt E, Stashak TS, Othic A: Update on topical wound medications. *Clin Tech Equine Pract* 3:164–172, 2004.

Farstvedt E, Stashak TS: Topical wound treatments and wound care products. In Stashak TS, Theoret CL, editors: *Equine Wound Management*, ed 2, Ames, IA, 2008, Wiley-Blackwell Publishing, pp 137–160.

AUTHORS: **CHRISTINE THÉORÊT** and **TED STASHAK**

EDITOR: **DAVID A. WILSON**

Differential Diagnosis

Abdominal Distension

Obesity
  Regional adiposity
Overconsumption of roughage
Pregnancy
  Fetal hydrops
  Ruptured prepubic tendon
Gas accumulation (tympany)
  Intestinal obstruction (strangulating or nonstrangulating)
Grain overload
  Ileus or dysmotility
  Increased abdominal fluid

  Peritonitis
  Congestive heart failure
  Hepatic disease
  Hypoproteinemia
Abdominal neoplasia
Uroperitoneum (foals)

AUTHOR: **SARA GOMEZ-IBANEZ**

Abnormal Peritoneal Fluid

Abnormal color
  Serosanguineous
    Blood contamination during abdominocentesis
    Strangulating obstruction
    Post-celiotomy or post-castration
    Hemoabdomen
    Splenocentesis
  Brown, red-brown, or green
    Enterocentesis (few or no white blood cells [WBCs] on cytology)
    Intestinal rupture (intracellular and extracellular bacteria on cytology)
  White, yellow-white, or pink
    Severe peritonitis (with markedly elevated WBC count)
    Chyloabdomen
Elevated total protein or nucleated cell count (NCC) (sample is often turbid)
  Modified transudate (protein 2–4 g/dL and/or NCC up to 7,500 cells/µL)
    Early or mild intestinal inflammation
      Nonstrangulating obstruction
      Enteritis or enterocolitis
      Early strangulating obstruction (often serosanguineous)

  Exudate (protein >3 mg/dL and/or nucleated cell count >7,500 cells/µL)
    Moderate intestinal inflammation
      Nonstrangulating obstruction of longer duration
      Consider sand impaction
      Strangulating obstruction (usually serosanguineous in color)
  Exudate (nucleated cell count >20,000 cells/µL—indicative of septic peritonitis)
    RECOMMEND CULTURE AND SENSITIVITY
    Primary peritonitis (usually monomicrobial infection)
    Bowel perforation or rupture (mixed bacterial population ± feed material)
    Late or severe strangulating obstruction
Elevated peritoneal fluid lactate (two times or more than the serum value)
  Strangulating obstruction
  Severe enteritis

AUTHOR: **SARA GOMEZ-IBANEZ**

Anemia, Nonregenerative

Iron deficiency
  Chronic hemorrhage
  Nutritional deficiency (rare)
Chronic disease
  Chronic infection/inflammation
  Pleuritis/pneumonia
  Peritonitis/enteritis
  Bacterial endocarditis
  Internal abscess
  Chronic viral disease (e.g., equine infectious anemia [EIA])

Neoplasia
Endocrine disorders
Bone marrow failure
  Myelophthisis
  Myeloproliferative disease
  Bone marrow toxins
  Phenylbutazone
  Chloramphenicol
  Radiation
  Idiopathic pancytopenia

Miscellaneous conditions
   Administration of human recombinant erythropoietin
   Chronic hepatic disease
   Chronic renal disease
   Recent hemorrhage or hemolysis

From Sellon DC, Wise LN: Disorders of the hematopoietic system. In Reed SM, Bayly WM, Sellon DC (eds). *Equine Internal Medicine,* ed 3. St Louis, 2010, Saunders, pp 730–776.

Ataxia, Spinal

Differential Diagnosis

Common Causes	Major Diagnostic Tests
Cervical compressive myelopathy	Cervical radiography, myelogram
Equine protozoal myeloencephalitis	Western blot, IFAT
Equine herpesvirus-1 myeloencephalopathy	PCR, titers, virus isolation
West Nile encephalitis	IgM capture ELISA, PRNT
Trauma	Radiography, nuclear scintigraphy, ultrasound, MRI, CT, CSF analysis
Equine degenerative myeloencephalopathy	Rule out other causes, serum vitamin E levels
Neoplasia	CSF analysis, rule out other causes
Rabies	Rule out other causes
	Postmortem FA testing of brain
Less Common Causes	
Eastern and Western equine encephalitis	ELISA, titers, virus isolation
Occipitoatlantoaxial malformation	Age, breed, radiographs
Vertebral osteomyelitis, diskospondylitis, spinal abscess	CSF analysis, culture, radiography, nuclear scintigraphy
Diskospondylosis	Radiography, nuclear scintigraphy
	Rule out bacterial diskospondylitis
Cervical vertebral spinal hematoma, intervertebral disk disease	Radiographs, myelogram, CT, rule out other causes
Synovial cyst, arachnoid cyst	Radiographs, myelography, CT, MRI
Verminous meningoencephalitis	Rule out other causes
Strongylus vulgaris	CSF (eosinophilic leukocytosis supportive)
Halicephalobus gingivalis	CBC (eosinophilia supportive)
Setaria spp.	
Draschia megastoma	
Others	
Equine infectious anemia	Coggins test (agar gel immunodiffusion), ELISA
Aortic-iliac thrombosis	Rectal palpation
Cauda equina neuritis or Polyneuritis equi	Rule out other causes
Toxic Agents	
Stinging nettles	
Ivermectin, moxidectin	
Ionophores	
Moldy corn	
Locoism	
Sorghum, rye grass, dallis grass	
Heavy metals (lead, arsenic)	
Crotalaria	
Fluphenazine	
Propylene glycol	

CBC, complete blood count; *CSF,* cerebrospinal fluid; *CT,* computed tomography; *ELISA,* enzyme-linked immunosorbent assay; *FA,* fluorescent antibody; *IFAT,* indirect fluorescent antibody test; *IgM,* immunoglobulin M; *MRI,* magnetic resonance imaging; *PCR,* polymerase chain reaction; *PRNT,* plaque reduction neutralization test.
From Seino KK: Spinal ataxia. In Reed SM, Bayly WM, Sellon DC (eds). *Equine Internal Medicine,* ed 3. St Louis, 2010, Saunders, 135–138.

Bitting Problems

Soft tissue origin
  Tongue lacerations
  Foreign bodies trapped within the mouth
  Pinched soft tissue at commissures of mouth
  Mucosal irritation at interdental space
Bony/tooth origin
  Mandibular periostitis following overlying mucosal irritation
  Presence of wolf teeth (anecdotal evidence only)
  Dental fractures (anecdotal evidence only)

Others
  Lameness
  Back pain
  Temporomandibular disorders (anecdotal evidence only)

AUTHOR: **JAMES L. CARMALT**

Cardiac Murmurs

Differential Diagnosis

Auscultatory Finding		Likely Diagnosis	Diagnostic Plan
Left side Systolic murmur	PMI over basal area (aortic and pulmonary valve area) Early or midsystolic Usually <Grade III/VI	Functional murmur	None
	PMI over apical area (mitral valve area) Often holo- or pansystolic Grade I–VI/VI	Mitral regurgitation	If:>Grade III/VI or arrhythmia or resting HR >45 bpm or poor performance Then: ECHO and ± exercise ECG
Diastolic murmur	PMI over apical area (mitral valve area) Early diastolic Often musical quality	"2-year-old squeak," mostly seen in conditioned young horses but can be seen at an older age as well	None
	PMI over basal area (aortic valve) but may radiate toward the apex and over the entire thorax May also be heard from the right side of the thorax Often musical quality Holo- or pandiastolic Often >Grade III/VI	Aortic regurgitation	If: Horse >15 years old and sinus rhythm, normal HR, normal exercise tolerance, normal clinical exam Then: Regular monitoring If in doubt: ECHO If: Horse <15 years old or resting HR >45 bpm or arrhythmia or bounding pulses Then: ECHO and exercise ECG
Right side Systolic murmur	PMI over apical area (tricuspid valve) Grade I–VI/VI	Tricuspid regurgitation	Often no significant effect on performance If in doubt: ECHO
	PMI ventrally to tricuspid valve, just above the sternal border Often pansystolic Often >Grade IV/VI NOTE: Often a holosystolic murmur at the pulmonary valve is also heard due to relative pulmonic stenosis	Ventricular septal defect	ECHO
Diastolic murmur	PMI over basal area	Aortic regurgitation	See aortic regurgitation above

Overview of the most commonly auscultated cardiac murmurs in horses and suggestions for further diagnostics. For more detailed description of these diseases, see the relevant chapters. *ECG*, electrocardiography; *ECHO*, echocardiography; *HR*, heart rate; *PMI*, point of maximal intensity.

AUTHOR: **RIKKE BUHL**

Cardiac Murmurs, Causes

Differential Diagnosis

Cardiac Murmur	Lesion Identified by Echocardiography, Catheterization, or Necropsy
Functional murmurs*	No identifiable lesions
Congenital heart disease murmurs	Defect(s) in the atrial or ventricular septa, patent ductus arteriosus, atresia/stenosis of the tricuspid or pulmonic valve, valve stenosis, other malformations of the heart
Mitral regurgitation	High-level training, degenerative thickening of the valve, bacterial endocarditis, mitral valve prolapse into left atrium, rupture of a chorda tendinea, dilated-hypokinetic ventricle (dilated cardiomyopathy), papillary muscle lesion or dysfunction, valvulitis, malformation
Tricuspid regurgitation	High-level training,[†] same causes as for as mitral regurgitation, also pulmonary hypertension from severe left-sided heart failure or chronic respiratory disease
Aortic regurgitation	Degeneration of the aortic valve, congenital fenestration of the valve, bacterial endocarditis,[‡] aortic prolapse into a ventricular septal defect or the left ventricle, flail aortic valve leaflet, valvulitis, malformation, ruptured aorta or aortic sinus of Valsalva
Pulmonary insufficiency	Bacterial endocarditis,[‡] pulmonary hypertension, flail pulmonic valve leaflet, valvulitis, malformation, rupture of the pulmonary artery
Murmur associated with vegetative endocarditis	Insufficiency of the affected valve[‡]

Modified from Bonagura JD: Clinical evaluation and management of heart disease. *Equine Vet Educ* 2:31–37, 1990.

*Functional murmur may be innocent (unknown cause) or physiologic (suspected physiologic cause). Functional murmurs are common in foals and trained athletes (athletic murmur), associated with fever and high sympathetic nervous system activity (pain, stress, sepsis), and often are heard in anemic horses. Functional murmurs depend on the physiologic state and can be altered by changing the heart rate. Such dynamic auscultation is useful in detecting functional murmurs.

[†]Doppler echocardiography can identify "silent" regurgitation across a right-sided cardiac valve in some horses; this is probably a normal finding of no clinical significance.

[‡]Anatomic stenosis generally is caused by a large vegetation and also should be associated with a diastolic murmur of valvular insufficiency; increased flow across the valve, even in the absence of a true stenosis, may generate a murmur of "relative" valvular stenosis (eg, with aortic regurgitation a systolic ejection murmur may occur because of an increased stroke volume).

Cardiovascular Disease

Congenital cardiac malformation
  Simple systemic-to-pulmonary shunts (left to right)
    Atrial septal defect
    Ventricular septal defect
      Paramembranous defect
      Ventricular inlet defect
      Subarterial (subpulmonic) defect
      Muscular defect
    Patent ductus arteriosus
  Patent foramen ovale (permitting right-to-left shunting)
  Valvular dysplasia
    Mitral stenosis/atresia
    Pulmonic stenosis (bicuspid pulmonary valve)
    Pulmonary atresia (leading to a right-to-left shunt)
    Tricuspid stenosis/atresia (leading to a right-to-left shunt)
    Aortic stenosis/insufficiency (bicuspid or quadricuspid valve)
  Subaortic rings with stenosis
  Tetralogy of Fallot
  Pulmonary atresia with ventricular septal defect (pseudo-truncus arteriosus)
  Double-outlet right ventricle
  Subaortic stenosis
  Hypoplastic left side of the heart
  Other complex malformations
Valvular heart disease causing valve insufficiency or stenosis
  Congenital valve malformation
  Semilunar valve fenestrations causing valve insufficiency
  Degenerative (fibrosis) or myxomatous disease causing valve insufficiency
  Valvular prolapse
  Bacterial endocarditis causing valve insufficiency with or without stenosis
  Rupture of a chorda tendinea causing mitral or tricuspid valve insufficiency
  Rupture of a valve leaflet causing flail leaflet and valve insufficiency
  Noninfective valvulitis
  Valvular regurgitation following dilation of the heart or a great vessel
  Papillary muscle dysfunction causing valvular insufficiency
Myocardial disease
  Idiopathic dilated cardiomyopathy: ventricular dilation and myocardial contractility failure
  Myocarditis
  Myocardial fibrosis
    Ischemic (embolic?) myocardial fibrosis
    Parasitic (*Strongylus*) embolization
  Myocardial degeneration/necrosis
    Myocardial ischemia
    Myocardial infarction
    Toxic injury (eg, monensin)
    Nutritional deficiencies (eg, selenium deficiency)
  Myocardial neoplasia
    Lymphosarcoma
    Melanoma

Hemangioma/hemangiosarcoma
Pulmonary carcinoma
Infiltrative myocardial disease (eg, amyloidosis)
Pericardial disease
Pericardial effusion with or without cardiac tamponade
Infective: bacterial or viral
Idiopathic pericardial effusion
Constrictive pericardial disease
Mass lesion (intrapericardial or extrapericardial) compressing the heart
Pulmonary hypertension and cor pulmonale
Pulmonary hypertension following left-sided heart disease
Pulmonary vascular disease following left-to-right shunt
Immature pulmonary circulation
Primary bronchopulmonary or pulmonary vascular disease
Alveolar hypoxia with reactive pulmonary arterial vasoconstriction
Severe acidosis
Pulmonary thromboembolism

Cardiac arrhythmias
Atrial arrhythmias
Junctional (nodal) arrhythmias
Ventricular arrhythmias
Conduction disturbances
Vascular diseases
Congenital vascular lesions
Rupture of the aorta, pulmonary artery, or systemic artery
Aneurysm of the aortic sinus of Valsalva
Aortic or aortoiliac degenerative disease
Arteritis
Infective
Immune-mediated
(Jugular) Venous thrombosis/thrombophlebitis
Pulmonary embolism
Mass lesion or tumor obstructing blood flow
Aorto-iliac thrombosis

From Bonagura JD, Reef VB, Schwarzwald CC: Cardiovascular diseases. In Reed SM, Bayly WM, Sellon DC (eds). *Equine Internal Medicine*, ed 3. St Louis, 2010, Saunders, pp 372–487.

Cardiovascular Association of Poor Performance

Arrhythmias
Atrial premature complexes
Ventricular premature complexes
Atrial fibrillation
Supraventricular tachycardia
Ventricular tachycardia
Advanced second-degree atrioventricular block
Complete third-degree atrioventricular block
Congenital, valvular, or myocardial heart diseases associated with murmurs
Ventricular septal defect
Mitral regurgitation
Tricuspid regurgitation
Aortic regurgitation

Cardiomyopathy with secondary atrioventricular valvular regurgitation
Occult heart disease
Pericardial disease
Cardiomyopathy or myocarditis
Ischemic myocardial disease (?)
Vascular disorders
Aortic-iliac thrombosis
Jugular vein thrombosis/thrombophlebitis (bilateral)
Aortic root rupture (aorto-cardiac fistula)
Peripheral vein thrombosis/thrombophlebitis

From Bonagura JD, Reef VB, Schwarzwald CC: Cardiovascular diseases. In Reed SM, Bayly WM, Sellon DC (eds). *Equine Internal Medicine*, ed 3. St Louis, 2010, Saunders, pp 372–487.

Cervical Defects

Persistent/chronic endometrial infection: Endometrial infections may be found secondary to a cervical defect, but should be diagnosed and treated prior to surgical intervention. Endometrial infections can also be the cause of infertility independent of cervical defects.

Endometrial/periglandular fibrosis: Chronic inflammation/infections may lead to extensive periglandular fibrosis that may impede maintenance of pregnancy in the mare. If a cervical defect is diagnosed, an endometrial biopsy may assist in determining the extent of endometrial damage and give a prognosis if the mare may conceive and carry a foal to term.

Ascending placentitis (pregnancy): Mares that become pregnant and have a cervical defect may present with ascending placentitis. The defect cannot be diagnosed or treated during pregnancy, but treatment for the duration of the pregnancy with appropriate antibiotics, antiinflammatory medications, and uterine quiescent medications will be necessary.

AUTHOR: **CHELSEA MAKLOSKI**

Colic in the Adult Horse

Gastrointestinal causes
Large intestine
  Displacement
    Left dorsal displacement of the large colon (nephro-splenic)
    Right dorsal displacement of the large colon
  Large colon volvulus
  Obstruction
    Cecal, large colon, or small colon impaction
    Enterolith, fecalith, or phytobezoar
    Intussusception
    Mass
  Inflammation
    Colitis or typhlitis
  Nonstrangulating infarction
Small Intestine
  Obstruction
    Strangulating obstruction (see *Small Intestinal DIstension* in this section for exhaustive list)
    Foreign body
    Ileal impaction
    Intussusception
    Nonstrangulating infarction

Anterior enteritis
  Inflammatory bowel disease
Stomach
  Gastric ulcers
  Gastric impaction
  Gastric emptying disorder
Nongastrointestinal causes
Primary peritonitis
Abdominal abscess
Kidney or urinary tract disease
  Pyelonephritis
  Cystic or urethral calculi
  Urinary tract infection
Hepatic disease
  Cholangiohepatitis
  Hepatic encephalopathy
Reproductive tract disorders
  Uterine torsion
  Impending abortion (or parturition)
  Testicular torsion
  Epididymitis
  Inguinal hernia

Decreased Fecal Output

Decreased intake
Low-bulk diet, such as complete pellets only
Cecal, large colon, or small colon impaction
  Foreign body
  Phytobezoar

Fecalith or enterolith
Ileus
Grass sickness

AUTHOR: **SARA GOMEZ-IBANEZ**

Diarrhea in Foals

Nursing foals
Rotavirus
Necrotizing enterocolitis (*C. difficile, C. perfringens, Bacteroides fragilis*)
Salmonellosis
Enterotoxigenic *E. coli*
Cryptosporidium
Lactose intolerance
"Foal heat" diarrhea
Gastric ulcers

Weanlings and yearlings (also see adult causes)
Lawsonia intracellularis
Rhodococcus equi enterocolitis
Parasitism
Gastric ulcers

AUTHOR: **SARA GOMEZ-IBANEZ**

Diarrhea, Neonatal

Noninfectious
  Foal heat diarrhea
  Mechanical enterocolitis (pica)
  Dietary (milk replacer intolerance, lactase deficiency)
  Necrotizing enterocolitis
  Peripartum asphyxia associated (hypoxic-ischemic disease, dystocia, premature placental separation)
  Gastric ulcers
Infectious
  Clostridium difficile
  Clostridium perfringens

Salmonellosis
Enterotoxigenic *E. coli*
Rotavirus
Adenovirus (severe combined immunodeficiency [SCID] foals especially)
Cryptosporidium parvum

AUTHOR: **PHOEBE A. SMITH**

Draining Tracts from Jaw

Soft tissue origin
  Foreign body
  Sialo-cutaneous fistula
  Abscess
  Severe cellulitis ± dermatitis (eg, *Staphylococcus aureus* infection or dermatophycosis)

Bony origin
  Mandibular fracture
  Oro-cutaneous fistula
  Sequestrum
Swelling originating from internal structures
  Periapical infection: Tooth

AUTHOR: **JAMES L. CARMALT**

Dysphagia, Gastrointestinal

Structural causes
  Oral, lingual, or pharyngeal foreign body
  Dental disease
  Esophageal obstruction
    Feed impaction
    Stricture
  Pharyngeal obstruction
    Retropharyngeal lymphadenopathy
    Retropharyngeal mass
    Guttural pouch tympany
  Abnormal anatomy
    Cleft palate
    Subepiglottic cyst
    Fractured mandible
Functional causes
  Neurologic (central)
    Equine protozoal myelitis
    Viral encephalitis
    Cerebral trauma
    Toxic neuropathy (eg, yellow star thistle)

Neurologic (peripheral)
  Toxic neuropathy (eg, lead poisoning)
Guttural pouch pathology
  Empyema
  Mycosis
  Tympany
Neuromuscular
  Botulism
  Organophosphate poisoning
  Grass sickness
Muscular
  White muscle disease (foals)

AUTHOR: **SARA GOMEZ-IBANEZ**

DIFFERENTIAL DIAGNOSES

Edema, Peripheral or Ventral: Common Causes

Congestive heart failure
Valvular disease
Myocarditis
Monensin toxicosis
Vasculitis
Equine viral arteritis
Equine ehrlichiosis
Purpura hemorrhagica
Equine infectious anemia
Venous obstruction and congestion
Catheter-related thrombophlebitis
Disseminated intravascular coagulation
Tight bandages
Tumors
Immobility
Cellulitis
Staphylococcal
Clostridial
Counterirritant application
Lymphatic obstruction
Ulcerative lymphangitis
Lymphadenitis (*Streptococcus equi, Corynebacterium pseudotuberculosis*)

Lymphosarcoma
Tumors
Hypoalbuminemia
Parasitism
Pleural and peritoneal effusions
Protein loss (gastrointestinal, renal, or wounds)
Inadequate production (starvation)
Hemodilution (subsequent to hemorrhage)
Shock
Hemorrhagic
Endotoxic
Pleuritis
Late-term pregnancy
Prepubic tendon rupture
Starvation
Inadequate intake
Malabsorption

From Hinchcliff KW: Edema. In Reed SM, Bayly WM, Sellon DC (eds). *Equine Internal Medicine*, ed 3. St Louis, 2010, Saunders, pp 131–134.

Equine Diarrhea Differentials and Diagnostic Tests in Adults and Foals

Differential Diagnosis

NEONATES/FOALS		ADULTS	
Infectious	**Noninfectious**	**Infectious**	**Noninfectious**
Bacterial	Foal heat diarrhea	Bacterial	Dietary
Clostridium perfringens type A, B, C	Dietary	*Salmonella*	Teeth abnormalities
Clostridium difficile		*Clostridium difficile*	Neoplasia
Lawsonia intracellularis		*Aeromonas*	Right dorsal colitis
Salmonella		*Listeria monocytogenes*	Enteritis
Rhodococcus equi		Rickettsial	Cantharidin toxicosis
Clostridium piliforme		*Neorickettsia risticii*	NSAID toxicity
Aeromonas		Parasitic	
Bacteroides		Cyathostomiasis	
Viral		Protozoal	
Rotavirus		*Giardia*	
Coronavirus		*Cryptosporidium*	
Parasitic		Endotoxemia	
Strongyloidosis		Fungal	
Protozoal		Histoplasmosis	
Cryptosporidium			
Giardia			
Sepsis			
Endotoxemia			

NSAID, nonsteroidal antiinflammatory drug.

Summary of Diagnostics for the Most Common Causes of Diarrhea in Foals and Adults

	C. difficile	C. perfringens	Salmonella enteritidis	Lawsonia intracellularis	Neorickettsia risticii	Parasites
Sample to submit	Feces (collect and send in anaerobic culturette)	Feces (collect and send in anaerobic culturette)	Feces	Feces and serum	Feces, buffy coat, serum	Feces
Test run	1. ELISA 2. Cytotoxicity assay 3. Gram stain	1. Anaerobic culture 2. PCR 3. Gram stain	Culture PCR	1. PCR 2. ELISA	1. PCR (feces, buffy coat) 2. IFA (serum)	Fecal
Testing for	1. Toxin A & B 2. Toxin B 3. Organism	1. Organism 2. Toxin 3. Organism	Organism	1. Organism 2. Antibodies	Organism	Eggs and larvae

ELISA, enzyme-linked immunosorbent assay; IFA, indirect fluorescent antibody; PCR, polymerase chain reaction.

AUTHOR: **MELISSA BOURGEOIS**

Esophageal Disorders

Differential Diagnosis

Disorder	Presenting Complaints	Diagnosis	Treatment
Acquired Disorders			
Choke	Nasal discharge of saliva and food, retching, excessive salivation, cough, sweating, extension of head and neck	Passage of a nasogastric tube, endoscopy	Medical and surgical treatment options as described in Esophageal Obstruction in Section I text
Foreign bodies	Acute or recurrent choke	Endoscopy, radiography	Manual retrieval or removal, endoscopic removal, surgery
External compression	Acute or recurrent choke	Endoscopy, radiography, ultrasound	Removal of the obstructive mass
Muscular hypertrophy	No clinical signs observed in most affected horses; may predispose to esophageal diverticula	Incidental finding at necropsy	None
Gastroesophageal reflux disease	Inappetence, bruxism, ptyalism, colic, gastric reflux, weight loss, exercise intolerance	Esophageal and gastric endoscopy	Correct primary problem, decrease gastric acidity, gastric protectants, surgery
Stricture	Recurrent choke, weight loss	Endoscopy, contrast radiography	Bougienage, surgery
Diverticula*	Recurrent choke, weight loss	Endoscopy, contrast radiography	Surgery
Perforation, trauma	Salivation, bruxism, cough, nasal discharge, sepsis	Endoscopy	Enteral feeding, supportive care
Megaesophagus*	Recurrent choke, intermittent food and saliva from nares, pneumonia, weight loss, colic	Endoscopy, contrast radiography	Nutritional modification as described in text
Neoplasia	Recurrent choke, weight loss	Endoscopy, biopsy	Surgical resection
Granulation tissue	Recurrent choke, swelling in the region of the cervical esophagus	Endoscopy, biopsy	Laser surgical resection
Congenital Disorders			
Tubular duplication of the esophagus	Young horse, mass caudal to mandible, dyspnea, dysphagia, nasal regurgitation of food and saliva	Radiography and ultrasonography of mass, endoscopy, contrast radiography	Surgical excision
Cystic duplication of the esophagus	Young horse, mass in cervical or throatlatch area, recurrent choke, bruxism, excessive salivation, nasal regurgitation of saliva and feed, weight loss	Endoscopy, ultrasonography, aspiration of cyst, contrast radiography	Surgical excision, marsupialization of cyst
Vascular ring anomaly	Cervical swelling after introduction to solid feed, chronic respiratory disease	Endoscopy, contrast radiography, computed tomography, magnetic resonance imaging	Surgical correction

Continued

DIFFERENTIAL DIAGNOSES

Differential Diagnosis—cont'd

Disorder	Presenting Complaints	Diagnosis	Treatment
Congenital stenosis	Nasal regurgitation of milk, cough	Endoscopy, contrast radiography	Dietary management as described in text
Ectasia	Nasal regurgitation of milk	Histologic evaluation	None described

From Sanchez LC: Esophageal diseases. In Reed SM, Bayly WM, Sellon DC (eds). *Equine Internal Medicine,* ed 3. St Louis, 2010, Saunders, pp 830–838.

*May occur as congenital or acquired lesions.

Esophageal Obstruction

Differential Diagnosis

Category	Differential	Examples
Intraluminal	Foreign body Feed material	Apples, potatoes
Extramural	Neoplasia Vascular ring anomaly Granuloma	Squamous cell carcinoma, lymphoma Persistent right aortic arch
Intramural	Esophageal abscess Granuloma Neoplasia Cysts Diverticula Stenosis	Squamous cell carcinoma, leiomyosarcoma Intramural cysts, duplication cysts
Functional disorders	Dehydration Exhaustion Pharmacologic Primary megaesophagus Esophagitis Autonomic dysautonomia Vagal neuropathies	Acepromazine, detomidine Congenital ectasia

From Sanchez LC: Esophageal diseases. In Reed SM, Bayly WM, Sellon DC (eds). *Equine Internal Medicine,* ed 3. St Louis, 2010, Saunders, pp 830–838.

Facial Swelling

Soft tissue origin
Foreign body
Neoplasia
Squamous cell carcinoma
Melanoma
Sarcoid
Sialolith
Abscess
Bony origin
Fibroma
Suture line exostosis
Bone cyst
Facial fracture ± sequestrum

Swelling originating from internal structures
Paranasal sinus cyst
Primary or secondary sinusitis
Periapical infection: Tooth
Osteoma
Normal eruption cysts ("bumps")

AUTHOR: **JAMES L. CARMALT**

Failure of Passive Transfer

Maternal causes
  Premature lactation
    Placentitis
    Twins
    Premature placental separation
  Poor colostral quality
    Maiden mares
    Older mares
  Failure of lactation
    Aglactia
    Fescue toxicosis

Foal causes
  Failure to ingest colostrums
    Weakness
    Prematurity
    Musculoskeletal deformity
    Perinatal asphyxia syndrome
  Failure to absorb colostrums
    Prematurity
    Necrotizing enterocolitis

From Sellon DC, Wilkins PA: Failure of passive transfer. In Reed SM, Bayly WM, Sellon DC (eds). *Equine Internal Medicine,* ed 3. St Louis, 2010, Saunders, pp 1335–1336.

Fungal Diseases

Differential Diagnosis

Disease	Common Causative Agents	Clinical Signs
Superficial Infections		
Dermatophytosis	*Microsporum* and *Trichophyton* spp.	Circular patches or hair loss, crusting and scaling, urticaria, papules
Piedra	*Piedraia* spp. or *Trichosporon beigelii*	Black or white filamentous nodules on hair shaft
Intermediate Infections		
Sporotrichosis	*Sporothrix schenckii*	Papules and nodules occur along lymphatics; nodules may ulcerate, become thickened, and drain a thick brown to red-colored exudate
Phaeohyphomycosis (chronic, subcutaneous fungal infection caused by pigmented opportunistic fungi)	*Hormodendrum, Drechslera, Phialophora, Curvularia, Cladosporium*	Single or multiple nodules; lesions may be grossly or microscopically pigmented, nonpruritic, nonpainful, and cool to the touch
Mycetoma (chronic subcutaneous infection)	Filamentous bacterial organisms and opportunistic fungi	Single or multiple nodular lesions are present; ulcerated, draining tracts are common; mycetomata discharge tissue grains in contrast to phaeohyphomycosis, which does not

From Rees CA: Disorders of the skin. In Reed SM, Bayly WM, Sellon DC (eds). *Equine internal medicine*, ed. 3. St. Louis, 2010, Saunders, pp 682–729.

Gastric Reflux

Anterior enteritis
  Duodenitis/proximal jejunitis
Small intestinal obstruction
  Ileal impaction
  Strangulating obstruction
  Small intestinal foreign body
    Phytobezoar
    Trichobezoar
  Small intestinal obstruction secondary to large intestinal distension or displacement
Gastric obstruction
  Gastric impaction
  Gastric emptying defect

  Gastric foreign body
    Phytobezoar
    Trichobezoar
Dysmotility
  Postoperative ileus
  Grass sickness
Peritonitis

AUTHOR: **SARA GOMEZ-IBANEZ**

Hematuria

Blood clots in the bladder of neonatal foals
Cantharidiasis (blister beetle toxicosis)
  Alfalfa hay feeding
  Clinicopathologic abnormalities include hyperkalemia, hypocalcemia, hypomagnesemia, and azotemia
Cystitis
Exercise-induced hematuria
Glomerulonephritis
Hemoglobinuria
  Increased mean corpuscular hemoglobin (MCH), mean corpuscular hemoglobin concentration (MCHC)
  Serum is discolored due to hemolysis
Idiopathic hematuria
  Reported primarily in Arabians
Myoglobinuria
  Elevated creatine kinase (CK), aspartate aminotransferase (AST), and lactate dehydrogenase (LDH) activity
  Serum is not discolored
Neoplasia
Nonsteroidal antiinflammatory drug toxicity
Pigmenturia
  Plant (red and white clover) and drug (rifampin, phenothiazine, nitazoxanide, phenazopyridine, doxycycline) derived urinary pigments

Polycystic kidney disease
  Ultrasonographic examination of the kidneys may show multiple hypoechoic cystic structures
Pyelonephritis
Pyrocatechin
  An oxidizing agent normally found in urine
Urethral rent
  Hematuria at the end of urination in geldings
  Endoscopic examination reveals a 5- to 10-mm linear defect on the convex surface of the urethra, distal to the openings of the bulbourethral glands, near the level of the ischial arch
Urolithiasis
  Hematuria after exercise indicates cystic calculi
Vascular anomaly
  Color-flow Doppler ultrasonography for diagnosis

Schumacher J: Hematuria and pigmenturia of horses. *Vet Clin N Am Equine Pract* 23:655, 2007.

AUTHORS: JOHN SCHUMACHER and **BRYAN M. WALDRIDGE**

Hemolysis

Infectious diseases
  Piroplasmosis
  Equine infectious anemia (EIA)
Immune-mediated disease
  Autoimmune disease
  Bacterial infection
    Clostridium perfringens
    Streptococcal infections
  Viral infection
    EIA
  Neoplasia
    Lymphosarcoma
  Drug reaction
    Penicillin
  Neonatal isoerythrolysis
Oxidative Injury
  Phenothiazine
  Onion

Red maple leaf
Familial methemoglobinemia
Iatrogenic conditions
  Hypotonic solutions
  Hypertonic saline
Miscellaneous conditions
  Hepatic disease
  Hemolytic uremic syndrome
  Disseminated intravascular coagulation (DIC)
Other toxicities
  Intravenous dimethyl sulfoxide
  Bacterial toxins (*Clostridium*)
  Oak
  Burn injury

From Sellon DC, Wise LN: Disorders of the Hematopoietic System. In Reed SM, Bayly WM, Sellon DC (eds). *Equine Internal Medicine*, ed 3. St Louis, 2010, Saunders, pp 730–776.

Hemorrhage

Degenerative disorders
  Vessel rupture
    Aorta
    Middle uterine artery

Anomalies
  Idiopathic hematuria in geldings and stallions
  Coagulation abnormalities
    Genetic platelet function disorders
    Coagulation factor disorders (von Willebrand's disease)

Neoplastic conditions
    Paranasal sinus and skull neoplasia
    Urogenital (renal, ureteral, bladder, uterine, perineal) neoplasia
    Abdominal organ neoplasia
Inflammatory
    Infectious
        Guttural pouch mycosis (*Aspergillis* species)
        Pneumonia
        Pleuritis
        Paranasal sinus infection
        Pyelonephritis
        Cystitis
        Urolithiasis
        Abdominal abscess (*Streptococcus equi*)
    Parasitic
        Verminous arteritis
        Gastrointestinal and ectoparasites
    Noninfectious
        Gastrointestinal ulceration
        Hepatic failure (lack of coagulation factors)
        Envenomation
        Systemic inflammatory response syndrome
Immune disorders
    Granulomatous enteritis

Trauma
    Exercise-induced pulmonary hemorrhage
    Head trauma, skull fracture
    Ventral straight muscle (longus capitus and rectus capitus ventralis muscle) rupture
        Poll trauma
    Thoracic trauma
    Rib fracture
    Abdominal trauma
        Splenic rupture
        Hepatic fracture
        Mesenteric vessel rupture
    Iatrogenic trauma
        Surgery
        Nasogastric intubation
        Percutaneous biopsy
    Wounds
    Foreign bodies
Toxicity
    Nonsteroidal antiinflammatory medications (right dorsal colitis)
    Rodenticides
    Heparin overdose
    High-dose colloid administration (hetastarch or dextran)

AUTHOR: **AMELIA MUNSTERMAN**

Hepatic Disease, Acute

Theiler's disease (Serum-associated hepatitis)
Hyperlipemia/hepatic lipidosis
Tyzzer's disease
Cholangiohepatitis
Acute biliary obstruction
    Cholelithiasis
    Colon displacement
    Hepatic torsion
Parasitic hepatitis
    Parascaris equorum
    Large *Strongyles*
    Echinococcus granulosa
Toxic hepatopathy
    Plants

Mycotoxins
    Chemicals
    Drugs
    Iron
Viral hepatitis
    Equine infectious anemia
    Equine herpesvirus type 1
    Equine viral arteritis
    Giant cell hepatopathy

Barton MH: Diseases of the liver. In Reed SM, Bayly WM, Sellon DC (eds). *Equine Internal Medicine,* ed 3. St Louis, 2010, Saunders, pp 939–975.

AUTHOR: **MICHELLE HENRY BARTON**

Hepatic Disease, Chronic

Pyrrolizidine alkaloid toxicity
Clover poisoning
Chronic active hepatitis
Cholelithiasis
Gastroduodenal obstruction
Abscess
Neoplasia
    Metastatic infiltration of the liver
    Cholangiocarcinoma
    Hepatocellular carcinoma
    Hepatoblastoma
    Mixed hamartoma

Amyloidosis
Chronic hypoxia
Congenital or heritable—may be acute or chronic
    Portosystemic shunt
    Biliary atresia
    Hyperammonemia of Morgans

Barton MH: Diseases of the liver. In Reed SM, Bayly WM, Sellon DC (eds). *Equine Internal Medicine,* ed 3. St Louis, 2010, Saunders, pp 939–975.

AUTHOR: **MICHELLE HENRY BARTON**

Hypersalivation (Ptyalism)

Esophageal obstruction
Slaframine toxicosis (from ingesting mold on red clover)
Lesions of the oral cavity and tongue
　Grass awns or other foreign body
　Vesicular lesions
　Laceration
　Abscess

Dysphagia (see above for more exhaustive list) In particular:
　Pharyngitis
　Botulism
　Grass sickness
Gastric ulceration (especially in foals)

AUTHOR: **SARA GOMEZ-IBANEZ**

Hypoxemia

Hypoxia-oxygen responsive
　Iatrogenic (reduced inspired oxygen content)
　　Anesthetic circuit malfunction
　Environmental
　　High altitudes
Hypoventilation (ventilation/perfusion ratio <1): Oxygen responsive
　Neurogenic
　　Anesthesia, head trauma, central nervous system neoplasia, edema, or infection
　Musculoskeletal
　　Botulism, tetanus, paralytic medications
　Pulmonary
　　Pneumothorax, pleural effusion, flail chest
　Mechanical
　　Upper airway obstruction, laryngeal hemiplegia
　Iatrogenic
　　Anesthetic circuit malfunction, anesthetic overdose
Reduced diffusion: Oxygen responsive
　Pulmonary disease
　　Pneumonia, pulmonary edema or fibrosis, recurrent airway obstruction, acute respiratory distress syndrome, or acute lung injury

Ventilation/perfusion mismatch (ventilation/perfusion ratio >1):
　Oxygen responsive
　Positional
　　Prolonged recumbency
Vascular shunt: Oxygen resistant
　Pulmonary
　　Atelectasis, pneumonia, pulmonary edema, neoplasia
　Cardiovascular
　　Tetralogy of Fallot, patent foramen ovale, patent ductus arteriosis

SUGGESTED READING

Chevalier H, et al: Pulmonary dysfunction in adult horses in the intensive care unit. *Clin Tech Eq Pract* 2(2):165–177, 2003.
Wilkins PA: Disorders of foals. In Reed SM, Bayly WM, Sellon DC (eds). *Equine Internal Medicine*, ed 3. St Louis, 2010, Saunders, pp 1338–1339.

AUTHOR: **AMELIA MUNSTERMAN**

Icterus in the Neonatal Foal

Hemolytic anemia: As seen with neonatal isoerythrolysis
Sepsis: Often accompanied by leukopenia, left shift, injected mucous membranes, hypoperfusion
Anorexia: Elevation in indirect bilirubin
Equine herpesvirus type 1 infection: Also see weakness at birth, neurologic signs, leukopenia

Tyzzer's Disease: Also see profound hypoglycemia, acute liver failure

AUTHOR: **PHOEBE A. SMITH**

Inappetence

Gastrointestinal discomfort (colic)
  Gastric ulcers
  Small intestinal distension
  Gastric dilation
  Impaction (any type)
Fever
Infection
  Pneumonia
  Enterocolitis
  Peritonitis

Severe pain
Noninfectious systemic disease
  Neoplasia
  Renal disease
  Heart failure
  Liver failure
  Recurrent airway obstruction

AUTHOR: **SARA GOMEZ-IBANEZ**

Lameness in the Neonate

Septic arthritis
Septic physitis
Fracture (don't forget the third phalanx or pelvis)
Soft tissue injuries (strains or sprains)

Congenital flexural deformity
Congenital malformation of musculoskeletal system

AUTHOR: **ELIZABETH M. SANTSCHI**

Large Intestinal Distension

Gas accumulation (tympany)
Obstruction
  Cecal impaction
  Large colon impaction
  Small colon impaction
  Enterolith
  Fecalith
  Phytobezoar
  Mass
  Meconium impaction (foals)

Displacement
  Right dorsal displacement of the large colon
  Left dorsal displacement of the large colon (nephrosplenic)
  Large colon volvulus
Other
  Cecal dysfunction
  Mesocolic rupture (post-foaling)
  Nonstrangulating infarction

AUTHOR: **SARA GOMEZ-IBANEZ**

Lower Airway Disorders That May Be Associated with Respiratory Distress in Adult Horses

Pulmonary disorders
  Pulmonary edema
  Diffuse interstitial pneumonia
  Aspiration pneumonia
  Abscessing or coalescing bronchopneumonia
  Acute respiratory distress syndrome
  Silicosis
  Smoke inhalation

Extrapulmonary disorders
  Pleural effusion
  Intrathoracic hemorrhage
  Pneumothorax

From Barr B: Support of respiratory function. In Reed SM, Bayly WM, Sellon DC (eds). *Equine Internal Medicine*, ed 3. St Louis, 2010, Saunders, pp 265–269.

Melena

Any source of mucosal inflammation, erosion, or ulceration
  Gastric ulcers
  Right dorsal colitis
  Intestinal neoplasia
  Enteritis or enterocolitis

Ingested blood
  Traumatic nasogastric intubation
  Hemorrhage from respiratory tract
Hemorrhage occurring distal to the right dorsal colon may appear as hematochezia

AUTHOR: **SARA GOMEZ-IBANEZ**

Muscle Disease

Myopathies associated with rhabdomyolysis, creatine kinase (CK) typically high (eg, >2,000 IU)
  Polysaccharide storage myopathy: Most likely diagnosis in any horse that has "tied up"
  Recurrent exertional rhabdomyolysis: May be a cause of tying up in Thoroughbreds
  Streptococcal-associated myopathy: Rhabdomyolysis and rapid muscle atrophy in young Quarter horses and draft horses exposed to streptococcus or other respiratory disease; purpura hemorrhagica causing infarctive myopathy in any age or breed
  Selenium deficiency myopathy (masticatory myopathy): Adult horses with severe selenium deficiency—targets masticatory muscles; severe acute disease can cause recumbency
  Toxic myopathy: Ionophore exposure, plant toxicity
  Pasture-associated myopathy: Unknown cause; must rule out other possible causes of rhabdomyolysis
Myopathies and denervating diseases associated with weakness, CK typically low (eg, <2,000 IU)
  Polysaccharide storage myopathy: especially in draft-related horses
  Equine motor neuron disease: Long-term (e.g., 1 year or more) severe vitamin E deficiency—little or no grass pasture, alfalfa products, or vitamin E supplementation
  Botulism

Hyperkalemic periodic paralysis: CK should be normal; episodic weakness; myotonic discharges on electromyogram (EMG); DNA test diagnostic
Myopathies and denervating diseases associated with abnormal gait
  Polysaccharide storage myopathy: Unexplained hind limb lameness, shivers, or stiff gait
  Neuropathy: Causing fibrotic myopathy or stringhalt; generalized short-strided gait in equine motor neuron disease
  Myotonic dystrophy-like myopathy: Young horses, progressive muscle hypertrophy and stiff gait, myotonic discharges on EMG
Myopathies and denervating diseases associated with symmetric muscle atrophy
  Equine motor neuron disease: See above
  Polysaccharide storage myopathy
  Streptococcal-associated rhabdomyolysis: See above
  Pituitary pars intermedia dysfunction (Cushing's disease)
  Selenium deficiency myopathy: masticatory muscles or tongue

SUGGESTED READING

Valentine BA, McGavin MD: Skeletal muscle. In McGavin MD, Zachary JF (eds). *Pathologic Basis of Veterinary Disease*. St Louis, 2010, Mosby Elsevier, pp 996–1039.

AUTHOR: **BETH A. VALENTINE**

Muscle Disease: Problem-Based Approach

Disorders are grouped according to similar clinical appearance. (No category is mutually exclusive. Disorders are grouped by most common clinical presentation. The reader is directed to the text for more extensive discussion for each disorder or disease.)

Profound muscle cramping with exercise, tying-up syndrome, increased plasma/serum creatine kinase (CK) activity after exercise
  Horses with inborn myopathy (inborn error of metabolism)
    Recurrent exertional rhabdomyolysis in Thoroughbreds
    Polysaccharide storage myopathy in Quarter Horses and draft horses
    Idiopathic chronic exertional rhabdomyolysis
    Mitochondrial myopathy (also has lactic acidosis)

  Horses without inborn myopathy
    Overexertion
    Vitamin E or selenium deficiency
    Electrolyte depletion
Horses with altered gait but without inborn myopathy and without muscle cramping; with or without elevated CK
  Acute: Muscle strain, sprain, tear
  Chronic: Fibrotic myopathy
Muscle weakness
  Hyperkalemic periodic paralysis (intermittent)
  Myotonia congenita and myotonia dystrophica (worsens with exercise)
  Equine motor neuron disease (worsens when standing still)

Equine polysaccharide storage myopathy in draft horses (can be progressive over time; rule out shivers as a differential diagnosis)

Muscle wasting

Generalized, may be accompanied by mild elevations in CK activity

Equine motor neuron disease

Streptococcal immune-mediated myositis: Mediated by IgG

Cachectic atrophy

Disuse atrophy

Endocrine; equine Cushing's syndrome

Segmental

Neurogenic

Disuse atrophy

Fibrotic myopathy

Posthealing of severe trauma

Acute rhabdomyolysis, swollen painful musculature, with or without recumbency, with or without death

Severe, acute exercise-related rhabdomyolysis as above

Malignant hyperthermia/postanesthetic myopathy

Clostridial myonecrosis

Sarcocystis spp

Streptococcal immune-mediated myositis; Henoch-Schönlein purpura

Aortic-iliac thrombosis

Toxic plants

Cassia occidentalis

White snakeroot

Ionophore toxicity (may also present as chronic heart failure without a history of acute rhabdomyolysis)

Disorders of the neonate

White muscle disease/nutritional myodegeneration

Foal rhabdomyolysis

Glycogen branching enzyme deficiency

Arthrogryposis

Miscellaneous disorders

Atypical myoglobinuria

Postanesthetic myasthenia

Polymyopathy

Abscesses

Tumors

From MacLeay JM: Disorders of the musculoskeletal system. In Reed SM, Bayly WM, Sellon DC (eds). *Equine Internal Medicine*, ed 3. St Louis, 2010, Saunders, pp 488–544.

Myodegeneration, Nutritionally Related

Atypical myoglobinuria

Botulism

Cerebellar diseases

Colic

Equine motor neuron disease

Equine rhabdomyolysis syndrome

Medullary diseases, such as herpesvirus type 1 and myelitis

Muscular dystrophy

Purpura hemorrhagica

Rabies

Septic polyarthritis

Spinal cord diseases

Suppurative meningitis

Tetanus

Tick paralysis

Trauma

Various causes of dysphagia (eg, cleft palate, ulcers, and peripheral damage to certain cranial nerves)

Various causes of dyspnea (eg, pneumonia and cardiac disease)

From MacLeay JM: Disorders of the musculoskeletal system. In Reed SM, Bayly WM, Sellon DC (eds). *Equine Internal Medicine*, ed 3. St Louis, 2010, Saunders, pp 488–544.

Myopathy

Classification of equine myopathies according to cause

Neurogenic: May be hereditary or environmental in origin, acquired, or congenital

Disorders of anterior horn cells

Disorders of motor nerve roots

Peripheral neuropathies

Disorders of neuromuscular transmission

Botulism

Tetanus

Tick paralysis

Myogenic

Inborn errors of metabolism—genetic

Disorders of carbohydrate metabolism

Polysaccharide storage myopathy in Quarter Horses

Polysaccharide storage myopathy in draft horses

Polysaccharide storage myopathy in Warmblood Horses

Glycogen branching enzyme deficiency

Disorders of lipid metabolism

Multiple acyl-CoA dehydrogenase deficiency (MADD)

Disorders of purine metabolism—no known disorders in the horse

Mitochondrial enzyme deficiencies

Complex I: Nicotinamide adenine dinucleotide (NADH) CoQ reductase deficiency

Channelopathies, aberrations of ion and electrolyte flux

Paramyotonias and myotonias

Hyperkalemic periodic paralysis (paramyotonia)

Myotonia congenita (myotonia)

Myotonia dystrophica (myotonia)

Recurrent exertional rhabdomyolysis in Thoroughbreds

Idiopathic chronic exertional rhabdomyolysis (may be reclassified as additional diseases are identified)

Acquired

Traumatic

Fibrotic myopathy

Gastrocnemius muscle rupture

Serratus ventralis muscle rupture

Inflammatory
Sore or pulled muscles
Infectious
Bacterial
Clostridial myonecrosis
Streptococcus spp
Abscessation
Autoimmune
Purpura hemorrhagica
Immunoglobulin G mediated
Immunoglobulin A mediated (Henoch-Schönlein purpura)
Staphylococcus spp
Corynebacterium pseudotuberculosis
Viral
Parasitic
Sarcocystis spp
Trichinella spiralis
Circulatory
Postanesthetic myositis
Aortic-iliac thrombosis
Nutritional
Vitamin E deficiency; equine motor neuron disease, equine degenerative myelopathy

Nutritional myodegeneration (white muscle disease); vitamin E with and without selenium deficiency
Malnutrition
Electrolyte deficiency
Cachectic atrophy after chronic disease
Exercise-related, overexertion, and the exhausted horse syndrome
Toxic
Cassia occidentalis
White snakeroot
Ionophores
Endocrine
Equine Cushing's syndrome
Hypothyroidism (unsubstantiated)
Disuse atrophy
Malignancy: Muscle tumors
Miscellaneous or idiopathic
Atypical myoglobinuria/pasture associated myopathy
Postanesthetic myasthenia

From MacLeay JM: Disorders of the musculoskeletal system. In Reed SM, Bayly WM, Sellon DC (eds). *Equine Internal Medicine,* ed 3. St Louis, 2010, Saunders, pp 488–544.

Neonatal Colic

Meconium impaction: Hard dry feces in rectum, enema delivers feces, abdominal bloating, large impaction in mid-abdomen can be seen via transabdominal ultrasound, abdominal radiography reveals gas in large colon and cecum and mass in transverse colon.

Atresia coli: No feces ever passed, even with enema, abdominal bloating, gas-filled colon apparent on abdominal radiography with no soft tissue mass, rectal positive contrast material or rectal endoscopy ends in blind sac. Abdominal exploratory is confirmatory.

Enteritis: Diarrhea and fever, nasogastric reflux, low peripheral white blood cell counts, transabdominal ultrasound reveals distended and perhaps thickened small intestine that has uncoordinated, swirling motility, abdominal radiography reveals mildly distended loops of small intestine with gas accumulation.

Small intestinal volvulus: Can have signs similar to enteritis and be difficult to differentiate, and enteritis can precede volvulus. Abdominal radiography reveals severely distended loops of small intestine with gas accumulation, and transabdominal ultrasound reveals distended small intestine that has very little motility and can exhibit particle sedimentation. Abdominal exploratory is confirmatory.

Overo lethal white syndrome (OLWS): All white or nearly white foals from breeds with white skin patches (includes American Paint Horses, Quarter Horses, and American Miniature Horses), no feces ever passed, mucus only, abdominal bloating, transabdominal ultrasound reveals distended small intestine, abdominal radiography reveals small and large intestinal distension. Carrier status of OLWS mutation in mare and stallion supports diagnosis.

Uroperitoneum: Abdominal bloating, some fecal passage, poor urine passage, hyponatremia and hypochloremia, hyperkalemia and acidosis, transabdominal ultrasound reveals fluid accumulation in the peritoneal cavity, abdominal paracentesis reveals clear fluid with high creatinine concentration.

AUTHOR: **ELIZABETH M. SANTSCHI**

Neoplasia of the Gastrointestinal Tract

Esophagus
Squamous cell carcinoma
Stomach
Adenocarcinoma
Gastric polyp
Leiomyosarcoma
Lymphoma (lymphosarcoma)
Squamous cell carcinoma

Small Intestine
Adenocarcinoma
Adenomatous polyposis
Ganglioneuroma
Intestinal carcinoid
Leiomyoma
Leiomyosarcoma
Lipoma
Lymphoma (lymphosarcoma)
Neurofibroma

Cecum
- Adenocarcinoma
- Intestinal myxosarcoma
- Stromal tumor

Large Colon
- Adenocarcinoma
- Lipomatosis
- Lymphoma (lymphosarcoma)
- Neurofibroma

Small Colon
- Lipoma
- Lipomatosis
- Leiomyoma

Rectum
- Leiomyosarcoma
- Lipoma
- Lymphoma (lymphosarcoma)
- Polyps

Peritoneum
- Disseminated leiomyomatosis
- Mesothelioma
- Omental fibrosarcoma

From Zimmel DN: Neoplasia of the alimentary tract in Reed SM, Bayly WM, Sellon DC (eds). *Equine Internal Medicine,* ed 3. St Louis, 2010, Saunders, pp 892–895.

Neoplasia of the Oral Cavity

Odontogenic tumors (originates from dental tissue)
- Ameloblastoma
- Ameloblastic odontoma
- Cementoma
- Complex odontoma
- Compound odontoma
- Fibro-myxoma
- Odontoblastoma

Osteogenic tumors (originates from bone)
- Leiomyosarcoma
- Myxoma
- Osteoma
- Osteosarcoma

Soft tissue tumors
- Epulis
- Fibrous dysplasia
- Hemangiosarcoma
- Juvenile ossifying fibroma
- Melanoma
- Papilloma
- Sarcoid
- Salivary adenocarcinoma
- Squamous cell carcinoma

Tongue
- Chondrosarcoma
- Lymphosarcoma
- Multiple myeloma
- Rhabdomyosarcoma
- Paraneoplastic bullous stomatitis

From Zimmel DN: Neoplasia of the alimentary tract. In Reed SM, Bayly WM, Sellon DC (eds). *Equine Internal Medicine,* ed 3. St Louis, 2010, Saunders, pp 892–895.

Neurologic Disease of Neonatal Foals

Hypoxic-ischemic encephalopathy (perinatal asphyxia syndrome, neonatal maladjustment syndrome, dummy foal): Signs present at birth or develop during first 72 hours of life; signs vary widely, but may include abnormal mentation, decreased affinity for the dam, blindness, seizures

Central nervous system (CNS) trauma

Peripheral nerve injuries

Narcolepsy/cataplexy syndromes: Recognized especially in American Miniatures, Morgans, Suffolks, and Shetlands

Hydrocephalus: Dullness, compulsive walking, head pressing, seizures, ataxia

Bacterial meningitis: Definitely diagnosed with cerebrospinal fluid (CSF) sampling

Cerebellar abiotrophy: Seen in Arabian and Oldenburg foals, intention tremors, wide-base stance

Occipitoatlantoaxial malformation: Inherited in Arabians, random in other breeds, tetraparesis and ataxia of all limbs, head tilt, unusual neck carriage may be present

Lavender foal syndrome: Inherited in Arabians, especially Egyptian Arabians, foals cannot stand or right themselves, opisthotonic, paddling, seizures

Juvenile epilepsy of Arabians: Age of onset birth to 2 to 3 months of age, self-limiting

Botulism: Trembling, milk from mouth and nares when nursing, increased time spent recumbent, blank facial expression, mydriasis

Tetanus: Rapid progression of muscular rigidity and hyperresponsiveness to stimuli, occurs with poor dam vaccination and with failure of passive transfer

AUTHOR: **PHOEBE A. SMITH**

Ovarian Enlargement: Pathologic

Pathologically enlarged ovaries can result from several types of ovarian neoplasia or from ovarian hematomas. In most cases of neoplasia, a presumptive diagnosis may be made by transrectal palpation and ultrasonography and endocrine profiling; however, definitive diagnosis is made by histopathology.

Granulosa cell tumor (GCT)/Granulosa-theca cell tumor (GTCT)
  GCT is the most common tumor of the equine ovary.
  The affected ovary is enlarged and firm, and the ovulation fossa is usually not palpable; the contralateral ovary is almost always small and inactive. Rarely, bilateral tumors have been reported.
  Ultrasonography of the affected ovary reveals a multicystic, honeycombed structure, but the tumor may also be present as a solid mass or as a single large cyst.
  Behavioral abnormalities (stallion-like behavior, persistent estrus, or persistent anestrus) and/or infertility are common clinical features; behavioral changes are attributed to hormone production by the tumor.
  Serum inhibin is elevated in 90% of cases, testosterone in 50% to 60% of cases and progesterone is <1.0 ng/mL (Stabenfelt et al., 1979; McCue, 1992); measurements of inhibin (>0.7 ng/mL), testosterone (>50–100 ng/mL), and progesterone (<1.0 ng/mL) are suggestive of GCT (McCue, 2007).
  GCT/GTCT is the only ovarian abnormality in the mare associated with inactivity of the contralateral ovary. In rare cases where the mare continues to cycle on the contralateral ovary, the tumors are thought to be in the early stages of development.

Teratoma
  Teratoma is the second most common tumor of the equine ovary, but is rare.
  Teratomas contain two or more germinal cell layers and may contain a variety of tissue types, including hair, skin, bone, muscle, etc.
  Ultrasonography of the affected ovary varies depending on the tissues types present.
  Teratomas are most commonly diagnosed in young mares (<5 years).
  Unlike the GCT/GTCT, the teratoma is hormonally inactive and therefore is not associated with behavioral changes.
  The unaffected ovary is usually normal and the mare continues to cycle.

Cystadenoma
  Cystadenomas are very rare tumors of the ovarian surface epithelium.
  Cystadenomas are not hormonally active; however, testosterone is sometimes elevated.
  The unaffected ovary is usually normal and the mare continues to cycle and may become pregnant.

The ultrasonographic appearance of a cystadenoma may include one to many cystlike structures.

Dysgerminoma
  Dysgerminomas are very rare germ cell tumors.
  Dysgerminomas are not hormonally active and do not affect the contralateral ovary.
  Dysgerminomas, unlike other ovarian neoplasms, have a high tendency to metastasize.
  Ultrasonographic appearance of dysgerminoma has not been described in the horse.

Other ovarian tumors
  Other ovarian tumors are rare but melanomas, epitheliomas, hemangiomas adenocarcinomas, arrhenoblastomas, and hemoblastomas have been reported.

Hematoma
  Ovarian hematomas vary in size and could reach sizes of 20 cm in diameter or larger.
  On ultrasound exam, the appearance is usually uniformly echogenic and may organize into mottled blood clots after several days.
  Ovarian hematomas will gradually reduce in size over time; complete resolution may take several weeks; occasionally, a hematoma will fail to completely resolve and may become calcified.
  The contralateral ovary is normal and the mare usually continues to cycle.
  The mare's endocrine profile is normal.
  Hematomas are believed to form following excessive hemorrhage into the follicular lumen following ovulation. The existence of a true ovarian hematoma is somewhat questionable and the finding may, in fact, represent a hemorrhagic anovulatory follicle. See persistent anovulatory follicle/hemorrhagic anovulatory follicle for further information.

SUGGESTED READING

McCue PM: Equine granulosa cell tumors. *Proc Am Assoc Equine Practnr* 38:587–593, 1992.
McCue PM, et al: Granulosa cell tumors of the equine ovary. *Vet Clin N Am Pract Equine* 22:799–817, 2006.
McCue PM: Ovarian abnormalities. In Samper JC, Pycock JF, McKinnon AO (eds). *Current Therapy in Equine Reproduction.* St Louis, 2007, Saunders, pp 87–92.
Stabenfelt GH, et al: Clinical findings, pathologic changes and endocrinological secretory patterns in mares with ovarian tumors. *J Reprod Fert* 27(Suppl):277–285, 1979.

AUTHOR: **CATHERINE A. DeLUCA**

Patent Urachus

Superficial umbilical stump infection (all umbilical conditions can be differentiated by diagnostic ultrasound of the structures)
Urachitis (inflammation or infection)

Infection of the umbilical arteries or veins
Generalized septicemia or other septic processes (pneumonia, enteritis)

AUTHOR: **ELIZABETH M. SANTSCHI**

Periarticular Swelling in Foals

Strain or sprain of periarticular soft tissues
Septic arthritis
Septic physitis
Cellulitis

Edema
Congenital malformation of joint
Articular fracture

AUTHOR: **ELIZABETH M. SANTSCHI**

Photosensitization

Primary photosensitizers
Ammi majus (bishop's weed): Contains furocoumarins
Avena fatua (oatgrass)
Brassica (rape)
Cooperia pedunculata
Cymopterus watsonii (spring parsley): Contains furocoumarins
Erodium (trefoil)
Fagopyrum sagittatum (buckwheat): Contains the naphthodianthrone derivative fagopyrin
Hypericum perforatum (St. John's wort, Klamath weed): Contains the naphthodianthrone derivative hypericin
Perennial ryegrass
Ricinus communis (castor bean)
Rutaceae
Trifolium (clover)
Umbelliferae
Secondary or hepatogenous photosensitizers
Agave lecheguilla (lecheguilla)
Blue-green algae
Brachiaria brizantha
Brassia hyssopifolia
Brassica napus (cultivated rape)
Holocalyx glaziovii

Lantana spp
Lippia rehmanni
Myoporum laetum (ngaio)
Narthecium ossifragum (bog asphodel)
Nolina texana (sacahuiste)
Panicum spp (panic grass, kleingrass)
Pithomyces chartarum and *Periconia minutissima*
Senecio spp (ragwort, groundsel)
Tetradymia canescens (gray horsebrush)
Tetradymia glabrata (spineless horsebrush)
Tribulus terrestris (puncturevine)
Other photosensitizers
Avena (oats)
Euphorbia maculata (milk purslane)
Kochia scoparia (summer cyprus, fireweed)
Medicago (alfalfa)
Polygonum spp (smartweed)
Sorghum vulgare (Sudan grass)
Trifolium (clover)
Vicia spp (vetches)

From Talcott P: Toxicologic problems. In Reed SM, Bayly WM, Sellon DC (eds). *Equine Internal Medicine*, ed 3. St Louis, 2010, Saunders, pp 1364–1416.

Polyuria/Polydipsia

Acute renal failure
Chronic renal failure
Diabetes insipidus
  Affected horses are unable to concentrate urine with water deprivation
Diabetes mellitus
Endotoxemia and/or sepsis
Iatrogenic polyuria
  Excessive intravenous or enteral fluid therapy
  Diuretic, α_2 agonist, or corticosteroid administration
Equine metabolic syndrome
  Overweight horses with abnormal fat deposits
  Normal dexamethasone suppression or thyrotropin-releasing hormone response test

Pituitary pars intermedia dysfunction
  Older horses with hirsutism
  Abnormal dexamethasone suppression or thyrotropin-releasing hormone response test
Psychogenic salt consumption
Psychogenic water drinking
  Stalled, meal-fed horses with decreased access to forage
  Affected horses are able to concentrate urine with water deprivation

SUGGESTED READING

McKenzie EC: Polyuria and polydipsia in horses. *Vet Clin N Am Pract Equine* 23:641–653, 2007.

AUTHOR: **BRYAN M. WALDRIDGE**

Postpartum Emergencies

Genital

Retained fetal membranes
Toxic metritis
Postpartum hemorrhage
Uterine rupture
Uterine prolapse
Intussusception of the uterine horn
Necrotic vaginitis
Vaginal evisceration

Nongenital

Colon torsion
Gastric or small intestinal ileus
Intestinal or mesenteric rupture or trauma
Rectal prolapse
Diaphragmatic rupture
Bladder rupture
Bladder eversion
Bladder prolapse
Lactation tetany

AUTHOR: **MARIA S. FERRER**

Pruritus

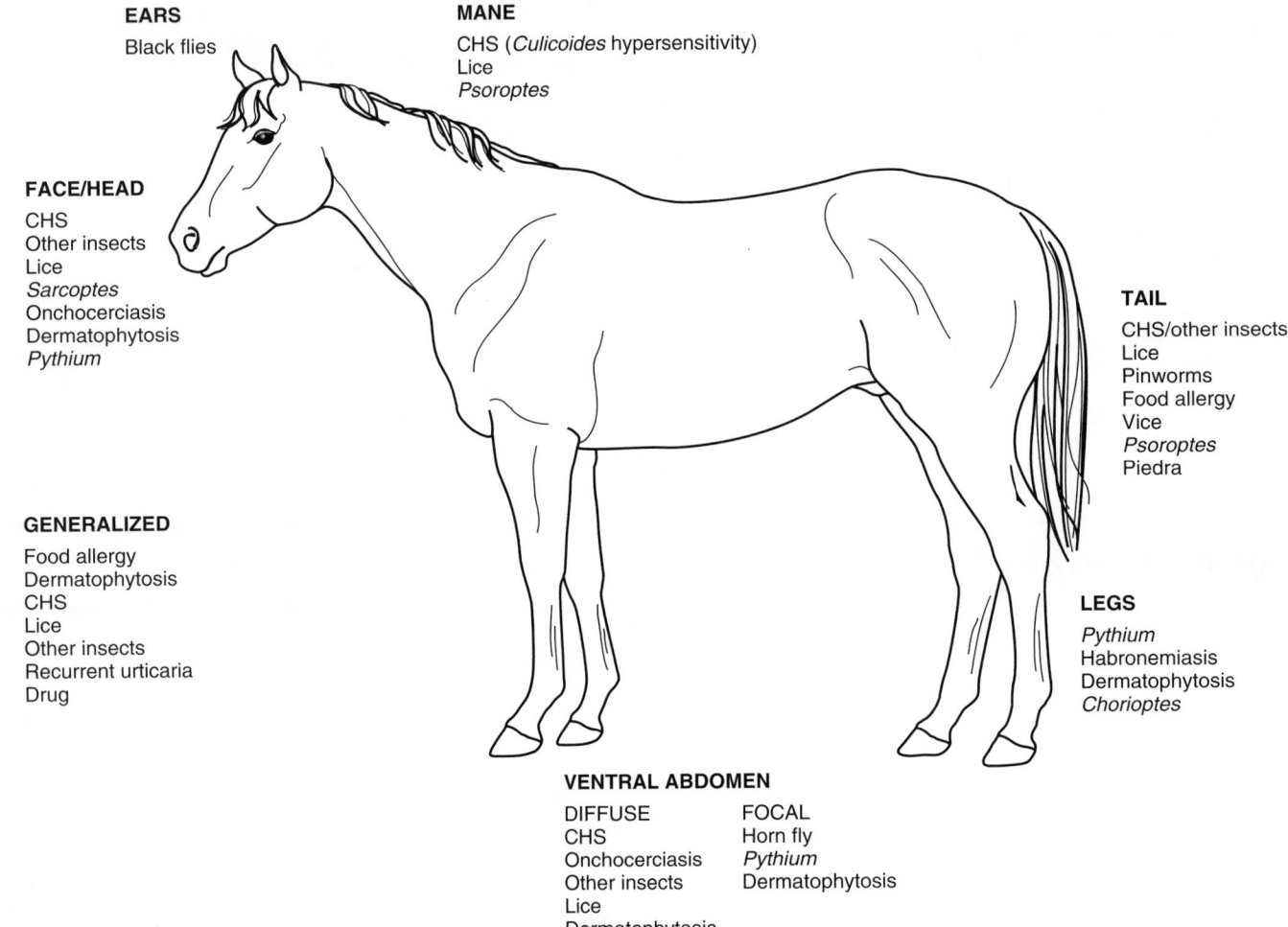

EARS

Black flies

MANE

CHS (*Culicoides* hypersensitivity)
Lice
Psoroptes

FACE/HEAD

CHS
Other insects
Lice
Sarcoptes
Onchocerciasis
Dermatophytosis
Pythium

TAIL

CHS/other insects
Lice
Pinworms
Food allergy
Vice
Psoroptes
Piedra

GENERALIZED

Food allergy
Dermatophytosis
CHS
Lice
Other insects
Recurrent urticaria
Drug

LEGS

Pythium
Habronemiasis
Dermatophytosis
Chorioptes

VENTRAL ABDOMEN

DIFFUSE
CHS
Onchocerciasis
Other insects
Lice
Dermatophytosis

FOCAL
Horn fly
Pythium
Dermatophytosis

From Rees CA: Disorders of the skin. In Reed SM, Bayly WM, Sellon DC (eds). *Equine Internal Medicine,* ed 3. St Louis, 2010, Saunders, pp 682–729.

Rhabdomyolysis

Acorn poisoning
Anthrax
Arthritis (joint pain)
Back problems
Botulism
Castration sequelae
Colic
Cystitis
Hernia
Iliac thrombosis
Inguinal/popliteal lymphadenitis

Laminitis
Nephritis
Pleuritis
Postexhaustion syndrome
Proximal limb lameness
Spinal cord disease
Tetanus
Tick paralysis

From MacLeay JM: Disorders of the musculoskeletal system. In Reed SM, Bayly WM, Sellon DC (eds). *Equine Internal Medicine*, ed 3. St Louis, 2010, Saunders, pp 488–544.

Seizures, Known and Suspected Causes in Horses Younger Than 1 Year

Differential Diagnosis

Classification	Extracranial	Intracranial	Diagnostic Aids*
Anomalies (congenital)		Hydrocephalus, Hydranencephaly, Benign epilepsy	1–6,8 11
Metabolic	Hypoxia, hyponatremia, hypoglycemia, hyperkalemia		2–4,8,11
Toxic	Organophosphates Strychnine Metaldehyde	Moldy corn Locoweed	2–6 9–11
Traumatic		Brain trauma Lightning	2–4 5,6,8,10,11
Vascular		Neonatal maladjustment syndrome (vascular accidents)	2–6
Infectious	Septicemia Endotoxemia Fever Tetanus Botulism	Bacterial meningitis Cerebral abscesses Rabies Viral encephalitis	2–4 5–9 11

*1, breed; 2, onset; 3, clinical course; 4, physical examination; 5, neurologic examination; 6, clinical pathology: cerebrospinal fluid analysis; 7, serologic testing; 8, radiology (computed tomography scan, ultrasound, radiographs); 9, toxicologic testing; 10, electrodiagnostics (electroencephalography [EEG], electromyelography [EMG]); 11, pathologic examination.

From Reed SM: Seizures, narcolepsy, and cataplexy. In Reed SM, Bayly WM, Sellon DC (eds). *Equine internal medicine*, ed. 3. St Louis, 2010, Saunders, pp 572–578.

Seizures, Known and Suspected Causes in Horses Older Than 1 Year

Differential Diagnosis

Classification	Extracranial	Intracranial	Diagnostic Aids*
Metabolic	Hepatoencephalopathy, hypomagnesemia, hypocalcemia, uremia, hyperlipidemia		2–6,11
Toxic	Organophosphates Strychnine Metaldehyde	Moldy corn Locoweed Bracken fern Lead, arsenic, mercury Rye grass	2–6 9–11

Continued

Differential Diagnosis—cont'd

Classification	Extracranial	Intracranial	Diagnostic Aids*
Traumatic		Brain trauma	8,10,11
Vascular		*Strongylus vulgaris*	2–4
		Cerebral thromboembolism	5,6,11
		Intracarotid injection	
Tumor		Neoplasia	2–5
		Hemarthroma	6,8,10,11
		Cholesterol granuloma	
Infectious		Cerebral abscess	1,3–6
		Rabies	7,8,12,13
		Tetanus	
		Arbovirus encephalitides	
		Mycotic cryptococcosis	
		Protozoal encephalomyelitis	

*1, breed; 2, onset; 3, clinical course; 4, physical examination; 5, neurologic examination; 6, clinical pathology: cerebrospinal fluid analysis; 7, serologic testing; 8, radiology (computed tomography scan, ultrasound, radiographs); 9, toxicologic testing; 10, electrodiagnostics (electroencephalography [EEG], electromyelography [EMG]); 11, pathologic examination.
From Reed SM: Seizures, narcolepsy, and cataplexy. In Reed SM, Bayly WM, Sellon DC (eds). *Equine Internal Medicine*, ed 3. St Louis, 2010, Saunders, pp 572–578.

Small Intestinal Distension

Ileus
  Anterior enteritis
  Postoperative ileus
  Peritonitis
  Grass sickness
Obstruction
  Strangulating lesions
    Volvulus
    Pedunculated lipoma
    Epiploic foramen entrapment
  Gastrosplenic ligament incarceration
  Mesenteric rent
  Mesodiverticular band
  Inguinal hernia
  Foreign body
  Ileal impaction
  Ascarid impaction
  Intussusception
  Nonstrangulating infarction

AUTHOR: **SARA GOMEZ-IBANEZ**

Sudden Cardiovascular Death

Electric disorders of the heart (arrhythmias)
  Ventricular tachycardia, flutter, or fibrillation
  Complete atrioventricular block
  Asystole
Toxic injury to the heart
  Acute myocardial failure
  Anesthetics
  Drug- or toxin-induced arrhythmia
  Toxic plants
  Myocardial toxins
  Systemic toxin secondarily affecting the heart
Cardiac tamponade
  Bacterial pericarditis
  Idiopathic pericarditis
  Viral pericarditis
  Trauma
Hemorrhage
  Rupture of the heart (with cardiac tamponade)
  Rupture of the aorta or pulmonary artery (with or without cardiac tamponade)
  Arterial rupture
  Middle uterine artery
  Mesenteric, omental, or other large arteries
  Severe pulmonary hemorrhage
  Rupture of the spleen or liver
  Brain hemorrhage
Embolism
  Carotid air embolism
  Coronary embolism or thrombosis
Electrocution
  Lightning
  Alternating current electrocution
Cardiac trauma
  Cardiac catheterization or needle puncture of a ventricle leading to ventricular fibrillation
  Penetrating thoracic wound

From Bonagura JD, Reef VB, Schwarzwald CC: Cardiovascular diseases. In Reed SM, Bayly WM, Sellon DC (eds). *Equine Internal Medicine*, ed 3. St Louis, 2010, Saunders, pp 372–487.

Thrombocytopenia

Decreased platelet production
  Hereditary defects
  Myelophthisis
  Myeloproliferative disease
  Idiopathic pancytopenia
  Myelosuppressive drugs
    Phenylbutazone
    Chloramphenicol
    Estrogens
    Trichlorethylene-extracted soybean meal
  Irradiation
Increased platelet use
  Intravascular coagulation
    Disseminated intravascular coagulation (DIC)
    Localized
      Hemolytic uremic syndrome
      Hemangioma
  Hemorrhage
  Thrombosis
Platelet sequestration
  Splenomegaly

Increased platelet destruction
  Infectious diseases
    Equine infectious anemia (EIA)
    Anaplasma phagocytophilum
  Immune-mediated diseases
    Autoimmune disease
    Systemic lupus erythematosus
    Idiopathic disease
    Secondary disease
    Neoplasia (lymphosarcoma)
    Bacterial infection
    Viral infection
    Drugs
    Neonatal alloimmune disease
  Drugs or toxins
  Snakebites
Laboratory error

From Sellon DC, Wise LN: Disorders of the hematopoietic system. In Reed SM, Bayly WM, Sellon DC (eds). *Equine Internal Medicine*, ed 3. St Louis, 2010, Saunders, pp 730–776.

Toxins: Differential Diagnoses

Table 1: Equine Toxins Listed by Clinical Sign and System Affected

Toxins are listed under systems most commonly affected or signs most commonly observed in horses in North America. After identifying possible differentials, go to Table 2 for description of other signs possible for each toxicant.

Abortions		Anemia	
Plants	*Allium* spp (onions, other)	Plants	*Alliums* spp (onions, others)
	Hoary alyssum		Bracken fern, horsetails
	Locoweeds		Sweet clover, moldy
	Lupine		Mushrooms
	Sudan/sorghum		Mustards
	White snakeroot, rayless goldenrod		Red maple
Mycotoxins	Fescue, endophyte-infected	Mycotoxins	Aflatoxins
Drugs	Glucocorticoids	Animals	Pit viper snakes
	Estrogens	Drugs	Vitamin K_3
	Prostaglandins		Phenothiazines
	Vitamin A		Penicillins
Metals/minerals	Iodine	Pesticides	Anticoagulant rodenticides
	Molybdenum	Metals/minerals	Iron
Other	Carbon monoxide		Lead
	Nitrate, chlorate		Mercury
	Any toxins causing anoxia	Other	Phenols
			Propylene glycol

Table 1: Equine Toxins Listed by Clinical Sign and System Affected—cont'd

Blindness

Plants	Alsike and red clover
	Cocklebur
	Milkvetches
	Bracken fern, horsetails
Drugs	Ivermectin, moxidectin
Pesticides	Metaldehyde
Metals/minerals	Lead
	Sodium, water deprivation

Bone Marrow Effects

Drugs	Chloramphenicol
	Estrogens
	Griseofulvin
	NSAIDs
	Sulfonamides

Cardiovascular

Plants	Avocado
	Cardiac glycoside plants
	Cyanogenic glycoside plants
	Death camas
	Gossypol
	Grayanotoxin plants
	Jimson weed
	Milkweeds
	Monkshood
	Mushrooms
	Nightshades
	White snakeroot, rayless goldenrod
	Yew
Animals	Blister beetles
	Pit vipers
	Bufo toads
Drugs	Amitraz
	Cardiac-glycoside drugs
	Illicit drugs
	Phenothiazines
	Tilmicosin
	Xylazine
Pesticides	4-aminopyridine
	Cholecalciferol, vitamin D_3
	Sodium fluoroacetate (1080)
Metals/minerals	Fluoride
	Selenium
Other	Ionophores
	Methylxanthines
	Non-protein nitrogen (urea)

Central Nervous System

Plants	Alsike and red clover
	Amanita mushrooms
	Black locust
	Bracken fern, horsetails
	Buckeye
	Buttercups
	Carolina allspice
	Carolina jessamine
	Chinaberry
	Cocklebur
	Death camas
	Grayanotoxin plants
	Kentucky coffee tree
	Golden chain tree
	Jimson weed
	Lathyrus
	Locoweeds
	Mayapple
	Milkweeds
	Milkvetches
	Monkshood
	Mushrooms
	Nicotine, tobacco
	Nightshades
	Pigweed
	Poison hemlock
	Sagebrush
	Soluble oxalates
	Stipa
	Water hemlock
	White snakeroot, rayless goldenrod
	Yellow star thistle, Russian knapweed
Mycotoxins	Fumonisin
	Tremorgenic forages
Animals	Bufo toads
	Mojave rattlesnakes and other neurotoxic snakes
Microorganisms	Botulinum toxin
	Tetanus
	Anatoxin-a (blue-green algae toxin)
	Anatoxin-a(s) (blue-green algae toxin)
Drugs	Amitraz
	Atropine
	Barbiturates
	Bronchodilators
	Fluoroquinolones
	Illicit drugs
	Ivermectin, moxidectin
	Metronidazole
	Phenothiazines
	Tilmicosin

Table 1: Equine Toxins Listed by Clinical Sign and System Affected—cont'd

Central Nervous System—cont'd

Pesticides	4-aminopyridine
	Anticholinesterase insecticides
	Cholecalciferol
	Metaldehyde
	Organochlorine insecticides
	Pyrethrins/pyrethroids
	Sodium fluoroacetate (1080)
	Starlicide
	Strychnine
	Zinc phosphide
Metals/minerals	Fluoride
	Iron
	Lead
	Mercury
	Sodium, water deprivation
Other	Carbon dioxide
	Carbon monoxide
	Ethanol
	Ethylene glycol
	Hydrogen sulfide
	Non-protein nitrogen (urea)
	Propylene glycol
	Turpentine

Coagulopathy

Plants	Sweet clover, moldy
Mycotoxins	Aflatoxins
Animals	Pit viper snakes
Drugs	Anticoagulant drugs
	NSAIDs
Pesticides	Anticoagulant rodenticides
Metals/minerals	Iron
Other	Any toxins causing severe liver damage

Dermatologic

Plants	Alsike and red clover
	Milkvetches
	Panicum spp
	Photosensitizing plants
	Pyrrolizidine alkaloid plants
	Seleniferous plants
	Vetch (*Vicia*)
Mycotoxins	Stachybotryotoxins
Animals	Brown recluse spider
Microorganisms	Microcystin (blue-green algae toxin)
Drugs	Glucocorticoids
	Sulfonamides
	Tetracycline
Pesticides	Paraquat
	Pyrethrins/pyrethroids
Metals/minerals	Arsenic
	Fluoride
	Iodine
	Molybdenum
	Selenium

Dermatologic—cont'd

Other	Acid and alkali
	Chromates
	Detergents, concentrated
	Pine oil
	Phenols
	Turpentine

Gastrointestinal

Plants	*Amanita* mushrooms
	Black locust
	Bracken fern
	Buckeye
	Buttercups
	Castor bean
	Cardiac glycoside plants
	Chinaberry
	Cocklebur
	Coffee senna
	Death camas
	Euphorbia spp
	Grayanotoxin plants
	Hoary alyssum
	Jimson weed
	Mayapple
	Milkweeds
	Mushrooms
	Nightshades
	Oak
	Poison hemlock
	Pokeweed
	Rosary pea
	Soluble oxalates
	Yew
Mycotoxins	Aflatoxins
	Citrinin, ochratoxin
	Slaframine
	Stachybotryotoxins
Animals	Blister beetles
Microorganisms	Anatoxin-a(s) (blue-green algae toxin)
	Mycrocystin (blue-green algae toxin)
Drugs	Amitraz
	Atropine
	Cardiac glycoside drugs
	Chloramphenicol, florfenicol
	Erythromycin
	Fluoroquinolones
	Glucocorticoids
	Lincomycin, clindamycin
	NSAIDs
	Tetracyclines
	Vitamin K_3

Continued

Table 1: Equine Toxins Listed by Clinical Sign and System Affected—cont'd

Gastrointestinal—cont'd

Pesticides	Anticholinesterase insecticides
	Chlorophenoxy herbicides
	Cholecalciferol, vitamin D$_3$
	Glyphosate herbicides
	Sodium fluoroacetate (1080)
	Metaldehyde
	Paraquat
	Zinc phosphide
Metals/minerals	Arsenic
	Cadmium
	Iron
	Lead
	Mercury
	Sodium
Other	Acid and alkali
	Chromates
	Detergents, concentrated
	Ethanol
	Fertilizers
	Ionophores
	Methylxanthines
	Nitrate, chlorate
	Pine oil
	Phenols
	Propylene glycol
	Turpentine

Hooves

Plants	Black walnut
	Hoary alyssum
	Seleniferous plants
Mycotoxins	Ergot alkaloids
	Fescue, endophyte-infected
Metals/minerals	Selenium

Liver

Plants	Alsike and red clover
	Amanita mushrooms
	Castor bean
	Cockleburs
	Pyrrolizidine alkaloid plants
	Lantana
	Mushrooms
	Panicum spp
Mycotoxins	Aflatoxins
	Fumonisin
Microorganisms	Microcystin (blue-green algae toxin)
Drugs	NSAIDs
	Sulfonamides
Pesticides	Metaldehyde
	Paraquat, diquat
Metals/minerals	Iron
Other	Phenols

Mammary

Plants	Avocado
Mycotoxins	Ergot alkaloids
	Fescue, endophyte-infected
Drugs	Estrogenic drugs

Methemoglobinemia

Plants	*Allium* spp (onions, other)
	Red maple
	Mushrooms
Pesticides	Starlicide
Other	Naphthalene
	Nitrate, chlorate
	Phenols

Musculoskeletal and Dental

Plants	Coffee senna
	Lathyrus spp
	Hypochaeris spp
	White snakeroot, rayless goldenrod
Animals	Gila monster
Drugs	Fluoroquinolones
	Tetracyclines
	Vitamin A
Metals/minerals	Cadmium
	Fluoride
	Iron
	Zinc
Other	Ionophores
	Methylxanthines
	Also see Teratogens

Neuromuscular Dysfunction, Including Paresis or Paralysis

Plants	Buckeye
	Bracken fern
	Chinaberry
	Cocklebur
	Death camas
	Hypochaeris
	Monkshood
	Lathyrus
	Locoweeds
	Milkweeds
	Milk vetches
	Mushrooms
	Nicotine, tobacco
	Nightshades
	Sudan/sorghum
	Tremorgenic forages
	White snakeroot, rayless goldenrod
	Yellow star thistle, Russian knapweed
Animals	Black widow spider
	Bufo toads
	Mojave rattlesnakes, other neurotoxic snakes
	Tick paralysis

Table 1: Equine Toxins Listed by Clinical Sign and System Affected—cont'd

Neuromuscular Dysfunction, Including Paresis or Paralysis—cont'd

Microorganisms	Anatoxin-a (blue-green algae toxin)
	Anatoxin-a(s) (blue-green algae toxin)
	Botulinum toxin
	Tetanus
Drugs	Aminoglycosides
Pesticides	Anticholinesterase insecticides
	Metaldehyde
	Organochlorine insecticides
	Starlicide
	Strychnine
Metals/minerals	Lead
	Mercury
	Selenium
	Zinc
Other	Ionophores
	Non-protein nitrogen (urea)

Oral Lesions

Plants	Buckeye
	Buttercups
	Euphorbia
Mycotoxins	Slaframine
	Stachybotryotoxins
Animals	Blister beetles
Metals/minerals	Mercury
Other	Acid, alkali
	Detergents, concentrated
	Pine oil
	Phenols
	Turpentine

Photosensitization

Plants	Alsike and red clover
	Alfalfa
	Lantana
	Panicum spp
	1° photosensitizing plants
	Pyrrolizidine alkaloid plants
	Sudan/sorghum
	Wheat
Microorganisms	Microcystin (blue-green algae toxin)
Drugs	Tetracyclines
	Sulfonamides
Other	Also any toxin causing liver failure

Rapid/Sudden Death

Plants	Castor bean
	Cocklebur
	Cardiac-glycoside plants
	Cyanogenic glycoside plants
	Death camas
	Gossypol
	Jimson weed
	Milkweeds
	Monkshood
	Mushrooms
	Nicotine, tobacco
	Poison hemlock
	Red maple
	Water hemlock
	White snakeroot, rayless goldenrod
	Yew
Animals	Blister beetles
	Bufo toads
	Pit viper snakes
Mycotoxins	Fumonisin
Microorganisms	Anatoxin-a (blue-green algae toxin)
	Anatoxin-a(s) (blue-green algae toxin)
	Botulinum toxin
Drugs	Insulin
	Illicit drugs
	Potassium
	Penicillins (anaphylaxis)
	Tilmicosin
Pesticides	4-aminopyridine
	Anticholinesterase insecticides
	Anticoagulant rodenticides
	Metaldehyde
	Sodium fluoroacetate (1080)
	Strychnine
	Zinc phosphide
Metals/minerals	Arsenic
	Iron
	Selenium
Other	Carbon dioxide
	Carbon monoxide
	Hydrogen sulfide
	Ionophores
	Nitrogen dioxide

Table 1: Equine Toxins Listed by Clinical Sign and System Affected—cont'd

Renal, Urinary

Plants	*Allium* spp (onions, others)
	Amanita mushrooms
	Cocklebur
	Mayapple
	Mushrooms
	Oak
	Oleander (see cardiac-glycoside plants)
	Pigweed
	Soluble oxalates
	Sudan/sorghum
	Red maple
	Vitamin D-containing plants (Cestrum diurnum)
	White snakeroot, rayless goldenrod
Mycotoxins	Citrinin, ochratoxin, patulin
Animals	Blister beetles
	Pit viper snakes
Drugs	Aminoglycosides
	NSAIDs
	Sulfonamides
	Tetracyclines
	Vitamin K_3
Pesticides	Cholecalciferol, vitamin D_3
	Metaldehyde
	Paraquat, diquat
Metals/minerals	Arsenic
	Cadmium
	Mercury
	Zinc
Other	Ethylene glycol
	Pine oil
	Phenols
	Turpentine
	Also any toxins causing hemoglobinuria, or myoglobinuria

Reproduction

Plants	Hoary alyssum
	Locoweeds
	Phytoestrogenic plants
Mycotoxins	Ergot alkaloids
	Fescue, endophyte-infected
Drugs	Anabolic steroids
	Estrogens
	Prostaglandins
	Also see Abortions
	Also see Teratogens

Respiratory, Including Upper Airway

Plants	Avocado
	Cyanogenic glycoside plants
	Death camas
	Mushrooms
Microorganisms	Botulinum toxin
	Tetanus

Respiratory, Including Upper Airway—cont'd

Pesticides	Anticholinesterase insecticides
	Paraquat
	Strychnine
	Zinc phosphide
Metals/minerals	Lead
	Iodine
	Zinc
Other	Ammonia
	Carbon dioxide
	Carbon monoxide
	Petroleum products
	Hydrogen sulfide
	Pine oil
	Phenols

Salivation, Excessive

Plants	Buttercup
	Cardiac glycoside plants
	Chinaberry
	Cocklebur
	Euphorbia
	Grayanotoxin plants
	Mayapple
	Monkshood
	Mushrooms
	Nettles
	Nicotine, tobacco
Mycotoxins	Slaframine
Microorganisms	Anatoxin a(s) (blue-green algae toxin)
	Botulinum toxin
Animals	Bufo toads
	Blister beetles
Drugs	Ivermectin, moxidectin
Pesticides	4-aminopyridine
	Anticholinesterase insecticides
	Metaldehyde
	Glyphosate
Metals/minerals	Arsenic
	Fluoride
	Iodine
	Lead
Other	Acid, alkali
	Detergents, concentrated
	Fertilizers

Seizures

Plants	Bracken fern, horse tails
	Buckeye
	Cyanogenic glycoside plants
	Grayanotoxin plants
	Jimson weed
	Milkweeds
	Mushrooms
	Nicotine, tobacco
	Nightshades
	Water hemlock

Table 1: Equine Toxins Listed by Clinical Sign and System Affected—cont'd

Seizures—cont'd		Tremors	
Mycotoxins	Tremorgenic forages	Plants	Alsike and red clover
Animals	Bufo toads		Bracken fern, horsetails
Microorganisms	Anatoxin-a (blue-greenalgae toxin)		Buttercups
	Anatoxin-a(s) (blue-green algae toxin)		Cardiac glycoside plants
	Tetanus		Cocklebur
Drugs	Illicit drugs		Death camas
	Metronidazole		Milkweeds
	Tilmicosin		Jimson weed
Pesticides	4-aminopyridine		Mushrooms
	Anticholinesterase insecticides		Nicotine, tobacco
	Metaldehyde		Nightshades
	Organochlorines		Pigweed
	Sodium fluoroacetate (1080)		Poison hemlock
	Strychnine		White snakeroot, rayless goldenrod
	Zinc phosphide	Mycotoxins	Anatoxin-a (blue-green algae toxin)
Metals/minerals	Iron		Anatoxin-a(s) (blue-green algae toxin)
	Lead		Tremorgenic forages
	Sodium	Microorganism	Botulinum toxin
Other	Carbon monoxide	Drugs	Cardiac glycoside drugs
	Ethylene glycol	Pesticides	4-aminopyridine
	Hydrogen sulfide		Anticholinesterase insecticides
	Methylxanthines		Metaldehyde
	Also, any toxins causing anoxia; can occur during terminal stages of many poisons		Pyrethrins/pyrethroids
			Organochlorine insecticides
			Sodium fluoroacetate (1080)
		Metals/minerals	Iron
Teratogens			Sodium
Plants	Locoweeds	Other	Ionophores
	Lupine		Methylxanthines
	Nicotine, tobacco		Nitrate fertilizers
	Poison hemlock		Non-protein nitrogen (urea)
	Sudan/sorghum		Phenols
Mycotoxins	Fescue, endophyte-infected		
Drugs	Corticosteroids		
	Griseofulvin		
	Vitamin A		

NSAIDs, nonsteroidal antiinflammatory drugs.

AUTHOR: CYNTHIA L. GASKILL

Table 2: Equine Toxins Listed Alphabetically

Descriptions of possible signs that can occur with these toxic substances in horses. Not all signs will be seen in every case. Presence of specific signs and severity of signs depends on dose, route of exposure, stage of intoxication, and individual animal variation.

Toxic Substance	Clinical Signs
Acid and alkali	Dysphagia, salivation, anorexia, colic, oral or dermal lesions, dyspnea, laryngeal edema and swelling
Aflatoxins	Acute high dose: Anorexia, depression, ataxia, weakness, dyspnea, colic, tachycardia, bloody diarrhea with mucus, seizures. Chronic: Liver damage, weight loss, rough coat, anemia, jaundice, anorexia, depression, coagulopathy
Alfalfa (*Medicago*)	Photosensitization. Legumes can contain phytoestrogens that cause reproductive problems.
Allium spp	Examples: Onions, garlic, leeks, shallots, chives. Anorexia, ataxia, lethargy, recumbency, tachycardia, tachypnea, dyspnea, hemolytic anemia, pale or icteric membranes, diarrhea, methemoglobinemia, hemoglobinuria, strong odor to breath, abortion, Heinz bodies, 2° renal damage
Alsike and red clover (*Trifolium*)	Liver damage, anorexia, weight loss, grinding of teeth, yawning, tremors, icterus, hepatoencephalopathy, depression, wandering, head pressing, ataxia, blindness, colic, dysphagia, recumbency, excitation, coma, 2° photosensitization. Legumes can contain phytoestrogens that cause reproductive problems.

Continued

Table 2: Equine Toxins Listed Alphabetically—cont'd

Toxic Substance	Clinical Signs
Amanita mushrooms	Colic, diarrhea, acute hepatotoxicity, lethargy, icterus, ataxia, seizures, coma, renal damage, and multiorgan failure
Aminoglycosides	Nephrotoxicity, ototoxicity, neuromuscular blockade
4-aminopyridine (Avitrol)	Salivation, hyperexcitability, tremors, incoordination, seizures, arrhythmias, sweating, fear, fluttering of third eyelid; may walk backwards. Rapid death may occur.
Amitraz	Depression, disorientation, ataxia, bradycardia, coma, seizures, hypothermia, ileus, colic, large colon impaction
Ammonia gas	Exposure to ammonia from animal waste: Lacrimation, dyspnea, coughing, nasal discharge. Anhydrous ammonia gas exposure much more dangerous: Acute death, apnea, laryngospasm, corneal damage, severe respiratory tract damage
Anabolic steroids	Behavioral changes including aggression, decreased testicular size and spermatogenesis, delayed onset of puberty, suppressed ovulation, early embryonic death, masculinization, other reproductive effects. Abrupt cessation of chronic anabolic steroid use can cause weight loss, anorexia, muscle wasting, laminitis, poor hair coat, adrenal insufficiency
Anatoxin-a (blue-green algae toxin)	Muscle tremors, rigidity, lethargy, respiratory distress, seizures. Rapid death can occur.
Anatoxin-a(s) (blue-green algae toxin)	Salivation, frequent urination and defecation, lacrimation, colic, diarrhea, tremors, dyspnea, convulsions. Rapid death can occur.
Anticholinesterase insecticides	Examples: Organophosphates, carbamates. Varying degrees of muscarinic, nicotinic, and CNS signs. Restlessness, colic, salivation, lacrimation, frequent urination and defecation, diarrhea, ataxia, tremors, muscle fasciculations, weakness, paresis, dyspnea, bronchoconstriction, bronchorrhea, hyperactivity, seizures. Rapid death can occur.
Anticoagulant rodenticides	Examples: Warfarin, brodifacoum, bromadiolone, chlorophacinone, difethialone, diphacinone, and many others. Coagulopathy. Signs depend upon location of bleeding. Bleeding can be localized or widespread. Signs include lethargy, anorexia, weakness, dyspnea, lameness, bruising with ecchymoses, petechiae, frank hemorrhage from nose or rectum, hematuria, seizures, paralysis, other neurologic signs, pale membranes. Abortion. Unusual color to feces (color of bait) can sometimes be noted.
Arsenic	Salivation, colic, abdominal pain, diarrhea (green, watery black, or bloody), weakness, depression, ataxia, weak pulse, shock, hypotension, recumbency, dehydration, acidosis, tremors, respiratory distress, hyperemic membranes, renal damage. Rapid death can occur.
Atropine	Ileus, colic, excitation or sedation, dry membranes, tachycardia, mydriasis, visual disturbances
Avocado (*Persea*)	Cardiopulmonary signs, noninfectious mastitis, agalactia, colic, diarrhea, edema of ventral abdomen, head, and neck, respiratory edema, hydrothorax
Barbiturates	Overdose: CNS depression, respiratory depression, apnea, coma, death
Black locust (*Robinia*)	Anorexia, abdominal pain, diarrhea, colic, hemorrhagic gastroenteritis; depression or excitation, head pressing, weakness, posterior paresis, mydriasis, blindness, arrhythmias, diaphragmatic flutter
Black walnut (*Juglans*)	Laminitis, often in herd outbreaks. Reluctance to move, depression, hyperthermia, tachycardia, tachypnea, edema of lower limbs, increased coronary band and hoof temperature, pounding digital pulses, respiratory signs may be seen.
Black widow spider (*Latrodectus*)	Muscle fasciculations, rigidity, abdominal pain, ataxia, ascending paralysis, dyspnea, elevated CK
Blister beetles	Depression, colic, restlessness, sweating, congested membranes, tachycardia, tachypnea, pollakiuria, diarrhea, shock, oral lesions, salivation, "thumps," stiff gait, muscle fasciculations, hypocalcemia, hypomagnesemia. Rapid death can occur.
Botulinum toxin	Progressive flaccid paralysis, weakness, ataxia, ileus, constipation, weakness of muscles of tail, tongue, paralysis of third eyelid, tremors, twitch in triceps area, difficulty prehending and swallowing food, anorexia, salivation, tremors (foals). Distended bladder and constipation/impaction of large bowel can be palpated rectally. Recumbency, paddling, respiratory paralysis. Rapid death with no other signs can occur.
Bracken fern (*Pteridium*), Horsetail (*Equisetum*)	Anorexia, unthrifty appearance, weight loss, weakness, depression, tremors, ataxia, incoordination, tremors, wide crouching stance, posterior paralysis, recumbency, seizures, opisthotonus
β$_2$ agonist bronchodilators	Tachycardia, sweating, excitement, tremors. Paradoxical bronchoconstriction is possible.
Brown recluse spider (Loxosceles)	Skin lesion developing into enlarging necrotic lesion
Buckeye, horse chestnut (*Aesculus*)	Colic, diarrhea, oral irritation, depression or excitation, ataxia, stiff gait, twitches, incoordination, spasms, seizures, recumbency, opisthotonos, head flopping. Red urine may be seen.
Bufo toads	Convulsions, ataxia, hyperemic membranes, salivation, arrhythmias, seizures. Rapid death can occur.
Buttercups (*Ranunculus* spp)	Blistering, erythema, swelling of muzzle and lips, salivation, GI irritation, colic, diarrhea, weakness, hematuria, tremors, seizures
Cadmium	Acute: Colic, anorexia, diarrhea Chronic: Osteochondrosis, osteoporosis, lameness, swollen joints, unthriftiness, renal damage
Carbon dioxide	Staggering, collapse, coma, death if high concentrations
Carbon monoxide	Lethargy, weakness, incoordination, cherry-red membranes initially, dyspnea, coma, terminal spasms, acute death. Abortion can occur.
Cardiac glycoside drugs	Examples: Digoxin, digitoxin. Colic, diarrhea, anorexia, cardiac arrhythmias, weakness, hyperkalemia
Cardiac glycoside-containing plants	Examples: Oleander, laurel, dogbane, foxglove, lily of the valley, some milkweeds, and others. Sudden death, depression, anorexia, diarrhea (can be profuse, bloody), colic, weakness, salivation, sweating, arrhythmias, cold extremities, pale membranes, lethargy, mydriasis, tremors, frequent urination, cyanosis, seizures, dyspnea, coma, cardiac damage, hyperkalemia. Renal damage can occur with oleander ingestion.

Table 2: Equine Toxins Listed Alphabetically—cont'd

Toxic Substance	Clinical Signs
Carolina allspice (*Calycanthus fertilis*)	Hyperexcitability, recumbency, muscle spasms resulting in extensor rigidity, opisthotonus, seizures
Carolina jessamine (*Gelsemium sempervirens*)	Incoordination, weakness, recumbency, respiratory paralysis
Castor bean (*Ricinus*)	Depression, abdominal pain, watery diarrhea (can be bloody), colic, incoordination, sweating, muscle spasms, tachycardia, tachypnea, hemorrhagic gastroenteritis, liver damage
Chinaberry (*Melia*)	Diarrhea with or without blood, colic, anorexia, salivation, ataxia, excitement or depression, seizures, paresis, coma, tachycardia or bradycardia, mydriasis or miosis, dyspnea, pulmonary edema, oliguria, muscle rigidity, opisthotonus. Rapid death can occur.
Chloramphenicol, florfenicol	Anorexia, diarrhea, colitis. Can interfere with metabolism and clearance of other drugs. Chronic use: Anemia, pancytopenia, bone marrow suppression
Chlorophenoxy herbicides	Examples: 2,4-D, MCPA, MCPP, dicamba. If exposure to concentrated product occurs, can see GI irritation, colic, diarrhea
Cholecalciferol, vitamin D_3	Calcification of tissues, hypercalcemia, hyperphosphatemia, anorexia, depression, diarrhea (sometimes bloody), PU/PD, renal failure, arrhythmias
Citrinin, ochratoxin, patulin	Colic, diarrhea (can be bloody), depression, anorexia, dehydration, hyperthermia, conjunctivitis, PU/PD, renal damage
Cocklebur (*Xanthium*)	Depression, colic, anorexia, salivation, dyspnea, tremors, extensor rigidity, spasmodic contractions of limbs and neck muscles, seizures, paddling, recumbency, coma, hyperexcitability, blindness, renal damage, hepatic necrosis, hepatoencephalopathy, depression, weakness, prostration, opisthotonus, coma, profound hypoglycemia. Rapid death can occur.
Coffee senna, sicklepod (*Senna*)	Diarrhea, then constipation. Muscle weakness, decreased muscle tone, slow gait, recumbency while remaining bright and alert and eating, myoglobinuria, very elevated CK, AST
Cyanogenic glycoside-containing plants	Examples: *Prunus* spp such as wild cherry, choke cherry; elderberry, Johnson grass, sorghum, Sudan, and many other plants. Sudden death. Seizures, respiratory distress, flaring nostrils, involuntary urination and defecation, tremors, ataxia, coma, shock, respiratory failure, cherry red color to membranes and blood initially. Rapid death can occur.
Day-blooming jessamine (*Cestrum diurnum*)	Weight loss, depression, weakness, infertility, anorexia, arrhythmias, stiff gait, lameness, humped up appearance, grazing on knees, recumbency, hypercalcemia, hyperphosphatemia, tissue calcification, renal damage
Death camas (*Zigadenus*)	Depression, salivation, ataxia, tremors, incoordination, dyspnea, miosis, bradycardia, cyanosis, weakness, hypothermia, colic, collapse, coma. Rapid death can occur.
Detergents, concentrated	Colic, diarrhea, oral or dermal lesions
Ergot alkaloids	Agalactia, prolonged gestation, dystocia, abortion, retained placenta, neonatal mortality, infertility, gangrene of extremities, laminitis, heat intolerance
Erythromycin	Diarrhea, colitis (can be severe in adults), hyperthermia, local reaction and pain if given IM
Estrogens	Bone marrow toxicity, leukopenia, thrombocytopenia, aplastic anemia, infertility, irregular estrus, endometrial hyperplasia, pyometra, abortion, feminization
Ethanol	Ataxia, lethargy, sedation, hypothermia, metabolic acidosis, respiratory depression, coma, death
Ethylene glycol	Depression, ataxia, polydipsia, acidosis, anorexia, renal failure, coma, terminal convulsions
Euphorbia spp	Example: Spurges, leafy spurge. Irritation and blistering of mouth and skin, salivation, colic, diarrhea (sometimes bloody), collapse
Fertilizers	Oral lesions, salivation, colic, and diarrhea (also: methemoglobinemia if contains nitrates—see nitrate fertilizers. Iron toxicity if contains iron. If contains calcium cyanamide, can see ataxia, dyspnea, shock, hypotension)
Fescue: endophyte-infected tall fescue	Also endophyte-infected rye straw. Agalactia, lack of udder development, prolonged gestation, abortion, dystocia and complications of dystocia, increased embryonic death, fetal asphyxia, weakness, dysmaturity, hypothyroid, stillbirths, failure of passive transfer, premature placental separation, retained placenta, thickened edematous placenta, red bag presentation, fertility problems, laminitis, altered thermoregulation, sweating
Fluoride	Acute poisoning: Excitement, seizures, urinary incontinence, weakness, salivation, depression, cardiac failure, death. Chronic poisoning: Skeletal and teeth abnormalities, lameness, arched back, stiffness, dry hair coat, rough skin
Fluoroquinolones	Colic, diarrhea, seizures, articular cartilage lesions, arthropathy and lameness in foals
Fumonisin	Leukoencephalomalacia, sudden onset abnormal behavior, hyperexcitability, aimless circling, head pressing, repetitive motions, paresis, facial paralysis, ataxia, blindness, depression, coma, seizures. Dyspnea can be seen. High doses: Also liver damage, icterus, petechiae, coagulopathy, swelling of lips/muzzle. Dyspnea, cyanosis may be seen. Rapid death can occur.
Gila monster	Pain and bleeding at bite site, tissue necrosis, secondary infection, muscle fasciculations regionally
Glucocorticoids	Adverse effects vary with drug. Adrenal suppression, laminitis, PU/PD, abortion, GI ulceration, immunosuppression
Glyphosate herbicides	Example: Roundup™. If exposure to concentrated products occurs, can see salivation, colic, diarrhea, anorexia, lethargy
Golden chain tree (*Laburnum anagyroides*)	Anorexia, excitement, weakness, muscle tremors, ataxia, seizures, colic
Gossypol	Effects of gossypol are not well documented in horses. Effects seen in other animals include sudden death, chronic heart failure, fluid in chest and abdominal cavities, anorexia, ill thrift, poor hair coat.
Grayanotoxin-containing plants	Examples: Rhododendron, azalea, laurels, pieris, mountain pieris, fetter bush, others. Depression, salivation, colic, diarrhea, arrhythmias, tachypnea, hyperthermia, hypotension, sweating, weakness, ataxia, lateral recumbency, seizures, opisthotonus, aspiration pneumonia

Continued

Table 2: Equine Toxins Listed Alphabetically—cont'd

Toxic Substance	Clinical Signs
Griseofulvin	Bone marrow suppression and GI signs may be possible but not documented in horses. Teratogenic effects reported in horses include microphthalmia, brachygnathia, and other effects.
Hoary alyssum (*Berteroa*)	Lethargy, hyperthermia, edema of distal limbs, laminitis, colic, diarrhea, early parturition or late-term abortion, scrotal and testicular edema, intravascular hemolysis, hemorrhagic gastroenteritis, shock, dehydration, renal failure, endotoxemia, DIC in severe cases
Hydrogen sulfide	Lacrimation, dyspnea, pulmonary edema, cyanosis, seizures, apnea, collapse with respiratory paralysis at high concentrations
Hypochaeris spp	Examples: Spotted cat's ear, hairy cat's ear, flatweed. Stringhalt: Sudden involuntary flexion and delayed extension of hocks, especially when backing or turning. Stumbling. Legs strike abdomen during flexion.
Illicit stimulant drugs	Examples: Many drugs including cocaine, amphetamines, PCP, LSD. Signs vary depending on drug and dosage, but may include restlessness, hyperactivity, bizarre behavior, hypersalivation, tachycardia, arrhythmias, tremors, mydriasis, hyperthermia, ataxia, seizures, death
Insulin	Possible signs might include hypoglycemia, weakness, muscle fasciculation, ataxia, bizarre behavior, coma, death
Iodine	Lacrimation, salivation, cough, dry skin, anorexia, tachycardia, abortion, infertility, goiter, decreased immune response. Foals: Weakness and goiter
Ionophores	Feed refusal, weakness, ataxia, incoordination, tremors, hesitance to move, tachycardia, congested membranes, tremors, arrhythmias, hypotension, hyperpnea, sweating, recumbency, jugular pulse, pitting edema, seizures, and death. Persistent cardiac damage: Unthriftiness, poor performance, exercise intolerance, pitting edema, arrhythmias, sudden death
Iron	Anorexia, lethargy, depression, dyspnea, GI corrosive effects, colic, bloody diarrhea, hypotension, shock, hypovolemia, cardiac damage, hepatic necrosis, icterus, metabolic acidosis, coagulopathy, lethargy, hepatic encephalopathy, hyperglycemia, coma, seizures, tremors, head pressing, ataxia, anemia, thrombocytopenia, lymphopenia
Ivermectin, moxidectin	Depression, mydriasis, tremors, ataxia, salivation, blindness, muscle fasciculations, flaccid lips, coma. Urinary bladder rupture in foals may occur
Jimson weed (*Datura stramonium*)	CNS excitation or depression, anorexia, weakness, decreased urination, hyperthermia, tachycardia, dry mucus membranes, mydriasis, visual impairment, GI atony and impaction, gas accumulation, gastric dilation and rupture, colic, diarrhea, seizures, death
Kentucky coffee tree (*Gymnocladus dioica*)	Colic, diarrhea, hypotension, bradycardia, seizures, death
Lantana	Liver damage, 2° photosensitization
Lathyrus spp	Examples: Wild pea, singletary pea, vetchling; also chick peas. Stilted gait, weakness, lameness, laryngeal hemiplegia, spastic paraparesis, hind limb paralysis
Lead	Peripheral neuropathy, weight loss, depression, ataxia, dysphagia, dysphonia, roaring, laryngeal paralysis, facial nerve deficits, seizures, anemia, nucleated red blood cells, basophilic stippling, blindness, GI signs, aspiration pneumonia
Lidocaine	Muscle fasciculations, ataxia, depression, seizures
Lincomycin, clindamycin	Pseudomembranous colitis, colic, diarrhea
Locoweeds (*Astragalus, Oxytropis*)	Depression (can be severe), weight loss, circling, incoordination, tremors, ataxia, unpredictable behavior, falling over backward, rearing, weakness, blindness, coma, convulsions; congenital abnormalities such as crooked legs in foals; abortion and other reproductive effects; vacuoles in peripheral lymphocytes. Locoweeds also can accumulate selenium.
Lupine (*Lupinus*)	Teratogenic: Arthrogryposis, scoliosis, kyphosis, torticollis, and cleft palate. (Also lupinosis: liver damage, myopathy—1° Australia)
Mayapple (*Podophyllum*)	Anorexia, diarrhea, colic, salivation, lacrimation, hyperthermia, ataxia, paralysis, coma, renal damage
Mercury	Renal damage, stomatitis, diarrhea, dehydration, shock. Alkyl mercurial compounds (found in some fungicides) can cause skin lesions, conjunctivitis, stomatitis, weakness, depression, ataxia, incoordination, paresis, tachycardia, tachypnea, blindness, anemia, anorexia, proprioceptive deficits, paralysis, and coma. Rapid death can occur.
Metaldehyde	Salivation, restlessness, agitation, ataxia, tremors, twitching, nystagmus, hyperpnea, hyperthermia, hyperesthesia, sweating, tachycardia, convulsions, dyspnea, colic, liver damage, renal damage, DIC, blindness
Methylxanthines	Examples: Caffeine, theobromine, theophylline. Restlessness, hyperactivity, tachycardia, tachypnea, tremors, seizures, arrhythmias, colic, diarrhea, weakness, agitation, behavioral abnormalities
Metronidazole	Neurotoxicity, ataxia, lethargy, anorexia, nystagmus, seizures
Microcystin (blue-green algae toxin)	Hepatotoxicity, lethargy, diarrhea, colic, weakness, pale membranes, death. 2° photosensitization can occur in survivors.
Milkweeds (*Asclepias*)	Cardiotoxic or neurotoxic depending on the plant species. Colic, diarrhea, restlessness, incoordination, weakness, tremors, muscle fasciculations, apprehension, hyperthermia, sweating, mydriasis, cardiac arrhythmias, seizures, head pressing, paddling. Rapid death can occur.
Milkvetches (*Astragalus*)	Neuromuscular abnormalities, abnormal gait, rear limb proprioceptive defects, paresis or paralysis; goose-stepping, reluctance to back up, weakness, temporary blindness, rough dull haircoat
Mojave rattlesnake (*Crotalus scutulatus*)	Neurologic deficits, paralysis
Molybdenum	Abortion, 2° copper deficiency
Monkshood (*Aconitum*)	Restlessness, salivation, weakness, arrhythmias, dyspnea, lateral recumbency. Rapid death can occur.
Mushrooms with GI effects	Colic, abdominal pain, diarrhea, weakness, sweating

Table 2: Equine Toxins Listed Alphabetically—cont'd

Toxic Substance	Clinical Signs
Mushrooms with hallucinogenic effects	Bizarre mentation, mydriasis, agitation or depression, incoordination, tremors, recumbency
Mushrooms with muscarinic effects	Lacrimation, miosis, salivation, sweating, colic, bradycardia, bronchorrhea, frequent urination, diarrhea
Mustards (*Brassica*)	Depression, anemia, hemoglobinemia, hemoglobinuria, pale or icteric membranes
Napthalene	Signs might include colic, diarrhea, anorexia, hemolytic anemia, icterus, pale membranes, hematuria, renal damage, but cases have not been reported in horses.
Nicotine, tobacco (*Nicotiana*)	Excitement, tremors, seizures, tachypnea, salivation, lacrimation, diarrhea, colic, ataxia, staggering, followed by weakness, depression, tachycardia, recumbency, coma, paralysis, death by respiratory paralysis. Sudden death can occur. Teratogenic effects include arthrogryposis, scoliosis, kyphosis, torticollis, and cleft palate.
Nightshades (*Solanum*)	Examples: black, bittersweet, and silverleaf nightshades; horse nettles, others. Anorexia, salivation, abdominal pain, colic, diarrhea, mydriasis, depression, weakness, tremors, progressive paralysis, prostration, seizures
Nitrate, chlorate	Weakness, ataxia, tachycardia, tremors, methemoglobinemia, colic, diarrhea, dyspnea, collapse, convulsions, abortion. Rapid death can occur.
Non-protein nitrogen (urea)	Restlessness, tremors, dyspnea, frequent urination and defecation, stiffness, colic, arrhythmias, head pressing. Rapid death can occur.
NSAIDs (nonsteroidal antiinflammatory drugs)	Colic, anorexia, oral and GI ulcers, renal damage, diarrhea with blood, liver damage
Oak (*Quercus*)	Colic, anorexia, depression, abdominal pain, constipation or diarrhea (sometimes bloody), hemoglobinuria, hematuria, icterus, tachycardia, tachypnea, renal damage, dehydration. Acorn husks may be seen in feces.
Oleander (*Nerium*)	See "Cardiac glycoside-containing plants"
Organochlorine insecticides	Example: Endosulfan. Salivation, agitation, hyperexcitability, incoordination, tremors, seizures, opisthotonus, clamped jaws, paddling, hyperthermia
Panicum spp	Examples: Switchgrass, Kleingrass, panic grass. Liver damage, photosensitization, depression, pruritus, anorexia, icterus, dark urine, photophobia
Paraquat	Oral or dermal lesions, colic, renal damage, liver damage, delayed onset of pulmonary damage and respiratory signs, death
Penicillins	Anaphylactic reactions, hemolytic anemia, thrombocytopenia. Procaine toxicosis: Excitation, tremors, incoordination, apnea
Petroleum products	Anorexia, weight loss, diarrhea, lethargy, unthriftiness, depression, ataxia, laminitis, seizures, aspiration pneumonia, hepatic and renal damage, death. Possibly abortions and infertility
Phenothiazines	Sedation or excitement, sweating, trembling, tachypnea, tachycardia, seizures, decreased hematocrit, hypotension, cardiovascular collapse, penile prolapse. If given intra-arterially, can see severe CNS excitement or depression, seizures, and death.
Phenols	Oral and GI burns, dermal burns, laryngeal edema, salivation, mydriasis, weakness, nasal discharge, tremors, seizures, coma, arrhythmias, diarrhea, hypotension, liver damage, renal damage, respiratory irritation and dyspnea, methemoglobinemia, hemolytic anemia
1° photosensitizing plants	Examples: Bishop's weed, Dutchman's breeches, spring parsley, cow parsnip, St. John's wort, buckwheat. 1° photosensitization, photophobia, conjunctivitis, diarrhea, intravascular hemolysis, anemia
2° photosensitizing plants	See "Pyrrolizidine alkaloid containing plants"
Phytoestrogenic plants	Examples: Clover, alfalfa, vetches, other legumes. Infertility, abnormal estrus cycles, feminization, cystic hyperplasia
Pigweed (*Amaranthus*)	Depression, weakness, tremors, incoordination, renal damage, hypocalcemia
Pine oil	Oral or dermal lesions, depression, arrhythmias, diarrhea, renal damage, aspiration pneumonia, hypotension, respiratory depression, ataxia, myoglobinuria
Pit vipers	Examples: Rattlesnakes, copperheads, and water moccasins (cottonmouths). Pain, swelling regionally and at bite site, puncture wounds, ecchymoses, petechiation, tissue necrosis, sloughing, coagulopathy, dyspnea from swelling of muzzle; shock, hypotension, tachycardia, lethargy, colic, muscle fasciculations, salivation, cardiac arrhythmias, persistent cardiac damage, elevated CK, echinocytes, thrombocytopenia. Later sloughing of tissues, chronic heart damage. Rapid death can occur.
Poison hemlock (*Conium*)	Apprehension, weakness, tremors, ataxia, staggering, salivation, tachycardia, cold extremities, mydriasis, frequent urination and defecation, strong odor to breath, depression, recumbency, coma. Teratogenic: Arthrogryposis, scoliosis, kyphosis, torticollis, and cleft palate have been reported in other species
Pokeweed (*Phytolacca*)	Colic, diarrhea, salivation, anorexia
Potassium	Overdose: Cardiac arrhythmias, cardiovascular arrest, muscular weakness, death
Prostaglandins	Sweating, diarrhea, colic; incoordination, ataxia, dyspnea, abortion
Propylene glycol	Colic, salivation, sweating, ataxia, circling, depression, metabolic acidosis, recumbency, shallow breathing, cyanosis, strong odor
Pyrethrin/pyrethroid insecticides	Paresthesia, salivation, tremors, restlessness
Pyrrolizidine alkaloid-containing plants (2° photosensitizers)	Examples: *Senecio, Crotalaria, Amsinckia, Cynoglossum, Echium, Heliotropium*. Acute: Acute liver failure, anorexia, depression, icterus, edema, ascites Chronic: Rough haircoat, depression, anorexia, chronic liver failure: icterus, ascites, emaciation, hepatoencephalopathy, head pressing, behavioral changes; 2° photosensitization, photophobia, conjunctivitis

Continued

Table 2: Equine Toxins Listed Alphabetically—cont'd

Toxic Substance	Clinical Signs
Red maple (*Acer*)	Depression, anorexia, weakness, methemoglobinemia, hemolysis, icterus, anemia, hemoglobinuria, dark urine, tachypnea, dyspnea, tachycardia, cyanosis, abortion, Heinz bodies, spherocytosis, 2° renal damage. Sudden death can occur.
Rifampin	Stains everything red; red urine, feces, tears, sweat, and saliva. When combined with erythromycin, can cause diarrhea and enterocolitis, hyperthermia, and acute respiratory distress. IV rifampin can cause depression, sweating, hemolysis, anorexia.
Rosary pea (*Abrus*)	Diarrhea, colic, hemorrhagic gastroenteritis
Sagebrush (*Artemisia*)	Unpredictable behavior, nervousness, depression, circling, incoordination, strong odor to breath
Selenium	Acute: Anorexia, depression, weakness, dyspnea, strong odor to breath, rapid death Chronic: Lameness, hoof overgrowth and deformation, hoof wall cracks, hair loss/breakage and discoloration
Slaframine	Examples: Moldy red clover and other legumes. Excessive salivation, anorexia, diarrhea, colic, frequent urination, lacrimation, bradycardia, decreased milk production, dehydration
Sodium	Colic, diarrhea, weakness, dehydration, tremors, seizures, blindness, behavioral changes. Elevated serum sodium and chloride
Sodium fluoroacetate (1080)	Staggering, sweating, tremors, colic, diarrhea, acidosis, hyperesthesia, arrhythmias, seizures, extensor rigidity, sudden death
Soluble oxalates	Examples: Beets, dock, halogeton, lamb's quarter, greasewood, rhubarb. Depression, anorexia, twitching, colic, grinding teeth, ataxia, diarrhea, bradycardia, salivation, weakness, incoordination, recumbency, coma, seizures, renal damage, hypocalcemia
Stachybotryotoxins	Salivation, erythema and edema and erosions of nose, lips, buccal mucosa, tongue; colic, diarrhea, hyperthermia, neutropenia, thrombocytopenia
Starlicide (3-CPT)	Methemoglobinemia, depression, flaccid paralysis, hypothermia
Stipa (needlegrass)	Sluggish, dragging feet, difficult to arouse, head held low, staggering, sweating
Strychnine	Ataxia, stiffness beginning with face, neck, and limbs; severe muscle spasms, seizures, anxiety, tachypnea, salivation, generalized seizures, opisthotonus, clamped jaws, hyperthermia, extensor rigidity, impaired respirations
Sudan grass (*Sorghum*)	Photosensitization. Neuropathy: Weakness and ataxia of hind legs, collapsing when backed; urinary incontinence with dribbling of urine, scalding of perineum and hind legs; hematuria, thick atonic bladder, tail flaccidity, dilation of rectum, fecal accumulation in rectum. Alert, normal appetite, respirations, and heart rate. Cystitis and ascending pyelonephritis can develop. Continuously open and close vulva in females, penis relaxed and extended in males. Abortion. Teratogenic: Foals born weak or with arthrogryposis
Sulfonamides	Renal damage, liver damage, coagulopathy, blood dyscrasias, bone marrow suppression, diarrhea. Teratogenic at high doses; abortion. IV use: Hypotension, collapse. Combined with pyrimethamine: neurologic signs, ataxia, dysphagia, facial nerve paralysis
Sweet clover (*Melilotus*), moldy	Coagulopathy, blood loss, hematomas, epistaxis, hemorrhage, colic, anemia, pale membranes. Signs depend on where bleeding occurs. Abortion
Tetanus	Muscle stiffness, elevated third eyelid, abnormal blink, elevated tail, flared nostrils, saw-horse stance, clamped jaws, dysphagia, aphagia; finally recumbent, convulsions, contraction of muscles of respiration, death
Tetracyclines	Renal damage, affect on developing teeth and bone, colitis. IV: Hypotension and collapse. Possibly photosensitivity, blood dyscrasias
Tick paralysis	Reported in horses in Australia, not in North America at this time. Progressive general paralysis, ataxia, recumbency, flaccid tail, flaccid anus, weak facial muscles
Tilmicosin	Tachypnea, seizures, ataxia, acute death
Tremorgenic forages	Examples: Perennial rye grass, Dallisgrass, bahia grass, Bermuda grass. Fine tremors of head and neck, tremors, stiffness, ataxia, incoordination, hypermetria, seizures and opisthotonus after minimal stimulation, behavioral changes. Episodic
Tropane alkaloids	Examples: Jimson weed (*Datura*), Belladonna (*Atropa*), bindweed (*Convolvulus*). Anorexia, weight loss, mydriasis, thirst, wandering, blindness, restlessness, twitching, incoordination, paralysis, delirium, dry membranes, GI stasis, colic, tachycardia, tachypnea, seizures
Turpentine	Oral or dermal lesions, depression, dyspnea, pulmonary edema if aspirated, colic, ataxia, agitation
Vetch (*Vicia*)	Dermatitis with papular swellings, plaques, exudation, crusting, pruritus. Lesions start on neck, tailhead, and udder and then progress. Granulomatous inflammation of organs. Weight loss, anorexia, hyperthermia, subcutaneous edema. Differs from photosensitization in that lesions are not restricted to white pigmented areas.
Vitamin A	Anorexia, lameness, abortion, bone abnormalities
Vitamin K₃	Colic, depression, anorexia, hemolytic anemia, hematuria, renal damage
Vitamin D-containing plants	Example: Day-blooming jessamine (*Cestrum diurnum*). See "Day-blooming jessamine."
Water hemlock (*Cicuta*)	Apprehension, salivation, teeth grinding, chewing motions, frequent urination and defecation, mydriasis, ataxia, incoordination, muscle ticks progressing to muscle contractions, lateral recumbency, seizures, coma. Rapid death can occur.
Wheat (*Triticum*)	Photosensitization

Table 2: Equine Toxins Listed Alphabetically—cont'd

Toxic Substance	Clinical Signs
White snakeroot (*Eupatorium*). Also Rayless goldenrod (*Isocoma pluriforma*)	Depression, sluggishness, reluctance to move, stiffness, ataxia, wide-based stance, crossed rear legs, tremors (especially flank and hind legs), weakness, recumbency, sweating, mydriasis, injected sclera and conjunctiva, myoglobinuria, arrhythmias. Tremors quiet when horse is relaxed; increase when forced to move. Constipation, anorexia, salivation, urinary incontinence, dyspnea, coma, renal damage, strong odor to breath. Markedly elevated CK, myoglobinuria. Abortions may occur. Toxin transferred in milk. Rapid death can occur.
Xylazine	Muscle tremors, bradycardia, partial A-V block and other cardiac arrhythmias, sweating, hypotension.
Yellow star thistle (*Centaurea*), Russian knapweed (*Acroptilon repens*)	Nigropallidal encephalomalacia: acute onset dysphagia, cannot eat or drink; submerse muzzle deep in water, hypertonic facial muscles, dehydrated, weigh loss, depressed, somnolent. Brief periods of agitation, excitation. Head hanging low, pitting edema of head/neck. Excessive chewing, food dribbling from mouth, yawning, tongue protruding, curling of lips, ulceration of tongue and lips. Aimless circling, ataxia, tremors, proprioceptive deficits, weakness, aspiration pneumonia
Yew (*Taxus*)	Sudden death. Lethargic, tremors, arrhythmias, atonic lips and tail, weak pulses, ataxia, paresis, dyspnea, collapse, recumbency, rapid death
Zinc	Unthrifty, lameness, lateral recumbency, reluctance to rise or move, stiff, ached back, arthritis, osteochondrosis, joint effusion, laryngeal paralysis, skeletal abnormalities, nephrocalcinosis
Zinc phosphide, aluminum phosphide	Anorexia, depression, rapid wheezy respirations, dyspnea, sweating, colic, tremors, ataxia, weakness, recumbency, hypoxia, struggling, hyperesthesia, arrhythmias. Rapid death can be seen.

AST, aspartate aminotransferase; *A-V,* atrioventricular; *CK,* creatinine kinase; *CNS,* central nervous system; *DIC,* disseminated intravascular coagulation; *GI,* gastrointestinal; *PU/PD,* polyuria and polydipsia.

AUTHOR: **CYNTHIA L. GASKILL**

Upper Airway Disorders That May Be Associated with Respiratory Distress in Adult Horses

Nasal disorders
Trauma, foreign body
Hemorrhage or hematoma
Neoplasia
Abscess

Pharyngeal disorders
Neoplasia
Cyst
Dorsal displacement of soft palate
Trauma, foreign body
Abscess

Laryngeal disorders
Laryngeal paralysis
Laryngeal hemiplegia
Trauma, foreign body
Edema
Arytenoid chondritis
Epiglottitis

Miscellaneous
Guttural pouch enlargement
Head edema

From Barr B: Support of respiratory function. In Reed SM, Bayly WM, Sellon DC (eds). *Equine Internal Medicine,* ed 3. St Louis, 2010, Saunders, pp 265–269.

Urinary Incontinence

Cauda equina syndrome
Cystitis/sabulous urolithiasis
Urinalysis reveals pyuria, hematuria, and bacteriuria
Cystolithiasis
Hematuria, especially after exercise
Cystoscopy, ultrasound, or rectal examination should demonstrate urolithiasis
Dystocia or foaling injuries
Ectopic ureter
Fillies: Usually found within the vaginal vault
Colts: Usually found in the pelvic urethra

Equine degenerative myelopathy
Profound symmetrical ataxia and weakness without muscle wasting or loss of cutaneous sensation
Decreased serum vitamin E concentration
Equine herpesvirus type 1 myelitis
Loss of tail tone and perineal sensation, hind limb paresis, ataxia
Fever and herd outbreaks are possible
Positive polymerase chain reaction (PCR) on whole blood or nasal swab

DIFFERENTIAL DIAGNOSES

Xanthochromic cerebrospinal fluid with increased total protein concentration and normal nucleated cell count

Equine motor neuron disease

Loss of antigravity muscles and prolonged periods of recumbency without weakness

Affected horses stand with their legs gathered beneath them "horse balancing on a ball"

Biopsy of sacrocaudalis dorsalis muscle or ventral branch of the spinal accessory nerve

Equine protozoal myeloencephalopathy

Asymmetric ataxia and other neurologic deficits

Antibodies in cerebrospinal fluid against *Sarcocystis neurona* or *Neospora hughesi*

Hypoestrogenism

Older mares

Illicit tail blocking

Injection of alcohol or other demyelinating substances into the sacrococcygeal space

Neoplasia

Polyneuritis equi

Perineal hypalgesia, loss of tail tone and areflexia, and loss of anal tone

May also have cranial nerve deficits

Sacral or coccygeal trauma

Sorghum cystitis

Sudan grass toxicity

Urachal diverticulum

Foals

Can be visualized with ultrasonography or cystoscopy

SUGGESTED READING

Bayly WM: Urinary incontinence and bladder dysfunction. In Reed SM, Bayly WM, Sellon DC (eds). *Equine Internal Medicine*, ed 3. St Louis, 2010, Saunders, pp 1224–1227.

AUTHORS: **PETER R. MORRESEY** and **KELLY L. KALF**

Weight Loss

Inadequate caloric intake

Miscalculated or poor quality diet

Unable to access food source due to lameness or herd situation

Poor dentition

Dysphagia

Poor appetite

Stress

Gastric ulcers

Picky eater

Inadequate absorption of nutrients

Parasites

Inflammatory or infiltrative conditions of the intestine

Granulomatous enterocolitis

Lymphocytic/plasmacytic enterocolitis

Eosinophilic enterocolitis

Neoplasia of the gastrointestinal tract

Protein-losing enteropathy

Parasitism

Gastrointestinal ulceration

Diarrhea

Neoplasia

Noninfectious systemic disease

Neoplasia

Pituitary pars intermedia dysfunction (equine Cushing's disease)

Chronic renal disease

Recurrent airway obstruction

Heart failure

Liver failure

Infection

Pneumonia

Enterocolitis

Bacterial endocarditis

Peritonitis

AUTHOR: **SARA GOMEZ-IBANEZ**

Laboratory Tests

Acanthocytes

BASIC INFORMATION

DEFINITION

Acanthocytes are spiculated erythrocytes. They have 2 to 10 projections that are often blunted or clubbed on their ends. The projections are of variable length and often irregularly spaced on the cell.

SYNONYM(S)

Spur cells

TYPICAL NORMAL RANGE (US UNITS; SI UNITS)

Rare to none

PHYSIOLOGY

The mechanism of acanthocyte formation in animals is not entirely certain, and there may be more than one mechanism depending on the condition they are associated with.

CAUSES OF ABNORMALLY HIGH LEVELS Acanthocytes are rarely noted on equine blood smears. In other species, they have most commonly been associated with hepatic and splenic disorders and with hemangiosarcoma. They also have been associated with glomerulonephritis and lymphoma.

SPECIMEN AND PROCESSING CONSIDERATIONS

LAB ARTIFACTS THAT MAY INTERFERE WITH READINGS OF LEVELS OF THIS SUBSTANCE (AND HOW—ARTIFICIALLY ELEVATED VS. DEPRESSED) Acanthocytes must be differentiated from echinocytes, which generally have many short, sharp projections that are relatively evenly spaced on the cell. Echinocyte formation often is an artifact of sample handling or slide preparation, but pathologic echinocytosis in horses has been associated with hyponatremia and hypochloremia, strenuous exercise, reaction to phenothiazine administration, hemolytic anemia due to clostridial infection, and snake envenomation. Inadequate filling of EDTA (purple top) blood collection tubes may result in artifactual formation of spiculated cells, which may be difficult to differentiate from acanthocytes and/or echinocytes.

AUTHOR: **MARLYN S. WHITNEY**

EDITOR: **CHARLES WIEDMEYER**

Activated Clotting Time (ACT)

BASIC INFORMATION

DEFINITION

Screening coagulation test of the surface-induced (intrinsic) and common pathways.

SYNONYM(S)

Activated coagulation time
ACT

TYPICAL NORMAL RANGE (US UNITS; SI UNITS)

Measurements reported in seconds. Prolonged when there is about a 90% to 95% decrease in activity of a single factor. Laboratory, instrument, and species-specific reference intervals must be used. Values in healthy newborn foals (<24 hours old) may be greater than reference intervals established for adults.

PHYSIOLOGY

Blood is drawn into a vacuum tube containing siliceous (diatomaceous) earth, which activates the surface-induced pathway. The blood is mixed by five inversions, and the tube is incubated at 37° C for 60 seconds. The tube is then checked every 5 to 10 seconds for the first evidence of clot formation.

CAUSES OF ABNORMALLY HIGH LEVELS Decreased production (liver disease, vitamin K antagonism or absence), increased factor inactivation and consumption (disseminated intravascular coagulation [DIC]), dilution of factors (massive transfusions of plasma-poor fluids), hereditary factor defects, factor inhibition (heparin therapy). Severe thrombocytopenia may also cause a prolonged result due to decreased phospholipid availability.

NEXT DIAGNOSTIC STEP TO CONSIDER IF LEVELS HIGH
- Confirm with more sensitive test of surface induced and common pathways.
- Platelet count

DRUG EFFECTS ON LEVELS Increased by heparin

SPECIMEN AND PROCESSING CONSIDERATIONS

LAB ARTIFACTS THAT MAY INTERFERE WITH READINGS OF LEVELS OF THIS SUBSTANCE (AND HOW—ARTIFICIALLY ELEVATED VS. DEPRESSED) Modifications of the protocol may affect expected values. Variations have related to syringe versus vacuum collection, incubation temperature, length of initial incubation period, and frequency of inspection for clots. End point is subject to observer variability.

SAMPLE FOR COLLECTION (TYPE OF SPECIMEN, COLOR TUBE) AND ANY SPECIAL SPECIMEN HANDLING NOTES Prewarmed to 37° C tube of siliceous earth (gray top, with large granules) filled with whole blood

PEARLS Considered an insensitive test. Carriers of hemophilia cannot be detected by activated partial thromboplastin time (aPTT) because the decrease in factor activity is approximately 50%.

AUTHOR: **BRITTON GRASPERGE**

EDITOR: **CHARLES WIEDMEYER**

Activated Partial Thromboplastin Time (aPTT)

BASIC INFORMATION

DEFINITION

Screening coagulation test of the surface-induced (intrinsic) and common pathways

SYNONYM(S)

Partial thromboplastin time (PTT)
aPTT
APTT

TYPICAL NORMAL RANGE (US UNITS; SI UNITS)

Measurements reported in seconds. Prolonged when there is about a 70% decrease in activity of a single factor. Laboratory, instrument, and species-specific reference intervals must be used. Values in healthy newborn foals (<24 hours old) may be greater than reference intervals established for adults.

PHYSIOLOGY

Measures the time in seconds required for fibrin clot formation in citrated plasma after addition of a contact activator of the surface-induced pathway, a phospholipid that substitutes for platelet-derived phospholipid, and calcium.

CAUSES OF ABNORMALLY HIGH LEVELS Decreased production (liver disease, vitamin K antagonism or absence), increased factor inactivation and consumption (disseminated intravascular coagulation [DIC]), dilution of factors (massive transfusions of plasma-poor fluids), hereditary factor defects, factor inhibition (heparin therapy)

NEXT DIAGNOSTIC STEP TO CONSIDER IF LEVELS HIGH Measurement of individual factors if hereditary disease is suspected

CAUSES OF ABNORMALLY LOW LEVELS Not reliable for detecting hypercoagulability

DRUG EFFECTS ON LEVELS
- Increased by heparin and aspirin
- Oxyglobin interferes with optical detection of clot formation.

SPECIMEN AND PROCESSING CONSIDERATIONS

LAB ARTIFACTS THAT MAY INTERFERE WITH READINGS OF LEVELS OF THIS SUBSTANCE (AND HOW—ARTIFICIALLY ELEVATED VS. DEPRESSED)
- Decrease: Contamination with tissue factor during sampling, overfilling citrate tube
- Increase: Lipemia, hemolysis, and icterus interfere with optical detection of clot formation; incomplete filling of citrate tube; old specimen

SAMPLE FOR COLLECTION (TYPE OF SPECIMEN, COLOR TUBE) AND ANY SPECIAL SPECIMEN HANDLING NOTES Obtain sample via minimally traumatic phlebotomy. Collect specimen in citrate (blue top) tube. Fill to ratio of nine parts blood to one part citrate (2.7 mL blood in a 3-mL citrate tube).

PEARLS Carriers of hemophilia cannot be detected by aPTT because the decrease in factor activity is approximately 50%.

AUTHOR: **BRITTON GRASPERGE**

EDITOR: **CHARLES WIEDMEYER**

ACTH (Adrenocorticotropic Hormone), Endogenous/Baseline

BASIC INFORMATION

DEFINITION

Polypeptide hormone secreted by the anterior pituitary gland (adenohypophysis) in response to corticotropin-releasing hormone (CRH) secreted by the hypothalamus.

SYNONYM(S)

Corticotropin

TYPICAL NORMAL RANGE (US UNITS; SI UNITS)

Horses: 18.68 ± 6.79 pg/mL (mean $\pm$ SD); ponies: 8.35 ± 2.92 pg/mL. Limited information regarding normal plasma ACTH concentrations in ponies; some sources suggest plasma ACTH is lower (5.4–11.2 pg/mL) in ponies compared to horses. It is important to consider the time of year (seasonal variation) when interpreting plasma ACTH concentrations. In normal horses and ponies, it has been shown that plasma ACTH concentrations are significantly higher in September than in January and May. To convert pg/mL to pmol/L multiply pg/mL by 0.22.

PHYSIOLOGY

In response to stress and/or illness, the hypothalamus releases CRH. CRH stimulates release of ACTH from the anterior pituitary gland. ACTH is derived from the proteolytic fragmentation of the large prohormone, proopiomelanocortin (POMC). ACTH stimulates release of cortisol and aldosterone by the adrenal glands. Increasing levels of circulating cortisol inhibit secretion of CRH and ACTH (negative-feedback system).

CAUSES OF ABNORMALLY HIGH LEVELS Pituitary pars intermedia dysfunction (PPID)/equine pituitary Cushing's syndrome, exercise induced/stressful transport, autumn (specifically September), abrupt cessation of chronic glucocorticoid administration (eg, racing horses), adrenal exhaustion/turn-out syndrome, primary hypoadrenocorticism (rare)

NEXT DIAGNOSTIC STEP TO CONSIDER IF LEVELS HIGH Rule out stressful travel and/or excessive exercise; determine treatment history (glucocorticoid administration); signalment, clinical signs, and high ACTH level may be sufficient for a diagnosis of PPID; additional diagnostics, for example, dexamethasone suppression test, may be warranted.

CAUSES OF ABNORMALLY LOW LEVELS Iatrogenic hypoadrenocorticism (chronic glucocorticoid administration), functional adrenal cortical tumor (rare)

NEXT DIAGNOSTIC STEP TO CONSIDER IF LEVELS LOW Rule out sampling error (see "Lab Artifacts" section), ACTH stimulation test.

IMPORTANT INTERSPECIES DIFFERENCES See "Typical Normal Range" section.

SPECIMEN AND PROCESSING CONSIDERATIONS

LAB ARTIFACTS THAT MAY INTERFERE WITH READINGS OF LEVELS OF THIS SUBSTANCE (AND HOW—ARTIFICIALLY ELEVATED VS. DEPRESSED) Decreased: Storage in a glass tube, increased temperatures/thawing of specimen

SAMPLE FOR COLLECTION (TYPE OF SPECIMEN, COLOR TUBE) AND ANY SPECIAL SPECIMEN HANDLING NOTES Collect blood (2–5 mL) in a purple-top EDTA tube (either plastic or siliconized glass). Chill the whole blood and separate plasma within 3 hours of drawing. Transfer plasma to a plastic tube. Freeze specimen if not shipping immediately. Specimens should be shipped on ice so they arrive chilled (at or below 60° F) or frozen.

PEARLS: ACTH is very labile in whole blood and serum; therefore, increased temperatures will give falsely low values. ACTH also binds to glass resulting in falsely low values. Plasma needs to be transferred and stored in plastic tubes.

AUTHOR: **MICHELLE CORA**

EDITOR: **CHARLES WIEDMEYER**

Albumin

BASIC INFORMATION

DEFINITION

Albumin is the major single protein found in serum.

TYPICAL NORMAL RANGE (US UNITS; SI UNITS)

2.8 to 4.8 g/dL (28–48 g/L); varies slightly between reference laboratories. Young animals often have lower concentrations.

PHYSIOLOGY

Albumin is synthesized by hepatocytes, and it is a negative acute phase protein. Albumin is the major contributor to plasma colloidal osmotic pressure, and it serves as a transport protein for ions, bilirubin, fatty acids, thyroxine, drugs, and many other substances.

CAUSES OF ABNORMALLY HIGH LEVELS Dehydration

NEXT DIAGNOSTIC STEP TO CONSIDER IF LEVELS HIGH Assess hydration status; if normal recheck albumin values.

CAUSES OF ABNORMALLY LOW LEVELS Decreased synthesis (inflammation, liver disease, malabsorptive and maldigestive diseases), increased loss (blood loss, protein-losing nephropathies or enteropathies, severe exudative skin lesions or burns), hemodilution (excess fluid administration, edematous disorders)

NEXT DIAGNOSTIC STEP TO CONSIDER IF LEVELS LOW Review history and physical exam and assess for presence of hepatic, renal, or intestinal tract disorders. Assess in conjunction with hematocrit, total protein, globulins (albumin:globulin ratio), fibrinogen, liver enzymes, and renal function. If a cause cannot be determined, then additional testing could include urine protein-to-creatinine ratio, fecal flotation, ultrasound, or biopsies.

SPECIMEN AND PROCESSING CONSIDERATIONS

DRUG EFFECTS ON LEVELS See "Lab Artifacts."

LAB ARTIFACTS THAT MAY INTERFERE WITH READINGS OF LEVELS OF THIS SUBSTANCE (AND HOW—ARTIFICIALLY ELEVATED VS. DEPRESSED)

- False increase: Test reagent (bromcresol green [BCG]) may bind to globulin when albumin is very low and globulins are high.
- False decreases: Use of human testing reagents may underestimate albumin (if sample is submitted to a human medical laboratory rather than a veterinary laboratory); some anticonvulsants and antibiotics can competitively bind BCG.

SAMPLE FOR COLLECTION (TYPE OF SPECIMEN, COLOR TUBE) AND ANY SPECIAL SPECIMEN HANDLING NOTES Serum (red top) or lithium heparin plasma (green top); contact reference laboratory for their preference. Allow specimen to clot (red top only), centrifuge, collect serum or plasma, refrigerate, ship on ice.

AUTHOR: **BRIDGET C. GARNER**

EDITOR: **CHARLES WIEDMEYER**

LABORATORY TESTS

Albuminuria and Proteinuria

BASIC INFORMATION

DEFINITION

The presence of excess protein and/or albumin in urine

TYPICAL NORMAL RANGE (US UNITS; SI UNITS)

Approximately 2 mg/dL to 36 mg/dL with wet chemistry instrument methods and negative or trace on dipstick methods

PHYSIOLOGY

- The glomerular capillary wall restricts the filtration of most plasma proteins on the basis of protein weight and protein charge. Small (<68,000 d) electrically neutral or positively charged proteins are more readily filtered. In most healthy animals, the proteins that pass the glomerular filter are resorbed in the proximal tubules. Albumin is negatively charged and too large (69,000 d) to filter through the normal glomerulus.

- A small amount of albumin and Tamm-Horsfall protein, a mucoprotein secreted by the tubular and collecting duct cells, makes up most of the protein found in the urine of healthy animals.

CAUSES OF ABNORMALLY HIGH LEVELS

- Prerenal (overflow): Caused by fever, stress, hemoglobinuria, myoglobinuria, and paraproteinuria
- Glomerular proteinuria: Caused by increased glomerular permeability due

to autoimmune destruction, glomerulonephritis, and amyloidosis
- Tubular proteinuria: Caused by decreased protein resorption due to congenital or acquired proximal tubular diseases. This is a rare cause of proteinuria in horses.
- Hemorrhagic or inflammatory proteinuria
- Inflammation in regions other than the urinary tract may cause trace proteinuria.
- Transient postexercise proteinuria is common at submaximal and maximal levels of exertion.
- False-positive reaction (see later)

NEXT DIAGNOSTIC STEP TO CONSIDER IF LEVELS HIGH
- Examine the urine sediment for evidence of inflammation or hemorrhage.
- Examine serum for evidence of hemolysis.
- Measure serum protein for evidence of hyperproteinemia, hyperglobulinemia, or hypoalbuminemia.
- Urine protein-to-creatinine ratio

DRUG EFFECTS ON LEVELS False increases in protein detected via sulfosalicylic acid (SSA) precipitation method may occur after administration of iodine-based contrast media, sulfisoxazole, and very large doses of penicillin.

SPECIMEN AND PROCESSING CONSIDERATIONS

LAB ARTIFACTS THAT MAY INTERFERE WITH READINGS OF LEVELS OF THIS SUBSTANCE (AND HOW—ARTIFICIALLY ELEVATED VS. DEPRESSED)
- False increases (via dipstick method) may occur with pigmenturia, highly alkaline urine (pH >8.0), moderately alkaline urine if highly concentrated, and active urine sediments.
- In order to attribute proteinuria to hemorrhage alone, the dipstick heme reaction must be greater than or equal to 3+ and hematuria should be visible grossly.
- False decreases (via dipstick method) may occur if a protein other than

albumin (Bence Jones proteinuria) is present.
- False decreases via SSA precipitation method may occur if urine is highly alkaline (pH >8.0).
- False increases (via SSA precipitation method) may occur after administration of iodine-based contrast media, sulfisoxazole, very large doses of penicillin, and coprecipitation of crystals because of the low pH of SSA.

SAMPLE FOR COLLECTION (TYPE OF SPECIMEN, COLOR TUBE) AND ANY SPECIAL SPECIMEN HANDLING NOTES Midstream urine collection in a clean container

PEARLS Dipstick measurements of proteinuria are often overestimated due to the highly concentrated and alkaline nature of horse urine. If this method of assessing proteinuria is used, results should be interpreted together with urine specific gravity and pH.

AUTHOR: **LAURA C. CREGAR**

EDITOR: **CHARLES WIEDMEYER**

Alkaline Phosphatase (ALP)

BASIC INFORMATION

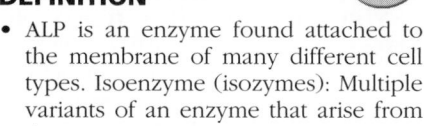

DEFINITION
- ALP is an enzyme found attached to the membrane of many different cell types. Isoenzyme (isozymes): Multiple variants of an enzyme that arise from the same gene
- Induced enzyme: Membrane-bound enzymes (not cytoplasmic) with increased activity attributed to cholestasis, drug, or hormonal effects

SYNONYM(S)
ALP

TYPICAL NORMAL RANGE (US UNITS; SI UNITS)
75 to 220 IU/L

PHYSIOLOGY
On cell membrane of almost all tissues, very wide reference interval and is of limited utility. Unknown function and multiple isoenzymes induced in a variety of diseases. Most circulating ALP is the

hepatic isozyme, followed by the bone isoenzyme. Very little intestinal ALP is in circulation. Placental form is present only in late pregnancy.

CAUSES OF ABNORMALLY HIGH LEVELS
- Hepatic isoenzyme: Increased mostly with cholestatic diseases. Inducible with excessive stress, pituitary pars intermedia dysfunction (equine Cushing's disease) or corticosteroid therapy
- Bone isoenzyme: Increased with increased osteoblastic activity (young growing animals, bony lysis, proliferative bone lesions, primary or secondary hyperparathyroidism)
- Placental isoenzyme: late pregnancy

NEXT DIAGNOSITC STEP TO CONSIDER IF LEVELS HIGH
- Complete blood count/serum chemistry profile and serum bile acid concentration
- Radiographs (bony lesions)
- Ultrasonography (for pregnancy)

CAUSES OF ABNORMALLY LOW LEVELS Insignificant

SPECIMEN AND PROCESSING CONSIDERATIONS

LAB ARTIFACTS THAT MAY INTERFERE WITH READINGS OF LEVELS OF THIS SUBSTANCE (AND HOW—ARTIFICIALY ELEVATED VS. DEPRESSED) Hemolysis may decrease results. Bilirubinemia may increase or decrease results depending on the analyzer.

SAMPLE FOR COLLECTION (TYPE OF SPECIMEN, COLOR TUBE) AND ANY SPECIAL SPECIMEN HANDLING NOTES Serum, quickly separated from the clot and refrigerated. ALP activity decreased 3% to 6% daily at room and refrigerator temperatures. Stable for 1 month frozen

PEARLS

Generally ALP is not useful in horses. Isoenzyme analysis may be helpful but is no longer commercially available.

AUTHOR: **PAULA M. KRIMER**

EDITOR: **CHARLES WIEDMEYER**

Ammonia

BASIC INFORMATION

DEFINITION

- Ammonia: NH₃ is toxic, non-ionized free ammonia that readily permeates cell membranes.
- Ammonium: NH₄⁺ (ammonium ion) is nontoxic ionized circulating ammonium that does not readily permeate cell membranes.
- Urea: A highly water-soluble neutral (not acidic or basic) nitrogenous molecule necessary for disposal of nitrogenous waste in mammals.

TYPICAL NORMAL RANGE (US UNITS; SI UNITS)

13 to 108 μg/dL (7.63–63.4 μmol/L)

PHYSIOLOGY

Ammonia is derived from bacterial enzymatic action on ingested amino acids. It is absorbed from the gastrointestinal tract and delivered through the portal vein to the liver, which converts most of it into urea. At physiologic blood pH, ammonia is ionized to form the ammonium ion (NH₄⁺), which does not permeate cell membranes. Ammonia (NH₃) can diffuse into cells and negatively affects cell function. When there is liver failure or impaired hepatic function, less ammonia is converted to urea or ammonium ion, resulting in decreased blood urea nitrogen (BUN) concentrations and increased toxic ammonia (NH₃) concentrations. Dietary protein affects circulating levels, but variation between individuals is generally greater than dietary effects.

CAUSES OF ABNORMALLY HIGH LEVELS

- Mostly hepatic insufficiency (chronic fibrosing hepatitis, cirrhosis, severe single toxic or infectious insult) in adults
- Colic or "enteric hyperammonemia" (combination of increased bacterial production and increased gut permeability that occurs despite normal hepatic function.
- Congenital portosystemic venous shunts (rare) and urea cycle enzyme deficiency (Morgan foals, very rare)

NEXT DIAGNOSTIC STEP TO CONSIDER IF LEVELS HIGH

- Complete blood count/serum chemistry profile
- Serum bile acids concentration for evidence of hepatic insufficiency or acute hepatic insult
- Coagulation profile
- Transabdominal ultrasonography and liver biopsy
- Dye clearance test for hepatic function
- Congenital portosystemic shunts diagnosed with ultrasonography, liver biopsy, operative mesenteric portography, or nuclear hepatic scintigraphy

CAUSES OF ABNORMALLY LOW LEVELS Insignificant

DRUG EFFECTS ON LEVELS Lactulose will lower ammonia concentrations.

SPECIMEN AND PROCESSING CONSIDERATIONS

LAB ARTIFACTS THAT MAY INTERFERE WITH READINGS OF LEVELS OF THIS SUBSTANCE (AND HOW—ARTIFICIALLY ELEVATED VS. DEPRESSED) Poor venipuncture, partial filling of an evacuation tube, background ammonia (ie, barn odors) and any exposure to cigarette smoke (laboratory technician, horse handler, or veterinarian is a smoker) will falsely increase ammonia.

SAMPLE FOR COLLECTION (TYPE OF SPECIMEN, COLOR TUBE) AND ANY SPECIAL SPECIMEN HANDLING NOTES Lithium heparin glass tube, filled completely. Labile: Put specimen immediately on ice, centrifuge in less than 15 minutes, and analyze immediately to prevent artificial increases. In EDTA, whole blood can be refrigerated for up to 6 hours. Plasma can be frozen but must remain frozen until received by laboratory.

PEARLS: Postmortem evaluation of cerebrospinal fluid (CSF) and aqueous humor ammonia can be used to document hyperammonemia.

AUTHOR: **PAULA M. KRIMER**

EDITOR: **CHARLES WIEDMEYER**

Anemia, Nonregenerative

BASIC INFORMATION

DEFINITION

Decreased red blood cell (RBC) mass (anemia) due to decreased RBC production

SYNONYM(S)

Nonresponding or nonresponsive anemia

TYPICAL NORMAL RANGE (US UNITS; SI UNITS)

- Hematocrit: 27% to 43% (0.27–0.43 L/L)
- Hemoglobin: 10.1 to 16.1 g/dL (101–161 g/L)
- RBC count: 6.0 to 10.4 × 10⁶/μL (6.0–10.4 × 10¹²/L)

PHYSIOLOGY

The bone marrow is unable to respond to the need to produce new erythrocytes as old ones are lost. This may occur due to ineffective erythropoiesis (defects in normal maturation of erythrocytes) or due to hypoplasia of the erythroid cells in the marrow (hypoplastic anemia).

CAUSES OF ABNORMALLY LOW LEVELS Causes of nonregenerative anemia include:

- Nutritional deficiencies (iron, vitamin B₁₂, folate, or copper)
- Chronic blood loss resulting in depletion of iron stores and subsequent iron deficiency
- Chronic inflammation
- Infection or neoplasia (the so-called anemia of chronic disease or anemia of inflammation)

- Equine ehrlichiosis
- Equine viral arteritis
- Myelophthisis
- Myeloproliferative or lymphoproliferative disease
- Chronic renal disease
- Chronic hepatic disease
- Exposure to bone marrow toxins such chloramphenicol or phenylbutazone
- Lead toxicosis
- Radiation toxicosis
- Endocrinopathies

In occasional cases of immune-mediated destruction of erythrocytes (immune-mediated hemolytic anemia), the immune response is directed at erythroid precursor cells in the bone marrow and the expected regenerative response to hemolysis (see section on regenerative anemia) does not occur. This results in so-called pure red cell aplasia and may occur after repeated administration of recombinant human erythropoietin (EPO).

NEXT DIAGNOSTIC STEP TO CONSIDER IF LEVELS LOW A careful clinical history should be obtained and a thorough physical examination should be carried out. Causes of regenerative anemia (blood loss or hemolysis) should be ruled out. A blood smear should be evaluated to check for morphologic abnormalities such as hypochromasia, microcytosis, macrocytosis, presence of *Ehrlichia* morulae, evidence of inflammation, or the presence of neoplastic cells. A serum biochemistry profile should be done to evaluate for renal or hepatic disease. In some cases, a bone marrow examination may be helpful to establish that the anemia is truly nonregenerative and is also sometimes helpful for determining a cause. If iron deficiency is suspected, serum iron, total iron binding capacity (TIBC), and ferritin levels can be used for confirmation (iron deficiency is expected to result in decreased serum iron and ferritin levels and cause an increase in TIBC).

AUTHOR: **MARLYN S. WHITNEY**

EDITOR: **CHARLES WIEDMEYER**

Anemia, Regenerative

BASIC INFORMATION

DEFINITION

Anemia is decreased erythrocyte (red blood cell [RBC]) mass, as identified by decreases in hematocrit, hemoglobin, and RBC count. Regenerative anemias are those in which the bone marrow is responding properly in an attempt to correct the anemia and are due to blood loss or hemolysis (premature destruction of RBCs).

SYNONYM(S)

Responding or responsive anemia.

TYPICAL NORMAL RANGE (US UNITS; SI UNITS)

- Hematocrit: 27% to 43% (0.27–0.43 L/L)
- Hemoglobin: 10.1 to 16.1 g/dL (101–161 g/L)
- RBC count: 6.0 to 10.4×10^6 /μL ($6.0–10.4 \times 10^{12}$/L)

PHYSIOLOGY

Regenerative anemia occurs due to blood loss or premature destruction of erythrocytes (hemolysis). Decreased tissue oxygenation stimulates erythropoietin production, which stimulates the bone marrow to increase RBC production.

CAUSES OF ABNORMALLY LOW LEVELS

- As stated previously, regenerative anemia occurs due to blood loss or hemolysis.
- Causes of blood loss include traumatic loss, loss to parasites that feed on blood, blood loss into the gastrointestinal or urogenital tracts from bleeding lesions such as tumors or ulcerations, and blood loss due to disorders of hemostasis.
- Causes of hemolytic anemia include immune-mediated destruction of RBCs (including neonatal isoerythrolysis and reaction to an incompatible blood transfusion), oxidative damage to RBCs (eg, red maple leaf, onion, rye grass, *Brassica* spp, or phenothiazine toxicosis; one known case of glucose-6-phosphate dehydrogenase deficiency), RBC parasitism, severe hypophosphatemia, snake envenomation, hypotonic fluid administration, and RBC fragmentation due to microangiopathy (eg, vasculitis or disseminated intravascular coagulation).

NEXT DIAGNOSTIC STEP TO CONSIDER IF LEVELS LOW

- Complete blood count including a blood smear examination to look for RBC shape changes or parasites
- Physical examination for icterus (may occur in association with hemolytic anemia) or evidence of external blood loss or ectoparasites
- Fecal examination (check for frank or occult blood, parasites)
- Serum biochemistry panel, urinalysis (check for hematuria as a cause of blood loss)
- Hemoglobinuria may occur in some cases of hemolytic anemia.
- Bone marrow examination is not usually necessary for regenerative anemia; usually a source of blood loss or evidence of hemolysis can be found via physical examination, history taking (eg, possible exposure to toxins), and/or results of other laboratory tests.

IMPORTANT INTERSPECIES DIFFERENCES Horses with regenerative anemia may exhibit greater degrees of variability in erythrocyte size (greater anisocytosis) than healthy horses. In most species, regenerative anemia is identified by the presence of increased reticulocytes (immature RBC) in the circulating blood (reticulocytosis). Because horses with regenerative anemia do not release reticulocytes into circulation, reticulocytosis cannot be used to identify a regenerative response in this species. Serial hematocrit measurement or bone marrow examination may be necessary to differentiate between regenerative and non-regenerative anemia. Finding a source of blood loss or evidence of hemolysis may obviate the need for a bone marrow examination, unless appropriate treatment for the blood loss or hemolysis does not result in recovery from the anemia. The erythrocyte regenerative capability of the horse is not as great as for some other domestic species, so complete recovery from severe blood loss or hemolysis may take 4 to 12 weeks (regeneration tends to take longer for blood loss anemias than for hemolytic anemias).

AUTHOR: **MARLYN S. WHITNEY**

EDITOR: **CHARLES WIEDMEYER**

Anion Gap

BASIC INFORMATION

DEFINITION

A calculated value, using the formula $[(Na^{2+} + K^+) - (Cl^- + HCO_3^-)]$, that can aid in determining the cause of acid-base abnormalities

TYPICAL NORMAL RANGE (US UNITS; SI UNITS)

Approximately 5 to 15 mEq/L. Reference ranges may change among different laboratories. Clinically normal, 2- to 7-week-old foals may have a higher anion gap compared with adults (difference of 4–5 mEq/L).

PHYSIOLOGY

Because total cations equal total anions in the blood, the anion gap indirectly represents the difference between unmeasured anions and unmeasured cations (UA − UC). In health, major unmeasured anions include albumin, phosphates, sulfates, and small organic acids; unmeasured cations include calcium, magnesium, and gamma globulins. The latter are rarely ever increased enough to decrease the anion gap.

CAUSES OF ABNORMALLY HIGH LEVELS
Lactic acidosis (lactate), uremic acids, ketoacids (acetoacetate, β-hydroxybutyrate), and ethylene glycol and propylene glycol metabolites

NEXT DIAGNOSTIC STEP TO CONSIDER IF LEVELS HIGH
Measure lactate concentrations, evaluate renal function (blood urea nitrogen [BUN], creatinine, and electrolytes with concurrent urinalysis), and review history of ethylene glycol or propylene glycol exposure. Propylene glycol has similar gross appearance as mineral oil and has been mistakenly administered.

CAUSES OF ABNORMALLY LOW LEVELS
Uncommon and usually clinically insignificant. Causes include hypoalbuminemia and, rarely, markedly increased cations such as calcium and globulins. Saline or hypertonic saline fluid administration may also cause a decrease in anion gap due to hyperchloremia.

DRUG EFFECTS ON LEVELS
- Increased anion gap can be seen with mistaken administration of propylene glycol and may possibly follow sodium citrate and sodium penicillin treatments. Decreased anion gap can be seen with potassium bromide treatment (may cause pseudohyperchloremia).
- Hypertonic saline or saline fluid administration may also cause a decrease in anion gap due to hyperchloremia.

SPECIMEN AND PROCESSING CONSIDERATIONS

LAB ARTIFACTS THAT MAY INTEFERE WITH READINGS OF LEVELS OF THIS SUBSTANCE (AND HOW—ARTIFICALLY ELEVATED VS. DEPRESSED)
Lipemia and hemolysis may interfere with the measurement of the electrolytes included in the anion gap calculation and alter the anion gap value.

SAMPLE FOR COLLECTION (TYPE OF SPECIMEN, COLOR TUBE) AND ANY SPECIAL SPECIMEN HANDLING NOTES
Heparinized plasma for chemistry analysis including electrolytes is used by most laboratories. For bench-top and point of care analyzers (eg, NOVA and iSTAT, respectively) heparinized whole blood or plasma should be used according to the manufacturer instruction.

PEARLS
Anion gap is very helpful in differentiating secretional from titrational metabolic acidosis. Secretional metabolic acidosis has a normal anion gap; it is caused by bicarbonate loss, typically due to gastrointestinal disease with diarrhea. Titrational metabolic acidosis has an increased anion gap; it is caused by organic acid accumulation and their titration by bicarbonate. Additionally, increased anion gap in face of normal or alkaline blood pH may suggest a mixed acid-base disturbance with a component of metabolic acidosis.

AUTHOR: **SHIR GILOR**

EDITOR: **CHARLES WIEDMEYER**

Antithrombin (AT)

BASIC INFORMATION

DEFINITION

Major inhibitor of coagulation enzymes, most importantly thrombin, factor IXa, and factor Xa

SYNONYM(S)

Antithrombin III (ATIII)
AT

TYPICAL NORMAL RANGE (US UNITS; SI UNITS)

Expressed as percent activity compared to species-specific plasma pool. Has also been reported in U/mL or U/dL. Laboratory, instrument, and species-specific reference intervals must be used.

PHYSIOLOGY

Produced primarily by hepatocytes. Binds to and inactivates thrombin, thus preventing conversion of fibrinogen to fibrin. AT activity is markedly enhanced in the presence of circulating unfractionated heparin or heparan sulfate on endothelial cells. Plasma added to a reagent containing heparin, excess thrombin or factor Xa, and the corresponding chromogen-labeled substrate for thrombin or Xa.

CAUSES OF ABNORMALLY HIGH LEVELS
Insignificant

CAUSES OF ABNORMALLY LOW LEVELS
Decreased production (hepatic disease, hyperestrogenism), loss (protein-losing nephropathy, protein-losing enteropathy, severe hemorrhage), consumption (disseminated intravascular coagulation [DIC], sepsis)

NEXT DIAGNOSTIC STEP TO CONSIDER IF LEVELS LOW
Evaluation of complete blood count and serum biochemistry to determine most likely etiology

IMPORTANT INTERSPECIES DIFFERENCES
Neonatal foals have been shown to have plasma AT activities that are substantially lower than adult values.

DRUG EFFECTS ON LEVELS
Decreased by heparin administration

SPECIMEN AND PROCESSING CONSIDERATIONS

LAB ARTIFACTS THAT MAY INTERFERE WITH READINGS OF LEVELS OF THIS SUBSTANCE (AND HOW—ARTIFICIALLY ELEVATED VS. DEPRESSED May be overestimated in some thrombin chromogenic assays because heparin cofactor II activity may be detected in addition.

SAMPLE FOR COLLECTION (TYPE OF SPECIMEN, COLOR TUBE) AND ANY SPECIAL SPECIMEN HANDLING NOTES Obtain sample via minimally traumatic phlebotomy. Collect specimen in citrate (blue top) tube. Fill to ratio of nine parts blood to one part citrate (2.7-mL blood in a 3-mL citrate tube).

AUTHOR: BRITTON GRASPERGE

EDITOR: CHARLES WIEDMEYER

Arginase

BASIC INFORMATION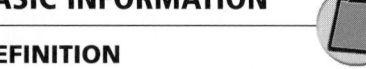

DEFINITION

Leakage enzyme: Soluble cytoplasmic enzymes released into circulation after increased membrane permeability (sublethal cellular injury or cellular necrosis)

TYPICAL NORMAL RANGE (US UNITS; SI UNITS)

0 to 14 IU/L

PHYSIOLOGY

Arginase is a leakage enzyme necessary for protein catabolism and excretion that is relatively specific to the liver. The degree of increase is generally proportional to the number of injured hepatocytes; very high values suggest acute hepatocellular damage. It has a brief half-life and levels return to normal before aspartate aminotransferase (AST); consistently increased values suggest ongoing and active hepatocellular damage.

CAUSES OF ABNORMALLY HIGH LEVELS

• Marked increases in acute hepatitis (equine herpesvirus type 1, embolic bacterial diseases, Tyzzer's disease (*Clostridium piliformis*), hepatotoxins such as pyrrolizidine alkaloids, Theiler's disease (serum hepatitis), and chronic active hepatitis
• Mild increases in cholestasis and hyperlipemia syndrome

NEXT DIAGNOSTIC STEP TO CONSIDER IF LEVELS HIGH

• Vaccination history (serum hepatitis)
• Complete blood count/serum chemistry profile, serum bile acids, and urinalysis to rule out hyperlipemia syndrome and hepatitis/hepatic necrosis
• Transabdominal ultrasound and liver biopsy to identify specific liver pathology or etiology

CAUSES OF ABNORMALLY LOW LEVELS Insignificant

DRUG EFFECTS ON LEVELS Increased: benzimidazole anthelmintics

SPECIMEN AND PROCESSING CONSIDERATIONS

LAB ARTIFACTS THAT MAY INTERFERE WITH READINGS OF LEVELS OF THIS SUBSTANCE (AND HOW—ARTIFICIALLY ELEVATED VS. DEPRESSED) Hemolysis can cause increases due to intraerythrocyte arginase.

SAMPLE FOR COLLECTION (TYPE OF SPECIMEN, COLOR TUBE) AND ANY SPECIAL SPECIMEN HANDLING NOTES Serum, quickly separated from clot. Extremely labile; stable 5 hours room temperature, less than 24 hours refrigerated and 48 hours frozen. If immediate onsite evaluation is not possible, serum should be frozen and mailed on ice packs to nearby laboratory.

PEARLS Arginase is specific for liver disease in horses but is not as sensitive an indicator as AST. Due to its instability, very few laboratories offer this test.

AUTHOR: PAULA M. KRIMER

EDITOR: CHARLES WIEDMEYER

Aspartate Aminotransferase (AST)

BASIC INFORMATION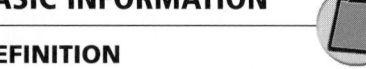

DEFINITION

Leakage enzyme: Soluble cytoplasmic enzymes released into circulation after increased membrane permeability (sublethal cellular injury or cellular necrosis).

SYNONYM(S)

Previously known as serum glutamic oxaloacetic transaminase (SGOT)

TYPICAL NORMAL RANGE (US UNITS; SI UNITS)

226 to 366 IU/L

PHYSIOLOGY

AST is a nonspecific leakage enzyme involved in protein catabolism. It is found in all tissues especially skeletal myocytes, myocardiocytes, and hepatocytes. It has a half-life over 18 hours, longer than most other liver indicators and creatine kinase (CK). The degree of increase is generally proportional to the number of injured cells; very high values suggest acute hepatocellular damage or rhabdomyolysis.

CAUSES OF ABNORMALLY HIGH LEVELS Sublethal injury, hypoxia, or necrosis of muscle (strenuous exercise, bacterial myonecrosis, exertional rhabdomyolysis, and nutritional myodegeneration of vitamin E/selenium deficiency) or hepatocytes (infectious hepatitis including Tyzzer's disease and toxic hepatopathy, chronic passive congestion)

• Hyperlipemia syndrome
• Intravascular hemolysis (release from erythrocytes)

NEXT DIAGNOSTIC STEP TO CONSIDER IF LEVELS HIGH

• Complete blood count for evidence of hemolytic anemia
• Serum chemistry profile (including creatine phosphokinase), serum bile acids, and urinalysis for evidence of hyperlipemia syndrome, hepatitis/hepatic necrosis, or rhabdomyolysis

- Transabdominal ultrasonography and liver biopsy to identify specific liver pathology or etiology
- Echocardiography or electrocardiogram and serum cardiac troponin I for cardiac disease

CAUSES OF ABNORMALLY LOW LEVELS: Insignificant

SPECIMEN AND PROCESSING CONSIDERATIONS

LAB ARTIFACTS THAT MAY INTERFERE WITH READINGS OF LEVELS OF THIS SUBSTANCE (AND HOW—ARTIFICIALLY ELEVATAED VS. DEPRESSED) Hemolysis will increase values due to presence of AST in erythrocytes, even if hemolysis is not visible. Lipemia will increase values and marked bilirubinemia will decrease values. Hyperammonemia or increased glutamate dehydrogenase (GLD) can artificially decrease AST.

SAMPLE FOR COLLECTION (TYPE OF SPECIMEN, COLOR TUBE) AND ANY SPECIAL SPECIMEN HANDLING NOTES Serum, immediately separated from the clot and refrigerated. Immediate separation is vital to reduce contamination by erythrocytes. Stable at all temperatures.

PEARLS AST is not a reliable indicator of hepatic disease in horses and most commonly is significantly increased with muscle disease. Pituitary adenomas can cause hypercortisolemia or decreased antidiuretic hormone production, either of which can cause increased AST (and sorbitol dehydrogenase (SDH) and gamma-glutamyl transpeptidase [GGT]) along with dilute urine.

AUTHOR: **PAULA M. KRIMER**

EDITOR: **CHARLES WIEDMEYER**

Baermann Test

BASIC INFORMATION

DEFINITION

A test to detect parasite larvae in feces

TYPICAL NORMAL RANGE (US AND IU UNITS)

Results are reported as positive or negative for larvae often with a genus identification.

PHYSIOLOGY

This test is based upon the active migration of larvae out of feces when warm water is added. The feces, contained within gauze, are placed in a funnel, which is connected to a short length of tubing that has a clamp at the end. After warm water is added to the funnel, the larvae migrate into the water and sink to the bottom of the tubing, where they are collected after several hours and then microscopically identified.

CAUSES OF ABNORMALLY HIGH LEVELS Nematodes shedding larvae

NEXT DIAGNOSTIC STEP TO CONSIDER IF LEVELS HIGH A positive result is definitive for infection.

CAUSES OF ABNORMALLY LOW LEVELS A negative test may result from sexually immature parasites or the intermittent shedding of larvae.

NEXT DIAGNOSTIC STEP TO CONSIDER IF LEVELS LOW Perform another Baermann on a new sample if no larvae are detected and parasite-associated disease is suspected.

DRUG EFFECTS ON LEVELS Drugs may reduce or eliminate parasite infection, resulting in few or no larvae shed.

SPECIMEN AND PROCESSING CONSIDERATIONS

SAMPLE FOR COLLECTION (TYPE OF SPECIMEN, COLOR TUBE) AND ANY SPECIAL SPECIMEN HANDLING NOTES A fresh fecal sample should be collected into a clean, dry container. If the test can not be performed within a few hours, refrigerate the fecal specimen. In older samples, larvae may hatch from embryonated eggs of *Strongyloides*. Freezing the fecal sample will kill the larvae.

PEARLS
- This test is usually done to detect the larvae of the lungworm, *Dictyocaulus*.
- Avoid collecting samples from the ground as free-living soil nematodes may contaminate the sample.
- May need to centrifuge the collected water sample, decant it, and then examine the sediment for larvae.

AUTHOR: **BRENDA T. BEERNTSEN**

EDITOR: **CHARLES WIEDMEYER**

Base Deficit or Excess (BDE)

BASIC INFORMATION

DEFINITION

The number of millimoles of acid or base required to titrate a liter of arterial blood to a pH of 7.4, with 100% saturation of oxygen, and a PCO_2 of 40 mm Hg at 38° C. It is calculated from PCO_2 and pH.

SYNONYM(S)

Base excess if value is positive
Base deficit if the value is negative

TYPICAL NORMAL RANGE (US UNITS; SI UNITS)

- Varies based on blood gas machine used:
  ○ For Istat (Heska) meters: −5 to 5 mmol/L
  ○ For Nova CCX: 0.1 to 6.0 mmol/L

PHYSIOLOGY

Used as an estimate of the metabolic component of acid-base analysis. It has been proposed that mitochondrial oxidative dysfunction results in reduced production of ATP, which leads to an accumulation of hydrogen ions and, therefore, an increased (more negative) base deficit.

CAUSES OF ABNORMALLY HIGH LEVELS Base excess: Metabolic alkalosis or hypoproteinemia

NEXT DIAGNOSTIC STEP TO CONSIDER IF LEVELS HIGH

- Consider remainder of blood gas analysis to determine cause.
- Low serum protein increases base excess due to an increased proportion of bicarbonate buffer.

CAUSES OF ABNORMALLY LOW LEVELS

- Base deficit: Metabolic acidosis
- Negative levels may correlate to lower oxygen utilization by the tissues, bicarbonate loss, or treatment with high chloride fluids.

NEXT DIAGNOSTIC STEP TO CONSIDER IF LEVELS LOW

- Anion gap and lactate measurements
  - Elevations indicate titration metabolic acidosis.
  - Normal levels indicate bicarbonate loss.

IMPORTANT INTERSPECIES DIFFERENCES Base excess calculated by blood gas machines utilizes a formula based on human proteins and their charges; small variations are inherent but are likely clinically insignificant.

DRUG EFFECTS ON LEVELS: Fluids containing large amounts of chloride (0.9% sodium chloride) or bicarbonate will alter the base deficit.

SPECIMEN AND PROCESSING CONSIDERATIONS

SAMPLE FOR COLLECTION (TYPE OF SPECIMEN, COLOR TUBE) AND ANY SPECIAL SPECIMEN HANDLING NOTES Samples for blood gas analysis are obtained anaerobically in arterial blood gas syringes or heparinized syringes and should be analyzed within 10 minutes of sampling (or placed on ice if sampling must be delayed).

PEARLS Base deficit may correlate to accumulating tissue debt and its severity may be related to prognosis for survival.

ADDITIONAL READING

Magdesian KG: Monitoring the critically ill equine patient. *Vet Clin N Am Pract Equine* 20:11–39, 2004.

Prittie J: Optimal endpoints of resuscitation and early goal-directed therapy. *J Vet Em Crit Care* 16(4):329–339, 2006.

AUTHOR: **AMELIA MUNSTERMAN**

EDITOR: **CHARLES WIEDMEYER**

Basophil (Basophilia, Basopenia)

BASIC INFORMATION

DEFINITION

Basophils are granulocytes that originate from the bone marrow. These cells have a lobulated nucleus and contain moderate numbers of basophilic granules.

SYNONYM(S)

baso

TYPICAL NORMAL RANGE (US UNITS; SI UNITS)

0.0 to $0.3 \times 10^3/\mu L$

PHYSIOLOGY

Basophils are the least numerous granulocyte and have functions similar to mast cells. They can release histamine in allergic reactions and type I hypersensitivity responses. They are involved in lipid metabolism via activation of lipoprotein lipase and have less effective antiparasitic activity than eosinophils. They often act in conjunction with eosinophils in performing various functions.

CAUSES OF ABNORMALLY HIGH LEVELS Elevations in basophils or basophilia usually accompany an eosinophilia and can be seen with long-standing IgE stimulation such as allergic responses or parasitic infestation. Also, during hyperlipidemic states can result in a basophilia in the absence of an eosinophilia.

NEXT DIAGNOSTIC STEP TO CONSIDER IF LEVELS HIGH Fecal floatation may be beneficial to rule out parasitic infestation.

CAUSES OF ABNORMALLY LOW LEVELS Basopenia is difficult to identify because many of the reference ranges for basophils extend to 0.

IMPORTANT INTERSPECIES DIFFERENCES The granules of equine basophils are more obvious than in the dog and cat.

SPECIMEN AND PROCESSING CONSIDERATIONS

SAMPLE FOR COLLECTION (TYPE OF SPECIMEN, COLOR TUBE) AND ANY SPECIAL SPECIMEN HANDLING NOTES Whole, anticoagulated blood is necessary for evaluation. Most commonly, EDTA or purple top tubes are used for complete blood count (CBC); however, sodium citrate (blue top tube) can also be used. If the blood cannot be evaluated immediately, preparation of a blood smear to preserve the integrity of red and white blood cell morphology is recommended.

AUTHOR: **ANNE BARGER**

EDITOR: **CHARLES WIEDMEYER**

Bicarbonate

BASIC INFORMATION

DEFINITION

Bicarbonate anion is a major blood plasma buffer and is part of the bicarbonate/carbonic acid buffering system.

SYNONYM(S)

HCO_3^-

TYPICAL NORMAL RANGE (US UNITS; SI UNITS)

Horses: Approximately 24 to 30 mEq/L (mEq/L = mmol/L)

PHYSIOLOGY

Gaseous carbon dioxide is dissolved in plasma and is hydrated to form carbonic acid (H_2CO_3) by carbonic anhydrase. Carbonic acid is ionized into bicarbonate and hydrogen ions. Changes in plasma pH depend on the ratio of dissolved HCO_3^- and CO_2. The goal of the bicarbonate/carbonic acid buffering system is to "neutralize" excess acid or base and keep the plasma pH within a normal range. In metabolic acidosis, bicarbonate binds excess hydrogen ions, thereby decreasing the amount of measurable HCO_3^-.

CAUSES OF ABNORMALLY HIGH LEVELS Metabolic alkalosis (causes: repeated evacuation of the stomach contents via nasogastric tube, proximal jejunitis-ileitis, excessive administration of bicarbonate or other alkalinizing agents, diuretic therapy, liver disease) or respiratory acidosis (causes: airway obstruction, pulmonary disease [pneumonia, pulmonary edema], pulmonary restrictive disease [pleural effusion, diaphragmatic hernia, pneumothorax, pulmonary fibrosis, chronic obstructive pulmonary disease], respiratory center depression [neurologic disease, narcotics, sedatives, inhalation anesthetics])

NEXT DIAGNOSTIC STEP TO CONSIDER IF LEVELS HIGH Evaluate a full arterial blood gas profile to differentiate between primary metabolic alkalosis (high pH, high HCO_3^-, normal to high PCO_2) or metabolic compensation for respiratory acidosis (low pH, normal to high HCO_3^-, high PCO_2). Examine for underlying cause (listed previously) of the acid/base disturbance.

CAUSES OF ABNORMALLY LOW LEVELS Metabolic acidosis (causes: increased anion gap [lactic acidosis, uremic acidosis, ketoacidosis, intoxication with other organic acids], bicarbonate loss [diarrhea, renal tubular acidosis]) or compensation for respiratory alkalosis (causes: tachypnea due to hypoxemia, [severe anemia, pulmonary disease, congestive heart failure], direct stimulation of central nervous system [central neurologic disease, gram-negative sepsis, hepatic disease, heat stroke, pain, fear], mechanical ventilation)

NEXT DIAGNOSTIC STEP TO CONSIDER IF LEVELS LOW Evaluate a full arterial blood gas profile to differentiate between primary metabolic acidosis (low pH, low HCO_3^-, normal to low PCO_2) or metabolic compensation for respiratory alkalosis (high pH, normal to low HCO_3^-, low PCO_2). Examine for underlying cause (listed previously) of the acid/base disturbance.

DRUG EFFECTS ON LEVELS Increases can be observed with administration of alkalinizing agents such as sodium bicarbonate or sodium acetate and use of diuretics such as furosemide.

SPECIMEN AND PROCESSING CONSIDERATIONS

LAB ARTIFACTS THAT MAY INTERFERE WITH READINGS OF LEVELS OF THIS SUBSTANCE (AND HOW—ARTIFICIALLY ELEVATED VS. DEPRESSED) Decreases can occur due to a delay in sample processing or exposure of the sample to air. See following for sample handling notes.

SAMPLE FOR COLLECTION (TYPE OF SPECIMEN, COLOR TUBE) AND ANY SPECIAL SPECIMEN HANDLING NOTES Bicarbonate is a calculated value determined as part of blood gas analysis. For blood gas analysis, a heparinized whole blood sample in a syringe free of air is recommended. Samples should be analyzed within 15 to 30 minutes of collection or stored in a capped air-free syringe and placed in an ice bath for up to 2 hours.

PEARLS Total carbon dioxide (TCO_2) is included on many serum chemistry panels and is a good estimator of plasma bicarbonate. HCO_3^- is the major contributor to TCO_2 though small amounts come from dissolved H_2CO_3 and carbamino acids. Although serum TCO_2 is generally 1 to 2 mEq/L higher than plasma HCO_3^-, it is considered a clinically accurate assessment of bicarbonate. If abnormal values of TCO_2 are present, follow up with blood gas analysis is recommended to further assess the acid/base status of the patient.

AUTHOR: **KIMBERLY WEBER**

EDITOR: **CHARLES WIEDMEYER**

Bilirubin

BASIC INFORMATION

DEFINITION

- Bilirubin (total): The major pigment created from the breakdown of hemoglobin, myoglobin, peroxidases, and cytochromes
- Unconjugated bilirubin (free or indirect-reacting): Water-insoluble bilirubin bound to albumin
- Conjugated bilirubin (direct-reacting): Water-soluble bilirubin that has been conjugated with glucuronic acid in the liver
- Cholestasis: The accumulation in the blood of components secreted in the bile, including bilirubin, and causing icterus/jaundice
- Liver function test: Changes in blood concentrations of substances normally processed or produced by the liver that are used to evaluate liver function
- Porphyrins: Water-soluble, nitrogenous biologic pigments complexed to metals including hemoglobin, myoglobin, and cytochromes

TYPICAL NORMAL RANGE (US UNITS; SI UNITS)

- Total bilirubin: 1.0 to 2.0 mg/dL (7.1–34.2 μmol/L)
- Unconjugated bilirubin: 0.2 to 2.0 mg/dL (3.42–34.2 μmol/L)
- Conjugated bilirubin: 0 to 0.4 mg/dL (0–6.84 μmol/L)

PHYSIOLOGY

Bilirubin is produced by hepatic, splenic, and marrow phagocytes from the catabolism of hemoglobin in senescent red cells, myoglobin, and cytochromes. Bound to albumin, unconjugated bilirubin is transported to the liver where hepatocytes conjugate it with glucuronic acid to produce conjugated bilirubin for excretion in the bile. In the gastrointestinal tract, some of the excreted bilirubin is reduced to urobilinogens or oxidized to stercobilinogens, and the rest is reabsorbed. Some is excreted in the urine as yellow urobilin. Renal tubular epithelium can produce bilirubin when there is hemoglobinuria; otherwise, bilirubin is not normally present in the urine of horses.

CAUSES OF ABNORMALLY HIGH LEVELS

- Prehepatic (increases in unconjugated bilirubin) from anorexia, intravascular or extravascular hemolytic anemia or severe rhabdomyolysis. Certain drugs can also increase the unconjugated bilirubin fraction (especially heparin, steroids). There is one report of persistent hyperbilirubinemia due to failure of bilirubin conjugation (Gilbert's syndrome) in a Thoroughbred.

- Hepatic hyperbilirubinemia (increases in both unconjugated and conjugated bilirubin) is due to acute hepatitis (infectious, inflammatory, toxic, hyperlipidemia, or idiopathic) or chronic diseases (chronic active hepatitis, pyrrolizidine alkaloid toxicity, cholelithiasis).
- Posthepatic hyperbilirubinemia (conjugated bilirubin greater than 30% of total bilirubin concentration) is due to bile duct obstruction (cholelithiasis, hepatic fibrosis, neoplasia, or colon displacement).
- Neonates have increased serum bile acid concentrations for the first 2 to 3 weeks of life.

NEXT DIAGNOSTIC STEP TO CONSIDER IF LEVELS HIGH

- Complete blood count to rule out hemolytic anemia
- Serum chemistry profile, serum bile acids concentration, and urinalysis to rule out hyperlipemia syndrome, hepatic insufficiency, systemic inflammation, rhabdomyolysis, and Gilbert's syndrome
- Transabdominal ultrasonography to identify choleliths
- Rectal examination to identify colonic displacement

CAUSES OF ABNORMALLY LOW LEVELS Insignificant

DRUG EFFECTS ON LEVELS

- Decreased: phenobarbital
- Increased: corticosteroids, halothane, and heparin

SPECIMEN AND PROCESSING CONSIDERATIONS

LAB ARTIFACTS THAT MAY INTERFERE WITH READINGS OF LEVELS OF THIS SUBSTANCE (AND HOW—ARTIFICIALLY ELEVATED VS. DEPRESSED) Lipemia and hemolysis cause variable interference.

SAMPLE FOR COLLECTION (TYPE OF SPECIMEN, COLOR TUBE) AND ANY SPECIAL SPECIMEN HANDLING NOTES Serum, quickly separated from the clot and refrigerated. Temperature stable but very light-sensitive. Horses should not be fasted.

PEARLS Bilirubin is an insensitive and nonspecific indicator of liver disease. Neonates can have mildly to moderately increased unconjugated bilirubin concentrations. Anorexia is unlikely to cause elevations higher than 6 to 8 mg/dL (102.6–136.8 μmol/L). Conjugated bilirubin >30% of total bilirubin suggests cholestasis.

AUTHOR: **PAULA M. KRIMER**

EDITOR: **CHARLES WIEDMEYER**

Bilirubinuria

BASIC INFORMATION

DEFINITION

The presence of bilirubin in urine

TYPICAL NORMAL RANGE (US UNITS; SI UNITS)

Negative or trace in healthy animals

PHYSIOLOGY

Unconjugated bilirubin (Bu) is a byproduct of hemoglobin metabolism, and forms from the degradation of heme. Bu is conjugated in hepatocytes, and conjugated bilirubin (Bc) is excreted via the biliary system. If regurgitated into the plasma, Bc passes through the glomerulus and is excreted in the urine. Conjugated bilirubin is water soluble and therefore more likely to be passed in the urine than unconjugated bilirubin. Unconjugated bilirubin is bound to albumin and other carrier proteins and may appear in the urine if albuminuria or proteinuria is present.

CAUSES OF ABNORMALLY HIGH LEVELS

- Excessive bilirubin formation (hemolytic states, eg, Red Maple toxicity)
- Impaired hepatobiliary excretion of Bc
- Glomerular leakage of Bu with significant proteinuria
- Mild bilirubinuria may result from anorexia in horses.
- Bilirubinuria may precede hyperbilirubinemia due to the low renal threshold for bilirubin.
- False increases (see later)

NEXT DIAGNOSTIC STEP TO CONSIDER IF LEVELS HIGH Assess hematocrit and liver enzyme activity

SPECIMEN AND PROCESSING CONSIDERATIONS

LAB ARTIFACTS THAT MAY INTERFERE WITH READINGS OF LEVELS OF THIS SUBSTANCE (AND HOW—ARTIFICIALLY ELEVATED VS. DEPRESSED)

- False increases in bilirubin (via dipstick method) may be caused by indican, a product of tryptophan degradation by intestinal bacteria, and metabolites of etodolac, a nonsteroidal antiinflammatory drug.
- Bilirubin degradation occurs with exposure to UV light. Analysis of the urine within 30 minutes of sampling is recommended.
- Discolored urine may mask the test pad color change for bilirubin.

SAMPLE FOR COLLECTION (TYPE OF SPECIMEN, COLOR TUBE) AND ANY SPECIAL SPECIMEN HANDLING NOTES Midstream urine collection in a clean container

AUTHOR: **LAURA C. CREGAR**

EDITOR: **CHARLES WIEDMEYER**

Blood Gas Analysis

BASIC INFORMATION

DEFINITION

A method for evaluating blood pH, P_{CO_2}, P_{O_2}, bicarbonate (HCO_3^-), and calculated values such as base excess (BE)

SYNONYM(S)

Acid-base analysis

TYPICAL NORMAL RANGE (US UNITS; SI UNITS)

- Blood pH 7.36 to 7.44 (arterial), 7.33 to 7.41 (venous)
- P_{CO_2} (mm Hg) 37 to 49 (arterial), 46 to 64 (venous)
- P_{O_2} (mm Hg) 89 to 115 (arterial), 28.7 to 48.6 (venous)
- HCO_3^- (mmol/L) 23 to 30 (arterial), 31.6 to 37.7 (venous)
- Base excess (mmol/L) 6.4 to 12.3

PHYSIOLOGY

Maintenance of blood pH within a narrow range is dependent upon a variety of physiologic buffering systems. Of these systems is the bicarbonate buffering system. Blood HCO_3^- and P_{CO_2} are the main parameters used to detect abnormalities in the metabolic and respiratory components of this system respectively. Arterial p_{O_2} is used for evaluating respiratory function. Generally, interpretation of blood gas analysis focuses on first blood pH then closer examination of HCO_3^- and P_{CO_2} to determine if there is a metabolic or respiratory disturbance in physiologic buffering. BE is a calculated value used to confirm changes in the metabolic component of the disturbance.

CAUSES OF ABNORMALLY HIGH LEVELS See blood pH section.

CAUSES OF ABNORMALLY LOW LEVELS See blood pH section.

SPECIMEN AND PROCESSING CONSIDERATIONS

LAB ARTIFACTS THAT MAY INTERFERE WITH READINGS OF LEVELS OF THIS SUBSTANCE (AND HOW—ARTIFICIALLY ELEVATED VS. DEPRESSED) Exposure to room air will result in falsely increased P_{CO_2} and decreased P_{O_2}. Change in P_{CO_2} can alter blood pH levels.

SAMPLE FOR COLLECTION (TYPE OF SPECIMEN, COLOR TUBE) AND ANY SPECIAL SPECIMEN HANDLING NOTES Whole blood should be collected in a heparinized syringe, the needle capped to limit exposure to room air. Specimens should be analyzed as promptly as possible.

PEARLS

- Severe alterations in any of the blood gas parameters can be life threatening.
- Hand held and bench-top instrumentation for the analysis are available.
- Venous blood samples are adequate for determination of acid-base status but arterial blood is necessary to accurately assess respiratory function (ie, P_{O_2}).

AUTHOR and EDITOR: **CHARLES WIEDMEYER**

Blood pH

BASIC INFORMATION

DEFINITION

Blood pH is a measure of the blood's acidity or alkalinity.

TYPICAL NORMAL RANGE (US UNITS; SI UNITS)

Blood pH 7.36 to 7.44 (arterial), 7.33 to 7.41 (venous)

PHYSIOLOGY

The pH of any fluid is inversely related to the hydrogen ion concentration [H+]. Increased [H+] results in decreased pH, which is termed acidemia, and decreased [H+] results in increased pH termed alkalemia. Hydrogen ions are produced continually through body metabolic processes and either excreted through the kidneys or buffered.

CAUSES OF ABNORMALLY HIGH LEVELS Increases in blood pH indicate alkalemia. Increases can be a result of a respiratory (or metabolic) disturbance. Respiratory alkalosis is the result of alveolar hyperventilation. Hyperventilation (ie, decreased P_{CO_2}) causes removal of CO_2 and subsequent H+ faster than H+ is being produced. Hyperventilation can be caused by hypoxic states, stimulation of respiratory centers, or mechanical ventilation. Metabolic alkalosis (ie, increased HCO_3^- or increased base excess) is the state in which there is depletion of blood H+ or increases in HCO_3^-. Typical causes are loss of H+ through the gastrointestinal tract or kidney or administration of sodium bicarbonate.

NEXT DIAGNOSTIC STEP TO CONSIDER IF LEVELS HIGH Evaluate respiratory, neurologic, renal, and gastrointestinal systems. Review treatment history.

CAUSES OF ABNORMALLY LOW LEVELS Decreases in blood pH indicate acidosis. Decreases can be a result of a respiratory or metabolic disturbance. Respiratory acidosis occurs when there is alveolar hypoventilation resulting in the impaired ability to eliminate CO_2. Hypoventilation (ie, increased P_{CO_2}) can be caused by inhibition of the respiratory center through drugs or brainstem lesions, paralysis of the diaphragm, upper airway blockage, and respiratory disease that affects gas exchange (ie, pneumonia) or mechanical hypoventilation. Metabolic acidosis (ie, decreased HCO_3^- or decreased base excess) occurs when there is excess generation of H+ or loss of HCO_3^-. Common causes include lactic acidosis, ketoacidosis, renal failure, or gastrointestinal losses of HCO_3^- (ie, diarrhea).

NEXT DIAGNOSTIC STEP TO CONSIDER IF LEVELS LOW To evaluate metabolic acidosis, calculate anion gap to determine if the acidosis is the result of bicarbonate loss or presence of organic acids. Most common organic acids include lactate, ketones, or uremic acids (phosphates, sulfates, and citrates). Evaluate serum chemistry profile for evidence of muscle damage, renal disease, or metabolic abnormalities related to glucose homeostasis. Evaluate respiratory system (ie, pneumonia).

SPECIMEN AND PROCESSING CONSIDERATIONS

LAB ARTIFACTS THAT MAY INTERFERE WITH READING OF LEVELS OF THIS SUBSTANCE (AND HOW—ARTIFICIALLY ELEVATED VS. DEPRESSED) Delay in analysis may result in decreased blood pH.

SAMPLE FOR COLLECTION (TYPE OF SPECIMEN, COLOR TUBE) AND ANY SPECIAL SPECIMEN HANDLING NOTES Venous whole blood collected in heparinized tube and analyzed promptly.

PEARLS Disturbances in blood pH can be life threatening. Periodic monitoring during anesthesia, patients with severe respiratory disturbances or metabolic (eg, gastrointestinal) disturbances.

AUTHOR and EDITOR: **CHARLES WIEDMEYER**

Blood Typing

BASIC INFORMATION

DEFINITION

Blood typing is the identification of allelic antigens on the surface of erythrocytes.

TYPICAL NORMAL RANGE (US UNITS; SI UNITS)

- Blood systems are represented by upper case letters, while the factors are represented by lower case letters (eg, Ca). Blood groups are identified as being either positive or negative. Blood types Aa, Ca, and Qa appear to be the ones most important in the development of hemolytic reactions in blood transfusions and neonatal iso-erythrolysis.
- Approximately 10% of horses have naturally occurring alloantibodies. Typically, animals may have antibodies to the erythrocyte antigens they are lacking. Therefore if an animal is Aa and Ca negative, then it is possible that it has both anti-Aa and anti-Ca antibodies. An animal positive for

these antigens can be assumed to lack these antibodies. Alloantibodies may also be acquired following exposure to blood factor antigens following transfusions and pregnancy.

PHYSIOLOGY

There are eight major blood systems in the horse, seven of which are internationally recognized (A, C, D, K, P, Q, U). The T system is primarily of interest in research. Each blood type system is represented by a gene for which two or more alleles exist. These alleles encode for proteins, which are the factors, or antigenic sites, on erythrocytes. More than 30 factors are known to exist in horses.

SPECIMEN AND PROCESSING CONSIDERATIONS

SAMPLE FOR COLLECTION (TYPE OF SPECIMEN, COLOR TUBE) AND ANY SPECIAL SPECIMEN HANDLING NOTES EDTA anticoagulated whole blood (purple top) is required for blood typing.

PEARLS

- Blood typing is useful for identifying donors for blood transfusions.
- Blood typing may also be used to predict the development of neonatal isoerythrolysis through assessment of mare/stallion compatibility prior to breeding.
- The best equine blood donors are Aa, Ca, and Qa negative. These animals lack factor antigens that may react with preexisting patient alloantibodies. Additionally, these animals will not sensitize mares against antigens implicated in neonatal isoerythrolysis.
- Blood typing does not obviate the need for pretransfusion cross-matching of donor and recipient for evaluation of complete compatibility.

AUTHOR: **LAURA ANN SNYDER**

EDITOR: **CHARLES WIEDMEYER**

Blood Urea Nitrogen (BUN)

BASIC INFORMATION

DEFINITION

- Urea: A highly water-soluble neutral (not acidic or basic) nitrogenous molecule necessary for disposal of nitrogenous waste in mammals
- Blood urea nitrogen (BUN): Serum urea nitrogen (SUN) and BUN are the same concentration because urea nitrogen passively diffuses throughout total body water.
- Azotemia: An increase in blood nitrogen-containing compounds, especially urea nitrogen and creatinine

TYPICAL NORMAL RANGE (US UNITS; SI UNITS)

7 to 17 mmol/L, 10 to 24 mg/dL

PHYSIOLOGY

Most urea is synthesized by the liver from dietary ammonia created through gastrointestinal protein catabolism. Urea is highly water-soluble and passively diffuses throughout the total body water within 90 minutes. Most urea is excreted through the kidney via simple glomerular filtration. It is passively reabsorbed in the collecting ducts inversely to the rate of urine flow. A decreased glomerular filtra-

tion rate and decreased urine flow will allow for less filtration and more reabsorption, respectively, and increase BUN. Antidiuretic hormone (ADH) allows diffusion of urea from collecting tubules into the renal interstitium where it contributes to the medullary concentration gradient. Urea is also excreted in saliva, sweat, and the gastrointestinal tract; the latter is reabsorbed directly or as ammonia.

CAUSES OF ABNORMALLY HIGH LEVELS

- Prerenal causes due to increased protein catabolism (such as with small bowel hemorrhage, starvation, high-

protein diet, prolonged exercise, infection, and fever) or decreased renal perfusion (shock, endotoxemia, hypovolemia, dehydration, and cardiovascular disease).
- Foals may have spurious increases near birth.
- Renal azotemia can be acute or chronic (vasomotor nephropathy, toxins, interstitial nephritis, duodenitis/proximal jejunitis, hemolytic anemia/hemoglobinuria, or rhabdomyolysis/myoglobinuria).
- Postrenal azotemia is due to urinary obstruction (urethral calculi, nephroliths) or uroperitoneum.

NEXT DIAGNOSTIC STEP TO CONSIDER IF LEVELS HIGH
- Complete blood count/serum chemistry profile and urinalysis to differentiate prerenal (increased urine specific gravity and hemoconcentration), acute renal failure (anuria or oliguria, urinary casts, hypochloridemia, hyponatremia, hypocalcemia or hypercalcemia, metabolic acidosis, and occasional hyperkalemia), chronic renal failure (nonregenerative anemia, hyponatremia, hypochloremia, hypophospha-

temia, hypercalcemia, isosthenuria, proteinuria), urinary blockage (crystals, urine leukocytes, blood, and protein), and uroperitoneum (hyponatremia, hyperkalemia, hypochloremia, and abdominal effusion)
- Abdominocentesis to rule out uroperitoneum (abdominal fluid creatinine is at least twice as high as serum creatinine concentration)
- Urinary GGT fractional excretion >25 to confirm chronic renal failure
- Transabdominal ultrasonography, rectal examination, and/or renal biopsy

CAUSES OF ABNORMALLY LOW LEVELS
- Hepatic insufficiency
- Malnutrition (low-protein diet)
- Starvation (total caloric deficit)
- Anabolic steroids
- Neonates (high metabolic rate)

NEXT DIAGNOSTIC STEP TO CONSIDER IF LEVELS LOW
- Complete blood count/serum chemistry profile, serum bile acids concentration
- Hepatic ultrasonography and liver biopsy

DRUG EFFECTS ON LEVELS
- Decreased: anabolic steroids
- Increased: corticosteroids and tetracycline

SPECIMEN AND PROCESSING CONSIDERATIONS

LAB ARTIFACTS THAT MAY INTERFERE WITH READINGS OF LEVELS OF THIS SUBSTANCE (AND HOW—ARTIFICIALLY ELEVATED VS. DEPRESSED) Hyperammonemia can falsely elevate. Bilirubin, hemolysis, and ascorbic acid variably interfere.

SAMPLE FOR COLLECTION (TYPE OF SPECIMEN, COLOR TUBE) AND ANY SPECIAL SPECIMEN HANDLING NOTES Serum, quickly separated from the clot and refrigerated. Reagent strips can be used for estimation but are inaccurate. Stable.

PEARLS Moderate increases in BUN suggest renal failure; very high BUN suggests a prerenal component. Foals may have a transient spurious increase in BUN and low specific gravity.

AUTHOR: **PAULA M. KRIMER**

EDITOR: **CHARLES WIEDMEYER**

Bone Marrow Cytology and Biopsy

BASIC INFORMATION

DEFINITION

Bone marrow cytology is the microscopic evaluation of bone marrow aspirate slides or impression smears. Bone marrow core biopsies allow the microscopic evaluation of marrow tissue sections.

TYPICAL NORMAL RANGE (US UNITS; SI UNITS)

- Normal adult bone marrow ranges from 25% to 75% cellularity (hematopoietic cells) with the remainder comprised of adipose tissue. Immature animals are expected to have high marrow cellularity, and geriatric animals normally have lower cellularity.
- In addition to total marrow cellularity, the proportions of all main hematopoietic cell lines must be considered. The erythroid and granulocytic cell lines are evaluated in comparison to one another, with a granulocytic to erythroid (aka myeloid to erythroid) ratio calculated or estimated. Normal granulocytic to erythroid ratios in healthy animals are approximately 1:1. The

presence of a few to several megakaryocytes per large bone marrow particle is adequate for a bone marrow aspirate in a healthy individual.
- Normal bone marrow will display orderly, pyramidal maturation of hematopoietic cells with very low numbers of immature blasts and the largest concentration of more mature blood cells. Low numbers of lymphocytes, plasma cells, macrophages, and rare mast cells can be seen.
- Iron stores are subjectively assessed in bone marrow samples, with normal samples containing low numbers of hemosiderin-laden macrophages.

PHYSIOLOGY

Postnatal production of all major blood cell lines (erythroid, granulocytic, monocytic, and megakaryocytic) occurs within bone marrow. Sampling sites include the sternum, dorsal ribs, and ilium. Indications for bone marrow evaluation include persistent cytopenia(s), staging neoplasia, the presence of atypical cells in circulation, or unexplained persistent hypercalcemia or hyperglobulinemia. Bone marrow is a remarkably plastic tissue, capable of rapidly expanding the production of blood cell lines to meet

peripheral tissue needs and to maintain overall hematologic homeostasis. For this reason, bone marrow evaluation must be accompanied by concurrent or recent (within 24 hours) complete blood count (CBC) data for full interpretation.

CAUSES OF ABNORMALLY HIGH LEVELS

- An increase in marrow cellularity may be an appropriate response, may indicate inflammation within the marrow, or may represent neoplasia. Appropriate increases in marrow cellularity are as follows: An increased erythroid compartment in the face of blood loss or hemolytic anemia, an increased granulocytic compartment in the face of leukopenia or an inflammatory stimulus, and an increased concentration of megakaryocytes in the face of increased platelet consumption or destruction.
- Increased concentrations of any cell line can be seen with appropriate hyperplasia of that compartment, leukemia, or myelodysplastic syndromes.
- Lymphocyte and plasma cell concentrations may increase with antigenic stimulation or neoplasia (leukemia, leukemic phase of lymphoma, or multiple myeloma).

- The presence of any epithelial populations or of dysplastic spindle cells suggests metastatic or primary neoplasia.
- Iron stores may be increased as a result of increased iron intake (over-administration of iron supplements), anemia of chronic disease, or with hemolytic anemias.

NEXT DIAGNOSTIC STEP TO CONSIDER IF LEVELS HIGH Overall this is dependent on clinical signs and exact laboratory findings. Bone marrow biopsies can provide a better estimate of true marrow cellularity and can sometimes identify metastatic neoplasms earlier than bone marrow aspirate cytology. If neoplastic cells are present in marrow samples, additional stains can be employed to further differentiate the neoplastic cell type. Specialized laboratories can analyze bone marrow aspirates in EDTA tubes via flow cytometry for the same purpose.

CAUSES OF ABNORMALLY LOW LEVELS

- Minimally cellular bone marrow aspirate slides may be the result of suboptimal sampling technique, may indicate the presence of increased trabecular bone or fibrous tissue (myelofibrosis), or may reflect a truly hypoplastic marrow.

- True hypoplasia in one or more cell lines can occur with processes such as immune-mediated destruction of blood cell precursors, drug reactions, estrogen toxicity, anemia of chronic disease, and renal disease-associated anemia.
- Decreased iron stores are found in iron deficiency.

NEXT DIAGNOSTIC STEP TO CONSIDER IF LEVELS LOW Bone marrow biopsies of good quality can provide a better estimate of true marrow cellularity and can identify the presence of myelofibrosis or osteosclerosis.

SPECIMEN AND PROCESSING CONSIDERATIONS

SAMPLE FOR COLLECTION (TYPE OF SPECIMEN, COLOR TUBE) AND ANY SPECIAL SPECIMEN HANDLING NOTES

- Slides must be prepared immediately upon bone marrow aspiration for optimal sample quality. A small amount of EDTA should be drawn into the syringe prior to aspiration to help prevent blood clotting. The aspirated material can be dispensed directly on tilted glass slides or a Petri dish to allow the excess blood to drain away from the cellular marrow particles, which appear as white/tan flecks. If

using a Petri dish, these marrow particles can be gently transferred to glass slides via a pipette and spread in a "squash preparation" technique by placing a spreading slide on top of the sample and pulling the two slides apart. Multiple slides should be made and air-dried. It is prudent to check sample quality on at least one slide (assess whether or not there are marrow particles present) to ensure a diagnostic specimen is submitted to the laboratory.
- Bone marrow core biopsies can be gently rolled on glass slides to create impression smears for cytologic evaluation, if desired. The biopsy sample is then placed in a container of 10% formalin and submitted to a laboratory for further processing and evaluation.

PEARLS

- Current CBC data (within 24 hours of marrow sampling) must be available for review in conjunction with bone marrow aspirate slides or a bone marrow core biopsy for full interpretation.
- Bone marrow aspirate slides must be prepared immediately upon sample acquisition.

AUTHOR: **ANGELA B. ROYAL**

EDITOR: **CHARLES WIEDMEYER**

Calcium

BASIC INFORMATION

DEFINITION

- Mineral required for many essential intracellular and extracellular functions
- Main element for bone mineralization
- Present as free (also referred as ionized calcium), about 50%; anion bound (mainly to albumin, less to globulins), 40% to 45%; and non–protein bound, 5% to 10% to lactate, phosphate, or citrate

SYNONYM(S)

Ca^{2+} calcium
tCa^{2+} total calcium
iCa^{2+} ionized calcium (= fCa^{2+} free calcium)

TYPICAL NORMAL RANGE (US UNITS; SI UNITS)

10 to 13.5 mg/dL

PHYSIOLOGY

- Absorption from intestine mainly depends on the dietary calcium

content (not vitamin D, due to lack of 1α-hydroxylase in horses).
- Parathyroid hormone (PTH), calcitonin, and vitamin D regulate bone deposition and resorption.
- Kidney is the main route of excretion.

CAUSES OF ABNORMALLY HIGH LEVELS

- Hyperparathyroidism
- Hypercalcemia of malignancy (myeloma, gastric carcinoma, lymphoma, adrenocortical carcinoma, squamous cell carcinoma)
- Renal insufficiency/failure both acute and chronic
- Vitamin D toxicity (excessive supplementation, ingestion of certain plants: *Cestrum diurnum-jasmin, Solanum malacoxylon, or Ilisetum flavescens*)
- Rarely urinary bladder rupture in foals

NEXT DIAGNOSTIC STEP TO CONSIDER IF LEVELS HIGH Measure iCa^{2+}, PTH, PTHrp; measure phosphate and electrolyte levels; evaluate kidney function, exposure to vitamin D, presence of neoplasia

CAUSES OF ABNORMALLY LOW LEVELS

- Insufficient diet supply (all grain diets and diets high in oxalates: pangola, Setaria, kikuyu, greasewood)
- Primary hypoparathyroidism
- Hypoalbuminemia, hypoproteinemia
- Horses with colic due to different gastrointestinal (GI) disorders (GI disease associated with colic)
- Blister beetle poisoning
- Myopathies associated with transport, strenuous exercise
- Sweating (mainly decrease in fCa^{2+})
- Puerperal tetany in mares
- Acute renal failure
- Sepsis, endotoxemia

NEXT DIAGNOSTIC STEP TO CONSIDER IF LEVELS LOW Thorough history including diet, previous race/strenuous exercise, GI disease; measure PTH, phosphorus, serum albumin, magnesium levels

DRUG EFFECTS ON LEVELS

- Decrease: furosemide, sodium bicarbonate, steroids, calcium binding anticoagulants

- Increase: thiazide diuretics, calcium gluconate

SPECIMEN AND PROCESSING CONSIDERATIONS

LAB ARTIFACTS THAT MAY INTERFERE WITH READINGS OF LEVELS OF THIS SUBSTANCE (AND HOW—ARTIFICIALLY ELEVATED VS. DEPRESSED)

- False decrease: Use of calcium binding anticoagulants (oxalate, EDTA, citrate)
- False increase: Lipemia and hemolysis

SAMPLE FOR COLLECTION (TYPE OF SPECIMEN, COLOR TUBE) AND ANY SPECIAL SPECIMEN HANDLING NOTES

- Preferred is serum, sometimes heparinized plasma can be used.
- iCa^{2+} serum, heparinized plasma, heparinized whole blood, serum; necessary to be anaerobically processed
- iCa^{2+} stability: serum or heparinized plasma up to 4 days (room temperature), heparinized whole blood 9 hours (4° C), serum or plasma in glass tube 1 week (4° C), 6 weeks in (−20° C)
- Use calcium citrated heparin tubes or heparin less than 15 U/mL.

PEARLS

- Metabolic alkalosis leads to hypocalcemia.
- Metabolic acidosis leads to hypercalcemia.

AUTHOR: **IDA PIPERISOVA**

EDITOR: **CHARLES WIEDMEYER**

Casts in Urine Sediment

BASIC INFORMATION

DEFINITION

Cylindrical structures composed of proteins, intact cells, and/or cellular debris that form in renal tubular lumens and are shed in the urine.

TYPICAL NORMAL RANGE (US UNITS; SI UNITS)

Less than 1 hyaline or granular cast per low powered microscope field (100×) is considered normal; however, casts are rarely observed in equine urine sediment.

PHYSIOLOGY

- Tamm-Horsfall mucoprotein is secreted by the renal tubular and collecting duct epithelial cells. The conglutination of this protein into a cylindrical structure is known as a hyaline cast.
- Granular, lipid, and cellular casts form when cellular debris or cells in the renal tubules become trapped in the Tamm-Horsfall mucoprotein.
- Waxy casts are formed from the deterioration of granular casts and reflect chronic tubular disease.
- Casts composed of leukocytes or red blood cells indicate renal inflammation or hemorrhage, respectively.

CAUSES OF ABNORMALLY HIGH LEVELS Renal tubular degeneration, necrosis, hemorrhage, or inflammation

NEXT DIAGNOSTIC STEP TO CONSIDER IF LEVELS HIGH Assess renal function and evaluate history for exposure to renal toxins. A renal biopsy may be indicated in some cases.

DRUG EFFECTS ON LEVELS Gentamicin, amikacin, or other renal tubular toxins may cause granular or cellular casts.

SPECIMEN AND PROCESSING CONSIDERATIONS

LAB ARTIFACTS THAT MAY INTERFERE WITH READINGS OF LEVELS OF THIS SUBSTANCE (AND HOW—ARTIFICIALLY ELEVATED VS. DEPRESSED) Excessive sample mixing, high-speed centrifugation, and delay in examination may cause dissolution of casts and false-negative results.

SAMPLE FOR COLLECTION (TYPE OF SPECIMEN, COLOR TUBE) AND ANY SPECIAL SPECIMEN HANDLING NOTES Midstream urine collection in a clean container

PEARLS

- Casts are soluble in alkaline urine. Due to the alkaline nature of equine urine, casts are rarely seen in urine sediment.
- Mucous threads are common in equine urine and are often confused with casts. Mucous threads do not have well-delineated edges and often resemble twisted ribbons.

AUTHOR: **LAURA C. CREGAR**

EDITOR: **CHARLES WIEDMEYER**

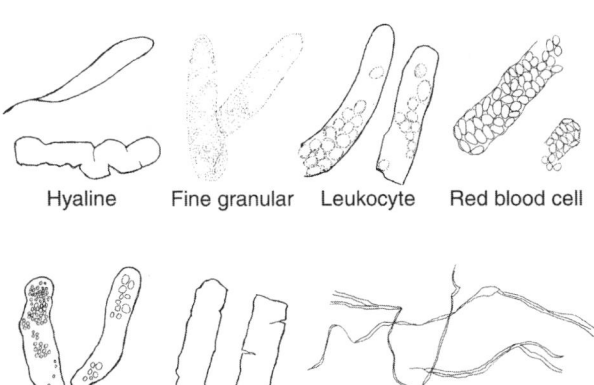

Hyaline   Fine granular   Leukocyte   Red blood cell

Fatty   Waxy   Mucous threads resembling casts

FIGURE 1 Casts commonly found in urine sediment smears. (From Cowell R, Tyler R: *Diagnostic Cytology and Hematology of the Dog and Cat,* ed 3. St Louis, MO: Mosby Elsevier, 2008.)

Cerebrospinal Fluid (CSF) Analysis

BASIC INFORMATION

DEFINITION

CSF analysis includes the determination of the fluid's physical characteristics (color, clarity, volume), total protein concentration, nucleated cell concentration, red blood cell concentration, and the microscopic evaluation of the cells present.

TYPICAL NORMAL RANGE (US UNITS; SI UNITS)

Normal CSF is clear and colorless. Total protein concentration is very low, with reports for normal equine CSF samples averaging approximately 90 mg/dL, and ranging up to about 120 mg/dL. Because protein is present in the mg/dL range rather than g/dL, protein determination is measured via microprotein assays rather than by a refractometer. Normal nucleated cell concentration ranges up to 8/μL; this is measured via a hemacytometer. The vast majority of nucleated cells present should be large and small mononuclear cells. Rare neutrophils may be seen in normal animals.

PHYSIOLOGY

CSF is a plasma ultrafiltrate that surrounds the brain and spinal cord, cushioning these organs and allowing for diffusion of nutrients and waste products. Due to the normally stringent blood-CSF barrier, CSF typically is minimally cellular and has very little protein. With any disruption of the blood-CSF barrier, the cell concentration and/or protein can increase. CSF can be sampled from the lumbosacral region (most common) or the atlanto-occipital space.

CAUSES OF ABNORMALLY HIGH LEVELS

- Elevated protein concentration with a normal cell count (sometimes referred to as albuminocytologic dissociation) can be seen with compromise of the blood-CSF barrier (eg, with vasculitis), hemorrhage, neoplasia, or with local production of immunoglobulins into the CSF.
- An elevation in the nucleated cell concentration (called pleocytosis) and/or in the proportion of granulocytes suggests inflammation. An elevation in protein concentration is often seen in conjunction with pleocytosis. Viral encephalitis can result in mononuclear pleocytosis or a mixed pleocytosis with increased granulocytes in addition to mononuclear cells. Bacterial meningitis/meningoencephalitis typically results in neutrophilic (suppurative) pleocytosis. Fungal, parasitic, and protozoal infections often yield mixed pleocytosis, sometimes with an increased number of eosinophils. Trauma, necrosis, or degeneration of CNS tissue can result in pleocytosis of any type, though in some cases pleocytosis will be lacking. Rarely, neoplasia may result in pleocytosis.
- The presence of red blood cells indicates either true pathologic hemorrhage or iatrogenic blood contamination. In slides prepared from fresh samples, the presence of erythrophagocytosis is evidence of true hemorrhage. Additionally, previous hemorrhage into CSF may result in xanthochromia, a yellow discoloration of the fluid.

NEXT DIAGNOSTIC STEP TO CONSIDER IF LEVELS HIGH This will be dependent upon clinical signs, history, and radiographic findings. If a bacterial or fungal process is suspected and no organisms are found cytologically, microbiologic culture of CSF is indicated. Serology or polymerase chain reaction (PCR) testing may be indicated to rule in or out other infectious diseases.

SPECIMEN AND PROCESSING CONSIDERATIONS

SAMPLE FOR COLLECTION (TYPE OF SPECIMEN, COLOR TUBE) AND ANY SPECIAL HANDLING NOTES CSF should be split into at least two aliquots if being sent to an outside laboratory: one in a purple top EDTA tube or red top tube for cell counts and total protein determination, and the other in a red top tube with an addition of autologous serum in a 1:1 ratio for cytologic evaluation. As CSF normally has a very minimal protein concentration, this addition of serum can improve the cell stability during transit. If microbiologic culture is desired, a third aliquot in a red top tube or in culture medium is recommended. Slides for cytologic evaluation must be prepared from concentrated CSF; these are often made in the laboratory upon sample arrival via cytocentrifugation. In-house methods for concentrating CSF have also been described. CSF must be shipped on ice but not frozen, preferably no longer then overnight to the laboratory.

PEARLS

- Fluid samples should be shipped to a laboratory overnight, on ice but not frozen.
- Microbiologic culture is recommended if bacterial or fungal disease is suspected but no organisms are found cytologically.

AUTHOR: **ANGELA B. ROYAL**

EDITOR: **CHARLES WIEDMEYER**

Chloride

BASIC INFORMATION

DEFINITION

- Hyperchloremia: Increased chloride concentration in the blood
- Normochloremia: Normal chloride concentration in the blood
- Hypochloremia: Decreased chloride concentration in the blood

SYNONYM(S)

Cl⁻

TYPICAL NORMAL RANGE (US UNITS; SI UNITS)

99 to 109 mEq/L; 99 to 109 mmol/L

PHYSIOLOGY

Chloride is the most significant anion in the extracellular fluid compartment. It is regulated by oral intake and renal reabsorption and secretion. Chloride is most commonly associated with proportionate changes in sodium concentration and is altered by the acid-base status of the animal. Chloride from HCl from the stomach mucosa is reabsorbed in the intestines.

CAUSES OF ABNORMALLY HIGH LEVELS

With proportional increases in sodium:
- Water deficit: Water deprivation, hyperventilation, fever, diarrhea, diuresis, diuretics, burns, renal disease, diabetes insipidus–central/nephrogenic
- Increased absorption: Salt poisoning, hypertonic saline administration
- Decreased excretion: Hyperaldosteronism

Without proportional increases in sodium:
- Metabolic acidosis, renal tubular acidosis, compensation for primary respiratory alkalosis.

NEXT DIAGNOSTIC STEP TO CONSIDER IF LEVELS HIGH Review history, clinical signs, complete blood count, biochemistry profile, urinalysis, and rectal examination. Blood gas analysis, urine fractional excretion for renal disease, water deprivation test/measure plasma vasopressin for diabetes insipidus, measure aldosterone concentration

CAUSES OF ABNORMALLY LOW LEVELS

With proportional decreases in sodium:
- Excessive sweating/salivation, nasogastric intubation, diarrhea, hemorrhage, fluid drainage, third-space loss, prolonged diuresis, hypoaldosteronism, hypoadrenocorticism

Without proportional decreases in sodium:
- Excessive sweating/salivation, metabolic alkalosis, compensation for respiratory acidosis, diuretics, adrenal insufficiency, metabolic acidosis with increased anion gap (ketoacidosis, lactic acidosis) volvulus, torsion, intestinal obstruction, nasogastric drainage
- Water excess due to congestive heart failure, hepatic cirrhosis, nephrotic syndrome, syndrome of inappropriate ADH secretion
- Water shift from intracellular fluid to extracellular fluid space: hyperglycemia, mannitol administration
- Chloride shift from intravascular to extravascular: uroperitoneum.

NEXT DIAGNOSTIC STEP TO CONSIDER IF LEVELS LOW Review history, clinical signs, complete blood count, biochemistry profile, urinalysis, and rectal examination. Abdominocentesis and thoracocentesis for third space loss, radiographic imaging, blood gas analysis, measure blood aldosterone concentration, adrenocorticotrophic hormone (ACTH) stimulation test for hypoadrenocorticism, measure plasma vasopressin concentration for syndrome of inappropriate secretion

DRUG EFFECTS ON LEVELS

- Decrease: Furosemide, thiazide diuretics
- Increase: Potassium bromide (artifactual increase)

SPECIMEN AND PROCESSING CONSIDERATIONS

LAB ARTIFACTS THAT MAY INTERFERE WITH READINGS OF LEVELS OF THIS SUBSTANCE (AND HOW—ARTIFICIALLY ELEVATED VS. DEPRESSED)

- Increase: Aged sample (dehydrated); potassium bromide or lactate if potentiometry used
- Decrease: Lipemia and hyperproteinemia

SAMPLE FOR COLLECTION (TYPE OF SPECIMEN, COLOR TUBE) AND ANY SPECIAL SPECIMEN HANDLING NOTES

- Serum preferred; plasma can be used
- Methodology: Potentiometry and spectrophotometry

PEARLS

- If chloride is shifting proportionally with sodium (sodium concentration minus chloride concentration should be between 25–50 mEq/L) consider similar causes to changes in sodium. If the change is disproportionate consider an acid-base abnormality.
- Normochloremia is important to notice especially if there is hypernatremia or hypobicarbonatemia (on blood gas analysis) or low total CO_2 (on biochemistry profile) because it suggests the presence of an increased anion gap, which can indicate the presence of unmeasured anions like lactic acids, ketoacids, uremia, and penicillin toxicity.

AUTHORS: **LAURA V. LANE** and **THERESA E. RIZZI**

EDITOR: **CHARLES WIEDMEYER**

Codocytes

BASIC INFORMATION

DEFINITION

Codocytes are bell-shaped erythrocytes that resemble targets when viewed on blood smears (in addition to the marginal ring of hemoglobin, a spot of hemoglobin is seen within the central pallor area due to a central bulge in the cell).

SYNONYM(S)

Target cell
Mexican hat cell

TYPICAL NORMAL RANGE (US UNITS; SI UNITS)

Rare to none

CAUSES OF ABNORMALLY HIGH LEVELS Codocytes are not commonly noted in equine blood. If present, they are probably difficult to recognize on blood smears, because equine erythrocytes generally do not exhibit a distinctive central pallor. In other species, codocyte formation has been associated with iron deficiency, regenerative anemia, and hepatic disease.

AUTHOR: **MARLYN S. WHITNEY**

EDITOR: **CHARLES WIEDMEYER**

Computed Tomography: Dental Disease

BASIC INFORMATION

DEFINITION

- Computed tomography (CT) images are cross sectional and depict variations in tissue density.
- Problems of superimposition of the skull on the dentition that are routinely encountered in dental radiography are largely eliminated using this modality.
- Provides relative density values for tissues that is measured in Hounsfield units (HU).

TYPICAL NORMAL RANGE (US UNITS; SI UNITS)

- CT allows for a complete evaluation of the internal architecture of the tooth, the supporting osseous structures, and associated paranasal sinuses.
  - Excellent contrast resolution allows differentiation of cementum, enamel and dentin, the dental lamina dura, and the surrounding alveolar bone.
  - Furthermore, the infundibulae and pulp horns can be clearly delineated and evaluated for the presence of disease.
- Enamel is the most dense dental tissue represented on CT as the whitest structure with the highest HU value.

- Appears as an undulating dense tissue that is present in the crown, reserve crown, and root that is denser than the alveolar bone lamina dura.
  - Surrounded by either dentin or cementum.
- Dentin
  - Primary, secondary, and tertiary dentin has a density on CT images that is intermediate to enamel and the soft tissues of the pulp chamber or the periodontal ligament.
  - Slightly more dense that the surrounding bone.
  - Primary dentin lies between the layers of internal and external enamel.
  - Secondary dentin lines the pulp cavities.
  - Reparative or tertiary dentine is produced by odontoblasts in response to insult.
- Pulp cavity: In the young horse the pulp cavity and apex will appear as a large and well-defined radiolucent space and as the tooth ages, this appearance is lost.
- Cementum
  - Surrounds the peripheral portions of the tooth including the reserve crown and root.

- Forms a functional unit with the periodontal ligament from a single functional unit, anchoring the tooth to the alveolar bone.
  - Found as a covering over the infundibula of the incisors and maxillary cheek teeth.
  - Radiographically and on CT images, the cementum is seen as slightly hypodense to enamel but more dense than the periodontal ligament, which should appear as a well defined, thin radiolucent (hypodense) line that is smoothly margined and follows the external surface of the tooth. Recognition of this line is critically important when assessing teeth for apical infections or periodontal disease.
- Pulp
  - Houses the vascular and nervous tissues of the tooth and is lined by odontoblasts.
  - Appears as hypodense (soft tissue dense) material.
  - Contiguous with the periodontal connective tissues at the apex of the tooth root.
  - Pulpar configuration is complex, particularly in the maxillary cheek teeth and the configuration in all teeth changes as the teeth age.

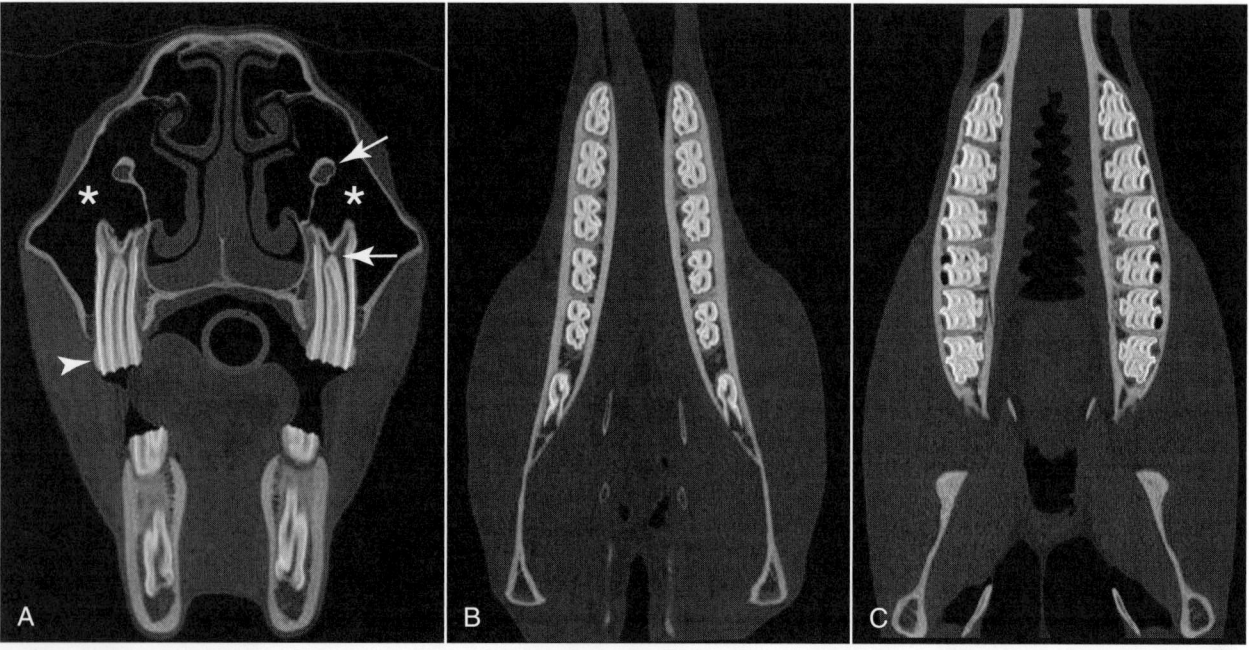

FIGURE 1 A, Transverse image through the '09 teeth. The elimination of superimposition makes the internal architecture of the teeth more clear. Cement can be identified on the external surface of the enamel (*white arrowhead at lower left*). Pulp is soft tissue that is relatively hypodense (*lower right arrow*). The infraorbital canal (*arrow at top right*) is identified as it courses through the maxillary sinuses (***). **B,** Dorsal plane reformatted image through the mandibular arcade. **C,** Dorsal plane reformatted image through the maxillary arcade.

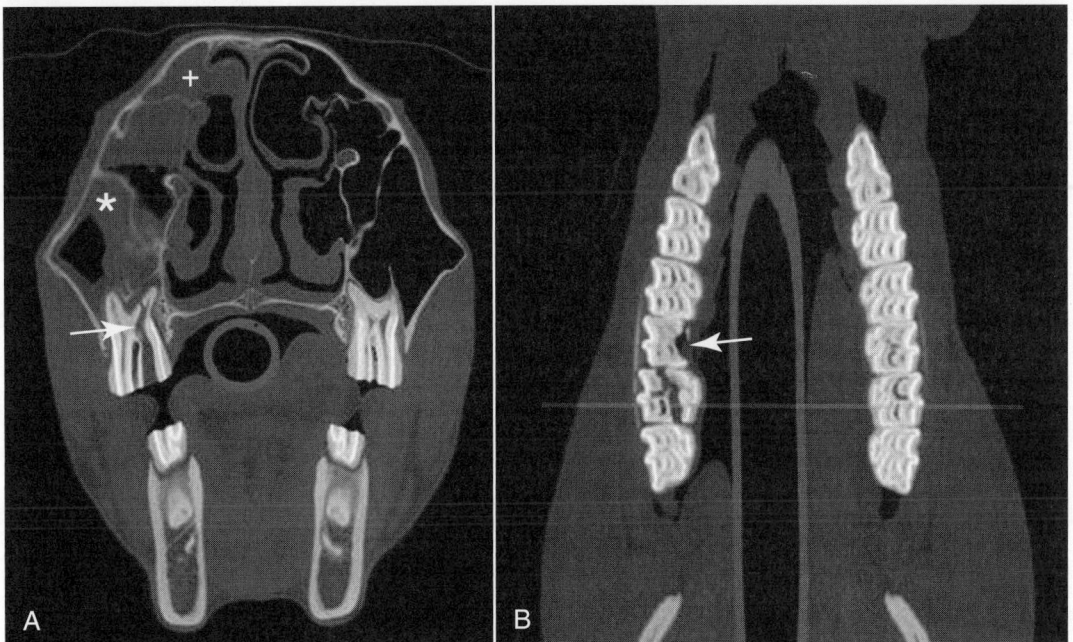

FIGURE 2 **A,** Transverse image made through the '10 teeth. A complete, displaced sagittal fracture is present through the 110 (*white arrow*). Fluid is accumulating in the caudal maxillary sinus (*) and the dorsal conchal sinus (+). The fluid lines appear to be inverted because the images are acquired with the horse in dorsal recumbency. There is disruption of the dental lamina dura and communication from the oral cavity to the caudal maxillary sinus through the fractured tooth. Gas is present within the infundibula. **B,** Dorsal plane reformatted image. The grey line demarcates the location of the transverse image. Note that the 109 is also fractured in a sagittal fashion on the lingual surface of the tooth (*white arrow*). Both fractures occur through lingual pulp cavities.

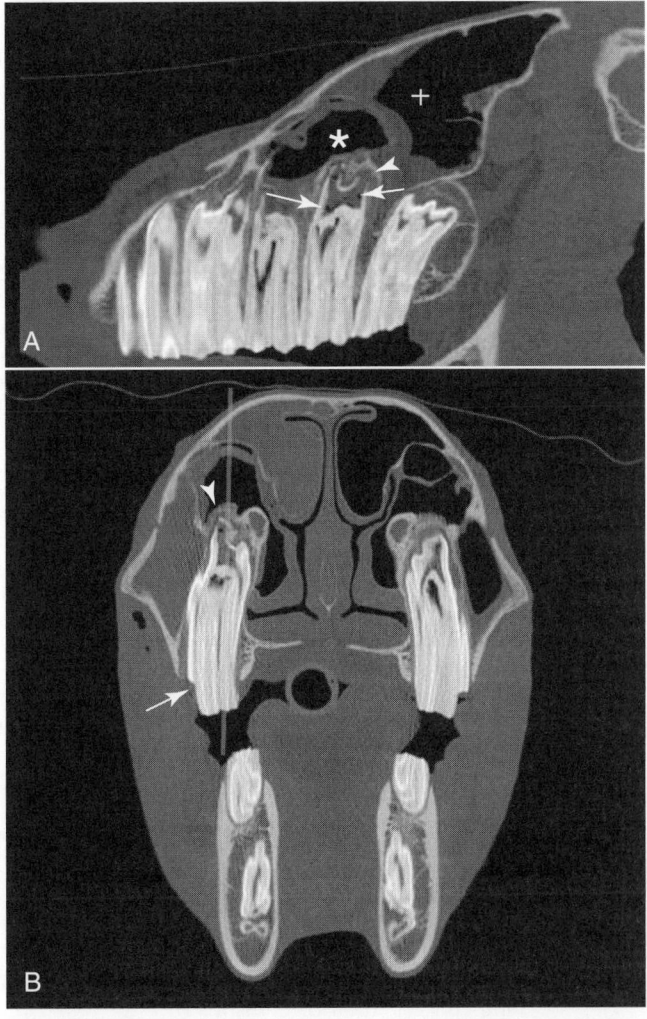

FIGURE 3 **A,** Sagittal reformatted image of endodontal disease of the 110 tooth of the maxillary arcade. There is soft tissue thickening of the mucosal surfaces of the rostral (*) and caudal (+) maxillary sinuses. There is gas present within the root, pulp, and alveolus of the tooth (*white arrows*). There is thickening of the lamina dura (*arrowhead*) and disruption of the interdental bone. **B,** Transverse image made through the '10 teeth. Similar to A small, buccal, incomplete fracture is present at the occlusal surface of the 110. This fracture communicates with the buccal pulp and is likely the source of the infection. The grey line demarcates the site of the sagittal plane image.

○ Age-related differences are very important to recognize when evaluating CT scans as well as radiographs.
- Lamina dura
  ○ A very dense shelf of bone that is attached to the periodontal ligament.
  ○ Outside the lamina dura is the alveolar bone, which is then surrounded by the trabecular bone of incisive bone, mandible, and maxilla. The bone will respond to both pathologic and physiologic processes

with sclerosis and periosteal proliferation.
  ○ Appears on radiographs as a thin and well-defined radio-opaque line.
  ○ Early changes secondary to infection involve loss of definition of the lamina dura and sclerosis of the surrounding alveolar bone.
- The overlying anatomy and the relationship of the cheek teeth to the paranasal sinuses complicates radiographic interpretation. Only a thin shelf of bone lies between the rostral maxillary sinuses and the caudal roots of the

fourth premolars and all of the roots of the first molars. Similarly, a thin shelf of bone lies between the caudal maxillary sinuses and the roots of the second and third molars. In the maxillary arcade, CT becomes particularly valuable. When overlying sinusitis or abscess formation can lead to the misinterpretation of lucencies or sclerotic change on radiographs, CT is able to delineate the differences through the elimination of superimposition.

AUTHOR: **SARAH M. PUCHALSKI**

Coombs' Test

BASIC INFORMATION

DEFINITION

Detection of erythrocyte associated immunoglobulins (IgG and IgM) and complement

SYNONYM(S)

May also be referred to as the direct antiglobulin test (DAT).

TYPICAL NORMAL RANGE (US UNITS; SI UNITS)

Results are most commonly reported as being either positive or negative. Some laboratories may report dilutions at which the test was positive/negative. Dilutions of the test are performed to optimize the concentration of reagent in the presence of the patient's erythrocytes. The dilutions at which a sample is positive do not correlate with the severity of disease.

PHYSIOLOGY

In the Coombs' test, the patient's washed erythrocytes are incubated with serial dilutions of a polyvalent Coombs' reagent (contains a mixture of anti-IgG, IgM, and

C3 complement protein antibodies). If immunoglobulins or complement proteins are present on erythrocytes, then cross linking and microscopically visible agglutination should occur.
CAUSES OF ABNORMALLY HIGH LEVELS Immune mediated hemolytic anemia (IMHA) results in a positive test. IMHA may be a primary autoimmune disease, secondary to drugs, infection, or neoplastic processes, or may be associated with the presence of alloantibodies in neonatal isoerythrolysis and blood transfusions.
NEXT DIAGNOSTIC STEP TO CONSIDER IF LEVELS HIGH Evaluate patient for clinical evidence of infection or neoplasia. Evaluation of blood smear for supportive erythrocyte morphologic changes, including ghost cells and spherocytes. Historical information such as drug administration and recent blood transfusion may also be helpful.
IMPORTANT INTERSPECIES DIFFERENCES Species-specific Coombs' reagent is necessary.
DRUG EFFECTS ON LEVELS Administration of glucocorticoids may cause false-negative results.

SPECIMEN AND PROCESSING CONSIDERATIONS

LAB ARTIFACTS THAT MAY INTERFERE WITH READINGS OF LEVELS OF THIS SUBSTANCE False negatives may be observed with prolonged sample storage resulting in detachment of antibodies or complement proteins, excessive washing of erythrocytes, or if only very low levels of antibody/complement proteins are present on erythrocytes.
SAMPLE FOR COLLECTION (TYPE OF SPECIMEN, COLOR TUBE) AND ANY SPECIAL SPECIMEN HANDLING NOTES EDTA anticoagulated whole blood (purple top). Samples should be analyzed as soon as possible and ideally within 24 hours, as antibody and complement elution may occur.

PEARLS

- A negative Coombs' test does not rule out IMHA. In these cases, IMHA likely exists if clinical findings, laboratory data, and response to therapy are supportive of the disease.
- The presence of spontaneous agglutination obviates the need for Coombs' testing as this is essentially the natural endpoint of the test.

AUTHOR: **LAURA ANN SNYDER**

EDITOR: **CHARLES WIEDMEYER**

Cortisol

BASIC INFORMATION

DEFINITION

- Hypercortisolemia: Increased circulating concentration of cortisol

- Hypocortisolemia: Decreased circulating concentration of cortisol

TYPICAL NORMAL RANGE (US UNITS; SI UNITS)

36 to 81 nmol/L; 1.30 to 2.93 µg/dL

PHYSIOLOGY

Cortisol is a glucocorticoid hormone produced by the adrenal cortex (zona fasciculata and zona reticularis) when stimulated by adrenocorticotropic hormone (ACTH) produced by the anterior lobe of the pituitary gland, which is in turn controlled by corticotropin-releasing hormone (CRH) released by the hypothalamus. Peak secretion of cortisol occurs in the morning in horses maintained in their usual environment; subsequently time of collection and management may be an important factor in interpreting test results. Systemically, cortisol has many effects including gluconeogenesis, protein catabolism, lipolysis, immune responses, and water balance. Cortisol is able to cross the cytoplasmic membrane and bind to receptor proteins in the cytoplasm. The cortisol-receptor complex then translocates to the nucleus where it initiates the synthesis of hormone and cytokine receptors as well as other proteins.

CAUSES OF ABNORMALLY HIGH LEVELS Primary elevations in circulating cortisol concentrations may be due to increased secretion of ACTH from the pituitary (most commonly associated with a functional adenoma) or increased secretion of cortisol from the adrenal glands (very rare in horses). In either case, both glands are unresponsive to the negative feedback mechanisms in place to maintain a homeostatic level of cortisol. Stress may also cause false elevations in circulating cortisol levels, as CRH secretion is also under nervous system control.

NEXT DIAGNOSTIC STEP TO CONSIDER IF LEVELS HIGH A baseline plasma ACTH concentration should be collected in an EDTA tube to be evaluated. Special handling of the sample is required as ACTH is very labile. Plasma should be removed from the erythrocyte mass, placed in a plastic tube (as ACTH can adhere to glass), and chilled or frozen (if the sample cannot be analyzed the day of collection).

CAUSES OF ABNORMALLY LOW LEVELS A low baseline concentration of cortisol can be due to either a decreased circulating level of ACTH due to pituitary gland destruction (via disease process or surgery) or atrophy of the adrenal glands. Additionally, exogenous long term administration of corticosteroids and anabolic steroids can lead to suppression of the hypothalamic-pituitary-adrenal (HPA) axis, causing a decreased circulating concentration of cortisol due to adrenal gland atrophy.

NEXT DIAGNOSTIC STEP TO CONSIDER IF LEVELS LOW A thorough investigation of the treatment history of the horse should be collected to determine if there has been any use of steroids. A baseline plasma ACTH concentration should be collected in an EDTA tube to be evaluated. Special handling is required as detailed previously. If circulating baseline ACTH concentrations are low, an ACTH stimulation test should be performed (see ACTH stimulation test, section II). This will assist in determining if the hypocortisolemia is due to a pituitary deficiency of ACTH or adrenal gland atrophy.

DRUG EFFECTS ON LEVELS Hypocortisolemia: Exogenously administered corticosteroids and anabolic steroids can affect the HPA axis.

SPECIMEN AND PROCESSING CONSIDERATIONS

LAB ARTIFACTS THAT MAY INTERFERE WITH READINGS OF LEVELS OF THIS SUBSTANCE (AND HOW—ARTIFICIALLY ELEVATED VS. DEPRESSED) Stability of cortisol concentrations is better in EDTA plasma samples than serum samples and better in cold samples. Hence, shipping EDTA plasma samples on ice is preferred.

SAMPLE FOR COLLECTION (TYPE OF SPECIMEN, COLOR TUBE) AND ANY SPECIAL SPECIMEN HANDLING NOTES EDTA (purple top tube) is preferred; serum may also be used.

PEARLS Hypocortisolemia is rare in horses, although adrenal insufficiency is increasingly recognized in critically ill, septic, neonatal patients. Hypercortisolemia is much more commonly recognized in middle aged horses, primarily in association with pars pituitary intermedia dysfunction (PPID) or Cushing's disease.

AUTHORS: **SHANE F. DeWITT** and **TANYA M. GRONDIN**

EDITOR: **CHARLES WIEDMEYER**

Creatine Kinase

BASIC INFORMATION

DEFINITION
A cytoplasmic enzyme found within skeletal, cardiac, and smooth myocytes. Brain and other tissue of the central nervous tissue contain high cytoplasmic CK activity. Most serum enzyme activity comes from skeletal muscle.

SYNONYM(S)
Creatine phosphokinase (CPK) is not an acceptable term for the enzyme.

TYPICAL NORMAL RANGE (US UNITS; SI UNITS)
109 to 456 U/L

PHYSIOLOGY
• CK is an essential enzyme for the production of energy for muscle contraction.

• CK catalyzes a reversible reaction in the transfer of PO_4 from creatine-PO_4 to ADP forming ATP.
• Increases in serum activity occur approximately 4 to 6 hours following muscle damage. The half-life of CK is approximately 2 hours in horses. Persistent elevations in serum CK levels indicate ongoing muscle damage.
• CK isoenzymes exist but have no clinical relevance.

CAUSES OF ABNORMALLY HIGH LEVELS Muscle damage from a variety of insults such as exertional rhabdomyolysis, seizures, neoplasms, nutritional (ie, vitamin E or selenium deficiency), hyperkalemic myopathy, inflammatory, toxic, or trauma. Damage to central nervous tissues is not known to contribute to serum activity.

NEXT DIAGNOSTIC STEP TO CONSIDER IF LEVELS HIGH Evaluate for muscle damage causes. Examine serum biochemistry analysis for changes in aspartate aminotransferase (AST) and lactate dehydrogenase (LDH). These values may offer clues as to the persistence of the muscle damage.

CAUSES OF ABNORMALLY LOW LEVELS Clinically insignificant

SPECIMEN AND PROCESSING CONSIDERATIONS

LAB ARTIFACTS THAT MAY INTERFERE WITH READINGS OF LEVELS OF THIS SUBSTANCE (AND HOW—ARTIFICIALLY ELEVATED VS. DEPRESSED) *In vitro* hemolysis may cause a false increase in CK levels.

SAMPLE FOR COLLECTION (TYPE OF SPECIMEN, COLOR TUBE) AND ANY SPECIAL SPECIMEN HANDLING NOTES Serum or plasma can be used for analysis. Dilution of sample may be necessary if values are markedly elevated.

AUTHOR and EDITOR: **CHARLES WIEDMEYER**

Creatinine

BASIC INFORMATION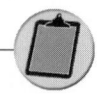

DEFINITION

Azotemia: An increase in blood nitrogen-containing compounds, especially urea nitrogen and creatinine

TYPICAL NORMAL RANGE (US UNITS; SI UNITS)

62 to 194 µmol/L, 0.7 to 2.2 mg/dL

PHYSIOLOGY

- Creatinine is a nonprotein nitrogenous substance derived from muscle creatine.
- Circulating levels vary with dietary intake of creatine and muscle mass.
- It distributes through all body water more slowly than urea.
- It is freely filtered through the glomeruli, not reabsorbed in the tubules, and excreted in urine. A decreased glomerular filtration rate will allow for less filtration resulting in increased levels of creatinine.
- It is a more sensitive indicator of azotemia than blood urea nitrogen (BUN).

CAUSES OF ABNORMALLY HIGH LEVELS

- Increases classified as prerenal, renal, and postrenal causes
- Prerenal due to decreased renal perfusion (shock, endotoxemia, hypovolemia, dehydration, and cardiovascular disease)
- Renal azotemia (acute or chronic) due to vasomotor nephropathy, toxins, interstitial nephritis, or less commonly duodenitis/proximal jejunitis, hemolytic anemia (hemoglobinuria), or rhabdomyolysis (myoglobinuria)

- Postrenal azotemia due to a urinary obstruction (usually urethral), nephroliths, or uroperitoneum

NEXT DIAGNOSTIC STEP TO CONSIDER IF LEVELS HIGH

- Complete blood count/serum chemistry profile and urinalysis to differentiate prerenal (increased urine specific gravity and hemoconcentration), acute renal failure (anuria or oliguria, urinary casts, hypochloridemia, hyponatremia, hypocalcemia or hypercalcemia, metabolic acidosis, and occasional hyperkalemia), chronic renal failure (nonregenerative anemia, hyponatremia, hypochloridemia, hypophosphatemia, hypercalcemia, isosthenuria, proteinuria), urinary blockage (crystals, urine leukocytes, blood, and protein), and uroperitoneum (hyponatremia, hyperkalemia, hypochloridemia, and abdominal effusion)
- Abdominocentesis to rule out uroperitoneum (abdominal fluid creatinine is at least twice as high as serum creatinine)
- Urinary gamma-glutamyl transpeptidase (GGT) fractional excretion >25 to confirm renal failure of mostly tubular origin
- Transabdominal ultrasonography, rectal examination, and/or renal biopsy

CAUSES OF ABNORMALLY LOW LEVELS

Muscle wasting (neurologic, malnutrition, or other underlying disease)

NEXT DIAGNOSTIC STEP TO CONSIDER IF LEVELS LOW

- Complete blood count/serum chemistry profile and urinalysis to rule out malabsorption or chronic disease

- Neurologic examination
- Electromyography and/or muscle biopsy

DRUG EFFECTS ON LEVELS: None known

SPECIMEN AND PROCESSING CONSIDERATIONS

LAB ARTIFACTS THAT MAY INTERFERE WITH READINGS OF LEVELS OF THIS SUBSTANCE (AND HOW—ARTIFICIALLY ELEVATED VS. DEPRESSED) High concentrations of chromogens (acetoacetate, glucose, ascorbic acid, uric acid, pyruvate, cephalosporins, and amino acids) can artificially increase. Hyperbilirubinemia can cause artificial decreases. Hemolysis may increase or decrease values.

SAMPLE FOR COLLECTION (TYPE OF SPECIMEN, COLOR TUBE) AND ANY SPECIAL SPECIMEN HANDLING NOTES Serum, quickly separated from the clot and refrigerated. Stable.

PEARLS Creatinine is a more specific indicator of renal glomerular filtration rate than BUN, which is more easily affected by nonrenal factors. Mild increases in creatinine, along with hyperkalemia and increased creatine kinase, are sometimes seen with hyperkalemic periodic paralysis or heavily muscled horses.

AUTHOR: **PAULA M. KRIMER**

EDITOR: **CHARLES WIEDMEYER**

Culture and Sensitivity, Bacterial

BASIC INFORMATION

DEFINITION

Submission of infected tissue or sample (eg, nasal discharge, fecal) for isolation and identification of potential pathogens and *in vitro* identification of appropriate antimicrobial agents (antibiotics) to which the isolated organism(s) are susceptible.

TYPICAL NORMAL RANGE (US UNITS; SI UNITS)

- Relevant bacterial isolates are reported in number (heavy, moderate, light) and identified by genus and species such as *Rhodococcus equi.*
- Susceptibility to antimicrobial agents is determined by standardized methods of agar disc diffusion (Kirby-Bauer) or by the broth microdilution method also known as minimum inhibitory concentration (MIC). Results, interpreted according to the National

Committee for Clinical Laboratory Standards, are reported as sensitive, intermediate, or resistant.

PHYSIOLOGY

Small quantities of submitted samples, discharge or tissues, are aseptically plated on enrichment and selective media to enhance the growth of suspected pathogen(s). Individual colonies are identified by morphologic features (form, elevation, and margins) and biochemical characteristics (hemolytic, lactose fer-

menter) in the initial steps of identification. Isolated pathogens are grown to specific levels and exposed to antimicrobial agents for determination of susceptibility to antimicrobial agents.
CAUSES OF ABNORMALLY HIGH LEVELS Bacterial infection or bacterial contamination
NEXT DIAGNOSTIC STEP TO CONSIDER IF LEVELS HIGH Select an appropriate antimicrobial agent based on experience, sensitivity, appropriate method of delivery (topical, enteral, parenteral), and site of infection.
CAUSES OF ABNORMALLY LOW LEVELS Insignificant
IMPORTANT INTERSPECIES DIFFERENCES Some organisms are commensal and normal flora in some species but pathogens in others. Some antibiotics are appropriate for one species of patient but toxic in another.

DRUG EFFECTS ON LEVELS Previous or concurrent therapy with antimicrobial agents, even if not the chemotherapeutic agent of choice may inhibit growth of microbes including potential pathogens. In some cases, such as when a bacteriostatic agent is used, a clinical laboratory may still be able to recover clinically important isolates if informed of the use of antimicrobial agents.

SPECIMEN COLLECTION AND PROCESSING CONSIDERATIONS
LAB ARTIFACTS THAT MAY INTERFERE WITH READINGS OF LEVELS OF THIS SUBSTANCE (AND HOW—ARTIFICIALLY ELEVATED VS. DEPRESSED) Contamination can occur during collection or by use of nonsterile containers or prolonged storage at room temperature or delays in shipment. Such contamination with nonrelevant organ-

isms may inhibit the growth of more fastidious organisms leading to reduced chances of their isolation.
SAMPLE FOR COLLECTION (TYPE OF SPECIMEN, COLOR TUBE) AND ANY SPECIAL SPECIMEN HANDLING NOTES Fresh tissue or fluids should be aseptically collected in a sterile container. Culture swab is acceptable for both aerobic and anaerobic cultures. If a streptococcal infection is suspected, Dacron is the best swab to use, as cotton swabs are somewhat inhibitory to preservation of streptococcal isolates.
PEARLS Be aware of and monitor for potential toxic effects of the antimicrobial agent toxicity by appropriate clinical monitoring and laboratory tests.

AUTHOR: **THOMAS J. REILLY**

EDITOR: **CHARLES WIEDMEYER**

Dental Radiography

BASIC INFORMATION

DEFINITION
Radiographs are two-dimensional of regional anatomy. Dental radiographs are complicated by superimposition of the skull and paranasal sinuses.

TYPICAL NORMAL RADIOGRAPHIC FINDINGS
Although teeth have a complicated internal architecture, their relationship to the mandible, incisive bone, and maxilla have similar characteristics.
- Cementum: The external surface of each tooth that operates as a single functional unit with the periodontal ligament
  ○ Appears as clearly demarcated radiolucent line that abuts the thin shelf of very dense bone termed the dental lamina dura.
- Lamina dura appears as a thin, well-defined radio-opaque line.
  ○ In the mandible, incisive bone, and rostral maxilla, the lamina dura is more opaque than the surrounding trabecular bone often term the alveolar bone. The caudal maxillary cheek teeth have reserve crown and roots that reside within the rostral and caudal maxillary sinuses.

  ○ The radiolucent periodontal ligament and the radiopaque lamina dura are readily evident in the normal horse (Figure 1).
- Because dental disease frequently results in infectious or inflammatory lesions of the sinuses and surrounding bone, these characteristics are pivotal in the accurate identification of abnormal teeth (Figure 2).
- Changes with advancing age
  ○ Particularly evident when evaluating the pulp horns and tooth roots (Figures 3 and 4).
  ○ In very young horses, the germinal tissue of the teeth appear as wide radiolucent zones with some evidence of radio-opaque dental tissue within the respective bones.
  ○ Pulp horns
    - With aging, the pulp horns become more well-defined and smaller.
    - All of the cheek teeth have more than one pulp horn; the pulp horns should appear as radiolucent, smoothly margined structures.
    - Comparison of one arcade to the contralateral arcade can be performed to identify changes in pulp horn and tooth root size and shape.

  - Abnormalities of pulp are particularly difficult to identify.
  - The pulp horns should be evaluated for size, shape, margination, and symmetry when compared to the ipsilateral and contralateral arcades.
  ○ Paranasal sinuses
    - Normally air filled
    - Appear to increase in internal volume as the horse ages due to the continual eruption of the cheek teeth.
    - When sinusitis develops as a result of maxillary cheek tooth abnormalities, it can appear as fluid lines or in more chronic cases, soft tissue accumulation.
    - The thin shelf of bone termed interdental bone is present between the reserve crown portions of adjacent teeth. This bone should be wedge-shaped tapering toward the occlusal surface of the teeth.
    - When chronic periodontal disease exists, particularly in the older horse, the interdental bone can become blunted as a result of osseous resorption.

AUTHOR: **SARAH M. PUCHALSKI**

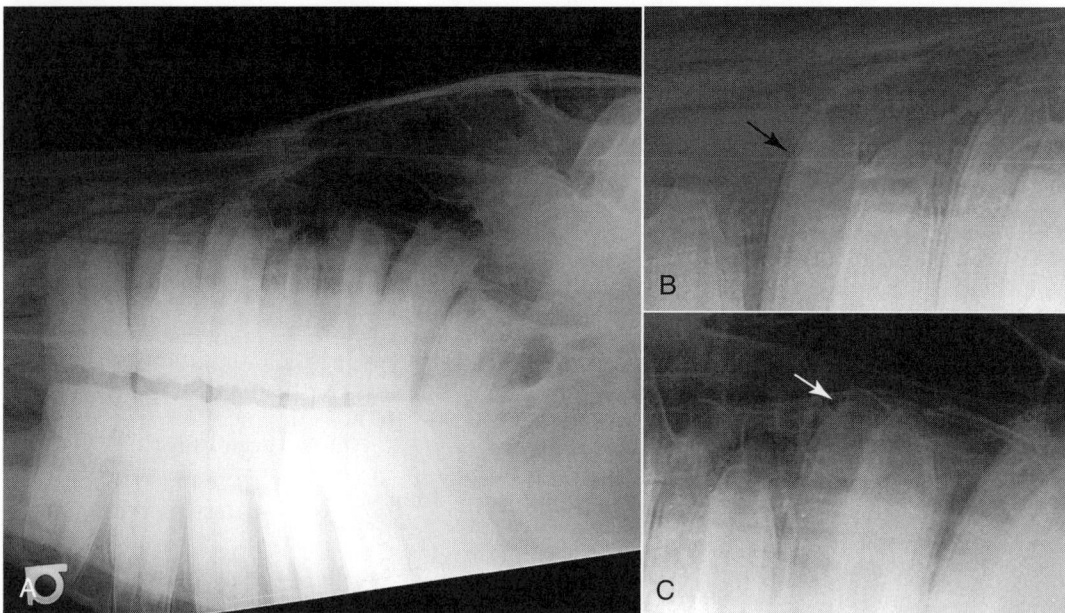

FIGURE 1 **A,** Normal maxillary oblique projection. **B,** The rostral maxillary cheek teeth are similar to mandibular cheek teeth where the thin radiolucent periodontal (*black arrow*) ligament is well defined and surrounded by the opaque lamina dura, which is surrounded by trabecular bone termed alveolar bone. **C,** The caudal maxillary cheek teeth have a visible thin radiolucent periodontal ligament (*white arrow*) surrounded by the lamina dura that is then surrounded by air of the maxillary sinuses.

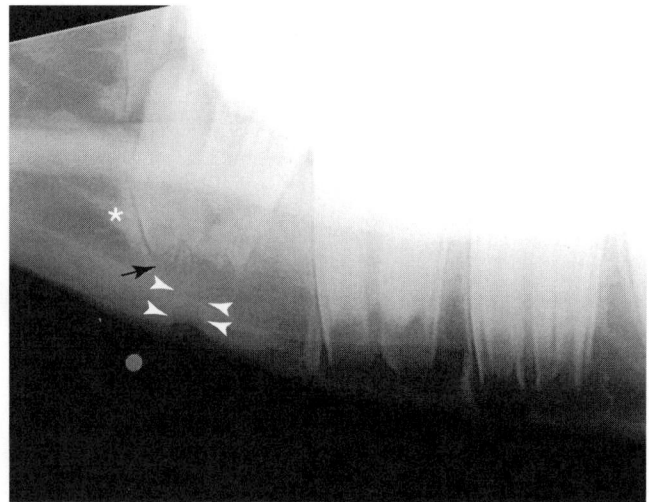

FIGURE 2 Infected mandibular #06. The exit point of the draining tract is marked with a radio-opaque BB. The draining tract extends from the periapical region of the tooth through the ventral cortex of the mandible (*white arrowheads*). There is loss of the lamina dura (black arrow) and surrounding alveolar bone sclerosis (*). These findings are consistent with apical infection and surrounding osteomyelitis.

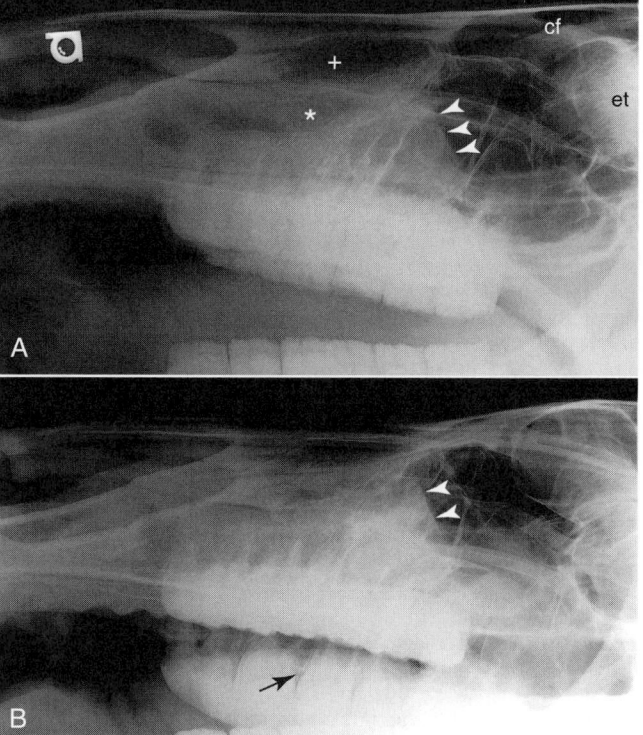

FIGURE 3 **A,** Open mouth lateral projection of an adult horse. There is fluid within the rostral maxillary sinus (*white arrowheads*). Consistent with this horse's age, the sinuses appear more spacious as the reserve crown erupts. +, dorsal conchal sinus; *, ventral conchal sinus; *cf*, conchofrontal or frontal sinus; *et*, ethmoturbinates. **B,** Open mouth oblique projection of the same horse. Note that the fluid of the rostral maxillary sinus obscures the apical region of the caudal maxillary cheek teeth complicating evaluation of the periodontal ligament and lamina dura. Open mouth projection allow for evaluation of the occlusal surfaces of the cheek teeth and interdental bone. There is blunting of the interdental bone of the opposite maxillary arcade (*black arrow*).

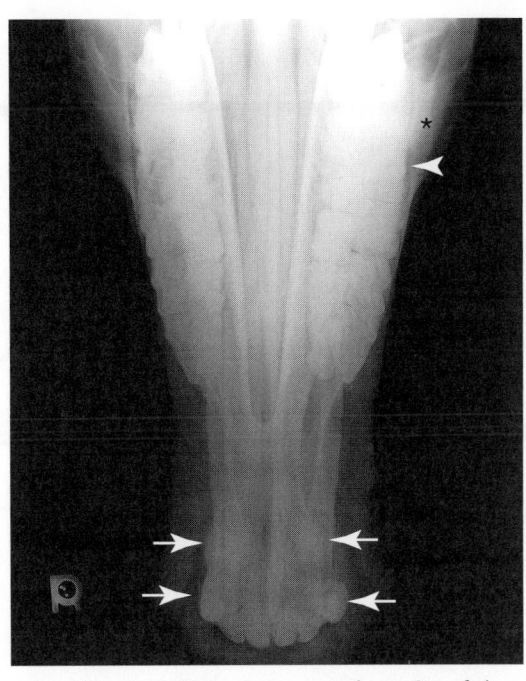

FIGURE 4 DV projection of the horse shown in Figure 3. There is increased opacity of the rostral maxillary sinus (*) with widening of the periodontal space surrounding the 209 (*white arrowhead*). There is an additional finding of cemental hyperplasia surrounding several canine and incisor teeth (*white arrows*).

Dermatophyte Culture

BASIC INFORMATION

DEFINITION

Examination of tissue or exudates for presence of fungal organisms

TYPICAL NORMAL RANGE (US UNITS; SI UNITS)

Reported as negative or as heavy, moderate, or light growth of organism along with identification. Culture period may take 1 to 2 weeks prior to report and up to 6 weeks for growth negative cultures.

PHYSIOLOGY

Laboratory conditions are set to enhance the growth of potential fungal pathogens allowing for their isolation and identification based on their growth characteristics, microscopic structure, and biochemical tests.

CAUSES OF ABNORMALLY HIGH LEVELS Fungal infections. Common equine fungal infections include dermatophytosis (*T. equinum, M. gypseum, and M. equinum*); aspergillosis (commonly associated with *Pseudomonas aeruginosa* infections of the cornea). Saprophytes may cause skin lesions and lead to systemic disease in immune-compromised hosts.

NEXT DIAGNOSTIC STEP TO CONSIDER IF LEVELS HIGH Culture is definitive, though depending on organism isolated, may take weeks.

DRUG EFFECTS ON LEVELS Corticosteroid therapy decreases patient's resistance to original pathogen and secondary bacterial or vial invaders.

SPECIMEN AND PROCESSING CONSIDERATIONS

LAB ARTIFACTS THAT MAY INTERFERE WITH READINGS OF LEVELS OF THIS SUBSTANCE (AND HOW—ARTIFICIALLY ELEVATED VS. DEPRESSED) False-negative results: Poor quality sample, improper media, or improper growth conditions may lead to false-negative results. Contamination may lead to false-positive results.

SAMPLE FOR COLLECTION (TYPE OF SPECIMEN, COLOR TUBE) AND ANY SPECIAL SPECIMEN HANDLING NOTES Dermatophytes: Hair plucked from affected areas should be submitted in dermatophyte test media or sterile dry containers. Tissues or exudates should be submitted in sterile dry container.

PEARLS Do not submit specimens for culture if strong suspicion for cryptococcosis, blastomycosis, histoplasmosis, or coccidioidomycosis as these agents are zoonotic and extremely hazardous to laboratory personnel. Serologic tests along with cytologic or histologic lesions are most appropriate for diagnosis.

AUTHOR: **THOMAS J. REILLY**

EDITOR: **CHARLES WIEDMEYER**

Eccentrocytes

BASIC INFORMATION

DEFINITION

Eccentrocytes are erythrocytes in which the hemoglobin is eccentrically located. On blood smears, the hemoglobin is seen to be concentrated on one side of the cell, leaving a clear area just inside the cell margin on the other side.

SYNONYM(S)

Hemi-ghosts, hemi-ghost erythrocytes

TYPICAL NORMAL RANGE (US UNITS; SI UNITS)

Rare to absent

PHYSIOLOGY

Eccentrocyte formation is the result of oxidative damage to erythrocyte membranes, leading to cross-linkage of membrane proteins. They may be seen in conjunction with Heinz bodies, which occur due to oxidative damage to hemoglobin. Eccentrocyte formation is usually associated with a toxic exposure, but rare cases may occur due to hereditary defects in the molecular milieu that acts to protect erythrocytes from oxidative damage (see later).

CAUSES OF ABNORMALLY HIGH LEVELS Eccentrocyte formation in horses may occur in association with red maple leaf toxicosis, wild onion toxicosis, or phenothiazine administration. Copper and zinc toxicosis could potentially cause eccentrocyte formation. In rare cases, hereditary defects in the mechanisms that act to protect erythrocytes from oxidative damage may result in eccentrocyte formation. Included here would be deficiencies of glucose-6-phosphate dehydrogenase, flavanone-adenine dinucleotide (FAD), glutathione, or glutathione reductase.

AUTHOR: **MARLYN S. WHITNEY**

EDITOR: **CHARLES WIEDMEYER**

Ehrlichiosis, Equine Granulocytic

BASIC INFORMATION

DEFINITION

- *Anaplasma phagocytophila* (formerly *Ehrlichia equi*)
- The etiologic agent of equine granulocytic ehrlichiosis (EGE); an infectious, noncontagious, seasonal disease, occurring primarily in the late fall, winter, and spring
- Found in membrane-lined vacuoles within the cytoplasm of equine granulocytes, particularly neutrophils and eosinophils.
- Morulae, the name for these inclusion bodies, composed of one or more coccoid or coccobacillary organisms and large granular aggregates. Morulae are typically visible under high magnification with light microscopy but may only be visible for a short period of time.
- Horses are usually aberrant hosts (infected after a tick bite) and unlikely to serve as reservoirs of disease as the presence of the organism in circulation appears to be limited only to the acute phase of the disease. Additionally, horses do not appear to serve as a zoonotic vector of disease for humans, which can become afflicted with human granulocytic ehrlichiosis (HGE).

SYNONYM(S)

Equine granulocytic ehrlichiosis (EGE)

TYPICAL NORMAL RANGE (US UNITS; SI UNITS)

There is no published normal range; a fourfold increase in acute versus convalescent titers is required for diagnosis.

PHYSIOLOGY

A. phagocytophila enters the dermis of affected hosts after tick bite inoculation and spreads via the lymphatics and blood to infect granulocytes. The organism then replicates within vacuoles in the target cell and is believed to initiate a cascade of localized pathologic inflammatory events after being sequestered in the spleen, liver, and lung within the granulocytes.

CAUSES OF ABNORMALLY HIGH LEVELS Elevations in serum antibody titer are typically due to either active infection or exposure to the etiologic agent of disease.

NEXT DIAGNOSTIC STEP TO CONSIDER IF LEVELS HIGH If the clinical signs are detected acutely, collection of a blood sample in an EDTA (purple top) tube for a buffy coat preparation may provide a quicker diagnosis via visualization of the characteristic morulae in the cytoplasm of equine granulocytes.

CAUSES OF ABNORMALLY LOW LEVELS Low antibody concentrations suggest lack of exposure to the causative agent of disease.

NEXT DIAGNOSTIC STEP TO CONSIDER IF LEVELS LOW Low levels suggest lack of exposure to the causative agent of disease and the need to consider other etiologic agents or pathologic processes as the source of the observed clinical disease.

SPECIMEN AND PROCESSING CONSIDERATIONS

SAMPLE FOR COLLECTION (TYPE OF SPECIMEN, COLOR TUBE) AND ANY SPECIAL SPECIMEN HANDLING NOTES Blood collected in an EDTA (purple top) tube for buffy coat preparation or serum in a red top tube

PEARLS The indirect fluorescent assay (IFA) antibody test is the most commonly used serologic assay. An enzyme-linked immunosorbent assay (ELISA) and Western immunoblot are also available. In either case, documentation of an increasing antibody titer is required to confirm active infection. A polymerase chain reaction (PCR) assay has recently become available which tests for organismal antigen in the blood sample. PCR has the advantage of being used as a single test.

AUTHORS: **SHANE F. DeWITT** and **TANYA M. GRONDIN**

EDITOR: **CHARLES WIEDMEYER**

Eosinophils (Eosinophilia, Eosinopenia)

BASIC INFORMATION

DEFINITION

Eosinophils are granulocytic cells that originate from the bone marrow and are associated with allergic or hypersensitivity responses or parasite infestation. Eosinophils have a segmented nucleus and contain many large eosinophilic granules.

SYNONYM(S)

Eos

TYPICAL NORMAL RANGE (US UNITS; SI UNITS)

0.1 to $0.8 \times 10^3/\mu L$

PHYSIOLOGY

Eosinophils have several functions. Eosinophils use a combination of antibody opsonization (IgE and IgG), perforin from T cells, complement, and hydrolytic enzymes from eosinophil granules to attack and kill helminthic parasites. Additionally, eosinophils are effector cells for asthma and other allergic diseases by elaborating proinflammatory mediators including platelet activating factor, leukotriene C4, and eicosanoids. Eosinophils can also modulate the inflammatory response by controlling the activities of mast cells and basophils.

CAUSES OF ABNORMALLY HIGH LEVELS

Elevations in eosinophil numbers or eosinophilia usually indicate parasitic hypersensitivity or paraneoplastic responses. Causes include enteric or lung parasites, allergic skin disease, lymphoma, or mast cell neoplasia.

NEXT DIAGNOSTIC STEP TO CONSIDER IF LEVELS HIGH

Fecal floatation is recommended to rule out parasitic infestation.

CAUSES OF ABNORMALLY LOW LEVELS

Decreased numbers of eosinophils, below the reference range or eosinopenia may occur as part of a stress response but is a fairly nonspecific response.

NEXT DIAGNOSTIC STEP TO CONSIDER IF LEVELS LOW

Evaluate the patient for systemic or chronic disease.

DRUG EFFECTS ON LEVELS

Glucocorticoids and other immunosuppressive drugs may cause an eosinopenia.

SPECIMEN AND PROCESSING CONSIDERATIONS

SAMPLE FOR COLLECTION (TYPE OF SPECIMEN, COLOR TUBE) AND ANY SPECIAL SPECIMEN HANDLING NOTES

Whole, anticoagulated blood is necessary for evaluation. Most commonly, ethylenediamine tetraacetic acid or purple top tubes are used for complete blood count (CBC); however, sodium citrate (blue top tube) can also be used. If the blood cannot be evaluated immediately, preparation of a blood smear, to preserve the integrity of red and white blood cell morphology is recommended.

AUTHOR: **ANNE BARGER**

EDITOR: **CHARLES WIEDMEYER**

Equine Infectious Anemia (EIA)

BASIC INFORMATION

DEFINITION

EIA is a bloodborne, viral infection of horses first described in 1843 in France. EIA virus (EIAV) is a lentivirus of the family Retroviridae, which is transmitted between horses via biting flies, most commonly of the Tabanus family (horseflies and deerflies). It is an enveloped, RNA virus. The insects serve only as a means of mechanical transfer and are not an indirect host in the life cycle of the virus, as the virus is not capable of reproducing in insect cells. Subsequently, there is a finite period of time that the virus will remain viable on the insect, allowing it to be transmitted to another horse. Being a lentivirus, once the horse is infected, it is persistently infected for life.

SYNONYM(S)

Swamp fever

TYPICAL NORMAL RANGE (US UNITS; SI UNITS)

Negative. Any positive result is indication of exposure and subsequent infection with the virus.

PHYSIOLOGY

- EIAV can survive in the host as either free viral particles or cell-associated. Upon encountering a susceptible host cell, EIAV binds to a glycoprotein receptor, termed equine lentivirus receptor 1, the viral envelope fuses with the cell membrane, and the virion is internalized. A viral reverse transcriptase enzyme results in production of viral DNA from the RNA genome, which is then inserted into the host cell genome, after translocating to the nucleus.
- The severity of clinical disease is most commonly correlated with circulating viral load. EIAV infects macrophages and endothelial cells most commonly. Subsequently, multiple tissues and organ systems are affected. Increased circulating concentrations of proinflammatory cytokines cause much of the observed clinical signs in acute cases. Most horses, however, are asymptomatic, silent carriers of the virus.

CAUSES OF ABNORMALLY HIGH LEVELS

Elevations in serum antibody titer are typically due to either active infection or exposure to the etiologic agent of disease.

NEXT DIAGNOSTIC STEP TO CONSIDER IF LEVELS HIGH

If the titer is positive, the state veterinarian needs to be contacted immediately. The next diagnostic step will be for the regulatory officials to repeat the EIA serologic testing using the agar gel immunodiffusion (AGID) test to confirm the result.

CAUSES OF ABNORMALLY LOW LEVELS

Low antibody concentrations suggest lack of exposure to the causative agent of disease.

NEXT DIAGNOSTIC STEP TO CONSIDER IF LEVELS LOW

Low levels suggest lack of exposure to the causative agent of disease and the need to consider other etiologic agents or pathologic processes as the source of the observed clinical disease.

SPECIMEN AND PROCESSING CONSIDERATIONS

SAMPLE FOR COLLECTION (TYPE OF SPECIMEN, COLOR TUBE) AND ANY SPECIAL SPECIMEN HANDLING NOTES Blood collected in a red top tube for recovery of serum.

PEARLS

- Currently four serologic tests are approved by the USDA.
  - AGID test
  - Competitive enzyme linked immunosorbent assay (cELISA)
  - Synthetic antigen ELISA (SA-ELISA)
  - Vira-CHEK ELISA

- The AGID test or Coggins test (named after Dr. Leroy Coggins who developed the test in the 1970s) is still considered the gold standard for diagnosis of EIA. The AGID tests for antibody against the EIAV gap p26 protein. The major downfall to the AGID test is that it requires 24 hours to perform the test.
- Both the cELISA and Vira-CHEK ELISA also test for the p26 protein, are more sensitive than the AGID, and only require minutes to perform the test, but are significantly less specific than the Coggins test. Subsequently, any

positive ELISA test needs to be confirmed by an AGID.
- The SA-ELISA tests for the p26 protein and an EIAV envelope gp45 protein. A positive result must also be confirmed with an AGID test.
- A Western blot (WB) test is also available as a means of detecting antibodies to EIAV, but is only used to diagnose cases where previous results have been contradictory. It is not considered an approved test by the USDA.

AUTHORS: SHANE F. DeWITT and **TANYA M. GRONDIN**

EDITOR: CHARLES WIEDMEYER

Erythrocytosis

BASIC INFORMATION

DEFINITION

An increase in the concentration of erythrocytes in the peripheral blood, characterized by increases in the hematocrit, red blood cell count (RBC) count, and hemoglobin level.

SYNONYM(S)

Polycythemia is the term formerly used for this condition, but erythrophagocytosis is now the preferred term.

TYPICAL NORMAL RANGE (US UNITS; SI UNITS)

- Hematocrit: 27% to 43% (0.27–0.43 L/L)
- Hemoglobin: 10.1 to 16.1 g/dL (101–161 g/L)
- Red blood cell count: 6.0 to 10.4 × 10^6/μL (6.0–10.4 × 10^{12}/L)

PHYSIOLOGY

Relative erythrocytosis does not involve an actual increase in the red cell mass in the body; it occurs due to hemoconcentration (as from dehydration or endotoxemia) or splenic contraction (ejection into the peripheral blood of erythrocytes stored in the spleen). Absolute (true) erythrocytosis is an actual increase in the total red cell mass of the body (see causes later).

CAUSES OF ABNORMALLY HIGH LEVELS Relative erythrocytosis occurs due to dehydration or endotoxemia (hemoconcentration) or excitement/exercise (splenic contraction). The vast majority of horses with erythrocytosis have the relative variety. Absolute (true) erythrocytosis can be a primary or secondary disorder. Secondary erythrocyto-

sis may be considered appropriate or inappropriate. Appropriate secondary erythrocytosis occurs in response to increased erythropoietin (EPO) levels resulting from sustained hypoxia. Causes of sustained hypoxia include cardiac disease such as congenital right to left cardiac shunts, severe pulmonary disease leading to poor oxygenation of the blood, and hyperthyroidism leading to a higher metabolic rate and thus an increased tissue demand for oxygen. Movement to a higher altitude or prolonged exercise training may cause erythrocytosis, but apparently not consistently. Secondary inappropriate erythrocytosis occurs in response to increased EPO production, which is occurring for some reason other than hypoxia. Possible causes include an EPO-producing renal cyst or neoplasm or an extrarenal neoplasm that is producing EPO or an EPO-like substance. Primary erythrocytosis is rare and is due to increased RBC production that is not occurring in response to EPO. A potential cause, probably very rare in horses, is a neoplastic disorder known as polycythemia vera, which involves neoplastic production of erythroid, myeloid, and megakaryocytic cells.

NEXT DIAGNOSTIC STEP TO CONSIDER IF LEVELS HIGH Breed and altitude should be taken into consideration in deciding if a horse has an elevation in its hematocrit, hemoglobin level, and RBC count. If the animal is excited, has been exercising, or has clinical evidence of dehydration and/or endotoxemia, the erythrocytosis is most likely relative. Erythrocytosis due to splenic contraction is transient (persists for less than an hour to several hours); that due to dehydration

resolves with rehydration. If relative erythrocytosis is ruled out, the patient should be evaluated for evidence of cardiac or pulmonary disease. Hyperthyroidism (due to oversupplementation of hypothyroid horses or rare naturally occurring cases due to functional thyroid adenocarcinoma) should be ruled out. Arterial blood gas analysis should reveal a decreased oxygen level in horses with appropriate secondary absolute erythrocytosis. Arterial blood oxygen levels are usually normal in animals with inappropriate secondary absolute erythrocytosis. Determination of EPO levels would be helpful for identifying horses with secondary absolute erythrocytosis, but equine EPO determination is not done in most veterinary diagnostic laboratories. A complete blood cell count (including blood smear evaluation) and a bone marrow examination should be helpful in identifying hematopoietic neoplasia.

IMPORTANT INTERSPECIES DIFFERENCES Horses are more likely than most other domestic species to experience erythrocytosis due to exercise or excitement, and light horse breeds are far more likely to be affected than draft breeds.

SPECIMEN AND PROCESSING CONSIDERATIONS

SAMPLE FOR COLLECTION (TYPE OF SPECIMEN, COLOR TUBE) AND ANY SPECIAL SPECIMEN HANDLING NOTES EDTA anticoagulated blood (purple-top tube) is used to determine the hematocrit, the hemoglobin level, and the RBC count.

AUTHOR: MARLYN S. WHITNEY

EDITOR: CHARLES WIEDMEYER

Estrogen

BASIC INFORMATION

DEFINITION
- Hyperestrogenemia: Increased circulating concentration of estrogen
- Hypoestrogenemia: Decreased circulating concentration of estrogen

SYNONYM(S)
Estradiol is the most commonly measured estrogen, except in pregnancy when estrone sulfate is evaluated.

TYPICAL NORMAL RANGE (US UNITS; SI UNITS)
- Geldings: <50 pg/mL
- Stallions: >400 pg/mL
- Nonpregnant mare: 0.1 to 3.6 ng/mL
- Pregnant mares (>100 days of gestation): >30 ng/mL

PHYSIOLOGY
- Estrogens are a group of steroid hormones and function as the primary female sex hormone. The three primary naturally occurring estrogens are estradiol (most potent naturally occurring estrogen), estriol, and estrone. They derived their name from their role in the estrus cycle.
- Estrogens are produced primarily by developing follicles in the ovaries, the corpus luteum (CL), and the placenta. Synthesis of estrogens starts in theca interna cells in the ovary, by the synthesis of androstenedione from cholesterol. Androstenedione then crosses the basal membrane into the surrounding granulosa cells, where it is converted to estrone or estradiol, either immediately or through testosterone, under the action of aromatase. Being lipophilic, estrogens enter all cells freely and interact with a cytoplasmic target cell receptor. The steroid receptor complex can then enter the nucleus and regulate gene transcription.
- Estrogens have numerous roles, but in most females, the primary role is involved with the reproductive cycle. Estrogen production from the developing follicle leads to the luteinizing hormone (LH) surge that results in ovulation. During diestrus, estrogen production from the CL (along with progesterone) prepare the endometrium for the possibility of an implanted embryo. During pregnancy, the majority of the estrogens are produced by the fetoplacental unit. Subsequently estrogen concentration can be used to indirectly assess the health of the pregnancy. Estrogens also play a vital role in parturition (increasing oxytocin receptors, promoting synthesis of prostaglandins).

CAUSES OF ABNORMALLY HIGH LEVELS
The sex of the individual being tested is important. Elevated concentrations in a supposedly castrated male horse would indicate the presence of functional testicular tissue. Elevated concentrations in a mare would suggest estrus or pregnancy depending on the concentration as outlined above. Otherwise, a functional neoplasia secreting estrogens would also need to be considered.

NEXT DIAGNOSTIC STEP TO CONSIDER IF LEVELS HIGH
In male horses, a human chorionic gonadotropin stimulation test should be performed if the male is supposedly castrated. In females, diagnostic rectal ultrasonography to evaluate the reproductive tract would be most useful in determining the stage of the reproductive cycle or the pregnancy status of the patient.

CAUSES OF ABNORMALLY LOW LEVELS
In male horses, low concentrations of estrogens would indicate the lack of testicular tissue. In females, particularly during pregnancy, decreased concentrations would indicate compromise of the fetoplacental unit and decreased estrogen production.

NEXT DIAGNOSTIC STEP TO CONSIDER IF LEVELS LOW
In pregnant females, diagnostic rectal or abdominal ultrasonography to evaluate the health of the pregnancy would be indicated.

SPECIMEN AND PROCESSING CONSIDERATIONS

SAMPLE FOR COLLECTION (TYPE OF SPECIMEN, COLOR TUBE) AND ANY SPECIAL SPECIMEN HANDLING NOTES
Collection of whole blood in a red top tube and separation of serum is ideal, although plasma can be used. Sample can then be refrigerated or frozen and shipped to a diagnostic laboratory with a cold pack.

PEARLS
- The embryo begins producing estrogens as early as day 12 and surpass prepregnancy estrogen concentrations between days 60 to 100 of gestation. Peak serum concentrations occur between day 180 to 240 of pregnancy, and then slowly decline to the end of pregnancy. Consequently, serum estrogen concentrations can be useful in determining pregnancy status from day 60 through term. As estrogen concentrations are increasing during early gestation (prior to day 60), false negatives may occur if sampled too early.
- Due to the fact that the testes of sexually mature stallions produce large amounts of estrogen, serum estrogen concentrations can also be used to detect the presence of testicular tissue.

AUTHORS: **SHANE F. DeWITT** and **TANYA M. GRONDIN**

EDITOR: **CHARLES WIEDMEYER**

Fecal Culture

BASIC INFORMATION

DEFINITION
Examination of fecal material for the presence of enteric bacterial pathogens

TYPICAL NORMAL RANGE (US UNITS; SI UNITS)
The results are reported as "no significant growth" or as heavy, moderate, or light growth of identified bacterial isolates. A common enteric bacterial pathogen, *Salmonella,* is often recovered only after primary and/or secondary enrichment and reported as such.

PHYSIOLOGY
There are multiple etiologies of diarrhea including systemic reasons, toxins, and infectious agents including viral and bacterial agents. Fecal samples submitted to a clinical laboratory are put under conditions to enhance the growth of potential bacterial pathogens allowing for their

isolation and identification based on their growth characteristics, morphologic, biochemical, and immunochemical properties.

CAUSES OF ABNORMALLY HIGH LEVELS Enteric infection: Common enteric pathogens include specific *Escherichia coli* strains, *Shigella* spp, *Yersinia* spp, *Campylobacter, Salmonella* spp, and less often obligate anaerobes including *Clostridium* spp.

NEXT DIAGNOSTIC STEP TO CONSIDER IF LEVELS HIGH Request antimicrobial agent susceptibility testing.

DRUG EFFECTS ON LEVELS Utilization of antimicrobial agents prior to acquisition of sample may inhibit growth of sensitive enteric pathogens.

SPECIMEN AND PROCESSING CONSIDERATIONS

LAB ARTIFACTS THAT MAY INTERFERE WITH READINGS OF LEVELS OF THIS SUBSTANCE (AND HOW—ARTIFICIALLY ELEVATED VS. DEPRESSED) False-negative results may occur if delay in setting up cultures, especially important to fastidious and strictly anaerobic organisms.

SAMPLE FOR COLLECTION (TYPE OF SPECIMEN, COLOR TUBE) AND ANY SPECIL SPECIMEN HANDLING NOTES Collect fresh fecal material into sterile container. If *Shigella, Campylobacter,* or *Clostridium* are suspected, special transport media may be required depending on the transport and process time for the

clinical laboratory. Contact laboratory for appropriate transport media. Although initial and primary enrichment may fail to produce growth of *Salmonella,* 7 days are required for final assessment of secondary enrichment.

PEARLS

- Most enteric pathogens are zoonotic and can cause disease in humans; specimen handling precautions are necessary to reduce the risk.
- Identification of certain fecal bacteria does not always indicate cause and effect relationship, presence of *E. coli* in fecal material is expected.

AUTHOR: **THOMAS J. REILLY**

EDITOR: **CHARLES WIEDMEYER**

Fecal Flotation

BASIC INFORMATION

DEFINITION

A test to detect parasite eggs, oocysts, or cysts in feces

TYPICAL NORMAL RANGE (US UNITS; SI UNITS)

Results are reported as positive or negative usually with a genus, species, or type (eg, strongyle) identification.

PHYSIOLOGY

Parasite eggs and cysts are concentrated in feces using a flotation solution that separates eggs/cysts from debris using the principle of buoyancy. After feces are mixed in a test tube with a flotation solution, a centrifugation step is used and the less dense parasite eggs/cysts will float at the top of the meniscus. These parasite stages are removed and examined microscopically. Because many parasite eggs and cysts will float efficiently in a solution that has a specific gravity (sg) of 1.2 to 1.3, flotation solutions, such as saturated sucrose (sg = 1.27), magnesium sulfate (sg = 1.2), or zinc sulfate (sg = 1.18), often are used.

CAUSES OF ABNORMALLY HIGH LEVELS Eggs and cysts from nematodes and protozoans inhabiting the gastrointestinal tract often will be observed.

NEXT DIAGNOSTIC STEP TO CONSIDER IF LEVELS HIGH A positive result is definitive for infection.

CAUSES OF ABNORMALLY LOW LEVELS A negative test may result from sexually immature parasites or the intermittent shedding of eggs/cysts.

NEXT DIAGNOSTIC STEP TO CONSIDER IF LEVELS LOW Perform a series of flotations on new samples if no eggs/cysts are observed and parasite-associated disease is suspected.

DRUG EFFECTS ON LEVELS Drugs may reduce or eliminate parasite infection, resulting in fewer or no eggs/cysts shed.

SPECIMEN AND PROCESSING CONSIDERATIONS

LAB ARTIFACTS THAT MAY INTERFERE WITH READINGS OF LEVELS OF THIS SUBSTANCE (AND HOW—ARTIFICIALLY ELEVATED VS. DEPRESSED) Use of certain kinds of flotation solutions may shrink/distort some cysts.

SAMPLE FOR COLLECTION (TYPE OF SPECIMEN, COLOR TUBE) AND ANY SPECIAL SPECIMEN HANDLING NOTES A fresh fecal sample should be collected into a clean, dry container. If the test can not be performed within a few hours, refrigerate the fecal specimen. For longer term storage, samples can be mixed with an equal volume of 10% buffered formalin prior to the flotation. Do not freeze the sample as it can distort or destroy parasite eggs/cysts.

PEARLS

- The centrifugation step considerably increases the sensitivity of the test.
- Check the specific gravity of the flotation solution using a hydrometer available from a scientific supply company.
- Avoid collecting samples from the ground as soil nematodes may contaminate the sample.
- Tapeworm eggs are often difficult to observe using the common flotation solutions.
- Occasionally, larvae may be observed in a flotation.

AUTHOR: **BRENDA T. BEERNTSEN**

EDITOR: **CHARLES WIEDMEYER**

Fibrinogen

BASIC INFORMATION

DEFINITION
Fibrinogen is a soluble plasma protein produced by hepatocytes.

TYPICAL NORMAL RANGE (US UNITS; SI UNITS)
Adults: 0.1 to 0.4 g/dL (1.0–4.0 g/L); varies slightly between reference laboratories. Values in healthy newborns (<24 hours) may be lower than adult reference intervals.

PHYSIOLOGY
Fibrinogen is important in coagulation, and it is a positive acute phase protein that increases with inflammation. Fibrinogen provides a substrate for fibrin formation and a matrix for migration of inflammatory-related cells.

CAUSES OF ABNORMALLY HIGH LEVELS
- Dehydration
- Inflammation: Increased fibrinogen production by the liver

NEXT DIAGNOSTIC STEP TO CONSIDER IF LEVELS HIGH Look for source of inflammation or dehydration: Perform minimum database (complete blood count, biochemistry panel, and urinalysis).

CAUSES OF ABNORMALLY LOW LEVELS
- Decreased synthesis by the liver
- Increased consumption by intravascular coagulation or increased fibrinogenolysis

NEXT DIAGNOSTIC STEP TO CONSIDER IF LEVELS LOW Assess for coagulation abnormalities or liver disease.

SPECIMEN AND PROCESSING CONSIDERATIONS
SAMPLE FOR COLLECTION (TYPE OF SPECIMEN, COLOR TUBE) AND ANY SPECIAL SPECIMEN HANDLING NOTES
- Heat-precipitation (estimate only): The difference in the total protein values (by refractometer) before and after removal of fibrinogen by heat precipitation and centrifugation in hematocrit tubes. This method is not sensitive enough to detect decreases in fibrinogen. Requires EDTA anticoagulated blood (purple-top tube).
- Thrombin clotting time (for more accurate quantification or to detect decreased fibrinogen). Requires citrate tube (blue top) centrifuged and plasma removed within 1 hour of collection.

PEARLS
- Total protein:fibrinogen ratio: Helps to differentiate hyperfibrinogenemia due to inflammation and dehydration.

$$plasma\ total\ protein\ (g/dL) \div fibrinogen\ (g/dL)$$

- Ratio >15: Normal animal or consistent with dehydration.
- Ratio <10: Inflammation is likely due to selective increase in fibrinogen.
- Ratio = 10 to 15: Dehydration or inflammation cannot be entirely ruled out.

AUTHOR: **BRIDGET C. GARNER**

EDITOR: **CHARLES WIEDMEYER**

Fibrinogen (Fibrin) Degradation Products/D-dimer

BASIC INFORMATION

DEFINITION
Fibrinogen (or fibrin) degradation products (FDPs) are fragments released following plasmin-mediated degradation of fibrinogen or fibrin. The D-dimer is a specific fragment formed only upon degradation of cross-linked fibrin.

SYNONYM(S)
Fibrin split products

TYPICAL NORMAL RANGE (US UNITS; SI UNITS)
- FDPs <10 µg/mL (serum) or <5 µg/mL (plasma)
- D-dimer usually <1000 ng/mL (plasma)

PHYSIOLOGY
Activation of the coagulation cascade results in thrombin generation, which in turn cleaves fibrinogen to form fibrin monomers. Cross-linked fibrin is the endpoint of the coagulation cascade. Plasmin (as part of the fibrinolytic pathway) degrades fibrin (and fibrinogen), resulting in FDPs. One of the specific FDPs is fragment D. Dimers of this fragment (D-dimer) are detected only upon degradation of cross-linked fibrin (indicating active coagulation and fibrinolysis).

CAUSES OF ABNORMALLY HIGH LEVELS
- Inflammatory and ischemic forms of colic
- Postcolic surgery
- Sepsis in foals
- Thrombosis
- Disseminated intravascular coagulation (DIC)
- Fibrinolysis during endurance racing, acute laminitis and colic
- FDPs also elevated with decreased hepatic clearance (severe liver disease)

NEXT DIAGNOSTIC STEP TO CONSIDER IF LEVELS HIGH
- Coagulation profile (prothrombin time [PT], activated partial thromboplastin time [aPTT], fibrinogen concentration, platelet count)
- Antithrombin III activity
- Thromboelastography (TEG)
- Evaluate for colic, laminitis, sepsis, or other conditions causing a hypercoagulable state

SPECIMEN AND PROCESSING CONSIDERATIONS
SAMPLE FOR COLLECTION (TYPE OF SPECIMEN, COLOR TUBE) AND ANY SPECIAL SPECIMEN HANDLING NOTES
- Plasma D-dimer and FDP assays: Blood collection in either EDTA (purple-top tube) or citrate (3.2%–3.8% sodium citrate at a ratio of nine parts blood to one part anticoagulant)
- Serum FDP assays: Blood collection in special tubes containing a fibrinolytic inhibitor (usually soybean trypsin inhibitor or aprotinin) and a procoagulant (thrombin or reptilase [*Bothrops atrox* venom])

PEARLS D-dimer is presumed to be a better indicator of fibrinolysis than FDPs. Serum FDP assay has low specificity and sensitivity in the diagnosis of DIC (many healthy horses have elevated serum FDPs), and some plasma FDP assays are unreliable in detecting equine FDPs.

AUTHOR: **JANELLE S. RENSCHLER**

EDITOR: **CHARLES WIEDMEYER**

Gamma Glutamyl Transferase/Transpeptidase (GGT)

BASIC INFORMATION

DEFINITION

Induced enzyme: Membrane-bound enzymes (not cytoplasmic) with increased activity attributed to cholestasis, drug, or hormonal effects

TYPICAL NORMAL RANGE (US UNITS; SI UNITS)

3 to 23 IU/L

PHYSIOLOGY

GGT is an inducible, membrane-bound enzyme found primarily in the biliary canalicular cells. GGT activity can also be found in renal tubular cells and pancreatic cells, and high concentrations can be found in the mammary epithelium in some species but not horses. It is involved in glutathione metabolism, amino acid absorption, and antioxidation.

CAUSES OF ABNORMALLY HIGH LEVELS

- GGT is induced with cholestasis or biliary hyperplasia. It is markedly increased with extrahepatic cholestasis (cholelithiasis and intestinal obstructive disease—particularly colonic displacement or stricture formation post duodenal ulceration).
- Mild to moderate increases occur with hepatocellular damage (hepatotoxins or infectious diseases) or chronic fibrosing hepatic diseases that cause cholestasis.
- GGT is normally mildly higher in training Thoroughbreds, neonates, and donkeys.

NEXT DIAGNOSTIC STEP TO CONSIDER IF LEVELS HIGH

- Complete blood count/serum chemistry profile and serum bile acids and urinalysis to rule out extrahepatic cholestasis and hepatitis/hepatic necrosis.
- Transabdominal ultrasonography to identify choleliths/colonic displacement and liver biopsy to identify specific liver pathology or etiology.

CAUSES OF ABNORMALLY LOW LEVELS Insignificant

DRUG EFFECTS ON LEVELS Increases:
Dexamethasone, prednisone, phenobarbital, rifampin, and benzimidazole anthelmintics

SPECIMEN AND PROCESSING CONSIDERATIONS

LAB ARTIFACTS THAT MAY INTERFERE WITH READINGS OF LEVELS OF THIS SUBSTANCE (AND HOW—ARTIFICIALLY ELEVATED VS. DEPRESSED) Increased bilirubin or hemolysis can falsely increase GGT with dry chemistry systems.

SAMPLE FOR COLLECTION (TYPE OF SPECIMEN, COLOR TUBE) AND ANY SPECIAL SPECIMEN HANDLING NOTES Serum, quickly separated from the clot, and refrigerated. Stable.

PEARLS GGT should be included in the minimal database of horses with suspected hepatic disease. Pituitary adenomas can cause hypercortisolemia or decreased antidiuretic hormone production, either of which can cause increased GGT (as well as aspartate aminotransferase [AST] and sorbitol dehydrogenase [SDH]) along with dilute urine. The half-life of GGT is long and blood levels may remain increased for several weeks following resolution of hepatic disease. Neonatal foals have greater serum GGT activities than adult horses. It is not related to uptake through the colostrum. Serum GGT activity is a better indicator of cholestasis than alkaline phosphatase.

AUTHOR: **PAULA M. KRIMER**

EDITOR: **CHARLES WIEDMEYER**

Globulins

BASIC INFORMATION

DEFINITION

Globulins are a heterogeneous group of large serum proteins other than albumin. These include clotting proteins, complement, many acute phase proteins, immunoglobulins, and lipoproteins.

TYPICAL NORMAL RANGE (US UNITS; SI UNITS)

Adults: 2.4 to 4.1 g/dL (24–41 g/L); variation occurs between reference laboratories. Foals may have lower values.

PHYSIOLOGY

Globulins are typically classified as alpha, beta, or gamma depending on their electrophoretic mobility.

CAUSES OF ABNORMALLY HIGH LEVELS Hemoconcentration, inflammation (especially chronic), B-lymphocyte neoplasia

NEXT DIAGNOSTIC STEP TO CONSIDER IF LEVELS HIGH Evaluate albumin:globulin (A:G) ratio. If A:G ratio is close to 1, then dehydration is likely. If A:G is <1 then increased globulin production is indicated (assuming albumin is normal). Protein electrophoresis may be pursued.

CAUSES OF ABNORMALLY LOW LEVELS Decreased globulin production (liver insufficiency); maldigestion/malabsorption; globulin loss as a consequence of blood loss, protein-losing enteropathies and nephropathies, or severe skin exudative lesions. In foals, consider failure of passive transfer or congenital immunodeficiencies (albumin should be normal).

NEXT DIAGNOSTIC STEP TO CONSIDER IF LEVELS LOW Evaluate for hemorrhage, renal or intestinal protein loss, liver insufficiency, malnutrition, and malabsorption. Measure foal IgG levels to evaluate for failure of passive transfer.

SPECIMEN AND PROCESSING CONSIDERATIONS

LAB ARTIFACTS THAT MAY INTERFERE WITH READINGS OF LEVELS OF THIS SUBSTANCE (AND HOW—ARTIFICIALLY ELEVATED VS. DEPRESSED) Globulin concentration is determined by subtraction: [total protein] − [albumin] = [globulin]; therefore errors in those values can lead to erroneous globulin values.

SAMPLE FOR COLLECTION (TYPE OF SPECIMEN, COLOR TUBE) AND ANY SPECIAL SPECIMEN HANDLING NOTES Serum (red-top tube) or lithium heparin plasma (green-top tube); contact reference laboratory for preference. Allow specimen to clot (red-top only), centrifuge, collect serum or plasma, refrigerate, ship on ice.

AUTHOR: **BRIDGET C. GARNER**

EDITOR: **CHARLES WIEDMEYER**

Glucose

BASIC INFORMATION

DEFINITION
A six-carbon monosaccharide that is the principle source of cellular energy and serves as an important metabolic intermediate

SYNONYM(S)
Blood sugar

TYPICAL NORMAL RANGE (US UNITS; SI UNITS)
62 to 134 mg/dL (3.44–7.44 mmol/L)

PHYSIOLOGY
Blood glucose homeostasis is maintained by the hormones insulin and glucagon.
CAUSES OF ABNORMALLY HIGH LEVELS Causes of hyperglycemia include diabetes mellitus, metabolic syndrome, hyperadrenocorticism, hyperpituitarism, acute abdominal disease (colic), and septicemia (early phases). Transient increases may occur postprandially; with endogenous epinephrine and/or glucocorticoid release; associated with such factors as fear, pain, stress, and transport; or with administration of dextrose-containing fluids.
NEXT DIAGNOSTIC STEP TO CONSIDER IF LEVELS HIGH Measure for glucosuria if possible. Utilize other diagnostic tests to confirm metabolic or infectious causes.
CAUSES OF ABNORMALLY LOW LEVELS Causes of hypoglycemia include chronic hepatic insufficiency, adrenocortical insufficiency, extreme or prolonged exertion, septicemia, starvation, malabsorption syndromes.
NEXT DIAGNOSTIC STEP TO CONSIDER IF LEVELS LOW Chemistry profile with special attention paid to liver function tests (ie, bile acids, ammonium, etc.)
DRUG EFFECTS ON LEVELS Drugs that may induce hyperglycemia include corticosteroids, xylazine, thiazides, and phenothiazine. Insulin administration can cause hypoglycemia.

SPECIMEN AND PROCESSING CONSIDERATIONS
LAB ARTIFACTS THAT MAY INTERFERE WITH READINGS OF LEVELS OF THIS SUBSTANCE (AND HOW—ARTIFICIALLY ELEVATED VS. DEPRESSED) Lipemia or hemolysis may cause artificially high readings, depending upon the methodology used and the severity of the lipemia or hemolysis.
SAMPLE FOR COLLECTION (TYPE OF SPECIMEN, COLOR TUBE) AND ANY SPECIAL SPECIMEN HANDLING NOTES Serum or heparinized plasma (harvested from a red-top or green-top tube, respectively) may be used for analysis. The serum or plasma should be harvested from the cells as soon as possible to avoid artifactual decreases due to *in vitro* glycolysis by blood cells.

AUTHOR: **MARLYN S. WHITNEY**

EDITOR: **CHARLES WIEDMEYER**

Glucosuria

BASIC INFORMATION

DEFINITION
Glucose in urine

SYNONYM(S)
Glycosuria

TYPICAL NORMAL RANGE (US UNITS; SI UNITS)
Negative in healthy horses

PHYSIOLOGY
Serum glucose is freely filtered by the glomerulus and subsequently reabsorbed from the ultrafiltrate by the proximal tubules. The reabsorption of glucose by the renal tubules is a saturable process, and serum glucose levels above 150 mg/dL result in more glucose in the ultrafiltrate than can be resorbed by the renal tubules.
CAUSES OF ABNORMALLY HIGH LEVELS
- Hyperglycemic glucosuria (eg, pituitary pars intermedia dysfunction [PPID], Cushing's disease, and rarely diestrus)
- Renal glucosuria (normoglycemic glucosuria) due to defective renal tubular resorption resulting from tubular abnormalities or damage
- False increase (see later)
NEXT DIAGNOSTIC STEP TO CONSIDER IF LEVELS HIGH Evaluate serum glucose concentration and renal parameters.
DRUG EFFECTS ON LEVELS
- False increases (via Clinitest copper-reduction method) may occur with cephalosporins and high concentrations of ascorbic acid.
- False increases may also occur with elevated progesterone levels and megestrol acetate.
- False decreases (via dipstick) may be caused by ascorbic acid.

SPECIMEN AND PROCESSING CONSIDERATIONS
LAB ARTIFACTS THAT MAY INTERFERE WITH READINGS OF LEVELS OF THIS SUBSTANCE (AND HOW—ARTIFICIALLY ELEVATED VS. DEPRESSED)
- False increases (via dipstick) may occur with contamination of hydrogen peroxide or bleach.
- False decreases (via dipstick) may occur with marked bilirubinuria,

ketones, highly concentrated samples, or cold urine.

SAMPLE FOR COLLECTION (TYPE OF SPECIMEN, COLOR TUBE) AND ANY SPECIAL SPECIMEN HANDLING NOTES Midstream urine collection in a clean container

PEARLS Urine should be at room temperature or warmer for enzymes in the reagent pad of the dipstick to work appropriately.

AUTHOR: **LAURA C. CREGAR**

EDITOR: **CHARLES WIEDMEYER**

Glutamate Dehydrogenase (GLD)

BASIC INFORMATION

DEFINITION

Leakage enzyme: Soluble cytoplasmic enzymes released into circulation after increased membrane permeability (sublethal cellular injury or cellular necrosis)

TYPICAL NORMAL RANGE (US UNITS; SI UNITS)

0 to 11.8 IU/L

PHYSIOLOGY

GLD is a mitochondrial enzyme involved in the citric acid cycle and amino acid metabolism that is relatively specific for hepatic disease in the horse. It is leaked after hepatocyte necrosis but not sublethal damage. GLD is most highly concentrated in centrilobular hepatocytes (zone 3) and is most affected by hypoxia and the majority of hepatotoxins.

CAUSES OF ABNORMALLY HIGH LEVELS

- Marked increases in acute hepatitis (equine herpesvirus type 1), embolic bacterial diseases, Tyzzer's disease (*Clostridium piliformis*), hepatotoxins such as pyrrolizidine alkaloids, Theiler's disease (aka serum hepatitis), and chronic active hepatitis
- Mild increases in cholestasis and hyperlipemia syndrome

NEXT DIAGNOSITC STEP TO CONSIDER IF LEVELS HIGH

- Vaccination history (serum hepatitis)
- Complete blood count/serum chemistry profile, serum bile acids, and urinalysis to rule out hyperlipemia syndrome and hepatitis/hepatic necrosis
- Transabdominal ultrasonography and liver biopsy to identify specific liver pathology or etiology

CAUSES OF ABNORMALLY LOW LEVELS Insignificant

DRUG EFFECTS ON LEVELS Increased: Benzimidazole anthelmintics

SPECIMEN AND PROCESSING CONSIDERATIONS

LAB ARTIFACTS THAT MAY INTERFERE WITH READINGS OF LEVELS OF THIS SUBSTANCE (AND HOW—ARTIFICIALLY ELEVATED VS. DEPRESSED) Increased bilirubin and hyperlipemia can falsely decrease values.

SAMPLE FOR COLLECTION (TYPE OF SPECIMEN, COLOR TUBE) AND ANY SPECIAL SPECIMEN HANDLING NOTES Serum, quickly separated from the clot and refrigerated. Stable 2 days at room temperature, 1 week refrigerated, and up to 6 months frozen

PEARLS GLD is mitochondrial and leaked after hepatocellular necrosis but not sublethal damage; hence inflammatory diseases are less likely to increase GLD than necrotic diseases. GLD is not widely available, partially due to poor assay precision and enzyme instability.

AUTHOR: **PAULA M. KRIMER**

EDITOR: **CHARLES WIEDMEYER**

Heinz Bodies

BASIC INFORMATION

DEFINITION

Heinz bodies are erythrocyte structures composed of precipitated denatured hemoglobin. On Wright's-stained blood smears, they appear as a rounded structure protruding from the margin of an erythrocyte or as a small somewhat refractile spot within the cell.

SYNONYM(S)

Erythrocyte refractile bodies

TYPICAL NORMAL RANGE (US UNITS; SI UNITS)

Rare to absent

PHYSIOLOGY

Heinz bodies are the result of oxidative damage to erythrocyte hemoglobin. They may be seen in conjunction with eccentrocytes, which are the result of oxidative damage to the erythrocyte membrane. Heinz body formation is a cause of hemolytic anemia. Heinz body hemolytic anemia is usually associated with a toxic exposure, but rare cases may result from hereditary defects in the molecular milieu that acts to protect erythrocytes from oxidative damage (see later).

CAUSES OF ABNORMALLY HIGH LEVELS Heinz body formation in horses has been associated with red maple leaf toxicosis, wild onion toxicosis, and phenothiazine administration. Copper and zinc toxicosis have caused Heinz body

formation in other species and might potentially do so in horses. In rare cases, hereditary defects in the mechanisms that act to protect erythrocytes from oxidative damage may result in Heinz body formation. Included here would be deficiencies of glucose-6-phosphate dehydrogenase, flavanone-adenine dinucleotide (FAD), glutathione, or glutathione reductase.

SPECIMEN AND PROCESSING CONSIDERATIONS

LAB ARTIFACTS THAT MAY INTERFERE WITH READINGS OF LEVELS OF THIS SUBSTANCE (AND HOW—ARTIFICIALLY ELEVATED VS. DEPRESSED) The presence of large numbers of Heinz bodies may cause falsely elevated hemoglobin reading on a complete blood count.

PEARLS New methylene blue (NMB) stains Heinz bodies dark blue, making them easier to identify on a blood smear. To make a NMB stained smear, mix a drop of whole EDTA-anticoagulated blood with a drop of NMB stain in a clean tube and let the mixture stand for 20 minutes. Place a small drop on a slide and use a spreader slide to make a blood smear in the usual manner. No additional staining is necessary to visualize Heinz bodies that might be present.

AUTHOR: **MARLYN S. WHITNEY**

EDITOR: **CHARLES WIEDMEYER**

Hematocrit

BASIC INFORMATION

DEFINITION

The percentage of blood volume made up of erythrocytes

SYNONYM(S)

Packed cell volume

TYPICAL NORMAL RANGE (US UNITS; SI UNITS)

27% to 43% (0.27–0.43 L/L)

PHYSIOLOGY

CAUSES OF ABNORMALLY HIGH LEVELS: An increase in hematocrit is called erythrocytosis (a previous term now falling into disfavor is polycythemia). An increase in hematocrit is usually a relative increase (does not involve an actual increase in the red cell mass of the body) due to dehydration, endotoxemia, or splenic contraction occurring in association with excitement or exercise. Absolute increases (these involve increased production of erythrocytes) are rare in horses, except perhaps those that train at high elevations. See the section on erythrocytosis for more detail.

NEXT DIAGNOSTIC STEP TO CONSIDER IF LEVELS HIGH If dehydration is present, reevaluate the hematocrit following rehydration. If the animal is excited or has been exercising, recheck the hematocrit when the animal is calm. See Erythrocytosis in this section for more detail.

CAUSES OF ABNORMALLY LOW LEVELS A decrease in hematocrit is characteristic of anemia. Anemia may be due to loss of erythrocytes (blood loss), destruction of erythrocytes (hemolysis), or due to inadequate production of erythrocytes by the bone marrow. See Regenerative Anemia and Nonregenerative Anemia in this section for more detail.

NEXT DIAGNOSTIC STEP TO CONSIDER IF LEVELS LOW Please see Regenerative Anemia and Nonregenerative Anemia in this section.

IMPORTANT INTERSPECIES DIFFERENCES Horses are more likely than most other domestic species to have an increased hematocrit due to splenic contraction.

SPECIMEN AND PROCESSING CONSIDERATIONS

LAB ARTIFACTS THAT MAY INTERFERE WITH READINGS OF LEVELS OF THIS SUBSTANCE (AND HOW—ARTIFICIALLY ELEVATED VS. DEPRESSED) Improper centrifugation may affect results when the microhematocrit tube method of determination is used (improper cell packing may result in an artifactually high hematocrit reading). Inadequate filling of the blood tube (see later) may result in an artifactually low reading. Inadequate mixing of blood prior to testing may cause false high or low values. Many blood analyzers calculate the hematocrit from the red blood cell (RBC) count and the analyzer determined erythrocyte mean cell volume. Erythrocyte clumping (agglutination) may cause a falsely low RBC count and/or a falsely high determination of mean corpuscular volume (MCV), thus inducing inaccuracy into the calculated hematocrit.

SAMPLE FOR COLLECTION (TYPE OF SPECIMEN, COLOR TUBE) AND ANY SPECIAL SPECIMEN HANDLING NOTES EDTA or heparin anticoagulated blood (purple-top or green-top tube, respectively) is used to determine the hematocrit, the hemoglobin level, and the RBC count. An EDTA tube is preferred if blood smear evaluation is also to be done, as EDTA-anticoagulated specimens usually provide better staining quality. Inadequate filling of EDTA tubes (less than half full) may result in artifactually low hematocrit readings.

PEARLS Excessive parenteral administration of fluids (overhydration, hemodilution) can decrease the hematocrit and give a false impression of anemia.

AUTHOR: **MARLYN S. WHITNEY**

EDITOR: **CHARLES WIEDMEYER**

Hematuria

BASIC INFORMATION

DEFINITION

Hematuria is blood or red blood cells present in the urine; it is associated with red to reddish brown turbid urine that clears after centrifugation leaving a red pellet in the bottom of the tube.

TYPICAL NORMAL RANGE (US UNITS; SI UNITS)

Voided sample: <8 red blood cells (RBCs/high-power field (hpf); catheterized sample: <5 RBCs/hpf

PHYSIOLOGY

Erythrocytes may appear in the urine from anywhere in the urogenital system or the collection process (catheterization). Hematuria will result in a positive blood test on a urine dipstick

CAUSES OF ABNORMALLY HIGH LEVELS Hematuria may be associated with trauma, hemorrhage, urolithiasis, inflammation, infection, toxemia, exercise, or neoplasia.

NEXT DIAGNOSTIC STEP TO CONSIDER IF LEVELS HIGH

- Determine at what time during micturition the hematuria occurred: Start of micturition suggests lesions in the lower urinary tract or genital tract; end or throughout micturition indicates urinary bladder or upper urinary tract disorders.
- Thorough physical examination with rectal palpation
- Complete blood count (CBC), serum biochemistry panel, or coagulation tests may help to differentiate some causes.
- Endoscopic examination of the urethra, bladder, and ureteral orifices
- Ultrasonographic examination or renal biopsy if lower urinary tract lesions are not present

SPECIMEN AND PROCESSING CONSIDERATIONS

LAB ARTIFACTS THAT MAY INTERFERE WITH READINGS OF LEVELS OF THIS SUBSTANCE (AND HOW—ARTIFICIALLY ELEVATED VS. DEPRESSED)

- Red blood cells may not be seen on examination of sediment due to rupture in dilute or alkaline urine or from delayed analysis; red blood cell ghosts may be visible.
- A positive for blood on urine dipstick can also be due to bilirubinuria, hemoglobinuria, myoglobinuria, or contamination of urine with oxidizing compounds (disinfectants such as bleach or iodine, or microbial or leukocyte peroxidase).

SAMPLE FOR COLLECTION (TYPE OF SPECIMEN, COLOR TUBE) AND ANY SPECIAL SPECIMEN HANDLING NOTES Samples should be refrigerated and analyzed as soon as possible.

PEARLS

- Equine urine can change color after urination and be falsely reported as hematuria.
- To differentiate hematuria from hemoglobinuria and myoglobinuria, which all have a positive blood test on a urine dipstick, evaluate the color of the supernatant after centrifugation of the urine; hematuria will have a clear supernatant, whereas hemoglobinuria and myoglobinuria will not. To differentiate hemoglobinuria from myoglobinuria, evaluate the plasma color; hemoglobinuria will have a pink to red plasma color, whereas myoglobinuria will not.

AUTHOR: **SARA A. HILL**

EDITOR: **CHARLES WIEDMEYER**

Hemoglobin

BASIC INFORMATION

DEFINITION

Hemoglobin is the oxygen-carrying molecule within erythrocytes (red blood cells [RBCs]). Hemoglobin determination is usually done as part of a complete blood count (CBC).

TYPICAL NORMAL RANGE (US UNITS; SI UNITS)

Hemoglobin: 10.1 to 16.1 g/dL (101–161 g/L)

PHYSIOLOGY

CAUSES OF ABNORMALLY HIGH LEVELS Hemoglobin is increased along with the hematocrit and RBC count in erythrocytosis.

CAUSES OF ABNORMALLY LOW LEVELS Hemoglobin is decreased along with the hematocrit and RBC count in anemia.

SPECIMEN AND PROCESSING CONSIDERATIONS

LAB ARTIFACTS THAT MAY INTERFERE WITH READINGS OF LEVELS OF THIS SUBSTANCE (AND HOW—ARTIFICIALLY ELEVATED VS. DEPRESSED) Lipemia is likely to cause artifactually high hemoglobin readings.

The presence of Heinz bodies may cause artifactually high readings on some hematology analyzers.

SAMPLE FOR COLLECTION (TYPE OF SPECIMEN, COLOR TUBE) AND ANY SPECIAL SPECIMEN HANDLING NOTES: EDTA- or heparin-anticoagulated whole blood (purple- and green-top blood collection tubes, respectively) is usually used for hemoglobin determination.

AUTHOR: **MARLYN S. WHITNEY**

EDITOR: **CHARLES WIEDMEYER**

Hemoglobinuria

BASIC INFORMATION

DEFINITION

Hemoglobinuria is the presence of hemoglobin in the urine; it is associated with red to amber colored transparent urine that remains pigmented after centrifugation.

TYPICAL NORMAL RANGE (US UNITS; SI UNITS)

Not present

PHYSIOLOGY

Free hemoglobin in the plasma splits into dimers that are immediately bound to haptoglobin and cleared by hepatocytes by the formation of bilirubin, iron, and amino acids or bound to macrophages. If haptoglobin is saturated, hemoglobin dimers accumulate in the plasma (hemoglobinemia) and pass through the glomerulus where they are resorbed and degraded by proximal tubule cells or excreted in the urine (hemoglobinuria). Hemoglobinuria will cause a positive blood test on a urine dipstick.

CAUSES OF ABNORMALLY HIGH LEVELS

- Severe intravascular hemolysis
- Hemoglobinuria may also be present in cases of hematuria in which red blood cells have lysed (as with dilute or alkaline samples or delayed processing); however, hemoglobinemia should be absent.

NEXT DIAGNOSTIC STEP TO CONSIDER IF LEVELS HIGH

- Complete blood count (CBC) with blood smear examination to evaluate for causes of hemolysis (ie, Heinz bodies, erythrocyte agglutination)
- Serum biochemistry panel to look for triggers of hemolytic anemia

SPECIMEN AND PROCESSING CONSIDERATIONS

LAB ARTIFACTS THAT MAY INTERFERE WITH READINGS OF LEVELS OF THIS SUBSTANCE (AND HOW—ARTIFICIALLY ELEVATED VS. DEPRESSED) A positive result for blood on a urine dipstick can also be due to bilirubinuria, myoglobinuria, hematuria, or contamination of urine with oxidizing compounds (disinfectants such as bleach or iodine, or microbial or leukocyte peroxidase).

SAMPLE FOR COLLECTION (TYPE OF SPECIMEN, COLOR TUBE) AND ANY SPECIAL SPECIMEN HANDLING NOTES Samples should be refrigerated and analyzed as soon as possible.

PEARLS Generally, to differentiate hemoglobinuria from myoglobinuria and hematuria, which all have a positive blood test on a urine dipstick, evaluate the color of the supernatant after centrifugation of the urine; hematuria will have a clear supernatant, whereas hemoglobinuria and myoglobinuria will not. To differentiate hemoglobinuria from myoglobinuria, evaluate the plasma color; hemoglobinuria will have a pink to red plasma color, whereas myoglobinuria will not.

AUTHOR: **SARA A. HILL**

EDITOR: **CHARLES WIEDMEYER**

Hemolysis

BASIC INFORMATION

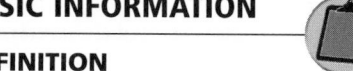

DEFINITION

Hemolysis is the disruption of erythrocyte membranes, which causes the release of hemoglobin. Hemolysis is also defined as erythrocyte necrosis and occurs at the end of every erythrocyte's life.

SYNONYM(S)

Erythrolysis

TYPICAL NORMAL RANGE (US UNITS; SI UNITS)

Plasma or serum will appear pink when the hemoglobin concentration exceeds 50 mg/dL.

PHYSIOLOGY

Hemolysis may occur *in vitro* or *in vivo*. *In vitro* hemolysis can result from the lysis of the red blood cells during collection and handling of the blood sample. *In vivo* hemolysis occurs if the rate of erythrocyte destruction is increased, thereby decreasing erythrocyte life span. Erythrocytes may be lysed within the vasculature (intravascular hemolysis) mainly in blood vessels and heart and it is clinically recognized by hemoglobinemia, hemoglobinuria, and decreased serum haptoglobin concentration. Erythrocytes may be also destroyed in macrophages (extravascular hemolysis or intracellular hemolysis) of the mononuclear phagocytic system of the spleen, liver, and bone marrow. Extravascular hemolysis does not cause hemoglobinemia and hemoglobinuria but usually causes hemolytic icterus (hyperbilirubinemia associated with bilirubinuria).

CAUSES OF ABNORMALLY HIGH LEVELS

In vivo hemolysis is present in conditions called hemolytic anemias. Causes of hemolytic anemias include:

- Immune-mediated erythrocyte destruction: Neonatal isoerythrolysis, incompatible blood transfusion, drugs including penicillin and heparin
- Hemoparasites: *Babesia* spp.
- Other infectious agents: *Leptospira, Ehrlichia, Clostridium,* equine infectious anemia virus
- Chemicals and plants: Red maple, Phenothiazine
- Fragmentation: Disseminated intravascular coagulation (DIC), vasculitis, uremia
- Hypo-osmolality: Hypotonic fluid administration
- Hypophosphatemia
- Liver failure: Hemolytic syndrome in horses with liver disease

NEXT DIAGNOSTIC STEP TO CONSIDER IF LEVELS HIGH Assess the underlying cause of hemolysis.

SPECIMEN AND PROCESSING CONSIDERATIONS

LAB ARTIFACTS THAT MAY INTERFERE WITH READINGS OF LEVELS OF THIS SUBSTANCE (AND HOW—ARTIFICIALLY ELEVATED VS. DEPRESSED) Slight hemolysis has little effect on most test values; however, moderate to severe hemolysis may directly interfere with spectrophotometric absorbance reading and alter the pH of reactions. Aspartate aminotransferase (AST) and lactate dehydrogenase (LDH) have higher activity within the erythrocytes compared with plasma, and their levels will be increased in either *in vivo* or *in vitro* hemolysis. Hemolysis may falsely increase the following analytes: AST, alanine transaminase (ALT), LDH, total bilirubin, glucose, calcium, phosphorus, total protein, albumin, magnesium, amylase, lipase, creatine kinase (CK), iron, hemoglobin, and mean corpuscular hemoglobin concentration (MCHC). On the other side, hemolysis may falsely decrease creatinine, alkaline phosphatase (ALP), potassium, packed cell volume (PCV), and mean corpuscular volume (MCV).

AUTHOR: **ROBERTA DI TERLIZZI**

EDITOR: **CHARLES WIEDMEYER**

Hypochromasia

BASIC INFORMATION

DEFINITION

Hypochromasia refers to the appearance on a Wright's-stained blood smear of erythrocytes containing less than the normal amount of hemoglobin. They are seen in association with anemia (hypochromic anemia). The cells do not stain as deeply as normal and they exhibit increased central pallor (there is a thinned rim of hemoglobin around the margin of the cell). When hypochromasia is present on blood smears, the mean corpuscular hemoglobin concentration (MCHC) is expected to be low. Hypochromic erythrocytes may be smaller than normal (microcytic), so the mean corpuscular volume (MCV) may also be decreased.

TYPICAL NORMAL RANGE (US UNITS; SI UNITS)

Erythrocytes from healthy horses do not exhibit hypochromasia. A reported normal range for MCHC in horses is 35.3% to 39.3%.

PHYSIOLOGY

CAUSES OF ABNORMALLY HIGH LEVELS Hypochromic anemia is usually due to iron deficiency. Lead toxicity may occasionally cause hypochromic anemia. Iron deficiency may be nutritional or due to chronic blood loss. Iron deficiency is uncommon to rare in horses, especially adult horses. Copper deficiency could potentially cause hypochromic anemia, but this probably rarely occurs in horses.

PEARLS In addition to exhibiting hypochromasia, blood smears from iron deficient animals may exhibit erythrocyte morphologic abnormalities, such as the presence of codocytes, keratocytes, schistocytes, and echinocytes.

AUTHOR: **MARLYN S. WHITNEY**

EDITOR: **CHARLES WIEDMEYER**

Icterus

BASIC INFORMATION

DEFINITION

Icterus is defined as the accumulation of bilirubin in plasma (hyperbilirubinemia) and tissues (sclera, skin, and mucous membranes). Icterus usually becomes evident when the plasma bilirubin concentration exceeds 1.5 mg/dL. Bilirubin is an orange-yellow pigment derived from the catabolism of heme.

SYNONYM(S)

Jaundice
Hyperbilirubinemia

TYPICAL NORMAL RANGE (US UNITS; SI UNITS)

0.0 to 0.4 mg/dL

PHYSIOLOGY

Hyperbilirubinemia occurs when the rate of bilirubin production (unconjugated) exceeds the rate of uptake by hepatocytes, or the rate of bilirubin formation (conjugated) in hepatocytes exceeds the rate of excretion in the bile.

CAUSES OF ABNORMALLY HIGH LEVELS
Diseases and conditions that cause icterus—hyperbilirubinemia include:
- Increased bilirubin production (unconjugated)
- Hemolytic (prehepatic) icterus especially seen in extravascular hemolysis
- Decreased bilirubin uptake by hepatocytes
- Fasting or anorexia (very common in horses) due to interference of fatty acids with unconjugated bilirubin uptake
- Decreased functional hepatic mass
- Decreased bilirubin conjugation
- Decreased excretion of bilirubin (conjugated) in bile
- Obstructive cholestasis in hepatic lipidosis, diabetes mellitus, inflammatory liver diseases, neoplasia, toxins
- Functional cholestasis (sepsis-associated cholestasis)

NEXT DIAGNOSTIC STEP TO CONSIDER IF LEVELS HIGH Identify the cause of icterus based on clinical signs and other laboratory data.

SPECIMEN AND PROCESSING CONSIDERATIONS

LAB ARTIFACTS THAT MAY INTERFERE WITH READINGS OF LEVELS OF THIS SUBSTANCE (AND HOW—ARTIFICIALLY ELEVATED VS. DEPRESSED) Severe hyperbilirubinemia may decrease the serum creatinine levels with some methods (Jaffe reaction). The presence of icterus also falsely decreases serum triglycerides and magnesium concentration and falsely increases serum alkaline phosphatase (ALP), phosphorus, total proteins and chlorides.

SAMPLE FOR COLLECTION (TYPE OF SPECIMEN, COLOR TUBE) AND ANY SPECIAL SPECIMEN HANDLING NOTES Serum is preferred (red-top tube). Ultraviolet lights degrade bilirubin. In direct sunlight, total bilirubin concentration may decrease up to 50% in 1 hour.

AUTHOR: **ROBERTA DI TERLIZZI**

EDITOR: **CHARLES WIEDMEYER**

Insulin

BASIC INFORMATION

DEFINITION

- Hyperinsulinemia: Increased circulating concentration of insulin
- Hypoinsulinemia: Decreased circulating concentration of insulin

TYPICAL NORMAL RANGE (US UNITS; SI UNITS)

0 to 35.9 pmol/L; 0 to 5 µU/mL

PHYSIOLOGY

Insulin is a polypeptide pancreatic hormone secreted by the beta cells of the islets of Langerhans. Preproinsulin is produced by ribosomes of the beta cells and quickly cleaved to proinsulin and stored in secretory granules of the Golgi complex. Proinsulin is then cleaved to form insulin, C-peptide, and split peptides. Insulin's primary role in the body involves the metabolism of carbohydrates and the regulation of glucose levels in the blood, by promoting the uptake, utilization, or storage of glucose by hepatocytes, myocytes, and adipocytes. Insulin promotes glucose uptake into myocytes and adipocytes via the glucose transporter GLUT-4 but is not required for other carriers. Insulin secretion is stimulated by increasing blood concentrations of glucose, growth hormone, glucagon, or amino acids. The sequence of the insulin molecule is highly conserved between species. Equine insulin has one amino acid difference from porcine insulin, which has one amino acid difference from human insulin.

CAUSES OF ABNORMALLY HIGH LEVELS

Elevations in circulating insulin concentrations are typically due to increased insulin production and release either due to hyperglycemia (appropriate response) or a functional beta cell neoplasia in the pancreas. Exogenously administered insulin will also falsely elevate baseline concentrations. Anti-insulin antibodies may result in a false elevation in insulin concentrations determined by certain assays.

NEXT DIAGNOSTIC STEP TO CONSIDER IF LEVELS HIGH

If the baseline circulating concentration of insulin is elevated, a serum glucose concentration should be determined. If the serum glucose concentration is below reference interval, an abdominal ultrasound should be performed in an attempt to visualize the pancreas and identify a mass. Therapeutic interventions should also be initiated to manage the hypoglycemia. If the serum glucose concentration is within reference interval or increased, the presence of an insulin antagonist (ie, cortisol) or peripheral insulin resistance should be suspected and investigated via a baseline serum cortisol concentration (if there is no history of exogenous corticosteroid administration) or a glucose tolerance test in euglycemic patients.

CAUSES OF ABNORMALLY LOW LEVELS

Decreased circulating insulin concentrations are due to decreased insulin production and release by the pancreatic beta cells. This is primarily a result of either destruction of pancreatic beta cells or pancreatic invasion by neoplasia or amyloid. The presence of circulating anti-insulin antibodies may also falsely decrease insulin concentrations.

NEXT DIAGNOSTIC STEP TO CONSIDER IF LEVELS LOW

A serum glucose concentration or urinalysis should be obtained to determine circulating concentration of glucose. Anti-insulin antibodies should also be evaluated.

DRUG EFFECTS ON LEVELS

Hyperinsulinemia: Alcohol, monoamine oxidase (MAO) inhibitors, beta-blockers like propranolol, salicylates like aspirin, and anabolic steroids

SPECIMEN AND PROCESSING CONSIDERATIONS

LAB ARTIFACTS THAT MAY INTERFERE WITH READINGS OF LEVELS OF THIS SUBSTANCE (AND HOW—ARTIFICIALLY ELEVATED VS. DEPRESSED) Delayed separation of the red cell mass from the serum sample may artificially decrease glucose concentrations due to erythrocyte metabolism, making it difficult to assess insulin concentrations.

SAMPLE FOR COLLECTION (TYPE OF SPECIMEN, COLOR TUBE) AND ANY SPECIAL SPECIMEN HANDLING NOTES Whole blood should be collected in a clot tube (red top); serum should be removed and refrigerated after the clot has formed. Ideally, a fasting sample is best for evaluating resting insulin concentrations. Fasting samples are difficult to obtain in most herbivores due to either fore or hindgut fermentation. Subsequently collection of a sample prior to morning feeding after "fasting" the animal overnight is usually adequate. A serum glucose concentration should be evaluated concurrently.

PEARLS There have been few reports of hypoinsulinemia in association with diabetes mellitus in horses. Hyperinsulinemia is a much more common clinical entity and is typically either associated with a cellular insulin resistance and circulating hyperglycemia as is seen in equine metabolic syndrome, or due to hypercortisolemia leading to hyperglycemia in association with pituitary pars intermedia dysfunction (equine Cushing's disease).

AUTHORS: **SHANE F. DeWITT** and **TANYA M. GRONDIN**

EDITOR: **CHARLES WIEDMEYER**

Keratocytes

BASIC INFORMATION

DEFINITION

Keratocytes are erythrocytes with one or two projections that may form as a result of rupture of a vacuole or hole within an erythrocyte. Their mechanism of formation is not entirely certain.

SYNONYM(S)

Helmet cells
Erythrocytes with one projection are sometimes described by the term "budding fragmentation."

TYPICAL NORMAL RANGE (US UNITS; SI UNITS)

Rare to none

PHYSIOLOGY

Keratocyte formation has been associated with mechanical damage to erythrocytes within the vasculature and with oxidative damage. They also may occur due to increased erythrocyte fragility, such as occurs with iron deficiency. They often are seen along with schistocytes. In the case of exposure to oxidant toxins, they may be seen in association with Heinz bodies and/or eccentrocytes.

CAUSES OF ABNORMALLY HIGH LEVELS Conditions associated with keratocyte formation include thrombotic disorders, diffuse intravascular coagulation, vasculitis, endocarditis and other cardiac disorders, glomerulonephritis, liver disease, myelofibrosis, hemangiosar-

coma, iron deficiency, and exposure to oxidant toxins such as from red maple leaf or onion ingestion.

AUTHOR: **MARLYN S. WHITNEY**

EDITOR: **CHARLES WIEDMEYER**

Lactate

BASIC INFORMATION

DEFINITION

Lactate is the organic anion of lactic acid. It is produced in excess during anaerobic metabolism as the end product of glycolysis. L-lactate is the predominating form present in mammals.

TYPICAL NORMAL RANGE (US UNITS; SI UNITS)

Depends on the instrument used and the method of sample collection. See your laboratory reference range.

PHYSIOLOGY

During normal metabolism and exercise, lactate is constantly produced via lactate dehydrogenase (LDH) in a variety of cells (eg, erythrocytes, gut, skeletal muscle). Increase in lactate leading to lactic acidosis does not occur until the rate of lactate production exceeds the rate of lactate removal. Lactate is primarily removed from the blood by the liver and kidneys, where it can be resynthesized into glucose.

CAUSES OF ABNORMALLY HIGH LEVELS

- Tissue hypoxia considered the most common. It can be caused by decreased tissue perfusion and shock (eg, hypovolemia associated with colic, endotoxemic shock, cardiogenic shock, and acute blood loss). It can also be caused by sustained heavy exercise.

- Conditions of adequate tissue oxygenation: Main differentials include increased lactic acid production by enteric organisms during carbohydrate overload and diarrhea. Other suggested causes include impaired hepatic clearance, lactate production by leukocytes in inflammation, and rare hereditary defects (pyruvate dehydrogenase deficiency, mitochondrial myopathy).
- Lactic acidosis can cause titrational acidosis (ie, decreased bicarbonate or TCO_2 with increased anion gap). Because lactate is not measured on routine biochemical profiles, it should be added when titrational acidosis is present.

SPECIMEN AND PROCESSING CONSIDERATIONS

LAB ARTIFACTS THAT MAY INTERFERE WITH READINGS OF LEVELS OF THIS SUBSTANCE (AND HOW—ARTFICIALLY ELEVATED VS. DEPRESSED) Increased: Delayed plasma harvest, venous stasis, increased PCV using Accutrend POC (PCV >40%) and Accusport (PCV >53%)

SAMPLE FOR COLLECTION (TYPE OF SPECIMEN, COLOR TUBE) AND ANY SPECIAL SPECIMEN HANDLING NOTES Analyzer dependent. For most wet chemistry blood gas analyzers such as Stat Profile Critical Care Xpress (Nova Biomedical, Waltham, MA) and ABL 605 (Radiometer, Copenhagen, Denmark), whole blood in heparin or sodium fluoride is the sample of choice. The sample

should be processed as soon as possible (preferably within 5–15 minutes) or stored on ice and processed within 60 minutes. Alternatively, plasma is quickly obtained by centrifugation, stored at 4°C and sent to the lab within 4 hours. Some reports suggest that lactate is stable for 4 hours at room temperature. Several point of care (POC) analyzers have been validated for use in horses such as Accusport for plasma and peritoneal fluid in horses with colic (sodium fluoride), Lactate Pro (heparinized whole blood) in horses with colic or in variable degrees of exercise and Accutrend for plasma (obtained from heparinized whole blood and less favorably for heparinized whole blood) in horses presented for different emergencies (mainly colic).

PEARLS Lactate concentration has been suggested as a useful prognostic indicator in horses with colic (lactate concentration >6.8 mmol/L suggests poor survival probability) and critically ill neonates. It is also suggested as a predictor of colonic viability and survival after 360-degree volvulus of the ascending colon (lactate concentration >7 mmol/L suggests poor prognosis). Peritoneal lactate concentration is a better indicator of intestinal ischemia than plasma lactate concentration and may be useful for prognostic purposes in horses with colic. Lactate is also helpful in training and standardized exercise testing of race horses.

AUTHOR: **SHIR GILOR**

EDITOR: **CHARLES WIEDMEYER**

Lactate Dehydrogenase (LDH)

BASIC INFORMATION

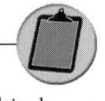

DEFINITION

Cytoplasmic enzyme found within hepatocytes, erythrocytes, and muscle (skeletal and cardiac)

TYPICAL NORMAL RANGE (US UNITS; SI UNITS)

147 to 581 U/L

PHYSIOLOGY

- Lactate dehydrogenase (LDH) catalyzes a reversible reaction that converts pyruvate to lactate at the end of anaerobic glycolysis.

- There are five isoenzymes of LDH present in various tissues that exist as tetramers. Identification of the isoenzymes that are causing the increase in serum activity can possibly increase the diagnostic sensitivity of the test but techniques to separate and identify the isoenzymes are not widely available.
- Because of its lack of tissue specificity, it is not a commonly used test but may offer supportive evidence of muscle or hepatocellular damage.

CAUSES OF ABNORMALLY HIGH LEVELS Increases can be the result of muscle damage, hepatocellular damage or necrosis, and hemolysis. Alone, LDH can be used as a screening test for liver or muscle damage.

NEXT DIAGNOSTIC STEP TO CONSIDER IF LEVELS HIGH
- Evaluate for muscle or liver damage.
- Examine serum biochemistry analysis for changes in aspartate aminotransferase (AST), creatine kinase (CK), or sorbitol dehydrogenase (SDH). These values may offer clues as to the tissue affected (ie, AST and CK for muscle damage, SDH for hepatocellular damage).
- Evaluate packed cell volume (PCV) or hematocrit (HCT) for evidence of hemolytic anemia.

CAUSES OF ABNORMALLY LOW LEVELS Clinically insignificant

SPECIMEN AND PROCESSING CONSIDERATIONS
LAB ARTIFACTS THAT MAY INTERFERE WITH READINGS OF LEVELS OF THIS SUBSTANCE (AND HOW—ARTIFICIALLY ELEVATAED VS. DEPRESSED) *In vitro* hemolysis can cause increases in LDH. Variation in assay temperature may alter LDH activity.
SAMPLE FOR COLLECTION (TYPE OF SPECIMEN, COLOR TUBE) AND ANY SPECIAL SPECIMEN HANDLING NOTES Serum or plasma

AUTHOR and EDITOR: **CHARLES WIEDMEYER**

Lipemia

BASIC INFORMATION

DEFINITION

Lipemia is the presence of excess fat (triglycerides) in the blood of a sufficient magnitude to impart a visible lactescent (milky) appearance to serum or plasma that does not resolve upon routine centrifugation. It is due to the presence in circulation of chylomicrons (CM) and/or excess very low density lipoprotein (VLDL) particles. It is characterized by hypertriglyceridemia, because CM and VLDL particles have a high triglyceride content. Serum or plasma samples with a triglyceride concentration of greater than 400 to 500 mg/dL (4.52–5.65 mmol/L) are likely to appear lipemic.

SYNONYM(S)

Lipidemia, hyperlipemia. Lipemia is sometimes used as a synonym for hyperlipidemia (synonym hyperlipoproteinemia), but the term is probably best reserved for those forms of hyperlipidemia/hyperlipoproteinemia that results in visible lactescence of serum and plasma.

TYPICAL NORMAL RANGE (US UNITS; SI UNITS)

Lipemia should not be evident in healthy horses, except perhaps following nursing in foals.

PHYSIOLOGY

CAUSES OF ABNORMALLY HIGH LEVELS Conditions involving negative energy balance favor lipolysis and are likely to result in hypertriglyceridemia. If the hypertriglyceridemia is of sufficient magnitude (greater than 400–500 mg/dL or 4.52–5.65 mmol/L), lipemia will be evident. Conditions causing negative energy balance include malnutrition, anorexia, stress, pregnancy, lactation, endotoxemia, and renal failure. Ponies, donkeys, and miniature horses are predisposed to become markedly hypertriglyceridemic under such conditions. Obesity is a predisposing factor to development of hypertriglyceridemia during metabolic stress. Equids with diabetes mellitus or metabolic syndrome are likely to be hypertriglyceridemic, as are those with hyperadrenocorticism (Cushing's-like syndrome, usually due to functional pituitary adenoma or adenomatous hyperplasia). Some such patients may develop lipemia. Transient hypertriglyceridemia may occur postprandially, especially in nursing foals.

DRUG EFFECTS ON LEVELS Corticosteroid administration may contribute to lipemia.

SPECIMEN AND PROCESSING CONSIDERATIONS

LAB ARTIFACTS THAT MAY INTERFERE WITH READINGS OF LEVELS OF THIS SUBSTANCE (AND HOW—ARTIFICIALLY ELEVATED VS. DEPRESSED) Lipemia can predispose to artifactual hemolysis during blood sample collection. Lipemia interferes with many laboratory tests. It is likely to cause artifactually high results for hemoglobin and mean corpuscular hemoglobin concentration (MCHC) on a complete blood count (CBC). It is likely to cause artifactually high estimates of the plasma protein level as determined by refractometry. Lipemia may have adverse effects on many serum/plasma biochemical tests. Specific effects depend upon the methodology used, the severity of the lipemia, and the laboratory's success in clearing lipemia prior to specimen analysis.

AUTHOR: **MARLYN S. WHITNEY**

EDITOR: **CHARLES WIEDMEYER**

Lymphocytes (Lymphocytosis, Lymphopenia)

BASIC INFORMATION

DEFINITION

Lymphocytes consist of T cells, B cells, and natural killer cells. These cells are an integral part of the humoral and cell-mediated immune response. Morphologically, these cells are small and round with a scant rim of basophilic cytoplasm with a round nucleus and a condensed chromatin pattern. Occasionally, these cells contain few eosinophilic cytoplasmic granules.

TYPICAL NORMAL RANGE (US UNITS; SI UNITS)

1.2 to $5.0 \times 10^3/\mu L$

PHYSIOLOGY

Lymphocytes have specific roles in the immune response as either effector cells or regulator cells. These cells can be further identified as T or B cells based on the presence of cellular antigens such as CD3 (T cell), CD79 or CD20 (B cells), CD4 (helper T cells), or CD8 (cytotoxic T cells). B cells are antibody producing cells and are important in the humoral immune response. T cells are the most predominant lymphocytes and have prominent roles as both effector and regulatory lymphocytes. Lymphoid cells can be identified in many different tissues in the body including lymph nodes, spleen, bone marrow, thymus, gastrointestinal (GI) tract, and respiratory tract. These cells have the ability to enter and exit lymphoid tissue and peripheral blood. Many of the other leukocytes such as neutrophils are unable to reenter the peripheral blood once they enter the tissue.

CAUSES OF ABNORMALLY HIGH LEVELS
Increases in lymphocytes or lymphocytosis can be transient secondary to epinephrine release with excitement or fear, or as part of an antigenic response. Presence of reactive lymphocytes are often seen in patients with chronic antigenic stimulation. Recently vaccinated animals will often have low numbers of circulating reactive lymphocytes. Patients with leukemia or lymphoma may have large or atypical lymphocytes in circulation or may have unusually high levels of lymphocytes (>30,000/µL).

NEXT DIAGNOSTIC STEP TO CONSIDER IF LEVELS HIGH
Evaluation of a peripheral blood smear is recommended to evaluate the morphology of the lymphocytes. Circulating reactive lymphocytes supports a diagnosis of antigenic stimulation. These cells are a little larger than small lymphocytes with a thin rim of deeply basophilic cytoplasm and a coarser chromatin pattern. If large, atypical lymphocytes with prominent nucleoli are identified in circulation, aspiration of bone marrow or lymphoid tissue is recommended to rule out lymphoma or leukemia. Lymphocytosis from excitement or fear secondary to epinephrine release are often transient so repeating of the complete blood count (CBC) when the patient is more calm may show a resolution of the lymphocytosis.

CAUSES OF ABNORMLLY LOW LEVELS
Decreased lymphocyte numbers or lymphopenia can be seen with a stress response, viral infection, endotoxemia, overwhelming bacterial infection, and immunodeficiency. Many inflammatory diseases may also result in a stress response so it is common to see lymphopenia with an inflammatory leukon as part of a stress response. Immunodeficiency is seen most commonly in young animals. Arabian foals with severe combined immunodeficiency (SCID) lack a normal IL-2 receptor and have abnormal lymphocyte numbers and function, and may have severe lymphopenia.

NEXT DIAGNOSTIC STEP TO CONSIDER IF LEVELS LOW
Evaluation of the patient for evidence of systemic inflammatory disease and fibrinogen measurement. If the patient is an Arabian foal, genetic testing may be beneficial.

IMPORTANT INTERSPECIES DIFFERENCES
Horses have higher numbers of circulating lymphocytes than dogs and cats so a lymphopenia may be more subtle in a stress response.

DRUG EFFECTS ON LEVELS
Glucocorticoids and other immunosuppressive drugs may cause a lymphopenia.

SPECIMEN AND PROCESSING CONSIDERATIONS

SAMPLE FOR COLLECTION (TYPE OF SPECIMEN, COLOR TUBE) AND ANY SPECIAL SPECIMEN HANDLING NOTES
Whole, anticoagulated blood is necessary for evaluation. Most commonly, ethylenediamine tetraacetic acid or purple-top tubes are used for CBC; however, sodium citrate (blue-top tube) can also be used. If the blood cannot be evaluated immediately, preparation of a blood smear, to preserve the integrity of red and white blood cell morphology is recommended. Blood smear examination is essential to identify reactive and atypical lymphocytes.

PEARLS
Evaluation of lymphocyte morphology can help identify the cause of a lymphocytosis. Presence of large cells with prominent nucleoli may help identify an underlying neoplastic process such as lymphoma or leukemia.

AUTHOR: **ANNE BARGER**

EDITOR: **CHARLES WIEDMEYER**

Macrocytosis

BASIC INFORMATION

DEFINITION

A macrocyte is an erythrocyte of greater than normal size. A significant increase in macrocytes (macrocytosis) may result in an increase in the average (mean) size of a patient's erythrocytes, as determined by visual inspection of a stained blood smear and/or determination of the erythrocyte mean corpuscular volume (MCV). The MCV is measured by many hematology analyzers. It also may be calculated from a spun hematocrit value and the red blood cell (RBC) count by use of the following formula: MCV (in femtoliters, fl) = (hematocrit × 10) / RBC count (in millions).

SYNONYM(S)

Mean corpuscular volume is a synonym for mean cell volume.

TYPICAL NORMAL RANGE (US UNITS; SI UNITS)

A reported normal range for MCV in the horse is 37 to 49 fl.

PHYSIOLOGY

CAUSES OF ABNORMALLY HIGH LEVELS Mild macrocytosis may occasionally occur during regenerative anemia in horses. High-dose heparin therapy has been reported to increase the MCV, though this may be an artifact of heparin-induced agglutination of erythrocytes.

SPECIMEN AND PROCESSING CONSIDERATIONS

LAB ARTIFACTS THAT MAY INTERFERE WITH READINGS OF LEVELS OF THIS SUBSTANCE (AND HOW—ARTIFICIALLY ELEVATED VS. DEPRESSED) Agglutination of erythrocytes may cause an artifactual increase in MCV.

Agglutination may occur in association with immune-mediated destruction of erythrocytes or due to high dose heparin therapy.

AUTHOR: **MARLYN S. WHITNEY**

EDITOR: **CHARLES WIEDMEYER**

Magnesium

BASIC INFORMATION

DEFINITION

- Hypermagnesemia: Increased magnesium concentration in the blood
- Normomagnesemia: Normal magnesium concentration in the blood
- Hypomagnesemia: Decreased magnesium concentration in the blood

SYNONYM(S)

Mg^{2+}

TYPICAL NORMAL RANGE (US UNITS; SI UNITS)

Equine: 2.2 to 2.8 mEq/L; 0.91 to 1.15 mmol/L

PHYSIOLOGY

Ionized magnesium accounts for 65% to 80% of total magnesium. The remainder is bound to albumin and globulin and therefore total serum magnesium is dependent on protein concentration. Magnesium is also stored in the bones and skeletal muscles. Dietary intake is the chief source of magnesium; it is absorbed in the distal small intestine and colon and reabsorbed in the kidneys. Absorption is enhanced by vitamin D and inhibited by dietary calcium and phosphate. Magnesium is excreted in feces and by the kidneys.

CAUSES OF ABNORMALLY HIGH LEVELS

- Decreased glomerular filtration rate (GFR); dehydration, renal failure
- Intracellular fluid (ICF) to extracellular fluid (ECF) shift: Hemolysis, severe rhabdomyolysis, acidosis
- Increased absorption: $MgSO_4$/Epsom salt overdose especially in conjunction with dioctyl sodium sulfosuccinate, excessive IV administration
- Other: Systemic inflammatory response syndrome

NEXT DIAGNOSTIC STEP TO CONSIDER IF LEVELS HIGH Review history, clinical signs, complete blood count, biochemistry profile, urinalysis, and rectal examination. Blood gas analysis, urine fractional clearance

CAUSES OF ABNORMALLY LOW LEVELS

- Loss: Endurance exercise, sweating
- Decreased absorption: Undernutrition, enterocolitis, colic, diarrhea, malabsorption, IV fluids deficient in magnesium, low magnesium diet/grass tetany, hypoparathyroidism
- Redistribution: Third space loss
- Increased excretion: Gentamicin administration, loop diuretics, osmotic diuresis, ketonuria
- ECF to ICF shift: Metabolic alkalosis
- Other: Endotoxemia, renal tubular acidosis, Cantharidin toxicosis (blister beetle), lactation tetany in Shetland mares

NEXT DIAGNOSTIC STEP TO CONSIDER IF LEVELS LOW Review history, clinical signs, complete blood count, biochemistry profile, urinalysis, and rectal examination. Abdominocentesis and thoracocentesis for third space loss; blood gas analysis, urine fractional clearance of magnesium for diet assessment; measure parathyroid hormone.

DRUG EFFECTS ON LEVELS Decreased: Gentamicin, furosemide

SPECIMEN AND PROCESSING CONSIDERATIONS

LAB ARTIFACTS THAT MAY INTERFERE WITH READINGS OF LEVELS OF THIS SUBSTANCE (AND HOW—ARTIFICIALLY ELEVATED VS. DEPRESSED)

- Increased: *In vitro* hemolysis, delayed separation of serum from clot
- Decreased: Hypoproteinemia

SAMPLE FOR COLLECTION (TYPE OF SPECIMEN, COLOR TUBE) AND ANY SPECIAL SPECIMEN HANDLING NOTES

- Serum preferred. Heparinized plasma can be used. Do not use anticoagulants that bind magnesium (Mg^{2+} EDTA, citrate, or oxalate) for magnesium assays.
- Methodology: Photometry and spectrometry

AUTHORS: **LAURA V. LANE** and **THERESA E. RIZZI**

EDITOR: **CHARLES WIEDMEYER**

Microcytosis

BASIC INFORMATION

DEFINITION

Microcytosis refers to the presence in the blood of significant numbers of erythrocytes that are smaller than normal (micro-

cytes), often resulting in a decrease in the mean corpuscular volume (MCV). Microcytes may be mixed with cells of normal size on the blood smear, resulting in increased variation in erythrocyte size (anisocytosis). Anemia associated with

microcytosis may be referred to as microcytic anemia.

TYPICAL NORMAL RANGE (US UNITS; SI UNITS)

A reported normal range for MCV in the horse is 37 to 49 fl.

PHYSIOLOGY

CAUSES OF ABNORMALLY LOW MCV LEVELS Iron deficiency is the most likely cause of microcytic anemia, but iron deficiency is uncommon to rare in horses, especially adult horses. Iron deficient erythrocytes are usually also hypochromic, and poikilocytosis (variability in erythrocyte shape) may be present. Copper deficiency is a potential cause of microcytosis. During the period from 2 weeks to 3 months of age, the MCV may be lower than the reference range for adult horses.

AUTHOR: **MARLYN S. WHITNEY**

EDITOR: **CHARLES WIEDMEYER**

Monocyte (Monocytosis, Monocytopenia)

BASIC INFORMATION

DEFINITION

Monocytes are produced in the bone marrow and descend from a bipotential cell that is common to neutrophils and monocytes. These cells are similar to neutrophils in size though they may appear a little larger because their cytoplasm can spread out on a glass slide. The nucleus may vary in shape from oval to reniform to lobulated.

SYNONYM(S)

Monos

TYPICAL NORMAL RANGE (US UNITS; SI UNITS)

0.1 to 0.8 × 103/μL

PHYSIOLOGY

When monocytes exit the peripheral blood, they become tissue macrophages. Macrophages are professional antigen presenting cells and have a vital role in the innate immune response. They present antigen via MHC II to T cells. They produce many cytokines which mediate the immune response such as interferon gamma, IL-12, IL-15, IL-1, IL-6 among others. Additionally, macrophages have marked phagocytic activity for removal of dead or damaged cells and engulfment and digestion of microorganisms including bacteria as well as some fungal organisms.

CAUSES OF ABNORMALLY HIGH LEVELS Monocytosis can occur with both acute and chronic disease and can accompany a peripheral neutrophilia.

NEXT DIAGNOSTIC STEP TO CONSIDER IF LEVELS HIGH Evaluate the patient for evidence of systemic disease. Examine the peripheral blood smear to make sure the cells being counted are actually monocytes.

CAUSES OF ABNORMALLY LOW LEVELS Monocytopenia is not a clinically significant observation.

IMPORTANT INTERSPECIES DIFFERENCES Monocytosis in dogs is part of a stress response; however, this is not a consistent finding in other species.

SPECIMEN AND PROCESSING CONSIDERATIONS

LAB ARTIFACTS THAT MAY INTERFERE WITH READINGS OF LEVELS OF THIS SUBSTANCE (AND HOW—ARTIFICIALLY ELEVATED VS. DEPRESSED) Circulation of large atypical blast cells can be misidentified as monocytes by automated counters.

SAMPLE FOR COLLECTION (TYPE OF SPECIMEN, COLOR TUBE) AND ANY SPECIAL SPECIMEN HANDLING NOTES Whole, anticoagulated blood is necessary for evaluation. Most commonly, ethylenediamine tetraacetic acid or purple-top tubes are used for complete blood count (CBC); however, sodium citrate (blue-top tube) can also be used. If the blood cannot be evaluated immediately, preparation of a blood smear to preserve the integrity of red and white blood cell morphology is recommended.

AUTHOR: **ANNE BARGER**

EDITOR: **CHARLES WIEDMEYER**

Myoglobinuria

BASIC INFORMATION

DEFINITION

Myoglobinuria is the presence of myoglobin (a low molecular weight heme protein found in muscle) in the urine; it is associated with red- to amber-colored transparent urine that remains pigmented after centrifugation.

TYPICAL NORMAL RANGE (US UNITS; SI UNITS)

Not present

PHYSIOLOGY

Myoglobin is released from damaged myocytes into the plasma. It is quickly cleared through the glomerulus where it is either reabsorbed by renal tubules or excreted in the urine. Myoglobin will cause a positive blood test on a urine dipstick.

CAUSES OF ABNORMALLY HIGH LEVELS: Myopathy caused by trauma, necrosis, ischemia, or toxic injury

NEXT DIAGNOSTIC STEP TO CONSIDER IF LEFELS HIGH

- Thorough physical exam to evaluate muscle injury or necrosis
- Complete blood count (CBC) and serum biochemical panel specifically looking at creatine kinase levels and evaluating for hemolysis
- An ammonium sulfate precipitation test may differentiate myoglobinuria from hemoglobinuria but is unreliable.

SPECIMEN AND PROCESSING CONSIDERATIONS

LAB ARTIFACTS THAT MAY INTERFERE WITH READINGS OF LEVELS OF THIS SUBSTANCE (AND HOW—ARTIFICIALLY ELEVATED VS. DEPRESSED) A positive result for blood on a urine dipstick can also be due to bilirubinuria, hemoglobinuria, hematuria, or contamination of urine with oxidizing compounds (disinfectants such as bleach or iodine, or microbial or leukocyte peroxidase).

SAMPLE FOR COLLECTION (TYPE OF SPECIMEN, COLOR TUBE) AND ANY SPECIAL SPECIMEN HANDLING NOTES Samples should be refrigerated and analyzed as soon as possible.

PEARLS Generally, to differentiate myoglobinuria from hemoglobinuria and hematuria, which all have a positive blood test on a urine dipstick, evaluate the color of the supernatant after centrifugation of the urine; hematuria will have a clear supernatant, whereas hemoglobinuria and myoglobinuria will not. To differentiate hemoglobinuria from myoglobinuria, evaluate the plasma color; hemoglobinuria will have a pink to red plasma color, whereas myoglobinuria will not.

AUTHOR: **SARA A. HILL**

EDITOR: **CHARLES WIEDMEYER**

Neospora hughesi

BASIC INFORMATION

DEFINITION

- *Neospora hughesi* is a newly identified intracellular coccidian parasite that has also been implicated in causing equine protozoal myeloencephalitis (EPM) in a small percentage of horses. In comparison to *Sarcocystis neurona*, the seroprevalence to *N. hughesi* is significantly lower.
- *N. hughesi* is a separate and unique organism from *N. caninum*, although the life cycle involving the reproductive stage occurring in the intestine of the definitive host and asexual stages forming cysts in tissues of the intermediate host is believed to be similar. Currently, the definitive and intermediate hosts have yet to be identified. Small rodents are believed to potentially play a role in the life cycle of the parasite. Horses are believed to be an aberrant host.

TYPICAL NORMAL RANGE (US UNITS; SI UNITS)

There is no published reference range.

PHYSIOLOGY

As the specific life cycle is yet to be determined, the exact pathophysiology is still to be determined but is believed to be similar to *S. neurona*.

CAUSES OF ABNORMALLY HIGH LEVELS Elevations in serum antibody titer are typically due to either active infection or exposure to the etiologic agent of disease.

NEXT DIAGNOSTIC STEP TO CONSIDER IF LEVELS HIGH Therapeutic intervention directed toward treating the clinical syndrome of EPM should be initiated.

CAUSES OF ABNORMALLY LOW LEVELS Low antibody concentrations suggest lack of exposure to the causative agent of disease.

NEXT DIAGNOSTIC STEP TO CONSIDER IF LEVELS LOW Low levels suggest lack of exposure to the causative agent of disease and the need to consider other etiologic agents or pathologic processes as the source of the observed clinical disease.

SPECIMEN AND PROCESSING CONSIDERATIONS

SAMPLE FOR COLLECTION (TYPE OF SPECIMEN, COLOR TUBE) AND ANY SPECIAL SPECIMEN HANDLING NOTES Collection of whole blood in a red top tube and separation of serum is ideal. Sample can then be refrigerated or frozen and shipped to a diagnostic laboratory with a cold pack.

PEARLS Currently there are Western immunoblot (WB), enzyme-linked immunosorbent assay (ELISA), and indirect fluorescent antibody (IFA) tests available for testing for *N. hughesi*. Currently testing is only performed at specific laboratories nationwide (USA). Please contact the laboratory prior to sending samples for testing.

AUTHORS: **SHANE F. DeWITT** and **TANYA M. GRONDIN**

EDITOR: **CHARLES WIEDMEYER**

Neutrophils (Neutrophilia, Neutropenia, Bands)

BASIC INFORMATION

DEFINITION

Neutrophils are the most common white blood cells in the horse. They are of granulocytic origin and are important in bacterial infection and the innate immune response. These cells have a lobulated nucleus, usually three to four lobules, and pale basophilic cytoplasm with poorly staining granules.

SYNONYM(S)

Segmented neutrophil
Segs
Polymorphonuclear neutrophil

TYPICAL NORMAL RANGE (US UNITS; SI UNITS)

2.9 to 8.5 × 10³/mL

PHYSIOLOGY

- Neutrophils originate from myeloid precursors in the bone marrow. There are three pools of cells in the bone marrow:
  - The proliferative pool, which consists of dividing cells, myeloblasts, promyelocytes, and myelocytes
  - The maturation pool, which consists of metamyelocytes and bands
  - The storage pool, which consists of mature neutrophils and some bands. This is the first group of cells to head out into the peripheral blood when needed.
- Within the peripheral blood, there are two pools, the circulating pool and the marginating pool:
  - The circulating pool are those cells that are counted in the complete blood count (CBC).
  - The marginating pool are cells that are preparing to leave the blood and enter the tissue.
- Neutrophils respond to chemotactic signals at sites of inflammation. In response to those signals, neutrophils rearrange their cytoskeleton, marginate, roll along the endothelium, adhere, and transmigrate to the tissue.

- In the tissue, neutrophil functions include phagocytosis, enzyme secretion for tissue degradation and antimicrobial activity, activation of NADPH oxidase to generate oxygen radicals, which decreases pH and assists in intracellular microbicidal activities. They also have immunoregulatory roles and produce proinflammatory cytokines such as IL-1, IL-6, IL-8, among others.

CAUSES OF ABNORMALLY HIGH LEVELS

- Increased numbers of neutrophils or neutrophilia can occur with any time of inflammatory stimulus or glucocorticoid (stress) response.
- Basic mechanisms of neutrophilia include:
  - Increased proliferation within the bone marrow
  - Marrow storage pool shift from marrow to peripheral blood
  - Shifting of the marginating pool to the circulating pool
  - Decreased egress into the tissues
- Bacterial infection, nonseptic inflammation, tissue necrosis, and immune-mediated disorders can all result in significant neutrophilia by increasing bone marrow proliferation and release of the storage pool into the peripheral blood.
- Neutrophilia as part of a stress response occurs by shifting the marginating pool to the circulating pool and decreasing egress of neutrophils into the tissue.
- Granulocytic leukemia may cause excessive bone marrow production.

NEXT DIAGNOSTIC STEP TO CONSIDER IF LEVELS HIGH Evaluation of a peripheral blood smear is essential to evaluate for presence of toxic changes in the cytoplasm of the neutrophils (cytoplasmic basophilia, Dohle bodies, azurophilic granules, and foamy cytoplasm) and to further evaluate for the presence of a left shift or bands. Band neutrophils are less mature neutrophils that have a horseshoe-shaped or band-shaped nucleus that lacks obvious segmentation. These cells are released into the peripheral blood when the tissue demand begins to exceed neutrophil availability within the bone marrow. This indicates a severe inflammatory response.

CAUSES OF ABNORMALLY LOW LEVELS A decrease in neutrophil numbers or neutropenia can occur with a severe inflammatory response such as severe enteritis (ie, salmonellosis), endotoxemia, severe injury, or decreased production from the bone marrow secondary to cytotoxic drugs or bone marrow disease.

NEXT DIAGNOSTIC STEP TO CONSIDER IF LEVELS LOW Evaluation of the patient for evidence of systemic inflammatory disease, fibrinogen, and examination of peripheral blood smear for presence of bands or toxic changes. If no evidence of inflammation is present, bone marrow aspiration may be indicated.

DRUG EFFECTS ON LEVELS Glucocorticoids may cause a mature neutrophilia. Sulfa drugs may cause neutropenia.

SPECIMEN AND PROCESSING CONSIDERATIONS

SAMPLE FOR COLLECTION (TYPE OF SPECIMEN, COLOR TUBE) AND ANY SPECIAL SPECIMEN HANDLING NOTES Whole, anticoagulated blood is necessary for evaluation. Most commonly, ethylenediamine tetraacetic acid or purple-top tubes are used for CBC; however, sodium citrate (blue-top tube) can also be used. If the blood cannot be evaluated immediately, preparation of a blood smear to preserve the integrity of red and white blood cell morphology is recommended. Blood smear examination is essential to identify the presence of bands (left shift) and toxic changes.

PEARLS Elevated fibrinogen is often a more sensitive indicator of inflammation in horses. Changes in the CBC are often subtle. Presence of bands in the peripheral blood is a significant finding.

AUTHOR: **ANNE BARGER**

EDITOR: **CHARLES WIEDMEYER**

Normal Indices for Cerebrospinal Fluid

Parameter	Levels
Color	Clear
Total protein (mg/dL)	AO = 62
	LS = 77
Glucose	80% of blood glucose
PH	7.34–7.4
WBC count (cells/μL)	<5
RBC count (cells/μL)	0–100
Creatinine kinase (IU/L)	4–24
Sodium (mmol/L)	140–145
Potassium (mmol/L)	2.5–5.1
Chloride (mmol/L)	106–112

AO, atlanto-occipital; *LS*, lumbosacral.

AUTHOR: **MAUREEN T. LONG**

EDITOR: **CHARLES WIEDMEYER**

Parathyroid Hormone (PTH)

BASIC INFORMATION

DEFINITION

- Hyperparathormonemia: Increased circulating concentration of parathyroid hormone
- Hypoparathormonemia: Decreased circulating concentration of parathyroid hormone

SYNONYM(S)

Parathormone

TYPICAL NORMAL RANGE (US UNITS; SI UNITS)

Less than 4.0 pmol/L or 40 pg/mL

PHYSIOLOGY

PTH is a polypeptide hormone secreted by the parathyroid gland that regulates the metabolism of calcium and phosphorus in the body. PTH acts on parathyroid hormone receptor in bones, the kidneys, and small intestine to regulate serum calcium concentration. In bone, PTH binds directly to osteoblasts, which stimulates them to increase their expression of receptor activator of nuclear factor kappa B ligand (RANKL), which can bind to osteoclast precursors containing RANK. The binding of RANKL to RANK stimulates these precursors to fuse, forming new osteoclasts which ultimately enhance the resorption of bone, resulting in increased serum calcium concentration. In the kidney, PTH enhances active reabsorption of calcium from the distal tubules and the thick ascending limb of the loop of Henle. Additionally, PTH upregulates 25-hydroxyvitamin D3 1-alpha-hydroxylase, the enzyme responsible for 1-alpha hydroxylation of 25-hydroxy vitamin D, converting vitamin D to its active form. This activated form of vitamin D affects the absorption of calcium in the intestine via calbindin. PTH is inactivated and degraded by the kidneys and liver. Increased concentrations of vitamin D and free calcium inhibit synthesis of PTH.

CAUSES OF ABNORMALLY HIGH LEVELS Increased circulating concentrations are typically due to increased production of PTH by either neoplastic cells or nonneoplastic parathyroid gland hyperplasia.

NEXT DIAGNOSTIC STEP TO CONSIDER IF LEVELS HIGH If neoplasia is suspected, imaging of the gland via ultrasound or radioisotope labeled nuclear scintigraphy would be indicated. In cases of suspected hyperplasia, serum biochemistry and dietary calcium intake should be evaluated to assess renal status and calcium balance.

CAUSES OF ABNORMALLY LOW LEVELS Decreased circulating concentrations of PTH are primarily due to either direct damage to the parathyroid glands or inhibition of PTH production due to hypervitaminosis D or nonparathyroid, hypercalcemic disorders (neoplasia producing parathyroid hormone related protein [PTHrp]).

NEXT DIAGNOSTIC STEP TO CONSIDER IF LEVELS LOW If decreased concentration is due to suspected damage to the gland, imaging of the gland via ultrasound or radioisotope labeled nuclear scintigraphy would be indicated. If the decreased concentration is due to suspected inhibition, serum concentrations of vitamin D and PTHrp should be determined.

SPECIMEN AND PROCESSING CONSIDERATIONS

LAB ARTIFACTS THAT MAY INTERFERE WITH READINGS OF LEVELS OF THIS SUBSTANCE (AND HOW—ARTIFICIALLY ELEVATED VS. DEPRESSED) Prolonged storage or delay between collection and processing may result in artificially decreased concentrations of PTH.

SAMPLE FOR COLLECTION (TYPE OF SPECIMEN, COLOR TUBE) AND ANY SPECIAL SPECIMEN HANDLING NOTES A whole blood sample collected in an ethylenediamine tetraacetic acid (EDTA, purple top) tube containing a protease inhibitor (aprotinin) is preferred as PTH is susceptible to proteolysis. Plasma or serum promptly separated from the cell mass and frozen for storage and transit is also acceptable.

PEARLS Serum total calcium and free ionized calcium concentrations should also be known when interpreting the serum PTH concentration.

AUTHORS: **SHANE F. DEWITT** and **TANYA M. GRONDIN**

EDITOR: **CHARLES WIEDMEYER**

Passive Transfer

BASIC INFORMATION

DEFINITION

- Measurement of the antibody (IgG) concentrations in the neonate to determine if adequate absorption of maternal antibodies has occurred following ingestion of colostrum.
- The radial immunodiffusion assay (RID) is considered to be the most accurate method for quantitative assessment of plasma IgG concentrations in foals. However, RID assay results typically have a 24-hour turnaround time, making them clinically impractical for critically ill foals.
- Most clinics utilize semiquantitative foal-side tests including turbidimetric immunoassays, latex agglutination tests, enzyme immunoassays, zinc sulfate turbidity tests, and glutaraldehyde coagulation tests. Though rapid and clinically applicable, these tests appear to be less reliable than the RID assay.

SYNONYM(S)

Neonatal immunoglobulin (IgG) levels

TYPICAL NORMAL RANGE (US UNITS; SI UNITS)

- Most foal-side tests are semiquantitative.
- <200 mg/dL = complete failure of passive transfer
- <400 mg/dL = failure of passive transfer
- 400 to 800 mg/dL = partial failure of passive transfer
- >800 mg/dL = adequate passive transfer

PHYSIOLOGY

Transplacental transfer of antibodies does not occur in horses and cattle.

These animals rely on immunoglobulin-rich colostrum in the early post-partum period. Failure of passive transfer (FPT) occurs when foals fail to consume or absorb sufficient amounts of colostrum during this critical period. Alternatively, FPT may occur if the mare produces poor quality colostrum or if colostrum is lost through premature leakage of milk. In the foal, specialized enterocytes responsible for immunoglobulin absorption are present within the small intestine. Immunoglobulin absorption is greatest in the first 6 to 8 hours of life. Absorption ceases at 24 to 36 hours as the specialized enterocytes are replaced by normal gastrointestinal epithelial cells. Because of the narrow window for colostrum absorption, IgG level testing at 8 to 12 hours is recommended. Tests performed during this window allow for oral supplementation with colostrum or a colostrum substitute in time for gastrointestinal absorption. Postsupplement IgG testing is recommended. Foals with FPT due to malabsorption of colostrum or identification after the 24- to 36-hour time period may require intravenous supplementation.

CAUSES OF ABNORMALLY LOW LEVELS
- Poor colostral quality in the mare (low IgG levels; <1000 mg/dL)
- Inadequate consumption of maternal colostrum: Inability or lack of desire to nurse in the foal and foal rejection by mare
- Premature lactation or milk loss in the mare
- Gastrointestinal malabsorption of ingested colostrum in the foal

IMPORTANT INTERSPECIES DIFFERENCES
- Foals have virtually no IgG in their plasma prior to colostrum ingestion. Calves, however, may have very low concentrations without ingesting colostrum. Reference intervals for failure of passive transfer have not been firmly established in calves. General guidelines for calves are:
  - >1000 mg/dL = evidence of passive transfer
  - <500 mg/dL = evidence of complete failure of passive transfer

SPECIMEN AND PROCESSING CONSIDERATIONS

LAB ARTIFACTS THAT MAY INTERFERE WITH READINGS OF LEVELS OF THIS SUBSTANCE (AND HOW—ARTIFICIALLY ELEVATEAD VS. DEPRESSED) Artifactual changes depend on the methodology utilized. Lipemia and hemolysis may falsely increase IgG levels if turbidity is measured via spectrophotometry. Additionally, zinc sulfate tests may underestimate IgG levels if they are greater than 400 mg/dL.

SAMPLE FOR COLLECTION (TYPE OF SPECIMEN, COLOR TUBE) AND ANY SPECIAL SPECIMEN HANDLING NOTES Most foal-side tests require either plasma (purple top) or serum (red top); whole blood (purple top) may also be utilized for some tests.

PEARLS
- Assessment of failure of passive transfer is best performed early (8–12 hours after birth) to allow for early intervention and proper medical management.
- Foal-side tests allow for rapid, semiquantitative assessment of IgG levels. IgG levels greater than 800 mg/dL are generally considered to be adequate.

AUTHOR: **LAURA ANN SNYDER**

EDITOR: **CHARLES WIEDMEYER**

Peritoneal Fluid Analysis

BASIC INFORMATION

DEFINITION
Complete peritoneal fluid analysis consists of determination of the fluid's physical characteristics (color, clarity, sample volume), total protein as estimated by a refractometer, nucleated cell concentration, red blood cell concentration, and the microscopic examination of direct and/or concentrated fluid slides. Additional tests are sometimes indicated.

TYPICAL NORMAL RANGE (US UNITS; SI UNITS)
- Normal peritoneal fluid is clear and watery. In horses, even normal animals will have enough peritoneal fluid volume for sample collection.
- Total protein is normally <2.5 g/dL. Nucleated cell concentration is usually <5,000/μL but can vary, with some normal horses reported as having up to 10,000/μL. The nucleated cells are predominantly neutrophils, fewer large mononuclear cells/macrophages, and even fewer mature lymphocytes.

Packed cell volume (PCV) of the fluid will be <1%.

PHYSIOLOGY
Peritoneal fluid is an ultrafiltrate of plasma, which serves as a lubricant around abdominal organs and allows the diffusion of electrolytes and other substances to and from the serosal surfaces of the abdominal cavity. This fluid is normally removed from the peritoneal cavity by lymphatics in proportion to the rate of production.

CAUSES OF ABNORMALLY HIGH LEVELS
- Increased peritoneal fluid volume, cell counts, and total protein can be seen for many different reasons. Increased plasma hydrostatic pressure, decreased plasma colloidal pressure, enteritis, rupture of a visceral organ, tissue ischemia/necrosis, neoplasia, lymphatic obstruction, or intraabdominal hemorrhage can increase all of these parameters to differing degrees.
- In general, effusions with the highest nucleated cell counts and total protein concentrations (exudates) will be seen

with inflammation related to gastrointestinal (GI) perforation or some nonseptic types of peritonitis, tissue necrosis/ischemia, or lymphatic obstruction related to neoplasia or inflammation.
- Effusions with lower cell counts and total proteins (transudates to modified transudates) can be seen as a result of hypoalbuminemia, congestive heart failure, portal hypertension, uroperitoneum, or neoplasia.
- The presence of red blood cells indicates either true pathologic hemorrhage or iatrogenic blood contamination. In slides prepared from fresh samples, the presence of erythrophagocytosis and sometimes hemosiderin-laden macrophages are evidence of true hemorrhage into the abdominal cavity.
- With effusions of any nature, reactive mesothelial cells are commonly found in peritoneal fluid samples. These can appear quite dysplastic, and in some cases these cells cannot be reliably differentiated from neoplastic cells.

- Occasionally enterocentesis occurs, in which gut contents themselves are sampled. These preparations will contain large numbers of bacteria, possibly GI protozoa, and digesta particles. It is important to note that intracellular bacteria should not be found, and the number of leukocytes present is often very low.

NEXT DIAGNOSTIC STEP TO CONSIDER IF LEVELS HIGH

- Bacterial culture and sensitivity are warranted anytime suppurative inflammation and/or an exudate are present. Bacterial culture is a more sensitive means of diagnosing bacterial peritonitis than simply looking for bacteria on a fluid smear.
- In suspected uroperitoneum cases, peritoneal fluid creatinine can be determined and compared to that of the plasma or serum. With acute bladder rupture, peritoneal fluid creatinine to blood creatinine ratio is often >2:1.
- Peritoneal fluid glucose concentrations <40 mg/dL (in fresh samples) or a difference of >50 mg/dL between glucose concentration of serum/plasma and peritoneal fluid are suggestive of but not definitive for septic peritonitis.

SPECIMEN AND PROCESSING CONSIDERATIONS

SAMPLE FOR COLLECTION (TYPE OF SPECIMEN, COLOR TUBE) AND ANY SPECIAL SPECIMEN HANDLING NOTES Ideally at least 3 mL of peritoneal fluid should be collected. The sample can be split between an EDTA purple-top tube for cell counts and cytologic evaluation, a red-top (clot) tube for culture and biochemical analysis as deemed necessary, and transport media for culture if desired. It is essential to prepare one or more direct smears ± concentrated smears of the peritoneal fluid as soon as possible after sample collection. These slides should be air-dried and submitted as is to a laboratory or stained with a Romanowsky-type stain (like Diff-Quik or Wright's-Giemsa) for in-house evaluation. All fluid submissions should be mailed overnight to a laboratory on ice, but not frozen, and packaged to prevent tube or slide breakage. Pertinent history and signalment should always be included.

PEARLS

- Fluid smears should be prepared as soon as possible after sample collection to include with fluid submission to a laboratory. If smears are not prepared quickly, *in vitro* phagocytosis of red blood cells or potentially bacterial contaminants can occur and would thus alter the interpretation of the fluid cytology.
- Fluid samples should be shipped to a laboratory overnight, on ice but not frozen.
- Enterocentesis can be distinguished from septic peritonitis by the lack of intracellular bacteria and typically low numbers of leukocytes found in enterocentesis samples.

AUTHOR: **ANGELA B. ROYAL**

EDITOR: **CHARLES WIEDMEYER**

Phosphorus

BASIC INFORMATION

DEFINITION

- Hyperphosphatemia: Increased phosphorous concentration in the blood
- Normophosphatemia: Normal phosphorous concentration in the blood
- Hypophosphatemia: Decreased phosphorous concentration in the blood

TYPICAL NORMAL RANGE (US UNITS; SI UNITS)

3.1 to 5.6 mEq/L; 1.00 to 1.81 mmol/L

PHYSIOLOGY

Organic phosphorous is found intracellularly, primarily as phospholipid. Inorganic phosphorous is found extracellularly complexed with cations and bound to protein. Phosphorous is primarily found in the skeleton bound to calcium as hydroxyapatite. It is the primary form of energy storage and transfer of adenosine triphosphate, adenosine diphosphate, adenosine monophosphate. Phosphorous in the extracellular fluid exists as a buffer pair $H_2PO_4^-$ and HPO_4^{2-} and plays a role in acid base balance. It is regulated by dietary factors, active metabolites of vitamin D, parathormone, and calcitonin. It is absorbed in the small and large intestines and reabsorbed/excreted by the kidneys.

CAUSES OF ABNORMALLY HIGH LEVELS

- Decreased urinary excretion: Decreased glomerular filtration rate (GFR) due to dehydration, acute renal failure, uroperitoneum, hypoparathyroidism
- Increased absorption: Increased ingestion, hypervitaminosis D, ischemic intestinal lesions
- Intracellular (ICF) to extracellular fluid (ECF) shift: Endurance exercise, acute rhabdomyolysis, hemolysis, tumor necrosis
- Other: Lactic acidosis

NEXT DIAGNOSTIC STEP TO CONSIDER IF LEVELS HIGH: Review history, clinical signs, complete blood count, biochemistry profile, urinalysis, and rectal examination. Abdominocentesis for uroperitoneum, imaging, blood gas analysis, urine fractional clearance of phosphorus for renal disease, measure parathyroid hormone concentration, measure vitamin D concentration

CAUSES OF ABNORMALLY LOW LEVELS

- Increased excretion: Chronic renal failure, acute renal failure, diuresis, hyperparathyroidism
- Decreased absorption: Decreased dietary intake, starvation, malabsorption

- ECF to ICF shift: Parenteral nutrition/increased glucose and insulin, respiratory alkalosis
- Other: Brassica toxicity, sepsis, hypercalcemia of malignancy, halothane anesthesia

NEXT DIAGNOSTIC STEP TO CONSIDER IF LEVELS LOW:

- Review history, clinical signs, complete blood count, biochemistry profile, urinalysis, and rectal examination. Blood gas analysis, urine fractional clearance for renal disease, imaging for primary tumor, measure parathyroid hormone

SPECIMEN AND PROCESSING CONSIDERATIONS

LAB ARTIFACTS THAT MAY INTERFERE WITH READINGS OF LEVELS OF THIS SUBSTANCE (AND HOW—ARTIFICIALLY ELEVATED VS. DEPRESSED)

- Increased: *In vitro* hemolysis, delayed removal of serum from clot, hyperbilirubinemia, and monoclonal gammopathies
- Decreased: Hyperbilirubinemia

SAMPLE FOR COLLECTION (TYPE OF SPECIMEN, COLOR TUBE) AND ANY SPECIAL SPECIMEN HANDLING NOTES

- Serum preferred, plasma can be used.
- Methodology: Photometry

AUTHORS: **LAURA V. LANE** and **THERESA E. RIZZI**

EDITOR: **CHARLES WIEDMEYER**

PEARLS

- Higher levels may normally be seen in juveniles.
- Acute hypophosphatemia can lead to intravascular hemolysis.

Platelets

BASIC INFORMATION

DEFINITION

- Thrombocytopenia/thrombopenia: Low number of circulating platelets
- Thrombocytosis/thrombocythemia: Increased number of circulating platelets
- Thrombopathia/thrombocytopathia: Abnormal platelet function, often in the presence of a normal platelet number

TYPICAL NORMAL RANGE (US UNITS; SI UNITS)

117,000 to 256,000/μL with no reported variation between breeds

PHYSIOLOGY

Platelets are made by megakaryocytes in the bone marrow, spleen, and lung. They are small, anuclear, discoid fragments of megakaryocyte cytoplasm that are sheared off during thrombopoiesis, rather than formed through stepwise mitosis. Their main function is in primary hemostasis, where they adhere to the site of vascular injury through interaction with von Willebrand factor (vWF) and various glycoprotein receptors. Once initial adhesion occurs, platelets bridge fibrinogen via exposed GP IIb-IIIa receptors and form a platelet plug. After the platelet plug is formed, a conformational change occurs, causing release of the platelet α and β granules, which contain various vasoactive compounds, clotting factors, and cytokines, thus promoting both the clotting and inflammatory cascades. As they also release numerous growth factors, platelets play a crucial role in wound healing. Equine platelets are typically smaller, paler staining, and more uniform, compared to those of other domestic species.

CAUSES OF ABNORMALLY HIGH LEVELS

- Physiologic (excitement causing splenic contraction)
- Primary thrombocytosis (rare myeloproliferative disorder, sometimes secondary to megakaryocytic leukemia)
- Secondary thrombocytosis (due to increased platelet production following cytokine release with inflammation, infection, anemia, leukopenia, and/or neoplasia or due to decreased removal by macrophages with excessive glucocorticoids)

NEXT DIAGNOSTIC STEP TO CONSIDER IF LEVELS HIGH

- Examine blood smear to confirm the increase
- Repeat complete blood count (CBC) in several hours (physiologic thrombocytosis is transient)
- Look for signs of inflammation on CBC (ie, neutrophilia with left shift, increased fibrinogen, increased globulins), along with signs of anemia or leukopenia
- If no explanation is apparent, consider primary thrombocytosis and examine bone marrow

CAUSES OF ABNORMALLY LOW LEVELS

- Decreased production
  - Immune-mediated with antibodies against megakaryocytes
  - Bone marrow hypoplasia secondary to certain drugs (estrogens), chemicals, mycotoxins, plant toxins (bracken fern), exposure to ionizing radiation
  - Myelophthisis
  - Equine infectious anemia (EIA) may directly infect and destroy hematopoietic cells
  - Hereditary bone marrow hypoplasia—familial in some Standardbreds
- Increased consumption (acute, severe hemorrhage or inflammation, disseminated intravascular coagulation [DIC])
- Increased destruction
  - Primary and secondary immune-mediated thrombocytopenia, sometimes secondary to heparin
  - DIC
  - Neoplasia
  - Idiopathic thrombocytopenic purpura
  - Potomac Horse fever (formerly Ehrlichiosis) reportedly causes decreased numbers via all of these mechanisms

Causes of Platelet Dysfunction (Thrombopathia/Thrombocytopathia)

- Hereditary/congenital problems with binding, granule release, and/or granule contents
  - Decreased prothrombinase in Thoroughbreds
  - Decreased GPIIb causing Glanzmann's thrombasthenia
  - Decreased adhesion factors (ie, von Willebrand's disease)
- Acquired inhibition/dysfunction
  - Nonsteroidal antiinflammatory drugs (NSAIDs) (COX-1 inhibitors)
  - Some calcium-channel blockers
  - Uremia
  - Hepatic cirrhosis
  - Leukemias
  - Crotalid envenomation

NEXT DIAGNOSTIC STEP TO CONSIDER IF LEVELS LOW

- Evaluate blood smear to confirm the decrease, making sure there are no blood parasites (ie, *Onchocerca cervicalis* microfilaria whose cuticle has been shown to induce platelet aggregation) or large platelet clumps at the feathered edge
- If no cause is evident, repeat the sample making sure there is clean venipuncture, adequate blood volume to anticoagulant ratio, and proper mixing of the sample prior to analysis
- Thorough history to exclude exposure to certain drugs (estrogens) and toxic plants (bracken fern)
- CBC and other diagnostics to look for infectious agents
- Coagulation profile to evaluate for bleeding and DIC
- If no explanation is apparent, evaluate bone marrow
- Next diagnostic step to consider if platelet dysfunction is suspected:
  - Repeat CBC and evaluate blood smear to confirm adequate platelet numbers
  - Exclude factor deficiencies with prothrombin time (PT), partial thromboplastin time (PTT)
  - If NSAID interference is suspected, withdraw the drug and repeat sampling after 48 hours
  - If no other cause of bleeding is evident, can do in-house platelet function tests (ie, buccal mucosal bleeding time)
  - Likely will require vWF assay, platelet aggregometry, and/or flow cytometry at a specialized laboratory for platelet function analysis

DRUG EFFECTS ON LEVELS
- Thrombocytosis: Corticosteroids (through splenic contraction)
- Thrombocytopenia: Chloramphenicol, sulfadiazine, estrogen, phenylbutazone, heparin (through a first exposure immune response)
- Thrombopathia: NSAIDs (COX-1 inhibitors), some calcium channel blockers

SPECIMEN AND PROCESSING CONSIDERATIONS

LAB ARTIFACTS THAT MAY INTERFERE WITH READINGS OF LEVELS OF THIS SUBSTANCE (AND HOW—ARTIFICIALLY ELEVATED VS. DEPESSED)
- False increases: Small particles (ie, lipid droplets or red blood cell [RBC] fragments) in circulation

- False decreases: Clumping, particularly in heparinized samples, tissue contamination during blood collection, increased platelet volume

SAMPLE FOR COLLECTION (TYPE OF SPECIMEN, COLOR TUBE) AND ANY SPECIAL SPECIMEN HANDLING NOTES
- EDTA (purple top) preferred; citrate (blue top) also acceptable
- Minimize tissue contamination and excessive trauma when collecting sample, to minimize clumping
- Ensure adequate blood to anticoagulant ratio and proper sample mixing

PEARLS

Consider thrombopathia if buccal mucosal bleeding time is prolonged, in the presence of normal platelet count and coagulation profile (PT, PTT). Be sure to exclude drug-induced platelet dysfunction prior to expensive, time-consuming platelet function testing.

AUTHOR: **MELINDA S. CAMUS**

EDITOR: **CHARLES WIEDMEYER**

Polymerase Chain Reaction (PCR)

BASIC INFORMATION

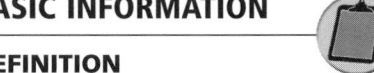

DEFINITION

PCR is a testing method that copies and amplifies the target nucleic acid (RNA or DNA) sequence. This method allows for the detection of very small amounts of the target organism by creating millions of copies, which are then able to be visually detected.

SYNONYM(S)

RT-PCR, TaqMan PCR, Real-time PCR are all variations.

TYPICAL NORMAL RANGE (US UNITS; SI UNITS)

Results are typically reported as positive or negative. Any positive means that the organism in question is present.

PHYSIOLOGY

IMPORTANT INTERSPECIES DIFFERENCES: PCR tests for the pathogen itself so the species of sample origin is not normally a factor.

SPECIMEN AND PROCESSING CONSIDERATIONS

LAB ARTIFACTS THAT MAY INTERFERE WITH READINGS OF LEVELS OF THIS SUBSTANCE (AND HOW—ARTIFICIALLY ELEVATED VS. DEPRESSED) Recent vaccination (within several weeks for tissue samples), especially with a modified live vaccine may

result in that organism being detected by PCR. PCR detects nucleic acid not intact organisms so noninfectious organisms may be detected, for example bacteria already killed by antibiotics. Inhibitors in certain sample types may cause false-negative results.

SAMPLE FOR COLLECTION (TYPE OF SPECIMEN, COLOR TUBE) AND ANY SPECIAL SPECIMEN HANDLING NOTES
- The type of sample required for PCR is based on the organ system affected.
- For enteric diseases (including *Clostridium, Salmonella, Lawsonia,* rotavirus, and *Neorickettsia risticii*—Potomac horse fever), fecal samples should be submitted. For the best chance of a successful diagnosis, small samples from 2 to 3 days should be sent as shedding can be intermittent.
- For respiratory diseases (including *Rhodococcus equi, Streptococcus equi,* strangles, influenza, and equine herpesvirus types 1 and 4), nasal swabs or transtracheal wash in combination with a blood sample in a purple-top tube (ethylenediamine tetraacetic acid anticoagulated blood) is the best sample submission. Local laboratories may have preferences on the type of swab used for nasal swab collection.
- For neurologic diseases (including West Nile virus, eastern equine encephalitis, western equine encephalitis), the preferred sample is brain or spinal fluid, which generally speaking

are used postmortem. A purple-top tube of whole blood can be used antemortem; however, the assays are much less sensitive when using blood samples. Regardless of the sample type they should be kept cold and shipped overnight on cold packs.

PEARLS
- PCR detects the presence of the organism being tested for, not just exposure, and can be helpful as a follow-up test to a positive serology result.
- The sensitivity of PCR can result in false positives, by picking up the presence of an organism in the environment or detecting a recent modified live vaccination. Nucleic acid sequencing can sometimes be used to determine if vaccine or a field strain is being detected.
- A differentiating real-time PCR assay for the EHV1 neurologic form has been developed; this is a special type of PCR that detects very small genetic changes between the two forms.
- The significance of a positive PCR must be interpreted alongside clinical observations. For example, most horses will have EHV1 but only a small percentage will develop clinically relevant disease. This must be considered when using PCR as a screening tool to determine health of animal for movement or purchase.

AUTHOR: **SUSAN SCHOMMER**

EDITOR: **CHARLES WIEDMEYER**

Polymerase Chain Reaction (PCR) Methods for Infectious and Genetic Diseases

Technique	Description	What Is a Positive Test	Advantage	Disadvantage
Conventional PCR	Basic amplification of target that is part of the genome originating from DNA	Gel-based test that in most laboratories is based on analysis of correct target by size only May be inherently inaccurate depending on system	Faster than culture of organism Does not require live organism in most cases	Slow and less sensitive than real-time Less automation available May be less specific if analysis of end product not performed
Conventional reverse transcription (rt) PCR	Basic amplification of target that is part of the genome originating from RNA An extra step is utilized before PCR, where a viral reverse transcription enzyme transcribes the RNA into cDNA for amplification.	Gel-based test that in most laboratories is based on analysis of correct target by size only May be inherently inaccurate depending on system	Faster than culture of organism Does not require live organism in most cases	Slow and less sensitive than real-time Less automation available May be less specific if analysis of end product not performed
Real-time PCR	Still basic PCR amplification, but coupled to a fluorochrome and light detection system The target is DNA.	The use of a probe in addition to primers provides specificity within the assay.	Very fast analysis Same cycle number is more sensitive than conventional PCR but still may be less sensitive than nested PCR. More specific because of probe that binds to generated target	Still can have contamination issues May have false-positive issues due to high sensitivity
Real-time reverse transcription (rt) PCR	Still basic PCR amplification, but coupled to a fluorochrome and light detection system The target is RNA where a viral reverse transcription enzyme transcribes the RNA into cDNA for PCR amplification.	The use of a probe in addition to primers provides specificity within the assay	Very fast analysis Same cycle number is more sensitive than conventional PCR More specific because of probe that binds to generated target	Still can have contamination issues May have false-positive issues due to high sensitivity

AUTHOR: **MAUREEN T. LONG**

EDITOR: **CHARLES WIEDMEYER**

Potassium

BASIC INFORMATION

DEFINITION

- Hyperkalemia: Increased potassium concentration in the blood
- Normokalemia: Normal potassium concentration in the blood
- Hypokalemia: Decreased potassium concentration in the blood

SYNONYM(S)

K$^+$

TYPICAL NORMAL RANGE (US UNITS; SI UNITS)

2.4 to 4.7 mEq/L; 2.4 to 4.7 mmol/L

PHYSIOLOGY

Potassium is critical for many biochemical cellular reactions. It is ingested daily and renal excretion is regulated by aldosterone. Potassium is also lost in feces and sweat. Most of the body's potassium is found intracellularly. Serum (extracellular) potassium is less than 2% of the whole body potassium.

CAUSES OF ABNORMALLY HIGH LEVELS

- Shift from intracellular fluid (ICF) to extracellular fluid (ECF): Metabolic acidosis, hyperkalemic periodic paralysis (HYPP) in Quarter Horses, vigorous exercise, muscle damage, severe cellular damage/tissue necrosis, intravascular hemolysis, and diabetes mellitus

- Decreased excretion: Renal insufficiency or failure, uroperitoneum, angiotensin-converting enzyme (ACE) inhibitors, Trimethoprim, hypoaldosteronism, hypoadrenocorticism
- Increased absorption: Administration of potassium-rich fluids

NEXT DIAGNOSTIC STEP TO CONSIDER IF LEVELS HIGH: Review history, clinical signs, complete blood count, biochemistry profile, urinalysis, and rectal examination. Abdominocentesis and fluid creatinine concentration for uroperitoneum, imaging, blood gas analysis, urine fractional clearance of potassium for renal disease, electromyography or DNA blood test for HYPP, adrenocorticotropic hormone (ACTH) stimulation test for hypoadrenocorticism

CAUSES OF ABNORMALLY LOW LEVELS

- Shift from ECF to ICF: Acute metabolic alkalosis, administration of insulin and/or glucose, endotoxemia
- Decreased absorption: Dietary deficiency, prolonged anorexia
- Increased excretion/loss/sequestration: Diarrhea, excessive sweating/salivation, peritonitis, furosemide or thiazide administration, post urethral obstruction diuresis, excessive and rapid bicarbonate administration, ketonuria, lactaturia, bicarbonaturia, renal tubular acidosis, hyperaldosteronism, ileus, torsion, volvulus
- Other: Endogenous release or exogenous administration of catecholamines

NEXT DIAGNOSTIC STEP TO CONSIDER IF LEVELS LOW Review history, clinical signs, complete blood count, biochemistry profile, urinalysis, and rectal examination. Urinary fractional clearance for whole body deficiency, abdominocentesis for peritonitis, blood gas analysis, measurement of aldosterone concentration

DRUG EFFECTS ON LEVELS

- Increase: Trimethoprim
- Decrease: Thiazide diuretics, furosemide

SPECIMEN AND PROCESSING CONSIDERATIONS

LAB ARTIFACTS THAT MAY INTERFERE WITH READINGS OF LEVELS OF THIS SUBSTANCE (AND HOW—ARTIFICIALLY ELEVATED VS. DEPRESSED)

- Increase: *In vitro* hemolysis, delayed serum separation from clot, leukocytosis, thrombocytosis
- Serum potassium will be slightly higher than plasma potassium due to platelet release of potassium during clotting.

SAMPLE FOR COLLECTION (TYPE OF SPECIMEN, COLOR TUBE) AND ANY SPECIAL SPECIMEN HANDLING NOTES

- Serum preferred. Do not use K3EDTA tubes.
- Methodology: Potentiometry and flame photometry

PEARLS

- Hypokalemia may only become apparent as fluids and electrolyte losses are replaced.
- Decreased dietary intake plus loss equals marked hypokalemia.
- Hypokalemia may not correlate or predict whole body potassium deficiency.
- Consider the acid-base status when interpreting abnormal potassium concentrations (movement of potassium between intracellular and extracellular compartments). If the acid-base status is normal, then serum potassium tends to reflect total body potassium.

AUTHORS: **LAURA V. LANE** and **THERESA E. RIZZI**

EDITOR: **CHARLES WIEDMEYER**

Potomac Horse Fever (PHF)

BASIC INFORMATION

DEFINITION

- An acute enterocolitis syndrome producing mild colic, fever, and diarrhea in horses
- Caused by Neorickettsia risticii (formerly Ehrlichia risticii), a gram-negative coccus.
- First recognized in 1979 along the Potomac River in Maryland and has subsequently been diagnosed worldwide.
- *N. risticii* is often found in membrane lined vacuoles within the cytoplasm of macrophages and glandular epithelial cells of the large intestine. Although commonly found in the cytoplasm, it is rarely visualized on peripheral blood smears.

SYNONYM(S)

Equine monocytic ehrlichiosis (EME), equine ehrlichial colitis

TYPICAL NORMAL RANGE (US UNITS; SI UNITS)

There are no published reference intervals for serology. A fourfold increase in titers between acute and convalescent blood samples is required for definitive diagnosis.

PHYSIOLOGY

Once *N. risticii* gains access to the host, it infects blood monocytes. Despite being actively phagocytized, the organism evades the monocytes natural defense mechanisms by inhibiting lysosomal fusion with phagosomes. The resultant clinical syndrome of diarrhea is believed to be due to loss of epithelial cell microvilli, reduction in electrolyte transport, and increased intracellular cyclic adenosine monophosphate in infected cells.

CAUSES OF ABNORMALLY HIGH LEVELS Elevations in serum antibody titer are typically due to either active infection or exposure to the etiologic agent of disease.

NEXT DIAGNOSTIC STEP TO CONSIDER IF LEVELS HIGH Therapeutic intervention directed toward treating the clinical syndrome of PHF should be initiated.

CAUSES OF ABNORMALLY LOW LEVELS Low antibody concentrations suggest lack of exposure to the causative agent of disease.

NEXT DIAGNOSTIC STEP TO CONSIDER IF LEVELS LOW Low levels suggest lack of exposure to the causative agent of disease and the need to consider other etiologic agents or pathologic processes as the source of the observed clinical disease.

SPECIMEN AND PROCESSING CONSIDERATIONS

SAMPLE FOR COLLECTION (TYPE OF SPECIMEN, COLOR TUBE) AND ANY SPECIAL SPECIMEN HANDLING NOTES Collection of whole blood in a red-top tube and separation of serum is ideal. Sample can then be refrigerated or frozen and shipped to a diagnostic laboratory with a cold pack.

PEARLS

- Serologic testing relies on either an enzyme-linked immunosorbent assay (ELISA) or indirect fluorescent antibody (IFA) titer. Both are of limited value as antibody concentrations are often not detectable for a prolonged period of time after the onset of clinical disease. Subsequently, paired serum samples to evaluate both an acute and convalescent titer are an absolute requirement for serologic diagnosis. Concern over the specificity of the IFA further complicates interpreting test results.
- Ideally, diagnosis should be based on isolation or detection of the organism from blood or feces. Visualization of the organism on a peripheral blood smear occurs rarely. Culture of the organism from cell culture is not routinely available and is time consuming. Recent development of polymerase

chain reaction (PCR) assays have decreased the turnaround time on diagnosis.

AUTHORS: **SHANE F. DeWITT** and **TANYA M. GRONDIN**

EDITOR: **CHARLES WIEDMEYER**

Progesterone

BASIC INFORMATION

DEFINITION

- Hyperprogesteronemia: Increased circulating concentration of progesterone
- Hypoprogesteronemia: Decreased circulating concentration of progesterone

TYPICAL NORMAL RANGE (US UNITS; SI UNITS)

For pregnant mares: 2.5 to 4 ng/mL

PHYSIOLOGY

- Progesterone, or 4-pregnene-3,20-dione, is a steroid hormone involved in the female reproductive cycle, pregnancy, and embryogenesis. It is synthesized from pregnenolone, a derivative of cholesterol, under the action of cholesterol side chain cleavage enzyme and 3-beta-hydroxysteroid dehydrogenase. Progesterone is also the precursor of the mineralocorticoid aldosterone and, after conversion to 17-hydroxyprogesterone, cortisol and androstenedione. Androstenedione can additionally be further modified to testosterone, estrone, and estradiol.
- Progesterone exerts its action primarily through the intracellular progesterone receptor. Once bound to the receptor, the complex translocates to the nucleus and binds directly to specific nucleotide sequences of the chromosomal DNA, altering transcriptional activity of certain genes. Additionally, progesterone has a number of physiologic effects that are amplified in the presence of estrogen. Estrogen, through estrogen receptors, upregulates the expression of progesterone receptors.
- The most important role for progesterone is involved with maintenance of pregnancy. In the pregnant mare, progesterone is produced from the primary corpus luteum until approximately day 40 of pregnancy, at which

time accessory corpora lutea (formed under the influence of pituitary follicle-stimulating hormone [FSH] and equine chorionic gonadotropin [eCG]) supplement the progesterone concentration. From approximately day 70, the placenta produces significant quantities of progesterone by metabolizing maternally derived cholesterol into progesterone. Subsequent to this, progesterone concentrations begin to decline at approximately 120 days (4 months) and will reach baseline concentrations by 180 days (6 months). Subsequently, progesterone concentrations for evaluating pregnancy may be of limited value after midgestation. At this point, pregnancy is being maintained by progesterone being secreted directly to the endometrium and myometrium by the allantochorion, hence circulating systemic concentrations are low. Progesterone is typically produced by ovarian luteal tissue in the nonpregnant mare, with low concentrations occurring during late diestrus and early estrus.

CAUSES OF ABNORMALLY HIGH LEVELS

In the nonpregnant mare, increased circulating concentrations of progesterone indicate the onset of estrus and the presence of functional luteal tissue on the ovaries during diestrus.

NEXT STEP TO CONSIDER IF LEVELS HIGH

Diagnostic rectal ultrasonography to evaluate the reproductive tract would be called for in an attempt to stage the reproductive cycle. Additionally, evaluation of the uterus could be performed to evaluate for early pregnancy.

CAUSES OF ABNORMALLY LOW LEVELS

During diestrus, as the luteal tissue regresses, progesterone concentrations will decrease normally. In the pregnant mare, decreasing concentrations of progesterone could imply an appropriate decreased production by the ovarian luteal tissue, or an inappropriate production of progesterone, indicating possible compromise of the pregnancy.

NEXT DIAGNOSTIC STEP TO CONSIDER IF LEVELS LOW:

A repeat progesterone concentration should be evaluated as single samples are often not useful. Additionally, ultrasonographic evaluation of the fetus should be performed to evaluate the health of the fetus and the placenta.

SPECIMEN AND PROCESSING CONSIDERATIONS

LAB ARTIFACTS THAT MAY INTERFER WITH READINGS OF LEVELS OF THIS SUBSTANCE (AND HOW—ARTIFICIALLY ELEVATED VS. DEPRESSED) Radioimmunoassay also detects 5 alpha-pregnanes from the utero fetoplacental unit after day 100.

SAMPLE FOR COLLECTION (TYPE OF SPECIMEN, COLOR TUBE) AND ANY SPECIAL SPECIMEN HANDLING NOTES Collection of whole blood in a red-top tube and separation of serum is ideal, although plasma can be used. Sample can then be refrigerated or frozen and shipped to a diagnostic laboratory with a cold pack. Serum progesterone concentrations are low during estrus and begin to increase within 12 to 24 hours of ovulation, subsequently peaking between 5 to 10 days postovulation.

PEARLS Progesterone concentrations may be used to determine the stage of the estrus cycle and to confirm that ovulation has occurred. Circulating progesterone concentration may also be used as an indirect method of pregnancy diagnosis in the mare; however, false positives are common. Single samples of peripheral blood progesterone concentration are difficult to interpret because repeated sampling of normal pregnant mares has revealed widely variable concentrations over short periods of time.

AUTHORS: **SHANE F. DeWITT** and **TANYA M. GRONDIN**

EDITOR: **CHARLES WIEDMEYER**

Protein Electrophoresis

BASIC INFORMATION

DEFINITION

Qualitative and quantitative determination of proteins, typically measured in serum, but may also be performed on cerebrospinal fluid (CSF) and urine. Proteins separate into four to six major groups (fractions) based on their rate of migration in an electric field. Protein charge and size determine migration rate.

TYPICAL NORMAL RANGE (US UNITS; SI UNITS)

- Albumin (2.6–3.7 g/dL; 26–37 g/L)
- Alpha 1 globulin (0.06–0.7 g/dL; 0.6–7 g/L)
- Alpha 2 globulin (0.3–1.3 g/dL; 3–13 g/L)
- Beta 1 globulin (0.4–1.6 g/dL; 4–16 g/L)
- Beta 2 globulin (0.3–0.9 g/dL; 3–9 g/L)
- Gamma globulin (0.6–1.9 g/dL; 6–19 g/L)
- Total serum protein (5.2–7.9 g/dL; 52–79 g/L)

PHYSIOLOGY

- Soluble body proteins can be divided into albumin and five globulin regions: Alpha 1, alpha 2, beta 1, beta 2, and gamma.
- The alpha 1, alpha 2, and beta 1 globulin fractions includes several acute phase proteins as well as others.
- The beta 2 fraction contains lipoproteins and complement.

- Some of the immunoglobulins (Ig) such as IgM and IgA can migrate in the beta regions, but the gamma globulin fraction can include IgG as well as IgA and IgM.
- An equine-specific immunoglobulin, IgG subclass T, can migrate in the alpha 2, beta, or gamma regions.
- An increased concentration of Ig is called a gammopathy. A narrow peak is a monoclonal gammopathy; this may include one Ig or a group of proteins migrating together. A broad based peak or multiple peaks is a polyclonal gammopathy.

CAUSES OF ABNORMALLY HIGH LEVELS

- Alpha globulin: Acute inflammation
- Beta globulin: Active liver disease, intestinal parasites
- Beta and gamma globulin (bridging): Chronic active hepatitis, lymphoma
- Gamma globulin (monoclonal gammopathy): Plasma cell neoplasia, B lymphocyte neoplasia, idiopathic
- Gamma globulin (polyclonal gammopathy): Chronic inflammation, equine infectious anemia

NEXT DIAGNOSTIC STEP TO CONSIDER IF LEVELS HIGH

- Monoclonal gammopathy: Assess for myeloma or B-cell neoplasia (including lymphoma and leukemia).
- Polyclonal gammopathy: Assess for inflammation, infection, immune mediated disease, liver disease or neoplasia.

CAUSES OF ABNORMALLY LOW LEVELS

- Albumin: Acute phase response, renal disease, liver insufficiency, gastrointestinal disease, blood loss, third spacing of proteinaceous fluid
- Globulins: Failure of passive transfer (foals), inherited or acquired immunodeficiency

NEXT DIAGNOSTIC STEP TO CONSIDER IF LEVELS LOW

Investigate albumin loss or decreased production; measure foal IgG; evaluate for inherited immunodeficiencies.

SPECIMEN AND PROCESSING CONSIDERATIONS

SAMPLE FOR COLLECTION (TYPE OF SPECIMEN, COLOR TUBE) AND ANY SPECIAL SPECIMEN HANDLING NOTES Serum from a red-top tube is preferred over plasma to prevent interference from fibrinogen, but urine or CSF can also be evaluated. Allow blood to clot, centrifuge, collect serum, refrigerate, and ship on ice.

PEARLS Equine serum often has a minor post albumin fraction (or shoulder) on the cathodal side of the albumin peak. This shoulder often becomes more prominent with hypoalbuminemia. A prominent post albumin fraction with or without hypoalbuminemia has been considered pathognomonic for liver disease in the horse (Figures 1 and 2).

AUTHOR: **BRIDGET C. GARNER**

EDITOR: **CHARLES WIEDMEYER**

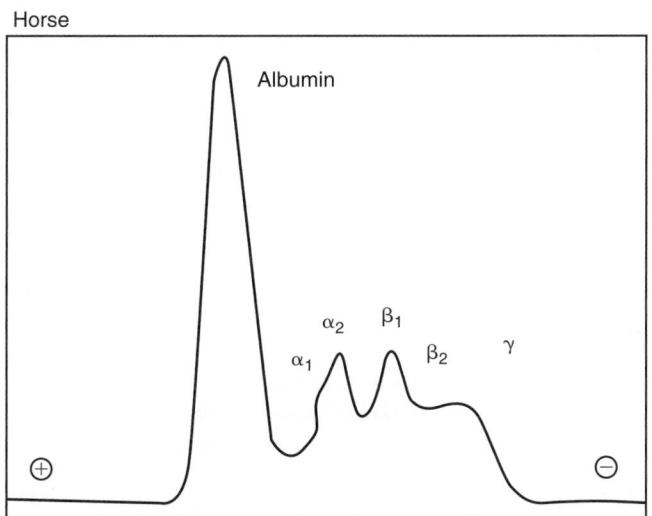

FIGURE 1 Electrophoresis tracing from a hypogammaglobulinemic foal with failure of passive transfer.

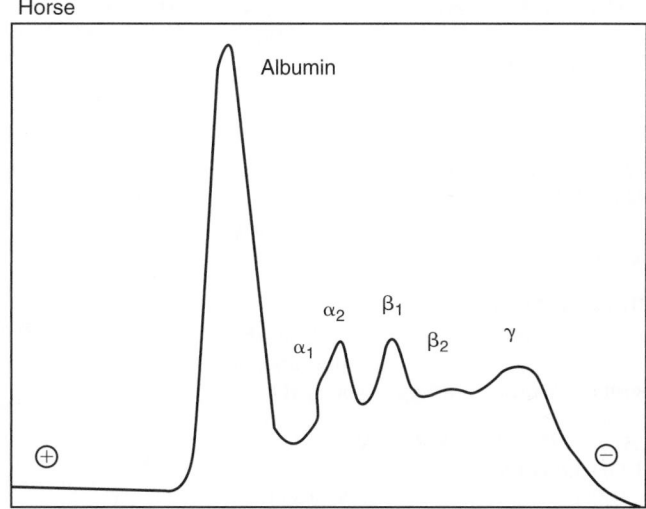

FIGURE 2 Electrophoresis tracing from a normal horse.

Prothrombin Time (PT)

BASIC INFORMATION

DEFINITION

Screening coagulation test of the tissue factor (extrinsic) and common pathways

SYNONYM(S)

One-stage prothrombin time (OSPT)
PT

TYPICAL NORMAL RANGE (US UNITS; SI UNITS)

Measurements reported in seconds. Prolonged when there is about a 70% decrease in activity of a single factor. Laboratory, instrument, and species specific reference intervals must be used. Values in healthy newborn foals (<24 hours old) may be greater than reference intervals established for adults.

PHYSIOLOGY

Measures the time in seconds required for fibrin clot formation in citrated plasma after addition of a Ca^{2+}-thromboplastin reagent (containing phospholipid and excess tissue factor) so that tissue factor will activate factor VII in the tissue factor pathway.

CAUSES OF ABNORMALLY HIGH LEVELS Decreased production (liver disease, vitamin K antagonism or absence [may be elevated more acutely than activated partial thromboplastin time (aPTT) due to vitamin K antagonism]), increased factor inactivation and consumption (DIC), dilution of factors (massive transfusions of plasma-poor fluids), hereditary factor defects, factor inhibition (FDPs, heparin therapy)

NEXT DIAGNOSTIC STEP TO CONSIDER IF LEVELS HIGH Measurement of individual factors if hereditary disease is suspected

CAUSES OF ABNORMALLY LOW LEVELS: Not reliable for detecting hypercoagulability

DRUG EFFECTS ON LEVELS Increased by heparin. Oxyglobin interferes with optical detection of clot formation.

SPECIMEN AND PROCESSING CONSIDERATIONS

LAB ARTIFACTS THAT MAY INTERFERE WITH READINGS OF LEVELS OF THIS SUBSTANCE (AND HOW—ARTIFICIALLY ELEVATED VS. DEPRESSED)

- Different thromboplastin reagents produce different results (some appear to be affected by protein induced by vitamin K absence [PIVKA], which inhibits *in vitro* coagulation).
- Decrease: Contamination with tissue factor during sampling, overfilling citrate tube.
- Increase: Lipemia, hemolysis, and icterus interfere with optical detection of clot formation, incomplete filling of citrate tube, old specimen.

SAMPLE FOR COLLECTION (TYPE OF SPECIMEN, COLOR TUBE) AND ANY SPECIAL SPECIMEN HANDLING NOTES Obtain sample via minimally traumatic phlebotomy. Collect specimen in citrate (blue top) tube. Fill to ratio of nine parts blood to one part citrate (2.7-mL blood in a 3-mL citrate tube).

PEARLS Used to monitor warfarin therapy with a target of PT approximately 1.5 to 2.0 times baseline

AUTHOR: **BRITTON GRASPERGE**

EDITOR: **CHARLES WIEDMEYER**

Pyuria

BASIC INFORMATION

DEFINITION

The presence of increased numbers of leukocytes in the urine sediment

TYPICAL NORMAL RANGE (US UNITS; SI UNITS)

A low number (<2 per 400× field) may be found in the urine of healthy animals.

PHYSIOLOGY

Leukocytes may enter the urine from the kidney, urinary bladder, urethra, and/or genital tract before or during micturition.

CAUSES OF ABNORMALLY HIGH LEVELS

- Inflammation of the urinary or genital tract
- False positives or increases (see later)

NEXT DIAGNOSTIC STEP TO CONSIDER IF LEVELS HIGH

- Assess the method of urine collection. If urine was obtained via free catch, consider collection via urethral catheter or midstream catch for further evaluation and localization of inflammation.
- Assess other urinalysis findings: pH and the presence of red blood cells and bacteria.
- Consider urine culture.

CAUSES OF ABNORMALLY LOW LEVELS

- Decreased neutrophil function associated with some systemic diseases (Cushing's) may reduce the number of leukocytes observed in the urine of a patient with inflammation of the urinary or genital tract.
- Very dilute urine may give the misleading appearance of low numbers of leukocytes in the urine of patients with urinary or genital tract inflammation.
- False negatives or decreases (via dipstick methods) may occur with elevated glucose concentrations (>3 g/dL) or high specific gravity.

DRUG EFFECTS ON LEVELS

- False positives (via dipstick methods) may occur with the presence of cephalexin and cephalothin.
- False negatives or decreases (via dipstick methods) may occur with high levels of tetracycline.

SPECIMEN AND PROCESSING CONSIDERATIONS

LAB ARTIFACTS THAT MAY INTERFERE WITH READINGS OF LEVELS OF THIS SUBSTANCE (AND HOW—ARTIFICIALLY ELEVATED VS. DEPRESSED)

- Leukocytes deteriorate in urine within a few hours, and prompt sample analysis is necessary for accurate assessment of pyuria.

- False-positive and false-negative readings for leukocytes via dipstick analysis have been noted in equine urine, and cytologic analysis of the urine sediment is preferable to diagnose pyuria in horses.

SAMPLE FOR COLLECTION (TYPE OF SPECIMEN, COLOR TUBE) AND ANY SPECIAL SPECIMEN HANDLING NOTES Midstream urine collection in a clean container

PEARLS

- Even in the absence of pyuria, a urine culture and sensitivity is indicated if the patient is suspected of having a

disease that reduces neutrophil function or causes dilute urine.

- For negative bacterial urine cultures with concurrent pyuria, consider the effects of antibiotics and fungal or algal urinary tract infections.

AUTHOR: **LAURA C. CREGAR**

EDITOR: **CHARLES WIEDMEYER**

Sarcocystic neurona

BASIC INFORMATION

DEFINITION

- *S. neurona* is an apicomplexan parasite that is the primary cause of equine protozoal myeloencephalitis (EPM).
- Oocysts of the parasite are passed in the feces of the infected definitive host (opossum) and undergoes sporogeny, releasing two sporocysts into the environment.
- In the natural life cycle, an intermediate host (possibly skunks, raccoon, nine-banded armadillo, domestic cat, or sea otter) then ingests a sporocyst, which releases sporozoites within the body of the intermediate host.
- The parasite then undergoes asexual reproduction resulting in the production of meronts.
- Merozoites emerge from the second-generation meronts and enter the mononucleate cells where they develop by endodyogeny.
- Subsequent generations of merozoites continue to develop throughout the body with the final asexual generation developing in the muscle tissue.
- These merozoites form metrocytes and initiate sarcocyst formation during which additional metrocytes are formed and develop into bradyzoites (that are infections for the definitive host).
- The cycle completes itself when the intermediate host is consumed by the definitive host, resulting in sexual reproduction of the parasite in the host's gut to create macro- and microgamonts.
- Fusion of a microgamont and macrogamont creates a zygote, which will develop into an oocyst.
- In the case of EPM, the horse is an aberrant host, and although recently it has been shown to develop sarcocysts

in rare cases, is not believed to act as an intermediate host. Horses are typically infected by grazing on contaminated pasture or ingesting contaminated feed.

TYPICAL NORMAL RANGE (US UNITS; SI UNITS)

There is no published reference interval. Results are typically reported as positive or negative (or variations thereof).

PHYSIOLOGY

The clinical syndrome of *S. neurona* typically manifests as asymmetric neurologic disease. Because the protozoa may infect any part of the central nervous system (CNS), almost any neurologic sign is possible, although clinical signs of spinal cord disease are much more common than signs of brain disease. The exact pathogenic mechanism of disease is unknown, but it is believed that the parasite causes damage during migration of merozoites throughout the body.

CAUSES OF ABNORMALLY HIGH LEVELS Elevations in serum antibody titer are typically due to either active infection or exposure to the etiologic agent of disease.

NEXT DIAGNOSTIC STEP TO CONSIDER IF LEVELS HIGH Therapeutic intervention directed toward treating the clinical syndrome of EPM should be initiated.

CAUSES OF ABNORMALLY LOW LEVELS Low antibody concentrations suggest lack of exposure to the causative agent of disease.

NEXT DIAGNOSTIC STEP TO CONSIDER IF LEVELS LOW Low levels suggest lack of exposure to the causative agent of disease and the need to consider other etiologic agents or pathologic processes as the source of the observed clinical disease.

SPECIMEN AND PROCESSING CONSIDERATIONS

SAMPLE FOR COLLECTION (TYPE OF SPECIMEN, COLOR TUBE) AND ANY SPECIAL SPECIMEN HANDLING NOTES Collection of whole blood in a red-top tube and separation of serum is ideal. Sample can then be refrigerated or frozen and shipped to a diagnostic laboratory with a cold pack.

PEARLS

- Serology for the diagnosis of EPM has been frustrating as many horses are seropositive for the disease.
- Western immunoblot (WIB) for detection of antibodies in either serum or cerebrospinal fluid (CSF) simply detects exposure to the disease, not necessarily active infection, although a positive immunoblot in the face of appropriate clinical signs is strongly suggestive. The test has inherently poor specificity, although sensitivity is better.
- Enzyme-linked immunosorbent assay (ELISA) direct against surface antigens (SAG) of *S. neurona* and indirect fluorescent antibody (IFA) test will hopefully increase diagnostic accuracy. Both the ELISA and IFA have shown improved sensitivity and specificity.
- The gold standard for diagnosis remains histopathologic identification of the offending organism.
- There is some concern that there may be cross-reactivity of the SAG; ELISA for *S. neurona* may cross react with *Neospora hughesi*. These tests can also be utilized to test CSF for EPM. Preliminary results suggest similar sensitivity and specificity as with serum.

AUTHORS: **SHANE F. DeWITT** and **TANYA M. GRONDIN**

EDITOR: **CHARLES WIEDMEYER**

LABORATORY TESTS

Schistocytes

BASIC INFORMATION

DEFINITION

Schistocytes are fragmented erythrocytes. They are irregular in shape and smaller than normal erythrocytes on blood smears.

SYNONYM(S)

Schizocytes
Red blood cell fragments

TYPICAL NORMAL RANGE (US UNITS; SI UNITS)

Rare to absent

PHYSIOLOGY

Schistocyte formation occurs most often due to mechanical damage to erythrocytes, usually as the result of turbulent blood flow, contact with roughened vascular surfaces, or shearing by intravascular fibrin strands. They also may occur in association with iron deficiency (iron deficient erythrocytes are fragile) or as a result of fragmentation of abnormal (and probably poorly deformable) erythrocytes such as acanthocytes and keratocytes.

CAUSES OF ABNORMALLY HIGH LEVELS Conditions associated with schistocyte formation include thrombotic disorders, diffuse intravascular coagulation, vasculitis, endocarditis and other cardiac disorders, glomerulonephritis, liver disease, myelofibrosis, hemangiosarcoma, and iron deficiency

AUTHOR: **MARLYN S. WHITNEY**

EDITOR: **CHARLES WIEDMEYER**

Serum Bile Acid (SBA) Concentration

BASIC INFORMATION

DEFINITION

- Bile: An alkaline liquid secreted by hepatocytes necessary for digestion
- Bile acids (bile salts): Cholesterol conjugates made by the liver and excreted in the bile
- Cholestasis: Any condition in which the flow of bile from the liver is blocked resulting in the accumulation in the blood of components normally secreted in the bile, including bile acids

TYPICAL NORMAL RANGE (US UNITS; SI UNITS)

- <15 μmol/L
- Radioimmunoassay: 8.2 ± 1.6 μmol/L
- Colorimetric method 5.0 to 28.0 μmol/L

PHYSIOLOGY

- Bile acids, synthesized by hepatocytes from cholesterol, are necessary for fat digestion and are the primary pathway for cholesterol metabolism. They are secreted in bile. Most (70%–95%) are reabsorbed in the small intestines, removed from portal blood by hepatocytes, and recycled (enterohepatic circulation).
- Bile acids are a test of liver function rather than hepatocellular damage, but contribute to hepatocellular damage when there is cholestasis.
- Bile is continuously secreted into the small intestine of horses, which do not have gall bladders, and only a single point in time sample is necessary for evaluation.
- A reduced total hepatic functional mass decreases bile acid recycling hence serum bile acids are a liver function test. Increases are highly specific to liver disease but not specific to etiology.

CAUSES OF ABNORMALLY HIGH LEVELS

- Cholestasis for any reason
- Hepatic insufficiency (acute or chronic hepatic disease).
- Portosystemic shunts
- Hyperlipemia syndrome
- Prolonged fasting causes mild increases
- Neonates have increased serum bile acid concentrations for the first 2 to 3 weeks of life.

NEXT DIAGNOSTIC STEP TO CONSIDER IF LEVELS HIGH

- Complete blood count/serum chemistry profile and urinalysis to rule out hepatic insufficiency, chronic hepatitis, and cholestasis
- Coagulation profile
- Transabdominal ultrasonography to rule out choleliths and evaluate liver
- Dye clearance test to evaluate liver function
- Liver biopsy to evaluate liver pathology

CAUSES OF ABNORMALLY LOW LEVELS Ileal malabsorption reduces enterohepatic recycling (rare).

NEXT DIAGNOSTIC STEP TO CONSIDER IF LEVELS LOW

- Complete blood count/serum chemistry profile and urinalysis to rule out malabsorption or signs of chronic disease and acid-base abnormalities
- Fecal examination and smear (steatorrhea)
- Oral lactose tolerance test in neonates
- D-glucose and D-xylose absorption test

DRUG EFFECTS ON LEVELS None

SPECIMEN AND PROCESSING CONSIDERATIONS

LAB ARTIFACTS THAT MAY INTERFERE WITH READINGS OF LEVELS OF THIS SUBSTANCE (AND HOW—ARTIFICIALLY ELEVATED VS. DEPRESSED) Lipemia and hemolysis cause variable interference.

SAMPLE FOR COLLECTION (TYPE OF SPECIMEN, COLOR TUBE) AND ANY SPECIAL SPECIMEN HANDLING NOTES Serum, quickly separated from the clot, and refrigerated. Stable.

PEARLS

Values >20 μmol/L suggest chronic liver disease, despite cholestasis. Neonates can have significantly increased values.

AUTHOR: **PAULA M. KRIMER**

EDITOR: **CHARLES WIEDMEYER**

Sodium

BASIC INFORMATION

DEFINITION

- Hypernatremia: Increased sodium concentration in the blood
- Normonatremia: Normal sodium concentration in the blood
- Hyponatremia: Decreased sodium concentration in the blood

SYNONYM(S)

Na^+

TYPICAL NORMAL RANGE (US UNITS; SI UNITS)

132 to 146 mEq/L; 132 to 146 mmol/L

PHYSIOLOGY

Sodium maintains extracellular fluid osmolality and extracellular fluid volume and is essential for renal water retention. The movement of sodium is frequently associated with movement of water. The rennin-angiotensin-aldosterone system in hypovolemia stimulates active sodium reabsorption. Osmolality increases and decreases thirst. Sodium is self-regulated via aldosterone.

CAUSES OF ABNORMALLY HIGH LEVELS

- Water loss or deprivation: Hyperventilating due to exercise, pulmonary disease, acidosis, severe anemia, fever, diarrhea, burns, renal disease, diabetes insipidus central/nephrogenic, water deprivation due to lack of source, dysphagia
- Increased sodium absorption: Hypertonic saline or sodium bicarbonate administration, salt poisoning
- Decreased excretion: Hyperaldosteronism

NEXT DIAGNOSTIC STEP TO CONSIDER IF LEVELS HIGH

- Review history, clinical signs, complete blood count, biochemistry profile, urinalysis, and rectal examination. Review hydration status via capillary refill time, moisture of mucous membranes, skin tent, pack cell volume, and total protein. Imaging, urine fractional clearance of sodium for renal disease, blood gas analysis, water deprivation test/measure plasma vasopressin concentration for diabetes insipidus, measure aldosterone concentration.
- Concurrent disease states can result in normonatremia
  - Dehydration with concurrent diarrhea, renal disease, osmotic diuresis, diuretics, sweating
  - Edema with concurrent congestive heart failure, hepatic cirrhosis, nephrotic syndrome

CAUSES OF ABNORMALLY LOW LEVELS

- Sodium loss/sequestration: Excessive sweat/salivation, diarrhea, protein-losing gastroenteropathy, colitis, nasogastric intubation, diuretics, prolonged diuresis, renal disease, ketonuria, lactaturia, bicarbonaturia, adrenal insufficiency, hypoaldosteronism, displacement, torsion, volvulus, obstruction, or ileus of the gastrointestinal tract
- Third space loss: Ascites, peritonitis, uroperitoneum, pleural drainage, hemorrhage
- Excess water: Sodium-poor fluid administration, excessive administration of 5% dextrose solution, psychogenic polydipsia syndrome, congestive heart failure, hepatic cirrhosis, nephrotic syndrome, syndrome of inappropriate antidiuretic hormone secretion
- Water shift from intracellular fluid (ICF) to extracellular fluid (ECF): Hyperglycemia, mannitol administration
- Sodium shift from ECF to ICF: Acute muscle damage, potassium depletion
- Sodium shift to ECF: Uroperitoneum
- Other: Iatrogenic or primary hyperadrenocorticism, stress

NEXT DIAGNOSTIC STEP TO CONSIDER IF LEVELS LOW

Review history, clinical signs, complete blood count, biochemistry profile, urinalysis, and rectal examination. Review hydration status via capillary refill time, moisture of mucous membranes, skin tent, pack cell volume, and total protein. Abdominocentesis and thoracocentesis for effusions; imaging; urine fractional clearance of sodium for renal disease, water deprivation test/measure plasma vasopressin for diabetes insipidus, dexamethasone suppression test for hyperadrenocorticism, adrenocorticotrophic hormone (ACTH) stimulation for adrenal exhaustion, measure aldosterone concentration

DRUG EFFECTS ON LEVELS

Decrease: Loop diuretics (furosemide, thiazide) osmotic diuretics (mannitol)

SPECIMEN AND PROCESSING CONSIDERATIONS

LAB ARTIFACTS THAT MAY INTERFERE WITH READINGS OF LEVELS OF THIS SUBSTANCE (AND HOW—ARTIFICIALLY ELEVATED VS. DEPRESSED)

- Increase: Aged (dehydrated) sample
- Decrease: Marked hyperlipidemia, hyperproteinemia, and hyperglycemia

SAMPLE FOR COLLECTION (TYPE OF SPECIMEN, COLOR TUBE) AND ANY SPECIAL SPECIMEN HANDLING NOTES

- Serum preferred; sodium heparin can be used. Avoid sodium EDTA.
- Methodology: Direct and indirect potentiometry and flame photometry

PEARLS

Interpret sodium levels with knowledge of hydration status.

AUTHORS: **LAURA V. LANE** and **THERESA E. RIZZI**

EDITOR: **CHARLES WIEDMEYER**

Sorbitol Dehydrogenase (SDH)

BASIC INFORMATION

DEFINITION

Leakage enzyme: Soluble cytoplasmic enzymes released into circulation after increased membrane permeability (sublethal cellular injury or cellular necrosis)

TYPICAL NORMAL RANGE (US UNITS; SI UNITS)

1.0 to 8.0 IU/L

PHYSIOLOGY

Sorbitol dehydrogenase is a rapid leakage enzyme essential for carbohydrate metabolism and is specific to the liver. The degree of increase is generally proportional to the number of injured hepatocytes; very high values suggest acute hepatitis. It has a short half-life of less than 12 hours and quickly returns to normal; consistently increased values suggest ongoing and active hepatocellular damage.

CAUSES OF ABNORMALLY HIGH LEVELS

- Marked increases in acute hepatitis (equine herpesvirus type 1, embolic bacterial diseases, Tyzzer's disease (*Clostridium piliformis*), hepatotoxins, Theiler's disease (serum hepatitis), cholangiohepatitis associated with ascending enteric bacteria, and chronic active hepatitis
- Mild to moderate increases in cholelithiasis, strangulating or obstructive gastrointestinal diseases, acute enterocolitis with endotoxemia, and hyperlipemia syndrome

NEXT DIAGNOSTIC STEP TO CONSIDER IF LEVELS HIGH

- Vaccination history (serum hepatitis)
- Complete blood count/serum chemistry profile, serum bile acids, and urinalysis to rule out extrahepatic cholestasis, hepatitis/hepatic necrosis, endotoxemia, and hyperlipemia syndrome
- Liver biopsy to identify specific liver pathology or etiology

CAUSES OF ABNORMALLY LOW LEVELS: Insignificant

DRUG EFFECTS ON LEVELS: Increases: Benzimidazole anthelmintics and halothane

SPECIMEN AND PROCESSING CONSIDERATIONS

LAB ARTIFACTS THAT MAY INTERFERE WITH READINGS OF LEVELS OF THIS SUBSTANCE (AND HOW—ARTIFICIALLY ELEVATED VS. DEPRESSED) Reference intervals are different for fresh serum and heparinized plasma; interpret carefully.

SAMPLE FOR COLLECTION (TYPE OF SPECIMEN, COLOR TUBE) AND ANY SPECIAL SPECIMEN HANDLING NOTES Serum, quickly separated from clot. Extremely labile; stable 5 hours at room temperature, less than 24 hours refrigerated and 48 hours frozen. If immediate on-site evaluation is not possible, serum should be frozen and mailed on ice packs to nearby laboratory.

PEARLS

- SDH is very specific for active liver damage in horses, but it has a short half-life and thus may not be readily available in all laboratories.
- Pituitary adenomas can cause hypercortisolemia or decreased antidiuretic hormone production, either of which can cause increased aspartate aminotransferase (AST) (and SDH and gamma-glutamyl transpeptidase [GGT]) along with dilute urine.

AUTHOR: **PAULA M. KRIMER**

EDITOR: **CHARLES WIEDMEYER**

Synovial Fluid Analysis

BASIC INFORMATION

DEFINITION

Synovial fluid analysis includes the determination of the fluid's physical properties (color, clarity, volume, viscosity), nucleated and red blood cell concentrations, total protein concentration, the cytologic evaluation of direct and/or concentrated smears, and in some cases performance of the mucin clot test.

SYNONYM(S)

Joint fluid analysis

TYPICAL NORMAL RANGE (US UNITS; SI UNITS)

- Normal synovial fluid is clear, pale yellow, viscous, and minimally cellular. Reported normal nucleated cell concentrations range up to greater than 2000/μL from some joints, but the majority of commonly sampled joints should have <500 to 1000 nucleated cells/μL.
- The nucleated cells are predominantly large and small mononuclear cells, with only very low numbers of neutrophils found in normal synovial fluid.
- Total protein ranges from approximately 1 to 3 g/dL and is commonly determined via a refractometer.

- If a mucin clot test is performed on normal fluid, a good clot should form upon mixture with 2.5% glacial acetic acid. Not all laboratories routinely perform this test. The results indicate a rough approximation of the synovial fluid viscosity or quality of the synovial fluid. The mucin clot test reflects the hyaluronate polymerization of the fluid.

PHYSIOLOGY

Synovial fluid is an ultrafiltrate of plasma, which lubricates joints and allows diffusion of electrolytes and other substances to and from the synovial and articular surfaces.

CAUSES OF ABNORMALLY HIGH LEVELS

- Increased concentrations of mononuclear cells and total protein are seen with degenerative joint disease and some traumatic joint disease. In these cases, the total nucleated cell count is typically <5000/μL.
- Increased concentrations of neutrophils and total protein are seen with septic synovitis, immune-mediated joint disease, acute traumatic joint disease, and following administration of some chemicals (therapeutics) into joints. Total nucleated cell counts are often >5000/μL these cases.

- The presence of red blood cells in synovial fluid indicates either true pathologic hemorrhage or iatrogenic blood contamination. In slides prepared from fresh samples, the presence of erythrophagocytosis and sometimes hemosiderin-laden macrophages are evidence of true hemorrhage into the joint.

NEXT DIAGNOSTIC STEP TO CONSIDER IF LEVELS HIGH Bacterial culture and sensitivity are indicated in suppurative (neutrophilic) synovitis, as microscopic detection of bacteria on fluid smears is an insensitive means of diagnosing septic synovitis.

CAUSES OF ABNORMALLY LOW LEVELS With any synovitis, viscosity of the fluid tends to decrease, and there may be poor clot formation on a mucin clot test.

SPECIMEN AND PROCESSING CONSIDERATIONS

SAMPLE FOR COLLECTION (TYPE OF SPECIMEN, COLOR TUBE) AND ANY SPECIAL SPECIMEN HANDLING NOTES Synovial fluid should be placed in EDTA purple-top tubes for analysis, and an aliquot may be placed in a red-top (clot) tube for microbiologic culture. If a mucin clot test is to be performed, an aliquot in a red-top or green-top (heparin) tube is required. Direct smears should be prepared as soon as possible after collection to include with the fluid submission to the laboratory. Fluid samples should be shipped overnight and on ice, but not frozen.

PEARLS

- Direct fluid smears should be prepared as soon as possible after sample collection to include with fluid submission to a laboratory. If smears are not prepared quickly, *in vitro* phagocytosis of red blood cells or potentially bacterial contaminants can occur and would thus alter the interpretation of the fluid cytology.
- Fluid samples should be shipped to a laboratory overnight, on ice but not frozen.
- If bacterial sepsis is suspected, fluid should be submitted for bacterial culture and sensitivity, as the microscopic examination for bacteria on fluid smears is a poorly sensitive means of diagnosing septic synovitis.

AUTHOR: **ANGELA B. ROYAL**

EDITOR: **CHARLES WIEDMEYER**

T4/Free T4

BASIC INFORMATION

DEFINITION

- Hyperthyroxinemia: Increased circulating concentration of thyroxine
- Hypothyroxinemia: Decreased circulating concentration of thyroxine

SYNONYM(S)

Thyroxine

TYPICAL NORMAL RANGE (US UNITS; SI UNITS)

- T4: 16.39 to 23.35 nmol/L
- Free T4: 10.15 to 12.95 pmol/L

PHYSIOLOGY

Thyroxine (or 3,5,3',5'-tetraiodothyronine) is the major hormone secreted by the follicular cells of the thyroid gland. T4 is transported in blood, the majority being protein bound, principally to thyroxine-binding globulin (TBG), and to a lesser extent transthyretin and serum albumin. T4 not bound to proteins is referred to as free T4 (fT4) and is the biologically active form. T4 is involved in controlling the rate of metabolic processes in the body and influencing physical development. fT4 enters most cells where it is converted to T3.

CAUSES OF ABNROMALLY HIGH LEVELS Typically due to a functional neoplasia of the thyroid gland resulting in increased production of the hormone. However, exogenous administration of thyroid-stimulating hormone (TSH) or thyroid-releasing hormone (TRH) could also cause a physiologic increase in circulating hormone concentrations as well as administration of iodide containing compounds.

NEXT DIAGNOSTIC STEP TO CONSIDER IF LEVELS HIGH Determination of fT4 would be crucial to evaluate the active component of the circulating thyroid hormone. Determination of fT4 concentration by equilibrium dialysis is considered the gold standard. Additionally, one may consider a fine needle aspirate or biopsy of the thyroid gland to assess any underlying pathologic conditions.

CAUSES OF ABNORMALLY LOW LEVELS Usually due to decreased production of T4 by the thyroid gland due to destruction of normal thyroid gland tissue. Additionally, hypothyroxinemia could be due to primary deficiency of TSH or TRH from the pituitary or hypothalamus, respectively, or a dietary iodine deficiency. Last, it is important to remember that many nonthyroidal diseases, exercise, exogenous drug administration, and dietary factors may have an effect on thyroid hormone production in the absence of thyroid gland disease. Rarely, congenital thyroid gland aplasia could also account for a decreased concentration.

NEXT DIAGNOSTIC STEP TO CONSIDER IF LEVELS LOW Performing a TSH stimulation test would be ideal, although equine-specific TSH is not currently available. Alternatively, a TRH stimulation test can be performed to evaluate the thyroid glands ability to produce thyroid hormones. Realize that use of a TRH simulation test does not rule out pituitary disease as a possible cause of hypothyroxinemia and actually relies on a functional pituitary to assess thyroid hormone production.

DRUG EFFECTS ON LEVELS: Hypothyroxinemia: Phenylbutazone, corticosteroids, sulfa drugs, iodine-containing compounds

SPECIMEN AND PROCESSING CONSIDERATIONS

SAMPLE FOR COLLECTION (TYPE OF SPECIMEN, COLOR TUBE) AND ANY SPECIAL SPECIMEN HANDLING NOTES Collection of either plasma in EDTA (purple top) or serum in red-top tubes is acceptable.

PEARLS Horses have a diurnal variation in T4 concentration with higher concentrations occurring in the late afternoon and the lowest concentrations in the early morning. Foals have increased thyroid hormone concentrations in comparison to adult horses. Primary thyroid gland disease is rare in horses.

AUTHORS: **SHANE F. DeWITT** and **TANYA M. GRONDIN**

EDITOR: **CHARLES WIEDMEYER**

Testosterone

BASIC INFORMATION

DEFINITION

- Hypertestosteronemia: Increased circulating concentration of testosterone
- Hypotestosteronemia: Decreased circulating concentration of testosterone

PHYSIOLOGY

- Testosterone or 17-beta-hydroxy-4-androstene-3-one is a steroid hormone from the androgen group. It is primarily secreted by the testes in the male and ovaries in the female, but small amounts are also secreted by the adrenal glands.

- In general, testosterone and other androgens promote protein synthesis and growth of those tissues with androgen receptors. More specifically, the effects of testosterone cause an increase in muscle mass and strength, an increase in bone density and strength and stimulation of linear growth. Additionally, it is the principal male sex hormone responsible for the development of secondary male sexual characteristics.
- Testosterone, similar to other steroid hormones, is derived from cholesterol. The testicle produces the largest amount of testosterone by Leydig cells. In females, thecal cells in the ovaries are also capable of producing testosterone, but in far smaller quantities than in males. Additionally, testosterone can be produced by the placenta and by the zona reticularis of the adrenal cortex in both sexes.
- The clinical effects of testosterone are the result of activation of the androgen receptor and by conversion of testosterone to estradiol with subsequent activation of certain estrogen receptors Most testosterone circulates in the blood bound to sex hormone binding globulin (SHBG). Free testosterone (T) is transported into the cytoplasm of target tissue cells, where it can bind to the androgen receptor, or can be reduced to 5α-dihydrotestosterone (DHT) by the cytoplasmic enzyme 5α reductase. DHT binds to the same androgen receptor with a greater affinity than testosterone (its androgenic potency is approximately 2.5 times that of testosterone). The steroid receptor complex then translocates to the nucleus and binds directly to spe-

cific nucleotide sequences of the chromosomal DNA, altering transcriptional activity of certain genes.
- Estradiol exerts its influence primarily in bones and brain tissue. Testosterone is aromatized under the action of aromatase to estradiol. Estradiol serves as the most important feedback signal to the hypothalamus.

TYPICAL NORMAL RANGE (US UNITS; SI UNITS)
- Nonpregnant mare: <45 pg/mL
- Gelding: <40 pg/mL
- Stallion: >100 pg/mL

CAUSES OF ABNORMALLY HIGH LEVELS Depending on the sex of the horse tested, elevated levels may be normal in stallions depending on seasonality. In supposedly castrated males, elevated circulating levels of testosterone are indicative of functional testicular tissue and may indicate the presence of a cryptorchid testicle. In intact, nonpregnant females, increased concentration of circulating testosterone would indicate an inappropriate increase in production by the thecal cells of the ovary, most likely in association with neoplasia (granulosa thecal cell tumor). In intact, pregnant females, an elevated concentration of testosterone could occur transiently in association with increased testosterone production by the placenta, but should not be used as a method of pregnancy diagnosis.

NEXT DIAGNOSTIC STEP TO CONSIDER IF LEVELS HIGH
- Gelding: Perform a human chorionic gonadotrophin (hCG) stimulation test by administering 10,000 IU of hCG. A two- to threefold increase in circulat-

ing testosterone concentration from baseline levels indicates the presence of a testicle.
- Nonpregnant mare: Rectal ultrasonography or palpation to evaluate the reproductive tract, with particular attention to the ovaries would be indicated. Collection of a blood sample for evaluation of the circulating concentration of inhibin would be indicated.

CAUSES OF ABNORMALLY LOW LEVELS Depending on the sex of the horse, a low concentration of testosterone may be normal (gelding). In a stallion, low circulating concentrations of testosterone would indicate decreased production from the testicle.

NEXT DIAGNOSTIC STEP TO CONSIDER IF LEVELS LOW Performing an hCG stimulation test would be indicated to assess the ability of the testicle to produce testosterone when stimulated.

SPECIMEN AND PROCESSING CONSIDERATIONS

SAMPLE FOR COLLECTION (TYPE OF SPECIMEN, COLOR TUBE) AND ANY SPECIAL SPECIMEN HANDLING NOTES Collection of whole blood in a red-top tube and separation of serum is ideal, although plasma can be used. Sample can then be refrigerated or frozen and shipped to a diagnostic laboratory with a cold pack.

PEARLS Serum testosterone concentration in young colts (<18 months of age) should be evaluated cautiously as their concentration can often be <100 pg/mL.

AUTHORS: **SHANE F. DeWITT** and **TANYA M. GRONDIN**

EDITOR: **CHARLES WIEDMEYER**

Thyroid-Stimulating Hormone (TSH)

BASIC INFORMATION

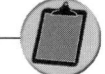

DEFINITION
- Hyperthyrotropinemia: Increased circulating concentration of TSH
- Hypothyrotropinemia: Decreased circulating concentration of TSH

SYNONYM(S)
Thyrotropin

TYPICAL NORMAL RANGE (US UNITS; SI UNITS)
There are no published reference intervals for equids. Inclusion of a blood sample from a clinically normal, nonaf-

fected horse may be useful for comparison purposes.

PHYSIOLOGY
TSH is released from the pituitary gland upon stimulation by thyroid-releasing hormone (TRH) from the hypothalamus. Both hormones are part of the thyroid-pituitary-hypothalamic axis, which regulates systemic thyroid hormone levels. TSH then goes on to stimulate the release of triiodothyronine (T3) and thyroxine (T4) from the thyroid gland. Administration of exogenous TSH assesses the ability of the thyroid gland to secrete T3 and T4, which should increase in concentration upon stimulation. TSH level

can also be assessed by administration of exogenous TRH which assesses the ability of the pituitary to secrete TSH.

CAUSES OF ABNORMALLY HIGH LEVELS Due to a defect in the thyroid gland leading to hypothyroidism, there is a lack of secretion of thyroid hormones and subsequently no negative feedback on the hypothalamus and pituitary, resulting in continued secretion of TRH and TSH in a homeostatic attempt to increase systemic concentrations of thyroid hormone.

NEXT DIAGNOSTIC STEP TO CONSIDER IF LEVELS HIGH Systemic concentration of T4, preferably free T4, should be determined.

CAUSES OF ABNORMALLY LOW LEVELS Primarily due to decreased stimulation from TRH, most likely resulting from negative feedback due to elevated circulating concentrations of thyroid hormone. Increased concentration of circulating thyroid hormones would most likely be due to a functional neoplasm of the thyroid gland. Alternatively, primary insult to the hypothalamus would result in decreased concentrations of TRH and subsequently low concentrations of TSH, although this would be very rare.

NEXT DIAGNOSTIC STEP TO CONSIDER IF LEVELS LOW A TRH stimulation test should be performed to assess the response of the pituitary to exogenously administered TRH. Additionally, systemic concentration of T4, preferably free T4, should be determined.

DRUG EFFECTS ON LEVELS Corticosteroids will potentially decrease TSH concentrations.

SPECIMEN AND PROCESSING CONSIDERATIONS

SAMPLE FOR COLLECTION (TYPE OF SPECIMEN, COLOR TUBE) AND ANY SPECIAL SPECIMEN HANDLING NOTES Collection of plasma in EDTA (purple top) or serum in red-top tubes is sufficient.

PEARLS Sufficient antigenic variation exists between species in the TSH molecule necessitating species-specific tests to be developed. Additionally, TSH is currently not available for clinical use in equine medicine. TRH is available and labeled for human medicine (not approved in horses), but relatively expensive.

AUTHORS: **SHANE F. DeWITT** and **TANYA M. GRONDIN**

EDITOR: **CHARLES WIEDMEYER**

Transtracheal Wash (TTW)

BASIC INFORMATION

DEFINITION

Transtracheal wash is a means of sampling the cells present in lower airways for cytologic evaluation.

TYPICAL NORMAL RANGE (US UNITS; SI UNITS)

In normal horse TTW, fluid macrophages predominate, with fewer lymphocytes, very low numbers of neutrophils, even fewer mast cells, and rare eosinophils observed. Low numbers of columnar respiratory epithelial cells and goblet cells can be found. Small amounts of purple mucinous material may be seen in the background. Environmental contaminants including some types of fungus and mold spores are relatively common findings in equine TTW samples, and must not be misinterpreted as evidence of true pathologic fungal infection.

PHYSIOLOGY

CAUSES OF ABNORMALLY HIGH LEVELS

- Increases in the proportion of neutrophils can be seen with primary or secondary bacterial infection. An increase in both neutrophils and macrophages is typically seen with chronic inflammatory airway disease, smoke inhalation, silicosis, fungal infection, or protozoal infection. With exercise-induced pulmonary hemorrhage, macrophages will contain phagocytized red blood cells and/or the hemoglobin breakdown products hemosiderin and hematoidin. An increased proportion of eosinophils and mast cells can be found with parasitic or allergic respiratory disease. Increased amounts of mucus in the background and in particular the presence of consolidated mucus plugs (Curschmann's spirals) suggest chronic lower airway disease with overproduction of mucus and distal airway plugging.

- The presence of mature squamous epithelial cells indicates oropharyngeal contamination of the sample. If oropharyngeal contamination is present, resident bacterial populations from that area are likely to be found in the background of the slides.

NEXT DIAGNOSTIC STEP TO CONSIDER IF LEVELS HIGH Infectious agents may or may not be seen with bacterial and fungal infections, and if these are suspected bacterial and/or fungal culture are indicated.

CAUSES OF ABNORMALLY LOW LEVELS Very low cellularity including a paucity of respiratory epithelial cells likely indicates a poor sample with suboptimal cell retrieval.

NEXT DIAGNOSTIC STEP TO CONSIDER IF LEVELS LOW Bronchoalveolar lavage may be considered so as to obtain a more directed sample from the location of interest.

SPECIMEN AND PROCESSING CONSIDERATIONS

SAMPLE FOR COLLECTION (TYPE OF SPECIMEN, COLOR TUBE) AND ANY SPECIAL SPECIMEN HANDLING NOTES Retrieved fluid should be placed in sterile red-top or plastic tubes without additives. Separate aliquots should be submitted for cytologic evaluation and bacterial/fungal culture. Direct or, preferably, concentrated smears should be prepared and air-dried as soon as possible after collection for cytologic analysis. Cell populations in TTW fluid are often fragile, so it is important to refrain from using excessive pressure when making slides. The fluid samples should be shipped to the laboratory on ice, overnight, in addition to prepared smears.

PEARLS
- Fluid smears should be prepared as soon as possible after sample collection to include with fluid submission to the laboratory. If smears are not prepared quickly, *in vitro* phagocytosis of red blood cells or potentially bacterial contaminants can occur and would thus alter the interpretation of the TTW cytology.
- Fluid samples should be shipped to a laboratory overnight, on ice but not frozen.
- Environmental contaminants including some types of fungus are somewhat common in equine TTW samples.

AUTHOR: **ANGELA B. ROYAL**

EDITOR: **CHARLES WIEDMEYER**

Triglyceride

BASIC INFORMATION

DEFINITION

A triglyceride (TG) molecule consists of a glycerol backbone esterified with three fatty acids. Triglycerides are the main constituent of vegetable and animal fats in the diet, and are the main constituent of the body's fat stores. Serum or plasma total TG concentrations may be determined to assess metabolic disorders.

SYNONYM(S)

Triacylglycerol
Triacylglyceride

TYPICAL NORMAL RANGE (US UNITS; SI UNITS)

6 to 54 mg/dL (0.07–0.61 mmol/L). This is the typical range for full-sized horses. Healthy ponies and donkeys may have higher triglyceride levels. Healthy donkeys have been reported to have levels as high as 290 mg/dL (3.28 mmol/L).

PHYSIOLOGY

TGs are not soluble in the aqueous environment of the bloodstream. For transport in the blood, they are carried by macromolecular particles called lipoproteins. The surface of lipoprotein particles is made up of proteins, free cholesterol, and phospholipids, oriented so as to be water soluble, and hydrophobic substances such as TG and esterified cholesterol are carried in the cores of the particles. Chylomicrons (CM) and very low density lipoprotein (VLDL) particles are the main TG carriers among the various types of lipoproteins, whereas low-density lipoproteins (LDL) and high-density lipoproteins (HDL) are mainly involved in transport of cholesterol. The CM particles carry dietary TG from the intestine to extrahepatic tissues such as muscle and adipose tissue. The VLDL particles carry TG made in the liver to extrahepatic tissues. Various disease states increase the amount of VLDL made by the liver and/or interfere with the clearance of CM or VLDL associated TG from the blood via uptake by muscle and/or adipose tissue. During conditions favoring lipolysis, nonesterified fatty acids (NEFAs) can be released from TG in the body's fat stores and used for energy production. Excess mobilized NEFAs beyond what can be oxidized for energy may be reesterified into TG molecules in the liver. Accumulation of excess TG in the liver results in hepatic lipidosis (fatty liver). The equine liver is efficient at forming and secreting VLDL particles so as to remove excess TG, but disorders leading to impaired extrahepatic removal of the TG from those VLDL particles leads to hypertriglyceridemia, which, at levels greater than 400 to 500 mg/dL (4.52–5.65 mmol/L), causes lipemia.

CAUSES OF ABNORMALLY HIGH LEVELS Conditions involving negative energy balance favor lipolysis and are likely to result in hypertriglyceridemia. Such conditions include malnutrition, anorexia, stress, pregnancy, lactation, endotoxemia, and renal failure. Ponies, donkeys, and miniature horses are pre-disposed to become markedly hypertriglyceridemic under such conditions. Obesity is a predisposing factor to development of hypertriglyceridemia during metabolic stress. Hypertriglyceridemia has been reported to occur within 3 days of fasting in horses. Equids with diabetes mellitus or metabolic syndrome are likely to be hypertriglyceridemic, as are those with hyperadrenocorticism (Cushing's-like syndrome, usually due to functional pituitary adenoma or adenomatous hyperplasia). Foals in the first 2 weeks of life have triglyceride levels higher than those of adults. Transient hypertriglyceridemia occurs postprandially in some species but this possibility is not much discussed in the equine literature, except in regard to its occurrence in nursing foals.

DRUG EFFECTS ON LEVELS Corticosteroids can cause hypertriglyceridemia. Thiazides and phenothiazine have also been implicated.

SPECIMEN AND PROCESSING CONSIDERATIONS

SAMPLE FOR COLLECTION (TYPE OF SPECIMEN, COLOR TUBE) AND ANY SPECIAL SPECIMEN HANDLING NOTES Serum or heparinized plasma (red-top or green-top blood collection tubes, respectively) may be used. For accurate results, lipemic serum should not be cleared prior to analysis for triglyceride levels.

AUTHOR: **MARLYN S. WHITNEY**

EDITOR: **CHARLES WIEDMEYER**

Troponins, Cardiac

BASIC INFORMATION

DEFINITION

Troponins are intracellular myocardial polypeptides expressed in cardiac and skeletal muscle that regulate excitation-contraction coupling. Cardiac troponins are a tissue-specific isoform expressed within cardiac muscle.

SYNONYM(S)

cTnI
cTnT
Troponins

TYPICAL NORMAL RANGE (US UNITS; SI UNITS)

- The normal range for cTnI is analyzer dependent; each laboratory should develop its own normal ranges.
- Normal range for cTnI in adult horses using a Stratus CS (Dade Behring), a fluorometric enzyme immunoassay analyzer, is <0.1 ng/mL.

PHYSIOLOGY

- Cardiac troponins are a group of intracellular, contractile proteins within the cardiomyocyte that are part of the troponin-tropomyosin regulatory complex. They regulate the calcium dependent interaction of actin and myosin during excitation-contraction coupling.
- The troponin complex is comprised of three distinct subunits. Troponin C (cTnC) binds calcium, troponin I (cTnI) is the inhibitory component that prevents interaction between actin and myosin until intracellular calcium is bound by troponin C, allowing heart muscle relaxation, and troponin T (cTnT) binds troponin I to the actin filament.
- Approximately 95% of cTnI exists as structurally bound, with ~5% in the cytosolic pool.

- Cardiac troponins are released into circulation with ischemia, necrosis, or damage to the cardiomyocyte.
- The cardiac troponins are well-conserved across mammalian species and have been used with increasing frequency to aid in the diagnosis of certain cardiac diseases.
- The cardiac isoforms of troponin I and T are specific for cardiac muscle because they are antigenically distinct from the skeletal muscle isoforms, showing minimal cross-reactivity. They are the preferred biochemical diagnostic tools for detecting certain myocardial diseases in people.
- Troponin C is not used clinically because of homology (cross reactivity) to other isoforms.
- In people, cardiac troponins are released into the circulation within 4 to 6 hours after myocardial injury or damage, and may persist for 1 to 2 weeks.
- cTnI has been studied the most in horses. Its half-life in horses is not known; however, it appears to be released within 3 to 4 hours of myocardial injury.

CAUSES OF ABNORMALLY HIGH LEVELS Tachydysrhythmia (particularly ventricular in origin), myocardial disease (secondary to toxins, infectious agents, nutritional disturbances, inflammatory lesions, trauma, and neoplasia), cardiomyopathy, congestive heart failure, prolonged strenuous exercise such as endurance racing, administration of pressor agents such as dobutamine or epinephrine, in association with certain gastrointestinal diseases

NEXT DIAGNOSTIC STEP TO CONSIDER IF LEVELS HIGH Complete cardiac workup (complete 2-D, M-mode, and Doppler echocardiography, electrocardiogram [ECG]), along with a complete blood count and serum biochemistry evaluation. If indicated, a 24-hour Holter monitor or telemetric monitoring of ECG should be done.

IMPORTANT INTERSPECIES DIFFERENCES In dogs and humans, serum levels of cTnI correlate with the extent of myocardial injury and may be used as a prognostic indicator. This has not been determined in horses.

SPECIMEN AND PROCESSING CONSIDERATIONS

SAMPLE FOR COLLECTION (TYPE OF SPECIMEN, COLOR TUBE) AND ANY SPECIAL SPECIMEN HANDLING NOTES
- Heparinized plasma (green-top tube), serum (red-top tube), or EDTA plasma (purple-top tube), depending on analyzer manufacturer specifications

- Plasma or serum is separated from red blood cells and refrigerated or frozen ($-20°$ C or $-80°$C) until analysis.

PEARLS
- In people, cTnI concentrations are superior to enzymatic tests (ie, isoenzymes of creatine kinase or lactate dehydrogenase), with increased sensitivity and specificity for cardiac injury.
- Sensitivity and specificity for various cardiac diseases in the horse are not known; however, based on utility in other species such as people and small animals, appears promising.
- cTnI is not useful as an indicator of cardiac disease in horses with mild to moderate valvular diseases.

SUGGESTED READING

Apple FS, et al: The diagnostic utility of cardiac biomarkers in detecting myocardial infarction. *Clin Cornerstone* 7:S25, 2005.

Durando MM, et al: Acute effects of short duration, maximal exercise on cardiac troponin I in healthy horses. *Equine and Comparative Exercise Physiology* 3:217, 2007.

La Vecchia L, et al: Cardiac troponin I as diagnostic and prognostic marker in severe heart failure. *Journal of Heart and Lung Transplantation* 19:644, 2000.

AUTHORS: **MARY M. DURANDO** and **CHARLES WIEDMEYER**

EDITOR: **CHARLES WIEDMEYER**

Urine Cortisol: Creatinine Ratio

BASIC INFORMATION

DEFINITION
- Hypercortisoluria: Increased cortisol concentration in the urine
- Hypocortisoluria: Decreased cortisol concentration in the urine

TYPICAL NORMAL RANGE (US UNITS; SI UNITS)
0.9 to 11.6×10^{-6}

PHYSIOLOGY
In theory, this diagnostic test is utilized to detect a hyperadrenal state. Use of the urine cortisol:creatinine ratio should provide more accurate results than a basal cortisol concentration as cortisol will accumulate in the urine over time, limiting the effects of diurnal variation by which cortisol is secreted in the horse. In horses, this test is used most commonly for adjunctive diagnosis of pituitary pars intermedia dysfunction (PPID).

CAUSES OF ABNORMALLY HIGH LEVELS Abnormally increased concentrations of cortisol in the urine would indicate either a hyperadrenal state or exogenous administration of corticosteroids.

NEXT DIAGNOSTIC STEP TO CONSIDER IF LEVELS HIGH If clinically indicated, a baseline adrenocorticotrophic hormone (ACTH) or cortisol concentration should be evaluated to further support the diagnostic findings. Also, a low dose dexamethasone suppression test could be performed to aid in the diagnosis of PPID, if suspected.

CAUSES OF ABNORMALLY LOW LEVELS Abnormally decreased concentrations of cortisol would indicate a hypoadrenal state, theoretically. Clinical hypoadrenal states or conditions in the horse are very unusual and would most likely be the result of abrupt cessation of prolonged exogenous corticosteroid therapy, not allowing the hypothalamic-pituitary-adrenal (HPA) axis the appropriate time to adjust.

NEXT DIAGNOSTIC STEP TO CONSIDER IF LEVELS LOW Baseline circulating cortisol concentration should be determined, including a possible ACTH stimulation test to ensure the functionality of the HPA axis. Exogenous corticosteroid therapy should be considered if clinically indicated.

SPECIMEN AND PROCESSING CONSIDERATIONS

SAMPLE FOR COLLECTION (TYPE OF SPECIMEN, COLOR TUBE) AND ANY SPECIAL SPECIMEN HANDLING NOTES A clean urine sample should be collected in a specimen container or a red-top tube.

PEARLS The major downfall to the use of this diagnostic test is that it has poor positive predictive value for pathologic hyperadrenal states as there are numerous physiologic states that will also cause increased cortisol secretion over time.

AUTHORS: **SHANE F. DeWITT** and **TANYA M. GRONDIN**

EDITOR: **CHARLES WIEDMEYER**

LABORATORY TESTS

Urine Crystals

BASIC INFORMATION

DEFINITION
Precipitation of salts forming crystals in the urine.

SYNONYM(S)
Crystalluria

TYPICAL NORMAL RANGE (US UNITS; SI UNITS)
- Reported as the number of crystals seen per low-power field (10×) with specific identification.
- Urine in healthy equine patients may contain marked numbers of calcium carbonate crystals. Low numbers of other crystals may also be seen.

PHYSIOLOGY
Salts resulting from normal and abnormal metabolic processes and some medications may precipitate in urine and form crystals if the concentration of the salts is sufficiently high and the urine is of appropriate pH. Some salts precipitate in an alkaline pH, while others precipitate in an acidic pH. Most crystals can be found in healthy animals. Due to the alkaline pH and high concentration of calcium and carbonate in equine urine, calcium carbonate crystals are frequently seen.

CAUSES OF ABNORMALLY HIGH LEVELS
- Abnormal or increased metabolic products
- High calcium diets (alfalfa) may favor the precipitation of calcium carbonate and calcium oxalate crystals.

NEXT DIAGNOSTIC STEP TO CONSIDER IF LEVELS HIGH Assess the diet and current medications.

DRUG EFFECTS ON LEVELS Sulfonamides are associated with crystalluria.

SPECIMEN AND PROCESSING CONSIDERATIONS

LAB ARTIFACTS THAT MAY INTERFERE WITH READINGS OF LEVELS OF THIS SUBSTANCE (AND HOW—ARTIFICIALLY ELEVATED VS. DEPRESSED) Dissolution of crystals may occur as urine pH changes after voiding and with prolonged storage. Conversely, crystal formation may occur *in vitro* with urine evaporation or refrigeration.

SAMPLE FOR COLLECTION (TYPE OF SPECIMEN, COLOR TUBE) AND ANY SPECIAL SPECIMEN HANDLING NOTES Midstream urine collection in a clean container

PEARLS Crystalluria is not a reliable indicator for the presence of urolithiasis; however, crystalluria is a risk factor for the formation of uroliths.

AUTHOR: **LAURA C. CREGAR**

EDITOR: **CHARLES WIEDMEYER**

Urinary Crystals

Name	Description	Significance
Struvite (magnesium ammonium phosphate)	Colorless prisms with three to six sides (coffin lid)	Common in mildly acidic to alkaline urine in normal dogs and cats; may be associated with struvite calculi and infection with urease-producing bacteria
Calcium oxalate (monohydrate)	Dumbbells or small spindles	May be normal (especially if delay in analysis after urine collection), or due to ethylene glycol intoxication; may be associated with oxalate calculi
Calcium oxalate (dihydrate)	Colorless envelopes or small stars	May be normal (especially if delay in analysis after urine collection), or due to ethylene glycol intoxication; may be associated with oxalate calculi
Calcium phosphate	Prisms (long) or amorphous	May be normal or associated with calculi
Ammonium urate	Yellow-brown "thorn apples"	Normal in dalmatians and English bulldogs; associated with hepatic insufficiency and portosystemic shunts; may be associated with urate calculi
Uric acid	Yellow to yellow-brown prisms, diamonds, or rosettes	Same as ammonium urate
Bilirubin	Golden-yellow to brown needles or granules	May be present in normal dogs with concentrated urine or may be due to bilirubinuria
Cystine	Colorless, flat hexagonal plates	Due to cystinuria; may be associated with calculi
Cholesterol	Colorless, flat, notched plates	May be found in normal dogs and cats
Hippuric acid	Prisms (four to six) sides with rounded corners	Uncertain; have been confused with calcium oxalate monohydrate crystals
Sulfonamide	Clear to brown eccentrically bound needles in sheaves	Associated with sulfonamide administration

Modified from Willard M, Tvedten H: *Small Animal Clinical Diagnosis by Laboratory Methods*, ed 4. St Louis, 2004, WB Saunders.

Urine Osmolality

BASIC INFORMATION

DEFINITION

The solute concentration of a solution that may be expressed as moles of solute or osmoles of solute particles per kilogram of solvent, mol/kg and osmol/kg, respectively.

TYPICAL NORMAL RANGE (US UNITS; SI UNITS)

600 to 1500 mOsm/kg, but is widely variable

PHYSIOLOGY

Sodium, chloride, and urea account for most of the osmotic activity in the urine. Large molecules (protein), cells, and casts contribute little to osmolality. The osmolality of urine is variable, and depends on the fluid and electrolyte balance of the body and the nitrogen content of the diet. In most urine samples, there is a linear relationship between urine specific gravity and osmolality.

PEARLS

- The ratio of urine osmolality (Uosm) to plasma osmolality (Posm) is useful to determine the ability of the kidneys to concentrate or dilute urine.
- A Uosm:Posm ratio greater than 1 indicates that the kidneys are able to concentrate urine.
- A Uosm:Posm ratio of 1 indicates that water and solute are being excreted in a state that is iso-osmotic with plasma.
- A Uosm:Posm ratio significantly less than 1 indicates the kidneys are able to dilute urine.

AUTHOR: **LAURA C. CREGAR**

EDITOR: **CHARLES WIEDMEYER**

Urine pH

BASIC INFORMATION

DEFINITION

The negative logarithm of urine hydrogen ion concentration

SYNONYM(S)

- Aciduria (urine pH <7.0)
- Alkalinuria (urine pH >7.0)

TYPICAL NORMAL RANGE (US UNITS; SI UNITS)

The majority of horses will have pH values equal to or greater than 7.0, and typically range from 7.5 to 8.5.

PHYSIOLOGY

Renal and extrarenal factors affect urine pH, including diet. Herbivores typically have alkaline urine unless they are consuming a milk diet.

CAUSES OF ABNORMALLY HIGH LEVELS Alkalinuria is expected in healthy herbivores.

CAUSES OF ABNORMALLY LOW LEVELS

- Aciduria is expected in herbivores on a milk diet.
- Acidosis (metabolic and less commonly respiratory) may cause urinary excretion of excess acid.
- Paradoxical aciduria associated with hypochloremic metabolic alkalosis
- Hypokalemia (hydrogen ion excretion in exchange for K^+ resorption in the distal tubules)
- Loop diuretic treatment (furosemide)
- Proximal renal tubular acidosis (if bicarbonate is depleted)
- Hydrogen production by some bacteria

NEXT DIAGNOSTIC STEP TO CONSIDER IF LEVELS LOW

Evaluate serum electrolyte and acid-base status (Na^+, K^+, Cl^-, HCO_3^-)

IMPORTANT INTERSPECIES DIFFERENCES Horses tend to have more alkaline urine than other veterinary species, particularly dogs and cats.

DRUG EFFECTS ON LEVELS Potassium wasting diuretics may result in renal K^+ conservation and excess H^+ excretion, causing aciduria.

SPECIMEN AND PROCESSING CONSIDERATIONS

LAB ARTIFACTS THAT MAY INTERFERE WITH READINGS OF LEVELS OF THIS SUBSTANCE

- High pH (>9.0) may cause a false positive urine protein (via dipstick).
- Pigmenturia (abnormal urine color) may interfere with visual interpretation of the color change on the dipstick reagent pad.
- Contamination of the dipstick pH reagent pad with buffer from an adjacent protein reagent pad may falsely decrease the urine pH result.

SAMPLE FOR COLLECTION (TYPE OF SPECIMEN, COLOR TUBE) AND ANY SPECIAL SPECIMEN HANDLING NOTES Midstream urine collection in a clean container

AUTHOR: **LAURA C. CREGAR**

EDITOR: **CHARLES WIEDMEYER**

Urine Specific Gravity

BASIC INFORMATION

DEFINITION

Urine specific gravity (USG) is a comparison of the density of urine to that of water. It is an estimate of urine osmolality (the solute concentration of a solution).

SYNONYM(S)

- Relative density
- Hyposthenuria: USG <1.008
- Isosthenuria: USG 1.008 to 1.014

TYPICAL NORMAL RANGE (US UNITS; SI UNITS)

1.020 to 1.050 assuming normal hydration status and no treatments that alter water resorption by the kidney

PHYSIOLOGY

The specific gravity of urine is dependent on the hydration status of the animal and the ability of the kidney to respond appropriately in order to dilute or concentrate urine over that of plasma.

CAUSES OF ABNORMALLY HIGH LEVELS

- Dehydration, marked proteinuria, and marked glucosuria
- Concentrated urine is commonly seen in horses fed a high percentage of hay and those living in hot environments.
- USG may be falsely increased 0.003 to 0.005 for every 1 g/dL of protein in the urine.
- USG may be falsely increased 0.004 to 0.005 for every 1 g/dL of glucose in the urine.

NEXT DIAGNOSTIC STEP TO CONSIDER IF LEVELS HIGH Assess hydration status.

CAUSES OF ABNORMALLY LOW LEVELS

- Marked hyposthenuria (USG 1.001–1.005) is rarely seen in horses; however, causes include psychogenic polydipsia, pituitary tumors, and diabetes insipidus.
- Hyposthenuria (USG <1.008) may be seen in horses with moderate kidney damage (when the ability to concentrate has been lost, but the ability to dilute has not) or with a high water content in the feed (nursing foals or horses at pasture).
- Isosthenuria (USG 1.008–1.014) occurs with renal disease (>75% nonfunctioning tubules or chronic renal failure), administration of diuretics (furosemide) and hypercalcemia.
- Hyposthenuria or isosthenuria in the face of dehydration or azotemia supports a diagnosis of renal disease.

NEXT DIAGNOSTIC STEP TO CONSIDER IF LEVELS LOW Assess hydration status and evaluate serum blood urea nitrogen (BUN), creatinine, phosphate, glucose, calcium, sodium, and potassium.

IMPORTANT INTERSPECIES DIFFERENCES Adults have greater concentrating ability than neonates.

DRUG EFFECTS ON LEVELS Diuretics will cause the USG to decrease.

SPECIMEN AND PROCESSING CONSIDERATIONS

LAB ARTIFACTS THAT MAY INTERFERE WITH READINGS OF LEVELS OF THIS SUBSTANCE (AND HOW—ARTIFICIALLY ELEVATED VS. DEPRESSED)

- A refractometer should be used for USG measurements. Specific gravity test pads on reagent strips are unreliable in equine urine. When using dipsticks to determine USG, the following will alter the reading:
  - pH of urine: The reagent strip underestimates USG in alkaline urine.
  - Protein: Urine with a reagent strip reading of 1+ to 2+ protein has an overestimated USG.
  - Ketones: Urine with a positive ketone reading (rare in horses) has an overestimated USG.

SAMPLE FOR COLLECTION (TYPE OF SPECIMEN, COLOR TUBE) AND ANY SPECIAL SPECIMEN HANDLING NOTES First urine sample voided (or collected via catheterization) before fluid therapy or immediately after institution of fluid treatment

PEARLS A wide range of USG can be found in clinically healthy or sick horses, and concurrent evaluation of hydration status, USG, and serum chemistry values are essential for proper interpretation. A USG without knowledge of these aspects is meaningless and collection of urine and serum at the same time is essential.

AUTHOR: **LAURA C. CREGAR**

EDITOR: **CHARLES WIEDMEYER**

Venous Oxygen Saturation/Venous Oxygen Tension

BASIC INFORMATION

DEFINITION

Venous oxygen saturation and venous oxygen tension are used as a reflection of tissue oxygenation to identify occult tissue oxygen debt. Mixed venous oxygen saturation and mixed venous oxygen tension, measured by a pulmonary artery catheter, are more accurate reflections of the venous oxygen content. Due to size restrictions, jugular venous blood is used to estimate mixed venous oxygen content in adult horses. Central venous samples are used in foals to estimate mixed venous oxygen content.

TYPICAL NORMAL RANGE (US UNITS; SI UNITS)

- Adult horses:
  - Normal jugular venous oxygen
    - 45.6 ± 4.7 mm Hg
  - Normal jugular oxygen saturation
    - 65% to 75%
- Foals (0–14 days of age):
  - Central venous oxygen content
    - 40.5 ± 0.4 mm Hg (recumbent)
    - 35.9 ± 0.4 mm Hg (upright)
  - Central venous oxygen saturation
    - 75%

PHYSIOLOGY

Mixed venous oxygen saturation and tension represent the oxygen remaining in the venous bloodstream after extraction of oxygen by the tissues.

CAUSES OF ABNORMALLY HIGH LEVELS Venous oxygen saturation and tension increase with impairment of oxygen extraction and utilization, typically due to mitochondrial dysfunction (ie, post-cardiac arrest, severe colitis).

Arterial oxygen content and delivery may be normal, with shunting occuring at the tissue level.

NEXT DIAGNOSTIC STEP TO CONSIDER IF LEVELS HIGH Determine the cause of systemic disease to provide definitive therapy. Determine values for other markers of reduced tissue perfusion (mean arterial pressure, venous lactate, central venous pressure, urine output) and optimize these parameters by increasing circulating fluid volume and cardiac output.

CAUSES OF ABNORMALLY LOW LEVELS Venous oxygen saturation and tension decrease as arterial oxygen delivery decreases (ie, reduced oxygen uptake by the lung), due to increased oxygen extraction by the tissues. Increased extraction in hypermetabolic states (ie, sepsis, seizures) may also reduce venous oxygen content, in the face of a normal arterial oxygen content.

NEXT DIAGNOSTIC STEP TO CONSIDER IF LEVELS LOW Continued low levels of venous oxygen despite fluid resuscitation indicate continued tissue oxygen debt. Determine values for other markers of reduced tissue perfusion (mean arterial pressure, venous lactate, central venous pressure, urine output) and optimize these parameters by increasing circulating fluid volume and cardiac output.

SPECIMEN AND PROCESSING CONSIDERATIONS

LAB ARTIFACTS THAT MAY INTERFERE WITH READINGS OF LEVELS OF THIS SUBSTANCE (AND HOW—ARTIFICIALLY ELEVATED VS. DEPRESSED)

- Exposure to room air will falsely increase oxygen levels.
- Increased time until sample assessment will falsely decrease oxygen.

SAMPLE FOR COLLECTION (TYPE OF SPECIMEN, COLOR TUBE) AND ANY SPECIAL SPECIMEN HANDLING NOTES

- Obtain an anaerobic sample, using a blood gas syringe, or 1-mL syringe rinsed with heparin, from the jugular vein in adults, and from a central venous line in foals.
- Samples should be analyzed immediately (within 10 minutes) on a blood gas meter for venous oxygen tension.
- Oxygen saturation is measured by infrared venous oximetry, available through a central venous catheter, or estimated by calculation from the oxyhemoglobin curve on most blood gas analyzers.

PEARLS: Jugular or cranial vena cava venous oxygen may be higher than $PcvO_2$ samples in shock or hypovolemia. Position may affect the correlation as well (sternal recumbency negatively affects this correlation).

SUGGESTED READING

Magdesian KG: Monitoring the critically ill equine patient. *Vet Clin N Am Equine Pract* 20:11–39, 2004.

Prittie J: Optimal endpoints of resuscitation and early goal-directed therapy. *J Vet Em Crit Care* 16(4):329–339, 2006.

AUTHOR: **AMELIA MUNSTERMAN**

EDITOR: **CHARLES WIEDMEYER**

West Nile Virus (WNV)

BASIC INFORMATION

DEFINITION

- A positive sense, single stranded, enveloped RNA virus, is a flavivirus of the family Flaviviridae.
- WNV is subcategorized as a member of the Japanese encephalitis virus group, which also includes St. Louis encephalitis virus.
- It is a vector borne virus, which is cycled between birds and ornithophilic mosquitos.
- WNV was first identified in 1937 from the blood of a woman in Uganda and since then has been the cause of several human epidemic and veterinary epizootics in northern Africa, southern Europe, and the Middle East. In 1999, WNV was identified as the cause of encephalomyelitis in several horses, birds, and humans in the United States. Subsequent to this, the virus has spread across the continental United States as well as portions of northern Mexico and southern Canada.
- House sparrows, crows, and birds of prey are the most common avian species affected.
- Horses and humans are aberrant hosts and appear to not be capable of amplification of the virus.

TYPICAL NORMAL RANGE (US UNITS; SI UNITS)

- Normal IgM titer should be negative or <1:4.
- There are no published reference intervals for serology. A fourfold increase in titers between acute and convalescent blood samples is required for definitive diagnosis.

PHYSIOLOGY

WNV is believed to infect susceptible cells (nervous tissue) through glycoprotein receptors followed by receptor-mediated endocytosis. Fusion of the viral envelope with the endosomal membrane results in release of the viral nucleoprotein and subsequent replication, translation, and release of new viral particles from the infected host cell.

CAUSES OF ABNORMALLY HIGH LEVELS Elevations in serum antibody titer are typically due to either active infection or exposure to the etiologic agent of disease.

NEXT DIAGNOSTIC STEP TO CONSIDER IF LEVELS HIGH Therapeutic intervention directed toward treating the clinical syndrome of WNV should be initiated.

CAUSES OF ABNORMALLY LOW LEVELS Low antibody concentrations suggest lack of exposure to the causative agent of disease.

NEXT DIAGNOSTIC STEP TO CONSIDER IF LEVELS LOW Low levels suggest lack of exposure to the causative agent of disease and the need to consider other etiologic agents or pathologic processes as the source of the observed clinical disease.

SPECIMEN AND PROCESSING CONSIDERATIONS

SAMPLE FOR COLLECTION (TYPE OF SPECIMEN, COLOR TUBE) AND ANY SPECIAL SPECIMEN HANDLING NOTES Ideal sample is serum separated from whole blood collected in a red-top tube.

PEARLS The most commonly utilized test is the IgM capture enzyme-linked immunosorbent assay (MAC-ELISA). Horses develop a very robust IgM response once exposed to the WNV that lasts approximately 6 weeks. As the diagnostic test is evaluating IgM in place of IgG, a positive test is indicative of recent exposure to the offending virus and subsequently active infection. The only other explanation for a positive titer is recent (within the previous 2 weeks) vaccination. Alternatively, a four-fold change in paired neutralizing antibody titers using the plaque reduction neutralizing test (PRNT) can also identify affected horses. Vaccination is more of a confounding variable in this instance as the process of vaccination will induce the formation of neutralizing antibody and complicate interpretation of the test results. Subsequently, use of the PRNT has decreased significantly with the introduction of WNV vaccines.

AUTHORS: **SHANE F. DeWITT** and **TANYA M. GRONDIN**

EDITOR: **CHARLES WIEDMEYER**

White Blood Cells

BASIC INFORMATION

DEFINITION

White blood cells consist of granulocytes (neutrophils, eosinophils, and basophils), monocytes, and lymphocytes. Occasionally, mast cells can be observed in the tissue and the peripheral blood.

SYNONYM(S)

Leukocytes

TYPICAL NORMAL RANGE (US UNITS; SI UNITS)

5 to 12 × 10^3/mL

PHYSIOLOGY

Leukocytes originate from the bone marrow and consist of granulocytic and mononuclear cells. These cells are important in both the innate and adaptive immune response. Characterization of increases and decreases of specific cells (neutrophils, eosinophils, basophils, lymphocytes, and monocytes) can help characterize how a patient is responding to a particular antigenic stimulus.

CAUSES OF ABNORMALLY HIGH LEVELS Causes of abnormally high levels or leukocytosis depend on which cell type is increased. An increase in neutrophils or neutrophilia may indicate a stress or inflammatory response. If there is an eosinophilia, parasitemia or a hypersensitivity response should be considered. Lymphocytosis can occur with immune stimulation, or associated with epinephrine release which can accompany excitement or exercise.

NEXT DIAGNOSTIC STEP TO CONSIDER IF LEVELS HIGH Evaluation of individual leukocytes should be utilized to better characterize the leukocytosis. Additionally, examination of a peripheral blood smear is recommended to evaluate the cellular morphology.

CAUSES OF ABNORMALLY LOW LEVELS A decrease in white blood cell numbers or leukopenia can occur with increased tissue demand as can be seen in severe inflammatory responses, endotoxemia, or bone marrow suppression.

NEXT DIAGNOSTIC STEP TO CONSIDER IF LEVELS LOW A 100-cell differential count is necessary to help further identify the cause of leukopenia; generally lymphopenia or neutropenia. Severe tissue demand is a common cause of neutropenia and generally the patient will have systemic evidence of disease. However, if no systemic cause is evident, bone marrow aspiration may be indicated.

SPECIMEN AND PROCESSING CONSIDERATIONS

SAMPLE FOR COLLECTION (TYPE OF SPECIMEN, COLOR TUBE) AND ANY SPECIAL SPECIMEN HANDLING NOTES Whole, anticoagulated blood is necessary for evaluation. Most commonly, ethylenediamine tetraacetic acid (purple-top tube) is used for complete blood count (CBC); however, sodium citrate (blue-top tube) can also be used. If the blood cannot be evaluated immediately, preparation of a blood smear to preserve the integrity of red and white blood cell morphology is recommended.

PEARLS Severe leukocytosis in horses is fairly uncommon and therefore evaluation of specific blood cells in the differential count is essential to appropriately interpret changes in the white blood cell count.

AUTHOR: **ANNE BARGER**

EDITOR: **CHARLES WIEDMEYER**

Clinical Algorithms

Abnormal Breathing

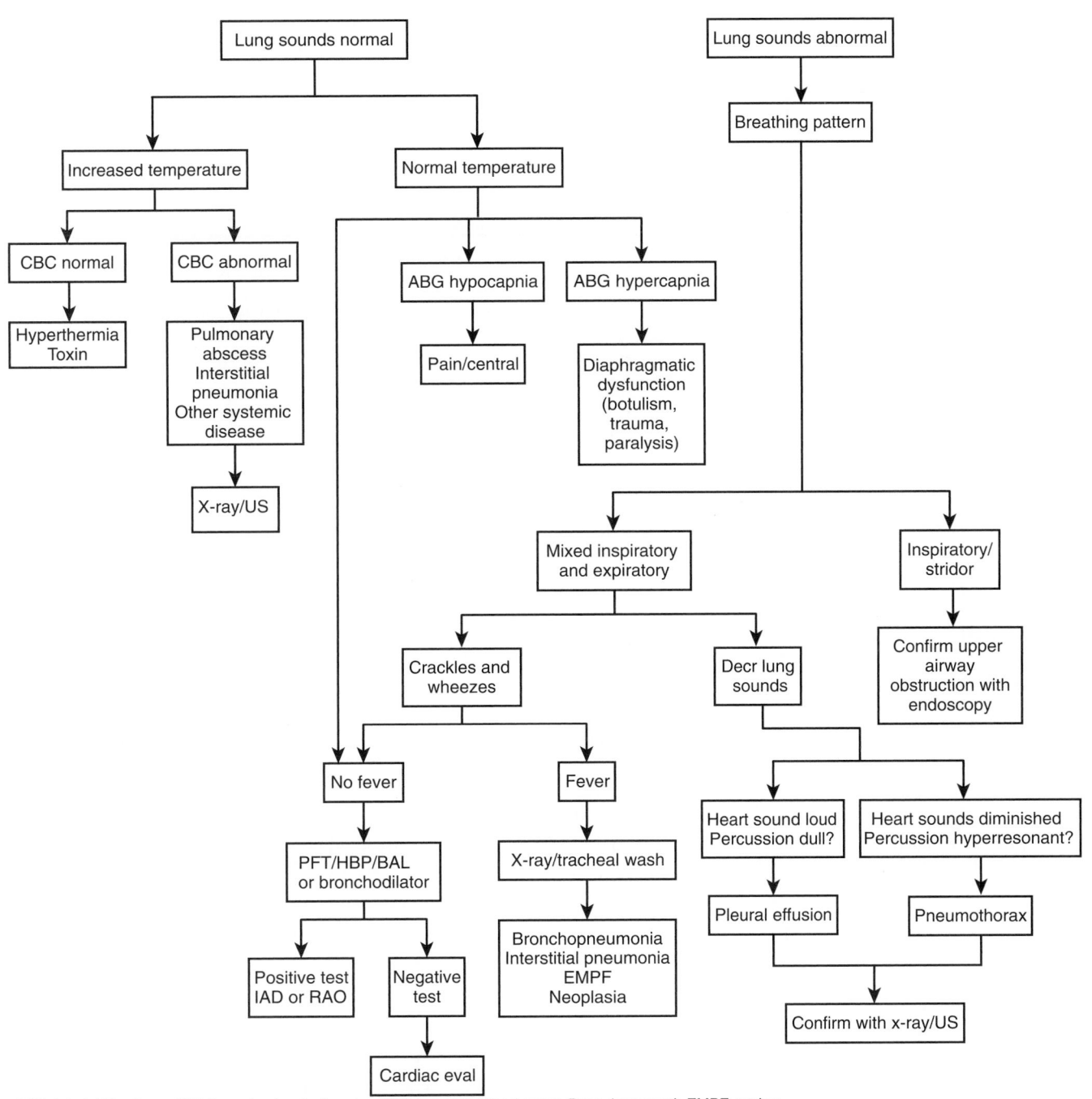

ABG, Arterial blood gas; *BAL,* bronchoalveolar lavage; *CBC,* complete blood count; *Decr,* decreased; *EMPF,* equine multinodular pulmonary fibrosis; *HBP,* high blood pressure; *IAD,* inflammatory airway disease; *PFT,* pulmonary function test; *RAO,* recurrent airway obstruction; *US,* ultrasound.

Author: **Melissa R. Mazan**

Arterial Blood Gas Samples: Assessment

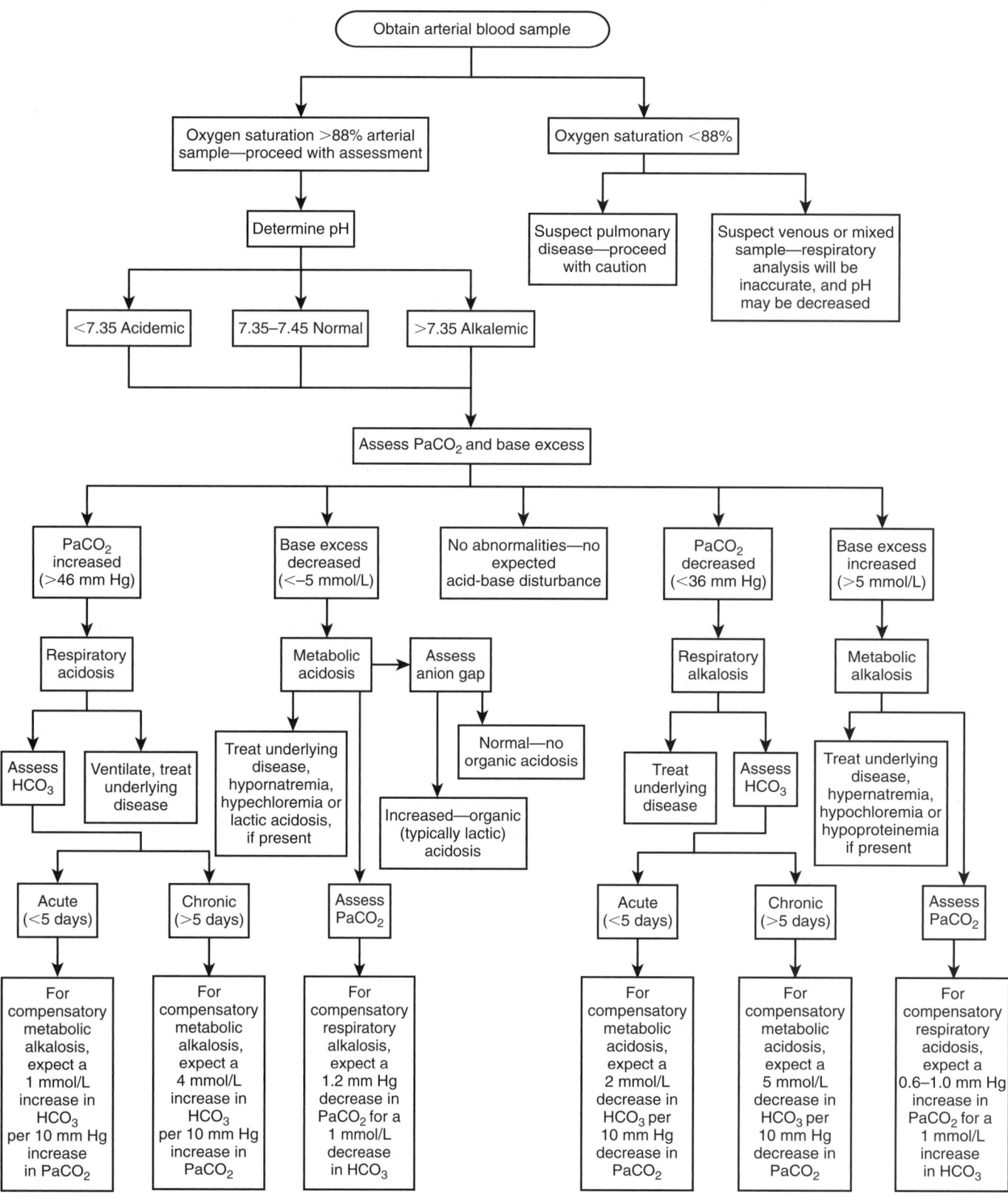

Obtain arterial blood sample

Oxygen saturation >88% arterial sample—proceed with assessment

Oxygen saturation <88%

Suspect pulmonary disease—proceed with caution

Suspect venous or mixed sample—respiratory analysis will be inaccurate, and pH may be decreased

Determine pH

<7.35 Acidemic

7.35–7.45 Normal

>7.35 Alkalemic

Assess $PaCO_2$ and base excess

$PaCO_2$ increased (>46 mm Hg)

Base excess decreased (<–5 mmol/L)

No abnormalities—no expected acid-base disturbance

$PaCO_2$ decreased (<36 mm Hg)

Base excess increased (>5 mmol/L)

Respiratory acidosis

Metabolic acidosis

Assess anion gap

Respiratory alkalosis

Metabolic alkalosis

Assess HCO_3

Ventilate, treat underlying disease

Treat underlying disease, hypornatremia, hypechloremia or lactic acidosis, if present

Normal—no organic acidosis

Increased—organic (typically lactic) acidosis

Treat underlying disease

Assess HCO_3

Treat underlying disease, hypernatremia, hypochloremia or hypoproteinemia if present

Acute (<5 days)

Chronic (>5 days)

Assess $PaCO_2$

Acute (<5 days)

Chronic (>5 days)

Assess $PaCO_2$

For compensatory metabolic alkalosis, expect a 1 mmol/L increase in HCO_3 per 10 mm Hg increase in $PaCO_2$

For compensatory metabolic alkalosis, expect a 4 mmol/L increase in HCO_3 per 10 mm Hg increase in $PaCO_2$

For compensatory respiratory alkalosis, expect a 1.2 mm Hg decrease in $PaCO_2$ for a 1 mmol/L decrease in HCO_3

For compensatory metabolic acidosis, expect a 2 mmol/L decrease in HCO_3 per 10 mm Hg decrease in $PaCO_2$

For compensatory metabolic acidosis, expect a 5 mmol/L decrease in HCO_3 per 10 mm Hg decrease in $PaCO_2$

For compensatory respiratory acidosis, expect a 0.6–1.0 mm Hg increase in $PaCO_2$ for a 1 mmol/L increase in HCO_3

If expected and actual values calculated for compensation do not match, look for evidence of a mixed acid-base disorder.

HCO_3, Bicarbonate; $PaCO_2$, arterial partial pressure of carbon doxide.

Author: **Amelia Munsterman**

Blindness, Acute and Gradual Onset

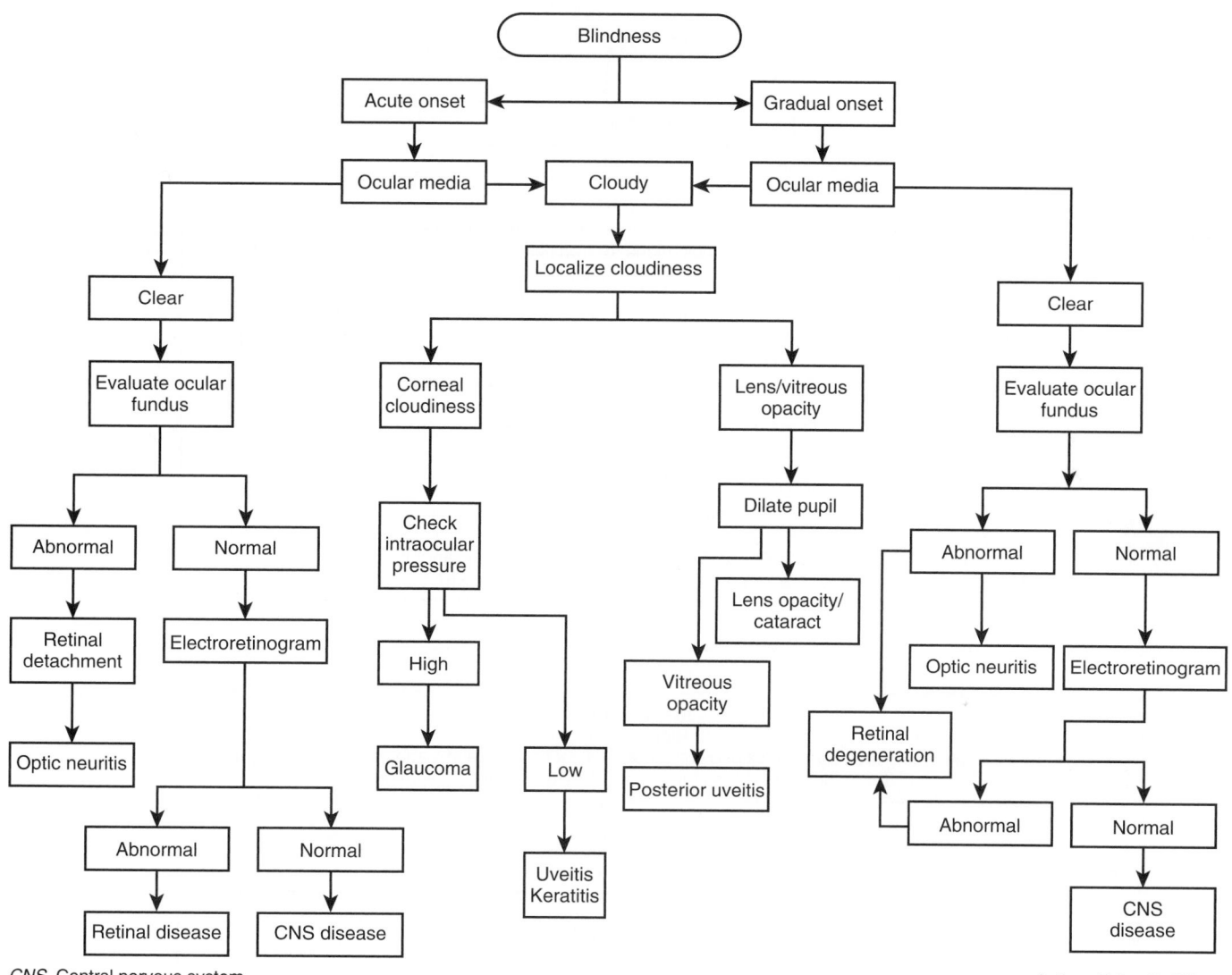

CNS, Central nervous system.

Author: **Brian C. Gilger**

Blood Transfusion in Adult Horses

Acute hemorrhagic shock

↓

Patient assessment

↓

Clinical Examination

Indications for transfusion:
Tachycardia (>60/min); tachypnea (>32/min), pale mucous membranes, sweating, trembling, colic, uncontrollable bleeding, cool extremities, systolic blood pressure <80 mm Hg, persistent hypotension after fluids, estimate of loss: >33% of estimated blood volume (critical volume)

↓

Clinicopathologic Examination

Packed cell volume <12%*
Hemoglobin <7 g/dL
Total plasma protein <4.0 g/dL
Venous L-lactate >4 mmol/L
PvO_2 <25 mm Hg
* PCV is an unreliable indicator in cases of acute hemorrhagic anemia. If low (<20%), this indicates severe hemorrhage and warrants immediate transfusion therapy.

↓

Compatability testing

1. Cross-matching (major and minor) or
2. Blood typing (if known)
In an emergency situation skip to collection and choose a healthy, adult gelding of the same breed (ideally) with no previous history of transfusion administration.

↓

Calculate estimated deficit

If signs of hypovolemic hemorrhagic shock are present, estimate at least >25% loss of blood volume.
If hemorrhage is external, calculate the blood loss by collecting blood into a container or weighing surgical sponges and calculating the loss in milliliters/minute.
Liters of blood lost can also be estimated by the following (if not acute hemorrhage):
((normal PCV - patient PCV)/normal PCV) × (0.08) × (patient weight in kg).
Goal is to administer 40% of blood lost

↓

Blood collection

Choose an appropriate anticoagulant depending on how soon the blood will be administered.
Draw blood in a sterile manner into plastic bag, rocking gently during collection.
Donor may require sedation and crystalloids depending on the volume removed.
Up to 20% of donor blood volume may be harvested.

↓

Begin administration

Use a blood administration set with filter; change the set every 3–4 L.
Start at 0.1 mL/kg for 10–15 minutes.
Monitor for signs of transfusion reaction...STOP if reaction occurs.
Continue at 20–30 mL/kg/hour until desired volume administered.
Monitor for signs of transfusion reaction...STOP if reaction occurs.

PCV, Packed cell volume.

Author: **Samuel Hurcombe**

Cardiac Auscultation

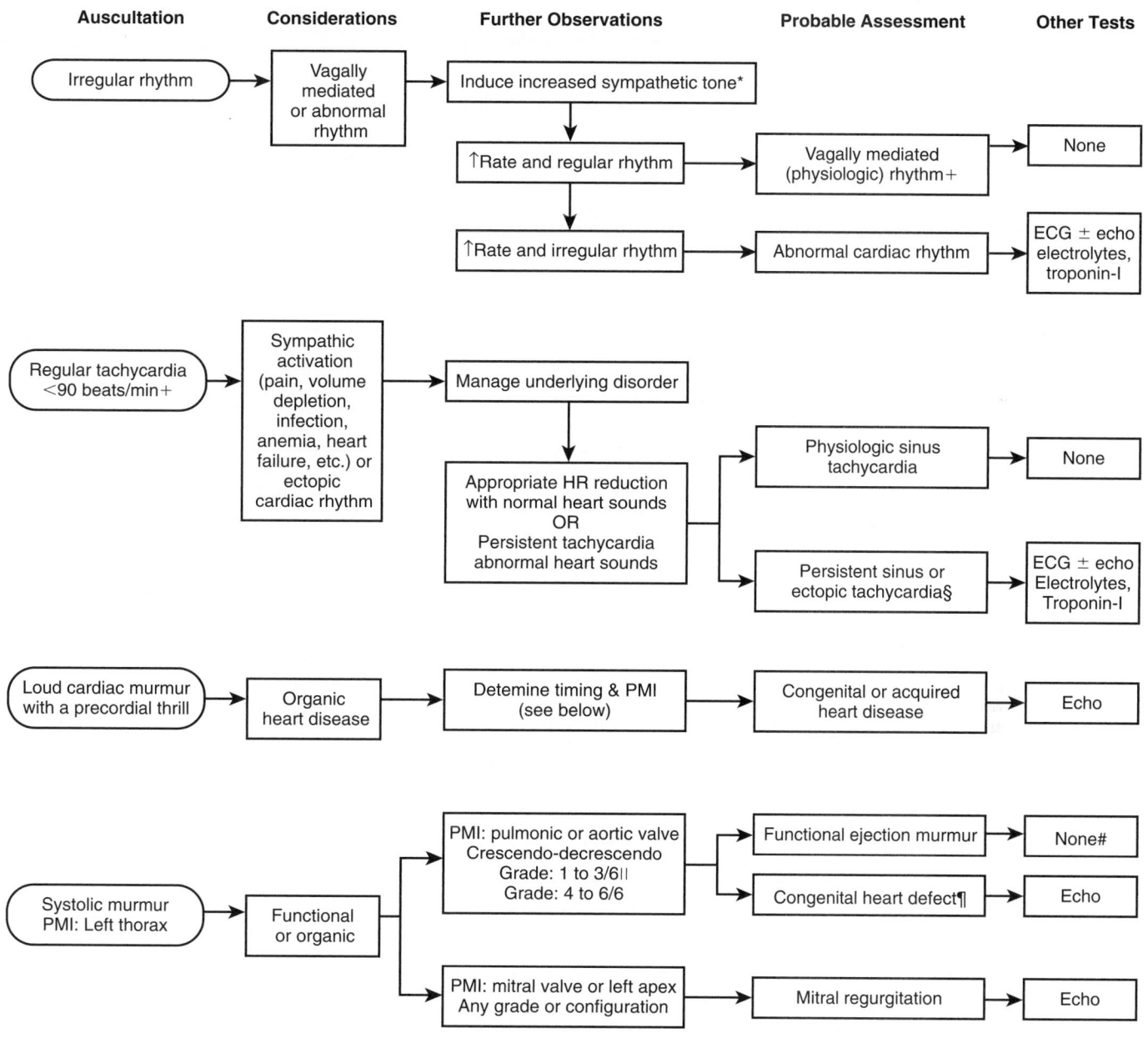

Auscultation	Considerations	Further Observations	Probable Assessment	Other Tests

Configuration: Refers to the phonocardiographic "shape" or a murmur, such as a plateau-shaped murmur that extends from the first sound through the second sound is termed holosystolic or pansystolic (e.g., mitral regurgitation or ventricular septal defect); a "diamond-shaped" murmur is crescendo-decrescendo in configuration (e.g., functional ejection); a "blowing" murmur that starts suddenly but dissipates gradually is decrescendo (e.g., aortic regurgitation), while a murmur that becomes progressively louder and then stops is crescendo in configuration (e.g., mitral regurgitation from mitral valve prolapse).

ECG: Perform an electrocardiogram to determine heart rhythm.

Echo: Perform an echocardiogram to identify abnormal structure, cardiac size, or function; Doppler studies are added to assess normal and abnormal blood flow patterns and are optimal for evaluating horses with cardiac murmurs; Doppler studies must be interpreted relative to auscultatory findings.

Grade: Intensity of the murmur on a 1 through 6 scale; in most systems a grade 5 or 6 murmur is accompanied by a precordial thrill.

HR: Heart rate.

Organic: Related to a structural lesion in the heart or great vessels.

PMI: Point of maximal murmur intensity.

Precordial thrill: The palpable thoracic vibration associated with a loud cardiac murmur. troponin-I: Serum level of inhibitory cardiac troponin or cTnI, a biomarker used to detect cardiomyocyte injury or necrosis.

Valve: Refers to the general valve area of auscultation.

Cont. on p. 980

CLINICAL ALGORITHMS

Cont. from p. 979

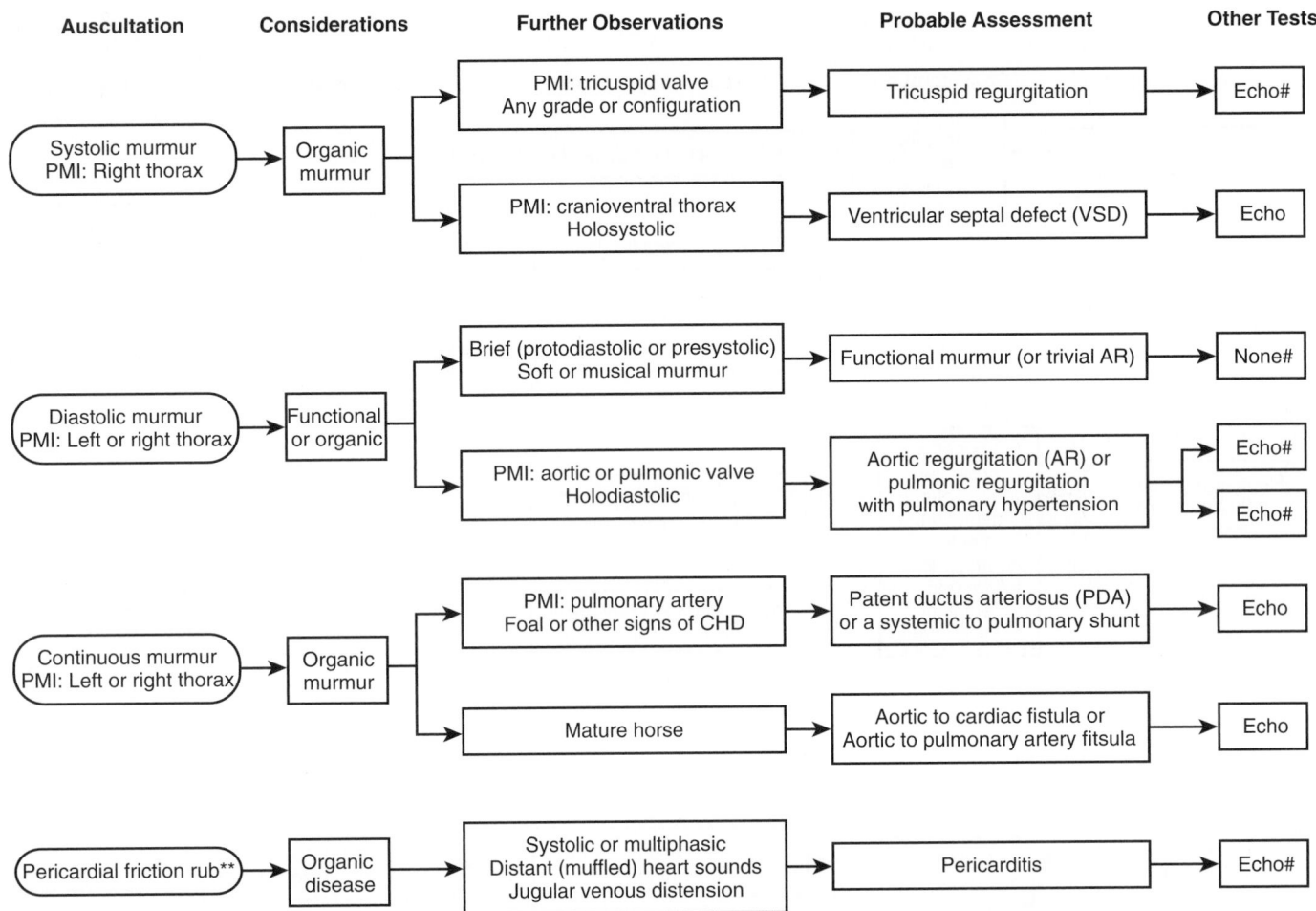

Auscultation	Considerations	Further Observations	Probable Assessment	Other Tests
Systolic murmur PMI: Right thorax	Organic murmur	PMI: tricuspid valve Any grade or configuration	Tricuspid regurgitation	Echo#
		PMI: cranioventral thorax Holosystolic	Ventricular septal defect (VSD)	Echo
Diastolic murmur PMI: Left or right thorax	Functional or organic	Brief (protodiastolic or presystolic) Soft or musical murmur	Functional murmur (or trivial AR)	None#
		PMI: aortic or pulmonic valve Holodiastolic	Aortic regurgitation (AR) or pulmonic regurgitation with pulmonary hypertension	Echo# / Echo#
Continuous murmur PMI: Left or right thorax	Organic murmur	PMI: pulmonary artery Foal or other signs of CHD	Patent ductus arteriosus (PDA) or a systemic to pulmonary shunt	Echo
		Mature horse	Aortic to cardiac fistula or Aortic to pulmonary artery fitsula	Echo
Pericardial friction rub**	Organic disease	Systolic or multiphasic Distant (muffled) heart sounds Jugular venous distension	Pericarditis	Echo#

* Endogenous sympathetic activity can be transiently increased by suddenly leading the horse in four or five tight circles or through trotting or lunging; the horse should be examined immediately after the activity has stopped.

† Vagally induced rhythms include sinus pause or arrest, sinoatrial block, sinus arrhythmia, and second-degree atrioventricular block.

‡ Resting tachycardia exceeding 90/min should be evaluated with an ECG to qualify the rhythm; the cut-off rate is arbitrary but clinically useful.

§ Ectopic rhythms include ectopic atrial tachycardia, junctional (nodal) tachycardia, and ventricular tachycardia.

‖ Functional murmurs due to ejection of blood into the great vessels often become transiently louder following an increase in sympathetic activity.

¶ Loud ejection murmurs over the semilunar valves and great vessels may indicate pulmonic stenosis or complex defects such as tetralogy of Fallot.

Judgment should be exercised regarding the need for echocardiography. An echocardiogram might be indicated in the prepurchase examination of any valuable foal or horse with a cardiac murmur, whereas echocardiography may not be indicated in an older horse with a soft murmur or AR or in a fit racehorse with a typical murmur of tricuspid regurgitation.

** Classical pericardial friction rubs are heard during systole, early diastole, and late diastole. Occasionally a functional presystolic murmur exhibits a frequency quality similar to a brief friction rub.

Author: **John D. Bonagura**

Cardiac Output and Blood Pressure

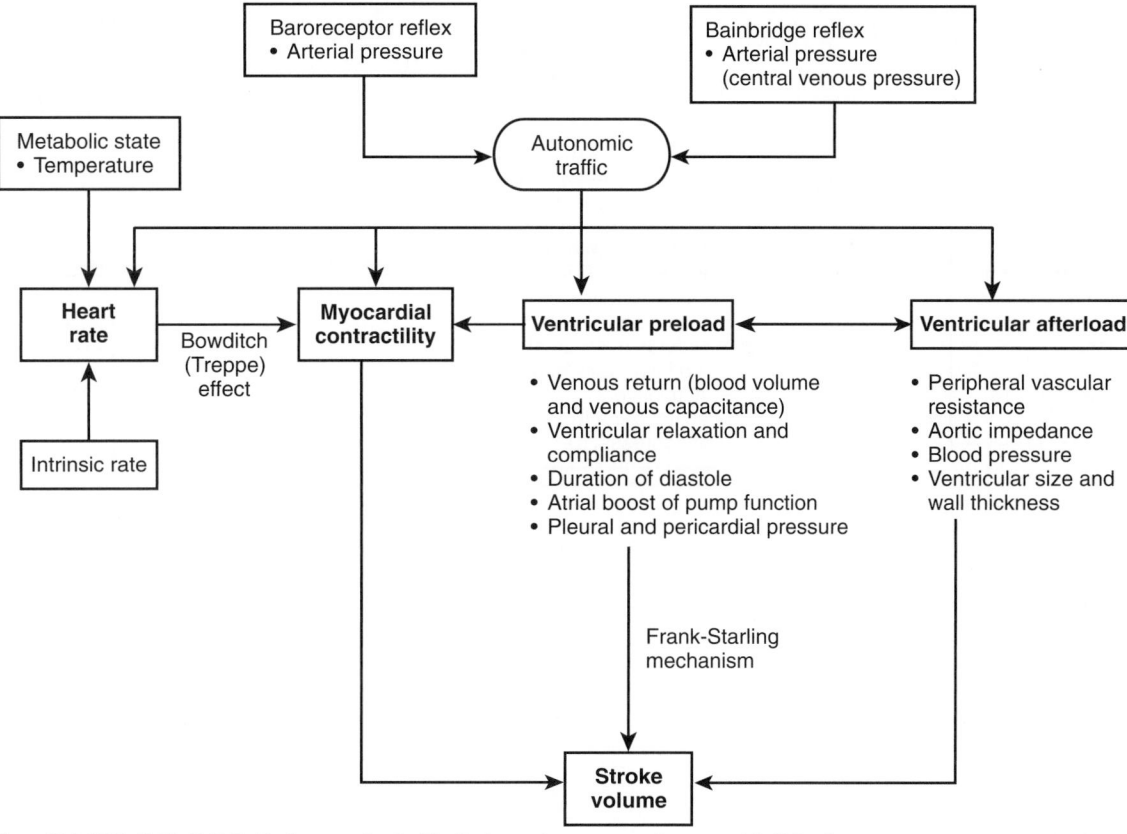

From Muir WW, Hubbell JAE. *Equine anesthesia: Monitoring and emergency therapy*, ed 2, St Louis, 2009, Saunders Elsevier, p 50.

Cardiopulmonary Cerebral Resuscitation (CPCR)

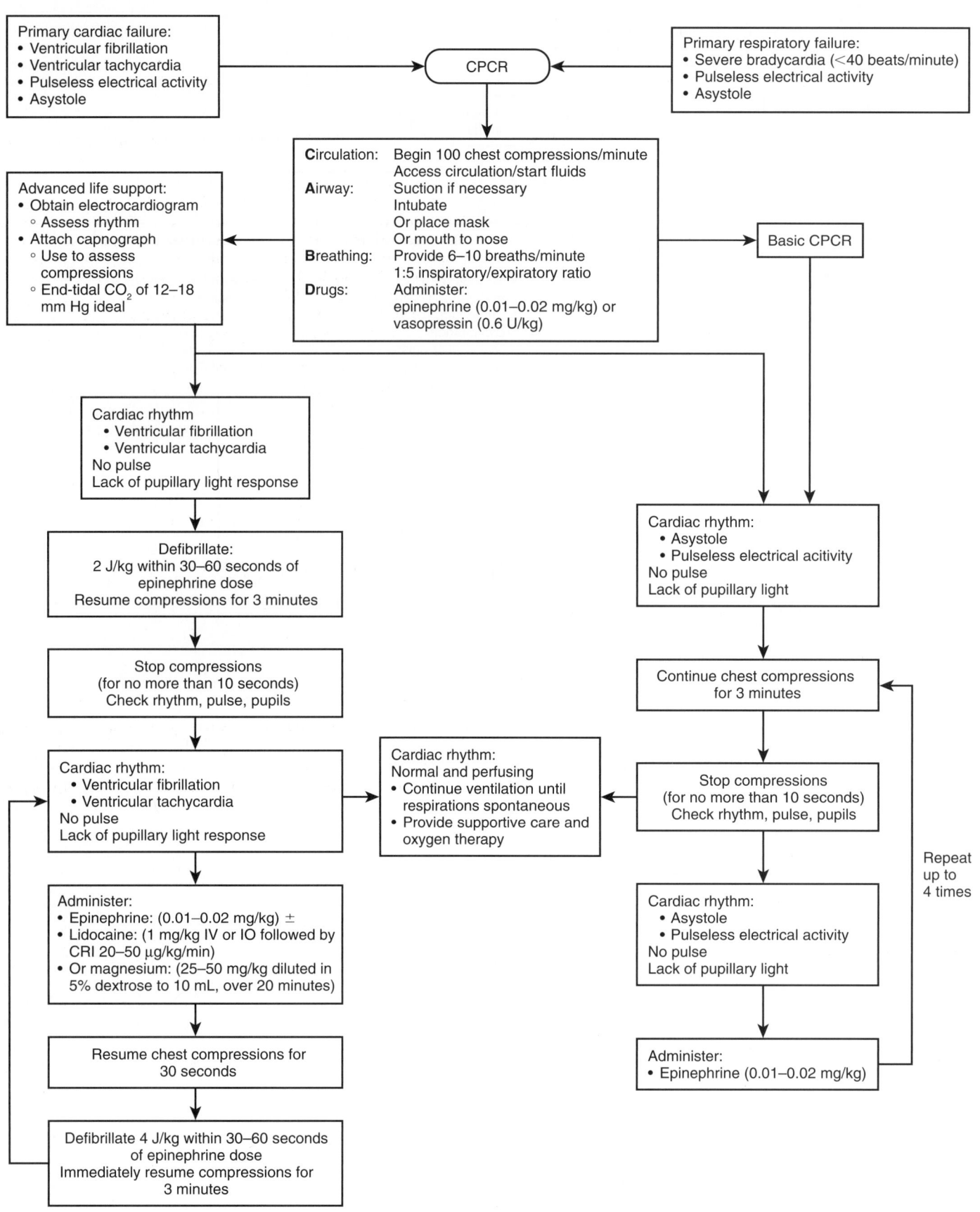

Primary cardiac failure:
- Ventricular fibrillation
- Ventricular tachycardia
- Pulseless electrical activity
- Asystole

CPCR

Primary respiratory failure:
- Severe bradycardia (<40 beats/minute)
- Pulseless electrical activity
- Asystole

Circulation: Begin 100 chest compressions/minute
Access circulation/start fluids
Airway: Suction if necessary
Intubate
Or place mask
Or mouth to nose
Breathing: Provide 6–10 breaths/minute
1:5 inspiratory/expiratory ratio
Drugs: Administer:
epinephrine (0.01–0.02 mg/kg) or
vasopressin (0.6 U/kg)

Advanced life support:
- Obtain electrocardiogram
  ○ Assess rhythm
- Attach capnograph
  ○ Use to assess compressions
  ○ End-tidal CO_2 of 12–18 mm Hg ideal

Basic CPCR

Cardiac rhythm
- Ventricular fibrillation
- Ventricular tachycardia
No pulse
Lack of pupillary light response

Defibrillate:
2 J/kg within 30–60 seconds of epinephrine dose
Resume compressions for 3 minutes

Stop compressions
(for no more than 10 seconds)
Check rhythm, pulse, pupils

Cardiac rhythm:
- Ventricular fibrillation
- Ventricular tachycardia
No pulse
Lack of pupillary light response

Cardiac rhythm:
Normal and perfusing
- Continue ventilation until respirations spontaneous
- Provide supportive care and oxygen therapy

Administer:
- Epinephrine: (0.01–0.02 mg/kg) ±
- Lidocaine: (1 mg/kg IV or IO followed by CRI 20–50 µg/kg/min)
- Or magnesium: (25–50 mg/kg diluted in 5% dextrose to 10 mL, over 20 minutes)

Resume chest compressions for 30 seconds

Defibrillate 4 J/kg within 30–60 seconds of epinephrine dose
Immediately resume compressions for 3 minutes

Cardiac rhythm:
- Asystole
- Pulseless electrical activity
No pulse
Lack of pupillary light

Continue chest compressions for 3 minutes

Stop compressions
(for no more than 10 seconds)
Check rhythm, pulse, pupils

Cardiac rhythm:
- Asystole
- Pulseless electrical activity
No pulse
Lack of pupillary light

Administer:
- Epinephrine (0.01–0.02 mg/kg)

Repeat up to 4 times

Author: **Amelia Munsterman**

Central Nervous System Trauma

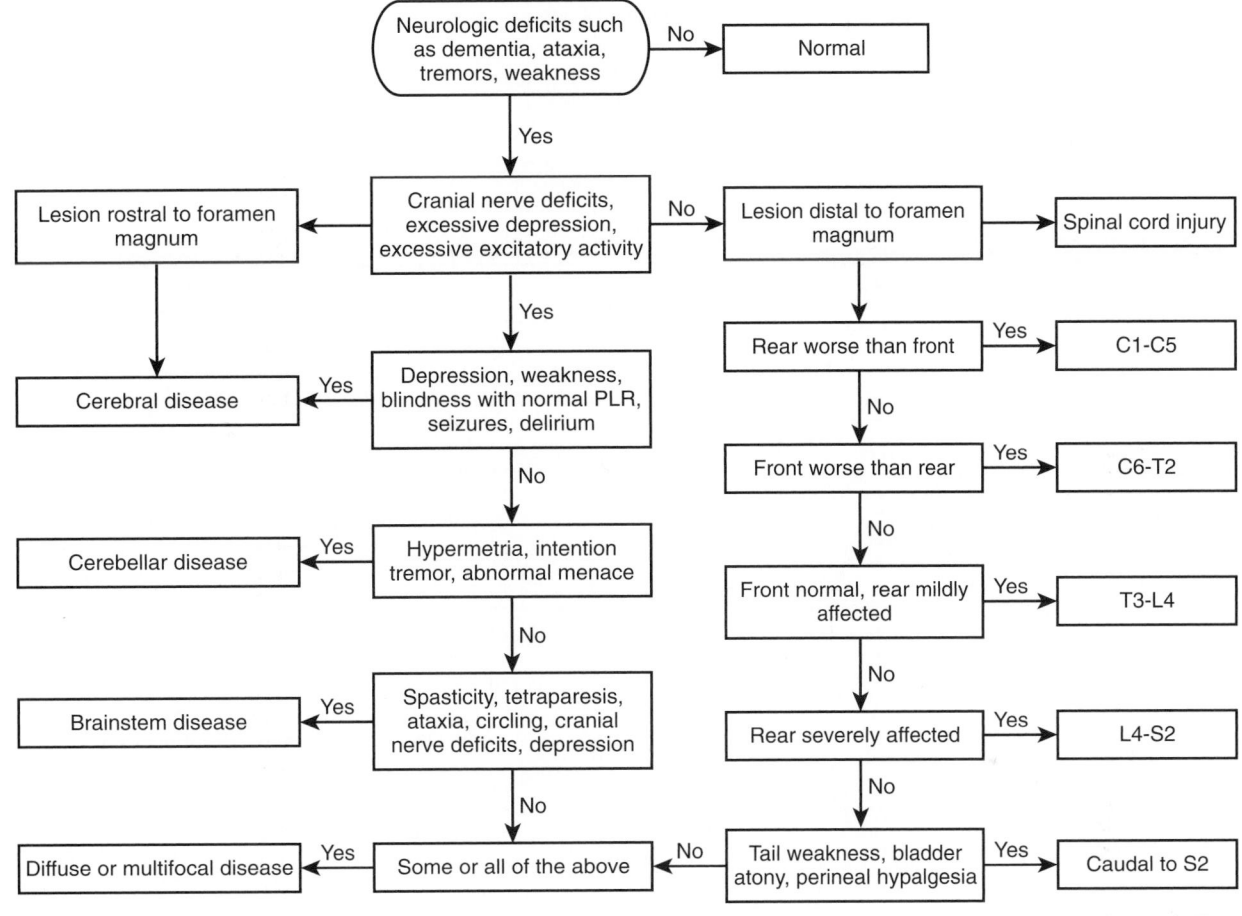

PLR, Pupillary light response.

Author: **Yvette S. Nout**

Corneal Ulcer

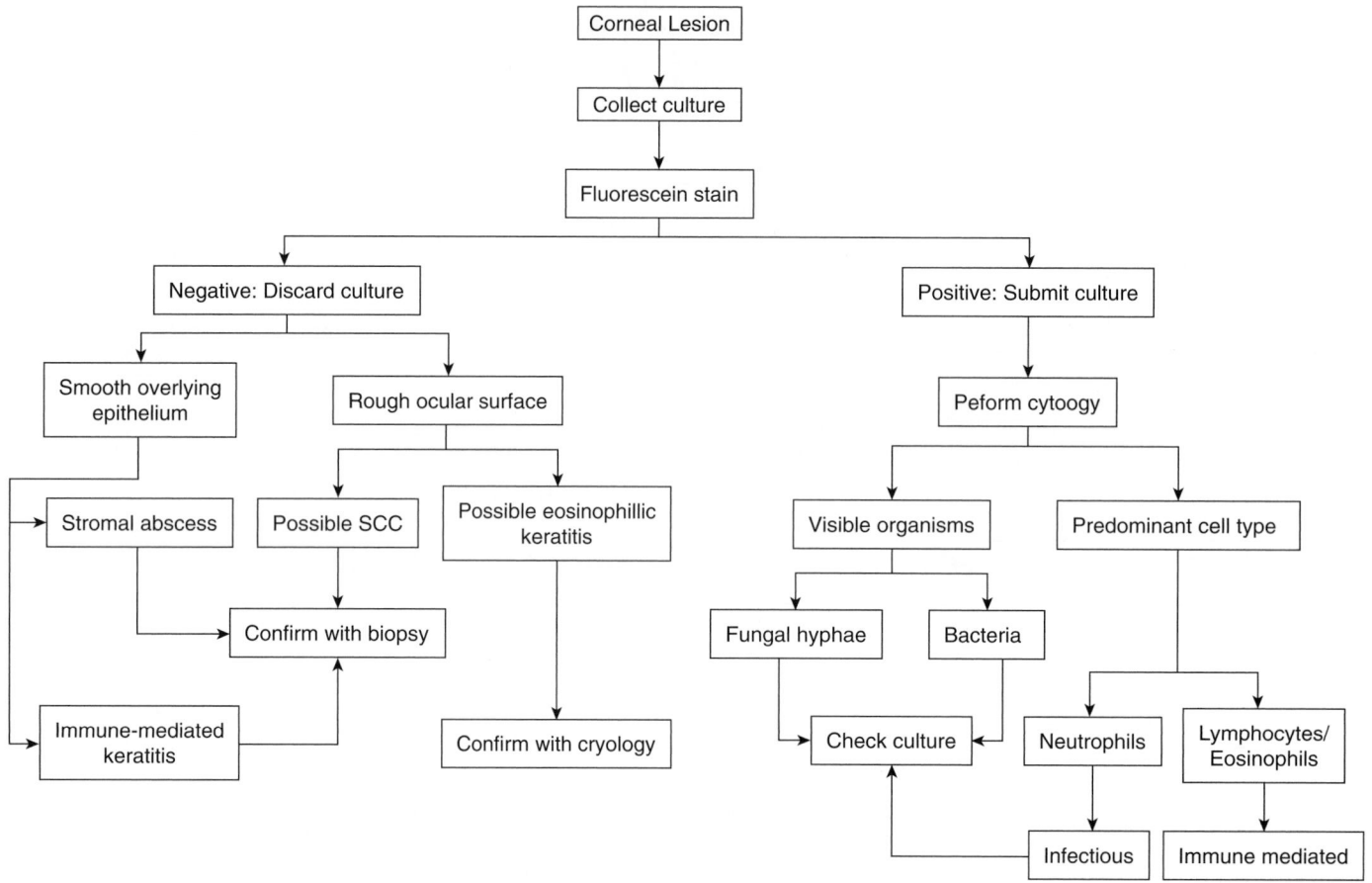

SCC, Squamous cell carcinoma.

Author: **Brian C. Gilger**

Cough

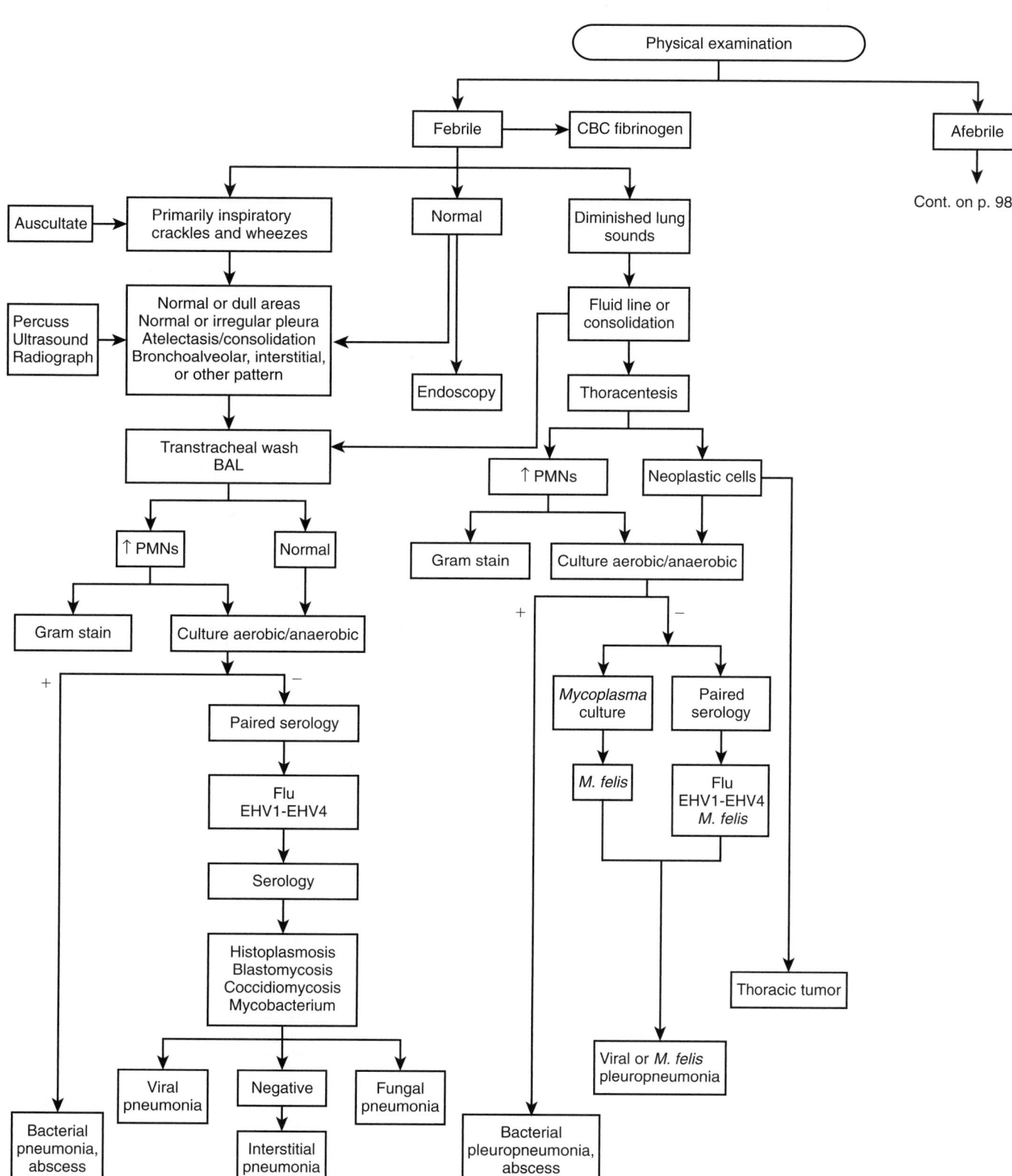

From Reed SJ, Bayly WM, Sellon DC: *Equine internal medicine*, ed 3, St Louis, 2010, Saunders Elsevier.

AEF, Arytenoepiglottic fold entrapment; *BAL*, bronchoalveolar lavage; *BAS*, basophils; *CBC*, complete blood count; *DDSP*, dorsal displacement of the soft palate; *DPPA*, displacement of the palatopharyngeal arch; *EIPH*, exercise-induced pulmonary hemorrhage; EOS, eosinophils; *EPM*, equine protozoal myelitis; *IAD*, inflammatory airway disease; *MC*, mast cells; *PMN*, polymorphonuclear leukocyte; *RAO*, recurrent airway obstruction; *TTA*, transtracheal aspirate.

Cont. on p. 986

CLINICAL ALGORITHMS

Cont. from p. 985

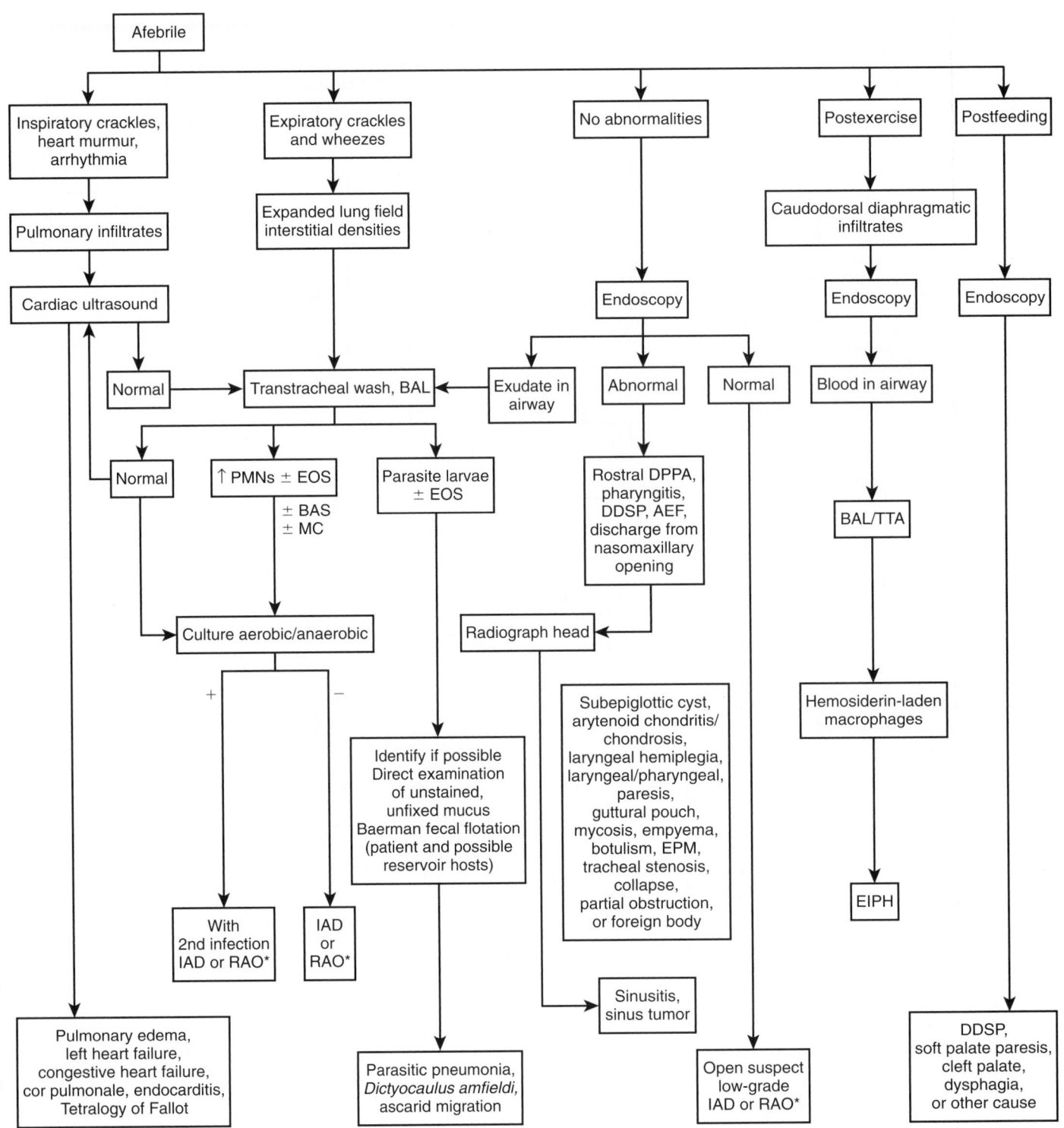

IAD, compared with RAO, is characterized by less neutrophilic inflammation and is more likely to have increased numbers of eosinophils, basophils, and monocytes in BAL fluid samples.

Dental Disease

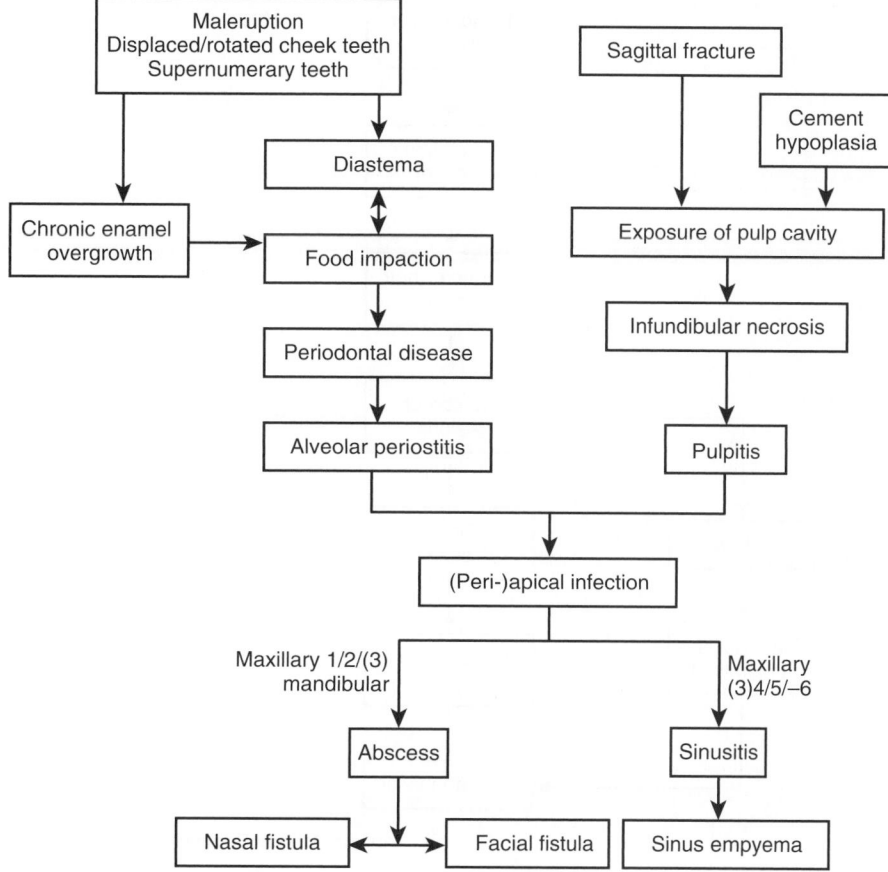

Baker G: *Equine dentistry,* ed 2, St. Louis, 2004, Saunders Elsevier.

Dermatophilosis

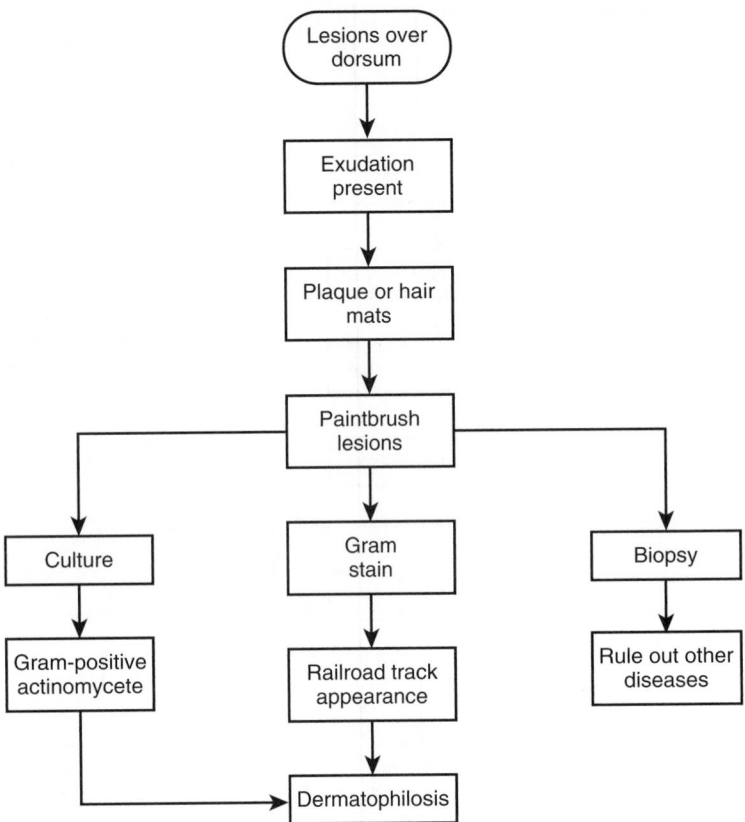

Author: **Alfredo Sanchez Londoño**

Dermatophytosis

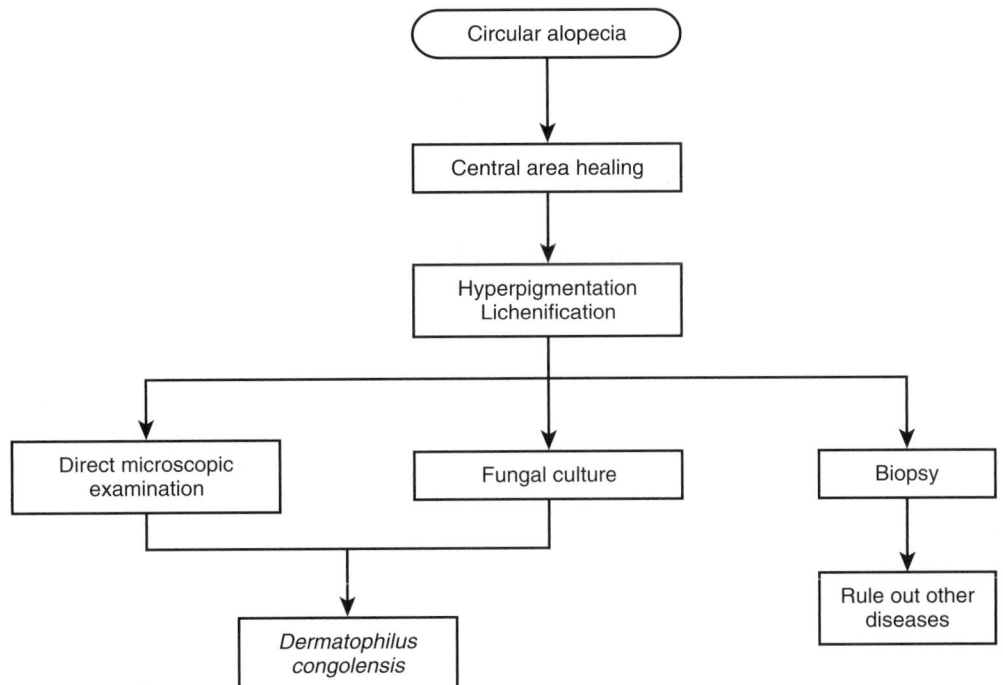

Author: **Alfredo Sanchez Londoño**

Electrocardiography/Arrhythmia

PART A

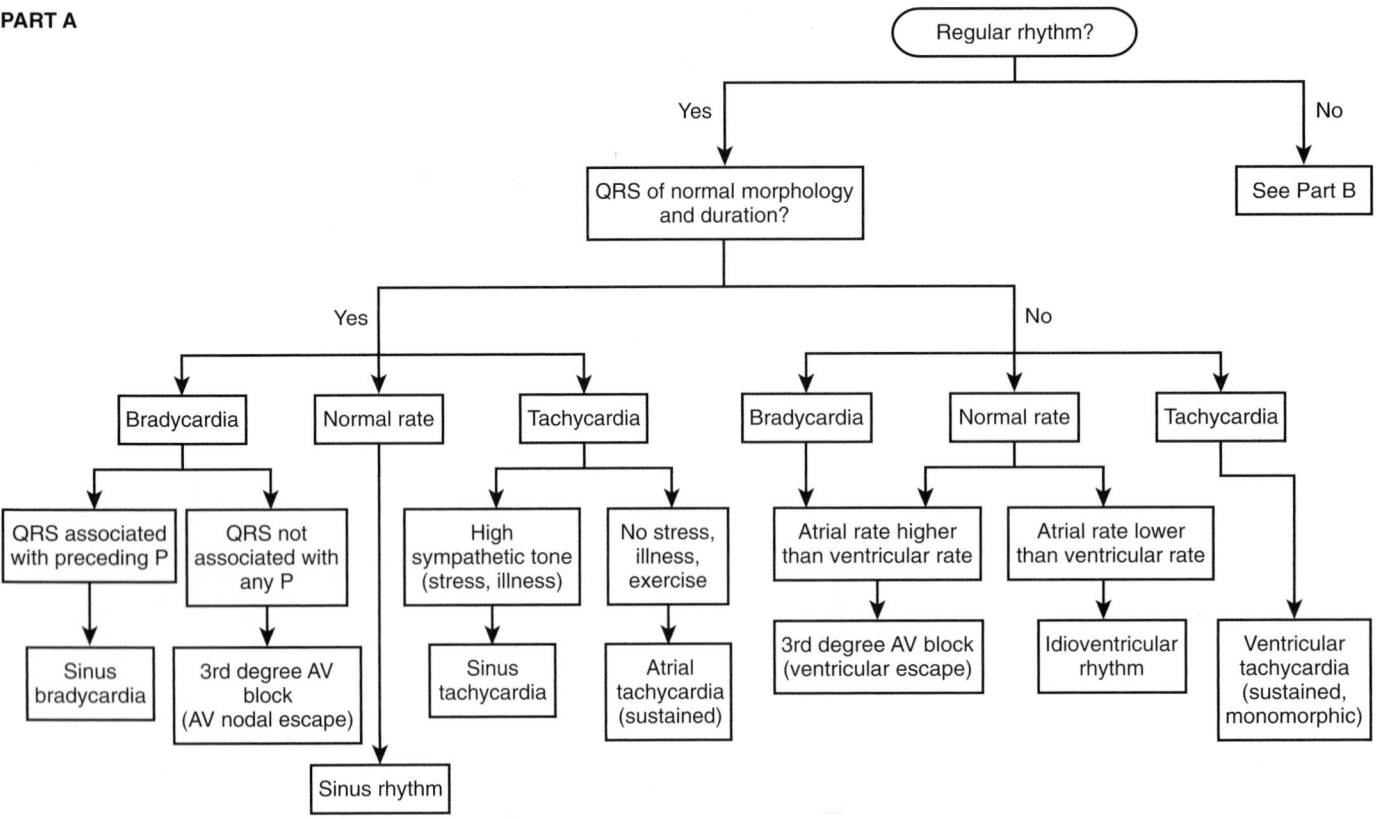

AV, Atrioventricular.

Author: **Gunther van Loon**

PART B

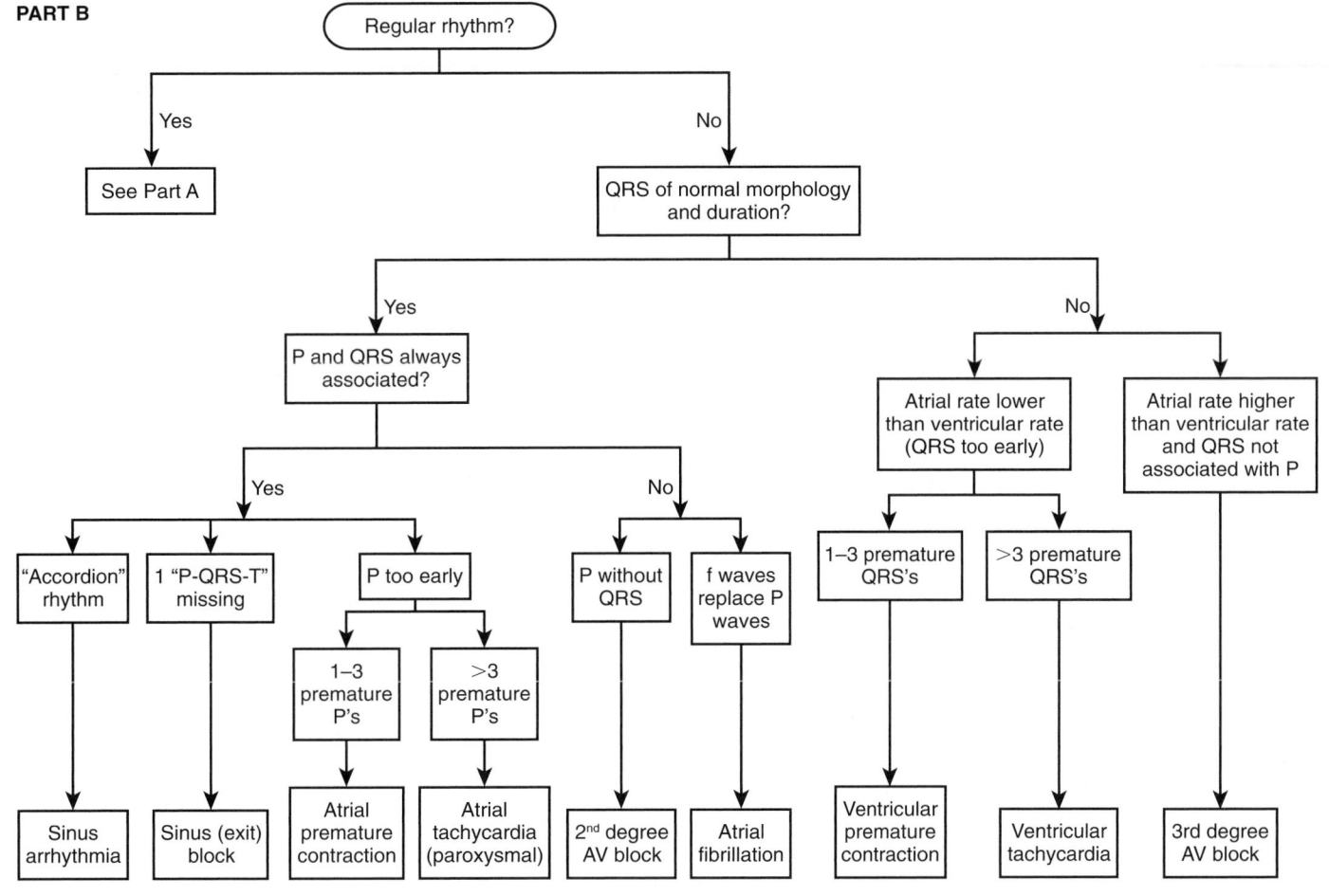

Author: **Gunther van Loon**

Epiphora

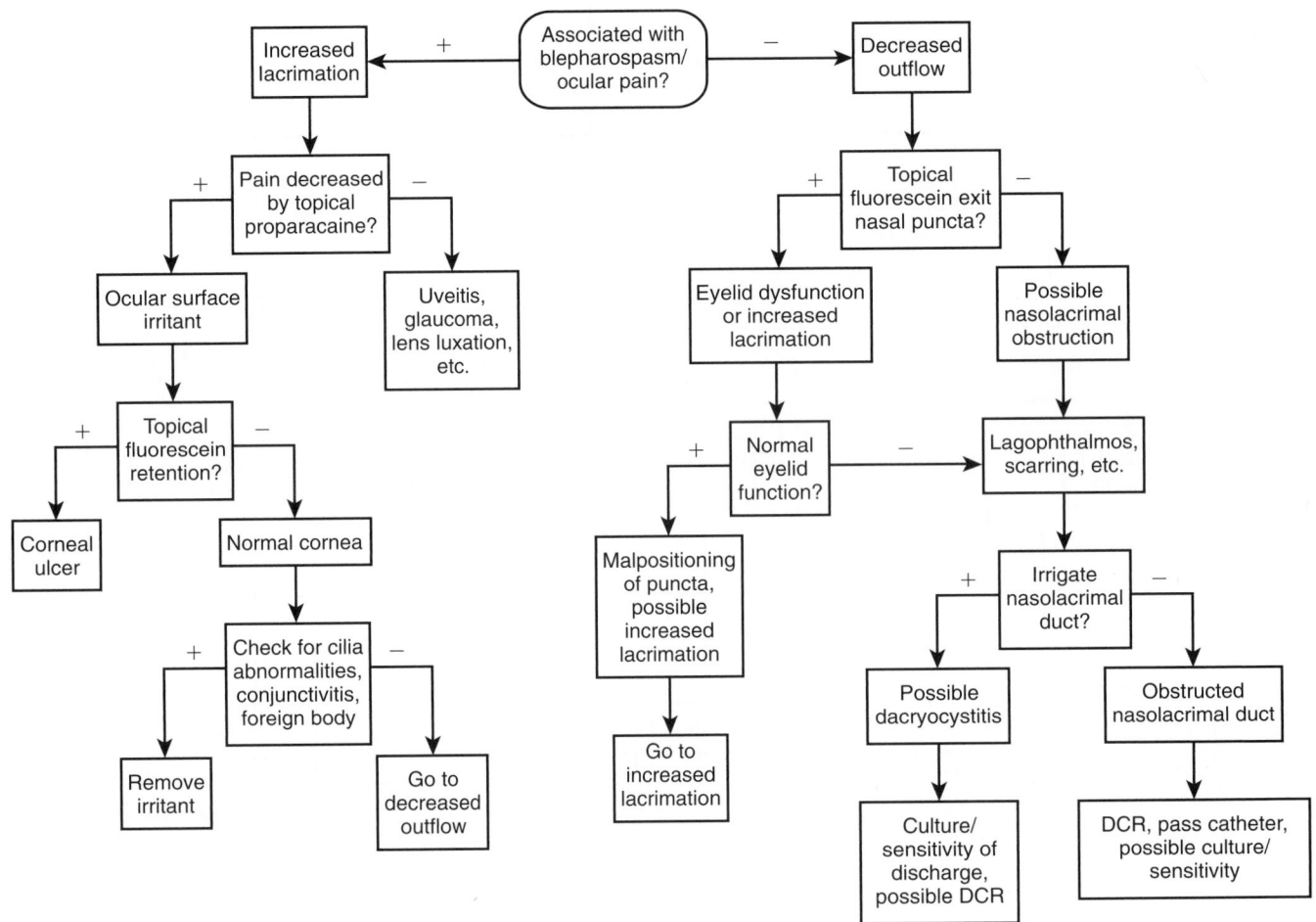

DCR, Dacryocystorhinography.
Gilger, B: *Equine ophthalmology*, ed 2, St Louis, 2010, Elsevier.

Failure to Cycle or Irregular Cycling

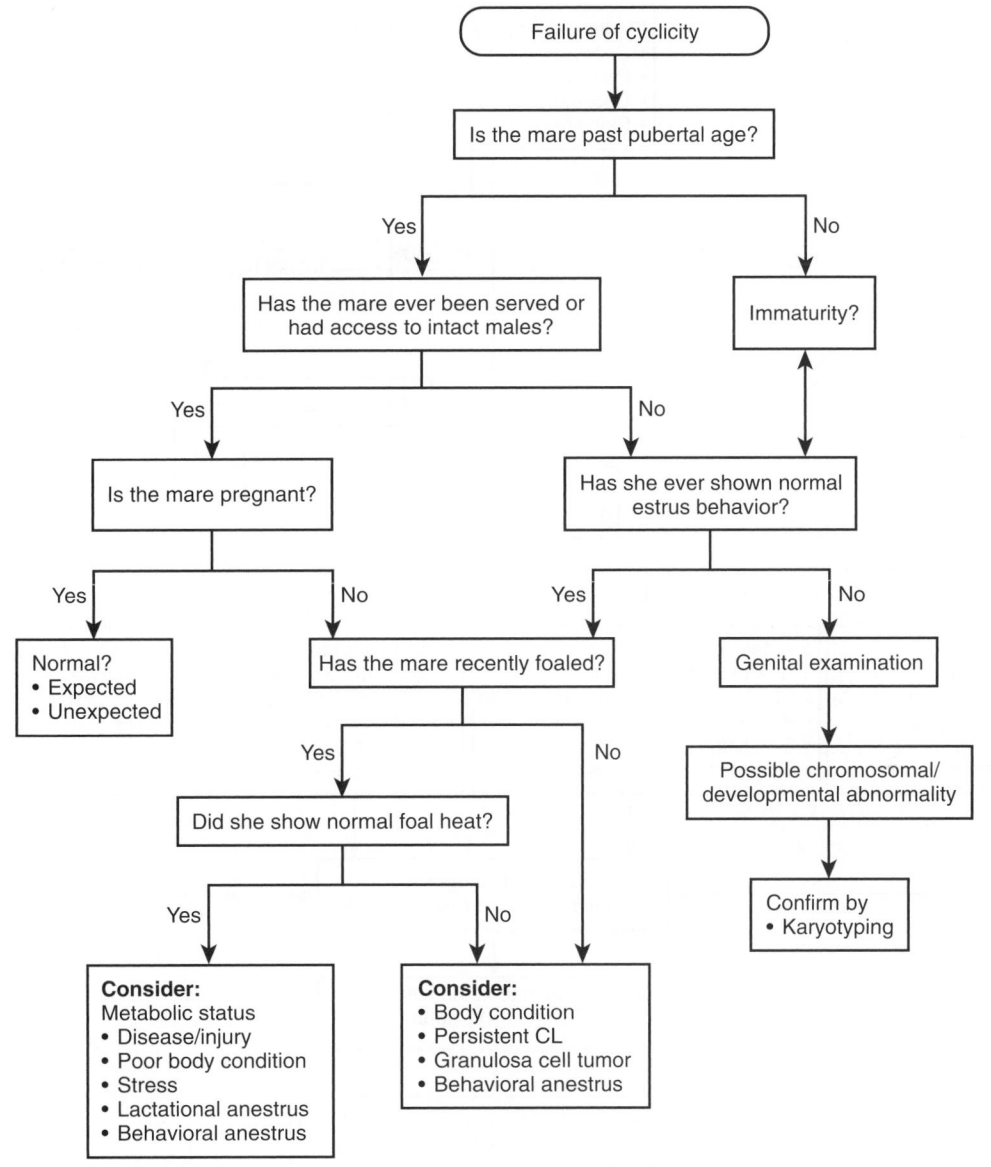

CL, Corpus luteum.
From Knottenbelt DC: *Equine stud farm medicine & surgery*, Philadelphia, 2003, Saunders Elsevier, p. 160.

Fluid Therapy: Basic Equine

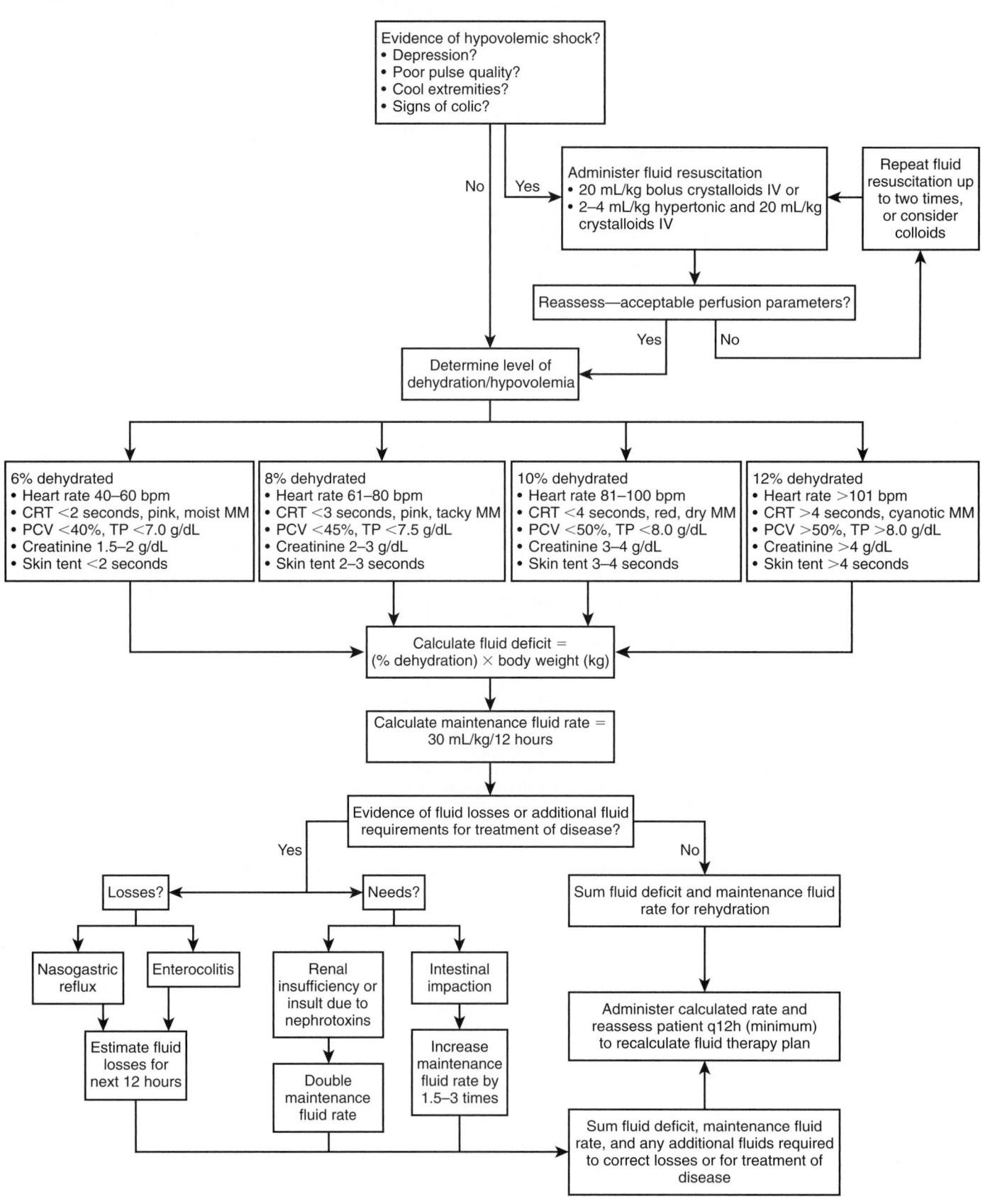

CRT, Capillary refill time; MM, mucous membranes;
PCV, packed cell volume; TP, total plasma protein.

Author: **Amelia Munsterman**

Hepatobiliary Disease in Adult Horses

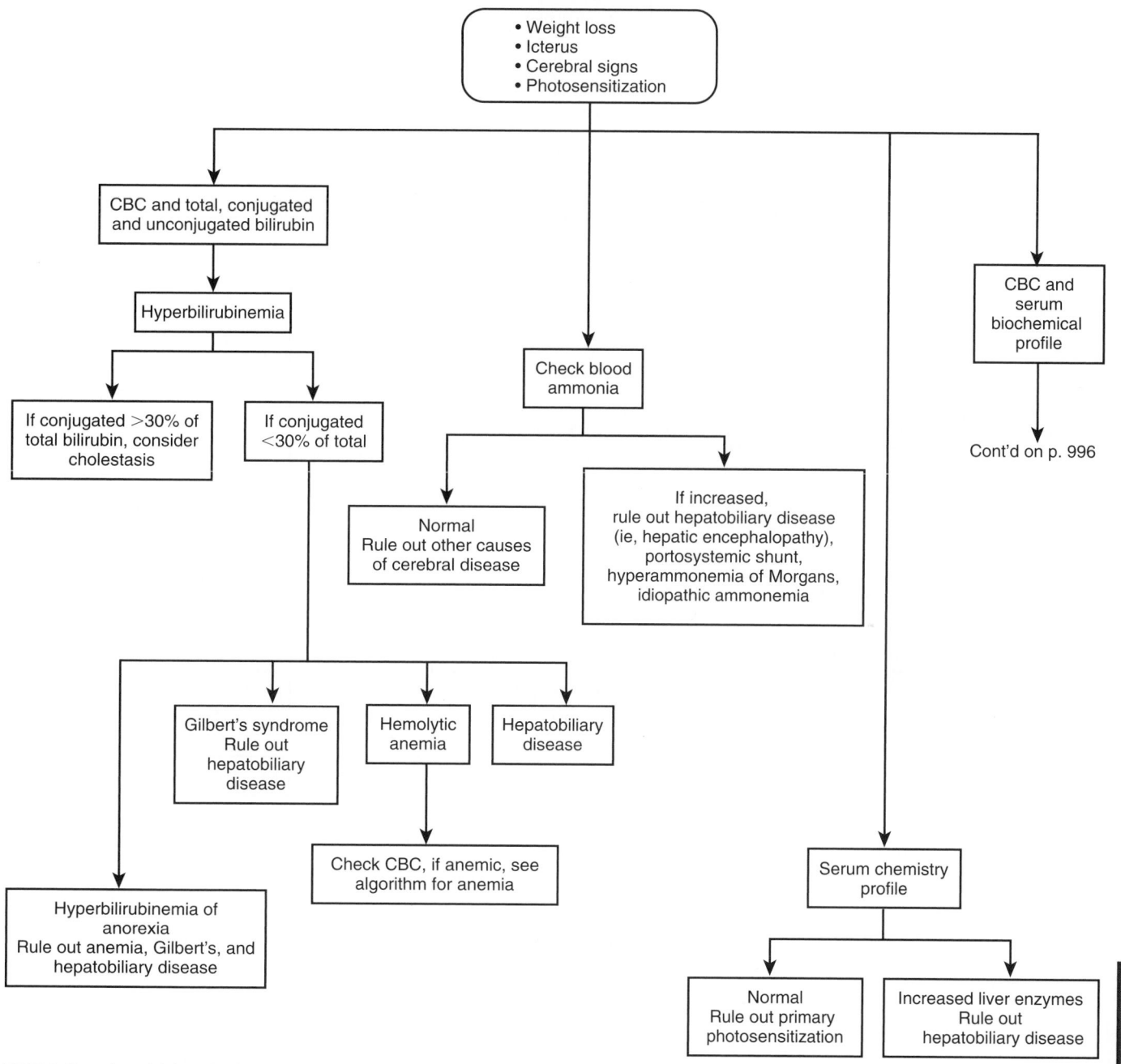

- Weight loss
- Icterus
- Cerebral signs
- Photosensitization

CBC and total, conjugated and unconjugated bilirubin

Hyperbilirubinemia

If conjugated >30% of total bilirubin, consider cholestasis

If conjugated <30% of total

Gilbert's syndrome
Rule out hepatobiliary disease

Hemolytic anemia

Hepatobiliary disease

Check CBC, if anemic, see algorithm for anemia

Hyperbilirubinemia of anorexia
Rule out anemia, Gilbert's, and hepatobiliary disease

Check blood ammonia

Normal
Rule out other causes of cerebral disease

If increased,
rule out hepatobiliary disease (ie, hepatic encephalopathy), portosystemic shunt, hyperammonemia of Morgans, idiopathic ammonemia

CBC and serum biochemical profile

Cont'd on p. 996

Serum chemistry profile

Normal
Rule out primary photosensitization

Increased liver enzymes
Rule out hepatobiliary disease

APTT, Activated partial thromboplastin time; *CBC*, complete blood count;
CHF, congestive heart failure; *IBD*, inflammatory bowel disease; *PPID*, pituitary pars intermedia dysfunction; *PT*, prothrombin time.

CLINICAL ALGORITHMS

Author: **Michelle Henry Barton**

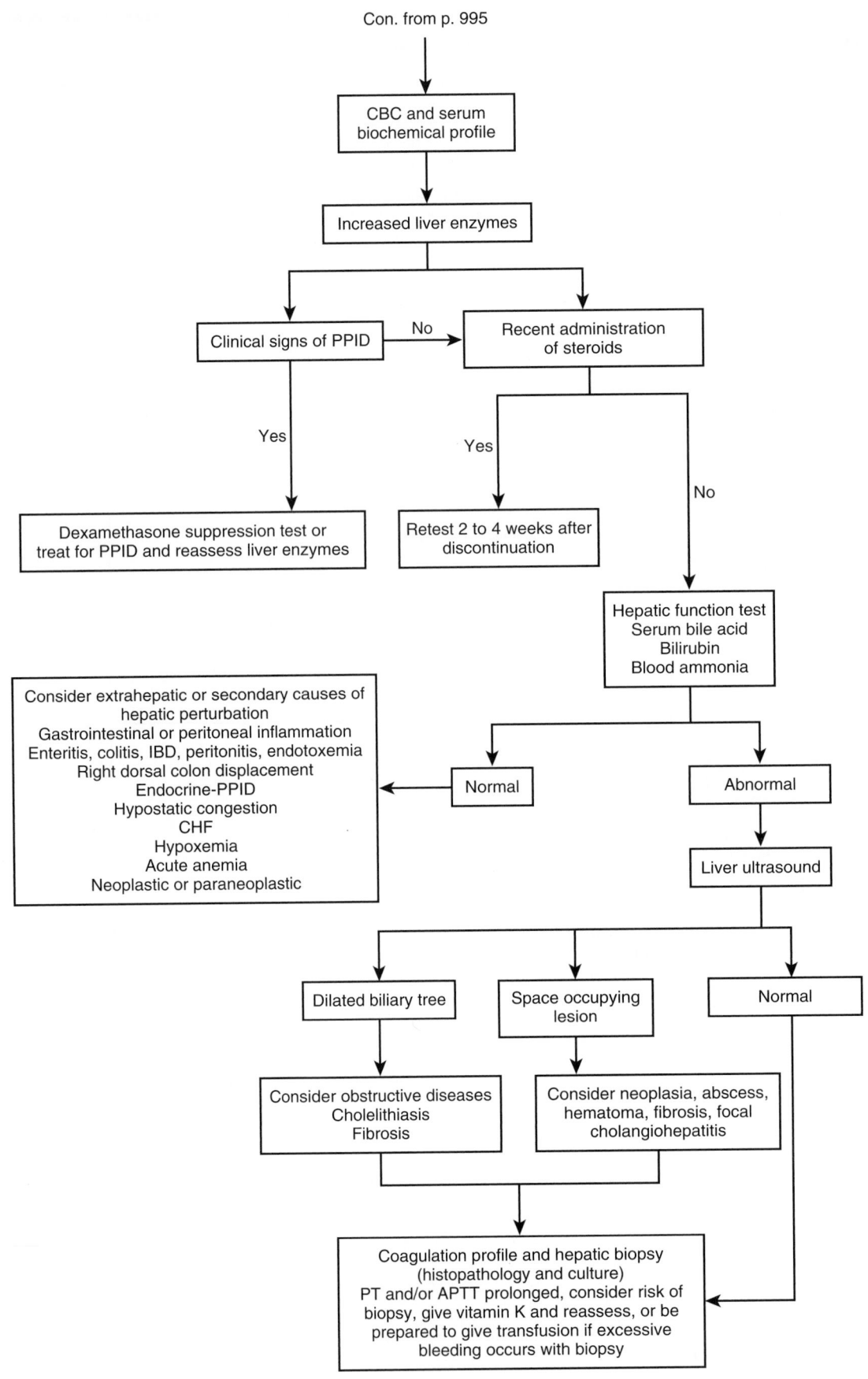

Con. from p. 995

CBC and serum
biochemical profile

Increased liver enzymes

Clinical signs of PPID — No → Recent administration
of steroids

Yes (from Clinical signs of PPID)

Dexamethasone suppression test or
treat for PPID and reassess liver enzymes

Yes (from Recent administration of steroids)

Retest 2 to 4 weeks after
discontinuation

No (from Recent administration of steroids)

Hepatic function test
Serum bile acid
Bilirubin
Blood ammonia

Consider extrahepatic or secondary causes of
hepatic perturbation
Gastrointestinal or peritoneal inflammation
Enteritis, colitis, IBD, peritonitis, endotoxemia
Right dorsal colon displacement
Endocrine-PPID
Hypostatic congestion
CHF
Hypoxemia
Acute anemia
Neoplastic or paraneoplastic

← Normal

Abnormal

Liver ultrasound

Dilated biliary tree

Space occupying
lesion

Normal

Consider obstructive diseases
Cholelithiasis
Fibrosis

Consider neoplasia, abscess,
hematoma, fibrosis, focal
cholangiohepatitis

Coagulation profile and hepatic biopsy
(histopathology and culture)
PT and/or APTT prolonged, consider risk of
biopsy, give vitamin K and reassess, or be
prepared to give transfusion if excessive
bleeding occurs with biopsy

Hypercalcemia

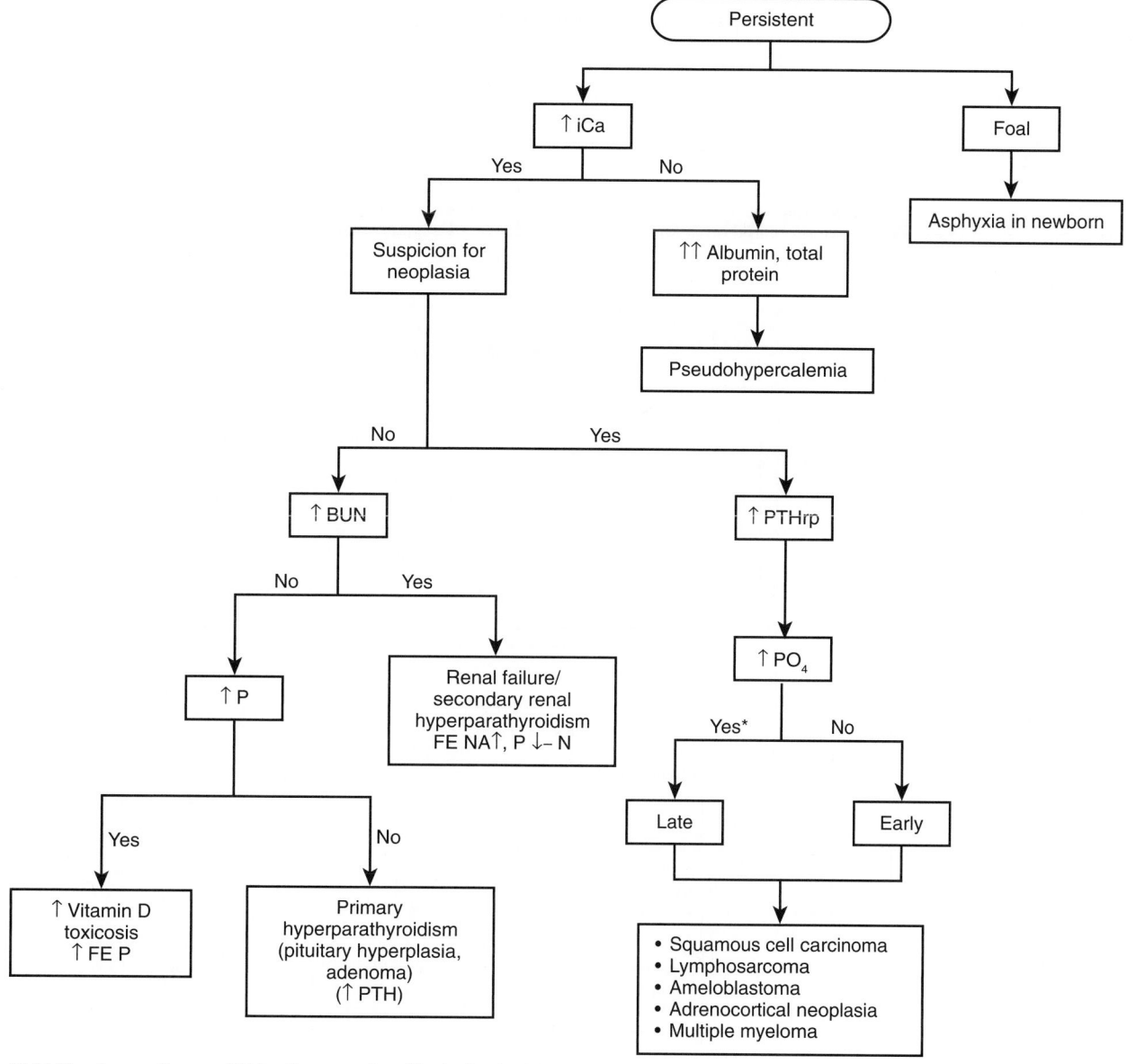

BUN, Blood urea nitrogen; FE, fraction excretion; iCa, ionized calcium; N, normal; Na, sodium; P, phosphorous; PO_4, phosphate including PO_4, HPO_4, H_2PO_4; PTH, parathyroid hormone.

*May cause mineralization and secondary renal failure later in disease course.

Author: **Ida Piperisova**

Hyperthermia

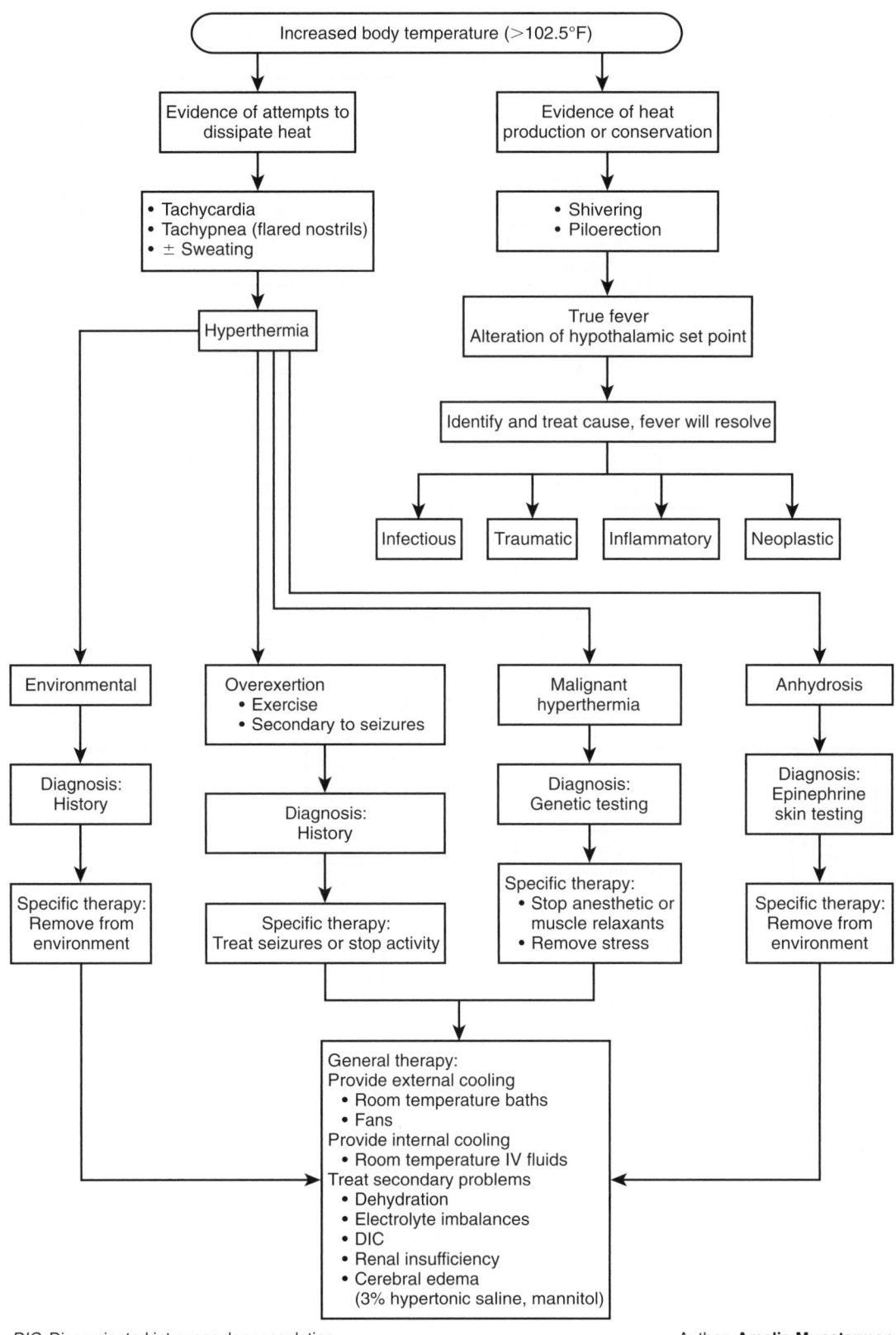

DIC, Disseminated intravascular coagulation.

Author: **Amelia Munsterman**

Hypocalcemia

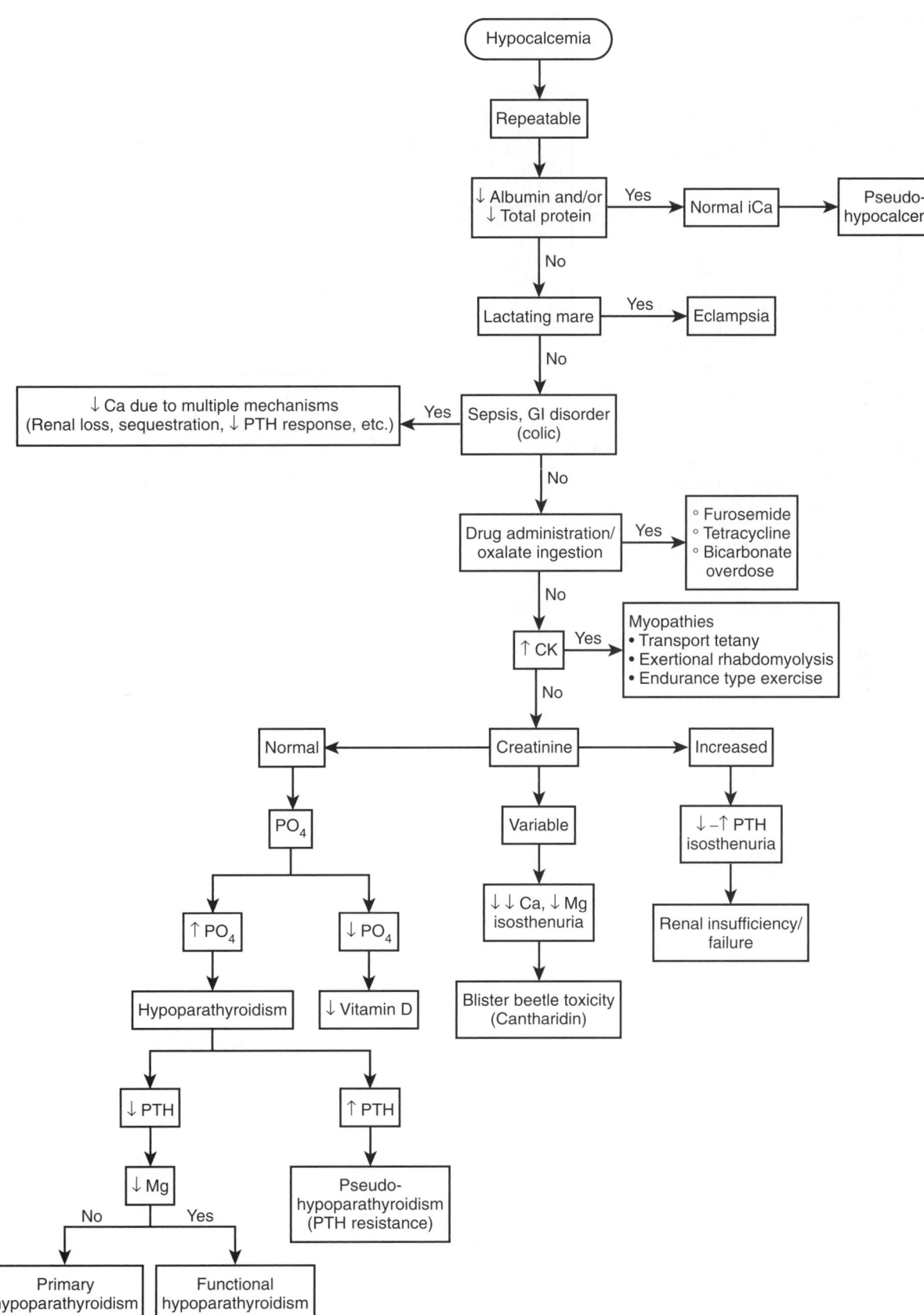

CK, Creatine kinase; iCA, ionized calcium; Mg, magnesium; PO_4, phosphate
(including PO_4, HPO_4, H_2PO_4); PTH, parathyroid hormone.

Author: **Ida Piperisova**

Infertility

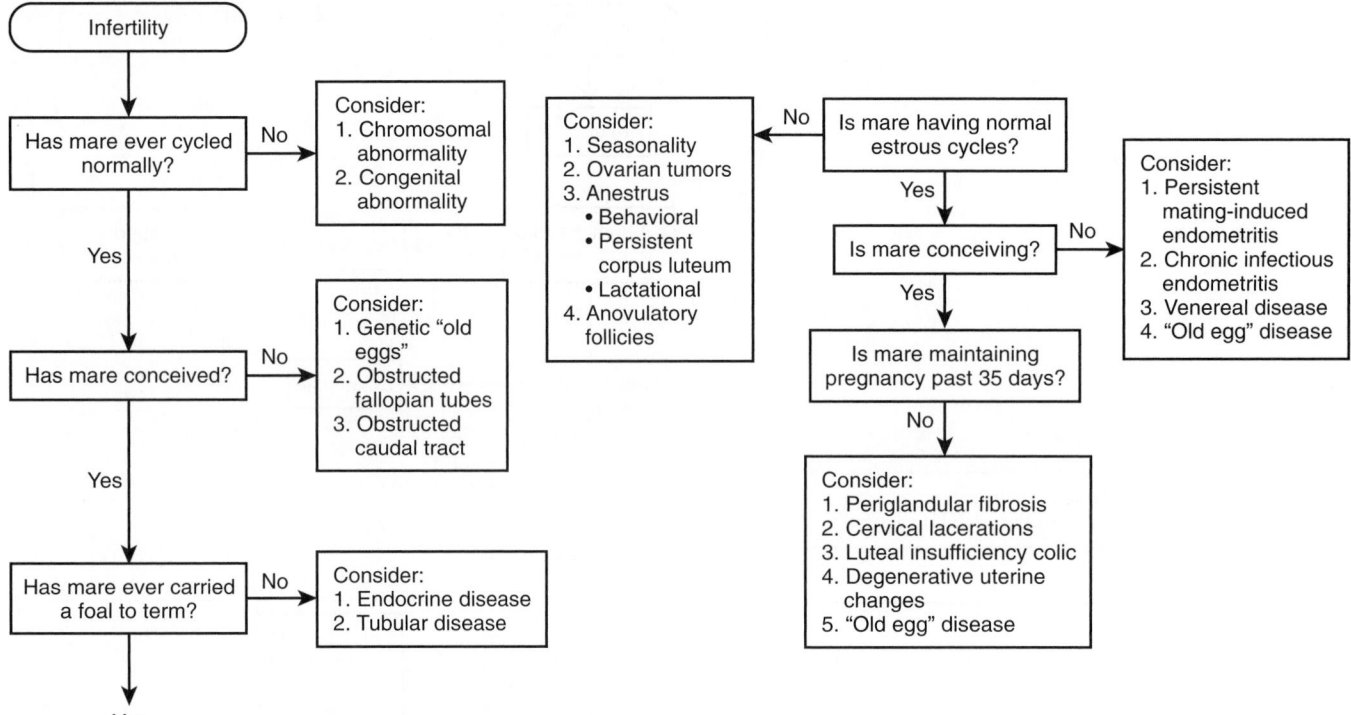

From Knottenbelt DC: *Equine stud farm medicine & surgery,* Philadelphia, 2003, Saunders Elsevier.

Interpretation of *S. equi* subsp. *equi* on Suspect Horse with Lymphadenopathy

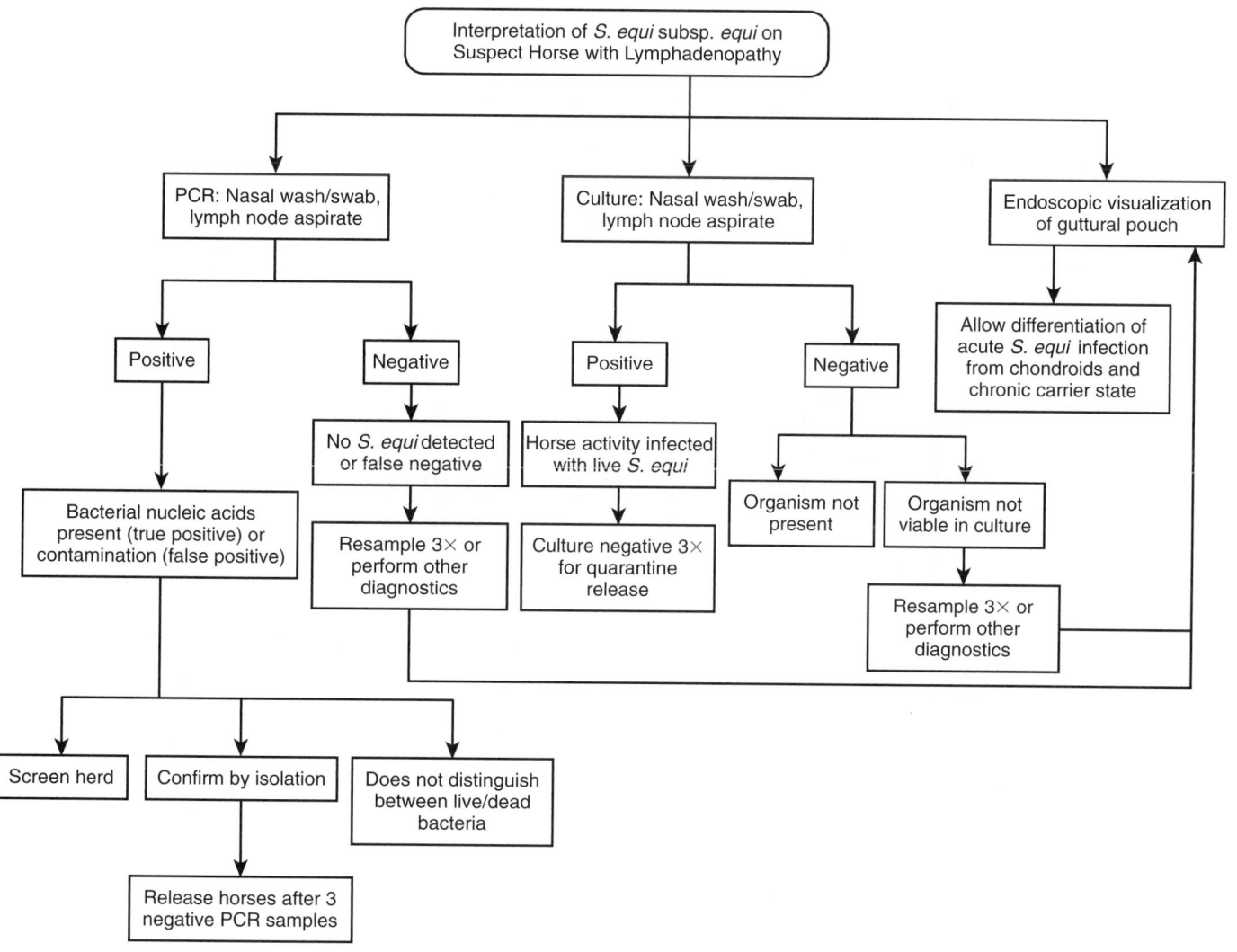

PCR, Polymerase chain reaction.

Author: **Maureen T. Long**

Localizing a Lesion in the Nervous System of a Recumbent Horse

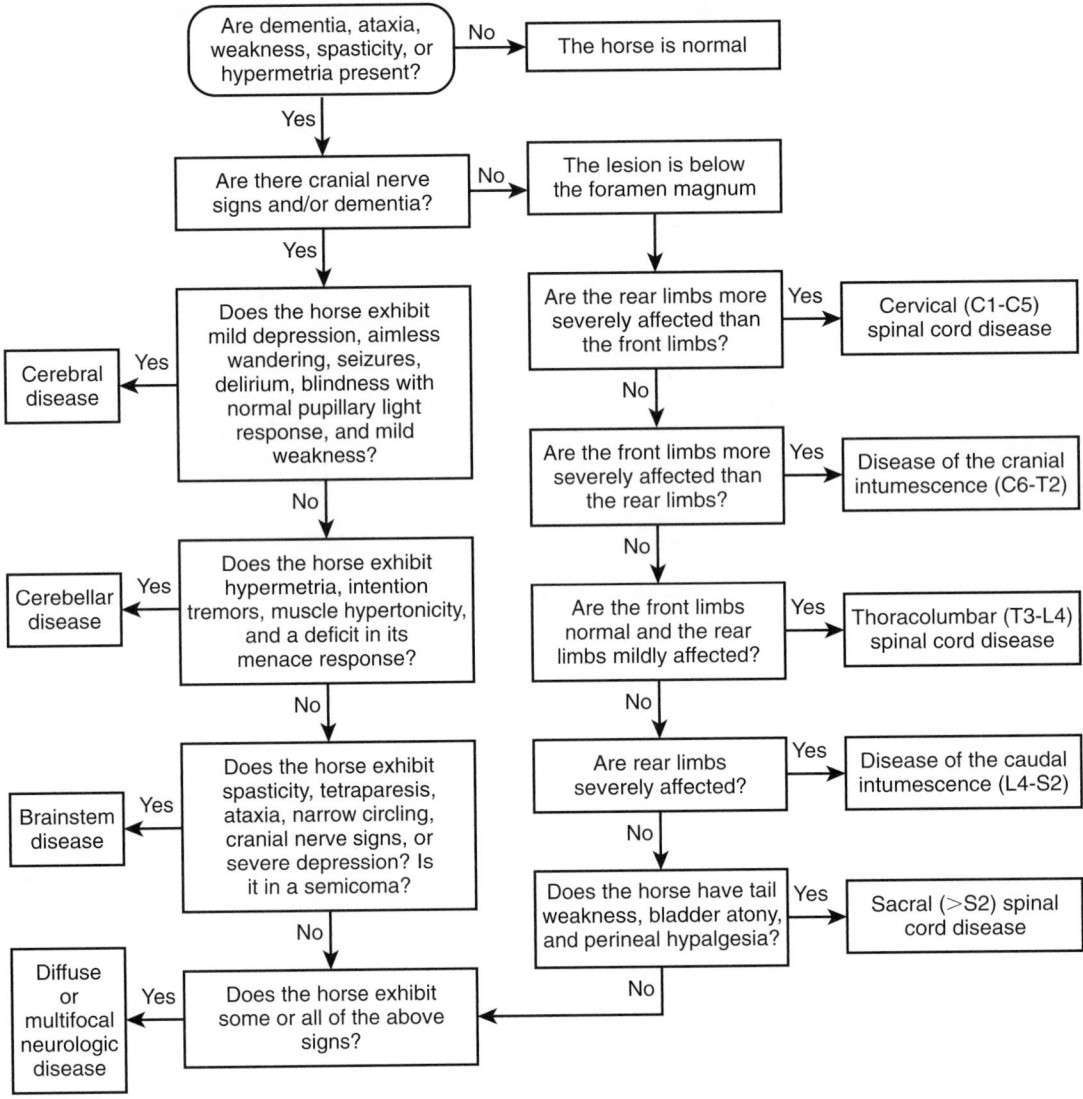

From Reed SJ, Bayly WM, Sellon DC: *Equine internal medicine*, ed 3, St Louis, 2010, Saunders Elsevier.

Mare Breeding Soundness Examination

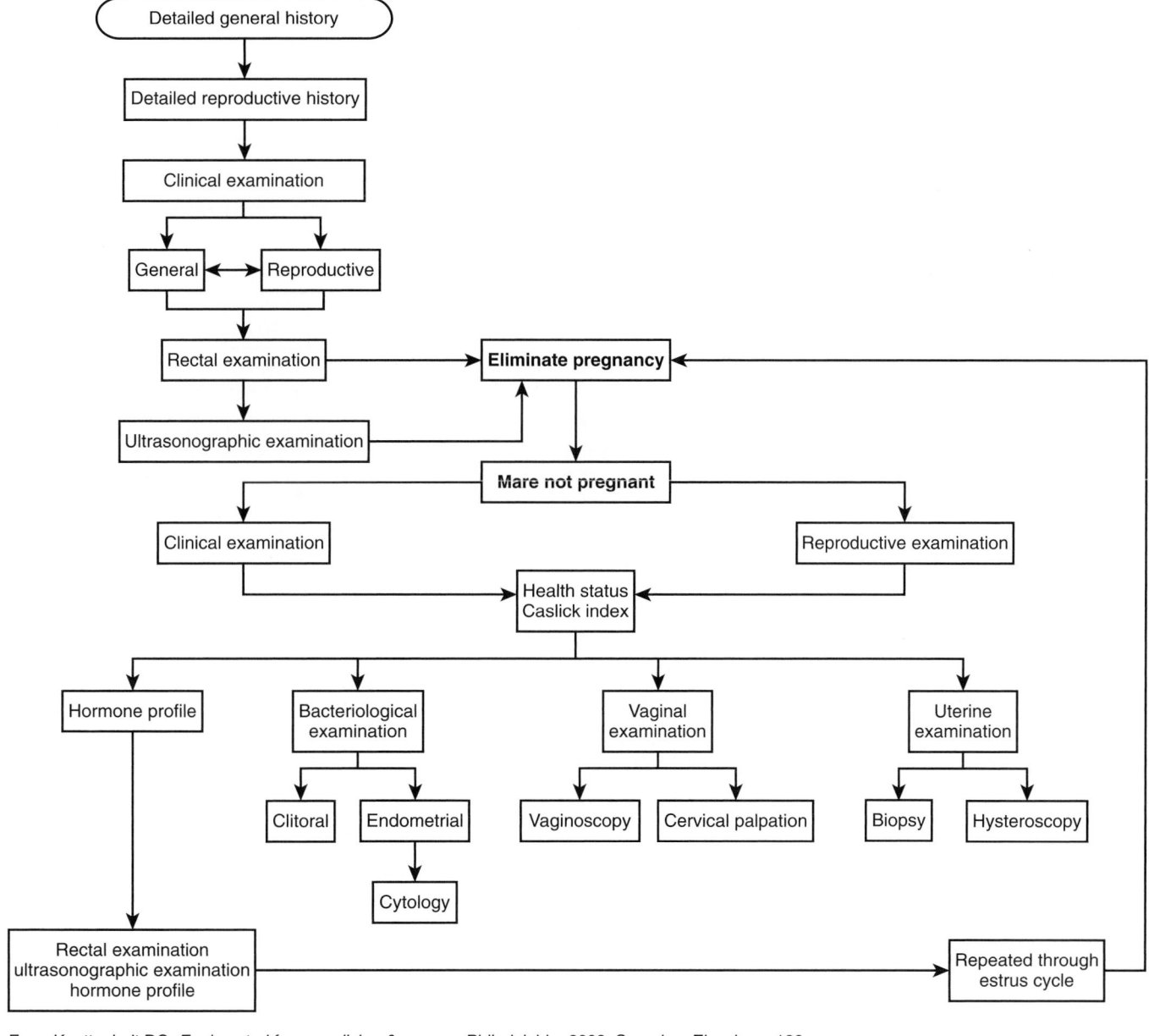

From Knottenbelt DC: *Equine stud farm medicine & surgery*, Philadelphia, 2003, Saunders Elsevier, p 129.

Mare Infertility Based on the Presence of Intrauterine Fluid

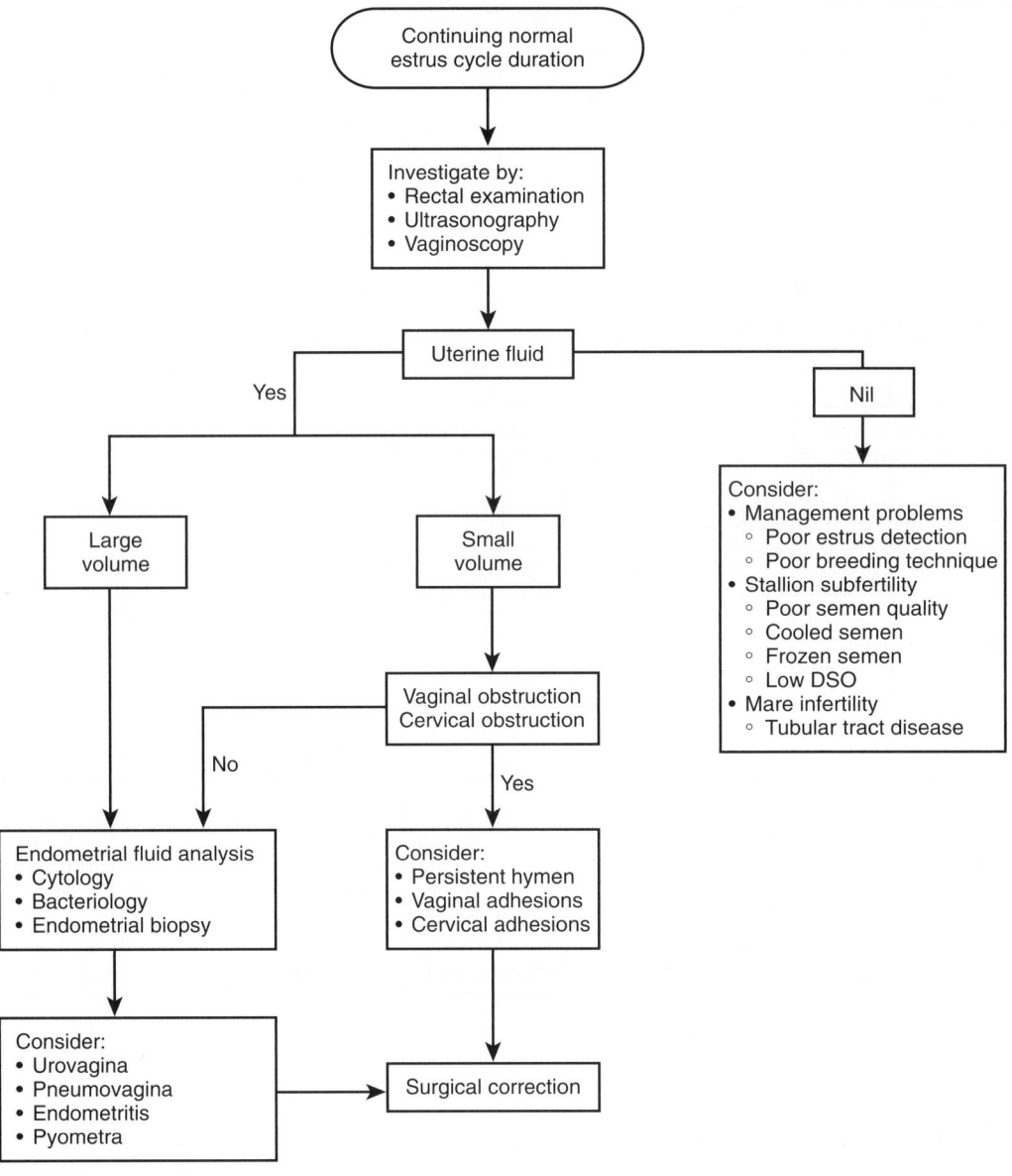

DSO, Daily sperm output.

From Knottenbelt DC: *Equine stud farm medicine & surgery,* Philadelphia, 2003, Saunders Elsevier.

Mare Infertility from a Perspective of Ovarian Size

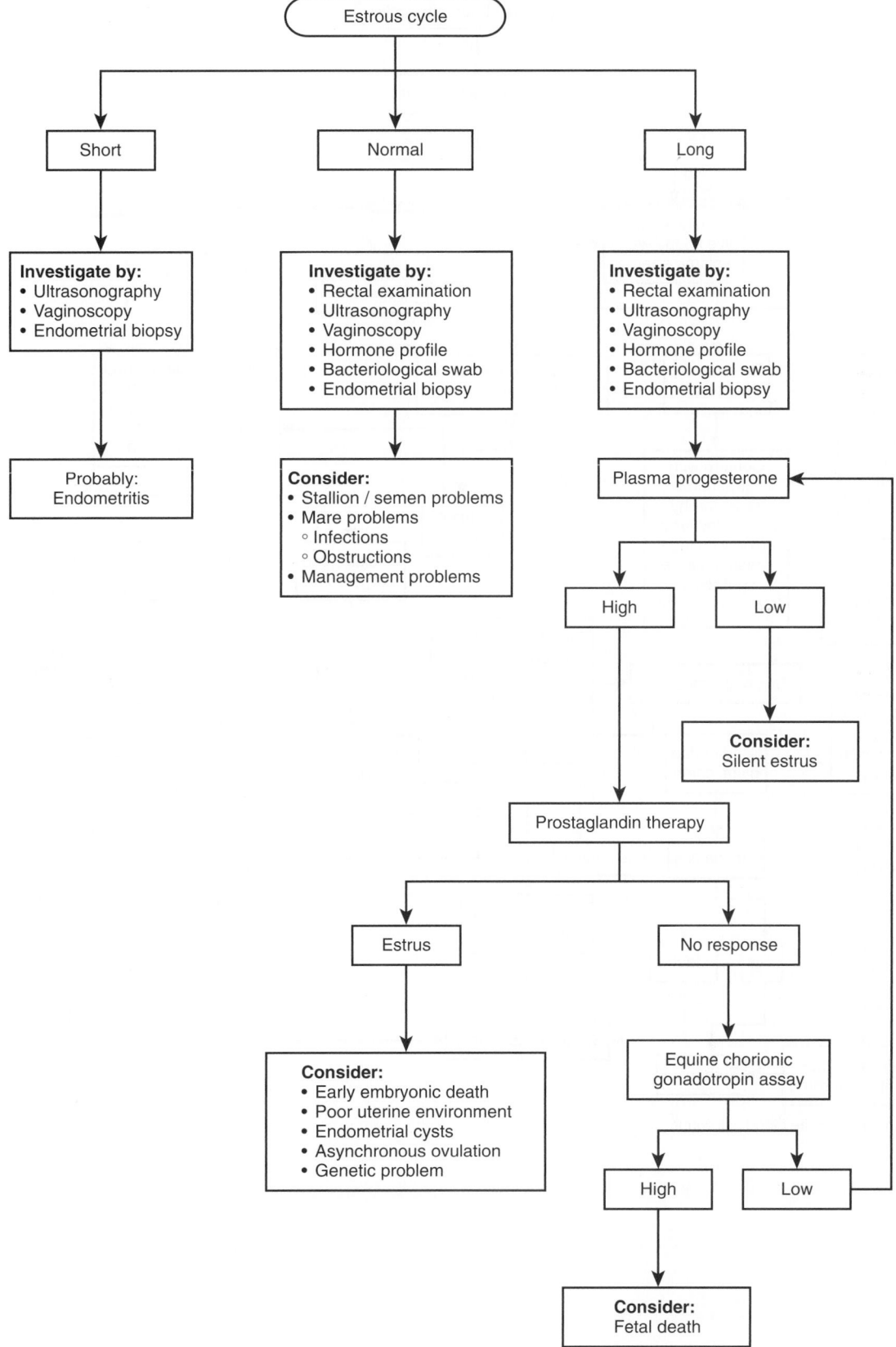

From Knottenbelt DC: *Equine stud farm medicine & surgery*, Philadelphia, 2003, Saunders Elsevier, p 159.

Neonatal Colic

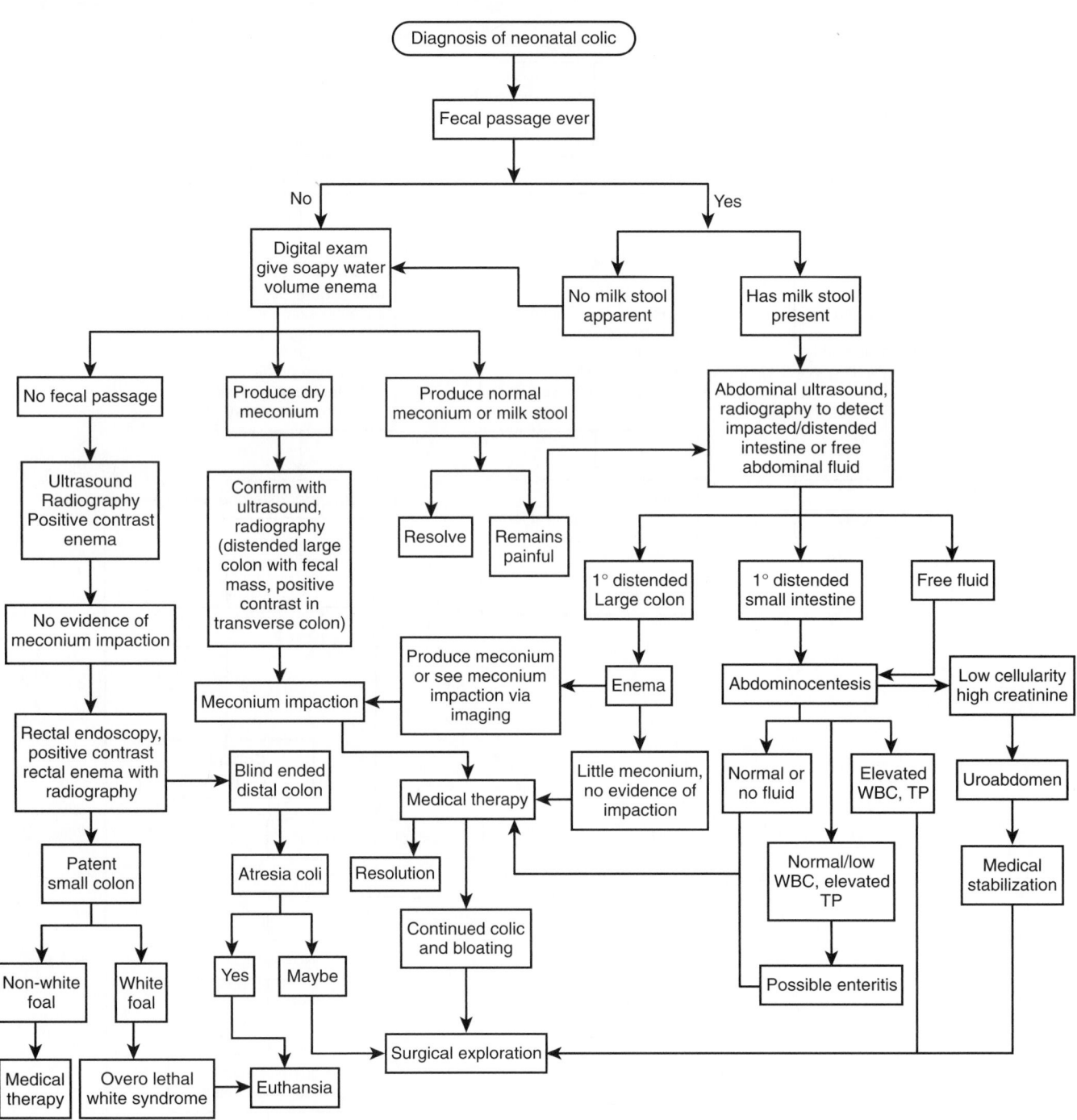

Diagnosis of neonatal colic

Fecal passage ever

No — Digital exam give soapy water volume enema

Yes — No milk stool apparent / Has milk stool present

No fecal passage
Ultrasound Radiography Positive contrast enema
No evidence of meconium impaction
Rectal endoscopy, positive contrast rectal enema with radiography
Patent small colon
Non-white foal / White foal
Medical therapy / Overo lethal white syndrome → Euthansia

Produce dry meconium
Confirm with ultrasound, radiography (distended large colon with fecal mass, positive contrast in transverse colon)
Meconium impaction
Blind ended distal colon
Atresia coli
Yes / Maybe → Euthansia

Produce normal meconium or milk stool
Resolve / Remains painful

Produce meconium or see meconium impaction via imaging
Medical therapy
Resolution
Continued colic and bloating
Surgical exploration

Abdominal ultrasound, radiography to detect impacted/distended intestine or free abdominal fluid
1° distended Large colon / 1° distended small intestine / Free fluid
Enema
Little meconium, no evidence of impaction
Abdominocentesis
Normal or no fluid / Elevated WBC, TP
Normal/low WBC, elevated TP
Possible enteritis
Low cellularity high creatinine
Uroabdomen
Medical stabilization

TP, Total protein; WBC, white blood cell count.

Author: **Elizabeth M. Santschi**

Neonatal Lameness

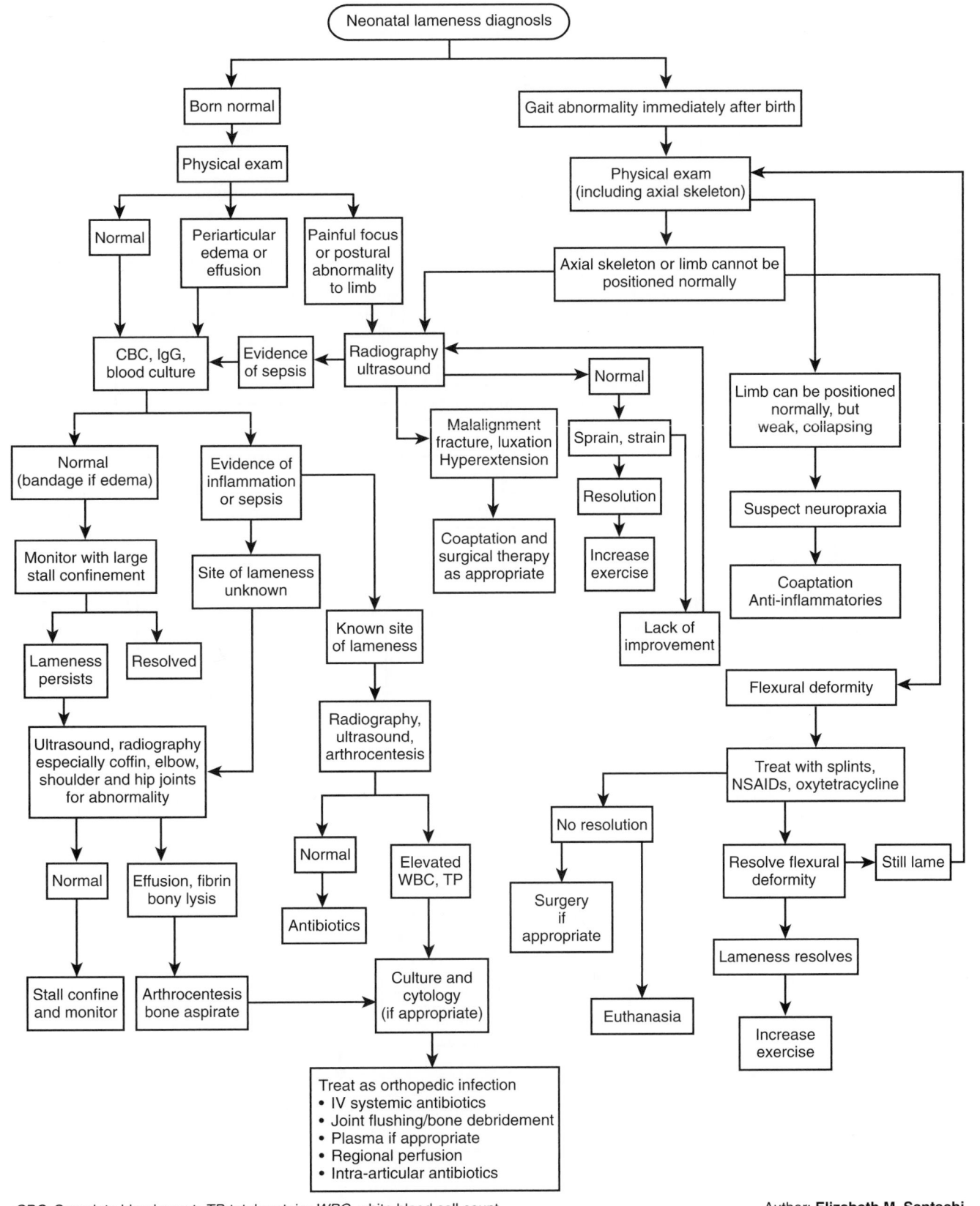

CBC, Complete blood count; TP, total protein; WBC, white blood cell count.

Author: **Elizabeth M. Santschi**

Neonatal Resuscitation Assessment

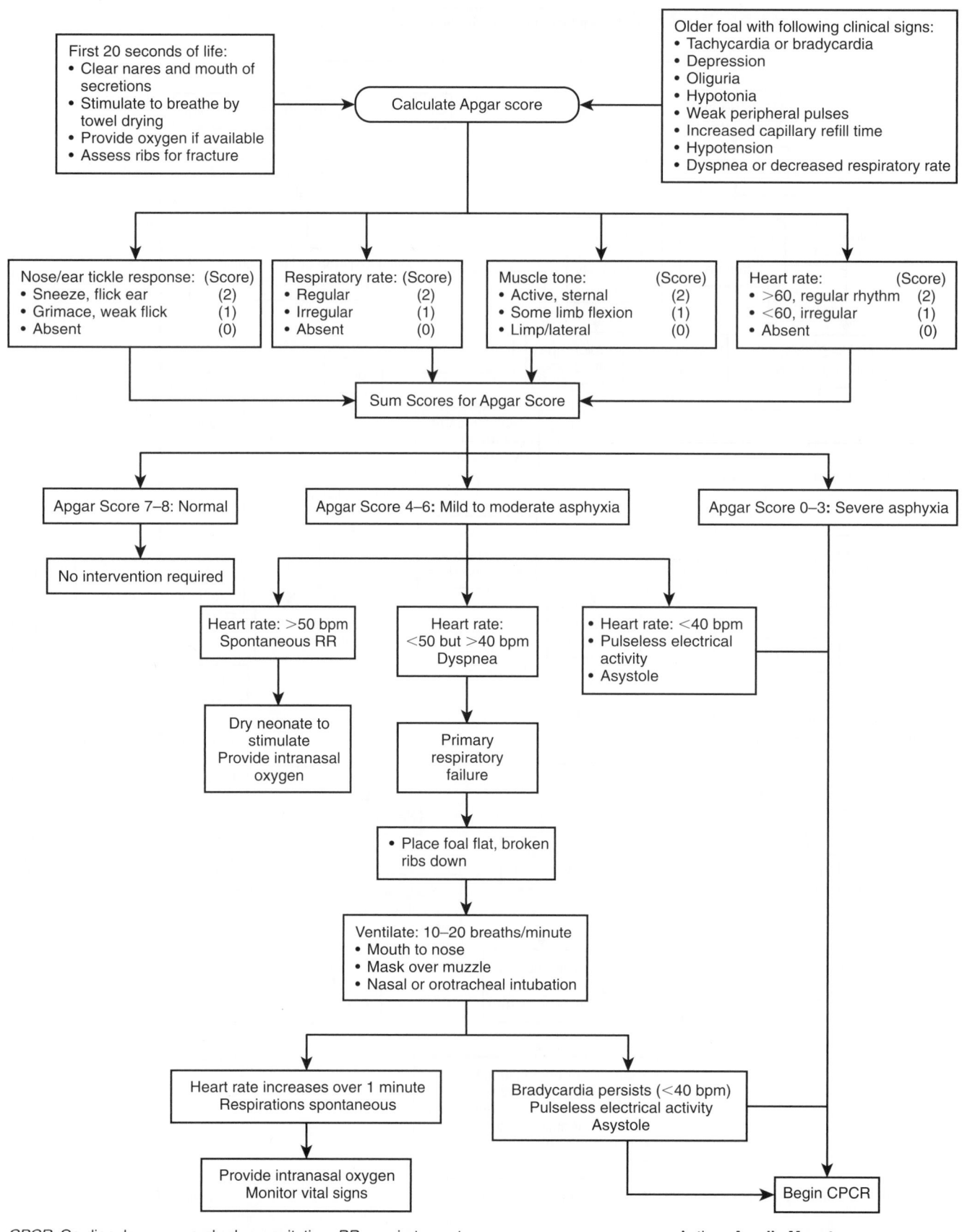

First 20 seconds of life:
- Clear nares and mouth of secretions
- Stimulate to breathe by towel drying
- Provide oxygen if available
- Assess ribs for fracture

Older foal with following clinical signs:
- Tachycardia or bradycardia
- Depression
- Oliguria
- Hypotonia
- Weak peripheral pulses
- Increased capillary refill time
- Hypotension
- Dyspnea or decreased respiratory rate

Calculate Apgar score

Nose/ear tickle response: (Score)
- Sneeze, flick ear (2)
- Grimace, weak flick (1)
- Absent (0)

Respiratory rate: (Score)
- Regular (2)
- Irregular (1)
- Absent (0)

Muscle tone: (Score)
- Active, sternal (2)
- Some limb flexion (1)
- Limp/lateral (0)

Heart rate: (Score)
- >60, regular rhythm (2)
- <60, irregular (1)
- Absent (0)

Sum Scores for Apgar Score

Apgar Score 7–8: Normal

Apgar Score 4–6: Mild to moderate asphyxia

Apgar Score 0–3: Severe asphyxia

No intervention required

Heart rate: >50 bpm
Spontaneous RR

Heart rate: <50 but >40 bpm
Dyspnea

- Heart rate: <40 bpm
- Pulseless electrical activity
- Asystole

Dry neonate to stimulate
Provide intranasal oxygen

Primary respiratory failure

- Place foal flat, broken ribs down

Ventilate: 10–20 breaths/minute
- Mouth to nose
- Mask over muzzle
- Nasal or orotracheal intubation

Heart rate increases over 1 minute
Respirations spontaneous

Bradycardia persists (<40 bpm)
Pulseless electrical activity
Asystole

Provide intranasal oxygen
Monitor vital signs

Begin CPCR

CPCR, Cardiopulmonary cerebral resuscitation; *RR,* respiratory rate.

Author: **Amelia Munsterman**

Nodular Dermatitis

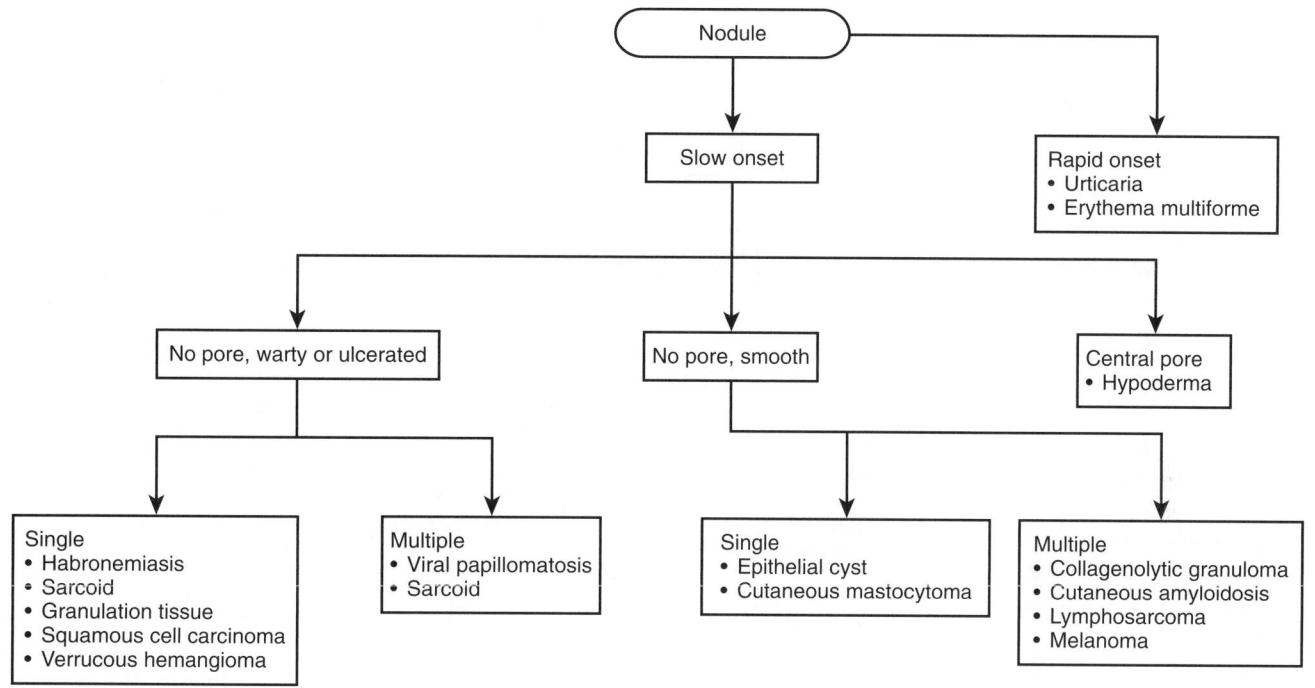

From Reed SJ, Bayly WM, Sellon DC: *Equine internal medicine*, ed 3, St. Louis, 2010, Saunders Elsevier.

Patent Urachus

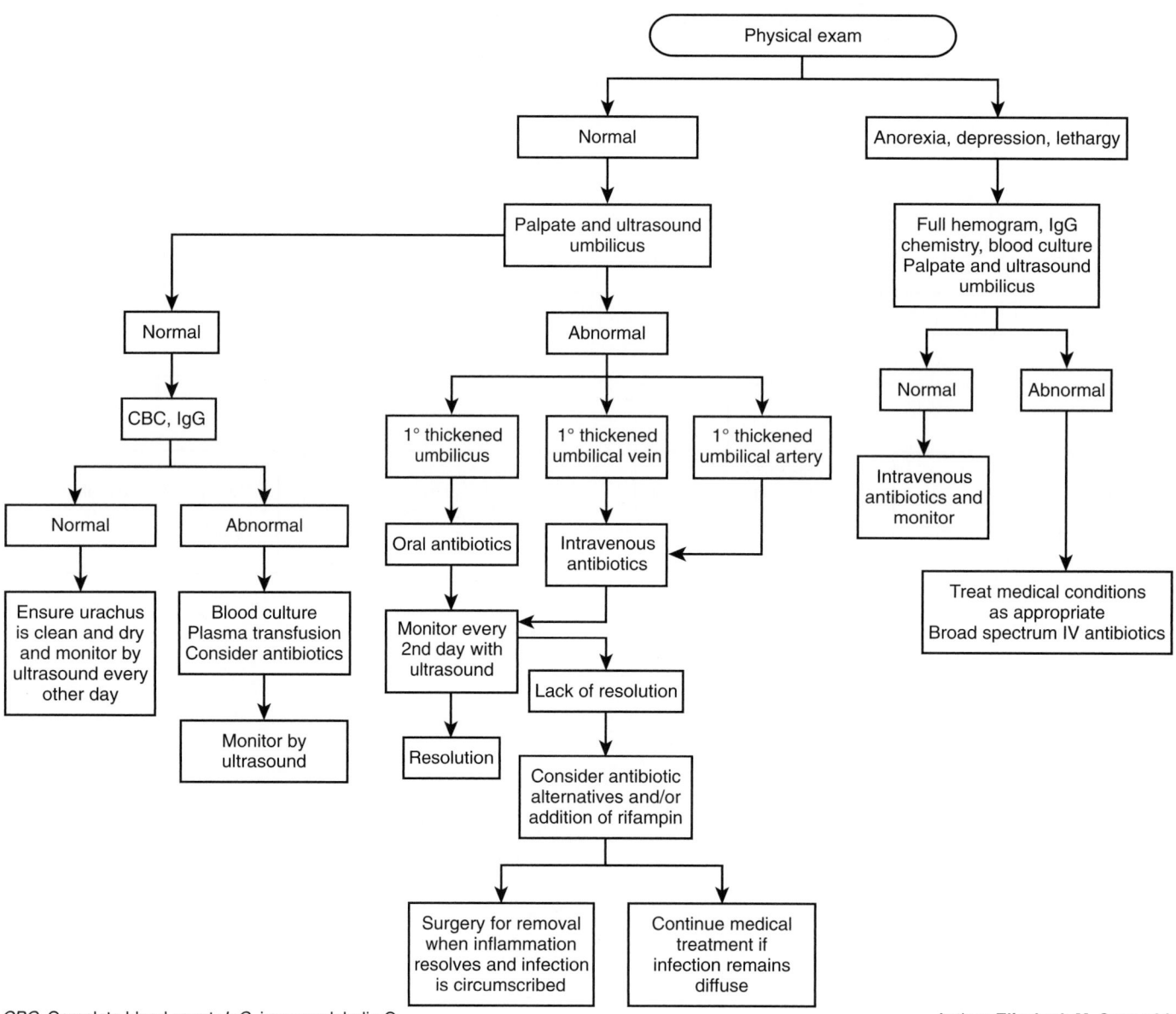

CBC, Complete blood count; *IgG,* immunoglobulin G.

Author: **Elizabeth M. Santschi**

Pemphigus

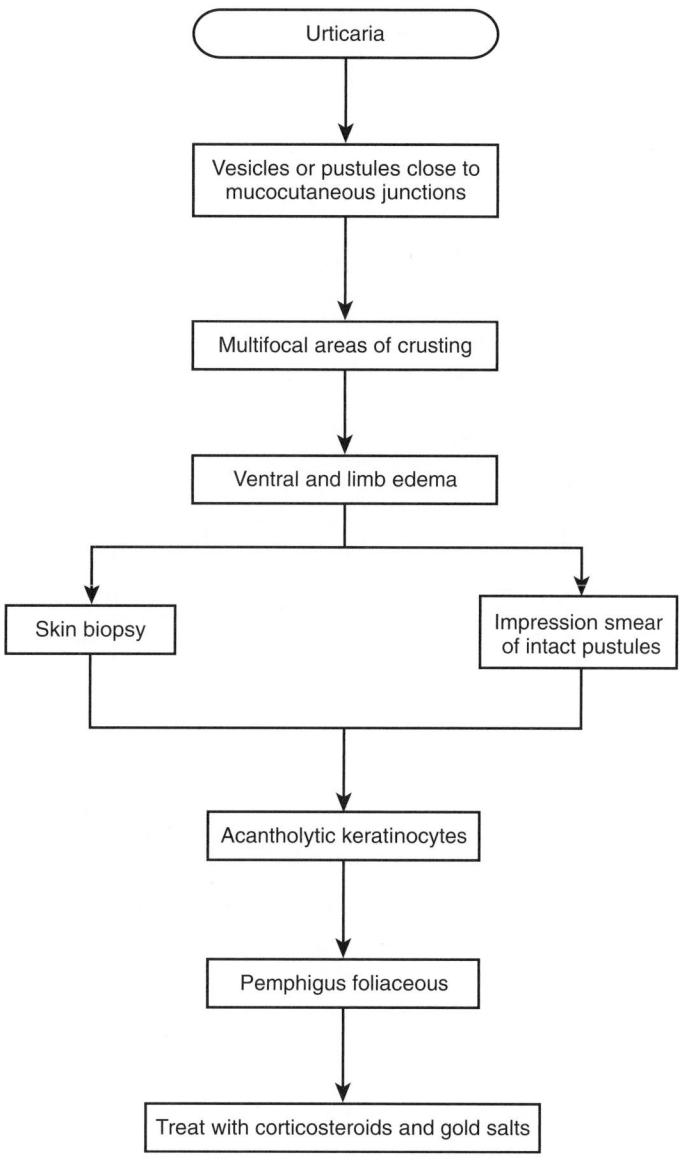

Author: **Alfredo Sanchez Londoño**

Pigmenturia from a Clinical Perspective

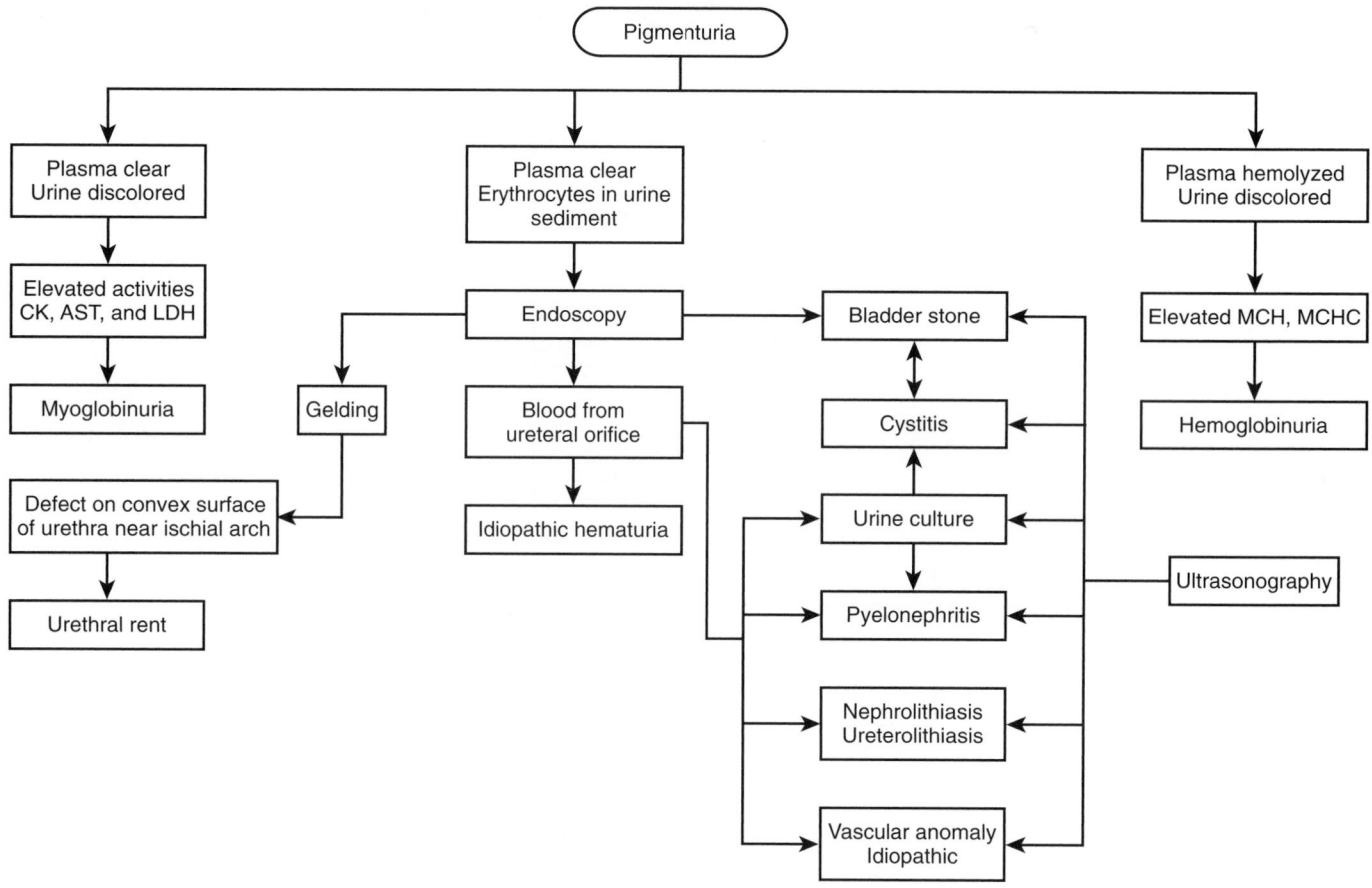

AST, Aspartate aminotransferase; CK, creatine kinase; LDH, lactate dehydrogenase; MCH, mean corpuscular hemoglobin; MCHC, mean corpuscular hemoglobin concentration.

Author: **Bryan M. Waldridge**

Pigmenturia from a Laboratory Perspective

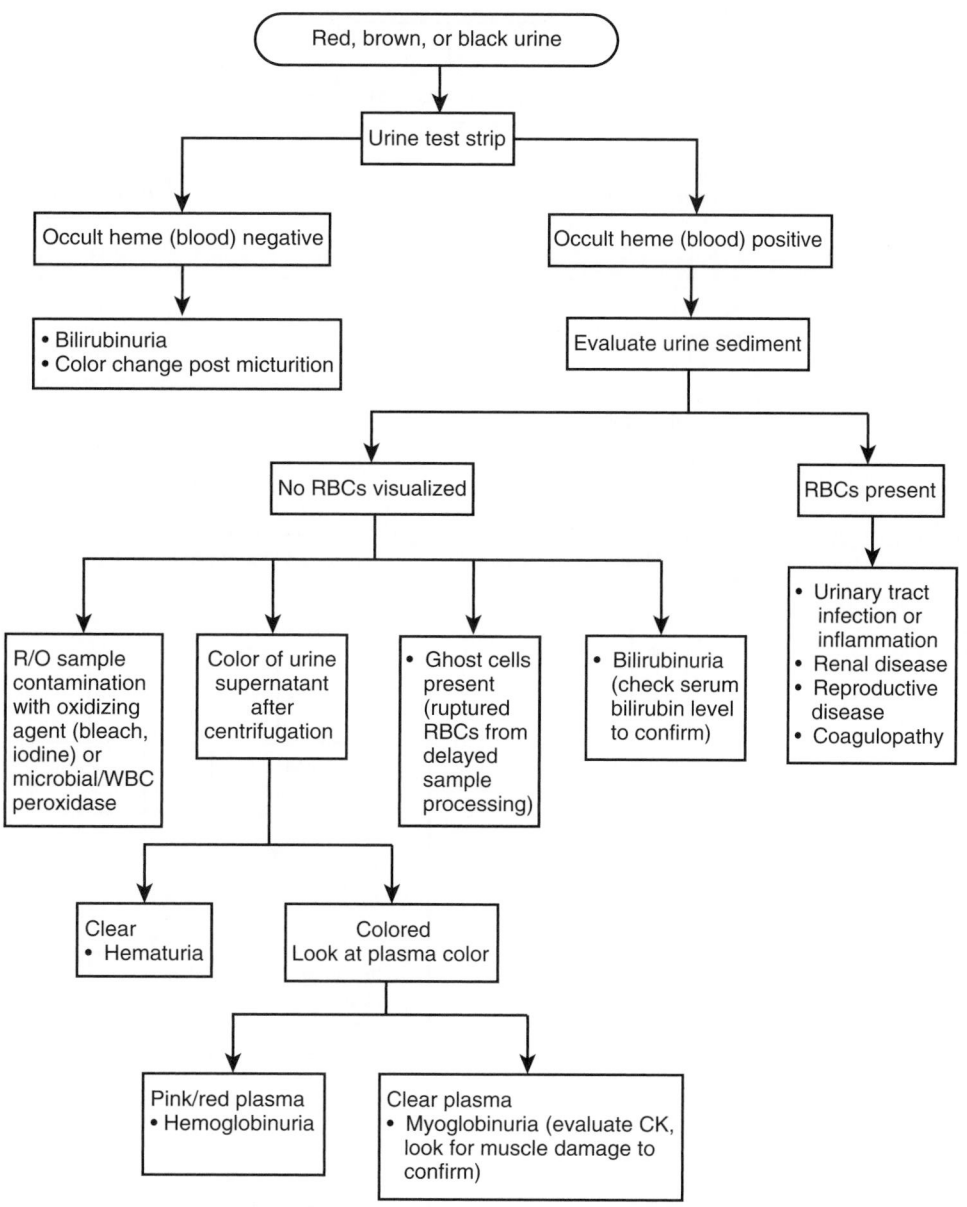

CK, Creatine kinase; RBC, red blood cells; WBC, white blood cells.

Author: **Sara A. Hill**

Polyuria/Polydipsia

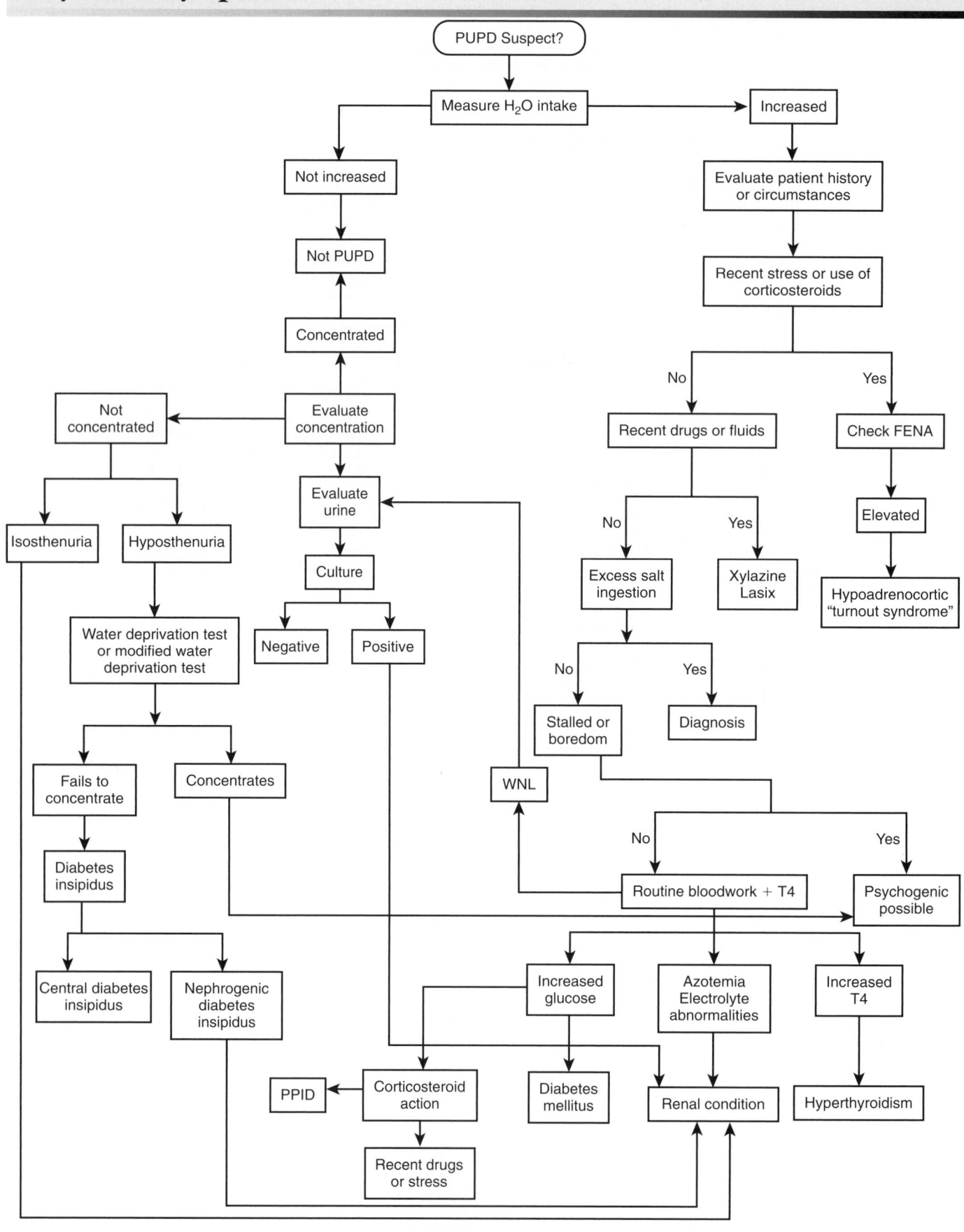

FENA, Fractional excretion of sodium; PPID, pituitary pars intermedia dysfunction; PUPD, polyuria and polydipsia; WNL, within normal limits.

Author: **Philip Johnson**

Proteinuria

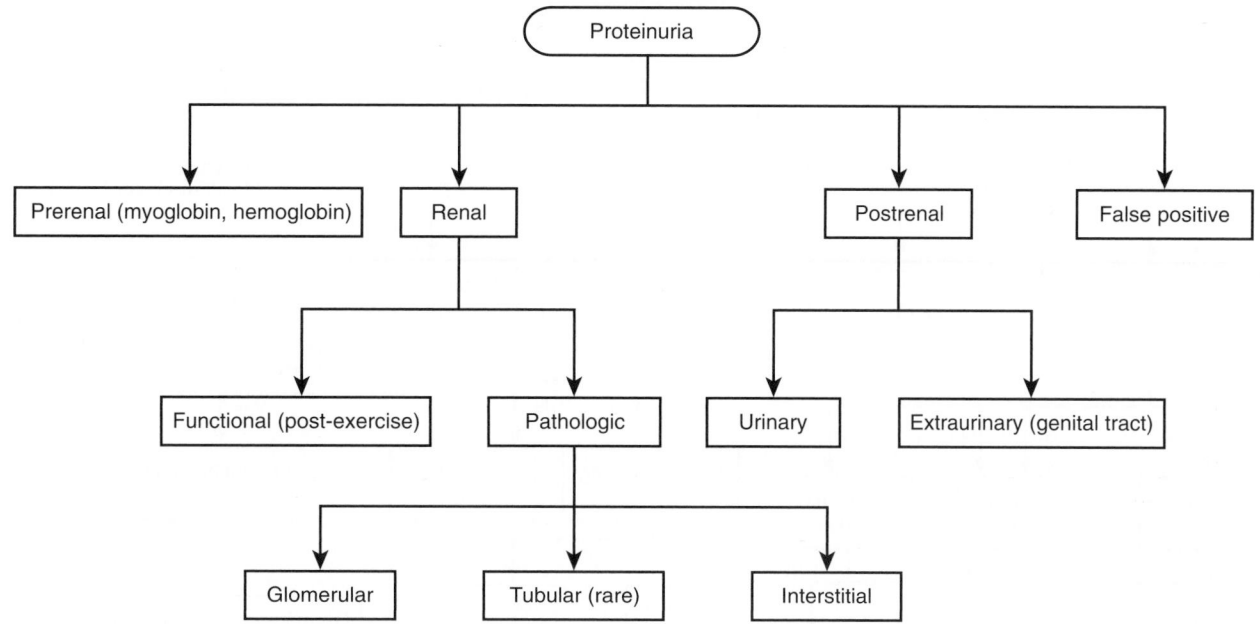

Note: Dipstick measurements of proteinuria are often overestimated due to the highly concentrated and alkaline nature of equine urine.

Author: **Charles Wiedmeyer**

Pruritus

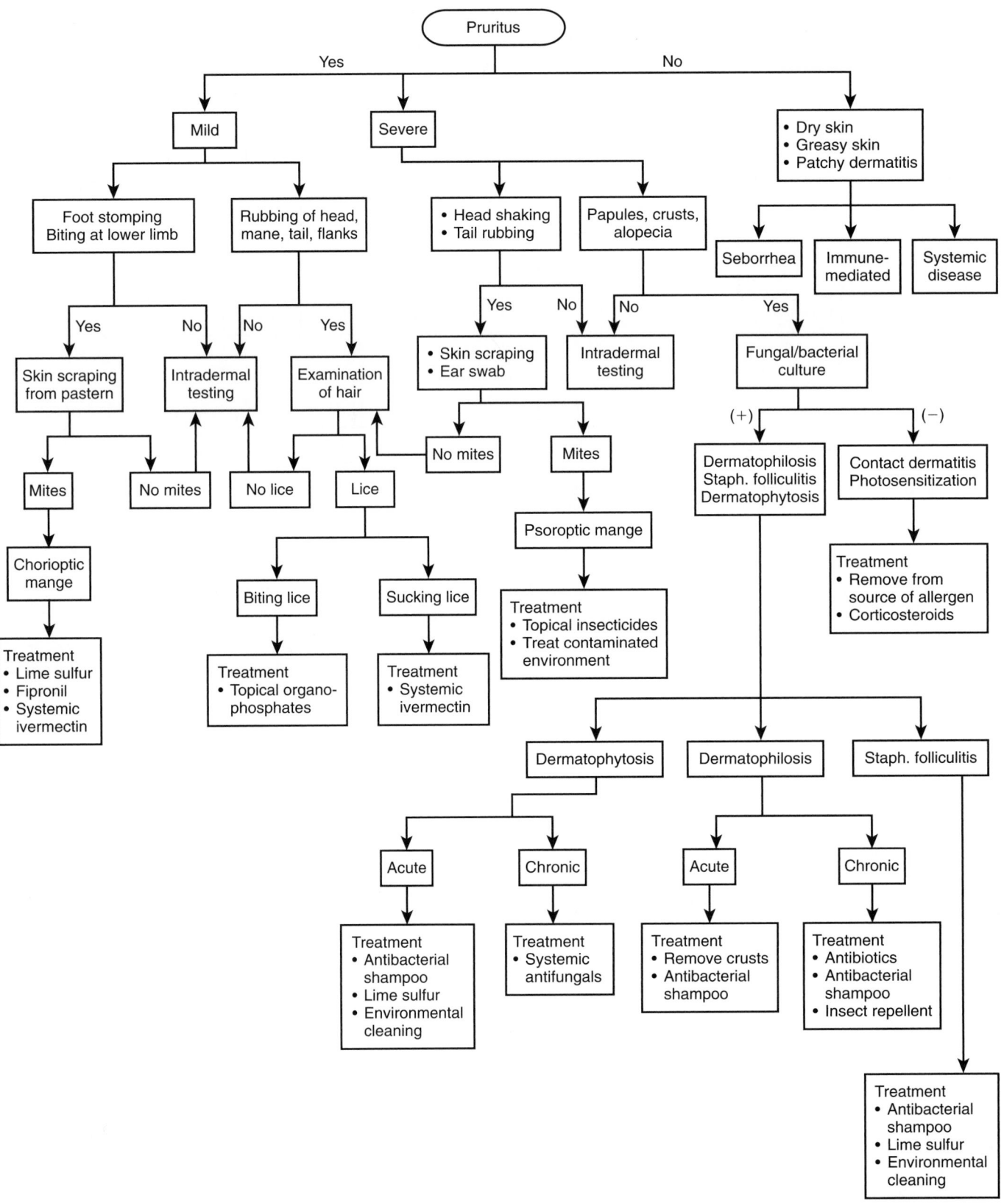

Author: **Alfredo Sanchez Londoño**

Renal Failure, Acute

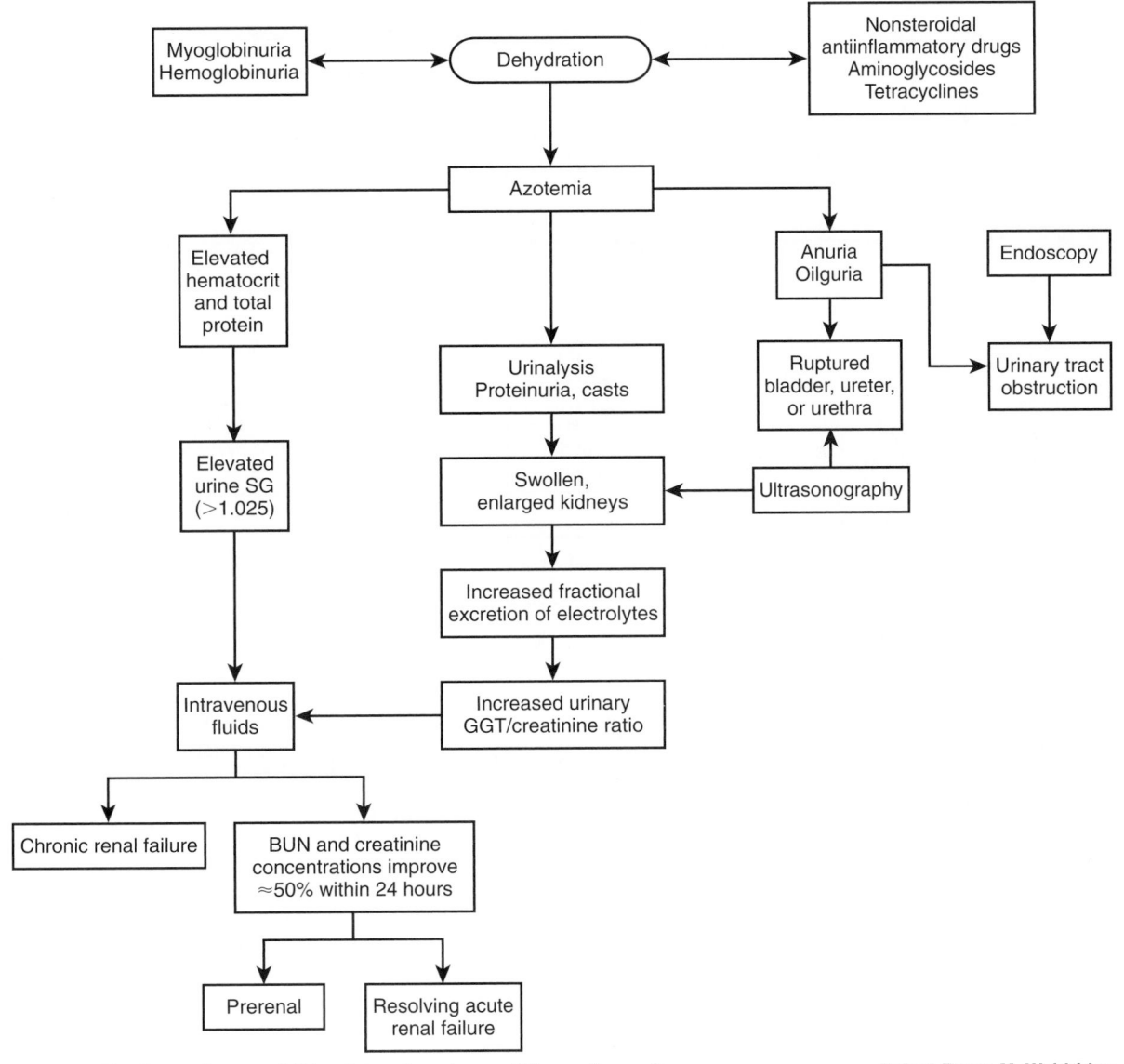

BUN, Blood urea nitrogen; *GGT*, γ-glutamyltransferase; *SG*, specific gravity.

Author: **Bryan M. Waldridge**

Renal Failure, Chronic

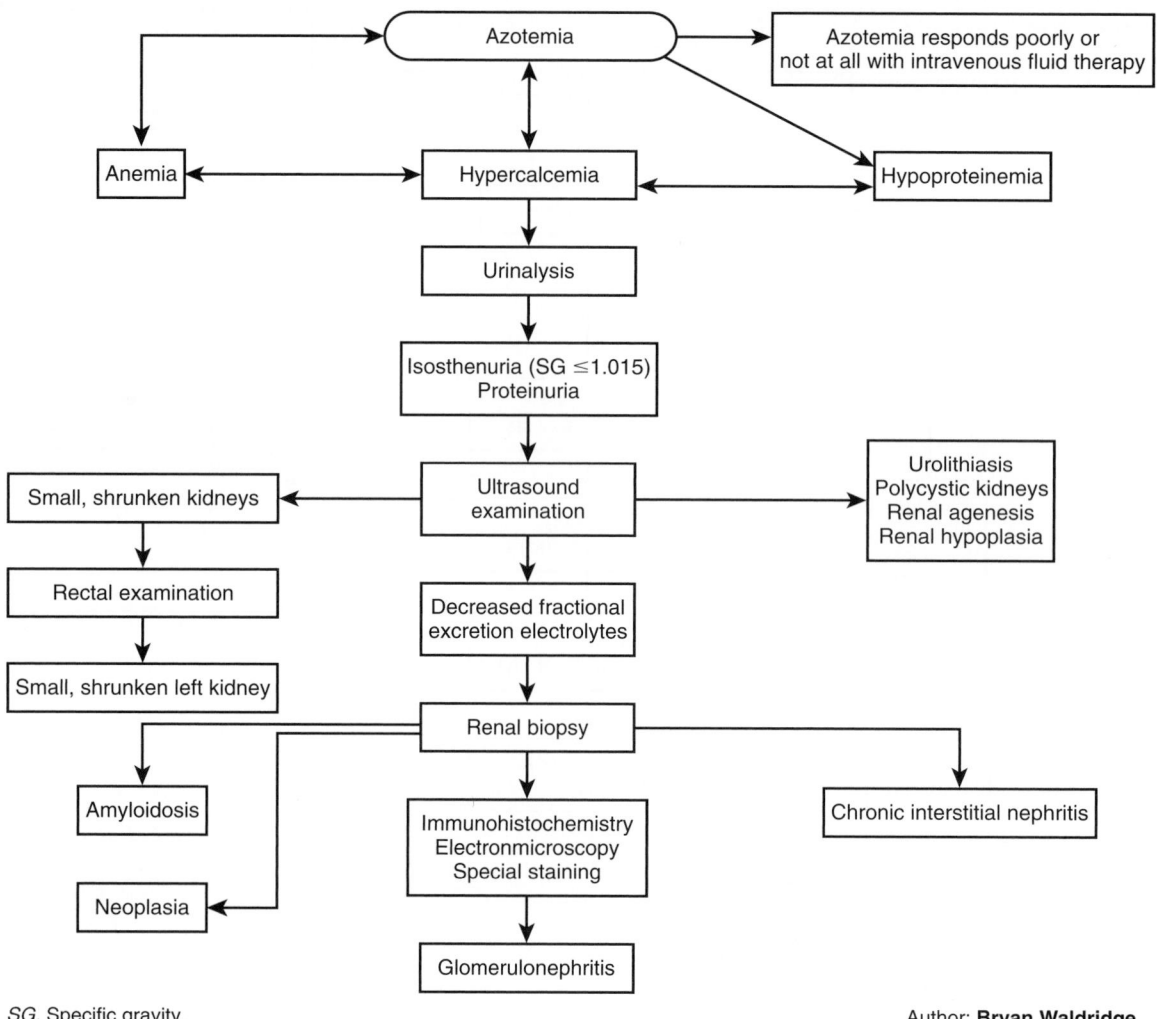

SG, Specific gravity.

Author: **Bryan Waldridge**

Scaling and Crusting Diseases

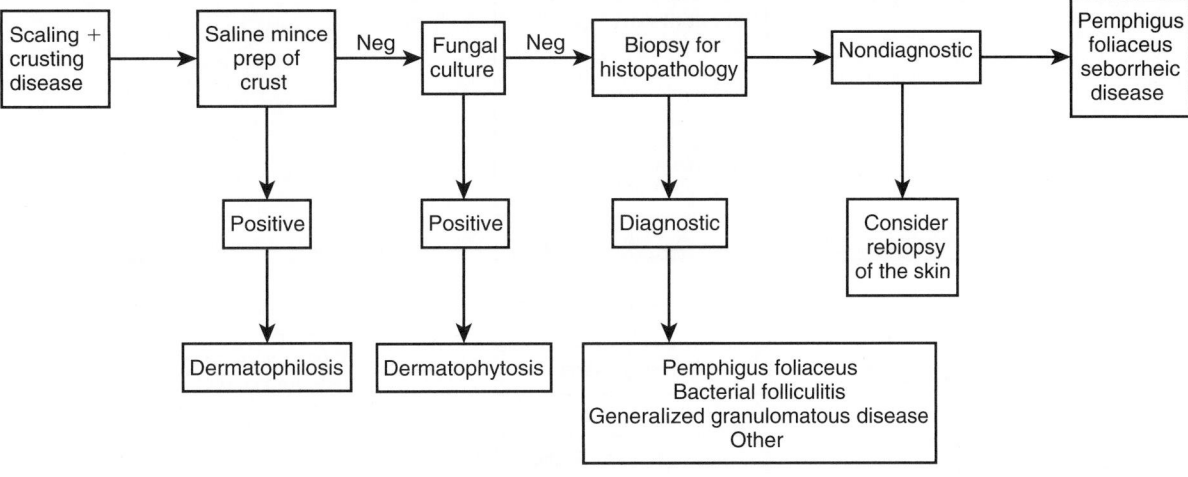

From Reed SJ, Bayly WM, Sellon DC: *Equine internal medicine*, ed 3, St Louis, 2010, Saunders Elsevier.

Seborrhea

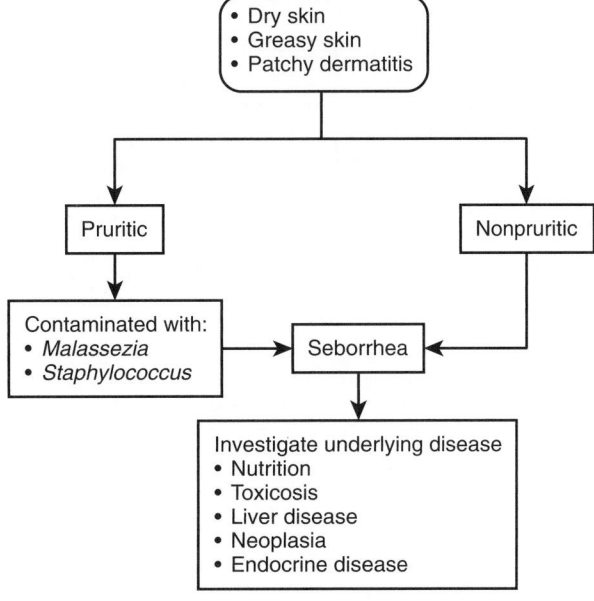

Author: **Alfredo Sanchez Londoño**

Spinal Ataxia

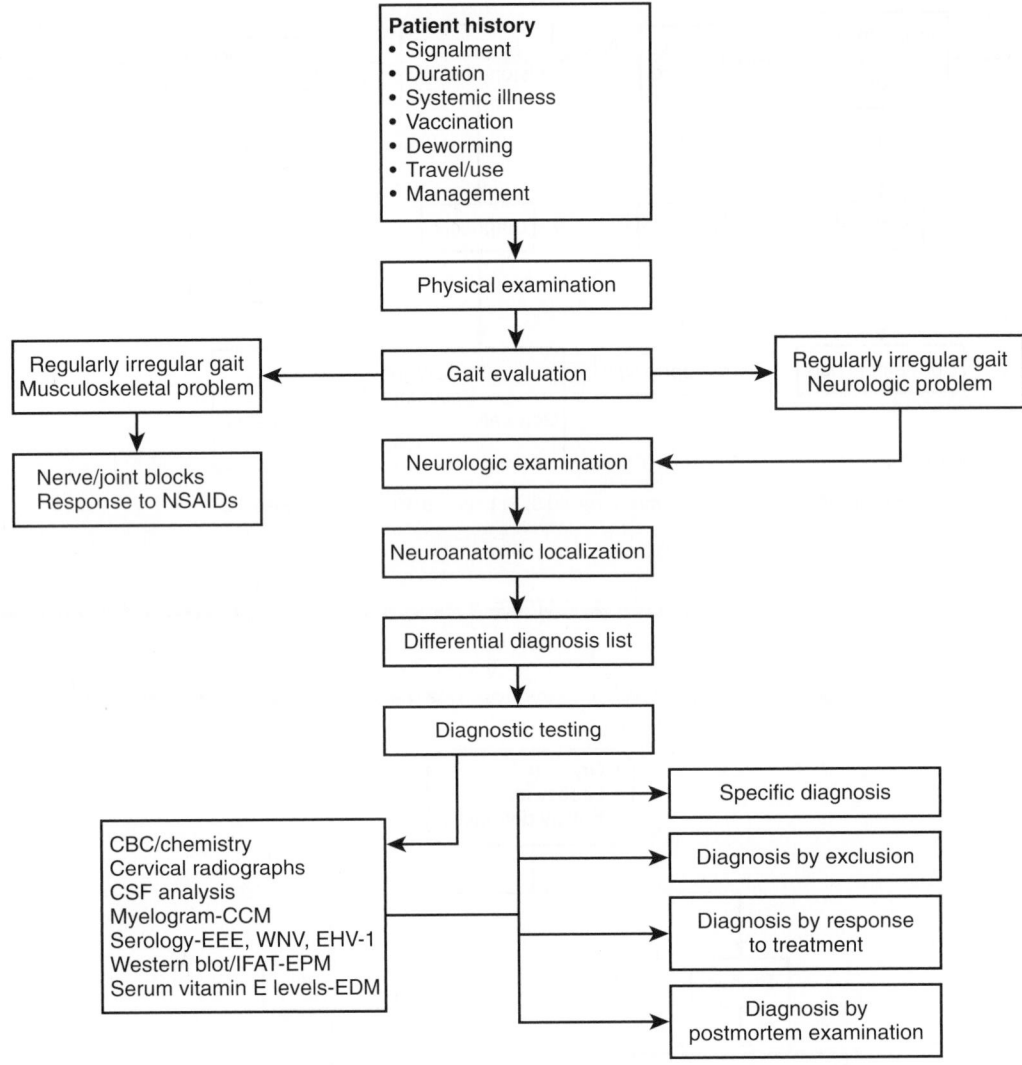

CBC, Complete blood count; CCM, cervical compressive myelopathy; CSF, cerebrospinal fluid; EDM, equine degenerative myeloencephalopathy; EEE, Eastern equine encephalitis; EHV-1, equine herpesvirus 1; IFAT-EPM, indirect fluorescent antibody test for equine protozoal myeloencephalitis; NSAIDs, nonsteroidal antiinflammatory drugs.
From Reed SJ, Bayly WM, Sellon DC: Equine internal medicine, ed 3, St Louis, 2010, Saunders Elsevier.

Staphylococcus Pyoderma

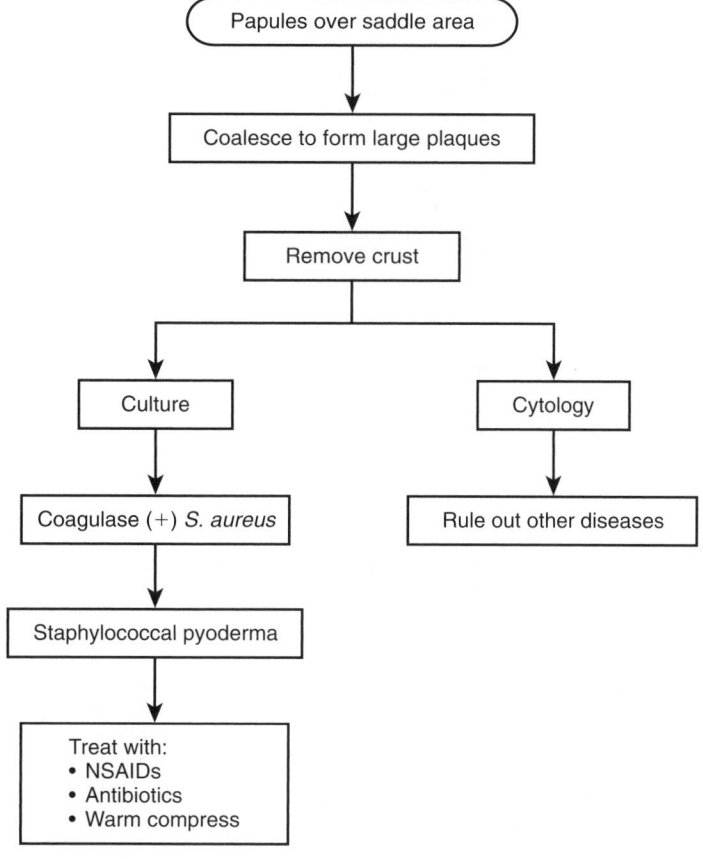

NSAIDs, Nonsteroidal antiinflammatory drugs.

Author: **Alfredo Sanchez Londoño**

Suspected Breeding Problem in the Mare

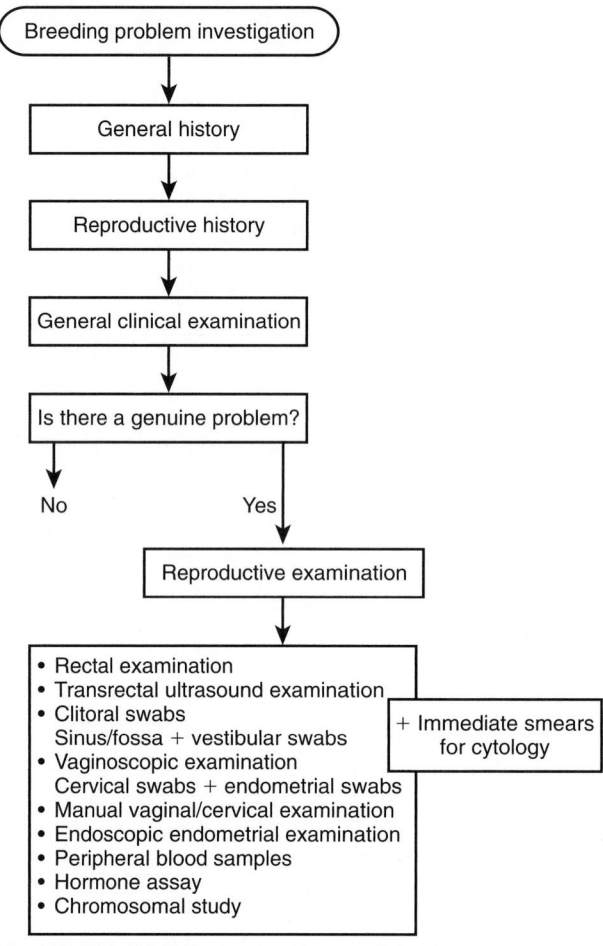

From Knottenbelt DC: Equine *stud farm medicine & surgery*,
Philadelphia, 2003, Saunders Elsevier, p 157.

Synovial Fluid Analysis

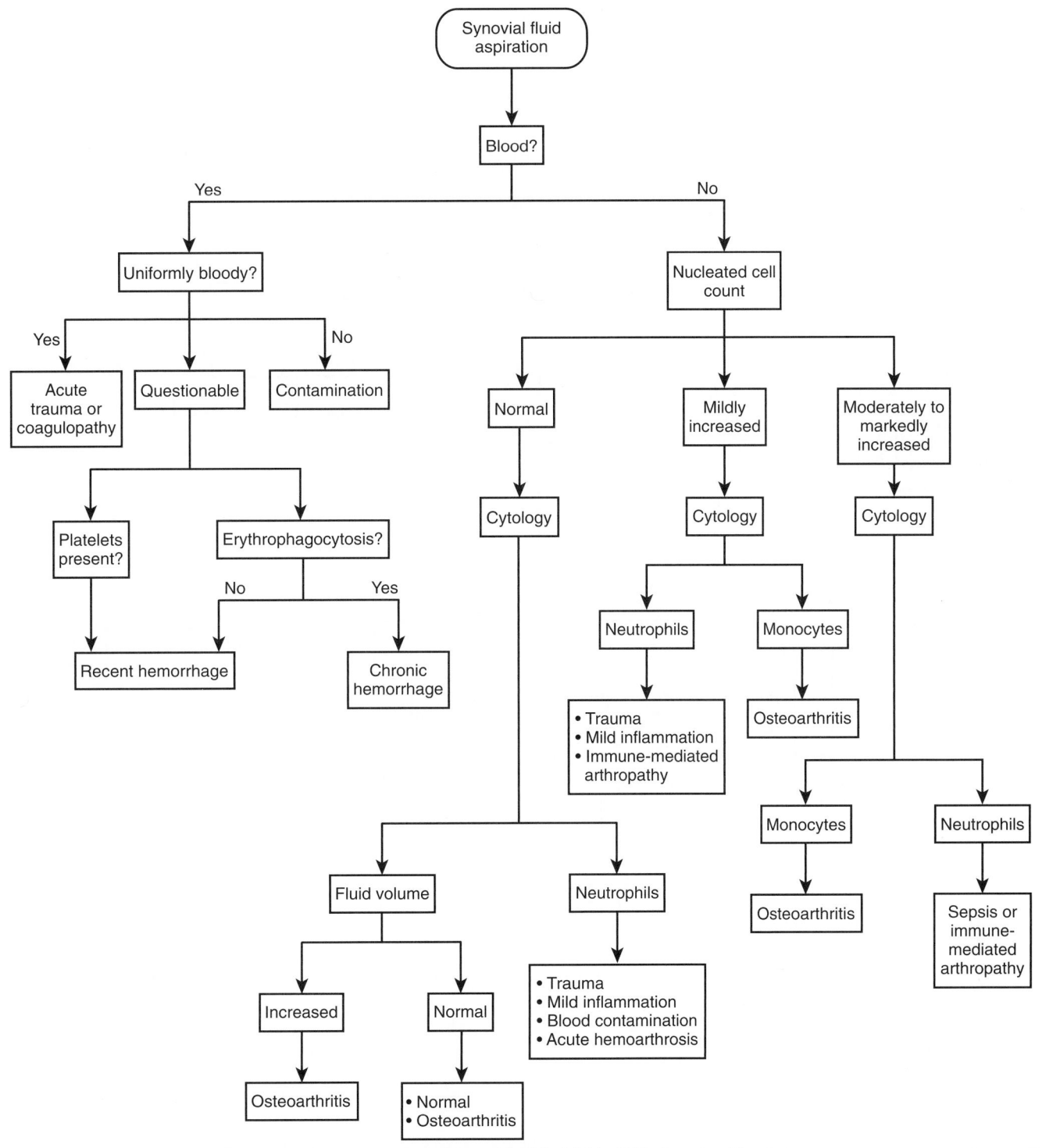

Modified from Ettinger SJ: *Textbook of veterinary internal medicine*, ed 7, Philadelphia, 2009, Saunders Elsevier.

Systemic Inflammatory Response Syndrome and Sepsis

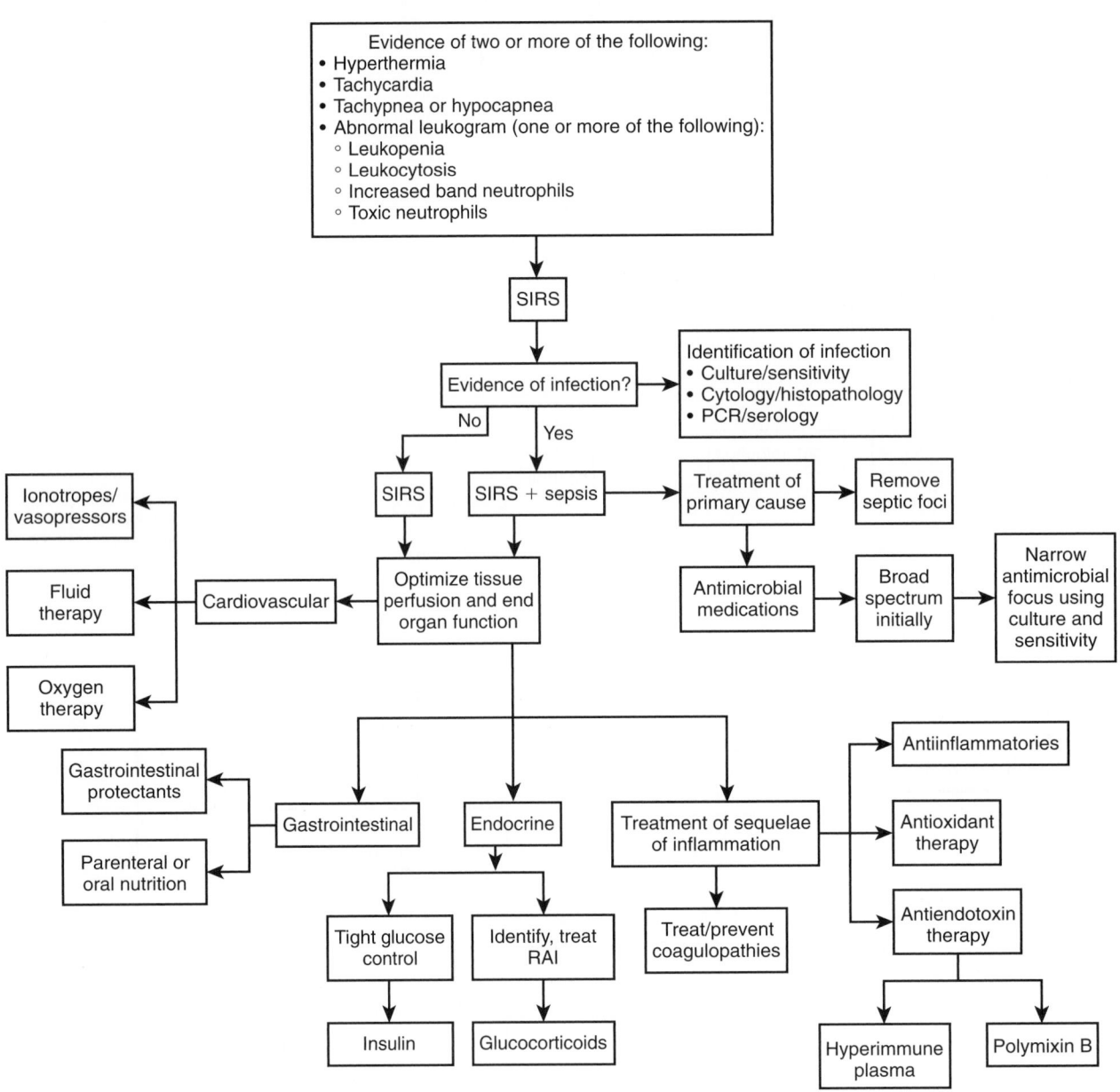

PCR, Polymerse chain reaction; *RAI,* relative adrenal insufficiency;
SIRS, systemic inflammatory response syndrome.

Author: **Amelia Munsterman**

Twin Pregnancy: Suspected or Confirmed

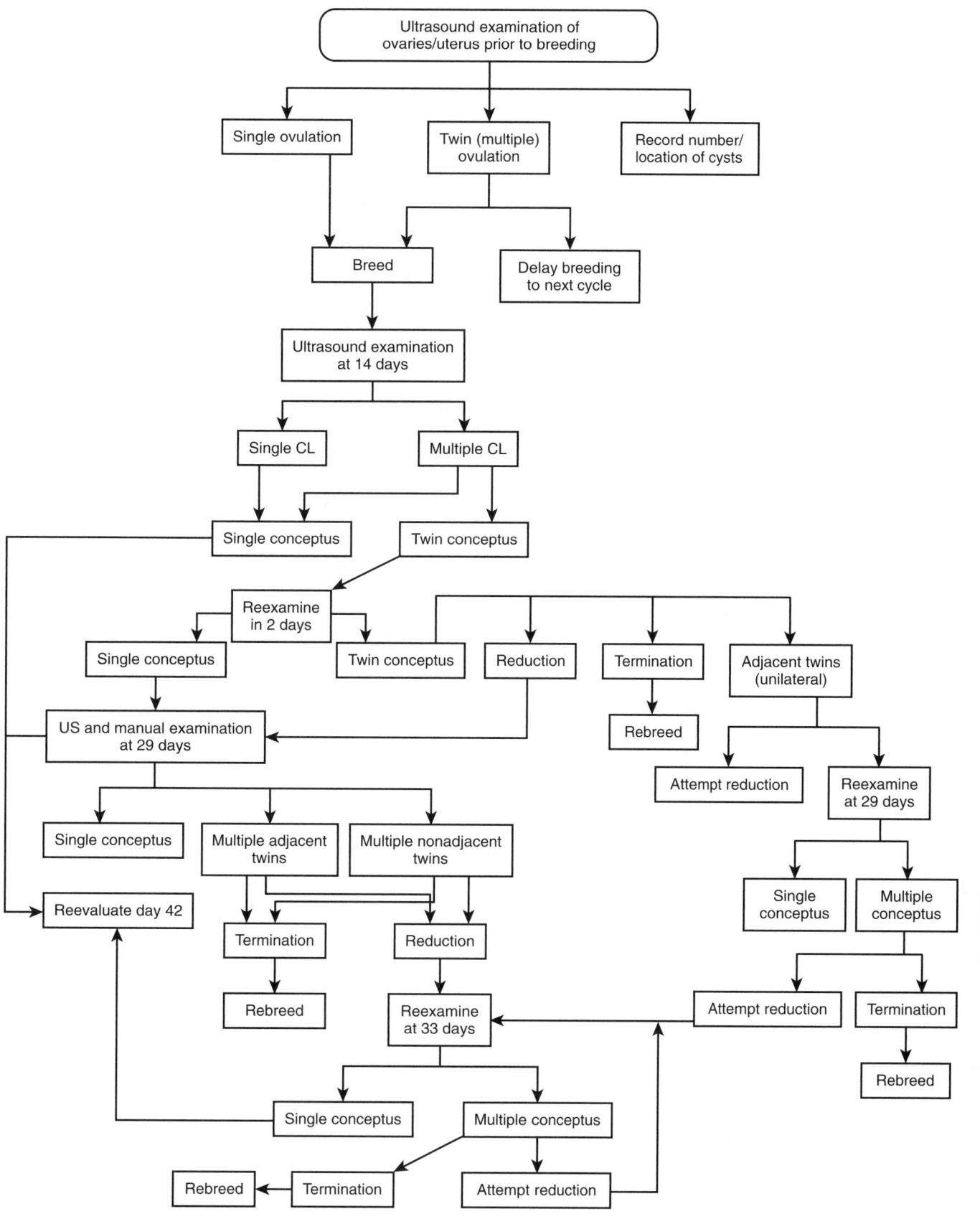

CL, Corpus luteum; US, ultrasound.
From Knottenbelt DC: *Equine stud farm medicine & surgery*, Philadelphia, 2003, Saunders Elsevier, p 248.

Urinary Incontinence

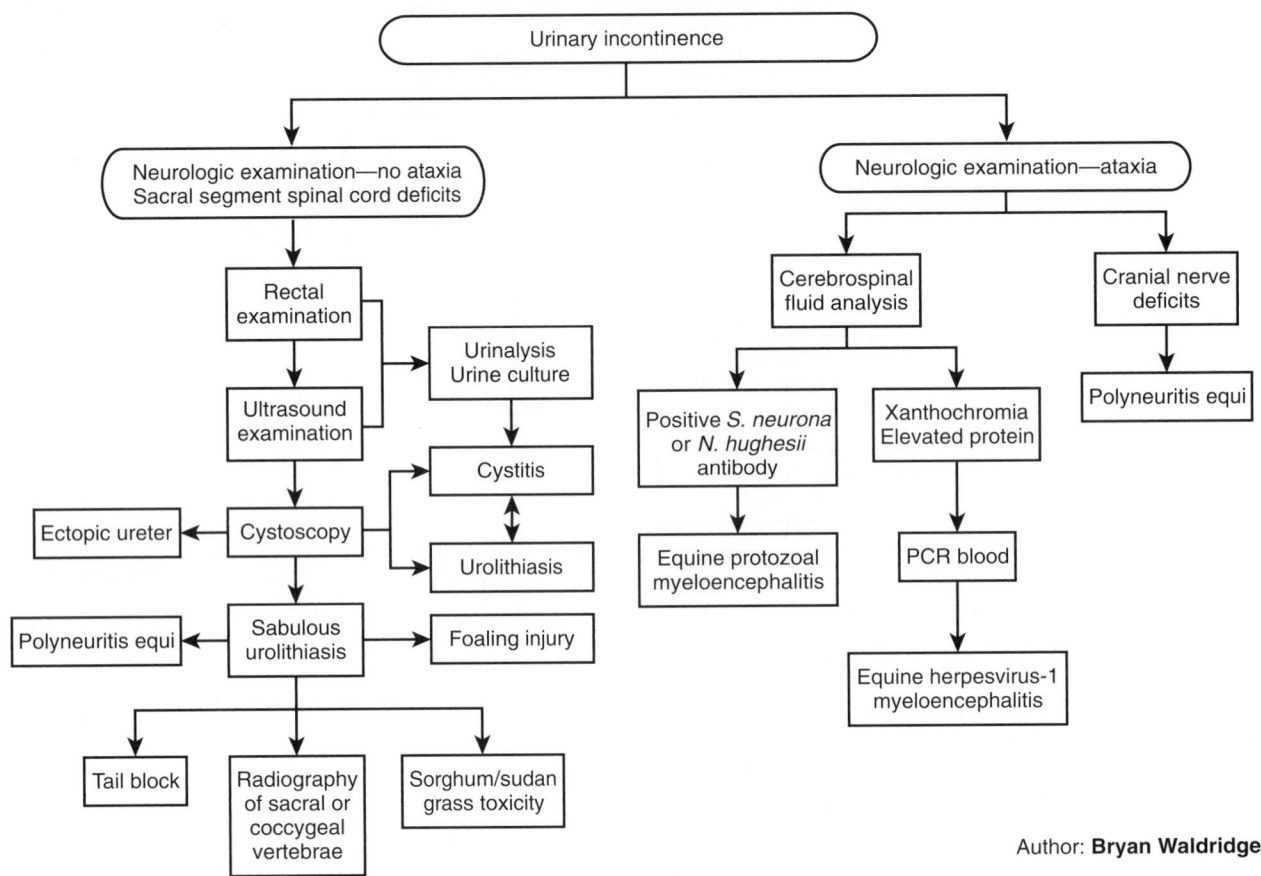

PCR, polymerase chain reaction.

Author: **Bryan Waldridge**

Uveitis, Acute and Chronic

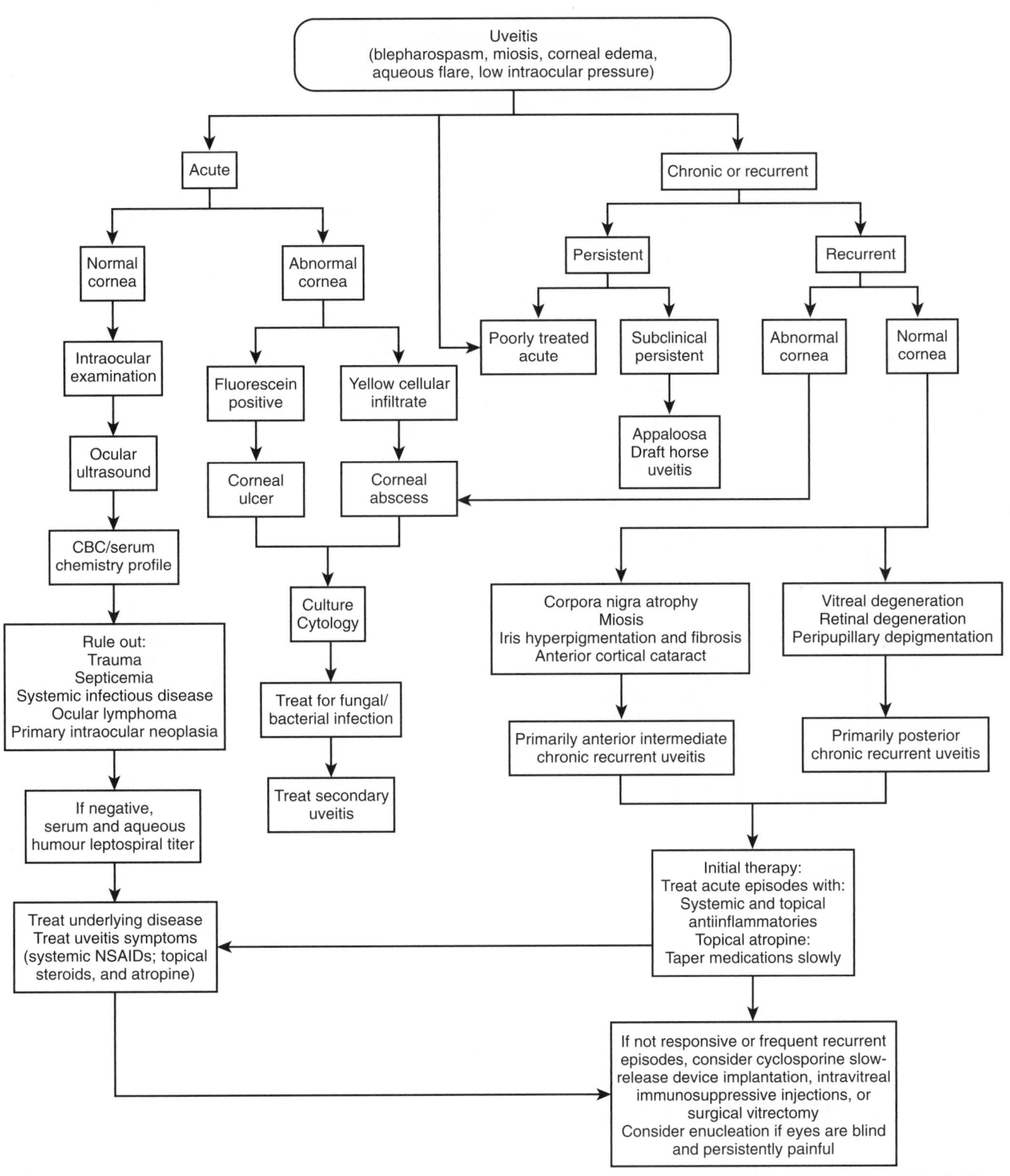

CBC, complete blood count; *NSAIDs,* nonsteroidal antiinflammatory drugs.

Author: **Brian C. Gilger**

Weak, Nonnursing Foal (Sepsis vs. HIE)

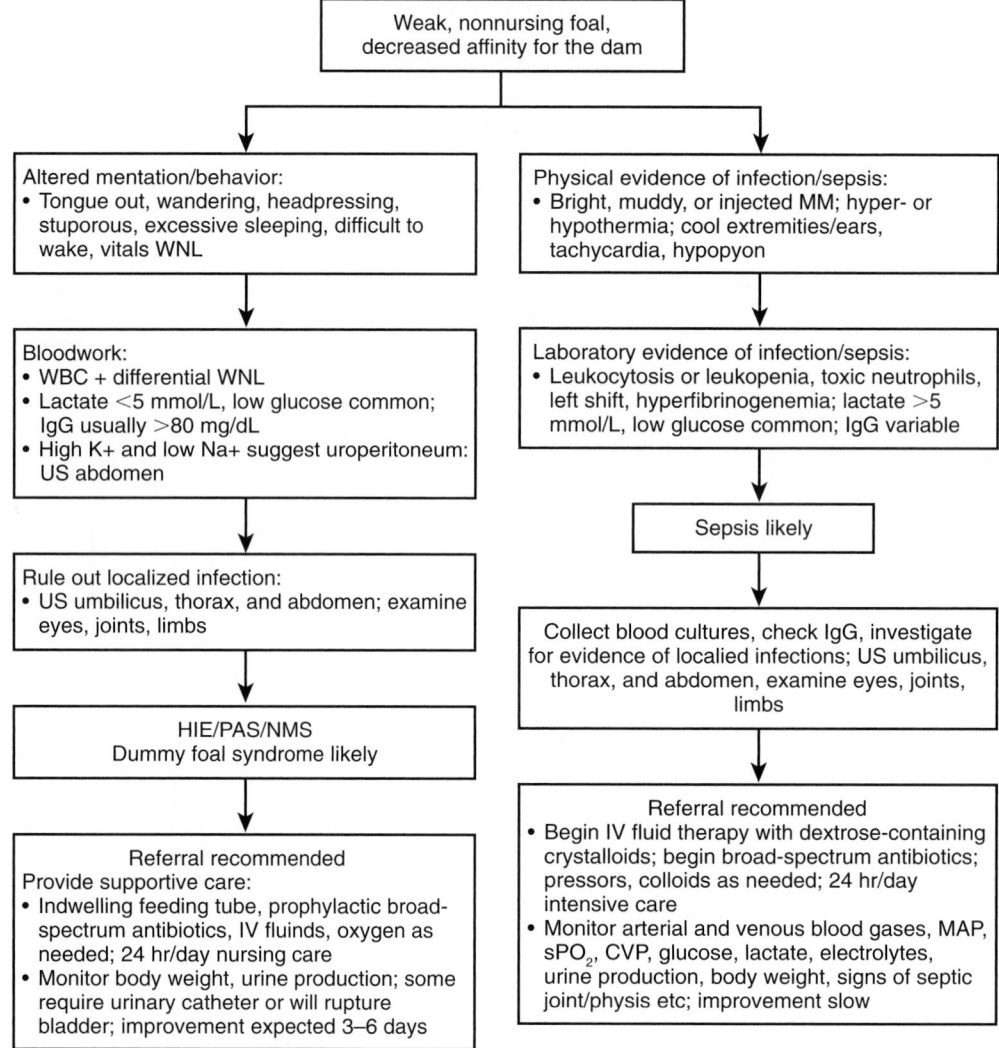

CVP, Central venous pressure; HIE, hypoxic ischemic encephalopathy; MAP, mean arterial pressure; MM, mucous membranes; NMS, neonatal maladjustment syndrome; PAS, perinatal asphyxia syndrome; sPO₂, pulse oximeter oxygen saturation; US, ultrasound; WNL, within normal limits.

Author: **Phoebe Smith**

SECTION VI

Drug Formulary

Drug Formulary

Drug	Class	Dose	Mechanism	Indication for Use	Potential Side Effects	Formulation
Acepromazine	Phenothiazine tranquilizer	0.02–0.066 mg/kg IV, IM, PO	Central blocking effects of dopamine. Peripheral alpha-adrenergic blocking effect causing vasodilation/hypotension	Sedative: suggested sedative for botulism; hypotensive resuscitation in hemorrhage; hypotensive dose for laminitis/renal failure	A reported side effect in stallions is priapism	10 mg/mL Promace 5-, 10- and 25-mg tablets Promace
Acetazolamide	Carbonic anhydrase inhibitor	2.5 mg/kg PO q12h	Diuretic effect causing renal loss of HCO_3 ion, which carries out NA, HOH, and K	Prevention of hyperkalemic periodic paralysis; decrease production of aqueous humor, making it useful to lower intraocular pressure for the treatment of glaucoma	None documented in horses	125- and 250-mg tablets: generic 500 mg per vial injectable: generic
Acetylcysteine solution 4%	Mucolytic	200 mL per rectum through Foley catheter and clamp for 20 minutes before evacuating the rectum	Reduces the viscosity of both purulent and nonpurulent secretions. The free sulfhydryl group on the drug is believed to reduce disulfide linkages in mucoproteins	Enema for meconium impaction	Not documented in horses	10% (100 mg/mL) and 20% (200 mg/mL) in 4-, 10-, and 30-mL vials: generic
Activated charcoal	Intestinal absorbent	1 g/kg as a slurry preferably administered via stomach tube or PO	Has a microporous structure that provides a large surface area on which a variety of compounds are absorbed	Endotoxemia secondary to colitis; adsorption of pesticides, pharmaceuticals, mycotoxins, phytotoxins, bacterial toxins, ethylene glycol and feed additives	Not documented in horses	Powder
Acyclovir	Antiviral	10 mg/kg IV q12h or 15–20 mg/kg PO q4–6h	Functions as a DNA polymerase inhibitor, DNA chain terminator, and can produce binding between viral DNA polymerase and the interrupted chain	Equine herpesvirus	Not documented in horses	400- and 800-mg tablets: generic 500 mg 10-mL vial 1000 mg 20-mL vial
Albuterol	Bronchodilator	Adult: 360–720 µg aerosolized q12h or q4h in severe respiratory distress Neonatal: 1 µg/kg aerosolized q12h or q4h depending on severity of respiratory distress Nebulization: 0.001 to 0.01 mg/kg q6–8h	β2 agonist causing the relaxation of bronchial, uterine, and vascular smooth muscle	Bronchoconstriction; small airway inflammation; chronic obstructive pulmonary disease	Not documented in horses	Aerosol: 90 µg per activation in 17-g canister 5 mg/mL inhalation solution

Continued

Drug	Class	Dose	Mechanism	Indication for Use	Potential Side Effects	Formulation
Altrenogest	Synthetic progestin	0.044 to 0.088 mg/kg PO q12h	Synthetic progestin	Regulation of estrus; behavior modification to help reduce libido and aggressive behavior in stallions; pregnancy maintenance when used early in pregnancy when there is concern of a dysfunctional corpus luteum; help maintain pregnancy in mares that have been exposed to endotoxin when treated at 0.088 mg/kg	Can be absorbed through unbroken skin; therefore, use gloves when administering	0.22% in oil solution in 150- and 1000-mL bottles; Regumate
Amikacin sulfate	Aminoglycoside antibiotic	21–25 mg/kg IV or IM SID Therapeutic drug monitoring is recommended to maintain a trough between 2–4 mg/mL	Inhibits protein synthesis by binding to the ribosomal 30S subunit interfering with mRNA synthesis. Bactericidal with its effect concentration dependent	Gram-negative infections	Nephrotoxic Ototoxic Aminoglycosides can also cause neuromuscular blockade	250 mg/mL in 48-mL bottles; Amiglyde-V
Aminocaproic acid	Hemostatic	40 mg/kg diluted in 1-L saline over 30–60 minutes; 20 mg/kg diluted in 1 L of saline over 30–60 minutes QID	Inhibits plasminogen activation resulting in inhibition of fibrinolysis. This is thought to aid in the stabilization of the clot but does not affect clot formation	Acute hemorrhage; exercise-induced pulmonary hemorrhage	Not documented in horses	250 mg/mL in 20-mL vials
Aminophylline	Bronchodilator and diuretic	5–10 mg/kg IV slowly diluted in at least 100 mL of 5% dextrose or normal saline; 5–15 mg/kg PO q6–12h	Phosphodiesterase inhibitor	Bronchoconstriction secondary to hyperreactive airways; oliguria	CNS excitement and gastrointestinal disturbances; use of cimetidine and erythromycin can potentiate the effects of aminophylline	25 mg/mL in 10- and 20-mL vials: generic 100, 200, and 225 mg tablets: generic
Amoxicillin	Antibiotic; aminopenicillin	10–30 mg/kg PO q8–12h (absorbed in foals). Do not use in adults.	Inhibits bacterial cell wall synthesis via binding to penicillin-binding proteins (PBPs). An amino side group makes it easier for the drug to penetrate gram-negative bacteria	Gram-positive infections	Gastrointestinal disturbances	Oral suspension 50 mg/mL in 100-, 150-, and 200-mL bottles: generic
Amphotericin B	Antifungal	0.3–0.5 mg/kg IV in 1 L of 5% dextrose over 1 hour q2days; 100–200 mg intrauterine direct injection into fungal granulomas	Binds ergosterol in the fungal cell membrane changing its barrier function	Systemic fungal infections; fungal endometritis; pythiosis	Nephrotoxicity	50-mg powder vial; Fungizone

Drug	Classification	Dosage	Action	Indications	Adverse Effects	Supply
Ampicillin	Antibiotic; aminopenicillin	20–40 mg/kg IV q6–8h	Inhibits bacterial cell wall synthesis via binding to PBPs. An amino side group makes it easier for the drug to penetrate gram-negative bacteria. Synergism with aminoglycosides	Gram-positive and some gram-negative infections	Gastrointestinal disturbances	1-, 2-, 3-, and 10-gram powder vials: generic
Aspirin (acetylsalicylic acid)	NSAID	10 mg/kg PO q24h or 17 mg/kg PO EOD	Irreversibly inhibits cyclooxygenase. Platelets are particularly susceptible to aspirin because they cannot regenerate cyclooxygenase.	Thromboembolic diseases: thrombophlebitis, laminitis, intestinal ischemia	Not documented in horses	325-mg tablets: generic
Atropine	Parasympatholytic	0.014–0.02 mg/kg IV or IM for bronchodilation. For organophosphate and carbamate toxicity, 0.2 mg/kg, ¼ IV and the remaining ¾ IM, repeated q1.5–4h, not to exceed 65 mg for the average horse 5–10 mg per joint	Competitively inhibits acetylcholine at muscarinic receptors of effector cells. The result is a decreased response to parasympathetic impulses	Bronchodilator anecdotally used in conjunction with steroids to reduce distended joints and tendon sheaths	Generally dose-related ileus and colic; ataxia and seizures; pupil dilation	2 mg/mL 100-mL vial and 0.5 mg/mL 30- and 100-mL vials: generic
Azithromycin	Azilide antibiotic	10 mg/kg PO for 5 days and then every other day; normally used in combination with Rifampin	Inhibits bacterial protein synthesis by binding to subunits of 50s ribosomes	*Rhodococcus equi* pneumonia; gram-positive infections	Hyperthermia (restrict exposure to sunlight); colitis	500-mg tablets or compounded suspensions
Baclofen	Muscle relaxant	0.4 mg/kg PO q8h	Unknown. Speculated to inhibit reflexes at the spinal level. It is an analog of GABA and may potentiate its activity.	Stringhalt	Not documented in horses	10- and 20-mg tablets
Beclomethasone	Corticosteroid	10–12 activations SID for 2 weeks then q48h or EOD for another 2 weeks. Continue q24h if signs reoccur. After 4 weeks: maintenance dose 8–12 activations q48h or EOD	Local antiinflammatory effect. The result is inhibition of leukocyte migration, lysosomal stabilization, and reversal of increased capillary permeability	Small airway inflammation; COPD	Not documented in horses	80 μg per activation; QVAR 80
Benztropine mesylate	Anticholinergic	0.4 mg/kg PO q8h	Centrally acting anticholinergic with antihistaminic properties	Priapism, acute fluphenazine toxicity	Not documented in horses	2-mg tablets: generic

Continued

Drug	Class	Dose	Mechanism	Indication for Use	Potential Side Effects	Formulation
Bethanechol	Parasympathomimetic	Prokinetic: 0.025 mg/kg SQ q8h Detrusor activity: 80–100 mg PO q8h	Structurally related to acetylcholine. Binds to and stimulates muscarinic receptors of the parasympathetic nervous system. It is not destroyed by acetylcholinesterase to the same degree as acetylcholine.	Ileus, neurogenic atony of the bladder	Salivation, diarrhea	5 mg/mL injectable solution 50-mg tablets
Bismuth subsalicylate	Intestinal protectant	Foal: 0.5–1 mL/kg PO q4–6h Adult: 1–2 L via NGT q12–24 h	Cleaved in the small intestine to bismuth carbonate and salicylate. Bismuth has protective, anti-endotin and weak antibacterial properties. Salicylate has anti-prostaglandin activity	Diarrhea	Impaction	Oral suspension: generic
Boldenone undecylenate	Anabolic steroid	1.1 mg/kg IM, may be repeated at 3-week intervals	Marked anabolic effect with lesser androgenic properties	Treating debilitated horses	Fertility in stallions (decreased sperm production and testicular weight); abnormal aggressive behavior	25 mg/mL in 10-mL vials; 50 mg/mL in 10- and 50-mL vials; Equipoise
Butorphanol tartrate	Analgesic/sedative	0.01–0.1 mg/kg IV or IM	Narcotic agonist-antagonist because it can either activate or block opiate receptors. 5–7 times the analgesic activity of morphine. Has an antitussive property	Analgesia/sedation	Transient ataxia; CNS excitement (head tossing, jittering, lip smacking)	10 mg/mL injectable solution in 50-mL vials
Caffeine	Stimulant	10 mg/kg PO; maintenance 2.5 mg/kg PO q12h	Xanthine that acts as a psychoactive drug	Respiratory stimulant for "dummy foals"	Excitement Tachycardia	100-mg caffeine tablets: generic
Carbamazepine	Anticonvulsant and analgesic	2–8 mg/kg PO q6–8h	Stabilizes the inactive state of the sodium channels therefore fewer of these channels are open making nerves and brain cells less excitable	Headshaking	Not documented in horses	4300-mg tablets or capsules: generic
Cefazolin	Cephalosporin antibiotic	11 mg/kg IV q6–8h	First-generation cephalosporin. Inhibits bacterial cell wall synthesis by binding to PBPs. More resistant to β-lactamases	Gram-positive infections	Colitis	5, 10, and 20-mg powder for injection
Cefepime	Antibiotic	Foals: 11 mg/kg IV q8h Adults: 2.2 mg/kg IV q8h	Fourth-generation cephalosporin. Inhibits bacterial cell wall synthesis by binding to PBPs. More resistant to β-lactamases	Foals with septicemia and other infections that appear resistant to more routine antibiotics	Colitis	1 g 10-mL solution or 2 g 20-mL solution

Drug	Class	Dose	Mechanism	Indication	Adverse effects	Formulation
Cefotaxime	Antibiotic	20–40 mg/kg IV q6h	Third-generation cephalosporin. Inhibits bacterial cell wall synthesis by binding to PBPs. More resistant to β-lactamases	Gram-negative meningitis; severe infections due to susceptible organisms	Colitis	1-g powder for injection vials
Cefpodoxime proxetil	Antibiotic	10 mg/kg PO q6–8h	Third-generation cephalosporin. Inhibits bacterial cell wall synthesis by binding to PBPs. More resistant to β-lactamases	Foals, broad-spectrum antibiotic	Diarrhea	Oral suspension 50 mg/5 mL; 100 mg/5 mL and tablets 100 mg and 200 mg
Ceftiofur	Antibiotic	Foals: 2.2–10 mg/kg IM, IV, SQ q6–24h Adults: 2.2 mg/kg IM, IV, SQ q12–24h	Third-generation cephalosporin. Inhibits bacterial cell wall synthesis by binding to PBPs. More resistant to β-lactamases	Gram-negative and gram-positive infections	Concerns about colitis in particular horses on the racetrack	1- and 4-g powder for injection. Stable for 7 days when refrigerated and 8 weeks when frozen
Cephalexin	Antibiotic	25 mg/kg PO QID	First-generation cephalosporin. Inhibits bacterial cell wall synthesis by binding to PBPs. More resistant to β-lactamases	Gram-positive infections	Diarrhea	500- and 750-mg capsules; oral suspension 250 mg/5 mL 200-mL bottle
Chloramphenicol	Antibiotic	(Palmitate oral) 40–50 mg/kg PO q6–8h (Sodium succinate parenteral) 25/mg kg IV q4–6h	Reversibly binds 50S ribosomal subunit. Bacteriocidal at higher doses	Aerobic and anaerobic infections; Lawsonia intracellularis; meningitis	Diarrhea/colitis; (humans) fatal aplastic anemia in humans due to its affinity for mitochondrial ribosomes in some mammalian cells	1-g tablets and 10-g powder injection vials
Cimetidine	Antiulcer medication	15–20 mg/kg PO q6h 6.6–10 mg/kg IV q6–8h Melanomas: 2.5 mg/kg PO q8h for 3 months	Histamine type 2 (H2) receptor antagonists. Competitively inhibits histamine's action at H2 receptor sites of gastric parietal cells	Gastric ulceration; melanomas: variable results	Not documented in horses	400- and 800-mg tablets; cimetidine HCL for injection 150 mg/mL 8-mL multidose vials
Cisapride	Prokinetic	0.1 mg/kg IM q8h or 60–100 mg/500 kg animal per rectum q2–6h	Enhances release of acetylcholine. Affects serotonin receptors (5HT). Stimulates motilin production	Ileus	Human product has been taken off the market due to cardiac arrhythmias and deaths in some patients. This has not been documented in horses. Macrolide antibiotics should be avoided as they can slow the metabolism of cisapride (as do other medications metabolized by cytochrome p450).	Compounding pharmacies

Continued

Drug	Class	Dose	Mechanism	Indication for Use	Potential Side Effects	Formulation
Cisplatin	Antineoplastic agent	1 mg per cubic cm intratumoral injection. Drug preparation: 10 mg cisplatin powder is mixed with 1 mL water. This mixture is mixed with 2 mL sesame oil using a two-way connector mixing between the two syringes. Cisplatin biodegradable beads are currently available.	Heavy metal complex. Cisplatin is cytotoxic to actively dividing cells because it binds to DNA causing intrastrand and interstrand cross linking.	Sarcoids; squamous cell carcinoma; some melanomas	Contraindicated in pregnant animals	Compounding pharmacies; biodegradable beads (Royer Biomedical, Maryland)
Clarithromycin	Antibiotic	7.5 mg/kg PO q12h. Recommended to be used with Rifampin.	A macrolide antibiotic that inhibits protein synthesis by binding to the 50S subunit of bacterial ribosomes	*Rhodococcus equi* infections in foals; *Lawsonia intracellularis* (in foals <500 pounds)	Hyperthermia (Keep animal out of direct sunlight); Colitis (Increased prevalence noted in animals > 500 pounds); DO NOT USE IN ADULT ANIMALS	500 mg tablets
Clebuterol	Bronchodilator	0.8–3.0 µg/kg PO q12h Start with 0.8 µg at first and then slowly increase by 0.8 µg increments if appropriate response is not noted	A β2 adrenergic agonist. Relaxes bronchial smooth muscle by action on the β2 adrenergic receptors. Improves mucociliary clearance	Small airway inflammation; COPD; have been used in ruminants as a tocolytic: effect on myometrium after oral dosing controversial	At higher end of the dose can affect beta-1 receptors causing: sweating, trembling, tachycardia, excitement. Do not use in pregnant mares near term due to its effects of relaxing the uterus	72.5 µg/mL syrup
Cloprostenol	Prostaglandin F2alpha analogue	250 µg IM abortion: Give q24h. Mare will usually abort in 3–5 days. Must be beyond 80 days pregnant	Causes regression of the corpus luteum and has stimulatory effect on uterine smooth muscle	Induce abortion; luteolysis; improve uterine clearance postbreeding (250 µg IM postbreeding)	Mild colic and sweating	250 µg/mL in 10 or 20-mL vials
Colchicine	Antifibrotic	0.3 mg/kg PO q12–24h	Also apparently blocks the synthesis and secretion of serum amyloid A by hepatocytes thereby preventing the formation of amyloid enhancing factor and preventing amyloid deposition. Has also been proposed for treating hepatic and renal fibrosis presumably by decreasing the formation of collagen	Amyloidosis; chronic hepatitis fibrosis; renal fibrotic disease	Not documented in horses	0.5- and 0.6-mg tablets
Cyproheptadine	Serotonin antagonist	0.3 mg/kg PO q12h	An antihistamine that also has anticholinergic and antiserotonin activity	Photic headshaking; equine Cushing's disease	Drowsiness	Compounding pharmacies

Drug	Classification	Dose	Mechanism of Action	Indication	Adverse Effects	Formulation
Dantrolene	Muscle relaxant (skeletal)	Prevention of exertional rhabdomyolysis (ER): 2–4 mg/kg PO q24h; Treatment of ER: 2.5 mg/kg IV in saline, slowly up to q6h (dantrolene sodium)	Decreases muscle contraction by interfering with the release of calcium from the sarcoplasmic reticulum	Treatment of ER; treatment of postanesthetic myopathy	Sedation: may increase when administered with other sedatives	100-mg capsules and for injection in 20-mg vials
Deslorelin	Synthetic hormone	1.5 mg/500 kg IM or 2.1-mg implant	A synthetic GnRH that induces ovulation by increasing endogenous LH	Induce ovulation; must have a follicle which is >30 mm. Approximately 84% given the medication will ovulate within 48 hours	If implant is not removed then will result in prolonged diestrus	Compounding pharmacies. The sale of the implant was discontinued in the United States in 2004 but remains in some countries.
Detomidine	Analgesic/sedative	0.01–0.02 mg/kg IV or IM	Alpha2 adrenergic agonist	Analgesia/sedation; analgesia via constant rate infusion	Ileus; excessive sedation: Do not use in neonates	10 mg/mL solution
Dexamethasone	Synthetic glucocorticoid	0.05–0.2 mg/kg PO, IV or IM q24h. Pars intermedia dysfunction testing: 20 mg IM and measure for cortisol levels 19 hours after administration	Antiinflammatory and immunosuppressive properties by inhibiting macrophage and leukocyte functions. This class also inhibits phospholipase A2, preventing the breakdown of arachidonic acid into prostaglandins and leukotrienes.	Antiinflammatory; allergic conditions; immunosuppression; shock/trauma	Laminitis Decreased renal Perfusion Excessive immunosuppression	2 and 4 mg/mL injection, various oral suspensions available through compounding pharmacies
Diazepam	Anticonvulsive/sedative	Foals: 5–15 mg IV or IM Adults: 15–30 mg IV	Benzodiazepine that enhances the inhibitory neurotransmitter gamma-aminobutyric acid (GABA). This class of medication binds to the GABA receptor at a "benzodiazepine binding site"	Anticonvulsant; preanesthesia medication; stallions breeding; may enhance sexual arousal and facilitate ejaculation. Use 0.05 mg/kg IV 15 minutes before breeding	Exceeding a dose of 0.2 mg/kg may produce sterna or lateral recumbency due to the medication's muscle relaxant properties	5 mg/mL injectable solution
Digoxin	Cardiac inotrope	Loading: 0.002–0.006 mg/kg IV or 0.06 mg/kg PO Maintenance: 0.01 mg/kg PO q12h	Increases myocardial contractility with increased cardiac output, increased diuresis with reduction of edema. Also has several electrocardiac effects including decreased conduction velocity through AV node and prolonged effective refractory period (ERP)	Congestive heart disease; supraventricular tachycardia; atrial fibrillation	Cardiac effects are seen before extracardiac effects (colic, anorexia and diarrhea). Cardiac effects may include worsening of heart failure, complete or incomplete heart block, multifocal premature ventricular contractions and ST segment changes	0.25 mg/mL solution and 0.5-mg tablets

Continued

Drug	Class	Dose	Mechanism	Indication for Use	Potential Side Effects	Formulation
Diphenhydramine	Antihistamine	0.5–1 mg/kg IV or IM	Antihistamine	Anaphylaxis, urticaria, fluphenazine toxicity	CNS excitement	10 or 50 mg/mL vials
Dimethyl sulfoxide	Antiinflammatory	0.5–1.0 g/kg q12–24h	Controversial; one mechanism for the antiinflammatory properties is its ability to scavenge oxygen radicals. Diuretic	CNS trauma; parenteral and topical antiinflammatory	Local irritation if given topically	900 mg to 1 g per mL solution and various gel formulations
Dinoprost tromethamine	Prostaglandin F2 alpha	0.02 mg/kg IV	PGF2 alpha causes increase in intracellular calcium due to control of gated calcium channels. Luteolysis is thought to occur due to cell death associated by high intracellular calcium levels.	Induce estrus (luteolysis): Give at least 4 days after ovulation 10 mg/500 kg animal. Estrus will occur in 2–4 days following treatment and ovulation will occur in 7–12 days; Abortion: Prior to day 35 one dose results in abortion in 2–3 days. After day 35 daily treatment for 3–5 days is required; postbreeding	Colic, sweating	5 mg/mL injectable solution
Dobutamine	Cardiac inotrope	250 mg in 500 mL 5% dextrose of saline solution results in 250 µg/mL solution. Administer 2–5 µg/kg/min (0.45 mL/kg/hr)	Direct beta-1 adrenergic agonist that results in increase stroke volume and cardiac output	Heart failure/shock; renal compromise secondary to hypotensive shock	Tachycardia, ectopic beats	12.5 mg/mL in 20-mL vials
Dopamine	Endogenous catecholamine	200 mg in 500 mL 5% dextrose or saline solution gives 200 µg/mL solutions. Administer 2–5 µg/kg/ minute (0.45 mL/kg/hr)	Dopamine is a precursor to norepinephrine and acts directly and indirectly (by releasing norepinephrine) on both alpha and beta 1 receptors. Dopamine also had dopaminergic effects. Low IV dose 0.5 to 2 µg/ min acts predominately on dopamine receptors and dilates renal, mesenteric, coronary, and intracerebral vasculature; 2–10 µg/min results in the stimulation of beta 1 receptors, which results in a positive inotropic activity.	Hypotensive shock; azotemia secondary to hypotension; vasopressor	Tachycardia, ectopic beats	40, 80, and 160 mg/ mL in 5-, 10- and 20-mL vials

Drug	Class	Dosage	Action	Adverse Effects	Formulation
Domperidone	Dopamine antagonist	1.14 mg/kg PO q12–24h	Dopamine antagonist. Dopamine mimetic agents (fescue alkaloids) cause a reduction in prolactin release. Domperidone is thought to block the effect of the alkaloids.	Not documented in horses	11% oral gel
			Fescue toxicosis (1.14 mg/kg PO q24h): Initiate 10 days prior to expected foaling date and continue up to foaling. Continue for 5 days after foaling if the mare is not producing milk adequately. Agalactia: Give q12h for 3–4 days and then q24h for at least 3 more days		
Doxapram	CNS stimulant	0.5 mg/kg IV	Stimulation of the medullary respiratory center and stimulation of chemoreceptors of the carotid and aortic regions	Convulsions and hyperventilation	20 mg/mL solution in 20-ml vials
			Respiratory stimulant		
Doxycycline	Antibiotic	10 mg/kg PO q12h	Inhibits protein synthesis by reversible binding to 30s ribosomal subunits	Intravenous administration has been reported to be fatal in horses; diarrhea; flexural laxity in neonates/foals	50- and 100-mg tablets
			Mainly gram-positive infections (including *Rhodococcus equi*; *Leptospirosis* and *Borrelia burgdorferi*; *Lawsonia Intracellularis*); inhibition of matrix metalloproteinase (MMP) activity. Anecdotal reports of low-dose doxycycline in horses with chronic laminitis and melting corneal ulcers—1–3 mg/kg PO q12h		
Enalapril	ACE inhibitor	1 mg/kg PO q24h or 0.5 mg/kg PO q12h	Inhibits conversion of Angiotensin I to Angiotensin II	Has been documented in humans to cause congenital malformations when given to pregnant women. This has not been documented in the mare. I have used in on several pregnant animals, which have foaled healthy animals with no indication of congenital lesions.	10- and 20-mg tablets
			Congestive heart disease		
Enrofloxacin	Fluoroquinolone antibiotic	6 mg/kg IV q24h; 7.5 mg/kg PO q24h	Inhibits DNA gyrase resulting in inhibition of DNA coiling and synthesis. Has significant postantibiotic effect	Cartilage damage in young animals; chemically induced arthropathy; flexural laxity	100 mg/mL intravenous solution; compounding pharmacies for oral suspension
			Gram-negative and *Staphylococcus* infections resistant to other antibiotics		

Continued

Drug	Class	Dose	Mechanism	Indication for Use	Potential Side Effects	Formulation
Epinephrine	Catecholamine	Foals: 0.5–1 mL of 1:1000 IV or IM during resuscitation. Can repeat every 5 to 10 minutes Adults: 5–10 mL of 1:1000 IV or IM for anaphylaxis	Catecholamine	Anaphylaxis and foal resuscitation	Can cause dangerous tachycardia and vasoconstriction	1:1000 (1 mg/mL) injectable solution
Erythromycin	Antibiotic	25 mg/kg PO q6–8h	Inhibits protein synthesis by binding to 50s ribosomes. Erythromycin stearate and erythromycin phosphate are the forms best absorbed by foals.	*Rhodococcus equi* infections; postoperative ileus; 0.5–2.2 mg/kg of erythromycin lactobionate IV q6h over 30–60 minutes diluted in 1 L of saline	Hyperthermia (do not expose to sunlight); diarrhea/colitis; do not use in adult horses because can cause fatal colitis	Compounding pharmacies
Etodolac	NSAID	23 mg/kg PO q12–24h	More selective for inhibition of cyclooxygenase 2 than cyclooxygenase 1. This indicates greater inhibition of the prostaglandins involved with pain and inflammation than those involved with cytoprotection of the GI tract and renal tissue	Alleviation of inflammation and pain associated with musculoskeletal disorders	Not documented in horses	300- and 400-mg tablets
Fentanyl transdermal	Narcotic analgesic	100 µg/hr patch: Change patch(es) every 2–3 days 1 patch for animals up to 250–750 pounds; 2 patches for 750–1200 pounds; 3 patches for 1200–1500 pounds. Note: Clip hair, do not scrub site	An opioid antagonist that acts primarily at the mu-receptors in the brain and spinal cord. Analgesic properties at least 100 times of morphine	Pain control. Especially good for visceral pain vs. somatic pain	Excessive sedation; ileus	100-µg transdermal patches
Firocoxib	NSAID	0.1 mg/kg PO q24h	Selective cyclooxygenase type 2 inhibitor	Osteoarthritis	Nephrotoxicity and GI/colonic ulceration	6.93-g paste syringe
Filgrastim	Granulocyte stimulating factor	300 µg SQ for a foal can repeat in 48 hours if needed 6 µg/kg SQ for an adult; repeat in 48 hours if needed	Regulates the production of neutrophils within the bone marrow and affects neutrophil progenitor proliferation	Idiopathic neutropenia in foals	Not noted in horses	300 µg injectable solution
Fluconazole	Azole antifungal	5 mg/kg PO q24h; Candidiasis: Loading dose of 8 mg/kg orally followed by 4 mg/kg q12–24h	Inhibition of fungal cytochrome P450 enzyme results in reduced synthesis of ergosterol in fungal cell membranes. The drug has less affinity for mammalian P450	Systemic fungal infections; conidiobolomycosis; fungal endometritis; fungal keratitis	Not documented in horses	200 mg tablets and 2 mg/mL injectable solution 100-mL vials

Flunixin meglumine	NSAID	1.1 mg/kg IV q8–24h	Modifies the inflammatory cascade by inhibiting the enzyme cyclooxygenase (COX), thus preventing the production from arachidonic acid. Flunixin has activity against COX 1 and COX 2 enzymes.	Colic-visceral pain; endotoxemia; musculoskeletal pain	IM dosing can result in fatal clostridial myositis; renal papillary necrosis; GI ulceration (stomach and right dorsal colon)	50 mg/mL injectable solution, granules, and paste
Fluorouracil	Antineoplastic	Case dependent; mares with vulva lesions may be treated daily for up to 3.7 months; males with tumors on the prepuce are treated topically 1 time every 2 weeks with the number of treatments ranging from 2 to 7	Interferes with the synthesis of DNA and to the lesser extent RNA. It does this by interrupting the formation of thymidine, an essential substrate for DNA synthesis.	Squamous cell carcinoma; sarcoids; fibrosarcoma	Not documented in horses	5% topical cream
Fluphenazine decanoate	Phenothiazine tranquilizer	0.06 mg/kg IM can be repeated in 3–4 weeks	Blocks post synaptic D2 dopamine receptors and presynaptic D2 autoreceptors within the limbic system. This results in decreased dopamine activity and synthesis.	Long-term tranquilization	Extrapyramidal signs (agitation, hypermetria, pawing, striking, stupor, etc.)	25 mg/mL injectable solution
Furosemide	Diuretic-saluretic	0.25–1 mg/kg IV	Loop diuretic that reduces the absorption of electrolytes in the ascending loop of Henle. Decreased reabsorption of sodium and chloride and increases excretion of potassium in the distal renal tubule.	EIPH (Give 4 hours before racing at a dose of 0.5 mg/kg IV) Treatment of edema, oliguria, acute heart failure: 0.5–3.0 mg/kg SC, IM, or IV q8–12h or as a bolus of 0.12 mg/kg IV, followed by a CRI at a rate of 0.12 mg/kg/hr; doses should be adjusted as needed to produce a diuretic effect.	Hypovolemia when used in excessive doses; hypokalemia	5% solution for injection (50 mg/mL)

Continued

Drug	Class	Dose	Mechanism	Indication for Use	Potential Side Effects	Formulation
Gabapentin	GABA analog	2.5–10 mg/kg PO q8h	Originally thought to act by increasing the concentration or receptor affinity of GABA in the CNS, which would explain its anticonvulsant and antianxiety effects as well as its effectiveness as a treatment for neuropathic pain. However, this theory is in question. More recent work has shown that gabapentin binds to $\alpha 2\delta$ subunits of voltage-dependent calcium channel complexes. Gabapentin acts in an inhibitory manner for these subunits.	Labeled for use in human medicine as an antiepileptic and for postherpetic neuralgia; neuropathic pain; refractory seizures in foals (400 mg PO q8h for 50–75 kg foal); laminitis	Abrupt discontinuation of treatment in humans has been associated with withdrawal-like symptoms (agitation and irritability), seizures and rebound pain	400- and 800-mg capsules
Gentamicin	Aminoglycoside antibiotic	6.6 mg/kg IV q24h	Actively moved across bacterial cell membranes by an oxygen dependent interaction of the drug with the LPS of gram-negative cell membranes. Once in the cell it binds to the 30s subunit of bacterial ribosomes inhibiting ribosomal protein synthesis. Postantibiotic effect	Gram-negative infections; regional limb perfusion usually one third of systemic dose diluted to 60 mL total volume	Nephrotoxic; ototoxic; aminoglycosides can also cause neuromuscular blockade	100 mg/mL injectable solution
Glycopyrrolate	Parasympatholytic	0.002–0.004 mg/kg IV	Competitively inhibits acetylcholine at postganglionic cholinergic (muscarinic) nerve terminals therefore inhibiting the action of acetylcholine on smooth muscle, cardiac muscle, exocrine glands. Does not cross blood brain barrier	Bronchodilator; arrhythmias (bradyarrhythmias due to increased parasympathetic tone)	Generally dose related; ileus and colic; ataxia and seizures (very rare: More commonly noted with atropine); pupil dilation	0.2 mg/mL solution
Griseofulvin	Antifungal	10 mg/kg PO q24h	Fungistatic medication that disrupts the mitotic spindle. It is concentrated in the stratum corneum.	Ringworm infection cause by the *Tricbophyton equinum* or *Microsporum gypseum*. Anecdotal evidence, topical therapy may be more important in controlling the spread of ringworm	Do not use in pregnant animals: Teratogenic	Oral powder 2.5 g/ scoop

Drug	Classification	Dosage	Action	Adverse Effects	Supply
Guaifenesin	Muscle relaxant/ anesthetic	110 mg/kg IV to affect and then slow drip: IV anesthesia "triple drip" is made by adding 500 mg xylazine and 1 g ketamine to 1 L of 5% guaifenesin. After induction with xylazine and ketamine, anesthesia is maintained with approximately 2 mL/ kg/hr. This protocol maintains anesthesia for approximately 25–45 minutes; 3 mg/kg Expectorant PO	Centrally blocking nerve impulses at the internuncial neurons on subcortical areas, brainstem, and spinal cord	Muscle relaxation/ anesthesia; expectorant	Increased incidence of thrombophlebitis in horses given 10% solution compared to 5%; paresis of respiratory muscles resulting in apneustic respiratory pattern and potential death (overdose)	5% and 10% IV solution
Heparin sodium	Anticoagulant	40–80 IU/kg SQ or IV q8h	Binds to antithrombin III, which inactivates thrombin preventing the conversion of fibrinogen to fibrin	Endotoxemia, DIC, laminitis, thrombophlebitis, GI disease, intraabdominal adhesions	Agglutination of red cells; bleeding	1000, 5000, and 10,000 U/mL injectable
Hetastarch (hydroxyethyl starch)	Colloid	10 mL/kg q36–48h IV	Acts like a plasma volume expander by increasing the oncotic pressure within the intravascular space similarly to either dextran or albumin. Maximum volume expansion occurs within a few minutes of the completion of infusion.	Hypovolemic patients secondary to hypoproteinemia	Increased cutaneous bleeding time has been reported in dogs and humans; thrombocytopenia secondary to dilutional effect; reduction of von Willebrand factor antigen, which may affect hemostasis	500 mL 6% hydroxyethyl starch
Human chorionic gonadotropin (hCG)	Hormone	Induce ovulation: 2500 IU units IV. Ovulation will occur in 24–48 hours. Determining cryptorchidism: 10,000 units of hCG IV. Blood sample prior to and 2 hours after administration. If a testicle is present there will be a 2- to 3-fold increase in testosterone. Cryptorchidism: Give 2500 IU 2 times a week for 4–6 weeks. 58% of cryptorchids will have a palpable testicle. Must have no anatomical obstruction before attempting	Has a clinical effect that is mainly that of LH. In females, LH effect enhances ovulation. In males, it stimulates the Leydig cells of the testis to produce androgens	Induce ovulation; cryptorchidism	Not described in the horse	1000 IU/mL following reconstitution

Continued

Drug	Class	Dose	Mechanism	Indication for Use	Potential Side Effects	Formulation
Hydralazine	Vasodilator	0.5–1.5 mg/kg PO q12h	Direct action on vascular smooth muscle and reduces peripheral resistance and blood pressure	Congestive heart disease	Transient weakness and lethargy	50- and 100-mg tablets
Hydroxyzine	Antihistamine	1 mg/kg PO q8–12h	Competes with histamine for the H1 receptor. Also seems to have some interaction with serotonin and acetylcholine.	Urticaria	Sedation for several days	50- and 100-mg tablets
Imipenem-cilastatin	Antibiotic	10–15 mg/kg IV diluted in fluids q6–8h	Inhibits cell wall synthesis by binding to PCPs	Severe systemic infections	Colitis/diarrhea	250 and 500 mg injectable solution
Imipramine	Tricyclic antidepressant	2 mg/kg PO	Potentiates dopamine, serotonin, and norepinephrine by blocking their reuptake at nerve terminals	Pharmacologically induced ejaculation: Treat 2 hours prior to semen ejaculation. At 2 hours give 0.4 mg/kg xylazine IV. Ejaculation is likely to occur in 1–2 minutes as the horse becomes sedated, or in 15–20 minutes as the effects of xylazine subsides. Urospermia: Controlled when given 4 hours prior to breeding. Speculated that drug may help with bladder neck closure during ejaculation. Narcolepsy: Give BID	Hyperexcitability, muscle fasciculations, hemolysis	25- and 50-mg tablets
Ipratropium bromide	Bronchodilator	5 activations (90 µg/ activation) q12h for a 500-kg horse; Therapeutic range from 0.5–3 µg/kg via aerosolization depending on severity of bronchoconstriction q8–12h	Anticholinergic (parasympatholytic). Bronchial smooth muscle contracts when levels of cyclic guanosine monophosphate (cGMP) increase due to muscarinic receptor (M3) stimulation by acetylcholine. This medication blocks M3 receptors. This mechanism is local and site specific; pronounced bronchodilation of the larger airways in the lung compared to β2 agonists that relax peripheral small airways	Small airway inflammation; COPD	Not noted in the horse. Little absorption from the respiratory or GI tracts	MDI delivers approximately 17–18 µg at the mouthpiece with each activation

Drug	Classification	Dose	Action	Indications for Use	Adverse Effects	Formulation
Isoxsuprine	Vasodilator	0.6 mg/kg PO q12h	Potent α-adrenoreceptor antagonist. At high concentrations it decreases blood viscosity and inhibits platelet aggregation; poor bioavailability 2.2%	Navicular disease and laminitis	None documented in the horse	10- and 20-mg tablets
Itraconazole	Antifungal	5–6 mg/kg PO q24h	Fungistatic triazole acts by altering the cellular membranes of susceptible fungi	Systemic fungal infections; good for aspergillosis	Hepatotoxicity	Compounded
Ivermectin	Anthelmintic	0.2 mg/kg PO	Interacts with GABA receptors of the parasite that results in paralysis. Does not cross the blood brain barrier in adult mammals	Deworming: small strongyles, pinworms, ascarids, *Habronema*, *Gastrophilus*, lungworms, *Strongyloides westeri*	Foals <1 month of age may exhibit CNS signs (blindness, depression, ataxia); ventral midline edema secondary to *Onchocerca* death	1.87% paste or 1% oral solution
Ketamine	General anesthetic	2.2 mg/kg IV (0.4–0.8 mg/kg/hr for analgesia)	Dissociative general anesthetic. Analgesia via stimulation of opiate receptors. NMDA receptor antagonist	IV anesthesia; analgesia via CRI	Administered without a sedative can cause muscular rigidity and seizures	100 mg/mL injectable solution
Ketoconazole	Antifungal	10 mg/kg PO q12h; questionable bioavailability in the horse	Fungistatic/fungicidal. Speculated to interfere with ergosterol synthesis which increases cell membrane permeability and causes secondary metabolic effects and growth inhibition; blocks thromboxane	Fungal infections; good for aspergillosis; small airway inflammation	GI disturbances; decreased serum testosterone levels in dogs when administered the medication. The hormone increased after medication discontinued; hepatotoxicity	200-mg tablets or compounded
Ketoprofen	NSAID	2.2. mg/kg IV q24h	Inhibits COX 1 and COX 2 and has been shown to inhibit lipoxygenase	Musculoskeletal inflammation	Gastric ulceration, nephrotoxicity	100 mg/mL injectable
Lidocaine	Local anesthetic	See "Indications for Use"	Nerve conduction is due to action potentials, which are generated by the movement of sodium ions through channels in the nerve membrane. Lidocaine is thought to block the movement of sodium ions through the channels	Ileus or systemic analgesia: 1.3 mg/kg as slow bolus and then 0.05 mg/kg/min as CRI. Epidural: 8 mL of 2% lidocaine in a 450-kg horse. Antiarrhythmic: (ventricular arrhythmia): 0.5–1 mg/kg IV every 5 minutes: Do not administer more than 4 mg/kg total dose	Drowsiness, ataxia, muscle tremors	2% injectable solution or 0.8% solution in 500-mL bags

Continued

Drug	Class	Dose	Mechanism	Indication for Use	Potential Side Effects	Formulation
Magnesium sulfate	Antiarrhythmic	Antiarrhythmic: Adult: 25–50 g/500 kg IV Diluted in 1 L of fluids given over 30 minutes; NMDA receptor antagonist (neonate): 20 mg/kg IV diluted in fluids q6–24h. Monitor magnesium levels if given over prolonged period of time or increased frequency	Decrease nerve conduction and NMDA receptor antagonist	Ventricular tachycardia; perinatal asphyxia	CNS drowsiness, bradycardia, respiratory depression, hypotension	50% injectable solution
Mannitol	Diuretic	0.5–1 g/kg IV q6–24h	Osmotic diuretic	Cerebral edema; oliguric acute renal disease; enhanced urinary excretion of some toxins	Dehydration, hypernatremia, controversy about using for cranial and spinal cord trauma if there is ongoing hemorrhage	20% solution
Methocarbamol	Skeletal muscle relaxant	25 mg/kg PO q12h (Range 25–75 mg/kg PO) OR 5–25 mg/kg IV slowly	Carbamate derivative of guaifenesin. Not really understood. It does not act directly on the contractile mechanism of the muscle	Muscle relaxation and sore backs	CNS depression, ataxia	500- and 750-mg tablets and 100 mg/mL injectable solution
Methylprednisolone acetate	Corticosteroid	100 mg IA (range 40–120 mg); 0.5 mg/kg IM	Inhibits the production of inflammatory mediators cyclooxygenase and lipoxygenase	Synovitis/osteoarthritis; allergic dermatitis	Nephrotoxicity and immune suppression	20, 40, and 80 mg/mL injectable vials
Metoclopramide	Prokinetic	0.1–0.2 mg/kg IV, SQ, IM q6–8h; 0.1–0.25 mg/kg PO q6h; 0.04 mg/kg/hr CRI IV	Enhancement of ACH release from postganglionic cholinergic neurons, dopamine and alpha-2 adrenergic antagonist	Intestinal ileus	Extrapyramidal signs: excessive stall walking, stupor or hyperexcitability	5 mg/mL injectable solution and 1 mg/mL oral syrup
Metronidazole	Antibiotic/ antiprotozoal	Adult: 15 mg/kg PO q6–8h Foals: 10 mg/kg PO q8–12h	Disrupts helical structure of DNA in susceptible organisms. Has some antiinflammatory properties	Anaerobic infections and clostridial enterocolitis	Anorexia, depression, hepatitis, and neurotoxicity	500-mg tablets
Midazolam	Anticonvulsant/ sedative	0.06–0.1 mg/kg IV or IM 2–6 mg/hr/50 kg	Benzodiazepam enhances the inhibitory neurotransmitter GABA, which results in hyperpolarization of the postsynaptic cell	Neonatal seizures	Respiratory arrest and depression	5 mg/mL injectable solution

Drug	Classification	Dosage	Mechanism of Action	Indications	Adverse Effects	How Supplied
Misoprostol	Prostaglandin E1 analog	2–5 µg/kg PO q6–12h	PGE1 (Misoprostol) is an antisecretory medication and cytoprotectant. It binds to prostaglandin receptors on gastric parietal cells resulting in decreased acid secretion. Cytoprotection is from increased mucosal blood flow producing bicarbonate, mucus, and increased epithelial turnover.	Treatment and prevention of gastrointestinal damage from NSAIDs; cervical dilation (200 µg tablet is softened in a small amount of saline or lubricating jelly and inserted into cervical canal	Seating, diarrhea, abdominal cramping, abortion	200-µg tablets
Moxidectin	Anthelmintic	0.4 mg/kg PO	Enhances the release of GABA at presynaptic neurons (hyperpolarization of the nerve terminals). Does not cross blood brain barrier	Deworming	Ataxia, depression. Do not use in foals <4 months of age	20 mg/mL oral gel
N-Butylscopolammonium bromide	Parasympatholytic	0.3 mg/mL IV	Occupies the muscarinic receptors sites of the effector cells, preventing acetylcholine from occupying these sites. A competitive inhibitor of acetylcholine at these sites	Spasmodic colic; facilitation of rectal exams; choke; meconium impactions: Given before administering acetylcysteine enemas	Increased HR posttreatment	20 mg/mL injectable solution
Naloxone	Narcotic antagonist	See "Indications for Use"	Competitive antagonist of opioids. Has affinity for the opioid receptors but no activity at these sites	Foals: Perinatal asphyxia : Give 4 mg IV; Hemorrhagic shock: Anecdotally in mares give 12–20 mg IV bolus; Stereotypic behavior: 0.03 mg/kg IV or IM	Increased signs of pain when endogenous opioids are antagonized	0.4 mg/mL injectable solution
Naproxen	NSAID	10 mg/kg PO q12h	Inhibits prostaglandin synthesis	Musculoskeletal pain	Nephropathy	500-mg tablets and 8-g packets containing 4-g of naproxen
Neostigmine	Parasympathomimetic	Foals: 1 mg SQ q1–2h (or to effect); has been given IV. Adult: Up to 6 mg SQ q1h; repeat as indicated	Cholinesterase inhibitor. Inhibits the breakdown of acetylcholine by the enzyme acetylcholinesterase	Cecal dysfunction; large colon ileus	Colic	1 mg/mL injectable solution
Nitazoxanide	Antiprotozoal	25 mg/kg PO q24h for the first 5 days and then 50 mg/kg PO q24h for 23 days	Interferes with pyruvate: ferredoxin oxidoreductase (PFOR) reaction, which is necessary for anaerobic energy metabolism	EPM	Fevers, diarrhea, colic, ulceration	Oral paste 320 mg/g

Continued

Drug	Class	Dose	Mechanism	Indication for Use	Potential Side Effects	Formulation
Omeprazole	Antiulcer medication	1–4 mg/kg PO q24h; 4 mg/kg loading dose for 28 days and then use 1 mg/kg as a maintenance	Inhibits H+/K+ ATPase, the energy source for the proton pump of parietal cells. The result is reduced acid secretion. Proton pump inhibitor	Gastric ulceration	None noted in the horse	Oral paste 2.28 g per syringe
Oxytetracycline	Antibiotic	6.6 mg/kg IV q12–24h diluted in 1 L of fluids	Inhibits protein synthesis by binding to receptors on the 30S subunit of the bacterial ribosome. Bacteriostatic	Bacterial infections; Potomac horse fever; equine granulocytic ehrlichiosis; Lyme disease; leptospirosis; flexural contraction in foals: Give 2.5–3.0 g in 1 L of fluids q24h	Nephrotoxicity; sudden death; flexural laxity; colitis	200 mg/mL injectable solution
Oxytocin	Hormone	See "Indications for Use"	Acts on oxytocin receptors of the mammary gland and uterus	Retained placenta: 20–30 units IM 60- to 90-minute intervals or 80–100 units added to 1 L of saline and given as a drip. If mare shows discomfort then the medication rate is slowed. Breeding management: Clearing fluid postbreeding. Give 4–8 hours after breeding; 10–20 units IM. Induction of parturition: 40–60 units IM produces a quiet, safe foaling within 1 hour. Prior determination of mares readiness for foaling is critical for the health of the foal. Choke: 0.11–0.22 units/kg Typical dose is 2.5–5 mL/450 kg	Colic, prolapsed uterus	20 USP units/mL injectable solution
Potassium penicillin	Antibiotic	22,000–50,000 IU/kg IV q6h	Affinity for proteins in the cell membranes of bacteria referred to as PBPs. These proteins are involved in the third and final step in cell wall synthesis	Gram-positive infections; leptospirosis	Colic; colitis; immune mediated anemia	20 million units powder injectable
Procaine penicillin	Antibiotic	20,000–40,000 IU/kg IM q12h	Affinity for proteins in the cell membranes of bacteria referred to as PBPs. These proteins are involved in the third and final step in cell wall synthesis	Gram-positive infections; leptospirosis	Colic; colitis; immune mediated anemia; procaine reactions: Immediate excitement and occasionally death	300,000 IU/mL injectable suspension

Drug	Class	Dose	Mechanism	Indication	Side Effects	Formulation
Pentoxifylline	Hemorheologic	7.5 mg/kg q8–12h PO or IV (IV must be diluted in 500–1000 mL of saline)	Methylxanthine derivative. Phosphodiesterase (PDE) inhibitor that increases red blood cell flexibility. PDE regulates cAMP and cGMP, which play a role in smooth muscle tone of airways. Inhibits endotoxin induced increase in TNF and IL-6. May decrease fibrosis of the liver and kidneys	Endotoxemia; placentitis; reactive airway disease; cholangiohepatitis; nephritis; laminitis	As with other methylxanthine can cause excitation if given rapidly IV	400-mg tablets; compounded oral and IV suspensions
Pergolide	Dopamine agonist	0.002–0.006 mg/kg PO q24h, up to 3 mg/day in adult horses	Dopamine receptor agonist	Pars intermedia dysfunction	Anorexia, diarrhea, depression	Compounding pharmacies
Phenazopyridine	Local anesthetic	4 mg/kg PO q8h	Unknown. Chemical that is excreted in the urine and causes local analgesia to the urinary tract	Stranguria secondary to bladder infections; postoperative bladder surgery	Will stain clothes and horse's hair coat if not properly given orally	Generic tablets
Phenobarbital	Barbiturate	8–16 mg/kg IV diluted in 50 mL saline over 20–30 minutes to effect. Maintenance: 5–10 mg/kg IV (as described above) q8h or 2–10 mg/kg PO q12h. Plasma concentration should be monitored: 5–15 µg/mL. Induces hepatic enzymes that over time will increase clearance; therefore dose may have to be increased	Depresses the motor centers of the cerebral cortex. Increases the seizure threshold by enhancing inhibitory postsynaptic effects of GABA	Anticonvulsant	Respiratory depression; bradycardia; hypotension	100-mg tablets or injectable 65 mg/mL, 130 mg/mL in 1-mL vials
Phenylbutazone	NSAID	2–6 mg/kg PO or IV q12–24h	Cyclooxygenase inhibitor. COX 1 and COX 2	Musculoskeletal inflammation and pain	Dose related; gastric and colonic ulcers; renal papillary necrosis; lowers T4 levels for up to 1 week after use; crosses the placenta and results in substantial concentration in neonates; concentration in milk is very low	1-g tablets, powder formula with 1-g scoop, Oral paste in 12 g/syringe and 200 mg/mL injectable 100-mL vials

Continued

Drug	Class	Dose	Mechanism	Indication for Use	Potential Side Effects	Formulation
Phenytoin	Anticonvulsant/muscle relaxant	15 mg/kg PO q24h Rhabdomyolysis: Initial loading dose of 6–8 mg/kg PO q12h for 3–5 days. If still experiencing rhabdomyolysis but is not drowsy then can increase dose by 1 mg/kg increments every 3–4 days to maximum dose of 10 mg/kg PO q12h (monitor serum levels). Neurologic disorders: 10 mg/kg PO q12h Need serum concentrations of 5–10 µg/mL for effect; Foals: 2.8–16.5 mg/kg PO q8h; *Hypochoeris radicata* (false dandelion) toxicity: 15 mg/kg PO q24h for 2 weeks	Acts on a number of ion channels within muscle and nerves including sodium and calcium channels. Phenytoin also affects triglyceride metabolism. Therapeutic levels vary so oral doses are adjusted by monitoring serum levels to achieve 8 µg/mL and not to exceed 12 µg/mL; stabilizes effects on synaptic junctions. Appears to work by the extrusion from neurons. The primary site of action is the motor cortex. Effects on muscle may be due to sodium flux at the sarcolemma or altering the neuromuscular junction.	Anticonvulsant, stringhalt, shivers, chronic rhabdomyolysis, digoxin-induced arrhythmias	Drowsiness and ataxia if the dose is too high and therefore should be decreased by 50%	100-mg oral capsules, 50-mg oral tablets and 50 mg/mL injectable vials
Phenylephrine	Sympathomimetic	20 mg in 1 L of saline over 10–15 minutes for an adult 500–600 kg animal 3 µg/kg/min over 15 minutes	Contraction of the spleen by up to 75%	Nephrosplenic contraction	Tachycardia; colic; restlessness; hemorrhage has been reported after use especially in older horses; contraction of the uterus and constriction of uterine vessels	10-mg injectable vials
Polymyxin B	Endotoxin-binding antibiotic	6000 U/kg IV q8–12h	Endotoxin-binding properties are due to the molecule binding to the lipid A region of endotoxins	Endotoxemia; endometritis: 1 million units infused into the uterus q24h for 3 days; good for *Pseudomonas*	Neurotoxin and nephrotoxic	500,000 IU injectable powder
Ponazuril	Antiprotozoal/anticoccidial	5–10 mg/kg PO q24h	Targets the "plastid" body, which is an organelle in *Sarcocystis neurona* and other members of the Apicomplexa phylum	EPM	Rapid kill of EPM organism resulting in worsening of neurologic signs	150 mg/g in oral paste
Praziquantel	Anticestodal anthelmintic	1.5 mg/kg PO	Causes immediate titanic contraction of the musculature. There is rapid vacuolization of the syncytial membrane. Increases cell permeability to calcium	Removal of tapeworms	No effects on pregnancy or spermatogenesis	In combination with ivermectin and moxidectin products

Drug	Class	Dose	Mechanism of Action	Indication	Adverse Effects/Cautions	Formulation
Prednisolone	Corticosteroid	1 mg/kg IV or PO q24h	Inhibits phospholipase A2 resulting in its antiinflammatory effect. Immunosuppression is mainly through the effects on leukocytes and macrophages. Direct effect on humoral immunity is minor.	CNS trauma; shock; COPD; allergic conditions	Excessive immunosuppression; laminitis; renal papillary necrosis; stomach/gastric ulceration	50-mg tablets, 100 mg and 500 mg for injection
Pyrantel pamoate/pyrantel tartrate	Anthelmintic	6.6 mg/kg PO	Cholinergic agonist affecting the nicotinic receptors of the parasite resulting in spastic paralysis	Routine deworming. Tapeworms (double dose)	Not noted in the horse	Oral paste 180 mg/mL or oral suspension 50 mg/mL
Pyrimethamine	Antiprotozoal	1 mg/kg PO q24h	Interfere with the production of folic acid by binding to dihydrofolate reductase, the enzyme required for the reduction of dihydrofolic acid to tetrafolic acid. High affinity for the protozoal enzyme	Used in combination with a sulfa for treatment of EPM	Do not supplement with folic acid: Paradoxically will cause folic acid deficiency: anemia, leukopenia, and glossitis Caution with pregnancy: Bone marrow hypoplasia, renal nephrosis, and epithelial dysplasia has been documented in mares treated with this medication and supplemented with folic acid	25-mg tablets and compound formulations
Quinapril	Vasodilator	120 mg PO q24h for 1000–1200 lb animal; 140 mg PO q24h for 1200–1400 lb animal	ACE inhibitor that results in decreased total peripheral resistance, pulmonary vascular resistance, mean arterial and right atrial pressures, and pulmonary capillary wedge pressure	Congestive heart disease associated with valvular disease	GI distress and hypotension	20- and 40-mg tablets
Quinidine sulfate	Antiarrhythmic	Adult horses: Loading dose of 20 g then 10 g increments q2h, dose to maximum of 60 g. Advise: Use stomach tube to administer. Horses hate the taste.	Class 1A antiarrhythmic. Depresses myocardial excitability, conduction velocity, and contractility. Will prolong the effective refractory period, which prevents the reentry phase. Also possesses anticholinergic activity that decreases vagal tone and may facilitate AV conduction.	Atrial fibrillation	GI effects: anorexia, diarrhea; nasal edema; urticaria; AV block; sudden death; multiform ventricular tachycardia	Quinidine sulfate 300-mg tablets

Continued

Drug	Class	Dose	Mechanism	Indication for Use	Potential Side Effects	Formulation
Ranitidine	Antiulcer medication	6.6 mg/kg PO q6–8h; 1.5 to 2 mg/kg IV q6–8h	Decreases gastric secretions of both HCl acid and gastrin by inhibiting histamine at the H2 receptor sites of parietal cells. Known as H2 receptor antagonist	Gastric ulcers. Not indicated as prophylactic use as antiulcer medication in critically ill foals. Studies have shown poor response to treatment.	Not noted in horses	150- and 300-mg tablets, compounded oral formulations and ranitidine HCl as 25 mg/mL injectable solutions
Reserpine	Catecholamine-depleting agent	0.006 mg/kg IM q2–3 weeks; 2.5 mg PO q24h (adult)	Depletes catecholamines and 5-hydroxytryptamine in the brain, adrenal medulla, and heart tissue. Reserpine causes norepinephrine to be released from storage granules in presynaptic adrenergic nerve terminals where it is then metabolized by MAO. The result is a decrease in sympathetic activity in both central and peripheral nervous system. May also stimulate prolactin release	Long-acting tranquilizer; agalactia	Depression; muscle trembling; bradycardia; miosis, upper eyelid ptosis; paraphimosis; colic; extrapyramidal neurologic signs; diarrhea: Noted 2–3 days after IM injection, which is usually self-limiting	0.25-mg tablets and 2.5 mg/mL solution for injection
Rifampin	Antibiotic	5 mg/kg PO q12h frequently used in combination with a macrolide to treat *R. equi* or *Lausonia*	Enters bacterial cell wall and inhibits RNA polymerase. It is generally bactericidal. Particularly effective in diseases with intracellular organisms because of its lipid solubility and entrance into neutrophils and macrophages	Gram-positive infections; *R. equi; Lausonia*	Diarrhea	Compounded oral suspensions and 300-mg capsules
Romifidine	Sedative/analgesic	40–120 µg/kg IV; 40 µg/kg provides analgesia for 30 minutes and sedation for 75 minutes; 120 µg/kg provides analgesia for 150 minutes and sedation for 3 hours	Alpha-2 adrenergic receptor agonist. Sedative aspect primarily due to activation of presynaptic alpha-2 receptors in the brainstem. Activation results in decreased release of norepinephrine. Stimulation of these receptors in the spinal cord results in analgesia and sedation.	Analgesia/sedation	Paradoxical excitation; decrease GI motility; bradycardia; initial increase in blood pressure followed by more prolonged decrease	10 mg/mL injectable solution

Drug	Classification	Dosage	Action	Indications	Comments	How Supplied
Selenium	Chemical element	0.06 mg/kg IM (if large dose divide into 2 separate sites). Repeat 3 days later and at 8–10 days	Essential micronutrient; antioxidant	Deficiency, white muscle disease in foals	Do not give IV: Can cause death	E-Se 2.5 mg Se and 68 U Vitamin E per mL
Sodium iodide	Iodine	70 mg/kg IV q24h (adult: one 20% solution 250-mL bottle a day)—sometimes followed by oral treatment with potassium iodide 20 mg/kg PO q24h for 4 weeks	Unknown, they are known to enhance phagocytic cells and inhibit neutrophil chemotaxis. These actions may be why they are used for their antigranulomatous effects.	Granulomatous infections (sporotrichosis, pythiosis, conidiobolomycosis, and basidiobolomycosis)	Lacrimation; cough; dry skin and scaling; inappetence; abortion has been reported in pregnant animals	20% solution in 250-mL bottles
Stanozolol	Anabolic steroid	0.55 mg/kg IM	Anabolic steroid	Use in debilitated horses with the goal of improving appetite and weight gain	Preferred by some practitioners because they feel there are less androgenic side effects. Report of adrenal insufficiency with long-term administration	50 mg/mL injectable solutions in 10- and 30-mL bottles
Sucralfate	Antiulcer medication	20 mg/kg PO q6h	A disaccharide (sucrose) aluminum hydroxide complex that in acid environment the sucrose (disaccharide) is freed from the aluminum and binds to anions of damaged GI epithelial cells forming a sticky viscous gel. Other properties such as increased blood flow via enhanced PG synthesis and binding of epidermal growth factor have been reported.	Gastric and right dorsal ulcerations	Minimally absorbed. No known side effects in horses. May interfere with absorption of other medications when given at the same time. Separate by 2 hours	1-g tablets or 1 g/10 mL oral suspensions
Tetracycline	Antibiotic	6.6 mg/kg IV q12–24h	Inhibits protein synthesis by reversible binding to 30s ribosomal subunits	Mainly gram-positive infections; *Leptospirosis* and *Borrelia burgdorferi*; *Lawsonia intracellularis*; inhibition of MMP activity	Rapid intravenous administration has been reported to be fatal in horses. Diarrhea. Flexural laxity in neonates/foals	200 mg/mL injectable solution (LA-200)

Continued

Drug	Class	Dose	Mechanism	Indication for Use	Potential Side Effects	Formulation
Ticarcillin	Antibiotic	50 mg/kg IV q6–8h (ticarcillin/clavulanate) 3–6 g intrauterine	Extended spectrum penicillin. Interferes with bacterial cell wall synthesis by binding to bacterial PBPs. The extended spectrum penicillins have greater activity against most gram-negative bacteria (especially *Pseudomonas*) due to their better penetration of the cell walls. This is due to a large polar group in the side chain of the antibiotic molecule.	Gram-positive and gram-negative systemic infections	Diarrhea	Ticarcillin disodium: 6-g vials for intrauterine infusion Ticarcillin/clavulanate 3.1-g powder for injection (vial)
Tolazoline	Alpha-1 and alpha-2 adrenergic antagonist	2–4 mg/kg IV	Alpha-1 and alpha-2 adrenergic antagonist	Reversal of xylazine, detomidine, and romifidine	Tachycardia, peripheral vasodilation, sweating, muscle fasciculations, hyperalgesia of lips, piloerection, death	100 mg/mL injectable solution
Triamcinolone acetonide	Synthetic glucocorticoid	0.02–0.04 mg/kg IM or IA	Primary mechanism for antiinflammatory effect is the stimulation of production of lipocortin. Lipocortin inhibits phospholipase A2, which decreases arachidonic acid. This results in decreased production of prostaglandins, thromboxane, leukotrienes, and chemotactic lipids. Immunosuppressive effects include mononuclear phagocytosis and cytokine production	Intra-articular therapy, COPD, allergic dermatitis	Laminitis	10 and 40 mg/mL injectable suspensions

Drug	Class	Dose	Mechanism	Indication	Adverse effects	Formulation
Trimethoprim (TMP)/sulfadiazine (SDZ)	Antibiotic	30 mg/kg PO q12–24h	This combination drug inhibits the production of folic acid at two steps. Trimethoprim inhibits the production of folate by binding to dihydrofolate reductase. It has high affinity for bacterial dihydrofolate reductase but a low affinity for the mammalian enzyme. Sulfadiazines are structurally similar to para amino benzoic acid (PABA) and are mistaken for PABA by bacteria in the folic acid production pathway.	Gram-positive and gram-negative bacterial infections	Diarrhea; reports of arrhythmias and death when given with detomidine; reports of death when given IV	Powder and paste formulations (67 mg trimethoprim and 333 mg sulfadiazine per g of powder) and 960-mg tablets (160 mg TMP/800 mg SDZ)
Trimethoprim/sulfamethoxazole	Antibiotic	30 mg/kg PO q12–24h	This combination drug inhibits the production of folic acid at two steps. Trimethoprim inhibits the production of folate by binding to dihydrofolate reductase. It has high affinity for bacterial dihydrofolate reductase but a low affinity for the mammalian enzyme. Sulfamethoxazole is structurally similar to PABA and are mistaken for PABA by bacteria in the folic acid production pathway.	Gram-positive and gram-negative bacterial infections	Diarrhea; reports of arrhythmias and death when given with detomidine; reports of death when given IV	960-mg tablets (160 mg TMP/800 mg sulfamethoxazole)
Valacyclovir	Antiviral	30 mg/kg PO q12h	Prodrug of acyclovir. This medication is converted to acyclovir via hepatic first-pass metabolism. Acyclovir once phosphorylated functions in three ways: DNA polymerase inhibitor, DNA chain terminator, binding between vital DNA polymerase and the interrupted chain	EHV-1 infection	None noted in the horse	500-mg tablet

Continued

Drug	Class	Dose	Mechanism	Indication for Use	Potential Side Effects	Formulation
Vancomycin	Antibiotic	6 mg/kg IV q8h; resistant *Clostridium difficile*. 4 mg/kg PO loading dose and then 2 mg/kg PO q6h. Regional limb perfusion: 300 mg in 60-mL saline	Inhibits bacterial cell wall synthesis by binding to precursor units of the cell wall. This occurs at different sites than β-lactam antibiotics. There is also an inhibition of RNA synthesis.	(Use as a last resort) *C. difficile* colitis, methicillin-resistant staphylococci	Nephrotoxicity and ototoxicity	500-mg and 1-g powder vials for injection (can give the injectable form orally)
Vitamin E	Nutrient	10–20 IU/kg PO q24h	Controls lipid peroxidation. The water soluble natural vitamin E has been shown to pass the blood brain barrier in clinically normal horses with levels detectable in the CSF.	Vitamin E deficiency; equine motor neuron disease; equine degenerative myeloencephalopathy; acute neurologic injury; rhabdomyolysis	Rare	Natural form has the ideal bioavailability compared to the synthetic form. Natural form is known as either D-alpha-tocopherol or D-alpha-tocopherol acetate
Xylazine	Sedative/analgesic	0.2–1 mg/kg IV; Epidural: combination of 1 mL xylazine with 5 mL 2% lidocaine	Alpha-2 adrenergic receptor agonist. Activation of these receptors decreases the release of neurotransmitters, particularly norepinephrine.	Analgesia; epidural anesthesia	Behavioral: Hypersensitivity around the hind quarters (kicking) may become aggressive around the handlers	100 mg/mL injectable solution
Yohimbine	Alpha-2 adrenergic antagonist	0.075–0.12 mg/kg IV	Alpha-2 adrenergic antagonist	Reversal of xylazine, detomidine, and romifidine	Death	5 mg/mL in 20-mL injectable vials

ACE, Angiotensin-converting enzyme; *ACH,* acetylcholine; *AV,* atrioventricular; *CNS,* central nervous system; *COPD,* chronic obstructive pulmonary disease; *CRI,* continuous rate infusion; *CSF,* cerebrospinal fluid; *DIC,* disseminated intravascular coagulation; *EHV-1,* equine herpesvirus type 1; *EIIPH,* exercise induced pulmonary hemorrhage; *EOD,* every other day; *EPM,* equine protozoal myeloencephalitis; *GI,* gastrointestinal; *GnRH,* gonadotropin-releasing hormone; *HR,* heart rate; *IA,* intra-articular; *LH,* luteinizing hormone; *LPS,* lipopolysaccharide; *MAO,* monoamine oxidase; *MDI,* metered dose inhaler; *NGT,* nasogastric tube; *NMDA,* N-methyl d-aspartate; *NSAID,* nonsteroidal antiinflammatory drug; *PBPs,* penicillin binding proteins; *PG,* prostaglandin; *TNF,* tumor necrosis factor.

Page numbers followed by "f" indicate figures, "t" indicate tables, and "b" indicate boxes.

A

Abdominal cavity, neoplasia of, 387–389
Abdominal distention
  colitis X and, 120
  differential diagnosis of, 859–861
  grain overload and, 229
  ischemia-reperfusion injury and, 306
Abdominal pain. *See also* Colic
  aortic aneurysm and, 34
  cecal intussusception and, 95
  nonstrangulating cecal infarction and, 100
Abdominal tap. *See* Abdominocentesis
Abdominocentesis, 220, 663–664
  in hepatic amyloidosis, 256
  in ischemia-reperfusion injury, 306
  in small intestinal intussusception, 551
  in small intestinal volvulus, 556
Abortion
  complications of, 196
  as estrus suppression treatment, 731
  methods for, 196
  spontaneous
    brucellosis and, 78
    coccidioidomycosis and, 114
    as early embryonic loss, 156
    equine herpesvirus and, 271–272
    equine infectious, 1–4
    equine viral arteritis and, 42
    fescue-related toxicosis and, 198
    hoary alyssum toxicosis and, 275
    listeriosis and, 342
    toxin-induced, 885t
Abscess
  of cecal wall, 95
  cerebral, 585f
  Corynebacterium pseudotuberculosis infection
      and, 128–129
  hepatic, 254–255
  internal
    coccidioidomycosis and, 114
    Corynebacterium pseudotuberculosis infection
        and, 128
  perirectal, 4–5
  pleural, 449
  pulmonary, 486f
  splenic, 573–574
  subsolar, 589–591
  testicular, 601
  ultrasound imaging of, 834f
  urachal, 620
Abuse, definition of, 785
Acanthocytes, 899–901
Acanthoma, papillary. *See* Papillomatosis, cutaneous
Acepromazine, 1031
  for black walnut toxicosis, 66
  for ileus, 289
Acer toxicosis, 885t. *See also* Red maple leaf
    toxicosis
Acetazolamide, 1031
Acetylcysteine enemas. *See* Enemas, retention/high
Acetylcysteine solution 4%, 1031
Acid ingestion, toxic effects of, 891t
Acidosis
  lactic, 942
    cyanide poisoning and, 134
  metabolic, 498
    acute colitis/diarrhea and, 118
    diarrhea of the neonatal foal and, 151
    hyperchloremia and, 919
    typhlitis and, 615
  renal tubular, 497–498
Aciduria, 969
Acinetobacter, presence in equine uterus, 167
Acremonium coenophialum, 198
Acriflavines, as photosensitization cause, 445
Acrosome reaction, 562, 568
Actinobacillosis, 5–6
  bronchopneumonia, 77
  cholangiohepatitis, 107

Actinobacillosis *(Continued)*
  endocarditis, 162
  peritonitis, 439
  pleuropneumonia, 448
  pyelonephritis, 478
Actinobacillus equilli infections, 573
Actinomyces, presence in equine uterus, 167
Activated charcoal, 804–806, 1031
  for acute colitis/diarrhea, 119
  for black walnut toxicosis, 66
  for cockleburr poisoning, 116
  in grain overload, 230
  for ivermectin toxicosis, 308
  for moxidectin toxicosis, 308
  for nightshade toxicosis, 402
  for nonsteroidal anti-inflammatory drug toxicity,
      405
  for organophosphate toxicosis, 415
Activated charcoal dressings, 848
Activated clotting time (ACT), 901
Activated macrophage supernatant (AMS), 849
Activated partial thromboplastin time (aPTT), 153, 902
Acute respiratory distress syndrome, 474
Acyclovir, 1031
  for equine herpesvirus-1 myeloencephalitis, 369
  for multinodular pulmonary fibrosis, 474
Adenocarcinoma
  pancreatic, 83
  of urinary tract, 396
Adenoma, of urinary tract, 396
(S)-Adenosylmethionine (SAMe), 261, 263
Adenovirus infections, 7–8, 295, 455–456
Adhesions
  abdominal, 8–9
  cervical, 102
Adipose tissue, insulin activity in, 303
Adrenal artery, rupture of, 250
Adrenal insufficiency, relative, 10–11
Adrenocorticotropic hormone (ACTH)
  in adrenal insufficiency, 10
  in Cushing syndrome, 132–133
  endogenous/baseline, 902–903
  interactions with cortisol, 922–923
  in polydipsia/polyuria, 463
Adrenocorticotropic hormone (ACTH) stimulation
      test, 10–11, 664
AeroHippus, 766f
AeroMask, 765f
Aeromonas infections, 258
Aflatoxin toxicosis, 11–12
African animal trypanosomiasis, 613
African horse sickness, 12–14, 224
Agalactia, 198–199
Aggressive behavior
  hepatic encephalopathy and, 256
  in stallions, 15
AGID test. *See* Coggins test
Air embolism, venous, 639–640
Airway disease, inflammatory, 297–298
Airway obstruction
  pulmonary hypertension and, 474
  recurrent, 16
  summer pasture-associated, 589–591
  upper, dorsal displacement of the soft palate
      and, 154–156
Albumin, 903, 957
Albuminuria, 903–904
Albuterol, 1031
Albuterol, for inflammatory airway disease, 157
Alfalfa/alfalfa hay, toxic effects of, 891t
  blister beetles and, 67–68, 67f
  enterolithiasis, 171
  hematuria, 243–244
  photosensitization, 445
Algal toxicosis, 17–19, 891t
  as photosensitization cause, 445
Alkali ingestion, toxic effects of, 891t
Alkaline phosphatase (ALP), 904
  in azoospermia, 564
  in oligozoospermia, 566

Alkalinuria, 969
Alkaloids, tropane, toxic effects of, 891t
Allergic inhalant dermatitis. *See* Dermatitis, atopic
Allium, toxic effects of, 891t
Aloe vera, 857
Alopecia
  areata, 19
  atopic dermatitis and, 143
  insect hypersensitivity and, 302
ALP. *See* Alkaline phosphatase (ALP)
Alpha globulin, 957
Alphaviruses, 395–396
Alsike clover, as toxicosis cause, 113, 891t
Altrenogest, 423, 1032
Aluminum phosphide, toxic effects of, 891t
Alveolar bone, 922
Amanitin toxicosis, 21–22
Ambulatory electrocardiography, 644, 742–743,
    743f
Ameblastoma, 412–413
American Association of Equine Practitioners,
    equine influenza vaccination
    recommendations of, 301
American miniature horses, hepatic lipidosis in, 258
American Paint horses. *See also* Paint horses
  neonatal isoerythrolysis in, 383
American Quarter horses, cryptorchidism in, 130
American Saddlebred horses. *See also* Saddlebred
    horses
  cryptorchidism in, 130
  inguinal hernia in, 267
Amianthium, 137, 138f
Amikacin, 856
  for endometritis, 165t
  for neonatal pneumonia, 454
Amikacin sulfate, 1032
Amino acids, 775–776
  as parenteral nutrient mixture component, 787
  requirements in older horses, 780
Aminocaproic acid, 1032
Aminocaproic acid, for hemorrhage, 249, 250
Aminoglycoside antibiotics
  for diarrhea of the neonatal foal, 151
  drug interactions of, 405
  plasma concentrations of, 695
  toxic effects of, 22–24, 609, 891t
Aminophylline, 1032
Amino Plex, 858
4-Aminopyridine, toxic effects of, 891t
Amiodarone, for ventricular tachycardia, 645
Amitraz, toxic effects of, 891t
Ammonia, 905
  neurotoxicity of, 257
Ammonia gas, toxic effects of, 891t
Ammonium urate urinary crystals, 968t
Amoxicillin, 1032
Amphotericin, 452
Amphotericin B, 1032
  for endometritis, 165t, 167t
  for histoplasmosis, 275
  for mucormycosis, 659
Ampicillin, 1033
Ampullae, plugged, 564–566, 568–569
Ampullitis, 482–483
Amsinckia, as photosensitization cause, 445
Amylase, in pancreatic fluid, 83
Amyloidosis, 24–25
  hepatic, 255
  myeloma and, 391
  protein-losing nephropathy and, 472
Amyotrophic lateral sclerosis, 364
Anabolic steroids
  effect on sperm quality, 563
  toxic effects of, 891t
Anagen defluxion, 25
Analgesia, perineural. *See* Dental nerve blocks
Analgesic therapy. *See also specific analgesics*
  for cecal tympany, 98
  for gastric ulcers, 223
  for grain overload, 230